Recommended Dietary Allowances (RDA) and Adequate Intakes (AI) for Vitamins

Age (yr)	Thiamin RDA (mg/day)	Riboflavin RDA (mg/day)	Niacin RDA (mg/day)[a]	Biotin AI (μg/day)	Pantothenic acid AI (mg/day)	Vitamin B_6 RDA (mg/day)	Folate RDA (μg/day)[b]	Vitamin B_{12} RDA (μg/day)	Choline AI (mg/day)	Vitamin C RDA (mg/day)	Vitamin A RDA (μg/day)[c]	Vitamin D RDA (μg/day)[d]	Vitamin E RDA (mg/day)[e]	Vitamin K AI (μg/day)
Infants														
0–0.5	0.2	0.3	2	5	1.7	0.1	65	0.4	125	40	400	10*	4	2.0
0.5–1	0.3	0.4	4	6	1.8	0.3	80	0.5	150	50	500	10*	5	2.5
Children														
1–3	0.5	0.5	6	8	2	0.5	150	0.9	200	15	300	15	6	30
4–8	0.6	0.6	8	12	3	0.6	200	1.2	250	25	400	15	7	55
Males														
9–13	0.9	0.9	12	20	4	1.0	300	1.8	375	45	600	15	11	60
14–18	1.2	1.3	16	25	5	1.3	400	2.4	550	75	900	15	15	75
19–30	1.2	1.3	16	30	5	1.3	400	2.4	550	90	900	15	15	120
31–50	1.2	1.3	16	30	5	1.3	400	2.4	550	90	900	15	15	120
51–70	1.2	1.3	16	30	5	1.7	400	2.4	550	90	900	15	15	120
>70	1.2	1.3	16	30	5	1.7	400	2.4	550	90	900	20	15	120
Females														
9–13	0.9	0.9	12	20	4	1.0	300	1.8	375	45	600	15	11	60
14–18	1.0	1.0	14	25	5	1.2	400	2.4	400	65	700	15	15	75
19–30	1.1	1.1	14	30	5	1.3	400	2.4	425	75	700	15	15	90
31–50	1.1	1.1	14	30	5	1.3	400	2.4	425	75	700	15	15	90
51–70	1.1	1.1	14	30	5	1.5	400	2.4	425	75	700	15	15	90
>70	1.1	1.1	14	30	5	1.5	400	2.4	425	75	700	20	15	90
Pregnancy														
≤18	1.4	1.4	18	30	6	1.9	600	2.6	450	80	750	15	15	75
19–30	1.4	1.4	18	30	6	1.9	600	2.6	450	85	770	15	15	90
31–50	1.4	1.4	18	30	6	1.9	600	2.6	450	85	770	15	15	90
Lactation														
≤18	1.4	1.6	17	35	7	2.0	500	2.8	550	115	1200	15	19	75
19–30	1.4	1.6	17	35	7	2.0	500	2.8	550	120	1300	15	19	90
31–50	1.4	1.6	17	35	7	2.0	500	2.8	550	120	1300	15	19	90

NOTES: For all nutrients, values for infants are AI. The glossary on the inside back cover defines units of nutrient measure.

[a]Niacin recommendations are expressed as niacin equivalents (NE), except for recommendations for infants younger than 6 months, which are expressed as preformed niacin.

[b]Folate recommendations are expressed as dietary folate equivalents (DFE).

[c]Vitamin A recommendations are expressed as retinol activity equivalents (RAE).

[d]Vitamin D recommendations are expressed as cholecalciferol and assume an absence of adequate exposure to sunlight.

[e]Vitamin E recommendations are expressed as α-tocopherol.

*Adequate Intake

Recommended Dietary Allowances (RDA) and Adequate Intakes (AI) for Minerals

Age (yr)	Sodium AI (mg/day)	Chloride AI (mg/day)	Potassium AI (mg/day)	Calcium RDA (mg/day)	Phosphorus RDA (mg/day)	Magnesium RDA (mg/day)	Iron RDA (mg/day)	Zinc RDA (mg/day)	Iodine RDA (μg/day)	Selenium RDA (μg/day)	Copper RDA (μg/day)	Manganese AI (mg/day)	Fluoride AI (mg/day)	Chromium AI (μg/day)	Molybdenum RDA (μg/day)
Infants															
0–0.5	120	180	400	200*	100	30	0.27	2	110	15	200	0.003	0.01	0.2	2
0.5–1	370	570	700	260*	275	75	11	3	130	20	220	0.6	0.5	5.5	3
Children															
1–3	1000	1500	3000	700	460	80	7	3	90	20	340	1.2	0.7	11	17
4–8	1200	1900	3800	1000	500	130	10	5	90	30	440	1.5	1.0	15	22
Males															
9–13	1500	2300	4500	1300	1250	240	8	8	120	40	700	1.9	2	25	34
14–18	1500	2300	4700	1300	1250	410	11	11	150	55	890	2.2	3	35	43
19–30	1500	2300	4700	1000	700	400	8	11	150	55	900	2.3	4	35	45
31–50	1500	2300	4700	1000	700	420	8	11	150	55	900	2.3	4	35	45
51–70	1300	2000	4700	1000	700	420	8	11	150	55	900	2.3	4	30	45
>70	1200	1800	4700	1000	700	420	8	11	150	55	900	2.3	4	30	45
Females															
9–13	1500	2300	4500	1300	1250	240	8	8	120	40	700	1.6	2	21	34
14–18	1500	2300	4700	1300	1250	360	15	9	150	55	890	1.6	3	24	43
19–30	1500	2300	4700	1000	700	310	18	8	150	55	900	1.8	3	25	45
31–50	1500	2300	4700	1000	700	320	18	8	150	55	900	1.8	3	25	45
51–70	1300	2000	4700	1200	700	320	8	8	150	55	900	1.8	3	20	45
>70	1200	1800	4700	1200	700	320	8	8	150	55	900	1.8	3	20	45
Pregnancy															
≤18	1500	2300	4700	1300	1250	400	27	12	220	60	1000	2.0	3	29	50
19–30	1500	2300	4700	1000	700	350	27	11	220	60	1000	2.0	3	30	50
31–50	1500	2300	4700	1000	700	360	27	11	220	60	1000	2.0	3	30	50
Lactation															
≤18	1500	2300	5100	1300	1250	360	10	14	290	70	1300	2.6	3	44	50
19–30	1500	2300	5100	1000	700	310	9	12	290	70	1300	2.6	3	45	50
31–50	1500	2300	5100	1000	700	320	9	12	290	70	1300	2.6	3	45	50

SOURCE: Data from the *Dietary Reference Intakes* series, National Academies Press, Copyright 1997, 1998, 2000, 2001, 2002, 2004, 2010, by the National Academies of Sciences. From Sizer/WHITNEY/PICHE. Nutrition, 2E.

Tolerable Upper Intake Levels (UL) for Vitamins

Age (yr)	Niacin (mg/day)[a]	Vitamin B_6 (mg/day)	Folate (µg/day)[a]	Choline (mg/day)	Vitamin C (mg/day)	Vitamin A (µg/day)[b]	Vitamin D (µg/day)	Vitamin E (mg/day)[c]
Infants								
0–0.5	—	—	—	—	—	600	25	—
0.5–1	—	—	—	—	—	600	37.5	—
Children								
1–3	10	30	300	1000	400	600	62.5	200
4–8	15	40	400	1000	650	900	75	300
9–13	20	60	600	2000	1200	1700	100	600
Adolescents								
14–18	30	80	800	3000	1800	2800	100	800
Adults								
19–70	35	100	1000	3500	2000	3000	100	1000
>70	35	100	1000	3500	2000	3000	100	1000
Pregnancy								
≤18	30	80	800	3000	1800	2800	100	800
19–50	35	100	1000	3500	2000	3000	100	1000
Lactation								
≤18	30	80	800	3000	1800	2800	100	800
19–50	35	100	1000	3500	2000	3000	100	1000

[a]The UL for niacin and folate apply to synthetic forms obtained from supplements, fortified foods, or a combination of the two.
[b]The UL for vitamin A applies to the preformed vitamin only.

[c]The UL for vitamin E applies to any form of supplemental α-tocopherol, fortified foods, or a combination of the two.

Tolerable Upper Intake Levels (UL) for Minerals

Age (yr)	Sodium (mg/day)	Chloride (mg/day)	Calcium (mg/day)	Phosphorus (mg/day)	Magnesium (mg/day)[d]	Iron (mg/day)	Zinc (mg/day)	Iodine (µg/day)	Selenium (µg/day)	Copper (µg/day)	Manganese (mg/day)	Fluoride (mg/day)	Molybdenum (µg/day)	Boron (mg/day)	Nickel (mg/day)	Vanadium (mg/day)
Infants																
0–0.5	—[e]	—[e]	1000	—	—	40	4	—	45	—	—	0.7	—	—	—	—
0.5–1	—[e]	—[e]	1500	—	—	40	5	—	60	—	—	0.9	—	—	—	—
Children																
1–3	1500	2300	2500	3000	65	40	7	200	90	1000	2	1.3	300	3	0.2	—
4–8	1900	2900	2500	3000	110	40	12	300	150	3000	3	2.2	600	6	0.3	—
9–13	2200	3400	3000	4000	350	40	23	600	280	5000	6	10	1100	11	0.6	—
Adolescents																
14–18	2300	3600	3000	4000	350	45	34	900	400	8000	9	10	1700	17	1.0	—
Adults																
19–50	2300	3600	2500	4000	350	45	40	1100	400	10,000	11	10	2000	20	1.0	1.8
51–70	2300	3600	2000	3000	350	45	40	1100	400	10,000	11	10	2000	20	1.0	1.8
>70	2300	3600	2000	3000	350	45	40	1100	400	10,000	11	10	2000	20	1.0	1.8
Pregnancy																
≤18	2300	3600	3000	3500	350	45	34	900	400	8000	9	10	1700	17	1.0	—
19–50	2300	3600	2500	3500	350	45	40	1100	400	10,000	11	10	2000	20	1.0	—
Lactation																
≤18	2300	3600	3000	4000	350	45	34	900	400	8000	9	10	1700	17	1.0	—
19–50	2300	3600	2500	4000	350	45	40	1100	400	10,000	11	10	2000	20	1.0	—

[d]The UL for magnesium applies to synthetic forms obtained from supplements or drugs only.
[e]Source of intake should be from human milk (or formula) and food only.

NOTE: An Upper Limit was not established for vitamins and minerals not listed and for those age groups listed with a dash (—) because of a lack of data, not because these nutrients are safe to consume at any level of intake. All nutrients can have adverse effects when intakes are excessive.

NELSON EDUCATION | *Canada's Learning Advantage*

CENGAGENOW

Just What You Need To Know And Do NOW!

CengageNOW™ is an online teaching and learning resource that provides more control in less time and delivers better student outcomes.

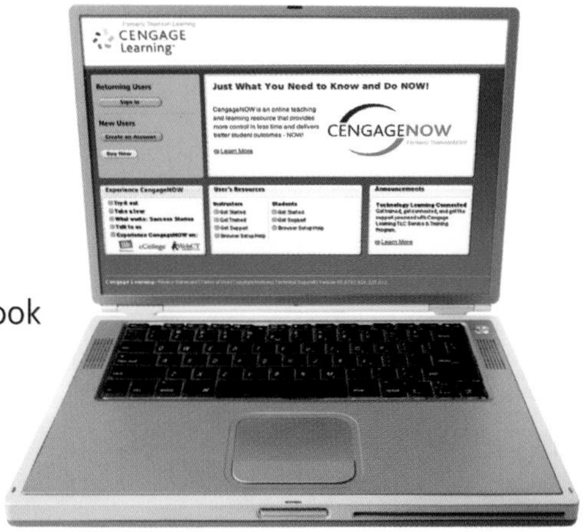
CENGAGE Learning
Just What You Need to Know and Do NOW!
CENGAGENOW

- ▶ **Teaching and Learning Resource**—Creating assignments, grading, quizzing, and tracking student outcomes.
- ▶ **More Control in Less Time**—Flexible assignment and grade book options to best suit your overall course plan.
- ▶ **Better Student Outcomes**—A diagnostic Personalized Study plan empowers students to master concepts, prepare for exams, and get a better grade.

Over 550,000 students have already taken advantage of CengageNOW, and here is what students and instructors are saying...

According to a survey of over 1300 student users:		According to a survey of over 250 instructors:	
80%	believed using CengageNOW helped them better understand key concepts in the course	**91%**	believed using CengageNOW helps students better understand key concepts
75%	believed using CengageNOW helped them be more prepared for exams	**86%**	believed using CengageNOW helps students be more prepared for exams
77%	believed using CengageNOW helped them get a better grade	**84%**	believed using CengageNOW helps students get a better grade
75%	would recommend CengageNOW to a friend	**76%**	would recommend CengageNOW to a colleague

Go to www.nelson.com/coursemaster to take a tour and learn more.

Nelson Education Ltd. 1120 Birchmount Road Toronto ON M1K 5G4
416 752 9448 or 1 800 268 2222 Fax 416 752 8101 or 1 800 430 4445 email: nelson.orderdesk@nelson.com **www.nelson.com**

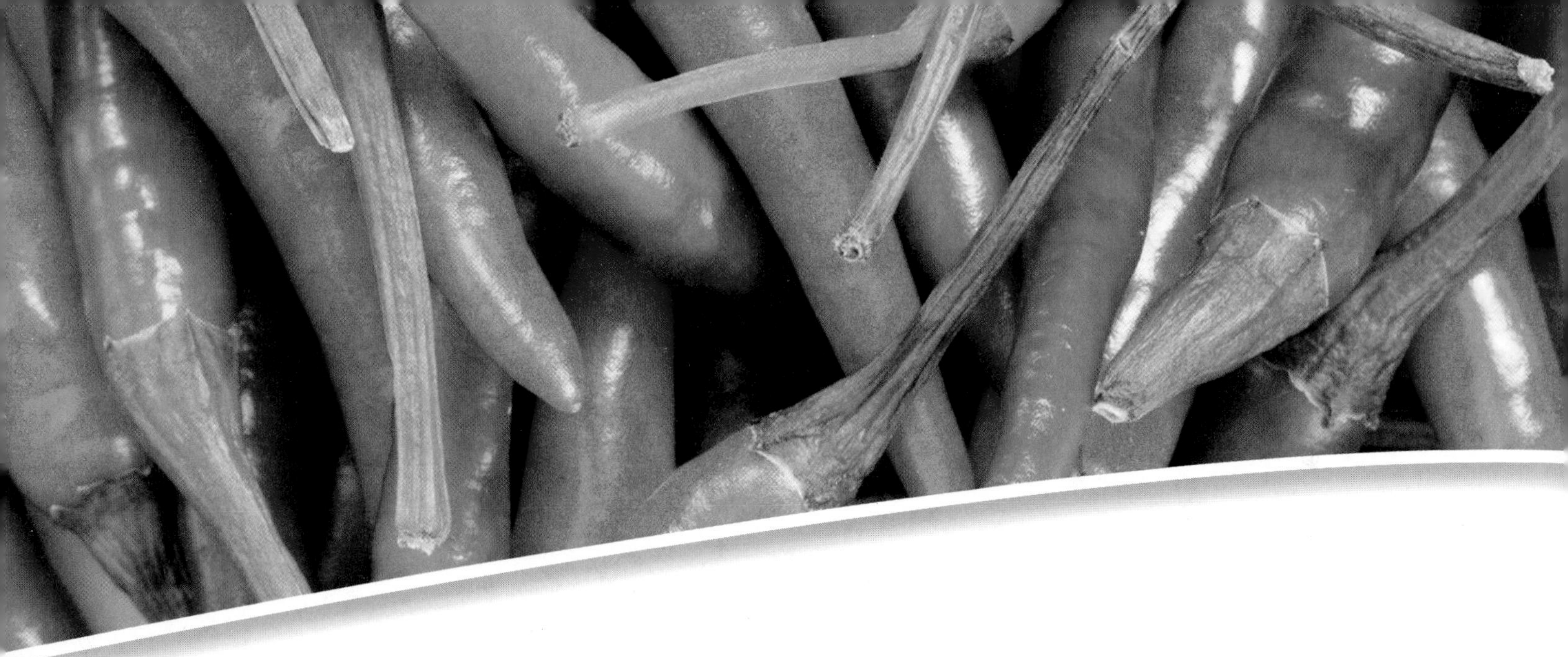

Understanding Nutrition

First Canadian Edition

ELLIE WHITNEY • Nutrition and Health Associates
SHARON RADY ROLFES • Nutrition and Health Associates
GAIL HAMMOND • University of British Columbia
LEONARD A. PICHÉ • Brescia University College

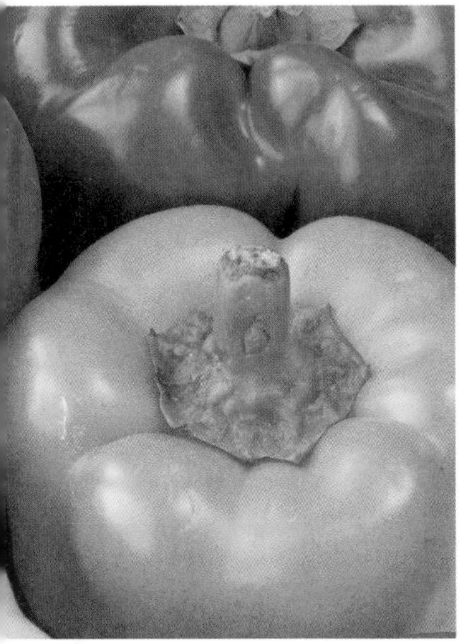

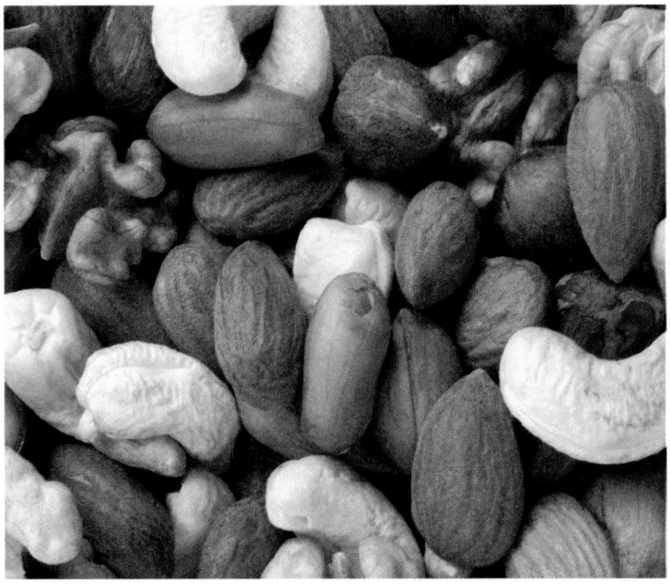

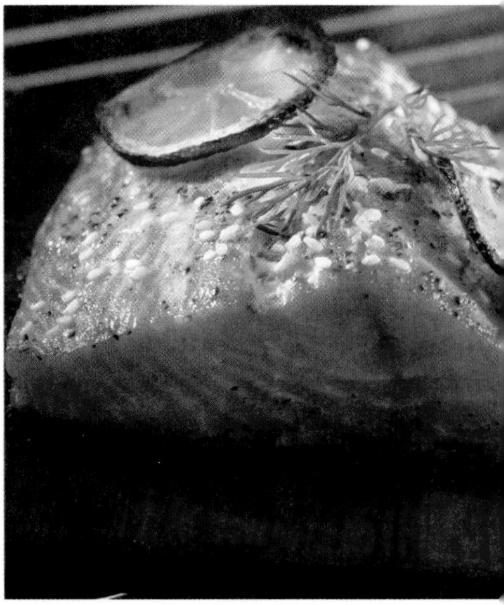

NELSON EDUCATION

NELSON EDUCATION

Understanding Nutrition, First Canadian Edition

by Ellie Whitney, Sharon Rady Rolfes, Gail Hammond, and Leonard A. Piché

Vice President, Editorial Higher Education:
Anne Williams

Publisher:
Paul Fam

Executive Editor:
Jackie Wood

Marketing Manager:
Alexis Hood

Senior Developmental Editor:
Mark Grzeskowiak

Photo Researcher and Permissions Coordinator:
Natalie Russell

Senior Content Production Manager:
Natalia Denesiuk Harris

Production Service:
Integra Software Services Pvt. Ltd.

Copy Editor:
Wendy Yano

Proofreader:
Integra Software Services Pvt. Ltd.

Indexer:
Integra Software Services Pvt. Ltd.

Manufacturing Manager:
Joanne McNeil

Design Director:
Ken Phipps

Managing Designer:
Franca Amore

Interior Design:
Hespenheide Design

Cover Design:
Dianna Little

Cover Image:
Masterfile

Compositor:
Integra Software Services Pvt. Ltd.

Printer:
RR Donnelley

Printed and bound in the United States of America
1 2 3 4 15 14 13 12

For more information contact Nelson Education Ltd., 1120 Birchmount Road, Toronto, Ontario, M1K 5G4. Or you can visit our Internet site at http://www.nelson.com

Library and Archives Canada Cataloguing in Publication Data

Understanding nutrition / Ellie Whitney ... [et al.]. — 1st Canadian ed.

Includes bibliographical references and index.
ISBN 978-0-17-650095-5

1. Nutrition—Textbooks.
I. Whitney, Eleanor Noss

QP141.U53 2012
613.2 C2011-908654-9

ISBN-13: 978-0-17-650095-5
ISBN-10: 0-17-650095-2

To the memory of my parents, Phyllis and Joseph, whose wisdom and love guide me in all that I do. To all students who inspire excellence in teaching and learning.

Gail Hammond

To my entire family, especially Roxanne, for letting me know in their own way that they do appreciate how important it really is from a health-standpoint to "Let the science of nutrition influence the art of eating."

Love, Len/Dad/Papa

About the Authors

Gail Hammond recently earned her doctoral degree in human nutrition at the University of British Columbia. Her qualitative study evaluated the use of a community-based participatory research approach to develop nutrition education resources on food choice and bone health by and for midlife women. Prior to entering her doctoral program, she was a community nutritionist and taught introductory nutrition as a sessional faculty member at UBC, a position that she continues in today. Integrating the scholarship of teaching and learning in nutrition education lies at the core of her work, and she is a graduate of the UBC Faculty Certificate Program on Teaching and Learning in Higher Education. Gail has published articles in peer-reviewed journals and is a reviewer for the *Canadian Journal of Dietetic Practice and Research* and the *Journal of Human Nutrition and Dietetics*. She is a Registered Dietitian and a member of the Dietitians of Canada and the College of Dietitians of British Columbia.

Leonard A. Piché received his PhD in human nutrition from the University of Guelph in 1987. He is a Full Professor in the Division of Foods & Nutritional Sciences, Brescia University College, and teaches basic and advanced undergraduate and graduate courses in nutrition. He is also an Adjunct Professor in the school of Kinesiology, University of Western Ontario. He is a member of seven professional national organizations. He was a contributor for two recent editions of *Mosby's Medical Dictionary,* a consultant for a Canadian edition of a high school food and nutrition textbook, and coauthor of a Canadianized university-level nutrition text. He has been involved in and coauthored peer-reviewed articles on experiments in humans looking at the relationship between diet and heart disease risk. He has provided feedback to Health Canada on more than 50 occasions regarding food- and nutrition-related issues. He was an advisor on three of Dietitians of Canada's online courses for health professionals. He has supervised the nutrient analysis of seven recipe books targeted at different segments of the general public. He has recently been involved, as a team member, in studies looking at children's beverage consumption and other factors that contribute to children's screen-related sedentary behaviours, which have resulted in peer-reviewed publications, of which he is coauthor. He was also a member (2006–2010) of the Expert Advisory Committee for Health Canada's Natural Health Products Directorate. His current areas of interest include local food maps, the nutrient content of restaurant foods, meals served to residents in long-term care, foods grown/produced in Canada, the bioactive components of functional foods, and sport supplement use by university students.

U.S. Authors

Ellie Whitney grew up in New York City and received her BA and PhD degrees in English and Biology at Radcliffe/Harvard University and Washington University, respectively. She has taught at both Florida State University and Florida A&M University, has written newspaper columns on environmental matters for the *Tallahassee Democrat,* and has authored almost a dozen college textbooks on nutrition, health, and related topics, many of which have been revised multiple times over the years. In addition to teaching and writing, she has spent the past three-plus decades exploring outdoor Florida and studying its ecology. Her latest book is *Priceless Florida: The Natural Ecosystems* (Pineapple Press, 2004).

Sharon Rady Rolfes received her MS in nutrition and food science from Florida State University. She is a founding member of Nutrition and Health Associates, an information resource centre that maintains a research database on over 1000 nutrition-related topics. Her other publications include the college textbooks *Understanding Normal and Clinical Nutrition* and *Nutrition for Health and Health Care* and a multimedia CD-ROM called *Nutrition Interactive*. In addition to writing, she occasionally teaches at Florida State University and serves as a consultant for various educational projects. Her volunteer work includes serving on the board of Working Well, a community initiative dedicated to creating a healthy workforce. She maintains her registration as a dietitian and membership in the American Dietetic Association.

Brief Contents

Contents

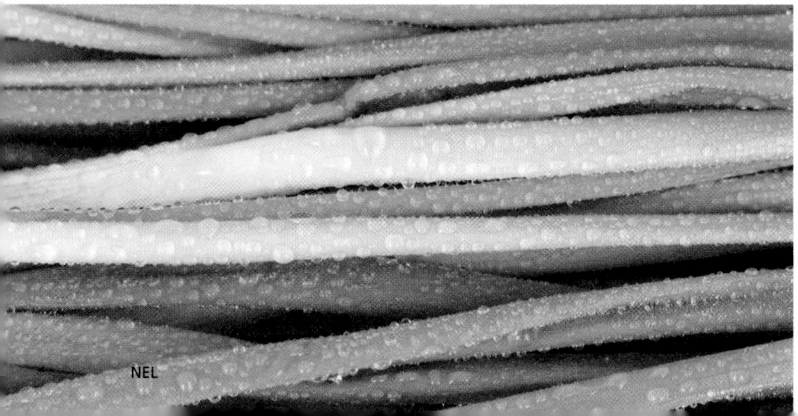

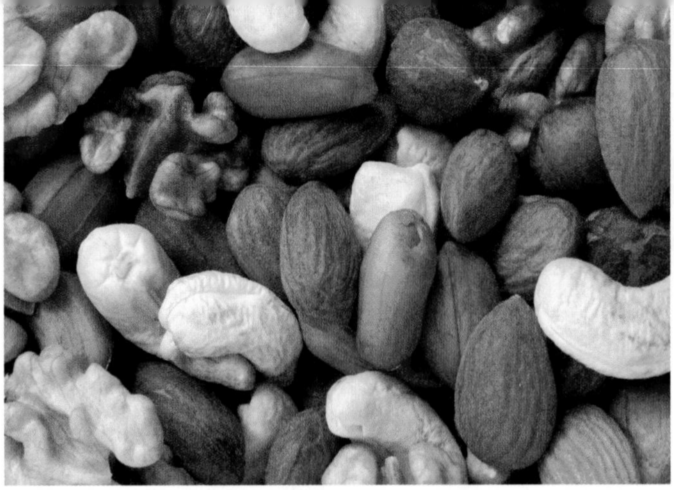

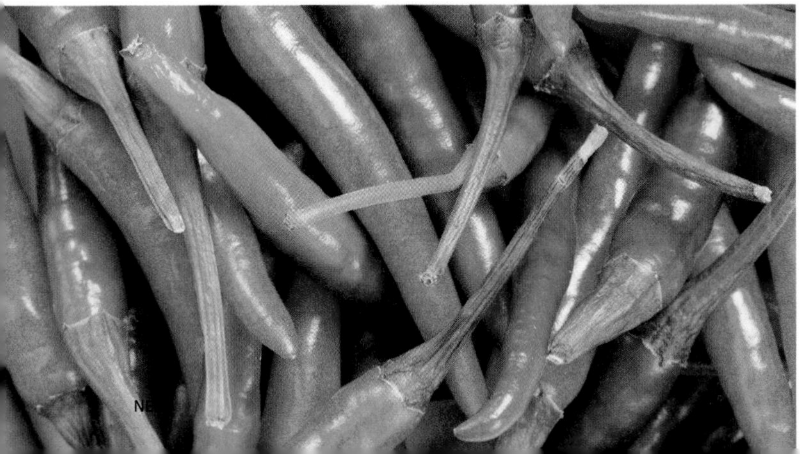

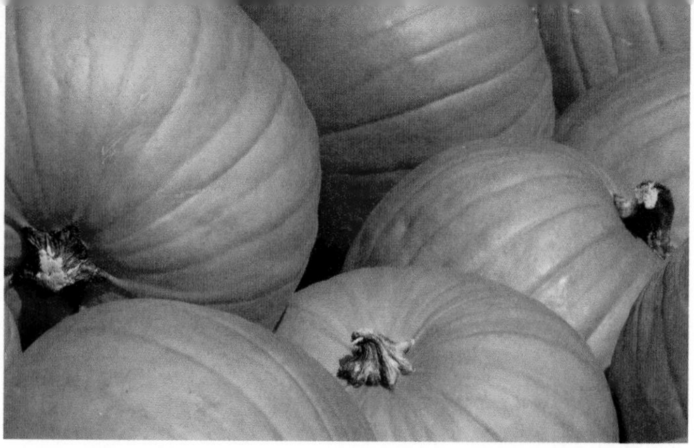

CHAPTER 16
Life Cycle Nutrition: Pregnancy and Lactation 505

CHAPTER 17
Life Cycle Nutrition: Infancy, Childhood, and Adolescence 543

CHAPTER 18
Life Cycle Nutrition: Adulthood and the Later Years 587

CHAPTER 19
Diet and Health 617

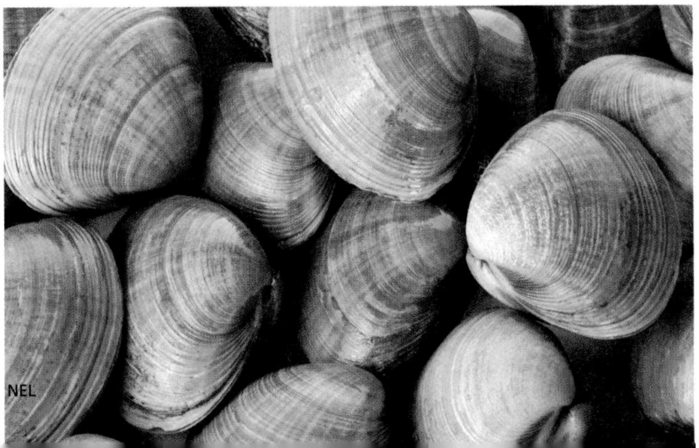

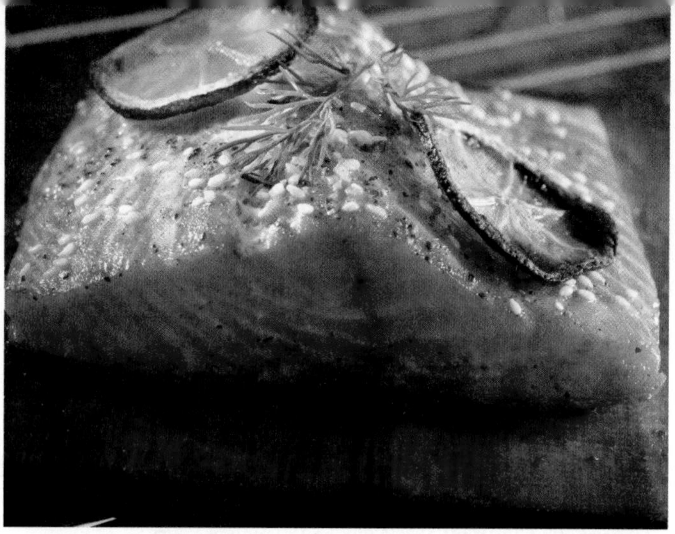

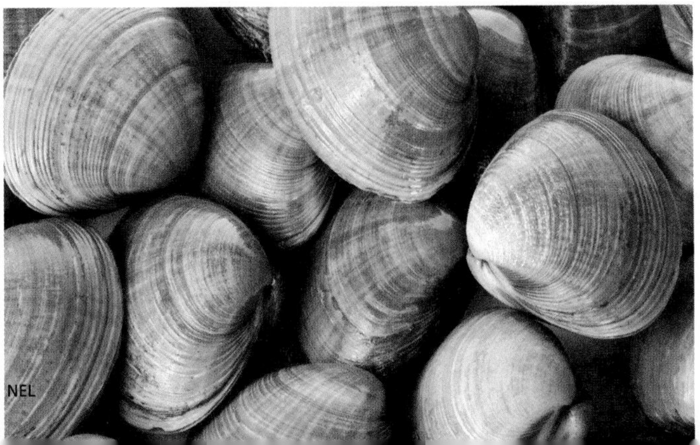

CHAPTER 20

Consumer Concerns about Foods and Water 659

CHAPTER 21

Hunger and the Global Environment 697

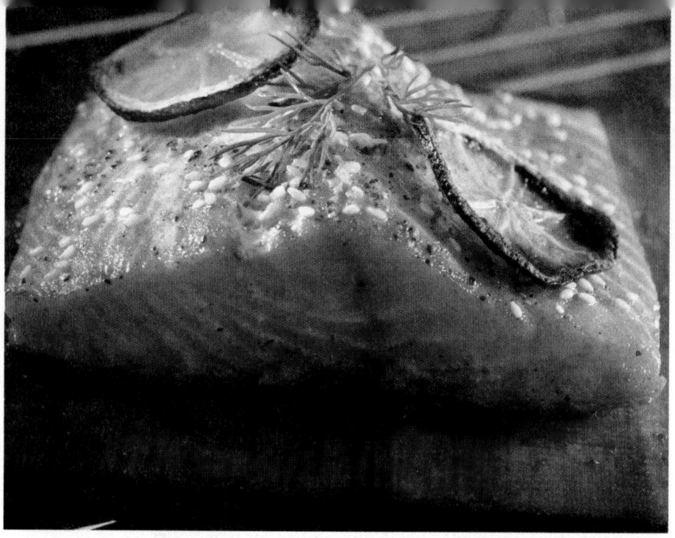

APPENDIX A

APPENDIX B

APPENDIX C

APPENDIX D

APPENDIX E

APPENDIX F

APPENDIX G

APPENDIX H

APPENDIX I

INSIDE COVERS

Preface

Nutrition is a science. The details of a nutrient's chemistry or a cell's biology can be overwhelming and confusing to some, but it needn't be. When the science is explained step by step and the facts are connected one by one, the details become clear and understandable. By telling stories about fat mice, using analogies of lamps, and applying guidance to groceries, we make the science of nutrition meaningful and memorable. That has been our mission since the first U.S. edition—to reveal the fascination of science and share the excitement of nutrition with readers. We have learned from the hundreds of professors and more than a million students who have used this book through the years that readers want an *understanding* of nutrition so that they can make healthy choices in their daily lives. We hope that this book serves you well.

A Book Tour of This Edition

The first Canadian edition of *Understanding Nutrition* presents the core information of an introductory nutrition course. The early chapters introduce the nutrients and their work in the body, and the later chapters apply that information to people's lives—describing the role of foods and nutrients in energy balance and weight control, in physical activity, in the life cycle, in disease prevention, in food safety, and in hunger.

The Chapters Chapter 1 begins by exploring why we eat the foods we do and continues with a brief overview of the nutrients, the science of nutrition, recommended nutrient intakes, assessment, and important relationships between diet and health. Chapter 2 describes the diet-planning principles and food guides used to create diets that support good health and includes instructions on how to read a food label. In Chapter 3, readers follow the journey of digestion and absorption as the body breaks down foods into nutrients and moves them into and around the body. Chapters 4 through 6 describe carbohydrates, fats, and proteins—their chemistry, metabolism, roles in the body, and places in the diet. Then Chapter 7 shows how the body derives energy from these three nutrients and their metabolic fate. Chapters 8 and 9 continue the story with a look at energy balance, the factors associated with weight maintenance, overweight and underweight, and the benefits and dangers of weight loss and weight gain. Chapters 10 through 14 complete the introductory lessons by describing the vitamins, the minerals, and water—their roles in the body, deficiency and toxicity symptoms, and sources.

The next seven chapters weave that basic information into practical applications, showing how nutrition influences people's lives. Chapter 15 describes how physical activity and nutrition work together to support fitness. Chapters 16, 17, and 18 present the special nutrient needs of people through the life cycle—pregnancy and lactation; infancy, childhood, and adolescence; and adulthood and the later years. Chapter 19 focuses on the dietary risk factors and recommendations associated with common chronic diseases, and Chapter 20 addresses consumer concerns about the safety of the food and water supply. Chapter 21 closes the book by examining hunger and the global environment.

The Highlights Every chapter is followed by a Highlight that provides readers with an in-depth look at a current, and often controversial, topic that relates to its companion chapter. New to this edition are two highlights: one that examines the scientific evidence behind some of the current controversies surrounding carbohydrates and their role in weight gain and weight loss; the other examines issues associated with fluid balance in the body, including the risks of too little and too much water.

Special Features The art and layout in this edition have been carefully designed to be inviting while enhancing student learning. In addition, special features help readers identify key concepts and apply nutrition knowledge. For example, when a new term is introduced, it is printed in **bold type**, and a definition is provided. These definitions often include pronunciations and derivations to facilitate understanding. The glossary at the end of the text includes all defined terms.

definition (DEF-eh-NISH-en): the meaning of a word.
- **de** = from
- **finis** = boundary

*Note: The headings below appear as depicted in the chapters to better help you familiarize yourself with the visual cues for the special features in this book.

Nutrition in Your Life

Each chapter begins with a Nutrition in Your Life section. These short paragraphs introduce the essence of the chapter in a friendly and familiar scenario.

Nutrition Portfolio

At the end of the chapter, a Nutrition Portfolio section revisits that message and prompts readers to consider whether their personal choices are meeting the dietary goals introduced in the chapter. New to this edition are instructions for using the Diet Analysis Plus computer program to complete this assignment.

IN SUMMARY **Each major section within a chapter concludes with a summary paragraph that reviews the key concepts. Similarly, summary tables cue readers to important reviews.**

Also featured in this edition are the *Dietary Guidance for Canadians* sections, which are introduced in Chapter 2 and presented throughout the text whenever their subjects are discussed. Look for the following design.

Dietary Guidance for Canadians

These guidelines provide science-based advice to promote health and to reduce the risk of chronic disease through diet and physical activity.

HOW TO Many of the chapters include "How To" sections that guide readers through problem-solving tasks. For example, the "How To" in Chapter 1 takes students through the steps of calculating energy intake from the grams of carbohydrate, fat, and protein in a food; another "How To" in Chapter 21 describes how to make environmentally friendly food-related choices.

TRY IT New to this edition are "Try It" activities that help readers practise the "How To" lessons. Additional activities can be found in CengageNOW, the online student study tool that accompanies this text.

Nutrition on the Net

Each chapter and many highlights conclude with Nutrition on the Net—a list of websites for further study of topics covered in the accompanying text. These lists do not imply an endorsement of the organizations or their programs. We have tried to provide reputable sources but cannot be responsible for the content of these sites. Read Highlight 1 to learn how to find reliable nutrition information on the Internet.

Study Cards New to this edition are Study Cards located at the back of the text—one for each chapter. Each study card presents a review list of the chapter's core concepts, and perhaps a table or figure to remind readers of key points. The backside of the study card provides essay and multiple-choice questions to help prepare students for exams.

The Appendixes The Appendixes are valuable references for a number of purposes. Appendix A summarizes background information on the hormonal and nervous systems, complementing Appendixes B and C on basic chemistry, the chemical structures of nutrients, and major metabolic pathways. Appendix D describes measures of protein quality. Appendix E provides detailed coverage of nutrition assessment, and Appendix F presents the estimated energy requirements for men and women at various levels of physical activity. Appendix G presents the Canadian meal-planning system, *Beyond the Basics: Meal Planning for Healthy Eating, Diabetes Prevention and Management.* Appendix H is Health Canada's *Nutrient Value of Some Common Foods.* Appendix I presents recommendations from the World Health Organization and food guidance for Americans, including the USDA key recommendations from the *Dietary Guidelines for Americans, 2010*; Food Patterns; and MyPlate icon.

The Inside Covers The inside covers put commonly used information at your fingertips. The inside front covers (pp. A–C) present the current nutrient recommendations from the latest Dietary Reference Intake Reports; the left inside back cover (p. Y) features the Canadian Daily Value Reference Standards used to calculate the % Daily Values (%DV) that appear on food labels and a glossary of nutrient measures; and the right inside back cover (p. Z) shows the suggested weight ranges for various heights. The pages immediately following the index (pp. W–X) assist readers with calculations and conversions between imperial and metric units of measurement.

Notable Changes in the First Canadian Edition

Because nutrition is an active science, staying current is paramount. To that end, this edition builds on the science of previous U.S. editions with the latest in nutrition research. Much has changed in the world of nutrition and in our daily lives since the first U.S. edition of *Understanding Nutrition.* The number of foods has increased dramatically—even as we spend less time than ever in the kitchen preparing meals. The connections between diet and disease have become more apparent—and consumer interest in making smart health choices has followed. More people are living longer and healthier lives. The science of nutrition has grown rapidly, with new "facts" emerging daily. In this first Canadian edition, as with all previous U.S. editions, every chapter has been revised to enhance learning by presenting current information accurately and attractively.

We have included relevant Canadian information throughout the text and reviewed and updated content in all chapters and highlights.

For individual chapters, we have included the following new features:

Chapter 1—An Overview of Nutrition

- Qualitative research in the science of nutrition
- Data from national nutrition surveys conducted in Canada
- Ten leading causes of death in Canada
- Factors contributing to deaths in Canada
- Accredited baccalaureate dietetics programs across Canada

Chapter 2—Planning a Healthy Diet

- *Eating Well with Canada's Food Guide*
- My Food Guide
- MyPlate (U.S. food guidance icon)
- Dietary guidance for Canadians
- Family members' meal plans aligned with *Eating Well with Canada's Food Guide*
- Culturally sensitive ethnic food choices for the Canadian context
- Canadian food labels
- Regulated health claims allowed on food packages in Canada

Chapter 3—Digestion, Absorption, and Transport

- Canadian prevalence of digestive problems

Chapter 4—The Carbohydrates: Sugars, Starches, and Fibres

- Guidelines for carbohydrate intake from Health Canada—for example, from the *Food Guide* and DRI reports
- Alternative sweeteners approved for use in Canada

Chapter 5—The Lipids: Triglycerides, Phospholipids, and Sterols

- Data from the 2007–2009 Canadian Community Health Measures survey (CHMS)—for example, for blood cholesterol
- Canadian Community Health Survey (CCHS) data on total fat, cholesterol, saturated fat, and *trans* fat intake
- *Food Guide* and DRI report recommendations for the intake of dietary total fat, saturated fat, and *trans* fats

Chapter 6—Protein: Amino Acids

- The latest food allergy labelling regulations (effective August 2012)
- CCHS data on protein intake
- A brief statement about protein quality and an example of how it is measured and a definition of the protein digestibility corrected amino acid score (PDCAAS), along with the latest DRI classification of indispensable, conditionally indispensable, and dispensable amino acids

Chapter 7—Metabolism: Transformations and Interactions

- Numerous points to help clarify the descriptions of various metabolic steps
- Canadian information on legal drinking age and tips for drinking responsibly

Chapter 8—Energy Balance and Body Composition

- New table showing factors that increase or decrease BMR
- Distribution of body weights in Canadian adults
- Canadian websites for eating disorders

Chapter 9—Weight Management: Overweight, Obesity, and Underweight

- *Eating Well with Canada's Food Guide* added to eating plans
- Dietary guidance for Canadians
- Canadian classifications for underweight, overweight, and obesity
- Canadian prevalence for underweight, overweight, and obesity (CCHS data)

Chapters 10–14 present a functional approach to the micronutrients.

Chapter 10—Nutrients for Energy Metabolism

- New figures of select nutrients used in energy metabolism showing the amounts found in foods sorted by food group and compared with the DRI
- Overview of the vitamins and minerals
- Canadian regulations for vitamin and mineral supplements

Chapter 11—Water and Electrolytes

- New figures showing the amounts of select electrolyte nutrients found in commonly consumed foods sorted by food group and compared with the DRI
- Canadian's electrolyte intakes from food (CCHS data)
- Map of water hardness across Canada
- New Highlight: Fluid Balance

Chapter 12—The Antioxidant Nutrients

- New figures showing the amounts of select antioxidant nutrients found in commonly consumed foods sorted by food group and compared with the DRI
- Map of selenium distribution across Canadian prairie soils

Chapter 13—Nutrients for Bone Health

- New figures showing the amounts of select bone health nutrients found in commonly consumed foods sorted by food group and compared with the DRI
- New section: About Bones
- Map of fluoridated public water supplies across Canada
- Canadian's intake of key bone health nutrients from food (CCHS data)

Chapter 14—Nutrients for Blood Health

- New figures showing the amounts of select blood health nutrients found in commonly consumed foods sorted by food group and compared with the DRI
- New section: About Blood

Chapter 15—Fitness: Physical Activity, Nutrients, and Body Adaptations

- 2011 *Canadian Physical Activity Guidelines* for adults
- Canadians, physical activity levels
- Discussion on nutrients of concern expanded to include calcium and vitamin D

Chapter 16—Life Cycle Nutrition: Pregnancy and Lactation

- Information and weblinks to Health Canada concerning prenatal nutrition (e.g., prenatal nutrition updates on folate, iron, and fish and omega-3 fatty acids), "Nutrition for Healthy Term Infants," and the Canada Prenatal Nutrition Program (CPNP)
- Information on breastfeeding rates, including more than two dozen additional references to Canadian documents about pregnancy and breastfeeding

Chapter 17—Life Cycle Nutrition: Infancy, Childhood, and Adolescence

- Canadian growth charts for infants and toddlers
- *Food Guide* Servings for children
- Statistics on childhood obesity
- 2011 *Canadian Physical Activity Guidelines* for children and adolescents
- Canadian BMI graphs for girls and boys 2–19 yrs
- Information about the Breakfast For Learning program and provincial school nutrition policies

Chapter 18—Life Cycle Nutrition: Adulthood and the Later Years

- Statistics on Canada's aging population
- Statistics on obesity of adults
- Calcium and fibre intakes
- The "new" vitamin D recommendations
- Nutrition screening tools for seniors
- 2011 *Canadian Physical Activity Guidelines* for adults and older adults

Chapter 19—Diet and Health

- Statistics on major chronic diseases (along with four dozen additional references about these chronic diseases)
- Canadian algorithm for estimating 10-year risk for heart disease
- Information on health claims on food and chronic diseases (e.g., plant sterols, oats, saturated and *trans* fats, sodium)
- Information on Natural Health Products databases, licensing, and labelling (along with weblinks to these databases and regulations)

Chapter 20—Consumer Concerns about Food and Water

- Information about the recent Listeriosis outbreak in Canada and the more recent *E. coli* outbreak in Europe
- Table of agencies that monitor Canada's food supply
- Information about the labelling of irradiated foods and which foods are allowed to be irradiated
- Information on the CFIA's pesticide monitoring program for domestic and imported fruits and vegetables
- New Canada Organic logo
- Examples of genetically modified foods sold in Canada
- Information about acrylamide, BPA, and bST
- Canada's freshwater supply and bottled water regulations

Chapter 21—Hunger and the Global Environment

- Information about food insecurity in Canada, including statistics on food bank use
- Information about how students can better understand their personal eating patterns using the Dietitians of Canada's online "eaTracker" software
- Information on local foods with weblinks to a national registry (presently eight provinces) of farmers' markets and to local food maps throughout Ontario
- Resources such as the David Suzuki Foundation to help all of us learn how to "eat for a healthy planet"

Ancillaries

Instructor Ancillaries

The **Nelson Education Teaching Advantage (NETA)** program delivers research-based instructor resources that promote student engagement and higher-order thinking to enable the success of Canadian students and educators.

Instructors today face many challenges. Resources are limited, time is scarce, and a new kind of student has emerged: one who is juggling school with work, has gaps in his or her basic knowledge, and is immersed in technology in a way that has led to a completely new style of learning. In response, Nelson Education has gathered a group of dedicated instructors to advise us on the creation of richer and more flexible ancillaries that respond to the needs of today's teaching environments.

The members of our editorial advisory board have experience across a variety of disciplines and are recognized for their commitment to teaching. They include

Norman Althouse, Haskayne School of Business, University of Calgary

Brenda Chant-Smith, Department of Psychology, Trent University

Scott Follows, Manning School of Business Administration, Acadia University

Jon Houseman, Department of Biology, University of Ottawa

Glen Loppnow, Department of Chemistry, University of Alberta

Tanya Noel, Department of Biology, York University

Gary Poole, Senior Scholar, Centre for Health Education Scholarship, and Associate Director, School of Population and Public Health, University of British Columbia

Dan Pratt, Department of Educational Studies, University of British Columbia

Mercedes Rowinsky-Geurts, Department of Languages and Literatures, Wilfrid Laurier University

David DiBattista, Department of Psychology, Brock University

Roger Fisher, PhD

In consultation with the editorial advisory board, Nelson Education has completely rethought the structure, approaches, and formats of our key textbook ancillaries. We've also increased our investment in editorial support for our ancillary authors. The result is the Nelson Education Teaching Advantage and its key components: *NETA Engagement, NETA Assessment,* and *NETA Presentation.* Each component includes one or more ancillaries prepared according to our best practices, and a document explaining the theory behind the practices.

NETA Engagement presents materials that help instructors deliver engaging content and activities to their classes. Instead of Instructor's Manuals that regurgitate chapter outlines and key terms from the text, NETA Enriched Instructor's Manuals (EIMs) provide genuine assistance to teachers. The EIMs answer questions like *What should students learn?, Why should students care?,* and *What are some common student misconceptions and stumbling blocks?* EIMs not only identify the topics that cause students the most difficulty, but also describe techniques and resources to help students master these concepts. Dr. Roger Fisher's *Instructor's Guide to Classroom Engagement (IGCE)* accompanies every Enriched Instructor's Manual. (Information about the NETA Enriched Instructor's Manual prepared for the first Canadian edition of *Understanding Nutrition* is included in the description of the IRCD below.)

NETA Assessment relates to testing materials: not just Nelson's Test Banks and Computerized Test Banks, but also in-text self-tests, Study Guides and web quizzes, and homework programs like CNOW. Under *NETA Assessment*, Nelson's authors create multiple-choice questions that reflect research-based best practices for constructing effective questions and testing not just recall but also higher-order thinking. Our guidelines were developed by David DiBattista, a 3M National Teaching Fellow whose recent research as a professor of psychology at Brock University has focused on multiple-choice testing. All Test Bank authors receive training at workshops conducted by Prof. DiBattista, as do the copyeditors assigned to each Test Bank. A copy of *Multiple Choice Tests: Getting Beyond Remembering*, Prof. DiBattista's guide to writing effective tests, is included with every Nelson Test Bank/Computerized Test Bank package. (Information about the NETA Test Bank prepared for the first Canadian edition of *Understanding Nutrition* is included in the description of the IRCD below.)

NETA Presentation has been developed to help instructors make the best use of PowerPoint® in their classrooms. With a clean and uncluttered design developed by Maureen Stone of StoneSoup Consulting, NETA Presentation features slides with improved readability, more multimedia and graphic materials, activities to use in class, and tips for instructors on the Notes page. A copy of *NETA Guidelines for Classroom Presentations* by Maureen Stone is included with each set of PowerPoint slides. (Information about the NETA PowerPoint® prepared for the first Canadian edition of *Understanding Nutrition* is included in the description of the IRCD below.)

IRCD

Key instructor ancillaries are provided on the *Instructor's Resource CD* (ISBN 978-0-17-661836-0), giving instructors the ultimate tool for customizing lectures and presentations. The IRCD includes

- **NETA Engagement:** The Enriched Instructor's Manual was written by Danny Pincivero, Department of Kinesiology, McMaster University. It is organized according to the textbook chapters and addresses eight key educational concerns, such as typical stumbling blocks student face and how to address them. Other features include worksheets, classroom activities, and solutions.
- **NETA Assessment**: The Test Bank was written by Rhona Hanning, School of Public Health and Health Systems, University of Waterloo. It includes over 2000 multiple-choice questions written according to NETA guidelines for effective construction and development of higher-order questions. Also included are essay and matching questions. Test Bank files are provided in Word format for easy editing and in PDF format for convenient printing, whatever your system.

  The Computerized Test Bank by ExamView® includes all the questions from the Test Bank. The easy-to-use ExamView software is compatible with Microsoft Windows and Mac. Create tests by selecting questions from the question bank, modifying these questions as desired, and adding new questions you write yourself. You can administer quizzes online and export tests to WebCT, Blackboard, and other formats.
- **NETA Presentation:** Microsoft® PowerPoint® lecture slides for every chapter have been created by Danielle Battram, Division of Food and Nutritional Sciences, Brescia University College. There is an average of 30–40 slides per chapter, many featuring key figures, tables, and photographs from the first Canadian edition of *Understanding Nutrition*. NETA principles of clear design and engaging content have been incorporated throughout.
- **Image Library:** This resource consists of digital copies of figures, short tables, and photographs used in the book. Instructors may use these jpegs to create their own PowerPoint presentations.
- **DayOne:** Day One—Prof InClass is a PowerPoint presentation that you can customize to orient your students to the class and their text at the beginning of the course.

Student Ancillaries

- **Diet Analysis Plus:** New to the first Canadian edition of *Understanding Nutrition* is the inclusion of Health Canada's *Nutrient Value of Some Common Foods* in Diet Analysis Plus.

  Dynamic and rewarding, the newly updated Diet Analysis Plus software encourages active learning by making it easier for students to track diet and activity through personalized profiles. The interactive nutrition labs respect diverse ways of learning and encourage students to practise in order to achieve concept mastery. With Diet Analysis Plus, students can analyze the nutritional value of the food they eat in order to adjust their diets to reach personal health goals—all while gaining a better understanding of how nutrition relates to, and impacts, their lives.

Diet Analysis Plus is integrated into all Cengage Learning Introductory Nutrition textbooks through activities in each chapter that show students how the chapter concepts relate to their diet and health goals. Instructors can use these activities for assignments or extra credit.

- **CengageNOW:** An intelligent, Web-based study system and course management tool, CengageNOW provides a completely integrated package of diagnostic quizzes, personalized study, animations, videos, case studies, and more—along with an Instructor Grade Book that automatically captures and tracks student progress. Pre-tests assess students' understanding of what they have read and direct them to further study of concepts they have not yet mastered using the interactive e-book and other online tools. New to this edition is a set of 17 videos covering more difficult concepts. Videos are available as pop-up tutors in the e-book and can be downloaded to an iPod or other portable device. The self-grading pre-tests and post-tests are also ideal for homework assignments, as results flow automatically into the built-in Instructor Grade Book. CengageNOW is also available in the WebCT® and Blackboard® platforms.

Students and Instructors

Visit the website to accompany *Understanding Nutrition*, First Canadian Edition, at http://understandingnutrition1e.nelson.com. This website contains flashcards, weblinks, and more.

Acknowledgments

Canadian Acknowledgments

We are grateful to Eleanor Noss Whitney and Sharon Rady Rolfes, authors of *Understanding Nutrition* in the United States, for providing a solid twelfth edition on which this text is based.

Special thanks to our executive editor, Jackie Wood, and our senior developmental editor, Mark Grzeskowiak, for their continual encouragement to ensure the highest quality in all facets of this book. Deep gratitude is extended to Natalia Denesiuk Harris and Wendy Yano for making sense of the final manuscript and to Natalie Russell for her photo research and permission clearance. Thank you, Alexis Hood, for your excellent work in marketing this text and providing support for the sales team. Many thanks to the authors of the supplements accompanying this book for helping to make it a well-rounded package for instructors and students. To our reviewers, a heartfelt thank-you for your many thoughtful ideas and suggestions in guiding the development of this first Canadian edition.

Gail Hammond
Len Piché
October 2011

U.S. Acknowledgments

We have taken great care to provide accurate information and have included many references at the end of each chapter and highlight. However, to keep the number of references manageable, many statements that appeared in previous editions with references now appear without them. All statements reflect current nutrition knowledge and the authors will supply references upon request. In addition to supporting text statements, the end-of-chapter references provide readers with resources for finding a good overview or more details on the subject. Nutrition is a fascinating subject, and we hope our enthusiasm for it comes through on every page.

To produce a book requires the coordinated effort of a team of people—and, no doubt, each team member has another team of support people as well. We salute, with a big round of applause, everyone who has worked so diligently to ensure the quality of this book.

We thank our partners and friends, Linda DeBruyne and Fran Webb, for their valuable consultations and contributions; working together over the past 25-plus years has been a most wonderful experience. We especially appreciate Linda's research assistance on several chapters. Special thanks to our colleagues Kathy Pinna for her insightful comments and Gail Hammond for her Canadian perspective. Thank you to Alex Rodriguez for her work on manuscript preparation and to James Gegenheimer for his assistance in creating informative tables and descriptive figures.

Our heartfelt thanks to our editorial team for their efforts in creating an outstanding nutrition textbook—Peggy Williams for her leadership and support; Nedah Rose for her thoughtful suggestions and efficient analysis of reviews; Trudy Brown and Jerilyn Emori for their management of this project; Laura McGinn for her energetic efforts in marketing; Lauren Tarson for her dedication in developing online animations and study tools; Bill Jentzen and Roberta Broyer for their assistance in obtaining permissions; and Elesha Feldman for her competent coordination of ancillaries.

We also thank Gary Hespenheide for creatively designing these pages; Joan Keyes for her diligent attention to the innumerable details involved in production; Roman Barnes for selecting photographs that deliver nutrition messages attractively; Susan Gall for copyediting more than 2000 manuscript pages; Pat Lewis for proofreading close to 1000 final text pages; and Ken Hassman for composing a thorough and useful index. To the hundreds of others involved in production and sales, we tip our hats in appreciation.

We are especially grateful to our friends and families for their continued encouragement and support. We also thank our many reviewers for their comments and contributions.

Ellie Whitney
Sharon Rady Rolfes
October 2009

Canadian Reviewers of Understanding Nutrition

Sebastian Boyas
University of Ottawa

Ingrid Brenner
Trent University

Tristaca Caldwell
Acadia University

Debbie Gurfinkel
University of Toronto

Rhona Hanning
University of Waterloo

Manuela Keeler
Niagara College

Paul Leblanc
Brock University

Norman Temple
Athabasca University

Linda Wykes
McGill University

U.S. Reviewers of Understanding Nutrition

Becky Alejandre
American River College

Janet B. Anderson
Utah State University

Sandra D. Baker
University of Delaware

Angelina Boyce
Hillsborough Community College

Lynn S. Brann
Syracuse University

Shalon Bull
Palm Beach Community College

Dorothy A. Byrne
University of Texas, San Antonio

John R. Capeheart
University of Houston, Downtown

Leah Carter
Bakersfield College

James F. Collins
University of Florida

Diane Curtis
Los Rios Community College District

Lisa K. Diewald
Montgomery County Community College

Kelly K. Eichmann
Fresno City College

Mary Flynn
Brown University

Sue Fredstrom
Minnesota State University, Mankato

Trish Froehlich
Palm Beach Community College

Stephen P. Gagnon
Hillsborough Community College

Jill Golden
Orange Coast College

Kathleen Gould
Towson University

Margaret Gunther
Palomar College

Charlene Hamilton
University of Delaware

D. J. Hennager
Kirkwood Community College

Catherine Hagen Howard
Texarkana College

Ernest B. Izevbigie
Jackson State University

Craig Kasper
Hillsborough Community College

Younghee Kim
Bowling Green State University

Rebecca A. Kleinschmidt
University of Alaska Southeast

Vicki Kloosterhouse
Oakland Community College

Donna M. Kopas
Pennsylvania State University

Susan M. Krueger
University of Wisconsin, Eau Claire

Melissa Langone
Pasco-Hernando Community College

Darlene M. Levinson
Oakland Community College, Orchard Ridge

Kimberly Lower
Collin County Community College

Melissa B. McGuire
Maple Woods Community College

Diane L. McKay
Tufts University

Anne Miller
De Anza College

Anahita M. Mistry
Eastern Michigan University

Mithia Mukutmoni
Sierra College

Steven Nizielski
Grand Valley State University

Jane M. Osowski
University of Southern Mississippi

Sarah Panarello
Yakima Valley Community College

Ryan Paruch
Tulsa Community College

Jill Patterson
Pennsylvania State University

Julie Priday
Centralia College

Kathy L. Sedlet
Collin County Community College

Melissa Shock
University of Central Arkansas

LuAnn Soliah
Baylor University

Kenneth Strothkamp
Lewis & Clark College

Andrea Villarreal
Phoenix College

Terry Weideman
Oakland Community College, Highland Lake

H. Garrison Wilkes
University of Massachusetts, Boston

Lynne C. Zeman
Kirkwood Community College

Maureen Zimmerman
Mesa Community College

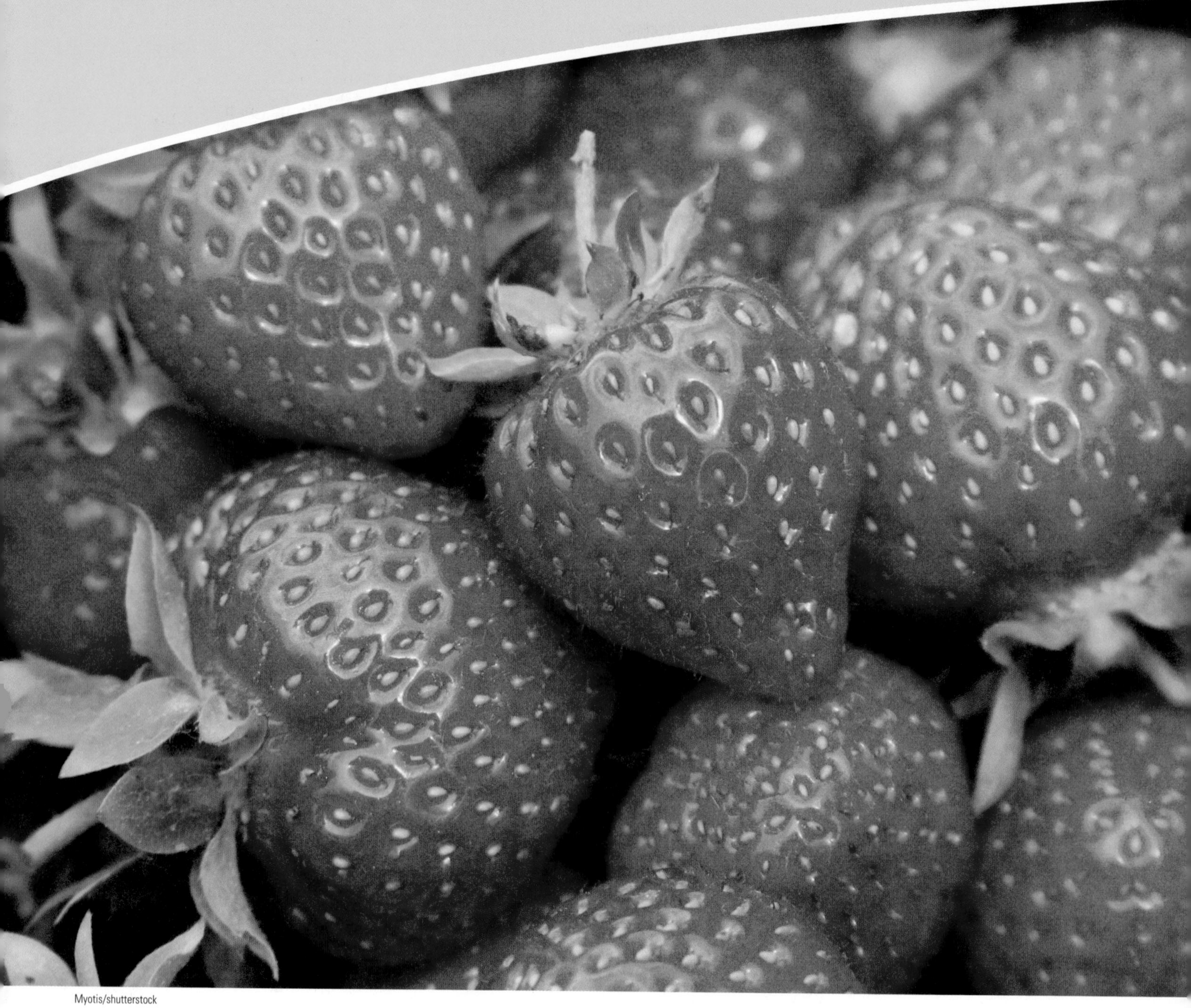

Myotis/shutterstock

Nutrition in Your Life

Believe it or not, you have probably eaten at least 20 000 meals in your life. Without any conscious effort on your part, your body uses the nutrients from those foods to make all its components, fuel all its activities, and defend itself against diseases. How successfully your body handles these tasks depends, in part, on your food choices. Nutritious food choices support healthy bodies.

CENGAGENOW™

Throughout this chapter, the CengageNOW logo indicates an opportunity for online self-study, linking you to interactive tutorials, activities, and videos to increase your understanding of chapter concepts.
www.cengage.com/sso

CHAPTER 1

An Overview of Nutrition

CHAPTER OUTLINE

Welcome to the world of **nutrition.** Although you may not always have been aware of it, nutrition has played a significant role in your life. And it will continue to affect you in major ways, depending on the **foods** you select.

Every day, several times a day, you make food choices that influence your body's health for better or worse. Each day's choices may benefit or harm your health only a little, but when these choices are repeated over years and decades, the rewards or consequences become major. That being the case, paying close attention to good eating habits now supports health benefits later. Conversely, carelessness about food choices can contribute to many chronic diseases ♦ prevalent in later life, including heart disease, diabetes, and cancer. Of course, some people will become ill or die young no matter what choices they make, and others will live long lives despite making poor choices. For the majority of us, however, the food choices we make each and every day will benefit or impair our health in proportion to the wisdom of those choices.

Although most people realize that their food habits affect their health, they often choose foods for other reasons. After all, foods bring to the table a variety of pleasures, traditions, and associations as well as nourishment. The challenge, then, is to combine favourite foods and fun times with a nutritionally balanced **diet**.

♦ In general, a **chronic disease** progresses slowly or with little change and lasts a long time. By comparison, an **acute disease** develops quickly, produces sharp symptoms, and runs a short course.
- **chronos** = time
- **acute** = sharp

Food Choices

People decide what to eat, when to eat, and even whether to eat in highly personal ways, often based on behavioural or social motives rather than on an awareness of nutrition's importance to health. A variety of food choices can support good health, and an understanding of human nutrition helps you make sensible selections more often.

Personal Preference As you might expect, the number one reason people choose foods is taste—they like certain flavours. Two widely shared preferences are for the sweetness of sugar and the savouriness of salt. Liking high-fat foods also appears to be a universally common preference. Other preferences might be for the hot peppers common in Mexican cooking or the curry spices of South

nutrition: the science of foods and the nutrients they contain, and of their actions within the body (including ingestion, digestion, absorption, transport, metabolism, and excretion). A broader definition includes the social, economic, cultural, and psychological implications of food and eating.

foods: products derived from plants or animals that can be taken into the body to yield energy and nutrients for the maintenance of life and the growth and repair of tissues.

diet: the foods and beverages a person eats and drinks.

Asian cuisine. Research suggests that genetics may influence taste perceptions and therefore food likes and dislikes.[1] Similarly, the hormones of pregnancy seem to influence food cravings and aversions (see Chapter 16).

Habit People sometimes select foods out of habit. They eat cereal every morning, for example, simply because they have always eaten cereal for breakfast. Eating a familiar food and not having to make any decisions can be comforting.

Ethnic Heritage or Tradition Among the strongest influences on food choices are ethnic heritage and tradition. People eat the foods they grew up eating. Every country, and in fact every region of a country, has its own typical foods and ways of combining them into meals. The "Canadian diet" includes many ethnic foods that originate in various countries, all adding variety to the diet.

Social Interactions Most people enjoy companionship while eating. It's fun to go out with friends for pizza or gelato. Chapter 9 describes how people tend to eat more food when socializing with others. Meals are often social events, and sharing food is part of hospitality—regardless of hunger signals. Social customs invite people to accept food or drink offered by a host or shared by a group.

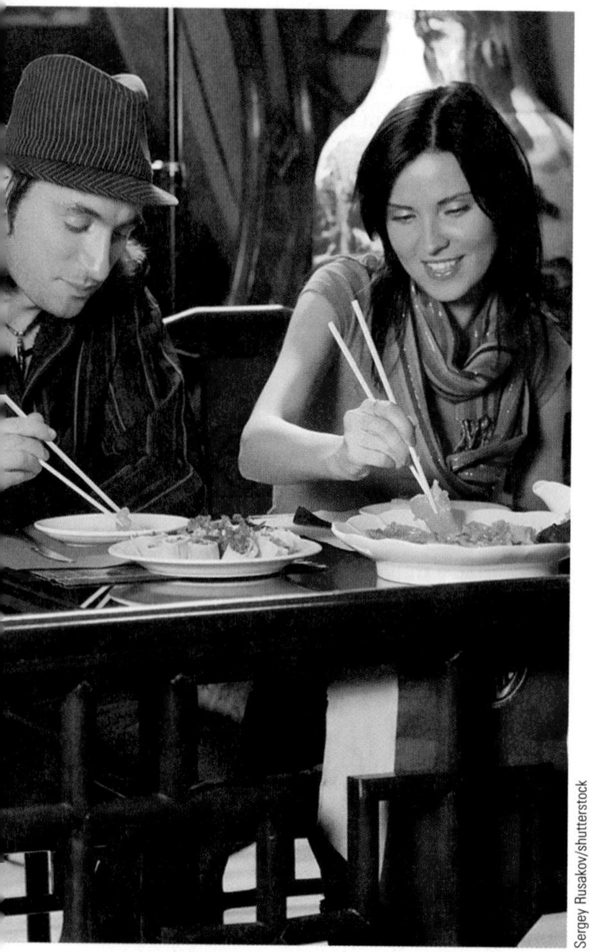
Sergey Rusakov/shutterstock

An enjoyable way to learn about other cultures is to taste their ethnic foods.

Availability, Convenience, and Economy People often eat foods that are accessible, quick and easy to prepare, and within their financial means. Consumers who value convenience frequently eat out, bring home ready-to-eat meals, or have food delivered. Even when they venture into the kitchen, they want to prepare a meal in 15 to 20 minutes, using less than a half dozen ingredients—and those "ingredients" are often semiprepared foods, such as canned soups. Those who frequently prepare their own meals eat fast-food less often and are more likely to meet dietary guidelines for fat, calcium, fruits, vegetables, and whole grains.[2]

Consumer emphasis on convenience limits food choices to the selections offered on menus and products designed for quick preparation. Whether decisions based on convenience meet a person's nutrition needs depends on the choices made. Eating a banana or a chocolate bar may be equally convenient, but the fruit provides more vitamins and minerals and less sugar and fat.

Rising food costs have shifted some consumers' priorities and changed their shopping habits. They are less likely to buy higher priced convenience foods and more likely to buy less-expensive store brand items and prepare home-cooked meals. In fact, about 70 percent of Canadian adults report eating breakfast and lunch at home four or more times a week and almost 90 percent report eating dinner at home four or more times a week.[3]

Positive and Negative Associations People tend to like particular foods associated with happy occasions—such as hot dogs at ball games or cake and ice cream at birthday parties. By the same token, people can develop aversions and dislike foods that they ate when they felt sick or that they were forced to eat as a child. By using foods as rewards or punishments, parents may inadvertently teach their children to like and dislike certain foods.

Emotions Some people cannot eat when they are emotionally upset. Others may eat in response to a variety of emotional stimuli—for example, to relieve boredom or depression or to calm anxiety. A depressed person may choose to eat rather than to call a friend. A person who has returned home from an exciting evening out may unwind with a late-night snack. These people may find emotional comfort, in part, because foods can influence the brain's chemistry and the mind's response. Carbohydrate and alcohol, for example, tend to calm, whereas protein and caffeine are more likely to activate. Eating in response to emotions can easily lead to overeating and obesity, but it may be appropriate at times. For example, sharing food at times of bereavement serves both the giver's need to provide comfort and the receiver's need to be cared for and to interact with others, as well as to take nourishment.

Values Food choices may reflect people's religious beliefs, political views, or environmental concerns. For example, some Christians forgo meat on Fridays during Lent (the period prior to Easter), Jewish law includes an extensive set of dietary rules that govern the use of foods derived from animals, and Muslims fast between sunrise and sunset during Ramadan (the ninth month of the Islamic calendar). Some vegetarians select foods based on their concern for animal rights. Concerned consumers may buy fruit that is fair-trade only. People may buy vegetables from local farmers to save the fuel and environmental costs of foods shipped from far away. They may also select foods packaged in containers that can be reused or recycled. Some consumers accept or reject foods that have been irradiated, grown organically, or genetically modified, depending on their approval of these processes (see Chapter and Highlight 20 for a complete discussion).

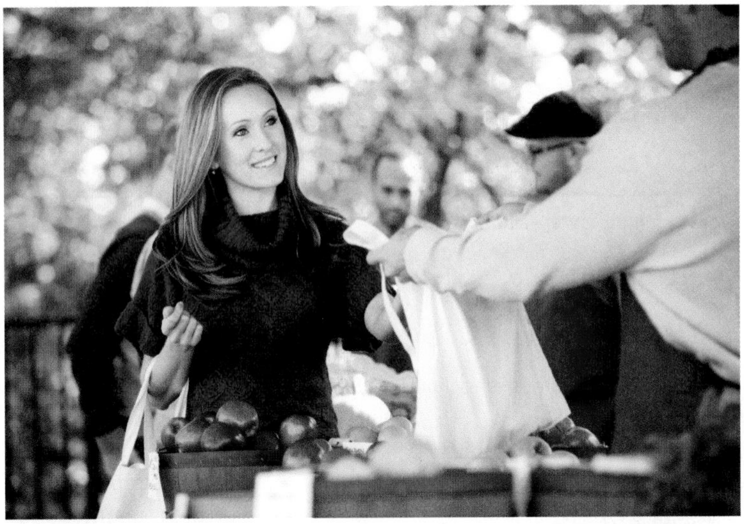

© Sean Locke/iStockphoto LP

To enhance your health, keep nutrition in mind when selecting foods. To protect the environment, shop at local markets and reuse cloth shopping bags.

Body Weight and Image Sometimes people select certain foods and supplements that they believe will improve their physical appearance and avoid those they believe might be detrimental. Such decisions can be beneficial when based on sound nutrition and fitness knowledge, but decisions based on fads or carried to extremes undermine good health, as pointed out in later discussions of eating disorders (Highlight 8) and dietary supplements commonly used by athletes (Highlight 15).

Nutrition and Health Benefits Finally, of course, many consumers make food choices that will benefit health. Food manufacturers and restaurant chefs have responded to scientific findings linking health with nutrition by offering an abundant selection of health-promoting foods and beverages. Foods that provide health benefits beyond their nutrient contributions are called **functional foods.**[4] Whole foods—as natural and familiar as oatmeal or tomatoes—are the simplest functional foods. In other cases, foods have been modified to provide health benefits, perhaps by lowering the fat contents. In still other cases, manufacturers have fortified foods by adding nutrients or **phytochemicals** that provide health benefits (see Highlight 14). ♦ Examples of these functional foods include orange juice fortified with calcium to help build strong bones and margarine made with a plant sterol that lowers blood cholesterol.

♦ Functional foods may include whole foods, modified foods, or fortified foods.

Consumers typically welcome new foods into their diets, provided that these foods are reasonably priced, clearly labelled, easy to find in the grocery store, and convenient to prepare. These foods must also taste good—as good as the traditional choices. Of course, a person need not eat any "special" foods to enjoy a healthy diet; many "regular" foods provide numerous health benefits as well. In fact, "regular" foods such as vegetables and fruit; whole grains; legumes; low-fat milk products; and lean meats, fish, and poultry are among the healthiest choices a person can make.

IN SUMMARY **A person selects foods for a variety of reasons. Whatever those reasons may be, food choices influence health. Individual food selections neither make nor break a diet's healthfulness, but the balance of foods selected over time can make an important difference to health.[5] For this reason, people are wise to think "nutrition" when making their food choices.**

The Nutrients

Biologically speaking, people eat to receive nourishment. Do you ever think of yourself as a biological being made of carefully arranged atoms, molecules, cells, tissues, and organs? Are you aware of the activity going on within your body even

functional foods: foods that contain physiologically active compounds that provide health benefits beyond their nutrient contributions; sometimes called *designer foods* or *nutraceuticals.*

phytochemicals (FIE-toe-KEM-ih-cals): nonnutrient compounds found in plant-derived foods that have biological activity in the body.
- **phyto** = plant

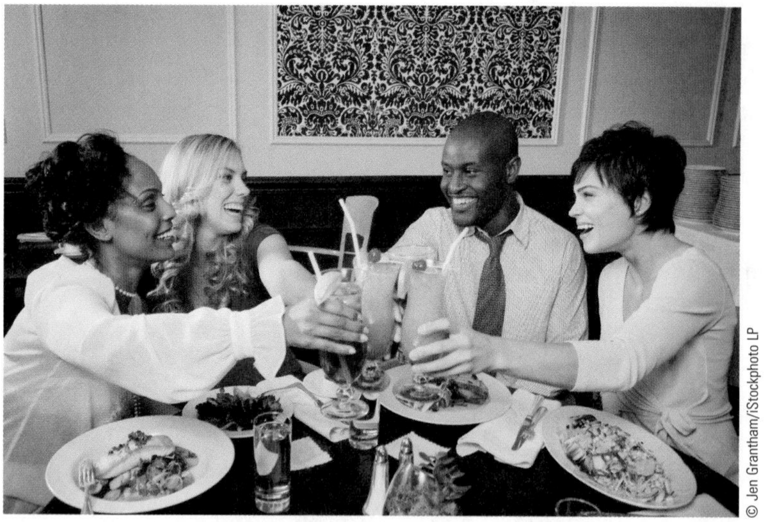
© Jen Grantham/iStockphoto LP

Foods bring pleasure—and nutrients.

as you sit still? The atoms, molecules, and cells of your body continuously move and change, even though the structures of your tissues and organs and your external appearance remain relatively constant. Your skin, which has covered you since your birth, is replaced entirely by new cells every seven years. The fat beneath your skin is not the same fat that was there a year ago. Your oldest red blood cell is only 120 days old, and the entire lining of your digestive tract is renewed every two to seven days.[6] To maintain your "self," you must continually replenish, from foods, the **energy** and the **nutrients** you deplete as your body maintains itself.

Nutrients in Foods and in the Body

Amazingly, our bodies can derive all the energy, structural materials, and regulating agents we need from the foods we eat. This section introduces the nutrients that foods deliver and shows how they participate in the dynamic processes that keep people alive and well.

Nutrient Composition of Foods Chemical analysis of a food such as a tomato shows that it is composed primarily of water (95 percent). Most of the solid materials are carbohydrates, lipids, ♦ and proteins. If you could remove these materials, you would find a tiny residue of vitamins, minerals, and other compounds. Water, carbohydrates, lipids, proteins, vitamins, and some of the minerals found in foods represent the six classes ♦ of nutrients—substances the body uses for the growth, maintenance, and repair of its tissues.

♦ As Chapter 5 explains, dietary lipids are fats and oils.

♦ Six classes of nutrients:
- Carbohydrates
- Lipids (fats)
- Proteins
- Vitamins
- Minerals
- Water

This book focuses mostly on the nutrients, but foods contain other compounds as well—fibres, phytochemicals, pigments, additives, alcohols, and others. Some are beneficial, some are neutral, and a few are harmful. Later sections of the book touch on these compounds and their significance.

Nutrient Composition of the Body A chemical analysis of your body would show that it is made of materials similar to those found in foods (see Figure 1-1).

FIGURE 1-1 Body Composition of Healthy-Weight Men and Women

The human body is made of compounds similar to those found in foods—mostly water (60 percent) and some fat (13 to 21 percent for young men, 23 to 31 percent for young women), with carbohydrate, protein, vitamins, minerals, and other minor constituents making up the remainder. (Chapter 8 describes the health hazards of too little or too much body fat.)

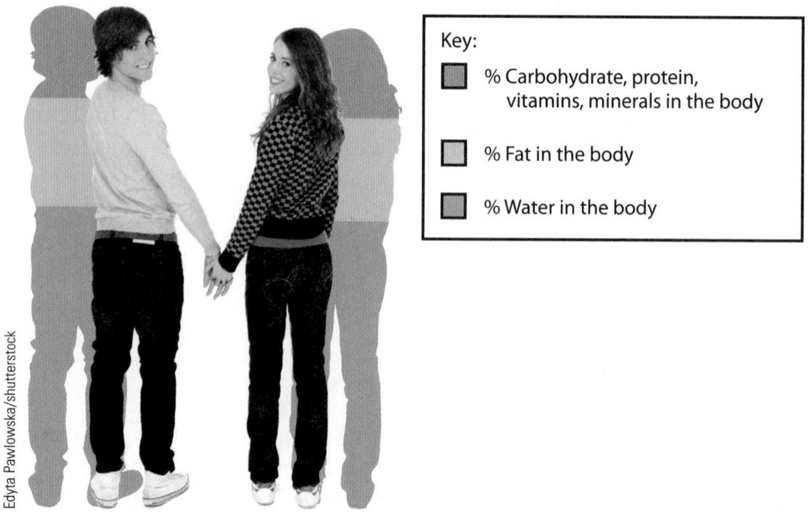
Key:
% Carbohydrate, protein, vitamins, minerals in the body
% Fat in the body
% Water in the body
Edyta Pawlowska/shutterstock

energy: the capacity to do work. The energy in food is chemical energy. The body can convert this chemical energy to mechanical, electrical, or heat energy.

nutrients: chemical substances obtained from food and used in the body to provide energy, structural materials, and regulating agents to support growth, maintenance, and repair of the body's tissues. Nutrients may also reduce the risks of some diseases.

A healthy 70 kilogram (150-pound) body contains about 42 kilograms (90 pounds) of water and about 10 to 20 kilograms (20 to 45 pounds) of fat. The remaining kilograms are mostly protein, carbohydrate, and the major minerals of the bones. Vitamins, other minerals, and incidental extras constitute a fraction of a kilogram.

Chemical Composition of Nutrients The simplest of the nutrients are the minerals. Each mineral is a chemical element; its atoms are all alike. As a result, its identity never changes. For example, iron may have different electrical charges, but the individual iron atoms remain the same when they are in a food, when a person eats the food, when the iron becomes part of a red blood cell, when the cell is broken down, and when the iron is lost from the body by excretion. The next simplest nutrient is water, a compound made of two elements—hydrogen and oxygen. Minerals and water are chemically **inorganic** nutrients, which means they do not contain carbon.

The other four classes of nutrients (carbohydrates, lipids, proteins, and vitamins) are more complex. In addition to hydrogen and oxygen, they all contain carbon, an element found in all living things. They are therefore called chemically **organic** nutrients (meaning, literally, "alive"). This chemical definition of *organic* differs from the agricultural definition. As Chapter 20 explains, *organic farming* refers to growing crops and raising livestock according to standards set by the Organic Products Regulations (2009) in the *Canada Agricultural Products Act.* Protein and some vitamins also contain nitrogen and may contain other elements such as sulphur as well (see Table 1-1).

Essential Nutrients The body can make some nutrients, but it cannot make all of them. Also, it makes some in insufficient quantities to meet its needs and, therefore, we must obtain these nutrients from foods. The nutrients that foods must supply are **essential nutrients.** When used to refer to nutrients, the word *essential* means more than just "necessary"; it means "needed from outside the body"—normally, from foods.

The Energy-Yielding Nutrients: Carbohydrate, Fat, and Protein

In the body, three organic nutrients can be used to provide energy: carbohydrate, fat, and protein. ♦ In contrast to these **energy-yielding nutrients,** vitamins, minerals, and water do not directly yield energy in the human body.

Energy Measured in kCalories The energy released from carbohydrate, fat, and protein can be measured in **calories**—tiny units of energy so small that a single apple provides tens of thousands of them. To ease calculations, energy is expressed in 1000-calorie metric units known as kilocalories (shortened to kcalories, but

TABLE 1-1 Elements in the Six Classes of Nutrients

Notice that organic nutrients contain carbon.

	Carbon	Hydrogen	Oxygen	Nitrogen	Minerals
Inorganic nutrients					
Minerals					✓
Water		✓	✓		
Organic nutrients					
Carbohydrate	✓	✓	✓		
Lipid (fat)	✓	✓	✓		
Protein[a]	✓	✓	✓	✓	
Vitamins[b]	✓	✓	✓		

[a]Some proteins also contain the mineral sulphur.
[b]Some vitamins contain nitrogen; some contain minerals.

♦ Carbohydrate, fat, and protein are sometimes called **macronutrients** because the body requires them in relatively large amounts (many grams daily). In contrast, vitamins and minerals are **micronutrients,** required only in small amounts (milligrams or micrograms daily).

inorganic: not containing carbon or pertaining to living things.
- **in** = not

organic: in chemistry, a substance or molecule containing carbon-carbon bonds or carbon-hydrogen bonds. This definition excludes coal, diamonds, and a few carbon-containing compounds that contain only a single carbon and no hydrogen, such as carbon dioxide (CO_2), calcium carbonate ($CaCO_3$), magnesium carbonate ($MgCO_3$), and sodium cyanide (NaCN).

essential nutrients: nutrients a person must obtain from food because the body cannot make them for itself in sufficient quantity to meet physiological needs; also called **indispensable nutrients.** About 40 nutrients are currently known to be essential for human beings.

energy-yielding nutrients: the nutrients that break down to yield energy the body can use:
- Carbohydrate
- Fat
- Protein

calories: units by which energy is measured. Food energy is measured in *kilocalories* (1000 calories equal 1 kilocalorie), abbreviated **kcalories** or **kcal.** One kcalorie is the amount of energy necessary to raise the temperature of 1 kilogram (kg) of water 1°C. The scientific use of the term *kcalorie* is the same as the popular use of the term *calorie.* On food labels, the energy content of a food is listed as Calories (with a capital "C"), meaning kcalories.

♦ The international unit for measuring food energy is the **joule,** a measure of *work* energy. To convert kcalories to kilojoules, multiply by 4.2; to convert kilojoules to kcalories, multiply by 0.24.

commonly called "calories"). When you read in popular books or magazines that an apple provides "100 calories," it actually means 100 kcalories. This book uses the term **kcalorie** and its abbreviation **kcal** throughout, as do other scientific books and journals. ♦ The accompanying "How To" provides a few tips on "thinking metric."

HOW TO Think Metric

Like other scientists, nutrition scientists use metric units of measure. In Canada, we use the metric system; however, often with food we use Imperial measures (e.g., cup, tablespoon, teaspoon). This "How To" box reminds us how to think metric when encountering Imperial measures. Scientists measure food energy in kilocalories, people's height in centimetres, people's weight in kilograms, and the weights of foods and nutrients in grams, milligrams, or micrograms. For ease in using these measures, it helps to remember that the prefixes on the grams imply 1000. For example, a *kilo*gram is 1000 grams, a *milli*gram is 1/1000 of a gram, and a *micro*gram is 1/1000 of a milligram.

Most food labels and many recipe books provide "dual measures," listing both household measures, such as cups, tablespoons, and teaspoons, and metric measures, such as millilitres, litres, and grams.

To facilitate communication, many members of the international scientific community have adopted a common system of measurement—the International System of Units (SI). In addition to using metric measures, the SI establishes common units of measurement. For example, the SI unit for measuring food energy is the joule (not the kcalorie). A joule is the amount of energy expended when 1 kilogram is moved 1 metre by a force of 1 Newton. The joule is thus a measure of *work* energy, whereas the kcalorie is a measure of *heat* energy. While many scientists and journals report their findings in kilojoules (kJ), many others, particularly those in North America, use kcalories (kcal). To convert energy measures from kcalories to kilojoules, multiply by 4.2. For example, a 50-kcalorie cookie provides 210 kilojoules:

$$50 \text{ kcal} \times 4.2 = 210 \text{ kJ}$$

Exact conversion factors for these and other units of measure are in the Aids to Calculation section on the last two pages of the book.

CENGAGENOW™
For additional practice log on to **www.cengage.com/sso.**

Volume: Litres (L)

1 L = 1000 millilitres (mL)
0.95 L = 1 quart
1 mL = 0.03 fluid ounces
240 mL = 1 cup*

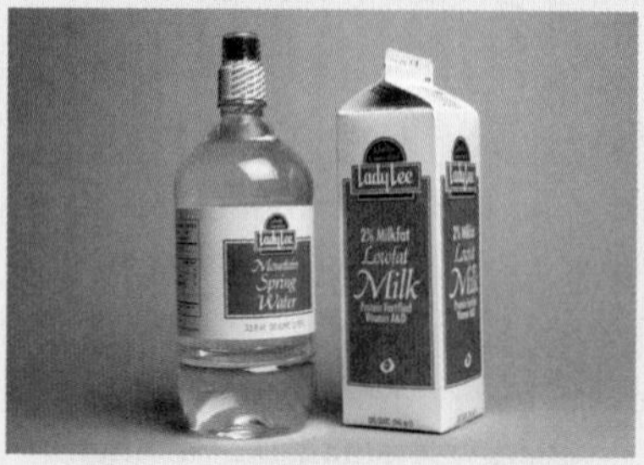
Lady Lee
Mountain Spring Water
Lady Lee
2% Milkfat
Lowfat
Milk
© Felicia Martinez/PhotoEdit

A litre of liquid is approximately one quart. Four litres are only about 5 percent more than a gallon.

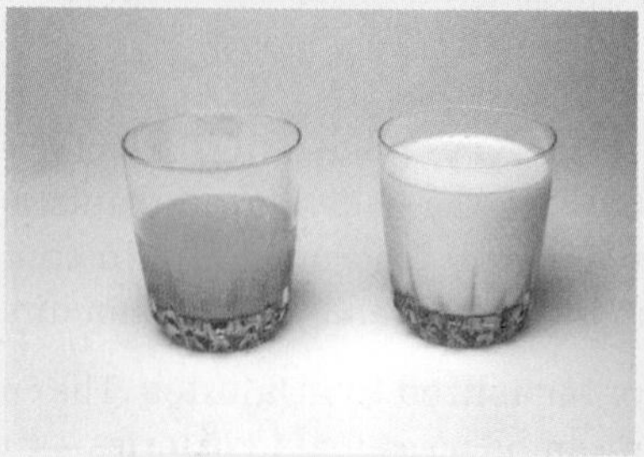
© Felicia Martinez/PhotoEdit

One cup is about 240 millilitres; a half-cup of liquid is about 120 millilitres.

Weight: Grams (g)

1 g = 1000 milligrams (mg)
1 g = 0.04 ounce (oz)
1 oz = 28.35 g (or 30 g)
100 g = 3½ oz
1 kilogram (kg) = 1000 g
1 kg = 2.2 pounds (lb)
454 g = 1 lb

A kilogram is slightly more than 2 lb; conversely, a pound is about ½ kg.

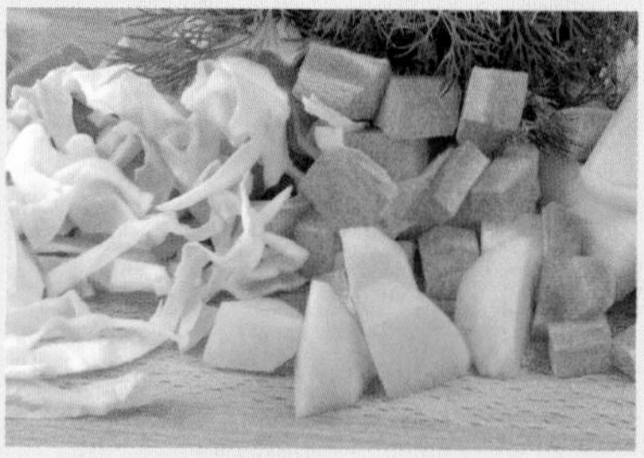
Kamila i Wojtek Cyganek/shutterstock

A half-cup of vegetables weighs about 100 grams; one pea weighs about ½ gram.

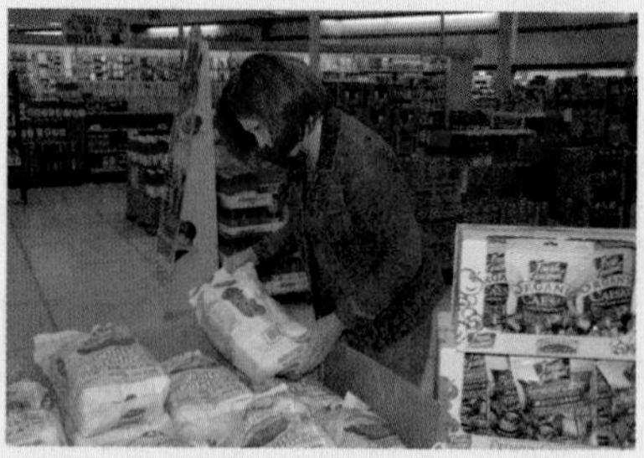
© Jennifer Brown/Alamy

A 2 kilogram bag of potatoes weighs about 5 pounds, and an 80-kilogram person weighs 176 pounds.

*250 mL is more commonly used to convert 1 cup to metric mL, though 240 mL is more accurate.

TRY IT Convert your body weight from pounds to kilograms and your height from inches to centimetres.

HOW TO Calculate the Energy Available from Foods

To calculate the energy available from a food, multiply the number of grams of carbohydrate, protein, and fat by 4, 4, and 9, respectively. Then add the results together. For example, 1 slice of bread with 15 millilitres (1 Tbsp) of peanut butter on it contains 16 grams carbohydrate, 7 grams protein, and 9 grams fat:

16 g carbohydrate × 4 kcal/g =	64 kcal
7 g protein × 4 kcal/g =	28 kcal
9 g fat × 9 kcal/g =	81 kcal
Total =	173 kcal

From this information, you can calculate the percentage of kcalories each of the energy nutrients contributes to the total. To determine the percentage of kcalories from fat, for example, divide the 81 fat kcalories by the total 173 kcalories:

81 fat kcal ÷ 173 total kcal = 0.468 (rounded to 0.47)

Then multiply by 100 to get the percentage:

0.47 × 100 = 47%

Dietary recommendations that urge people to limit fat intake to 20 to 35 percent of kcalories refer to the *day's total energy intake*, not to individual foods. Still, if the proportion of fat in each food choice throughout a day exceeds 35 percent of kcalories, then the day's total surely will, too. Knowing that this snack provides 47 percent of its kcalories from fat alerts a person to the need to make lower-fat selections at other times that day.

1 tablespoon (15 mL) is abbreviated 1 Tbsp

CENGAGENOW™
For additional practice log on to **www.cengage.com/sso.**

TRY IT Calculate the energy available from a bean burrito with cheese (55 grams carbohydrate, 15 grams protein, and 12 grams fat). Determine the percentage of kcalories from each of the energy nutrients.

TABLE 1-2 kCalorie Values of Energy Nutrients[a]

Nutrients	Energy (kcal/g)
Carbohydrate	4
Fat	9
Protein	4

NOTE: Alcohol contributes 7 kcalories per gram that can be used for energy, but it is not considered a nutrient because it interferes with the body's growth, maintenance, and repair.
[a]For those using kilojoules: 1 g carbohydrate = 17 kJ; 1 g protein = 17 kJ; 1 g fat = 37 kJ; and 1 g alcohol = 29 kJ.

Energy from Foods The amount of energy a food provides depends on how much carbohydrate, fat, and protein it contains. ♦ When completely broken down in the body, a gram of carbohydrate yields about 4 kcalories of energy; a gram of protein also yields 4 kcalories; and a gram of fat yields 9 kcalories (see Table 1-2). The accompanying "How To" explains how to calculate the energy available from foods.

Because fat provides more energy per gram, it has a greater **energy density** than either carbohydrate or protein. Figure 1-2 (p. 10) compares the energy density of two breakfast options, and later chapters describe how considering a food's energy density can help with weight management. ♦ Energy density differs from **nutrient density**, which refers to foods that deliver the most nutrients for the least food energy. Chapter 2 describes nutrient density in the context of planning a healthy diet.

One other substance contributes energy—alcohol. Alcohol, however, is not considered a nutrient. Unlike the essential nutrients, alcohol does not sustain life. In fact, it interferes with the growth, maintenance, and repair of the body. Its only common characteristic with nutrients is that it yields energy (7 kcalories per gram) when metabolized in the body.

Most foods contain all three energy-yielding nutrients, as well as vitamins, minerals, water, and other substances. For example, meat contains water, fat, vitamins, and minerals as well as protein. Bread contains water, a trace of fat, a little protein, and some vitamins and minerals in addition to its carbohydrate. Only a few foods are exceptions to this rule—the common ones being sugar (pure carbohydrate) and oil (essentially pure fat).

Energy in the Body The body uses the energy-yielding nutrients to fuel all its activities. When the body uses carbohydrate, fat, or protein for energy, the bonds between the nutrient's atoms break. As the bonds break, they release energy. ♦ Some of this energy is released as heat, but some is used to send electrical impulses through the brain and nerves, to synthesize body compounds, and

♦ The energy-yielding nutrients:
- Carbohydrate
- Fat
- Protein

♦ Foods with a high energy density help with weight gain, whereas those with a low energy density help with weight loss.

♦ The processes by which nutrients are broken down to yield energy or used to make body structures are known as **metabolism** (defined and described further in Chapter 7)

energy density: a measure of the energy a food provides relative to the amount of food (kcalories per gram).

nutrient density: a measure of the nutrients a food provides relative to the energy it provides. The more nutrients and the fewer kcalories, the higher the nutrient density.

FIGURE 1-2 Energy Density of Two Breakfast Options Compared

Gram for gram and bite for bite, foods with a high energy density deliver more kcalories than foods with a low energy density. Both of these breakfast options provide 500 kcalories, but the cereal with milk, fruit salad, scrambled egg, turkey sausage, and toast with jam offers three times as much food as the doughnuts (based on weight); it has a lower energy density than the doughnuts. Selecting a variety of foods also helps to ensure nutrient adequacy.

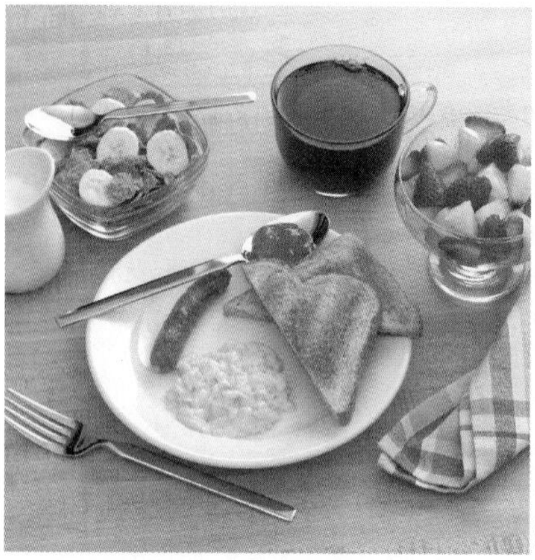

© Matthew Farruggio

LOWER ENERGY DENSITY
This 450-gram breakfast delivers 500 kcalories, for an energy density of 1.1 (500 kcal ÷ 450 g = 1.1 kcal/g).

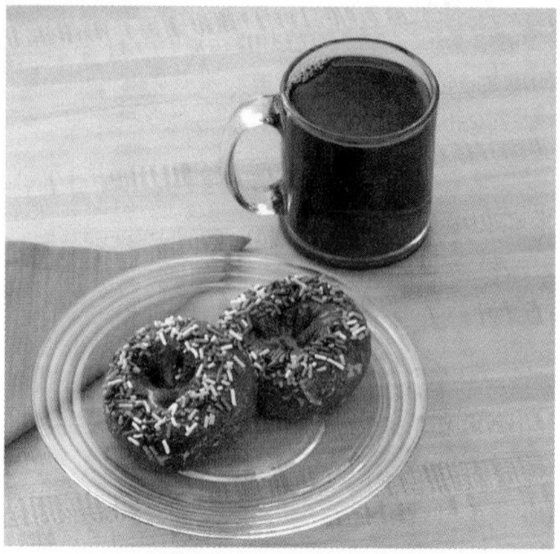

© Matthew Farruggio

HIGHER ENERGY DENSITY
This 144-gram breakfast delivers 500 kcalories, for an energy density of 3.5 (500 kcal ÷ 144 g = 3.5 kcal/g).

to move muscles. Thus the energy from food supports every activity from quiet thought to vigorous sports.

If the body does not use these nutrients to fuel its current activities, it converts them into storage compounds (such as body fat) to be used between meals and overnight when energy supplies run low. If more energy is consumed than expended, the result is an increase in energy stores and weight gain. Similarly, if less energy is consumed than expended, the result is a decrease in energy stores and weight loss.

When consumed in excess of energy needs, alcohol, too, can be converted to body fat and stored. When alcohol contributes a substantial portion of the energy in a person's diet, the harm it does far exceeds the problems of excess body fat. (Highlight 7 describes the effects of alcohol on health and nutrition.)

Other Roles of Energy-Yielding Nutrients In addition to providing energy, carbohydrates, fats, and proteins provide the raw materials for building the body's tissues and regulating its many activities. In fact, protein's role as a fuel source is relatively minor compared to its other roles and to the other two energy-yielding nutrients. Proteins are found in structures such as the muscles and skin and help to regulate activities such as digestion and energy metabolism. (Chapter 6 presents a full discussion on proteins.)

The Non-Energy-Yielding Nutrients: Vitamins, Minerals, and Water

The vitamins, minerals, and water do not directly yield energy, but support the production of energy from the three energy-yielding nutrients.

The Vitamins The **vitamins** are also organic, but they do not provide energy. Instead, they facilitate the release of energy from carbohydrate, fat, and protein and participate in numerous other activities throughout the body.

Each of the 13 vitamins has its own special roles to play.* One vitamin helps the eyes to see in dim light, another helps protect the lungs from air pollution, and still another helps make the sex hormones—among other things. When you cut yourself, one vitamin helps stop the bleeding and another helps repair the skin.

vitamins: organic, essential nutrients required in small amounts by the body for health.

*The water-soluble vitamins are vitamin C and the eight B vitamins: thiamin, riboflavin, niacin, vitamins B_6 and B_{12}, folate, biotin, and pantothenic acid. The fat-soluble vitamins are vitamins A, D, E, and K.

Vitamins busily help replace old red blood cells and the lining of the digestive tract. Almost every action in the body requires the assistance of vitamins.

Vitamins can function only if they are intact, but because they are complex organic molecules, they are vulnerable to destruction by heat, light, and chemical agents. This is why the body handles them carefully and why nutrition-wise cooks do, too. The strategies of cooking vegetables at moderate temperatures for short times and using small amounts of water help to preserve the vitamins.

The Minerals In the body, some **minerals** are put together in orderly arrays in such structures as bones and teeth. Minerals are also found in the fluids of the body, which influences fluid balance and distribution. Whatever their roles, minerals do not yield energy.

Only 16 minerals are known to be essential in human nutrition.* Others are being studied to determine whether they play significant roles in the human body. Still other minerals, such as lead, are environmental contaminants that displace the nutrient minerals from their workplaces in the body, disrupting body functions. The problems caused by contaminant minerals are described in Chapter 14.

Because minerals are inorganic, they are indestructible and need not be handled with the special care that vitamins require. Minerals can, however, be bound by substances that interfere with the body's ability to absorb them. They can also be lost during food-refining processes or during cooking when they leach into water that is discarded.

Water Water provides the environment in which nearly all the body's activities are conducted. It participates in many metabolic reactions and supplies the medium for transporting vital materials to cells and carrying waste products away from them. Water is discussed fully in Chapter 11, but it is mentioned in every chapter. If you watch for it, you cannot help but be impressed by water's participation in all life processes.

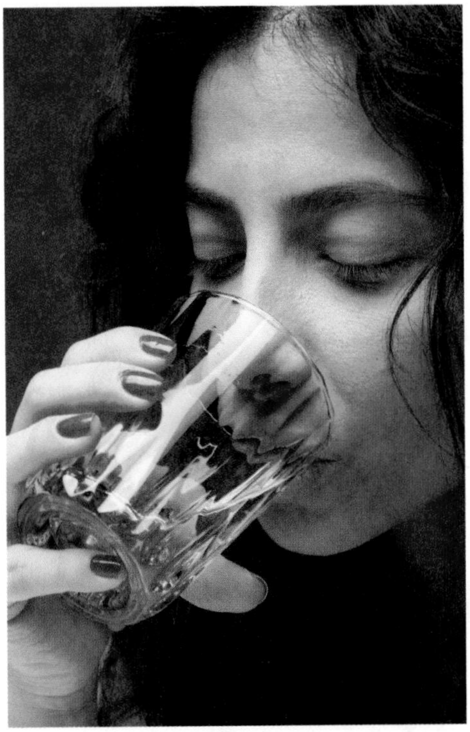
© emreogan/iStockphoto

Water itself is an essential nutrient and naturally carries minerals, usually in small amounts.

IN SUMMARY **Foods provide nutrients—substances that support the growth, maintenance, and repair of the body's tissues. The six classes of nutrients include:**

- **Carbohydrates**
- **Lipids (fats)**
- **Proteins**
- **Vitamins**
- **Minerals**
- **Water**

Foods rich in the energy-yielding nutrients (carbohydrate, fat, and protein) provide the major materials for building the body's tissues and yield energy for the body's use or storage. Energy is measured in kcalories. Vitamins, minerals, and water facilitate a variety of activities in the body.

Without exaggeration, nutrients provide the physical and metabolic basis for nearly all that we are and all that we do. The next section introduces the science of nutrition with emphasis on the research methods scientists have used in uncovering the wonders of nutrition.

The Science of Nutrition

The science of nutrition is the study of the nutrients and other substances in foods and the body's handling of them. Its foundation depends on several other sciences, including biology, biochemistry, and physiology. As sciences go, nutrition is young, but as you can see from the size of this book, much has happened in nutrition's short life. And it is currently experiencing a tremendous growth spurt as scientists apply knowledge gained from sequencing the human **genome**. The integration of nutrition, genomics, and molecular biology has opened a whole new world of study called **nutritional genomics**—the science of how nutrients affect the activities of genes and how genes affect the interactions between diet and disease.[7] Highlight 6

minerals: inorganic elements. Some minerals are essential nutrients required in small amounts by the body for health.

genome (GEE-nome): the complete set of genetic material (DNA) in an organism or a cell. The study of genomes is called **genomics.**

nutritional genomics: the science of how nutrients affect the activities of genes **(nutrigenomics)** and how genes affect the interactions between diet and disease **(nutrigenetics).**

*The major minerals are calcium, phosphorus, potassium, sodium, chloride, magnesium, and sulphur. The trace minerals are iron, iodine, zinc, chromium, selenium, fluoride, copper, and manganese.

♦ A personal account of an experience or event is an **anecdote** and is not accepted as reliable scientific information.

- **anekdotos** = unpublished

describes how nutritional genomics is shaping the science of nutrition, and examples of nutrient–gene interactions appear throughout later sections of the book.

Conducting Research Consumers may depend on personal experience or reports from friends ♦ to gather information on nutrition, but researchers use different scientific methodologies to guide their work. Research can be broadly categorized into quantitative and qualitative inquiry. Quantitative studies collect and interpret numerical data based on a stated hypothesis, whereas qualitative studies collect and interpret narrative data and generate hypotheses. Although nutrition is a relatively young discipline as a science, quantitative research has dominated research designs in the past. Qualitative research is increasingly contributing to our understanding of different aspects of nutrition, such as making food choices and accessing adequate nutritious food.

Quantitative Research As Figure 1-3 shows, quantitative research begins with a problem or a question. For example, "What foods or nutrients might protect

FIGURE 1-3 The Quantitative Scientific Method

Quantitative research scientists typically follow the scientific method outlined here. Note that most research generates new questions, not final answers. Thus the sequence begins anew, and research continues in a somewhat cyclical way.

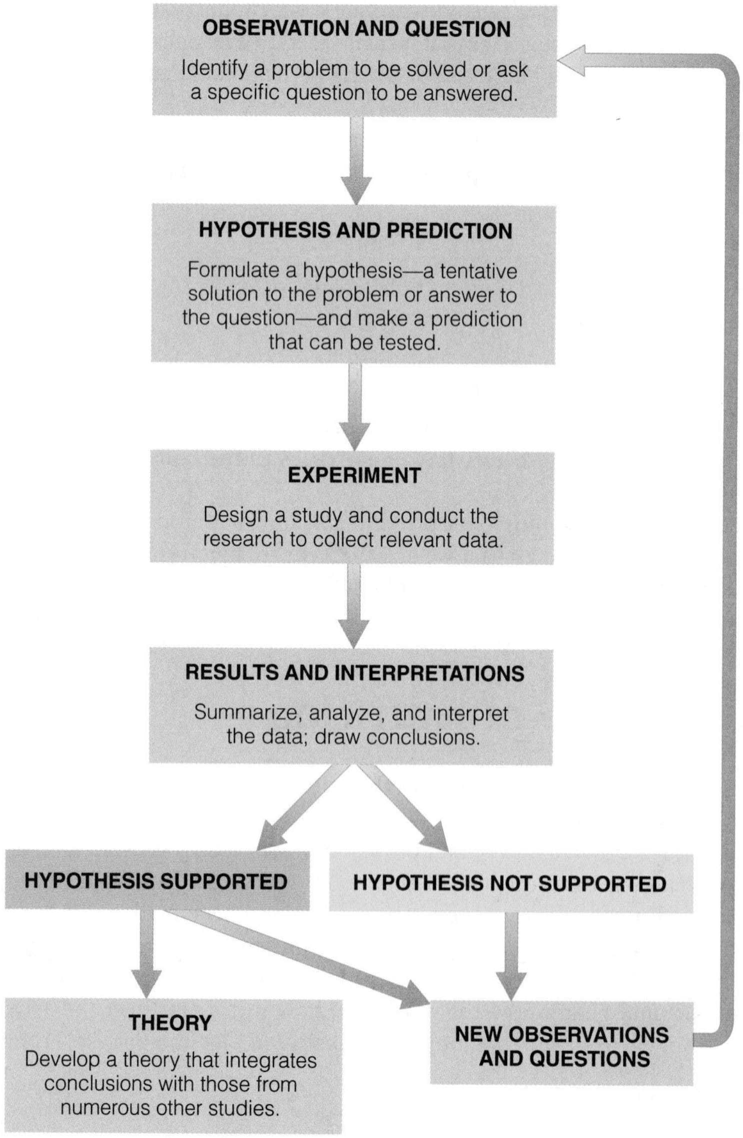
OBSERVATION AND QUESTION
Identify a problem to be solved or ask a specific question to be answered.
HYPOTHESIS AND PREDICTION
Formulate a hypothesis—a tentative solution to the problem or answer to the question—and make a prediction that can be tested.
EXPERIMENT
Design a study and conduct the research to collect relevant data.
RESULTS AND INTERPRETATIONS
Summarize, analyze, and interpret the data; draw conclusions.
HYPOTHESIS SUPPORTED
HYPOTHESIS NOT SUPPORTED
THEORY
Develop a theory that integrates conclusions with those from numerous other studies.
NEW OBSERVATIONS AND QUESTIONS

TABLE 1-3 Strengths and Weaknesses of Research Designs

Type of Research	Strengths	Weaknesses
Epidemiological studies determine the incidence and distribution of diseases in a population. Epidemiological studies include cross-sectional, case-control, and cohort (see Figure 1-4).	• Can narrow down the list of possible causes • Can raise questions to pursue through other types of studies	• Cannot control variables that may influence the development or the prevention of a disease • Cannot prove cause and effect
Laboratory-based studies explore the effects of a specific variable on a tissue, cell, or molecule. Laboratory-based studies are often conducted in test tubes (in vitro) or on animals (in vivo).	• Can control conditions • Can determine effects of a variable	• Cannot apply results from test tubes or animals to human beings
Human intervention or **clinical trials** involve human beings who follow a specified regimen.	• Can control conditions (for the most part) • Can apply findings to some groups of human beings	• Cannot generalize findings to all human beings • Cannot use certain treatments for clinical or ethical reasons

against the common cold?" In search of an answer, scientists make an educated guess (**hypothesis**) such as "foods rich in vitamin C reduce the number of common colds." Then they systematically conduct research studies to collect data that will test the hypothesis (see the glossary for definitions of research terms). Because each type of study has strengths and weaknesses, some provide stronger evidence than others (see Table 1-3). Some examples of various types of research designs are presented in Figure 1-4 (p. 14).

In attempting to discover whether a nutrient relieves symptoms or cures a disease, researchers deliberately manipulate one variable (e.g., the amount of vitamin C in the diet) and measure any observed changes (perhaps the number of colds). As much as possible, all other conditions are held constant. The following paragraphs illustrate how this is accomplished.

Controls In studies examining the effectiveness of vitamin C, researchers typically divide the **subjects** into two groups. One group (the **experimental group**) receives a vitamin C supplement, and the other (the **control group**) does not. Researchers observe both groups to determine whether one group has fewer, milder, or shorter colds than the other. The following discussion describes some of the pitfalls inherent in an experiment of this kind and ways to avoid them.

In sorting subjects into two groups, researchers must ensure that each person has an equal chance of being assigned to either the experimental group or the control group. This is accomplished by **randomization**; that is, the subjects are chosen randomly from the same population by flipping a coin or some other

GLOSSARY OF RESEARCH TERMS

blind experiment: an experiment in which the subjects do not know whether they are members of the experimental group or the control group.

control group: a group of individuals similar in all possible respects to the experimental group except for the treatment. Ideally, the control group receives a placebo while the experimental group receives a real treatment.

correlation (CORE-ee-LAY-shun): the simultaneous increase, decrease, or change in two variables. If A increases as B increases, or if A decreases as B decreases, the correlation is *positive*. (This does not mean that A causes B or vice versa.) If A increases as B decreases, or if A decreases as B increases, the correlation is *negative*. (This does not mean that A prevents B or vice versa.) Some third factor may account for both A and B.

double-blind experiment: an experiment in which neither the subjects nor the researchers know which subjects are members of the experimental group and which are serving as control subjects, until after the experiment is over.

experimental group: a group of individuals similar in all possible respects to the control group except for the treatment. The experimental group receives the real treatment.

hypothesis (hi-POTH-eh-sis): an unproven statement that tentatively explains the relationships between two or more variables.

peer review: a process in which a panel of scientists rigorously evaluates a research study to assure that the scientific method was followed.

placebo (pla-SEE-bo): an inert, harmless medication given to provide comfort and hope; a sham treatment used in controlled research studies.

placebo effect: a change that occurs in response to expectations about the effectiveness of a treatment that actually has no pharmaceutical effects.

randomization (RAN-dom-ih-ZAY-shun): a process of choosing the members of the experimental and control groups without bias.

replication (REP-lih-KAY-shun): repeating an experiment and getting the same results.

subjects: the people or animals participating in a research project.

theory: a tentative explanation that integrates many and diverse findings to further the understanding of a defined topic.

validity (va-LID-ih-tee): having the quality of being founded on fact or evidence.

variables: factors that change. A variable may depend on another variable (e.g., a child's height depends on his age), or it may be independent (e.g., a child's height does not depend on the colour of her eyes). Sometimes both variables correlate with a third variable (a child's height and eye colour both depend on genetics).

FIGURE 1-4 Examples of Research Designs

EPIDEMIOLOGICAL STUDIES

CROSS-SECTIONAL STUDIES

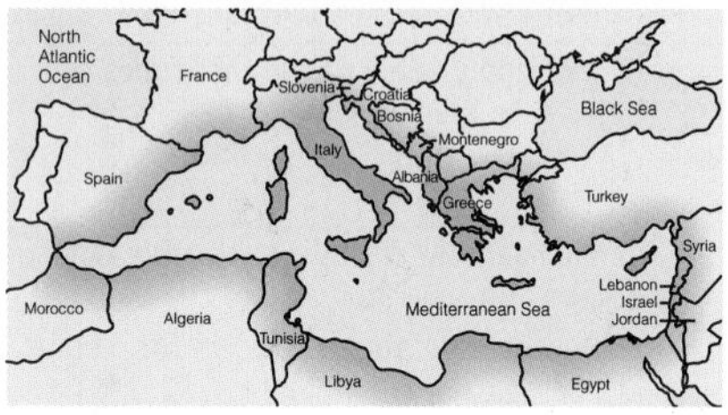
North Atlantic Ocean
France
Slovenia
Croatia
Bosnia
Montenegro
Black Sea
Italy
Albania
Greece
Turkey
Spain
Syria
Lebanon
Israel
Jordan
Morocco
Algeria
Mediterranean Sea
Tunisia
Libya
Egypt

Researchers observe how much and what kinds of foods a group of people eat and how healthy those people are. Their findings identify factors that might influence the incidence of a disease in various populations.

Example. Many people in the Mediterranean region drink more wine, eat more fat from olive oil, and yet have a lower incidence of heart disease than northern Europeans and North Americans.

CASE-CONTROL STUDIES

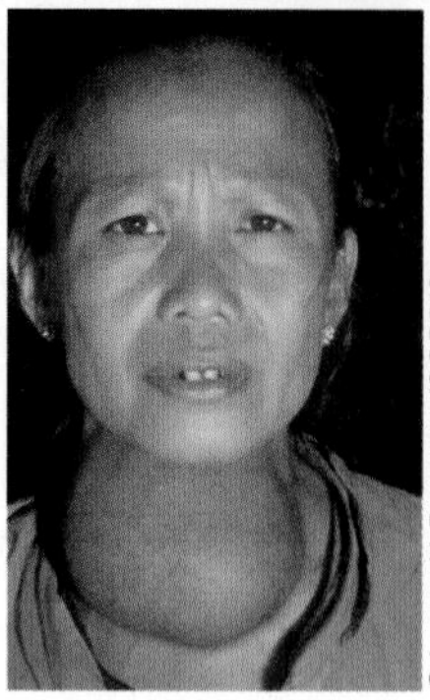

© Lester V. Bergman/CORBIS

Researchers compare people who do and do not have a given condition such as a disease, closely matching them in age, gender, and other key variables so that differences in other factors will stand out. These differences may account for the condition in the group that has it.

Example. People with goiter lack iodine in their diets.

COHORT STUDIES

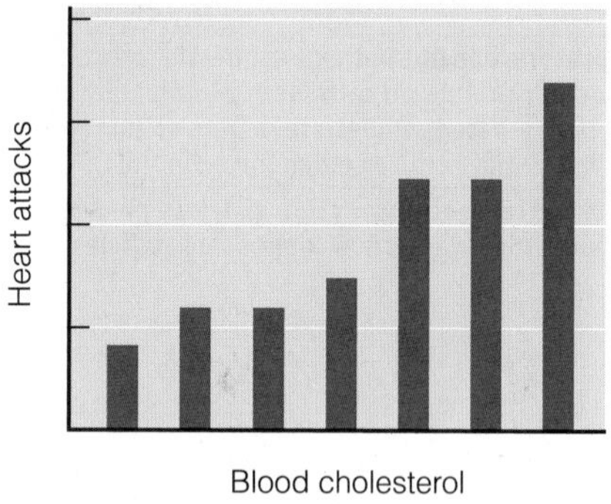
Heart attacks
Blood cholesterol

Researchers analyze data collected from a selected group of people (a cohort) at intervals over a certain period of time.

Example. Data collected periodically over the past several decades from over 5000 people randomly selected from the town of Framingham, Massachusetts, in 1948 have revealed that the risk of heart attack increases as blood cholesterol increases.

EXPERIMENTAL STUDIES

LABORATORY-BASED ANIMAL STUDIES

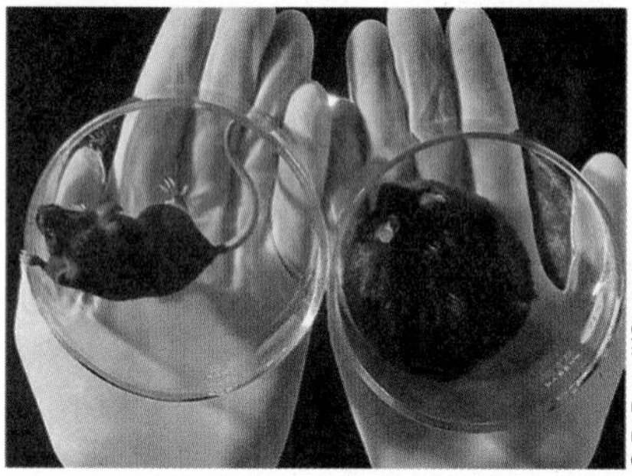

© R. Benali/Getty Images

Researchers feed animals special diets that provide or omit specific nutrients and then observe any changes in health. Such studies test possible disease causes and treatments in a laboratory where all conditions can be controlled.

Example. Mice fed a high-fat diet eat less food than mice given a lower-fat diet, so they receive the same number of kcalories—but the mice eating the fat-rich diet become severely obese.

LABORATORY-BASED IN VITRO STUDIES

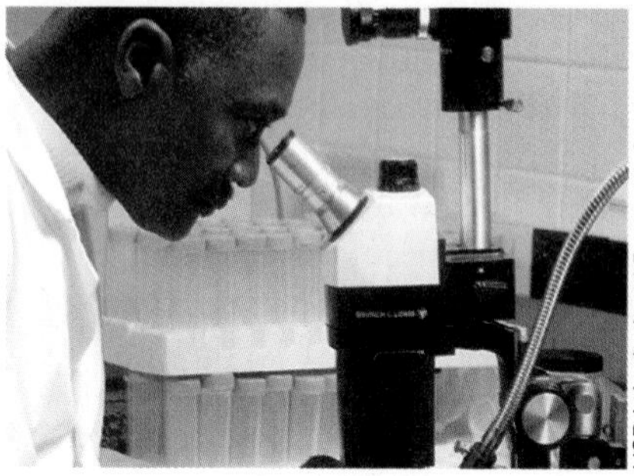

USDA Agricultural Research Service

Researchers examine the effects of a specific variable on a tissue, cell, or molecule isolated from a living organism.

Example. Laboratory studies find that fish oils inhibit the growth and activity of the bacteria implicated in ulcer formation.

HUMAN INTERVENTION (OR CLINICAL) TRIALS

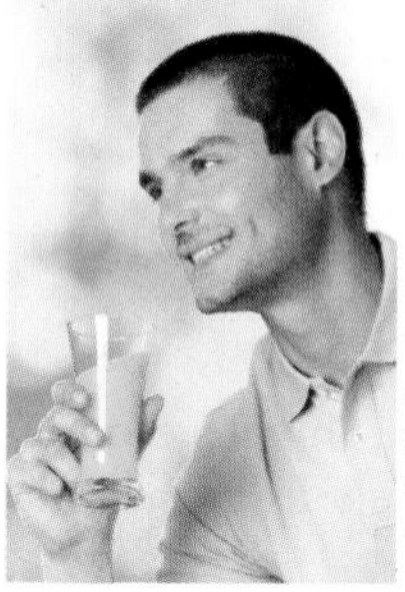

vgstudio/shutterstock

Researchers ask people to adopt a new behaviour (e.g., eat a citrus fruit, take a vitamin C supplement, or exercise daily). These trials help determine the effectiveness of such interventions on the development or prevention of disease.

Example. Heart disease risk factors improve when men receive fresh-squeezed orange juice daily for two months compared with those on a diet low in vitamin C—even when both groups follow a diet high in saturated fat.

method involving chance. Randomization helps to ensure that the two groups are "equal" and that observed differences reflect the treatment and not other factors.[8]

Importantly, the two groups of people must be similar and must have the same track record with respect to colds to rule out the possibility that observed differences in the rate, severity, or duration of colds might have occurred anyway. If, for example, the control group would normally catch twice as many colds as the experimental group, then the findings prove nothing.

In experiments involving a nutrient, the diets of both groups must also be similar, especially with respect to the nutrient being studied. If those in the experimental group were receiving less vitamin C from their usual diet, then any effects of the supplement may not be apparent.

Sample Size To ensure that chance variation between the two groups does not influence the results, the groups must be large. For example, if one member of a group of five people catches a bad cold by chance, he will pull the whole group's average toward bad colds; but if one member of a group of 500 catches a bad cold, she will not unduly affect the group average. Statistical methods are used to determine whether differences between groups of various sizes support a hypothesis.

Placebos If people who take vitamin C for colds *believe* it will cure them, their chances of recovery may improve. Taking anything believed to be beneficial may hasten recovery. This phenomenon, the result of expectations, is known as the **placebo effect.** In experiments designed to determine vitamin C's effect on colds, this mind-body effect must be rigorously controlled. Severity of symptoms is often a subjective measure, and people who believe they are receiving treatment may report less-severe symptoms.

One way experimenters control for the placebo effect is to give pills to all participants. Those in the experimental group, for example, receive pills containing vitamin C, and those in the control group receive a **placebo**—pills of similar appearance and taste containing an inactive ingredient. This way, the expectations of both groups will be equal. It is not necessary to convince all subjects that they are receiving vitamin C, but the extent of belief or unbelief must be the same in both groups. A study conducted under these conditions is called a **blind experiment**—that is, the subjects do not know (are blind to) whether they are members of the experimental group (receiving treatment) or the control group (receiving the placebo).

Double Blind When both the subjects and the researchers do not know which subjects are in which group, the study is called a **double-blind experiment.** Being fallible human beings and having an emotional and sometimes financial investment in a successful outcome, researchers might record and interpret results with a bias in the expected direction. To prevent such bias, the pills are coded by a third party, who does not reveal to the experimenters which subjects are in which group until all results have been recorded.

Analyzing Research Findings

Research findings must be analyzed and interpreted with an awareness of each study's limitations. Scientists must be cautious about drawing any conclusions until they have accumulated a body of evidence from multiple studies that have used various types of research designs. As evidence accumulates, scientists begin to develop a **theory** that integrates the various findings and explains the complex relationships.

Correlations and Causes Researchers often examine the relationships between two or more **variables**—for example, daily vitamin C intake and the number of colds or the duration and severity of cold symptoms. Importantly, researchers must be able to observe, measure, or verify the variables selected. Findings sometimes suggest no **correlation** between variables (regardless of the amount of vitamin C consumed, the number of colds remains the same). Other times, studies find either a **positive correlation** (the more vitamin C, the more colds) or a **negative correlation** (the more vitamin C, the fewer colds). Notice that in a positive correlation, both variables change in the same direction, regardless of whether the direction is "more" or "less"—"the more vitamin C, the more colds" is a positive correlation, just as is "the less vitamin C, the fewer colds." In a negative correlation, the two variables change in opposite directions: "the less vitamin C, the more colds" or "the more vitamin C, the fewer colds." Also notice that a positive correlation does not necessarily reflect a desired outcome, nor does a negative correlation always reflect an unwanted outcome.

Correlational evidence proves only that variables are associated, not that one is the cause of the other. People often jump to conclusions when they notice

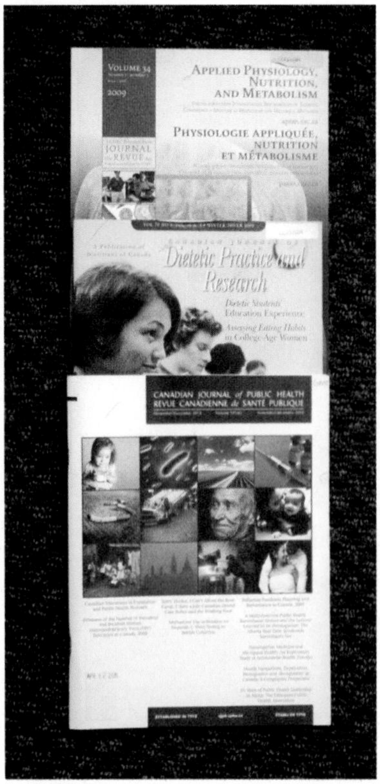
APPLIED PHYSIOLOGY, NUTRITION, AND METABOLISM
PHYSIOLOGIE APPLIQUÉE, NUTRITION ET MÉTABOLISME
Dietetic Practice and Research
CANADIAN JOURNAL of PUBLIC HEALTH
REVUE CANADIENNE de SANTÉ PUBLIQUE

Dick Hemingway

Knowledge about the nutrients and their effects on health comes from scientific studies.

correlations, but their conclusions are often wrong. To actually prove that A causes B, scientists have to find evidence of the *mechanism*—that is, an explanation of how A might cause B.

Cautious Conclusions When researchers record and analyze the results of their experiments, they must exercise caution in their interpretation of the findings. For example, in an epidemiological study, scientists may use a specific segment of the population—say, men 18 to 30 years old. When the scientists draw conclusions, they are careful not to generalize the findings to all people. Similarly, scientists performing research studies using animals are cautious in applying their findings to human beings. Conclusions from any one research study are always tentative and take into account findings from studies conducted by other scientists as well. As evidence accumulates, scientists gain confidence about making recommendations that affect people's health and lives. Still, their statements are worded cautiously, such as "A diet high in fruits and vegetables *may* protect against *some* cancers."

Quite often, as scientists approach an answer to one research question, they raise several more questions, so future research projects are never lacking. Further scientific investigation then seeks to answer questions such as "What substance or substances within fruits and vegetables provide protection?" If those substances turn out to be the vitamins found so abundantly in fresh produce, then "How much is needed to offer protection?" "How do these vitamins protect against cancer?" "Is it their action as antioxidant nutrients?" "If not, might it be another action or even another substance that accounts for the protection fruits and vegetables provide against cancer?" (Highlight 12 explores the answers to these questions and reviews recent research on antioxidant nutrients and disease.)

Publishing Research

The findings from a research study are submitted to a board of reviewers composed of other scientists who rigorously evaluate the study to assure that the scientific method was followed—a process known as **peer review**. The reviewers critique the study's hypothesis, methodology, statistical significance, and conclusions. They also note the funding source, recognizing that financial support may bias scientific conclusions.[9] If the reviewers consider the conclusions to be well supported by the evidence—that is, if the research has **validity**—they endorse the work for publication in a scientific journal where others can read it. This raises an important point regarding information found on the Internet: much gets published without the rigorous scrutiny of peer review. Consequently, readers must assume greater responsibility for examining the data and conclusions presented—often without the benefit of journal citations. Highlight 1 offers guidance in determining whether website information is reliable. Table 1-4 describes the parts of a typical research article.

Even when a new finding is published or released to the media, it is still only preliminary and not very meaningful by itself. Other scientists will need to confirm or disprove the findings through **replication**. To be accepted into the body of nutrition knowledge, a finding must stand up to rigorous, repeated testing

TABLE 1-4 Parts of a Research Article

- *Abstract.* The abstract provides a brief overview of the article.
- *Introduction.* The introduction clearly states the purpose of the current study.
- *Review of literature.* A comprehensive review of the literature reveals all that science has uncovered on the subject to date.
- *Methodology.* The methodology section defines key terms and describes the instruments and procedures used in conducting the study.
- *Results.* The results report the findings and may include tables and figures that summarize the information.
- *Conclusions.* The conclusions drawn are those supported by the data and reflect the original purpose as stated in the introduction. Usually, they answer a few questions and raise several more.
- *References.* The references reflect the investigator's knowledge of the subject and should include a list of relevant studies (including key studies several years old as well as current ones).

in experiments performed by several different researchers. What we "know" in nutrition results from years of replicating study findings. Communicating the latest finding in its proper context without distorting or oversimplifying the message is a challenge for scientists and journalists alike.

With each report from scientists, the field of nutrition changes a little—each finding contributes another piece to the whole body of knowledge. People who know how science works understand that single findings, like single frames in a movie, are just small parts of a larger story. Over years, the picture of what is "true" in nutrition gradually changes, and dietary recommendations change to reflect the current understanding of scientific research. Highlight 5 provides a detailed look at how dietary fat recommendations have evolved over the past several decades as researchers have uncovered the relationships between the various kinds of fat and their roles in supporting or harming health.

Qualitative Research Qualitative approaches to conducting nutrition research are gaining in popularity and provide a complementary alternative to quantitative studies. Qualitative research seeks to understand real world complexities in a way that uses narrative data, rather than numerical data. Generally, qualitative inquiry develops theory by purposively recruiting a small number of participants to gain a deep understanding of *why* and *how* certain phenomena occur, whereas quantitative research tends toward recruiting a large number of subjects to generate statistical results based on *what* has occurred.

When qualitative researchers study phenomena they start with general research questions and choose methodological approaches that are congruent with answering their questions, such as individual interviews, focus groups, participant observation, and photovoice. Researchers simultaneously collect and analyze data using an iterative process until saturation of the data is achieved, that is when no new knowledge is gained. Because each researcher is an integral instrument in this interpretive process, it is important for qualitative researchers to explicate how their stances shape their research when disseminating their findings for peer-review. Table 1-5 lists several qualitative research methodologies, each with a unique purpose.

TABLE 1-5 Examples of Qualitative Methodologies and Purposes

Methodology	Purpose
Grounded theory	To explain core processes in a given situation
Phenomenology	To explain the essence of individual experiences
Participatory research	To create an action agenda
Case study research	To explore a unique phenomenon in depth
Ethnography	To understand people and their culture

IN SUMMARY **Scientists learn about nutrition by conducting research that uses quantitative or qualitative designs and methods. In designing quantitative studies, researchers randomly assign control and experimental groups, seek large sample sizes, provide placebos, and remain blind to treatments. Their findings must be reviewed and replicated by other scientists before being accepted as valid. Qualitative studies seek to improve our understanding of why and how certain phenomena occur by selectively recruiting small numbers of people and using individual or group interviews, observation, and other methods to critically analyze their experiences of a certain phenomenon. Like quantitative research, qualitative research is also under scrutiny from external reviewers before publication.**

The characteristics of well-designed research have enabled scientists to study many phenomena related to food and the actions of nutrients in the body. Such research has laid the foundation for quantifying how much of each nutrient the body needs.

Dietary Reference Intakes

Using the results of thousands of research studies, nutrition experts have produced a set of standards that define the amounts of energy, nutrients, other dietary components, and physical activity that best support health. These recommendations are called **Dietary Reference Intakes (DRI)**, and they reflect the collaborative

Dietary Reference Intakes (DRI): a set of nutrient intake values for healthy people in Canada and the United States. These values are used for planning and assessing diets and include:
- Estimated Average Requirements (EAR)
- Recommended Dietary Allowances (RDA)
- Adequate Intakes (AI)
- Tolerable Upper Intake Levels (UL)

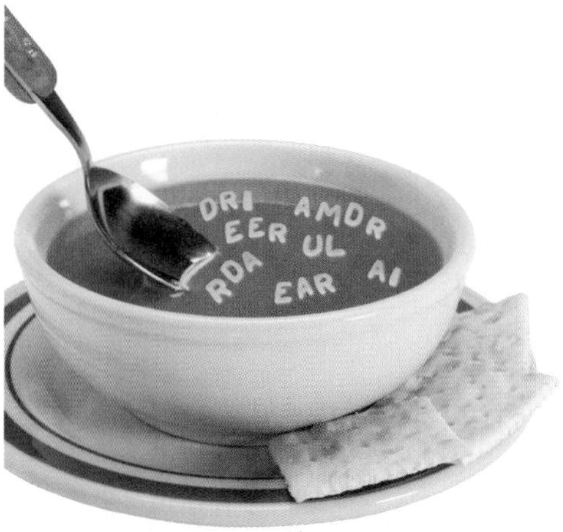
DRI
AMDR
EER
UL
RDA
AI
EAR

© Photodisc/Getty Images

Don't let the DRI "alphabet soup" of nutrient intake standards confuse you. Their names make sense when you learn their purposes.

efforts of researchers in both Canada and the United States.*[10] The inside front covers of this book provide a handy reference for DRI values.

Establishing Nutrient Recommendations

The DRI Committee consists of highly qualified scientists who base their estimates of nutrient needs on careful examination and interpretation of scientific evidence. These recommendations apply to healthy people and may not be appropriate for people with diseases that increase or decrease nutrient needs. The next several paragraphs discuss specific aspects of how the committee goes about establishing the values that make up the DRI:

- Estimated Average Requirements (EAR)
- Recommended Dietary Allowances (RDA)
- Adequate Intakes (AI)
- Tolerable Upper Intake Levels (UL)

Estimated Average Requirements (EAR) The committee reviews hundreds of research studies to determine the **requirement** for a nutrient—how much is needed in the diet. The committee selects a different criterion for each nutrient based on its roles in supporting various activities in the body and in reducing disease risks.[11]

An examination of all the available data reveals that each person's body is unique and has its own set of requirements. Men differ from women, and needs change as people grow from infancy through old age. For this reason, the committee clusters its recommendations for people into groups based on age and gender. Even so, the exact requirements for people of the same age and gender are likely to be different. For example, person A might need 40 units of a particular nutrient each day; person B might need 35; and person C, 57. Looking at enough people might reveal that their individual requirements fall into a symmetrical distribution, with most near the midpoint and only a few at the extremes (see the left side of Figure 1-5). Using this information, the committee

FIGURE 1-5 Estimated Average Requirements (EAR) and Recommended Dietary Allowances (RDA) Compared

Each square in the graphs below represents a person with unique nutritional requirements. (The text discusses three of these people—A, B, and C.) Some people require only a small amount of nutrient X and some require a lot. Most people, however, fall somewhere in the middle.

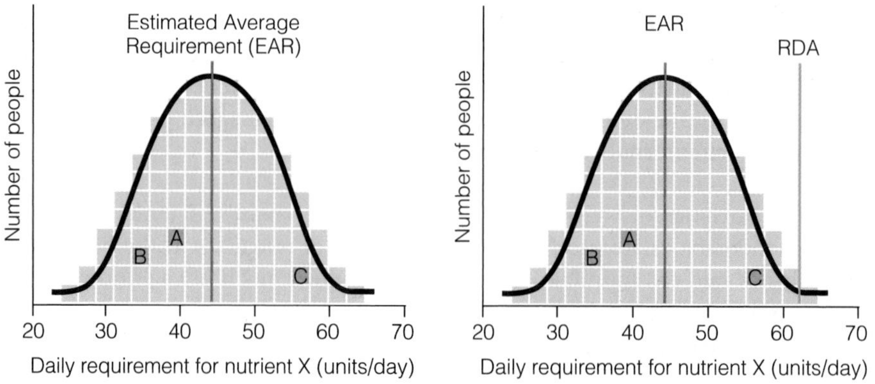
Estimated Average Requirement (EAR)
Number of people
A
B
C
20 30 40 50 60 70
Daily requirement for nutrient X (units/day)
EAR
RDA
Number of people
A
B
C
20 30 40 50 60 70
Daily requirement for nutrient X (units/day)

The Estimated Average Requirement (EAR) for a nutrient is the amount that covers half of the population (shown here by the red line).

The Recommended Dietary Allowance (RDA) for a nutrient (shown here in green) is set well above the EAR, covering about 98% of the population.

requirement: the lowest continuing intake of a nutrient that will maintain a specified criterion of adequacy.

*The DRI reports are produced by the U.S. Food and Nutrition Board, Institute of Medicine of the National Academies, with active involvement of scientists from Canada and the United States.

determines an **Estimated Average Requirement (EAR)** for each nutrient—the average amount that appears sufficient for half of the population. In Figure 1-5, the Estimated Average Requirement is shown as 45 units.

Recommended Dietary Allowances (RDA) Once a nutrient *requirement* is established, the committee must decide what intake to *recommend* for everybody—the **Recommended Dietary Allowance (RDA).** As you can see by the distribution in Figure 1-5, the Estimated Average Requirement (shown in the figure as 45 units) is probably closest to everyone's need. However, if people consumed exactly the average requirement of a given nutrient each day, half of the population would develop deficiencies of that nutrient—in Figure 1-5, for example, person C would be among them. Recommendations are therefore set high enough above the Estimated Average Requirement to meet the needs of most healthy people.

Small amounts above the daily requirement do no harm, whereas amounts below the requirement may lead to health problems. When people's nutrient intakes are consistently **deficient** (less than the requirement), their nutrient stores decline, and over time this decline leads to poor health and deficiency symptoms. Therefore, to ensure that the nutrient RDA meet the needs of as many people as possible, the RDA are set near the top end of the range of the population's estimated requirements.

In this example, a reasonable RDA might be 63 units a day (see the right side of Figure 1-5). Such a point can be calculated mathematically so that it covers about 98 percent of a population. Almost everybody—including person C whose needs were higher than the average—would be covered if they met this dietary goal. Relatively few people's requirements would exceed this recommendation, and even then, they wouldn't exceed by much.

Adequate Intakes (AI) For some nutrients, such as calcium, there is insufficient scientific evidence to determine an Estimated Average Requirement (which is needed to set an RDA). In these cases, the committee establishes an **Adequate Intake (AI)** instead of an RDA. An AI reflects the average amount of a nutrient that a group of healthy people consume. Like the RDA, the AI may be used as a nutrient goal for individuals.

Although both the RDA and the AI serve as nutrient intake goals for individuals, their differences are noteworthy. An RDA for a given nutrient is based on enough scientific evidence to expect that the needs of almost all healthy people will be met. An AI, on the other hand, must rely more heavily on scientific judgments because sufficient evidence is lacking. The percentage of people covered by an AI is unknown; an AI is expected to exceed average requirements, but it may cover more or fewer people than an RDA would cover (if an RDA could be determined). For these reasons, AI values are more tentative than RDA. The table on the inside front cover identifies which nutrients have an RDA and which have an AI. Later chapters present the RDA and AI values for the vitamins and minerals.

Tolerable Upper Intake Levels (UL) As mentioned earlier, the recommended intakes for nutrients are generous, and they do not necessarily cover every individual for every nutrient. Nevertheless, it is probably best not to exceed these recommendations by very much or very often. Individual tolerances for high doses of nutrients vary, and somewhere above the recommended intake is a point beyond which a nutrient is likely to become toxic.[12] This point is known as the **Tolerable Upper Intake Level (UL).** Only nutrients with strong scientific evidence to indicate adverse effects are assigned a UL. It is naïve—and inaccurate—to think of recommendations as minimum amounts. A more accurate view is to see a person's nutrient needs as falling within a range, with marginal and danger zones both below and above it (see Figure 1-6).

Paying attention to upper levels is particularly useful in guarding against the overconsumption of nutrients, which may occur when people use large-dose dietary supplements and fortified foods regularly. Later chapters discuss the dangers associated with excessively high intakes of vitamins and minerals, and the inside front cover (p. C) presents tables of upper levels for selected nutrients.

FIGURE 1-6 Inaccurate versus Accurate View of Nutrient Intakes

The RDA or AI for a given nutrient represents a point that lies within a range of appropriate and reasonable intakes between toxicity and deficiency. Both of these recommendations are high enough to provide reserves in times of short-term dietary inadequacies, but not so high as to approach toxicity. Nutrient intakes above or below this range may be equally harmful.

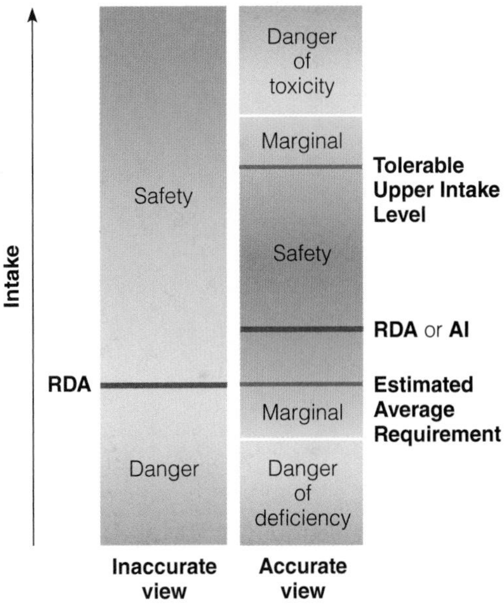
Intake
Safety
RDA
Danger
Inaccurate view
Danger of toxicity
Marginal
Safety
Marginal
Danger of deficiency
Accurate view
Tolerable Upper Intake Level
RDA or AI
Estimated Average Requirement

Estimated Average Requirement (EAR): the average daily amount of a nutrient that will maintain a specific biochemical or physiological function in half the healthy people of a given age and gender group.

Recommended Dietary Allowance (RDA): the average daily amount of a nutrient considered adequate to meet the known nutrient needs of practically all healthy people; a goal for dietary intake by individuals.

deficient: the amount of a nutrient below which almost all healthy people can be expected, over time, to experience deficiency symptoms.

Adequate Intake (AI): the average daily amount of a nutrient that appears sufficient to maintain a specified criterion; a value used as a guide for nutrient intake when an RDA cannot be determined.

Tolerable Upper Intake Level (UL): the maximum daily amount of a nutrient that appears safe for most healthy people and beyond which there is an increased risk of adverse health effects.

Establishing Energy Recommendations

In contrast to the RDA and AI values for nutrients, the recommendation for energy is not generous. Excess energy cannot be readily excreted and is eventually stored as body fat. These reserves may be beneficial when food is scarce, but they can also lead to obesity and its associated health consequences.

Estimated Energy Requirement (EER) The energy recommendation—called the **Estimated Energy Requirement (EER)**—represents the average dietary energy intake (kcalories per day) that will maintain energy balance in a person who has a healthy body weight ♦ and level of physical activity. Balance is key to the energy recommendation. Enough energy is needed to sustain a healthy and active life, but too much energy can lead to weight gain and obesity. Because *any* amount in excess of energy needs will result in weight gain, no upper level for energy has been determined.

♦ Reference adults:
- Men: 19–30 yr, 177 cm, and 70 kg (5 ft 10 in, and 154 lb)
- Women: 19–30 yr, 163 cm, and 57 kg (5 ft 4 in, and 126 lb)

Acceptable Macronutrient Distribution Ranges (AMDR) People don't eat energy directly; they derive energy from foods containing carbohydrates, fats, and proteins. Each of these three energy-yielding nutrients contributes to the total energy intake, and those contributions vary in relation to one another. The DRI Committee has determined that the composition of a diet that provides adequate energy and nutrients and reduces the risk of chronic diseases is:

- 45 to 65 percent kcalories from carbohydrate
- 20 to 35 percent kcalories from fat
- 10 to 35 percent kcalories from protein

These values are known as **Acceptable Macronutrient Distribution Ranges (AMDR)**.

Using Nutrient Recommendations

Although the intent of nutrient recommendations seems simple, they are the subject of much misunderstanding and controversy. Perhaps the following facts will help put them in perspective:

1. Estimates of adequate energy and nutrient intakes apply to *healthy* people. They need to be adjusted for malnourished people or those with medical problems who may require supplemented or restricted dietary intakes.
2. *Recommendations* are not minimum requirements, nor are they necessarily optimal intakes for all individuals. Recommendations can target only "most" of the people and cannot account for individual variations in nutrient needs—yet. Given the recent explosion of knowledge about genetics, the day may be fast approaching when nutrition scientists will be able to determine an individual's optimal nutrient needs.[13] Until then, registered dietitians ♦ and other qualified health professionals can help determine if recommendations should be adjusted to meet individual needs.
3. Most nutrient goals are intended to be met through diets composed of a variety of *foods* whenever possible. Because foods contain mixtures of nutrients and nonnutrients, they deliver more than just those nutrients covered by the recommendations. Excess intakes of vitamins and minerals are unlikely when they come from foods rather than dietary supplements.
4. Recommendations apply to *average* daily intakes. Trying to meet the recommendations for every nutrient every day is difficult and unnecessary. The length of time over which a person's intake can deviate from the average without risk of deficiency or overdose varies for each nutrient, depending on how the body uses and stores the nutrient. For most nutrients (such as thiamin and vitamin C), deprivation would lead to rapid development of deficiency symptoms (within days or weeks); for others (such as vitamin A and vitamin B_{12}), deficiencies would develop more slowly (over months or years).
5. Each of the DRI categories serves a unique purpose. For example, the Estimated Average Requirements are most appropriately used to develop and evaluate nutrition programs for *groups* such as schoolchildren or military personnel. The RDA (or AI if an RDA is not available) can be used to set

♦ A **registered dietitian (RD)** is a university-educated food and nutrition specialist who is qualified to evaluate people's nutritional health and needs. See Highlight 1 for more on what constitutes a nutrition expert.

Estimated Energy Requirement (EER): the average dietary energy intake that maintains energy balance and good health in a person of a given age, gender, weight, height, and level of physical activity.

Acceptable Macronutrient Distribution Ranges (AMDR): ranges of intakes for the energy-yielding nutrients that provide adequate energy and nutrients and reduce the risk of chronic diseases.

goals for *individuals*. Tolerable Upper Intake Levels serve as a reminder to keep nutrient intakes below amounts that increase the risk of toxicity—not a common problem when nutrients derive from foods, but a real possibility for some nutrients if supplements are used regularly.

With these understandings, professionals can use the DRI for a variety of purposes.

Comparing Nutrient Recommendations At least 40 different nations and international organizations have published nutrient standards similar to those used in Canada and the United States. Slight differences may be apparent, reflecting differences both in the interpretation of the data from which the standards were derived and in the food habits and physical activities of the populations they serve.

Many countries use the recommendations developed by two international groups: FAO (Food and Agriculture Organization) and WHO (World Health Organization). ♦ The FAO/WHO recommendations are considered sufficient to maintain health in nearly all healthy people worldwide.

♦ Nutrient recommendations from FAO/WHO are provided in APPENDIX I.

IN SUMMARY **The Dietary Reference Intakes (DRI) are a set of nutrient intake values that can be used to plan and evaluate diets for healthy people. The Estimated Average Requirement (EAR) defines the amount of a nutrient that supports a specific function in the body for half of the population. The Recommended Dietary Allowance (RDA) is based on the Estimated Average Requirement and establishes a goal for dietary intake that will meet the needs of almost all healthy people. An Adequate Intake (AI) serves a similar purpose when an RDA cannot be determined. The Estimated Energy Requirement (EER) defines the average amount of energy intake needed to maintain energy balance, and the Acceptable Macronutrient Distribution Ranges (AMDR) define the proportions contributed by carbohydrate, fat, and protein to a healthy diet. The Tolerable Upper Intake Level (UL) establishes the highest amount that appears safe for regular consumption.**

Nutrition Assessment

What happens when a person doesn't get enough or gets too much of a nutrient or energy? If the deficiency or excess is significant over time, the person experiences symptoms of **malnutrition.** With a deficiency of energy, the person may develop the symptoms of **undernutrition** by becoming extremely thin, losing muscle tissue, and becoming prone to infection and disease. With a deficiency of a nutrient, the person may experience skin rashes, depression, hair loss, bleeding gums, muscle spasms, night blindness, or other symptoms. With an excess of energy, the person may become obese and vulnerable to diseases associated with **overnutrition** such as heart disease and diabetes. With a sudden nutrient overdose, the person may experience hot flashes, yellowing skin, a rapid heart rate, low blood pressure, or other symptoms. Similarly, over time, regular intakes in excess of needs may also have adverse effects.

Malnutrition symptoms—such as diarrhea, skin rashes, and fatigue—are easy to miss because they resemble the symptoms of other diseases. But a person who has learned how to use assessment techniques to detect malnutrition can identify when these conditions are caused by poor nutrition and can recommend steps to correct it. This discussion presents the basics of nutrition assessment; many more details are offered in later chapters and in APPENDIX E.

malnutrition: any condition caused by excess or deficient food energy or nutrient intake or by an imbalance of nutrients.
- **mal** = bad

undernutrition: deficient energy or nutrients.

overnutrition: excess energy or nutrients.

nutrition assessment: a comprehensive analysis of a person's nutrition status that uses health, socioeconomic, drug, and diet histories; anthropometric measurements; physical examinations; and laboratory tests.

Nutrition Assessment of Individuals To prepare a **nutrition assessment,** a registered dietitian or other trained health-care professional uses:

- Historical information
- Anthropometric measurements

- Physical examinations
- Laboratory tests

Each of these methods involves collecting data in various ways and interpreting each finding in relation to the others to create a total picture.

Historical Information One step in evaluating nutrition status is to obtain information about a person's history with respect to health status, socioeconomic status, drug use, and diet. The health history reflects a person's medical record and may reveal a disease that interferes with the person's ability to eat or the body's use of nutrients. The person's family history of major diseases is also noteworthy, especially for conditions such as heart disease that have a genetic tendency to run in families. Economic circumstances may show a financial inability to buy enough nutritious foods or inadequate kitchen facilities in which to prepare them. Social factors such as marital status, ethnic background, and educational level also influence food choices and nutrition status. A drug history, including all prescribed and over-the-counter medications, may highlight possible interactions that lead to nutrient deficiencies (as described in Highlight 18). A diet history that examines a person's intake of foods, beverages, and dietary supplements may reveal either a surplus or inadequacy of nutrients or energy.

To take a diet history, the assessor collects data about the foods a person eats. The data may be collected by recording the foods the person has eaten over a period of 24 hours, as was done for the 2004 Canadian Community Healthy Survey. Data may also be collected in three-day food records, or for longer periods of time, such as weeks, months, or a year, in which case food frequency questionnaires are often used. The record must be fairly typical of the person's diet, and portion sizes must be recorded accurately. To determine the amounts of nutrients consumed, the assessor usually enters the foods and their portion sizes into a computer using a diet analysis program. This step can also be done manually by looking up each food in a table of food composition such as APPENDIX H in this book. The assessor then compares the calculated nutrient intakes with the DRI to determine the probability of adequacy (see Figure 1-7).[14] Alternatively, the diet history might be compared against standards such as *Eating Well with Canada's Food Guide* (described in Chapter 2).

anthropometric (AN-throw-poe-MET-rick): relating to measurement of the physical characteristics of the body, such as height and weight.
- **anthropos** = human
- **metric** = measuring

FIGURE 1-7 Using the DRI to Assess the Dietary Intake of a Healthy Individual

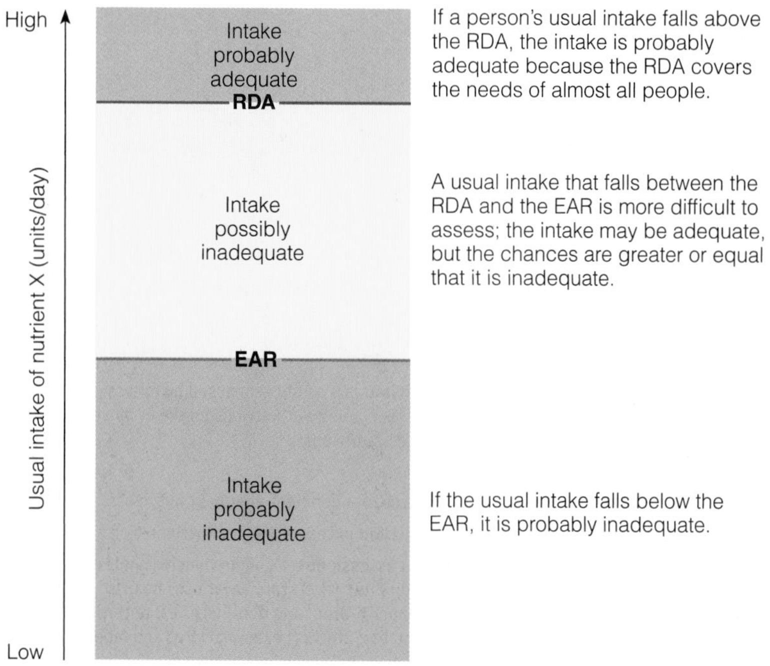
High
Low
Usual intake of nutrient X (units/day)
Intake probably adequate
RDA
Intake possibly inadequate
EAR
Intake probably inadequate
If a person's usual intake falls above the RDA, the intake is probably adequate because the RDA covers the needs of almost all people.
A usual intake that falls between the RDA and the EAR is more difficult to assess; the intake may be adequate, but the chances are greater or equal that it is inadequate.
If the usual intake falls below the EAR, it is probably inadequate.

An estimate of energy and nutrient intakes from a diet history, when combined with other sources of information, can help confirm or rule out the *possibility* of suspected nutrition problems. A sufficient intake of a nutrient does not guarantee adequacy, and an insufficient intake does not always indicate a deficiency. Such findings, however, warn of possible problems.

Anthropometric Measurements A second technique that may help to reveal nutrition problems is taking **anthropometric** measurements such as those of height and weight. The assessor compares a person's measurements with standards specific for gender and age or with previous measures on the same individual. (Chapter 8 presents information on body weight and its standards, and APPENDIX E includes growth charts for children.)

Measurements taken periodically and compared with previous measurements reveal patterns and indicate trends in a person's overall nutrition status, but they provide little information about specific nutrients. Instead, measurements out of line with expectations may reveal such problems as growth failure in children, wasting or swelling of body tissues in adults, and obesity—conditions that may reflect energy or nutrient deficiencies or excesses.

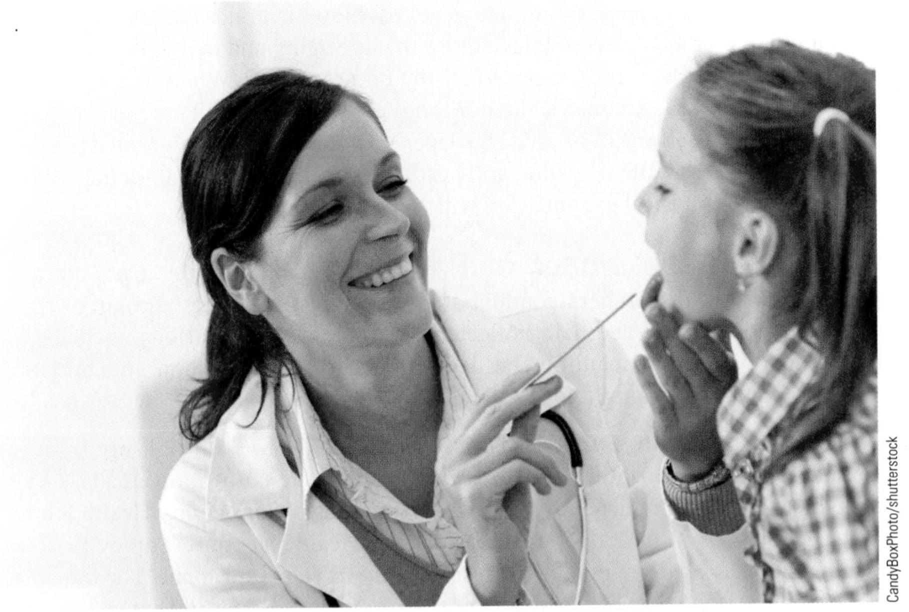
CandyBoxPhoto/shutterstock

A peek inside the mouth provides clues to a person's nutrition status. An inflamed tongue may indicate a deficiency of one of the B vitamins, and mottled teeth may reveal fluoride toxicity, for example.

Physical Examinations A third nutrition assessment technique is a physical examination looking for clues to poor nutrition status. Visual inspection of the hair, eyes, skin, posture, tongue, and fingernails can provide such clues. The examination requires skill because many physical signs reflect more than one nutrient deficiency or toxicity—or even nonnutrition conditions. Like the other assessment techniques, a physical examination alone does not yield firm conclusions. Instead, physical examinations reveal possible imbalances that must be confirmed by other assessment techniques, or they confirm results from other assessment measures.

Laboratory Tests A fourth way to detect a developing deficiency, imbalance, or toxicity is to take samples of blood or urine, analyze them in the laboratory, and compare the results with normal values for a similar population. Laboratory tests are most useful in uncovering early signs of malnutrition before symptoms appear. In addition, they can confirm suspicions raised by other assessment methods.

Iron, for Example The mineral iron can be used to illustrate the stages in the development of a nutrient deficiency and the assessment techniques useful in detecting them. The **overt**, or outward, signs of an iron deficiency appear at the end of a long sequence of events. Figure 1-8 describes what happens in the body as a nutrient deficiency progresses and shows which assessment methods can reveal those changes.

First, the body has too little iron—either because iron is lacking in the person's diet (a **primary deficiency**) or because the person's body doesn't absorb enough, excretes too much, or uses iron inefficiently (a **secondary deficiency**). A diet history provides clues to primary deficiencies; a health history provides clues to secondary deficiencies.

Next, the body begins to use up its stores of iron. At this stage, the deficiency might be described as a **subclinical deficiency**. It exists as a **covert** condition, and although it might be detected by laboratory tests, outward signs are not yet apparent.

overt (oh-VERT): out in the open and easy to observe.
- **ouvrir** = to open

primary deficiency: a nutrient deficiency caused by inadequate dietary intake of a nutrient.

secondary deficiency: a nutrient deficiency caused by something other than an inadequate intake such as a disease condition or drug interaction that reduces absorption, accelerates use, hastens excretion, or destroys the nutrient.

subclinical deficiency: a deficiency in the early stages, before the outward signs have appeared.

covert (KOH-vert): hidden, as if under covers.
- **couvrir** = to cover

FIGURE 1-8 Stages in the Development of a Nutrient Deficiency

Internal changes precede outward signs of deficiencies. However, outward signs of sickness need not appear before a person takes corrective measures. Laboratory tests can help determine nutrient status in the early stages.

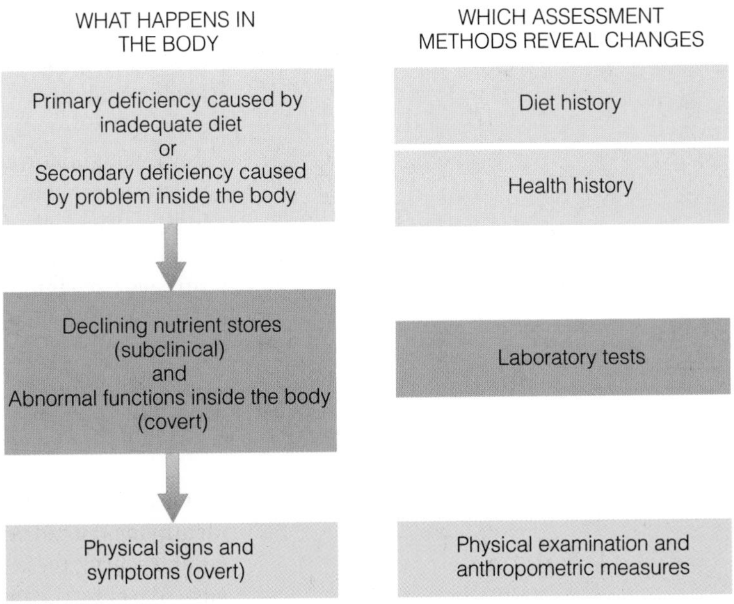
WHAT HAPPENS IN THE BODY
WHICH ASSESSMENT METHODS REVEAL CHANGES
Primary deficiency caused by inadequate diet or Secondary deficiency caused by problem inside the body
Diet history
Health history
Declining nutrient stores (subclinical) and Abnormal functions inside the body (covert)
Laboratory tests
Physical signs and symptoms (overt)
Physical examination and anthropometric measures

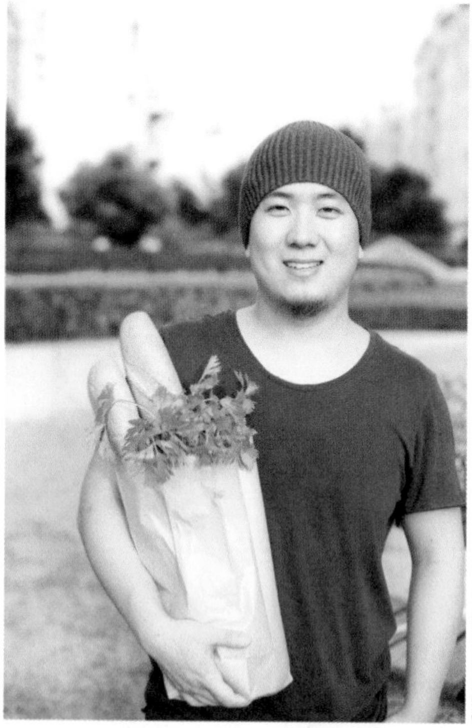

© iPandastudio/iStockphoto

Surveys provide valuable information about the kinds of foods people eat.

Finally, the body's iron stores are exhausted. Now, it cannot make enough iron-containing red blood cells to replace those that are aging and dying. Iron is needed in red blood cells to carry oxygen to all the body's tissues. When iron is lacking, fewer red blood cells are made, the new ones are pale and small, and every part of the body feels the effects of oxygen shortage. Now the overt symptoms of deficiency appear—weakness, fatigue, pallor, and headaches, reflecting the iron-deficient state of the blood. A physical examination will reveal these symptoms.

Nutrition Assessment of Populations

To assess a population's nutrition status, researchers conduct surveys using techniques similar to those used on individuals. The data collected are then used by various agencies for numerous purposes, including the development of national food and nutrition public policies, programs, and health goals.

National Nutrition Surveys Despite the lack of a formal program of population-based nutrition surveillance in Canada, the Nutrition Canada Survey was the first to be conducted in 1970–72; the Canadian Community Health Survey, Cycle 2.2, followed in 2004; and the Canadian Health Measures Survey in 2007. Each survey has used a nationally representative sample of Canadians. The Canadian Community Health Survey, Cycle 2.2, provided timely, reliable, and extensive information on Canadians' dietary intakes, which is being used to inform public policies and programs, among other purposes. For example, scientists use the information to establish research priorities. The food industry uses these data to guide decisions in public relations and product development. The Dietary Reference Intakes and other major reports that examine the relationships between diet and health depend on information collected from these nutrition surveys. These data also provide the basis for developing and monitoring national health goals. Findings from the Canadian Health Measures Survey, which collected physical, blood, and urine measurements of Canadians, are being used to determine relationships between health status and risk of disease and to identify emerging public health issues.

National Trends What do we eat in Canada and how has it changed over the past 40 years? The short answer to both questions is "a lot." We eat more meals away from home, particularly at fast-food restaurants. We eat larger portions. We drink more sweetened beverages and eat more energy-dense, nutrient-poor foods such as candy and chips. We snack frequently. Despite these dietary habits, our energy intake has fallen slightly over the past decade; however, declining physical activity at work has also occurred, which may help to explain an increased incidence of overweight and obesity.[15] Overweight and obesity, in turn, profoundly influence our health—as the next section explains.

IN SUMMARY **People become malnourished when they get too little or too much energy or nutrients. Deficiencies, excesses, and imbalances of nutrients lead to malnutrition diseases. To detect malnutrition in individuals, health-care professionals use a combination of four nutrition assessment methods. Reviewing historical information on diet and health may suggest a possible nutrition problem. Laboratory tests may detect a possible nutrition problem in its earliest stages, whereas anthropometric measurements and physical examinations pick up on the problem only after it causes symptoms. National surveys use similar assessment methods to measure people's food consumption and to evaluate the nutrition status of populations.**

Diet and Health

Foods play a vital role in supporting health.[16] Early nutrition research focused on identifying the nutrients in foods that would prevent such common diseases as rickets and scurvy, the vitamin D– and vitamin C–deficiency diseases. With this knowledge, developed countries have successfully defended against nutrient deficiency diseases. World hunger and nutrient deficiency diseases still pose a major health threat in developing countries, however, but not because of a lack of nutrition knowledge (as Chapter 21 explains). More recently, nutrition research has focused on **chronic diseases** associated with energy and nutrient excesses. Once thought to be "rich countries' problems," chronic diseases have now become epidemic in developing countries as well—contributing to three out of five deaths worldwide.[17]

Chronic Diseases

Table 1-6 lists the ten leading causes of death in Canada. These "causes" are stated as if a single condition such as heart disease caused death, but most chronic diseases arise from multiple factors over many years. A person who died of heart disease may have been overweight, had high blood pressure, been a cigarette smoker, and spent years eating a diet high in saturated fat and getting too little exercise.

Of course, not all people who die of heart disease fit this description, nor do all people with these characteristics die of heart disease. People who are overweight might die from the complications of diabetes instead, or those who smoke might die of cancer. They might even die from something totally unrelated to any of these factors such as an automobile accident. Still, statistical studies have shown that certain conditions and behaviours are linked to certain diseases.

Notice that Table 1-6 highlights four of the top six causes of death as having a link with diet. As knowledge about these diet and disease relationships has grown, the death rates for three of these—cancer, heart disease, and stroke—has decreased; however, death rates for diabetes—a chronic disease closely associated with obesity—has increased.[18]

TABLE 1-6 Ten Leading Causes of Death, Canada, 2005

	Percentage of Total Deaths
1. **Cancer**	**29.3**
2. **Heart disease**	**22.4**
3. **Stroke**	**6.1**
4. Respiratory disease	4.6
5. Accidents	4.1
6. **Diabetes**	**3.4**
7. Influenza and pneumonia	2.5
8. Alzheimer's disease	2.5
9. Suicide	1.6
10. Kidney disease	1.6

NOTE: The diseases highlighted in bold have relationships with diet.
SOURCE: Statistics Canada, Leading Causes of Death in Canada, 84-215-XWE2009000, March 2009; http://www.statcan.gc.ca/bsolc/olc-cel/olc-cel?catno=84-215-x&lang=eng

Risk Factors for Chronic Diseases

Factors that increase or reduce the *risk* of developing chronic diseases can be identified by analyzing statistical data. A strong association between a **risk factor** and a disease means that when the factor is present, the *likelihood* of developing the disease increases. It does not mean that all people with the risk factor will develop the disease. Similarly, a lack of risk factors does not guarantee freedom from a given disease. On the average, though, the more risk factors in a person's life, the greater that person's chances of developing the disease. Conversely, the fewer risk factors in a person's life, the better the chances for good health.

Risk Factors Persist Risk factors tend to persist over time. Without intervention, a young adult with high blood pressure will most likely continue to have high blood pressure as an older adult, for example. Thus, to minimize the damage, early intervention is most effective.

Risk Factors Cluster Risk factors tend to cluster. For example, a person who is obese may be physically inactive, have high blood pressure, and have high blood cholesterol—all risk factors associated with heart disease. Intervention that focuses on one risk factor often benefits the others as well. For example, physical activity can help reduce weight. Physical activity and weight loss will, in turn, help to lower blood pressure and blood cholesterol.

Risk Factors in Perspective The most prominent risk factor contributing to premature death in Canada is tobacco use, ♦ followed by diet and activity patterns, and alcohol use (see Table 1-7).[19] Risk factors such as smoking, poor dietary habits, physical inactivity, and alcohol consumption are personal behaviours that can be changed. Decisions to not smoke, to eat a well-balanced diet, to engage in regular physical activity, and to drink alcohol in moderation (if at all) improve the likelihood that a person will enjoy good health. Other risk factors, such as genetics, gender, and age, also play important roles in the development of chronic diseases, but they cannot be changed. Health recommendations acknowledge the influence of such factors on the development of disease, but they must focus on the factors that are changeable. For Canadians who do not smoke or drink alcohol excessively, the one choice that can influence long-term health prospects more than any other is diet.

TABLE 1-7 Risk Factors for Chronic Disease in Canada

Factors
Daily/occasional smoking
Heavy drinking
Low fruit/vegetable consumption
Inactivity
Obesity

SOURCE: Adapted from Statistics Canada, Leading Causes of Death in Canada, 84-215-XWE2009000, March 2009; http://www.statcan.gc.ca/bsolc/olc-cel/olc-cel?catno=84-215-x&lang=eng

♦ Cigarette smoking is responsible for one of every five deaths in Canada each year.

chronic diseases: diseases characterized by a slow progression and long duration. Examples include heart disease, cancer, and diabetes.

risk factor: a condition or behaviour associated with an elevated frequency of a disease but not proved to be causal. Leading risk factors for chronic diseases include obesity, cigarette smoking, high blood pressure, high blood cholesterol, physical inactivity, and a diet high in saturated fats and low in vegetables, fruits, and whole grains.

IN SUMMARY **Within the range set by genetics, a person's choice of diet influences long-term health. Diet has no influence on some diseases but is linked closely to others. Personal life choices, such as engaging in physical activity and using tobacco or alcohol, also affect health for the better or worse.**

The next several chapters provide many more details about nutrients and how they support health. Whenever appropriate, the discussion shows how diet influences each of today's major diseases. Dietary recommendations appear again and again, as each nutrient's relationships with health are explored. Most people who follow the recommendations will benefit and can enjoy good health into their later years.

Nutrition Portfolio

Each chapter in this book ends with simple Nutrition Portfolio activities that invite you to review key messages and consider whether your personal choices are meeting the dietary goals introduced in the text. By using the information you are recording in Diet Analysis Plus, the dietary tracking software that accompanies this text, and keeping a journal of these Nutrition Portfolio assignments, you can examine how your knowledge and behaviours change as you progress in your study of nutrition.

Your food choices play a key role in keeping you healthy and reducing your risk of chronic diseases.

After you have recorded at least one day's foods in Diet Analysis Plus, please look at that day's choices and record your answers to the following in your journal:

- Identify the factors that most influence your food choices for meals and snacks.
- List the chronic disease risk factors and conditions (listed in the definition of *risk factors*, p. 25) that you have.
- Describe lifestyle changes you can make to improve your chances of enjoying good health.

Diet Analysis PLUS **To complete this exercise, go to your Diet Analysis Plus at www.cengage.com/sso.**

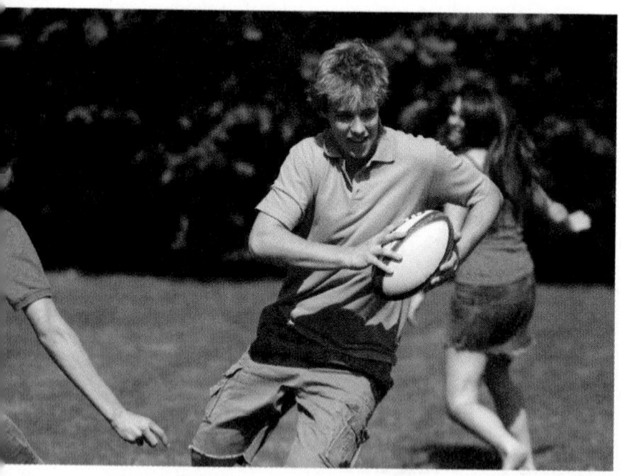

Physical activity can be both fun and beneficial.

Nutrition on the Net

CENGAGENOW™
For further study of topics covered in this chapter, log on to **www.cengage.com/sso.**

- Search for "nutrition" at Health Canada's and Public Health Agency of Canada's websites: **www.hc-sc.gc.ca** and **www.phac-aspc.gc.ca**
- Review the Dietary Reference Intakes: **www.nap.edu/topics.php?topic=380**
- Review nutrition recommendations from the Food and Agriculture Organization and the World Health Organization: **www.fao.org** and **www.who.int**
- Learn about the Canadian Community Health Survey: **www.hc-sc.gc.ca/fn-an/surveill/nutrition/commun/cchs_focus-volet_escc-eng.php**
- Find health information from the U.S. Centers for Disease Control and Prevention: **www.cdc.gov/healthyliving**

References

1. B. J. Tepper, Nutritional implications of genetic taste variation: The role of PROP sensitivity and other taste phenotypes, *Annual Review of Nutrition* 28 (2008): 367–388; A. A. Bachmanov and G. K. Beauchamp, Taste receptor genes, *Annual Review of Nutrition* 27 (2007): 389–414; A. El-Sohemy and coauthors, Nutrigenomics of taste—Impact on food preferences and food production, *Forum of Nutrition* 60 (2007): 176–182; K. Keskitalo and coauthors, Same genetic components underlie different measures of sweet taste preference, *American Journal of Clinical Nutrition* 86 (2007): 1663–1669; M. R. Yeomans and coauthors, Human hedonic responses to sweetness: Role of taste genetics and anatomy, *Physiology and Behavior* 91 (2007): 264–273; A. Knaapila and coauthors, Food neophobia shows heritable variation in humans, *Physiology and Behavior* 91 (2007): 573–578; D. R. Reed, T. Tanaka, and A. H. McDaniel, Diverse tastes: Genetics of sweet and bitter perception, *Physiology and Behavior* 88 (2006): 215–226.
2. N. Larson and coauthors, Food preparation by young adults is associated with better diet quality, *Journal of the American Dietetic Association* 106 (2006): 2001–2007.
3. Canadian Council of Food and Nutrition, Tracking Nutrition Trends VII, 2008, www.ccfn.ca/in_action/trends.asp, accessed August 22, 2010.
4. Dietitians of Canada, What are functional foods and nutraceuticals? www.dietitians.ca/Nutrition-Resources-A-Z/Fact-Sheet-Pages%28HTML%29/Miscellaneous/Functional-foods-and-nutraceuticals.aspx, accessed November 3, 2011; Position of the American Dietetic Association: Functional foods, *Journal of the American Dietetic Association* 104 (2004): 814–826.
5. Dietitians of Canada, Nutrition, Healthy Eating and Heart Health, www.dietitians.ca/Nutrition-Resources-A-Z/Fact-Sheet-Pages%28HTML%29/Heart-Health/ Nutrition,-Healthy-Eating-and-Heart-Health.aspx; Dietitians of Canada, Nutrition, Healthy Eating and Cancer, www.dietitians.ca/Nutrition-Resources-A-Z/Fact-Sheet-Pages%28HTML%29/Cancer/Nutrition,-Healthy-Eating-and-Cancer.aspx, accessed November 3, 2011.
6. C. Crosnier, D. Stamataki, and J. Lewis, Organizing cell renewal in the intestine: Stem cells, signals and combinatorial control, *Nature Reviews: Genetics* 7 (2006): 349–359.
7. A. El-Sohemy, The science of nutrigenomics, *Health Law Reviews* 16 (2008): 5–8; L. Afman and M. Müller, Nutrigenomics: From molecular nutrition to prevention of disease, *Journal of the American Dietetic Association* 106 (2006): 569–576; J. Ordovas and V. Mooser, Nutrigenomics and nutrigenetics, *Current Opinion in Lipidology* 15 (2005): 101–108.
8. R. B. D'Agostino, Jr. and R. B. D'Agostino, Sr., Estimating treatment effects using observational data, *Journal of the American Medical Association* 297 (2007): 314–316.
9. L. I. Lesser and coauthors, Relationship between funding source and conclusion among nutrition-related scientific articles, *PLoS Medicine* 4 (2007): 0001–0006.
10. S. I. Barr, Introduction to Dietary Reference Intakes in dietary assessment and planning, *Applied Physiology, Nutrition and Metabolism* 31 (2006): 61–65; Committee on Dietary Reference Intakes, *Dietary Reference Intakes for Water, Potassium, Sodium, Chloride, and Sulfate* (Washington, D.C.: National Academies Press, 2005); Committee on Dietary Reference Intakes, *Dietary Reference Intakes for Energy, Carbohydrate, Fiber, Fat, Fatty Acids, Cholesterol, Protein, and Amino Acids* (Washington, D.C.: National Academies Press, 2005); Committee on Dietary Reference Intakes, *Dietary Reference Intakes for Vitamin A, Vitamin K, Arsenic, Boron, Chromium, Copper, Iodine, Iron, Manganese, Molybdenum, Nickel, Silicon, Vanadium, and Zinc* (Washington, D.C.: National Academies Press, 2001); Committee on Dietary Reference Intakes, *Dietary Reference Intakes for Vitamin C, Vitamin E, Selenium, and Carotenoids* (Washington, D.C.: National Academies Press, 2000); Committee on Dietary Reference Intakes, *Dietary Reference Intakes for Thiamin, Riboflavin, Niacin, Vitamin B_6, Folate, Vitamin B_{12}, Pantothenic Acid, Biotin, and Choline* (Washington, D.C.: National Academies Press, 1998); Committee on Dietary Reference Intakes, *Dietary Reference Intakes for Calcium, Phosphorus, Magnesium, Vitamin D, and Fluoride* (Washington, D.C.: National Academies Press, 1997).
11. R. M. Russell, Current framework for DRI development: What are the pros and cons? *Nutrition Reviews* 66 (2008): 455–458.
12. C. L. Taylor, Highlights of "a model for establishing upper levels of intake for nutrients and related substances: Report of a joint FAO/WHO technical workshop on nutrient risk assessment, May 26, 2005," *Nutrition Reviews* 65 (2007): 31–38.
13. P. J. Stover, Influence of human genetic variation on nutritional requirements, *American Journal of Clinical Nutrition* 83 (2006): 436S–442S.
14. S. I. Barr, Applications of Dietary Reference Intakes in dietary assessment and planning, *Applied Physiology, Nutrition and Metabolism* 31 (2006): 66–73.
15. Statistics Canada. Food statistics, 2009. Catalogue no. 21-020-X. (2010); C. E. Juneau and L. Potvin. Trends in leisure-, transport-, and work-related physical activity in Canada 1994–2005. *Preventive Medicine* 51 (2010): 384–386.
16. D. R. Jacobs and L. C. Tapsell, Food, not nutrients, is the fundamental unit in nutrition, *Nutrition Reviews* 65 (2007): 439–450.
17. B. M. Popkin, Global nutrition dynamics: The world is shifting rapidly toward a diet linked with noncommunicable disease, *American Journal of Clinical Nutrition* 84 (2006): 289–298.
18. Statistics Canada, Ten leading causes of death, Canada, 2004 and 2005, www.statcan.gc.ca/pub/84-215-x/2009000/tbl/tbl1-eng.htm, accessed July 23, 2010.
19. Health Canada. Canadian Tobacco Use Monitoring Survey, www.hc-sc.gc.ca/hc-ps/tobac-tabac/research-recherche/stat/ctums-esutc_2008-eng.php, accessed July 22, 2010.

Nutrition Information and Misinformation—On the Net and in the News

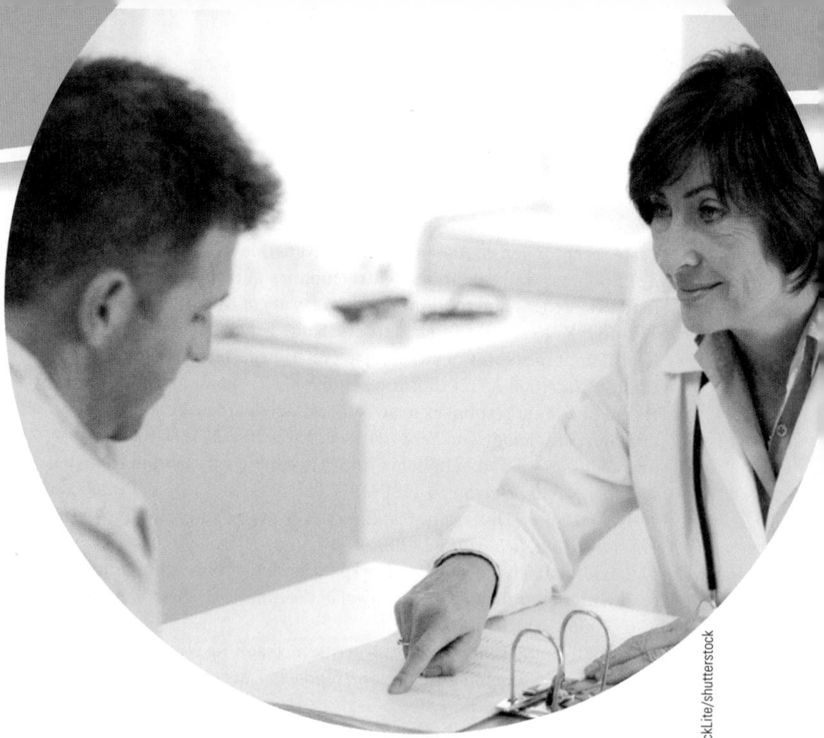

How can people distinguish valid nutrition information from misinformation? One excellent approach is to notice *who* is providing the information. The "who" behind the information is not always evident, though, especially in the world of electronic media. Keep in mind that *people* develop CDs and DVDs and create websites on the Internet, just as people write books and report the news. In all cases, consumers need to determine whether the person is qualified to provide nutrition information.

This highlight begins by examining the unique potential as well as the problems of relying on the Internet and the media for nutrition information. It continues with a discussion of how to identify reliable nutrition information that applies to all resources, including the Internet and the news. (The accompanying glossary defines related terms.)

Nutrition on the Net

Got a question? The **Internet** has an answer. The Internet offers endless opportunities to obtain high-quality information, but it also delivers an abundance of incomplete, misleading, or inaccurate information.[1] Simply put: anyone can publish anything.

With hundreds of millions of **websites** on the **World Wide Web,** searching for nutrition information can be an overwhelming experience—much like walking into an enormous bookstore with millions of books, magazines, newspapers, and videos. And like a bookstore, the Internet offers no guarantees of the accuracy of the information found there—much of which is pure fiction.

When using the Internet, keep in mind that the quality of health-related information available covers a broad range. You must evaluate websites for their accuracy, just like every other source. The accompanying "How To" provides tips for determining whether a website is reliable.

One of the most trustworthy sites used by scientists and others is the National Library of Medicine's PubMed, which provides free access to more than 10 million abstracts (short descriptions) of research papers published in scientific journals around the world. Many abstracts provide links to websites where full articles are available. Figure H1-1 (p. 30) introduces this valuable resource.

GLOSSARY

accredited: approved; in the case of dietetic programs certified by Dietitians of Canada.

dietetic technician: a person who often works under the supervision of a dietitian. Qualifications for a dietetic technician vary: many require a four-year undergraduate degree in human nutrition or a community college diploma in food service management.

dietitian: a person trained in nutrition, food science, and diet planning. See also *registered dietitian.*

Dietitians of Canada (DC): the professional organization of dietitians in Canada. The American equivalent is the American Dietetic Association.

fraudulent: the promotion, for financial gain, of devices, treatments, services, plans, or products (including diets and supplements) that alter or claim to alter a human condition without proof of safety or effectiveness.

Internet (the Net): a worldwide network of millions of computers linked together to share information.

licence to practise: permission under provincial law, granted on meeting specified criteria, to use a certain title (such as dietitian) and offer certain services.

misinformation: false or misleading information.

nutritionist: a person who specializes in the study of nutrition. Note that this definition does not specify qualifications and may apply not only to registered dietitians but also to self-described experts whose training is questionable.

public health dietitians: dietitians who specialize in providing nutrition services through organized community efforts.

RD: see *registered dietitian.*

registered dietitian (RD): a person who has completed a minimum of a bachelor's degree from an accredited university, has completed approved course work and a supervised practice program, has passed a national examination, and maintains registration through continuing professional education.

registration: listing; with respect to health professionals, listing with a professional organization that requires specific course work, experience, and passing of an examination.

websites: Internet resources composed of text and graphic files, each with a unique URL (Uniform Resource Locator) that names the site (e.g., www.dietitians.ca).

World Wide Web (the Web, commonly abbreviated **www**)**:** a graphical subset of the Internet.

Did you receive the e-mail warning about Costa Rican bananas causing the disease "necrotizing fasciitis"? If so, you've been scammed by Internet misinformation. When nutrition information arrives in unsolicited e-mails, be suspicious if:

- The person sending it to you didn't write it and you cannot determine who did or if that person is a nutrition expert.
- The phrase "Forward this to everyone you know" appears.
- The phrase "This is not a hoax" appears because chances are good that it is.
- The news is sensational and you've never heard about it from legitimate sources.
- The language is emphatic and the text is sprinkled with capitalized words and exclamation marks.
- No references are given or, if present, are of questionable validity when examined.
- The message has been debunked on websites such as **www.quackwatch.org** or **urbanlegends.about.com**.

HOW TO Determine Whether a Website Is Reliable

To determine whether a website offers reliable nutrition information, ask the following questions:

- **Who?** Who is responsible for the site? Is it staffed by qualified professionals? Look for the authors' names and credentials. Have experts reviewed the content for accuracy?
- **When?** When was the site last updated? Because nutrition is an ever-changing science, sites need to be dated and updated frequently.
- **Where?** Where is the information coming from? The three letters following the dot in a Web address identify the site's affiliation. Addresses ending in "ca" (Canada), "edu" (educational institute), and "org" (organization) generally provide reliable information; "com" (commercial) sites represent businesses and, depending on their qualifications and integrity, may or may not offer dependable information.
- **Why?** Why is the site giving you this information? Is the site providing a public service or selling a product? Many commercial sites provide accurate information, but some do not. When money is the prime motivation, be aware that the information may be biased.

If you are satisfied with the answers to all of the previous questions, then ask this final question:

- **What?** What is the message, and is it in line with other reliable sources? Information that contradicts common knowledge should be questioned. Many reliable sites provide links to other sites to facilitate your quest for knowledge, but this provision alone does not guarantee a reputable intention. Be aware that any site can link to any other site without permission.

TRY IT Visit a nutrition website and answer the five "W" questions to determine whether it is a reliable resource.

Nutrition in the News

Consumers get much of their nutrition information from Internet websites, television news, and magazine articles, which have heightened awareness of how diet influences the development of diseases. Consumers benefit from news coverage of nutrition when they learn to make lifestyle changes that will improve their health. Sometimes, however, popular reports mislead consumers and create confusion. They often tell a lopsided story based on a few testimonials instead of presenting the results of research studies or a balance of expert opinions.

Tight deadlines and limited understanding sometimes make it difficult to provide a thorough report. Hungry for the latest news, the media often report scientific findings prematurely—without benefit of careful interpretation, replication, and peer review. Usually, the reports present findings from a single, recently released study, making the news current and controversial. Consequently, the public receives diet and health news quickly, but not always in perspective. Reporters may twist inconclusive findings into "meaningful discoveries" when pressured to write catchy headlines and sensational stories.

As a result, "surprising new findings" seem to contradict one another, and consumers feel frustrated and betrayed. Occasionally, the reports are downright false, but more often the apparent contradictions are simply the normal result of science at work. A single study contributes to the big picture, but when viewed alone, it can easily distort the image. To be meaningful, the conclusions of any study must be presented cautiously within the context of other research findings.

Identifying Nutrition Experts

Regardless of whether the medium is electronic, print, or video, consumers need to ask whether the person behind the information is qualified to speak on nutrition. If the creator of an Internet website recommends eating three pineapples a day to lose weight, a trainer at the gym praises a high-protein diet, or a health-store clerk suggests an herbal supplement, should you believe these people? Can you distinguish between accurate news reports and infomercials on television? Have you noticed that many televised nutrition messages are presented by celebrities, athletes, psychologists, food editors, and chefs—that is, almost anyone except a **dietitian**? When you are confused or need sound dietary advice, whom should you ask?

Physicians and Other Health-care Professionals

Many people turn to physicians or other health-care professionals for dietary advice, expecting them to know about all health-related matters. But are they the best sources of accurate and current information on nutrition? In a recent survey, many Canadian medical students expressed low satisfaction with the time given to nutrition instruction in their medical training.[2] Currently, no national standards exist for including nutrition education in medical schools across Canada. This leads to varying amounts of required or elective nutrition instruction at different schools.

Most health-care professionals appreciate the connections between health and nutrition. Those who have specialized in clinical nutrition are especially well qualified to speak on the subject. Few, however, have the time or experience to develop diet plans and provide detailed diet instructions for clients. Often they wisely refer clients to a qualified nutrition expert—a **registered dietitian (RD).**

FIGURE H1-1 PUBMED (www.pubmed.gov): Internet Resource for Scientific Nutrition References

The U.S. National Library of Medicine's PubMed website offers tutorials to help teach beginners to use the search system effectively. Often, simply visiting the site, typing a query in the "Search for" box, and clicking "Go" will yield satisfactory results.

For example, to find research concerning calcium and bone health, typing "calcium bone" nets more than 30 000 results. Try setting limits on dates, types of articles, languages, and other criteria to obtain a more manageable number of abstracts to peruse.

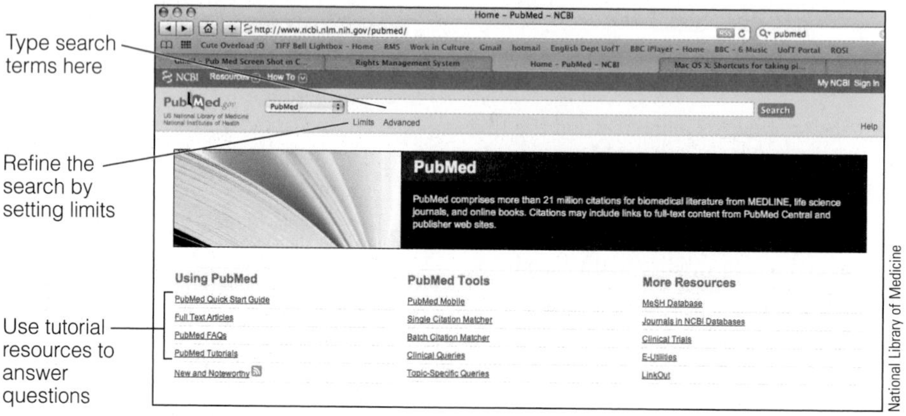
Type search terms here
Refine the search by setting limits
Use tutorial resources to answer questions
PubMed
Using PubMed
PubMed Tools
More Resources

National Library of Medicine

Registered Dietitian (RD)

A registered dietitian (RD) has the educational background necessary to deliver reliable nutrition advice and care.[3] To become an RD, a person must earn an undergraduate degree requiring about 120 credit hours in nutrition, food science, and other related subjects; complete a clinical internship or the equivalent; pass a national examination administered by the **Dietitians of Canada**; and maintain up-to-date knowledge and **registration** by participating in continuing education activities such as attending seminars, taking courses, or conducting research.

In Canada, the designated title and initials for dietitians vary by province (see Table H1-1). Provincial government legislation determines the professional designation for health-care professionals who practise in each province. Provinces have established colleges or organizations under their health professions legislation to ensure that the public receives quality nutritional care. Dietitians are registered (have a **licence to practise**) through a college or provincial regulatory body. The public can take complaints about dietetic practice to the college or regulatory body. Provincial colleges and regulatory bodies exist for the purpose of ensuring public safety. These regulatory bodies:

- monitor the competence of members (e.g., mandatory continuing education);
- protect the public from unsafe or unethical dietetic practice;
- protect the use of regulated title designation and initials (e.g., RD); and
- review the professional conduct of members based on complaints, and discipline members where appropriate.

All provinces include the word "dietitian" or "diététiste" in the title. The title **nutritionist** or variations (e.g., certified nutritionist, registered nutritionist) are not protected titles in most provinces. Some alternative educational programs qualify their graduates as "registered nutritional consulting practitioners," "certified nutritionists," "certified nutritional consultants," or "certified nutrition therapists"—terms that sound authoritative but lack the credentials of an RD. In fact, even Eddie, an English cocker spaniel, was able to obtain a certificate of membership from the American Association of Nutritional Consultants.[4]

Dietitians perform a multitude of duties in many settings in most communities. They work in the food industry, pharmaceutical companies, home health agencies, long-term care institutions, private practice, public health departments, research centres, education settings, fitness centres, and hospitals. Depending on their work settings, dietitians can assume a number of different job responsibilities and positions. In hospitals, administrative dietitians manage the foodservice system; clinical dietitians provide client care; and nutrition support team dietitians coordinate

TABLE H1-1 Provincial Designations for Dietitian

Province	Designation	Organization and Contact Information
Alberta	Dietitian, Registered Dietitian (RD), or Registered Nutritionist	College of Dietitians of Alberta www.collegeofdietitians.ab.ca
British Columbia	Dietitian or Registered Dietitian (RD)	The College of Dietitians of British Columbia www.collegeofdietitiansbc.org
Manitoba	Dietitian or Registered Dietitian (RD)	College of Dietitians of Manitoba www.manitobadietitians.ca
New Brunswick	Registered Dietitian (RD) or Registered Dietitian-Nutritionist (RDN)	New Brunswick Association of Dietitians www.adnb-nbad.com
Newfoundland and Labrador	Dietitian or Registered Dietitian (RD)	Newfoundland and Labrador College of Dietitians www.nlcd.ca
Nova Scotia	Dietitian, Nutritionist, or Professional Dietitian (PDt)	The Nova Scotia Dietetic Association www.nsdassoc.ca
Ontario	Registered Dietitian (RD) or Diététiste Professionnelle (DtP)	College of Dietitians of Ontario www.cdo.on.ca
Prince Edward Island	Dietitian, Diététiste, Registered Dietitian (RD), Professional Dietitian (PDt), or Diététiste Professionnelle (DtP)	The Prince Edward Island Dietitians Registration Board 153 Spring Street Summerside, PE C1N 3G2 Phone: 902-436-2438
Quebec	Diététiste Professionnelle (DtP), Nutritionniste, Professional Dietitian (PDt), or Registered Dietitian (RD)	Ordre professionnel des diététistes du Québec www.opdq.org
Saskatchewan	Dietitian, Professional Dietitian (PDt), or Registered Dietitian (RD)	Saskatchewan Dietitians Association www.saskdietitians.org

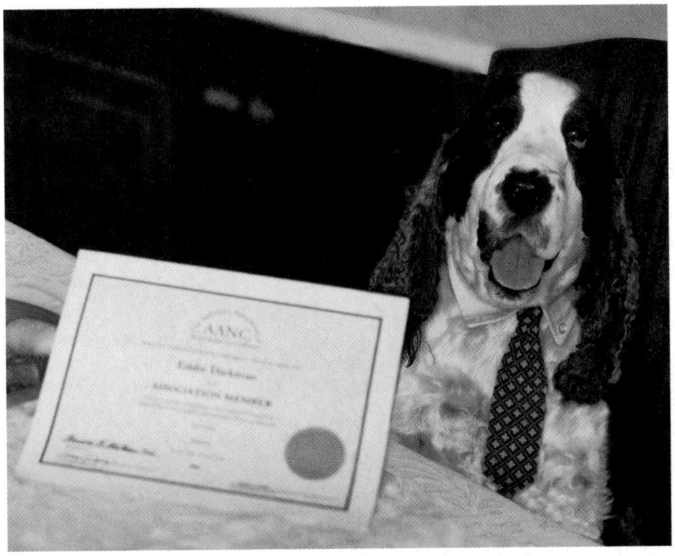
AANC

© Courtesy of eatright.org

Eddie displays his membership certificate to an association of nutritional consultants. His human companion, Connie Diekman, is a registered dietitian and past president of the American Dietetic Association.

nutrition care with other health-care professionals. In the food industry, dietitians conduct research, develop products, and market services.

Public health dietitians who work in government-funded agencies play a key role in delivering nutrition services to people in the community. Among their many roles, public health dietitians help plan, coordinate, and evaluate food assistance programs; act as consultants to other agencies; manage finances; and much more.

Dietetic Technician

In some facilities, a **dietetic technician** assists registered dietitians in both administrative and clinical responsibilities. A dietetic technician has been educated and trained to work under the guidance of a registered dietitian.

Other Dietary Employees

In addition to the dietetic technician, other dietary employees may include clerks, aides, cooks, porters, and assistants. These dietary employees do not have extensive formal training in nutrition, and their ability to provide accurate information may be limited.

Identifying Fake Credentials

In contrast to registered dietitians, thousands of people obtain fake nutrition degrees and claim to be nutrition consultants or doctors of "nutrimedicine." These and other such titles may sound meaningful, but most of these people lack the established credentials and training of a Dietitians of Canada-sanctioned dietitian. If you look closely, you can see signs of their fake expertise.

Consider educational background, for example. The minimum standards of education for a dietitian specify a bachelor's degree in human nutrition and food science or related fields from an **accredited** college or university. Such a degree generally requires 5 years of study. In contrast, a fake nutrition expert may display a degree from a 6-month course. Such a degree simply falls short. In some cases, businesses posing as schools offer even less—they sell certificates to anyone who pays the fees. To obtain these "degrees," a candidate need not attend any classes, read any books, or pass any examinations.

To safeguard educational quality and ensure that an educational institute provides complete and accurate schooling, dietetic programs across Canada are accredited by the Dietitians of Canada. Refer to the Dietitians of Canada website for a list of accredited Baccalaureate programs in Dietetic Education and Dietetic Internship/Practicum. Unfortunately, fake nutrition degrees are available from schools "accredited" by phony accrediting agencies. Acquiring false credentials is especially easy today, with **fraudulent** businesses operating via the Internet.

Knowing the qualifications of someone who provides nutrition information can help you determine whether that person's advice might be harmful or helpful. Don't be afraid to ask for credentials. Table H1-2 lists credible sources of nutrition information.

Red Flags of Nutrition Quackery

Figure H1-2 features eight red flags consumers can use to identify nutrition **misinformation.** Sales of unproven and dangerous products have always been a concern, but the Internet now provides merchants with an easy and inexpensive way to reach millions of customers around the world. Because of the difficulty in regulating the Internet, fraudulent and illegal sales of medical products have hit a bonanza. As is the case with the air, no one owns the Internet, and similarly, no one has control over the pollution. Countries have different laws regarding sales of drugs, dietary supplements, and other health products, but applying these laws to the Internet marketplace is almost impossible. Even if illegal activities could be defined and identified, finding the person responsible for a particular website is not always possible. Websites can open and close in a blink of a cursor. Now, more than ever, consumers must heed the caution "Buyer beware."

In summary, when you hear nutrition news, consider its source. Ask yourself these two questions: Is the person providing the information qualified to speak on nutrition? Is the information based on valid scientific research? If not, find a better source. After all, your health depends on it.

TABLE H1-2 Credible Sources of Nutrition Information

Government agencies, volunteer associations, consumer groups, and professional organizations provide consumers with reliable health and nutrition information. Credible sources of nutrition information include:

- Nutrition and food science departments at a university or community college
- Local agencies such as the health department
- Federal government health agencies such as:
  - Health Canada — **www.hc-sc.gc.ca**
  - Public Health Agency of Canada — **www.phac-aspc.gc.ca**
  - Canadian Food Inspection Agency — **www.inspection.gc.ca**
- Volunteer health agencies such as:
  - Canadian Cancer Society — **www.cancer.ca**
  - Canadian Diabetes Association — **www.diabetes.ca**
  - Heart and Stroke Foundation of Canada — **www.heartandstroke.com**
- Reputable consumer groups such as:
  - Canadian Council of Food and Nutrition — **www.ccfn.ca**
  - International Food Information Council — **www.foodinsight.org**
- Professional health organizations such as:
  - Dietitians of Canada — **www.dietitians.ca**
  - Canadian Medical Association — **www.cma.ca**
  - American Dietetic Association — **www.eatright.org**
- Journals such as:
  - *Canadian Journal of Dietetic Practice and Research* — **www.dcjournal.ca**
  - *Journal of the American Dietetic Association* — **www.adajournal.org**
  - *Nutrition Reviews* — **www.ilsi.org**
  - *Journal of Nutrition Education and Behavior* — **www.jneb.org**

FIGURE H1-2 Red Flags of Nutrition Quackery

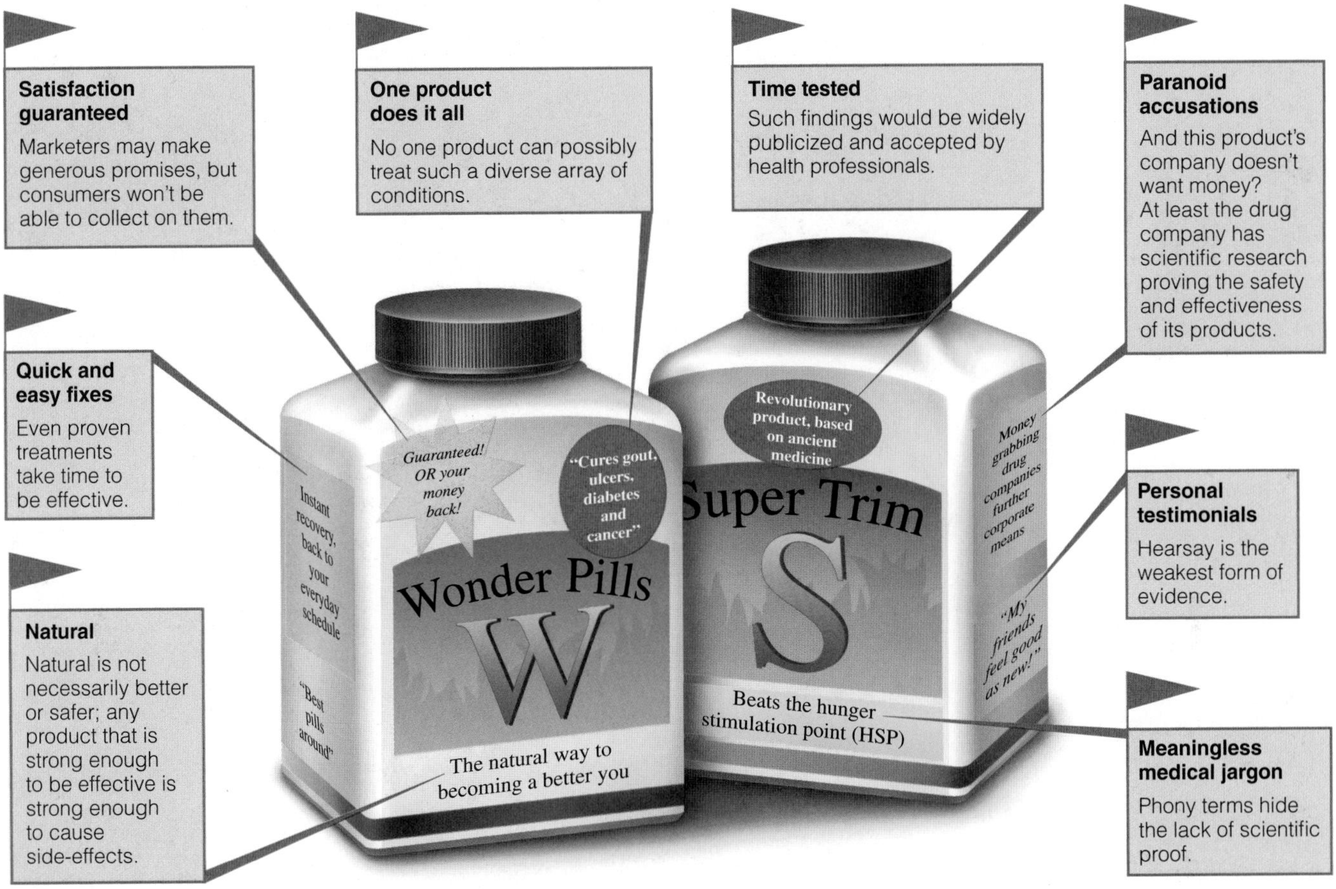
Satisfaction guaranteed
Marketers may make generous promises, but consumers won't be able to collect on them.
One product does it all
No one product can possibly treat such a diverse array of conditions.
Time tested
Such findings would be widely publicized and accepted by health professionals.
Paranoid accusations
And this product's company doesn't want money? At least the drug company has scientific research proving the safety and effectiveness of its products.
Quick and easy fixes
Even proven treatments take time to be effective.
Personal testimonials
Hearsay is the weakest form of evidence.
Natural
Natural is not necessarily better or safer; any product that is strong enough to be effective is strong enough to cause side-effects.
Meaningless medical jargon
Phony terms hide the lack of scientific proof.
Guaranteed! OR your money back!
"Cures gout, ulcers, diabetes and cancer"
Instant recovery, back to your everyday schedule
"Best pills around"
Wonder Pills
W
The natural way to becoming a better you
Revolutionary product, based on ancient medicine
Super Trim
S
Money grabbing drug companies further corporate means
"My friends feel good as new!"
Beats the hunger stimulation point (HSP)

Nutrition on the Net

CENGAGENOW™
For further study of topics covered in this Highlight, log on to **www.cengage.com/sso**.

- Find a registered dietitian in your area from the Dietitians of Canada: **www.dietitians.ca**
- Find out whether a school is properly accredited for a dietetics degree from the Dietitians of Canada: **www.dietitians.ca/Career/Education.aspx**
- Find reliable research articles: **www.pubmed.gov**
- Visit the National Council Against Health Fraud: **www.ncahf.org**
- Find useful and reliable health information from the Health on the Net Foundation: **www.hon.ch**
- Learn more about quackery from Stephen Barrett's Quackwatch: **www.quackwatch.org**

References

1. Position of the American Dietetic Association: Food and nutrition misinformation, *Journal of the American Dietetic Association* 106 (2006): 601–607.
2. L. M. Gramlich and coauthors, Medical students' perceptions of nutrition education in Canadian universities, *Applied Physiology, Nutrition, and Metabolism* 35 (2010): 336–343.
3. Dietitians of Canada, A career in nutrition, standards of practice. www.dietitians.ca/Downloadable-Content/Public/standards_practice.aspx, accessed September 10, 2011.
4. Who's dishing out your nutrition advice? Consumers beware: Make sure your source is a registered dietitian. www.eatright.org/Media/content.aspx?id=1568, accessed September 10, 2011.

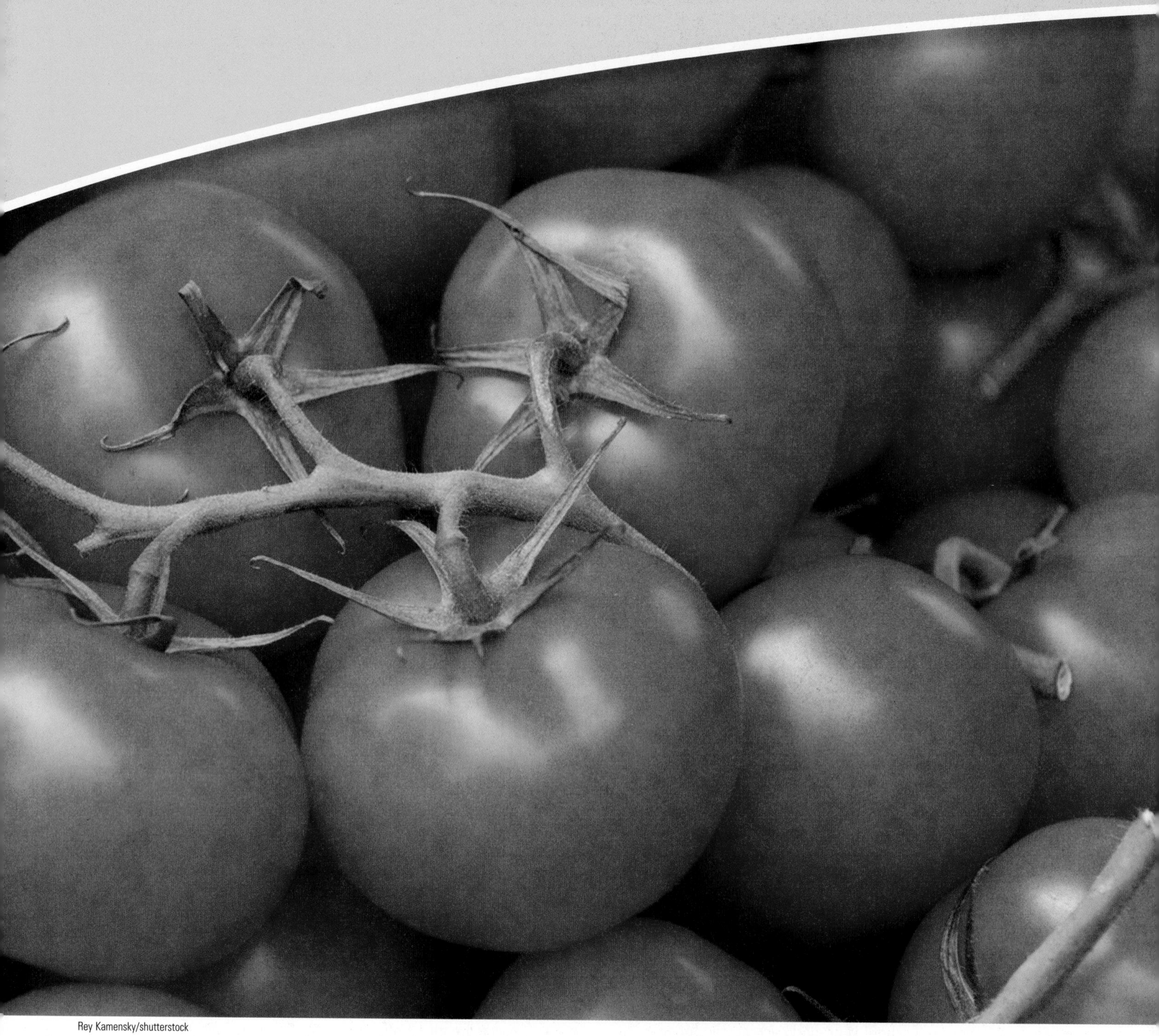

Rey Kamensky/shutterstock

CENGAGENOW™

Throughout this chapter, the CengageNOW logo indicates an opportunity for online self-study, linking you to interactive tutorials, activities, and videos to increase your understanding of chapter concepts.
www.cengage.com/sso

Nutrition in Your Life

You make food choices—deciding what to eat and how much to eat—more than 1000 times every year. We eat so frequently that it's easy to choose a meal without giving any thought to its nutrient contributions or health consequences. Even when we want to make healthy choices, we may not know which foods to select or how much to consume. With a few tools and tips, you can learn to plan a healthy diet.

CHAPTER

2

Planning a Healthy Diet

CHAPTER OUTLINE

Chapter 1 explains that the body's many activities are supported by the nutrients delivered by the foods people eat. Food choices made over years influence the body's health, and consistently poor choices increase the risks of developing chronic diseases. This chapter shows how a person can select from the tens of thousands of available foods to create a diet that supports good health. Fortunately, most foods provide several nutrients, so one trick for wise diet planning is to select a combination of foods that deliver a full array of nutrients. This chapter begins by introducing the diet-planning principles that assist people in selecting foods that will deliver nutrients without excess energy (kcalories).

Diet-Planning Principles

How well you nourish yourself does not depend on the selection of any one food. Instead, it depends on the selection of many different foods at numerous meals over days, months, and years. Diet-planning principles are key concepts to keep in mind whenever you are selecting foods—whether shopping at the grocery store, choosing from a restaurant menu, or preparing a home-cooked meal.

Basic Principles

Diet planners have developed several ways to select foods. Whatever plan or combination of plans they use, though, they keep in mind the six basic diet-planning principles ♦ listed in the margin.

Adequacy **Adequacy** means that the diet provides sufficient energy and enough of all the nutrients to meet the needs of healthy people. Take the essential nutrient iron, for example. Because the body loses some iron each day, people have to replace it by eating foods that contain iron. A person whose diet fails to provide enough iron-rich foods may develop the symptoms of iron-deficiency anemia: the person may feel weak, tired, and listless; have frequent headaches; and find that even the smallest amount of muscular work brings disabling fatigue. To prevent these deficiency symptoms, a person must include foods that supply adequate iron. The same is true for all the other essential nutrients introduced in Chapter 1.

Balance The art of balancing the diet involves consuming enough—but not too much—of foods across the major food groups. The essential minerals calcium and

♦ Basic diet-planning principles:
- Adequacy
- Balance
- kCalorie (energy) control
- Nutrient density
- Moderation
- Variety

adequacy (dietary): providing all the essential nutrients, fibre, and energy in amounts sufficient to maintain health.

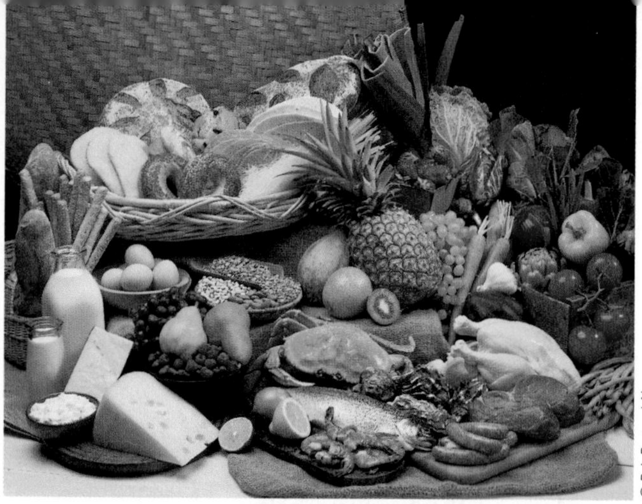
© Rob Bartee / Alamy

To ensure an adequate and balanced diet, eat a variety of foods daily, choosing different foods from each food group.

iron, taken together, illustrate the importance of dietary **balance.** Meats, fish, and poultry are rich in iron but poor in calcium. Conversely, milk and milk products are rich in calcium but poor in iron. Use some meat or meat alternatives for iron; use some milk and milk products for calcium; and save some space for other foods, too, because a diet consisting of milk and meat alone would not be adequate. ♦ For the other nutrients, people need to consume whole grains, **legumes**, vegetables, and fruits.

♦ Balance in the diet helps to ensure adequacy.

kCalorie (Energy) Control Designing an adequate diet within a reasonable kcalorie allowance requires careful planning. Once again, balance plays a key role. The amount of energy coming into the body from foods should balance with the amount of energy being used by the body to sustain its metabolic and physical activities. Upsetting this balance leads to gains or losses in body weight. The discussion of energy balance and weight control in Chapters 8 and 9 examines this issue in more detail, but one key to **kcalorie control** is to select foods of high **nutrient density.**

Nutrient Density To eat well without overeating, select nutrient-dense foods—that is, foods that deliver the most nutrients for the least food energy.[1] Consider foods containing calcium, for example. You can get about 300 milligrams of calcium from either 50 grams (1½ ounces) of cheddar cheese or 250 millilitres (1 cup) of skim (fat-free) milk, but the cheese delivers about twice as much food energy (kcalories) as the milk. The skim milk, then, is twice as calcium dense as the cheddar cheese; it offers the same amount of calcium for half the kcalories. Both foods are excellent choices for adequacy's sake alone, but to achieve adequacy while controlling kcalories, ♦ skim milk is the better choice. Alternatively, a person could select a low-fat cheddar cheese with its kcalories similar to skim milk. The many bar graphs that appear in Chapters 10 through 14 highlight the most nutrient-dense choices, and the accompanying "How To" describes how to compare foods based on nutrient density.

♦ Nutrient density promotes adequacy and kcalorie control.

Just as a financially responsible person pays for rent, food, clothes, and tuition on a limited budget, healthy people obtain iron, calcium, and all the other essential nutrients on a limited energy (kcalorie) allowance. Success depends on getting many nutrients for each kcalorie "dollar." For example, a can of pop and a handful of grapes may both provide about the same number of kcalories, but the grapes deliver many more nutrients. A person who makes nutrient-dense choices, such as fruit instead of pop, can meet daily nutrient needs on a lower energy budget. Such choices support good health.

Foods that are notably low in nutrient density—such as potato chips, candy, and soft drinks—are sometimes called **empty-kcalorie foods.** The kcalories these foods provide are called "empty" because they deliver energy (from sugar, fat, or both) with little, or no, protein, vitamins, or minerals.

The concept of nutrient density is relatively simple when examining the contributions of one nutrient to a food or diet. With respect to calcium, milk ranks high and meats rank low. With respect to iron, meats rank high and milk ranks low. But it is a more complex task to answer the question, which food is more nutritious? To answer that question, we need to consider several nutrients—including nutrients that may harm health as well as those that may be beneficial. Ranking foods based on their overall nutrient composition is known as **nutrient profiling.**[2] Researchers have yet to agree on an ideal way to rate foods based on the nutrient profile, but when they do, nutrient profiling will be quite useful in helping consumers identify nutritious foods and plan healthy diets.[3]

♦ Moderation contributes to adequacy, balance, and kcalorie control.

balance (dietary): providing foods in proportion to one another and in proportion to the body's needs.

legumes: plants of the lentil, bean and pea family, with seeds that are rich in protein compared with other plant-derived foods

kcalorie (energy) control: management of food energy intake.

nutrient density: a measure of the nutrients a food provides relative to the energy it provides. The more nutrients and the fewer kcalories, the higher the nutrient density.

empty-kcalorie foods: a popular term used to denote foods that contribute energy but lack protein, vitamins, and minerals.

nutrient profiling: ranking foods based on their nutrient composition.

moderation (dietary): providing enough but not too much of a substance.

Moderation Foods rich in fat and sugar provide enjoyment and energy but relatively few nutrients. In addition, they promote weight gain when eaten in excess. A person practising **moderation** ♦ eats such foods only on occasion and regularly selects foods low in solid fats and added sugars, a practice that automatically

HOW TO Compare Foods Based on Nutrient Density

One way to evaluate foods is simply to notice their nutrient contribution *per serving:* 250 millilitres (1 cup) of milk provides about 300 milligrams of calcium, and 125 millilitres (½ cup) of fresh, cooked turnip greens provides about 100 milligrams. Thus a serving of milk offers three times as much calcium as a serving of turnip greens. To get 300 milligrams of calcium, a person could choose either 250 millilitres (1 cup) of milk or 375 millilitres (1½ cups) of turnip greens.

Another valuable way to evaluate foods is to consider their nutrient density—their nutrient contribution *per kcalorie.* Skim (fat-free) milk delivers about 85 kcalories with its 300 milligrams of calcium. To calculate the nutrient density, divide milligrams by kcalories:

$$\frac{300 \text{ mg calcium}}{85 \text{ kcal}} = 3.5 \text{ mg per kcal}$$

Do the same for the fresh turnip greens, which provide 15 kcalories with the 100 milligrams of calcium:

$$\frac{100 \text{ mg calcium}}{15 \text{ kcal}} = 6.7 \text{ mg per kcal}$$

The more milligrams per kcalorie, the greater the nutrient density. Turnip greens are more calcium-dense than milk. They provide more calcium *per kcalorie* than milk, but milk offers more calcium *per serving.* Both approaches offer valuable information, especially when combined with a realistic appraisal. What matters most is which are you more likely to consume—375 millilitres of turnip greens or 250 millilitres of milk? You can get 300 milligrams of calcium from either, but the greens will save you about 40 kcalories (the savings would be even greater if you usually use whole milk).

Keep in mind, too, that calcium is only one of the many nutrients that foods provide. Similar calculations for protein, for example, would show that skim milk provides more protein both *per kcalorie* and *per serving* than turnip greens—that is, milk is more protein dense. Combining variety with nutrient density helps to ensure the adequacy of all nutrients.

CENGAGENOW™
For additional practice log on to **www.cengage.com/sso.**

TRY IT Compare the thiamin density of 90 grams (3 ounces) of lean t-bone steak (174 kcalories, 0.09 milligrams thiamin) with 125 millilitres (½ cup) of fresh cooked broccoli (27 kcalories, 0.05 milligrams thiamin).

improves nutrient density. Returning to the example of cheddar cheese versus skim milk, the skim milk not only offers the same amount of calcium for less energy, but it also contains far less fat than the cheese.

Variety A diet may have all of the virtues just described and still lack **variety**, if a person eats the same foods day after day. People should select foods from each of the food groups daily and vary their choices within each food group from day to day for several reasons. First, different foods within the same food group contain different arrays of nutrients. Among the fruits, for example, strawberries are especially rich in vitamin C while apricots are rich in vitamin A. Variety improves nutrient adequacy.[4] Second, no food is guaranteed to be entirely free of substances that, in excess, could be harmful. The strawberries might contain trace amounts of one contaminant, the apricots another. By alternating fruit choices, a person will ingest very little of either contaminant. (Contamination of foods is discussed in Chapter 20.) Third, as the adage goes, variety is the spice of life. A person who eats beans frequently can enjoy pinto beans in Mexican burritos today, garbanzo beans in a Greek salad tomorrow, and baked beans with barbecued chicken on the weekend. Eating nutritious meals need never be boring.

variety (dietary): eating a wide selection of foods within and among the major food groups.

IN SUMMARY A well-planned diet delivers adequate nutrients, a balanced array of nutrients, and an appropriate amount of energy. It is based on nutrient-dense foods, moderate in substances that can be detrimental to health, and varied in its selections.

Diet-Planning Guides

To plan a healthy diet, ♦ a person needs tools as well as knowledge. Among the most widely used tools for diet planning are **food group plans** that build a diet from clusters of foods that are similar in nutrient content and other important attributes. Thus each food group represents a set of nutrients that differs somewhat from the nutrients supplied by the other groups. Selecting foods from each of the groups eases the task of creating an adequate and balanced diet. The most widely used food group plan in Canada is *Eating Well with Canada's Food Guide*, or simply called the *Food Guide*. Another popular plan is *Dietary Approaches to Stop Hypertension* (DASH), which is presented in Chapters 13 and 19.

Eating Well with Canada's Food Guide

Canadians are encouraged to adopt a balanced eating plan as promoted in *Eating Well with Canada's Food Guide* (Figure 2-1). As shown in the rainbow image on the cover of the *Food Guide*, foods are categorized into four major groups, ♦ with each arc of the rainbow representing a relative proportion of food intake. In order of most to least intake, the four food groups are Vegetables and Fruit, Grain Products, Milk and Alternatives, and Meat and Alternatives. Foods are categorized into the food groups based on nutrient profile, a common agricultural origin, typical dietary use of foods, and how foods have been traditionally classified. Although the nutrient content of foods in each group can vary, each group provides a range of notable nutrients (see Table 2-1). This provides flexibility in diet planning because a person can select any food from a food group, and receive a similar range of nutrients. For example, when making selections from the Grain Products group, you can choose rice, bread, or cereal and obtain carbohydrate, folate, and iron. Importantly, foods in a food group provide not only notable nutrients, but smaller amounts of other nutrients and phytochemicals as well.

FIGURE 2-1 ***Eating Well with Canada's Food Guide***

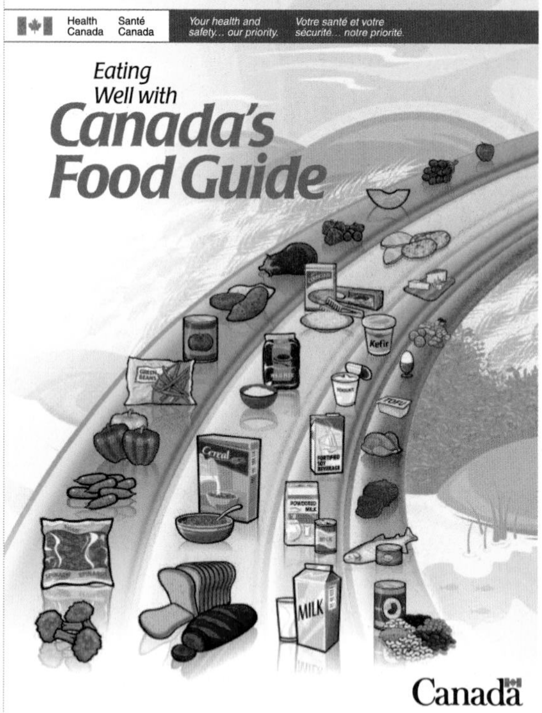
Health Canada
Santé Canada
Your health and safety... our priority.
Votre santé et votre sécurité... notre priorité.
Eating Well with
Canada's
Food Guide
MILK
Canada

SOURCE: Canada's Food Guide. Health Canada, 2007. Reproduced with the permission of the Minister of Health, 2011.

♦ A healthy diet:

- Emphasizes a variety of vegetables, fruits, whole grains, fat-free and low-fat milk products and alternatives, and lean meats, poultry, fish, eggs, legumes, nuts, and seeds.
- Is low in saturated and *trans* fats, cholesterol, salt (sodium), and added sugars.
- Stays within your daily energy needs to maintain your healthy body weight.
- Includes 30 to 45 millilitres (2 to 3 Tbsp) of unsaturated fat each day.
- Emphasizes drinking water regularly as a way to quench your thirst.

♦ The four food groups:

- Vegetables and fruit
- Grain products
- Milk and alternatives
- Meat and alternatives

food group plans: diet-planning tools that sort foods into groups based on nutrient content and other common attributes (e.g., commodity group, common use) and then specify that people should eat certain amounts of foods from each group.

TABLE 2-1 Notable Nutrients in the Food Groups

The type of food that people eat is just as important as the amount. That's why *Eating Well with Canada's Food Guide* provides guidance on specific types of foods to choose from each food group. Each food group provides notable nutrients among a variety of many nutrients.

Food group	Notable nutrients
Vegetables and Fruit	• These foods notably contribute carbohydrate, fibre, folate, vitamin A, vitamin C, vitamin K, magnesium, and potassium.
Grain Products	• These foods notably contribute carbohydrate, fibre, folate, thiamin, riboflavin, niacin, magnesium, and iron.
Milk and Alternatives	• These foods notably contribute protein, riboflavin, vitamin A, vitamin D, vitamin B_{12}, calcium, magnesium, phosphorus, potassium, and zinc.
Meat and Alternatives	• Meat, poultry, fish, and eggs notably contribute protein, thiamin, niacin, vitamin B6, vitamin B_{12}, iron, magnesium, potassium, and zinc; legumes, nuts, and seeds notably contribute protein, fibre, folate, thiamin, vitamin E, iron, magnesium, potassium, and zinc.

Eating Well with Canada's Food Guide also encourages people to choose foods lower in fat, sugar, and salt. Guidance to support these choices includes:

- Choose vegetables and fruits prepared with little or no added fat, sugar, or salt.
- Choose grain products that are lower in fat, sugar, or salt.
- Select lower-fat milk alternatives.
- Select lean meat and alternatives prepared with little or no added fat or salt.
- Limit foods and beverages high in calories, fat, sugar, or salt.

Guidance is also given to:

- Include a small amount of unsaturated fat each day.
- Satisfy your thirst with water.
- Enjoy a variety of foods from the four food groups.

Dietary Guidance for Canadians

Meet recommended intakes within your energy needs by adopting a balanced eating pattern such as *Canada's Food Guide* or the DASH eating plan. (The DASH eating plan is presented in Chapters 13 and 19.)

Recommended Number of *Food Guide* Servings per Day The inside of the *Food Guide* shows the recommended daily number of servings for each food group to meet nutrient and energy needs of most Canadians 2 years of age and older (Figure 2-2). *Food Guide* servings are presented in three age categories for children and in six different gender and age groupings for teens and adults. If you are an active person, you may need to increase your number of servings from the food groups. Estimated daily kcalorie needs for sedentary, low-active, and active men and women are shown in Table 2-2. ♦ Sample menus meeting the recommended servings from each food group for people of different ages and activity levels are provided in Table 2-3 on page 40. Determine how many servings in each food group are recommended for you and think of ways in which you could meet your recommended servings.

What Is One *Food Guide* Serving? To help you estimate your daily food intake, the serving sizes recommended in the *Food Guide* are given in metric units (e.g., mL, g) and common household units (e.g., cup, Tbsp) (Figure 2-3, p. 41). To put the *Food Guide* into action, use a measuring cup, tablespoon, teaspoon, or other measuring device to answer questions like these: ♦ What portion of a cup is a small handful of grapes? Is a "helping" of mashed potatoes more or less than 125 millilitres (half a cup)? What volume of cereal do you typically pour into a bowl? How many grams or ounces is the steak at your favourite restaurant? How many millilitres (cups) of milk does your glass hold? Compare the measures of what you eat with the single serving sizes provided in the *Food Guide* to estimate the number of daily servings you consume from each food group.

Make Each *Food Guide* Serving Count... By knowing how many servings are recommended from each food group and how big single servings actually are, you can make food choices that fit with the balanced eating plan promoted in Canada's *Food Guide*. Because each food group supplies notable nutrients, by choosing the types of foods recommended in the key messages for each food group you can make the most of your food selections.

Regardless of whether you are at school, at home, or out with friends, following the key messages will provide you with the nutrients most often lacking in the diets of Canadians or limit an excessive intake of other nutrients (Figure 2-4, p. 41). For example, all vegetables in the Vegetables and Fruit food group provide an array of nutrients, but some vegetables are especially good sources of certain vitamins, minerals, and beneficial phytochemicals. ♦ Dark green vegetables deliver the B vitamin folate and orange vegetables provide vitamin A. For this reason the *Food Guide* recommends that Canadians *eat at least one dark green and one orange vegetable each day.* A key message for the Grain Products group is to make at least half of your grain products whole grain. This recommendation helps Canadians increase their intake of fibre and B vitamins. For the Milk and Alternatives group,

FIGURE 2-2 Recommended Number of *Food Guide* Servings per Day

Recommended Number of Food Guide Servings per Day

	Children			Teens		Adults			
Age in Years	2–3	4–8	9–13	14–18		19–50		51+	
Sex	Girls and Boys			Females	Males	Females	Males	Females	Males
Vegetables and Fruit	4	5	6	7	8	7–8	8–10	7	7
Grain Products	3	4	6	6	7	6–7	8	6	7
Milk and Alternatives	2	2	3–4	3–4	3–4	2	2	3	3
Meat and Alternatives	1	1	1–2	2	3	2	3	2	3

The chart above shows how many Food Guide Servings you need from each of the four food groups every day.

Having the amount and type of food recommended and following the tips in *Canada's Food Guide* will help:

- Meet your needs for vitamins, minerals and other nutrients.
- Reduce your risk of obesity, type 2 diabetes, heart disease, certain types of cancer and osteoporosis.
- Contribute to your overall health and vitality.

SOURCE: Canada's Food Guide. Health Canada, 2007. Reproduced with the permission of the Minister of Health, 2011.

TABLE 2-2 Estimated kCalorie Needs for Adults

	Sedentary[a]	Low Active[b]	Active[c]
Women			
17–18 yr	1750	2100	2400
19–30 yr	1900	2100	2350
31–50 yr	1800	2000	2250
51–70 yr	1650	1850	2100
71+ yr	1550	1750	2000
Men			
17–18 yr	2450	2900	3300
19–30 yr	2500	2700	3000
31–50 yr	2350	2600	2900
51–70 yr	2150	2350	2650
71+ yr	2000	2200	2500

[a]Sedentary describes a lifestyle that includes only the activities typical of day-to-day life (e.g., household work, walking to the bus).
[b]Typical daily living activities plus 30 to 60 minutes of daily moderate activity (e.g., walking at 5 to 7 km/h). NOTE: In addition to gender, age, and activity level, energy needs vary with height and weight (see Chapter 8 and APPENDIX F).
[c]Active describes a lifestyle that includes activities typical of day-to-day life, plus at least 60 minutes of daily moderate activity.
SOURCE: Canadian Nutrient File. Health Canada, 2008. Reproduced with the permission of the Minister of Health, 2011.
NOTE: Canadian median heights and weights were used to calculate these values, however, energy needs vary with height and weight (see Chapter 8 and APPENDIX F).

TABLE 2-3 Family Members' Meal Plans Using *Eating Well with Canada's Food Guide*

	Jessica, age 18 Low active	Marc, age 22 Active	Sylvia, age 48 Sedentary	Lucas, age 51 Low active
***Food Guide* servings**				
Vegetables & Fruit	7	8–10	7–8	7
Grain Products	6	8	6–7	7
Milk & Alternatives	3–4	2	2	3
Meat & Alternatives	2	3	2	3
Meals				
Breakfast	30 g (125 mL) bran flake cereal with 30 mL (2 Tbsp) raisins and 125 mL (1/2 cup) 1% milk, 1 (medium) peach	60 g (500 mL) cold cereal with 250 mL (1 cup) 1% milk, 1 (medium) banana	2 whole-wheat waffles (90 g) with 30 mL (2 Tbsp) strawberry compote, 375 mL (1 1/2 cup) skim caffè latte	Omelette with 125 mL (1/2 cup) spinach, 60 mL (1/4 cup) mushrooms, and 30 mL (2 Tbsp) black olives, 500 mL (2 cups) skim caffè latte
Snack	3 (medium) prune plums	1 whole-wheat bagel with 30 mL (2 Tbsp) almond butter	15 g (1 Tbsp) each of roasted almonds, dried cranberries, and raisins	1 (medium) banana and 30 mL (2 Tbsp) walnuts
Lunch	Black bean burrito made with 1 corn tortilla, 125 mL (1/2 cup) shredded lettuce, 1/2 avocado, 100 mL (1/3 cup) salsa, and 30 g (2 Tbsp) Cheddar cheese, 250 mL (1 cup) 1% milk, 1 (medium) banana	1 submarine sandwich made with smoked turkey, onions, tomato, lettuce, jalapeno peppers, low-fat mayonnaise, regular soft drink (355 mL), potato chips (28 g package)	45 g (1 1/2 oz) grilled chicken breast with 375 mL (1 1/2 cups) mixed greens, 30 g (2 Tbsp) sunflower seeds, and 30 mL (2 Tbsp) salad dressing, 375 mL (1 1/2 cups) skim caffè latte	625 mL (2 1/2 cups) pasta salad made with beef, broccoli, bean sprouts, and soy-ginger dressing, 250 mL coffee with 15 mL (1 Tbsp) cream
Snack	3 stoned wheat crackers with 30 mL (2 Tbsp) hummus	1 (medium) apple	60 mL (1/4 cup) baby carrots, 500 mL (2 cups) Earl Grey tea	1 (medium) apple
Dinner	75 g (2 1/2 oz) broiled chicken breast, 175 mL (3/4 cup) cooked brown rice, 250 mL (1 cup) steamed mixed vegetables (broccoli, yams, and carrots), 25 mL (1 1/2 Tbsp) salad dressing, 250 mL (1 cup) water, 175 g (3/4 cup) 1% yogurt with 125 mL (1/2 cup) mixed berries	375 g (1 1/2 cup) pork and vegetable lo mein, 250 mL (1 cup) steamed mixed vegetables (peas, corn, and carrots), 375 mL (1 1/2 cups) 1% milk, 1 piece (155 g) of apple pie, 250 mL (1 cup) Earl Grey tea	375 mL (1 1/2 cup) homemade vegetarian black bean chili, 1 slice (35 g) of whole-wheat bread, 375 mL (1 1/2 cups) mixed greens salad with 30 mL (2 Tbsp) vinaigrette salad dressing, 125 mL (1/2 cup) steamed butternut squash, 250 mL (1 cup) skim milk, baked pear (medium) with 175 g (3/4 cup) skim vanilla yogurt	90 g (3 oz) grilled Coho salmon, 250 mL (1 cup) baby potatoes roasted with carrots, 125 mL (1/2 cup) roasted Brussels sprouts, 125 mL (1/2 cup) roasted yams, 250 mL (1 cup) cooked wild rice
Snack	1 slice (35 g) whole-grain toast with 15 mL (1 Tbsp) jam	3 whole-grain crackers (15 g) with 25 g (3/4 oz) Swiss cheese	500 mL (2 cups) air-popped popcorn, 1 (medium) nectarine	1 slice (50 g) of date loaf with 2 (100 g) fresh figs
Calories (total)	2108	3023	1815	2350
Calories from fat	580	952	444	620
Calories from saturated and *trans* fat	147	219	69	111

♦ Chapter 8 explains how to determine energy needs. For an approximation of your energy needs, turn to the DRI Estimated Energy Requirement (EER) on the inside front cover

emphasis is placed on consuming lower fat options: *Drink skim, 1%, or 2% milk each day.* And, in the Meat and Alternatives group, Canadians are encouraged to *have meat alternatives such as beans, lentils, and tofu more often.* Because legumes are often substituted for animal-based foods they are included in the Meat and Alternatives food group. As well as being excellent sources of fibre and the B vitamin folate, legumes contribute protein, iron, and zinc, which are similar notable nutrients provided by meats, fish, and poultry. Familiarize yourself with these key messages to help you make the most of your food choices.

In addition to the key messages of limiting a regular intake of high fat foods, specifically richer sources of saturated and *trans* fats, advice on oils and fats is to select small amounts of oil-based sources more often than solid or hydrogenated

FIGURE 2-3 What Is One *Food Guide* Serving?

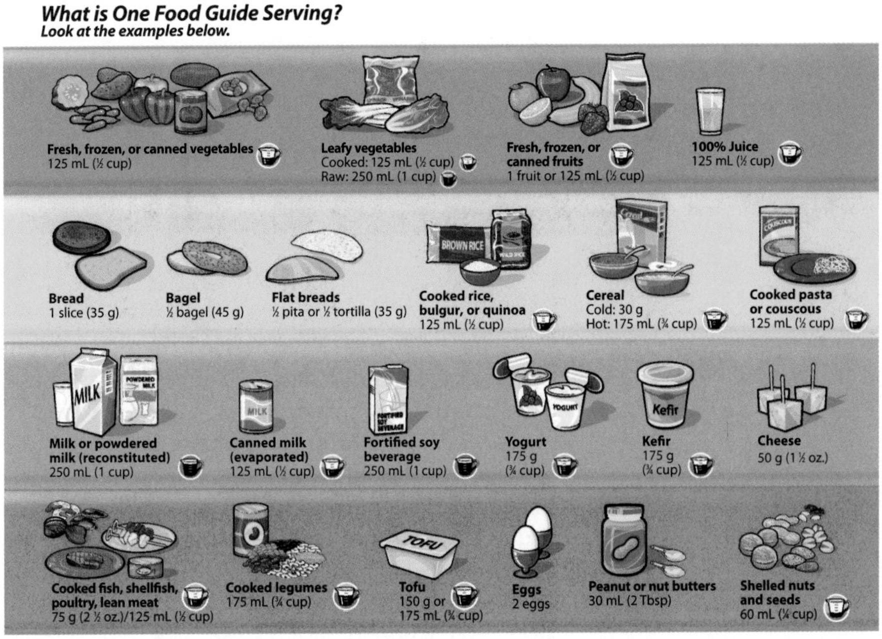
What is One Food Guide Serving?
Look at the examples below.
Fresh, frozen, or canned vegetables
125 mL (½ cup)
Leafy vegetables
Cooked: 125 mL (½ cup)
Raw: 250 mL (1 cup)
Fresh, frozen, or canned fruits
1 fruit or 125 mL (½ cup)
100% Juice
125 mL (½ cup)
Bread
1 slice (35 g)
Bagel
½ bagel (45 g)
Flat breads
½ pita or ½ tortilla (35 g)
Cooked rice, bulgur, or quinoa
125 mL (½ cup)
Cereal
Cold: 30 g
Hot: 175 mL (¾ cup)
Cooked pasta or couscous
125 mL (½ cup)
Milk or powdered milk (reconstituted)
250 mL (1 cup)
Canned milk (evaporated)
125 mL (½ cup)
Fortified soy beverage
250 mL (1 cup)
Yogurt
175 g
(¾ cup)
Kefir
175 g
(¾ cup)
Cheese
50 g (1 ½ oz.)
Cooked fish, shellfish, poultry, lean meat
75 g (2 ½ oz.)/125 mL (½ cup)
Cooked legumes
175 mL (¾ cup)
Tofu
150 g or
175 mL (¾ cup)
Eggs
2 eggs
Peanut or nut butters
30 mL (2 Tbsp)
Shelled nuts and seeds
60 mL (¼ cup)

SOURCE: Canada's Food Guide. Health Canada, 2007. Reproduced with the permission of the Minister of Health, 2011.

♦ For quick and easy estimates, visualize each serving as being about the size of a common object:
- 250 mL (1 cup) vegetables or fruits = a baseball
- 60 mL (1/4 cup) dried fruits or nuts = a golf ball
- 75–90 g (3 oz) meat = a deck of cards
- 30 mL (2 Tbsp) peanut butter = a ping pong ball
- 50 g (1½ oz) cheese = 4 stacked dice
- 125 mL (1/2 cup) ice cream = a racquetball
- 4 small cookies = 4 poker chips

♦ **Phytochemicals** are the nonnutrient compounds found in plant-derived foods that have biological activity in the body

fat sources (Figure 2-5, p. 42). Even though these choices are rich in kcalories, a small amount is recommended to provide nutrients that are lacking in other foods but are needed for good health (see Highlight 5). This will help you to consume enough of the essential fatty acids required for normal body functions.

A cornerstone principle of eating well is to consume a variety of foods from each food group. With more variety in your diet, you will enjoy a diversity of tastes, textures, and colours and improve the likelihood of reaching adequate nutrient intake.

Water is essential to life, even more so than food! Water is distributed throughout the body, so whenever possible try to satisfy your thirst with water. Your body will thank you for it.

Advice for Different Ages and Stages... As we grow and age, certain nutrients become of particular importance. As shown in Figure 2-6 (p. 42), the *Food Guide* advises all types of nutritious foods are suitable for children; a multivitamin supplement including folic acid is recommended for all women who could become pregnant, are pregnant, or are breastfeeding; a multivitamin supplement with the mineral iron is recommended for all pregnant women; extra energy is recommended for women who are pregnant or breastfeeding; and in addition to eating a healthy diet, a daily vitamin D supplement of 400 IU (10 μg) is recommended for everyone over the age of 50 years.

Eat Well and Be Active Today and Every Day! Making the most of your food choices is important for adequate energy and nutrient intake. Being active every day burns the calories that you consume and allows you to achieve and maintain a healthy body weight and better health overall (Figure 2-7, p. 43).

FIGURE 2-4 Make Each *Food Guide* Serving Count...

Make each Food Guide Serving count...
wherever you are – at home, at school, at work or when eating out!

- **Eat at least one dark green and one orange vegetable each day.**
  - Go for dark green vegetables such as broccoli, romaine lettuce, and spinach.
  - Go for orange vegetables such as carrots, sweet potatoes, and winter squash.
- **Choose vegetables and fruit prepared with little or no added fat, sugar, or salt.**
  - Enjoy vegetables steamed, baked, or stir-fried instead of deep-fried.
- **Have vegetables and fruit more often than juice.**

- **Make at least half of your grain products whole grain each day.**
  - Eat a variety of whole grains such as barley, brown rice, oats, quinoa, and wild rice.
  - Enjoy whole grain breads, oatmeal, or whole wheat pasta.
- **Choose grain products that are lower in fat, sugar, or salt.**
  - Compare the Nutrition Facts table on labels to make wise choices.
  - Enjoy the true taste of grain products. When adding sauces or spreads, use small amounts.

- **Drink skim, 1%, or 2% milk each day.**
  - Have 500 mL (2 cups) of milk every day for adequate vitamin D.
  - Drink fortified soy beverages if you do not drink milk.
- **Select lower fat milk alternatives.**
  - Compare the Nutrition Facts table on yogurts or cheeses to make wise choices.

- **Have meat alternatives such as beans, lentils, and tofu often.**
- **Eat at least two Food Guide Servings of fish each week.***
  - Choose fish such as char, herring, mackerel, salmon, sardines, and trout.
- **Select lean meat and alternatives prepared with little or no added fat or salt.**
  - Trim the visible fat from meats. Remove the skin on poultry.
  - Use cooking methods such as roasting, baking, or poaching that require little or no added fat.
  - If you eat luncheon meats, sausages, or prepackaged meats, choose those lower in salt (sodium) and fat.

SOURCE: Canada's Food Guide. Health Canada, 2007. Reproduced with the permission of the Minister of Health, 2011.

FIGURE 2-5 **Advice on Types of Fat, Eating a Variety of Foods, and Quenching Your Thirst with Water**

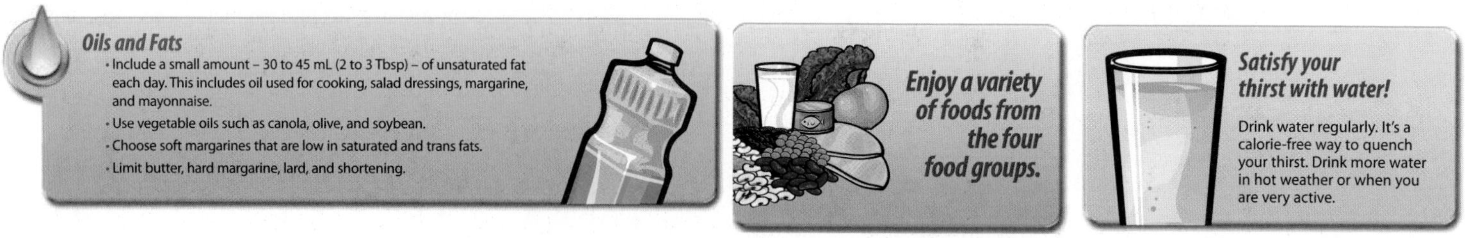
Oils and Fats
• Include a small amount – 30 to 45 mL (2 to 3 Tbsp) – of unsaturated fat each day. This includes oil used for cooking, salad dressings, margarine, and mayonnaise.
• Use vegetable oils such as canola, olive, and soybean.
• Choose soft margarines that are low in saturated and trans fats.
• Limit butter, hard margarine, lard, and shortening.
Enjoy a variety of foods from the four food groups.
Satisfy your thirst with water!
Drink water regularly. It's a calorie-free way to quench your thirst. Drink more water in hot weather or when you are very active.

FIGURE 2-6 **Advice for Different Ages and Stages...**

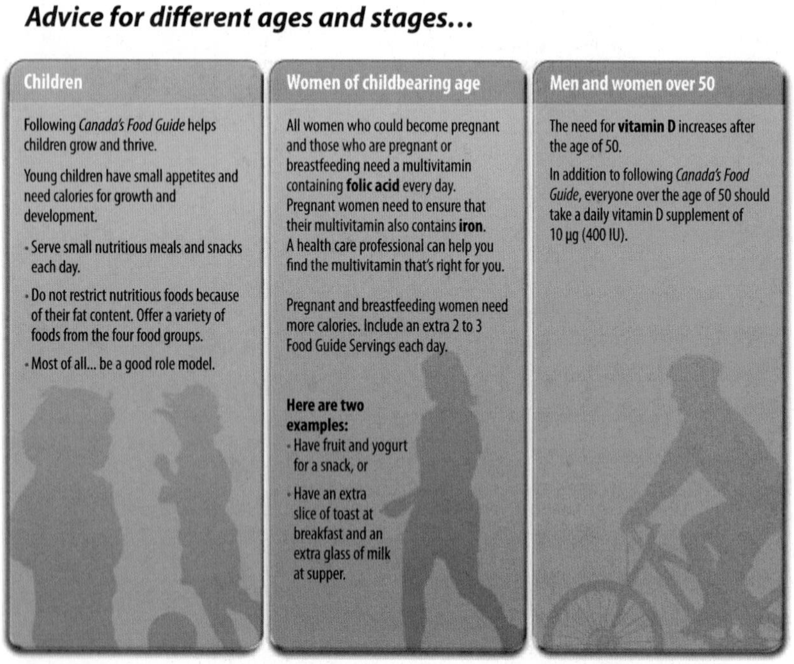
Advice for different ages and stages...
Children
Following Canada's Food Guide helps children grow and thrive.
Young children have small appetites and need calories for growth and development.
• Serve small nutritious meals and snacks each day.
• Do not restrict nutritious foods because of their fat content. Offer a variety of foods from the four food groups.
• Most of all... be a good role model.
Women of childbearing age
All women who could become pregnant and those who are pregnant or breastfeeding need a multivitamin containing folic acid every day. Pregnant women need to ensure that their multivitamin also contains iron. A health care professional can help you find the multivitamin that's right for you.
Pregnant and breastfeeding women need more calories. Include an extra 2 to 3 Food Guide Servings each day.
Here are two examples:
• Have fruit and yogurt for a snack, or
• Have an extra slice of toast at breakfast and an extra glass of milk at supper.
Men and women over 50
The need for vitamin D increases after the age of 50.
In addition to following Canada's Food Guide, everyone over the age of 50 should take a daily vitamin D supplement of 10 μg (400 IU).

By now you may have noticed the messages in *Canada's Food Guide* help you meet the six basic diet-planning principles previously described on pages 35–37. Go ahead and practise applying these basic principles when making your food choices. For comparison purposes, the United States Department of Agriculture Food Patterns and MyPlate are presented in APPENDIX I.

Dietary Guidance for Canadians

Consume a variety of nutrient-dense foods and beverages within and across the four food groups while choosing foods that limit the intake of calories, saturated and *trans* fats, cholesterol, added sugars, and salt.

Ethnic Food Choices People can use *Canada's Food Guide* and still enjoy a diverse array of culinary styles by sorting ethnic foods into their appropriate food groups. For example, a person eating South Asian foods would find okra and mango in the Vegetables and Fruit group, chapatis in the Grain Products group, yogurt in the Milk and Alternatives group, and lamb and chickpeas in the Meat and Alternatives group. Health Canada recognizes the multicultural makeup of Canada and publishes *Eating Well with Canada's Food Guide* in 10 different languages in addition to English and French. Table 2-4 (p. 44) features some ethnic food choices.

Vegetarian Diets Vegetarian diets rely mainly on plant foods: grains, vegetables, legumes, fruits, seeds, and nuts. Some vegetarian diets include eggs, milk products, or both. People who do not eat meats or milk products can still use *Canada's Food Guide* to create an adequate diet because each group includes plant-based foods.[5] Highlight 2 defines vegetarian terms and provides details on planning healthy vegetarian diets.

Mixtures of Foods Some foods—such as casseroles, soups, and sandwiches—fall into two or more food groups. With a little practice, users can learn to see these mixtures of foods as items from various food groups. For example, a grilled chicken fajita represents four different food groups: the onions, lettuce, bell peppers, and tomatoes from the Vegetables and Fruit group; the tortilla from the Grain Products group; the cheese from the Milk and Alternatives group; and the chicken from the Meat and Alternatives group. You may need to use half and double servings to estimate your daily total. *Eating Well with Canada's Food Guide* provides an example of how to count *Food Guide* servings in a meal.

My Food Guide Health Canada created an online interactive educational tool called My Food Guide (p. 45) that allows Canadians to personalize the Food Guide by entering the foods they consume. My Food Guide was designed to encourage consumers to make healthy food and physical activity choices every day. The recommendations in My Food Guide are supportive of, and consistent with, several other recommendations to control obesity and chronic diseases such as diabetes, heart disease, and cancer.[6]

The My Food Guide website ♦ helps consumers assess the types and amounts of foods to eat each day based on their age, gender, and activity level.[7] In addition to creating a personal plan, consumers are offered tips to help them improve their dietary and lifestyle practices.

FIGURE 2-7 Eat Well and Be Active Today and Every Day!

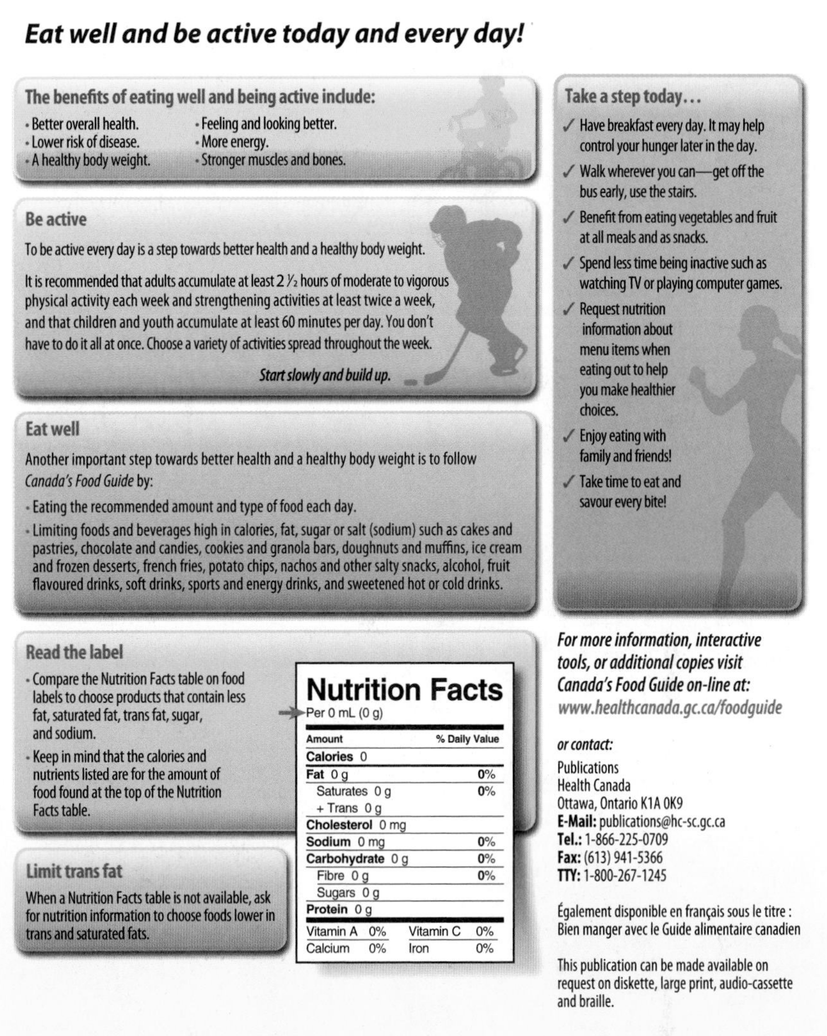
Eat well and be active today and every day!
The benefits of eating well and being active include:
• Better overall health.
• Lower risk of disease.
• A healthy body weight.
• Feeling and looking better.
• More energy.
• Stronger muscles and bones.
Be active
To be active every day is a step towards better health and a healthy body weight.
It is recommended that adults accumulate at least 2 ½ hours of moderate to vigorous physical activity each week and strengthening activities at least twice a week, and that children and youth accumulate at least 60 minutes per day. You don't have to do it all at once. Choose a variety of activities spread throughout the week.
Start slowly and build up.
Eat well
Another important step towards better health and a healthy body weight is to follow Canada's Food Guide by:
• Eating the recommended amount and type of food each day.
• Limiting foods and beverages high in calories, fat, sugar or salt (sodium) such as cakes and pastries, chocolate and candies, cookies and granola bars, doughnuts and muffins, ice cream and frozen desserts, french fries, potato chips, nachos and other salty snacks, alcohol, fruit flavoured drinks, soft drinks, sports and energy drinks, and sweetened hot or cold drinks.
Take a step today...
✓ Have breakfast every day. It may help control your hunger later in the day.
✓ Walk wherever you can—get off the bus early, use the stairs.
✓ Benefit from eating vegetables and fruit at all meals and as snacks.
✓ Spend less time being inactive such as watching TV or playing computer games.
✓ Request nutrition information about menu items when eating out to help you make healthier choices.
✓ Enjoy eating with family and friends!
✓ Take time to eat and savour every bite!
Read the label
• Compare the Nutrition Facts table on food labels to choose products that contain less fat, saturated fat, trans fat, sugar, and sodium.
• Keep in mind that the calories and nutrients listed are for the amount of food found at the top of the Nutrition Facts table.
Nutrition Facts
Per 0 mL (0 g)
Amount % Daily Value
Calories 0
Fat 0 g 0%
Saturates 0 g 0%
+ Trans 0 g
Cholesterol 0 mg
Sodium 0 mg 0%
Carbohydrate 0 g 0%
Fibre 0 g 0%
Sugars 0 g
Protein 0 g
Vitamin A 0% Vitamin C 0%
Calcium 0% Iron 0%
Limit trans fat
When a Nutrition Facts table is not available, ask for nutrition information to choose foods lower in trans and saturated fats.
For more information, interactive tools, or additional copies visit Canada's Food Guide on-line at:
www.healthcanada.gc.ca/foodguide
or contact:
Publications
Health Canada
Ottawa, Ontario K1A 0K9
E-Mail: publications@hc-sc.gc.ca
Tel.: 1-866-225-0709
Fax: (613) 941-5366
TTY: 1-800-267-1245
Également disponible en français sous le titre : Bien manger avec le Guide alimentaire canadien
This publication can be made available on request on diskette, large print, audio-cassette and braille.

SOURCE: Canada's Food Guide. Health Canada, 2011. Reproduced with the permission of the Minister of Health, 2011.

Recommendations versus Actual Intakes *Eating Well with Canada's Food Guide* and My Food Guide were developed to help people choose a balanced and healthful diet. Are consumers actually eating according to these recommendations? The short answer is "not really." In general, consumers are not selecting the most nutrient-dense items from the food groups. Instead, they are consuming too many foods high in solid fats and added sugars—soft drinks, desserts, whole milk products, and fatty meats.[8] They are also not selecting the suggested quantities from each of the food groups, typically eating too few vegetables, fruit, whole grains, and milk products.

Canada's Food Guide for First Nations, Inuit, and Métis *Canada's Food Guide for First Nations, Inuit, and Métis* (p. 45) complements the guidance provided in *Eating Well with Canada's Food Guide* but is tailored to reflect the values of First Nations, Inuit, and Métis peoples across Canada. On the cover, the circular design is meaningful to many Aboriginal cultures, with the core image representing traditional foods and food gathering activities and the outer circle representing the inclusion of store-bought foods in a healthy eating pattern. On the inside, recommended daily amounts and types of foods from the four food groups are given, and the back page provides guidance on limiting food and beverage choices that are high calorie, fat, sugar, and salt and on making the most of food choices for specific groups of people. The First Nations, Inuit and Métis *Food Guide* is available in Inuktitut, Ojibwe, Plains Cree, and Woods Cree language, in addition to English.

♦ My Food Guide can be found on the Health Canada Food and Nutrition website, under *Canada's Food Guide* link: www.hc-sc.gc.ca

USDA MyPlate and Food Patterns The USDA MyPlate visual (see p. 44) is intended to remind Americans to consume more nutrient-dense foods and less of other types of foods while striving to achieve a healthy balance between calories consumed and those expended. The MyPlate icon is based on the USDA Food Patterns that recommend daily amounts of foods from each of five food groups ♦, subgroups, and oils to meet people's nutrient needs. APPENDIX I provides details of the USDA Food Patterns for 12 different calorie levels.

♦ Five food groups from the USDA MyPlate:
- Fruits
- Vegetables
- Grains
- Meat and legumes
- Milk

TABLE 2-4 Ethnic Food Choices

	Vegetables & Fruit	Grain Products	Milk & Alternatives	Meat & Alternatives
Asian 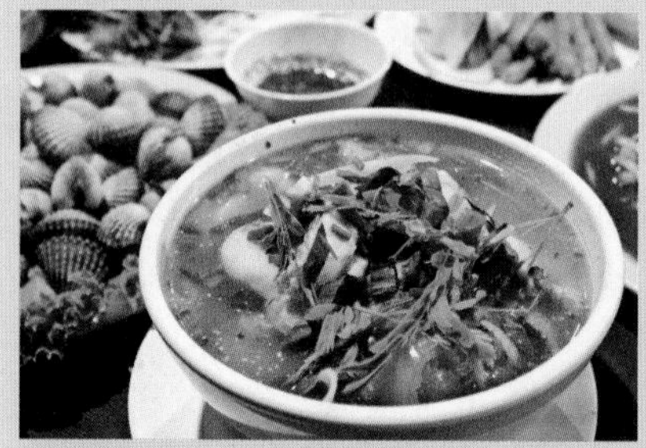 Getideaka/shutterstock	Baby corn, bamboo shoots, chayote, bok choy, gai lan, sugar peas, mushrooms, water chestnuts, kelp, guava, kumquat, lychee, persimmon, melon, mandarin oranges	Rice, noodles, millet	Often excluded	Soybeans and soy products (e.g., fortified soy beverage, tempeh, tofu), squid, duck, eggs, pork, poultry, fish and other seafood, peanuts, cashews
Mediterranean 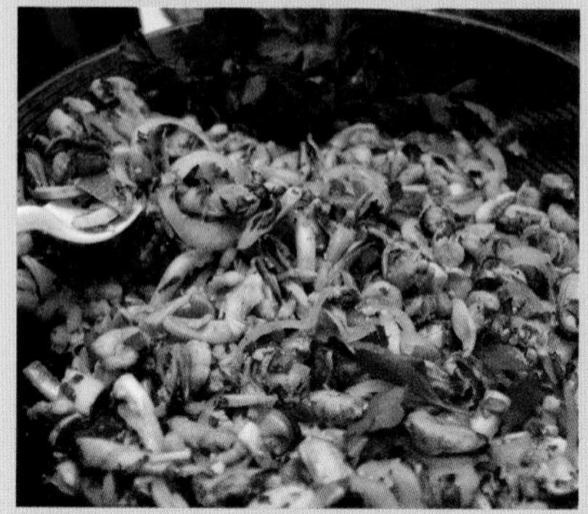 © Stephan Zabel/iStockphoto	Eggplant, tomatoes, peppers, cucumbers, grape leaves, olives, grapes, figs	Pita bread, pasta, rice, couscous, polenta, bulgur, focaccia	Cheeses: ricotta, provolone, parmesan, feta, mozzarella and goat, yogurt	Fish and other seafood, lamb, chicken, beef, pork, gyros, sausage, lentils, fava beans
South Asian 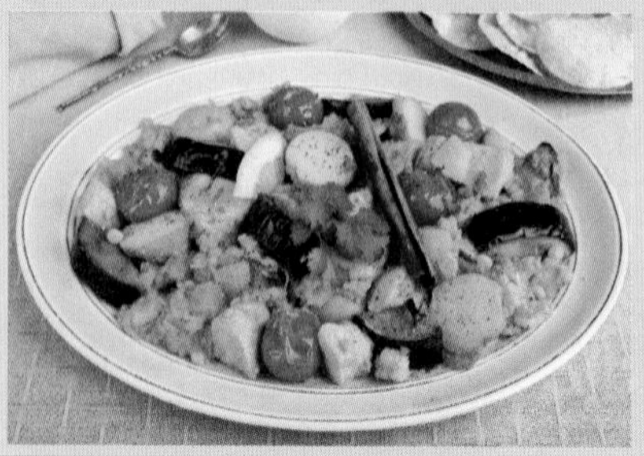 photos.com	Potatoes, peas, onions, cauliflower, spinach, okra, eggplant, cucumber, raisins, dates, bananas, mango, papaya	Rice, chapati, roti, naan, paratha	Yogurt, paneer	Lentils, chickpeas, fish, chicken, lamb, goat

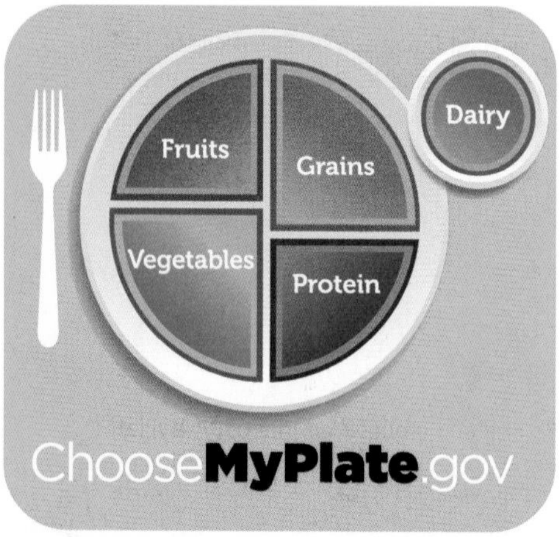
Fruits
Grains
Dairy
Vegetables
Protein
ChooseMyPlate.gov
USDA, ChooseMyPlate.gov

Using the familiar place setting, MyPlate reminds Americans how to eat healthfully from the five food groups.

Exchange Lists Food group plans are particularly well suited to help a person achieve dietary adequacy, balance, and variety. **Exchange lists** provide additional help in achieving kcalorie control and moderation. Originally developed as a meal-planning guide for people with diabetes, exchange lists have proved useful for general diet planning as well.

Canada's Food Guide sorts foods primarily by nutrient content and commodity group, whereas exchange lists sort foods according to their energy-yielding nutrient content. A popular meal-planning guide in Canada, *Beyond the Basics: Meal Planning for Healthy Eating, Diabetes Prevention and Management,* uses an exchange system to sort foods into food groups and defines specific portion sizes. As a result of using energy nutrients to sort foods, foods do not always appear on the exchange list where you might first expect to find them. For example, in *Beyond the Basics*, cheeses are grouped with Meat and Alternatives because, like meats, cheeses contribute energy from protein and fat but provide negligible carbohydrate. In *Canada's Food Guide*, cheeses are grouped with Milk and Alternatives because of their calcium content.

For similar reasons, the Grains and Starches list in *Beyond the Basics* contains starchy vegetables such as corn, potatoes, and sweet potatoes. Likewise, avocados

My Food Guide: Customize your own personalized version of *Canada's Food Guide*.

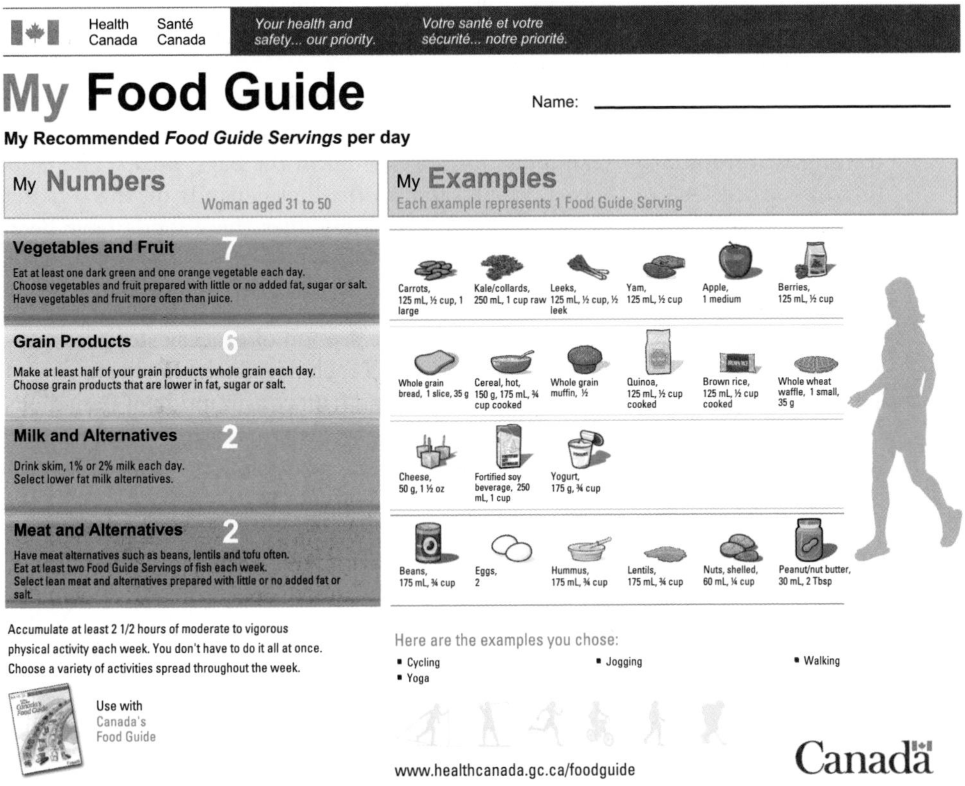
Health Canada Santé Canada
Your health and safety... our priority.
Votre santé et votre sécurité... notre priorité.
My Food Guide
Name:
My Recommended Food Guide Servings per day
My Numbers
Woman aged 31 to 50
My Examples
Each example represents 1 Food Guide Serving
Vegetables and Fruit 7
Eat at least one dark green and one orange vegetable each day.
Choose vegetables and fruit prepared with little or no added fat, sugar or salt.
Have vegetables and fruit more often than juice.
Carrots, 125 mL, ½ cup, 1 large
Kale/collards, 250 mL, 1 cup raw
Leeks, 125 mL, ½ cup, ½ leek
Yam, 125 mL, ½ cup
Apple, 1 medium
Berries, 125 mL, ½ cup
Grain Products 6
Make at least half of your grain products whole grain each day.
Choose grain products that are lower in fat, sugar or salt.
Whole grain bread, 1 slice, 35 g
Cereal, hot, 150 g, 175 mL, ¾ cup cooked
Whole grain muffin, ½
Quinoa, 125 mL, ½ cup cooked
Brown rice, 125 mL, ½ cup cooked
Whole wheat waffle, 1 small, 35 g
Milk and Alternatives 2
Drink skim, 1% or 2% milk each day.
Select lower fat milk alternatives.
Cheese, 50 g, 1 ½ oz
Fortified soy beverage, 250 mL, 1 cup
Yogurt, 175 g, ¾ cup
Meat and Alternatives 2
Have meat alternatives such as beans, lentils and tofu often.
Eat at least two Food Guide Servings of fish each week.
Select lean meat and alternatives prepared with little or no added fat or salt.
Beans, 175 mL, ¾ cup
Eggs, 2
Hummus, 175 mL, ¾ cup
Lentils, 175 mL, ¾ cup
Nuts, shelled, 60 mL, ¼ cup
Peanut/nut butter, 30 mL, 2 Tbsp
Accumulate at least 2 1/2 hours of moderate to vigorous physical activity each week. You don't have to do it all at once. Choose a variety of activities spread throughout the week.
Here are the examples you chose:
Cycling
Jogging
Walking
Yoga
Use with Canada's Food Guide
www.healthcanada.gc.ca/foodguide
Canada

My Food Guide. Health Canada, 2008. Reproduced with the permission of the Minister of Health, 2011

do not appear on the Fruit list but are classified on the Fat list because their fat content makes them more similar to oil than to grapes. Rather than being grouped with Meat and Alternatives, nuts and seeds are also categorized on the Fat list to remind users of their high fat content. It is clear from these few examples that using the energy-yielding characteristics of foods to form food groups provides people with another way to make healthy food choices. To learn more about this useful diet-planning tool, study APPENDIX G, which provides details of the *Beyond the Basics* exchange system.

exchange lists: diet-planning tools that organize foods by their proportions of carbohydrate, fat, and protein. Foods on any single list can be used interchangeably.

Putting the Plan into Action

When you are ready to put a diet plan into action, you will want to be familiar with each food group and the number of servings recommended for you. You will also want to practise estimating serving sizes of foods to be able to compare the number of servings that you consume to what is recommended in the *Food Guide*. Use the key messages to make nutrient-dense choices that help you get all the nutrients you need and keep your kcalories under control.

According to 2004 Canadian Community Health Survey data, 50 percent of Canadian adults did not meet the minimum daily servings of vegetables and fruits, and more than 25 percent of Canadians aged 31 to 50 obtained greater than 35 percent of their total calories from fat.[9] We all make countless food-related decisions daily—whether we have a plan or not—but following a plan such as *Canada's Food Guide*, which incorporates health recommendations and diet-planning principles, can help you make wise food decisions.

Eating Well with Canada's Food Guide - First Nations, Inuit and Métis provides guidance on healthy eating that respects the values, traditions, and food choices of these cultures.

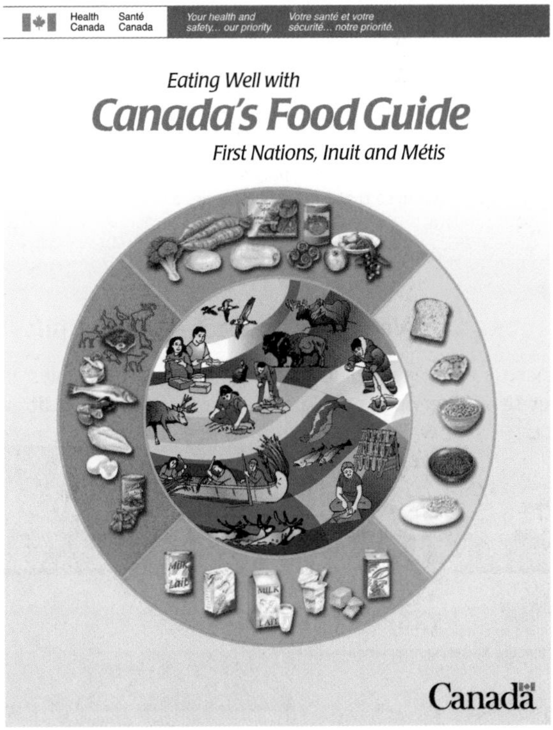
Health Canada Santé Canada
Your health and safety... our priority.
Votre santé et votre sécurité... notre priorité.
Eating Well with
Canada's Food Guide
First Nations, Inuit and Métis
Canada

Eating Well with Canada's Food Guide: First Nations, Inuit and Métis. Health Canada, 2010. Reproduced with the permission of the Minister of Health, 2011.

From Guidance to Groceries

Dietary recommendations emphasize nutrient-rich foods such as vegetables and fruit; whole grains; low-fat milk and milk alternatives; and lean meats, fish, and poultry, and legumes and other meat alternatives. You can design such a diet for yourself, but how do you begin? Start with the foods you enjoy eating. Then try to make improvements, little by little. When shopping, think of the food groups and choose nutrient-dense foods within each group.

Be aware that many of the 50 000 food options available today are **processed foods** that have lost valuable nutrients and gained sugar, fat, and salt as they were transformed from farm-fresh foods to those found in the bags, boxes, and cans that line grocery-store shelves. Their value in the diet depends on the starting food and how it was prepared or processed. Sometimes these foods have been **fortified** to improve their nutrient contents.

Vegetables and Fruit Posters in the produce section of grocery stores encourage consumers to eat more vegetables and fruits each day. Such efforts are part of a national campaign to increase the vegetable and fruit consumption of Canadians (see Figure 2-8). To help consumers remember to eat a variety of vegetables and fruits, the Mix It Up! campaign provides practical tips, such as selecting at least one serving from each of five colours—red, yellow-orange, green, blue-purple, and white-tan-brown—every day.

Choose fresh vegetables often, especially dark green leafy and yellow-orange vegetables like spinach, broccoli, carrots, and yams. Cooked or raw, vegetables are good sources of vitamins, minerals, and fibre. Frozen and canned vegetables without added salt are acceptable alternatives to fresh. To control fat, energy, and sodium intakes, limit putting butter and salt on vegetables.

Choose fresh fruits often, especially citrus fruits and yellow-orange fruits like cantaloupes and peaches. Frozen, dried, and canned fruits without added sugar are acceptable alternatives to fresh. Fruits supply valuable vitamins, minerals, fibres, and phytochemicals. They add flavours, colours, and textures to meals, and their natural sweetness makes them enjoyable as snacks or desserts.

Fruit juices are healthy beverages but lack dietary fibre compared with whole fruits. Whole fruits satisfy the appetite better than juices, thereby helping people to limit food energy intakes. For people who need extra food energy, though, 100 percent fruit juices are a good choice. Be aware that sweetened fruit "drinks" or "-ades" contain mostly water, sugar, and a little juice for flavour. Some may have been fortified with vitamin C or calcium but lack any other significant nutritional value.

processed foods: foods that have been treated to change their physical, chemical, microbiological, or sensory properties.

fortified: the addition to a food of nutrients that were either not originally present or present in insignificant amounts. Fortification can be used to correct or prevent a widespread nutrient deficiency or to balance the total nutrient profile of a food.

refined: the process by which the coarse parts of a food are removed. When wheat is refined into flour, the bran, germ, and husk are removed, leaving only the endosperm.

enriched: the addition to a food of nutrients that were lost during processing so that the food will meet a specified standard.

Dietary Guidance for Canadians

Choose a variety of vegetables and fruits each day. In particular, regularly choose dark green and orange vegetables and whole fruits more often than juice. Consuming vegetables and fruits helps you stay within your energy needs.

FIGURE 2-8 Veggies and Fruit—Mix It Up!!

Because everyone benefits from eating more vegetables and fruit, the Mix It Up! campaign (www.5to10aday.com) encourages consumers to eat several servings of a variety of vegetables and fruit every day.

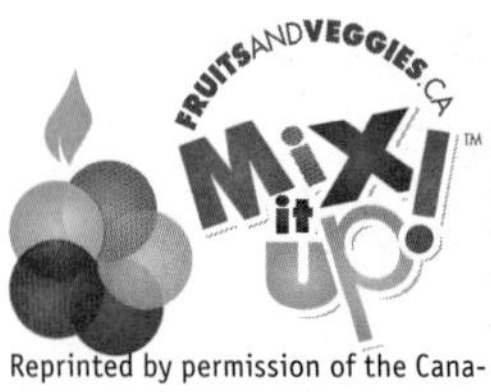

Reprinted by permission of the Canadian Produce Marketing Association

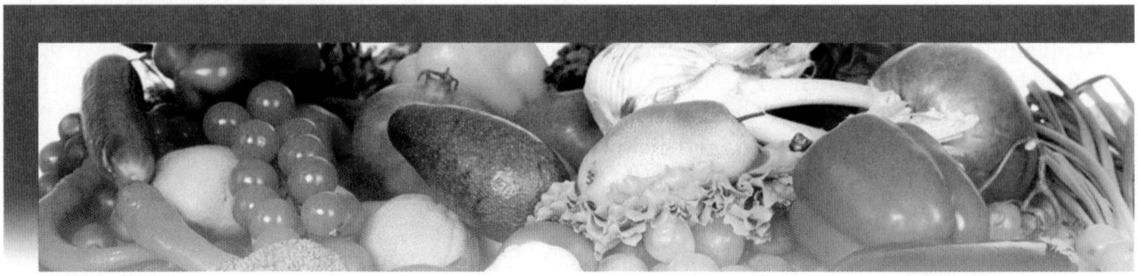

Poznyakov/shutterstock

Grains Products When shopping for grain products, you will find them described as *refined, enriched,* or *whole grain.* These terms refer to the milling process and the making of grain products, and they have different nutrition implications (see Figure 2-9). **Refined** foods may have lost many nutrients during processing; **enriched** products may have had some nutrients added back; and **whole-grain** products may be rich in fibre and all the nutrients found in the original grain. ♦ As such, whole-grain products support good health and should account for at least half of your daily intake of grain products.[10] Adding more whole grains to the diet can be as easy as eating oatmeal for breakfast and popcorn for a snack or substituting brown rice for white rice and whole-wheat bread for white bread. To find whole-grain products, read food labels and select those that name a whole grain first in the ingredient list. Products described as "multi-grain" or "stone-ground" are usually *not* whole-grain products. Brown colour is also not a useful hint, but fibre content often is.

♦ Examples of whole grains:
- Amaranth
- Barley
- Buckwheat
- Bulgur
- Corn (and popcorn)
- Couscous
- Millet
- Oats (and oatmeal)
- Quinoa
- Rice (brown or wild)
- Whole rye
- Whole wheat

Dietary Guidance for Canadians

In general, at least half of your daily intake of grain products should come from whole grains.

---

whole grain: a grain that maintains the same relative proportions of starchy endosperm, germ, and bran as the original (all but the husk); not refined.

FIGURE 2-9 A Wheat Plant

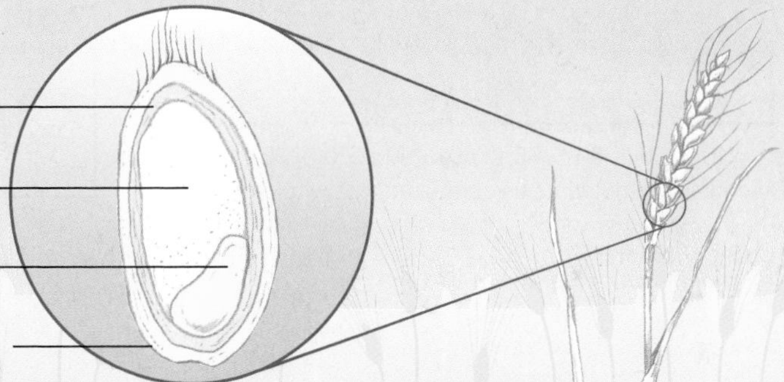

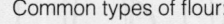

The protective coating of **bran** around the kernel of grain is rich in nutrients and fibre.

The **endosperm** contains mostly starch and some protein.

The **germ** is the seed that grows into a wheat plant, so it is especially rich in vitamins and minerals to support new life.

The outer **husk** (or **chaff**) is the inedible part of a grain.

Whole-grain products contain much of the germ and bran, as well as the endosperm; that is why they are so nutritious. Refined grain products contain only the endosperm. Even with nutrients added back, they are not as nutritious as whole-grain products, as Figure 2-10 shows.

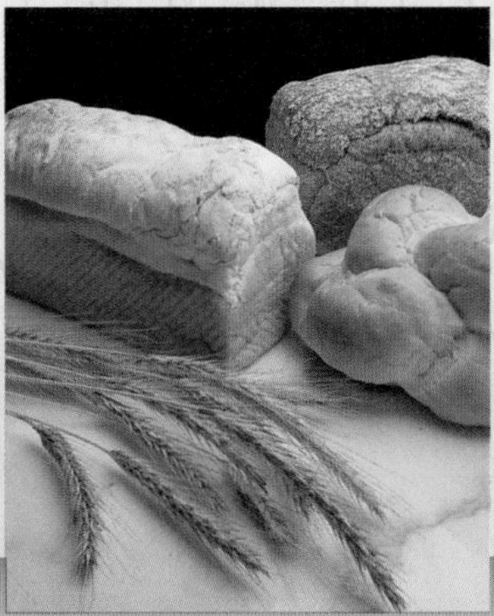

DUSAN ZIDAR/shutterstock

Common types of flour:

- **Refined flour:** finely ground endosperm that is enriched with nutrients and bleached for whiteness; also called *white flour, enriched flour, enriched white flour, or* simply *flour.*
- **Wheat flour:** any flour made from the endosperm of the wheat kernel.
- **Whole-wheat flour:** any flour made from the entire wheat kernel.

The difference between *white flour* and *white wheat* is noteworthy. Typically, *white flour* refers to refined flour (as defined above). Most flour—whether refined, or whole wheat—is made from red wheat. Whole-grain products made from red wheat are typically brown and full flavoured.

To capture the health benefits of whole grains for consumers who prefer white bread, manufacturers have been experimenting with a white variety of wheat called *white wheat.* Whole-grain products made from white wheat provide all the nutrients and fibre of a whole grain with a light colour and natural sweetness. Read labels carefully—white bread is a whole-grain product only if it is made from whole white wheat.

FIGURE 2-10 Nutrients in Bread

Whole-grain bread is more nutritious than other breads, even enriched bread. For iron, thiamin, riboflavin, niacin, and folate, enriched bread provides about the same quantities as whole-grain bread. For fibre and the other nutrients (those shown here as well as those not shown), enriched bread provides less than whole-grain bread.

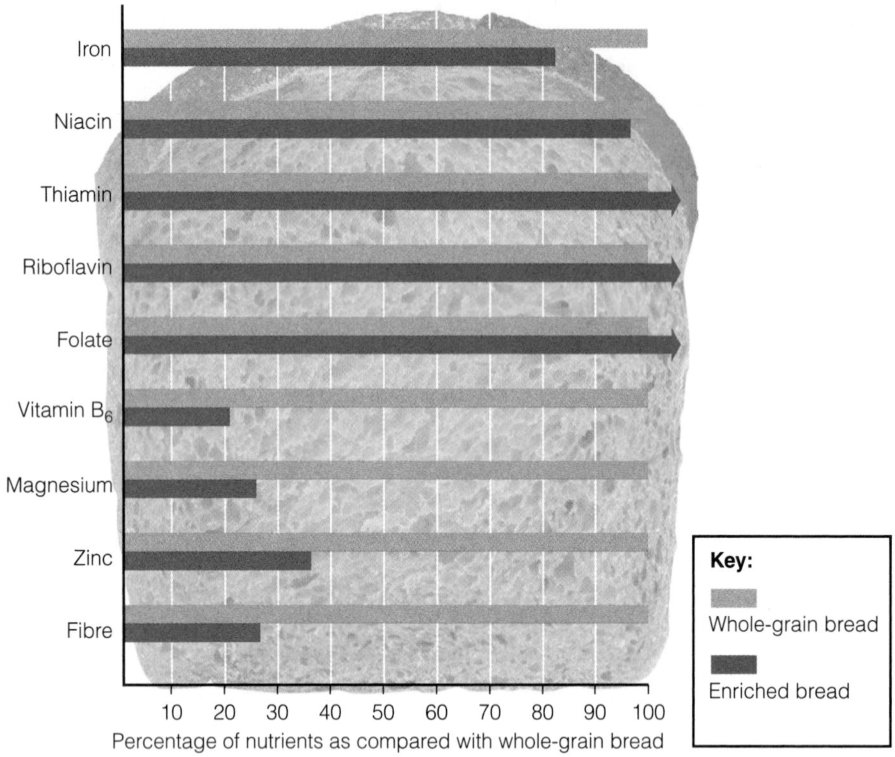
Iron
Niacin
Thiamin
Riboflavin
Folate
Vitamin B6
Magnesium
Zinc
Fibre
10 20 30 40 50 60 70 80 90 100
Percentage of nutrients as compared with whole-grain bread
Key:
Whole-grain bread
Enriched bread

When it became a common practice to refine the wheat flour used for bread by milling it and throwing away the bran and the germ, consumers suffered from a loss of many nutrients. In 1975, Canada introduced mandatory enrichment of grain products with the vitamins thiamin, riboflavin, and niacin and the mineral iron. In 1998, legislation was amended to include folic acid, a form of the vitamin folate, which is considered essential in the prevention of some birth defects. Grain products that have been refined, such as rice, wheat pastas like macaroni and spaghetti, and cereals (both cooked and ready-to-eat types), have subsequently been enriched. ♦ Food labels must specify that products have been enriched and include the enrichment nutrients in the ingredients list.

Enrichment doesn't make a slice of bread rich in these added nutrients, but people who eat several slices a day obtain significantly more of these nutrients than they would from unenriched bread. Even though the enrichment of flour helps to prevent deficiencies of these nutrients, it fails to compensate for losses of many other nutrients and fibre. As Figure 2-10 shows, whole-grain items still outshine the enriched ones. Only whole-grain flour contains all of the nutritive portions of the grain. Whole-grain products, such as brown rice and oatmeal, provide more nutrients and fibre and contain less salt and sugar than flavoured, processed rice or sweetened cereals.

♦ Grain enrichment nutrients:

- Iron
- Thiamin
- Riboflavin
- Niacin
- Folate

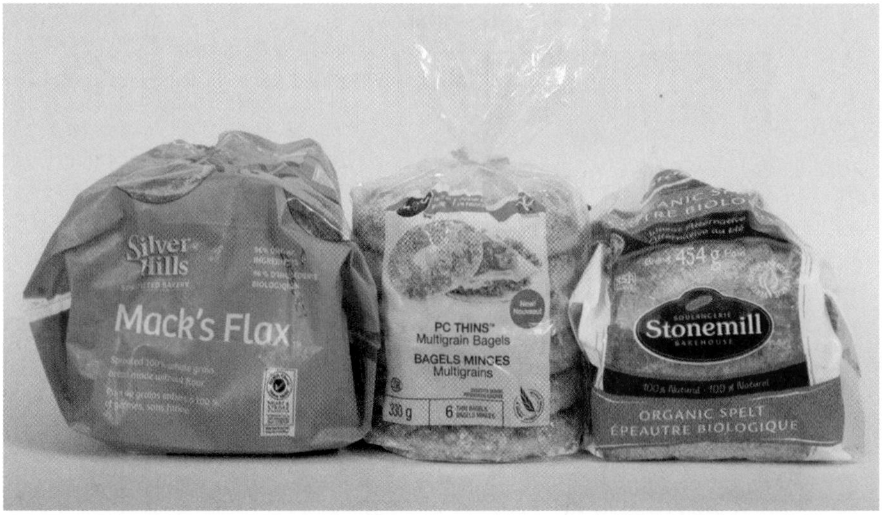
Silver Hills
Mack's Flax
PC THINS™
Multigrain Bagels
BAGELS MINCES
Multigrains
330 g
Stonemill
ORGANIC SPELT
ÉPEAUTRE BIOLOGIQUE

Dick Hemingway

When shopping for bread, look for the descriptive words *whole grain* or *whole wheat* and check the fibre content on the Nutrition Facts table of the label—the more fibre, the more likely the bread is a whole-grain product. You can also look for whole grain in the ingredient list.

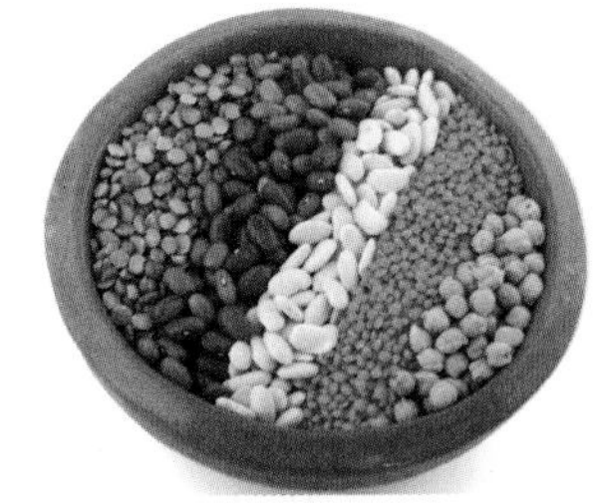
Ivonne Wierink/shutterstock

Combining legumes with foods from other food groups creates delicious meals.

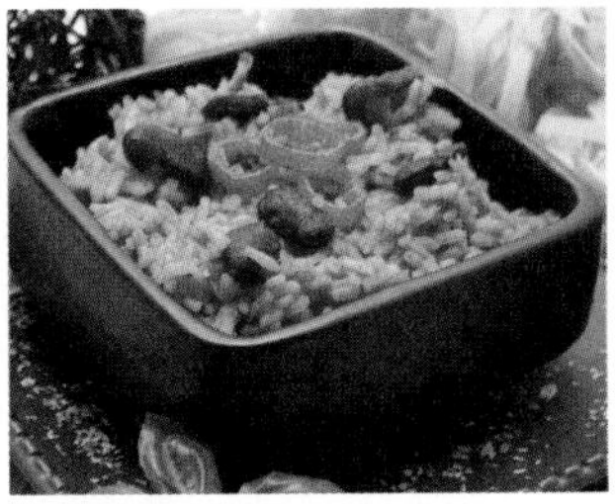
Silvia Bogdanski/shutterstock

Add rice to red beans for a hearty meal.

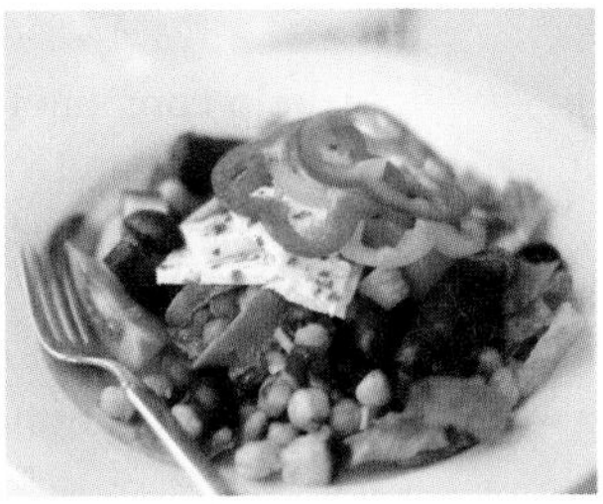
Quentin Bacon/Getty Images

Enjoy a Greek salad topped with garbanzo beans for a little ethnic diversity.

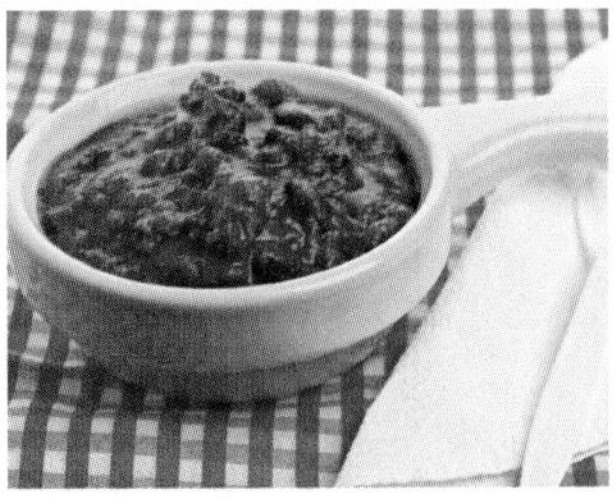
© Debbi Smirnoff/iStockphoto

A bit of meat and lots of spices turn kidney beans into chili con carne.

Speaking of cereals, ready-to-eat breakfast cereals are some of the most highly fortified foods on the market. Like an enriched food, a fortified food has had nutrients added during processing, but in a fortified food, the added nutrients may not have been present in the original product. Some breakfast cereals made from refined flour and fortified with high doses of vitamins and minerals are actually more like dietary supplements disguised as cereals than they are like whole grains. They may be nutritious—with respect to the nutrients added—but they still may fail to convey the full spectrum of nutrients that a whole-grain food or a mixture of such foods might provide. Still, fortified foods help people meet their vitamin and mineral needs.

Milk and Alternatives Shoppers find a variety of fortified foods in the dairy case. Examples are milk, to which vitamins A and D have been added, and plant-based beverages, ♦ such as soy beverage to which calcium, vitamin D, vitamin B_{12}, and other vitamins and minerals have been added. In addition, shoppers may find **imitation foods** (such as 'cheese' products), **substitute foods** (such as egg substitutes), and **functional foods** ♦ (such as margarine with added plant sterols). As food technology advances, many such foods offer alternatives to traditional choices that may help people who want to reduce their fat and cholesterol intakes. Chapter 5 provides other examples.

When shopping, choose skim ♦ or 1% milk, and low-fat yogurt, and cheeses. Such selections help consumers meet their vitamin and mineral needs within their energy and fat allowances. Milk products are important sources of calcium, but can provide too much sodium and fat if not selected with care.

Dietary Guidance for Canadians

Consume two to four daily servings of skim or 1% milk or equivalent milk products.

Meat and Alternatives Meat, fish, and poultry provide essential minerals, such as iron and zinc, and abundant B vitamins as well as protein. Legumes are low in fat and provide protein, iron, zinc, and fibre. ♦ To buy and prepare these foods without excess energy, fat, and sodium takes a little knowledge and planning. When shopping in the meat department, choose fish, poultry, and lean cuts of beef and pork named "round" or "loin" (as in top round or pork tenderloin). As a guide, "prime" and "choice" cuts generally have more fat than "select" cuts. Restaurants usually serve prime cuts. Ground beef, even "lean" ground beef, derives most of its food energy from fat. Have the butcher trim and grind a lean round steak instead. Alternatively, **textured vegetable protein** can be used instead of ground beef in a casserole, spaghetti sauce, or chili, saving fat kcalories.

Weigh meat after it is cooked and the bones and fat are removed. In general, 110 grams (4 ounces) of raw meat is equal to about 85 grams (3 ounces) of cooked meat. Some examples of 85 gram portions of meat include 1 medium pork chop, ½ chicken breast, or 1 steak or hamburger about the size of a deck of cards. To keep fat intake moderate, bake, roast, broil, grill, or braise meats (but do not fry them in fat); trim visible fat before cooking; remove the skin from poultry after cooking; and drain fat after cooking. Chapter 5 offers many additional strategies for moderating fat intake.

♦ Be aware that not all plant-based beverages have been fortified. Read labels carefully.

♦ **Functional foods** contain physiologically active compounds that provide health benefits beyond their nutrient contributions.

♦ Milk descriptions:
- Skim milk = fat-free, nonfat, zero-fat, or no-fat
- 1% milk = Low-fat milk
- 2% milk = Reduced-fat milk or less-fat

♦ Legumes include a variety of peas, beans, and lentils:
- Adzuki beans
- Black beans
- Black-eyed peas
- Fava beans
- Garbanzo beans
- Great northern beans
- Kidney beans
- Lentils
- Lima beans
- Navy beans
- Peanuts
- Pinto beans
- Soybeans
- Split peas

imitation foods: foods that substitute for and resemble another food in flavour, texture, appearance, and nutritional value. On food labels, the word "imitation" must appear as part of the common name, such as "imitation crab."

substitute foods: foods that have the same nutritional value as another food, but are not physically similar, such as simulated whole egg products.

textured vegetable protein: processed soybean protein used in vegetarian products such as soy burgers.

IN SUMMARY Food group plans such as *Eating Well with Canada's Food Guide* help consumers select the types and amounts of foods to provide adequacy, balance, and variety in the diet. They make it easier to plan a diet that includes a balance of vegetables and fruits, grain products, milk and alternatives, and meat and alternatives. In making any food choice, remember to view the food in the context of your total diet. The combination of many different foods provides the abundance of nutrients that is so essential to a healthy diet.

Food Labels

Many consumers read food labels to help them make healthy choices.[11] In Canada, food labelling is regulated under the Food and Drugs Act and Food and Drug Regulations. While Health Canada developed the nutrition labelling regulations, it is the Canadian Food Inspection Agency (CFIA) that enforces the food labelling regulations. The Consumer Packaging and Labelling Act and Regulations also apply to food packaging and labels. All current regulations for labelling requirements and making nutrition claims are described in the *Guide to Food Labelling and Advertising*.[12] Food labels appear on virtually all processed foods, and posters or brochures provide similar nutrition information for fresh meats, fruits, and vegetables (see Figure 2-11). A few foods need not carry nutrition labels: those contributing few nutrients, such as plain coffee, tea, and spices; those produced by small businesses, such as jams sold at farmers' markets; and those prepared and sold in the same establishment. Some producers of these items, however,

FIGURE 2-11 **Example of a Food Label**

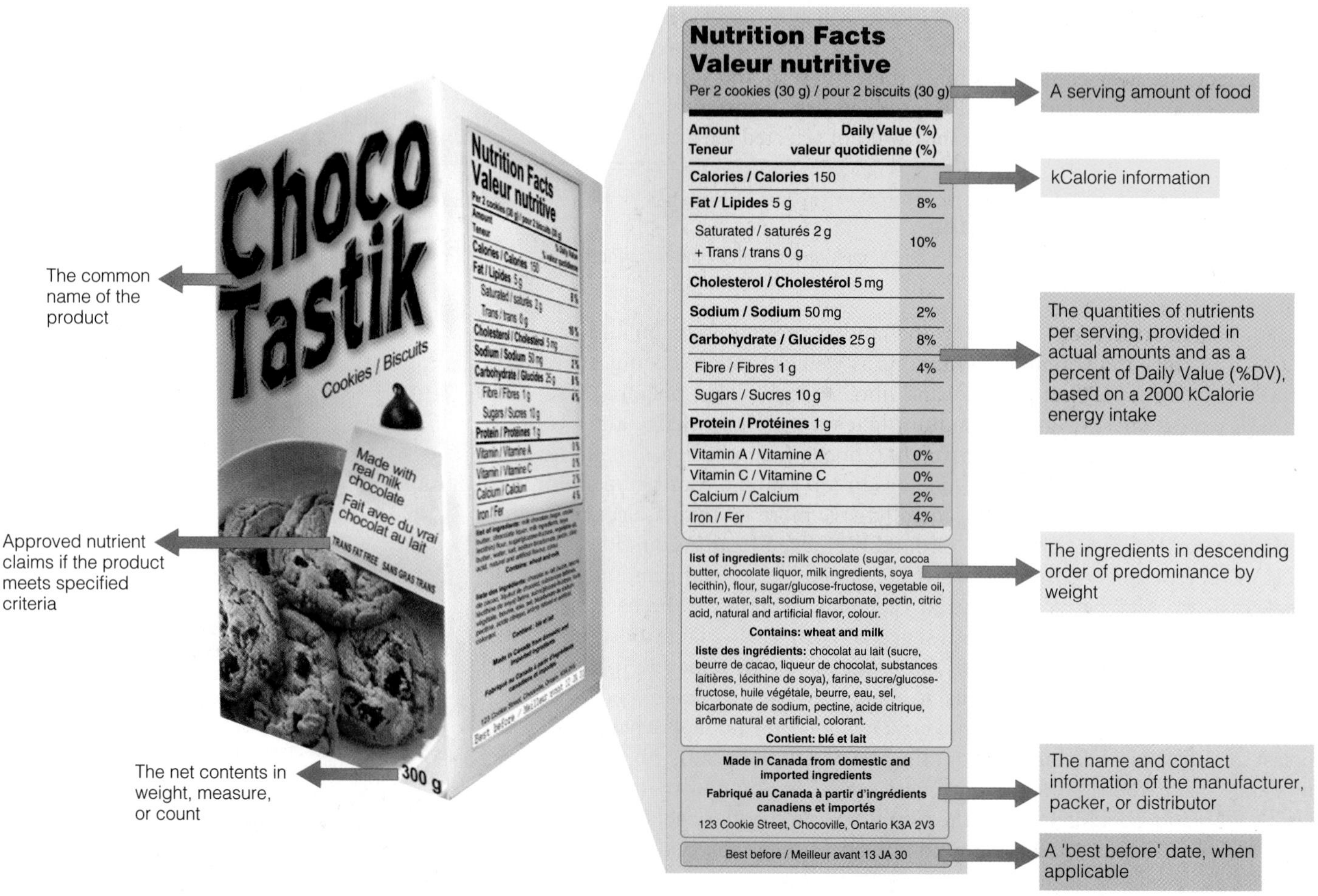
Choco Tastik
Cookies / Biscuits
Made with real milk chocolate
Fait avec du vrai chocolat au lait
TRANS FAT FREE SANS GRAS TRANS
300 g
The common name of the product
Approved nutrient claims if the product meets specified criteria
The net contents in weight, measure, or count
Nutrition Facts
Valeur nutritive
Per 2 cookies (30 g) / pour 2 biscuits (30 g)
Amount Daily Value (%)
Teneur valeur quotidienne (%)
Calories / Calories 150
Fat / Lipides 5 g 8%
Saturated / saturés 2 g
+ Trans / trans 0 g 10%
Cholesterol / Cholestérol 5 mg
Sodium / Sodium 50 mg 2%
Carbohydrate / Glucides 25 g 8%
Fibre / Fibres 1 g 4%
Sugars / Sucres 10 g
Protein / Protéines 1 g
Vitamin A / Vitamine A 0%
Vitamin C / Vitamine C 0%
Calcium / Calcium 2%
Iron / Fer 4%
list of ingredients: milk chocolate (sugar, cocoa butter, chocolate liquor, milk ingredients, soya lecithin), flour, sugar/glucose-fructose, vegetable oil, butter, water, salt, sodium bicarbonate, pectin, citric acid, natural and artificial flavor, colour.
Contains: wheat and milk
liste des ingrédients: chocolat au lait (sucre, beurre de cacao, liqueur de chocolat, substances laitières, lécithine de soya), farine, sucre/glucose-fructose, huile végétale, beurre, eau, sel, bicarbonate de sodium, pectine, acide citrique, arôme natural et artificial, colorant.
Contient: blé et lait
Made in Canada from domestic and imported ingredients
Fabriqué au Canada à partir d'ingrédients canadiens et importés
123 Cookie Street, Chocoville, Ontario K3A 2V3
Best before / Meilleur avant 13 JA 30
A serving amount of food
kCalorie information
The quantities of nutrients per serving, provided in actual amounts and as a percent of Daily Value (%DV), based on a 2000 kCalorie energy intake
The ingredients in descending order of predominance by weight
The name and contact information of the manufacturer, packer, or distributor
A 'best before' date, when applicable

voluntarily use labels. Even markets selling nonpackaged items voluntarily present nutrient information, either in brochures or on signs posted at the point of purchase. Restaurants need not supply complete nutrition information for menu items. Keep in mind that restaurants tend to serve extra-large portions—two to three times standard serving sizes. A "low-fat" ice cream, for example, may have only 3 grams of fat per 125 millilitres (½ cup), but you may be served 500 millilitres (2 cups) for a total of 12 grams of fat and all their accompanying kcalories. There are three main sections of nutrition information on a food label: the Nutrition Facts Table, the Ingredient List, and Claims, which can be nutrient or health-based. Food manufacturers also provide the company contact information.

TABLE 2-5 Household and Metric Measures

- 1 teaspoon (tsp) = 5 millilitre (mL)
- 1 tablespoon (Tbsp) = 15 mL
- 1 cup (c) = 240 mL
- 1 fluid ounce (fl oz) = 30 mL
- 1 ounce (oz) = 28 grams (g)

NOTE: The Aids to Calculation section at the back of the book provides additional weights and measures.

Nutrition Facts Table

A wealth of information is provided in the Nutrient Facts table: a serving size is declared, absolute amounts (grams, milligrams) of the core nutrients are given, and relative amounts (percent Daily Value) of most core nutrients are provided.

Serving Sizes Because labels present nutrient information based on one serving, they must identify the size of the serving. Canada's Food and Drug Regulations stipulate food manufacturers must use a serving size that falls within a specified range for similar products. For example, a serving size range for bread is 25–70 grams (1–2 slices). The food manufacturer indicates a serving size on the Nutrition Facts table that provides information about the product inside the packaging and falls within the allowable range. The quantity declared is the basis for all information provided in the table. It is important to note the serving size is declared for the product as it is sold (i.e., before preparation, when it is required). Preparing the product with other ingredients will alter the nutritional composition. The same serving size must be used wherever it appears on the packaging (e.g., Nutrition Facts table, directions for use). Serving sizes are expressed in both common household measures, such as cups, and metric measures, such as millilitres, to accommodate users of both types of measures (see Table 2-5).

When examining the nutrition facts on a food label, consumers need to compare the serving size on the label with how much they actually eat and adjust their calculations accordingly. For example, if the serving size is four cookies and you eat only two, then you need to cut the nutrient and kcalorie values in half; similarly, if you eat eight cookies, then you need to double the values. Notice, too, that small bags or individually wrapped items, such as chips or chocolate bars, may contain more than a single serving. The total number of servings per container is listed just below the serving size.

Be aware that serving sizes on food labels are not always the same as those in *Canada's Food Guide*. For example, a serving of rice on a food label is 250 millilitres (1 cup), whereas in the *Food Guide* it is 125 millilitres (½ cup). Unfortunately, this discrepancy, coupled with each person's own perception (oftentimes misperception) of serving sizes, sometimes creates confusion for consumers trying to follow recommendations.

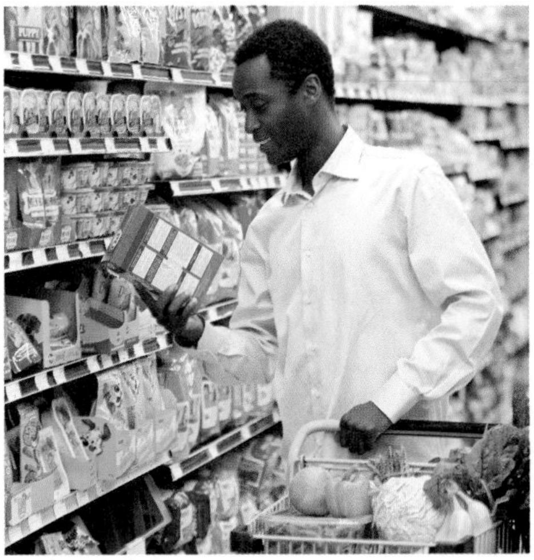

Fuse/Getty Images

Consumers read food labels to learn about the nutrient contents of a food or to compare similar foods.

Nutrition Facts In addition to the serving size, Canada's Food and Drug Regulations require that the Nutrition Facts table on a food label presents nutrient information in two ways—in absolute quantities (such as grams) and as percentages of standards called the **Daily Values**. The Nutrition Facts table must provide the nutrient amount, **percent Daily Value**, or both, for the following:

- Total food energy (kcalories)
- Food energy from fat (kcalories)
- Total fat (grams and percent Daily Value)
- Saturated and *trans* fat (grams and percent Daily Value)
- Cholesterol (milligrams and [optional] percent Daily Value)
- Sodium (milligrams and percent Daily Value)
- Total carbohydrate, which includes starch, sugar, and fibre (grams and percent Daily Value)
- Dietary fibre (grams and percent Daily Value)

Daily Values (DV): reference values developed specifically for use on food labels.

percent Daily Value (%DV): the percentage of a Daily Value recommendation found in a specified serving of food for key nutrients based on a 2000-kcalorie diet.

TABLE 2-6 Daily Values for Food Labels

Food labels must present the "% Daily Value" for these nutrients.

Food Component	Daily Value
Fat	65 g
Saturated fat	20 g
Cholesterol	300 mg
Carbohydrate (total)	300 g
Fibre	25 g
Sodium	2400 mg
Potassium	3500 mg
Vitamin C	60 mg
Vitamin A	1000 RE
Calcium	1100 mg
Iron	14 mg

NOTE: Daily Values were established for adults and children more than 2 years old. The values for energy-yielding nutrients are based on 2000 kcalories a day.

- Sugars, which includes both those naturally present in and those added to the food (grams)
- Protein (grams)

The labels must also present nutrient content information as a percent Daily Value for the following vitamins and minerals:

- Vitamin A
- Vitamin C
- Iron
- Calcium

At minimum, information for 13 different nutrients and kcalories is found on the Nutrition Facts table.

The Daily Values Table 2-6 presents the Daily Value standards for nutrients that are required to provide this information. Food labels list the amount of a nutrient in a product as a percentage of its Daily Value. Comparing nutrient amounts against the Daily Values helps make the numbers more meaningful to consumers. A person reading a food label might wonder, for example, whether 1 milligram of iron or calcium is a little or a lot. As Table 2-6 shows, the Daily Value for iron is 14 milligrams, so 1 milligram of iron is enough to notice—it is more than 5 percent, and that is what the food label will say. But because the Daily Value for calcium on food labels is 1100 milligrams, 1 milligram of calcium is insignificant, and the food label will read "0%."

The Daily Values reflect dietary recommendations for nutrients and dietary components that have important relationships with health. The "% Daily Value" column on a label provides a ballpark estimate of how individual foods contribute to the total diet. It compares key nutrients in a serving of food with the goals of a person consuming 2000 kcalories per day. A 2000-kcalorie diet is considered about right for sedentary younger women, active older women, and sedentary older men. Young children and sedentary older women may need fewer kcalories. The "% Daily Value" column on all labels applies only to a 2000-kcalorie diet. A 2500-kcalorie diet is considered about right for many men, teenage boys, and active younger women. People who are exceptionally active may have still higher energy needs.

People who consume 2000 kcalories a day can add up the "% Daily Values" for a particular nutrient to see how their intake of packaged foods fits with recommendations. Remember, foods without labels (e.g., fresh vegetables and fruit) also contribute to your daily nutrient intake. People who require more or less than 2000 kcalories daily must do some calculations to see how foods compare with their personal nutrition goals. They can use the suggestions presented in the accompanying "How To" feature.

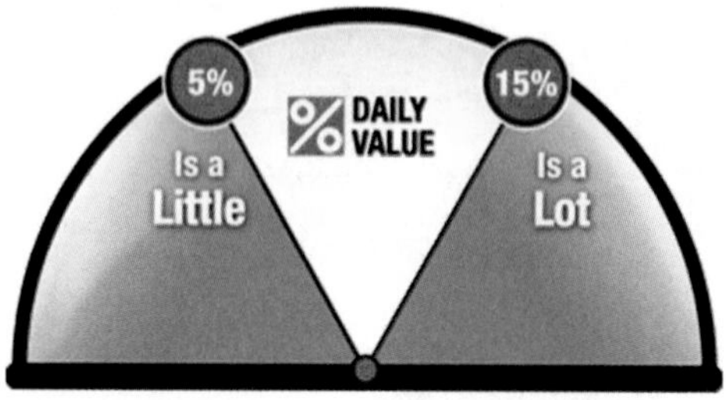
5%
Is a
Little
% DAILY VALUE
15%
Is a
Lot

Comparing between two different foods that may contain 'a little' or 'a lot' of a nutrient is easy when using % Daily Values.

Daily Values help consumers see easily whether a food contributes "a little" or "a lot" of a nutrient. ♦ For example, the "% Daily Value" column on a package of frozen macaroni and cheese may say 20 percent for fat. This tells the consumer that each serving of this food contains about 20 percent of the day's allotted 65 grams of fat. A person consuming 2000 kcalories a day could simply keep track of the percentages of Daily Values from foods eaten during a day and try not to exceed 100 percent. Be aware that for some nutrients (such as fat and sodium) you will want to select foods with a low "% Daily Value" and for others (such as calcium and fibre) you will want a high "% Daily Value." To determine whether a particular food is a wise choice, a consumer needs to consider its place in the diet among all the other foods eaten during the day. It is up to you to choose products that are higher in the nutrients you want more of (e.g., calcium, iron, fibre, or vitamin C) and lower in the nutrients you want to consume less (e.g., fat, saturated and trans fat, or sodium).

♦ % Daily Values:
- ≥25% = very high or excellent source
- ≥15% = high or good source
- ≥5% = source or contains

The percent Daily Value allows consumers to quickly compare the nutrient content of similar products. For example, a consumer might discover that frozen macaroni and cheese has a Daily Value for fat of 20 percent, whereas macaroni and cheese prepared from a boxed mix has a Daily Value of 15 percent. By comparing labels, consumers who are concerned about their fat intakes can make informed decisions.

The Daily Values used on labels are based on two reference points: Recommended Daily Intakes, which pertain to most vitamins and minerals; and

HOW TO Calculate Personal Daily Values

The Daily Values on food labels are designed for a 2000-kcalorie intake, but you can calculate a personal set of Daily Values based on your energy allowance. Consider a 1500-kcalorie intake, for example. To calculate a daily upper goal for fat, multiply energy intake by 30 percent:

$$1500 \text{ kcal} \times 0.30 \text{ kcal from fat} = 450 \text{ kcal from fat}$$

If you prefer to count grams of fat, you can divide this 450 kcalories from fat by 9 kcalories per gram to determine the goal in grams:

$$450 \text{ kcal from fat} \div 9 \text{ kcal/g} = 50 \text{ g fat}$$

Alternatively, you can calculate that 1500 kcalories is 75 percent of the 2000-kcalorie intake used for Daily Values:

$$1500 \text{ kcal} \div 2000 \text{ kcal} = 0.75$$
$$0.75 \times 100 = 75\%$$

Then, instead of trying to achieve 100 percent of the Daily Value, a person consuming 1500 kcalories will aim for 75 percent. Similarly, a person consuming 2800 kcalories would aim for 140 percent:

$$2800 \text{ kcal} \div 2000 \text{ kcal} = 1.40 \text{ or } 140\%$$

CENGAGENOW™
For additional practice log on to **www.cengage.com/sso**.

TRY IT Calculate the Daily Values for a 1800-kcalorie diet and revise the Daily Value percentages on the cereal label found on p. 50.

GLOSSARY OF TERMS ON FOOD LABELS

GENERAL TERMS

free: "nutritionally trivial" and unlikely to have a physiological consequence; synonyms include *without, no,* and *zero*. A food that does not contain a nutrient naturally may make such a claim, but only as it applies to all similar foods (e.g., "applesauce, a fat-free food").

good source of: the product provides 15 percent or more of the Daily Value for a given nutrient per serving; synonymous with *high in*.

high in: 15 percent or more of the Daily Value for a given nutrient per serving; synonymous with *good source*.

less: at least 25 percent less of a given nutrient or kcalories than the comparison food (see individual nutrients); synonymous with *reduced*.

light or **lite:** restricted to foods that meet the criteria for "reduced in fat" or "reduced in energy"; any use of the term other than as defined must specify what it is referring to (e.g., "light in colour" or "light in texture").

organic: on food labels, that at least 95 percent of the product's ingredients have been grown and processsed according to the Canadian Organic Products Regulations.

ENERGY

energy free: fewer than 5 kcalories per serving; synonyms include *Calorie-free* and *zero energy*.

low in energy: 40 kcalories or less per serving; synonyms include low Calorie and little energy.

reduced in energy: at least 25 percent fewer kcalories per reference amount of the comparison food; synonyms include *reduced Calories, less energy, and lower in energy*.

FAT AND CHOLESTEROL[a]

percent fat-free: may be used only if the product meets the definition of *low fat* or *fat-free* and must reflect the amount of fat in 100 grams (e.g., a food that contains 2.5 grams of fat per 50 grams can claim to be "95 percent fat-free").

fat-free: less than 0.5 gram of fat per serving; synonyms include *zero-fat, no-fat,* and *nonfat*.

low in fat: 3 grams or less fat per serving; synonyms include *low fat* and *little fat*.

reduced in fat: food contains at least 25 percent less fat than the comparison food; synonyms include *fat-reduced, less fat* and *lower fat*.

saturated fat-free: less than 0.2 gram of saturated fat and 0.2 gram of *trans* fat per serving.

low saturated fat: 2 grams or less of saturated and *trans* fat combined per serving.

less saturated fat: at least 25 percent less saturated fat and the content of *trans* fat is not higher than the reference amount of the comparison food.

***trans* fat-free:** less than 0.2 gram of *trans* fat per serving and is low in saturated fat.

cholesterol-free: less than 2 milligrams cholesterol per serving and low saturated fat per serving.

low cholesterol: 20 milligrams or less cholesterol per serving and is low in saturated fat.

reduced cholesterol: food contains at least 25 percent less cholesterol than the comparison food, and is low in saturated fat; synonyms include *lower in cholesterol* and *less cholesterol*.

extra lean: meat or poultry that has not been ground or aquatic animal that contains 7.5 percent or less fat by weight; ground meat or poultry can contain a maximum of 10 percent fat.

lean: meat or poultry that has not been ground or aquatic animal that contains 10 percent or less fat by weight; ground meat or poultry can contain a maximum of 17 percent fat.

CARBOHYDRATES: FIBRE AND SUGAR

source of fibre: 2 grams or more fibre per serving.

high source of fibre: 4 grams or more fibre per serving.

very high source of fibre: 6 grams or more fibre per serving.

sugar-free: less than 0.5 gram of sugar per serving and is energy-free.

reduced in sugar: food contains at least 25 percent less sugars totalling at least 5 grams per serving compared to a similar food.

SODIUM

sodium-free and **salt-free:** less than 5 milligrams of sodium per serving.

low sodium: 140 milligrams or less per serving.

reduced in sodium or salt: contains at least 25 percent less sodium per serving than a similar reference food.

lightly salted: contains at least 50% less sodium than the sodium added to a similar reference food.

[a]All cholesterol claims are prohibited when the food contains more than 2 grams saturated fat and *trans* fat combined per serving.

TABLE 2-7 Examples of Diet-related Health Claims on Food Labels

Disease Risk Reduction Claims

...with respect to stroke and heart disease:

- A healthy diet containing foods high in potassium and low in sodium may reduce the risk of high blood pressure, a risk factor for stroke and heart disease. (Naming the food) is sodium-free.

...with respect to osteoporosis:

- A healthy diet with adequate calcium and vitamin D, and regular physical activity, help to achieve strong bones and may reduce the risk of osteoporosis. (Naming the food) is an excellent source of calcium and vitamin D.

...with respect to heart disease:

- A healthy diet low in saturated and *trans* fats may reduce the risk of heart disease. (Naming the food) is low in saturated and *trans* fats.

...with respect to cancer:

- A healthy diet rich in a variety of vegetables and fruits may help reduce the risk of some types of cancer.

...with respect to dental caries:

- Non-fermentable carbohydrates may help reduce dental caries.
- Won't cause cavities.
- Does not promote tooth decay.
- Does not promote dental caries.
- Non-cariogenic.

Function Claims

...with respect to coarse wheat bran:

- (Naming the serving) of (naming the product) contains 7 grams (or naming the amount if more than 7 grams) of fibre from coarse wheat bran, which promotes laxation.

...with respect to green tea:

- Consumption of (250 mL [1 cup] optional) green tea helps to protect blood lipids from oxidation.

...with respect to psyllium:

- (Naming the serving) of (naming the product) provides (naming the amount) of fibre from psyllium seed. Consuming 3.5 grams of fibre from psyllium seed (daily) promotes regularity.

Nutrient Function Claims

- Protein helps build and repair body tissues.
- Carbohydrate supplies energy.
- Fat aids in the absorption of fat-soluble vitamins.
- Calcium aids in the formation and maintenance of bones and teeth.
- Iron is a factor in red blood cell formation.
- Vitamin E is a dietary antioxidant.
- Vitamin A aids in maintaining the health of skin and membranes.

General Health Claims

The nonspecific nature of messages that promote healthy eating, for example, those found in *Eating Well with Canada's Food Guide* are considered general health claims. These messages include:

- Eat at least one dark green and one orange vegetable each day.
- Have vegetables and fruits more often than juice.
- Make at least half of your grain products whole grain each day.
- Drink skim, 1%, or 2% milk each day.
- Have meat alternatives such as beans, lentils, and tofu often.
- Eat at least two *Food Guide* Servings of fish each week.
- Include a small amount of unsaturated fat each day.
- Satisfy your thirst with water.

Reference Standards, which apply to fat, saturated and trans fat, cholesterol, carbohydrates, fibre, sodium, and potassium.[13]

Ingredient List With few exceptions (e.g., single-serving packages), packaged foods must list all ingredients—including additives used to preserve or enhance foods, such as vitamins and minerals added to enrich or fortify products. The ingredients are listed on the label in descending order of predominance by weight. Knowing that the first ingredient predominates by weight, consumers can obtain important information. Compare these products, for example:

- A beverage powder that contains "sugar, citric acid, natural flavours..." versus a juice that contains "water, tomato concentrate, concentrated juices of carrots, celery...."
- A cereal that contains "puffed milled corn, sugar, corn syrup, molasses, salt..." versus one that contains "100 percent rolled oats."
- A canned fruit that contains "sugar, apples, water" versus one that contains simply "apples, water."

In each of these comparisons, consumers can see that the second product is more nutrient dense.

Claims **Diet-related Nutrient Claims** Have you noticed phrases such as "good source of fibre" on a box of cereal or "excellent source of calcium" on a package of cheese? These and other **diet-related nutrient claims** may be used on labels as long as they meet regulated criteria set forth in Canada's Food and Drug Regulations. For example, in addition to having less than 2 milligrams of cholesterol, a "cholesterol-free" product may not contain more than 2 grams of saturated fat and *trans* fat combined per serving. The glossary on page 53 defines nutrient terms on food labels, including criteria for foods described as "low," "reduced," and "free." When nutrients have been added to enriched or fortified products, they must appear in the ingredients list.

Diet-related Health Claims A **diet-related health claim** implies a relationship exists between the consumption of a food and health. In Canada, health claims have been categorized into three groups: disease risk reduction, function, and general health claims. Table 2-7 provides examples of diet-related health claims that are permitted in Canada.

- *Disease Risk Reduction Claims:* These statements make clear well-established links between a nutrient or other component in a food and reduction in risk of developing a diet-related disease in the context of the total diet.
- *Function Claims:* These statements claim well-established benefits from consuming a nutrient or other component in a food on normal biological functions in the body. Function claims cannot make statements about disease. Nutrient function claims are a subset that describe well-established roles for energy or other nutrients essential to maintaining good health.
- *General Health Claims:* These are broad claims that provide dietary guidance or promote general health through healthy eating. They do not pertain to specific or general disease or health effects or conditions.

Consumer Education Because labels are valuable only if people know how to use them, Health Canada has designed resources to educate consumers. Try the Interactive Nutrition Label: Get the Facts and its associated quiz (see Nutrition on the Net). Consumers who understand how to read labels are best able to apply the information to achieve and maintain healthful dietary practices.[14]

TABLE 2-8 From Guidance to Groceries

Dietary Guidance	*Eating Well with Canada's Food Guide*	Food Labels
Adequate nutrients within energy needs	Select the recommended amount and type of food from each food group at an energy level appropriate to your energy needs.	Look for foods that describe their vitamin, and mineral contents as a *good source* or *high in*. Look for foods that describe their fibre contents as *source of* or *high source*.
Weight management	Select nutrient-dense foods and beverages within and across the food groups. Limit foods and beverages that are high in calories, fat, added sugar, or salt.	Look for foods that describe their energy contents as *free, low, reduced, light,* or *less*.
Physical activity	Be physically active by engaging in 150 minutes of moderate- to vigorous-intensity activity per week and strengthening activities at least twice a week. Children and teenagers should aim for 60 minutes of moderate- to vigorous-intensity physical activity a day, as well as vigorous and strengthening activities at least 3 days per week.	
Food groups to encourage	Select a variety of vegetables and fruits each day. Make at least half of your grain selections whole grains. Select skim (fat-free) or 1% (low-fat) milk products. Choose meat alternatives such as beans, lentils and tofu often.	Look for foods that describe their fibre contents as *source of* or *high source*. Look for foods that provide at least 15 percent of the Daily Value for fibre, vitamin A, vitamin C, iron, and calcium from a variety of sources.
Fats	Choose foods within each food group that are lean, low in fat, or fat-free. Choose foods within each food group that have little added fat.	Look for foods that describe their fat, saturated fat, *trans* fat, and cholesterol contents as *free, less in, low, light, reduced in, lean,* or *extra lean*. Look for foods that provide no more than 5 percent of the Daily Value for fat, and cholesterol and no more than 10 percent of the Daily Value for saturated fat and *trans* fat combined.
Carbohydrates	Choose fibre-rich vegetables, fruits, and whole grains often. Choose foods and beverages within each food group that have little added sugars.	Look for foods that describe their sugar contents as *free* or *reduced in*. A food may be high in sugar if its ingredients list begins with or contains several of the following: *sugar, liquid sugar, dextrose, dextrin, sucrose, fructose, maltose, lactose, honey, syrup, corn syrup, high-fructose corn syrup, molasses, evaporated cane juice,* or *fruit juice concentrate*.
Sodium and potassium	Choose foods within each food group that are low in salt or sodium. Choose potassium-rich foods such as vegetables and fruits.	Look for foods that describe their salt and sodium contents as *free, low in,* or *reduced in*. Look for foods that provide no more than 5 percent of the Daily Value for sodium.
Alcoholic beverages	Use sensibly and in moderation (no adult should consume more than 2 drinks a day: women less than 9 drinks a week and men less than 14).	*Light* beverages contain less alcohol than regular versions.

Table 2-8 shows how general dietary guidance, key messages in *Eating Well with Canada's Food Guide*, and food labels coordinate with one another. Consumers can use *Canada's Food Guide* and food labels in conjunction with the *Canadian Physical Activity Guidelines* (see p. 471) to guide their healthy eating and physical activities. The purpose of these resources is to deliver simple messages that will motivate consumers to make small changes in their eating and physical activity habits to yield big rewards. Through the use of these resources, Canadians can make wise choices that will improve their overall health and reduce their risk for developing chronic disease.

IN SUMMARY **Food labels provide consumers with information they need to select foods that will help them meet their nutrition and health goals. When labels contain relevant information presented in a standardized, easy-to-read format, consumers are well prepared to plan and create healthful diets.**

This chapter provides the links to go from dietary guidance to buying groceries and offers helpful tips for selecting nutritious foods. For additional information on foods, including organic foods, irradiated foods, genetically modified foods, and more, turn to Chapter 20.

diet-related nutrient claims: statements that characterize the quantity of a nutrient in a food.

diet-related health claims: statements that characterize the relationship between a nutrient or other component in a food and a disease or health-related condition.

Nutrition Portfolio

The secret to making healthy food choices is learning to incorporate key messages found in *Eating Well with Canada's Food Guide* into your decision-making process.

Go to Diet Analysis Plus and choose one of the days on which you have tracked your diet for the entire day. Choose the MyPlate Report and, looking at it, record in your journal the answers to the following:

- How do the foods you consumed on the day you have chosen stack up with the daily goals (the percentages) in the MyPlate breakdown? Which food groups are over- or under-represented?
- Think about your choices within each food group for the day you recorded. Are they typical of the foods you choose from day to day? Are there simple and realistic ways to enhance the variety in your diet?
- Write yourself a letter describing the dietary changes you can make to improve your chances of enjoying good health.

Diet Analysis PLUS **To complete this exercise, go to your Diet Analysis Plus at www.cengage.com/sso.**

Nutrition on the Net

CENGAGENOW™
For further study of topics covered in this chapter, log on to **www.cengage.com/sso.**

- Try your hand at the Interactive Nutrition Label and Quiz and find information on Canada's nutrition guidelines and food labels: **www.hc-sc.gc.ca/fn-an/label-etiquet/nutrition/index-eng.php**
- Learn more about *Eating Well with Canada's Food Guide* and My Food Guide: **www.hc-sc.gc.ca/fn-an/food-guide-aliment/index-eng.php**
- Learn more about food labelling from the Canadian Food Inspection Agency: **www.inspection.gc.ca/english/fssa/labeti/guide/toce.shtml**
- Learn about American food labels by searching for "food labels" at the International Food Information Council: **www.foodinsight.org**

References

1. Practice paper of the American Dietetic Association: Nutrient density: Meeting nutrient goals within calorie needs, *Journal of the American Dietetic Association* 107 (2007): 860–869; A. Drewnowski, Defining nutrient density: Development and validation of the nutrient rich foods index, *Journal of the American College of Nutrition* 28 (2009): 421S-426S; G. D. Miller, A. Drewnowski, V. Fulgoni, R. P. Heaney, J. King, E. Kennedy, It is time for a positive approach to dietary guidance using nutrient density as a basic principle, *Journal of Nutrition* 139 (2009): 1198–1202.
2. A. Drewnowski and V. Fulgoni III, Nutrient profiling of foods: Creating a nutrient-rich food index, *Nutrition Reviews* 66 (2008): 23–39.
3. N. Darmon and coauthors, Nutrient profiles discriminate between foods according to their contribution to nutritionally adequate diets: A validation study using linear programming and the SAIN,LIM system, *American Journal of Clinical Nutrition* 89 (2009): 1227–1236; E. Kennedy, Food rating systems, diet quality, and health, *Nutrition Reviews* 66 (2008): 21–22.
4. S. P. Murphy and coauthors, Simple measures of dietary variety are associated with improved dietary quality, *Journal of the American Dietetic Association* 106 (2006): 425–429.
5. Position of the American Dietetic Association: Vegetarian diets, *Journal of the American Dietetic Association* 109 (2009): 1266–1282; Position of the American Dietetic Association and Dietitians of Canada: Vegetarian diets, *Canadian Journal of Dietetic Practice and Research* 64 (2003): 62–81.
6. S. W. Katamay, K. A. Esslinger, M. Vigneault, J. L. Johnston, B. A. Junkins, L. G. Robbins, I. V. Sirois, E. M. Jones-McLean, A. F. Kennedy, M. A. A. Bush, D. Brulé and C. Martineau, *Eating Well with Canada's Food Guide* (2007): Development of the food intake pattern, *Nutrition Reviews* 65 (2007): 155-166; Joint World Health Organization/Food and Agriculture Organization of the United Nations Expert Consultation on *Diet, Nutrition and the Prevention of Chronic Diseases. Diet, Nutrition and the Prevention of Chronic Diseases: Report of a Joint WHO/FAO Expert Consultation (WHO technical report series no. 916)*. Geneva: World Health Organization (2003). www.who.int/dietphysicalactivity/publications/trs916/en/, accessed September 1, 2011; M. A. A. Bush, C. Martineau, J. A. Pronk, D. Brulé, *Eating Well with Canada's Food Guide:* "A tool for the times," *Canadian Journal of Dietetic Practice and Research* 68 (2007): 92–96.
7. Health Canada, My Food Guide (2007). www.hc-sc.gc.ca/fn-an/food-guide-aliment/myguide-monguide/index-eng.php, accessed September 1, 2011.
8. D. Garriguet, Canadians' eating habits, *Health Reports* 19 (2007): 17–32.
9. D. Garriguet, Canadians' eating habits, *Health Reports* 18 (2007): 17–32.
10. V. S. Malik and F. B. Hu, Dietary prevention of atherosclerosis: Go with whole grains, *American Journal of Clinical Nutrition* 85 (2007): 1444–1445.
11. Tracking Nutrition Trends VII, Canadian Council of Food and Nutrition. www.ccfn.ca/in_action/archive.asp, accessed September 24, 2010.
12. Canadian Food Inspection Agency, Guide to food labelling and advertising. www.inspection.gc.ca/english/fssa/labeti/guide/toce.shtml, accessed September 1, 2011.
13. Canadian Food Inspection Agency, Guide to food labelling and advertising, Chapter 6 – The elements within the Nutrition Facts table (2010). www.inspection.gc.ca/english/fssa/labeti/guide/ch6e.shtml, accessed September 1, 2011.
14. M. R. L'Abbé, L. Dumais, E. Chao, and B. Junkins, Health claims on foods in Canada, *Journal of Nutrition* 138 (2008): 1221S-1227S; Health Canada, Managing health claims for foods in Canada: towards a modernized framework (2007). www.hc-sc.gc.ca/fn-an/consult/_man-gest_health_claims-allegations_sante/index-eng.php, accessed September 1, 2011.

HIGHLIGHT 2

Vegetarian Diets

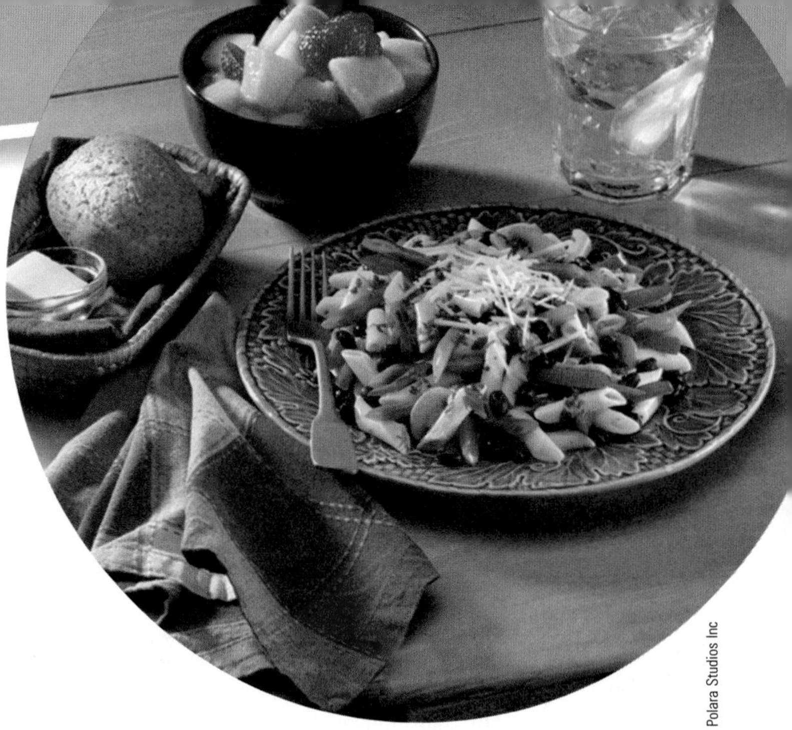

© Polara Studios Inc

The waiter presents this evening's specials: a fresh spinach salad topped with mandarin oranges, raisins, and sunflower seeds, served with a bowl of pasta smothered in a mushroom and tomato sauce and topped with grated parmesan cheese. Then this one: a salad made of chopped parsley, scallions, celery, and tomatoes mixed with bulgur wheat and dressed with olive oil and lemon juice, served with a spinach and feta cheese pie. Do these meals sound good to you? Or is something missing... a pork chop or chicken breast, perhaps?

Would vegetarian fare be acceptable to you some of the time? Most of the time? Ever? Perhaps it is helpful to recognize that dietary choices fall along a continuum—from one end, where people eat no meat or foods of animal origin, to the other end, where they eat generous quantities daily. Meat's place in the diet has been the subject of much research and controversy, as this highlight will reveal. One of the missions of this highlight, in fact, is to identify the *range* of meat intakes most compatible with health. The health benefits of a primarily vegetarian diet seem to have encouraged many people to eat more vegetarian meals. The popular press refers to these "part-time vegetarians" who eat small amounts of meat, fish, or poultry from time to time as "flexitarians."

People who choose to exclude meat and other animal-derived foods from their diets today do so for many of the same reasons the Greek philosopher Pythagoras cited in the sixth century BC: physical health, ecological responsibility, and philosophical concerns. They might also cite world hunger issues, economic reasons, ethical concerns, or religious beliefs as motivating factors. Whatever their reasons—and even if they don't have a particular reason—people who exclude meat will be better prepared to plan well-balanced meals if they understand the nutrition and health implications of vegetarian diets.

Vegetarians generally are categorized, not by their motivations, but by the foods they choose to exclude (see the accompanying glossary). Some people exclude red meat only; some also exclude chicken or fish; others also exclude eggs; and still others exclude milk and milk products as well. In fact, finding agreement on the definition of the term *vegetarian* is a challenge.

As you will see, though, the foods a person *excludes* are not nearly as important as the foods a person *includes* in the diet. Vegetarian diets that include a variety of whole grains, vegetables, legumes, nuts, and fruits offer abundant complex carbohydrates and fibre, an assortment of vitamins and minerals, a mixture of phytochemicals, and little fat—characteristics that reflect current dietary recommendations aimed at promoting health and reducing obesity. Each of these foods—whole grains, vegetables, legumes, nuts, and fruits—independently reduces the risk for several chronic diseases. This highlight examines the health benefits and potential problems of vegetarian diets and shows how to plan a well-balanced vegetarian diet. Highlight 21 includes a discussion of the environmental benefits of a plant-based diet.[1]

Health Benefits of Vegetarian Diets

Research on the health implications of vegetarian diets would be relatively easy if vegetarians differed from other people only in not eating meat. Many vegetarians, however, have also adopted lifestyles that may differ from many **omnivores:** they often use no tobacco or illicit drugs, use little (if any) alcohol, and are

GLOSSARY

lacto-vegetarians: people who include milk and milk products, but exclude meat, poultry, fish, seafood, and eggs from their diets.
- **lacto** = milk

lacto-ovo-vegetarians: people who include milk, milk products, and eggs, but exclude meat, poultry, fish, and seafood from their diets.
- **ovo** = egg

macrobiotic diet: a philosophical approach of eating mostly plant-based foods such as whole grains, legumes, and vegetables, with small amounts of fish, fruits, nuts, and seeds.
- **macro** = large, great
- **biotic** = life

meat replacements: products formulated to look and taste like meat, fish, or poultry; usually made of textured vegetable protein.

omnivores: people who have no formal restriction on the eating of any foods.
- **omni** = all
- **vores** = to eat

tempeh (TEM-pay): a fermented soybean food, rich in protein and fibre.

tofu (TOE-foo): a curd made from soybeans, rich in protein and often fortified with calcium; used in many Asian and vegetarian dishes in place of meat.

vegans (VEE-gans): people who exclude all animal-derived foods (including meat, poultry, fish, eggs, and dairy products) from their diets; also called **pure vegetarians, strict vegetarians,** or **total vegetarians.**

vegetarians: a general term used to describe people who exclude meat, poultry, fish, or other animal-derived foods from their diets.

physically active. Researchers must account for these lifestyle differences before they can determine which aspects of health correlate just with diet. Even then, *correlations* merely reveal what health factors *go with* the vegetarian diet, not what health effects may be *caused by* the diet. Despite these limitations, research findings suggest that well-planned vegetarian diets offer sound nutrition and health benefits to adults.[2] Dietary patterns that include very little, if any, meat may even increase life expectancy.

Weight Control

In general, weight gains are lowest for those eating the fewest animal-derived foods.[3] Vegetarians tend to maintain a lower and healthier body weight than nonvegetarians.[4] Vegetarians' lower body weights correlate with their high intakes of fibre and low intakes of fat. Because obesity impairs health in a number of ways, this gives vegetarians a health advantage.

Blood Pressure

Vegetarians tend to have lower blood pressure and lower rates of hypertension than nonvegetarians.[5] Appropriate body weight helps to maintain a healthy blood pressure, as does a diet low in total fat and saturated fat and high in fibre, fruits, vegetables, and soy protein.[6] Lifestyle factors also influence blood pressure: smoking and alcohol intake raise blood pressure, and physical activity lowers it.

Heart Disease

The incidence of heart disease and related deaths is slightly lower for vegetarians than for nonvegetarians, which could partly be explained by their avoidance of meat.[7] The dietary factor most directly related to heart disease is saturated animal fat, and in general, vegetarian diets are lower in total fat, saturated fat, and cholesterol than typical meat-based diets. The fats common in plant-based diets—the monounsaturated fats of olives, seeds, and nuts and the polyunsaturated fats of vegetable oils—are associated with a decreased risk of heart disease. Furthermore, vegetarian diets are generally higher in dietary fibre, antioxidant vitamins, and phytochemicals—all factors that help control blood lipids and protect against heart disease.

Many vegetarians include soy products such as **tofu** in their diets. Soy products may help to protect against heart disease because they contain polyunsaturated fats, fibre, vitamins, and minerals, and little saturated fat.[8] Even when intakes of energy, protein, carbohydrate, total fat, saturated fat, unsaturated fat, alcohol, and fibre are the same, people eating meals based on tofu have lower blood cholesterol and triglyceride levels than those eating meat. Some research suggests that soy protein and phytochemicals may be responsible for some of these health benefits (as Highlight 14 explains in greater detail).[9]

Cancer

Vegetarians have a significantly lower rate of cancer than the general population. Their low cancer rates may be due to their high intakes of vegetables and fruits (as Highlight 12 explains). In fact, the ratio of vegetables to meat may be the most relevant dietary factor responsible for cancer prevention.[10]

Some scientific findings indicate that vegetarian diets are associated not only with lower cancer mortality in general, but also with lower incidence of cancer at specific sites as well, most notably, colon cancer.[11] People with colon cancer seem to eat more meat, more saturated fat, and fewer vegetables than do people without colon cancer. High-protein, high-fat, low-fibre diets create an environment in the colon that promotes the development of cancer in some people. A high-meat diet has been associated with cancers of the esophagus, stomach, lungs, and liver as well as increased mortality.[12]

Other Diseases

In addition to obesity, hypertension, heart disease, and cancer, vegetarian diets may help prevent diabetes, osteoporosis, diverticular disease, gallstones, and rheumatoid arthritis.[13] These health benefits of a vegetarian diet depend on wise diet planning.

Vegetarian Diet Planning

The vegetarian has the same meal-planning task as any other person—using a variety of foods to deliver all the needed nutrients within an energy allowance that maintains a healthy body weight (as discussed in Chapter 2). Vegetarians who include milk products and eggs can meet recommendations for most nutrients about as easily as nonvegetarians. Such diets provide enough energy, protein, and other nutrients to support the health of adults and the growth of children and adolescents.

Vegetarians who exclude milk products and eggs can select legumes, nuts, and seeds and products made from them, such as peanut butter, **tempeh,** and tofu, from the Meat and Alternatives group. Those who do not use milk can use soy "milk"—a product made from soybeans that provides similar nutrients if fortified with calcium, vitamin D, vitamin B_{12}, and other vitamins and minerals (see Figure H2-1 on p. 59). Similarly, "milks" made from rice, almonds, and oats are reasonable alternatives, if adequately fortified.

Eating Well with Canada's Food Guide can be used for planning vegetarian diets: each food group contains plant-based foods. In addition, several food guides have been developed specifically for vegetarian diets. They all address the particular nutrition concerns of vegetarians but differ slightly. When selecting from the Vegetables and Fruit group, vegetarians should emphasize particularly good sources of calcium and iron, respectively. Green leafy vegetables, for example, provide almost five times as much calcium per serving as other vegetables. Similarly, dried fruits deserve special notice because they deliver six times as much iron as other fruits. The Milk and Alternatives group features fortified soy beverage for those who do not use Milk and Alternatives, cheese,

FIGURE H2-1 **1% Milk and Soy Milk Compared**

1% Milk

Nutrition Facts	
Serving Size 1 cup (250 mL)	
Amount Per Serving	% Daily Value
Calories 110	
Total Fat 2.5 g	4%
Saturated Fat 1.5 g	8%
Trans Fat 0 g	
Cholesterol 15 mg	
Sodium 130 mg	5%
Total Carbohydrate 13 g	4%
Dietary Fibre 0 g	0%
Sugars 12 g	
Protein 8 g	
Vitamin A 10% • Vitamin C 0%	
Calcium 30% • Iron 0%	
Vitamin D 45%	

Soy "Milk"

Nutrition Facts	
Serving Size 1 cup (250 mL)	
Amount Per Serving	% Daily Value
Calories 100	
Total Fat 4 g	6%
Saturated Fat 0.5 g	3%
Trans Fat 0 g	
Cholesterol 0 mg	
Sodium 120 mg	5%
Total Carbohydrate 8 g	3%
Dietary Fibre 1 g	4%
Sugars 6 g	
Protein 7 g	
Vitamin A 10% • Vitamin C 0%	
Calcium 30% • Iron 6%	
Vitamin D 30%	

or yogurt. The Meat and Alternatives group includes legumes, soy products, nuts, and seeds. Including 30 to 45 millilitres (2 to 3 Tbsp) of oil (e.g., cooking oil, salad dressing) or unsaturated fat (e.g., soft margarine) each day will contribute healthy fats to your diet. To ensure adequate intakes of vitamin B_{12}, vitamin D, and calcium, vegetarians need to select fortified foods or use supplements daily. *Eating Well with Canada's Food Guide* is flexible enough that most people can use it: people who have adopted various vegetarian diets, those who want to make the transition to a vegetarian diet, and those who simply want to include more plant-based meals in their diets.

Most vegetarians easily obtain large quantities of the nutrients that are abundant in plant foods: carbohydrate, fibre, thiamin, folate, vitamin B_6, vitamin C, vitamin A, and vitamin E. A vegetarian food guides can help to ensure adequate intakes of the main nutrients vegetarian diets might otherwise lack: protein, iron, zinc, calcium, vitamin B_{12}, vitamin D, and omega-3 fatty acids. Table H2-1 (p. 60) presents good vegetarian sources of these key nutrients.

Protein

The protein RDA for vegetarians is the same as for others, although some have suggested that it should be higher because of the lower digestibility of plant proteins. **Lacto-ovo-vegetarians,** who use animal-derived foods such as milk and eggs, receive high-quality proteins and are likely to meet their protein needs. Even those who adopt only plant-based diets are likely to meet protein needs provided that their energy intakes are adequate and the protein sources varied.[14] The proteins of whole grains, legumes, seeds, nuts, and vegetables can provide adequate amounts of all the amino acids. An advantage of many vegetarian sources of protein is that they are generally lower in saturated fat than meats and are often higher in fibre and richer in some vitamins and minerals.

Vegetarians sometimes use **meat replacements** made of textured vegetable protein (soy protein). These foods are formulated to look and taste like meat, fish, or poultry. Many of these products are fortified to provide the vitamins and minerals found in animal sources of protein. A wise vegetarian learns to use a variety of whole, unrefined foods often and commercially prepared foods less frequently. Vegetarians may also use soy products such as tofu to bolster protein intake.

Iron

Getting enough iron can be a problem even for meat eaters, and those who eat no meat must pay special attention to their iron intake. The iron in plant foods such as legumes, dark green leafy vegetables, iron-fortified cereals, and whole-grain breads and cereals is poorly absorbed. Because iron absorption from a vegetarian diet is low, the iron RDA for vegetarians is higher than for others (see Chapter 14 for more details).

Fortunately, the body seems to adapt to a vegetarian diet by absorbing iron more efficiently. Furthermore, iron absorption is enhanced by vitamin C, and vegetarians typically eat many vitamin C–rich fruits and vegetables. Consequently, vegetarians suffer no more iron deficiency than other people do.

Zinc

Zinc is similar to iron in that meat is its richest food source, and zinc from plant sources is not well absorbed. In addition, soy, which is commonly used as a meat alternative in vegetarian meals, interferes with zinc absorption. Nevertheless, most vegetarian adults are not zinc deficient. Perhaps the best advice to vegetarians regarding zinc is to eat a variety of nutrient-dense foods; include whole grains, nuts, and legumes such as black-eyed peas, pinto beans, and kidney beans; and maintain an adequate energy intake. For those who include seafood in their diets, oysters, crabmeat, and shrimp are rich in zinc.

Calcium

The calcium intakes of **lacto-vegetarians** are similar to those of the general population, but people who use no milk products risk deficiency. Careful planners select calcium-rich foods, such as calcium-fortified juices soy beverages, in ample quantities regularly. This advice is especially important for children and adolescents. Soy formulas for infants are fortified with calcium and can be used in cooking, even for adults. Other good calcium sources include figs, some legumes, some green vegetables such as broccoli and turnip

TABLE H2-1 Good Vegetarian Sources of Key Nutrients

	Food Groups					
Nutrients	*Grains*	*Vegetables*	*Fruits*	*Protein-rich foods*	*Milk*	*Oils*
Protein	Whole grains[a]			Legumes, seeds, nuts, soy products (tempeh, tofu, veggie burgers)[a] Eggs (for ovo-vegetarians)	Milk, cheese, yogurt (for lacto-vegetarians)	
Iron	Fortified cereals, enriched and whole grains	Dark green leafy vegetables (spinach, turnip greens)	Dried fruits (apricots, prunes, raisins)	Legumes (black-eyed peas, kidney beans, lentils)		
Zinc	Fortified cereals, whole grains			Legumes (garbanzo beans, kidney beans, navy beans), nuts, seeds (pumpkin seeds)	Milk, cheese, yogurt (for lacto-vegetarians)	
Calcium	Fortified cereals	Dark green leafy vegetables (bok choy, broccoli, collard greens, kale, mustard greens, turnip greens, watercress)	Fortified juices, figs	Fortified soy products, nuts (almonds), seeds (sesame seeds)	Milk, cheese, yogurt (for lacto-vegetarians) Fortified soy beverages	
Vitamin B_{12}	Fortified cereals			Eggs (for ovo-vegetarians) Fortified soy products	Milk, cheese, yogurt (for lacto-vegetarians) Fortified soy beverages	
Vitamin D					Milk, cheese, yogurt (for lacto-vegetarians) Fortified soy beverages	
Omega-3 Fatty acids				Flaxseed, walnuts, soybeans		Flaxseed oil, walnut oil, soybean oil

[a]As Chapter 6 explains, many plant proteins do not contain all the essential amino acids in the amounts and proportions needed by human beings. To improve protein quality, vegetarians can eat grains and legumes together, for example, although it is not necessary if protein intake is varied and energy intake is sufficient.

greens, some nuts such as almonds, certain seeds such as sesame seeds, and calcium-set tofu.* The choices should be varied because calcium absorption from some plant foods may be limited (as Chapter 13 explains).

Vitamin B_{12}

The requirement for vitamin B_{12} is small, but this vitamin is found only in animal-derived foods. Consequently, vegetarians, in general, and **vegans** who eat no foods of animal original, in particular, may not get enough vitamin B_{12} in their diets.[15] Fermented soy products such as tempeh may contain some vitamin B_{12} from the bacteria, but unfortunately, much of the vitamin B_{12} found in these products may be an inactive form. Seaweeds such as nori and chlorella supply some vitamin B_{12}, but not much, and excessive intakes of these foods can lead to iodine toxicity. To defend against vitamin B_{12} deficiency, vegans must rely on vitamin B_{12}–fortified sources (such as soy beverages or meat analogues) or supplements. Without vitamin B_{12}, the nerves suffer damage, leading to such health consequences as loss of vision.

*Calcium salts are often added during processing to coagulate the tofu. Tofu made with other salts will not be a source of calcium.

Vitamin D

The vitamin D status of vegetarians is similar to that of nonvegetarians.[16] People who do not use vitamin D–fortified foods and do not receive enough exposure to sunlight to synthesize adequate vitamin D may need supplements to defend against bone loss. This is particularly important for infants, children, and older adults. In northern climates during winter months, young children on vegan diets can readily develop rickets, the vitamin D–deficiency disease. Canadian adults over the age of 50 should take a daily supplement containing 10 micrograms (400 IU) vitamin D.

Omega-3 Fatty Acids

Chapter and Highlight 5 describe the health benefits of unsaturated fats, most notably the omega-3 fatty acids commonly found in fatty fish. A diet that includes some meat and fish provides more omega-3 fatty acids than a vegetarian diet.[17] To obtain sufficient amounts of omega-3 fatty acids, vegetarians need to consume flax meal, walnuts, soybeans, and their oils.

Healthy Food Choices

In general, adults who eat vegetarian diets have lowered their risks of mortality and several chronic diseases, including obesity, high blood pressure, heart disease, and cancer. But there is nothing mysterious or magical about the vegetarian diet. The quality of the diet depends not on whether it includes meat, but on whether the other food choices are nutritionally sound. A diet that includes ample, vegetables, fruits, whole grains, legumes, nuts, and seeds is higher in fibre, antioxidant vitamins, and phytochemicals and lower in saturated fats than meat-based diets. Variety is key to nutritional adequacy in a vegetarian diet. Restrictive plans that limit selections to a few grains and vegetables cannot possibly deliver a full array of nutrients.

Vegetarianism is not a religion like Buddhism or Hinduism, but merely an eating plan that selects plant foods to deliver needed nutrients. That said, some vegetarians choose to follow a **macrobiotic diet.** Those following a macrobiotic diet select natural, organic foods and embrace a Zen-like spirituality. In other words, a macrobiotic diet represents a way of life, not just a meal plan. A macrobiotic diet emphasizes whole grains, legumes, and vegetables, with small amounts of fish, fruits, nuts, and seeds. Practices include selecting locally grown foods, eating foods in their most natural state, and balancing cold, sweet, and passive foods with hot, salty, and aggressive ones. Some items, such as processed foods, alcohol, hot spices, and potatoes, are excluded from the diet. Early versions of the macrobiotic diet followed a progression that ended with the "ultimate" diet of brown rice and water—a less-than-nutritiously balanced diet. Today's version reflects a modified vegetarian approach with an appreciation of how foods can enhance health. With careful planning, a macrobiotic diet can provide an array of nutrients that support good health.

If not properly balanced, any diet—vegetarian, macrobiotic, or otherwise—can lack nutrients. Poorly planned vegetarian diets typically lack iron, zinc, calcium, vitamin B_{12}, and vitamin D; without planning, the meat eater's diet may lack vitamin A, vitamin C, folate, and fibre, among others. Quite simply, the negative health aspects of any diet, including vegetarian diets, reflect poor diet planning. Careful attention to energy intake and specific problem nutrients can ensure adequacy.

Keep in mind, too, that diet is only one factor influencing health. Whatever a diet consists of, its context is also important: no smoking, alcohol consumption in moderation (if at all), regular physical activity, adequate rest, and medical attention when needed all contribute to a healthy life. Establishing these healthy habits early in life seems to be the most important step one can take to reduce the risks of later diseases (as Highlight 17 explains).

Nutrition on the Net

CENGAGENOW™
For further study of topics covered in this chapter, log on to **www.cengage.com/sso**.

- Search for "vegetarian" at Health Canada's website: **www.hc-sc.gc.ca**
- Find a list of U.S. resources about vegetarian nutrition at the Food and Nutrition Information Center's website: **www.nal.usda.gov/fnic/pubs/bibs/gen/vegetarian07.pdf**
- Visit the Vegetarian Resource Group: **www.vrg.org**

References

1. B. M. Popkin, Reducing meat consumption has multiple benefits for the world's health, *Archives of Internal Medicine* 169 (2009): 543–545.
2. G. E. Fraser, Vegetarian diets: What do we know of their effects on common chronic diseases? *American Journal of Clinical Nutrition* 89 (2009): 1607S–1612S; S. E. Berkow and N. Barnard, Vegetarian diets and weight status, *Nutrition Reviews* 64 (2006): 175–188; T. J. Key, P. N. Appleby, and M. S. Rosell, Health effects of vegetarian and vegan diets, *Proceedings of the Nutrition Society* 65 (2006): 35–41; Position of the American Dietetic Association: Vegetarian diets, *Journal of the American Dietetic Association* 109 (2009): 1266–1282; J. L. Bedford and S. I. Barr, Diets and selected lifestyle practices of self-defined adult vegetarians from a population-based sample suggest they are more "health conscious," *International Journal of Behavioral Nutrition and Physical Activity* 2 (2005): 4 doi:10.1186/1479-5868-2-4. www.ijbnpa.org/content/2/1/4, accessed September 1, 2011.
3. M. Rosell and coauthors, Weight gain over 5 years in 21,966 meat-eating, fish-eating, vegetarian, and vegan men and women in EPIC-Oxford, *International Journal of Obesity* 30 (2006): 1389–1396.
4. Berkow and Barnard, 2006; P. K. Newby, K. L. Tucker, and A. Wolk, Risk of overweight and obesity among semivegetarian, lactovegetarian, and vegan women, *American Journal of Clinical Nutrition* 81 (2005): 1267–1274.
5. V. H. Myers and C. M. Champagne, Nutritional effects on blood pressure, *Current Opinion in Lipidology* 18 (2007): 20–24.
6. S. E. Berkow and N. D. Barnard, Blood pressure regulation and vegetarian diets, *Nutrition Reviews* 63 (2005): 1–8.
7. J. Chang-Claude and coauthors, Lifestyle determinants and mortality in German vegetarians and health-conscious persons: Results of a 21-year follow-up, *Cancer Epidemiology, Biomarkers, and Prevention* 14 (2005): 963–968.
8. F. M. Sacks and coauthors, Soy protein, isoflavones, and cardiovascular health: An American Heart Association Science Advisory for professionals from the Nutrition Committee, *Circulation* 113 (2006): 1034–1044.
9. D. Lukaczer and coauthors, Effect of a low glycemic index diet with soy protein and phytosterols on CVD risk factors in postmenopausal women, *Nutrition* 22 (2006): 104–113; B. L. McVeigh and coauthors, Effect of soy

protein varying in isoflavone content on serum lipids in healthy young men, *American Journal of Clinical Nutrition* 83 (2006): 244–251.
10. M. Kapiszewska, A vegetable to meat consumption ratio as a relevant factor determining cancer preventive diet: The Mediterranean versus other European countries, *Forum of Nutrition* 59 (2006): 130–153.
11. M. H. Lewin and coauthors, Red meat enhances the colonic formation of the DNA adduct O6-carboxymethyl guanine: Implications for colorectal cancer risk, *Cancer Research* 66 (2006): 1859–1865.
12. R. Sinha and coauthors, Meat intake and mortality: A prospective study of over half a million people, *Archives of Internal Medicine* 169 (2009): 562–571; A. J. Cross and coauthors, A prospective study of red and processed meat intake in relation to cancer risk, *PLoS Medicine* 4 (2007): 1973–1984.
13. C. Leitzmann, Vegetarian diets: What are the advantages? *Forum of Nutrition* 57 (2005): 147–156; G. E. Fraser, Vegetarian diets: What do we know of their effects on common chronic diseases? *American Journal of Clinical Nutrition* 89 (2009): 1607S–1612S.
14. Position of the American Dietetic Association, 2009.
15. I. Elmadfa and I. Singer, Vitamin B-12 and homocysteine status among vegetarians: A global perspective, *American Journal of Clinical Nutrition* 89 (2009): 1693S–1698S.
16. J. Chan, K. Jaceldo-Siegl, and G. E. Fraser, Serum 25-hydroxyvitamin D status of vegetarians, partial vegetarians, and nonvegetarians: The Adventist Health Study, *American Journal of Clinical Nutrition* 89 (2009): 1686S–1692S.
17. I. Mangat, Do vegetarians have to eat fish for optimal cardiovascular protection? *American Journal of Clinical Nutrition* 89 (2009): 1597S–1601S; N. Mann and coauthors, Fatty acid composition of habitual omnivore and vegetarian diets, *Lipids* 41 (2006): 637–646.

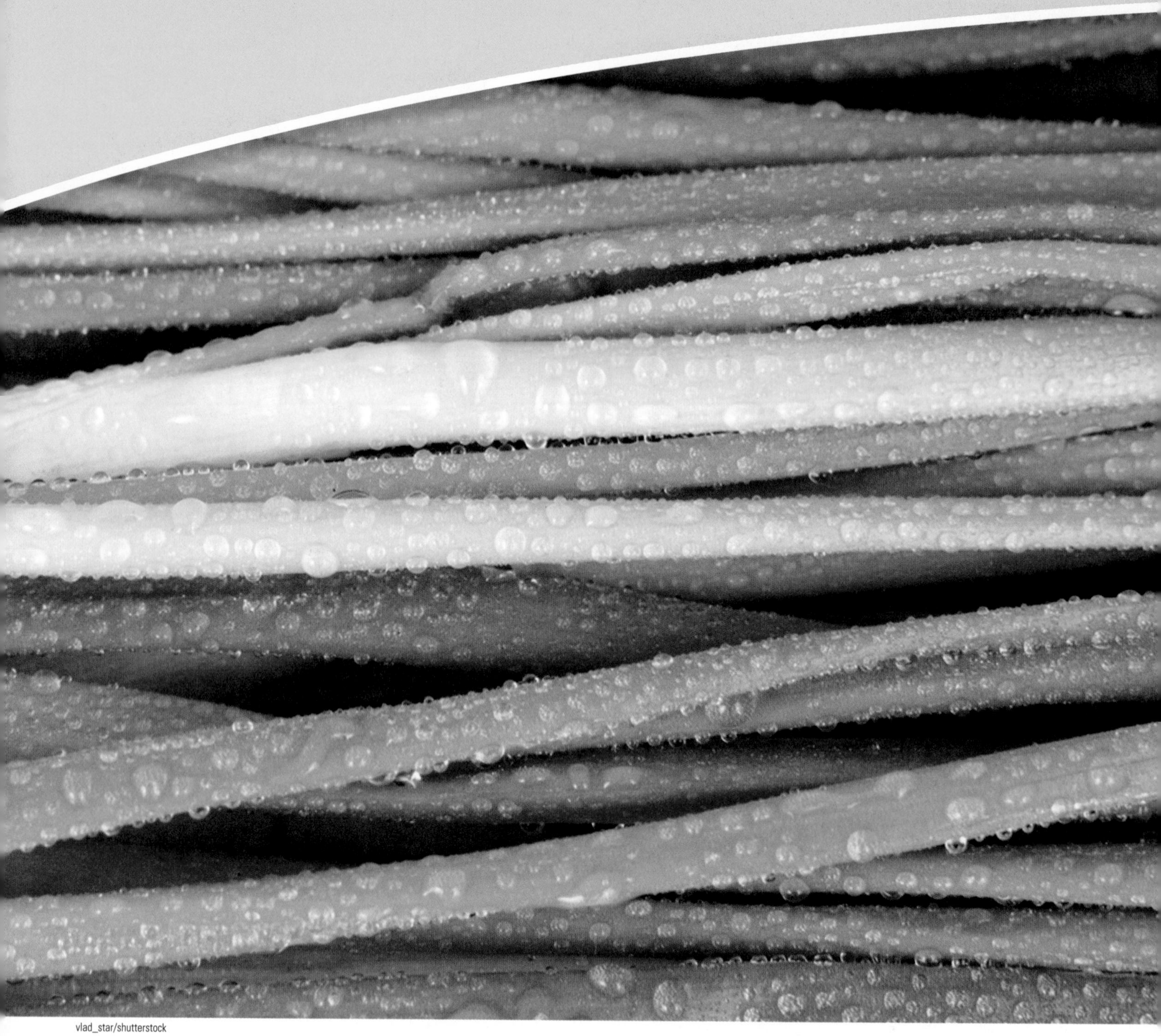

vlad_star/shutterstock

Nutrition in Your Life

CENGAGENOW™

Throughout this chapter, the CengageNOW logo indicates an opportunity for online self-study, linking you to interactive tutorials, activities, and videos to increase your understanding of chapter concepts.
www.cengage.com/sso

Have you ever wondered what happens to the food you eat after you swallow it? Or how your body extracts nutrients from food? Have you ever marvelled at how it all just seems to happen? Follow foods as they travel through the digestive system. Learn how a healthy digestive system takes whatever food you give it—whether sirloin steak and potatoes or tofu and Brussels sprouts—and extracts the nutrients that will nourish the cells of your body.

CHAPTER 3

Digestion, Absorption, and Transport

CHAPTER OUTLINE

This chapter follows the journey that breaks down foods into the nutrients featured in the later chapters. Then it follows the nutrients as they are absorbed through the intestinal cells and travel into the body to do their work. This introduction presents a general overview of the processes common to all nutrients; later chapters discuss the specifics of digesting and absorbing individual nutrients.

Digestion

Digestion is the body's ingenious way of breaking down foods into nutrients in preparation for **absorption.** In the process, it overcomes many challenges without any conscious effort. Consider these challenges:

1. Human beings breathe, eat, and drink through their mouths. Air taken in through the mouth must go to the lungs; food and liquid must go to the stomach. The throat must be arranged so that swallowing and breathing don't interfere with each other.
2. Below the lungs lies the diaphragm, a dome of muscle that separates the upper half of the major body cavity from the lower half. Food must pass through this wall to reach the stomach.
3. The materials within the digestive tract should be kept moving forward, slowly but steadily, at a pace that permits all reactions to reach completion.
4. To move through the system, food must be lubricated with fluids. Too much would form a liquid that would flow too rapidly; too little would form a paste too dry and compact to move at all. The amount of fluids must be regulated to keep the intestinal contents at the right consistency to move along smoothly.
5. Before the digestive enzymes can work, foods must be broken down into small particles and suspended in enough liquid so that every particle is accessible. Once digestion is complete and the needed nutrients have been absorbed out of the GI tract and into the body, the system must excrete the remaining waste. Excreting all the water along with the solid residue, however, would be both wasteful and messy. Some water must be withdrawn to leave a solid enough waste product to be smooth and easy to pass.

digestion: the process by which food is broken down into absorbable units.
- **digest** = take apart

absorption: the uptake of nutrients by the cells of the small intestine for transport into either the blood or the lymph.
- **absorb** = suck in

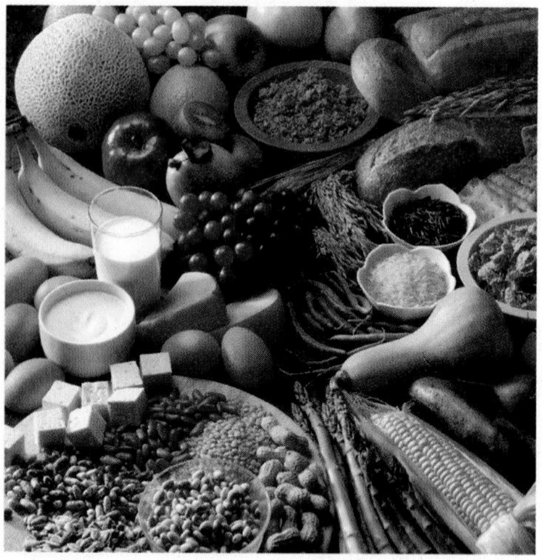

© Joe Pellegrini

The process of digestion breaks down all kinds of *foods* into *nutrients*.

6. Human digestive enzymes are designed to digest carbohydrate, fat, and protein. The cells of the GI tract are also made of carbohydrate, fat, and protein. These cells need to be protected against the powerful digestive juices that they secrete.
7. Once waste matter has reached the end of the GI tract, it must be excreted, but it would be inconvenient and embarrassing if this function occurred continuously. Evacuation needs to occur periodically.

The following sections show how the body elegantly and efficiently handles these challenges. Each section follows the GI tract from one end to the other—first describing its anatomy, then its muscular actions, and finally its secretions.

Anatomy of the Digestive Tract

The **gastrointestinal (GI) tract** is a flexible muscular tube that extends from the mouth, through the esophagus, stomach, small intestine, large intestine, and rectum to the anus. Figure 3-1 traces the path followed by food from one end to the other. In a sense, the human body surrounds the GI tract. The inner space within the GI tract, called the **lumen**, is continuous from one end to the other. (GI anatomy terms appear in boldface type and are defined in the accompanying glossary.) Only when a nutrient or other substance finally penetrates the GI tract's wall does it enter the body proper; many materials pass through the GI tract without being digested or absorbed.

♦ The process of chewing is called **mastication** (mass-tih-KAY-shun).

Mouth The process of digestion begins in the **mouth**. During chewing, ♦ teeth crush large pieces of food into smaller ones, and fluids from foods, beverages, and salivary glands blend with these pieces to ease swallowing. Fluids also help dissolve the food so that the tongue can taste it; only particles in solution can react with taste buds. When stimulated, the taste buds detect one, or a combination, of the four basic taste sensations: sweet, sour, bitter, and salty. Some scientists also include the flavour associated with monosodium glutamate, sometimes called *savoury* or its Asian name, *umami* (oo-MOM-ee). In addition to these chemical triggers, aroma, texture, and temperature also affect a food's flavour. In fact, the sense of smell is thousands of times more sensitive than the sense of taste.

gastrointestinal (GI) tract: the digestive tract. The principal organs are the stomach and intestines.

- **gastro** = stomach
- **intestinalis** = intestine

digestive system: all the organs and glands associated with the ingestion and digestion of food.

The tongue provides taste sensations and moves food around the mouth, facilitating chewing and swallowing. When a mouthful of food is swallowed, it passes through the **pharynx**, a short tube that is shared by both the **digestive system** and the respiratory system. To bypass the entrance to the lungs, the **epiglottis** closes

GLOSSARY OF GI ANATOMY TERMS

These terms are listed in order from start to end of the digestive system.

lumen (LOO-men): the space within a vessel, such as the intestine.

mouth: the oral cavity containing the tongue and teeth.

pharynx (FAIR-inks): the passageway leading from the nose and mouth to the larynx and esophagus, respectively.

epiglottis (epp-ih-GLOTT-iss): cartilage in the throat that guards the entrance to the trachea and prevents fluid or food from entering it when a person swallows.

- **epi** = upon (over)
- **glottis** = back of tongue

esophagus (ee-SOFF-ah-gus): the food pipe; the muscular conduit from the mouth to the stomach.

sphincter (SFINK-ter): a circular muscle surrounding, and able to close, a body opening. Sphincters are found at specific points alon g the GI tract and regulate the flow of food particles.

- **sphincter** = band (binder)

esophageal (ee-SOF-ah-GEE-al) **sphincter:** a sphincter muscle at the upper or lower end of the esophagus. The *lower esophageal sphincter* is also called the *cardiac sphincter*.

stomach: a muscular, elastic, saclike portion of the digestive tract that grinds and churns swallowed food, mixing it with acid and enzymes to form chyme.

pyloric (pie-LORE-ic) **sphincter:** the circular muscle that separates the stomach from the small intestine and regulates the flow of partially digested food into the small intestine; also called *pylorus* or *pyloric valve*.

- **pylorus** = gatekeeper

small intestine: a 3-metre length of small-diameter intestine that extends from the pyloric sphincter to the ileocecal sphincter and is the major site of digestion of food and absorption of nutrients. Its segments are the duodenum, jejunum, and ileum.

gallbladder: the organ that stores and concentrates bile. When it receives the signal that fat is present in the duodenum, the gallbladder contracts and squirts bile through the bile duct into the duodenum.

pancreas: a gland that secretes digestive enzymes and juices into the duodenum. (The pancreas also secretes hormones into the blood that help to maintain glucose homeostasis.)

duodenum (doo-oh-DEEN-um, doo-ODD-num): the top portion of the small intestine (about "12 fingers' breadth" long in ancient terminology).

- **duodecim** = twelve

jejunum (je-JOON-um): the first two-fifths of the small intestine beyond the duodenum.

ileum (ILL-ee-um): the last segment of the small intestine, accounting for about half the length of the small intestine.

ileocecal (ill-ee-oh-SEEK-ul) **sphincter:** the sphincter separating the small and large intestines.

large intestine or **colon** (COAL-un): about 1.5 metres of large-diameter intestine; the lower portion of intestine that completes the digestive process. Its segments are the ascending colon, the transverse colon, the descending colon, and the sigmoid colon.

- **sigmoid** = shaped like the letter S (sigma in Greek)

appendix: a narrow blind sac extending from the beginning of the colon that stores lymph cells.

rectum: the muscular terminal part of the intestine, extending from the sigmoid colon to the anus.

anus (AY-nus): the terminal outlet of the GI tract.

off the airway so that choking doesn't occur when swallowing, thus resolving the first challenge. (Choking is discussed on pp. 84–85.) After a mouthful of food has been chewed and swallowed, it is called a **bolus**.

Esophagus to the Stomach The **esophagus** has a **sphincter** muscle at each end. During a swallow, the upper **esophageal sphincter** opens. The bolus then slides down the esophagus, which passes through a hole in the diaphragm (challenge 2) to the **stomach**. The lower esophageal sphincter ♦ at the entrance to the stomach

♦ The lower esophageal sphincter is also called the *cardiac sphincter* because of its proximity to the heart.

bolus (BOH-lus): a portion; with respect to food, the amount swallowed at one time.
- **bolos** = lump

FIGURE 3-1 The Gastrointestinal Tract

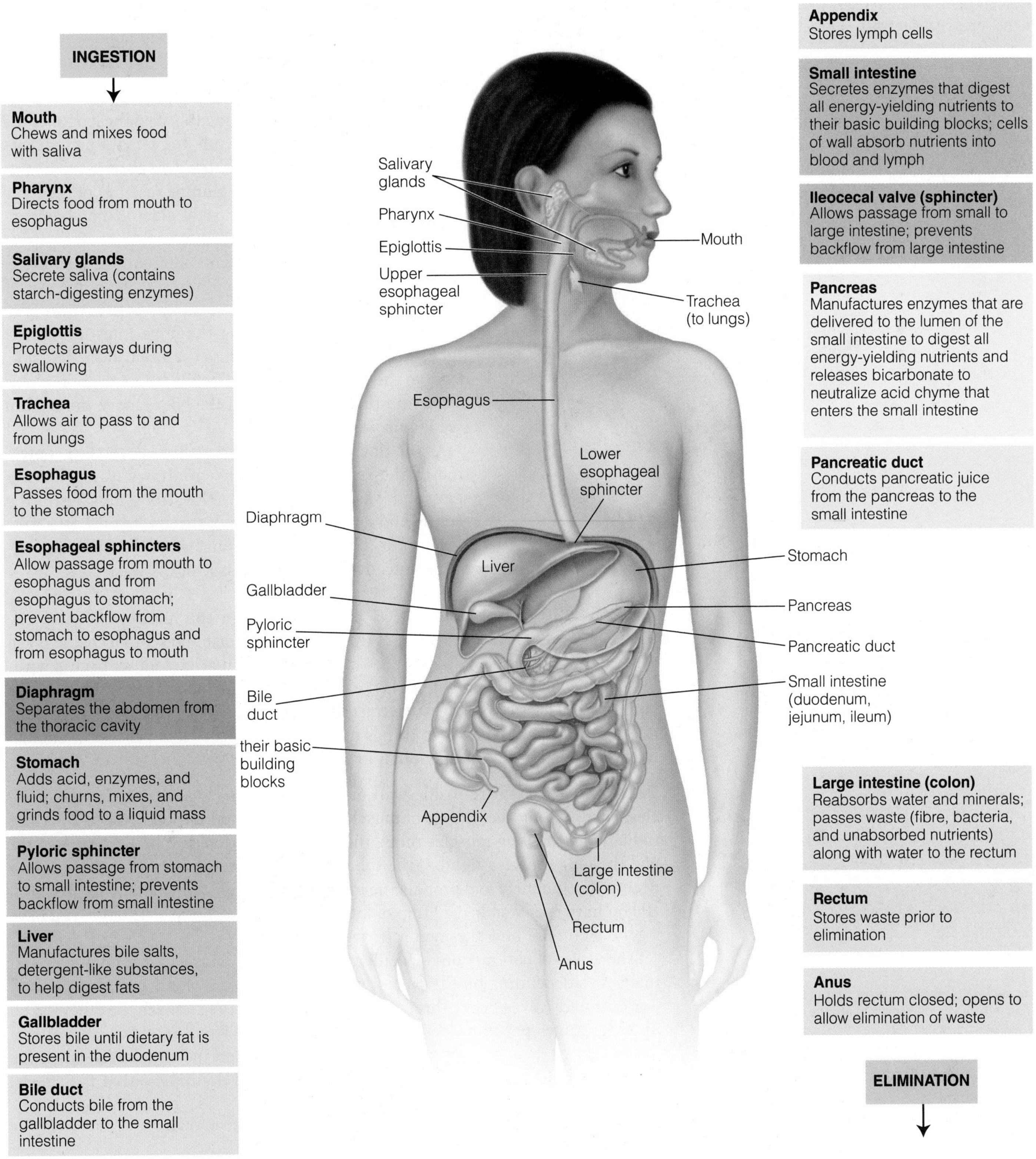
INGESTION
Mouth
Chews and mixes food with saliva
Pharynx
Directs food from mouth to esophagus
Salivary glands
Secrete saliva (contains starch-digesting enzymes)
Epiglottis
Protects airways during swallowing
Trachea
Allows air to pass to and from lungs
Esophagus
Passes food from the mouth to the stomach
Esophageal sphincters
Allow passage from mouth to esophagus and from esophagus to stomach; prevent backflow from stomach to esophagus and from esophagus to mouth
Diaphragm
Separates the abdomen from the thoracic cavity
Stomach
Adds acid, enzymes, and fluid; churns, mixes, and grinds food to a liquid mass
Pyloric sphincter
Allows passage from stomach to small intestine; prevents backflow from small intestine
Liver
Manufactures bile salts, detergent-like substances, to help digest fats
Gallbladder
Stores bile until dietary fat is present in the duodenum
Bile duct
Conducts bile from the gallbladder to the small intestine
Salivary glands
Pharynx
Epiglottis
Upper esophageal sphincter
Mouth
Trachea (to lungs)
Esophagus
Lower esophageal sphincter
Diaphragm
Liver
Stomach
Gallbladder
Pancreas
Pyloric sphincter
Pancreatic duct
Bile duct
Small intestine (duodenum, jejunum, ileum)
their basic building blocks
Appendix
Large intestine (colon)
Rectum
Anus
Appendix
Stores lymph cells
Small intestine
Secretes enzymes that digest all energy-yielding nutrients to their basic building blocks; cells of wall absorb nutrients into blood and lymph
Ileocecal valve (sphincter)
Allows passage from small to large intestine; prevents backflow from large intestine
Pancreas
Manufactures enzymes that are delivered to the lumen of the small intestine to digest all energy-yielding nutrients and releases bicarbonate to neutralize acid chyme that enters the small intestine
Pancreatic duct
Conducts pancreatic juice from the pancreas to the small intestine
Large intestine (colon)
Reabsorbs water and minerals; passes waste (fibre, bacteria, and unabsorbed nutrients) along with water to the rectum
Rectum
Stores waste prior to elimination
Anus
Holds rectum closed; opens to allow elimination of waste
ELIMINATION

closes behind the bolus so that it proceeds forward and doesn't slip back into the esophagus (challenge 3). The stomach retains the bolus for a while in its upper portion. Little by little, the stomach transfers the food to its lower portion, adds juices to it, and grinds it to a semiliquid mass called **chyme.** Then, bit by bit, the stomach releases the chyme through the **pyloric sphincter**, which opens into the **small intestine** and then closes behind the chyme.

FIGURE 3-2 The Colon

The colon begins with the ascending colon rising upward toward the liver. It becomes the transverse colon as it turns and crosses the body toward the spleen. The descending colon turns downward and becomes the sigmoid colon, which extends to the rectum. Along the way, the colon mixes the intestinal contents, absorbs water and salts across the colon wall, and forms stools.

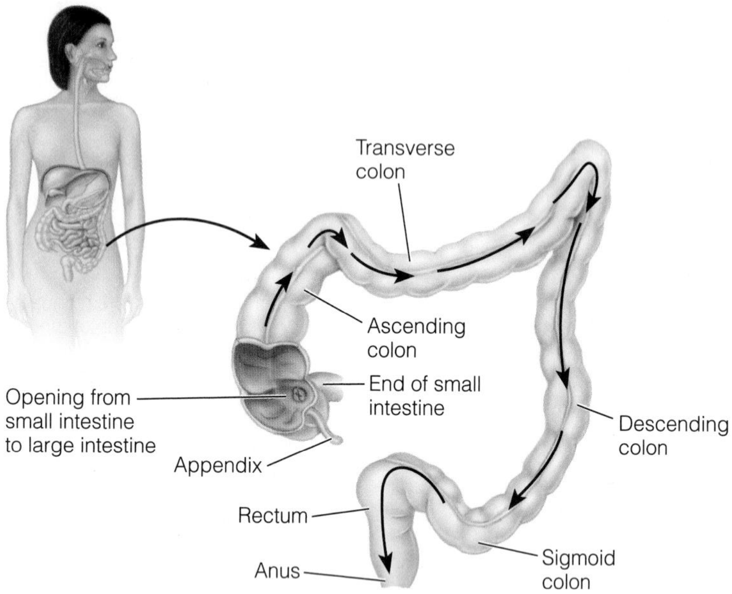
Transverse colon
Ascending colon
End of small intestine
Opening from small intestine to large intestine
Appendix
Descending colon
Rectum
Anus
Sigmoid colon

Small Intestine At the beginning of the small intestine, the chyme bypasses the opening from the common bile duct, which is dripping fluids (challenge 4) into the small intestine from two organs outside the GI tract—the **gallbladder** and the **pancreas.** The chyme travels on down the small intestine through its three segments—the **duodenum**, the **jejunum**, and the **ileum**—almost 3 metres of tubing coiled within the abdomen.*

Large Intestine (Colon) Having travelled the length of the small intestine to the distal ileum, the remaining contents arrive at another sphincter (challenge 3 again): the **ileocecal sphincter**, located at the beginning (cecum) of the **large intestine (colon)** in the lower right side of the abdomen. Upon entering the colon, the contents pass another opening. Should any intestinal contents slip into this opening, it would end up in the **appendix**, a blind sac about the size of your little finger. Normally, the contents bypass this opening, however, and travel along the large intestine up the right side of the abdomen, across the front to the left side, down to the lower left side, and finally below the other folds of the intestines to the back of the body, above the **rectum** (see Figure 3-2).

As the intestinal contents pass through the large intestine to the rectum, the colon withdraws water, leaving semisolid waste (challenge 5). The strong muscles of the rectum and anal canal hold back this waste until it is time to defecate. Then the rectal muscles relax (challenge 7), and the two sphincters of the **anus** open to allow passage of the waste.

The Muscular Action of Digestion

In the mouth, chewing, the addition of saliva, and the action of the tongue transform food into a coarse mash that can be swallowed. After swallowing, all the activity that follows occurs without much conscious thought. As is the case with so much else that happens in the body, the muscles of the digestive tract meet internal needs without any conscious effort on your part. They keep things moving ♦ at just the right pace, slow enough to get the job done and fast enough to make progress.

♦ The ability of the GI tract muscles to move is called **motility** (moh-TIL-ih-tee).

Peristalsis The entire inside wall of the GI tract is ringed with circular muscles. Surrounding these rings of muscle are longitudinal muscles. When the rings tighten and the long muscles relax, the tube is constricted. When the rings relax and the long muscles tighten, the tube bulges. This action—called **peristalsis**—occurs continuously and propels the intestinal contents along (challenge 3 again). (If you have ever watched a lump of food pass along the body of a snake, you have a good picture of how these muscles work.)

The waves of contraction normally ripple along the GI tract at varying rates and intensities depending on the part of the GI tract and on whether food is present. For example, waves occur three times per minute in the stomach, but they speed up to ten times per minute when chyme reaches the small intestine. Just after a meal is eaten, the waves are slow and continuous; when the GI tract is empty, the intestine is quiet except for periodic bursts of powerful rhythmic waves. Peristalsis,

chyme (KIME): the semiliquid mass of partly digested food released by the stomach into the duodenum.
- **chymos** = juice

peristalsis (per-ih-STALL-sis): wavelike muscular contractions of the GI tract that propel its contents along.
- **peri** = around
- **stellein** = wrap

*The small intestine is almost two and a half times shorter in living adults than it is at death, when muscles are relaxed and elongated.

along with sphincter muscles located at key places, keeps things moving along. Factors such as stress, medicines, and medical conditions may interfere with normal GI tract contractions.

Stomach Action The stomach has the thickest walls and strongest muscles of all the GI tract organs. In addition to the circular and longitudinal muscles, it has a third layer of diagonal muscles that also alternately contracts and relaxes (see Figure 3-3). These three sets of muscles work to break apart the bolus that you swallowed and force the chyme downward, but the pyloric sphincter usually remains tightly closed, preventing the chyme from passing into the duodenum of the small intestine. As a result, the chyme is churned and forced down, hits the pyloric sphincter, and remains in the stomach. Meanwhile, the stomach wall releases gastric juices. When the chyme is completely liquefied with gastric juices, the pyloric sphincter opens briefly, about three times a minute, to allow small portions of chyme to pass through. At this point, the chyme no longer resembles food in the least.

Segmentation The circular muscles of the intestines rhythmically contract and squeeze their contents (see Figure 3-4). These contractions, called

FIGURE 3-3 Stomach Muscles

The stomach has three layers of muscles.

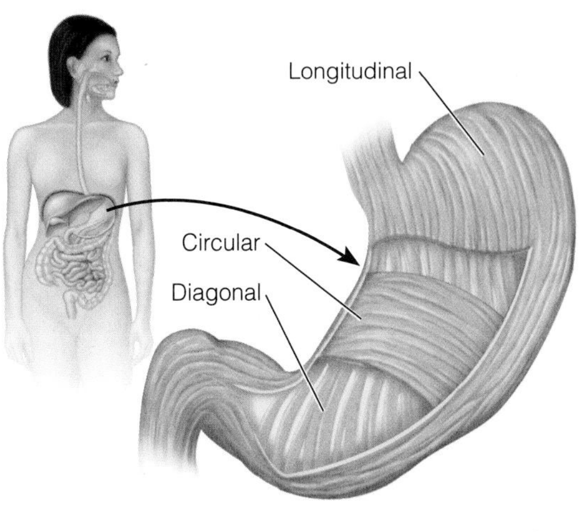
Longitudinal
Circular
Diagonal

FIGURE 3-4 Peristalsis and Segmentation

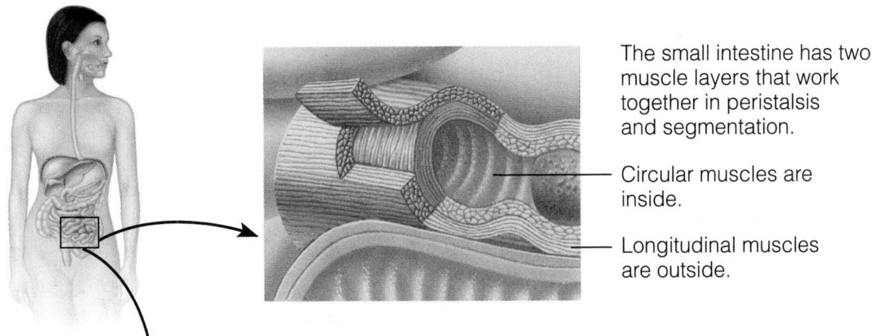
The small intestine has two muscle layers that work together in peristalsis and segmentation.
Circular muscles are inside.
Longitudinal muscles are outside.

Peristalsis

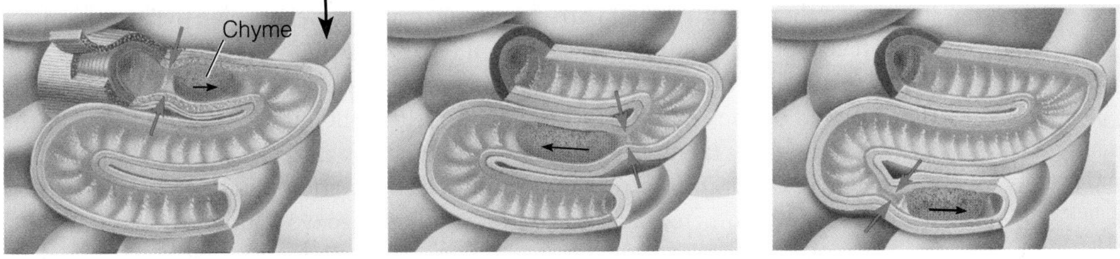
Chyme

The inner circular muscles contract, tightening the tube and pushing the food forward in the intestine.

When the circular muscles relax, the outer longitudinal muscles contract, and the intestinal tube is loose.

As the circular and longitudinal muscles tighten and relax, the chyme moves ahead of the constriction.

Segmentation

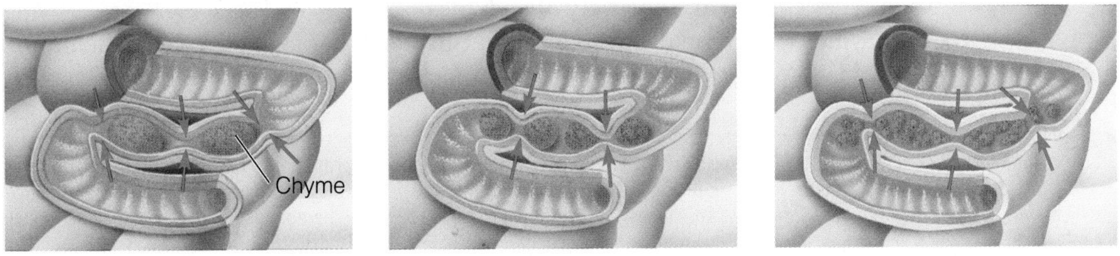
Chyme

Circular muscles contract, creating segments within the intestine.

As each set of circular muscles relaxes and contracts, the chyme is broken up and mixed with digestive juices.

These alternating contractions, occurring 12 to 16 times per minute, continue to mix the chyme and bring the nutrients into contact with the intestinal lining for absorption.

FIGURE 3-5 **An Example of a Sphincter Muscle**

When the circular muscles of a sphincter contract, the passage closes; when they relax, the passage opens.

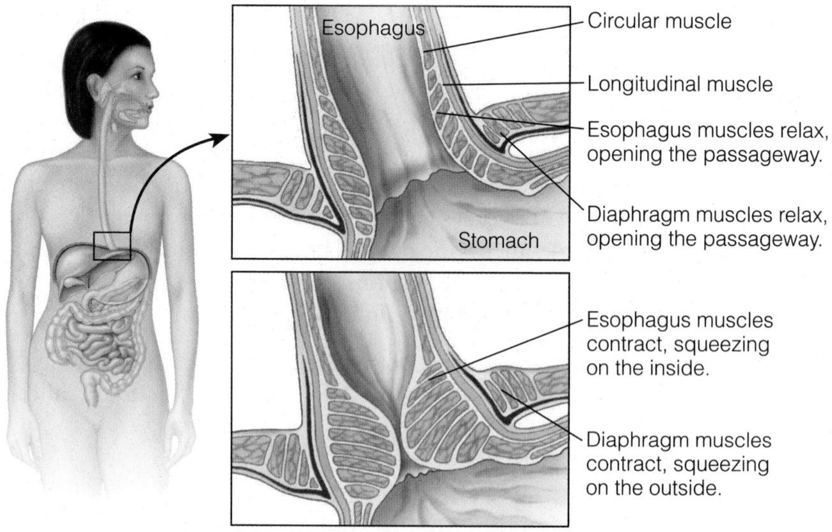
Esophagus
Circular muscle
Longitudinal muscle
Esophagus muscles relax, opening the passageway.
Diaphragm muscles relax, opening the passageway.
Stomach
Esophagus muscles contract, squeezing on the inside.
Diaphragm muscles contract, squeezing on the outside.

segmentation, further break apart food particles to mix the chyme and promote close contact with the digestive juices and the absorbing cells of the intestinal walls before letting the contents move slowly along. Figure 3-4 illustrates peristalsis and segmentation.

Sphincter Contractions Sphincter muscles periodically open and close, allowing the contents of the GI tract to move along at a controlled pace (challenge 3 again). At the top of the esophagus, the upper esophageal sphincter opens in response to swallowing. At the bottom of the esophagus, the lower esophageal sphincter (sometimes called the *cardiac sphincter* because of its proximity to the heart) prevents **reflux** of the stomach contents. At the bottom of the stomach, the pyloric sphincter, which stays closed most of the time, holds the chyme in the stomach long enough for it to be thoroughly mixed with gastric juice and liquefied. The pyloric sphincter also prevents the intestinal contents from backing up into the stomach. At the end of the small intestine, the ileocecal sphincter performs a similar function, allowing the contents of the small intestine to empty into the large intestine. Finally, the tightness of the rectal muscle acts as a kind of safety device; together with the two sphincters of the anus, it prevents continuous elimination (challenge 7). Figure 3-5 illustrates how sphincter muscles contract and relax to close and open passageways.

The Secretions of Digestion

The breakdown of food into nutrients requires secretions from five different organs: the salivary glands, the stomach, the pancreas, the liver (via the gallbladder), and the small intestine. These secretions enter the GI tract at various points along the way, bringing an abundance of water (challenge 4) and a variety of enzymes.

Enzymes ♦ are formally introduced in Chapter 6, but for now a simple definition will suffice. An enzyme is a protein that facilitates a chemical reaction—making

♦ All enzymes and some hormones are proteins, but enzymes are not hormones. Enzymes facilitate the making and breaking of bonds in chemical reactions; hormones act as chemical messengers, sometimes regulating enzyme action.

segmentation (SEG-men-TAY-shun): a periodic squeezing or partitioning of the intestine at intervals along its length by its circular muscles.

reflux: a backward flow.
- **re** = back
- **flux** = flow

GLOSSARY OF DIGESTIVE ENZYMES

-ase (AZE): a word ending denoting an enzyme. The word beginning often identifies the compounds the enzyme works on. Examples include:
- **carbohydrase** (KAR-boe-HIGH-draze), an enzyme that hydrolyzes carbohydrates.
- **lipase** (LYE-paze), an enzyme that hydrolyzes lipids (fats).
- **protease** (PRO-tee-aze), an enzyme that hydrolyzes proteins.

digestive enzymes: proteins found in digestive juices that act on food substances, causing them to break down into simpler compounds.

hydrolysis (high-DROL-ih-sis): a chemical reaction in which a major reactant is split into two products, with the addition of a hydrogen atom (H) to one and a hydroxyl group (OH) to the other (from water, H_2O). (The noun is **hydrolysis;** the verb is **hydrolyze.**)
- **hydro** = water
- **lysis** = breaking

a molecule, breaking a molecule apart, changing the arrangement of a molecule, or exchanging parts of molecules. As a **catalyst**, the enzyme itself remains unchanged. The enzymes involved in digestion facilitate a chemical reaction known as **hydrolysis**—the addition of water *(hydro)* to break *(lysis)* a molecule into smaller pieces. The glossary on p. 70 describes how to identify some of the common **digestive enzymes** and related terms; later chapters introduce specific enzymes. When learning about enzymes, it helps to know that the word ending ***-ase*** denotes an enzyme. Enzymes are often identified by the organ they come from and the compounds they work on. *Gastric lipase,* for example, is a stomach enzyme that acts on lipids, whereas *pancreatic lipase* comes from the pancreas (and also works on lipids).

Saliva The **salivary glands,** shown in Figure 3-6, squirt just enough **saliva** to moisten each mouthful of food so that it can pass easily down the esophagus (challenge 4). (Digestive **glands** and their secretions are defined in the glossary below.) The saliva contains water, salts, mucus, and enzymes that initiate the digestion of carbohydrates. Saliva also protects the teeth and the linings of the mouth, esophagus, and stomach from substances that might cause damage.

Gastric Juice In the stomach, **gastric glands** secrete **gastric juice**, a mixture of water, enzymes, and **hydrochloric acid**, which acts primarily in protein digestion. The acid is so strong that it causes the sensation of heartburn if it happens to reflux into the near-neutral pH of the esophagus. Highlight 3, following this chapter, discusses heartburn, ulcers, and other common digestive problems.

The strong acidity of the stomach prevents bacterial growth and kills most bacteria that enter the body with food. It would destroy the cells of the stomach as well, but for their natural defences. To protect themselves from gastric juice, the cells of the stomach wall secrete **mucus**, a thick, slippery, white substance that coats the cells, protecting them from the acid, enzymes, and disease-causing bacteria that might otherwise cause harm (challenge 6).

Figure 3-7 (p. 72) shows how the strength of acids is measured—in **pH** ♦ units. Note that the acidity of gastric juice registers below 2 on the pH scale—stronger than vinegar. The stomach enzymes work most efficiently in the stomach's strong acid, but the salivary enzymes, which are swallowed with food, do not work in acid this strong. Consequently, the salivary digestion of carbohydrates gradually ceases when the stomach acid penetrates each newly swallowed bolus of food. Once in the stomach, salivary enzymes just become other proteins to be digested.

Pancreatic Juice and Intestinal Enzymes By the time food leaves the stomach, digestion of all three energy nutrients (carbohydrates, fats, and proteins) has begun, and the action gains momentum in the small intestine. There the pancreas contributes digestive juices by way of ducts leading into the duodenum. The **pancreatic juice** contains enzymes that act on all three energy nutrients, and the cells of the intestinal wall also possess digestive enzymes on their surfaces.

FIGURE 3-6 The Salivary Glands

The salivary glands secrete saliva into the mouth to begin the chemical process of digestion. Given the short time food is in the mouth, salivary enzymes contribute little to digestion.

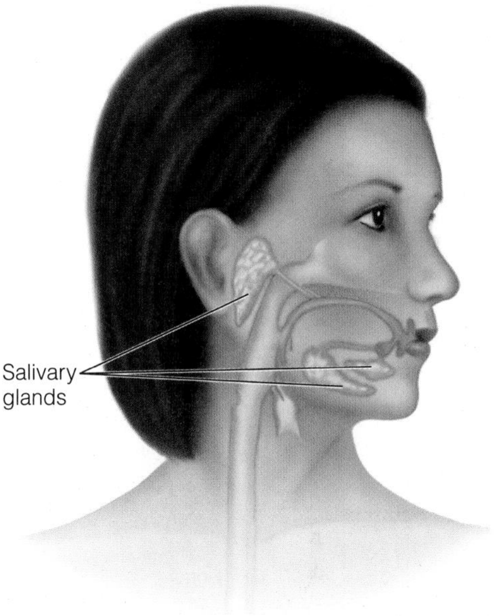
Salivary
glands

♦ The lower the pH, the higher the H^+ ion concentration and the stronger the acid. A pH above 7 is alkaline, or base (a solution in which OH^- ions predominate).

catalyst (CAT-uh-list): a compound that facilitates chemical reactions without itself being changed in the process.

pH: the unit of measure expressing a substance's acidity or alkalinity.

GLOSSARY OF DIGESTIVE GLANDS AND THEIR SECRETIONS

These terms are listed in order from start to end of the digestive tract.

glands: cells or groups of cells that secrete materials for special uses in the body. Glands may be *exocrine* (EKS-oh-crin) *glands,* secreting their materials "out" (into the digestive tract or onto the surface of the skin), or *endocrine* (EN-doe-crin) *glands,* secreting their materials "in" (into the blood).
- **exo** = outside
- **endo** = inside
- **krine** = to separate

salivary glands: exocrine glands that secrete saliva into the mouth.

saliva: the secretion of the salivary glands. Its principal enzyme begins carbohydrate digestion.

gastric glands: exocrine glands in the stomach wall that secrete gastric juice into the stomach.
- **gastro** = stomach

gastric juice: the digestive secretion of the gastric glands of the stomach.

hydrochloric acid: an acid composed of hydrogen and chloride atoms (HCl) that is normally produced by the gastric glands.

mucus (MYOO-kus): a slippery substance secreted by cells of the GI lining (and other body linings) that protects the cells from exposure to digestive juices (and other destructive agents). The lining of the GI tract with its coat of mucus is a **mucous membrane.** (The noun is **mucus;** the adjective is **mucous.**)

liver: the organ that manufactures bile. (The liver's many other functions are described in Chapter 7.)

bile: an emulsifier that prepares fats and oils for digestion; an exocrine secretion made by the liver, stored in the gallbladder, and released into the small intestine when needed.

emulsifier (ee-MUL-sih-fire): a substance with both water-soluble and fat-soluble portions that promotes the mixing of oils and fats in a watery solution.

pancreatic (pank-ree-AT-ic) **juice:** the exocrine secretion of the pancreas, containing enzymes for the digestion of carbohydrate, fat, and protein as well as bicarbonate, a neutralizing agent. The juice flows from the pancreas into the small intestine through the pancreatic duct. (The pancreas also has an endocrine function, the secretion of insulin and other hormones.)

bicarbonate: an alkaline compound with the formula HCO_3 that is secreted from the pancreas as part of the pancreatic juice. (Bicarbonate is also produced in all cell fluids from the dissociation of carbonic acid to help maintain the body's acid–base balance.)

FIGURE 3-7 The pH Scale

A substance's acidity or alkalinity is measured in pH units. The pH is the negative logarithm of the hydrogen ion concentration. Each increment represents a tenfold increase in concentration of hydrogen particles. This means, for example, that a pH of 2 is 1000 times stronger than a pH of 5.

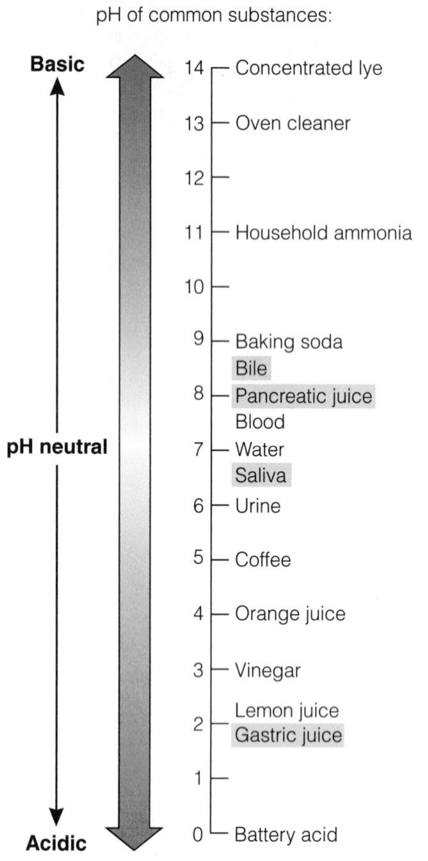
pH of common substances:
Basic
pH neutral
Acidic
14 Concentrated lye
13 Oven cleaner
12
11 Household ammonia
10
9 Baking soda
Bile
8 Pancreatic juice
Blood
7 Water
Saliva
6 Urine
5 Coffee
4 Orange juice
3 Vinegar
Lemon juice
2 Gastric juice
1
0 Battery acid

In addition to digestive enzymes, the pancreatic juice contains sodium **bicarbonate**, which is basic or alkaline—the opposite of the stomach's acid (review Figure 3-7). The pancreatic juice thus neutralizes the acidic chyme arriving in the small intestine from the stomach. From this point on, the chyme remains at a neutral or slightly alkaline pH. The enzymes of both the intestine and the pancreas work best in this environment.

Bile **Bile** also flows into the duodenum. The **liver** continuously produces bile, which is then concentrated and stored in the gallbladder. The gallbladder squirts the bile into the duodenum of the small intestine when dietary fat arrives there. Bile is not an enzyme; it is an **emulsifier** that brings fats into suspension in water so that enzymes can break them down into their component parts. A summary box of digestive secretions and their actions is presented below.

The Final Stage At this point, the three energy-yielding nutrients—carbohydrate, fat, and protein—have been digested and are ready to be absorbed. Some vitamins and minerals are altered slightly during digestion, but most are absorbed as they are. Undigested residues, such as some fibres, are not absorbed. Instead, they continue through the digestive tract, carrying some minerals, bile acids, additives, and contaminants out of the body. This semisolid mass helps exercise the GI muscles and keep them strong enough to perform peristalsis efficiently. Fibre also retains water, accounting for the consistency of **stools.**

By the time the contents of the GI tract reach the end of the small intestine, little remains but water, a few dissolved salts and body secretions, and undigested materials such as fibre (with some fat, cholesterol, and a few minerals bound to it). All of this remaining matter enters the large intestine (colon).

In the colon, intestinal bacteria ferment some fibres, producing water, gas, and small fragments of fat that provide energy for the cells of the colon. The colon itself retrieves all materials that the body can recycle—water and dissolved salts. The waste that is finally excreted has little or nothing of value left in it. The body has extracted all that it can use from the food. Figure 3-8 summarizes digestion by following a sandwich through the GI tract and into the body.

IN SUMMARY **As Figure 3-1 shows, food enters the mouth and travels down the esophagus and through the upper and lower esophageal sphincters to the stomach, then through the pyloric sphincter to the small intestine, on through the ileocecal sphincter to the large intestine, past the appendix to the rectum, ending at the anus. The wavelike contractions of peristalsis and the periodic squeezing of segmentation keep things moving at a reasonable pace. Along the way, secretions from the salivary glands, stomach, pancreas, liver (via the gallbladder), and glands in the wall of the small intestine deliver fluids and digestive enzymes.**

Summary of Digestive Secretions and Their Major Actions

Organ or Gland	Target Organ	Secretion	Action
Salivary glands	Mouth	Saliva	Fluid eases swallowing; salivary enzyme breaks down some *carbohydrate*.*
Gastric glands	Stomach	Gastric juice	Fluid mixes with bolus; hydrochloric acid uncoils *proteins;* enzymes digest proteins; mucus protects stomach cells.*
Pancreas	Small intestine	Pancreatic juice	Bicarbonate neutralizes acidic gastric juices; pancreatic enzymes digest *carbohydrates, fats,* and *proteins.*
Liver	Gallbladder	Bile	Bile stored until needed.
Gallbladder	Small intestine	Bile	Bile emulsifies *fat* so that enzymes can have access to digest it.
Intestinal (crypt) glands	Small intestine	Intestinal juice	Intestinal enzymes digest *carbohydrate, fat,* and *protein* fragments; mucus protects the intestinal wall.

*Saliva and gastric juice also contain lipases, but most fat breakdown occurs in the small intestine.

stools: waste matter discharged from the colon; also called *feces* (FEE-seez).

FIGURE 3-8 The Digestive Fate of a Sandwich

To review the digestive processes, follow a peanut butter and banana sandwich on whole-wheat, sesame seed bread through the GI tract. As the graph on the right illustrates, digestion of the energy nutrients begins in different parts of the GI tract, but all are ready for absorption by the time they reach the end of the small intestine.

CENGAGENOW™
Animated! figure
www.cengage.com/sso

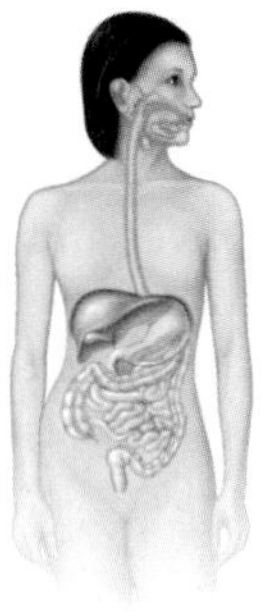

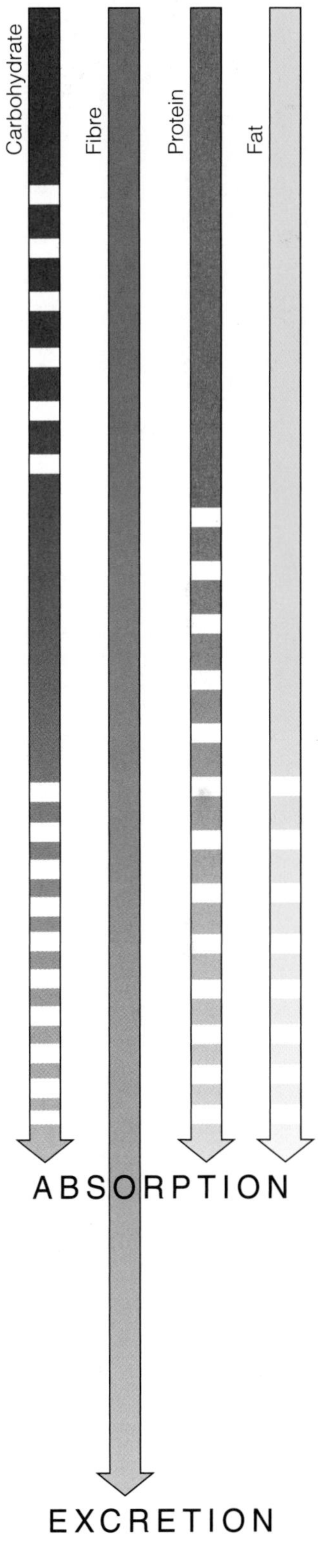
Carbohydrate
Fibre
Protein
Fat
ABSORPTION
EXCRETION

MOUTH: CHEWING AND SWALLOWING, WITH LITTLE DIGESTION

Carbohydrate digestion begins as the salivary enzyme starts to digest the starch from the bread and peanut butter.
Fibre covering on the sesame seeds is crushed by the teeth, which exposes the nutrients inside the seeds to the upcoming digestive enzymes.

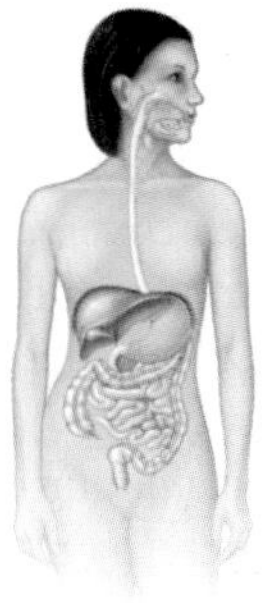

STOMACH: COLLECTING AND CHURNING, WITH SOME DIGESTION

Carbohydrate digestion continues until the mashed sandwich has been mixed with the gastric juices; the stomach acid of the gastric juices inactivates the salivary enzyme, and carbohydrate digestion ceases.
Proteins from the bread, seeds, and peanut butter begin to uncoil when they mix with the gastric acid, making them available to the gastric protease enzymes that begin to digest proteins.
Fat from the peanut butter forms a separate layer on top of the watery mixture.

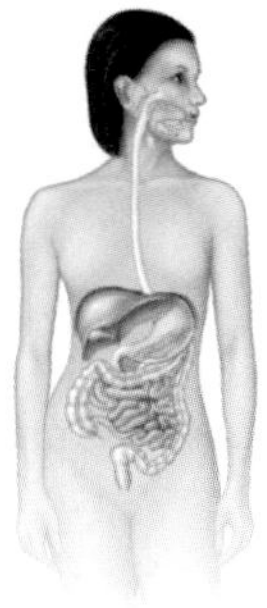

SMALL INTESTINE: DIGESTING AND ABSORBING

Sugars from the banana require so little digestion that they begin to traverse the intestinal cells immediately on contact.
Starch digestion picks up when the pancreas sends pancreatic enzymes to the small intestine via the pancreatic duct. Enzymes on the surfaces of the small intestinal cells complete the process of digesting starch into basic sugar units that can be absorbed through the intestinal cell walls and into the hepatic portal vein.
Fat from the peanut butter and seeds is emulsified with the watery digestive fluids by bile. Now the pancreatic and intestinal lipases can begin to digest the fat to smaller fragments that can be absorbed through the cells of the small intestinal wall and into the lymph.
Protein digestion depends on the pancreatic and intestinal proteases. Single amino acids and small fragments of protein are liberated and absorbed through the cells of the small intestinal wall but only single amino acids are absorbed into the hepatic portal vein.
Vitamins and minerals are absorbed.

Note: Sugars and starches are members of the carbohydrate family.

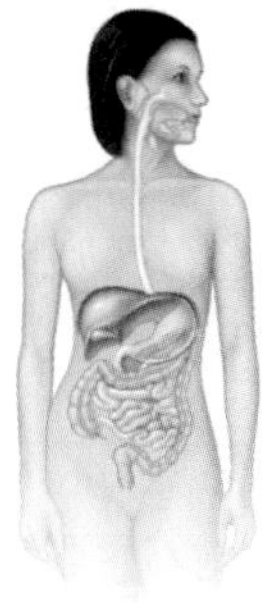

LARGE INTESTINE: REABSORBING AND ELIMINATING

Fluids and some minerals are absorbed.
Some fibres from the seeds, whole-wheat bread, peanut butter, and banana are partly fermented by the bacteria living in the large intestine, and some of these products are absorbed.
Most fibres pass through the large intestine and are excreted as feces; some fat, cholesterol, and minerals bind to fibre and are also excreted.

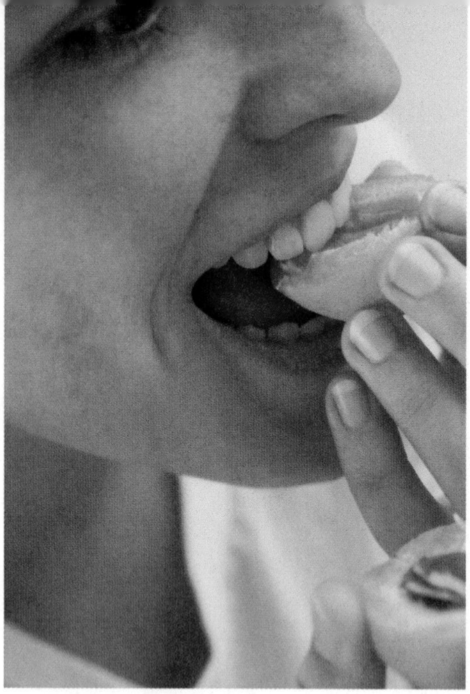
Foodcollection/Getty Images

Food must first be digested and absorbed before the body can use it.

Absorption

Within three or four hours after a person has eaten a dinner of beans and rice (or spinach lasagne, or steak and potatoes) with vegetable, salad, beverage, and dessert, the body must find a way to absorb the molecules derived from carbohydrate, protein, and fat digestion—and the vitamin and mineral molecules as well. Most absorption takes place in the small intestine, one of the most elegantly designed organ systems in the body. Within its 3-metre length, which provides a surface area equivalent to a tennis court, the small intestine traps and absorbs the nutrient molecules. To remove the absorbed molecules rapidly and provide room for more to be absorbed, a rush of circulating blood continuously washes the underside of this surface, carrying the absorbed nutrients away to the liver and other parts of the body. Figure 3-9 describes how most nutrients are absorbed by simple diffusion, facilitated diffusion, or active transport. Later chapters provide details on specific nutrients. Before following nutrients through the body, we must look more closely at the anatomy of the absorptive system.

Anatomy of the Absorptive System

The inner surface of the small intestine looks smooth and slippery, but when viewed through a microscope, it turns out to be wrinkled into hundreds of folds. Each fold is contoured into thousands of fingerlike projections, as numerous as the hairs on velvet fabric. These small intestinal projections are the **villi.** A single villus, magnified still more, turns out to be composed of hundreds of intestinal (absorptive) cells, each covered with its own microscopic hairs, the **microvilli** (see Figure 3-10). In the crevices between the villi lie the **crypt glands**—tubular glands that secrete the intestinal juices into the small intestine. Nearby **goblet cells** secrete mucus.

The villi are in constant motion. Each villus is lined by a thin sheet of muscle, so it can wave, squirm, and wriggle like the tentacles of a sea anemone. Any nutrient molecule small enough to be absorbed is trapped among the microvilli that coat the intestinal cells, and then it is drawn into the cells. Some partially digested nutrients are caught in the microvilli, digested further by enzymes there, and then absorbed into the cells.

villi (VILL-ee, VILL-eye): fingerlike projections from the folds of the small intestine; singular *villus.*

microvilli (MY-cro-VILL-ee, MY-cro-VILL-eye): tiny, hairlike projections on each intestinal cell of every villus that can trap nutrient particles and transport them into the cells; singular *microvillus.*

crypt (KRIPT) **glands:** tubular glands that lie between the intestinal villi and secrete intestinal juices into the small intestine.

goblet cells: cells of the GI tract (and lungs) that secrete mucus.

FIGURE 3-9 Absorption of Nutrients

Absorption of nutrients into intestinal cells typically occurs by simple diffusion, facilitated diffusion, or active transport. Occasionally, a large molecule is absorbed by *endocytosis*—a process in which the cell membrane engulfs the molecule, forming a sac that separates from the membrane and moves into the cell.

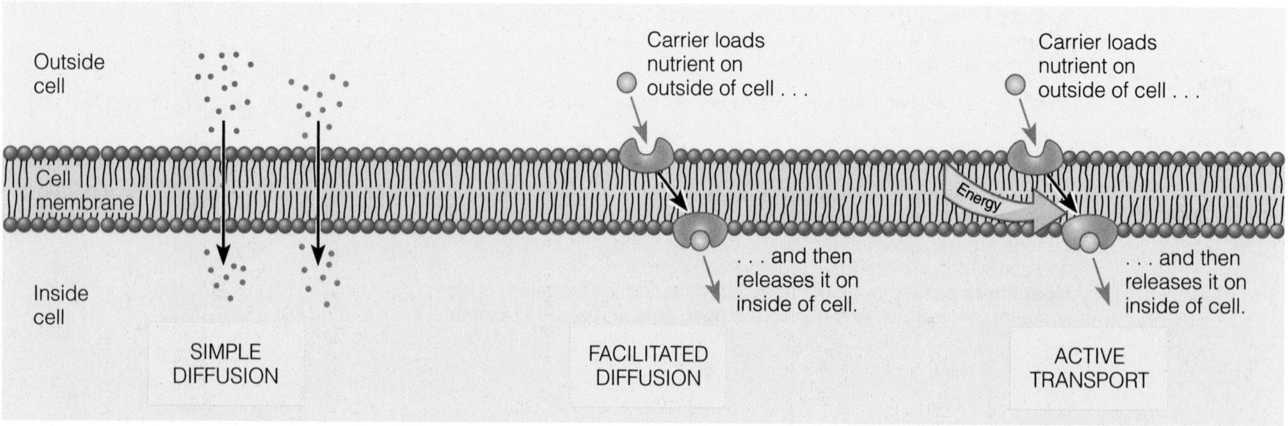
Outside cell
Cell membrane
Inside cell
SIMPLE DIFFUSION
Carrier loads nutrient on outside of cell . . .
. . . and then releases it on inside of cell.
FACILITATED DIFFUSION
Carrier loads nutrient on outside of cell . . .
Energy
. . . and then releases it on inside of cell.
ACTIVE TRANSPORT

Some nutrients (such as water and small lipids) are absorbed by simple diffusion. They cross into intestinal cells freely.

Some nutrients (such as the water-soluble vitamins) are absorbed by facilitated diffusion. They need a specific carrier to transport them from one side of the cell membrane to the other. (Alternatively, facilitated diffusion may occur when the carrier changes the cell membrane in such a way that the nutrients can pass through.)

Some nutrients (such as glucose and amino acids) must be absorbed actively. These nutrients move against a concentration gradient, which requires energy.

A Closer Look at the Intestinal (Absorptive) Cells The absorptive cells of the villi are among the most amazing in the body, for they recognize and select the nutrients the body needs and regulate their absorption. ♦ As already described, each absorptive cell of a villus is coated with thousands of microvilli, which project from the cell's membrane (Figure 3-10). In these microvilli, and in the membrane, lie hundreds of different kinds of enzymes and "pumps," which recognize and act on different nutrients. Descriptions of specific enzymes and "pumps" for

♦ The problem of food contaminants, which may be absorbed defencelessly by the body, is discussed in Chapter 20.

FIGURE 3-10 The Small Intestinal Villi

Absorption of nutrients into intestinal cells typically occurs by simple diffusion or active transport.

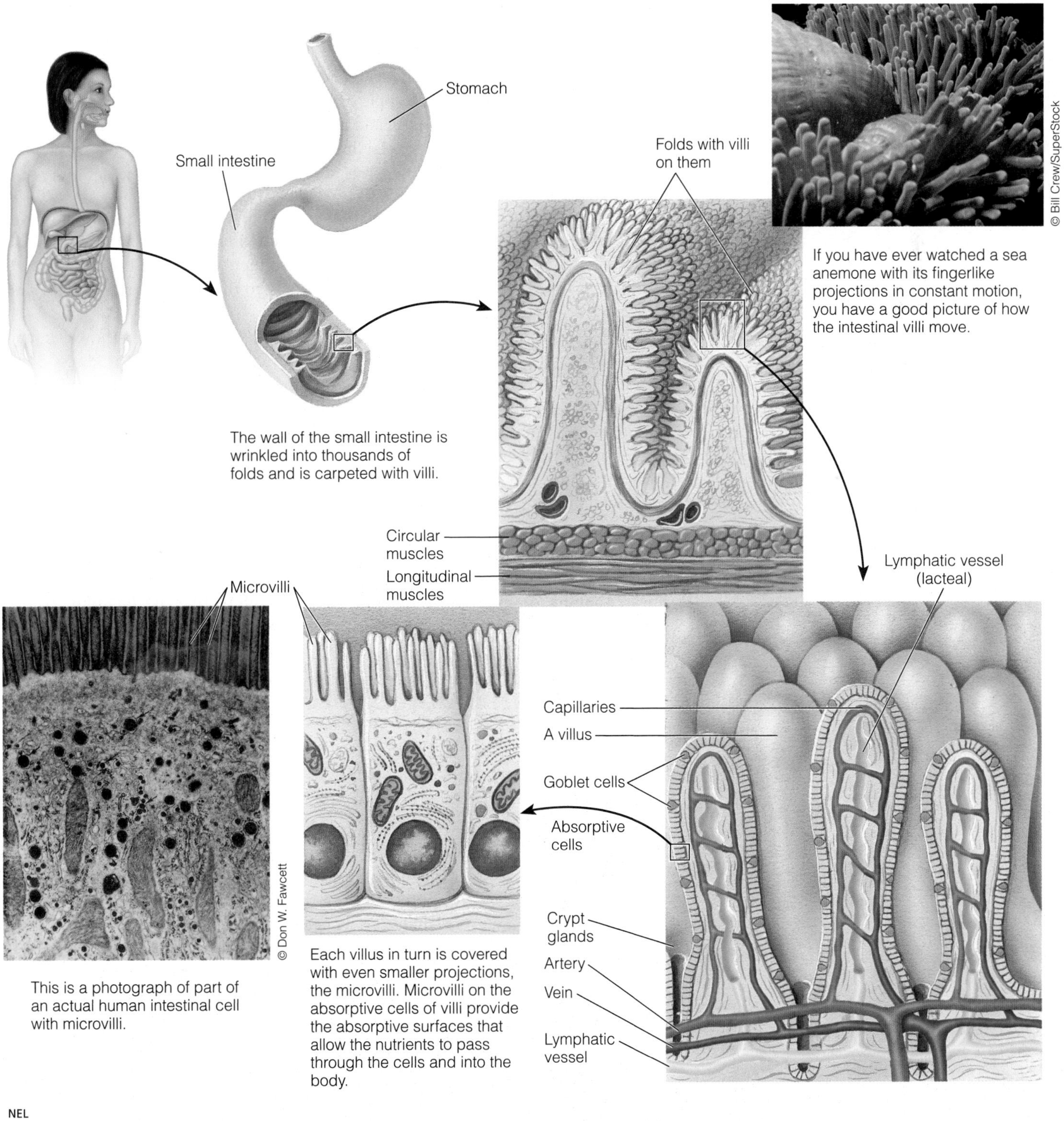
Stomach
Small intestine
Folds with villi on them
© Bill Crew/SuperStock
If you have ever watched a sea anemone with its fingerlike projections in constant motion, you have a good picture of how the intestinal villi move.
The wall of the small intestine is wrinkled into thousands of folds and is carpeted with villi.
Circular muscles
Longitudinal muscles
Lymphatic vessel (lacteal)
Microvilli
Capillaries
A villus
Goblet cells
Absorptive cells
Crypt glands
Artery
Vein
Lymphatic vessel
© Don W. Fawcett
This is a photograph of part of an actual human intestinal cell with microvilli.
Each villus in turn is covered with even smaller projections, the microvilli. Microvilli on the absorptive cells of villi provide the absorptive surfaces that allow the nutrients to pass through the cells and into the body.

each nutrient are presented in the following chapters where appropriate; the point here is that the cells are equipped to handle all kinds and combinations of foods and their nutrients.

Specialization in the GI Tract A further refinement of the system is that the cells of successive portions of the intestinal tract are specialized to absorb different nutrients. The nutrients that are ready for absorption early are absorbed near the top of the GI tract; those that take longer to be digested are absorbed farther down. Registered dietitians and medical professionals who treat digestive disorders learn the specialized absorptive functions of different parts of the GI tract so that if one part becomes dysfunctional, the diet can be adjusted accordingly.

The Myth of "Food Combining" The idea that people should not eat certain food combinations (e.g., fruit and meat) at the same meal, because the digestive system cannot handle more than one task at a time, is a myth. The art of "food combining" (which actually emphasizes "food separating") is based on this myth, and it represents faulty logic and a gross underestimation of the body's capabilities. In fact, the contrary is often true; foods eaten together can enhance each other's use by the body. For example, vitamin C in a pineapple or other citrus fruit can enhance the absorption of iron from a meal of beans and rice or other iron-containing foods. Many other instances of mutually beneficial interactions are presented in later chapters.

Preparing Nutrients for Transport When a nutrient molecule has crossed the absorptive cell of a villus, it enters either the bloodstream or the lymphatic system. Both transport systems supply vessels to each villus, as shown in Figure 3-10. The water-soluble nutrients including smaller products of fat digestion are released directly into the bloodstream and guided directly to the liver where their fate and destination will be determined.

The larger fats and the fat-soluble vitamins are insoluble in water, however, and blood is mostly water. The intestinal cells assemble many of the products of fat digestion into larger molecules. These larger molecules cluster together with special proteins, forming chylomicrons. ♦ Because these chylomicrons cannot pass into the blood **capillaries**, they are released into the lymphatic system instead; the chylomicrons move through the lymph and later enter the bloodstream at a point near the heart, thus bypassing the liver at first. Details follow.

♦ Chylomicrons (kye-lo-MY-cronz) are described in Chapter 5.

IN SUMMARY **The many folds and villi of the small intestine dramatically increase its surface area, facilitating nutrient absorption. Nutrients pass through the absorptive cells of the villi and enter either the blood (if they are water soluble or small fat fragments) or the lymph (if they are fat soluble).**

The Circulatory Systems

Once a nutrient has entered the bloodstream, it may be transported to any of the cells in the body, from the tips of the toes to the roots of the hair. The circulatory systems deliver nutrients wherever they are needed.

The Vascular System

The vascular, or blood circulatory, system is a closed system of vessels through which blood flows continuously, with the heart serving as the pump (see Figure 3-11). As the blood circulates through this system, it picks up and delivers materials as needed.

All the body tissues derive oxygen and nutrients from the blood and deposit carbon dioxide and other wastes back into the blood. The lungs exchange carbon dioxide (which leaves the blood to be exhaled) and oxygen (which enters the blood to be delivered to all cells). The digestive system supplies the nutrients. In the kidneys, wastes other than carbon dioxide are filtered out of the blood to be excreted in the urine.

capillaries (CAP-ill-aries): small vessels that branch from an artery. Capillaries connect arteries to veins. Exchange of oxygen, nutrients, and waste materials takes place across capillary walls.

FIGURE 3-11 The Vascular System

CENGAGENOW™
Animated! figure
www.cengage.com/sso

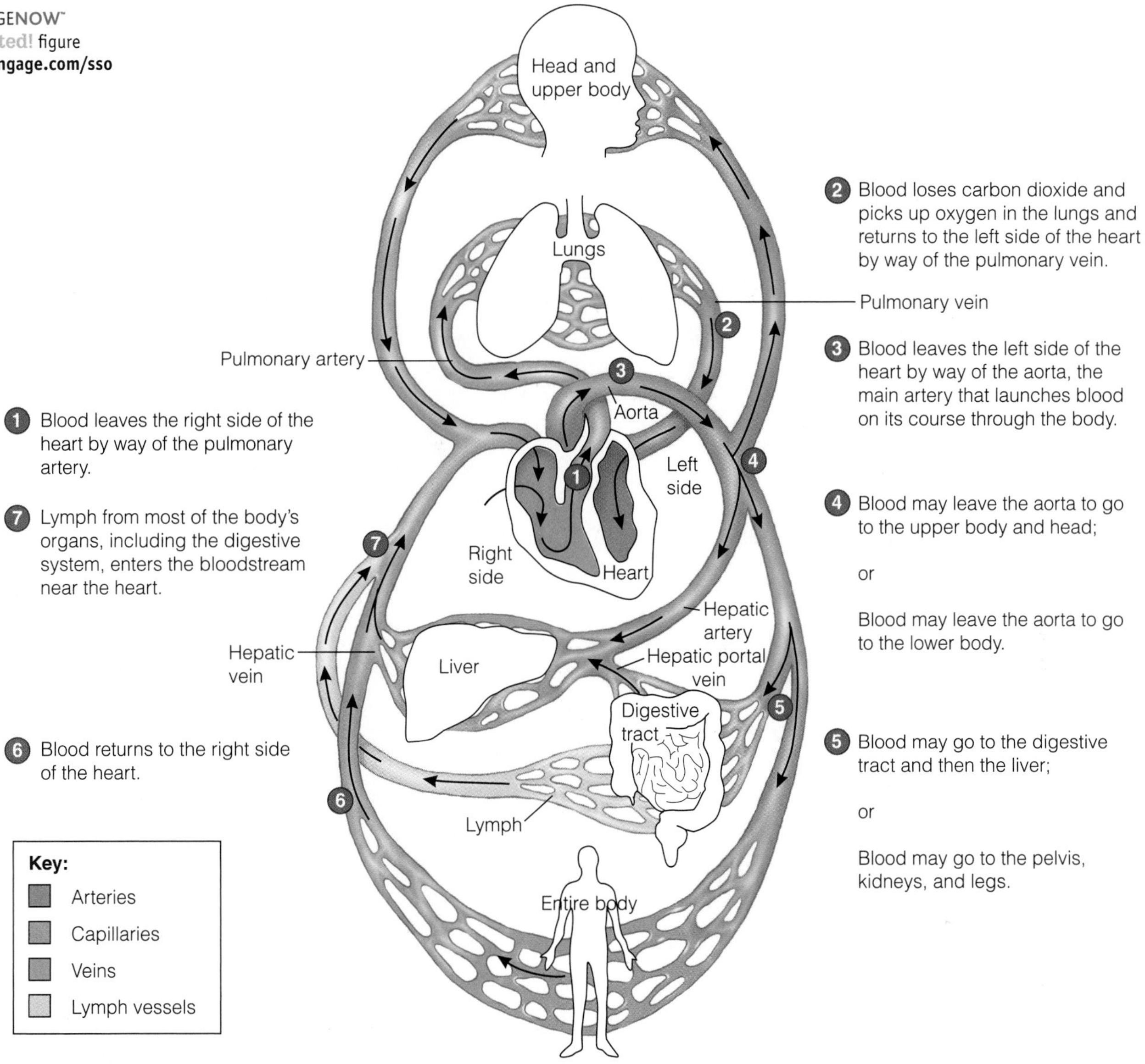
Head and upper body
Lungs
Pulmonary artery
Pulmonary vein
Aorta
Left side
Right side
Heart
Hepatic artery
Hepatic portal vein
Hepatic vein
Liver
Digestive tract
Lymph
Entire body
1 Blood leaves the right side of the heart by way of the pulmonary artery.
2 Blood loses carbon dioxide and picks up oxygen in the lungs and returns to the left side of the heart by way of the pulmonary vein.
3 Blood leaves the left side of the heart by way of the aorta, the main artery that launches blood on its course through the body.
4 Blood may leave the aorta to go to the upper body and head;
or
Blood may leave the aorta to go to the lower body.
5 Blood may go to the digestive tract and then the liver;
or
Blood may go to the pelvis, kidneys, and legs.
6 Blood returns to the right side of the heart.
7 Lymph from most of the body's organs, including the digestive system, enters the bloodstream near the heart.
Key:
Arteries
Capillaries
Veins
Lymph vessels

Blood leaving the right side of the heart circulates through the lungs and then back to the left side of the heart. The left side of the heart then pumps the blood out of the **aorta** through **arteries** to all systems of the body. The blood circulates in the capillaries, where it exchanges material with the cells and then collects into **veins**, which return it again to the right side of the heart. In short, blood travels this simple route:

- Heart to arteries to capillaries to veins to heart

The routing of the blood leaving the digestive system has a special feature. The blood is carried to the digestive system (as to all organs) by way of an artery, which (as in all organs) branches into capillaries to reach every cell. Blood leaving the digestive system, however, goes by way of a vein. The **hepatic portal vein** directs blood not back to the heart, but to another organ—the liver. This vein *again* branches into *capillaries* so that every cell of the liver has access to the blood. Blood leaving the liver then *again* collects into a vein, called the **hepatic vein**, which returns blood to the heart.

The route is:

- Heart to arteries to capillaries (in intestines) to hepatic portal vein to capillaries (in liver) to hepatic vein to heart

aorta (ay-OR-tuh): the large, primary artery that conducts blood from the heart to the body's smaller arteries.

arteries: vessels that carry blood from the heart to the tissues.

veins (VANES): vessels that carry blood to the heart.

hepatic portal vein: the vein that collects blood from the GI tract and conducts it to capillaries in the liver.
- **portal** = gateway

hepatic vein: the vein that collects blood from the liver capillaries and returns it to the heart.
- **hepatic** = liver

FIGURE 3-12 The Liver

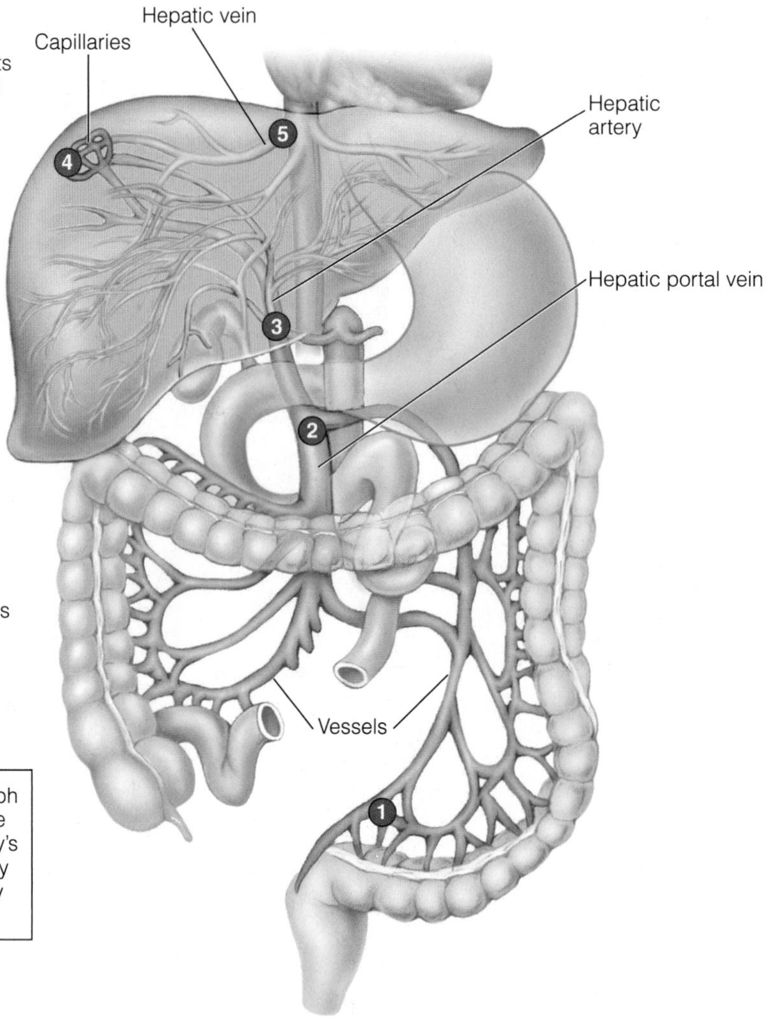
Hepatic vein
Capillaries
Hepatic artery
Hepatic portal vein
Vessels
1
2
3
4
5

1. Vessels gather up water-soluble nutrients and reabsorbed water and salts from all over the digestive tract.

Not shown here:
Parallel to these vessels (veins) are other vessels (arteries) that carry oxygen-rich blood from the heart to the intestines.

2. The vessels merge into the hepatic portal vein, which conducts all absorbed materials to the liver.

3. The hepatic artery brings a supply of freshly oxygenated blood (not loaded with nutrients) from the lungs to supply oxygen to the liver's own cells.

4. Capillaries branch all over the liver, making nutrients and oxygen available to all its cells and giving the cells access to nutrient-rich blood from the digestive system.

5. The hepatic vein gathers up blood in the liver and returns it to the heart.

In contrast, nutrients absorbed into lymph do not go to the liver first. They go to the heart, which pumps them to all the body's cells. The cells remove the nutrients they need, and the liver then has to deal only with the remnants.

Figure 3-12 shows the liver's key position in nutrient transport. An anatomist studying this system knows there must be a reason for this special arrangement. The liver's placement ensures that it will be first to receive the water-soluble nutrients absorbed from the GI tract. In fact, the liver has many jobs to do in preparing the absorbed nutrients for use by the body. It is the body's major metabolic organ.

In addition, the liver defends the body by detoxifying substances that might cause harm and preparing waste products for excretion. This is why, when people ingest poisons that succeed in passing the first barrier (the intestinal cells), the liver quite often suffers the damage—from viruses such as hepatitis, from drugs such as barbiturates or alcohol, from toxins such as pesticide residues, and from contaminants such as mercury. Perhaps, in fact, you have been undervaluing your liver, not knowing what heroic tasks it quietly performs for you.

♦ The lymphatic vessels of the intestine that take up nutrients and pass them to the lymph circulation are called **lacteals** (LACK-tee-als).

lymphatic (lim-FAT-ic) **system:** a loosely organized system of vessels and ducts that convey fluids toward the heart. The GI part of the lymphatic system carries the products of fat digestion into the bloodstream.

lymph (LIMF): a clear yellowish fluid that is similar to blood except that it contains no red blood cells or platelets. Lymph from the GI tract transports fat and fat-soluble vitamins to the bloodstream via lymphatic vessels.

thoracic (thor-ASS-ic) **duct:** the main lymphatic vessel that collects lymph and drains into the left subclavian vein.

subclavian (sub-KLAY-vee-an) **vein:** the vein that provides passage from the lymphatic system to the vascular system.

The Lymphatic System

The **lymphatic system** provides a one-way route for fluid from the tissue spaces to enter the blood. Unlike the vascular system, the lymphatic system has no pump; instead, **lymph** circulates *between* the cells of the body and collects into tiny vessels. The fluid moves from one portion of the body to another as muscles contract and create pressure here and there. Ultimately, much of the lymph collects in the **thoracic duct** behind the heart. The thoracic duct opens into the left **subclavian vein**, where the lymph enters the bloodstream. Thus nutrients from the GI tract that enter lymphatic vessels ♦ (large products of fat digestion and fat-soluble vitamins) ultimately enter the bloodstream, circulating through arteries, capillaries, and veins like the other nutrients, with a notable exception—they bypass the liver at first.

Once inside the vascular system, the nutrients can travel freely to any destination and can be taken into cells, then used as needed. What becomes of them is described in later chapters.

IN SUMMARY **Nutrients leaving the digestive system via the blood are routed directly to the liver before being transported to the body's cells. Those leaving via the lymphatic system eventually enter the vascular system but bypass the liver at first.**

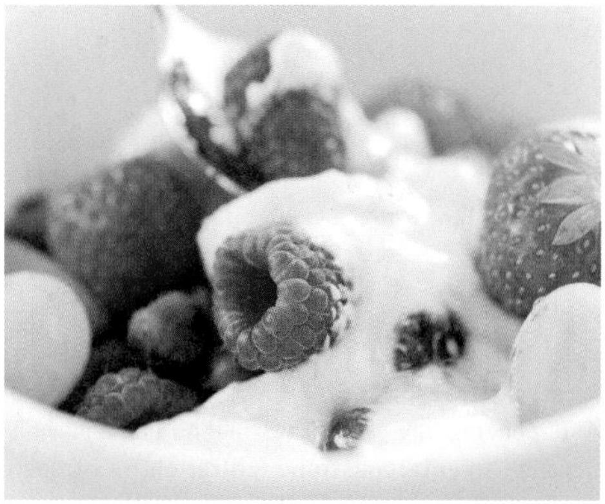

© Polara Studios

Eaten regularly, yogurt can alleviate common digestive problems.

The Health and Regulation of the GI Tract

This section describes the bacterial conditions and hormonal regulation of a healthy GI tract, but many factors ♦ can influence normal GI function. For example, peristalsis and sphincter action are poorly coordinated in newborns, so infants tend to "spit up" during the first several months of life. Older adults often experience constipation, in part, because the intestinal wall loses strength and elasticity with age, which slows GI motility. Diseases can also interfere with digestion and absorption and often lead to malnutrition. Lack of nourishment, in general, and lack of certain dietary constituents such as fibre, in particular, alter the structure and function of GI cells. Quite simply, GI tract health depends on adequate nutrition.

♦ Factors influencing GI function:
- Physical immaturity
- Aging
- Illness
- Nutrition

Gastrointestinal Bacteria

An estimated 10 trillion bacteria ♦ representing some 400 or more different species and subspecies live in a healthy GI tract. The prevalence of different bacteria in various parts of the GI tract depends on such factors as pH, peristalsis, diet, and other microorganisms. Besides processing food, the GI tract is a major immune organ protecting the body against harmful bacteria.[1] Beginning in the mouth, saliva produces immune bodies; in the stomach, relatively few microorganisms can survive the low pH and relatively rapid peristalsis; whereas the neutral pH and slow peristalsis of the lower small intestine and the large intestine permit the growth of a diverse and abundant bacterial population.[2]

♦ Bacteria in the intestines are sometimes referred to as **flora.**

Most bacteria in the GI tract are not harmful; in fact, they may actually be beneficial. Provided that the normal intestinal flora are thriving, infectious bacteria have a hard time establishing themselves to launch an attack on the system.

Diet is one of several factors that influence the body's bacterial population and environment. Consider **yogurt**, for example. Yogurt contains *Lactobacillus* and other living bacteria. These microorganisms are considered **probiotics** because they change the conditions and native bacterial colonies in the GI tract in ways that benefit health.[3] The potential GI health benefits of probiotics include helping to alleviate diarrhea, constipation, inflammatory bowel disease, ulcers, allergies, lactose intolerance, and infant colic; enhance immune function; and protect against colon cancer.[4] Some probiotics may have adverse effects under certain circumstances.[5] Research studies continue to explore how diet influences GI bacteria and which foods—with their probiotics—affect GI health. In addition, research studies are beginning to reveal several health benefits beyond the GI tract—such as improving blood pressure and immune responses.[6]

♦ Food components (such as fibre) that are not digested in the small intestine, but are used instead as food by bacteria to encourage their growth or activity are called **prebiotics.** A mixture of probiotics and prebiotics forms a **synbiotic.**

GI bacteria also ferment fibre and complex proteins.[7] ♦ In doing so, the bacteria produce nutrients such as short fragments of fat that the cells of the colon use for energy. Bacteria in the GI tract also produce several vitamins, ♦ although the amount is insufficient to meet the body's total need for these vitamins.[8]

♦ Vitamins produced by bacteria include:
- Biotin
- Folate
- Pantothenic acid
- Riboflavin
- Thiamin
- Vitamin B_6
- Vitamin B_{12}
- Vitamin K

yogurt: milk product that results from the fermentation of lactic acid in milk by *Lactobacillus bulgaricus* and *Streptococcus thermophilus.*

probiotics: living microorganisms found in foods and dietary supplements that, when consumed in sufficient quantities, are beneficial to health.
- **pro** = for
- **bios** = life

Gastrointestinal Hormones and Nerve Pathways

The ability of the digestive tract to handle its ever-changing contents illustrates an important physiological principle that governs the way all living things function—the principle of **homeostasis.** Simply stated, survival depends on body conditions staying about the same; if they deviate too far from the norm, the body must "do something" to bring them back to normal. The body's regulation of digestion is one example of homeostatic regulation. The body also regulates its temperature, its blood pressure, and all other aspects of its blood chemistry in similar ways.

Two intricate and sensitive systems coordinate all the digestive and absorptive processes: the hormonal (or endocrine) system and the nervous system. The coordination of these systems is illustrated in Figure 8-2 on page 244. Even before the first bite of food is taken, the mere thought, sight, or smell of food can trigger a response from these systems. Then, as food travels through the GI tract, it either stimulates or inhibits digestive secretions by way of messages that are carried from one section of the GI tract to another by both **hormones** ♦ and nerve pathways. (APPENDIX A presents a brief summary of the body's hormonal system and nervous system.)

♦ In general, any gastrointestinal hormone may be called an **enterogastrone** (EN-ter-oh-GAS-trone), but the term often refers specifically to the **gastric inhibitory peptide** that slows motility and inhibits gastric secretions.

Notice that the kinds of regulation described next are all examples of *feedback* mechanisms. A certain condition demands a response. The response changes that condition, and the change then cuts off the response. Thus the system is self-correcting. Examples follow:

- *The stomach normally maintains a pH between 1.5 and 1.7. How does it stay that way?* Food entering the stomach stimulates cells in the stomach wall to release the hormone **gastrin.** Gastrin, in turn, stimulates the stomach glands to secrete the components of hydrochloric acid. When pH 1.5 is reached, the acid itself turns off the gastrin-producing cells. They stop releasing gastrin, and the glands stop producing hydrochloric acid. Thus the system adjusts itself, as Figure 3-13 shows.

  Nerve receptors in the stomach wall also respond to the presence of food and stimulate the gastric glands to secrete juices and the muscles to contract. As the stomach empties, the receptors are no longer stimulated, the flow of juices slows, and the stomach quiets down.

FIGURE 3-13 An Example of a Negative Feedback Loop

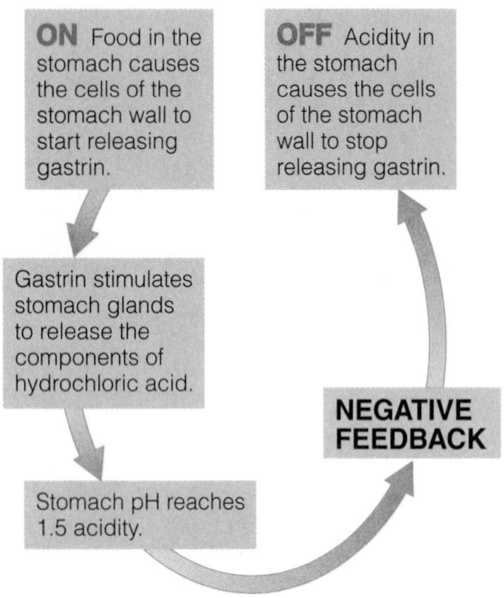
ON Food in the stomach causes the cells of the stomach wall to start releasing gastrin.
OFF Acidity in the stomach causes the cells of the stomach wall to stop releasing gastrin.
Gastrin stimulates stomach glands to release the components of hydrochloric acid.
NEGATIVE FEEDBACK
Stomach pH reaches 1.5 acidity.

- *The pyloric sphincter opens to let out a little chyme, then closes again. How does it know when to open and close?* When the pyloric sphincter relaxes, acidic chyme slips through. The cells of the pyloric muscle on the intestinal side sense the acid, causing the pyloric sphincter to close tightly. Only after the chyme has been neutralized by pancreatic bicarbonate and the juices surrounding the pyloric sphincter have become alkaline can the muscle relax again. This process ensures that the chyme will be released slowly enough to be neutralized as it flows through the small intestine. This is important because the small intestine has less of a mucous coating than the stomach does and so is not as well protected from acid.
- *As the chyme enters the small intestine, the pancreas adds bicarbonate to it so that the intestinal contents always remain at a slightly alkaline pH. How does the pancreas know how much to add?* The presence of chyme stimulates the cells of the duodenum wall to release the hormone **secretin** into the blood. When secretin reaches the pancreas, it stimulates the pancreas to release its bicarbonate-rich juices. Thus, whenever the duodenum signals that acidic chyme is present, the pancreas responds by sending bicarbonate to neutralize it. When the need has been met, the cells of the duodenum wall are no longer stimulated to release secretin, the hormone no longer flows through the blood, the pancreas no longer receives the message, and it stops sending pancreatic juice. Nerves also regulate pancreatic secretions.
- *Pancreatic secretions contain a mixture of enzymes to digest carbohydrate, fat, and protein. How does the pancreas know how much of each type of enzyme to provide?* This is one of the most interesting questions physiologists have asked. Clearly, the pancreas does know what its owner has been eating, and it secretes enzyme mixtures tailored to handle the food mixtures that have been arriving recently (over the last several days). Enzyme activity changes proportionately in response to the amounts of carbohydrate, fat, and protein in the diet. If a

homeostasis (HOME-ee-oh-STAY-sis): the maintenance of constant internal conditions (such as blood chemistry, temperature, and blood pressure) by the body's control systems. A homeostatic system is constantly reacting to external forces to maintain limits set by the body's needs.

- **homeo** = the same
- **stasis** = staying

hormones: chemical messengers. Hormones are secreted by a variety of glands in response to altered conditions in the body. Each hormone travels to one or more specific target tissues or organs, where it elicits a specific response to maintain homeostasis.

gastrin: a hormone secreted by cells in the stomach wall. Target organ: the glands of the stomach. Response: secretion of gastric acid.

secretin (see-CREET-in): a hormone produced by cells in the duodenum wall. Target organ: the pancreas. Response: secretion of bicarbonate-rich pancreatic juice.

person has been eating mostly carbohydrates, the pancreas makes and secretes mostly carbohydrases; if the person's diet has been high in fat, the pancreas produces more lipases; and so forth. Presumably, hormones from the GI tract, secreted in response to meals, keep the pancreas informed as to its digestive tasks. The day or two lag between the time a person's diet changes dramatically and the time digestion of the new diet becomes efficient explains why dietary changes can "upset digestion" and should be made gradually.

- *Why don't the digestive enzymes damage the pancreas?* The pancreas protects itself from harm by producing an inactive form of the enzymes. ♦ It releases these proteins into the small intestine where they are activated to become enzymes. In pancreatitis, the digestive enzymes become active within the infected pancreas, causing inflammation and damaging the delicate pancreatic tissues.
- *When fat is present in the intestine, the gallbladder contracts to squirt bile into the intestine to emulsify the fat. How does the gallbladder get the message that fat is present?* Fat in the intestine stimulates cells of the intestinal wall to release the hormone **cholecystokinin (CCK)**. This hormone travels by way of the blood to the gallbladder and stimulates it to contract, which releases bile into the small intestine. Cholecystokinin also travels to the pancreas and stimulates it to secrete its juices, which releases bicarbonate and enzymes into the small intestine. Once the fat in the intestine is emulsified and enzymes have begun to work on it, the fat no longer provokes release of the hormone, and the message to contract is cancelled. (By the way, fat emulsification can continue even after a diseased gallbladder has been surgically removed because the liver can deliver bile directly to the small intestine.)
- *Fat and protein take longer to digest than carbohydrate does. When fat or protein is present, intestinal motility slows to allow time for its digestion. How does the intestine know when to slow down?* Cholecystokinin is released in response to fat or protein in the small intestine. In addition to its role in fat emulsification and digestion, cholecystokinin slows GI tract motility. Slowing the digestive process helps to maintain a pace that allows all reactions to reach completion. Hormonal and nervous mechanisms like these account for much of the body's ability to adapt to changing conditions.

Table 3-1 summarizes the actions of these three GI hormones. Gastrin, secretin, and cholecystokinin are among the most studied GI hormones, but the GI tract releases more than 20 hormones.[9] In addition to assisting with digestion and absorption, many of these hormones regulate food intake and influence satiation. ♦ Current research is focusing on the roles these hormones may play in the development of obesity and its treatments (more details provided in Chapter 8).[10]

Once a person has started to learn the answers to questions like these, it may be hard to stop. Some people devote their whole lives to the study of physiology. For now, however, these few examples illustrate how all the processes throughout

♦ The inactive precursor of an enzyme is called a **zymogen** (ZYE-mo-jen).
- **zym** = concerning enzymes
- **gen** = to produce

♦ As Chapter 8 explains, **satiation** is the feeling of satisfaction and fullness that occurs during a meal and halts eating.

cholecystokinin (COAL-ee-SIS-toe-KINE-in), or **CCK:** a hormone produced by cells of the intestinal wall. Target organ: the gallbladder. Response: release of bile and slowing of GI motility.

TABLE 3-1 The Primary Actions of Selected GI Hormones

Hormone	Responds to	Secreted from	Stimulates	Response
Gastrin	Food in the stomach	Stomach wall	Stomach glands	Hydrochloric acid secreted into the stomach
Secretin	Acidic chyme in the small intestine	Duodenal wall	Pancreas	Bicarbonate-rich juices secreted into the small intestine
Cholecystokinin	Fat or protein in the small intestine	Intestinal wall	Gallbladder	Bile secreted into the duodenum
			Pancreas	Bicarbonate- and enzyme-rich juices secreted into the small intestine

the digestive system are precisely and automatically regulated without any conscious effort.

IN SUMMARY **A diverse and abundant bacteria population supports GI health. The regulation of GI processes depends on the coordinated efforts of the hormonal system and the nervous system. Together, digestion and absorption break down foods into nutrients for the body's use.**

The System at Its Best

This chapter describes the anatomy of the digestive tract on several levels: the sequence of digestive organs, the cells and structures of the villi, and the selective machinery of the cell membranes. The intricate architecture of the digestive system makes it sensitive and responsive to conditions in its environment. Several different kinds of GI tract cells confer specific immunity against intestinal diseases such as inflammatory bowel disease. In addition, secretions from the GI tract—saliva, mucus, gastric acid, and digestive enzymes—not only help with digestion, but also defend against foreign invaders. Together the GI's team of bacteria, cells, and secretions defend the body against numerous challenges.

One indispensable condition is good health of the digestive system itself. Like all the other organs of the body, the GI tract depends on a healthy supply of blood. The cells of the GI tract become weak and inflamed when blood flow is diminished, as may occur in heart disease when arteries become clogged or blood clots form. Just as a diminished blood flow to the heart or brain can cause a heart attack or stroke, respectively, too little blood to the intestines ♦ can also be damaging—or even fatal.

♦ A diminished blood flow to the intestines is called **intestinal ischemia** (is-KEY-me-ah) and is characterized by abdominal pain, forceful bowel movements, and blood in the stool.

The health of the digestive system is also affected by such lifestyle factors as sleep, physical activity, and state of mind. Adequate sleep allows for repair and maintenance of tissue and removal of wastes that might impair efficient functioning. Activity promotes healthy muscle tone. Mental state influences the activity of regulatory nerves and hormones; for healthy digestion, mealtimes should be relaxed and tranquil. Pleasant conversations and peaceful environments during meals ease the digestive process.

Another factor in GI health is the kind of foods eaten. Among the characteristics of meals that promote optimal absorption of nutrients are those mentioned in Chapter 2: balance, moderation, variety, and adequacy. Balance and moderation require having neither too much nor too little of anything. For example, too much fat can be harmful, but some fat is beneficial in slowing down intestinal motility and providing time for absorption of some of the nutrients that are slow to be absorbed.

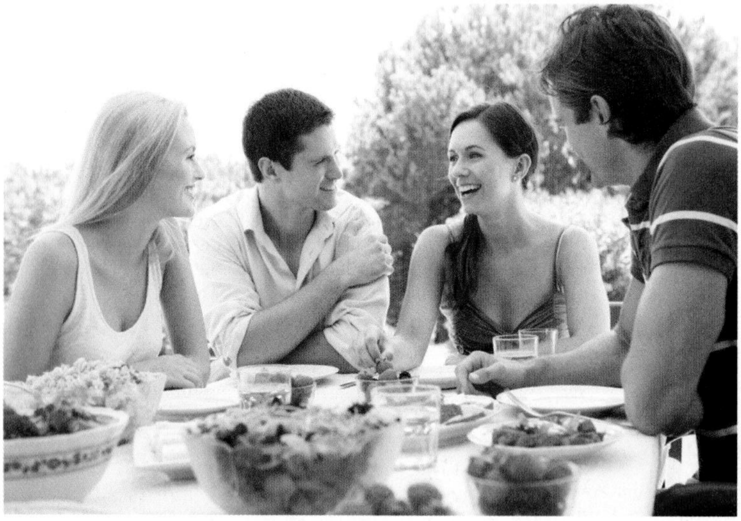

Monkey Business Images/shutterstock

Nourishing foods and pleasant conversations support a healthy digestive system.

Variety is important for many reasons, but one is that some food constituents interfere with nutrient absorption. For example, some compounds common in high-fibre foods such as whole-grain cereals, certain leafy green vegetables, and legumes bind with minerals. To some extent, then, the minerals in those foods may become unavailable for absorption. These high-fibre foods are still valuable, but they need to be balanced with a variety of other foods that can provide the minerals.

As for adequacy—in a sense, this entire book is about dietary adequacy. A diet must provide all the essential nutrients, fibre, and energy in amounts sufficient to maintain health. But here, at the end of this chapter, is a good place to emphasize the interdependence of the nutrients. It could almost be said that every nutrient depends on every other. All the nutrients work together, and all are present in the cells of a healthy digestive tract. To maintain health and promote the functions of the GI tract, make balance, moderation, variety, and adequacy features of your everyday food choices.

Nutrition Portfolio

A digestive system that is well cared for most of the time can adjust to handle almost any diet or combination of foods with ease on occasion.

Go to Diet Analysis Plus and choose one of the days on which you have tracked your diet for the entire day. Choose the day you thought you ate most poorly, and looking at it, record in your journal answers to the following:

- Describe the physical and emotional environment that typically surrounds your meals, including how it affects you and how it might be improved.
- Did you experience any GI discomforts on that day? Do you experience any GI discomforts regularly? If so, which of the foods that you ate might have contributed to your discomfort? What can you do to prevent or alleviate GI problems in the future? Use Table H3-1 (p. 90) as a guide.
- List any changes you can make in your eating habits to promote overall GI health.

Diet Analysis PLUS **To complete this exercise, go to your Diet Analysis Plus at www.cengage.com/sso.**

Nutrition on the Net

CENGAGENOW™
For further study of topics covered in this chapter, log on to **www.cengage.com/sso.**

- Visit the Canadian Digestive Health Foundation website for information about different digestive disorders: **www.cdhf.ca**
- Learn more about gastrointestinal diseases from the Canadian Society of Intestinal Research: **www.badgut.org**
- Visit the patient information section of the American College of Gastroenterology: **www.acg.gi.org**

References

1. B. Corthësy, Secretory immunoglobulin A: Well beyond immune exclusion at mucosal surfaces, *Immunopharmacology & Immunotoxicology* (2009): 174–179.
2. P. B. Eckburg and coauthors, Diversity of the human intestinal microbial flora, *Science* 308 (2005): 1635–1638.
3. C. C. Chen and W. A. Walker, Probiotics and prebiotics: Role in clinical disease states, *Advances in Pediatrics* 52 (2005): 77–113.
4. J. Rafter and coauthors, Dietary synbiotics reduce cancer risk factors in polypectomized and colon cancer patients, *American Journal of Clinical Nutrition* 85 (2007): 488–496; F. Savino and coauthors, *Lactobacillus reuteri* (American type culture collection strain 55730) versus simethicone in the treatment of infantile coli: A prospective randomized study, *Pediatrics* 119 (2007): e124; S. Santosa, E. Farnworth, and P. J. H. Jones, Probiotics and their potential health claims, *Nutrition Reviews* 64 (2006): 265–274; F. Guarner and coauthors, Should yoghurt cultures be considered probiotic? *British Journal of Nutrition* 93 (2005): 783–786.
5. J. Ezendam and H. van Loveren, Probiotics: Immunomodulation and evaluation of safety and efficacy, *Nutrition Reviews* 64 (2006): 1–14.
6. N. G. Hord, Eukaryotic-microbiota crosstalk: Potential mechanisms for health benefits of prebiotics and probiotics, *Annual Review of Nutrition* 28 (2008): 215–231; I. Lenoir-Wijnkoop and coauthors, Probiotic and prebiotic influence beyond the intestinal tract, *Nutrition Reviews* 65 (2007): 469–489; M. Liong, Probiotics: A critical review of their potential role as antihypertensives, immune modulators, hypocholesterolemics, and perimenopausal treatments, *Nutrition Reviews* 65 (2007): 316–328.
7. J. M. Wong and coauthors, Colonic health: Fermentation and short chain fatty acids, *Journal of Clinical Gastroenterology* 40 (2006): 235–243.
8. H. M. Said and Z. M. Mohammed, Intestinal absorption of water-soluble vitamins: An update, *Current Opinion Gastroenterology* 22 (2006): 140–146.
9. K. G. Murphy, W. S. Dhillo, and S. R. Bloom, Gut peptides in the regulation of food intake and energy homeostasis, *Endocrine Reviews* 27 (2006): 719–727.
10. D. E. Cummings and J. Overduin, Gastrointestinal regulation of food intake, *Journal of Clinical Investigation* 117 (2007): 13–23.

HIGHLIGHT 3

Common Digestive Problems

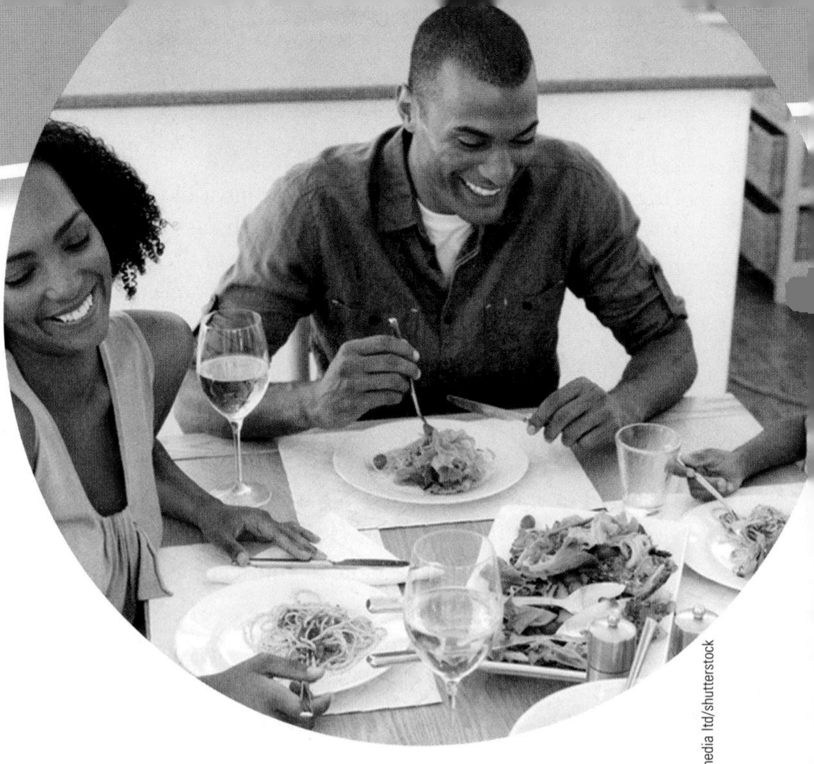

wavebreakmedia ltd/shutterstock

The facts of anatomy and physiology presented in Chapter 3 permit easy understanding of some common problems that occasionally arise in the digestive tract. Food may slip into the airways instead of the esophagus, causing choking. **Bowel** movements may be loose and watery, as in diarrhea, or painful and hard, as in constipation. Some people have problems with swallowing (**dysphagia**), others complain about belching, and others are bothered by intestinal gas. Sometimes people develop medical problems such as ulcers. This highlight describes some of the symptoms of these common digestive problems and suggests strategies for preventing them (the accompanying glossary defines the relevant terms). Sometimes problems can be caused by changes in digestive processes, such as lactose intolerance, which is discussed in Chapter 4.

Choking

A person chokes when a piece of food slips into the **trachea** and becomes lodged so securely that it cuts off breathing (see Figure H3-1). Without oxygen, the person may suffer brain damage or

GLOSSARY

acid controllers: medications used to prevent or relieve indigestion by suppressing production of acid in the stomach; also called *H2 blockers*. Common brands include Pepcid AC, Tagamet HB, Zantac 75, and Axid AR.

antacids: medications used to relieve indigestion by neutralizing acid in the stomach. Common brands include Alka-Seltzer, Maalox, Rolaids, and Tums.

belching: the expulsion of gas from the stomach through the mouth.

bowel: an alternative term for intestine, the *small bowel* refers to the small intestine and the *large bowel* refers to the large intestine or colon.

celiac disease (CEE-lee-ac): allergy to gluten, a protein found in wheat, rye, triticale, and barley that damages the villi and increases risk for malnutrition.

colonic irrigation: the popular, but potentially harmful practice of "washing" the large intestine with a powerful enema machine.

constipation: the condition of having infrequent or difficult bowel movements.

Crohn's disease: a type of **inflammatory** bowel disease of unknown cause resulting in abdominal pain, cramping, diarrhea, constipation, and bloody stools. Managed with medications and a dietary plan, but has no cure.

defecate (DEF-uh-cate): to move the bowels and eliminate waste.

- **defaecare** = to remove dregs

diarrhea: the frequent passage of watery bowel movements.

diverticula (dye-ver-TIC-you-la): sacs or pouches that develop in the weakened areas of the intestinal wall (like bulges in an inner tube where the tire wall is weak).

- **divertir** = to turn aside

diverticulitis (DYE-ver-tic-you-LYE-tis): infected or inflamed diverticula.

- **itis** = infection or inflammation

diverticulosis (DYE-ver-tic-you-LOH-sis): the condition of having diverticula. About one in every six people in Western countries develops diverticulosis in middle or later life.

- **osis** = condition

dysphagia: a commonly used term to describe problems with swallowing

enemas: solutions inserted into the rectum and colon to stimulate a bowel movement and empty the lower large intestine.

gastroesophageal reflux: the backflow of stomach acid into the esophagus, causing damage to the cells of the esophagus and the sensation of heartburn. **Gastroesophageal reflux disease (GERD)** is characterized by symptoms of reflux occurring two or more times a week.

heartburn: a burning sensation in the chest area caused by backflow of stomach acid into the esophagus.

Heimlich (HIME-lick) **manoeuvre (abdominal thrust manoeuvre):** a technique for dislodging an object from the trachea of a choking person (see Figure H3-2); named for the physician who developed it.

hemorrhoids (HEM-oh-royds): painful swelling of the veins surrounding the rectum.

hiccups (HICK-ups): repeated cough-like sounds and jerks that are produced when an involuntary spasm of the diaphragm muscle sucks air down the windpipe; also spelled *hiccoughs*.

inflammatory bowel disease: immune-engaged intestinal diseases of unknown cause, including **Crohn's disease** and **ulcerative colitis.**

indigestion: incomplete or uncomfortable digestion, usually accompanied by pain, nausea, vomiting, heartburn, intestinal gas, or belching.

- **in** = not

irritable bowel syndrome: an intestinal disorder of unknown cause. Symptoms include abdominal discomfort and cramping, diarrhea, constipation, or alternating diarrhea and constipation.

larynx (LAIR-inks): the entryway to the trachea that contains the vocal cords; also called the *voice box* (see Figure H3-1).

laxatives: substances that loosen the bowels and thereby prevent or treat constipation.

mineral oil: a purified liquid derived from petroleum and used to treat constipation.

peptic ulcer: a lesion in the mucous membrane of either the stomach (a gastric ulcer) or the duodenum (a duodenal ulcer).

- **peptic** = concerning digestion

trachea (TRAKE-ee-uh): the airway from the larynx to the lungs; also called the *windpipe*.

ulcer: a lesion of the skin or mucous membranes characterized by inflammation and damaged tissues. See also *peptic ulcer*.

ulcerative colitis (ko-LYE-tis): a type of **inflammatory bowel disease** of unknown cause resulting in sores and inflammation of the rectum and colon. Abdominal pain and cramping, diarrhea, and frequent false urges to defecate often restrict people's activities.

vomiting: expulsion of the contents of the stomach up through the esophagus to the mouth.

FIGURE H3-1 Normal Swallowing and Choking

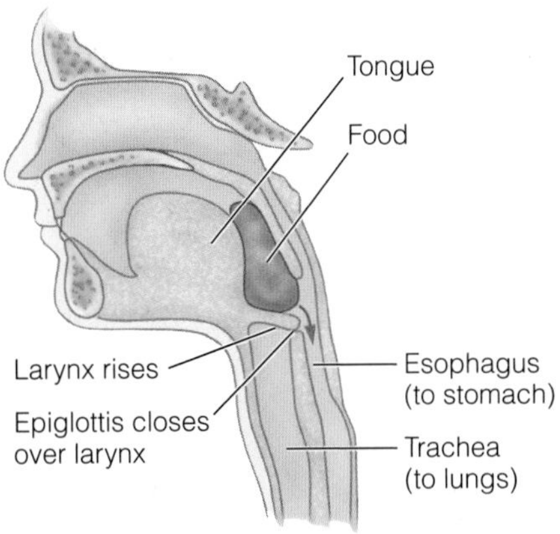
Tongue
Food
Larynx rises
Esophagus
(to stomach)
Epiglottis closes
over larynx
Trachea
(to lungs)

Swallowing. The epiglottis closes over the larynx, blocking entrance to the lungs via the trachea. The red arrow shows that food is heading down the esophagus normally.

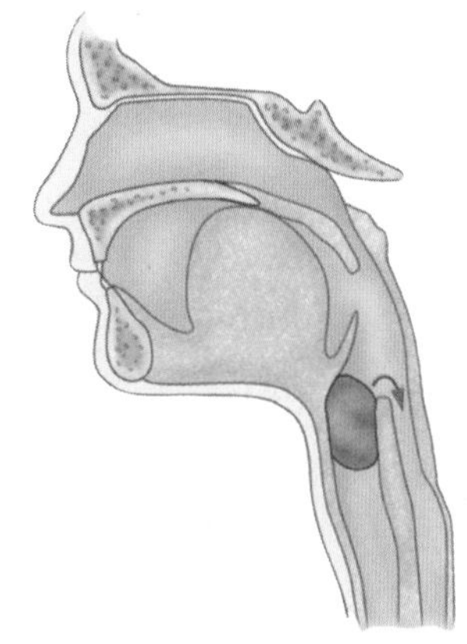

Choking. A choking person cannot speak or gasp because food lodged in the trachea blocks the passage of air. The red arrow points to where the food should have gone to prevent choking.

die. For this reason, it is imperative that everyone learns to recognize a person grabbing his or her own throat as the international signal for choking (shown in Figure H3-2) and act promptly.

The choking scenario might read like this. A person is dining in a restaurant with friends. A chunk of food, usually meat, becomes lodged in his trachea so firmly that he cannot make a sound. No sound can be made because the **larynx** is in the trachea and makes sound only when air is pushed across it. Often he chooses to suffer alone rather than "make a scene in public." If he tries to communicate distress to his friends, he must depend on pantomime. The friends are bewildered by his antics and become terribly worried when he "faints" after a few minutes without air. They call for an ambulance, but by the time it arrives, he is dead from suffocation.

To help a person who is choking, first ask this critical question: "Can you make any sound at all?" If so, relax. You have time to decide what you can do to help. Whatever you do, *do not* hit him on the back—the particle may become lodged more firmly in his air passage. If the person cannot make a sound, shout for help and perform the **Heimlich manoeuvre** (described in Figure H3-2). You would do well to take a lifesaving course and practise these techniques because you will have no time for hesitation if you are called upon to perform this death-defying act.

Almost any food can cause choking, although some are cited more often than others: chunks of meat, hot dogs, nuts, whole grapes, raw carrots, marshmallows, hard or sticky candies, gum, popcorn, and peanut butter. These foods are particularly difficult for young children to safely chew and swallow. Suffocation and choking injuries are the leading cause of injury death for infants less than one year of age and the fourth-leading cause of injury hospitalization. Each year in Canada, approximately 63 deaths and nearly 800 hospitalizations among children and youth under 20 years of age are due to suffocation and choking injuries.[1] Always remain alert to the dangers of choking whenever young children are eating. To prevent choking, cut food into small pieces, chew thoroughly before swallowing, don't talk or laugh with food in your mouth, and don't eat when breathing hard.

Vomiting

Another common digestive mishap is **vomiting.** Vomiting can be a symptom of many different diseases or may arise in situations that upset the body's equilibrium, such as air or sea travel. For whatever reason, the contents of the stomach are propelled up through the esophagus to the mouth and expelled.

FIGURE H3-2 First Aid for Choking

The first-aid strategy most likely to succeed is abdominal thrusts, sometimes called the Heimlich manoeuvre. Only if all else fails, open the person's mouth by grasping both his tongue and lower jaw and lifting. Then, and *only* if you can see the object, use your finger to sweep it out and begin rescue breathing.

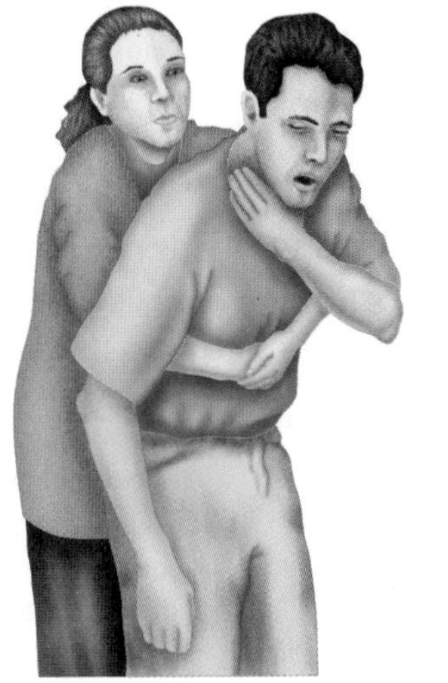

The universal signal for choking is when a person grabs his throat. It alerts others to the need for assistance. If this happens, stand behind the person, and wrap your arms around him. Place the thumb side of one fist snugly against his body, slightly above the navel and below the rib cage. Grasp your fist with your other hand and give him a sudden strong hug inward and upward. Repeat thrusts as necessary.

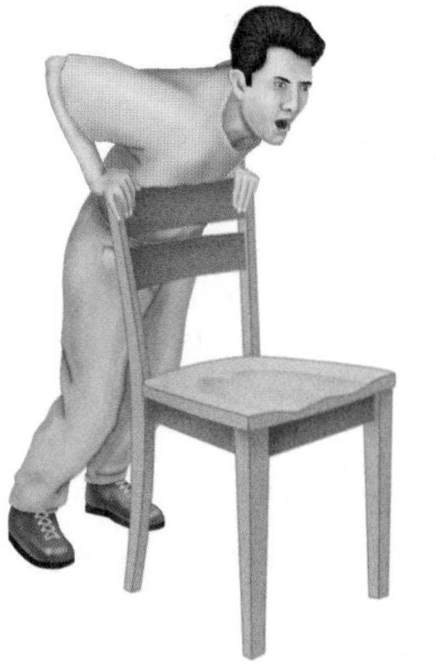

If you are choking and need to self-administer first aid, place the thumb side of one fist slightly above your navel and below your rib cage, grasp the fist with your other hand, and then press inward and upward with a quick motion. If this is unsuccessful, quickly press your upper abdomen over any firm surface such as the back of a chair, a countertop, or a railing.

If vomiting continues long enough or is severe enough, the muscular contractions will extend beyond the stomach and carry the contents of the duodenum, with its green bile, into the stomach and then up the esophagus. Although certainly unpleasant and wearying for the nauseated person, vomiting such as this is no cause for alarm. Vomiting is one of the body's adaptive mechanisms to rid itself of something irritating. The best advice is to rest and drink small amounts of liquids as tolerated until the nausea subsides.

A physician's care may be needed, however, when large amounts of fluid are lost from the GI tract, causing dehydration. With massive fluid loss from the GI tract, all of the body's other fluids redistribute themselves so that, eventually, fluid is taken from every cell of the body. Leaving the cells with the fluid are salts that are absolutely essential to the life of the cells, and they must be replaced. Replacement is difficult if the vomiting continues, and intravenous feedings of saline and glucose may be necessary while the physician diagnoses the cause of the vomiting and begins corrective therapy.

In an infant, vomiting is likely to become serious early in its course, and a physician should be contacted soon after onset. Infants have more fluid between their body cells than adults do, so more fluid can move readily into the digestive tract and be lost from the body. Consequently, the body water of infants becomes depleted and their body salt balance upset faster than in adults.

Self-induced vomiting, such as occurs in bulimia nervosa, also has serious consequences. In addition to fluid and salt imbalances, repeated vomiting can cause irritation and infection of the pharynx, esophagus, and salivary glands; erosion of the teeth and gums; and dental caries. The esophagus may rupture or tear, as may the stomach. Sometimes the eyes become red from pressure during vomiting. Bulimic behaviour reflects underlying psychological problems that require intervention. (Bulimia nervosa is discussed fully in Highlight 8.)

Projectile vomiting is also serious. The contents of the stomach are expelled with such force that they leave the mouth in a wide arc like a bullet leaving a gun. This type of vomiting requires immediate medical attention.

Diarrhea

Diarrhea is characterized by frequent, loose, watery stools. Such stools indicate that the intestinal contents have moved too quickly through the intestines for fluid absorption to take place, or that water has been drawn from the cells lining the intestinal tract and added to the food residue. Like vomiting, diarrhea can lead to considerable fluid and salt losses, but the composition of the fluids is different. Stomach fluids lost in vomiting are highly acidic, whereas intestinal fluids lost in diarrhea are nearly neutral. When fluid losses require medical attention, correct replacement is crucial.

Diarrhea is a symptom of various medical conditions and treatments. It may occur abruptly in a healthy person as a result of infections (such as food poisoning) or as a side-effect of medications. When used in large quantities, food ingredients such as the sugar alternative sorbitol and the fat alternative olestra may also cause diarrhea in some people. If a food is responsible, then that food must be omitted from the diet, at least temporarily. If medication is responsible, a different medicine, when possible, or a different form (injectable versus oral, for example) may alleviate the problem.

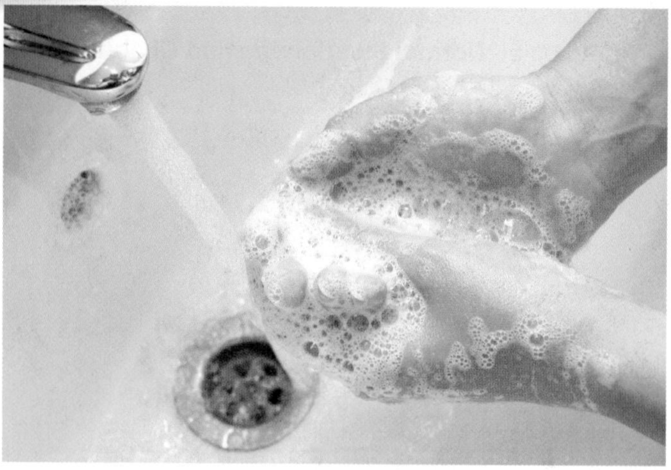

Voronin76/shutterstock

Personal hygiene (such as regular hand washing with soap and water) and safe food preparation are easy and effective steps to take in preventing diarrheal diseases.

Diarrhea may also occur as a result of disorders of the GI tract, such as irritable bowel syndrome, celiac disease, inflammatory bowel disease, and cystic fibrosis. **Irritable bowel syndrome** is one of the most common GI disorders, affecting five million Canadians, and is characterized by frequent or severe abdominal discomfort and a disturbance in the motility of the GI tract.[2] In most cases, GI contractions are stronger and last longer than normal, forcing intestinal contents through quickly and causing gas, bloating, and diarrhea. In some cases, however, GI contractions are weaker than normal, slowing the passage of intestinal contents and causing constipation. The exact cause of irritable bowel syndrome is not known, but researchers believe stress, genetics, and abnormal signals from the neurotransmitter serotonin are involved.[3] The condition seems to worsen for some people when they eat certain foods or during stressful events. These triggers seem to aggravate symptoms but not cause them. Dietary treatment hinges on identifying and avoiding individual foods that aggravate symptoms; small meals may also be beneficial. Probiotics appear to be efficacious in relieving symptoms of irritable bowel syndrome in some individuals.[4] Other effective treatments include dietary fibre, antispasmodic drugs, and peppermint oil.[5]

People with **celiac disease** have an immune-mediated response to gluten, a protein that is found in wheat, rye, triticale, and barley grains and grain products. Pure and uncontaminated oats are tolerated in limited amounts by many people with celiac disease; however, most oats sold in North America are cross-contaminated with grains that contain gluten. It is therefore important for people with gluten sensitivity to ensure that the oats they purchase are gluten-free. The gluten-induced inflammatory response reduces the number of digestive enzymes at the brush border and damages the intestinal cells causing the villi to flatten. With less surface area available for nutrient absorption and limited digestion of proteins, carbohydrates, and fats, the risk of malabsorption increases for these nutrients and many vitamins and minerals, and often results in symptoms of bloating, cramping, and diarrhea. To prevent further damage, people with celiac disease must eliminate foods that contain gluten from their diets. Current research estimates that up to 1 percent of Canadians have celiac disease.[6]

Inflammatory Bowel Disease (IBD) refers to two disorders caused by inflammation and ulceration of the intestines: **Crohn's disease** and **ulcerative colitis.** Crohn's disease can strike anywhere in the gastrointestinal tract, but commonly occurs in the ileum and upper part of the colon. On the other hand, ulcerative colitis is mostly localized in the colon and rectum. The cause of IBD is not known but the symptoms can have distressing effects on people's lives. People with IBD often experience symptoms of abdominal pain and cramping, diarrhea, bloody diarrhea, bouts of constipation, nausea, and vomiting leading to decreased food intake, weight loss, and increased risk of anemia. In addition, people with ulcerative colitis often experience false urges to defecate, which can limit their ability to engage in everyday activities. Although there is no cure for IBD, specific medications are useful in controlling the symptoms and a dietary plan usually including vitamin and mineral supplements helps to reduce the risk of malnutrition. Current estimates indicate 0.5 percent of the Canadian population has IBD.[7]

Cystic fibrosis is a genetic disorder that causes an overabundant secretion of mucous affecting the lungs and digestive tract, effectively blocking the release of digestive enzymes from the pancreas and preventing them from reaching the lumen of the small intestine. With limited digestion of the macronutrients, malnutrition can result. To minimize the effects of malabsorption, people with cystic fibrosis are often prescribed vitamin and mineral supplements and enterically coated pancreatic enzymes to take just before eating meals or snacks.

Treatment for diarrhea depends on cause and severity, but it always begins with rehydration.[8] Mild diarrhea may subside with simple rest and extra liquids (such as clear juices and soups) to replace fluid losses. If diarrhea is bloody or if it worsens or persists—especially in an infant, young child, elderly person, or person with a compromised immune system—call a physician. Severe diarrhea can be life threatening.

Constipation

Like diarrhea, **constipation** describes a symptom, not a disease. Each person's GI tract has its own cycle of waste elimination, which depends on its owner's health and state of hydration, the type of food eaten, when it was eaten, and when the person takes time to **defecate.** What's normal for some people may not be normal for others. Some people have bowel movements three times a day; others may have them three times a week. The symptoms of constipation include straining during bowel movements, hard stools, and infrequent bowel movements (fewer than three per week). Abdominal discomfort, headaches, backaches, and the passing of gas sometimes accompany constipation.

Often a person's lifestyle may cause constipation. Being too busy to respond to the defecation signal is a common complaint. If a person receives the signal to defecate and ignores it, the signal may not return for several hours. In the meantime, fluids continue to be withdrawn from the fecal matter, so when the person does defecate, the stools are dry and hard. In such a case, a person's daily regimen may need to be revised to allow time to have a bowel movement when the body sends its signal. One possibility is to go to bed earlier in order to rise earlier, allowing ample time for a leisurely breakfast and a movement.

Although constipation usually reflects lifestyle habits, in some cases it may be a side-effect of medication or may reflect a medical problem such as tumours that are obstructing the passage of waste. If discomfort is associated with passing fecal matter, seek medical advice to rule out disease. Once this has been done, simple treatments, such as increased fibre, fluids, and exercise, are recommended before the use of medications.[9]

One dietary measure along with adequate fluid intake that may be appropriate is to increase dietary fibre to 20 to 25 grams per day gradually over the course of a week or two. Fibres found in fruits, vegetables, and whole grains help to prevent constipation by increasing fecal mass. In the GI tract, fibre attracts water, creating soft, bulky stools that stimulate bowel contractions to push the contents along. These contractions strengthen the intestinal muscles. The improved muscle tone, together with the water content of the stools, eases elimination, reducing the pressure in the rectal veins and helping to prevent **hemorrhoids.** Chapter 4 provides more information on fibre's role in maintaining a healthy colon and reducing the risks of colon cancer and diverticulosis. **Diverticulosis** is a condition in which the intestinal walls develop bulges in weakened areas, most commonly in the colon (see Figure H3-3). These bulging pockets, known as **diverticula,** can worsen constipation, entrap feces, and become painfully infected and inflamed **(diverticulitis).**[10] Treatment may require hospitalization, antibiotics, or surgery.

Drinking plenty of water in conjunction with eating high-fibre foods also helps to prevent constipation. The increased bulk physically stimulates the upper GI tract, promoting peristalsis throughout. Similarly, physical activity improves the muscle tone and motility of the digestive tract. As little as 30 minutes of physical activity a day can help prevent or alleviate constipation.

Eating prunes—or "dried plums" as some have renamed them—can also be helpful. Prunes are high in fibre and also contain a laxative substance.* If a morning defecation is desired, a person can drink prune juice at bedtime; if the evening is preferred, the person can drink prune juice with breakfast.

These suggested changes in lifestyle or diet should correct chronic constipation without the use of **laxatives, enemas,** or **mineral oil,** although television commercials often try to persuade people otherwise. One of the fallacies often perpetrated by advertisements is that one person's successful use of a product is a good recommendation for others to use that product. As

*This substance is dihydroxyphenyl isatin.

FIGURE H3-3 Diverticula in the Colon

Diverticula may develop anywhere along the GI tract, but they are most common in the colon.

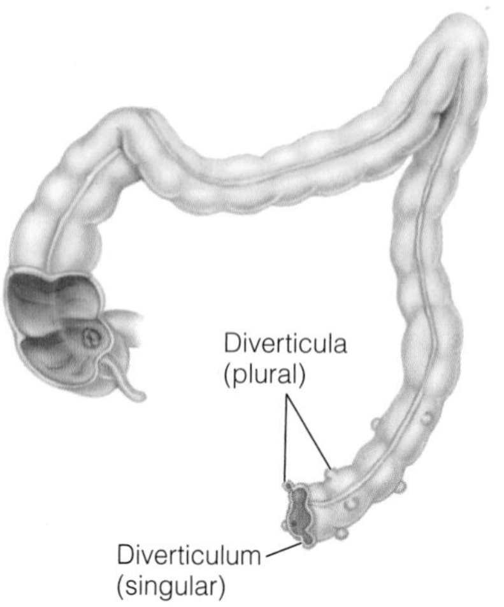
Diverticula
(plural)
Diverticulum
(singular)

a matter of fact, even dietary recommendations to relieve constipation may work for one person but may worsen the constipation of another. For instance, increasing fibre intake stimulates peristalsis and helps the person with a sluggish colon. Some people, though, have a spastic type of constipation, in which peristalsis promotes strong contractions that close off a segment of the colon and prevent passage; for these people, increasing fibre intake would be exactly the wrong thing to do.

A person who seems to need products such as laxatives frequently should seek a physician's advice. One potentially harmful but currently popular practice is **colonic irrigation**—the internal washing of the large intestine with a powerful enema machine. Such an extreme cleansing is not only unnecessary, but it can be hazardous, causing illness and death from equipment contamination, electrolyte depletion, and intestinal perforation. Less extreme practices can cause problems, too. Frequent use of laxatives and enemas can lead to dependency; upset the body's fluid, salt, and mineral balances; and, in the case of mineral oil, interfere with the absorption of fat-soluble vitamins. Mineral oil dissolves the vitamins but is not itself absorbed. Instead, it is excreted from the body, carrying the vitamins with it.

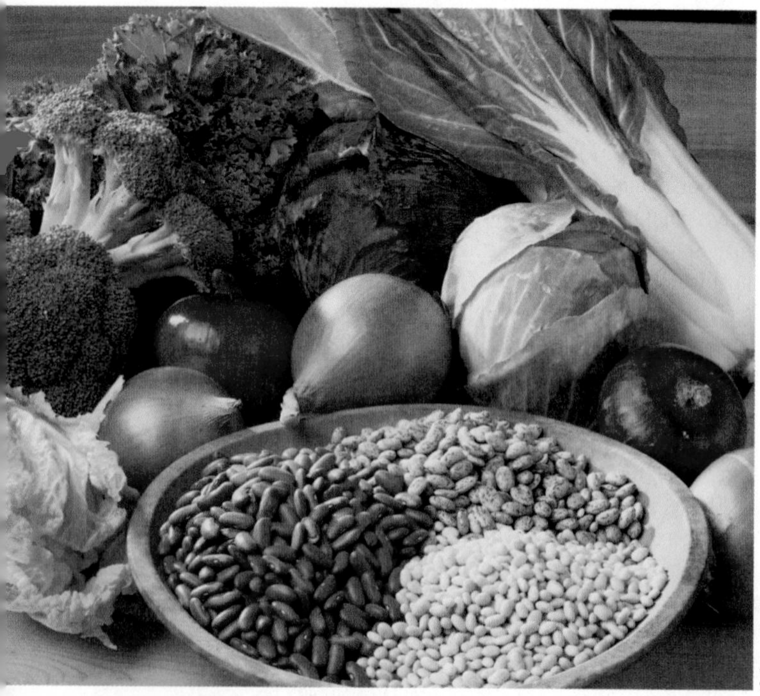

© Polara Studios, Inc.

People troubled by intestinal gas need to determine which foods bother them and then eat those foods in moderation.

Belching and Gas

Many people complain of problems that they attribute to excessive gas. For some, **belching** is the complaint. Others blame intestinal gas for abdominal discomforts and embarrassment. Most people believe that the problems occur after they eat certain foods. This may be the case with intestinal gas, but belching results from swallowing air. The best advice for belching seems to be to eat slowly, chew thoroughly, and relax while eating.

Everyone swallows a little bit of air with each mouthful of food, but people who eat too fast may swallow too much air and then have to belch. Ill-fitting dentures, carbonated beverages, and chewing gum can also contribute to the swallowing of air with resultant belching. Occasionally, belching can be a sign of a more serious disorder, such as gallbladder disease or a peptic ulcer.

People who eat or drink too fast may also trigger **hiccups,** the repeated spasms that produce a cough-like sound and jerky movement. Normally, hiccups soon subside and are of no medical significance, but they can be bothersome. The most effective cure is to hold the breath for as long as possible, which helps to relieve the spasms of the diaphragm.

Although expelling intestinal gas can be a humiliating experience, it is quite normal. (People who experience painful bloating from malabsorption diseases, however, require medical treatment.) Healthy people expel several hundred millilitres of intestinal gas several times a day. Almost all (99 percent) of the gases expelled—nitrogen, oxygen, hydrogen, methane, and carbon dioxide—are odourless. The remaining "volatile" gases are the infamous ones.

Foods that produce gas usually must be determined individually. The most common offenders are foods rich in the carbohydrates—sugars, starches, and fibres. When partially digested carbohydrates reach the large intestine, bacteria ferment (bacterial digestion) them, giving off gas as a by-product. People can test foods suspected of forming gas by omitting them individually for a trial period to see if there is any improvement.

Heartburn and "Acid Indigestion"

Almost everyone has experienced **heartburn** at one time or another, usually soon after eating a meal. On average, five million Canadians experience heartburn and/or acid regurgitation at least once a week.[11] Medically known as **gastroesophageal reflux,** heartburn is the painful sensation a person feels behind the breastbone when the lower esophageal sphincter allows the stomach contents to reflux into the esophagus (see Figure H3-4).[12] This may happen if a person eats or drinks too much (or both). Tight clothing and even changes of position (lying down, bending over) can cause it, too, as can some medications and smoking. Weight gain and overweight increase the frequency, severity, and duration of heartburn symptoms.[13] A defect of the sphincter muscle itself is a possible, but less common, cause.

If heartburn is not caused by an anatomical defect, treatment is fairly simple. To avoid such misery in the future, the person needs to learn to eat less at a sitting, chew food more thoroughly, and eat more slowly. Additional strategies are presented in Table H3-1 on the next page.

As far as "acid indigestion" is concerned, recall from Chapter 3 that the strong acidity of the stomach is a desirable condition—television commercials for **antacids** and **acid controllers** notwithstanding. People who overeat or eat too quickly are likely to suffer from **indigestion.** The muscular reaction of the stomach to unchewed lumps or to being overfilled may be so violent that it upsets normal peristalsis. When this happens, overeaters may taste the stomach acid and feel pain. Responding to advertisements, they may reach for antacids or acid controllers. Both of these drugs were originally designed to treat GI illnesses such as ulcers. As is true of most over-the-counter medicines, antacids and acid controllers should be used only infrequently for occasional heartburn; they may mask or cause problems if used regularly. Acid-blocking drugs weaken the defensive mucous barrier of the GI tract, thereby increasing the risks of infections such as pneumonia, especially in vulnerable populations like the elderly. Instead of self-medicating, people who suffer from frequent and regular bouts of heartburn and indigestion should try the strategies presented in Table H3-1 (p. 90). If problems continue, they may need to see a physician, who can prescribe specific medication to control gastroesophageal reflux. Without treatment, the repeated splashes of acid can severely damage the cells of the esophagus, creating a condition known as Barrett's esophagus. At that stage, the risk of cancer in the throat or esophagus increases dramatically.[14] To repeat, if symptoms persist, see a doctor—don't self-medicate.

Ulcers

Ulcers are another common digestive problem, affecting an estimated 800 000 to 1 million Canadians.[15] An **ulcer** is a lesion (a sore), and a **peptic ulcer** is a lesion in the lining of the stomach (gastric ulcers) or the duodenum of the small intestine (duodenal ulcers). The compromised lining is left unprotected and exposed to gastric juices, which can be painful. In some cases, ulcers can cause internal bleeding. If GI bleeding is excessive, iron deficiency may develop. Ulcers that perforate the GI lining can pose life-threatening complications.

FIGURE H3-4 Gastroesophageal Reflux

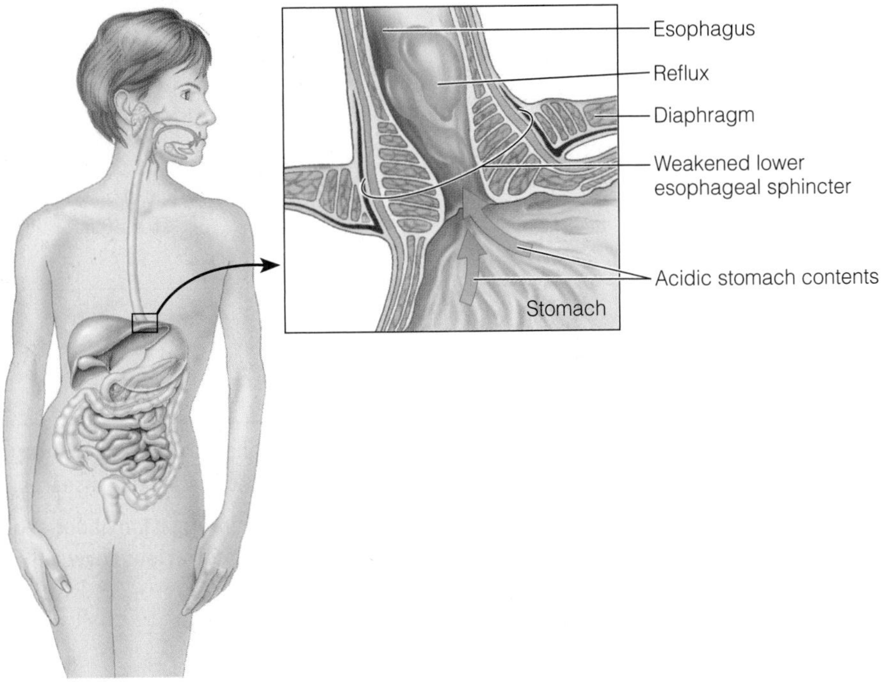
Esophagus
Reflux
Diaphragm
Weakened lower esophageal sphincter
Acidic stomach contents
Stomach

Many people naïvely believe that an ulcer is caused by stress or spicy foods, but this is not the case. The stomach lining in a healthy person is well protected by its mucous coat. What, then, causes ulcers to form?

Three major causes of ulcers have been identified: bacterial infection with *Helicobacter pylori* (commonly abbreviated *H. pylori*); the use of certain anti-inflammatory drugs such as aspirin, ibuprofen, and naproxen; and disorders that cause excessive gastric acid secretion. Most commonly, ulcers develop in response to *H. pylori* infection. The cause of the ulcer dictates the type of medication used in treatment. For example, people with ulcers caused by infection receive antibiotics, whereas those with ulcers caused by medicines discontinue their use.[16] All treatment plans aim to relieve pain, heal the ulcer, and prevent recurrence.

The regimen for ulcer treatment is to treat for infection, eliminate any food that routinely causes indigestion or pain, and avoid coffee and caffeine- and alcohol-containing beverages. Both regular and decaffeinated coffee stimulate acid secretion and so aggravate *existing* ulcers.

Ulcers and their treatments highlight the importance of not self-medicating when symptoms persist. People with *H. pylori* infection often take over-the-counter acid controllers to relieve the pain of their ulcers when, instead, they need physician-prescribed antibiotics. Suppressing gastric acidity not only fails to heal the ulcer, but it also actually worsens inflammation during an *H. pylori* infection. Furthermore, *H. pylori* infection has been linked with stomach cancer, making prompt diagnosis and appropriate treatment essential.[17]

Table H3-1 summarizes strategies to prevent or alleviate common GI problems. Many of these problems reflect hurried lifestyles. For this reason, many of their remedies require that people slow down and take the time to eat leisurely; chew food thoroughly to prevent choking, heartburn, and acid indigestion; rest until vomiting and diarrhea subside; and heed the urge to defecate. In addition, people must learn how to handle life's day-to-day problems and challenges without overreacting and becoming upset; learn how to relax, get enough sleep, and enjoy life. Remember, "what's eating you" may cause more GI distress than what you eat.

TABLE H3-1 Strategies to Prevent or Alleviate Common GI Problems

GI Problem	Strategies
Choking	• Take small bites of food. • Chew thoroughly before swallowing. • Don't talk or laugh with food in your mouth. • Don't eat when breathing hard.
Diarrhea	• Rest. • Drink fluids to replace losses. • Call for medical help if diarrhea persists.
Constipation	• Eat a high-fibre diet. • Drink plenty of fluids. • Exercise regularly. • Respond promptly to the urge to defecate.
Belching	• Eat slowly. • Chew thoroughly. • Relax while eating.
Intestinal gas	• Eat bothersome foods in moderation.
Heartburn	• Eat small meals. • Drink liquids between meals. • Sit up while eating; elevate your head when lying down. • Wait 3 hours after eating before lying down. • Wait 2 hours after eating before exercising. • Refrain from wearing tight-fitting clothing. • Avoid foods, beverages, and medications that aggravate your heartburn. • Refrain from smoking cigarettes or using tobacco products. • Lose weight if overweight.
Ulcer	• Take medicine as prescribed by your physician. • Avoid coffee and caffeine- and alcohol-containing beverages. • Avoid foods that aggravate your ulcer. • Minimize aspirin, ibuprofen, and naproxen use. • Refrain from smoking cigarettes.

Nutrition on the Net

CENGAGENOW™

For further study of topics covered in this Highlight, log on to **www.cengage.com/sso**.

- Visit the Canadian Digestive Health Foundation website for information sheets and personal stories from people living with a wide range of different digestive disorders: **www.cdhf.ca**
- Visit the Canadian Society of Intestinal Research website for information on intestinal diseases: **www.badgut.com**
- Find helpful information about celiac disease from the Canadian Celiac Association: **www.celiac.ca**

- Read the resources Shelley Case, a registered dietitian, author, speaker, and expert on celiac disease has on her website: **www.glutenfreediet.ca**
- Find information on cystic fibrosis from Cystic Fibrosis Canada: **www.cysticfibrosis.ca**
- Read or download consumer-friendly information on Crohn's disease and ulcerative colitis from the Crohn's and Colitis Foundation of Canada: **www.ccfc.ca**
- Visit the Digestive Diseases section of the National Institute of Diabetes and Digestive and Kidney Diseases: **www.niddk.nih.gov/health/health.htm**
- Visit the patient information section of the American College of Gastroenterology: **www.acg.gi.org**
- Learn more about *H. pylori* from the Helicobacter Foundation: **www.helico.com**

References

1. Brant County Health Unit, Preventing choking and suffocation (2010). www.bchu.org/content/view/1018/372/, accessed September 2, 2011.
2. E. A. Mayer, Irritable bowel syndrome, *New England Journal of Medicine* 358 (2008): 1692–1699; Canadian Digestive Health Foundation, Digestive disorders statistics (2010). www.cdhf.ca/digestive-disorders/statistics.shtml; accessed September 2, 2011.
3. A. Foxx-Orenstein, IBS—Review and what's new, *Medscape General Medicine* 8 (2006): 20.
4. P. Moayyedi, A. C. Ford, N. J. Talley, F. Cremonini, A. E. Foxx-Orenstein, L. J. Brandt, and E. M. M. Quigley, The efficacy of probiotics in the treatment of irritable bowel syndrome: A systematic review. *Gut* 59 (2009): 325-332.
5. A. C. Ford and coauthors, Effect of fibre, antispasmodics, and peppermint oil in the treatment of irritable bowel syndrome: Systematic review and meta-analysis, *British Journal of Medicine* 337 (2008): a2313.
6. Canadian Society of Intestinal Research, Celiac disease. www.badgut.org/information-centre/celiac-disease.html, accessed September 2, 2011.
7. Canadian Society of Intestinal Research, Inflammatory bowel disease. www.badgut.org/information-centre/inflammatory-bowel-disease.html, accessed September 2, 2011.
8. L. R. Schiller, Management of diarrhea in clinical practice: Strategies for primary care physicians, *Reviews in Gastroenterological Disorders* 7 (2007): S27–S38.
9. J. F. Johanson, Review of the treatment options for chronic constipation, *Medscape General Medicine* 9 (2007): 25.
10. D. O. Jacobs, Diverticulitis, *New England Journal of Medicine* 357 (2007): 2057–2066; H. Salzman and D. Lillie, Diverticular disease: Diagnosis and treatment, *American Family Physician* 72 (2005): 1229–1234.
11. Canadian Digestive Health Foundation, 2010.
12. P. J. Kahrilas, Gastroesophageal reflux disease, *New England Journal of Medicine* 359 (2008): 1700–1707.
13. B. C. Jacobson and coauthors, Body-mass index and symptoms of gastroesophageal reflux in women, *New England Journal of Medicine* 354 (2006): 2340–2348.
14. M. J. Schuchert and J. D. Luketich, Management of Barrett's esophagus, *Oncology (Williston Park)* 21 (2007): 1382–1389.
15. Canadian Digestive Health Foundation, Peptic ulcers (2009). www.cdhf.ca/digestive-disorders/peptic-ulcer.shtml, accessed September 2, 2011.
16. N. Vakil and D. Vaira, Sequential therapy for *Helicobacter pylori*—Time to consider making the switch? *Journal of the American Medical Association* 300 (2008): 1346–1347.
17. A. T. Axon, Relationship between *Helicobacter pylori* gastritis, gastric cancer and gastric acid secretion, *Advances in Medical Sciences* 52 (2007): 55–60.

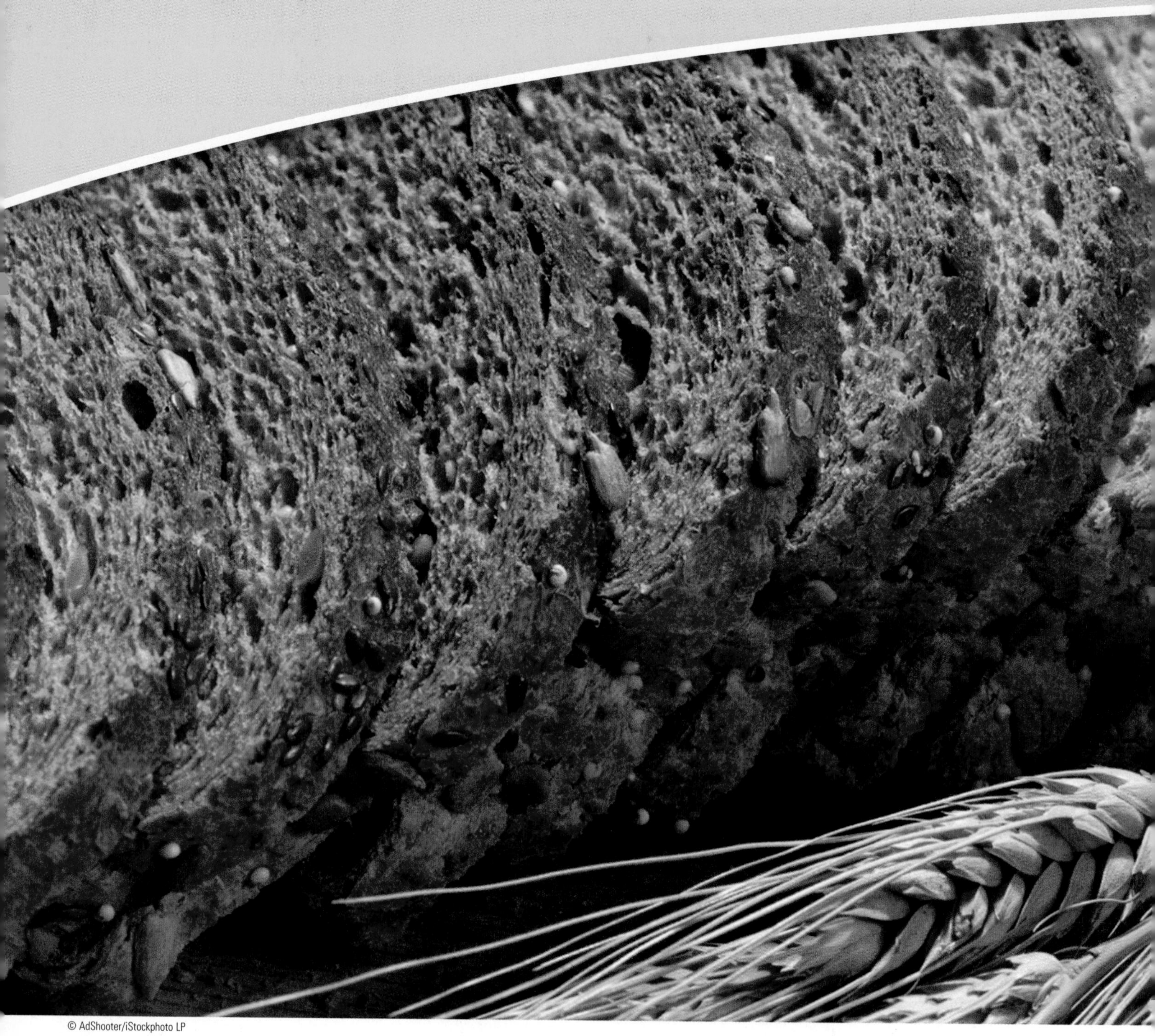

© AdShooter/iStockphoto LP

Nutrition in Your Life

CENGAGENOW™

Throughout this chapter, the CengageNOW logo indicates an opportunity for online self-study, linking you to interactive tutorials, activities, and videos to increase your understanding of chapter concepts.
www.cengage.com/sso

Whether you are studying for an exam or daydreaming about your next vacation, your brain needs carbohydrate to power its activities. Your muscles need carbohydrate to fuel their work, too, whether you are racing up the stairs to class or moving on the dance floor to your favourite music. Where can you get carbohydrate? Are some foods healthier choices than others? As you will learn from this chapter, whole grains, vegetables, legumes, and fruits naturally deliver ample carbohydrate and fibre with valuable vitamins and minerals and little or no fat. Milk products typically lack fibre, but they also provide carbohydrate along with an assortment of vitamins and minerals.

CHAPTER

4

The Carbohydrates: Sugars, Starches, and Fibres

CHAPTER OUTLINE

A student, quietly studying a textbook, is seldom aware that within his brain cells, billions of glucose molecules are splitting to provide the energy that permits him to learn. Yet glucose provides nearly all of the energy the human brain uses daily. Similarly, a marathon runner, bursting across the finish line in an explosion of sweat and triumph, seldom gives credit to the glycogen fuel her muscles have devoured to help her finish the race. Yet, together, these two **carbohydrates**—glucose and its storage form glycogen—provide about half of all the energy muscles and other body tissues use. The other half of the body's energy comes mostly from fat.

People don't eat glucose and glycogen directly. When they eat foods rich in carbohydrates, their bodies receive glucose for immediate energy and convert some glucose into glycogen for reserve energy. All plant foods—whole grains, vegetables, legumes, and fruits—provide ample carbohydrates. Milk also contains carbohydrates.

Many people mistakenly think of carbohydrates as "fattening" and avoid them when trying to lose weight. Such a strategy may be helpful if the carbohydrates are the concentrated sugars of soft drinks, candies, and cookies, but it is counterproductive if the carbohydrates are from whole grains, vegetables, and legumes. As the next section explains, not all carbohydrates are created equal.

The Chemist's View of Carbohydrates

The dietary carbohydrate family includes:[1] ♦

- Monosaccharides: single sugars
- Disaccharides: sugars composed of pairs of monosaccharides
- Polysaccharides: large molecules composed of chains of monosaccharides

To understand the structure of carbohydrates, look at the units of which they are made. The monosaccharides most important in nutrition ♦ each contain 6 carbon atoms, 12 hydrogens, and 6 oxygens (written in shorthand as $C_6H_{12}O_6$).

♦ Monosaccharides and disaccharides (the sugars) are sometimes called **simple carbohydrates,** and the polysaccharides (starches and fibres) are sometimes called **complex carbohydrates.**

♦ Most of the monosaccharides important in nutrition are *hexoses*, sugars with six atoms of carbon and the formula $C_6H_{12}O_6$.
- **hex** = six

carbohydrates: compounds composed of carbon, oxygen, and hydrogen arranged as monosaccharides or multiples of monosaccharides. Most, but not all, carbohydrates have a ratio of one carbon molecule to one water molecule: $(CH_2O)_n$.
- **carbo** = carbon (C)
- **hydrate** = with water (H_2O)

FIGURE 4-1 Atoms and Their Bonds

The four main types of atoms found in nutrients are hydrogen (H), oxygen (O), nitrogen (N), and carbon (C).

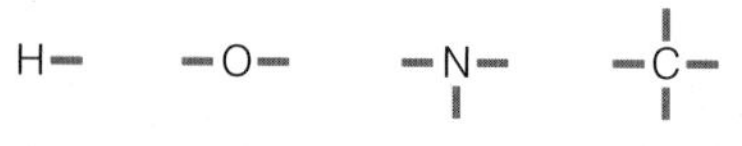
1
2
3
4

Each atom has a characteristic number of bonds it can form with other atoms.

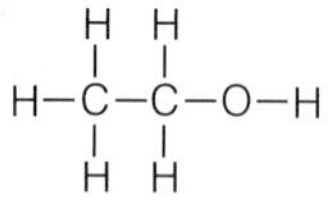

Notice that in this simple molecule of ethyl alcohol, each H has one bond, O has two, and each C has four.

FIGURE 4-2 Chemical Structure of Glucose

On paper, the structure of glucose has to be drawn flat, but in nature the five carbons and oxygen are roughly in a plane. The atoms attached to the ring carbons extend above and below the plane.

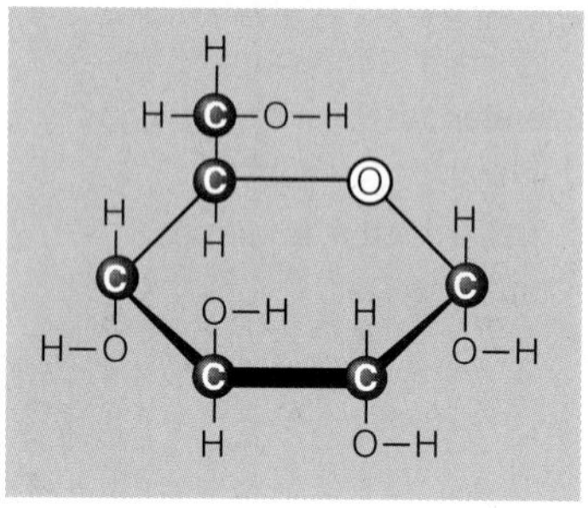

Each atom can form a certain number of chemical bonds with other atoms:

- Carbon atoms, four
- Nitrogen atoms, three
- Oxygen atoms, two
- Hydrogen atoms, only one

Chemists represent the bonds as lines between the chemical symbols (such as C, N, O, and H) that stand for the atoms (see Figure 4-1).

Atoms form molecules in ways that satisfy the bonding requirements of each atom. Figure 4-1 includes the structure of ethyl alcohol, the active ingredient of alcoholic beverages, as an example. The two carbons each have four bonds represented by lines; the oxygen has two; and each hydrogen has one bond connecting it to other atoms. Chemical structures always bond according to these rules.

The following list of the most important **sugars** in nutrition symbolizes them as hexagons and pentagons of different colours.* Three are monosaccharides:

- Glucose
- Fructose
- Galactose

Three are disaccharides:

- Maltose (glucose + glucose)
- Sucrose (glucose + fructose)
- Lactose (glucose + galactose)

Monosaccharides

The three **monosaccharides** important in nutrition all have the same numbers and kinds of atoms, but in different arrangements. These chemical differences account for the differing sweetness of the monosaccharides. A pinch of purified glucose on the tongue gives only a mild sweet flavour, and galactose hardly tastes sweet at all. Fructose, however, is as intensely sweet as honey and, in fact, is the sugar primarily responsible for honey's sweetness.

Glucose Chemically, **glucose** is a larger and more complicated molecule than the ethyl alcohol shown in Figure 4-1, but it obeys the same rules of chemistry: each carbon atom has four bonds; each oxygen, two bonds; and each hydrogen, one bond. Figure 4-2 illustrates the chemical structure of a glucose molecule.

The diagram of a glucose molecule shows all the relationships between the atoms and proves simple on examination, but chemists have adopted even simpler ways to depict chemical structures. Figure 4-3 presents the chemical structure of glucose in a more simplified way by combining or omitting several symbols—yet it conveys the same information.

Commonly known as blood sugar, glucose serves as an essential energy source for all the body's activities. Its significance to nutrition is tremendous. Later sections explain that glucose is one of the two sugars in every disaccharide and the unit from which the polysaccharides are made almost exclusively. One of these polysaccharides, starch, is the chief food source of energy for all the world's people; another, glycogen, is an important storage form of energy in the body. Glucose reappears frequently throughout this chapter and all those that follow.

Fructose **Fructose** is the sweetest of the sugars. Curiously, fructose has exactly the same chemical formula as glucose—$C_6H_{12}O_6$—but its structure differs (see Figure 4-4). The arrangement of the atoms in fructose stimulates the taste buds on the tongue to produce the sweet sensation. Fructose occurs naturally in fruits and honey; other sources include products such as soft drinks, ready-to-eat cereals, and desserts that have been sweetened with high-fructose corn syrup (defined on p. 109).

*Fructose is shown as a pentagon, but like the other monosaccharides, it has six carbons (as you will see in Figure 4-4).

sugars: monosaccharides and disaccharides.

monosaccharides (mon-oh-SACK-uh-rides): carbohydrates of the general formula $C_nH_{2n}O_n$ that typically form a single ring. See APPENDIX C for the chemical structures of the monosaccharides.

- **mono** = one
- **saccharide** = sugar

glucose (GLOO-kose): a monosaccharide; sometimes known as *blood sugar* or *dextrose*.

- **ose** = carbohydrate
- = glucose

fructose (FRUK-tose or FROOK-tose): a monosaccharide; sometimes known as *fruit sugar* or *levulose*. Fructose is found abundantly in fruits, honey, and saps.

- **fruct** = fruit
- = fructose

FIGURE 4-3 Simplified Diagrams of Glucose

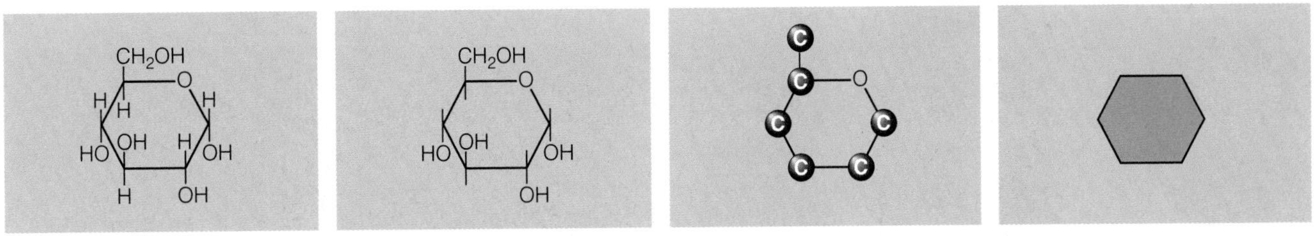

The lines representing some of the bonds and the carbons at the corners are not shown.

Now the single hydrogens are not shown, but lines still extend upward or downward from the ring to show where they belong.

Another way to look at glucose is to notice that its six carbon atoms are all connected.

In this and other illustrations throughout this book, glucose is represented as a blue hexagon.

Galactose The monosaccharide **galactose** occurs naturally as a single sugar in only a few foods. Galactose has the same numbers and kinds of atoms as glucose and fructose in yet another arrangement. Figure 4-5 shows galactose beside a molecule of glucose for comparison.

Disaccharides

The **disaccharides** are pairs of the three monosaccharides just described. Glucose occurs in all three; the second member of the pair is fructose, galactose, or another glucose. These carbohydrates—and all the other energy nutrients—are put together and taken apart by similar chemical reactions: condensation and hydrolysis.

Condensation To make a disaccharide, a chemical reaction known as **condensation** links two monosaccharides together (see Figure 4-6 on p. 96). A hydroxyl (OH) group from one monosaccharide and a hydrogen atom (H) from the other combine to create a molecule of water (H_2O). The two originally separate monosaccharides link together with a single oxygen (O).

Hydrolysis To break a disaccharide in two, a chemical reaction known as hydrolysis ♦ occurs (see Figure 4-7 on p. 96). A molecule of water splits to provide the H and OH needed to complete the resulting monosaccharides. Hydrolysis reactions commonly occur during digestion.

Maltose The disaccharide **maltose** consists of two glucose units. Maltose is produced whenever starch breaks down—as happens in human beings during

♦ A **hydrolysis** reaction splits a molecule into two, with H added to one and OH to the other (from water); Chapter 3 explained that hydrolysis reactions break down molecules during digestion

galactose (ga-LAK-tose): a monosaccharide; part of the disaccharide lactose.

•  = galactose

disaccharides (dye-SACK-uh-rides): pairs of monosaccharides linked together. See APPENDIX C for the chemical structures of the disaccharides.

• **di** = two

condensation: a chemical reaction in which water is released as two reactants combine to form one larger product.

maltose (MAWL-tose): a disaccharide composed of two glucose units; sometimes known as *malt sugar*.

• 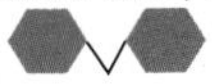 = maltose

FIGURE 4-4 Two Monosaccharides: Glucose and Fructose

Can you see the similarities? If you learned the rules in Figure 4-3, you will be able to "see" 6 carbons (numbered), 12 hydrogens (those shown plus one at the end of each single line), and 6 oxygens in both these compounds.

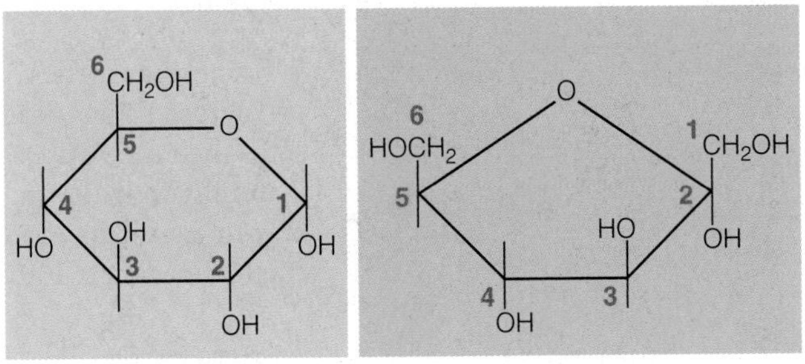

Glucose

Fructose

FIGURE 4-5 Two Monosaccharides: Glucose and Galactose

Notice the similarities and the difference (highlighted in red) between glucose and galactose. Both have 6 carbons, 12 hydrogens, and 6 oxygens, but the position of one OH group differs slightly.

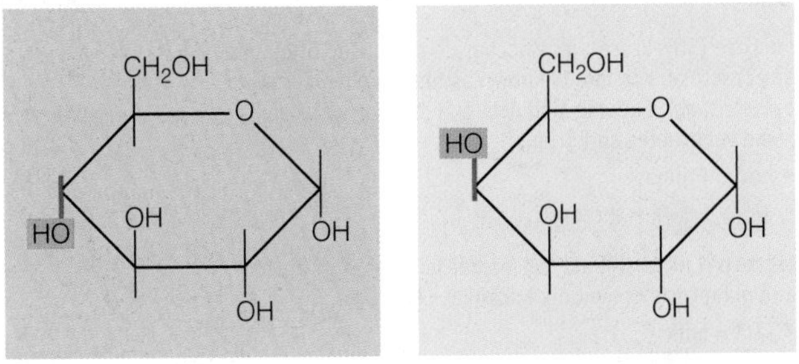

Glucose

Galactose

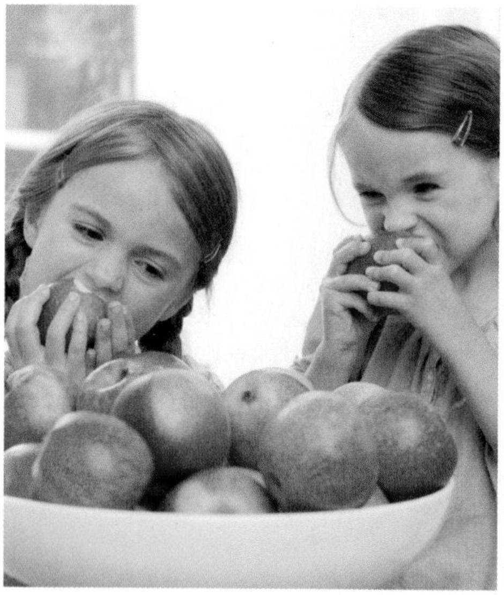

Fruits package their sugars with fibres, vitamins, and minerals, making them a sweet and healthy snack.

FIGURE 4-6 Condensation of Two Monosaccharides to Form a Disaccharide

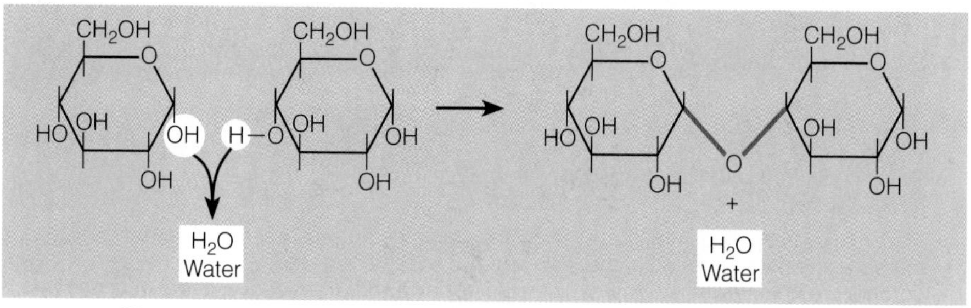
CH_2OH
O
HO
OH
H–O
H_2O
Water
+

Glucose + glucose → Maltose

An OH group from one glucose and an H atom from another glucose combine to create a molecule of H_2O.

The two glucose molecules bond together with a single O atom to form the disaccharide maltose.

carbohydrate digestion. It also occurs during the fermentation process that yields alcohol. Maltose is only a minor constituent of a few foods, most notably barley.

Sucrose Fructose and glucose together form **sucrose.** Because the fructose is accessible to the taste receptors, sucrose tastes sweet, accounting for some of the natural sweetness of fruits, vegetables, and grains. To make table sugar, sucrose is refined from the juices of sugarcane and sugar beets, then granulated. (Raw sugar is less refined and is the sugar that remains after the juice of sugarcane has been evaporated. There is little difference from it and the more refined table sugar.) Depending on the extent to which it is refined, the product becomes the familiar brown, white, and powdered sugars available at grocery stores.

Lactose The combination of galactose and glucose makes the disaccharide **lactose**, the principal carbohydrate of milk. Known as milk sugar, lactose contributes half of the energy (kcalories) provided by skim milk.

IN SUMMARY **The carbohydrates are made of carbon (C), oxygen (O), and hydrogen (H). Each of these atoms can form a specified number of chemical bonds: carbon forms four, oxygen forms two, and hydrogen forms one. Six sugars are important in nutrition. The three monosaccharides (glucose, fructose, and galactose) all have the same chemical formula ($C_6H_{12}O_6$), but their structures differ. The three disaccharides (maltose, sucrose, and lactose) are pairs of monosaccharides, each containing a glucose paired with one of the three monosaccharides. The sugars derive primarily from plants, except for**

FIGURE 4-7 Hydrolysis of a Disaccharide

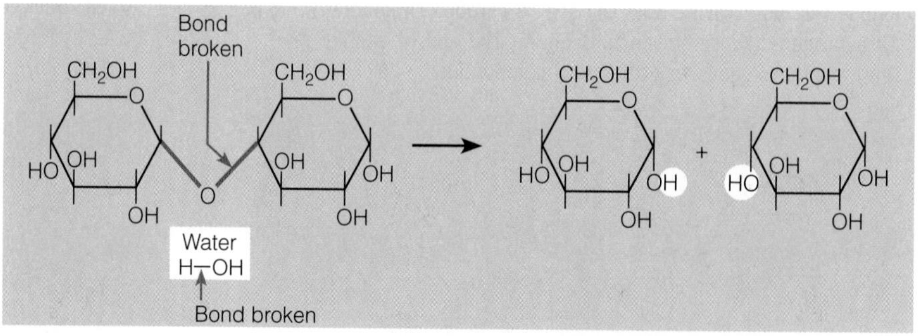
Bond broken
CH_2OH
O
HO
OH
Water
H–OH
Bond broken
+

Maltose → Glucose + glucose

The disaccharide maltose splits into two glucose molecules with H added to one and OH to the other (from the water molecule).

sucrose (SUE-krose): a disaccharide composed of glucose and fructose; commonly known as *table sugar, beet sugar,* or *cane sugar.* Sucrose also occurs in many fruits and some vegetables and grains.

- **sucro** = sugar
- 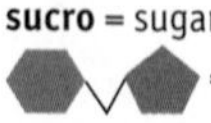 = sucrose

lactose (LAK-tose): a disaccharide composed of glucose and galactose; commonly known as *milk sugar.*

- **lact** = milk
- 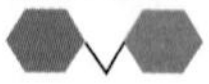 = lactose

lactose and its component galactose, which come from milk and milk products. Two monosaccharides can be linked together by a condensation reaction to form a disaccharide and water. A disaccharide, in turn, can be broken into its two monosaccharides by a hydrolysis reaction using water.

Polysaccharides

In contrast to the sugars just mentioned—the monosaccharides glucose, fructose, and galactose and the disaccharides maltose, sucrose, and lactose—the **polysaccharides** contain many glucose units and, in some cases, a few other monosaccharides strung together. Three types of polysaccharides are important in nutrition: glycogen, starches, and fibres.

Glycogen is a storage form of energy in the body; starch is the storage form of energy in plants; and fibres provide structure in stems, trunks, roots, leaves, and skins of plants. Both glycogen and starch are built of glucose units; fibres are composed of a variety of monosaccharides and other carbohydrate derivatives.

Glycogen

Glycogen is found to only a limited extent in meats and not at all in plants.* For this reason, food is not a significant source of this carbohydrate. However, glycogen performs an important role in the body: it stores glucose for future use. Glycogen is made of many glucose molecules linked together in highly branched chains (see the left side of Figure 4-8). When the hormonal message "release energy" arrives at the glycogen storage sites in a liver or muscle cell, enzymes respond by attacking the many branches of glycogen simultaneously, making a surge of glucose available.**

Starches

The human body stores glucose as glycogen, but plant cells store glucose as **starches**—long, branched or unbranched chains of hundreds or thousands of glucose molecules linked together (see the middle and right side of Figure 4-8). These giant starch molecules are packed side by side in grains such as wheat or rice, in root crops and tubers such as yams and potatoes, and in legumes such as peas and beans. When you eat the plant, your body hydrolyzes the starch to glucose and uses the glucose for its own energy purposes.

*Glycogen in animal muscles rapidly hydrolyzes after slaughter.

**Normally, liver cells produce glucose from glycogen to be sent *directly* to the blood; muscle cells can also produce glucose from glycogen, but must use it themselves. Muscle cells can restore the blood glucose level *indirectly*, however, as Chapter 7 explains.

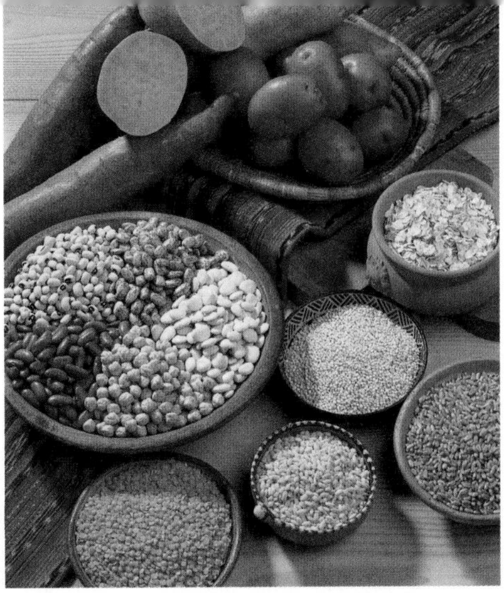

© Polara Studios, Inc.

Major sources of starch include grains (such as rice, wheat, millet, rye, barley, and oats), legumes (such as kidney beans, black-eyed peas, pinto beans, navy beans, and garbanzo beans), tubers (such as potatoes), and root crops (such as yams and cassava).

polysaccharides: compounds composed of many monosaccharides linked together. An intermediate string of three to ten monosaccharides is an *oligosaccharide*.

- **poly** = many
- **oligo** = few

glycogen (GLY-ko-jen): an animal polysaccharide composed of glucose; manufactured and stored in the liver and muscles as a storage form of glucose. Glycogen is not a significant food source of carbohydrate and is not counted as a dietary carbohydrate in foods.

- **glyco** = glucose
- **gen** = gives rise to

starches: plant polysaccharides composed of glucose.

FIGURE 4-8 Glycogen and Starch Molecules Compared (Small Segments)

These units would have to be magnified millions of times to appear at the size shown in this figure. For details of the chemical structures, see APPENDIX C.

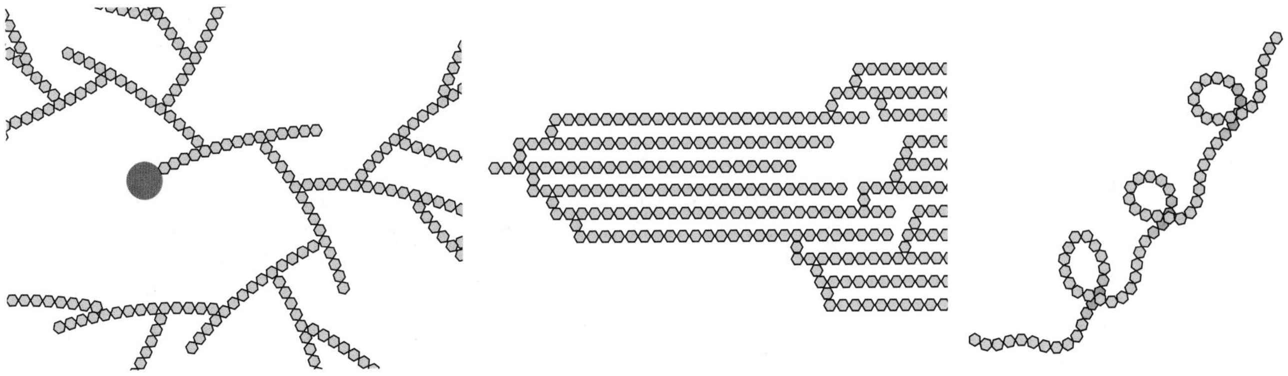

Glycogen

Starch (amylopectin)

Starch (amylose)

A glycogen molecule contains hundreds of glucose units in highly branched chains. Each new glycogen molecule needs a special protein for the attachment of the first glucose (shown here in red).

A starch molecule contains hundreds of glucose molecules in either occasionally branched chains (amylopectin) or unbranched chains (amylose).

FIGURE 4-9 Starch and Cellulose Molecules Compared (Small Segments)

The bonds that link the glucose molecules together in cellulose are different from the bonds in starch (and glycogen). Human enzymes cannot digest cellulose. See APPENDIX C for chemical structures and descriptions of linkages.

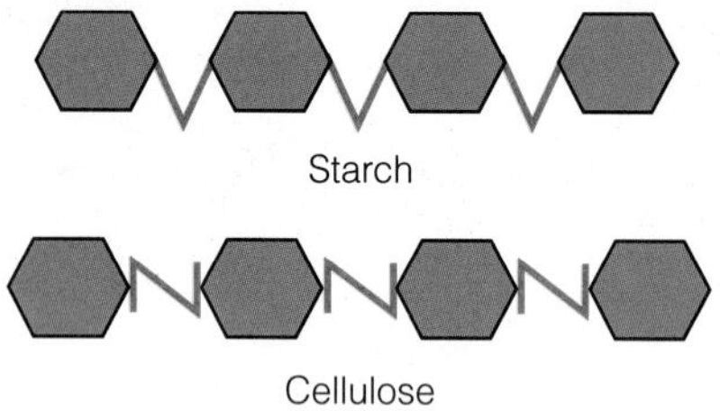
Starch
Cellulose

All starchy foods come from plants. Grains are the richest food source of starch, providing much of the food energy for people all over the world—rice in Asia; wheat in Canada, the United States, and Europe; corn in much of Central and South America; and millet, rye, barley, and oats elsewhere. Legumes and tubers are also important sources of starch. Some starch, such as that of cooked beans, digests more slowly and releases its glucose later in the digestion process. Less digestible starch, called **resistant starch**, is technically a kind of fibre and may behave similarly in the body. The starch of raw potatoes, for example, resists digestion; so does the resistant starch that forms during overheating of foods and the starch tucked inside the unbroken hulls of swallowed seeds. Some resistant starch may be digested, but slowly, and most remains intact until the bacteria of the colon eventually break it down. The rate of starch digestion may affect the body's handling of its glucose, as a later section explains.

Fibres **Dietary fibres** are the structural parts of plants and thus are found in all plant-derived foods—vegetables, fruits, whole grains, and legumes. Most dietary fibres are polysaccharides. As mentioned earlier, starches are also polysaccharides, but dietary fibres differ from starches in that the bonds between their monosaccharides cannot be broken down by digestive enzymes in the body. For this reason, dietary fibres are often described as *nonstarch polysaccharides*.* Figure 4-9 illustrates the difference in the bonds that link glucose molecules together in starch with those found in the fiber cellulose. Because dietary fibres pass through the body, they contribute no monosaccharides, and therefore little or no energy.

Even though most foods contain a variety of fibres, researchers often sort dietary fibres into two groups according to their solubility. Such distinctions help to explain their actions in the body.

Some dietary fibres dissolve in water (**soluble fibres**), form gels (**viscous**), and are easily digested by bacteria in the colon (**fermentable**). Commonly found in oats, barley, legumes, and citrus fruits, soluble fibres are most often associated with protecting against heart disease and diabetes by lowering blood cholesterol and glucose levels, respectively.[2]

Other fibres do not dissolve in water (**insoluble fibres**), do not form gels (nonviscous), and are less readily fermented. Found mostly in whole grains (bran) and vegetables, insoluble fibres promote bowel movements, alleviate constipation, and prevent diverticular disease.[3]

As mentioned, *dietary fibres* occur naturally in plants. When these fibres have been extracted from plants or are manufactured and then added to foods or used in supplements, they are called *functional fibres*—if they have beneficial health effects. Cellulose in cereals, for example, is a dietary fibre, but when consumed as a supplement to alleviate constipation, cellulose is considered a functional fibre. *Total fibre* refers to the sum of dietary fibres and functional fibres.

A few starches are classified as dietary fibres. Known as resistant starches, these starches escape digestion and absorption in the small intestine. Starch may resist digestion for several reasons, including the body's efficiency in digesting starches and the food's physical properties. Resistant starch is common in whole or partially milled grains, legumes, and just-ripened bananas. Cooked potatoes, pasta, and rice that have been chilled also contain resistant starch. Similar to insoluble fibres, resistant starch may support a healthy colon.[4]

Phytic acid is not a dietary fibre, but it is often found in the same foods. Because of this close association, researchers have been unable to determine whether it is the dietary fibre, the phytic acid, or both, that binds with minerals, preventing their absorption. This binding presents a risk of mineral deficiencies, but the risk is minimal when total fibre intake is reasonable (less than 40 grams a day) and mineral intake adequate. The nutrition consequences of mineral losses are described further in Chapters 13 and 14.

resistant starch: starch that, for the most part, escapes digestion and absorption in the small intestine of healthy people.

dietary fibres: in plant foods, the *nonstarch polysaccharides* that are not digested by human digestive enzymes, although some are digested by GI tract bacteria. Dietary fibres include cellulose, hemicelluloses, pectins, gums, and mucilages as well as the nonpolysaccharides lignins, cutins, and tannins.

soluble fibres: nonstarch polysaccharides that dissolve in water to form a gel. An example is pectin from fruit, which is used to thicken jellies.

viscous: a gel-like consistency.

fermentable: the extent to which bacteria in the GI tract can break down fibres to fragments that the body can use.*

insoluble fibres: nonstarch polysaccharides that do not dissolve in water. Examples include the tough, fibrous structures found in the strings of celery and the skins of corn kernels.

phytic (FYE-tick) **acid:** a nonnutrient component of plant seeds; also called *phytate* (FYE-tate). Phytic acid occurs in the husks of grains, legumes, and seeds and is capable of binding minerals such as zinc, iron, calcium, magnesium, and copper in insoluble complexes in the intestine, which the body excretes unused.

*Dietary fibres are fermented by bacteria in the colon to short-chain fatty acids, which are absorbed and metabolized by cells in the GI tract and liver (Chapter 5 describes fatty acids).

*The nonstarch polysaccharide fibres include cellulose, hemicelluloses, pectins, gums, and mucilages. Fibres also include some *nonpolysaccharides* such as lignins, cutins, and tannins.

IN SUMMARY The polysaccharides are chains of monosaccharides and include glycogen, starches, and dietary fibres. Both glycogen and starch are storage forms of glucose—glycogen in the body, and starch in plants—and both yield energy for human use. The dietary fibres also contain glucose (and other monosaccharides), but their bonds cannot be broken by human digestive enzymes, so they yield little, if any, energy. The following summarizes the carbohydrate family of compounds.

The Carbohydrate Family

- Monosaccharides
  Glucose
  Fructose
  Galactose
- Disaccharides
  Maltose (glucose + glucose)
  Sucrose (glucose + fructose)
  Lactose (glucose + galactose)
- Polysaccharides:
  Glycogen[a]
  Starches (amylose and amylopectin)
  Fibres (soluble and insoluble)

[a]Glycogen is a polysaccharide, but not a dietary source of carbohydrate.

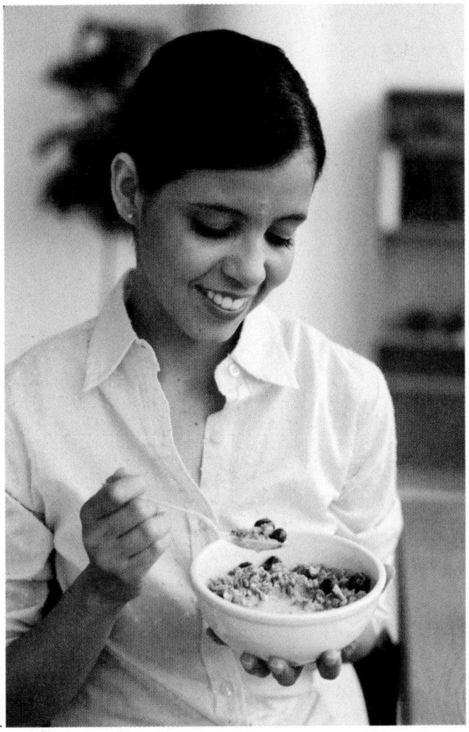

photos.com

When a person eats carbohydrate-rich foods, the body receives a valuable commodity—glucose.

Digestion and Absorption of Carbohydrates

The ultimate goal of digestion and absorption of sugars and starches is to break them into small molecules—chiefly glucose—that the body can absorb and use. The large starch molecules require extensive breakdown; the disaccharides need only be broken once and the monosaccharides not at all. The details follow.

Carbohydrate Digestion

Figure 4-10 (p. 100) traces the digestion of carbohydrates through the GI tract. When a person eats foods containing starch, enzymes hydrolyze the long chains to shorter chains, ♦ the short chains to disaccharides, and, finally, the disaccharides to monosaccharides. This process begins in the mouth.

♦ The short chains of glucose units that result from the breakdown of starch are known as *dextrins*. The word sometimes appears on food labels because dextrins can be used as thickening agents in processed foods.

In the Mouth In the mouth, thoroughly chewing high-fibre foods slows eating and stimulates the flow of saliva. The salivary enzyme **amylase** starts to work, hydrolyzing starch to shorter polysaccharides and to the disaccharide maltose. In fact, you can taste the change if you chew a piece of starchy food like a cracker and hold it in your mouth for a few minutes without swallowing it—the cracker begins tasting sweeter as the enzyme acts on it. Because food is in the mouth for a relatively short time, very little carbohydrate digestion takes place there; it begins again in the small intestine.

In the Stomach The swallowed bolus ♦ mixes with the stomach's acid and protein-digesting enzymes, which inactivate salivary amylase. Thus the role of salivary amylase in starch digestion is relatively minor. To a small extent, the stomach's acid continues breaking down starch, but its juices contain no enzymes to digest carbohydrate. Fibres linger in the stomach and delay gastric emptying, thereby providing a feeling of fullness and **satiety**.

♦ A **bolus** is a portion of food swallowed at one time.

♦ In general, the word ending **-ase** identifies an enzyme, and the beginning of the word identifies the molecule that the enzyme works on.

In the Small Intestine The small intestine performs most of the work of carbohydrate digestion. A major carbohydrate-digesting enzyme, pancreatic amylase, enters the intestine via the pancreatic duct and continues breaking down the polysaccharides to shorter glucose chains and maltose. The final step takes place on the outer membranes of the intestinal cells. There specific enzymes ♦ break down specific disaccharides:

amylase (AM-ih-lace): an enzyme that hydrolyzes amylose (a form of starch). Amylase is a **carbohydrase,** an enzyme that breaks down carbohydrates.

satiety (sah-TIE-eh-tee): the feeling of fullness and satisfaction that occurs after a meal and inhibits eating until the next meal. Satiety determines how much time passes between meals.

- **sate** = to fill

FIGURE 4-10 Carbohydrate Digestion in the GI Tract

STARCH

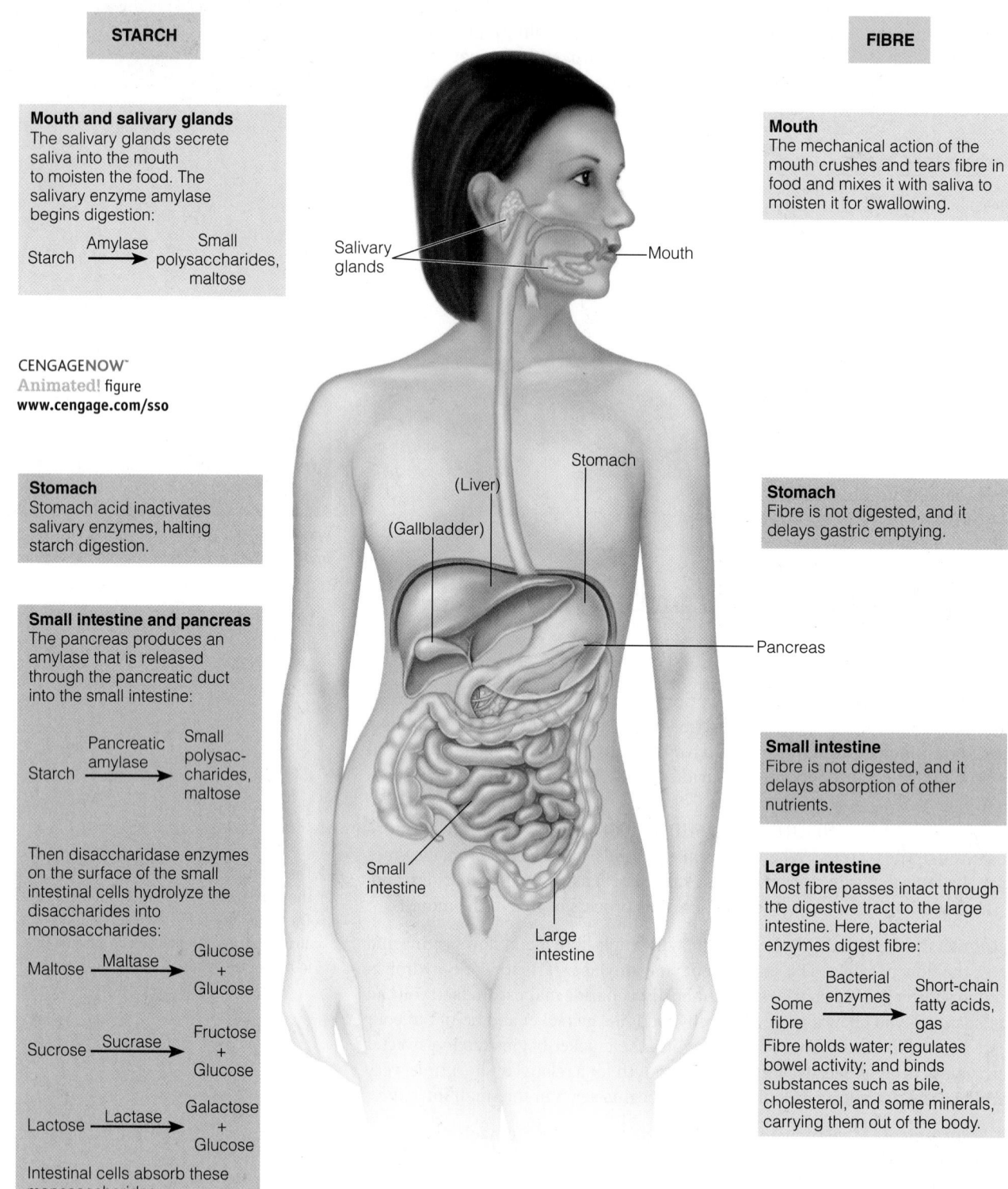

Mouth and salivary glands
The salivary glands secrete saliva into the mouth to moisten the food. The salivary enzyme amylase begins digestion:

Starch —Amylase→ Small polysaccharides, maltose

CENGAGENOW™
Animated! figure
www.cengage.com/sso

Stomach
Stomach acid inactivates salivary enzymes, halting starch digestion.

Small intestine and pancreas
The pancreas produces an amylase that is released through the pancreatic duct into the small intestine:

Starch —Pancreatic amylase→ Small polysaccharides, maltose

Then disaccharidase enzymes on the surface of the small intestinal cells hydrolyze the disaccharides into monosaccharides:

Maltose —Maltase→ Glucose + Glucose

Sucrose —Sucrase→ Fructose + Glucose

Lactose —Lactase→ Galactose + Glucose

Intestinal cells absorb these monosaccharides.

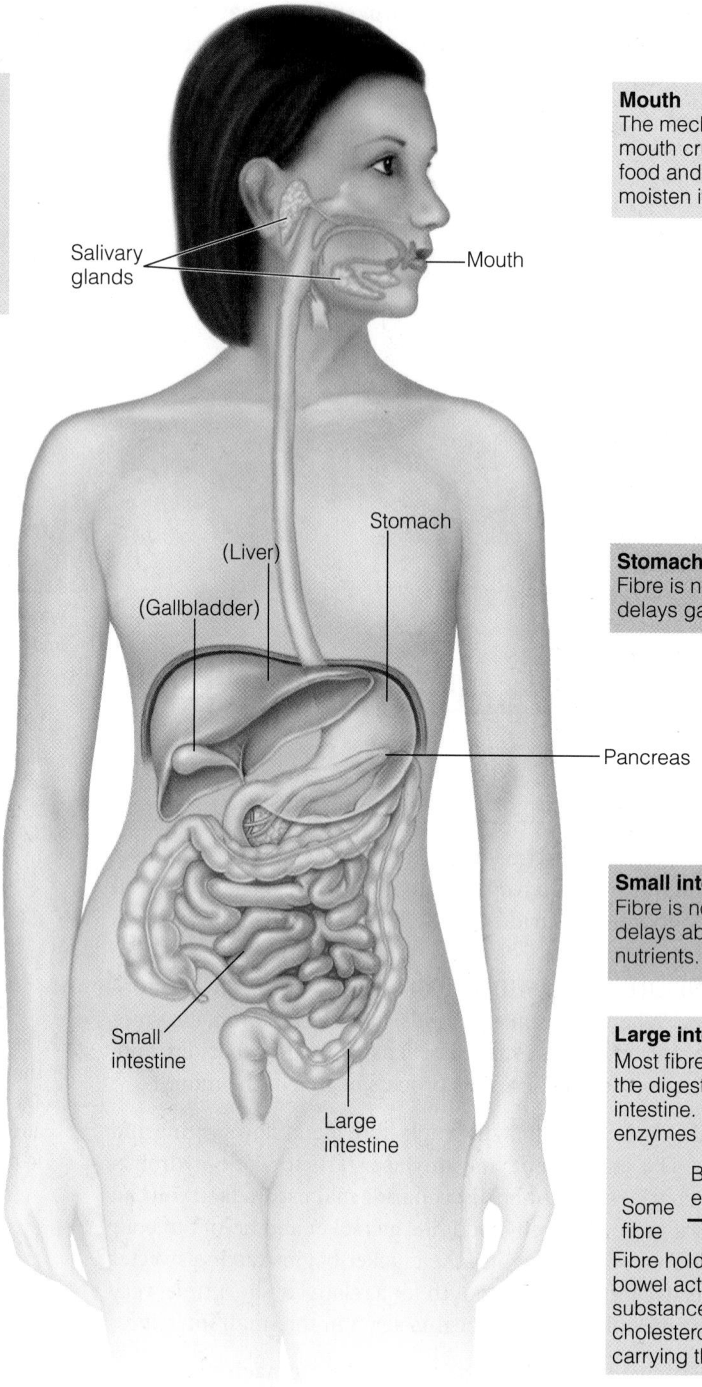
Salivary glands
Mouth
Stomach
(Liver)
(Gallbladder)
Pancreas
Small intestine
Large intestine

FIBRE

Mouth
The mechanical action of the mouth crushes and tears fibre in food and mixes it with saliva to moisten it for swallowing.

Stomach
Fibre is not digested, and it delays gastric emptying.

Small intestine
Fibre is not digested, and it delays absorption of other nutrients.

Large intestine
Most fibre passes intact through the digestive tract to the large intestine. Here, bacterial enzymes digest fibre:

Some fibre —Bacterial enzymes→ Short-chain fatty acids, gas

Fibre holds water; regulates bowel activity; and binds substances such as bile, cholesterol, and some minerals, carrying them out of the body.

- **Maltase** breaks maltose into two glucose molecules.
- **Sucrase** breaks sucrose into one glucose and one fructose molecule.
- **Lactase** breaks lactose into one glucose and one galactose molecule.

At this point, all polysaccharides and disaccharides have been broken down to monosaccharides—mostly glucose molecules, with some fructose and galactose molecules as well.

maltase: an enzyme that hydrolyzes maltose.
sucrase: an enzyme that hydrolyzes sucrose.
lactase: an enzyme that hydrolyzes lactose.

In the Large Intestine Within one to four hours after a meal, all the sugars and most of the starches have been digested. ♦ Only the fibres remain in the digestive tract. Fibres in the large intestine attract water, which softens the stools for passage without straining. Also, bacteria in the GI tract ferment some fibres. This process generates water, gas, and short-chain fatty acids (described in Chapter 5).* The cells of the colon use these small fat molecules for energy. Metabolism of short-chain fatty acids also occurs in the cells of the liver. Fibres, therefore, can contribute some energy (1.5 to 2.5 kcalories per gram), depending on the extent to which they are broken down by bacteria and the fatty acids are absorbed. How much energy fibre contributes to a person's daily intake remains unclear.[5]

♦ Starches and sugars are called *available carbohydrates* because human digestive enzymes break them down for the body's use. In contrast, fibres are called *unavailable carbohydrates* because human digestive enzymes cannot break their bonds.

Carbohydrate Absorption

Glucose is unique in that it can be absorbed to some extent through the lining of the mouth, but for the most part, nutrient absorption takes place in the small intestine. Glucose and galactose enter the cells lining the small intestine by active transport; fructose is absorbed by facilitated diffusion, which slows its entry and produces a smaller rise in blood glucose. Likewise, unbranched chains of starch are digested slowly and produce a smaller rise in blood glucose than branched chains, which have many more places for enzymes to attack and release glucose rapidly (review Figure 4-8 on p. 97).

As the blood from the small intestine circulates through the liver, cells there take up fructose and galactose and convert them to other compounds, most often to glucose, as shown in Figure 4-11. Thus all disaccharides provide at least one glucose molecule directly, and they can provide another one indirectly—through the conversion of fructose and galactose to glucose in the liver.

IN SUMMARY **In the digestion and absorption of carbohydrates, the body breaks down starches into the disaccharide maltose. Maltose and the other disaccharides (lactose and sucrose) from foods are broken down into monosaccharides, which are absorbed. When these monosaccharides arrive at the liver, they are converted mostly to glucose to provide energy for the cells' work. The fibres help to regulate the passage of food through the GI system and slow the absorption of glucose, but they contribute little, if any, energy.**

*The short-chain fatty acids produced by GI bacteria are primarily acetic acid, propionic acid, and butyric acid.

FIGURE 4-11 Absorption of Monosaccharides

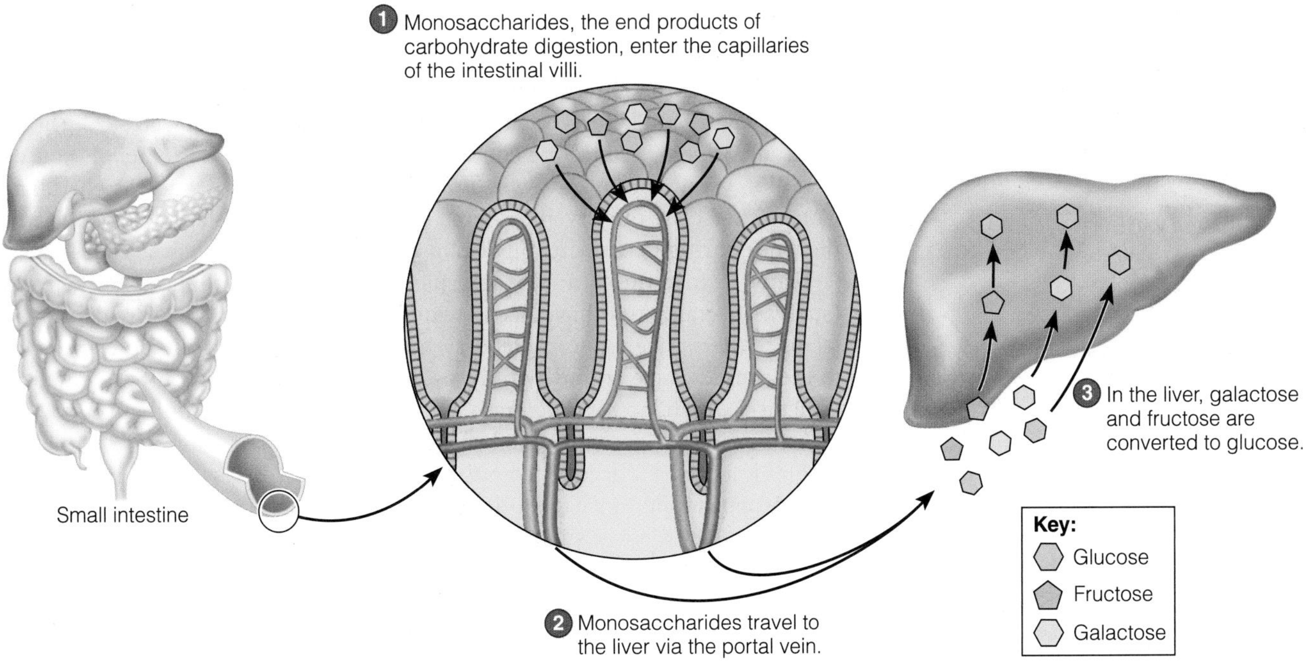
1 Monosaccharides, the end products of carbohydrate digestion, enter the capillaries of the intestinal villi.
Small intestine
2 Monosaccharides travel to the liver via the portal vein.
3 In the liver, galactose and fructose are converted to glucose.
Key:
Glucose
Fructose
Galactose

Lactose Intolerance Normally, the intestinal cells produce enough of the enzyme lactase to ensure that the disaccharide lactose found in milk is both digested and absorbed efficiently. Lactase activity is highest immediately after birth, as befits an infant whose first and only food for a while will be breast milk or infant formula. In the great majority of the world's populations, lactase activity declines dramatically during childhood and adolescence to about 5 to 10 percent of the activity at birth. Only a relatively small percentage (about 30 percent) of the people in the world retain enough lactase to digest and absorb lactose efficiently throughout adult life.

Symptoms When more lactose is consumed than the available lactase can handle, lactose molecules remain in the intestine undigested, attracting water and causing bloating, abdominal discomfort, and diarrhea—the symptoms of **lactose intolerance.** The undigested lactose becomes food for intestinal bacteria, which multiply and produce irritating acid and gas, further contributing to the discomfort and diarrhea.

Causes As mentioned, lactase activity commonly declines with age. **Lactase deficiency** may also develop when the intestinal villi are damaged by disease, certain medicines, prolonged diarrhea, or malnutrition. Depending on the extent of the intestinal damage, lactose malabsorption may be temporary or permanent. In extremely rare cases, an infant is born with a lactase deficiency, making feeding a challenge.

Prevalence The prevalence ♦ of lactose intolerance varies widely among ethnic groups, indicating that the trait is genetically determined.[6] The prevalence of lactose intolerance is lowest among Scandinavians and other northern Europeans and highest among Aboriginal peoples and Southeast Asians. Although data on lactose intolerance are not readily available for Canada, an estimated 30 to 50 million people in the United States are lactose intolerant.

♦ Estimated prevalence of lactose intolerance:
- 80% Southeast Asians
- 80% Aboriginal peoples
- 75% African Americans
- 70% Mediterranean peoples
- 60% Inuits
- 50% Hispanics
- 20% Caucasians
- 10% Northern Europeans

Dietary Changes Managing lactose intolerance requires some dietary changes, although total elimination of milk products usually is not necessary. Excluding all milk products from the diet can lead to nutrient deficiencies because these foods are a major source of several nutrients, notably the mineral calcium, vitamin D, and the B vitamin riboflavin. Fortunately, many people with lactose intolerance can consume foods containing up to 6 grams of lactose (125 mL or ½ cup milk) without symptoms. The most successful strategies are to increase intake of milk products gradually, take them with other foods in meals, and spread their intake throughout the day. In addition, yogurt containing live bacteria seems to improve lactose intolerance.[7] A change in the type, number, and activity of GI bacteria—not the reappearance of the missing enzyme—accounts for the ability to adapt to milk products.[8] Importantly, most lactose-intolerant individuals need to *manage* their dairy consumption rather than *restrict* it.

In many cases, lactose-intolerant people can tolerate fermented milk products such as yogurt and **kefir.** The bacteria in these products digest lactose for their own use, thus reducing the lactose content. Even when the lactose content is equivalent to milk's, yogurt produces fewer symptoms. Hard cheeses, such as cheddar, and cottage cheese are often well tolerated because most of the lactose is removed with the whey during manufacturing. Lactose continues to diminish as cheese ages.

Many lactose-intolerant people use commercially prepared milk products (such as Lactaid) that have been treated with an enzyme that breaks down the lactose. Alternatively, they take enzyme tablets with meals or add enzyme drops to their milk. The enzyme hydrolyzes much of the lactose in milk to glucose and galactose, which lactose-intolerant people can absorb without ill effects.

Because people's tolerance to lactose varies widely, lactose-restricted diets must be highly individualized. A completely lactose-free diet can be difficult because lactose appears not only in milk and milk products but also as an ingredient in many nondairy foods ♦ such as breads, cereals, breakfast drinks, salad dressings, and cake mixes. People on strict lactose-free diets need to read labels and avoid foods that include milk, milk solids, whey (milk liquid), and casein (milk protein, which may contain traces of lactose). They also need to check all medications

♦ Lactose in selected foods:

Whole-wheat bread, 1 slice	0.5 g
Dinner roll, 1	0.5 g
Cheese, 1 oz	
Cheddar	0.5 g
Parmesan or cream	0.8 g
Doughnut (cake type), 1	1.2 g
Chocolate bar, 1 oz	2.3 g
Sherbet, 1 c	4.0 g
Cottage cheese (2%), 1 c	7.5 g
Ice cream, 1 c	9.0 g
Milk, 1 c	12.0 g
Yogurt (2%), 1 c	15.0 g

NOTE: Yogurt is often enriched with nonfat milk solids, which increase its lactose content to a level higher than milk's.

lactose intolerance: a condition that results from inability to digest the milk sugar lactose; characterized by bloating, gas, abdominal discomfort, and diarrhea. Lactose intolerance differs from milk allergy, which is caused by an immune reaction to the protein in milk.

lactase deficiency: a lack of the enzyme required to digest the disaccharide lactose into its component monosaccharides (glucose and galactose).

kefir (keh-FUR): a fermented milk created by adding *Lactobacillus acidophilus* and other bacteria that break down lactose to glucose and galactose, producing a sweet, lactose-free product.

with the pharmacist because 20 percent of prescription drugs and 5 percent of over-the-counter drugs contain lactose as a filler.

People who consume few or no milk products must take care to meet riboflavin, vitamin D, and calcium needs. Later chapters on the vitamins and minerals offer help with finding good nonmilk sources of these nutrients.

IN SUMMARY **Lactose intolerance is a common condition that occurs when there is insufficient lactase to digest the disaccharide lactose found in milk and milk products. Symptoms include GI distress. Because treatment requires limiting milk intake, other sources of riboflavin, vitamin D, and calcium must be included in the diet.**

Glucose in the Body

The primary role of the available carbohydrates in the body is to supply the cells with glucose for energy. Starch contributes most to the body's glucose supply, but as explained earlier, any of the monosaccharides can also provide glucose.

Scientists have long known that providing energy is glucose's primary role in the body, but they have recently uncovered additional roles that glucose and other sugars perform in the body. ♦ When sugar molecules adhere to the body's protein and fat molecules, the consequences can be dramatic. Sugars attached to a protein change the protein's shape and function; when they bind to lipids in a cell's membranes, sugars alter the way cells recognize one another. ♦

♦ The study of sugars is known as *glycobiology*.

♦ These combination molecules are known as *glycoproteins* and *glycolipids*, respectively.

A Preview of Carbohydrate Metabolism

Glucose plays the central role in carbohydrate metabolism. This brief discussion provides just enough information about carbohydrate metabolism to illustrate that the body needs and uses glucose as a chief energy nutrient. Chapter 7 provides a full description of energy metabolism, and Chapter 10 shows how the B vitamins participate.

Storing Glucose as Glycogen The liver stores about one-third of the body's total glycogen and releases glucose into the bloodstream as needed. After a meal, blood glucose rises, and liver cells link the excess glucose molecules by condensation reactions into long, branching chains of glycogen. When blood glucose falls, the liver cells break glycogen by hydrolysis reactions into single molecules of glucose and release them into the bloodstream. Thus a limited amount of glucose becomes available to supply energy to the brain and other tissues regardless of whether the person has eaten recently. Muscle cells can also store glucose as glycogen (the other two-thirds), but they hoard most of their supply, using some of the energy in the glucose molecules just for themselves during exercise. The brain maintains a small amount of glycogen, which is thought to provide an emergency energy reserve during times of severe glucose deprivation.

Glycogen holds water and, therefore, is rather bulky. The body can store only enough glycogen to provide energy for relatively short periods of time—less than a day during rest and a few hours at most during exercise. For its long-term energy reserves, for use over days or weeks of food deprivation, the body uses its abundant, water-free fuel, fat, as Chapter 5 describes.

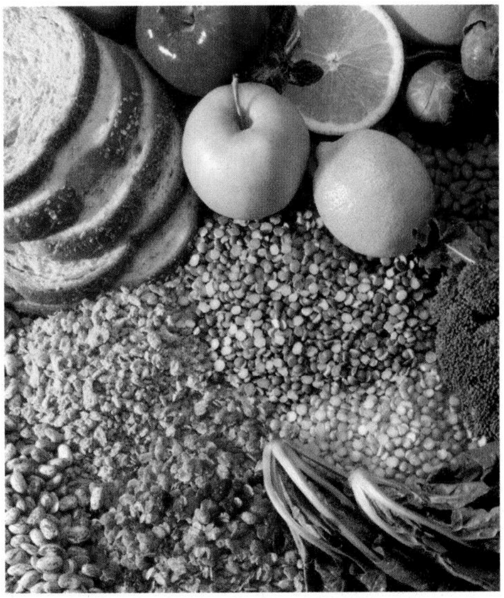

Brian Leatart/Getty Images

The carbohydrates of grains, vegetables, fruits, and legumes supply most of the energy in a healthful diet.

Using Glucose for Energy Glucose fuels the work of most of the body's cells. Inside a cell, enzymes break glucose in half. These halves can be put back together to make glucose, or they can be further broken down into even smaller fragments (never again to be reassembled to form glucose). The small fragments can yield energy when broken down completely to carbon dioxide and water (see Chapter 7).

As mentioned, the liver's glycogen stores last only for hours, not for days. To keep providing glucose to meet the body's energy needs, a person has to eat dietary carbohydrate frequently. Yet people who do not always attend faithfully to their bodies' carbohydrate needs still survive. How do they manage without glucose from dietary carbohydrate? Do they simply draw energy from the other two

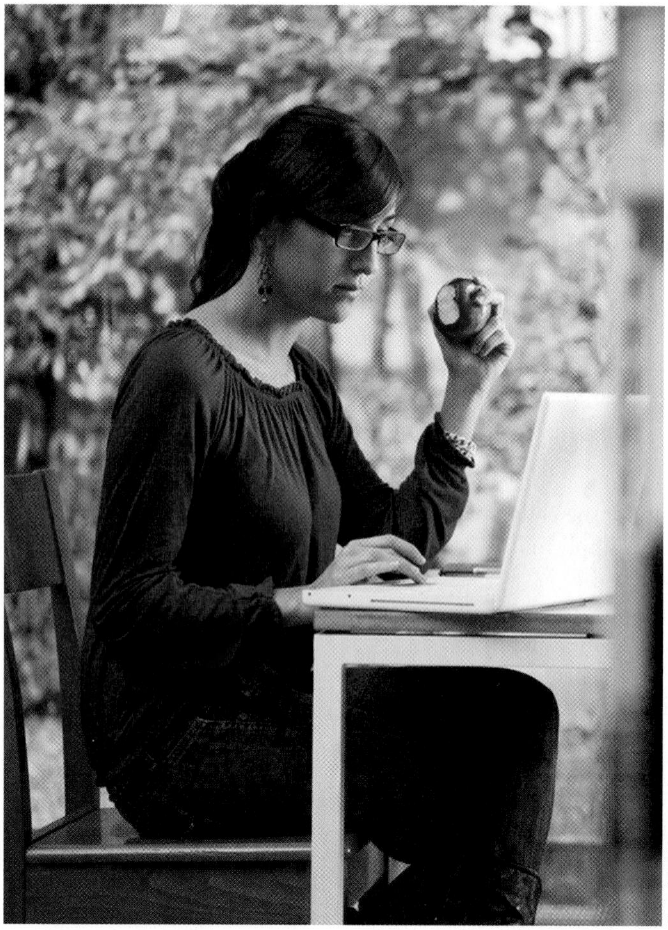
Diego Cervo/shutterstock

The brain uses glucose as its primary fuel for energy.

energy-yielding nutrients, fat and protein? They do draw energy from them, but not simply.

Making Glucose from Protein Glucose is the preferred energy source for brain cells, other nerve cells, and red blood cells. The amino acids of protein can be converted to glucose to some extent, but amino acids and proteins have jobs of their own that no other nutrient can perform. Fat cannot be converted to glucose to any significant extent. Thus, when a person does not replenish depleted glycogen stores by eating carbohydrate, body proteins are broken down to make glucose to fuel the brain and other special cells. These body proteins derive primarily from the liver and skeletal muscles.

The conversion of protein to glucose is called **gluconeogenesis**—literally, the making of new glucose. Only adequate dietary carbohydrate can prevent this use of protein for energy, and this role of carbohydrate is known as its **protein-sparing action.**

Making Ketone Bodies from Fat Fragments An inadequate supply of carbohydrate can shift the body's energy metabolism in a precarious direction. With less carbohydrate providing glucose to meet the brain's energy needs, fat takes an alternative metabolic pathway; instead of entering the main energy pathway, fat fragments combine with one another, forming **ketone bodies.** Ketone bodies provide an alternate fuel source during starvation, but when their production exceeds their use, they accumulate in the blood, causing **ketosis.** Because most ketone bodies are acidic, ketosis disturbs the body's normal **acid–base balance.** (Chapter 7 explores ketosis and the metabolic consequences of low-carbohydrate diets further.)

To spare body protein and prevent ketosis, the body needs at least 50 to 100 grams of carbohydrate a day. Dietary recommendations urge people to select abundantly from carbohydrate-rich foods to provide for considerably more.

Using Glucose to Make Fat After meeting its immediate energy needs and filling its glycogen stores to capacity, the body must find a way to handle any extra glucose. When glucose is abundant, energy metabolism shifts to use more glucose instead of fat. If that isn't enough to restore glucose balance, the liver breaks glucose into smaller molecules and puts them together into the more permanent energy-storage compound—fat. Thus, when carbohydrate is abundant, fat is either conserved (by using more carbohydrate in the fuel mix) or created (by using excess carbohydrate to make body fat). The fat then travels to the fatty tissues of the body for storage. Unlike the liver cells, which can store only enough glycogen to meet less than a day's energy needs, fat cells can store seemingly unlimited quantities of fat.

The Constancy of Blood Glucose

Every body cell depends on glucose for its fuel to some extent, and the cells of the brain and the rest of the nervous system depend almost exclusively on glucose for their energy. The activities of these cells never cease, and they have limited ability to store glucose. Day and night, they continually draw on the supply of glucose in the fluid surrounding them. To maintain the supply, a steady stream of blood moves past these cells bringing more glucose from either the small intestine (food) or the liver (via glycogen breakdown or gluconeogenesis).[9]

Maintaining Glucose Homeostasis To function optimally, the body must maintain blood glucose within limits that permit the cells to nourish themselves. If blood glucose falls below normal, ♦ a person may become dizzy and weak; if it

♦ Normal blood glucose (fasting): 4–6 mmol/L (published values vary slightly).

gluconeogenesis (gloo-ko-nee-oh-JEN-ih-sis): the making of glucose from a noncarbohydrate source (described in more detail in Chapter 7).
- **gluco** = glucose
- **neo** = new
- **genesis** = making

protein-sparing action: the action of carbohydrate (and fat) in providing energy that allows protein to be used for other purposes.

ketone (KEE-tone) **bodies:** the metabolic products of the incomplete breakdown of fat when glucose is not available in the cells.

ketosis (kee-TOE-sis): an undesirably high concentration of ketone bodies in the blood and urine.

acid–base balance: the equilibrium in the body between acid and base concentrations (see Chapter 11).

FIGURE 4-12 Maintaining Blood Glucose Homeostasis

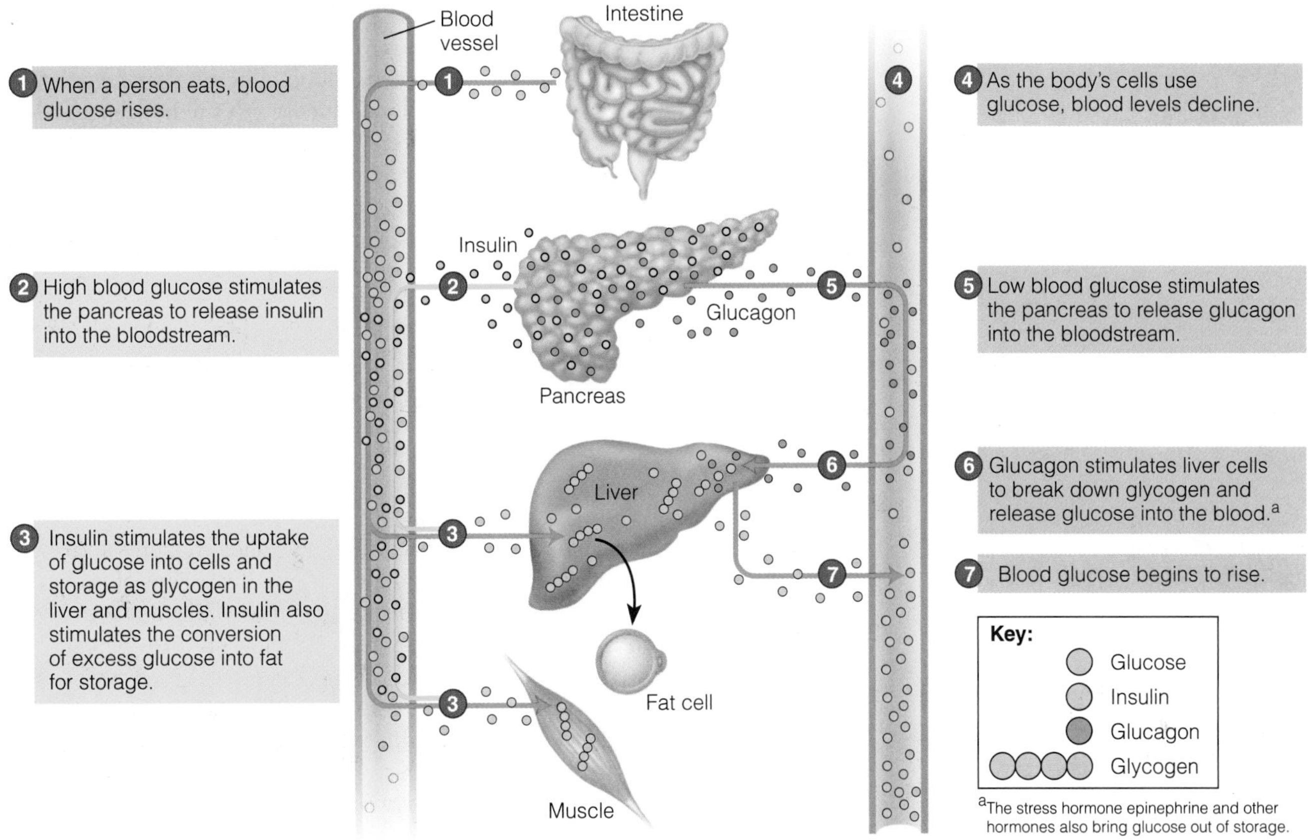

1 When a person eats, blood glucose rises.
2 High blood glucose stimulates the pancreas to release insulin into the bloodstream.
3 Insulin stimulates the uptake of glucose into cells and storage as glycogen in the liver and muscles. Insulin also stimulates the conversion of excess glucose into fat for storage.
Blood vessel
Intestine
Insulin
Pancreas
Glucagon
Liver
Fat cell
Muscle
4 As the body's cells use glucose, blood levels decline.
5 Low blood glucose stimulates the pancreas to release glucagon into the bloodstream.
6 Glucagon stimulates liver cells to break down glycogen and release glucose into the blood.a
7 Blood glucose begins to rise.
Key:
Glucose
Insulin
Glucagon
Glycogen

[a]The stress hormone epinephrine and other hormones also bring glucose out of storage.

rises above normal, a person may become fatigued. Left untreated, fluctuations to the extremes—either high or low—can be fatal.

The Regulating Hormones Blood glucose homeostasis ♦ is regulated primarily by two hormones: *insulin,* which helps to move glucose from the blood into some tissues, and *glucagon,* which brings glucose out of storage in the liver when necessary. Figure 4-12 depicts these hormonal regulators at work.

After a meal, as blood glucose rises, special cells of the pancreas respond by secreting **insulin** into the blood.* In general, the amount of insulin secreted corresponds with the rise in glucose. As the circulating insulin contacts the receptors on the body's other cells, the receptors respond by stimulating a series of reactions that result in ushering glucose from the blood into the cells. Most of the cells take only the glucose they can use for energy right away, but the liver and muscle cells can assemble the small glucose units into long, branching chains of glycogen for storage. The liver cells can also convert extra glucose to fat for export to other cells. Thus elevated blood glucose returns to normal levels as excess glucose is stored as glycogen and fat.

When blood glucose falls (as occurs between meals), other special cells of the pancreas respond by secreting **glucagon** into the blood.** Glucagon raises blood glucose by signalling the liver to break down its glycogen stores and release glucose into the blood for use by all the other body cells.

Another hormone that signals the liver cells to release glucose is the "fight-or-flight" hormone, **epinephrine.** When a person experiences stress, epinephrine acts quickly to ensure that all the body cells have energy fuel in emergencies.

♦ **Homeostasis** is the maintenance of constant internal conditions by the body's control systems.

insulin (IN-suh-lin): a hormone secreted by special cells in the pancreas in response to (among other things) increased blood glucose concentration. The primary role of insulin is to control the transport of glucose from the bloodstream into the muscle and fat cells.

glucagon (GLOO-ka-gon): a hormone that is secreted by special cells in the pancreas in response to low blood glucose concentration and elicits release of glucose from liver glycogen stores.

epinephrine (EP-ih-NEFF-rin): a hormone of the adrenal gland that modulates the stress response; formerly called *adrenaline*. When administered by injection, epinephrine counteracts anaphylactic shock by opening the airways and maintaining heartbeat and blood pressure.

*The *beta* (BAY-tuh) *cells*, one of several types of cells in the pancreas, secrete insulin in response to elevated blood glucose concentration.
**The *alpha cells* of the pancreas secrete glucagon in response to low blood glucose.

Among its many roles in the body, epinephrine works to release glucose from liver glycogen to the blood.

Balancing within the Normal Range The maintenance of normal blood glucose ordinarily depends on two processes. When blood glucose falls below normal, food can replenish it, or in the absence of food, glucagon can signal the liver to break down glycogen stores. When blood glucose rises above normal, insulin can signal the cells to take in glucose for energy. Eating balanced meals at regular intervals helps the body maintain a happy medium between the extremes. Balanced meals that provide abundant carbohydrates, including fibres, and a little fat help to slow down the digestion and absorption of carbohydrate so that glucose enters the blood gradually.

Falling outside the Normal Range The influence of foods on blood glucose has given rise to the oversimplification that foods *govern* blood glucose concentrations. Foods do not; the body does. In some people, however, blood glucose regulation fails. When this happens, either of two conditions can result: diabetes or hypoglycemia. People with these conditions need to plan their diets and physical activities to help maintain their blood glucose within a normal range.

♦ Blood glucose (fasting):
- Prediabetes: 6.1–6.9 mmol/L
- Diabetes: ≥7.0 mmol/L

Fasting blood tests are repeated to confirm a diagnosis. Blood glucose levels higher than normal, but below the diagnosis of diabetes, is sometimes called **prediabetes.**

Diabetes In **diabetes**, blood glucose rises after a meal and remains above normal levels ♦ because insulin is either inadequate or ineffective. Thus *blood* glucose is central to diabetes, but *dietary* carbohydrate does not cause diabetes. Furthermore, the Canadian Diabetes Association indicates that up to 10 percent of total energy from sucrose (sugar) is acceptable.

There are two main types of diabetes. In **type 1 diabetes**, the less common type, the pancreas fails to produce insulin. Although the exact cause is unclear, some research suggests that in genetically susceptible people, certain viruses activate the immune system to attack and destroy cells in the pancreas as if they were foreign cells. In **type 2 diabetes**, the more common type of diabetes, the cells fail to respond effectively to insulin. This condition tends to occur as a consequence of obesity. As the incidence of obesity in Canada has risen in recent decades, the incidence of diabetes has followed. This trend is most notable among children and adolescents as obesity among the nation's youth reaches epidemic proportions. Because obesity can precipitate type 2 diabetes, the best preventive measure is to maintain a healthy body weight.

Concentrated sweets are not strictly excluded from the diabetic diet as they once were; they can be eaten in limited amounts with meals as part of a healthy diet. Chapter 16 describes the type of diabetes that develops in some women during pregnancy (gestational diabetes), and Chapter 19 gives full coverage to type 1 and type 2 diabetes and their associated problems.

Hypoglycemia In healthy people, blood glucose rises after eating and then gradually falls back into the normal range. The transition occurs without notice. Should blood glucose drop below normal, a person would experience the symptoms of **hypoglycemia**: weakness, rapid heartbeat, sweating, anxiety, hunger, and trembling. Most commonly, hypoglycemia is a consequence of poorly managed diabetes: too much insulin, strenuous physical activity, inadequate food intake, or illness that causes blood glucose levels to plummet.

Hypoglycemia in healthy people is rare. Most people who experience hypoglycemia need only adjust their diets by replacing refined carbohydrates with fibre-rich carbohydrates and ensuring an adequate protein intake at each meal. In addition, smaller meals eaten more frequently may help. Hypoglycemia caused by certain medications, pancreatic tumours, overuse of insulin, alcohol abuse, uncontrolled diabetes, or other illnesses requires medical intervention.

diabetes (DYE-uh-BEET-eez): a chronic disorder of carbohydrate metabolism, usually resulting from insufficient or ineffective insulin.

type 1 diabetes: the less common type of diabetes in which the pancreas fails to produce insulin.

type 2 diabetes: the more common type of diabetes in which the cells fail to respond to insulin.

hypoglycemia (HIGH-po-gly-SEE-me-ah): an abnormally low blood glucose concentration.

glycemic (gly-SEEM-ic) **response:** the extent to which a food raises the blood glucose concentration and elicits an insulin response.

The Glycemic Response The **glycemic response** refers to how quickly glucose is absorbed after a person eats, how high blood glucose rises, and how quickly it returns to normal. Slow absorption, a modest rise in blood glucose, and a smooth return to normal are desirable (a low glycemic response). Fast absorption, a surge

FIGURE 4-13 **Glycemic Index of Selected Foods**

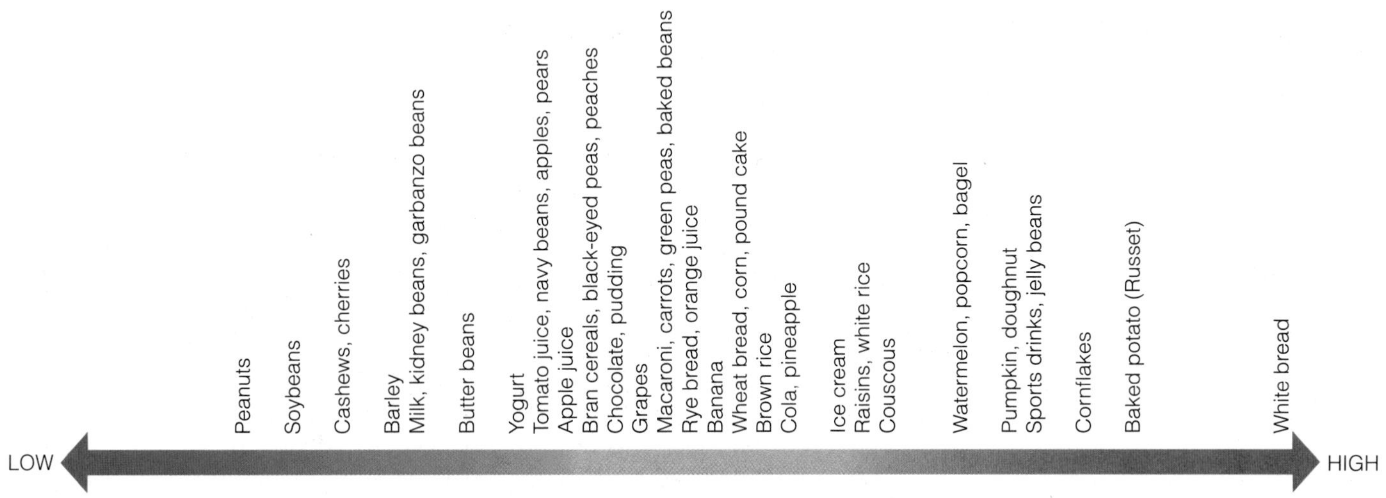
LOW
Peanuts
Soybeans
Cashews, cherries
Barley
Milk, kidney beans, garbanzo beans
Butter beans
Yogurt
Tomato juice, navy beans, apples, pears
Apple juice
Bran cereals, black-eyed peas, peaches
Chocolate, pudding
Grapes
Macaroni, carrots, green peas, baked beans
Rye bread, orange juice
Banana
Wheat bread, corn, pound cake
Brown rice
Cola, pineapple
Ice cream
Raisins, white rice
Couscous
Watermelon, popcorn, bagel
Pumpkin, doughnut
Sports drinks, jelly beans
Cornflakes
Baked potato (Russet)
White bread
HIGH

in blood glucose, and an overreaction that plunges glucose below normal are less desirable (a high glycemic response). Different foods have different effects on blood glucose.

The rate of glucose absorption is particularly important to people with diabetes, who may benefit from limiting foods that produce too great a rise, or too sudden a fall, in blood glucose.[10] To aid their choices, they may be able to use the **glycemic index**, a method of classifying foods according to their potential to raise blood glucose relative to a standard dose of glucose. ♦ Figure 4-13 ranks selected foods by their glycemic index.[11] ♦ Some studies have shown that selecting foods with a low glycemic index is a practical way to improve glucose control.[12]

♦ A related term, *glycemic load,* reflects both the glycemic index and the amount of carbohydrate.

♦ Glycemic index generalizations:

- Low: Legumes, milk products
- Moderate: Whole grains, fruits
- High: Processed foods made from refined flour such as snack foods, breads, ready-to-eat cereals

Lowering the glycemic index of the *diet* may improve blood lipids and reduce the risk of heart disease as well.[13] A low glycemic diet may also help with weight management, although research findings are mixed.[14]

Researchers debate whether selecting foods based on the glycemic index is practical or offers any real health benefits.[15] Those opposing the use of the glycemic index argue that it is not sufficiently supported by scientific research. The glycemic index has been determined for relatively few foods, and when the glycemic index has been established, it is based on an average of multiple tests with wide variations in their results. Values vary because of differences in the physical and chemical characteristics of foods, testing methods of laboratories, and digestive processes of individuals.[16]

Furthermore, the practical utility of the glycemic index is limited because this information is neither provided on food labels nor intuitively apparent. Indeed, a food's glycemic index is not always what one might expect. Ice cream, for example, is a high-sugar food but produces less of a glycemic response than baked potatoes, a high-starch food. Perhaps most relevant to real life, a food's glycemic effect differs depending on plant variety, food processing, cooking method, and whether it is eaten alone or with other foods. Most people eat a variety of foods, cooked and raw, that provide different amounts of carbohydrate, fat, and protein—all of which influence the glycemic index of a meal.

Paying attention to the glycemic index may not be necessary because current guidelines already suggest many low glycemic index choices: whole grains, legumes, vegetables, fruits, and milk products. In addition, eating frequent, small meals spreads glucose absorption across the day and thus offers similar metabolic advantages to eating foods with a low glycemic response. People wanting to follow a low glycemic diet should be careful not to adopt a low-carbohydrate diet as well. Highlight 4 explores the controversies surrounding low-carbohydrate and high glycemic diets.

glycemic index: a method of classifying foods according to their potential for raising blood glucose.

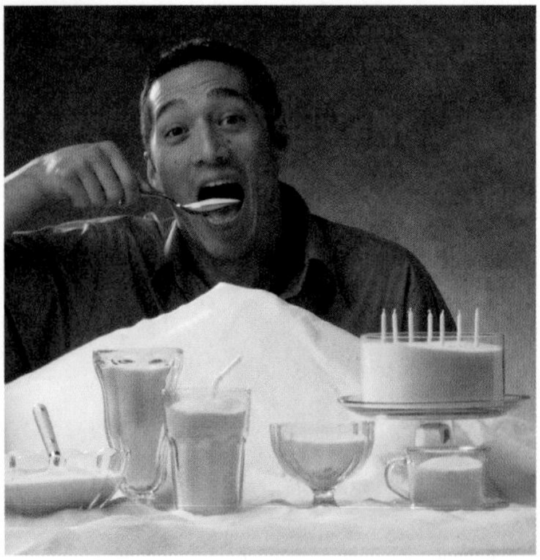

Polara Studios, Inc.

More than half of the added sugars in our diet come from soft drinks and table sugar, but baked goods, fruit drinks, ice cream, candy, and breakfast cereals also make substantial contributions.

The glycemic index, and its mathematical offshoot **glycemic load** (GI of a food item multiplied by the amount of available carbohydrate it contains), may be meaningful to people with diabetes who must take steps to regulate their blood glucose. A theory states that the lower the glycemic load of the diet, the less glucose builds up in the blood, and, therefore, the less insulin is needed to maintain normal blood glucose concentrations. Evidence also suggests that a low glycemic load may even help control body weight by ensuring a steady flow of glucose into the bloodstream and extend feelings of fullness. In contrast, a rapid rise in blood glucose seems to promote overeating in some overweight people and may lead to the increased presence of a marker of cardiovascular disease risk. New research is focusing on differences in the rate of blood glucose clearance by the tissues rather than absorption as a key factor in glycemic load.

The concept of glycemic load offers an accounting of both a food's glycemic index and its carbohydrate content. For example, in laboratory tests, 50 grams of carbohydrate from boiled carrots ranks in the middle of the glycemic index scale, indicating a moderate capacity for elevating blood glucose. However, the glycemic index fails to reveal that a typical 125 mL (1/2 cup) serving of carrots presents the body with only 8 grams of absorbable carbohydrate—to receive a test portion of 50 grams requires eating more than 750 mL (3 cups) of boiled carrots at a sitting. Therefore, the *glycemic load* of a serving of carrots is low, a point often overlooked. In addition, nutritional scientists are concerned about access to recent glycemic index and glycemic load values for all the new food products pouring onto the market and that manufacturers may adjust the carbohydrate content of and re-formulate familiar foods, thus necessitating their re-evaluation in terms of glycemic index or glycemic load. Today, the utility of the glycemic index or glycemic load for reducing weight or risks of diseases remains uncertain.

IN SUMMARY **Dietary carbohydrates provide glucose that can be used by the cells for energy, stored by the liver and muscles as glycogen, or converted into fat if intakes exceed needs. All of the body's cells depend on glucose; those of the central nervous system are especially dependent on it. Without glucose, the body is forced to break down some of its available protein tissues to make glucose and to alter energy metabolism to make ketone bodies from fats. Blood glucose regulation depends primarily on two pancreatic hormones: insulin to move glucose from the blood into the cells when levels are high and glucagon to free glucose from liver glycogen stores and release it into the blood when levels are low. The glycemic index measures how blood glucose responds to foods relative to a standard amount of glucose.**

Health Effects and Recommended Intakes of Sugars

Almost everyone finds pleasure in sweet foods—after all, the taste preference for sweets is inborn. To a child, the sweeter the food, the better. In adults, this preference is somewhat diminished, but most adults still enjoy an occasional sweet food or beverage. In North America, the natural sugars of milk, fruits, vegetables, and grains account for about half of the sugar intake; the other half consists of concentrated sugars that have been refined and added to foods for a variety of purposes. ♦ The use of **added sugars** has risen steadily over the past several decades, both in North America and around the world, with soft drinks and sugared fruit drinks accounting for most of the increase. These added sugars assume various names on food labels: sucrose, invert sugar, corn sugar, corn syrups and solids, high-fructose corn syrup, and honey. A food is likely to be high in added sugars if its ingredient list starts with any of the sugars named in the accompanying glossary or if it includes several of them.

♦ As an additive, sugar:
- Enhances flavour
- Supplies texture and colour to baked goods
- Provides fuel for fermentation, causing bread to rise or producing alcohol
- Acts as a bulking agent in ice cream and baked goods
- Acts as a preservative in jams
- Balances the acidity of tomato- and vinegar-based products

glycemic load a mathematical expression of both the glycemic index and the carbohydrate content of a food, meal, or diet (glycemic index multiplied by grams carbohydrate).

added sugars: sugars and syrups used as an ingredient in the processing and preparation of foods such as breads, cakes, beverages, jellies, and ice cream as well as sugars eaten separately or added to foods at the table.

Health Effects of Sugars In moderate amounts, sugars add pleasure to meals without harming health. In excess, however, they can be detrimental in two ways. One, sugars can contribute to nutrient deficiencies by supplying energy (kcalories) without providing nutrients. Two, sugars can contribute to tooth decay.

Nutrient Deficiencies Empty-kcalorie foods that contain lots of added sugars such as cakes, candies, and soft drinks provide the body with glucose and energy, but few, if any, other nutrients. By comparison, foods such as whole grains, vegetables, legumes, and fruits that contain some natural sugars and lots of starches and fibres also provide protein, vitamins, and minerals.

A person spending 200 kcalories of a day's energy allowance on a 480 millilitre (16 oz) soft drink gets little of value for those kcalories. In contrast, a person using 200 kcalories on three slices of whole-wheat bread gets 9 grams of protein, 6 grams of fibre, plus several of the B vitamins with those kcalories. For the person who wants something sweet, a reasonable compromise might be two slices of bread with a teaspoon of jam on each. The amount of sugar a person can afford to eat depends on how many **discretionary kcalories** are available beyond those needed to deliver indispensable vitamins and minerals.

By following *Canada's Food Guide* and making careful food selections, a typical adult can obtain all the needed nutrients within an allowance of about 1500 kcalories. Some people have more generous energy allowances. For example, an active teenage boy may need as many as 3000 kcalories a day. If he eats mostly nutritious foods, then he may have discretionary kcalories available for soft drinks and other "extras." In contrast, an inactive older woman who is limited to fewer than 1500 kcalories a day can afford to eat only the most nutrient-dense foods—with few, or no, discretionary kcalories available.

Some people believe that because honey is a natural food, it is nutritious—or, at least, more nutritious than sugar.* A look at their chemical structures reveals the truth. Honey, like table sugar, contains glucose and fructose. The primary difference is that in table sugar the two monosaccharides are bonded together as the disaccharide sucrose, whereas in honey some of them are free. Whether a person eats monosaccharides individually, as in honey, or linked together, as in table sugar, they end up the same way in the body: as glucose and fructose.

Honey does contain a few vitamins and minerals, but not many. Honey is denser than crystalline sugar, too, so it provides more energy per spoonful. Table 4-1 (p. 110) shows that honey and white sugar are similar nutritionally—and both fall short of milk, legumes, fruits, grains, and vegetables. Honey may offer some health benefits, however: it seems to relieve nighttime coughing in

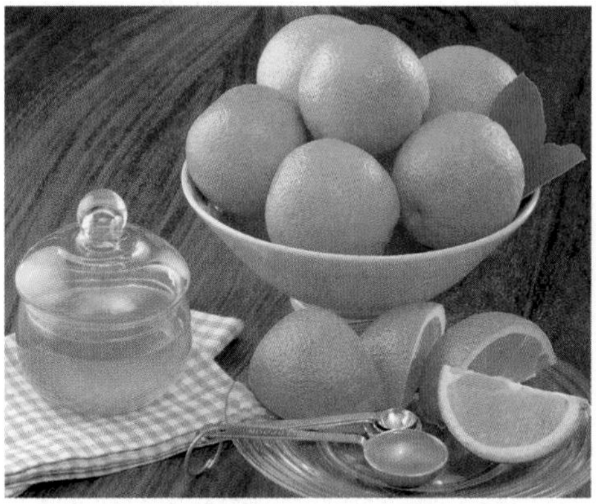

You receive about the same amount and kinds of sugars from an orange as from a tablespoon of honey, but the packaging makes a big nutrition difference.

discretionary kcalories: the kcalories remaining in a person's energy allowance after consuming enough nutrient-dense foods to meet all nutrient needs for a day.

*Honey should never be fed to infants because of the risk of botulism. Chapters 17 and 20 provide more details.

GLOSSARY OF ADDED SUGARS

brown sugar: refined white sugar crystals to which manufacturers have added molasses syrup with natural flavour and colour; 91 to 96 percent pure sucrose.

confectioners' sugar: finely powdered sucrose, 99.9 percent pure.

corn sweeteners: corn syrup and sugars derived from corn.

corn syrup: a syrup made from cornstarch that has been treated with acid, high temperatures, and enzymes that produce glucose, maltose, and dextrins. See also *high-fructose corn syrup (HFCS)*.

dextrose: an older name for glucose.

granulated sugar: crystalline sucrose; 99.9 percent pure.

high-fructose corn syrup (HFCS): a syrup made from cornstarch that has been treated with an enzyme that converts some of the glucose to the sweeter fructose; made especially for use in processed foods and beverages, where it is the predominant sweetener. With a chemical structure similar to sucrose, HFCS has a fructose content of 42, 55, or 90 percent, with glucose making up the remainder.

honey: sugar (mostly sucrose) formed from nectar gathered by bees. An enzyme splits the sucrose into glucose and fructose. Composition and flavour vary, but honey always contains a mixture of sucrose, fructose, and glucose.

invert sugar: a mixture of glucose and fructose formed by the hydrolysis of sucrose in a chemical process; sold only in liquid form and sweeter than sucrose. Invert sugar is used as a food additive to help preserve freshness and prevent shrinkage.

levulose: an older name for fructose.

maple sugar: a sugar (mostly sucrose) purified from the concentrated sap of the sugar maple tree.

molasses: the thick brown syrup produced during sugar refining. Molasses retains residual sugar and other by-products and a few minerals; blackstrap molasses contains significant amounts of calcium and iron.

raw sugar: the first crop of crystals harvested during sugar processing. Raw sugar cannot be sold in Canada or the United States because it contains too much filth (dirt, insect fragments, and the like). Sugar sold as "raw sugar" domestically has actually gone through more than half of the refining steps.

turbinado (ter-bih-NOD-oh) **sugar:** sugar produced using the same refining process as white sugar, but without the bleaching and anticaking treatment. Traces of molasses give turbinado its sandy colour.

white sugar: pure sucrose or "table sugar," produced by dissolving, concentrating, and recrystallizing raw sugar.

TABLE 4-1 Sample Nutrients in Sugar and Other Foods

The indicated portion of any of these foods provides approximately 100 kcalories. Notice that for a similar number of kcalories and grams of carbohydrate, milk, legumes, fruits, grains, and vegetables offer more of the other nutrients than do the sugars.

	Size of 100 kcal Portion	Carbohydrate (g)	Protein (g)	Calcium (mg)	Iron (mg)	Vitamin A (µg)	Vitamin C (mg)
Foods							
Milk, 1% low-fat	250 mL (1 cup)	12	8	300	0.1	144	2
Kidney beans	125 mL (½ cup)	20	7	30	1.6	0	2
Apricots	6	24	2	30	1.1	554	22
Bread, whole-wheat	1½ slices	20	4	30	1.9	0	0
Broccoli, cooked	500 mL (2 cups)	20	12	188	2.2	696	148
Sugars							
Sugar, white	30 mL (2 Tbsp)	24	0	trace	trace	0	0
Molasses, blackstrap	38 mL (2½ Tbsp)	28	0	343	12.6	0	0.1
Cola beverage	250 mL (1 cup)	26	0	6	trace	0	0
Honey	23 mL (1½ Tbsp)	26	trace	2	0.2	0	trace

FIGURE 4-14 Dental Caries

Dental caries begins when acid dissolves the enamel that covers the tooth. If not repaired, the decay may penetrate the dentin and spread into the pulp of the tooth, causing inflammation, abscess, and possible loss of the tooth.

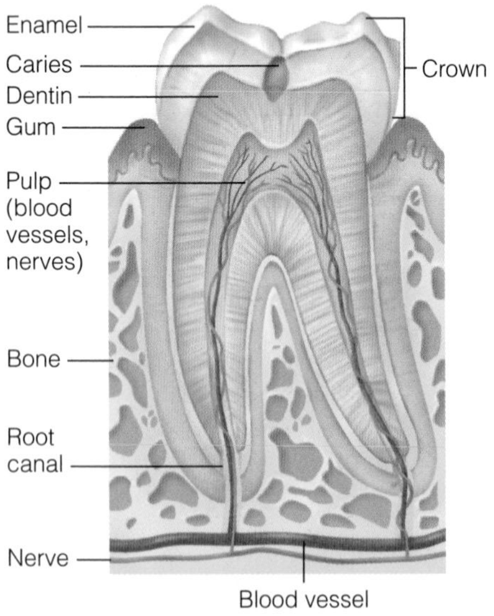
Enamel
Caries
Dentin
Gum
Crown
Pulp (blood vessels, nerves)
Bone
Root canal
Nerve
Blood vessel

children and reduce the severity of mouth ulcers in cancer patients undergoing chemotherapy or radiation.[17]

While the body cannot distinguish whether fructose and glucose derive from honey or table sugar, this is not to say that all sugar sources are alike. Some sugar sources are more nutritious than others. Consider a fruit, say, an orange. The fruit may give you the same amounts of fructose and glucose and the same number of kcalories as a spoonful of sugar or honey, but the packaging is more valuable nutritionally. The fruit's sugars arrive in the body diluted in a large volume of water, packaged in fibre, and mixed with essential vitamins, minerals, and phytochemicals.

As these comparisons illustrate, the significant difference between sugar sources is not between "natural" honey and "purified" sugar but between concentrated sugars and the dilute, naturally occurring sugars that sweeten foods. You can suspect an exaggerated nutrition claim when someone asserts that one product is more nutritious than another because it contains honey.

Added sugars contribute to nutrient deficiencies by displacing nutrients.[18] For nutrition's sake, the appropriate attitude to take is not that sugar is "bad" and must be avoided, but that nutritious foods must come first. If nutritious foods crowd sugar out of the diet, that is fine—but not the other way around. As always, balance, variety, and moderation guide healthy food choices.

Dental Caries Sugars from foods and from the breakdown of starches in the mouth can contribute to tooth decay. Bacteria in the mouth ferment the sugars and, in the process, produce an acid that erodes tooth enamel (see Figure 4-14), causing **dental caries**, or tooth decay. People can eat sugar without this happening, though, for much depends on how long foods stay in the mouth. Sticky foods stay on the teeth longer and continue to yield acid longer than foods that are readily cleared from the mouth. For that reason, sugar in a juice consumed quickly, for example, is less likely to cause dental caries than sugar in a pastry. By the same token, the sugar in sticky foods such as dried fruits can be more detrimental than its quantity alone would suggest.

Another concern is how often people eat sugar. Bacteria produce acid for 20 to 30 minutes after each exposure. If a person eats three pieces of candy at one time, the teeth will be exposed to approximately 30 minutes of acid destruction. But, if the person eats three pieces at half-hour intervals, the time of exposure increases to 90 minutes. Likewise, slowly sipping a sugary sports beverage may be more harmful than drinking quickly and clearing the mouth of sugar. Nonsugary foods can help remove sugar from tooth surfaces; hence, it is better to eat sugar with meals

dental caries: decay of teeth.
- **caries** = rottenness

than between meals. Foods such as milk and cheese may be particularly helpful in protecting against dental caries by neutralizing acids, stimulating salivary flow, inhibiting bacterial activity, and promoting remineralization of damaged enamel.[19]

Beverages such as soft drinks, orange juice, and sports drinks not only contain sugar but also have a low pH. These acidic drinks can erode tooth enamel and may explain why the prevalence of dental erosion is growing steadily.[20]

The development of caries depends on several factors: the bacteria that reside in **dental plaque**, the saliva that cleanses the mouth, the minerals that form the teeth, and the foods that remain after swallowing. For most people, good oral hygiene will prevent ♦ dental caries. In fact, regular brushing (twice a day, with a fluoride toothpaste) and flossing may be more effective in preventing dental caries than restricting sugary foods. Still nutrition is a key component of dental health.[21] *Canada's Food Guide* recommends limiting foods and beverages high in sugar.

What about Sugar and Behaviour? Many years ago, claims began appearing that eating sugary foods caused children to become unruly and adolescents and adults to exhibit antisocial and even criminal behaviour. Science has since put the "sugar-behaviour" theory to rest, but many teachers, parents, grandparents, and others still believe that some children react behaviourally to sugar.

Recommended Intakes of Sugars

Because added sugars deliver kcalories but few or no nutrients, *Canada's Food Guide* recommends that "Another important step towards better health and a healthy body weight is ... limiting foods and beverages high in calories ... sugar," such as those shown in the margin. ♦ But also remember that the DRI reports recommend that Canadians consume 130 grams of carbohydrate per day and the *Food Guide* recommends that we "Make at least half your grain products whole grain each day."[22]

Estimating the *added* sugars in a diet is not always easy for consumers. Food labels list the *total* grams of the sugars a food provides, but this total reflects both added sugars and those occurring naturally in foods. To help estimate sugar and energy intakes accurately, the list in the margin ♦ shows the amounts of concentrated sweets that are equivalent to 5 millilitres (1 tsp) of white sugar. These sugars all provide *about* 5 grams of carbohydrate and *about* 20 kcalories per 5 millilitres. Some are lower (16 kcalories for table sugar), and others are higher (22 kcalories for honey), but a 20-kcalorie average is an acceptable approximation. For a person who uses ketchup liberally, it may help to remember that 15 millilitres (1 Tbsp) of ketchup supplies about 5 millilitres (1 tsp) of sugar.

The DRI Committee did not publish an Upper Level for sugar, but as mentioned, excessive intakes can interfere with sound nutrition and dental health. Few people can eat lots of sugary treats and still meet all of their nutrient needs without exceeding their kcalorie allowance. Specifically, the DRI suggests that added sugars should account for no more than 25 percent of the day's total energy intake.[23] When added sugars occupy this much of a diet, however, intakes from the four food groups usually fall below recommendations. For a person consuming 2000 kcalories a day, 25 percent represents 500 kcalories (that is, 125 grams, or 31 teaspoons) from concentrated sugars—and that's a lot of sugar. ♦ Perhaps an athlete in training whose energy needs are high can afford the added sugars from sports drinks without compromising nutrient intake, but most people do better by limiting their use of added sugars. The World Health Organization (WHO) and the Food and Agriculture Organization (FAO) suggest restricting consumption of added sugars to less than 10 percent of total energy.

IN SUMMARY **Sugars pose no major health threat except for an increased risk of dental caries. Excessive intakes, however, may displace needed nutrients and fibre and may contribute to obesity when energy intake exceeds needs. A person deciding to limit daily sugar intake should recognize that not all sugars need to be restricted, just concentrated sweets, which are relatively empty of other nutrients and high in kcalories. Sugars that occur naturally in fruits, vegetables, and milk are acceptable.**

♦ To prevent dental caries:
- Limit between-meal juices and snacks containing sugars and starches.
- Brush with a fluoride toothpaste and floss teeth regularly.
- If brushing and flossing are not possible, at least rinse with water.
- Get a dental checkup regularly.

♦ *Canada's Food Guide* recommends that we limit our intake of the following:
- chocolate and candies
- fruit-flavoured drinks
- soft drinks
- sports and energy drinks
- sweetened hot or cold beverages

♦ 5 mL (1 tsp) white sugar =
- 5 mL (1 tsp) brown sugar
- 5 mL (1 tsp) candy
- 5 mL (1 tsp) corn sweetener or corn syrup
- 5 mL (1 tsp) honey
- 5 mL (1 tsp) jam or jelly
- 5 mL (1 tsp) maple sugar or maple syrup
- 5 mL (1 tsp) molasses
- 45 mL soft drink
- 15 mL (1 Tbsp) ketchup

♦ For perspective, each of these concentrated sugars provides about 500 kcal:
- 1200 mL cola
- 125 mL (1/2 cup) honey
- 125 jelly beans
- 23 marshmallows
- 150 mL (30 tsp) sugar

How many kcalories from sugar does your favourite beverage or snack provide?

dental plaque: a gummy mass of bacteria that grows on teeth and can lead to dental caries and gum disease.

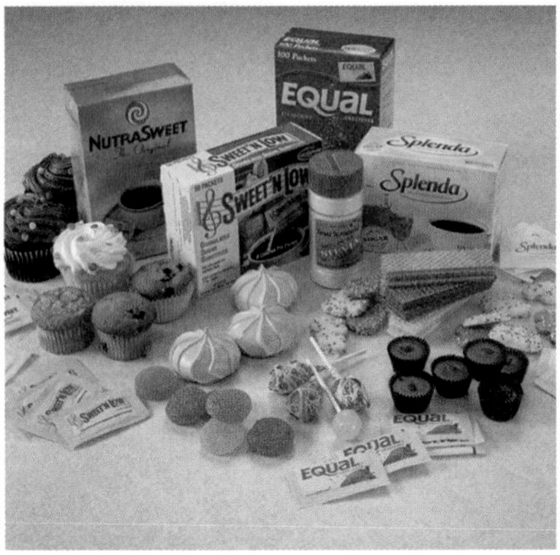
EQUAL
NUTRASWEET
Splenda
SWEET'N LOW

© Matthew Farruggio

Consumers use artificial sweeteners to help them limit kcalories and minimize sugar intake.

Alternative Sweeteners

To control weight gain, blood glucose, and dental caries, many consumers turn to alternative sweeteners to help them limit kcalories and minimize sugar intake. In doing so, they encounter three sets of alternative sweeteners: artificial sweeteners, herbal products, and sugar alcohols.

Artificial Sweeteners

Artificial sweeteners are sometimes called **nonnutritive sweeteners** because they provide virtually no energy. Table 4-2 (pp. 113–114) provides general details about each of the sweeteners. Chapter 9 includes a discussion of their use in weight control, and Chapter 20 focuses on some of the safety issues surrounding their use. ♦ Considering that all substances are toxic at some dose, it is little surprise that large doses of artificial sweeteners (or their components or metabolic by-products) may have adverse effects. The question to ask is whether their ingestion is safe for human beings in quantities people normally use (and potentially abuse). A number of these sweeteners including acesulfame-potassium, aspartame, sucralose, and saccharin are considered safe for pregnant women, although it is recommended that they use them sparingly.

♦ The estimated amount of a sweetener that individuals can safely consume each day over the course of a lifetime without adverse effect is known as the **Acceptable Daily Intake (ADI).**

Stevia—An Herbal Product

The herb stevia derives from a plant whose leaves have long been used by the people of South America to sweeten their beverages. Food manufacturers are not allowed to add stevia to foods in Canada, but it can be sold as an item on its own and added to Natural Health Products (NHPs) as a sweetening agent.[24] In the U.S., however, it was recently granted the status of "generally recognized as safe"; stevia can now be used as an additive in a variety of foods and beverages.

Sugar Alcohols

Some "sugar-free" or reduced-kcalorie products contain sugar alcohols. The **sugar alcohols** (or polyols) provide bulk and sweetness in cookies, hard candies, sugarless gums, jams, and jellies. These products claim to be "sugar-free" on their labels, but in this case, "sugar-free" does not mean free of kcalories. Sugar alcohols do provide kcalories, but fewer than their carbohydrate cousins, the sugars. Because sugar alcohols yield energy, they are sometimes referred to as **nutritive sweeteners.** Table 4-2 includes their energy values. Sugar alcohols occur naturally in fruits and vegetables; manufacturers also use sugar alcohols in many processed foods to add bulk and texture, to provide a cooling effect or taste, to inhibit browning from heat, and to retain moisture.

Sugar alcohols evoke a low glycemic response. The body absorbs sugar alcohols slowly; consequently, they are slower to enter the bloodstream than other sugars. Common side effects include intestinal gas, abdominal discomfort, and diarrhea.

The real benefit of using sugar alcohols is that they do not contribute to dental caries. Bacteria in the mouth cannot metabolize sugar alcohols as rapidly as sugar. Sugar alcohols are therefore valuable in chewing gums, breath mints, and other products that people keep in their mouths for a while. Figure 4-15 (p. 114) presents labelling information for products using sugar alternatives. For example, nutrition labelling regulations permit a health claim for the role of sugar alcohols related to dental caries. The following examples of claims would be acceptable: "Won't cause cavities" and "Does not promote tooth decay" on items such as gum that contain sugar alcohols.[25]

Health Canada's website has up-to-date information on sugar substitutes.[26] When used in moderation, these sweeteners will do no harm. In fact, they may even help, by providing an alternative to sugar for people with diabetes, by inhibiting caries-causing bacteria, and by limiting energy intake. People may find it appropriate to use any of the sweeteners at times: artificial sweeteners, herbal products, sugar alcohols, and sugar itself.

artificial sweeteners: sugar substitutes that provide negligible, if any, energy; sometimes called *nonnutritive sweeteners*.

nonnutritive sweeteners: sweeteners that yield no energy (or insignificant energy in the case of aspartame).

sugar alcohols: sugarlike compounds that can be derived from fruits or commercially produced from dextrose; also called *polyols*. Sugar alcohols are absorbed more slowly than other sugars and metabolized differently in the human body; they are not readily utilized by ordinary mouth bacteria. Examples are *maltitol, mannitol, sorbitol, xylitol, isomalt,* and *lactitol*.

nutritive sweeteners: sweeteners that yield energy, including both sugars and sugar alcohols.

TABLE 4-2 Alternative Sweeteners

(See the legend at the end of this table for the trade names for individual sweeteners.)

Sweetener	Chemical Composition	Body's Response	Relative Sweetness[a]	Energy (kcal/g)	Acceptable Daily Intake (ADI) and (Estimated Equivalent[b])	Approval Status
			Artificial Sweeteners			
Acesulfame potassium or Acesulfame K[c] (AY-sul-fame)	Potassium salt	Not digested or absorbed	200	0	15 mg/kg body weight[d] (30 cans diet pop)	Approved for use in Canada the United States
Aspartame[e] (ah-SPAR-tame or ASS-par-tame)	Amino acids (phenyl-alanine and aspartic acid) and a methyl group	Digested and absorbed	200	4[f]	40 mg/kg body weight[g] (18 cans diet pop)	Approved for use in Canada and the United States; warning for PKU
Cyclamate (SIGH-kla-mate)	Sodium or calcium salt of cyclamic acid	Incompletely absorbed; absorbed cyclamate is excreted unchanged; unabsorbed cyclamate may be metabolized by bacteria in the GI tract	30	0	11 mg/kg body weight (8 cans of diet pop)	Approved for use in Canada, but currently restricted to use as a tabletop sweetener
Neotame (NEE-oh-tame)	Aspartame with an additional side group attached	Not digested or absorbed	8000	0	2 mg/kg bw/day	Approved for use in Canada
Saccharin[h] (SAK-ah-ren)	Benzoic sulfimide	Rapidly absorbed and excreted	450	0	5 mg/kg body weight (10 packets of sweetener)	Approved for use in the United States; currently, restricted use as a tabletop sweetener in Canada
Sucralose[i] (SUE-kra-lose)	Sucrose with Cl atoms instead of OH groups	Not digested or absorbed	600	0	8.8 mg/kg body weight (6 cans diet pop)	Approved for use in Canada and the United States
Tagatose[j] (TAG-ah-tose)	Monosaccharide similar in structure to fructose; naturally occurring or derived from lactose	Mostly not absorbed; some short-chain fatty acids absorbed	0.8	1.5	80 mg/kg bw/day	Approved for use in the United States; it is GRAS[k] approved
			Herbal Sweeteners			
Stevia[l] (STEE-vee-ah)	Glycosides found in the leaves of the *Stevia rebaudiana* herb	Digested and absorbed	300	0	4 mg/kg body weight	Approved for use in Natural Health Prod-ucts (NHPs); GRAS approved
			Sugar Alcohols			
Erythritol	Sugar alcohol	Partially absorbed in small intestine; unab-sorbed sugar alcohols may be metabolized by bacteria in the GI tract	0.7	0.2	1000 mg/kg bw/day—[m]	Approved for use in Canada; GRAS approved
Isomalt	Sugar alcohol	Partially absorbed in small intestine; unab-sorbed sugar alcohols may be metabolized by bacteria in the GI tract	0.5	2.0	—[m]	Approved for use in Canada; GRAS approved
Lactitol	Sugar alcohol	Partially absorbed in small intestine; unab-sorbed sugar alcohols may be metabolized by bacteria in the GI tract	0.4	2.0	—[m]	Approved for use in Canada; GRAS approved
Maltitol	Sugar alcohol	Partially absorbed in small intestine; unab-sorbed sugar alcohols may be metabolized by bacteria in the GI tract	0.9	2.1	—[m]	Approved for use in Canada; GRAS approved

(continued)

Sweetener	Chemical Composition	Body's Response	Relative Sweetness[a]	Energy (kcal/g)	Acceptable Daily Intake (ADI) and (Estimated Equivalent[b])	Approval Status
			Sugar Alcohols			
Mannitol	Sugar alcohol	Partially absorbed in small intestine; unabsorbed sugar alcohols may be metabolized by bacteria in the GI tract	0.7	1.6	—[m]	Approved for use in Canada and the United States
Sorbitol	Sugar alcohol	Partially absorbed in small intestine; unabsorbed sugar alcohols may be metabolized by bacteria in the GI tract	0.5	2.6	—[m]	Approved for use in Canada; GRAS approved
Xylitol	Sugar alcohol	Partially absorbed in small intestine; unabsorbed sugar alcohols may be metabolized by bacteria in the GI tract	1.0	2.4	—[m]	Approved for use in Canada and the United States

[a]Relative sweetness is determined by comparing the approximate sweetness of a sugar substitute with the sweetness of pure sucrose, which has been defined as 1.0. Chemical structure, temperature, acidity, and other flavours of the foods in which the substance occurs all influence relative sweetness.
[b]Based on a person weighing 70 kg (154 lb).
[c]Marketed under the trade names Sunett, Sweet One.
[d]Recommendations from the World Health Organization limit acesulfame-K intake to 9 mg per kilogram of body weight per day.
[e]Marketed under the trade names NutraSweet, Equal, NatraTaste, Canderel.
[f]Aspartame provides 4 kcal per gram, as does protein, but because so little is used, its energy contribution is negligible. In powdered form, it is sometimes mixed with lactose, however, so a 1 g packet may provide 4 kcal.
[g]Recommendations from the World Health Organization and in Europe and Canada limit aspartame intake to 40 mg per kilogram of body weight per day.
[h]Marketed under the trade names Sweet'N Low, Necta Sweet.
[i]Marketed under the trade names Splenda, SucraPlus.
[j]Marketed under the trade names Nutralose, Nutrilatose, Tagatesse.
[k]GRAS = food additives that are generally recognized as safe. First established by the U.S. FDA in 1958, the GRAS list is subject to revision as new facts become known.
[l]Marketed under the trade names Sweetleaf, Purevia, Truvia, Honey Leaf.
[m]An ADI is "not specified" for sugar alcohols, indicating the highest safety category.

IN SUMMARY All three types of alternative sweeteners (artificial sweeteners, the herbal product/natural health product stevia, sugar alcohols), when used in moderation, may help some individuals manage their weight and blood sugar levels, while some may also be used to help prevent cavities. Note: It is becoming more and more common to see blends of these sweeteners in kcalorie-reduced beverages and food products.

FIGURE 4-15 **Sugar Alternatives on Food Labels**

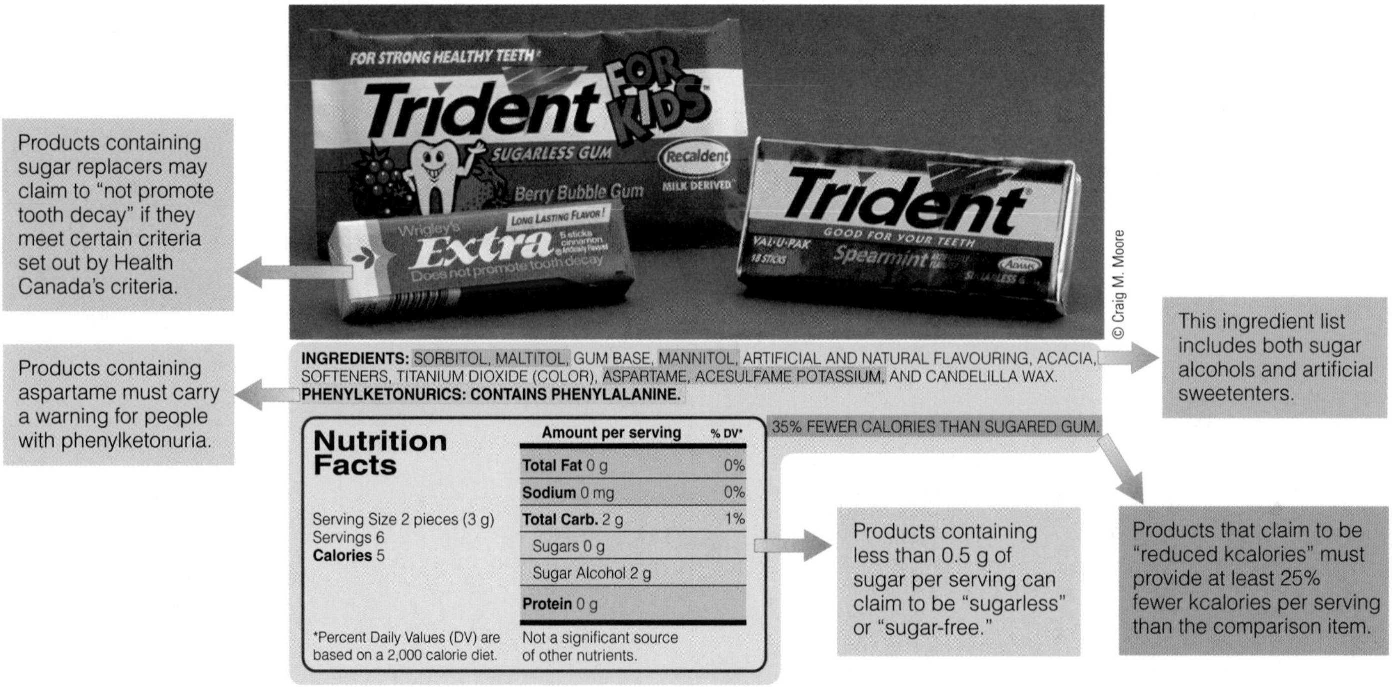
Products containing sugar replacers may claim to "not promote tooth decay" if they meet certain criteria set out by Health Canada's criteria.
Products containing aspartame must carry a warning for people with phenylketonuria.
This ingredient list includes both sugar alcohols and artificial sweetenters.
Products containing less than 0.5 g of sugar per serving can claim to be "sugarless" or "sugar-free."
Products that claim to be "reduced kcalories" must provide at least 25% fewer kcalories per serving than the comparison item.
FOR STRONG HEALTHY TEETH
Trident FOR KIDS
SUGARLESS GUM
Berry Bubble Gum
Recaldent
MILK DERIVED
Wrigley's Extra
LONG LASTING FLAVOR!
Does not promote tooth decay
Trident
GOOD FOR YOUR TEETH
VAL-U-PAK
18 STICKS
Spearmint
© Craig M. Moore
INGREDIENTS: SORBITOL, MALTITOL, GUM BASE, MANNITOL, ARTIFICIAL AND NATURAL FLAVOURING, ACACIA, SOFTENERS, TITANIUM DIOXIDE (COLOR), ASPARTAME, ACESULFAME POTASSIUM, AND CANDELILLA WAX.
PHENYLKETONURICS: CONTAINS PHENYLALANINE.
35% FEWER CALORIES THAN SUGARED GUM.
Nutrition Facts
Serving Size 2 pieces (3 g)
Servings 6
Calories 5
Amount per serving
% DV*
Total Fat 0 g 0%
Sodium 0 mg 0%
Total Carb. 2 g 1%
Sugars 0 g
Sugar Alcohol 2 g
Protein 0 g
*Percent Daily Values (DV) are based on a 2,000 calorie diet.
Not a significant source of other nutrients.

Health Effects and Recommended Intakes of Starch and Fibres

Carbohydrates and fats are the two major sources of energy in the diet. When one is high, the other is usually low—and vice versa. A diet that provides abundant carbohydrates (45 to 65 percent of energy intake) and some fat (20 to 35 percent of energy intake) within a reasonable energy allowance best supports good health. To increase carbohydrates in the diet, focus on whole grains, vegetables, legumes, and fruits—foods noted for their starch, fibres, and naturally occurring sugars.

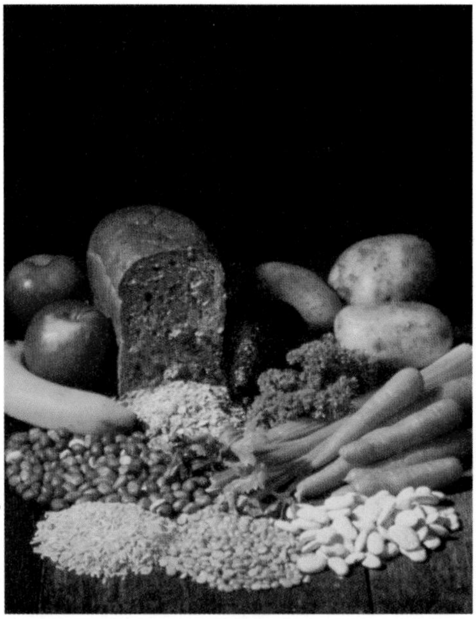
Andrew McClenaghan / Photo Researchers, Inc

Foods rich in starch and fibre offer many health benefits.

Health Effects of Starch and Fibres

In addition to starch, fibres, and natural sugars, whole grains, vegetables, legumes, and fruits supply valuable vitamins and minerals and little or no fat. The following paragraphs describe some of the health benefits of diets that include a variety of these foods daily.

Heart Disease Unlike high-carbohydrate diets rich in sugars that can alter blood lipids to favour heart disease, those rich in whole grains and soluble fibres may protect against heart disease and stroke, by lowering blood pressure, improving blood lipids, and reducing inflammation.[27] Such diets are low in animal fat and cholesterol and high in dietary fibres, vegetable proteins, and phytochemicals—all factors associated with a lower risk of heart disease. (The role of animal fat and cholesterol in heart disease is discussed in Chapter 5. The role of vegetable proteins in heart disease is presented in Chapter 6. The benefits of phytochemicals in disease prevention are featured in Highlight 14.)

Oatmeal was the first food recognized for its ability to reduce cholesterol and the risk of heart disease.[28] Foods rich in soluble fibres (such as oat bran, barley, and legumes) lower blood cholesterol ♦ by binding with bile acids (which are made from cholesterol) in the GI tract and thereby increasing their excretion. Consequently, the liver must use its cholesterol to make new bile acids. In addition, the bacterial by-products of fibre fermentation in the colon also inhibit cholesterol synthesis in the liver. The net result is lower blood cholesterol.

♦ Consuming 5 to 10 grams of soluble fibre daily reduces blood cholesterol by 3 to 5 percent. For perspective, 125 mL (½ cup) dry oat bran provides 8 grams of fibre, and 250 mL (1 cup) cooked barley or 125 mL (½ cup) cooked legumes provides about 6 grams of fibre.

Several researchers have speculated that fibre may also exert its effect by displacing fats in the diet. Whereas this is certainly helpful, even when dietary fat is low, fibres exert a separate and significant cholesterol-lowering effect. In other words, a high-fibre diet helps to decrease the risk of heart disease independent of fat intake.

Diabetes High-fibre foods—especially whole grains—play a key role in reducing the risk of type 2 diabetes.[29] When soluble fibres trap nutrients and delay their transit through the GI tract, glucose absorption is slowed, which helps to prevent the glucose surge and rebound that seem to be associated with diabetes onset.

GI Health Dietary fibres may enhance the health of the large intestine. The healthier the intestinal walls, the better they can block absorption of unwanted constituents. Insoluble fibres such as cellulose (as in cereal brans, fruits, and vegetables) increase stool weight, easing passage, and reduce transit time. In this way, the fibres help to alleviate or prevent constipation.

Taken with ample fluids, fibres help to prevent several GI disorders. Large, soft stools ease elimination for the rectal muscles and reduce the pressure in the lower bowel, making it less likely that rectal veins will swell (hemorrhoids). Fibre prevents compaction of the intestinal contents, which could obstruct the appendix and permit bacteria to invade and infect it (appendicitis). In addition, fibre stimulates the GI tract muscles so that they retain their strength and resist bulging out into pouches known as diverticula (illustrated in Figure H3-3 on p. 88).[30]

Cancer Many, but not all, research studies suggest that increasing dietary fibre protects against colon cancer.[31] When the largest study of diet and cancer to date examined the diets of more than a half million people in ten countries for four and a half years, the researchers found an inverse association between dietary fiber and colon cancer. People who ate the most dietary fibre (35 grams per day) reduced their risk of colon cancer by 40 percent compared with those who ate the least fibre (15 grams per day). Importantly, the study focused on dietary fiber, not fibre supplements or additives, which lack valuable nutrients and phytochemicals that also help protect against cancer. Plant foods—vegetables, fruits, and whole-grain products—reduce the risks of colon and rectal cancers.

Fibres may help prevent colon cancer by diluting, binding, and rapidly removing potential cancer-causing agents from the colon. In addition, soluble fibres stimulate bacterial fermentation of resistant starch and fibre in the colon, a process that produces short-chain fatty acids that lower the pH. These small fat molecules activate cancer-killing enzymes and inhibit inflammation in the colon.[32]

Weight Management High-fibre and whole-grain foods may help a person to maintain a healthy body weight. Foods rich in fibres tend to be low in fat and added sugars and can therefore prevent weight gains and promote weight loss by delivering less energy ♦ per bite.[33] In addition, as fibres absorb water from the digestive juices, they swell, creating feelings of fullness, lowering food intake, and delaying hunger.[34]

♦ Remember:
- Carbohydrate: 4 kcal/g
- Fat: 9 kcal/g

Many weight-loss products on the market today contain bulk-inducing fibres such as methylcellulose, but buying pure fibre compounds like this is neither necessary nor advisable. Instead of fibre supplements, consumers should select whole grains, legumes, fruits, and vegetables. High-fibre foods not only add bulk to the diet but are economical and nutritious as well.

Dietary fibre provides numerous health benefits.[35] Table 4-3 below summarizes fibre characteristics, food sources, actions in the body, and health benefits.

Harmful Effects of Excessive Fibre Intake Despite fibre's benefits to health, a diet excessively high in fibre also has a few drawbacks. A person who has a small capacity and eats mostly high-fibre foods may not be able to take in enough food to meet energy or nutrient needs. The malnourished, the elderly, and young children adhering to all-plant (vegan) diets are especially vulnerable to this problem.

Launching suddenly into a high-fibre diet can cause temporary bouts of abdominal discomfort, gas, and diarrhea and, more seriously, can obstruct the GI tract. To prevent such complications, a person adopting a high-fibre diet can take the following precautions:

- Increase fibre intake gradually over several weeks to give the GI tract time to adapt.
- Drink plenty of liquids to soften the fibre as it moves through the GI tract.
- Select fibre-rich foods from a variety of sources—fruits, vegetables, legumes, and whole-grain breads and cereals.

TABLE 4-3 Dietary Fibres: Their Characteristics, Food Sources, and Health Effects in the Body

Fibre Characteristics	Major Food Sources	Actions in the Body	Health Benefits
Soluble, viscous, more fermentable • Gums and mucilages • Pectins • Psyllium[a] • Some hemicelluloses	Whole-grain products (barley, oats, oat bran, rye), fruits (apples, citrus), legumes, seeds and husks, vegetables; also extracted and used as food additives	• Lower blood cholesterol by binding bile • Slow glucose absorption • Slow transit of food through upper GI tract • Hold moisture in stools, softening them • Yield small fat molecules after fermentation that the colon can use for energy	• Lower risk of heart disease • Lower risk of diabetes
Insoluble, nonviscous, less fermentable • Cellulose • Lignins • Psyllium[a] • Resistant starch • Many hemicelluloses	Brown rice, fruits, legumes, seeds, vegetables (cabbage, carrots, Brussels sprouts), wheat bran, whole grains; also extracted and used as food additives	• Increase fecal weight and speed fecal passage through colon • Provide bulk and feelings of fullness	• Alleviate constipation • Lower risks of diverticulosis, hemorrhoids, and appendicitis • May help with weight management

[a]Psyllium, a fibre laxative and cereal additive, has both soluble and insoluble properties.

Some fibres can limit the absorption of nutrients by speeding the transit of foods through the GI tract and by binding minerals. When mineral intake is adequate, however, a *reasonable* intake of high-fibre foods (less than 40 grams a day) does not compromise mineral balance.

Clearly, fibre is like most nutrients in that "more" is "better" only up to a point. Again, the key dietary goals are balance, moderation, and variety.

IN SUMMARY **Adequate intake of fibre:**

- **Fosters weight management**
- **Lowers blood cholesterol**
- **May help prevent colon cancer**
- **Helps prevent and control diabetes**
- **Helps prevent and alleviate hemorrhoids**
- **Helps prevent appendicitis**
- **Helps prevent diverticulosis**

Excessive intake of fibre:

- **Displaces energy- and nutrient-dense foods**
- **Causes intestinal discomfort and distention**
- **May interfere with mineral absorption**

Recommended Intakes of Starch and Fibres

The DRI suggests that carbohydrates provide about half (45 to 65 percent) of the energy requirement. ♦ A person consuming 2000 kcalories a day should therefore have 900 to 1300 kcalories of carbohydrate, or about 225 to 325 grams. ♦ This amount is more than adequate to meet the RDA ♦ for carbohydrate, which is set at 130 grams per day, based on the average minimum amount of glucose used by the brain.[36]

When it established the Daily Values that appear on food labels, Health Canada used a 60 percent of kcalories guideline in setting the Daily Value ♦ for carbohydrate at 300 grams per day. For most people, this means increasing total carbohydrate intake. To this end, the *Food Guide* encourages people to choose a variety of whole grains, vegetables, fruits, and legumes daily.

♦ Acceptable Macronutrient Distribution Ranges (AMDR):
- Carbohydrate: 45–65%
- Fat: 20–35%
- Protein: 10–35%

♦ The Aids to Calculation section at the end of this book explains how to solve such problems.

♦ RDA for carbohydrate:
- 130 g/day

♦ Daily Value:
- 300 g carbohydrate (based on 60% of 2000 kcal diet)

Dietary Guidance for Canadians

Choose fibre-rich fruits, vegetables, and whole grains often.

Recommendations for fibre ♦ suggest the same foods just mentioned: whole grains, vegetables, fruits, and legumes, which also provide minerals and vitamins. Health Canada set the Daily Value ♦ for fibre at 25 grams, rounding up from the recommended 11.5 grams per 1000 kcalories for a 2000-kcalorie intake. The DRI recommendation is slightly higher, at 14 grams per 1000-kcalorie intake—roughly 25 (for young adult females) to 35 (for young adult males) grams of dietary fibre daily. These recommendations are about two times higher than the usual intake in the Canada.[37] An effective way to add fibre while lowering fat is to substitute plant sources of proteins (legumes) for animal sources (meats). Table 4-4 (p. 118) presents a list of fibre sources.

Because high-fibre foods are so filling, they are not likely to be eaten in excess. Too much fibre can cause GI problems for some people, but it generally does not have adverse effects in most healthy people. For these reasons, an upper level ♦ has not been set for fibre.

♦ To increase your fibre intake:
- Eat raw vegetables.
- Eat fresh and dried fruit for snacks.
- Add legumes to soups, salads, and casseroles.
- Eat whole-grain breads that contain ≥3 g fibre per serving.
- Eat whole-grain cereals that contain ≥5 g fibre per serving.
- Eat fruits (such as pears) and vegetables (such as potatoes) with their skins.

♦ Daily Value:
- 25 g fibre (based on 11.5 g/1000 kcal)

♦ U.S. National Cancer Institute advises ≤35 g/day. World Health Organization advises ≤40 g/day.

From Guidance to Groceries

A diet following the *Food Guide*, which includes several servings of fruits, vegetables, and whole grains daily, can easily supply the recommended amount of carbohydrates and fibre. In selecting high-fibre foods, keep in mind the principle of variety. The fibres in oats lower cholesterol,

TABLE 4-4 Fibre in Selected Foods

Grains

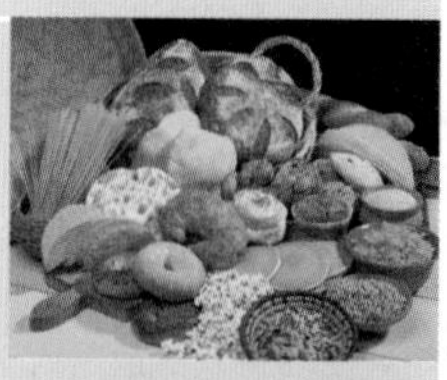

© Polara Studios, Inc.

Whole-grain products provide about 1 to 2 g (or more) of fibre per serving:

- 1 slice whole-wheat, pumpernickel, rye bread
- 30 grams ready-to-eat cereal (100% bran cereals contain 10 g or more)
- 125 mL (1/2 cup) cooked barley, bulgur, grits, oatmeal

Vegetables

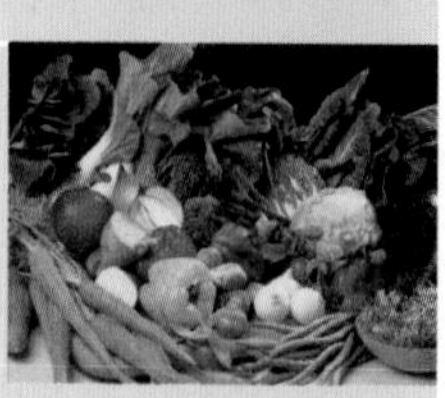

© Polara Studios, Inc.

Most vegetables contain about 2 to 3 g of fibre per serving:

- 250 mL (1 cup) raw bean sprouts
- 125 mL (1/2 cup) cooked broccoli, Brussels sprouts, cabbage, carrots, cauliflower, collards, corn, eggplant, green beans, green peas, kale, mushrooms, okra, parsnips, potatoes, pumpkin, spinach, sweet potatoes, swiss chard, winter squash
- 125 mL (1/2 cup) chopped raw carrots, peppers

Fruit

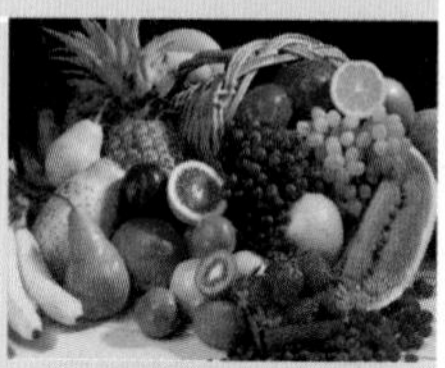

© Polara Studios, Inc.

Fresh, frozen, and dried fruits have about 2 g of fibre per serving:

- 1 medium apple, banana, kiwi, nectarine, orange, pear
- 125 mL (1/2 cup) applesauce, blackberries, blueberries, raspberries, strawberries
- Fruit juices contain very little fibre

Legumes

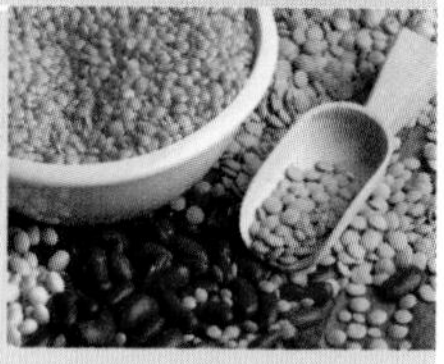

© MKucova/iStockphoto

Many legumes provide about 6 to 8 g of fibre per serving:

- 125 mL (1/2 cup) cooked baked beans, black beans, black-eyed peas, kidney beans, navy beans, pinto beans

Some legumes provide about 5 g of fibre per serving:

- 125 mL (1/2 cup) cooked garbanzo beans, great northern beans, lentils, lima beans, split peas

NOTE: APPENDIX H provides fibre grams for more than 2000 foods.

whereas those in bran help promote GI tract health. (Review Table 4-3 to see the diverse health effects of various fibres.)

Grain Products Thirty grams of most foods in the Grain Products group (for example, one slice of bread) provides about 15 grams of carbohydrate, mostly as starch. Be aware that some foods in this group, especially snack crackers and baked goods such as biscuits, croissants, and muffins, contain added sugars, added fat, or both. When selecting from the Grain Products group, be sure to include at least half as whole-grain products (see Figure 4-16). The "three are key" message may help consumers to remember to choose a whole-grain cereal for breakfast, a whole-grain bread for lunch, and a whole-grain pasta or rice for dinner. ♦

♦ Some food labels include information about the whole-grain contents.

Vegetables and Fruit The amount of carbohydrate a serving of vegetables provides depends primarily on its starch content. Starchy vegetables—125 millilitres (1/2 cup) of cooked corn, peas, or potatoes—provide about 15 grams of carbohydrate per serving. A serving of most other *nonstarchy* vegetables—such as 125 millilitres (1/2 cup) of broccoli, green beans, or tomatoes—provides about 5 grams. A typical fruit serving—a medium size banana, apple, or orange or 125 millilitres (1/2 cup) of most canned or fresh fruit—contains an average of about 15 grams of carbohydrate, mostly as sugars, including the fruit sugar fructose. Fruits vary greatly in their water and fibre contents and, therefore, in their sugar concentrations.

Milks and Alternatives A serving (250 mL or 1 cup) of milk or yogurt provides about 12 grams of carbohydrate. Cottage cheese provides about 6 grams of carbohydrate per 250 millilitres, but most other cheeses contain little, if any, carbohydrate.

Meats and Alternates With two exceptions, foods in the Meat and Alternatives group deliver almost no carbohydrate to the diet. The exceptions are nuts, which provide a little starch and fibre along with their abundant fat, and legumes, which provide an abundance of both starch and fibre. Just 125 millilitres (1/2 cup) serving of legumes provides about 20 grams of carbohydrate, a third from fibre.

♦ To calculate starch grams using the first label in Figure 4-16:
15 g total – 4 g (dietary fibre + sugars) = 11 g starch

Read Food Labels Food labels list the amount, in grams, of *total* carbohydrate—including starch, fibres, and sugars—per serving (review Figure 4-16). Fibre grams are also listed separately, as are the grams of sugars. (With this information, you can calculate starch grams ♦ by subtracting the grams of fibres and sugars from the total carbohydrate.) Sugars reflect both added sugars and those that occur naturally in foods. Total carbohydrate and dietary fibre are also expressed as "% Daily Values" for a person consuming 2000 kcalories; there is no Daily Value for sugars.

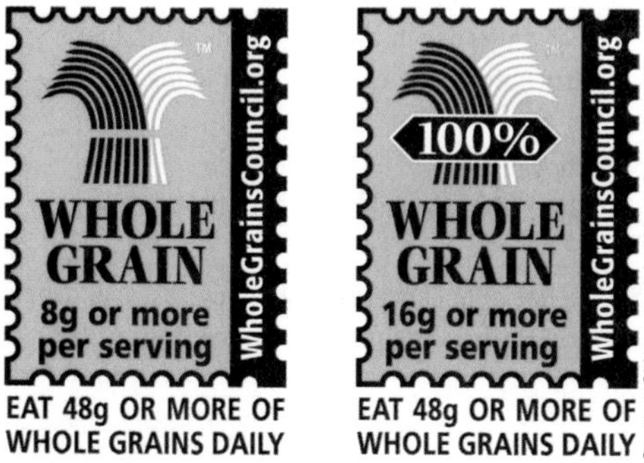
WholeGrainsCouncil.org
WHOLE GRAIN
8g or more per serving
EAT 48g OR MORE OF WHOLE GRAINS DAILY
WholeGrainsCouncil.org
100%
WHOLE GRAIN
16g or more per serving
EAT 48g OR MORE OF WHOLE GRAINS DAILY

Courtesy Oldways and the Whole Grains Council, www.wholegrainscouncil.org

Some food labels use a "whole-grain stamp" to help consumers identify whole-grain foods.

IN SUMMARY **Clearly, a diet rich in starches and fibres supports efforts to control body weight and prevent heart disease, cancer, diabetes, and GI disorders. For these reasons, recommendations urge people to eat plenty of whole grains, vegetables, legumes, and fruits—enough to provide 45 to 65 percent of the daily energy intake from carbohydrate.**

FIGURE 4-16 Bread Labels Compared

Although breads may appear similar, their ingredients vary widely. Breads made mostly from whole-grain flours provide more benefits to the body than breads made of enriched, refined, wheat flour.

Some "high-fibre" breads may contain purified cellulose or more nutritious whole grains. "Low-carbohydrate" breads may be regular white bread, thinly sliced to reduce carbohydrates per serving, or may contain soy flour, barley flour, or flaxseed to reduce starch content.

A trick for estimating a bread's content of a nutritious ingredient, such as whole-grain flour, is to read the ingredients list (ingredients are listed in order of predominance). Bread recipes generally include one teaspoon of salt per loaf. Therefore, when a bulky nutritious ingredient, such as whole grain, is listed after the salt, you'll know that less than a teaspoonful of the nutritious ingredient was added to the loaf—not enough to significantly improve the nutrient value of one slice of bread.

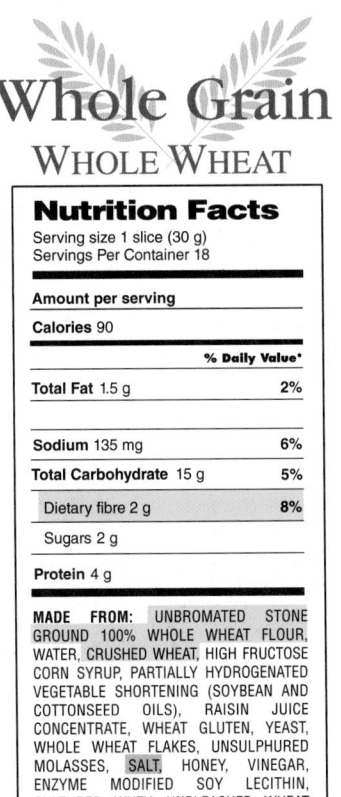

Whole Grain
WHOLE WHEAT

Nutrition Facts	
Serving size 1 slice (30 g)	
Servings Per Container 18	
Amount per serving	
Calories 90	
	% Daily Value*
Total Fat 1.5 g	2%
Sodium 135 mg	6%
Total Carbohydrate 15 g	5%
Dietary fibre 2 g	8%
Sugars 2 g	
Protein 4 g	

MADE FROM: UNBROMATED STONE GROUND 100% WHOLE WHEAT FLOUR, WATER, CRUSHED WHEAT, HIGH FRUCTOSE CORN SYRUP, PARTIALLY HYDROGENATED VEGETABLE SHORTENING (SOYBEAN AND COTTONSEED OILS), RAISIN JUICE CONCENTRATE, WHEAT GLUTEN, YEAST, WHOLE WHEAT FLAKES, UNSULPHURED MOLASSES, SALT, HONEY, VINEGAR, ENZYME MODIFIED SOY LECITHIN, CULTURED WHEY, UNBLEACHED WHEAT FLOUR AND SOY LECITHIN.

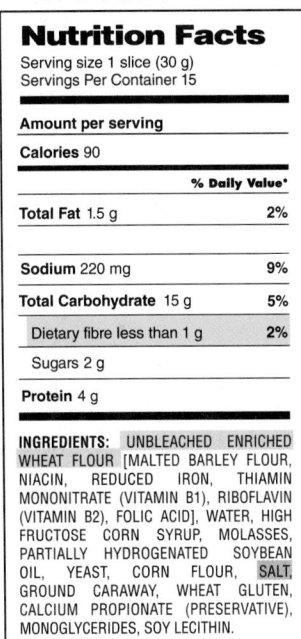

Natural
Wheat Bread

Nutrition Facts	
Serving size 1 slice (30 g)	
Servings Per Container 15	
Amount per serving	
Calories 90	
	% Daily Value*
Total Fat 1.5 g	2%
Sodium 220 mg	9%
Total Carbohydrate 15 g	5%
Dietary fibre less than 1 g	2%
Sugars 2 g	
Protein 4 g	

INGREDIENTS: UNBLEACHED ENRICHED WHEAT FLOUR [MALTED BARLEY FLOUR, NIACIN, REDUCED IRON, THIAMIN MONONITRATE (VITAMIN B1), RIBOFLAVIN (VITAMIN B2), FOLIC ACID], WATER, HIGH FRUCTOSE CORN SYRUP, MOLASSES, PARTIALLY HYDROGENATED SOYBEAN OIL, YEAST, CORN FLOUR, SALT, GROUND CARAWAY, WHEAT GLUTEN, CALCIUM PROPIONATE (PRESERVATIVE), MONOGLYCERIDES, SOY LECITHIN.

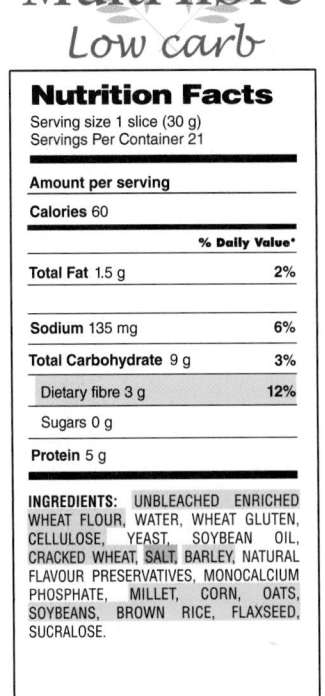

Multi-fibre
Low carb

Nutrition Facts	
Serving size 1 slice (30 g)	
Servings Per Container 21	
Amount per serving	
Calories 60	
	% Daily Value*
Total Fat 1.5 g	2%
Sodium 135 mg	6%
Total Carbohydrate 9 g	3%
Dietary fibre 3 g	12%
Sugars 0 g	
Protein 5 g	

INGREDIENTS: UNBLEACHED ENRICHED WHEAT FLOUR, WATER, WHEAT GLUTEN, CELLULOSE, YEAST, SOYBEAN OIL, CRACKED WHEAT, SALT, BARLEY, NATURAL FLAVOUR PRESERVATIVES, MONOCALCIUM PHOSPHATE, MILLET, CORN, OATS, SOYBEANS, BROWN RICE, FLAXSEED, SUCRALOSE.

In today's world, there is one other reason why plant foods rich in complex carbohydrates and natural sugars are a better choice than animal foods or foods high in concentrated sugars: in general, less energy and fewer resources are required to grow and process plant foods than to produce sugar or foods derived from animals. Chapter 21 takes a closer look at the environmental impacts of food production and use.

Nutrition Portfolio

Foods that derive from plants—whole grains, vegetables, legumes, and fruits—naturally provide ample carbohydrates and fibre with little or no fat. Refined foods often contain added sugars and fat.

Go to Diet Analysis Plus and choose one of the days on which you have tracked your diet for the entire day. Go to the Intake Spreadsheet report. Scroll down until you see: carb (g).

- Which of your foods for this day were highest in carbohydrate? Which of these foods also contain added sugars and fats? List better alternatives.
- List the types and amounts of grain products you ate on that day, making note of which are whole-grain or refined foods and how your choices could include more whole-grain options.

- List the types and amounts of fruits and vegetables you ate on that day, making note of how many are dark green, orange, or deep yellow, how many are starchy or legumes, and how your choices could include more of these options.
- Describe choices you can make in selecting and preparing foods and beverages to lower your intake of added sugars.

Diet Analysis PLUS

To complete this exercise, go to your Diet Analysis Plus at www.cengage.com/sso.

Nutrition on the Net

CENGAGENOW™

For further study of topics covered in this chapter, log on to **www.cengage.com/sso.**

- Learn more about lactose intolerance from the National Institute of Diabetes and Digestive and Kidney Diseases: **http://digestive.niddk.nih.gov/ddiseases/pubs/lactoseintolerance**
- Search for "sugar substitutes" at Health Canada, Food and Nutrition: **www.hc-sc.gc.ca**
- Search for "sugars" and "fiber" at the International Food Information Council site: **www.foodinsight.org**
- Learn more about dental caries from the Canadian Dental Association: **www.cda-adc.ca**
- Learn more about diabetes from the Canadian Diabetes Association: **www.diabetes.ca**

References

1. J. H. Cummings and A. M. Stephen, Carbohydrate terminology and classification, *European Journal of Clinical Nutrition* 61 (2007): S5–S18.
2. L. Van Horn and coauthors, The evidence for dietary prevention and treatment of cardiovascular disease, *Journal of the American Dietetic Association* 108 (2008): 287–331; M. O. Weickert and A. F. Pfeiffer, Metabolic effects of dietary fiber consumption and prevention of diabetes, *Journal of Nutrition* 138 (2008): 439–442; N. R. Sahyoan and coauthors, Whole-grain intake is inversely associated with metabolic syndrome and mortality in older adults, *American Journal of Clinical Nutrition* 83 (2006): 124–131.
3. J. R. Korzenik, Case closed? Diverticulitis: Epidemiology and fiber, *Journal of Clinical Gastroenterology* 40 (2006): S112–S116.
4. M.Nofrarías and coauthors, Long-term intake of resistant starch improves colonic mucosal integrity and reduces gut apoptosis and blood immune cells, *Nutrition* 23 (2007): 861–870.
5. Committee on Dietary Reference Intakes, *Dietary Reference Intakes: Energy, Carbohydrate, Fiber, Fat, Fatty Acids, Cholesterol, Protein, and Amino Acids* (Washington, D.C.: National Academies Press, 2005).
6. C. C. Robayo-Torres and B. L. Nichols, Molecular differentiation of congenital lactase deficiency from adult-type hypolactasia, *Nutrition Reviews* 65 (2007): 95–98; A. K. Campbell, J. P. Waud, and S. B. Matthews, The molecular basis of lactose intolerance, *Science Progress* 88 (2005): 157–202.
7. F. Guarner and coauthors, Should yoghurt cultures be considered probiotic? *British Journal of Nutrition* 93 (2005): 783–786.
8. T. He and coauthors, Effects of yogurt and bifidobacteria supplementation on the colonic microbiotia in lactose-intolerant subjects, *Journal of Applied Microbiology* 104 (2008): 595–604.
9. J. Wahren and K. Ekberg, Splanchnic regulation of glucose production, *Annual Review of Nutrition* 27 (2007): 329–345.
10. G. Riccardi, A. A. Rivellese, and R. Giacco, Role of glycemic index and glycemic load in the healthy state, in prediabetes, and in diabetes, *American Journal of Clinical Nutrition* 87 (2008): 269S–274S.
11. K. Foster-Powell, S.H.A. Holt, and J. C. Brand-Miller, International table of glycemic index and glycemic load values: 2002, *American Journal of Clinical Nutrition* 76 (2002): 5–56.
12. G. Livesey and coauthors, Glycemic response and health—A systematic review and meta-analysis: Relations between dietary glycemic properties and health outcomes, *American Journal of Clinical Nutrition* 87 (2008): 258S–268S; Canadian Diabetes Association Clinical Practice Expert Committee, Canadian Diabetes Association 2008 clinical practice guidelines for the prevention and management of diabetes in Canada, *Canadian Journal of Diabetes* 32 (2008): S1–S201.
13. A. W. Barclay and coauthors, Glycemic index, glycemic load, and chronic disease risk: A meta-analysis of observational studies, *American Journal of Clinical Nutrition* 87 (2008): 627–637; J. Howlett and M. Ashwell, Glycemic response and health: Summary of a workshop, *American Journal of Clinical Nutrition* 87 (2008): 212S–216S; A. Mosdøl and coauthors, Dietary glycemic index and glycemic load are associated with high-density-lipoprotein cholesterol at baseline but not with increased risk of diabetes in the Whitehall II study, *American Journal of Clinical Nutrition* 86 (2007): 988–994; T. L. Halton and coauthors, Low-carbohydrate-diet score and the risks of coronary heart disease in women, *New England Journal of Medicine* 355 (2006): 1991–2002; C. B. Ebbeling and coauthors, Effects of an ad libitum low-glycemic load diet on cardiovascular disease risk factors in obese young adults, *American Journal of Clinical Nutrition* 81 (2005): 976–982; S. Dickinson and J. Brand-Miller, Glycemic index, postprandial glycemia and cardiovascular disease, *Current Opinion in Lipidology* 16 (2005): 69–75.
14. C. B. Ebbeling and coauthors, Effects of a low-glycemic load vs low-fat diet in obese young adults: A randomized trial, *Journal of the American Medical Association* 297 (2007): 2092–2102; K. C. Maki and coauthors, Effects of a reduced-glycemic-load diet on body weight, body composition, and cardiovascular disease risk markers in overweight and obese adults, *American Journal of Clinical Nutrition* 85 (2007): 724–734; R. Sichieri and coauthors, An 18-mo randomized trial of a low-glycemic-index diet and weight change in Brazilian women, *American Journal of Clinical Nutrition* 86 (2007): 707–713; A. Flint and coauthors, Glycemic and insulinemic responses as determinants of appetite in humans, *American Journal of Clinical Nutrition* 84 (2006): 1365–1373; H. Hare-Bruun, A. Flint, and B. L. Heitmann, Glycemic index and glycemic load in relation to changes in body weight, body fat distribution, and body composition in adult Danes, *American Journal of Clinical Nutrition* 84 (2006): 871–879; M. A. Pereira, Weighing in on glycemic index and body weight, *American Journal of Clinical Nutrition* 84 (2006): 677–679; G. Livesey, Low-glycaemic diets and health: Implications for obesity, *Proceedings of the Nutrition Society* 64 (2005): 105–113.
15. H. Hare-Bruun and coauthors, Should glycemic index and glycemic load be considered in dietary recommendations? *Nutrition Reviews* 66 (2008): 569–590.

16. T.M.S. Wolever and coauthors, Measuring the glycemic index of foods: Interlaboratory study, *American Journal of Clinical Nutrition* 87 (2008): 247S–257S.
17. H. V. Worthington, J. E. Clarkson, and O. B. Eden, Interventions for preventing oral mucositis for patients with cancer receiving treatment, *Cochrane Database of Systematic Reviews* 4 (2007): CD000978; I. M. Paul and coauthors, Effect of honey, dextromethorphan, and no treatment on nocturnal cough and sleep quality for coughing children and their parents, *Archives of Pediatric and Adolescent Medicine* 161 (2007): 1140–1146.
18. A. Bhargava and A. Amialchuk, Added sugars displaced the use of vital nutrients in the National Food Stamp Program Survey, *Journal of Nutrition* 137 (2007): 453–460.
19. K. J. Cross, N. L. Huq, and E. C. Reynolds, Casein phosphopeptides in oral health: Chemistry and clinical applications, *Current Pharmaceutical Design* 13 (2007): 793–800; B. T. Amaechi and S. M. Higham, Dental erosion, Possible approaches to prevention and control, *Journal of Dentistry* 33 (2005): 243–252.
20. T. Jaeggi and A. Lussi, Prevalence, incidence and distribution of erosion, *Monographs in Oral Science* 20 (2006): 44–65; S. Wongkhantee and coauthors, Effect of acidic food and drinks on surface hardness of enamel, dentine, and tooth-coloured filling materials, *Journal of Dentistry* 34 (2006): 214–220; W. K. Seow and K. M. Thong, Erosive effects of common beverages on extracted premolar teeth, *Australian Dental Journal* 50 (2005): 173–178.
21. Position of the American Dietetic Association: Oral health and nutrition, *Journal of the American Dietetic Association* 107 (2007): 1418–1428.
22. Committee on Dietary Reference Intakes, 2002; Health Canada, *Eating Well with Canada's Food Guide* (2007). www.hc-sc.gc.ca/fn-an/food-guide-aliment/index-eng.php, accessed September 2, 2011.
23. Committee on Dietary Reference Intakes, 2005.
24. Health Canada, Notice—Revised Guidelines for the Use of Stevia in Natural Health Products (2009). www.hc-sc.gc.ca/dhp-mps/prodnatur/legislation/docs/notice-avis-stevia-eng.php, accessed September 2, 2011.
25. Canadian Food Inspection Agency, Summary Table of Disease Risk Reduction Claims, Table 8-1 (2009). www.inspection.gc.ca/english/fssa/labeti/guide/ch8e.shtml#tab8-1, accessed September 2, 2011.
26. Health Canada, Food and Nutrition, Sugar substitutes. www.hc-sc.gc.ca/fn-an/securit/addit/sweeten-edulcor/index-eng.php, accessed September 2, 2011.
27. M. T. Streppel and coauthors, Dietary fiber intake in relation to coronary heart disease and all-cause mortality over 40 y: The Zutphen Study, *American Journal of Clinical Nutrition* 88 (2008): 1119–1125; M. F. Chong, B. A. Fielding, and K. N. Frayn, Metabolic interaction of dietary sugars and plasma lipids with a focus on mechanisms and de novo lipogenesis, *Proceedings of the Nutrition Society* 66 (2007): 52–59; P. B. Mellen, T. F. Walsh, and D. M. Herrington, Whole grain intake and cardiovascular disease: A meta-analysis, *Nutrition, Metabolism and Cardiovascular Diseases* (2007): 283–290; R. Solà and coauthors, Effects of soluble fiber (*Plantago ovata* husk) on plasma lipids, lipoproteins, and apolipoproteins in men with ischemic heart disease, *American Journal of Clinical Nutrition* 85 (2007): 1157–1163; M. K. Jenson and coauthors, Whole grains, bran and germ in relation to homocysteine and markers of glycemic control, lipids, and inflammation, *American Journal of Clinical Nutrition* 83 (2006): 275–283.
28. M. B. Andon and J. W. Anderson, State of the art reviews: The oatmeal-cholesterol connection: 10 Years later, *American Journal of Lifestyle Medicine* 2 (2008): 51–57.
29. Jenson and coauthors, 2006.
30. D. O. Jacobs, Diverticulitis, *New England Journal of Medicine* 357 (2007): 2057–2066; H. Salzman and D. Lillie, Diverticular disease: Diagnosis and treatment, *American Family Physician* 72 (2005): 1229–1234.
31. A. Schatzkin and coauthors, Dietary fiber and whole-grain consumption in relation to colorectal cancer in the NIH-AARP Diet and Health Study, *American Journal of Clinical Nutrition* 85 (2007): 1353–1360; S. Bingham, Symposium on "Plant foods and public health": The fibre-folate debate in colo-rectal cancer, *Proceedings of the Nutrition Society* 65 (2006): 19–23; K. B. Michels and coauthors, Fiber intake and incidence of colorectal cancer among 76,947 women and 47,279 men, *Cancer Epidemiology Biomarkers and Prevention* 14 (2005): 842–849; Y. Park and coauthors, Dietary fiber intake and risk of colorectal cancer, *Journal of the American Medical Association* 294 (2005): 2849–2857.
32. D. J. Rose and coauthors, Influence of dietary fiber on inflammatory bowel disease and colon cancer: Importance of fermentation pattern, *Nutrition Reviews* 65 (2007): 51–62.
33. L. A. Tucker and K. S. Thomas, Increasing total fiber intake reduces risk of weight and fat gains in women, *Journal of Nutrition* 139 (2009): 567–581.
34. R. A. Samra and G. H. Anderson, Insoluble cereal fiber reduces appetite and short-term food intake and glycemic response to food consumed 75 min later by healthy men, *American Journal of Clinical Nutrition* 86 (2007): 972–979.
35. J. W. Anderson and coauthors, Health benefits of dietary fiber, *Nutrition Reviews* 67 (2009): 188–205.
36. Committee on Dietary Reference Intakes, 2005.
37. Health Canada, Food and Nutrition, Canadian Community Health Survey 2.2, Nutrition Focus (2004). www.hc-sc.gc.ca/fn-an/surveill/nutrition/commun/cchs_focus-volet_escc-eng.php#p1, accessed September 2, 2011.

HIGHLIGHT 4

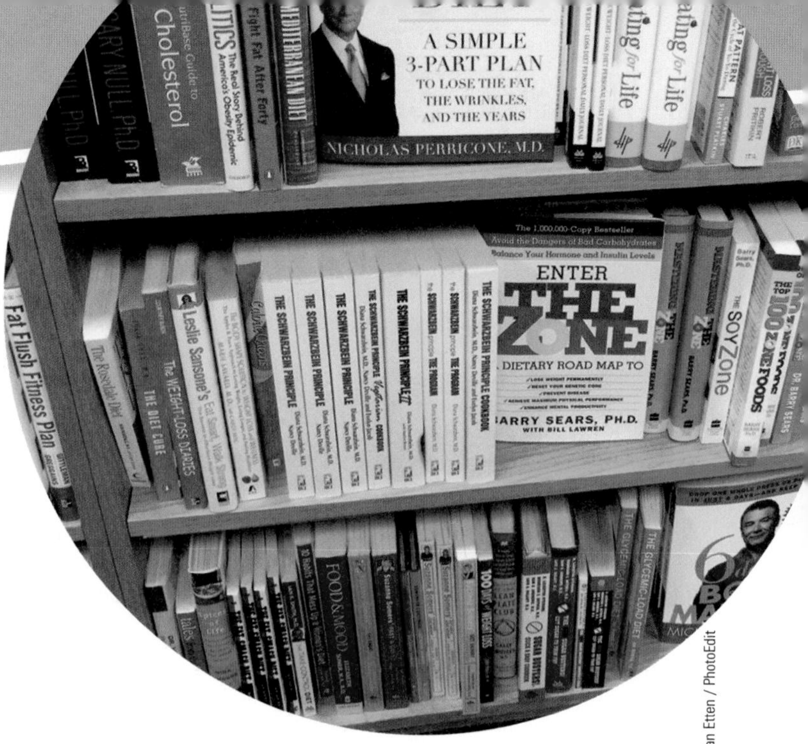
Cholesterol
Fight Fat After Forty
MEDITERRANEAN DIET
A SIMPLE
3-PART PLAN
TO LOSE THE FAT,
THE WRINKLES,
AND THE YEARS
NICHOLAS PERRICONE, M.D.
Fat Flush Fitness Plan
THE SCHWARZBEIN PRINCIPLE
ENTER
THE
ZONE
A DIETARY ROAD MAP TO
ARRY SEARS, PH.D.
SoyZone
FOOD & MOOD

Carbs, kCalories, and Controversies

Carbohydrate-rich foods are easy to like. Mashed potatoes, warm muffins, blueberry pancakes, freshly baked bread, and tasty rice or pasta dishes tempt most people's palates. In recent years, such homey foods have been blamed for causing weight gain and harming health. Popular writers have persuaded consumers that carbohydrates are "bad."[1] In contrast, the *Food Guide* urges people to consume plenty of fruits, vegetables, legumes, and whole grains—all carbohydrate-rich foods.

Do carbohydrate-rich foods cause obesity and related health problems?[2] Should people "cut carbs" to lose weight and protect their health? Many popular diet books espouse a carbohydrate-restricted or carbohydrate-modified diet. Some claim that all or some types of carbohydrates are bad. Some go so far as to equate carbohydrates with toxic poisons or addictive drugs. "Bad" carbohydrates—such as sugar, white flour, and potatoes—are considered evil because they are absorbed easily and raise blood glucose. The pancreas then responds by secreting insulin—and insulin is touted as the real villain responsible for our nation's epidemic of obesity. Whether restricting overall carbohydrate intake or replacing certain "bad" carbohydrates with "good" carbohydrates, many of these popular diets tend to distort the facts. This highlight examines the scientific evidence behind some of the current controversies surrounding carbohydrates and their kcalories.

Macronutrient kCalorie Contributions

The incidence of obesity in North America has risen dramatically over the past several decades.[3] Popular diet books often blame carbohydrates for this increase in obesity. One way researchers can explore whether the amount of carbohydrate in the diet contributes to increases in body weight over time is by reviewing national food statistics. Figure H4-1 presents a summary of estimated available energy from macronutrients (carbohydrates, fat, and protein) data over the past three decades. Since the 1970s, kcalories available from carbohydrates, fats and protein have remained virtually unchanged.[4]

A closer look at the data reveals that, while the percentage of kcalories from the three energy nutrients remained about the same, total daily energy available increased significantly. In general, as food became more readily available, consumers began to eat more than they had in the past.[5] Since the 1970s, total energy available to Canadians has increased by about 100–200 kcalories a day (see Figure H4-2).[6] Also, while physical activity levels of adult Canadians increased by approximately 10 percent since the mid 1990s only about half were considered to be at least moderately active in 2008.[7] In addition, and yet to be fully explained, is the fact that adult obesity has also increased over the last couple decades (see Figure H4-3).

Might too many carbohydrates in the diet be to blame for weight gains? Interestingly, epidemiological studies find an *inverse* relationship between carbohydrate intake and body weight.[8] Those with the highest carbohydrate intake have the lowest body weight and vice versa. Dietary fibre, which favours a healthy body weight, explains some but not all of this relationship.

FIGURE H4-1 **Macronutrients Available per capita over Time**

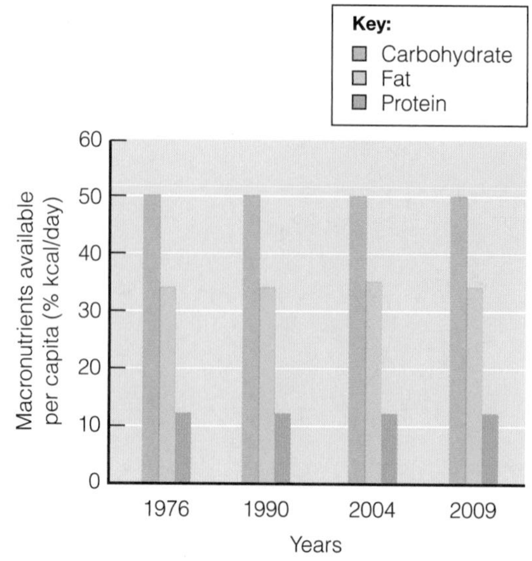
Key:
Carbohydrate
Fat
Protein
Macronutrients available per capita (% kcal/day)
0
10
20
30
40
50
60
1976
1990
2004
2009
Years

SOURCE: Modified from Statistics Canada. *Table 003-0080 – Nutrients in the food supply, by source of nutritional equivalent and commodity, annual (milligrams unless otherwise noted)*, CANSIM (database), Using E-STAT (distributor). http://estat.statcan.gc.ca/cgi-win/cnsmcgi.exe?Lang=E&EST-Fi=EStat/English/CII_1-eng.htm(accessed: September 16, 2011).

FIGURE H4-2 Daily Energy Intake over Time

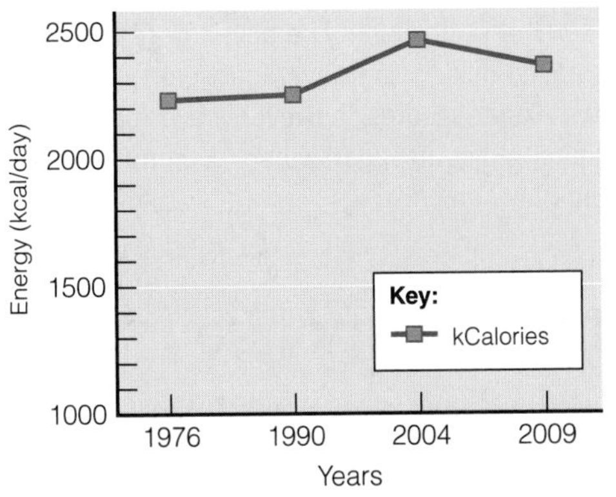
2500
2000
1500
1000
Energy (kcal/day)
Key:
kCalories
1976
1990
2004
2009
Years

SOURCE: Modified from Statistics Canada. *Table 003-0080 – Nutrients in the food supply, by source of nutritional equivalent and commodity, annual (milligrams unless otherwise noted)*, CANSIM (database), Using E-STAT (distributor). http://estat.statcan.gc.ca/cgi-win/cnsmcgi.exe?Lang=E&EST-Fi=EStat/English/CII_1-eng.htm(accessed: September 16, 2011).

FIGURE H4-3 Increases in Obesity (18 Years and Older)

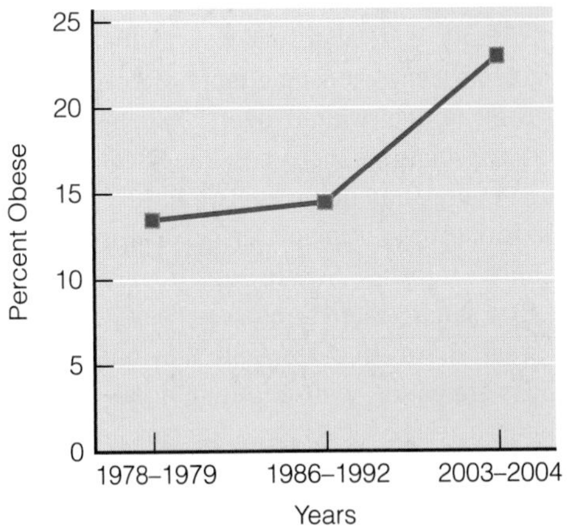
25
20
15
10
5
0
Percent Obese
1978–1979
1986–1992
2003–2004
Years

SOURCE: Modified from Statistics Canada. Health Reports Vol 17 (3) 2006 http://www.statcan.gc.ca/studies-etudes/82-003/archive/2006/9276-eng.pdf.

Might a low-carbohydrate diet support weight losses? Studies report that people following low-carbohydrate diets do lose weight.[9] In fact, they lose more than people following conventional high-carbohydrate, low-fat diets—but only for the first six months. Their later gains make up the difference, so total weight loss is no different after one year.[10] For the most part, weight loss is similar for people following either a low-carbohydrate diet or a high-carbohydrate diet.[11] This is an important point. Weight losses reflect restricted kcalories—not the proportion of energy nutrients in the diet.[12] Any diet can produce weight loss, at least temporarily, if energy intake is restricted.

Sugars' Share in the Problem

Over the past several decades, as obesity rates increased sharply, consumption of added sugars in North America reached an all-time high—much of it because high-fructose corn syrup use, especially in beverages, surged.[13] High-fructose corn syrup is composed of fructose and glucose in a ratio of roughly 50:50. Compared with sucrose, high-fructose corn syrup is less expensive, easier to use, and more stable. In addition to being used in beverages, high-fructose corn syrup sweetens candies, baked goods, and hundreds of other foods. While Canadians are consuming approximately 20 percent of their total energy intake as sugars (i.e., total sugar intake) "a 2011 estimate indicates that Canadians are consuming between 10–13 percent of their total kcalories as added sugars."[14]

Although the use of high-fructose corn syrup sweetener parallels unprecedented increases in the incidence of obesity, does it mean that the increasing sugar intakes are responsible for the increase in body fat and its associated health problems?[15] Excess sugar in the diet may be associated with more fat on the body.[16] When eaten in excess of need, energy from added sugars contributes to body fat stores, just as excess energy from other sources does.[17] Added sugars provide excess energy, raising the risk of weight gain.[18] When total energy intake is controlled, however, *moderate* amounts of sugar do not *cause* obesity. Yet moderating sugar intake can be a challenge. Some claim sugar is addictive. Others assert sugary beverages are particularly easy to swallow and make it difficult for the body to regulate appetite control and energy metabolism.

Cravings and Addictions

Do sugars cause cravings and addictions? Foods in general, and carbohydrates and sugars more specifically, are not physically addictive in the ways that drugs are. Yet some people describe themselves as having "carbohydrate cravings" or being "sugar addicts." One frequently noted theory is that people seek carbohydrates as a way to increase their levels of the brain neurotransmitter serotonin, which elevates mood. Interestingly, when those with self-described carbohydrate cravings indulge, they tend to eat more of everything; the percentage of energy from carbohydrates remains unchanged.

One reasonable explanation for the carbohydrate cravings that some people experience involves the self-imposed labelling of a food as both "good" and "bad"—that is, one that is desirable but should be eaten with restraint. Restricting intake heightens the desire further (a "craving"). Then "addiction" is used to explain why resisting the food is so difficult and, sometimes, even impossible. But the "addiction" is not physiological or pharmacological.

Simple to Swallow

One added sugar in particular—the liquid high-fructose corn syrup—is used to sweeten beverages. In general, the energy intake of people who drink soft drinks, fruit punches, and other sugary beverages is greater than those who choose differently. Adolescents, for example, who drink as much as 770 millilitres (26 fl oz) or more (about two cans) of sugar-sweetened soft drinks daily, consume 400 more kcalories a day than teens who don't.

Not too surprisingly, they also tend to weigh more.[19] Overweight children and adolescents consume more sweet desserts and soft drinks than their normal-weight peers.[20] Review of the research confirms that consuming sugary beverages correlates with both increased food energy and being overweight.[21]

The liquid form of sugar in soft drinks makes it especially easy to overconsume kcalories. Swallowing liquid kcalories requires little effort. The sugar kcalories of sweet beverages also cost less than many other energy sources, and they are widely available. Also, beverages are energy-dense, providing more than 150 kcalories per 355 millilitre (12 fl oz) can, and many people drink several cans a day. The convenience, economy, availability, and flavours of sugary foods and beverages make overconsumption especially likely.

Limiting selections of foods and beverages high in added sugars can be an effective weight-loss strategy, especially for people whose excess kcalories come primarily from added sugars. Replacing a can of cola with a glass of water every day, for example, can help a person lose half a kilogram (or at least not gain it) in one month.[22] That may not sound like much, but it adds up to more than 10 pounds a year, for very little effort.

Appetite Control

Recall from earlier in this Chapter that glucose stimulates the release of insulin from the pancreas. Insulin, in turn, sets off a sequence of hormonal actions that suppress the appetite.[23] (Appetite regulation is discussed fully in Chapter 8.) Fructose, in contrast, does not stimulate the release of insulin, and therefore does not suppress appetite. Theoretically, then, eating lots of fructose would never satisfy a person's appetite. Although this idea sounds plausible, a major flaw exists: people don't typically eat pure fructose. They eat sucrose or high-fructose corn syrup, and both of these sugars contain sufficient glucose to stimulate the release of insulin and suppress appetite accordingly.

Whether the meal or snack is liquid or solid may also affect appetite. Even when kcaloric intake is the same, a fresh apple suppresses appetite more than apple juice.[24] Consequently, beverages can influence weight gains both by providing energy and by not satisfying hunger.

Energy Regulation

One explanation of why it is so easy to overconsume sugary beverages is that perhaps the body's energy regulation system cannot detect the kcalories of sugar in liquid form. Consequently, a person would not compensate for energy excesses by reducing food intake at other times. A research study tested this hypothesis by giving students 450 kcalories' worth of either solid sugars (roughly 40 jelly beans) or liquid sugars (about three 355 mL cans of soft drinks) to consume daily whenever they chose.[25] Sure enough, the energy intake from other foods during "jelly-bean weeks" was lower—the students ate less food to compensate for the kcalories received from the jelly beans. By comparison, energy intake from other foods during the "soft-drink weeks" did *not* decrease—the students ate their meals without compensating for the kcalories in the beverages. Consequently, body weight increased during the beverage weeks, but not during the candy weeks. Other studies, however, have found no differences between liquid and solid sugars when examining appetite, energy intake, or body weight.[26]

Insulin's Response

Several popular diet books hold insulin responsible for the obesity problem and advocate a low glycemic diet as the weight-loss solution. Yet, among nutrition researchers, controversy continues to surround the questions of whether insulin promotes weight gain or a low glycemic diet fosters weight loss.[27]

Recall that just after a meal, blood glucose rises and insulin responds. How high insulin levels surge may influence whether the body stores or uses its glucose and fat supplies.[28] What does insulin do? Among its roles, insulin facilitates the transport of glucose into the cells, the storage of fatty acids as fat, and the synthesis of cholesterol. It is an anabolic hormone that builds and stores. True—but there's more to the story. Insulin is only one of many factors involved in the body's metabolism of nutrients and regulation of body weight.

Furthermore, as Chapter 4's discussion of the glycemic index pointed out, the glycemic effect of a particular food varies (see Figure 4-13 on p. 107)—diet books often mislead people by claiming that each food has a set glycemic effect. The glycemic effect of a food depends on how the food is ripened, processed, and cooked; the time of day the food is eaten; the other foods eaten with it; and the presence or absence of certain diseases such as type 2 diabetes in the person eating the food.[29]

Most importantly, insulin is critical to maintaining health, as any person with type 1 diabetes can attest. Insulin causes problems only when a person develops insulin resistance—that is, when the body's cells do not respond to the large quantities of insulin that the pancreas continues to pump out in an effort to get a response. Insulin resistance is a major health problem—but it is not caused by carbohydrate, or by protein, or by fat. It results from being overweight. Importantly, when a person loses weight, insulin response improves, regardless of the diet.

The Glycemic Index and Body Weight

As this chapter mentions, the glycemic index identifies foods that raise blood glucose and stimulate insulin secretion. What is the relationship between a diet's glycemic index and fat storage? Studies find that diets with a high glycemic index are positively associated with body weight.[30] Because fructose does not stimulate insulin secretion, it has a low glycemic index.[31] Yet some research suggests that fructose favours the fat-making pathways and impairs the fat-clearing pathways in the body.[32] As the liver busily makes lipids, its handling of glucose becomes unbalanced and insulin resistance develops.[33] Research is beginning to find links between high fructose intake and prediabetes and the metabolic syndrome.[34]

Might a low glycemic diet foster weight loss?[35] When obese people followed one of three low-kcalorie diets—high glycemic diet, low glycemic diet, or high-fat diet—for 9 months, they all lost about 10 kilograms (20 lbs).[36] Furthermore, insulin sensitivity improved for all of them. Other studies confirm that overweight people experience similar weight losses on a low-kcalorie diet regardless of whether it has a high or a low glycemic index.[37] In other words, all low-kcalorie diets support weight loss; defining the type or amount of carbohydrate does not enhance losses. A low glycemic meal may, however, prompt less energy intake at the next meal.[38]

Clearly, if kcalories are low, obese people on either a low glycemic diet or a traditional low-fat diet can lose weight. Overweight people can lose as much or more weight by emphasizing low glycemic foods as they can by following a typical low-fat, portion-controlled weight-loss diet.[39]

The Individual's Response to Foods

The body's insulin response depends not only on a food, but also on a person's metabolism. Some people react to dietary carbohydrate with a low insulin response. Others have a high insulin response. One study reports that increases in body weight over 6 years were similar in people following either a high-carbohydrate diet or a low-carbohydrate diet. But those with a high insulin response gained more weight, especially when they were on a high-carbohydrate diet.[40] By the same token, for those with a higher insulin response, weight loss may be greater on a low glycemic diet.[41]

How energy is stored after a meal depends in part on how the body responds to insulin. After eating a high-carbohydrate meal, normal-weight people who are insulin resistant tend to synthesize about half as much glycogen in muscles and make about twice as much fat in the liver as people who are insulin sensitive.[42] Some research suggests that restricting carbohydrate intake may improve glucose control, insulin response, and blood lipids.[43]

In Summary

As might be expected given the similarity in their chemical composition, high-fructose corn syrup and sucrose produce similar effects in appetite control and energy metabolism.[44] In fact, high-fructose corn syrup is more like sucrose than it is like fructose. Furthermore, people don't eat pure fructose; they eat foods and drink beverages that contain added sugars—either high-fructose corn syrup or sucrose. Limiting these sugars is a helpful strategy when trying to control body weight, but restricting all carbohydrates would be unwise.

The quality of the diet suffers when carbohydrates are restricted.[45] Without fruits, vegetables, and whole grains, low-carbohydrate diets lack not only carbohydrate, but fibre, vitamins, minerals, and phytochemicals as well—all dietary factors protective against disease.[46] The DRI recommends that carbohydrates contribute between 45 and 65 percent of daily energy intake. Intakes within this range can support healthy body weight and do not contribute to obesity—when total energy intake is appropriate. Similarly, added sugars increase energy intake, but need not contribute to obesity—when total energy intake is appropriate.

Research results on the glycemic index of diets are mixed, but when results are clear, a low glycemic diet has the greatest advantages. A low glycemic meal seems to curb appetite and limit energy intake of the next meal. Low glycemic diets are also more likely to be rich in nutrients and fibre than high glycemic diets.[47] A healthy diet includes a variety of carbohydrate-rich sources: whole-grain cereals, vegetables, legumes, and fruits.[48]

Nutrition on the Net

CENGAGENOW™
For further study of topics covered in this chapter, log on to **www.cengage.com/sso**.

- Learn more about how to make better food and activity choices from Dietitians of Canada with the help of their online eaTracker program: **www.eatracker.ca**
- Use Health Canada's online version of the Canadian Nutrient File to find out the energy and nutrient content of the foods you eat: **www.hc-sc.gc.ca/fn-an/nutrition/fiche-nutri-data/index-eng.php**
- Use the Dietitians of Canada and GSI Canada's online interactive website to find out the nutrient content of common foods in your diet: **http://www.eatwise.ca**
- Find out more about what Canadians are eating: **www.hc-sc.gc.ca/fn-an/surveill/nutrition/commun/art-nutr-eng.php**
- Find out more about guidelines for choosing a weight management program from Dietitians of Canada: **www.dietitians.ca/Nutrition-Resources-A-Z/Fact-Sheet-Pages(HTML)/Weight-Loss-and-Control/Guidelines-for-Choosing-a-Weight-Loss-Program.aspx**

References

1. G. A. Bray, Viewpoint: *Good Calories, Bad Calories* by Gary Taubes, *Obesity Reviews* 9 (2008): 251–263.
2. D. B. Allison and R. D. Mattes, Nutritively sweetened beverage consumption and obesity: The need for solid evidence on a fluid issue, *Journal of the American Medical Association* 301 (2009): 318–320.
3. K. Langlois, D. Garriguet, and L. Findlay, Diet composition and obesity among Canadian adults, *Health Reports* 20:4 (2009). Statistics Canada, Catalogue no. 82-003-XPE. www.statcan.gc.ca/pub/82-003-x/82-003-x2009004-eng.pdf#page=13, accessed September 15, 2011; C. L. Ogden and coauthors, Prevalence of overweight and obesity in the United States, 1999–2004, *Journal of the American Medical Association* 295 (2006): 1549–1555.
4. Statistics Canada, Table 003-0080 – Nutrients in the food supply, by source of nutritional equivalent and commodity, annual (milligrams unless otherwise noted), CANSIM (database), using E-STAT (distributor). http://estat.statcan.gc.ca/cgi-win/cnsmcgi.exe?Lang=E&EST-Fi=EStat/English/CII_1-eng.htm, accessed September 16, 2011.
5. Statistics Canada, Table 003-0080.
6. Statistics Canada, Table 003-0080.
7. Canadian Fitness and Lifestyle Research Institute, 2008 Physical Activity Monitor. http://72.10.49.94/node/82, accessed September 17, 2011.
8. G. A. Gaesser, Carbohydrate quantity and quality in relation to body mass index, *Journal of the American Dietetic Association* 107 (2007): 1768–1780.
9. A. Astrup, T. M. Larsen, and A. Harper, Atkins and other low-carbohydrate diets: Hoax or an effective tool for weight loss? *The Lancet* 364 (2004): 897–899; E. C. Westman and coauthors, Effect of 6-month adherence to a very low carbohydrate diet program, *American Journal of Medicine* 113 (2002): 30–36.
10. C. Erlanson-Albertsson and J. Mei, The effect of low carbohydrate on energy metabolism, *International Journal of Obesity* 29 (2005): S26–S30; L. Stern and coauthors, The effects of low-carbohydrate versus conventional weight loss diets in severely obese adults: One-year follow-up of a randomized trial, *Annals of Internal Medicine* 140 (2004): 778–785; G. D. Foster and coauthors, A randomized trial of a low-carbohydrate diet for obesity, *New England Journal of Medicine* 348 (2003): 2082–2090.
11. I. Shai and coauthors, Weight loss with a low-carbohydrate, Mediterranean, or low-fat diet, *New England Journal of Medicine* 359 (2008): 229–241; R. F. Kushner and B. Doerfier, Low-carbohydrate, high-protein diets revisited, *Current Opinion in Gastroenterology* 24 (2008): 198–203; A. K. Halyburton and coauthors, Low- and high-carbohydrate weight-loss diets have similar effects on mood but not cognitive performance, *American Journal of Clinical Nutrition* 86 (2007): 580–587; T. McLaughlin and coauthors, Effects of moderate variations in macronutrient composition on weight loss and reduction in cardiovascular disease risk in obese, insulin-resistant adults, *American Journal of Clinical Nutrition* 84 (2006): 813–821.
12. F. M. Sacks and coauthors, Comparison of weight-loss diets with different compositions of fat, protein, and carbohydrates, *New England Journal of Medicine* 360 (2009): 859-873; R. M. van Dam and J. C. Seidell, Carbohydrate intake and obesity, *European Journal of Clinical Nutrition* 61 (2007): S75–S99.
13. V. S. Malik, M. B. Schulze, and F. B. Hu, Intake of sugar-sweetened beverages and weight gain: A systematic review, *American Journal of Clinical Nutrition* 84 (2006): 274–288.
14. Canadian Sugar Institute, Sugars consumption (2011). www.sugar.ca/english/healthprofessionals/sugarsconsumption.cfm#intakes, accessed September 28, 2011; Statistics Canada, Sugar consumption of Canadians of all ages (September 2011). www.statcan.gc.ca/pub/82-003-x/2011003/article/11540-eng.htm, accessed September 28, 2011.
15. G. A. Bray, How bad is fructose? *American Journal of Clinical Nutrition* 86 (2007): 895–896; R. Dhingra and coauthors, Soft drink consumption and risk of developing cardiometabolic risk factors and the metabolic syndrome in middle-aged adults in the community, *Circulation* 116 (2007): 480–488; R. J. Johnson and coauthors, Potential role of sugar (fructose) in the epidemic of hypertension, obesity and the metabolic syndrome, diabetes, kidney disease, and cardiovascular disease, *American Journal of Clinical Nutrition* 86 (2007): 899–906; S. C. Larsson, L. Bergkvist, and A. Wolk, Consumption of sugar and sugar-sweetened foods and the risk of pancreatic cancer in a prospective study, *American Journal of Clinical Nutrition* 84 (2006): 1171–1176.
16. J. N. Davis and coauthors, Associations of dietary sugar and glycemic index with adiposity and insulin dynamics in overweight Latino youth, *American Journal of Clinical Nutrition* 86 (2007): 1331–1338.
17. R. A. Forshee and coauthors, A critical examination of the evidence relating high fructose corn syrup and weight gain, *Critical Reviews in Food Science and Nutrition* 47 (2007): 561–582.
18. L. R. Vartanian, M. B. Schwartz, and K. D. Brownell, Effects of soft drink consumption on nutrition and health: A systematic review and meta-analysis, *American Journal of Public Health* 97 (2007): 667–675.
19. R. Dhingra and coauthors, Soft drink consumption and risk of developing cardiometabolic risk factors and the metabolic syndrome in middle-aged adults in the community, *Circulation* 116 (2007): 480–488; L. R. Vartanian, M. B. Schwartz, and K. D. Brownell, Effects of soft drink consumption on nutrition and health: A systematic review and meta-analysis, *American Journal of Public Health* 97 (2007): 667–675.
20. I. Aeberli and coauthors, Fructose intake is a predictor of LDL particle size in overweight schoolchildren, *American Journal of Clinical Nutrition* 86 (2007): 1174–1178.
21. A. Drewnowski and F. Bellisle, Liquid kcalories, sugar, and body weight, *American Journal of Clinical Nutrition* 85 (2007): 651–661; V. S. Malik, M. B. Schulze, and F. B. Hu, Intake of sugar-sweetened beverages and weight gain: A systematic review, *American Journal of Clinical Nutrition* 84 (2006): 274–288.
22. L. Chen and coauthors, Reduction in consumption of sugar-sweetened beverages is associated with weight loss: The PREMIER trial, *American Journal of Clinical Nutrition* 89 (2009): 1299–1306.
23. K. J. Melanson and coauthors, High-fructose corn syrup, energy intake, and appetite regulation, *American Journal of Clinical Nutrition* 88 (2008): 1738S–1744S.
24. R. D. Mattes and W. W. Campbell, Effects of food form and timing of ingestion on appetite and energy intake in lean young adults and in young adults with obesity, *Journal of the American Dietetic Association* 109 (2009): 430–437.
25. D. P. DiMeglio and R. D. Mattes, Liquid versus solid carbohydrate: Effects on food intake and body weight, *International Journal of Obesity and Related Metabolic Disorders* 24 (2000): 794–800.
26. T. Akhavan and G. H. Anderson, Effects of glucose-to-fructose ratios in solutions on subjective satiety, food intake, and satiety hormones in young men, *American Journal of Clinical Nutrition* 86 (2007): 1354–1363; K. J. Melanson and coauthors, Effects of high-fructose corn syrup and sucrose consumption on circulating glucose, insulin, leptin, and ghrelin on appetite in normal weight-women, *Nutrition* 23 (2007): 103–112S; S. Soenen and M. S. Weterterp-Plantenga, No differences in satiety or

energy intake after high-fructose corn syrup, sucrose, or milk preloads, *American Journal of Clinical Nutrition* 86 (2007): 1586–1594.

27. R. Clemens and P. Pressman, Clinical value of glycemic index unclear, *Food Technology* 58 (2004): 18; M. A. Pereira and coauthors, Effects of a low-glycemic load diet on resting energy expenditure and heart disease risk factors during weight loss, *Journal of the American Medical Association* 292 (2004): 2482–2490; A. Raben, Should obese patients be counselled to follow a low-glycaemic index diet? No, *Obesity Reviews* 3 (2002): 245–256; D. B. Pawlak, C. B. Ebbeling, and D. S. Ludwig, Should obese patients be counselled to follow a low-glycaemic index diet? Yes, *Obesity Reviews* 3 (2002): 235–243.
28. M. A. Pereira, Weighing in on glycemic index and body weight, *American Journal of Clinical Nutrition* 84 (2006): 677–679.
29. F. X. Pi-Sunyer, Glycemic index and disease, *American Journal of Clinical Nutrition* 76 (2002): 290S–298S.
30. H. Hare-Bruun, A. Flint, and B. L. Heitmann, Glycemic index and glycemic load in relation to changes in body weight, body fat distribution, and body composition in adult Danes, *American Journal of Clinical Nutrition* 84 (2006): 871–879.
31. M. S. Segal, E. Gollub, and R. J. Johnson, Is the fructose index more relevant with regards to cardiovascular disease than the glycemic index? *European Journal of Nutrition* 46 (2007): 406–417.
32. E. J. Parks and coauthors, Dietary sugars stimulate fatty acid synthesis in adults, *Journal of Nutrition* 138 (2008): 1039–1046; M. F. Chong, B. A. Fielding, and K. N. Frayn, Mechanisms for the acute effect of fructose on postprandial lipemia, *American Journal of Clinical Nutrition* 85 (2007): 1511–1520; Bray, 2007; Bantle, 2006; P. J. Havel, Dietary fructose: Implications for dysregulation of energy homeostasis and lipid/carbohydrate metabolism, *Nutrition Reviews* 63 (2005): 133–157.
33. K. A. Lê and L. Tappy, Metabolic effects of fructose, *Current Opinion in Clinical and Metabolic Care* 9 (2006): 469–475.
34. A. Miller and K. Adeli, Dietary fructose and the metabolic syndrome, *Current Opinion in Gastroenterology* 24 (2008): 204–209.
35. J. Brand-Miller and coauthors, Carbohydrates: The good, the bad and the whole grain, *Asia Pacific Journal of Clinical Nutrition* 17 (2008): 16–19.
36. S. K. Raatz and coauthors, Reduced glycemic index and glycemic load diets do not increase the effects of energy restriction on weight loss and insulin sensitivity in obese men and women, *Journal of Nutrition* 135 (2005): 2387–2391.
37. R. Sichieri and coauthors, An 18-mo randomized trial of a low-glycemic-index diet and weight change in Brazilian women, *American Journal of Clinical Nutrition* 86 (2007): 707–713; S. K. Das and coauthors, Long-term effects of 2 energy-restricted diets differing in glycemic load on dietary adherence, body composition, and metabolism in CALERIE: A 1-y randomized controlled trial, *American Journal of Clinical Nutrition* 85 (2007): 1023–1030.
38. A. Flint and coauthors, Glycemic and insulinemic responses as determinants of appetite in humans, *American Journal of Clinical Nutrition* 84 (2006): 1365–1373.
39. K. C. Maki and coauthors, Effects of a reduced-glycemic-load diet on body weight, body composition, and cardiovascular disease risk markers in overweight and obese adults, *American Journal of Clinical Nutrition* 85 (2007): 724–734.
40. J. P. Chaput and coauthors, A novel interaction between dietary composition and insulin secretion: Effects on weight gain in the Quebec Family Study, *American Journal of Clinical Nutrition* 87 (2008): 303–309.
41. C. B. Ebberling and coauthors, Effects of a low-glycemic load vs low-fat diet in obese young adults: A randomized trial, *Journal of the American Medical Association* 297 (2007): 2092–2102.
42. K. F. Petersen and coauthors, The role of skeletal muscle insulin resistance in the pathogenesis of the metabolic syndrome, *Proceedings of the National Academy of Sciences* 104 (2007): 12587-12594.
43. R. J. Wood and M. L. Fernandez, Carbohydrate-restricted versus low-glycemic-index diets for the treatment of insulin resistance and metabolic syndrome, *Nutrition Reviews* 67 (2009): 179–183; J. S. Volek and R. D. Feinman, Carbohydrate restriction improves the features of metabolic syndrome. Metabolic syndrome may be defined by the response to carbohydrate restriction, *Nutrition and Metabolism* 2 (2005): 31–47.
44. K. J. Melanson and coauthors, High-fructose corn syrup, energy intake, and appetite regulation, *American Journal of Clinical Nutrition* 88 (2008): 1738S–1744S.
45. L. S. Greene-Finestone and coauthors, Adolescents' low-carbohydrate-density diets are related to poorer dietary intakes, *Journal of the American Dietetic Association* 105 (2005): 1783–1788; E. T. Kennedy and coauthors, Popular diets: Correlation to health, nutrition, and obesity, *Journal of the American Dietetic Association* 101 (2001): 411–420.
46. W. Cunningham and D. Hyson, The skinny on high-protein, low-carbohydrate diets, *Preventive Cardiology* 9 (2006): 166–171.
47. Pereira, 2006.
48. Van Dam and Seidell, 2007.

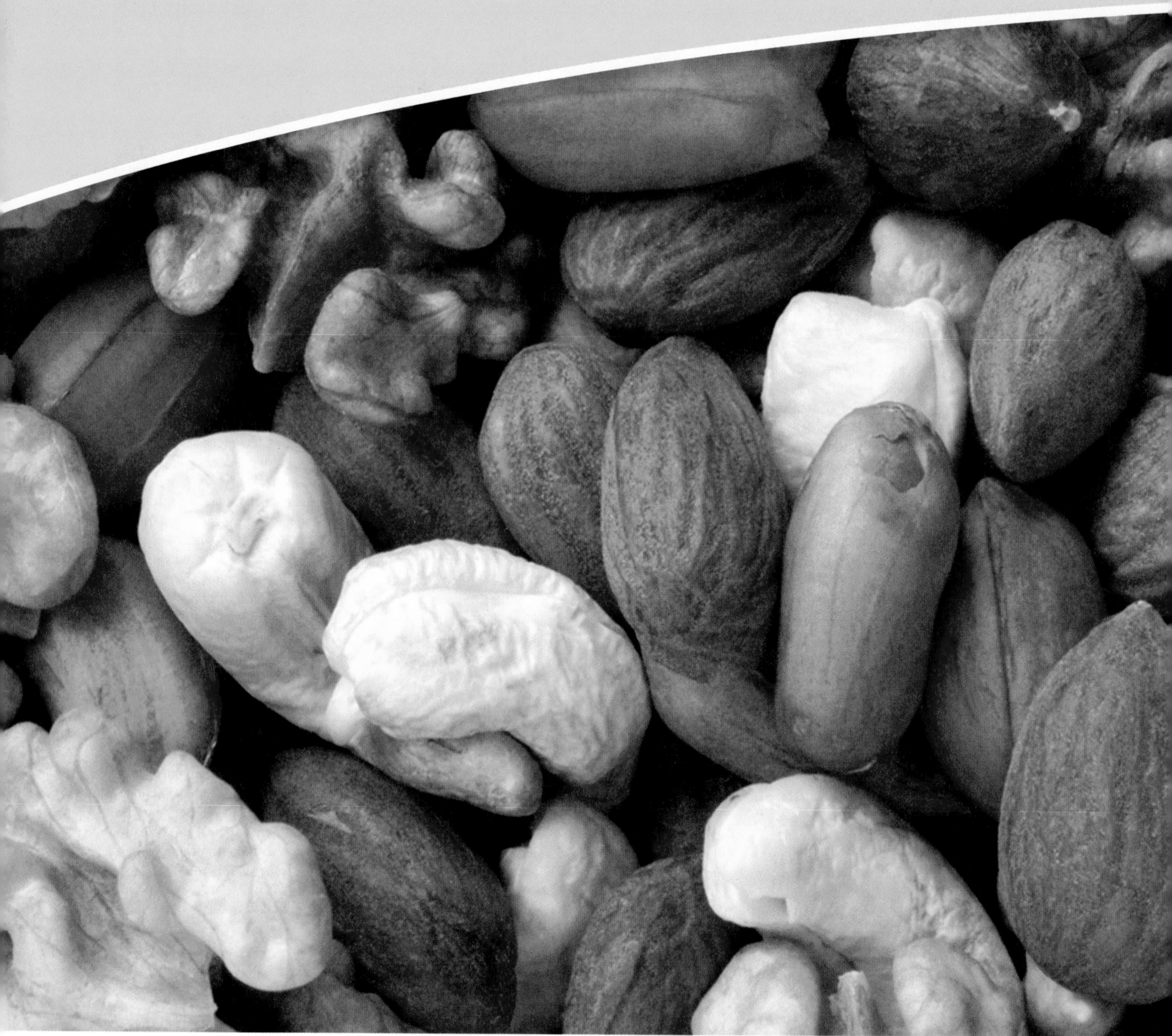

Olga Popova/shutterstock

Nutrition in Your Life

CENGAGENOW™

Throughout this chapter, the CengageNOW logo indicates an opportunity for online self-study, linking you to interactive tutorials, activities, and videos to increase your understanding of chapter concepts.
www.cengage.com/sso

Most likely, you know what you don't like about body fat, but do you appreciate how it insulates you against the cold or powers your hike around a lake? And what about food fat? You're right to credit fat for providing the delicious flavours and aromas of buttered popcorn and fried chicken—and to criticize it for contributing to the weight gain and heart disease so common today. The challenge is to strike a healthy balance of enjoying some fat, but not too much. Learning which kinds of fats are beneficial and which are most harmful will help you make wise decisions.

CHAPTER 5

The Lipids: Triglycerides, Phospholipids, and Sterols

CHAPTER OUTLINE

Most people are surprised to learn that fat has some virtues. Only when people consume either too much or too little fat, or too much of some kinds of fat, does poor health develop. It is true, though, that in our society of abundance, people are likely to consume too much fat.

Fat refers to the class of nutrients known as **lipids**. The lipid family includes triglycerides (**fats** and **oils**), phospholipids, and sterols. The triglycerides ♦ are most abundant, both in foods and in the body.

♦ Of the lipids in foods, 95% are fats and oils (triglycerides); of the lipids stored in the body, 99% are triglycerides.

The Chemist's View of Fatty Acids and Triglycerides

Like carbohydrates, lipids are composed of carbon (C), hydrogen (H), and oxygen (O). Because lipids have many more carbons and hydrogens in proportion to their oxygens, they can supply more energy per gram than carbohydrates can (Chapter 7 provides details).

The many names and relationships in the lipid family can seem overwhelming—like meeting a friend's extended family for the first time. To ease the introductions, this chapter first presents each of the lipids from a chemist's point of view using both words and diagrams. Then the chapter follows the lipids through digestion and absorption and into the body to examine their roles in health and disease. For people who think more easily in words than in chemical symbols, this *preview* of the upcoming chemistry may be helpful:

1. Every triglyceride contains one molecule of glycerol and three fatty acids (basically, chains of carbon atoms).
2. Fatty acids may be 4 to 24 (even numbers of) carbons long, the 18-carbon ones being the most common in foods and especially noteworthy in nutrition.
3. Fatty acids may be saturated or unsaturated. Unsaturated fatty acids may have one or more points of unsaturation. (That is, they may be *mono*unsaturated or *poly*unsaturated.)

lipids: a family of compounds that includes triglycerides, phospholipids, and sterols. Lipids are characterized by their insolubility in water. (Lipids also include the fat-soluble vitamins, described in Chapter 11.)

fats: lipids that are solid at room temperature (77°F or 25°C).

oils: lipids that are liquid at room temperature (77°F or 25°C).

4. Of special importance in nutrition are the polyunsaturated fatty acids whose *first* point of unsaturation is next to the third carbon (known as omega-3 fatty acids) or next to the sixth carbon (omega-6 fatty acids).
5. The 18-carbon fatty acids that fit this description are linolenic acid (omega-3) and linoleic acid (omega-6). Each is the primary member of a family of longer-chain fatty acids that help to regulate blood pressure, blood clotting, and other body functions important to health.

The paragraphs, definitions, and diagrams that follow present this information again in much more detail.

FIGURE 5-1 Acetic Acid

Acetic acid is a two-carbon organic acid.

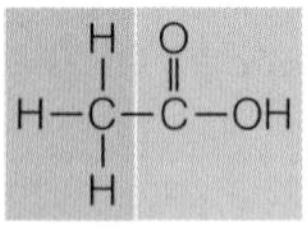
Methyl end
Acid end

Fatty Acids

A **fatty acid** is an organic acid—a chain of carbon atoms with hydrogens attached—that has an acid group (COOH) at one end and a methyl group (CH_3) at the other end. The organic acid shown in Figure 5-1 is acetic acid, the compound that gives vinegar its sour taste. Acetic acid is the shortest such acid, with a "chain" only two carbon atoms long. (Fatty acid and related terms are defined in the accompanying glossary.)

The Length of the Carbon Chain Most naturally occurring fatty acids contain even numbers of carbons in their chains—up to 24 carbons in length. This discussion begins with the 18-carbon fatty acids, which are abundant in our food supply. Stearic acid is the simplest of the 18-carbon fatty acids; the bonds between its carbons are all alike:

Stearic acid, an 18-carbon saturated fatty acid

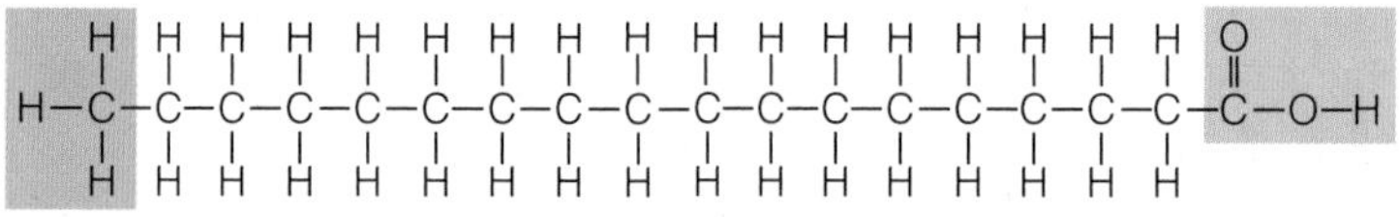

As you can see, stearic acid is 18 carbons long, and each atom meets the rules of chemical bonding described in Figure 4-1 on p. 94. The following structure also depicts stearic acid, but in a simpler way, with each "corner" on the zigzag line representing a carbon atom with two attached hydrogens:

Stearic acid (simplified structure)

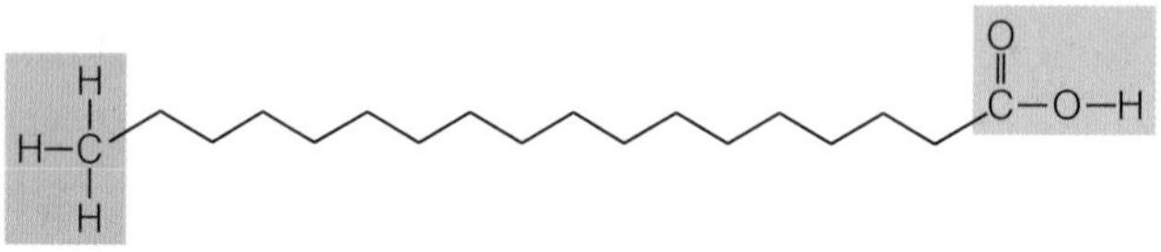

As mentioned, the carbon chains of fatty acids vary in length. The long-chain (12 to 24 carbons) fatty acids of meats, fish, and vegetable oils are most common in the diet. Smaller amounts of medium-chain (6 to 10 carbons) and short-chain (fewer than 6 carbons) fatty acids also occur, primarily in dairy products. (Tables C-1 and C-2 in APPENDIX C provide the names, chain lengths, and sources of fatty acids commonly found in foods.)

The Degree of Unsaturation Stearic acid (described and shown previously) is a **saturated fatty acid.** A saturated fatty acid is fully loaded with hydrogen atoms

GLOSSARY OF FATTY ACID TERMS

fatty acid: an organic compound composed of a carbon chain with hydrogens attached and an acid group (COOH) at one end and a methyl group (CH_3) at the other end.

monounsaturated fatty acid (MUFA): a fatty acid that lacks two hydrogen atoms and has one double bond between carbons—for example, oleic acid. A *monounsaturated oil or fat* is composed of triglycerides in which most of the fatty acids are monounsaturated.

- **mono** = one

point of unsaturation: the double bond of a fatty acid, where hydrogen atoms can easily be added to the structure.

polyunsaturated fatty acid (PUFA): a fatty acid that lacks four or more hydrogen atoms and has two or more double bonds between carbons—for example, linoleic acid (two double bonds) and linolenic acid (three double bonds). A *polyunsaturated oil or fat* is composed of triglycerides in which most of the fatty acids are polyunsaturated.

- **poly** = many

saturated fatty acid: a fatty acid carrying the maximum possible number of hydrogen atoms—for example, stearic acid. A *saturated fat* is composed of triglycerides in which most of the fatty acids are saturated.

unsaturated fatty acid: a fatty acid that lacks two or more hydrogen atoms and has at least one double bond between carbons (includes monounsaturated and polyunsaturated fatty acids). An *unsaturated fat* is composed of triglycerides in which most of the fatty acids are unsaturated.

and contains only single bonds between its carbon atoms. If two hydrogens were missing from the middle of the carbon chain, the remaining structure might be:

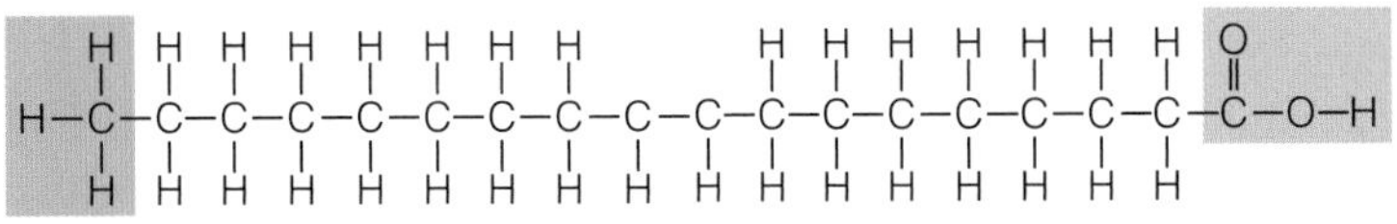

An impossible chemical structure

Such a compound cannot exist, however, because two of the carbons have only three bonds each, and every carbon must have four bonds. The two carbons therefore form a double bond:

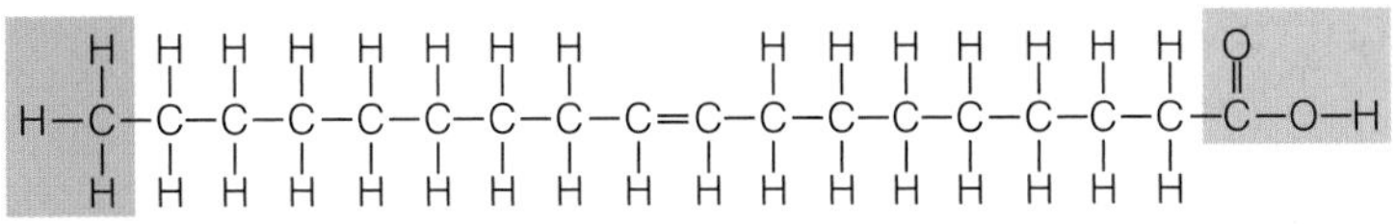

Oleic acid, an 18-carbon monounsaturated fatty acid; Canadian Community Health Survey (CCHS) 2.2 data reveal that young adults obtain about 12 percent of their total energy from oleic acid.

The same structure drawn more simply looks like this:*

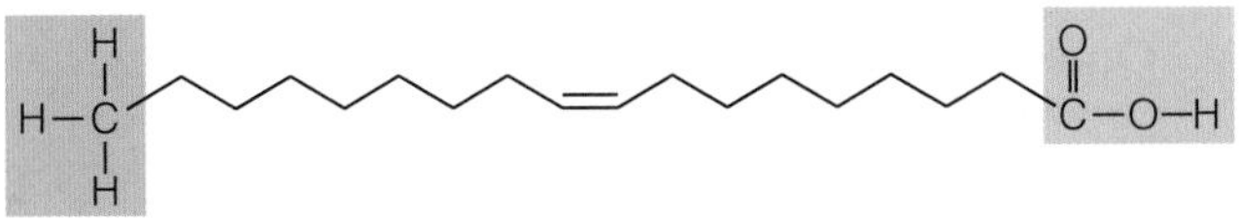

Oleic acid (simplified structure)

Although drawn straight here, the actual shape bends at the double bond (as shown in the left side of Figure 5-8 on p. 135). The double bond is a **point of unsaturation.** A fatty acid like this—with two hydrogens missing and a double bond—is an **unsaturated fatty acid.** This one is the 18-carbon **monounsaturated fatty acid** oleic acid, which is abundant in olive oil and canola oil.

A **polyunsaturated fatty acid** has two or more carbon-to-carbon double bonds. **Linoleic acid,** the 18-carbon fatty acid common in vegetable oils, lacks four hydrogens and has two double bonds:

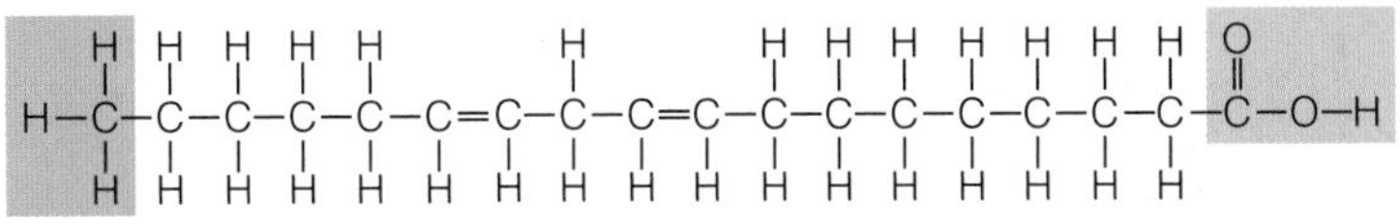

Linoleic acid, an 18-carbon polyunsaturated fatty acid

Drawn more simply, linoleic acid looks like this (though the actual shape would bend at the double bonds, as shown in the left side of Figure 5-8 on p. 135):

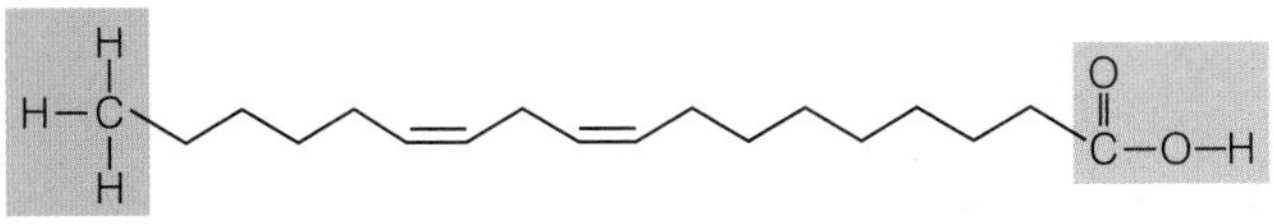

Linoleic acid (simplified structure)

A fourth 18-carbon fatty acid is **linolenic acid,** ♦ which has three double bonds. Table 5-1 presents the 18-carbon fatty acids. ♦

*Remember that each "corner" on the zigzag line represents a carbon atom with two attached hydrogens.

♦ See margin notes on page 150 for the DRI recommendations and CCHS data regarding linoleic and linolenic acids.

♦ Chemists use a shorthand notation to describe fatty acids. The first number indicates the number of carbon atoms; the second, the number of the double bonds. For example, the notation for stearic acid is 18:0.

TABLE 5-1 18-Carbon Fatty Acids

Name	Number of Carbon Atoms	Number of Double Bonds	Saturation	Common Food Sources
Stearic acid	18	0	Saturated	Most animal fats
Oleic acid	18	1	Monounsaturated	Olive, canola oils
Linoleic acid	18	2	Polyunsaturated	Sunflower, safflower, corn, and soybean oils
Linolenic acid	18	3	Polyunsaturated	Soybean and canola oils, flaxseed, walnuts

linoleic (lin-oh-LAY-ick) **acid:** an essential fatty acid with 18 carbons and two double bonds.

linolenic (lin-oh-LEN-ick) **acid:** an essential fatty acid with 18 carbons and three double bonds.

The Location of Double Bonds Fatty acids differ not only in the length of their chains and their degree of saturation, but also in the locations of their double bonds. Chemists identify polyunsaturated fatty acids by the position of the double bond nearest the methyl (CH_3) end of the carbon chain, which is described by an **omega** number. A polyunsaturated fatty acid with its first double bond three carbons away from the methyl end is an **omega-3 fatty acid.** Similarly, an **omega-6 fatty acid** is a polyunsaturated fatty acid with its first double bond six carbons away from the methyl end. Figure 5-2 compares two 18-carbon fatty acids—linolenic acid (an omega-3 fatty acid) and linoleic acid (an omega-6 fatty acid).

Monosaturated fatty acids tend to belong to the omega-9 group, with their first (and only) double bond nine carbons away from the methyl end. Oleic acid—the 18-carbon monounsaturated fatty acid common in olive oil mentioned earlier—is an omega-9 fatty acid. It is also the most predominant monounsaturated fatty acid in the diet.

FIGURE 5-2 Omega-3 and Omega-6 Fatty Acids Compared

The omega number indicates the position of the first double bond in a fatty acid, counting from the methyl (CH_3) end. Thus an omega-3 fatty acid's first double bond occurs three carbons from the methyl end, and an omega-6 fatty acid's first double bond occurs six carbons from the methyl end. The members of an omega family may have different lengths and different numbers of double bonds, but the first double bond occurs at the same point in all of them. These structures are drawn linearly here to ease counting carbons and locating double bonds, but their shapes actually bend at the double bonds, as shown in Figure 5-8 (p. 135).

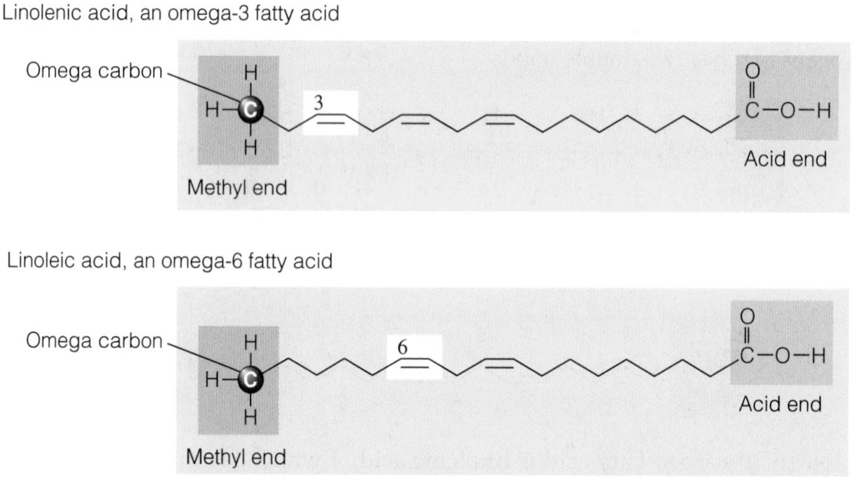
Linolenic acid, an omega-3 fatty acid
Omega carbon
3
Methyl end
Acid end
Linoleic acid, an omega-6 fatty acid
Omega carbon
6
Methyl end
Acid end

Triglycerides

Few fatty acids occur free in foods or in the body. Most often, they are incorporated into **triglycerides**—lipids composed of three fatty acids attached to a **glycerol** molecule. (Figure 5-3 presents a glycerol molecule.) To make a triglyceride, a series of condensation reactions combine a hydrogen atom (H) from the glycerol and a hydroxyl (OH) group from a fatty acid, forming a molecule of water (H_2O) and leaving a bond between the two molecules (see Figure 5-4). Most triglycerides contain a mixture of more than one type of fatty acid (as shown on the right side of Figure 5-4).

Degree of Unsaturation Revisited

The chemistry of a fatty acid—whether it is short or long, saturated or unsaturated, with its first double bond at carbon 3 or carbon 6—influences the characteristics of foods and the health of the body. A section later in this chapter explains how these features affect health; this section describes how the chemistry influences the fats and oils in foods.

Firmness The degree of unsaturation influences the firmness of fats at room temperature (see Figure 5-5). Generally speaking, most polyunsaturated vegetable

FIGURE 5-3 Glycerol

When glycerol is free, an OH group is attached to each carbon. When glycerol is part of a triglyceride, each carbon is attached to a fatty acid by a carbon-oxygen bond.

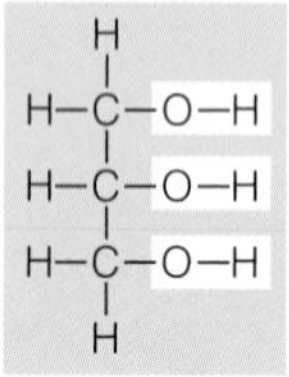

omega: the last letter of the Greek alphabet (ω), used by chemists to refer to the position of the first double bond from the methyl (CH_3) end of a fatty acid.

omega-3 fatty acid: a polyunsaturated fatty acid in which the first double bond is three carbons away from the methyl (CH_3) end of the carbon chain.

omega-6 fatty acid: a polyunsaturated fatty acid in which the first double bond is six carbons from the methyl (CH_3) end of the carbon chain.

triglycerides (try-GLISS-er-rides): the chief form of fat in the diet and the major storage form of fat in the body; composed of a molecule of glycerol with three fatty acids attached; also called *triacylglycerols* (try-ay-seel-GLISS-er-ols).*

- **tri** = three
- **glyceride** = of glycerol
- **acyl** = a carbon chain

glycerol (GLISS-er-ol): produced during carbohydrate metabolism is an alcohol composed of a three-carbon chain, which can serve as the backbone for a triglyceride.

- **ol** = alcohol

*Research scientists commonly use the term *triacylglycerols;* this book continues to use the more familiar term *triglycerides,* as do many other health and nutrition books and journals.

FIGURE 5-4 Condensation of Glycerol and Fatty Acids to Form a Triglyceride

To make a triglyceride, three fatty acids attach to glycerol in condensation reactions.

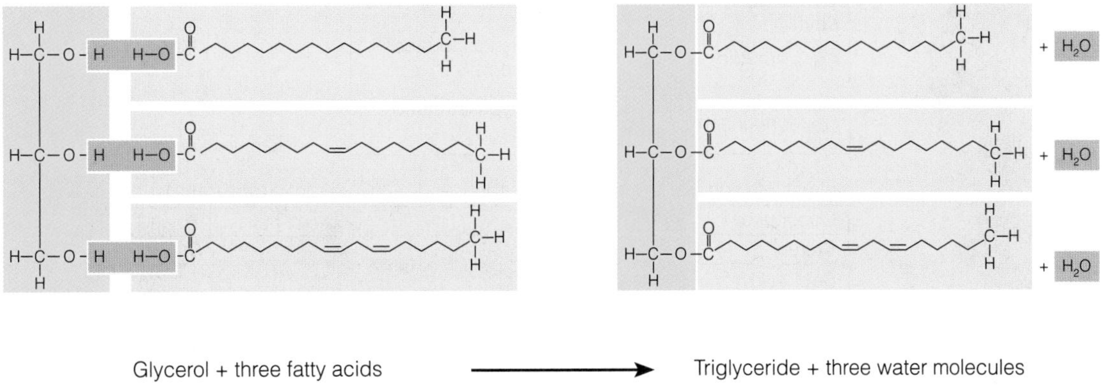
Glycerol + three fatty acids
Triglyceride + three water molecules
+ H_2O

An H atom from glycerol and an OH group from a fatty acid combine to create water, leaving the O on the glycerol and the C at the acid end of each fatty acid to form a bond.

Three fatty acids attached to a glycerol form a triglyceride and yield water. In this example, the triglyceride includes a saturated fatty acid, a monounsaturated fatty acid, and a polyunsaturated fatty acid, respectively.

FIGURE 5-5 Diagram of Saturated and Unsaturated Fatty Acids Compared

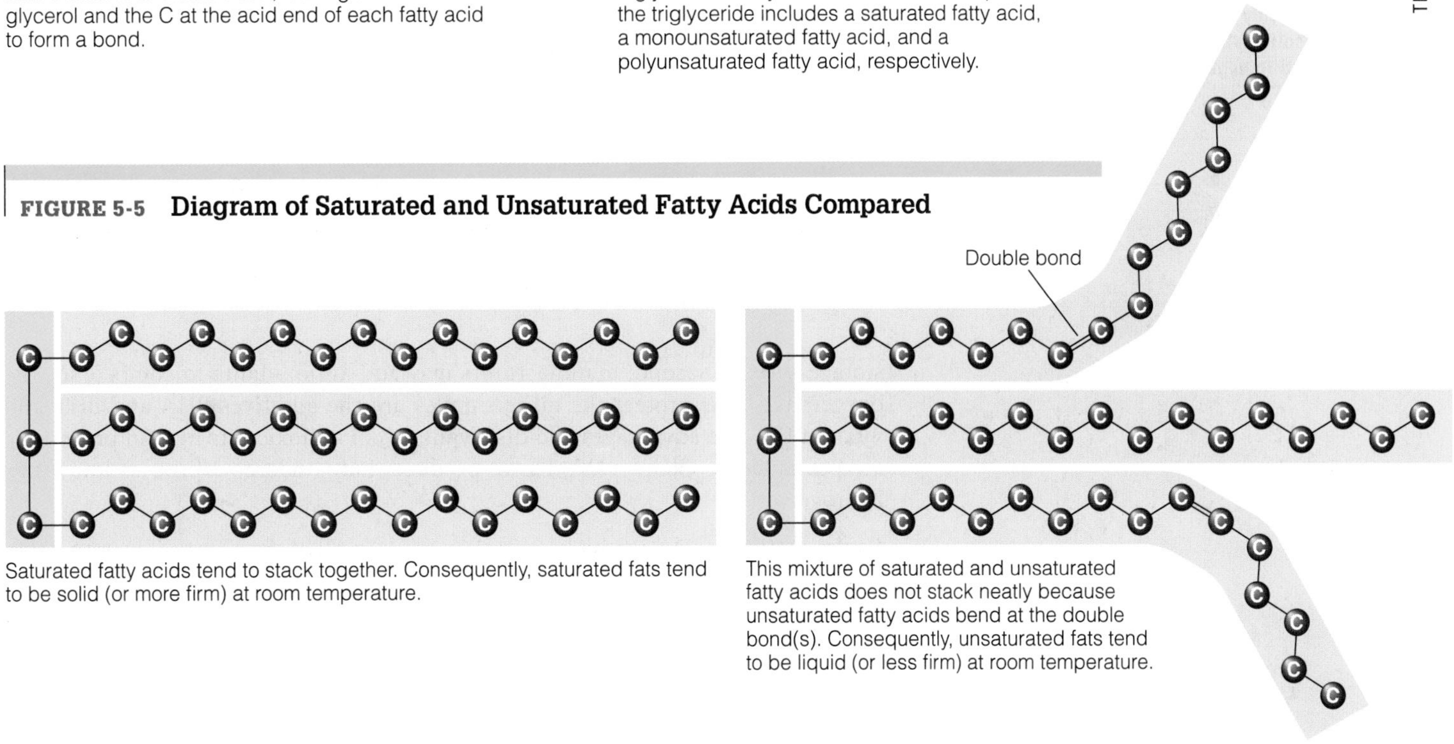
Double bond

Saturated fatty acids tend to stack together. Consequently, saturated fats tend to be solid (or more firm) at room temperature.

This mixture of saturated and unsaturated fatty acids does not stack neatly because unsaturated fatty acids bend at the double bond(s). Consequently, unsaturated fats tend to be liquid (or less firm) at room temperature.

oils are liquid at room temperature, and the more saturated animal fats are solid. Some vegetable oils—notably cocoa butter, palm oil, palm kernel oil, and coconut oil—are saturated; ♦ they are firmer than most vegetable oils because of their saturation, but softer than most animal fats because of their shorter carbon chains (8 to 14 carbons long). Generally, the shorter the carbon chain, the softer the fat is at room temperature. Fatty acid compositions of selected fats and oils are shown in Figure 5-6 (p. 134), and APPENDIX H provides the fat and fatty acid contents of many other foods.

♦ The food industry often refers to these saturated vegetable oils as the "tropical oils."

Stability Saturation also influences stability. All fats become spoiled when exposed to oxygen. The **oxidation** of fats produces a variety of compounds that smell and taste rancid. (Other types of spoilage can occur due to microbial growth.) Polyunsaturated fats spoil most readily because their double bonds are unstable; monounsaturated fats are slightly less susceptible. Saturated fats are most resistant to oxidation and thus least likely to become rancid.

Manufacturers can protect fat-containing products against rancidity in three ways—none of them perfect. First, products may be sealed in air-tight, nonmetallic containers, protected from light, and refrigerated—an expensive and inconvenient

oxidation (OKS-ee-day-shun): the process of a substance combining with oxygen; oxidation reactions involve the loss of electrons.

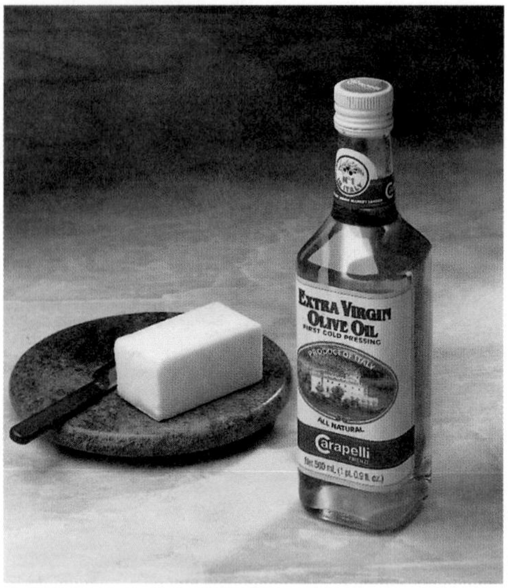
EXTRA VIRGIN
OLIVE OIL
FIRST COLD PRESSING
ALL NATURAL
Carapelli

© Polara Studios, Inc.

At room temperature, saturated fats (such as those commonly found in butter and other animal fats) are solid, whereas unsaturated fats (such as those found in vegetable oils) are usually liquid.

FIGURE 5-6 Comparison of Dietary Fats

Most fats are a mixture of saturated, monounsaturated, and polyunsaturated fatty acids.

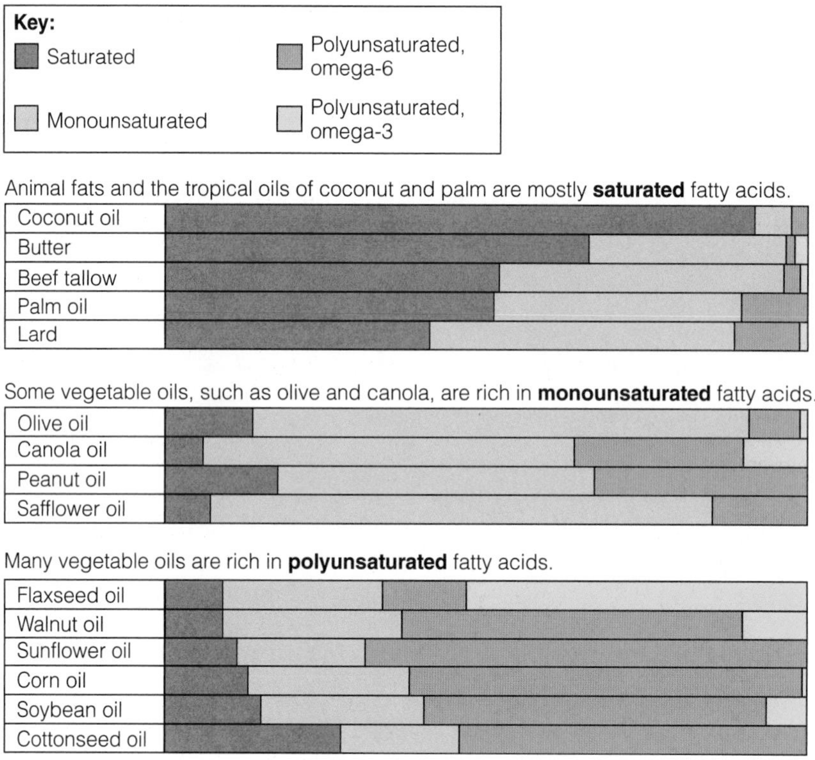
Key:
Saturated
Polyunsaturated, omega-6
Monounsaturated
Polyunsaturated, omega-3
Animal fats and the tropical oils of coconut and palm are mostly **saturated** fatty acids.
Coconut oil
Butter
Beef tallow
Palm oil
Lard
Some vegetable oils, such as olive and canola, are rich in **monounsaturated** fatty acids.
Olive oil
Canola oil
Peanut oil
Safflower oil
Many vegetable oils are rich in **polyunsaturated** fatty acids.
Flaxseed oil
Walnut oil
Sunflower oil
Corn oil
Soybean oil
Cottonseed oil

storage system. Second, manufacturers may add **antioxidants** to compete for the oxygen and thus protect the oil (examples are the additives BHA and BHT and vitamin E).* The advantages and disadvantages of antioxidants in food processing are presented in Chapter 20. Third, products may undergo a process known as hydrogenation.

Hydrogenation During **hydrogenation**, some or all of the points of unsaturation are saturated by adding hydrogen molecules. Hydrogenation offers two advantages. First, it protects against oxidation (thereby prolonging shelf life) by making polyunsaturated fats more saturated. Second, it alters the texture of foods by making liquid vegetable oils more solid (as in margarine and shortening). Hydrogenated fats improve the texture of foods, making margarines spreadable, pie crusts flaky, and puddings creamy.

Figure 5-7 illustrates the *total* hydrogenation of a polyunsaturated fatty acid to a saturated fatty acid. Total hydrogenation rarely occurs during food processing.

*BHA is butylated hydroxyanisole; BHT is butylated hydroxytoluene.

FIGURE 5-7 Hydrogenation

Double bonds carry a slightly negative charge and readily accept positively charged hydrogen atoms, creating a saturated fatty acid. Most often, fat is *partially* hydrogenated, creating a *trans*-fatty acid (shown in Figure 5-8).

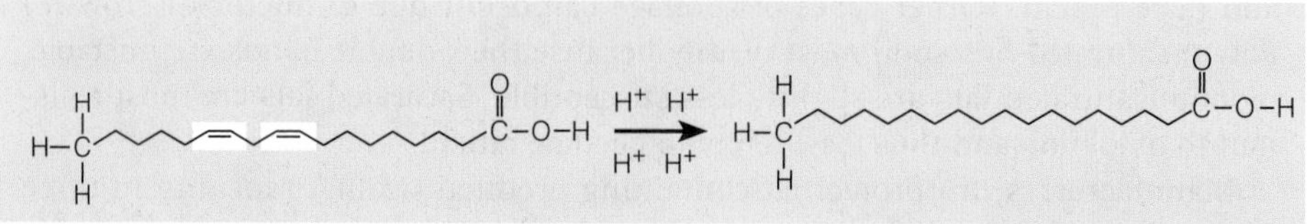
H⁺ H⁺
H⁺ H⁺

Polyunsaturated fatty acid (Linoleic acid)

Hydrogenated (saturated) fatty acid (Stearic acid)

antioxidants: as a food additive, preservatives that delay or prevent rancidity of fats in foods and other damage to food caused by oxygen.

hydrogenation (HIGH-dro-jen-AY-shun or high-DROJ-eh-NAY-shun): a chemical process by which hydrogens are added to monounsaturated or polyunsaturated fatty acids to reduce the number of double bonds, making the fats more saturated (solid) and more resistant to oxidation (protecting against rancidity). Hydrogenation produces *trans*-fatty acids.

FIGURE 5-8 ***Cis*- and *Trans*-Fatty Acids Compared**

This example shows the *cis* configuration for an 18-carbon monounsaturated fatty acid (oleic acid) and its corresponding *trans* configuration (elaidic acid).

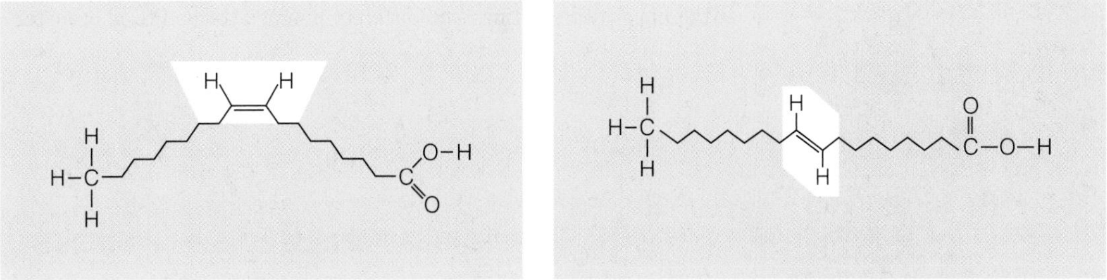

cis-fatty acid

A *cis*-fatty acid has its hydrogens on the same side of the double bond; *cis* molecules bend into a U-like formation. Most naturally occurring unsaturated fatty acids in foods are *cis*.

trans-fatty acid

A *trans*-fatty acid has its hydrogens on the opposite sides of the double bond; *trans* molecules are more linear. The *trans* form typically occurs in partially hydrogenated foods when hydrogen atoms shift around some double bonds and change the configuration from *cis* to *trans*.

Most often, a fat is *partially* hydrogenated, and some of the double bonds that remain after processing change their configuration from **cis** to ***trans***.

***Trans*-Fatty Acids** In nature, most double bonds are *cis*—meaning that the hydrogens next to the double bonds are on the same side of the carbon chain. Only a few fatty acids (notably a small percentage of those found in milk and meat products) naturally occur as ***trans*-fatty acids**—meaning that the hydrogens next to the double bonds are on opposite sides of the carbon chain (see Figure 5-8).* In the body, *trans*-fatty acids that derive from hydrogenation behave more like saturated fats than like unsaturated fats. The relationship between *trans*-fatty acids and heart disease has been the subject of much recent research, as a later section describes. In contrast, naturally occurring fatty acids that have a *trans* configuration, such as **conjugated linoleic acids**, may have health benefits.[1] Conjugated linoleic acids are not counted as *trans* fats on food labels.

IN SUMMARY **The predominant lipids both in foods and in the body are triglycerides: glycerol backbones with three fatty acids attached. Fatty acids vary in the length of their carbon chains, their degrees of unsaturation, and the location of their double bond(s). Those that are fully loaded with hydrogens are saturated; those that are missing hydrogens and therefore have double bonds are unsaturated (monounsaturated and polyunsaturated, including *trans*-fatty acids). The vast majority of triglycerides contain more than one type of fatty acid. Fatty acid saturation affects fats' physical characteristics and storage properties. Hydrogenation, which makes polyunsaturated fats more saturated, creates *trans*-fatty acids, altered fatty acids that may damage health in ways similar to those of saturated fatty acids.**

The Chemist's View of Phospholipids and Sterols

The preceding pages have been devoted to one of the classes of lipids, the triglycerides, and their component parts, glycerol and the fatty acids. The other lipids, the phospholipids and sterols, make up only 5 percent of the lipids in the diet but are major components of all cell membranes.

*For example, most dairy products contain less than 0.5 grams *trans* fat per serving.

cis: on the near side of; refers to a chemical configuration in which the hydrogen atoms are located on the same side of a double bond.

trans: on the other side of; refers to a chemical configuration in which the hydrogen atoms are located on opposite sides of a double bond.

***trans*-fatty acids:** fatty acids with hydrogens on opposite sides of the double bond.

conjugated linoleic acids: several fatty acids that have the same chemical formula as linoleic acid (18 carbons, two double bonds) but with different configurations (the double bonds occur on adjacent carbons). (These can occur naturally in milk and meat from cows.)

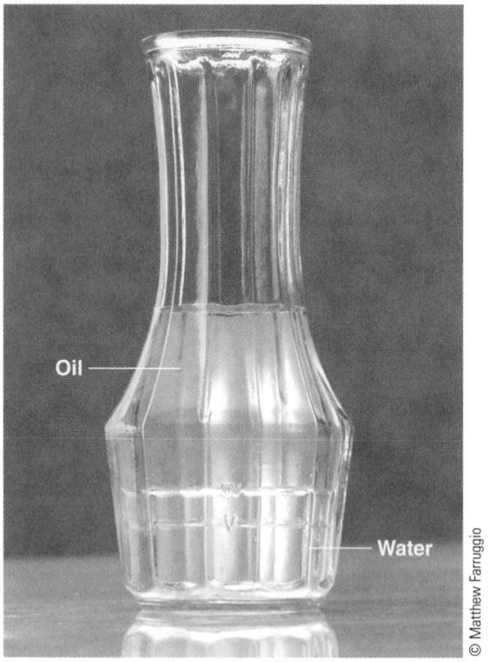
Oil
Water
© Matthew Farruggio

Without help from emulsifiers, fats and water don't mix.

FIGURE 5-9 Lecithin

Lecithin is one of the phospholipids. Notice that a molecule of lecithin is similar to a triglyceride but contains only two fatty acids. The third position is occupied by a phosphate group and a molecule of choline. Other phospholipids have different fatty acids at the upper two positions and different groups attached to phosphate.

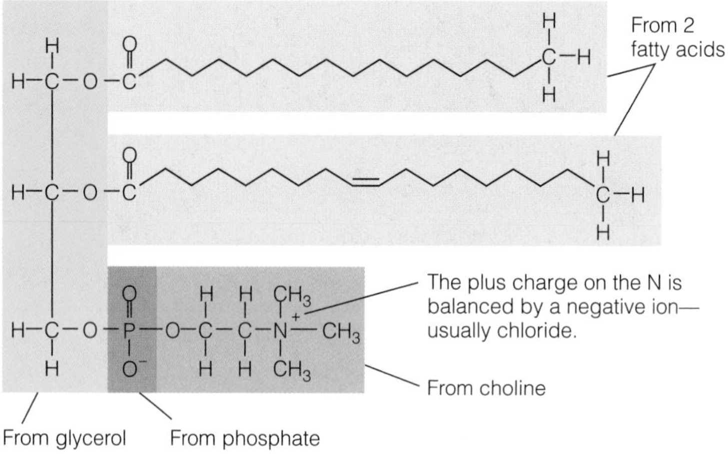
From 2 fatty acids
The plus charge on the N is balanced by a negative ion—usually chloride.
From choline
From glycerol
From phosphate

Phospholipids The best-known **phospholipid** is **lecithin** (see Figure 5-9). Notice that lecithin has one glycerol with two of its three attachment sites occupied by fatty acids like those in triglycerides. The third site is occupied by a phosphate group and a molecule of **choline**. The fatty acids make phospholipids soluble in fat; the phosphate group allows them to dissolve in water. Such versatility enables the food industry to use phospholipids as emulsifiers ♦ to mix fats with water in such products as mayonnaise and chocolate bars.

♦ **Emulsifiers** are substances with both water-soluble and fat-soluble portions that promote the mixing of oils and fats in watery solutions.

Phospholipids in Foods In addition to the phospholipids used by the food industry as emulsifiers, phospholipids are also found naturally in foods. The richest food sources of lecithin are eggs, liver, soybeans, wheat germ, and peanuts.

Roles of Phospholipids Lecithin and other phospholipids are major constituents of all of our cell membranes (see Figure 5-10). Because phospholipids are soluble in both water and fat, they can help fat-soluble substances, including vitamins and hormones, to pass easily in and out of cells. The phospholipids also act as emulsifiers in the body, helping to keep fats suspended in the blood and body fluids, and thus are also major components of the lipoproteins.

FIGURE 5-10 Phospholipids of a Cell Membrane

A cell membrane is made of phospholipids assembled into an orderly formation called a bilayer. The fatty acid "tails" orient themselves away from the watery fluid inside and outside of the cell. The glycerol and phosphate "heads" are attracted to the watery fluid.

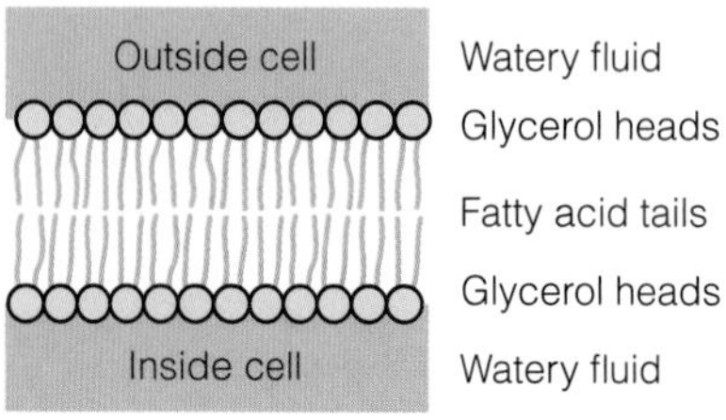
Outside cell
Inside cell
Watery fluid
Glycerol heads
Fatty acid tails
Glycerol heads
Watery fluid

Lecithin periodically receives attention in the popular press. Its advocates claim that it is a major constituent of cell membranes (true), that cell membranes are essential to the integrity of cells (true), and that consumers must therefore take lecithin supplements (false). The liver makes from scratch all the lecithin a person needs. As for lecithin taken as a supplement, the digestive enzyme lecithinase ♦ in the intestine hydrolyzes most of it before it passes into the body, so little lecithin reaches the tissues intact. In other words, lecithin is *not an essential nutrient;* it is just another lipid. Like other lipids, lecithin contributes 9 kcalories per gram—an unexpected "bonus" many people taking lecithin supplements fail to realize. Furthermore, large doses of lecithin may cause GI distress, sweating, and loss of

♦ The word ending **-ase** denotes an enzyme. Hence, lecithinase is an enzyme that works on lecithin.

phospholipid (FOS-foe-LIP-id): a compound similar to a triglyceride but having a phosphate group (a phosphorus-containing salt) and choline (or another nitrogen-containing compound) in place of one of the fatty acids.

lecithin (LESS-uh-thin): one of the phospholipids. Both nature and the food industry use lecithin as an emulsifier to combine water-soluble and fat-soluble ingredients that do not ordinarily mix, such as water and oil.

choline (KOH-leen): a nitrogen-containing compound found in foods and made in the body from the amino acid methionine. Choline is part of the phospholipid lecithin and the neurotransmitter acetylcholine.

appetite. Perhaps these symptoms can be considered beneficial—if they serve to warn people to stop taking lecithin supplements.

IN SUMMARY Phospholipids, including lecithin, have a unique chemical structure that allows them to be soluble in both water and fat. In the body, phospholipids are a major part of all of our cell membranes and lipoproteins; the food industry uses phospholipids as emulsifiers to mix fats with water.

Sterols

In addition to triglycerides and phospholipids, the lipids include the **sterols**, compounds with a multiple-ring structure.* The most famous sterol is **cholesterol**; Figure 5-11 shows its chemical structure.

Sterols in Foods Foods derived from both plants and animals contain sterols, but only those from animals contain cholesterol—meats, eggs, fish, poultry, and dairy products. Some people, confused about the distinction between dietary cholesterol and blood cholesterol, have asked which foods contain the "good" cholesterol. "Good" cholesterol is not a type of cholesterol found in foods, but it refers to the way the body transports cholesterol in the blood, as explained in a later section of this chapter.

Sterols other than cholesterol are naturally found in plants; thus, there is no cholesterol in plants or the vegetable oils derived from plants. Being structurally similar to cholesterol, plant sterols interfere with cholesterol absorption. By inhibiting cholesterol absorption, a diet rich in plant sterols lowers blood cholesterol levels.[2] Food manufacturers have fortified foods such as margarine with plant sterols, creating a functional food that helps to reduce blood cholesterol.[3] Health Canada has recently allowed a health claim to this effect on those foods that qualify for this claim.

Roles of Sterols Many vitally important body compounds are sterols. Among them are bile acids, the sex hormones (such as testosterone), the adrenal hormones (such as cortisol), and vitamin D, as well as cholesterol itself. Cholesterol in the body can serve as the starting material for the synthesis of these compounds (except Vitamin D) ♦ or as an important structural component of cell membranes; more than 90 percent of all the body's cholesterol resides in the cells. Despite popular impressions to the contrary, cholesterol is not a villain lurking in some evil foods—it is a compound the body makes and uses. ♦ Right now, as you read, your liver is manufacturing cholesterol from fragments of carbohydrate, protein, and fat. In fact, the liver makes about 800 to 1500 milligrams of cholesterol per day, ♦ thus contributing much more to the body's total than does the diet.

Cholesterol's harmful effects in the body occur when it accumulates in the artery walls and contributes to the formation of **plaque**. These plaque deposits lead to **atherosclerosis**, a disease that causes heart attacks and strokes. (Chapter 19 provides many more details.)

IN SUMMARY Sterols have a multiple-ring structure that differs from the structure of other lipids. In the body, sterols include cholesterol, bile, vitamin D, and some hormones. Animal-derived foods are rich sources of cholesterol.

To summarize, the members of the lipid family include:

- ***Triglycerides* (fats and oils), which are made of:**
  - ***Glycerol* (1 per triglyceride) and**
  - ***Fatty acids* (3 per triglyceride); depending on the number of double bonds, fatty acids may be:**
    - ***Saturated* (no double bonds)**
    - ***Monounsaturated* (one double bond)**
    - ***Polyunsaturated* (more than one double bond); depending on the location of the double bonds, polyunsaturated fatty acids may be:**
      - ***Omega-3* (first double bond 3 carbons away from methyl end)**
      - ***Omega-6* (first double bond 6 carbons away from methyl end)**
- ***Phospholipids* (such as lecithin)**
- ***Sterols* (such as cholesterol)**

*The four-ring core structure identifies a steroid; sterols are alcohol derivatives with a steroid ring structure.

FIGURE 5-11 Cholesterol

Fat-soluble vitamin D is synthesized using some of the steps in the metabolic pathway for cholesterol; notice the many structural similarities. The only difference is that cholesterol has a closed ring (highlighted in red), whereas vitamin D's is open, accounting for its vitamin activity. Notice, too, how different cholesterol is from the triglycerides and phospholipids.

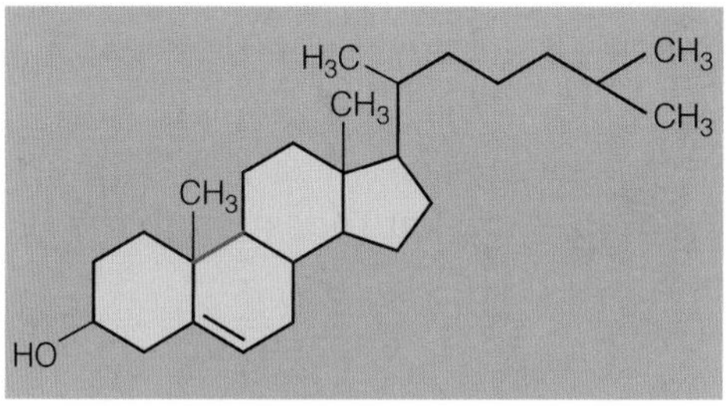
H3C
CH3
CH3
CH3
CH3
HO

Cholesterol

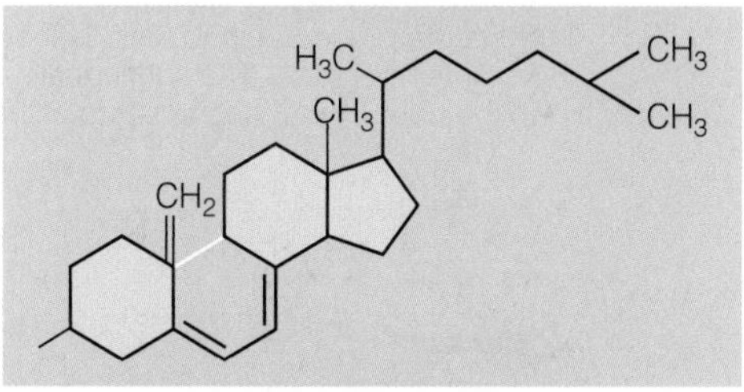
H3C
CH3
CH3
CH3
CH2

Vitamin D_3

♦ Compounds made from cholesterol:
- Bile acids
- Steroid hormones (testosterone, androgens, estrogens, progesterones, cortisol, cortisone, and aldosterone)

♦ The chemical structure is the same, but cholesterol that is made in the body is called **endogenous** (en-DOGDE-eh-nus), whereas cholesterol from outside the body (from foods) is called **exogenous** (eks-ODGE-eh-nus).
- **endo** = within
- **gen** = arising
- **exo** = outside (the body)

♦ For perspective, the Daily Value for cholesterol is 300 mg/day.

sterols (STARE-ols or STEER-ols): compounds containing a four-ring carbon structure with any of a variety of side chains attached.

cholesterol (koh-LESS-ter-ol): one of the sterols containing a four-ring carbon structure with a carbon side chain.

plaque (PLACK): an accumulation of fatty deposits, smooth muscle cells, and fibrous connective tissue that develops in the artery walls in atherosclerosis. Plaque associated with atherosclerosis is known as *atheromatous* (ATH-er-OH-ma-tus) *plaque.*

atherosclerosis (ATH-er-oh-scler-OH-sis): a type of artery disease characterized by plaques (accumulations of lipid-containing material) on the inner walls of the arteries (see Chapter 19).

Digestion, Absorption, and Transport of Lipids

hydrophobic (high-dro-FOE-bick): a term referring to water-fearing, or non-water-soluble, substances; also known as *lipophilic* (fat loving).

- **hydro** = water
- **phobia** = fear
- **lipo** = lipid
- **phile** = love

hydrophilic (high-dro-FIL-ick): a term referring to water-loving, or water-soluble, substances.

Each day, the GI tract receives, on average from the food we eat, 50 to 100 grams of triglycerides, 4 to 8 grams of phospholipids, and 200 to 350 milligrams of cholesterol. The body faces a challenge in digesting and absorbing these lipids. Fats are **hydrophobic**—that is, they tend to separate from the watery fluids of the GI tract—whereas the enzymes for digesting fats are **hydrophilic**. The challenge is keeping the fats mixed in the watery fluids of the GI tract.

Lipid Digestion

Figure 5-12 traces the digestion of fat through the GI tract. The goal of fat digestion is to dismantle triglycerides into small molecules that

FIGURE 5-12 Fat Digestion in the GI Tract

FAT

Mouth and salivary glands
Some hard fats begin to melt as they reach body temperature. The sublingual salivary gland in the base of the tongue secretes lingual lipase.

Stomach
The acid-stable lingual lipase initiates lipid digestion by hydrolyzing one bond of triglycerides to produce diglycerides and fatty acids. The degree of hydrolysis by lingual lipase is slight for most fats but may be appreciable for milk fats. The stomach's churning action mixes fat with water and acid. A gastric lipase accesses and hydrolyzes (only a very small amount of) fat.

Small intestine
Bile flows in from the gallbladder (via the common bile duct):

Fat —Bile→ Emulsified fat

Pancreatic lipase flows in from the pancreas (via the pancreatic duct):

Emulsified fat (triglycerides) —Pancreatic (and intestinal) lipase→ Monoglycerides, glycerol, fatty acids (absorbed)

Large intestine
Some fat and cholesterol, trapped in fibre, exit in feces.

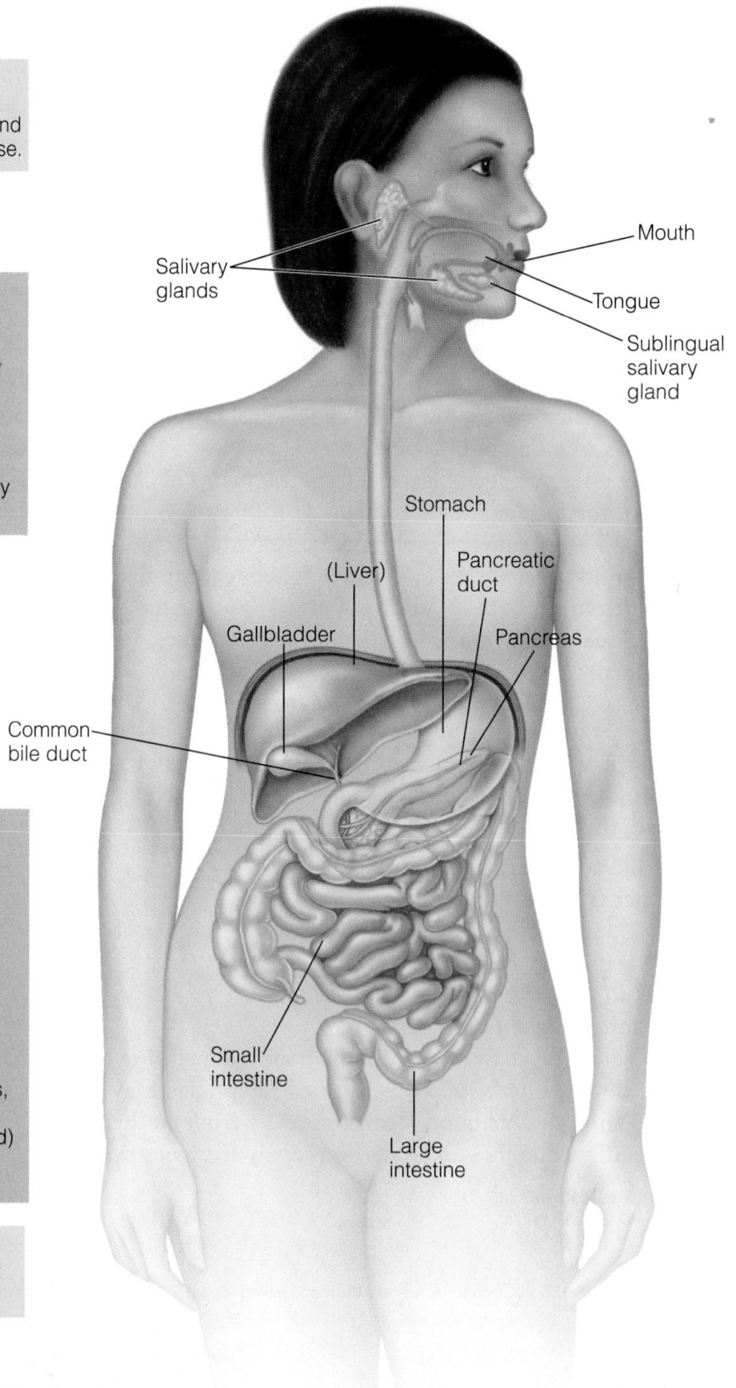
Mouth
Salivary glands
Tongue
Sublingual salivary gland
Stomach
(Liver)
Pancreatic duct
Gallbladder
Pancreas
Common bile duct
Small intestine
Large intestine

the body can absorb and use—namely, **monoglycerides**, fatty acids, and glycerol —because the body has no mechanism to allow the absorption of intact dietary triglycerides. The following paragraphs provide the details.

In the Mouth Fat digestion starts off slowly in the mouth. Some hard fats begin to melt as they reach body temperature. A salivary gland at the base of the tongue releases an enzyme (lingual lipase) ♦ that plays a minor role in fat digestion in adults but an active role in infants. In infants, this enzyme efficiently digests the short- and medium-chain fatty acids found in milk.

In the Stomach In a quiet stomach, fat would float as a layer above the watery components of swallowed food. But the strong muscle contractions of the stomach churn and propel the stomach contents toward the pyloric sphincter. Some chyme passes through the pyloric sphincter periodically, but the remaining partially digested food is propelled back into the body of the stomach. This churning grinds the solid pieces to finer particles, mixes the chyme, and disperses the fat into small droplets. These actions help to expose the fat for attack by the gastric lipase enzyme—an enzyme that performs best in the acidic environment ♦ of the stomach. Still, little fat digestion takes place in the stomach; most of the action occurs in the small intestine.

In the Small Intestine When fat enters the small intestine, it triggers the release of the hormone cholecystokinin (CCK), which signals the gallbladder to release its stores of bile. (Remember that the liver makes bile, and the gallbladder stores it until it is needed.) Among bile's many ingredients ♦ are bile acids, which are made in the liver from cholesterol and have a similar structure. In addition, bile acids often pair up with an amino acid (a building block of protein). The amino acid end is attracted to water, and the sterol end is attracted to fat (see Figure 5-13). This structure improves bile's ability to act as an emulsifier, drawing fat molecules into the surrounding watery fluids. There, the fats are fully digested as they encounter lipase enzymes from the pancreas and small intestine. The process of emulsification is diagrammed in Figure 5-14.

Most of the hydrolysis of triglycerides occurs in the small intestine. The major fat-digesting enzymes are pancreatic lipases; some intestinal lipases are also active. These enzymes remove one, then the other, of each triglyceride's

♦ An enzyme that hydrolyzes lipids is called a **lipase; lingual** refers to the tongue.

♦ The pH of the stomach is just below 2.

♦ In addition to bile acids and bile salts, bile contains cholesterol, phospholipids (especially lecithin), antibodies, water, electrolytes, and bilirubin and biliverdin (pigments resulting from the breakdown of heme).

monoglycerides: molecules of glycerol with one fatty acid attached. A molecule of glycerol with two fatty acids attached is a *diglyceride*.
- **mono** = one
- **di** = two

FIGURE 5-13 A Bile Acid

This is one of several bile acids the liver makes from cholesterol. It is then bound to an amino acid to improve its ability to form spherical complexes of emulsified fat (micelles). Most bile acids occur as bile salts, usually in association with sodium, but sometimes with potassium or calcium.

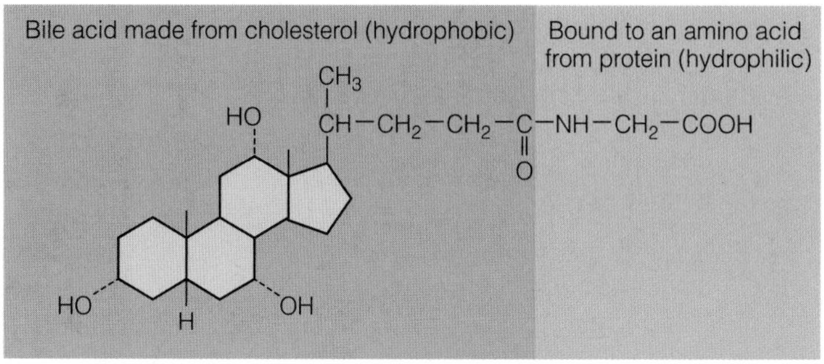
Bile acid made from cholesterol (hydrophobic)
Bound to an amino acid from protein (hydrophilic)
CH3
HO
CH—CH2—CH2—C—NH—CH2—COOH
O
HO
H
OH

FIGURE 5-14 Emulsification of Fat by Bile

Like bile, detergents are emulsifiers and work the same way, which is why they are effective in removing grease spots from clothes. Molecule by molecule, the grease is dissolved out of the spot and suspended in the water, where it can be rinsed away.

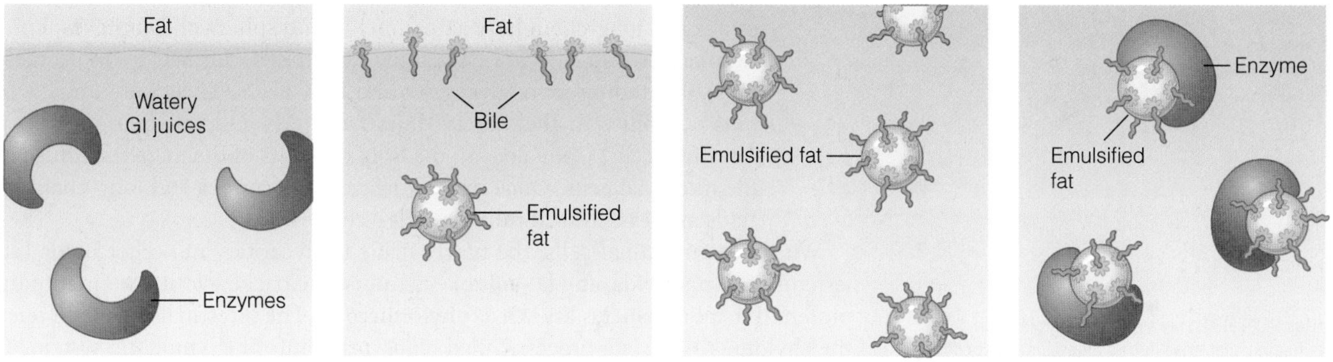
Fat
Watery GI juices
Enzymes
Fat
Bile
Emulsified fat
Emulsified fat
Enzyme
Emulsified fat

In the stomach, the fat and watery GI juices tend to separate. The enzymes in the GI juices can't get at the fat.

When fat enters the small intestine, the gallbladder secretes bile. Bile has an affinity for both fat and water, and acts as an emulsifier so it can bring the fat into the water.

Bile's emulsifying action converts large fat globules into small droplets that repel one another.

After emulsification, more fat is exposed to the enzymes, making fat digestion more efficient.

FIGURE 5-15 Digestion (Hydrolysis) of a Triglyceride

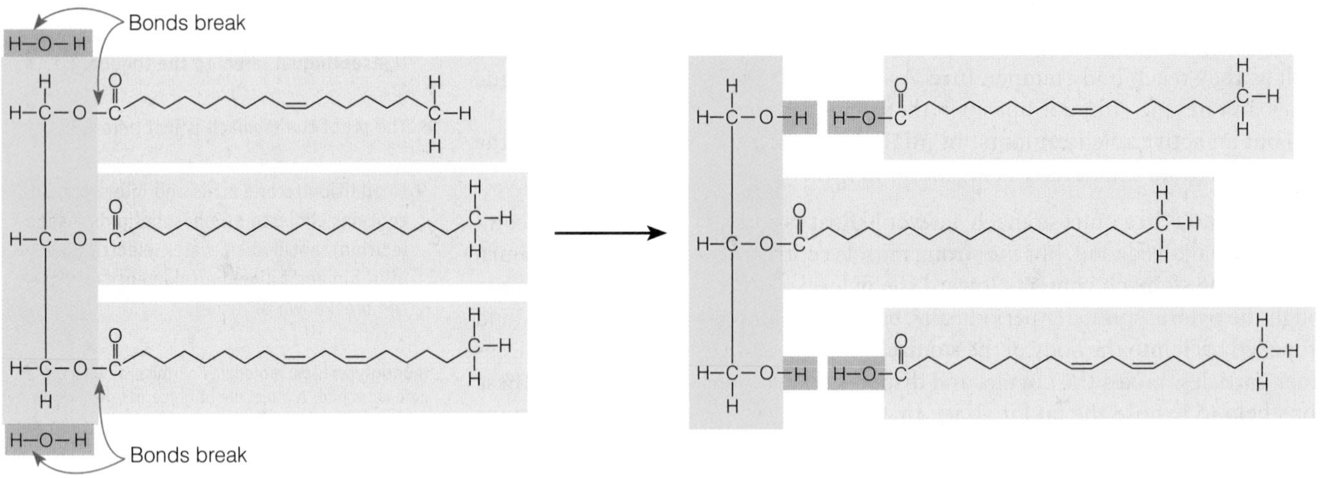
Bonds break
Bonds break

Triglyceride

The triglyceride and two molecules of water are split. The H and OH from water complete the structures of two fatty acids and leave a monoglyceride.

Monoglyceride + two fatty acids

These products may pass into the intestinal cells, but sometimes the monoglyceride is split with another molecule of water to give a third fatty acid and glycerol. Fatty acids, monoglycerides, and glycerol are absorbed into intestinal cells.

FIGURE 5-16 Enterohepatic Circulation

Most of the bile released into the small intestine is reabsorbed and sent back to the liver to be reused. This cycle is called the **enterohepatic circulation** of bile. Some bile is excreted.

- **enteron** = intestine
- **hepat** = liver

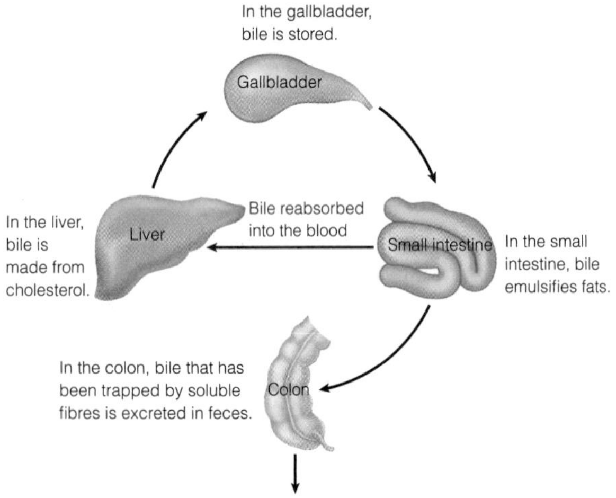
In the gallbladder, bile is stored.
Gallbladder
In the liver, bile is made from cholesterol.
Liver
Bile reabsorbed into the blood
Small intestine
In the small intestine, bile emulsifies fats.
In the colon, bile that has been trapped by soluble fibres is excreted in feces.
Colon

outer fatty acids (more than 70 percent of them are removed this way), leaving a monoglyceride. Occasionally, enzymes remove all three fatty acids, leaving a free molecule of glycerol. Hydrolysis of a triglyceride is shown in Figure 5-15.

Phospholipids are digested similarly—that is, their fatty acids are removed by hydrolysis. The two fatty acids and the remaining phospholipid fragment are then absorbed. Most sterols can be absorbed as is; if any fatty acids are attached, they are first hydrolyzed off.

Bile's Routes After bile enters the small intestine and emulsifies fat, it has two possible destinations, illustrated in Figure 5-16. Most of the bile is reabsorbed from the small intestine and recycled. The other possibility is that some of the bile can be trapped by dietary fibres in the large intestine and excreted. Because cholesterol is needed to make bile, the excretion of bile helps reduce blood cholesterol. As Chapter 4 explains, the dietary fibres most effective at lowering blood cholesterol this way are the soluble fibres commonly found in fruits, whole grains, and legumes.

Lipid Absorption

Figure 5-17 illustrates the absorption of lipids. Small molecules of digested triglycerides (glycerol and short- and medium-chain fatty acids) can diffuse easily into the intestinal cells; they are absorbed directly into the bloodstream. Larger molecules (the monoglycerides and long-chain fatty acids) merge into spherical complexes, known as **micelles.** Micelles are emulsified fat droplets formed by molecules of bile surrounding monoglycerides and fatty acids. This configuration permits solubility in the watery digestive fluids and transportation to the intestinal cells. Upon arrival, the lipid contents of the micelles diffuse into the intestinal cells. Once inside, the monoglycerides and long-chain fatty acids are reassembled into new triglycerides.

Within the intestinal cells, the newly made triglycerides and other lipids (cholesterol, phospholipids, and fat-soluble vitamins) are packed with protein into lipoprotein transport vehicles known as **chylomicrons.** The intestinal cells then release the chylomicrons (via a process called *pinocytosis*) into the lymphatic system. The chylomicrons glide through the lymph until they reach a point of entry into the bloodstream at the thoracic duct, a vein near the heart. (Recall from Chapter 3 that nutrients from the GI tract that enter the lymph system bypass the liver at first.) The blood carries these lipids to the rest of the body for immediate use or storage.

micelles (MY-cells): tiny spherical complexes of emulsified fat that arise during digestion; most contain bile salts and the products of lipid digestion, including fatty acids, monoglycerides, and cholesterol.

chylomicrons (kye-lo-MY-cronz): the class of lipoproteins that transport lipids from the intestinal cells to the rest of the body.

FIGURE 5-17 **Absorption of Fat**

The end products of fat digestion are mostly monoglycerides, some fatty acids, and very little glycerol. Their absorption differs depending on their size. (In reality, molecules of fatty acid are too small to see without a powerful microscope, whereas villi are visible to the naked eye.)

CENGAGENOW™
Animated! figure
www.cengage.com/sso

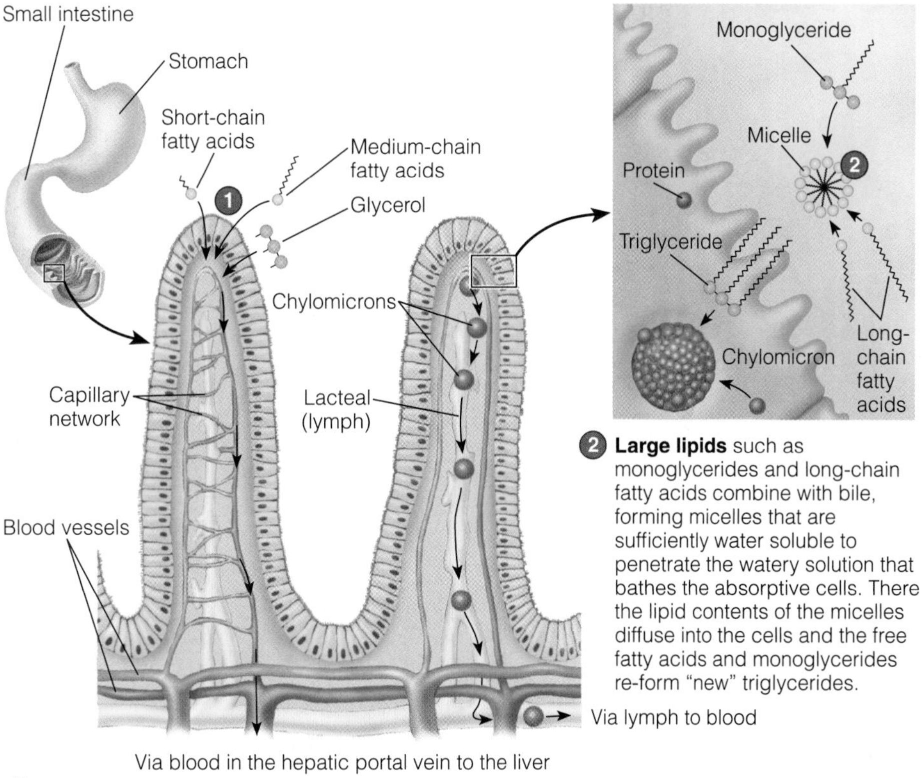
Small intestine
Stomach
Short-chain fatty acids
Medium-chain fatty acids
Glycerol
1
Chylomicrons
Capillary network
Lacteal (lymph)
Blood vessels
Monoglyceride
Micelle
2
Protein
Triglyceride
Chylomicron
Long-chain fatty acids
Via lymph to blood
Via blood in the hepatic portal vein to the liver

② **Large lipids** such as monoglycerides and long-chain fatty acids combine with bile, forming micelles that are sufficiently water soluble to penetrate the watery solution that bathes the absorptive cells. There the lipid contents of the micelles diffuse into the cells and the free fatty acids and monoglycerides re-form "new" triglycerides.

① **Glycerol and small lipids** such as short- and medium-chain fatty acids can move directly into the bloodstream.

A look at these lipids in the body reveals the kinds of fat the diet has been delivering.[4] The blood lipoproteins and red blood cell membranes, fat stores, and muscle cells of people who eat a diet rich in unsaturated fats, for example, contain more unsaturated fats than those of people who select a diet high in saturated fats.

IN SUMMARY **The body makes special arrangements to digest and absorb lipids. It provides the emulsifier bile to make them accessible to the fat-digesting lipases that dismantle triglycerides, mostly to monoglycerides and fatty acids, for absorption by the intestinal cells. The intestinal cells assemble freshly absorbed lipids (including "newly" formed triglycerides, fat-soluble vitamins, and cholesterol) into chylomicrons, lipid packages with protein escorts, for transport so that cells all over the body may select needed lipids from them.**

Lipid Transport

The chylomicrons are only one of several clusters of lipids and proteins that are used as transport vehicles for fats. As a group, these vehicles are known as **lipoproteins**, and they solve the body's challenge of transporting fat through the watery bloodstream. The body makes four main types of lipoproteins, distinguished by their size and density.* Each type contains different kinds and amounts of lipids and proteins. ♦ Figure 5-18 (p. 142) shows the relative compositions and sizes of the lipoproteins.

♦ The more lipids, the lower the density; the more proteins, the higher the density.

Chylomicrons The chylomicrons are the largest and least dense of the lipoproteins. They transport *diet*-derived lipids (mostly triglycerides) from the small

*Chemists can identify the various lipoproteins by their density. They place a blood sample below a thick fluid in a test tube and spin the tube in a centrifuge. The most buoyant particles (highest in lipids) rise to the top and have the lowest density; the densest particles (highest in proteins) remain at the bottom and have the highest density. Others distribute themselves in between.

lipoproteins (LIP-oh-PRO-teenz): clusters of lipids associated with proteins that serve as transport vehicles for lipids in the lymph and blood.

FIGURE 5-18 Sizes and Compositions of the Lipoproteins

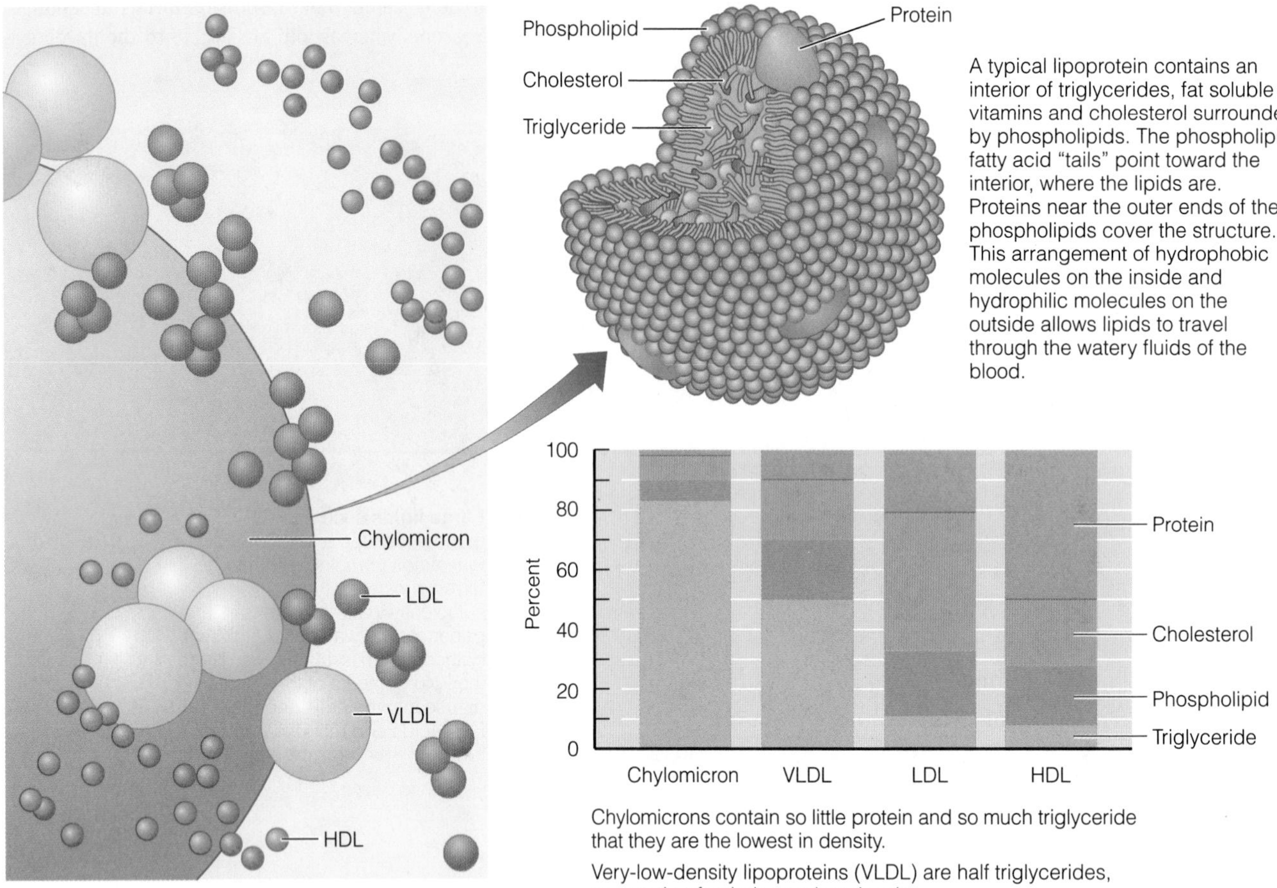
Phospholipid
Cholesterol
Triglyceride
Protein
Chylomicron
LDL
VLDL
HDL
100
80
60
40
20
0
Percent
Chylomicron
VLDL
LDL
HDL
Protein
Cholesterol
Phospholipid
Triglyceride

A typical lipoprotein contains an interior of triglycerides, fat soluble vitamins and cholesterol surrounded by phospholipids. The phospholipids' fatty acid "tails" point toward the interior, where the lipids are. Proteins near the outer ends of the phospholipids cover the structure. This arrangement of hydrophobic molecules on the inside and hydrophilic molecules on the outside allows lipids to travel through the watery fluids of the blood.

This solar system of lipoproteins shows their relative sizes. Notice how large the fat-filled chylomicron is compared with the others and how the others get progressively smaller as their proportion of fat declines and protein increases.

Chylomicrons contain so little protein and so much triglyceride that they are the lowest in density.

Very-low-density lipoproteins (VLDL) are half triglycerides, accounting for their very low density.

Low-density lipoproteins (LDL) are half cholesterol (bad cholesterol), accounting for their implication in heart disease.

High-density lipoproteins (HDL) are half protein (good cholesterol), accounting for their high density.

intestine (via the lymph system) to the rest of the body. Cells all over the body remove triglycerides from the chylomicrons as they pass by, so the chylomicrons get smaller and smaller (and become *chylomicron remnants*). Within 14 hours after absorption, most of the triglycerides have been depleted, and only a few remnants of protein, cholesterol, and phospholipid remain. Special protein receptors on the membranes of the liver cells recognize and remove these chylomicron remnants from the blood. After collecting the remnants, the liver cells first dismantle them and then either use or recycle the pieces.

VLDL (Very-Low-Density Lipoproteins) Meanwhile, in the liver—the most active site of lipid synthesis—cells are making cholesterol, fatty acids, and other lipid compounds. Ultimately, the lipids made in the liver and those collected from chylomicron remnants are packaged with proteins as **VLDL (very-low-density lipoproteins)** and shipped to other parts of the body.

As the VLDL travel through the body, cells remove triglycerides, causing the VLDL to shrink. As VLDL lose triglycerides, the proportion of lipids shifts. Cholesterol becomes the predominant lipid, and the lipoprotein density increases. The VLDL becomes an **LDL (low-density lipoprotein).*** This transformation explains why LDL contain few triglycerides but are loaded with cholesterol.

VLDL (very-low-density lipoprotein): the type of lipoprotein made primarily by liver cells to transport lipids to various tissues in the body; composed primarily of triglycerides (i.e., those derived from the diet and those synthesized by the liver from excess energy).

LDL (low-density lipoprotein): the type of lipoprotein derived from very-low-density lipoproteins (VLDL) as VLDL triglycerides are removed and broken down; composed primarily of cholesterol.

*Before becoming LDL, the VLDL are first transformed into intermediate-density lipoproteins (IDL), sometimes called VLDL remnants. About 50 percent of IDL may be picked up by the liver and rapidly broken down; those IDL that remain in circulation continue to deliver triglycerides to the cells and eventually become LDL. Researchers debate whether IDL are simply transitional particles or a separate class of lipoproteins; normally, IDL do not accumulate in the blood. Measures of blood lipids include IDL with LDL.

LDL (Low-Density Lipoproteins) The LDL ("bad cholesterol") circulate throughout the body, making their contents available to the cells of all tissues—muscles (including the heart muscle), fat stores, the mammary glands, and others. The cells take triglycerides, cholesterol, and phospholipids to build new membranes, make hormones or other compounds, or store for later use. Special LDL receptors on the liver cells play a crucial role in the control of blood cholesterol concentrations by removing LDL from circulation.

HDL (High-Density Lipoproteins) The liver makes **HDL** ("good cholesterol") to remove cholesterol from the cells and carry it back to the liver for recycling or disposal. In addition, HDL have anti-inflammatory properties that seem to keep atherosclerotic plaque from breaking apart and causing heart attacks.[5] Figure 5-19 summarizes lipid transport via the lipoproteins.

Health Implications The distinction between LDL and HDL has implications for the health of the heart and blood vessels. The blood cholesterol linked to heart disease is LDL cholesterol. As mentioned, HDL also carry cholesterol, but elevated HDL represent cholesterol returning ♦ from the rest of the body to the liver for breakdown and excretion. High LDL cholesterol is associated with a high risk of heart attack, whereas high HDL cholesterol seems to have a protective effect. This is why some people refer to LDL as "bad," and HDL as "good," cholesterol. ♦ Keep in mind that the cholesterol itself is the same, and that the differences between LDL and HDL reflect the *proportions* and *types* of lipids and proteins within them—not the type of cholesterol. The margin ♦ lists factors that influence LDL and HDL, and Chapter 19 provides many more details.

Not too surprisingly, numerous genes influence how the body handles the synthesis, transport, and degradation of lipids and lipoproteins. Much current research is focused on how nutrient–gene interactions may direct the progression of heart disease.

♦ The transport of cholesterol from the tissues to the liver is sometimes called *reverse cholesterol transport* or the *scavenger pathway.*

♦ Think of **H**DL as **H**ealthy and **L**DL as **L**ess healthy.

♦ Factors that lower LDL and/or raise HDL:
- Weight control
- Monounsaturated or polyunsaturated, instead of saturated, fat in the diet
- Soluble dietary fibres (see Chapter 4)
- Phytochemicals (see Highlight 14)
- *Moderate* alcohol consumption
- Physical activity

HDL (high-density lipoprotein): the type of lipoprotein that transports cholesterol back to the liver from the cells; composed primarily of protein.

FIGURE 5-19 Lipid Transport via Lipoproteins

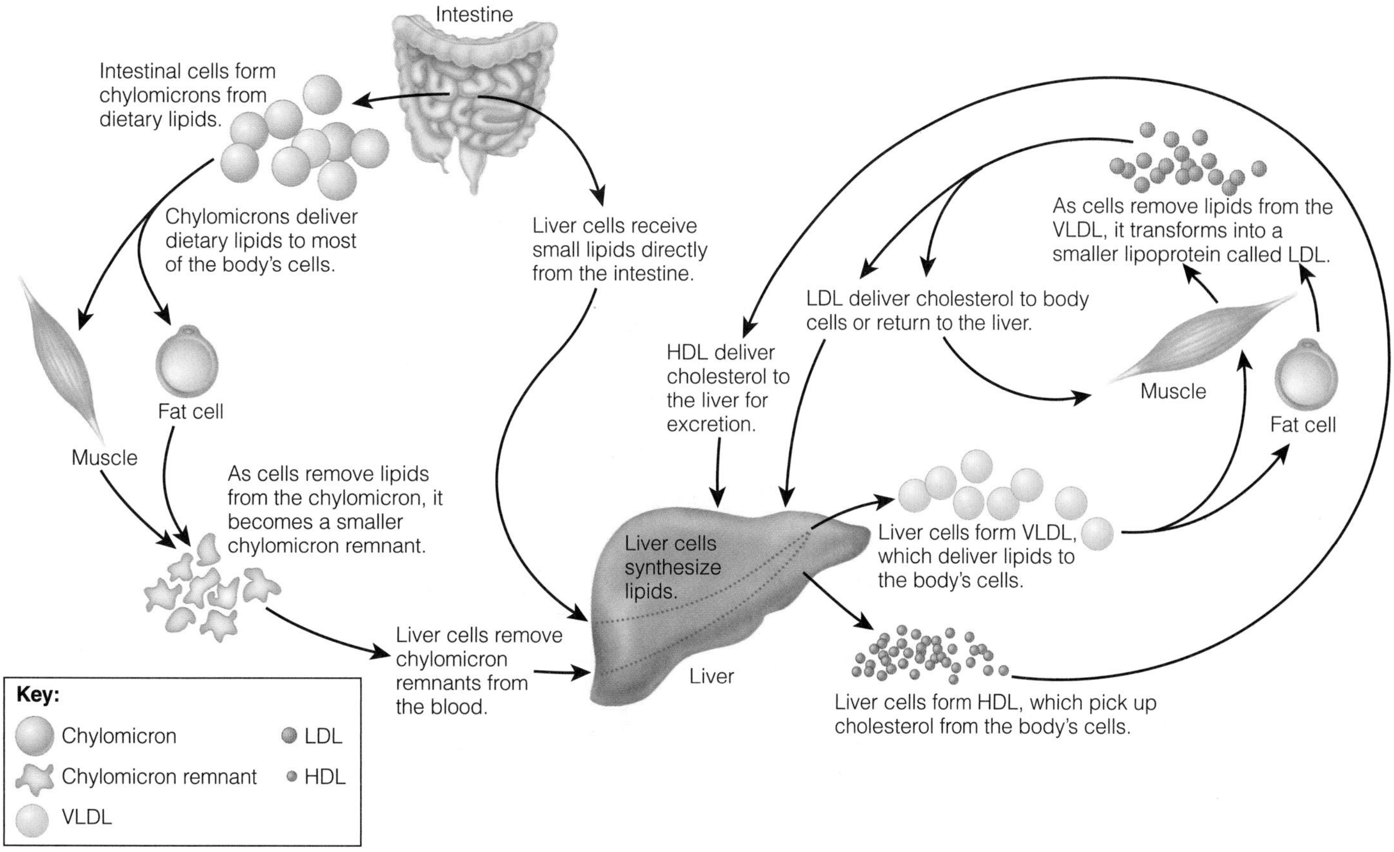
Intestine
Intestinal cells form chylomicrons from dietary lipids.
Chylomicrons deliver dietary lipids to most of the body's cells.
Fat cell
Muscle
As cells remove lipids from the chylomicron, it becomes a smaller chylomicron remnant.
Liver cells receive small lipids directly from the intestine.
Liver cells remove chylomicron remnants from the blood.
Liver cells synthesize lipids.
Liver
HDL deliver cholesterol to the liver for excretion.
LDL deliver cholesterol to body cells or return to the liver.
As cells remove lipids from the VLDL, it transforms into a smaller lipoprotein called LDL.
Muscle
Fat cell
Liver cells form VLDL, which deliver lipids to the body's cells.
Liver cells form HDL, which pick up cholesterol from the body's cells.
Key:
Chylomicron
Chylomicron remnant
VLDL
LDL
HDL

FIGURE 5-20 An Adipose Cell

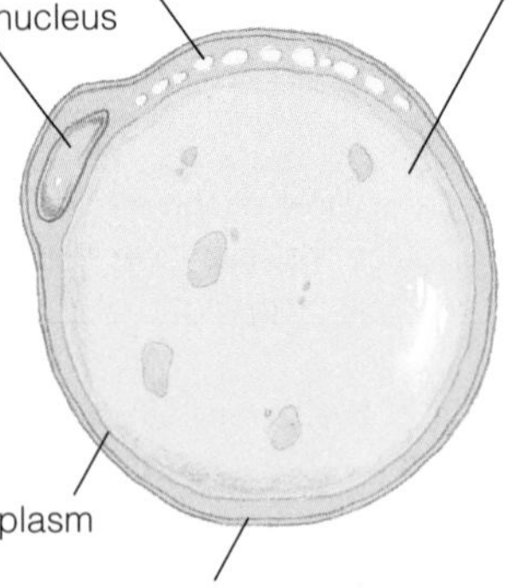
Newly imported triglycerides first form small droplets at the periphery of the cell, then merge with the large, central globule.
Large central globule of (pure) fat
Cell nucleus
Cytoplasm
As the central globule enlarges, the fat cell membrane expands to accommodate its swollen contents.

IN SUMMARY Lipoproteins transport lipids around the body. All four types of lipoproteins carry all classes of lipids (triglycerides, phospholipids, fat-soluble vitamins, and cholesterol), but the chylomicrons are the largest and contain mostly triglycerides; VLDL are smaller and are about half triglycerides; LDL ("bad cholesterol") are smaller still and contain mostly cholesterol; and HDL ("good cholesterol") are the densest and are rich in protein.

Lipids in the Body

In the body, lipids provide energy, insulate against temperature extremes, protect against shock, and maintain cell membranes. This section provides an overview of the roles of triglycerides and fatty acids and then of the metabolic pathways they can follow within the body's cells.

Roles of Triglycerides

First and foremost, the triglycerides—either from food or from the body's fat stores—provide the cells with energy. When a person dances all night, her dinner's triglycerides provide some of the fuel that keeps her moving. When a person loses his appetite, his stored triglycerides fuel much of his body's work until he can eat again.

Fat provides more than twice the energy of carbohydrate and protein, ♦ making it an extremely efficient storage form of energy. Unlike the liver's glycogen stores, the body's fat stores have virtually unlimited capacity, thanks to the special cells of the **adipose tissue.** Unlike most body cells, which can store only limited amounts of fat, the fat cells of the adipose tissue readily take up and store triglycerides. An adipose cell is depicted in Figure 5-20.

Adipose tissue is more than just a storage depot for fat. Adipose tissue actively secretes several hormones known as **adipokines**—proteins that help regulate energy balance and influence several body functions.[6] ♦ When body fat is markedly reduced or excessive, the type and quantity of adipokine secretions change, with consequences for the body's health.[7] Researchers are currently exploring how adipokines influence the links between obesity and chronic diseases such as type 2 diabetes, hypertension, and heart disease.[8] Obesity, for example, increases the release of an adipokine (resistin) that promotes inflammation and insulin resistance—factors that predict heart disease and diabetes.[9] Similarly, obesity decreases the release of an adipokine (adiponectin) that protects against inflammation, diabetes, and heart disease.[10]

Fat serves other roles in the body as well. Because fat is a poor conductor of heat, the layer of fat beneath the skin insulates the body from temperature extremes. Fat pads also serve as natural shock absorbers, providing a cushion for the bones and vital organs. Fat provides the structural material for cell membranes and participates in cell signalling pathways.

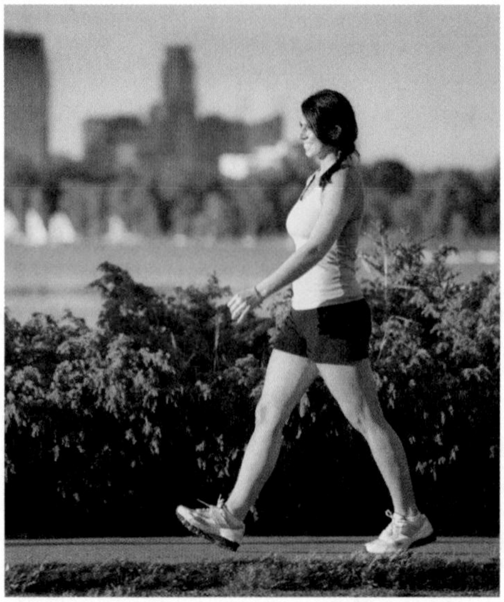
© YinYang/iStockphoto

Double thanks: The body's fat stores provide energy for a walk, and the heel's fat pads cushion against the hard pavement.

Essential Fatty Acids

The human body needs fatty acids, and it can make all but two of them—linoleic acid (the 18-carbon omega-6 fatty acid) and linolenic acid (the 18-carbon omega-3 fatty acid). These two fatty acids must be supplied by the diet and are therefore **essential fatty acids.** ♦ The cells do not possess

♦ Gram for gram, fat provides more than twice as much energy (9 kcal) as carbohydrate or protein (4 kcal).

♦ Examples of adipokines:
- Leptin
- Adiponectin
- Resistin
- Visfatin

♦ An **essential nutrient** is one that the body cannot make, or cannot make in sufficient quantities, to meet its physiological needs.

adipose (ADD-ih-poce) **tissue:** the body's fat tissue; consists of masses of triglyceride-storing cells.

adipokines: proteins synthesized and secreted by adipose cells.

essential fatty acids: fatty acids needed by the body that must be supplied by the diet because the body cannot make them. These are linoleic acid and linolenic acid.

the enzymes to make any of the primary omega-6 or omega-3 fatty acids from scratch, nor can they convert an omega-6 fatty acid to an omega-3 fatty acid or vice versa. Cells *can*, however, start with the primary 18-carbon member of an omega family and make the longer fatty acids of that family by forming double bonds (desaturation) and lengthening the chain two carbons at a time (elongation), as shown in Figure 5-21. This is a slow process because the omega-3 and omega-6 families compete for the same enzymes. Too much of a fatty acid from one family can create a deficiency of the other family's longer fatty acids, which becomes critical only when the diet fails to deliver adequate supplies. Therefore, the most effective way to maintain body supplies of all the omega-6 and omega-3 fatty acids is to obtain them directly from foods—most notably, from vegetable oils, seeds, nuts, fish, and other marine foods.

Linoleic Acid and the Omega-6 Family Linoleic acid is the primary member of the omega-6 fatty acid family and is an important component of membrane phospholipids. When the body receives linoleic acid from the diet, it can make other members of the omega-6 family—such as the 20-carbon polyunsaturated fatty acid **arachidonic acid.** Should a linoleic acid deficiency develop, arachidonic acid, and all other fatty acids that derive from linoleic acid, would also become essential and have to be obtained from the diet. ♦ Normally, vegetable oils and meats supply enough omega-6 fatty acids to meet the body's needs.

Linolenic Acid and the Omega-3 Family Linolenic acid is the primary member of the omega-3 fatty acid family and is an important component of membrane phospholipids.* Like linoleic acid, linolenic acid cannot be made in the body and must be supplied by foods. Given the 18-carbon linolenic acid, the body can make small amounts of the 20- and 22-carbon members of the omega-3 series, **eicosapentaenoic acid (EPA)** and **docosahexaenoic acid (DHA)**, respectively. These omega-3 fatty acids are found in the eyes and brain and are essential for normal growth and cognitive development.[11] They may also play an important role in the prevention and treatment of heart disease, as later sections explain.[12]

Eicosanoids The body uses arachidonic acid and EPA to make substances known as **eicosanoids.** Eicosanoids are a diverse group of compounds that are sometimes described as "hormonelike," but they differ from hormones in important ways. For one, hormones are secreted in one location and travel to affect cells all over the body, whereas eicosanoids appear to affect only the cells in which they are made or nearby cells in the same localized environment. For another, hormones elicit the same response from all their target cells, whereas eicosanoids often have different effects on different cells.

The actions of various eicosanoids sometimes oppose one another. For example, one causes muscles to relax and blood vessels to dilate, whereas another causes muscles to contract and blood vessels to constrict. Certain eicosanoids participate in the immune response to injury and infection, producing fever, inflammation, and pain. One of the ways aspirin relieves these symptoms is by slowing the synthesis of these eicosanoids.

Eicosanoids that derive from EPA differ from those that derive from arachidonic acid, with those from EPA providing greater health benefits. The EPA eicosanoids help lower blood pressure, reduce blood clot formation, protect against irregular heartbeats, and reduce inflammation.

Fatty Acid Deficiencies Most diets in Canada and the United States meet the minimum essential fatty acid requirement adequately (see margin note on page 144). Historically, deficiencies have developed only in infants and young children who have been fed fat-free milk and low-fat diets or in hospital clients who have been mistakenly fed formulas that provided no polyunsaturated fatty acids for long periods of time. Classic deficiency symptoms include growth retardation, reproductive failure, skin lesions, kidney and liver disorders, and subtle neurological and visual problems.

*This omega-3 linolenic acid is known as alpha-linolenic acid and is the fatty acid referred to in this chapter. Another fatty acid, also with 18 carbons and three double bonds, belongs to the omega-6 family and is known as gamma-linolenic acid.

FIGURE 5-21 The Pathway from One Omega-6 Fatty Acid to Another

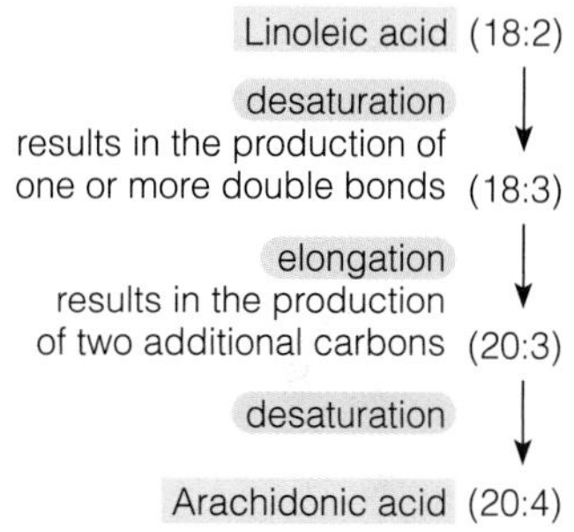
Linoleic acid (18:2)
desaturation
results in the production of one or more double bonds (18:3)
elongation
results in the production of two additional carbons (20:3)
desaturation
Arachidonic acid (20:4)

The first number indicates the number of carbons and the second, the number of double bonds. Similar reactions occur when the body makes the omega-3 fatty acids EPA and DHA from linolenic acid. Note: There is actually competition for some of the same enzymes when arachidonic acid (omega-6) and EPA or DHA (omega-3) are being synthesized.

♦ A nonessential nutrient (such as arachidonic acid) that must be supplied by the diet in special circumstances (as in a linoleic acid deficiency) is considered a **conditionally essential nutrient.**

arachidonic (a-RACK-ih-DON-ic) **acid:** an omega-6 polyunsaturated fatty acid with 20 carbons and four double bonds; present in small amounts in meat and other animal products and synthesized in the body from linoleic acid.

eicosapentaenoic (EYE-cossa-PENTA-ee-NO-ick) **acid (EPA):** an omega-3 polyunsaturated fatty acid with 20 carbons and five double bonds; present in fatty fish and synthesized in limited amounts in the body from linolenic acid.

docosahexaenoic (DOE-cossa-HEXA-ee-NO-ick) **acid (DHA):** an omega-3 polyunsaturated fatty acid with 22 carbons and six double bonds; present in fatty fish and synthesized in limited amounts in the body from linolenic acid.

eicosanoids (eye-COSS-uh-noyds): derivatives of 20-carbon fatty acids; biologically active compounds that help to regulate blood pressure, blood clotting, and other body functions. They include *prostaglandins* (PROS-tah-GLAND-ins), *thromboxanes* (throm-BOX-ains), and *leukotrienes* (LOO-ko-TRY-eens).

IN SUMMARY In the body, triglycerides:

- Provide energy
- Insulate against temperature extremes
- Protect against shock
- Help the body use carbohydrate and protein efficiently

Linoleic acid (18 carbons, omega-6) and linolenic acid (18 carbons, omega-3) are essential nutrients. They serve as structural parts of cell membranes and as precursors to the longer fatty acids that can make eicosanoids—powerful compounds that participate in blood pressure regulation, blood clot formation, and the immune response to injury and infection, among other functions. Because essential fatty acids are common in the diet and stored in the body, deficiencies are unlikely.

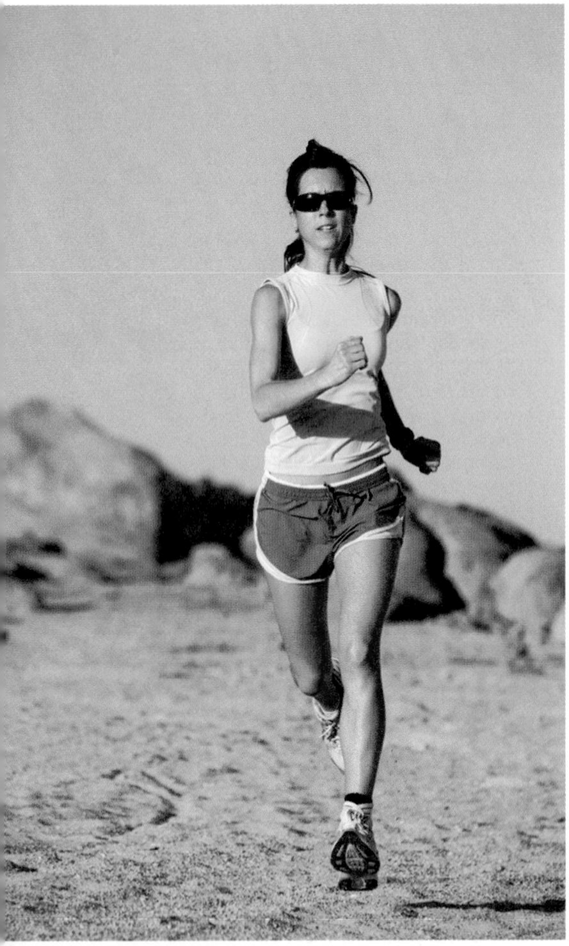
Photoroller

Fat supplies most of the energy during a long-distance run.

A Preview of Lipid Metabolism

This preview of fat metabolism describes how the cells store and release energy from fat. Chapter 7 provides details.

Storing Fat as Fat Adipose cells store fat after meals when a heavy traffic of chylomicrons and VLDL loaded with triglycerides passes by. An enzyme—**lipoprotein lipase (LPL)**—hydrolyzes triglycerides from lipoproteins, releasing fatty acids that enter the adipose cells. Inside the cells, other enzymes reassemble these lipids into triglycerides again for storage. Earlier, Figure 5-4 (page 133) showed how the body can make a triglyceride from glycerol and fatty acids. Triglycerides fill the adipose cells, storing a lot of energy in a relatively small space.

Using Fat for Energy Efficient energy metabolism depends on the energy nutrients—carbohydrate, fat, and protein—supporting one another. Glucose fragments combine with fat fragments during energy metabolism, and fat and carbohydrate help spare protein, providing energy so that protein can be used for other important tasks.

Fat supplies 60 percent of the body's ongoing energy needs during rest. During prolonged light to moderately intense exercise or extended periods of food deprivation, fat stores may make a slightly greater contribution to energy needs.

During energy deprivation, several lipase enzymes (most notably **hormone-sensitive lipase**) inside the adipose cells respond by dismantling stored triglycerides and releasing the glycerol and fatty acids directly into the blood.[13] Energy-hungry cells anywhere in the body can then capture these compounds and take them through a series of chemical reactions to yield energy, carbon dioxide, and water.

A person who fasts (drinking only water) will rapidly metabolize body fat. A half a kilogram (1 pound) of body fat provides 3500 kcalories, ♦ so you might think a fasting person who expends 2000 kcalories a day could lose more than one-quarter kilogram (1/2 pound) of body fat each day.* Actually, the person has to obtain some energy from lean tissue because the brain, nerves, and red blood cells need glucose. Also, the complete breakdown of fat requires carbohydrate or protein. Even on a total fast, a person cannot lose more than one-quarter kilogram (1/2 pound) of pure fat per day. Still, in conditions of forced starvation—say, during a siege or a famine—a fatter person can survive longer than a thinner person thanks to this energy reserve.

♦ 0.5 kg (1 lb) body fat = 3500 kcal

Although fat provides energy during a fast, it can provide very little glucose to give energy to the brain and nerves. Only the small glycerol molecule can be converted to glucose; fatty acids cannot be. (Figure 7-12 on p. 217 illustrates how only 3 of the 50 or so carbon atoms in a molecule of fat can yield glucose.) After prolonged glucose deprivation, brain and nerve cells develop the ability to derive about two-thirds of their minimum energy needs from the ketone bodies that the body makes from fat fragments. Ketone bodies cannot sustain life by themselves,

lipoprotein lipase (LPL): an enzyme that hydrolyzes triglycerides passing by in the bloodstream, which can then enter the cells, where they can be metabolized for energy or reassembled for storage.

hormone-sensitive lipase: an enzyme inside adipose cells that responds to the body's need for fuel by hydrolyzing triglycerides so that their parts (glycerol and fatty acids) escape into the general circulation and thus become available to other cells for fuel. The signals to which this enzyme responds include epinephrine and glucagon, which oppose insulin (see Chapter 4).

*The reader who knows that 1 pound = 454 grams and that 1 gram of fat = 9 kcalories may wonder why a pound of body fat does not equal 4086 (9 × 454) kcalories. The reason is that body fat contains some cell water and other materials; it is not quite pure fat.

however. As Chapter 7 explains, fasting for too long will cause death, even if the person still has ample body fat.

IN SUMMARY **The body can easily store unlimited amounts of fat if given excess, and this body fat is used for energy when needed. (Remember that the liver can also convert excess carbohydrate and protein into fat.) Fat breakdown requires simultaneous carbohydrate breakdown for maximum efficiency; without carbohydrate, fats break down to ketone bodies.**

Health Effects and Recommended Intakes of Lipids

Of all the nutrients, fat is most often linked with heart disease, some types of cancer, and obesity. Fortunately, the same recommendation can help with all of these health problems: choose a diet that is low in saturated fats, *trans* fats, and cholesterol and moderate in total fat.

Health Effects of Lipids

Hearing a physician say "Your blood lipid profile looks fine" is reassuring. The **blood lipid profile** ♦ reveals the concentrations of various lipids in the blood, notably triglycerides and cholesterol, and their lipoprotein carriers (VLDL, LDL, and HDL). This information alerts people to possible disease risks and perhaps to a need for changing their exercise and eating habits. Both the amounts and types of fat in the diet influence people's risk for disease.[14]

♦ Desirable blood lipid profile:
- Total cholesterol: <5.2 mmol/L
- LDL cholesterol: <2.5 mmol/L
- HDL cholesterol: ≥1.5 mmol/L
- Triglycerides: <1.7 mmol/L

Heart Disease Most people realize that elevated blood cholesterol is a major risk factor for **cardiovascular disease (CVD)**. Indeed, over 40 percent of Canadians between 20 and 79 years old are considered to have unhealthy blood cholesterol levels, according to the results of the 2007–2009 Canadian Community Health Measures (CHMS) survey.[15] Cholesterol accumulates in the arteries, restricting blood flow and raising blood pressure. The consequences are deadly; in fact, heart disease is the nation's number one killer of adults. Blood cholesterol level is often used to predict the likelihood of a person's suffering a heart attack or stroke; the higher the cholesterol, the earlier and more likely the tragedy. Much of the effort to prevent heart disease focuses on lowering blood cholesterol.

Risks from Saturated Fats As mentioned earlier, LDL cholesterol raises the risk of heart disease. Saturated fats are most often implicated in raising LDL cholesterol. In general, the more saturated fat in the diet, the more LDL cholesterol in the body. Not all saturated fats have the same cholesterol-raising effect, however. Most notable among the saturated fatty acids that raise blood cholesterol are lauric, myristic, and palmitic acids (12, 14, and 16 carbons, respectively). In contrast, stearic acid (18 carbons) does not seem to raise blood cholesterol.[16] However, making such distinctions may be impractical in diet planning because these saturated fatty acids typically appear together in the same foods. In addition to raising blood cholesterol, saturated fatty acids contribute to heart disease by promoting blood clotting.[17]

Fats from animal sources (meats and milk products), which also contain varying amounts of cholesterol, are the main sources of saturated fats ♦ in most people's diets.[18] Some vegetable fats (coconut and palm), which do not contain cholesterol (since plants do not make it), and hydrogenated fats provide smaller amounts of saturated fats. Selecting skinless poultry or fish and fat-free milk products helps to lower saturated fat intake and the risk of heart disease. Using nonhydrogenated margarine and unsaturated cooking oil is another simple change that can dramatically lower saturated fat intake.

♦ Major sources of saturated fats:
- Whole milk, cream, butter, cheese, ice cream
- Fatty cuts of beef and pork
- Coconut, palm, and palm kernel oils (the tropical oils and products containing them such as candies, pastries, pies, doughnuts, and cookies)

Risks from *Trans* Fats Research also suggests an association between dietary *trans*-fatty acids and heart disease.[19] In the body, *trans*-fatty acids alter blood cholesterol the same way some saturated fats do: they raise LDL cholesterol and, at

blood lipid profile: results of blood tests that reveal a person's total cholesterol, triglycerides, and various lipoproteins.

cardiovascular disease (CVD): a general term for all diseases of the heart and blood vessels. Atherosclerosis is the main cause of CVD. When the arteries that carry blood to the heart muscle become blocked, the heart suffers damage known as **coronary heart disease (CHD).**
- **cardio** = heart
- **vascular** = blood vessels

♦ Major sources of *trans* fats (e.g., foods made with partially hydrogenated vegetable oil):
- Cakes, cookies, doughnuts, pastry, crackers
- Meat and dairy products
- Margarine
- Deep-fried foods (vegetable shortening)
- Snack chips

♦ When selecting margarine, look for:
- Soft (liquid or tub) instead of hard (stick)
- ≤2 g saturated fat
- Liquid vegetable oil (not hydrogenated or partially hydrogenated) as first ingredient
- "*Trans* fat free"

♦ Major sources of cholesterol:
- Eggs
- Milk products
- Meat, poultry, shellfish

♦ Major sources of monounsaturated fats:
- Olive oil, canola oil, peanut oil
- Avocados

♦ Major sources of polyunsaturated fats:
- Vegetable oils (safflower, sesame, soy, corn, sunflower)
- Nuts and seeds

♦ For a brief history on canola oil, see "What Is Canola Oil?" at www.canolainfo.org

♦ Major sources of omega-3 fats:
- Vegetable oils (canola, soybean, flaxseed)
- Walnuts, flaxseeds
- Fatty fish (mackerel, salmon, sardines)

high intakes, lower HDL cholesterol.[20] Limiting the intake of *trans*-fatty acids can improve blood cholesterol and lower the risk of heart disease. To that end, many restaurants and manufacturers have taken steps to eliminate or greatly reduce *trans* fats in foods.[21] The average daily intake of *trans*-fatty acids in Canada is about 3.4 grams per day (~1.4 percent of Total Energy)—mostly from products that have been hydrogenated. ♦

Reports on *trans*-fatty acids raise the question whether margarine or butter is a better choice for heart health. The American Heart Association has stated that because butter is rich in both saturated fat and cholesterol whereas margarine is made from vegetable fat with no dietary cholesterol, margarine is still preferable to butter. Be aware that soft margarines (liquid or tub) ♦ are less hydrogenated and relatively lower in *trans*-fatty acids; consequently, they do not raise blood cholesterol as much as the saturated fats of butter or the *trans* fats of hard (stick) margarines do. Many manufacturers are now offering nonhydrogenated margarines that are "*trans* fat free." The last section of this chapter describes how to read food labels and compares butter and margarines. Whichever you decide to use, remember to use them sparingly.

Risks from Cholesterol Although its effect is not as strong as that of saturated fat or *trans* fat, dietary cholesterol also raises blood cholesterol and increases the risk of heart disease. To maximize the effect on blood cholesterol, limit dietary cholesterol as well.

Recall that cholesterol is found in all foods derived from animals. Consequently, eating less fat from meats, eggs, and milk products helps lower dietary cholesterol intake ♦ (as well as total and saturated fat intakes).

Most foods that are high in cholesterol are also high in saturated fat, but eggs are an exception. An egg contains only 1 gram of saturated fat but just over 200 milligrams of cholesterol—roughly one-third of what your body makes each day. For people with a healthy lipid profile, eating one egg a day is not detrimental. People with high blood cholesterol, however, may benefit from limiting daily cholesterol intake to less than 200 milligrams.[22] When eggs are included in the diet, other sources of cholesterol may need to be limited on that day. Eggs are a valuable part of the diet because they are inexpensive, useful in cooking, and a source of high-quality protein and other nutrients. Low saturated fat, high omega-3 fat eggs are now available, and food manufacturers have produced several fat-free, cholesterol-free egg substitutes.

Benefits from Monounsaturated Fats and Polyunsaturated Fats Replacing both saturated and *trans* fats with monounsaturated ♦ and polyunsaturated ♦ fats may be the most effective dietary strategy in preventing heart disease.[23] The lower rate of heart disease among people in the Mediterranean region of the world is often attributed to their liberal use of olive oil, a rich source of monounsaturated fatty acids. Olive oil, especially virgin olive oil, also delivers valuable phytochemicals that help to protect against heart disease.[24] Replacing saturated fats with the polyunsaturated fatty acids of other vegetable oils also lowers blood cholesterol. Highlight 5 examines various types of fats and their roles in supporting or harming heart health. Note: Both Figure 5-6 (page 134) and the margin notes on this page reveal that canola oil ♦ contains significant amounts of both monounsaturated fats and omega-3 fats.

Benefits from Omega-3 Fats Research on the different types of fats has spotlighted the beneficial effects of the omega-3 ♦ polyunsaturated fatty acids in reducing the risks of heart disease and stroke.[25] Regular consumption of omega-3 fatty acids helps to prevent blood clots, protect against irregular heartbeats, and lower blood pressure, especially in people with hypertension or atherosclerosis.[26] In addition, omega-3 fatty acids support a healthy immune system and defend against inflammatory disorders.[27]

Table 5-2 provides sources of omega-6 and omega-3 fatty acids. Fatty fish are among the best sources of omega-3 fatty acids, and Highlight 5 features their role in supporting heart health.[28] *Canada's Food Guide* recommends two servings of fish a week, with an emphasis on fatty fish (salmon, herring, and mackerel, for example).[29]

TABLE 5-2 Sources of Omega-3 and Omega-6 Fatty Acids

Omega-6	
Linoleic acid	Vegetable oils (corn, sunflower, safflower, soybean, cottonseed), poultry fat, nuts, seeds
Arachidonic acid	Meats, poultry, eggs (or can be made from linoleic acid)
Omega-3	
Linolenic acid	Oils (flaxseed, canola, walnut, wheat germ, soybean) Nuts and seeds (butternuts, flaxseeds, walnuts, soybean kernels) Vegetables (soybeans)
EPA and DHA	Human milk Pacific oysters and fish[a] (or can be made from linolenic acid)

[a]All fish contain some EPA and DHA; the amounts vary among species and within a species depending on such factors as diet, season, and environment (see Table H5-1 on p. 163).

Eating fish supports heart health, especially when combined with physical activity. When preparing fish, grill, bake, or broil, but do not fry. Fried fish does not benefit heart disease.[30] Fried fish from fast-food restaurants and frozen fried fish products are often low in omega-3 fatty acids and high in *trans*- and saturated fatty acids. Fish provides many minerals (except iron) and vitamins. Because fish is leaner than most other animal-protein sources, it can help with weight-loss efforts. The combination of losing weight and eating fish improves blood lipids even more effectively than can be explained by either the weight loss or the omega-3 fats of the fish.

Chapter 20 discusses the adverse consequences of mercury ♦ and other environmental contaminants common in some fish. To maximize the benefits and minimize the risks, most healthy people should eat two servings of fish a week.[31]

In addition to fish, other functional foods ♦ are being developed to help consumers improve their omega-3 fatty acid intake.[32] For example, hens fed flaxseed produce eggs rich in omega-3 fatty acids. Including even one enriched egg in the diet daily can significantly increase a person's intake of omega-3 fatty acids. Another option may be to select wild game or pasture-fed cattle or bison, which provide more omega-3 fatty acids and less saturated fat than grain-fed cattle.

Omega-3 fatty acids are also available in capsules of fish oil supplements. Routine supplementation, however, may not be for everyone.[33] High intakes of omega-3 polyunsaturated fatty acids may increase bleeding time, interfere with wound healing, raise LDL cholesterol, and suppress immune function.* Such findings reinforce the concept that too much of a good thing can sometimes be harmful. People with heart disease, however, may benefit from doses greater than can be achieved through diet alone. They should always consult a physician first because including supplements as part of a treatment plan may be contraindicated for some patients.[34] Because high intakes of omega-3 fatty acids can cause excessive bleeding, intakes should not exceed 3 grams a day without close medical supervision.[35]

♦ Fish relatively high in mercury:
- Tilefish (also called golden snapper or golden bass), swordfish, king mackerel, shark

Fish relatively low in mercury:
- Cod, haddock, pollock, salmon, sole, tilapia
- Most shellfish

♦ **Functional foods** contain physiologically active compounds that provide health benefits beyond basic nutrition. (See Highlight 14 for a full discussion.)

Omega-6 to Omega-3 Ratio Because omega-6 and omega-3 fatty acids compete for the same enzymes and their actions often oppose each other, researchers have studied whether there is an ideal ratio that best supports cardiovascular health. Suggested dietary ratios range from 5:1 to 10:1, but presently little scientific evidence supports such recommendations.[36] In fact, the emerging consensus is that the omega-6 to omega-3 ratio is of little value in improving health or predicting risk.[37] Simply increasing the amount of omega-3 fatty acids in the diet is most beneficial.[38] Reducing the amount of omega-6 fatty acids in the diet to "improve" the ratio is not beneficial, and could even be harmful.[39]

Cancer The evidence for links between dietary fats and cancer ♦ is less convincing than for heart disease. Dietary fat does not seem to *initiate* cancer development but, instead, may *promote* cancer once it has arisen.

♦ Other risk factors for cancer include smoking, alcohol, and environmental contaminants. Chapter 19 provides many more details about these risk factors and the development of cancer.

*Suppressed immune function is seen with daily intake of 0.9 to 9.4 grams EPA and 0.6 to 6.0 grams DHA for 3 to 24 weeks.

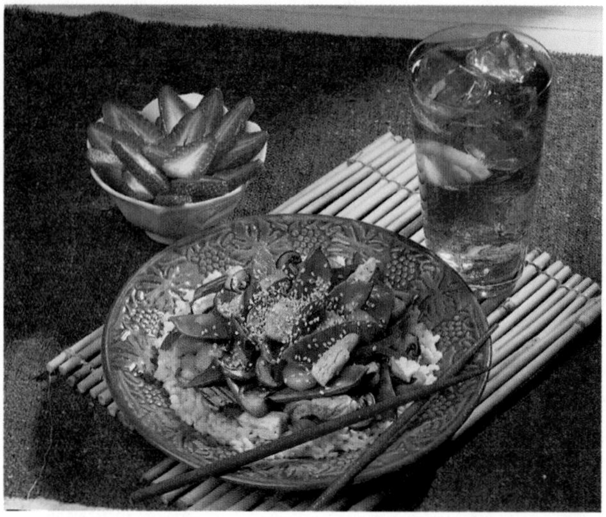
© Polara Studios, Inc.

Well-balanced, healthy meals provide some fat with an emphasis on monounsaturated and polyunsaturated fats.

The relationship between dietary fat and the risk of cancer differs for various types of cancers. In the case of breast cancer, evidence has been weak and inconclusive. Some studies indicate an association between dietary fat and breast cancer; more convincing evidence indicates that body fat contributes to the risk.[40] In the case of colon cancer, limited evidence suggests a harmful association with foods containing animal fats.

The relationship between dietary fat and the risk of cancer differs for various types and combinations of fats as well.[41] The increased risk in cancer from fat appears to be due primarily to saturated fats or dietary fat from meats (which is mostly saturated). Fat from milk or fish has not been implicated in cancer risk.[42] In fact, the omega-3 fatty acids of fatty fish may protect against some cancers, perhaps by suppressing inflammation.[43] Thus dietary advice to reduce cancer risks parallels that given to reduce heart disease risks: reduce saturated fats and increase omega-3 fatty acids, but evidence does not currently support omega-3 supplementation.

Obesity Fat contributes more than twice as many kcalories ♦ per gram as either carbohydrate or protein. Consequently, people who eat high-fat diets regularly may exceed their energy needs and gain weight, especially if they are inactive.[44] Because fat boosts energy intake, cutting fat from the diet can be an effective strategy in cutting kcalories. In some cases, though, choosing a fat-free food offers no kcalorie savings. Fat-free frozen desserts, for example, often have so much sugar added that the kcalorie count can be as high as in the regular-fat product. In this case, cutting fat and adding carbohydrate offers no kcalorie savings or weight-loss advantage. In fact, it may even raise energy intake and exacerbate weight problems. Later chapters revisit the role of dietary fat in the development of obesity.

♦ Fat is a more concentrated energy source than the other energy nutrients: 1 g carbohydrate or protein = 4 kcal, but 1 g fat = 9 kcal.

IN SUMMARY **High blood LDL cholesterol poses a risk of heart disease, and high intakes of saturated and *trans* fats, specifically, contribute most to high LDL. Omega-3 fatty acids appear to be protective.**

Recommended Intakes of Fat

Some fat in the diet is essential for good health, but too much fat, especially saturated and *trans* fat, increases the risks for chronic diseases. Defining the exact amount of fat, saturated fat, *trans* fat, or cholesterol that benefits health or begins to harm health, however, is not possible. For this reason, no RDA or Upper Level has been set. Instead, the DRI and Health Canada suggest a diet that is low in saturated fat, *trans* fat, and cholesterol and provides 20 to 35 percent of the daily energy intake from fat. ♦ These recommendations recognize that diets with up to 35 percent of kcalories from fat can be compatible with good health if energy intake is reasonable and saturated and *trans* fat intakes are low. When total fat exceeds 35 percent, saturated fat increases to unhealthy levels.[45] For a 2000-kcalorie diet, 20 to 35 percent represents 400 to 700 kcalories from fat (roughly 45 to 75 grams). Part of this fat allowance should provide for the essential fatty acids—linoleic acid and linolenic acid. For this reason, an Adequate Intake (AI) has been established for these two fatty acids. Recommendations suggest that linoleic acid ♦ provide 5 to 10 percent of the daily energy intake and linolenic acid ♦ 0.6 to 1.2 percent.[46]

To help consumers meet the dietary fat goals, Health Canada established Daily Values ♦ on food labels using 30 percent of energy intake as the guideline for fat and 10 percent for saturated fat. The Daily Value for cholesterol is 300 milligrams regardless of energy intake. There is no Daily Value for *trans* fat, but consumers should try to keep intakes as low as possible and within the 10 percent allotted for saturated fat. According to the CCHS 2.2 survey, diets in Canada provide about

♦ DRI and *Food Guide* recommendations for fat: 20 to 35% of energy intake (from mostly polyunsaturated and monounsaturated fat sources such as fish, nuts, and vegetable oils)

♦ Linoleic acid (omega-6) AI:
Men:
- 19–50 yr: 17 g/day (current intake is about 14 g/day)
- 51+ yr: 14 g/day

Women:
- 19–50 yr: 12 g/day (current intake is about 9.5 g/day)
- 51+ yr: 11 g/day

♦ Linolenic acid (omega-3) AI:
- Men: 1.6 g/day
- Women: 1.1 g/day

♦ Daily Values:
- 65 g fat (based on 30% of 2000 kcal diet)
- 20 g saturated fat (based on 10% of 2000 kcal diet)
- 300 mg cholesterol

30 percent of their total energy from fat, with saturated fat contributing about 10 percent of the total.[47] These data also reveal that cholesterol intakes in Canada average 220 milligrams a day for women and 345 for men.

Dietary Guidance for Canadians

- Dietary cholesterol, saturated fatty acids, and *trans*-fatty acids should be kept as low as possible while consuming a nutritionally adequate diet.

Canada's Food Guide has an Oils and Fats category ♦ and recommends we consume 30 to 45 millilitres (2 to 3 Tbsp) of unsaturated fat each day from vegetable oils and soft margarines.

♦ For perspective, 1 tsp oil = 5 g fat and provides about 45 kcal.

Although it is very difficult to do, some people actually manage to eat too little fat—to their detriment. Among them are people with eating disorders, described in Highlight 8, and athletes. Athletes following a diet too low in fat (less than 20 percent of total kcalories) fall short on energy, vitamins, minerals, and essential fatty acids as well as on performance.[48] As a practical guideline, it is wise to include the equivalent of at least 5 millilitres (1 tsp) of fat in every meal—a little peanut butter on toast or mayonnaise in tuna salad, for example. Dietary recommendations that limit fat are designed for healthy people over age 2; Chapter 17 discusses the fat needs of infants and young children.

As the photos in Figure 5-22 show, fat accounts for much of the energy in foods, and removing the fat from foods cuts energy and saturated fat intakes dramatically. To reduce dietary fat, eliminate fat as a seasoning and in cooking; remove the fat from high-fat foods; replace high-fat foods with low-fat alternatives; and

FIGURE 5-22 Cutting Fat Cuts kCalories—and Saturated Fat

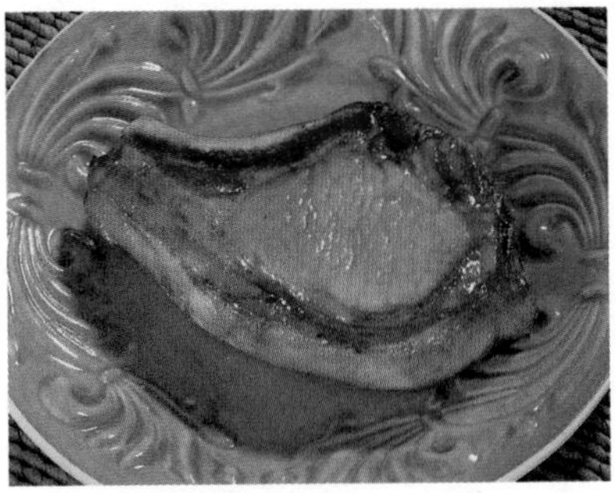
© Polara Studios, Inc.

Pork chop with fat (340 kcal, 19 g fat, 7 g saturated fat)

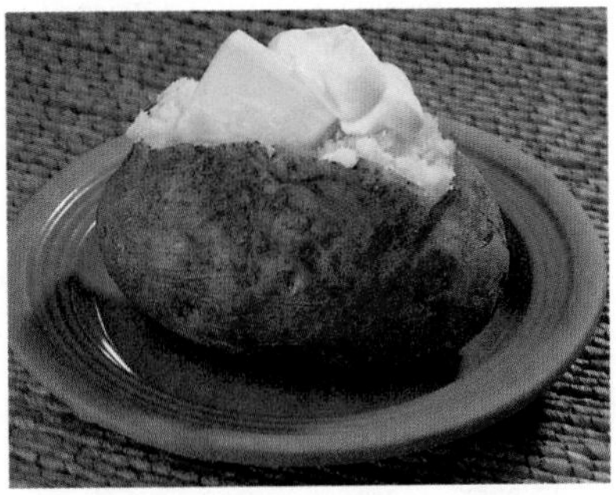
© Polara Studios, Inc.

Potato with 15 mL (1 Tbsp) butter and 15 mL (1 Tbsp) sour cream (350 kcal, 14 g fat, 10 g saturated fat)

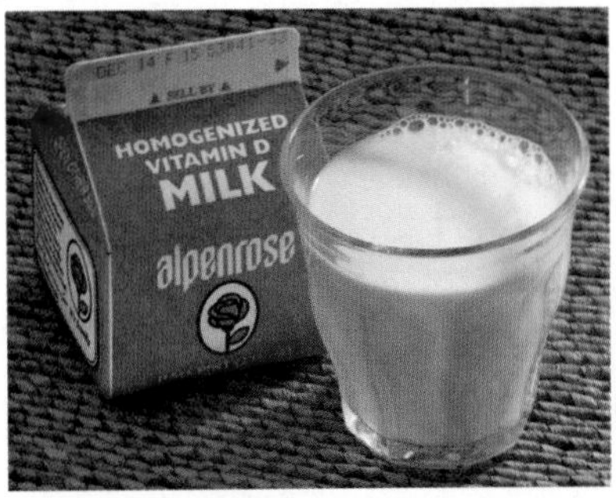
HOMOGENIZED
VITAMIN D
MILK
alpenrose
© Polara Studios, Inc.

Whole milk, 250 mL (1 c) (150 kcal, 8 g fat, 5 g saturated fat)

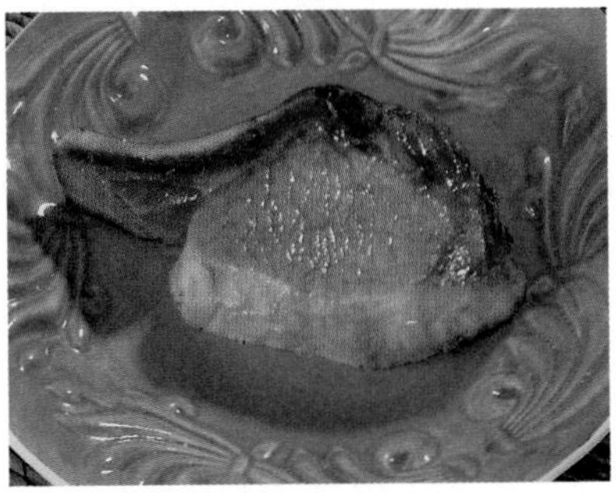
© Polara Studios, Inc.

Pork chop with fat trimmed off (230 kcal, 9 g fat, 3 g saturated fat)

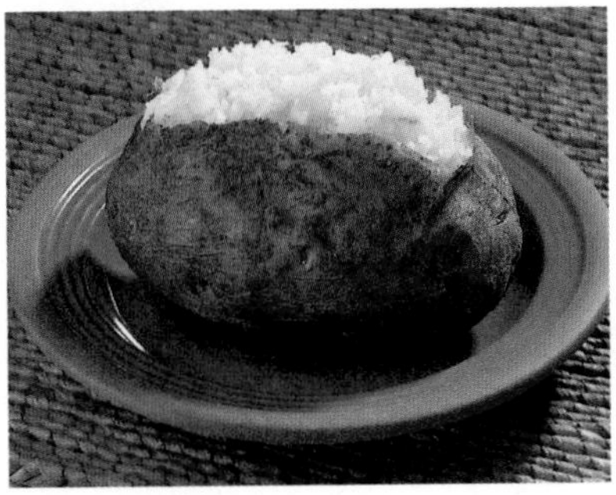
© Polara Studios, Inc.

Plain potato (200 kcal, <1 g fat, 0 g saturated fat)

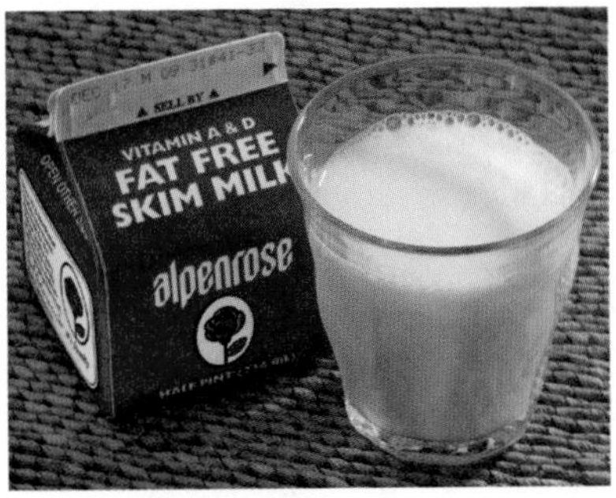
VITAMIN A & D
FAT FREE
SKIM MILK
alpenrose
© Polara Studios, Inc.

Skim milk, 250 mL (1 c) (90 kcal, <1 g fat, <1 g saturated fat)

emphasize whole grains, fruits, and vegetables. The accompanying "How To" suggests additional heart-healthy choices by food group.

From Guidance to Groceries Fats accompany protein in foods derived from animals, such as meat, fish, poultry, and eggs, and fats accompany carbohydrate in foods derived from plants, such as avocados and coconuts. Fats carry with them the four fat-soluble vitamins—A, D, E, and K—together with many

HOW TO Make Heart-Healthy Choices—by Food Group

Grain Products

- Select breads, cereals, and crackers that are low in saturated and *trans* fat (e.g., bagels instead of croissants).
- Prepare pasta with a tomato sauce instead of a cheese or cream sauce.

Vegetables and Fruit

- Enjoy the natural flavour of steamed vegetables (without butter) for dinner and fruits for dessert.
- Eat at least two vegetables (in addition to a salad) with dinner.
- Snack on raw vegetables or fruits instead of high-fat items like potato chips.
- Buy frozen vegetables without sauce.

Milk and Alternatives

- Switch from whole milk to 2%, from 2% to 1%, and from 1% to skim.
- Use fat-free and low-fat cheeses (such as part-skim ricotta and low-fat mozzarella) instead of regular cheeses.
- Use fat-free or low-fat yogurt or sour cream instead of regular sour cream.
- Use evaporated skim milk instead of cream.
- Enjoy fat-free frozen yogurt, sherbet, or ice milk instead of ice cream.

Meat and Alternatives

- Fat adds up quickly, even with lean meat; limit intake to about 175 grams(cooked weight) daily.
- Eat at least two servings of fish per week (particularly fish such as mackerel, lake trout, herring, sardines, and salmon).
- Choose fish, poultry, or lean cuts of pork or beef; look for unmarbled cuts named *round* or *loin* (eye of round, top round, bottom round, round tip, tenderloin, sirloin, centre loin, and top loin).
- Choose processed meats such as lunch meats and hot dogs that are low in saturated fat and cholesterol.
- Trim the fat from pork and beef; remove the skin from poultry.
- Grill, roast, broil, bake, stir-fry, stew, or braise meats; don't fry. When possible, place food on a rack so that fat can drain.
- Use lean ground turkey or lean ground beef in recipes; brown ground meats without added fat, then drain off fat.
- Select tuna, sardines, and other canned meats packed in water; rinse oil-packed items with hot water to remove much of the fat.
- Fill kabob skewers with lots of vegetables and slivers of meat; create main dishes and casseroles by combining a little meat, fish, or poultry with a lot of pasta, rice, or vegetables.
- Use legumes often.
- Eat a meatless meal or two weekly.
- Use egg substitutes in recipes instead of whole eggs or use two egg whites in place of each whole egg.

Oils and Fats

- Use butter or stick margarine sparingly; select soft margarines instead of hard margarines.
- Use fruit butters, reduced-kcalorie margarines, or butter replacers instead of butter.
- Use low-fat or fat-free mayonnaise and salad dressing instead of regular.
- Limit use of lard and meat fat.
- Limit use of products made with coconut oil, palm kernel oil, and palm oil (read labels on bakery goods, processed foods, popcorn oils, and nondairy creamers).
- Reduce use of hydrogenated shortenings and stick margarines and products that contain them (read labels on crackers, cookies, and other commercially prepared baked goods); use vegetable oils instead.

Miscellaneous

- Use a nonstick pan or coat the pan lightly with vegetable oil.
- Refrigerate soups and stews; when the fat solidifies, remove it before reheating.
- Use wine; lemon, orange, or tomato juice; herbs; spices; fruits; or broth instead of butter or margarine when cooking.
- Stir-fry in a small amount of oil; add moisture and flavour with broth, tomato juice, or wine.
- Use variety to enhance enjoyment of the meal: vary colours, textures, and temperatures—hot cooked versus cool raw foods—and use garnishes to complement food.
- Omit high-fat meat gravies and cheese sauces.
- Order pizzas with lots of vegetables, a little lean meat, and half the cheese.

SOURCE: Adapted from *Canada's Food Guide* and the *Third Report of the National Cholesterol Education Program (NCEP) Expert Panel on Detection, Evaluation, and Treatment of High Blood Cholesterol in Adults (Adult Treatment Panel III)*, NIH publication no. 02-5215 (Bethesda, MD: National Heart, Lung, and Blood Institute, 2002), pp. V-25–V-27.

CENGAGENOW™
For additional practice log on to **www.cengage.com/sso.**

TRY IT Compare the total kcalories, grams of fat, and percent kcalories from fat for 250 millilitres (1 cup) of whole milk, 2% milk, 1% milk, and skim milk.

of the compounds that give foods their flavour, texture, and palatability. Fat is responsible for the delicious aromas associated with sizzling bacon, hamburgers on the grill, onions being sautéed, and vegetables in a stir-fry. The essential oils of many spices are fat soluble. Of course, these wonderful characteristics lure people into eating too much from time to time. With careful selections, a diet following *Canada's Food Guide* can support good health and still meet fat recommendations.

Dietary Guidance for Canadians

When selecting and preparing meat, poultry, and milk or milk products, make choices that are lean, low-fat, or fat-free.

Meats and Alternates Many meats and meat alternates ♦ contain fat, saturated fat, and cholesterol but also provide high-quality protein and valuable vitamins and minerals. They can be included in a healthy diet if a person makes lean choices, prepares them using the suggestions outlined in the "How To" feature, and eats small portions. Selecting "free-range" meats from grass-fed instead of grain-fed livestock offers the nutrient advantages of being lower in fat, and the fat has more polyunsaturated fatty acids, including the omega-3 type. Another strategy to lower blood cholesterol is to prepare meals using soy protein instead of animal protein.[49]

Milks and Alternatives Like meats, milks and milk products ♦ should also be selected with an awareness of their fat, saturated fat, and cholesterol contents. Fat-free and low-fat milk products provide as much or more protein, calcium, and other nutrients as their whole-milk versions—but with little or no saturated fat. An interactive tool on Health Canada's website ♦ also helps Canadian better understand the concept of "a little" (5%) or "a lot" (15%) when choosing lower-fat foods using the % Daily Vales (%DV) on food labels. Selecting fermented milk products, such as yogurt, may also help to lower blood cholesterol.[50] These foods increase the population and activity of bacteria in the colon that use cholesterol.[51]

Vegetables, Fruits, and Grains Products Choosing vegetables, fruits, whole grains, and legumes also helps lower the saturated fat, cholesterol, and total fat content of the diet. Most vegetables and fruits naturally contain little or no fat. Although avocados and olives are exceptions, most of their fat is unsaturated, which is not harmful to heart health. Most grains contain only small amounts of fat. Consumers need to read food labels, though, because some grain *products* such as fried taco shells, croissants, and biscuits are high in saturated fat, and pastries, crackers, and cookies may be high in *trans* fats. Similarly, many people add butter, margarine, or cheese sauce to grains and vegetables, which raises their saturated- and *trans*-fat contents. Because fruits are often eaten without added fat, a diet that includes several servings of fruit daily can help a person meet the dietary recommendations for fat.

A diet rich in vegetables, fruits, whole grains, and legumes also offers abundant vitamin C, folate, vitamin A, vitamin E, and dietary fibre—all important in supporting health. Consequently, such a diet protects against disease by reducing saturated fat, cholesterol, and total fat as well as by increasing nutrients. It also provides valuable phytochemicals, which help defend against heart disease.

Invisible Fat *Visible* fat, such as butter and the fat trimmed from meat, is easy to see. *Invisible* fat is less apparent and can be present in foods in surprisingly high amounts. Invisible fat "marbles" a steak or is hidden in foods such as cheese. Any *fried* food contains abundant fat—potato chips, French fries, fried wontons, and fried fish. Many *baked* goods, too, are high in fat—pie crusts, pastries, crackers, biscuits, cornbread, doughnuts, sweet rolls, cookies, and cakes. Most chocolate bars deliver more kcalories from fat than from sugar. Even cream of mushroom soup prepared with water derives two-thirds of its energy from fat. Keep invisible fats in mind when making food selections.

Choose Wisely Consumers can find an abundant array of fresh, unprocessed foods that are naturally low in saturated fat, *trans* fat, cholesterol, and total fat. In addition,

♦ Very lean options:
- Chicken (white meat, no skin); cod, flounder, trout; tuna (canned in water); legumes

Lean options:
- Beef or pork "round" or "loin" cuts; chicken (dark meat, no skin); herring or salmon; tuna (canned in oil)

Medium-fat options:
- Ground beef, eggs, tofu

High-fat options:
- Sausage, bacon, luncheon meats, hot dogs, peanut butter, nuts

♦ Fat-free and low-fat options:
- Skim or 1% milk or yogurt (plain); fat-free and low-fat cheeses

Reduced-fat options:
- 2% milk, low-fat yogurt (plain)

High-fat options:
- Whole milk, regular cheeses

♦ Check out the "How to Choose" yogurt example provided in the Interactive Tools–Nutrition Labelling section on the Health Canada, Food and Nutrition website: www.hc-sc.gc.ca

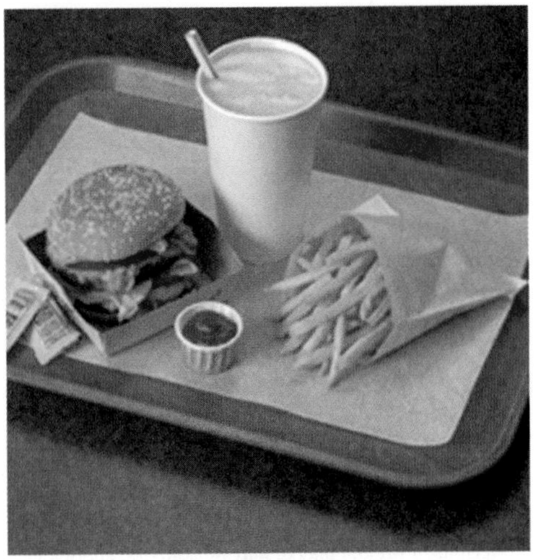

Beware of fast-food meals delivering too much fat, especially saturated fat. This double bacon cheeseburger, fries, and milk shake provide more than 1600 kcalories, with almost 90 grams of fat and more than 30 grams of saturated fat—far exceeding dietary fat guidelines for the entire day.

many familiar foods have been processed to provide less fat. For example, fat can be removed by skimming milk or trimming meats. Manufacturers can dilute fat by adding water or whipping in air. They can use skim milk in creamy desserts and lean meats in frozen entrées. Sometimes manufacturers simply prepare the products differently. For example, fat-free potato chips may be baked instead of fried. Beyond lowering the fat content, manufacturers have developed margarines fortified with plant sterols that lower blood cholesterol.*[52] (Highlight 14 explores these and other functional foods designed to support health.) Such choices make heart-healthy eating easy.

Dietary Guidance for Canadians

Limit intakes of fats and oils high in saturated and/or *trans*-fatty acids, and choose products low in such fats and oils.

To replace saturated fats with unsaturated fats, sauté foods in olive oil instead of butter, garnish salads with sunflower seeds instead of bacon, snack on mixed nuts instead of potato chips, use avocado instead of cheese on a sandwich, and eat salmon instead of steak. Table 5-3 shows how these simple substitutions can lower the saturated fat and raise the unsaturated fat in a meal. Highlight 5 provides more details about the benefits of healthy fats in the diet.

Fat Replacers Some foods are made with **fat replacers**—ingredients that provide some of the taste and texture of fats, but with fewer kcalories. Because the body may digest and absorb some of these fat replacers, they may contribute energy, although significantly less energy than fat's 9 kcalories per gram.

Some fat replacers are derived from carbohydrate, protein, or fat. Carbohydrate-based fat replacers are used primarily as thickeners or stabilizers in foods such as soups and salad dressings. Protein-based fat replacers provide a creamy feeling in the mouth and are often used in foods such as ice creams and yogurts. Fat-based replacers act as emulsifiers and are heat stable, making them most versatile in shortenings used in cake mixes and cookies.

Fat replacers offering the sensory and cooking qualities of fats but none of the kcalories are called **artificial fats.** A familiar example of an artificial fat that has been approved for use in the United States in snack foods such as potato chips, crackers, and tortilla chips is **olestra.** Olestra's chemical structure is similar to that of a regular fat (a triglyceride) but with important differences. A triglyceride is composed of a glycerol molecule with three fatty acids attached, whereas olestra is made of a sucrose molecule with six to eight fatty acids attached. Enzymes in the digestive tract cannot break the bonds of olestra, so unlike sucrose or fatty acids, olestra passes through the system unabsorbed. While Olestra has not been approved for use in foods in Canada, similar sucrose polyester fat replacers are allowed in Canadian foods.

*Margarines that lower blood cholesterol contain plant sterols and are marketed under the brand names Becel Pro.activ.

TABLE 5-3 Choosing Unsaturated Fat instead of Saturated Fat

Portion sizes have been adjusted so that each of these foods provides approximately 100 kcalories. Notice that for a similar number of kcalories and grams of fat, the first choices offer less saturated fat and more unsaturated fat.

Foods (100 kcal portions)	Saturated Fat (g)	Unsaturated Fat (g)	Total Fat (g)
Olive oil (15 mL/1Tbsp) vs butter (15 mL/1 Tbsp)	2 vs 7	9 vs 4	11 vs 11
Sunflower seeds (30 mL/2 Tbsp) vs bacon (2 slices)	1 vs 3	7 vs 6	8 vs 9
Mixed nuts (30 mL/2 Tbsp) vs potato chips (10 chips)	1 vs 2	8 vs 5	9 vs 7
Avocado (6 slices) vs cheese (1 slice)	2 vs 4	8 vs 4	10 vs 8
Salmon (60 g) vs steak (45 g)	1 vs 2	3 vs 3	4 vs 5
Totals	**7 vs 18**	**35 vs 22**	**42 vs 40**

fat replacers: ingredients that replace some or all of the functions of fat and may or may not provide energy.

artificial fats: zero-energy fat replacers that are chemically synthesized to mimic the sensory and cooking qualities of naturally occurring fats but are totally or partially resistant to digestion.

olestra: a synthetic fat made from sucrose and fatty acids that provides 0 kcalories per gram; also known as *sucrose polyester.*

HOW TO Calculate a Personal Daily Value for Fat

The % Daily Value for fat on food labels is based on 65 grams. To know how your intake compares with this recommendation, you can either count grams until you reach 65, or add the "% Daily Values" until you reach 100 percent—if your energy intake is 2000 kcalories a day. If your energy intake is more or less, you can calculate your personal daily fat allowance in grams. Suppose your energy intake is 1800 kcalories per day and your goal is 30 percent kcalories from fat. Multiply your total energy intake by 30 percent, then divide by 9:

$$1800 \text{ total kcal} \times 0.30 \text{ from fat} = 540 \text{ fat kcal}$$
$$540 \text{ fat kcal} \div 9 \text{ kcal/g} = 60 \text{ g fat}$$

(In familiar measures, 60 grams of fat is about the same as ⅔ stick of butter or 60 mL/¼ cup of oil.)

The accompanying table shows the numbers of grams of fat allowed per day for various energy intakes. With one of these numbers in mind, you can quickly evaluate the number of fat grams in foods you are considering eating.

CENGAGENOW™
For additional practice, log on to **www.cengage.com/sso.**

Energy (kcal/day)	20% kCal from Fat	35% kCal from Fat	Fat (g/day)
1200	240	420	27–47
1400	280	490	31–54
1600	320	560	36–62
1800	360	630	40–70
2000	400	700	44–78
2200	440	770	49–86
2400	480	840	53–93
2600	520	910	58–101
2800	560	980	62–109
3000	600	1050	67–117

TRY IT Calculate a personal daily fat allowance for a person with an energy intake of 2100 kcalories and a goal of 25 percent kcalories from fat.

The U.S. FDA's evaluation of olestra's safety addressed two questions. First, is olestra toxic? Research on both animals and human beings supports the safety of olestra as a partial replacement for dietary fats and oils, with no reports of cancer or birth defects. Second, does olestra affect either nutrient absorption or the health of the digestive tract? When olestra passes through the digestive tract unabsorbed, it binds with some of the fat-soluble vitamins A, D, E, and K and carries them out of the body, robbing the person of these valuable nutrients. To compensate for these losses, the FDA requires the manufacturer to fortify olestra with vitamins A, D, E, and K. Saturating olestra with these vitamins does not make the product a good source of vitamins, but it does block olestra's ability to bind with the vitamins from other foods. An asterisk in the ingredients list informs consumers that these added vitamins are "dietarily insignificant."

Some consumers experience digestive distress after eating olestra, such as cramps, gas, bloating, and diarrhea. The FDA initially required a warning label stating that "olestra may cause abdominal cramping and loose stools" and that it "inhibits the absorption of some vitamins and other nutrients" but has since concluded that such a statement is no longer warranted.

Consumers need to keep in mind that low-fat and fat-free foods still deliver kcalories. Alternatives to fat can help to lower energy intake and support weight loss only when they actually *replace* fat and energy in the diet.[53]

Read Food Labels Labels list total fat, saturated fat, *trans* fat, and cholesterol contents of foods per serving (see Figure 5-23 on p. 156). Because each package provides information for a single serving and because serving sizes are standardized, consumers can easily compare similar products.

Total fat, saturated fat, and cholesterol are also expressed as "% Daily Values" for a person consuming 2000 kcalories. People who consume more or less than 2000 kcalories daily can calculate their personal Daily Value for fat as described in the accompanying "How To" feature. *Trans* fats are combined with saturated fats when expressed as %DV on food labels.

FIGURE 5-23 **Butter and Margarine Labels Compared**

Food labels list the quantities and Daily Values for fat, saturated fat and *trans* fat combined, and optionally cholesterol. Information on polyunsaturated and monounsaturated fats is optional. Products that contain 0.5 g or less of *trans* fat and 0.5 g or less of saturated fat may claim "no *trans* fat." Similarly, products that contain 2 mg or less of cholesterol and 2 g or less of saturated fat may claim to be "cholesterol-free."

If the list of ingredients includes hydrogenated oils, you know the food contains *trans* fat. Chapter 2 explained that foods list their ingredients in descending order of predominance by weight. As you can see from this example, the closer "partially hydrogenated oils" is to the beginning of the ingredients list, the more *trans* fats the product contains. Notice that most of the fat in butter is saturated, whereas most of the fat in margarine is unsaturated; partially hydrogenated margarines tend to have more *trans* fat than hydrogenated liquid margarines.

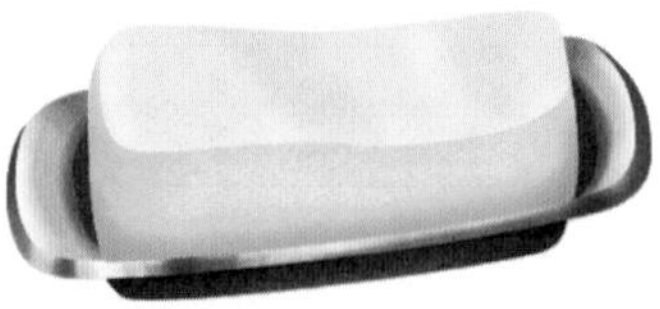

Butter

Nutrition Facts
Serving Size 1 Tbsp (14 g)
Servings per container about 32

Amount per serving	
Calories 100	
	%Daily Value*
Total Fat 11 g	17%
Saturated Fat 7 g / Trans Fat 0 g	37%
Cholesterol 30 mg	10%
Sodium 95 mg	4%
Total Carbohydrate 0 g	0%
Protein 0 g	
Vitamin A 8%	

Not a significant source of dietary fibre, sugars, vitamin C, calcium, and iron.

*Percent Daily Values are based on a 2000 calorie diet.

INGREDIENTS: Cream, salt.

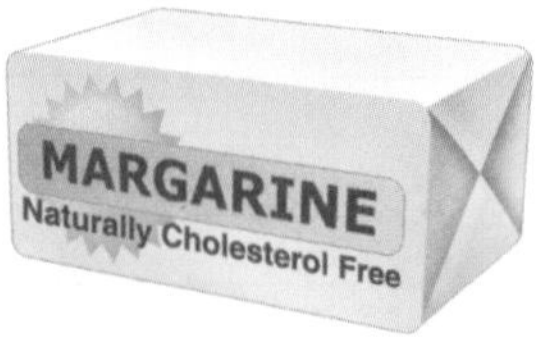
MARGARINE
Naturally Cholesterol Free

Margarine (stick)

Nutrition Facts
Serving Size 1 Tbsp (14 g)
Servings per container about 32

Amount per serving	
Calories 100	
	%Daily Value*
Total Fat 11 g	17%
Saturated Fat 2 g / Trans Fat 2.5 g	11%
Polyunsaturated Fat 3.5 g	
Monounsaturated Fat 2.5 g	
Cholesterol 0 mg	0%
Sodium 105 mg	4%
Total Carbohydrate 0 g	0%
Protein 0 g	
Vitamin A 10%	

Not a significant source of dietary fibre, sugars, vitamin C, calcium, and iron.

*Percent Daily Values are based on a 2000 calorie diet.

INGREDIENTS: Liquid soybean oil, partially hydrogenated soybean oil, water, buttermilk, salt, soy lecithin, sodium benzoate (as a preservative), vegetable mono and diglycerides, artificial flavour, vitamin A palmitate, coloured with beta carotene (provitamin A).

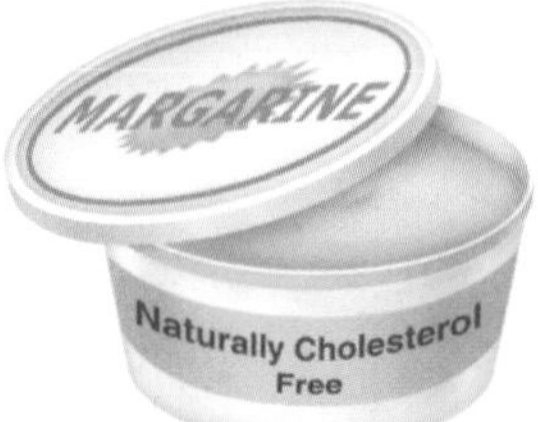
MARGARINE
Naturally Cholesterol Free

Margarine (tub)

Nutrition Facts
Serving size 1 Tbsp (14 g)
Servings per container about 32

Amount per serving	
Calories 100	
	%Daily Value*
Total Fat 11 g	17%
Saturated Fat 2.5 g / Trans Fat 2 g	13%
Polyunsaturated Fat 4 g	
Monounsaturated Fat 2.5 g	
Cholesterol 0 mg	0%
Sodium 80 mg	3%
Total Carbohydrate 0 g	0%
Protein 0 g	
Vitamin A 10%	

Not a significant source of dietary fibre, sugars, vitamin C, calcium, and iron.

*Percent Daily Values are based on a 2000 calorie diet.

INGREDIENTS: Liquid soybean oil, partially hydrogenated soybean oil, buttermilk, water, butter (cream, salt), salt, soy lecithin, vegetable mono and diglycerides, sodium benzoate added as a preservative, artificial flavour, vitamin A palmitate, coloured with beta carotene.

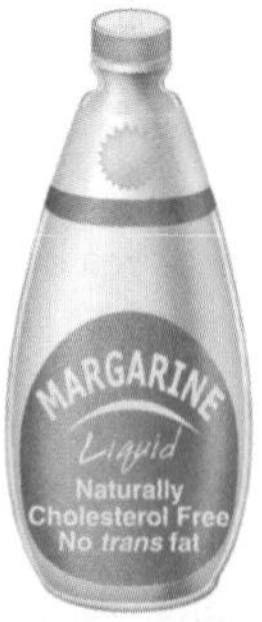
MARGARINE
Liquid
Naturally Cholesterol Free
No trans fat

Margarine (liquid)

Nutrition Facts
Serving size 1 Tbsp (14 g)
Servings per container about 24

Amount per serving	
Calories 70	
	%Daily Value*
Total Fat 8 g	13%
Saturated Fat 1.5 g / Trans Fat 0 g	7%
Polyunsaturated Fat 4.5 g	
Monounsaturated Fat 2 g	
Cholesterol 0 mg	0%
Sodium 110 mg	8%
Total Carbohydrate 0 g	0%
Protein 0 g	
Vitamin A 10%	

Not a significant source of dietary fibre, sugars, vitamin C, calcium, and iron.

*Percent Daily Values are based on a 2000 calorie diet.

INGREDIENTS: Liquid soybean oil, water, salt, hydrogenated cottonseed oil, vegetable monoglycerides and soy lecithin (emulsifiers), potassium sorbate and sodium benzoate (to preserve freshness), artificial flavour, phosphoric acid (acidulant), coloured with beta carotene (source of vitamin A), vitamin A palmitate.

Be aware that the "% Daily Value" for fat is not the same as "% kcalories from fat." This important distinction is explained in the accompanying "How To" feature. Because recommendations apply to average daily intakes rather than individual food items, food labels do not provide "% kcalories from fat." Still, you can get an idea of whether a particular food is high or low in fat.

IN SUMMARY **In foods, triglycerides:**

- **Deliver fat-soluble vitamins, energy, and essential fatty acids**
- **Contribute to the sensory appeal of foods and stimulate appetite**

HOW TO Understanding "% Daily Value"

The "% Daily Value" that is used on food labels to describe the amount of fat in a food is not the same as the "% kcalories from fat" that is used in dietary recommendations to describe the amount of fat in the diet. They may appear similar, but their difference is worth understanding. Consider, for example, a piece of lemon meringue pie that provides 140 kcalories and 12 grams of fat. Because the Daily Value for fat is 65 grams for a 2000-kcalorie intake, 12 grams represent about 18 percent:

$$12 \text{ g} \div 65 \text{ g} = 0.18$$
$$0.18 \times 100 = 18\%$$

The pie's "% Daily Value" is 18 percent, or almost one-fifth, of the day's fat allowance.

Uninformed consumers may mistakenly believe that this food meets recommendations to limit fat to "20 to 35 percent kcalories," but it doesn't—for the following reason. The pie's 12 grams of fat contribute 108 of the 140 kcalories, for a total of 77 percent kcalories from fat:

$$12 \text{ g fat} \times 9 \text{ kcal/g} = 108 \text{ kcal}$$
$$108 \text{ kcal} \div 140 \text{ kcal} = 77\%$$

Of course, if every selection throughout the day exceeds 35 percent kcalories from fat, you can be certain that the day's total intake will, too.

CENGAGENOW™
For additional practice log on to **www.cengage.com/sso.**

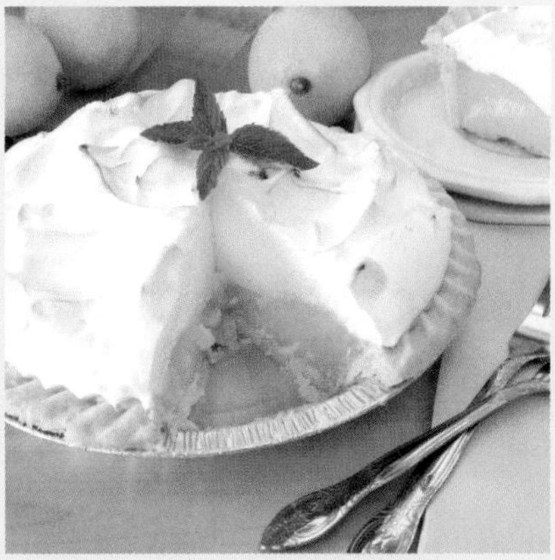

Darren K. Fisher/shutterstock

Whether a person's energy and fat allowance can afford a piece of lemon meringue pie depends on the other food and activity choices made that day.

TRY IT Calculate the percent Daily Value and the percent kcalories from fat for 125 millilitres (½ cup) of frozen yogurt that provides 115 kcalories and 4 grams of fat.

Although some fat in the diet is necessary, health authorities recommend a diet moderate in total fat and low in saturated fat, *trans* fat, and cholesterol. They also recommend replacing saturated fats with monounsaturated and polyunsaturated fats, particularly omega-3 fatty acids from foods such as fatty fish, not from supplements. Many selection and preparation strategies can help bring these goals within reach, and food labels help to identify foods consistent with these guidelines.

If people were to make only one change in their diets, they would be wise to limit their intakes of saturated fat. Sometimes these choices can be difficult, though, because fats make foods taste delicious. To maintain good health, must a person give up all high-fat foods forever—never again to eat marbled steak, hollandaise sauce, or gooey chocolate cake? Not at all. These foods bring pleasure to a meal and can be enjoyed as part of a healthy diet when eaten occasionally in small quantities; but they should not be everyday foods. The key dietary principle for fat is *moderation,* not *deprivation.* Appreciate the energy and enjoyment that fat provides, but take care not to exceed your needs.

Nutrition Portfolio

To maintain good health, eat enough, but not too much, fat and select the right kinds.

Go to Diet Analysis Plus and choose one of the days on which you have tracked your diet for the entire day. Go to the Intake Spreadsheet report. Scroll down until you see: fat (g), sat fat (g), mono fat (g), poly fat (g), and chol (g), which stand for grams of total fat, saturated fat, monounsaturated fat, polyunsaturated fat, and cholesterol, respectively. Use these columns to answer the following questions:

- List the types and amounts of fats and oils you ate on that day, making note of which are saturated, monounsaturated, or polyunsaturated and how your choices could include fewer saturated options.

- List the types and amounts of milk products, meats, fish, and poultry you eat daily, noting how your choices could include more low-fat options.
- Describe choices you can make in selecting and preparing foods to lower your intake of solid fats.

Diet Analysis PLUS **To complete this exercise, go to your Diet Analysis Plus at www.cengage.com/sso.**

Nutrition on the Net

CENGAGENOW™
For further study of topics covered in this chapter, log on to **www.cengage.com/sso.**

- Search for "fat" at the International Food Information Council website: **www.foodinsight.org**
- Find dietary strategies to prevent heart disease at the National Heart, Lung, and Blood Institute: **www.nhlbi.nih.gov**
- Visit the nutrition section, especially Face the Fats, of the American Heart Association: **www.heart.org**
- For more information about omega-3 fatty acids visit the DHA/EPA Omega-3 Institute's website: **www.dhaomega3.org**
- See Health Canada for more information about *trans*-fatty acids in Canada: **www.hc-sc.gc.ca/fn-an/nutrition/gras-trans-fats/index-eng.php**

References

1. Canadian Council of Food and Nutrition, Trans fats beyond June 2006—a CCFN watching brief (February 2008). www.canadiannutrition.ca/pdfs/Watching%20Brief%20on%20TRANS%20Fat%20-%20Feb25.pdf, accessed September 3, 2011. J. M. Chardigny and coauthors, Do *trans* fatty acids from industrially produced sources and from natural sources have the same effect on cardiovascular disease risk factors in healthy subjects? Results of the *trans* Fatty Acids Collaboration (TRANSFACT) study, *American Journal of Clinical Nutrition* 87 (2008): 558–566; M. A. Zulet and coauthors, Inflammation and conjugated linoleic acid: Mechanisms of action and implications for human health, *Journal of Physiology and Biochemistry* 61 (2005): 483–494.
2. M. B. Katan and coauthors, Efficacy and safety of plant sterols in the management of blood cholesterol levels, *Mayo Clinic Proceedings* 78:8 (2003): 965–978; S. Klingberg and coauthors, Inverse relation between dietary intake of naturally occurring plant sterols and serum cholesterol in northern Sweden, *American Journal of Clinical Nutrition* 87 (2008): 993–1001; Health Canada, Food and Nutrition, Plant sterols and blood cholesterol lowering (May 2010). www.hc-sc.gc.ca/fn-an/label-etiquet/claims-reclam/assess-evalu/phytosterols-eng.php, accessed September 3, 2011.
3. A. Breger, P. J. H. Jones, and S. S. Abumweis (Review) Plant sterols: Factors affecting their efficacy and safety as functional food ingredients, *Lipids in Health and Disease* 3:5 (2004): 1–19; J. Plat and R. P. Mensink, Plant stanol and sterol esters in the control of blood cholesterol levels: Mechanism and safety aspects, *American Journal of Cardiology* 96 (2005): 15D–22D.
4. Q. Sun and coauthors, Comparison between plasma and erythrocyte fatty acid content as biomarkers of fatty acid intake in U.S. women, *American Journal of Clinical Nutrition* 86 (2007): 74–81; W. S. Harris and coauthors, Comparison of the effects of fish and fish-oil capsules on the n-3 fatty acid content of blood cells and plasma phospholipids, *American Journal of Clinical Nutrition* 86 (2007): 1621–1625.
5. T. Hampton, New clues to HDL's benefits revealed, *Journal of the American Medical Association* 297 (2007): 1537.
6. T. Yamada and H. Katagiri, Avenues of communication between the brain and tissues/organs involved in energy homeostasis, *Endocrine Journal* 54 (2007): 497–505.
7. A. Garg, Adipose tissue dysfunction in obesity and lipodystrophy, *Clinical Cornerstone* 8 (2006): S7–S13.
8. G. Govindarajan, M. A. Alpert, and L. Tejwani, Endocrine and metabolic effects of fat: Cardiovascular implications, *American Journal of Medicine* 121 (2008): 366–370; G. Fantuzzi and T. Mazzone, Adipose tissue and atherosclerosis: Exploring the connection, *Arteriosclerosis, Thrombosis, and Vascular Biology* 27 (2007): 996–1003; P. Trayhurn, C. Bing, and I. S. Wood, Adipose tissue and adipokines: Energy regulation from the human perspective, *Journal of Nutrition* 136 (2006): 1935S–1939S; C. Bulcão and coauthors, The new adipose tissue and adipocytokines, *Current Diabetes Reviews* 2 (2006): 19–28; T. J. Guzik, D. Mangalat, and R. Korbut, Adipocytokines: Novel link between inflammation and vascular function? *Journal of Physiology and Pharmacology* 57 (2006): 505–528.
9. R. N. Redinger, The physiology of adiposity, *Journal of the Kentucky Medical Association* 106 (2008): 53–62; P. G. McTernan, C. M. Kusminski, and S. Kumar, Resistin, *Current Opinion in Lipidology* 17 (2006): 170–175.
10. Y. Okamoto and coauthors, Adiponectin: A key adipocytokine in metabolic syndrome, *Clinical Science* 110 (2006): 267–278.
11. M. A. Beydoun and coauthors, Plasma n-3 fatty acids and the risk of cognitive decline in older adults: The Atherosclerosis Risk in Communities Study, *American Journal of Clinical Nutrition* 85 (2007): 1103–1111; C. Dullemeijer and coauthors, n-3 Fatty acid proportions in plasma and cognitive performance in older adults, *American Journal of Clinical Nutrition* 86 (2007): 1479–1485; S. M. Innis, Dietary (n-3) fatty acids and brain development, *Journal of Nutrition* 137 (2007): 855–859; B. M. van Gelder and coauthors, Fish consumption, n-3 fatty acids, and subsequent 5-y cognitive decline in elderly men: The Zutphen Elderly Study, *American Journal of Clinical Nutrition* 85 (2007): 1142–1147; E. Nurk and coauthors, Cognitive performance among the elderly and dietary fish intake: The Hordaland Health Study, *American Journal of Clinical Nutrition* 86 (2007): 1470–1478; R. Uauy and A. D. Dangour, Nutrition in brain development and aging: Role of essential fatty acids, *Nutrition Reviews* 64 (2006): S24–S33; W. C. Heird and A. Lapillonne, The role of essential fatty acids in development, *Annual Review of Nutrition* 25 (2005): 549–571.
12. B. J. Holub, Clinical Nutrition, 4. Omega-3 fatty acids in cardiovascular care, *Canadian Medical Association* 166:5 (2002): 608–615; A. H. Stark, M. A. Crawford, and R. Reifen, Update on alpha-linolenic acid, *Nutrition Reviews* 66 (2008): 326–332; J. L. Breslow, n-3 Fatty acids and cardiovascular disease, *American Journal of Clinical Nutrition* 83 (2006): 1477S–1482S.
13. P. Arner and D. Langin, The role of neutral lipases in human adipose tissue lipolysis, *Current Opinion in Lipidology* 18 (2007): 246–250; R. E. Duncan and coauthors, Regulation of lipolysis in adipocytes,

Annual Review of Nutrition 27 (2007): 79–101; M. Rydén and coauthors, Comparative studies of the role of hormone-sensitive lipase and adipose triglyceride lipase in human fat cell lipolysis, *American Journal of Physiology—Endocrinology and Metabolism* 292 (2007): E1847–E1855.
14. P. J. Nestel and coauthors, Relation of diet to cardiovascular disease risk factors in subjects with cardiovascular disease in Australia and New Zealand: Analysis of the Long-Term Intervention with Pravastatin in Ischaemic Disease trial, *American Journal of Clinical Nutrition* 81 (2005): 1322–1329.
15. Statistics Canada, Fact sheet: Heart health and cholesterol levels of Canadians, 2007 to 2009. Results from the Canadian Health Measures Survey 2007 to 2009 (2010). www.statcan.gc.ca/pub/82-625-x/2010001/article/11136-eng.htm, accessed September 2, 2011.
16. S.E.E. Berry, G. J. Miller, and T.A.B. Sanders, The solid fat content of stearic acid–rich fats determines their postprandial effects, *American Journal of Clinical Nutrition* 85 (2007): 1486–1494.
17. J. Delgado-Lista and coauthors, Chronic dietary fat intake modifies the postprandial response of hemostatic markers to a single fatty test meal, *American Journal of Clinical Nutrition* 87 (2008): 317–322.
18. Position of the American Dietetic Association and Dietitians of Canada: Dietary fatty acids, *Journal of the American Dietetic Association* 107 (2007): 1599–1611.
19. D. Mozaffarian and coauthors, *Trans* fatty acids and cardiovascular disease, *New England Journal of Medicine* 354 (2006): 1601–1613.
20. J. E. Hunter, Dietary trans fatty acids: Review of recent human studies and food industry responses, *Lipids* 41 (2006): 967–992.
21. Health Canada, Food and Nutrition, Trans fat. www.hc-sc.gc.ca/fn-an/nutrition/gras-trans-fats/index-eng.php, accessed September 3, 2011; W. M. N. Ratneyake, M. R. Labbe, and D. Mozaffarian, Nationwide product reformulations to reduce trans fatty acids in Canada: When trans fat goes out, what goes in? *European Journal of Clinical Nutrition* 63 (2009): 808–811; W. M. N. Ratneyake and coauthors, Trans fatty acids: Current contents in Canadian foods and estimated intake levels for the Canadian population, *Journal of AOAC International* 92 (2009): 1258–1276; M. J. Albers and coauthors, 2006 Marketplace survey of *trans*–fatty acid content of margarines and butters, cookies and snack cakes, and savory snacks, *Journal of the American Dietetic Association* 108 (2008): 367–370; S. Borra and coauthors, An update of *trans*-fat reduction in the American diet, *Journal of the American Dietetic Association* 107 (2007): 2048–2050; S. Okie, New York to trans fats: You're out! *New England Journal of Medicine* 356 (2007): 2017–2021.
22. J. Genest and coauthors, 2009 Canadian Cardiovascular Society/Canadian guidelines for the diagnosis and treatment of dyslipidemia and prevention of cardiovascular disease in the adult—2009 recommendations, *Canadian Journal of Cardiology* 25:10 (2009) 567–579; Expert Panel on Detection, Evaluation, and Treatment of High Blood Cholesterol in Adults (Adult Treatment Panel III), *Third Report of the National Cholesterol Education Program* (NCEP), NIH publication no. 02–5215 (Bethesda, Md.: National Heart, Lung, and Blood Institute, 2002), p. v–10.
23. L. Berglund and coauthors, Comparison of monounsaturated fat with carbohydrates as a replacement for saturated fat in subjects with a high metabolic risk profile: Studies in the fasting and postprandial states, *American Journal of Clinical Nutrition* 86 (2007): 1611–1620; M. P. St-Onge and coauthors, Snack chips fried in corn oil alleviate cardiovascular disease risk factors when substituted for low-fat or high-fat snacks, *American Journal of Clinical Nutrition* 85 (2007): 1503–1510.
24. J. Ruano and coauthors, Intake of phenol-rich virgin olive oil improves the postprandial prothrombotic profile in hypercholesterolemic patients, *American Journal of Clinical Nutrition* 86 (2007): 341–346.
25. J. L. Breslow, n-3 Fatty acids and cardiovascular disease, *American Journal of Clinical Nutrition* 83 (2006): 1477S–1482S.
26. Breslow, 2006; P. J. H. Jones and V. W. Y. Lau, Effect of n-3 polyunsaturated fatty acids on risk reduction of sudden death, *Nutrition Reviews* 60 (2002): 407–413.
27. K. Fritsche, Fatty acids as modulators of the immune response, *Annual Review of Nutrition* 26 (2006): 45–73; S. M. Innis and K. Jacobson, Dietary lipids in early development and intestinal inflammatory disease, *Nutrition Reviews* 65 (2007): S188–S193; S. R. Shaikh and M. Edidin, Polyunsaturated fatty acids, membrane organization, T cells, and antigen presentation, *American Journal of Clinical Nutrition* 84 (2006): 1277–1289.
28. A. Philibert and coauthors, Fish intake and serum fatty acid profiles from freshwater fish, *American Journal of Clinical Nutrition* 84 (2006): 1299–1307.
29. Health Canada, Food and Nutrition, *Eating Well with Canada's Food Guide* (2007). www.hc-sc.gc.ca/fn-an/food-guide-aliment/index-eng.php, accessed September 3, 2011.
30. K. He and coauthors, Intakes of long-chain n-3 polyunsaturated fatty acids and fish in relation to measurement of subclinical atherosclerosis, *American Journal of Clinical Nutrition* 88 (2008): 1111–1118.
31. Health Canada, Healthy Living, Mercury and Human Health (2009). www.hc-sc.gc.ca/hl-vs/iyh-vsv/environ/merc-eng.php, accessed September 3, 2011. M. C. Nesheim and A. L. Yaktine, eds., Seafood, *Seafood Choices: Balancing Benefits and Risks* (Washington, D.C.: National Academies Press, 2007), p. 12; C. W. Levenson and D. M. Axelrad, Too much of a good thing? Update on fish consumption and mercury exposure, *Nutrition Reviews* 64 (2006): 139–145.
32. J. Whelan and C. Rust, Innovative dietary sources of n-3 fatty acids, *Annual Review of Nutrition* 26 (2006): 75–103.
33. P. M. Kris-Etherton and A. M. Hill, n-3 Fatty acids: Foods or supplements? *American Dietetic Association* 108 (2008): 1125–1130.
34. M. H. Raitt and coauthors, Fish oil supplementation and risk of ventricular tachycardia and ventricular fibrillation in patients with implantable defibrillators: A randomized control study, *Journal of the American Medical Association* 293 (2005): 2884–2891.
35. Fish and omega-3 fatty acids, www.americanheart.org, accessed 2009.
36. Committee on Dietary Reference Intakes, *Dietary Reference Intakes for Energy, Carbohydrate, Fiber, Fat, Fatty Acids, Cholesterol, Protein, and Amino Acids* (Washington, D.C.: National Academies Press, 2005).
37. J. C. Stanley and coauthors, UK Food Standards Agency Workshop report: The effects of the dietary n-6:n-3 fatty acid ratio on cardiovascular health, *British Journal of Nutrition* 98 (2007): 1305–1310; W. S. Harris, The omega-6/omega-3 ratio and cardiovascular disease risk: Uses and abuses, *Current Atherosclerosis Reports* 8 (2006): 453–459.
38. B. A. Griffin, How relevant is the ratio of dietary n-6 to n-3 polyunsaturated fatty acids to cardiovascular disease risk? Evidence from the OPTILIP study, *Current Opinion in Lipidology* 19 (2008): 57–62.
39. W. S. Harris and coauthors, Omega-6 fatty acids and risk for cardiovascular disease: A Science Advisory from the American Heart Association Nutrition Subcommittee of the Council on Nutrition, Physical Activity, and Metabolism; Council on Cardiovascular Nursing, and Council on Epidemiology and Prevention, *Circulation* 108 (2009): 902–907; W. C. Willett, The role of dietary n-6 fatty acids in the prevention of cardiovascular disease, *The Journal of Cardiovascular Medicine* 8 (2007): S42–S45.
40. A.C.M. Thiébaut and coauthors, Dietary fat and postmenopausal invasive breast cancer in the National Institutes of Health: AARP Diet and Health Study Cohort, *Journal of the National Cancer Institute* 99 (2007): 451–462; World Cancer Research Fund and American Institute for Cancer Research, *Food, Nutrition, Physical Activity, and the Prevention of Cancer: A Global Perspective,* www.dietandcancerreport.org, accessed, 2007.
41. E. Theodoratou and coauthors, Dietary fatty acids and colorectal cancer: A case-control study, *American Journal of Epidemiology* 166 (2007): 181–195; P. Bougnoux, B. Giraudeau, and C. Couet, Diet, cancer, and the lipidome, *Cancer Epidemiology Biomarkers and Prevention* 15 (2006): 416–421.
42. P. W. Parodi, Dairy product consumption and the risk of breast cancer, *Journal of the American College of Nutrition* 24 (2005): 556S–568S; J. Zhang and H. Kesteloot, Milk consumption in relation to incidence of prostate, breast, colon, and rectal cancers: Is there an independent effect? *Nutrition and Cancer* 53 (2005): 65–72.
43. R. S. Chapkin, D. N. McMurray, and J. R. Lupton, Colon cancer, fatty acids and anti-inflammatory compounds, *Current Opinion in Gastroenterology* 23 (2007): 48–54; A. Geelen and coauthors, Fish consumption, n-3 fatty acids, and colorectal cancer: A meta-analysis of prospective cohort studies, *American Journal of Epidemiology* 166 (2007): 1116–1125; J. Shannon and coauthors, Erythrocyte fatty acids and breast cancer risk: A case-control study in Shanghai, China, *American Journal of Clinical Nutrition* 85 (2007): 1090–1097; C. H. MacLean and coauthors, Effects of omega-3 fatty acids on cancer risk: A systematic review, *Journal of the American Medical Association* 295 (2006): 403–415.

44. Committee on Dietary Reference Intakes, 2005.
45. Committee on Dietary Reference Intakes, 2005.
46. Committee on Dietary Reference Intakes, 2005.
47. Health Canada, Food and Nutrition, Canadian Community Health Survey. www.hc-sc.gc.ca/fn-an/surveill/nutrition/commun/index-eng.php, accessed September 3, 2011.
48. Dietitians of Canada, American College of Sports Medicine, and the American Dietetic Association, Joint Position Paper, Nutrition and athletic performance (2008). www.dietitians.ca/Downloadable-Content/Public/noap-position-paper.aspx, accessed September 3, 2011.
49. C. W. Xiao, J. Mei, and C. M. Wood, Effect of soy proteins and isoflavones on lipid metabolism and involved gene expression, *Frontiers in Bioscience* 13 (2008): 2660–2673; K. Reynolds and coauthors, A meta-analysis of the effect of soy protein supplementation on serum lipids, *American Journal of Cardiology* 98 (2006): 633–640.
50. E. Fabian and I. Elmadfa, Influence of daily consumption of probiotic and conventional yoghurt on the plasma lipid profile in young healthy women, *Annals of Nutrition and Metabolism* 50 (2006): 387–393.
51. A. Dilmi-Bouras, Assimilation *(in vitro)* of cholesterol by yogurt bacteria, *Annals of Agricultural and Environmental Medicine* 13 (2006): 49–53.
52. M. B. Katan and coauthors, Efficacy and safety of plant sterols in the management of blood cholesterol levels, *Mayo Clinic Proceedings* 78: 8 (2003): 965–978; C. S. Patch, L. C. Tapsell, and P. G. Williams, Plant sterol/stanol prescription is an effective treatment strategy for managing hypercholesterolemia in outpatient clinical practice, *Journal of the American Dietetic Association* 105 (2005): 46–52.
53. Position of the American Dietetic Association: Fat replacers, *Journal of the American Dietetic Association* 105 (2005): 266–275.

High-Fat Foods—Friend or Foe?

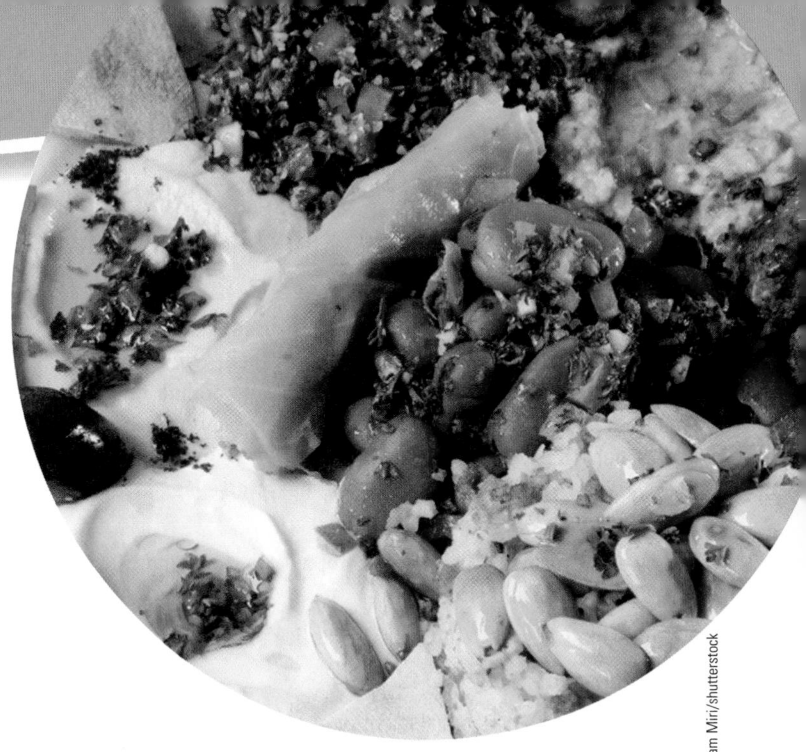

karam Miri/shutterstock

Eat less fat. Eat more fatty fish. Give up butter. Use margarine. Give up margarine. Use olive oil. Steer clear of saturated. Seek out omega-3. Stay away from *trans*. Stick with mono- and polyunsaturated. Keep fat intake moderate. Today's fat messages seem to be forever multiplying and changing. No wonder some people feel confused about dietary fat. The confusion stems in part from the complexities of fat and in part from the nature of recommendations. As Chapter 5 explained, *dietary fat* refers to several kinds of fats. Some fats support health whereas others impair it, and foods typically provide a mixture of fats in varying proportions. Researchers have spent decades sorting through the relationships among the various kinds of fat and their roles in supporting or harming health. Translating these research findings into dietary recommendations is challenging. Too little information can mislead consumers, but too much detail can overwhelm them. As research findings accumulate, recommendations slowly evolve and become more refined. Fortunately, that's where we are with fat recommendations today—refining them from the general to the specific. Though they may seem to be "forever multiplying and changing," in fact, they are becoming more meaningful.

This highlight begins with a look at the dietary guidelines for fat intake. It continues by identifying which foods provide which fats and presenting the Mediterranean diet, an example of a food plan that embraces the heart-healthy fats. It closes with strategies to help consumers choose the right amounts of the right kinds of fats for a healthy diet.

Guidelines for Fat Intake

Dietary recommendations for fat have shifted emphasis from lowering total fat, in general, to limiting saturated and *trans* fat, specifically. Instead of urging people to cut back on all fats, recommendations suggest carefully replacing the "bad" saturated fats with the "good" unsaturated fats and enjoying them in moderation.[1] The goal is to create a diet moderate in kcalories that provides enough of the fats that support good health, but not too much of those that harm health. (Turn to pp. 147–150 for a review of the health consequences of each type of fat.)

With these findings and goals in mind, the DRI Committee suggests a healthy range of 20 to 35 percent of energy intake from fat. This range appears to be compatible with low rates of heart disease, diabetes, obesity, and cancer.[2] Heart-healthy recommendations suggest that within this range, consumers should try to minimize their intakes of saturated fat, *trans* fat, and cholesterol and use monounsaturated and polyunsaturated fats instead.[3]

Asking consumers to limit their total fat intake is less than perfect advice, but it is straightforward—find the fat and cut back. Asking consumers to keep their intakes of saturated fats, *trans* fats, and cholesterol low and to use monounsaturated and polyunsaturated fats instead is more on target with heart health, but it also makes diet planning a bit more complicated. To make appropriate selections, consumers must first learn which foods contain which fats.

High-Fat Foods and Heart Health

Avocados, bacon, walnuts, potato chips, and mackerel are all high-fat foods, yet some of these foods have detrimental effects on heart health when consumed in excess, whereas others seem neutral or even beneficial. This section presents some of the accumulating evidence that helped to distinguish which high-fat foods belong in a healthy diet and which ones need to be kept to a minimum. As you will see, fat in the diet can be compatible with heart health, but only if the great majority of it is the unsaturated kind.

Cook with Olive Oil

As it turns out, the traditional diets of Greece and other countries in the Mediterranean region offer an excellent example of eating patterns that use "good" fats liberally. The primary fat in these diets is olive oil, which seems to play a key role in providing health benefits.[4] A classic study of the world's people, the Seven Countries Study, found that death rates from heart disease were strongly associated with diets high in saturated fats but only weakly linked with total fat.[5] In fact, the two countries with the highest fat intakes, Finland and the Greek island of Crete, had the highest (Finland) and lowest (Crete) rates of heart disease deaths. In both countries, the people consumed 40 percent or more of their kcalories from fat. Clearly, a high-fat diet was not the primary problem, so researchers refocused their attention on the *type* of fat. They began to notice the benefits of olive oil.

A diet that uses olive oil instead of other cooking fats, especially butter, stick margarine, and meat fats may offer numerous health benefits. Olive oil and other oils rich in monounsaturated fatty acids help to protect against heart disease, in part, by replacing dietary saturated fat and by:

- Lowering total and LDL cholesterol and not lowering HDL cholesterol or raising triglyceride[6]
- Lowering LDL cholesterol susceptibility to oxidation[7]
- Lowering blood-clotting factors[8]
- Providing phytochemicals that act as antioxidants (see Highlight 12)[9]
- Lowering blood pressure[10]
- Interfering with the inflammatory response[11]

When compared with other fats, olive oil seems to be a wise choice, but controlled clinical trials are too scarce to support population-wide recommendations to switch to a high-fat diet rich in olive oil. Importantly, olive oil is not a magic potion; drizzling it on foods does not make them healthier. Like other fats, olive oil delivers 9 kcalories per gram, which can contribute to weight gain in people who fail to balance their energy intake with physical activity. Its role in a healthy diet is to *replace* the saturated fats. Other vegetable oils, such as canola or safflower oil, are also generally low in saturated fats and high in unsaturated fats. For this reason, heart-healthy diets use these unsaturated vegetable oils as substitutes for the more saturated fats of butter, hydrogenated stick margarine, lard, or shortening.

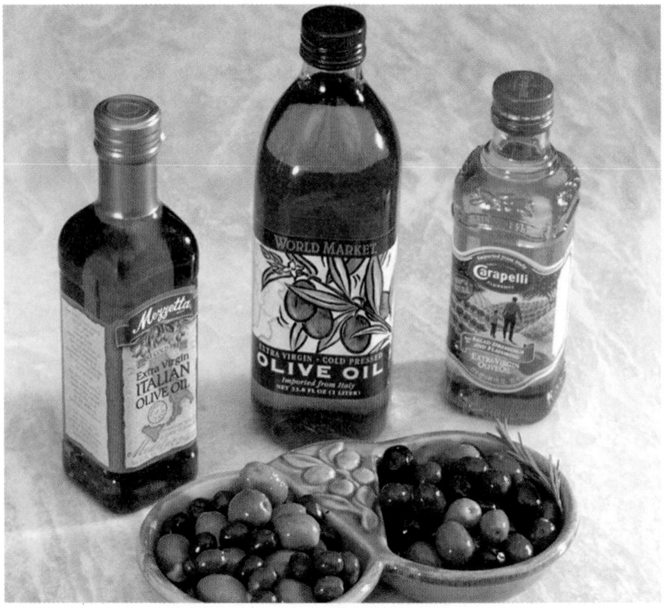
WORLD MARKET
OLIVE OIL
Carapelli
Extra Virgin ITALIAN OLIVE OIL

© Matthew Farruggio

Olives and their oil may benefit heart health.

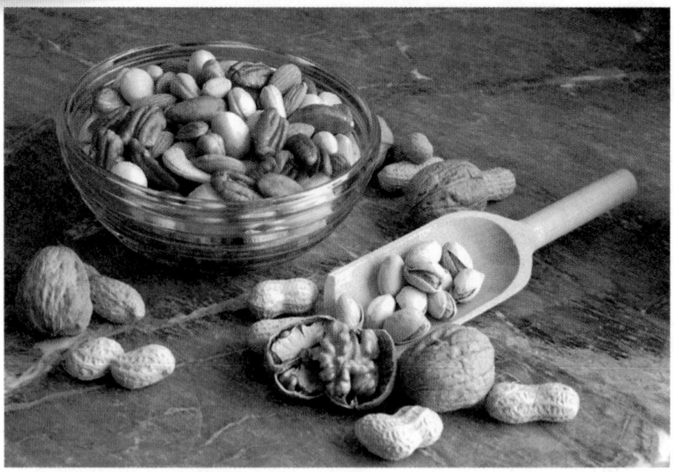

© Matthew Farruggio

For heart health, snack on a few nuts instead of potato chips. Because nuts are energy dense (high in kcalories per gram), it is especially important to keep portion size in mind when eating them.

(Remember that the tropical oils—coconut, palm, and palm kernel—are too saturated to be included with the heart-healthy vegetable oils.)

Nibble on Nuts

Tree nuts and peanuts are traditionally excluded from low-fat diets, and for good reasons. Nuts provide up to 80 percent of their kcalories from fat, and 60 millilitres (about ¼ cup or 30 grams) of mixed nuts provides more than 200 kcalories. In a recent review of the literature, however, researchers found that people who ate a 30 gram serving of nuts on five or more days a week had lower LDL cholesterol and a reduced risk of heart disease compared with people who consumed no nuts.[12] A smaller positive association was noted for any amount greater than one serving of nuts a week. The nuts in this study were those commonly eaten in North America: almonds, Brazil nuts, cashews, hazelnuts, macadamia nuts, pecans, pistachios, walnuts, and even peanuts. On average, these nuts contain mostly monounsaturated fat (59 percent), some polyunsaturated fat (27 percent), and little saturated fat (14 percent).

Including nuts may be a wise diet strategy against heart disease. Nuts may protect against heart disease because they provide:

- Monounsaturated and polyunsaturated fats in abundance, but few saturated fats
- Fibre, vegetable protein, and other valuable nutrients, including the antioxidant vitamin E (see Highlight 12)
- Phytochemicals that act as antioxidants (see Highlight 14)[13]
- Plant sterols

Before advising consumers to include nuts in their diets, however, a caution is in order. As mentioned, most of the energy nuts provide comes from fats. Consequently, they deliver many kcalories per bite. In studies examining the effects of nuts on heart disease, researchers carefully adjust diets to make room for the nuts without increasing the total kcalories—that is, they use nuts *instead of, not in addition to,* other foods (such as meats, potato chips, oils, margarine, and butter). Consumers who do not make similar replacements could end up gaining weight if they simply add nuts on top of their regular diets. Weight gain, in turn, elevates blood lipids and raises the risks of heart disease.

Feast on Fish

Research into the health benefits of the long-chain omega-3 polyunsaturated fatty acids (as mentioned earlier in Chapter 5) began with a simple observation: the native peoples of Alaska, northern Canada, and Greenland, who eat a traditional diet rich in omega-3 fatty acids, notably EPA and DHA, have a remarkably low rate of heart disease even though their diets are relatively high in fat.[14] These omega-3 fatty acids help to protect against heart disease by:[15]

- Reducing blood triglycerides
- Preventing blood clots
- Protecting against irregular heartbeats[16]
- Lowering blood pressure
- Defending against inflammation
- Serving as precursors to eicosanoids

For people with hypertension or atherosclerosis, these actions can be life saving.

Research studies have provided strong evidence that increasing omega-3 fatty acids in the diet supports heart health and lowers the rate of deaths from heart disease. For this reason, the Health Canada, the Canadian Cardiology Society, Dietitians of Canada, and numerous health authorities around the world recommend including fish in a heart-healthy diet. People who eat some fish each week can lower their risks of heart attack and stroke. Table H5-1 ranks commonly eaten fish by their omega-3 fatty acid content. Therefore, those who follow *Canada's Food Guide* recommendation to "Eat at least two *Food Guide* Servings of fish per week" from salmon, for example, might expect to obtain close to 1 gram of omega-3 fatty acids. This is in line with numerous health authorities in Canada and elsewhere.

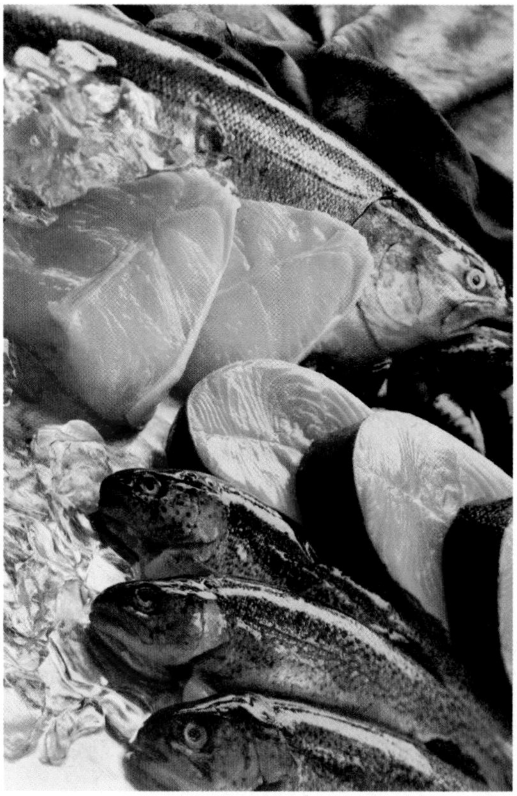

© ALEAIMAGE/iStockphoto

Fish is a good source of the omega-3 fatty acids.

TABLE H5-1 Omega-3 Fatty Acid Content of Commonly Eaten Fish

>500 mg per 100 gram Serving	150–500 mg per 100 gram Serving	<150 mg per 100 gram Serving
Bronzini	Black bass	Cod (Pacific)
Herring (Atlantic and Pacific)	Catfish (wild and farmed)	Corvina
Mackerel	Clam	Grouper
Oyster (Pacific)	Cod (Atlantic)	Lobster
Salmon (chinook, Coho, Copper River, farmed, pink, sockeye, wild Atlantic)	Crab (Alaskan king)	Mahi-mahi
Sardines	Croakers	Monkfish
Toothfish	Escolar	Red snapper
Trout (wild and farmed)	Flounder	Skate
	Haddock	Triggerfish
	Hake	Tuna
	Halibut	Wahoo
	Oyster (eastern and farmed)	
	Perch	
	Scallop	
	Shrimp (mixed varieties)	
	Sole	
	Swordfish	
	Tilapia (farmed)	

SOURCE: K. L. Weaver and coauthors, The content of favorable and unfavorable polyunsaturated fatty acids found in commonly eaten fish, *Journal of the American Dietetic Association* 108 (2008): 1178–1185; P. M. Kris-Etherton, W. S. Harris, and L. J. Appel, Fish consumption, fish oil, omega-3 fatty acids, and cardiovascular disease, *Circulation* 106 (2002): 2747–2757.

Fish is the best source of EPA and DHA in the diet, but it is also a major source of mercury, an environmental contaminant. Most fish contain at least trace amounts of mercury, but some have especially high levels. For this reason, Health Canada advises pregnant and lactating women, women of childbearing age who may become pregnant, and young children to include fish in their diets, but to avoid:

- Tilefish (also called golden snapper or golden bass), swordfish, king mackerel, marlin, and shark, etc.

And to limit average weekly consumption of:

- A variety of ocean fish and shellfish to 350 grams (cooked or canned)

- White (albacore) tuna to 175 grams (cooked or canned)

Commonly eaten seafood relatively low in mercury include shrimp, catfish, pollock, salmon, and canned light tuna.

In addition to the direct toxic effects of mercury, some (but not all) research suggests that mercury may diminish the health benefits of omega-3 fatty acids. Such findings serve as a reminder that our health depends on the health of our planet. The protective effect of fish in the diet is available, provided that the fish and their surrounding waters are not heavily contaminated. (Chapter 20 discusses the adverse consequences of mercury, and Chapter 21 presents the relationships between diet and the environment in more detail.)

In an effort to limit exposure to pollutants, some consumers choose farm-raised fish. Compared with fish caught in the wild, farm-raised fish tend to be lower in mercury, but they are also lower in omega-3 fatty acids. When selecting fish, keep the diet strategies of variety and moderation in mind. Varying choices and eating moderate amounts help to limit the intake of contaminants such as mercury.

High-Fat Foods and Heart Disease

The number one dietary determinant of LDL cholesterol is saturated fat. Figure H5-1 shows that each 1 percent increase in energy from saturated fatty acids in the diet may produce a 2 percent jump in heart disease risk by elevating blood LDL cholesterol. Conversely, reducing saturated fat intake by 1 percent can be expected to produce a 2 percent drop in heart disease risk by the same mechanism. Even a 2 percent drop in LDL represents a significant improvement for the health of the heart.[17] Like saturated fats, *trans* fats also raise heart disease risk by elevating LDL cholesterol. A heart-healthy diet limits foods rich in these two types of fat.

Limit Fatty Meats, Whole-Milk Products, and Tropical Oils

The major sources of saturated fats in the North American diet are fatty meats, whole milk products, tropical oils, and products made from any of these foods. To limit saturated fat intake, consumers must choose carefully among these high-fat foods. More than a third of the fat in most meats is saturated. Similarly, more than half of the fat is saturated in whole milk and other high-fat dairy products, such as cheese, butter, cream, half-and-half, cream cheese, sour cream, and ice cream. The tropical oils of palm, palm kernel, and coconut, which are rarely used by consumers in the kitchen, are used heavily by food manufacturers, and are commonly found in many commercially prepared foods.

When choosing meats, milk products, and commercially prepared foods, look for those lowest in saturated fat. Labels provide a useful guide for comparing products in this regard, and APPENDIX H lists the saturated fat in several thousand foods.

Even with careful selections, a nutritionally adequate diet will provide some saturated fat. Zero saturated fat is not possible even when experts design menus with the mission to keep saturated fat as low as possible.[18] Because most saturated fats come from animal foods, vegetarian diets can, and usually do, deliver fewer saturated fats than mixed diets.

Limit Hydrogenated Foods

Chapter 5 explains that solid shortening and margarine are made from vegetable oil that has been hardened through hydrogenation. This process both saturates some of the unsaturated fatty acids and introduces *trans*-fatty acids. Many convenience foods may still contain *trans* fats, including:

- Fried foods such as french fries, chicken, and other commercially fried foods
- Commercial baked goods such as cookies, doughnuts, pastries, breads, and crackers
- Snack foods such as chips
- Imitation cheeses

FIGURE H5-1 Potential Relationships among Dietary Saturated Fatty Acids, LDL Cholesterol, and Heart Disease Risk

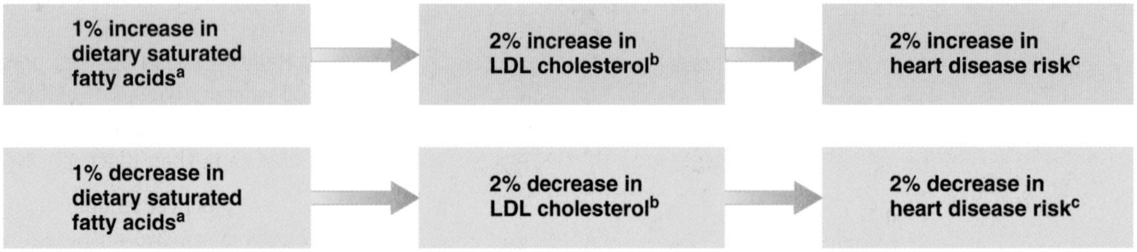
1% increase in dietary saturated fatty acids[a]
2% increase in LDL cholesterol[b]
2% increase in heart disease risk[c]
1% decrease in dietary saturated fatty acids[a]
2% decrease in LDL cholesterol[b]
2% decrease in heart disease risk[c]

[a]Percentage of change in total dietary energy from saturated fatty acids.
[b]Percentage of change in blood LDL cholesterol.
[c]Percentage of change in an individual's risk of heart disease; the percentage of change in risk may increase when blood lipid changes are sustained over time.
SOURCE: *Third Report of the National Cholesterol Education Program (NCEP) Expert Panel on Detection, Evaluation, and Treatment of High Blood Cholesterol in Adults (Adult Treatment Panel III)*, NIH publication no. 02-5215 (Bethesda, Md.: National Heart, Lung, and Blood Institute, 2002), pp. V-8 and II-4.

To keep *trans*-fat intake low, use these foods sparingly as an occasional taste treat.

Table H5-2 summarizes which foods provide which fats. Substituting unsaturated fats for saturated fats at each meal and snack can help protect against heart disease. Figure H5-2 (p. 166) compares two meals and shows how such substitutions can lower saturated fat and raise unsaturated fat—even when total fat and kcalories remain unchanged.

The Mediterranean Diet

The links between good health and traditional Mediterranean diets of the mid-1900s were introduced earlier with regard to olive oil. For people who eat these diets, the incidence of heart disease, some cancers, and other chronic inflammatory diseases is low, and life expectancy is high.[19]

Although each of the many countries that border the Mediterranean Sea has its own culture, traditions, and dietary habits, their similarities are much greater than the use of olive oil alone. In fact, no one factor alone can be credited with reducing disease risks—the association holds true only when the overall diet pattern is present. Apparently, each of the foods contributes small benefits that harmonize to produce either a substantial cumulative or a synergistic effect.

The Mediterranean diet features fresh, whole foods.[20] The people select crusty breads, whole grains, potatoes, and pastas; a variety of vegetables (including wild greens) and legumes; feta and mozzarella cheeses and yogurt; nuts; and fruits (especially grapes and figs). They eat some fish, other seafood, poultry, a few eggs, and little meat. Along with olives and olive oil, their principal sources of fat are nuts and fish; they rarely use butter or encounter hydrogenated fats. Consequently, traditional Mediterranean diets are:

- Low in saturated fat
- Very low in *trans* fat
- Rich in unsaturated fat
- Rich in complex carbohydrate and fibre
- Rich in nutrients and phytochemicals that support good health

As a result, lipid profiles improve, inflammation diminishes, and the risk of heart disease declines.[21]

People following the traditional Mediterranean diet can receive as much as 40 percent of a day's kcalories from fat, but their limited consumption of dairy products and meats provides less than 10 percent from saturated fats. In addition, because the animals in the Mediterranean region graze, the meat, dairy products, and eggs are richer in omega-3 fatty acids than those from animals fed grain. Other foods typical of the Mediterranean, such as wild

TABLE H5-2 Major Sources of Various Fatty Acids

Healthful Fatty Acids		
Monounsaturated	***Omega-6 polyunsaturated***	***Omega-3 polyunsaturated***
Avocado	Margarine (nonhydrogenated)	Fatty fish (herring, mackerel, salmon, tuna)
Oils (canola, olive, peanut, sesame)	Oils (corn, cottonseed, safflower, soybean)	Flaxseed
Nuts (almonds, cashews, filberts, hazelnuts, macadamia nuts, peanuts, pecans, pistachios)	Nuts (pine nuts, walnuts)	Nuts (walnuts)
Olives	Mayonnaise	
Peanut butter	Salad dressing	
Seeds (sesame)	Seeds (pumpkin, sunflower)	
Harmful Fatty Acids		
Saturated	***Trans***	
Bacon	Fried foods (hydrogenated shortening)	
Butter	Margarine (hydrogenated or partially hydrogenated)	
Chocolate	Nondairy creamers	
Coconut	Many fast foods	
Cream cheese	Shortening	
Cream, half-and-half	Commercial baked goods (including doughnuts, cakes, cookies)	
Lard	Many snackfoods (including microwave popcorn, chips, crackers)	
Meat		
Milk and milk products (whole)		
Oils (coconut, palm, palm kernel)		
Shortening		
Sour cream		

NOTE: Keep in mind that foods contain a mixture of fatty acids.

FIGURE H5-2 Two Meals Compared: Replacing Saturated Fat with Unsaturated Fat

Examples of ways to replace saturated fats with unsaturated fats include sautéing vegetables in olive oil instead of butter, garnishing salads with avocado and sunflower seeds instead of bacon and blue cheese, and eating salmon instead of steak. Each of these meals provides roughly the same number of kcalories and grams of fat, but the one on the left has almost four times as much saturated fat and only half as many omega-3 fatty acids.

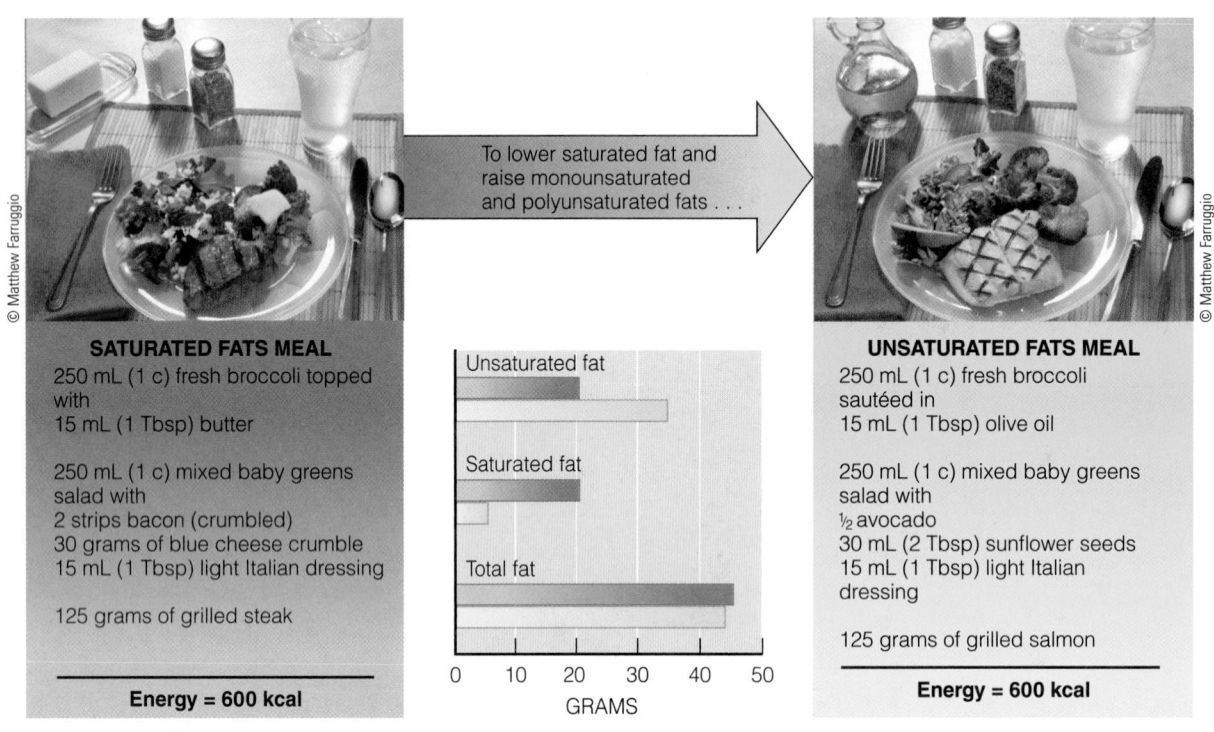

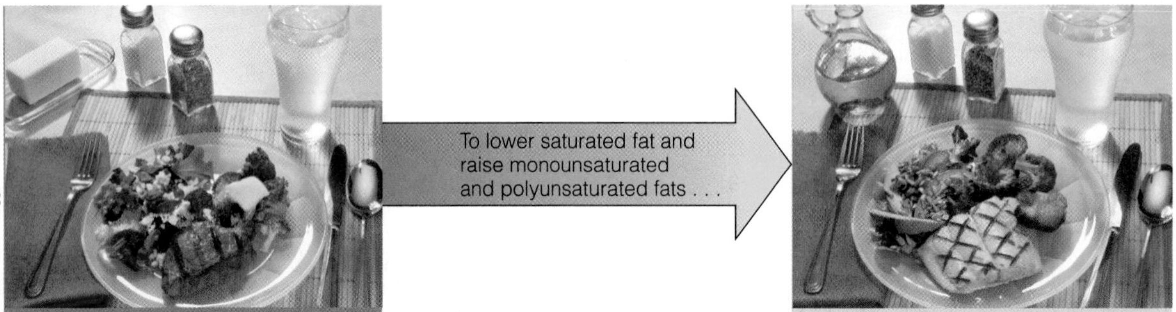
To lower saturated fat and
raise monounsaturated
and polyunsaturated fats . . .

© Matthew Farruggio

SATURATED FATS MEAL

250 mL (1 c) fresh broccoli topped with
15 mL (1 Tbsp) butter

250 mL (1 c) mixed baby greens salad with
2 strips bacon (crumbled)
30 grams of blue cheese crumble
15 mL (1 Tbsp) light Italian dressing

125 grams of grilled steak

Energy = 600 kcal

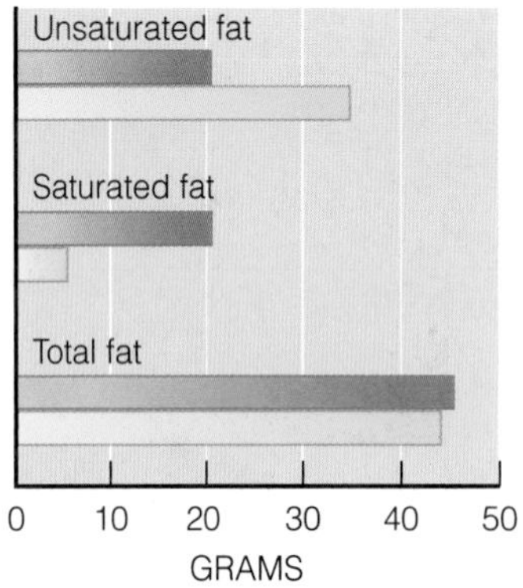
Unsaturated fat
Saturated fat
Total fat
0
10
20
30
40
50
GRAMS

UNSATURATED FATS MEAL

250 mL (1 c) fresh broccoli sautéed in
15 mL (1 Tbsp) olive oil

250 mL (1 c) mixed baby greens salad with
½ avocado
30 mL (2 Tbsp) sunflower seeds
15 mL (1 Tbsp) light Italian dressing

125 grams of grilled salmon

Energy = 600 kcal

© Matthew Farruggio

plants and snails, provide omega-3 fatty acids as well. All in all, the traditional Mediterranean diet has gained a reputation for its health benefits as well as its delicious flavours, but beware of the typical Mediterranean-style cuisine available in North American restaurants. It has been adjusted to popular tastes, meaning that it is often much higher in saturated fats and meats—and much lower in the potentially beneficial constituents—than the traditional fare. Unfortunately, it appears that people in the Mediterranean region who are replacing some of their traditional dietary habits with those of North America are losing the health benefits previously enjoyed.[22]

Conclusion

Are some fats "good," and others "bad" from the body's point of view? The saturated and *trans* fats indeed seem mostly bad for the health of the heart. Aside from providing energy, which unsaturated fats can do equally well, saturated and *trans* fats bring no indispensable benefits to the body. Furthermore, no harm can come from consuming diets low in them. Still, foods rich in these fats are often delicious, giving them a special place in the diet.

In contrast, the unsaturated fats are mostly good for the health of the heart when consumed in moderation. To date, their one proven fault seems to be that they, like all fats, provide abundant energy to the body and so may promote obesity if they drive kcalorie intakes higher than energy needs.[23] Obesity, in turn, often begets many body ills, as Chapter 8 makes clear.

When judging foods by their fatty acids, keep in mind that the fat in foods is a mixture of "good" and "bad," providing both saturated and unsaturated fatty acids. Even predominantly monounsaturated olive oil delivers some saturated fat. Consequently, even when a person chooses foods with mostly unsaturated fats, saturated fat can still add up if total fat is high. For this reason, fat must be kept below 35 percent of total kcalories if the diet is to be moderate in saturated fat. Even experts run into difficulty when attempting to create nutritious diets from a variety of foods that are low in saturated fats when kcalories from fat exceed 35 percent of the total.[24]

Does this mean that you must forever go without favourite cheeses, ice cream cones, or grilled steak? The famous chef Julia Child made this point about moderation:

> An imaginary shelf labelled INDULGENCES is a good idea. It contains the best butter, jumbo-size eggs, heavy cream, marbled steaks, sausages and pâtés, hollandaise and butter sauces, French butter-cream fillings, gooey chocolate cakes, and all those lovely items that demand disciplined rationing. Thus, with these items high up and almost out of reach, we are ever conscious that they are not everyday foods. They are for special occasions, and when that occasion comes we can enjoy every mouthful.
>
> —Julia Child, *The Way to Cook,* 1989

Additionally, food manufacturers have come to the assistance of consumers who wish to avoid the health threats of saturated and *trans* fats. Some companies now make margarine without *trans* fats, and many snack manufacturers have reduced the saturated and *trans* fats (and now in some cases there may even be zero *trans* fats) in their products and offer snack foods in 100-kcalorie packages. Other companies are following as consumers respond favourably.

Adopting some of the Mediterranean eating habits may serve those who enjoy a little more fat in the diet. Including vegetables, fruits, and legumes as part of a balanced daily diet is a good idea, as is *replacing* saturated fats such as butter, shortening, and meat fat with unsaturated fats such as olive oil and the oils from nuts and fish. These foods provide vitamins, minerals, and phytochemicals—all valuable in protecting the body's health. The authors of this book do not stop there, however. They urge you to reduce fats from convenience foods and fast foods; choose small portions of meats, fish, and poultry; and include fresh whole foods from all the food groups each day. Take care to select portion sizes that will best meet your energy needs. Also, exercise daily.

Nutrition on the Net

CENGAGENOW™

For further study of topics covered in this Highlight, log on to **www.cengage.com/sso**.

- Check out a Mediterranean food guide pyramid: **www.oldwayspt.org**

References

1. *Third Report of the National Cholesterol Education Program (NCEP) Expert Panel on Detection, Evaluation, and Treatment of High Blood Cholesterol in Adults (Adult Treatment Panel III),* publication NIH no. 02-5215 (Bethesda, Md.: National Heart, Lung, and Blood Institute, 2002); Committee on Dietary Reference Intakes, *Dietary Reference Intakes for Energy, Carbohydrate, Fiber, Fat, Fatty Acids, Cholesterol, Protein, and Amino Acids* (Washington, D.C.: National Academies Press, 2005).
2. Committee on Dietary Reference Intakes, 2005, p. 769.
3. American Heart Association Scientific statement: Diet and lifestyle recommendations revision 2006, *Circulation* 114 (2006): 82–96; *Third Report of the National Cholesterol Education Program (NCEP) Expert Panel on Detection, Evaluation, and Treatment of High Blood Cholesterol in Adults (Adult Treatment Panel III),* 2002; Committee on Dietary Reference Intakes, *Dietary Reference Intakes for Energy, Carbohydrate, Fiber, Fat, Fatty Acids, Cholesterol, Protein, and Amino Acids* (Washington, D.C.: National Academies Press, 2002, 2005).
4. M. A. Carluccio and coauthors, Vasculoprotective potential of olive oil components, *Molecular Nutrition and Food Research* 51 (2007): 1225–1234.
5. A. Keys, *Seven Countries: A Multivariate Analysis of Death and Coronary Heart Disease* (Cambridge: Harvard University Press, 1980).
6. M. I. Covas and coauthors, The effect of polyphenols in olive oil on the heart disease risk factors, *Annals of Internal Medicine* 145 (2006): 333–341.
7. M. Fitó, R. de la Torre, and M. I. Covas, Olive oil and oxidative stress, *Molecular Nutrition and Food Research* 51 (2007): 1215–1224; F. Visioli and coauthors, Virgin olive oil study (VOLOS): Vasoprotective potential of extra virgin olive oil in mildly dyslipidemic patients, *European Journal of Nutrition* 44 (2005): 121–127.
8. J. López-Miranda, Monounsaturated fat and cardiovascular risk, *Nutrition Reviews* 64 (2006): S2-S12.
9. J. Ruano and coauthors, Intake of phenol-rich virgin olive oil improves the postprandial prothrombotic profile in hypercholesterolemic patients, *American Journal of Clinical Nutrition* 86 (2007): 341–346; M. Covas and coauthors, The effect of polyphenols in olive oil on heart disease risk factors, *Annals of Internal Medicine* 145 (2006): 333–341.
10. B. M. Rasmussen and coauthors, Effects of dietary saturated, monounsaturated, and n-3 fatty acids on blood pressure in healthy subjects, *American Journal of Clinical Nutrition* 83 (2006): 221–226.
11. F. Pérez-Jiménez and coauthors, The influence of olive oil on human health: Not a question of fat alone, *Molecular Nutrition and Food Research* 51 (2007): 1199–1208.
12. A. E. Griel and P. M. Kris-Etherton, Tree nuts and the lipid profile: A review of clinical studies, *British Journal of Nutrition* 96 (2006): S68–S78; J. H. Kelly and J. Sabate, Nuts and coronary heart disease: An epidemiological perspective, *British Journal of Nutrition* 96 (2006): S61–S67.
13. P. E. Milbury and coauthors, Determination of flavonoids and phenolics and their distribution in almonds, *Journal of Agricultural and Food Chemistry* 54 (2006): 5027–5033.
14. A. Bersamin and coauthors, Westernizing diets influence fat intake, red blood cell fatty acid composition, and health in remote Alaskan native communities in the Center for Alaska Native Health Study, *Journal of the American Dietetic Association* 108 (2008): 266–273.
15. J. L. Breslow, n-3 Fatty acids and cardiovascular disease, *American Journal of Clinical Nutrition* 83 (2006): 1477S–1482S.
16. C. Chrysohoou and coauthors, Long-term fish consumption is associated with protection against arrhythmia in healthy persons in a Mediterranean region—The ATTICA study, *American Journal of Clinical Nutrition* 85 (2007): 1385–1391.
17. *Third Report of the National Cholesterol Education Program (NCEP) Expert Panel on Detection, Evaluation, and Treatment of High Blood Cholesterol in Adults (Adult Treatment Panel III),* 2002, pp. v-8.
18. Committee on Dietary Reference Intakes, 2005, p. 835.
19. M. De Lorgeril, Essential polyunsaturated fatty acids, inflammation, atherosclerosis and cardiovascular diseases, *Subcellular Biochemistry* 42 (2007): 283–297; D. Lairon, Intervention studies on Mediterranean diet and cardiovascular risk, *Molecular Nutrition and Food Research* 51

(2007): 1209–1214; L. Serra-Majem, B. Roman, and R. Estruch, Scientific evidence of interventions using the Mediterranean diet: A systematic review, *Nutrition Reviews* 64 (2006): S27–S47; C. Pitsavos and coauthors, Adherence to the Mediterranean diet is associated with total antioxidant capacity in healthy adults: The ATTICA study, *American Journal of Clinical Nutrition* 82 (2005): 694–699; M. Meydani, A Mediterranean-style diet and metabolic syndrome, *Nutrition Reviews* 63 (2005): 312–314.

20. J. M. Ordovas, J. Kaput, and D. Corella, Nutrition in the genomics era: Cardiovascular disease risk and the Mediterranean diet, *Molecular Nutrition and Food Research* 51 (2007): 1293–1299.
21. M. Fitó and coauthors, Effect of a traditional Mediterranean diet on lipoprotein oxidation, *Archives of Internal Medicine* 167 (2007): 1195–1203; K. Esposito, M. Ciotola, and D. Giugliano, Mediterranean diet, endothelial function and vascular inflammatory markers, *Public Health Nutrition* 9 (2006): 1073–1076.
22. P. A. Gilbert and S. Khokhar, Changing dietary habits of ethnic groups in Europe and implications for health, *Nutrition Reviews* 66 (2008): 203–215; F. Sofi and coauthors, Dietary habits, lifestyle, and cardiovascular risk factors in a clinically healthy Italian population: The "Florence" diet is not Mediterranean, *European Journal of Clinical Nutrition* 59 (2005): 584–591.
23. Committee on Dietary Reference Intakes, 2005, pp. 796–797.
24. Committee on Dietary Reference Intakes, 2005, pp. 799–802.

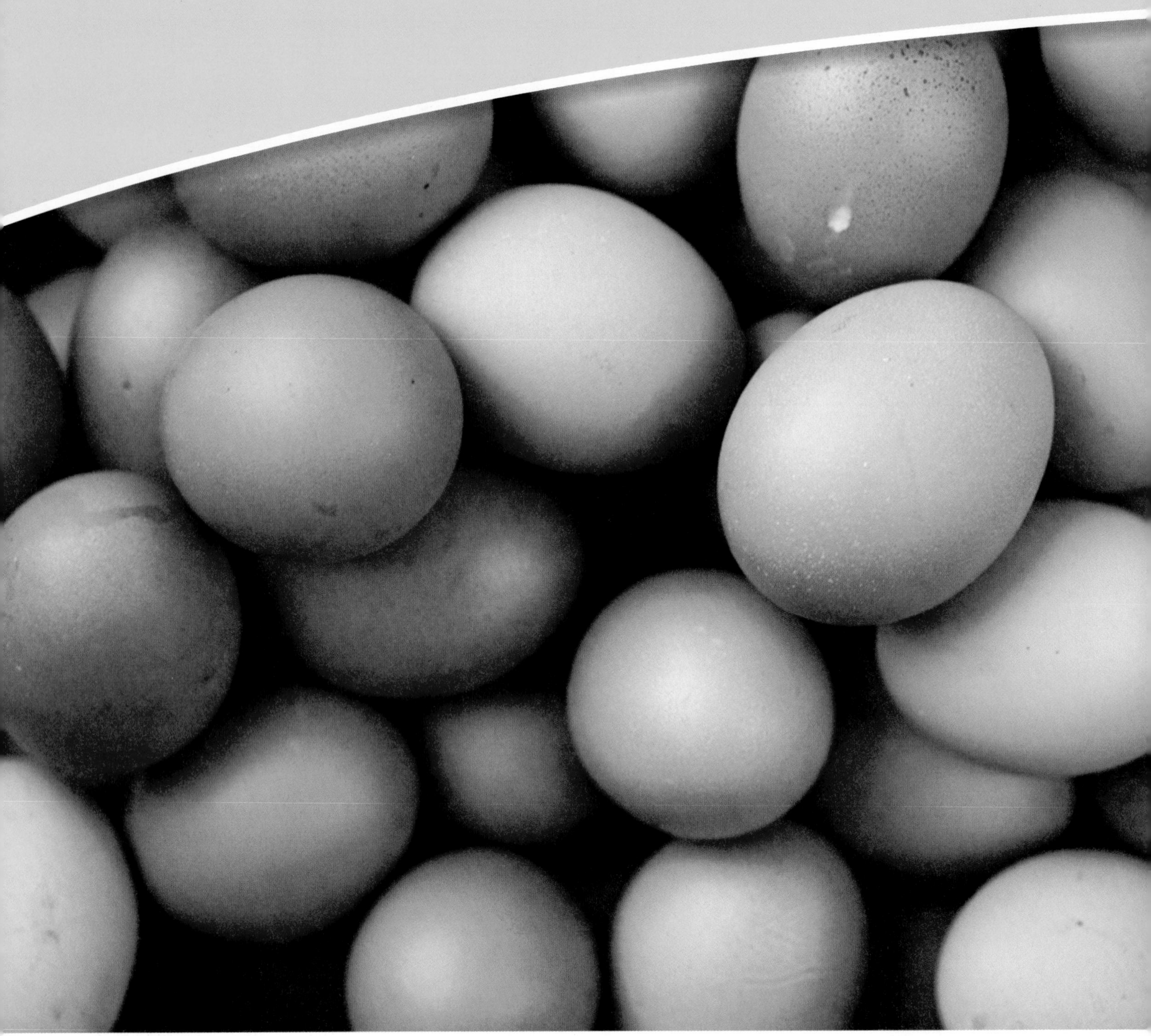

© howard Oates/iStockphoto

Nutrition in Your Life

CENGAGENOW™

Throughout this chapter, the CengageNOW logo indicates an opportunity for online self-study, linking you to interactive tutorials, activities, and videos to increase your understanding of chapter concepts.
www.cengage.com/sso

The versatility of proteins in the body is impressive. They help your muscles to contract, your blood to clot, and your eyes to see. They keep you alive and well by facilitating chemical reactions and defending against infections. Without them, your bones, skin, and hair would have no structure. No wonder they were named *proteins,* meaning "of prime importance." Does that mean proteins deserve top billing in your diet as well? Are the best sources of protein beef, beans, or broccoli? Learn which foods will supply you with enough, but not too much, high-quality protein.

CHAPTER

6

Protein: Amino Acids

CHAPTER OUTLINE

A few misconceptions surround the roles of protein in the body and the importance of protein in the diet. For example, people who associate meat with protein and protein with strength may eat steak to build muscles. Their thinking is only partly correct, however. Protein is a vital structural and working substance in all cells—not just muscle cells. To build strength, muscles cells need physical activity and all the nutrients—not just protein. Furthermore, protein is found in milk, eggs, legumes, and many grains and vegetables—not just meat. By overvaluing protein and overemphasizing meat in the diet, a person may mistakenly crowd out other, equally important nutrients and foods. As this chapter describes the various roles of protein in the body and food sources in the diet, keep in mind that protein is one of many nutrients needed to maintain good health.

The Chemist's View of Proteins

Chemically, **proteins** contain the same atoms as carbohydrates and lipids—carbon (C), hydrogen (H), and oxygen (O)—but proteins also contain nitrogen (N) atoms. These nitrogen atoms give the name *amino* (nitrogen containing) to the amino acids—the links in the chains of proteins.

Amino Acids

All **amino acids** have the same basic structure—a central carbon (C) atom with a hydrogen atom (H), an amino group (NH_2), and an acid group (COOH) attached to it. However, carbon atoms need to form four bonds, ♦ so a fourth attachment is necessary. This fourth site distinguishes each amino acid from the others. Attached to the central carbon at the fourth bond is a distinct atom, or group of atoms, known as the *side group* or *side chain* (see Figure 6-1 on p. 172).

Unique Side Groups The side groups on the central carbon vary from one amino acid to the next, making proteins more complex than either carbohydrates or lipids. A polysaccharide (starch, for example) may be several thousand units long, but each unit is a glucose molecule just like all the others. A protein, on the

♦ Reminder:
- H forms one bond.
- O forms two bonds.
- N forms three bonds.
- C forms four bonds.

proteins: compounds composed of carbon, hydrogen, oxygen, and nitrogen atoms, arranged into amino acids linked in a chain. Some amino acids also contain suphur atoms.

amino (a-MEEN-oh) **acids:** building blocks of proteins. Each contains an amino group, an acid group, a hydrogen atom, and a distinctive side group, all attached to a central carbon atom.

- **amino** = containing nitrogen

TABLE 6-1 Amino Acids

Proteins are made up of about 20 common amino acids. The second column lists the indispensable/essential amino acids for human beings (those the body cannot make—that must be provided in the diet). The third column lists the dispensable/nonessential amino acids. In special cases, some dispensable/nonessential amino acids may become conditionally essential (see first column). In a newborn, for example, only five amino acids are truly dispensable/nonessential; the other dispensable/nonessential amino acids are conditionally indispensable/essential until the metabolic pathways are developed enough to make those amino acids in adequate amounts.

Conditionally Indispensable/ Essential* Amino Acids		Indispensable/Essential Amino Acids		Dispensable/Nonessential Amino Acids	
Arginine	(ADJ-ih-neen)	Histidine	(HISS-tuh-deen)	Alanine	(AL-ah-neen)
Cysteine	(SIS-teh-een)	Isoleucine	(eye-so-LOO-seen)	Asparagine	(ah-SPAR-ah-geen)
Glutamine	(GLU-tah-meen)	Leucine	(LOO-seen)	Aspartic acid	(ah-SPAR-tic acid)
Glycine	(GLY-seen)	Lysine	(LYE-seen)	Glutamic acid	(GLU-tam-ic acid)
Proline	(PRO-leen)	Methionine	(meh-THIGH-oh-neen)	Serine	(SEER-een)
Tyrosine	(TIE-roe-seen)	Phenylalanine	(fen-il-AL-ah-neen)		
		Threonine	(THREE-oh-neen)		
		Tryptophan	(TRIP-toe-fan, TRIP-toe-fane)		
		Valine	(VAY-leen)		

* Required in the diet when unable to synthesize enough to meet the body's needs.

other hand, is made up of about 20 different amino acids, each with a different side group. Table 6-1 lists the amino acids most common in proteins.*

The simplest amino acid, glycine, has a hydrogen atom as its side group. A slightly more complex amino acid, alanine, has an extra carbon with three hydrogen atoms. Other amino acids have more complex side groups (see Figure 6-2 for examples). Thus, although all amino acids share a common structure, they differ in size, shape, electrical charge, and other characteristics because of differences in these side groups.

Dispensable/Nonessential Amino Acids More than half of the amino acids are *dispensable/nonessential,* ♦ meaning that the body can synthesize them for itself. Proteins in foods usually deliver these amino acids, but it is not essential that they do so. The body can make all **nonessential amino acids,** given nitrogen to form the amino group and fragments from carbohydrate to form the rest of the structure and an adequate amount of total energy.

*Besides the 20 common amino acids, which can all be components of proteins, others do not occur in proteins but can be found individually (e.g., taurine and ornithine). Some amino acids occur in related forms (e.g., proline can acquire an OH group to become hydroxyproline).

FIGURE 6-1 Amino Acid Structure

All amino acids have a central carbon with an amino group (NH_2), an acid group (COOH), a hydrogen (H), and a side group attached. The side group is a unique chemical structure that differentiates one amino acid from another.

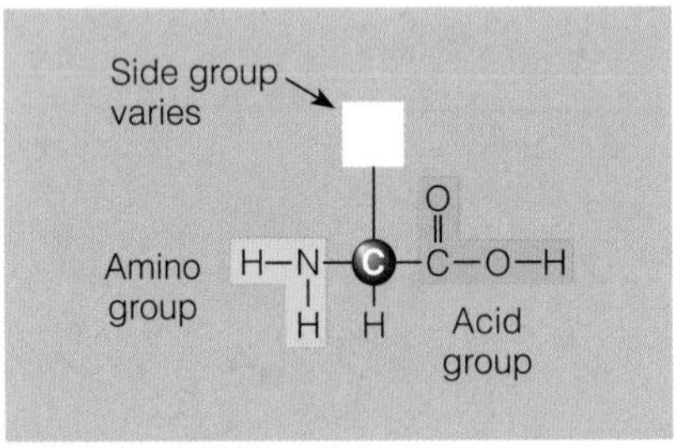
Side group varies
Amino group
Acid group

♦ Some researchers refer to essential amino acids as **indispensable** and to nonessential amino acids as **dispensable.**

nonessential amino acids: amino acids that the body can synthesize (see Table 6-1).

FIGURE 6-2 Examples of Amino Acids

Note that all amino acids have a common chemical structure but that each has a different side group. APPENDIX C presents the chemical structures of the 20 amino acids most common in proteins.

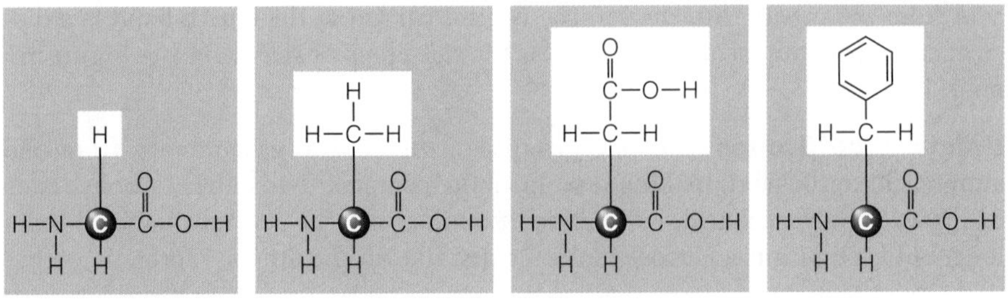

Glycine | Alanine | Aspartic acid | Phenylalanine

FIGURE 6-3 Condensation of Two Amino Acids to Form a Dipeptide

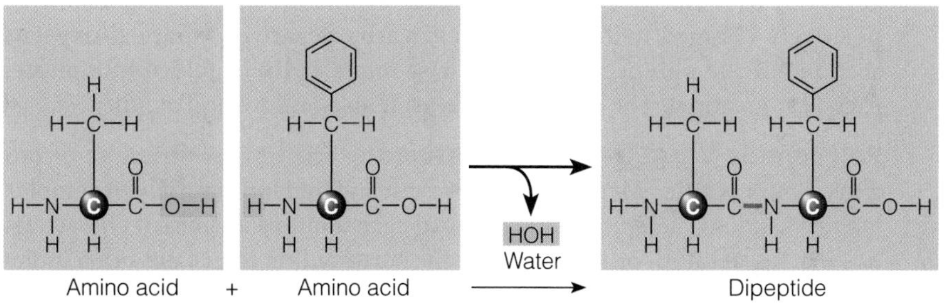
HOH
Water
Amino acid
+
Amino acid
Dipeptide

An OH group from the acid end of one amino acid and an H atom from the amino group of another join to form a molecule of water.

A peptide bond (highlighted in red) forms between the two amino acids, creating a dipeptide.

Indispensable/Essential Amino Acids There are nine amino acids that the human body either cannot make at all or cannot make in sufficient quantity to meet its needs. These nine amino acids must be supplied by the diet; they are *indispensable/essential.* The second column in Table 6-1 presents the **essential amino acids.**

Conditionally Essential Amino Acids Sometimes a nonessential amino acid becomes essential under special circumstances. For example, the body normally uses the essential amino acid phenylalanine to make tyrosine (a nonessential amino acid). But if the diet fails to supply enough phenylalanine, or if the body cannot make the conversion for some reason (as happens in the inherited disease phenylketonuria), then tyrosine becomes a **conditionally essential amino acid.**

Proteins

Cells link amino acids end-to-end in a variety of sequences to form thousands of different proteins. A **peptide bond** unites each amino acid to the next (see Figure 6-3).

Amino Acid Chains Condensation reactions (reactions that produce water, H_2O, as a by-product) connect amino acids, just as they combine two monosaccharides to form a disaccharide and three fatty acids with a glycerol to form a triglyceride. Two amino acids bonded together form a **dipeptide** (see Figure 6-3). By another such reaction, a third amino acid can be added to the chain to form a **tripeptide.** As additional amino acids join the chain, a **polypeptide** is formed. Most proteins are a few dozen to several hundred amino acids long. Figure 6-4 illustrates the protein insulin (a hormone).

FIGURE 6-4 Amino Acid Sequence of Human Insulin

Human insulin is a relatively small protein that consists of 51 amino acids in two short polypeptide chains. (For amino acid abbreviations, see APPENDIX C.) Two bridges link the two chains. A third bridge spans a section within the short chain. Known as *disulphide bridges,* these links always involve the amino acid cysteine (Cys), whose side group contains sulphur (S). Cysteines connect to each other when bonds form between these side groups.

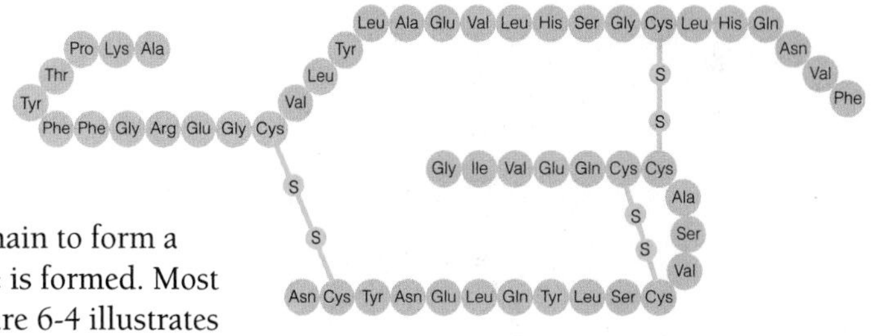
Leu Ala Glu Val Leu His Ser Gly Cys Leu His Gln
Pro Lys Ala
Tyr
Asn
Thr
Leu
Val
Tyr
Val
Phe
Phe Phe Gly Arg Glu Gly Cys
Gly Ile Val Glu Gln Cys Cys
Ala
Ser
Val
Asn Cys Tyr Asn Glu Leu Gln Tyr Leu Ser Cys
S

Amino Acid Sequence—Primary Structure The primary structure of a protein is determined by the sequence of amino acids. If a person could walk along a carbohydrate molecule like starch, the first stepping stone would be a glucose. The next stepping stone would also be a glucose, and it would be followed by a glucose, and yet another glucose. But if a person were to walk along a polypeptide chain, each stepping stone would be one of 20 different amino acids. The first stepping stone might be the amino acid methionine. The second might be an alanine. The third might be a glycine, the fourth a tryptophan, and so on. Walking along another polypeptide path, a person might step on a phenylalanine, then a valine, then a glutamine. In other words, amino acid sequences within proteins vary.

The amino acids can act somewhat like the letters in an alphabet. If you had only the letter *G*, all you could write would be a string of Gs: G–G–G–G–G–G–G. But with 20 different letters available, you can create poems, songs, and novels. Similarly, the 20 amino acids can be linked together in a variety of sequences—even more than are possible for letters in a word or words in a sentence. Thus the variety of possible sequences for polypeptide chains is tremendous.

essential amino acids: amino acids that the body cannot synthesize in amounts sufficient to meet physiological needs (see Table 6-1).

conditionally essential amino acid: an amino acid that is normally nonessential, but must be supplied by the diet in special circumstances when the need for it exceeds the body's ability to produce it (see Table 6-1).

peptide bond: a bond that connects the acid end of one amino acid with the amino end of another, forming a link in a protein chain.

dipeptide (dye-PEP-tide): two amino acids bonded together.

- **di** = two
- **peptide** = amino acid

tripeptide: three amino acids bonded together.

- **tri** = three

polypeptide: many (ten or more) amino acids bonded together.

- **poly** = many

FIGURE 6-5 The Structure of Hemoglobin

Four highly folded polypeptide chains form the globular hemoglobin protein.

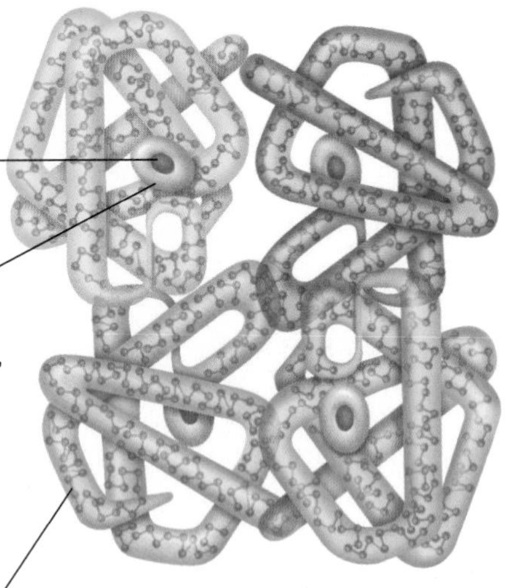
Iron
Heme, the nonprotein portion of hemoglobin, holds iron.
The amino acid sequence determines the shape of the polypeptide chain.

Polypeptide Shapes—Secondary Structure The secondary structure of proteins is determined not by chemical bonds as between the amino acids but by weak electrical attractions within the polypeptide chain. As positively charged hydrogens attract nearby negatively charged oxygens, sections of the polypeptide chain twist into a helix or fold into a pleated sheet, for example. These shapes give proteins strength and rigidity.

Polypeptide Tangles—Tertiary Structure The tertiary structure of proteins occurs as long polypeptide chains twist and fold into a variety of complex, tangled shapes. The unique side group of each amino acid gives it characteristics that attract it to, or repel it from, the surrounding fluids and other amino acids. Some amino acid side groups are attracted to water molecules; they are *hydrophilic*. Other side groups are repelled by water; they are *hydrophobic*. As amino acids are strung together to make a polypeptide, the chain folds so that its hydrophilic side groups are on the outer surface near water; the hydrophobic groups tuck themselves inside, away from water. Similarly, the disulphide bridges in insulin (see Figure 6-4) determine its tertiary structure. The extraordinary and unique shapes of proteins enable them to perform their various tasks in the body. Some form globular or spherical structures that can carry and store materials within them, and some, such as those of tendons, form linear structures that are more than ten times as long as they are wide. The intricate shape a protein finally assumes gives it maximum stability and its shape must be maintained in order for it to remain functional.

Multiple Polypeptide Interactions—Quaternary Structures Some polypeptides are functioning proteins just as they are; others need to associate with other polypeptides to form larger working complexes. The quaternary structure of proteins involves the interactions between two or more polypeptides. One molecule of **hemoglobin**—the large, globular protein molecule that, by the millions, packs the red blood cells and carries oxygen—is made of four associated polypeptide chains, each holding the mineral iron (see Figure 6-5).

Protein Denaturation When proteins are subjected to heat, acid, or other conditions that disturb their stability, they undergo **denaturation**—that is, they uncoil and lose their shapes and, consequently, also lose their ability to function. Past a certain point, denaturation is irreversible. Familiar examples of denaturation include the hardening of an egg when it is cooked, the curdling of milk when acid is added, and the stiffening of egg whites when they are whipped. In the body, proteins are denatured when they are exposed to stomach acid, which then allows it to become more digestible.

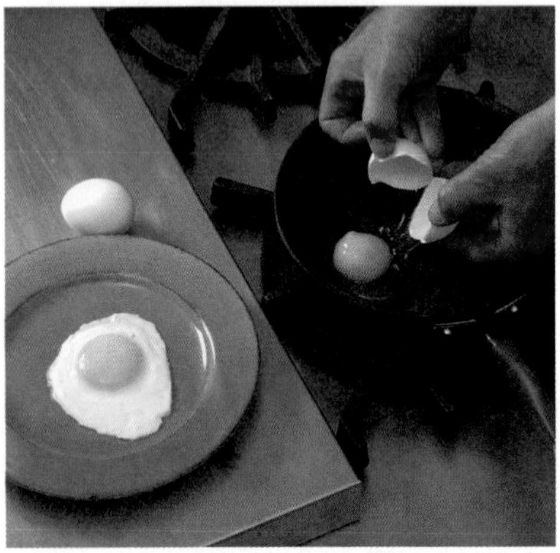

Cooking an egg denatures its proteins.

IN SUMMARY **Chemically speaking, proteins are more complex than carbohydrates or lipids; they are made of some 20 different amino acids, 9 of which the body cannot make (the indispensable/essential amino acids). Each amino acid contains an amino group, an acid group, a hydrogen atom, and a distinctive side group, all attached to a central carbon atom. Cells link amino acids together in a series of condensation reactions to create proteins. The distinctive sequence of amino acids in each protein determines its unique shape and function.**

Digestion and Absorption of Proteins

Proteins in foods do not become body proteins directly. Instead, they supply the amino acids from which the body makes its own proteins. When a person eats foods containing protein, enzymes break the long polypeptide strands into shorter strands, the short strands into tripeptides and dipeptides, and, finally, the tripeptides and dipeptides into individual amino acids.

Protein Digestion Figure 6-6 illustrates the digestion of protein through the GI tract. Proteins are crushed and moistened in the mouth, but the real action begins in the stomach.

hemoglobin (HE-moh-GLO-bin): the globular protein of the red blood cells that carries oxygen from the lungs to the cells throughout the body.
- **hemo** = blood
- **globin** = globular protein

denaturation (dee-NAY-chur-AY-shun): the change in a protein's shape and consequent loss of its function brought about by heat, agitation, acid, base, alcohol, heavy metals, or other agents.

FIGURE 6-6 Protein Digestion in the GI Tract

CENGAGENOW™ Animated! figure www.cengage.com/sso

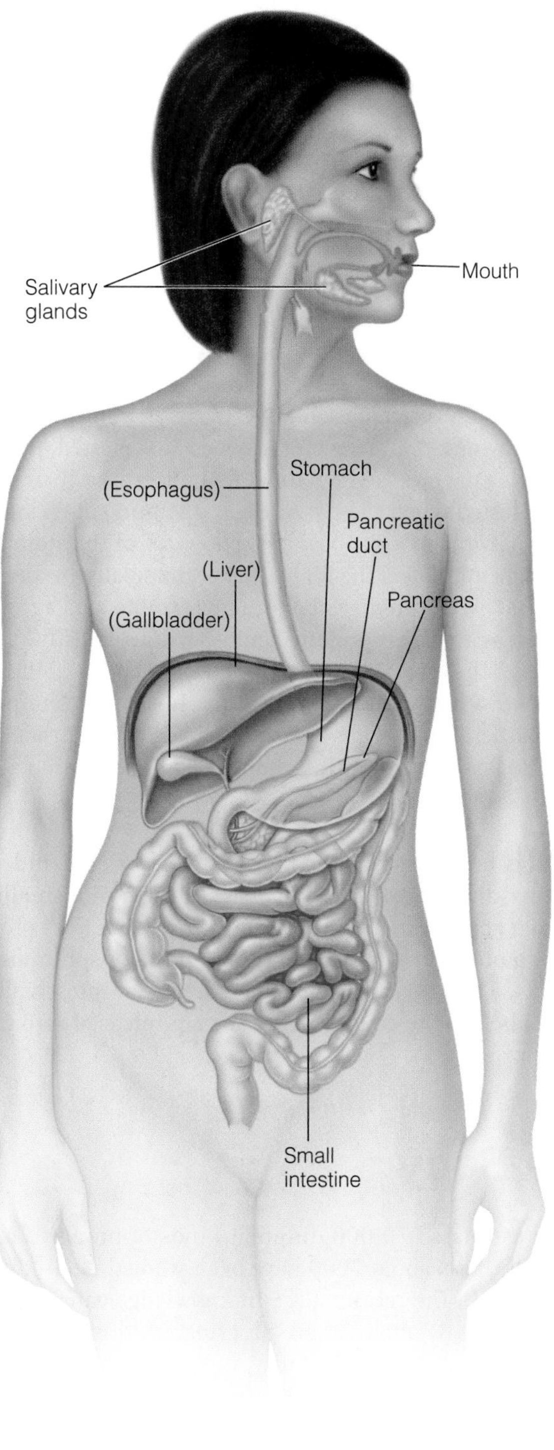
Salivary glands
Mouth
(Esophagus)
Stomach
Pancreatic duct
(Liver)
Pancreas
(Gallbladder)
Small intestine

PROTEIN

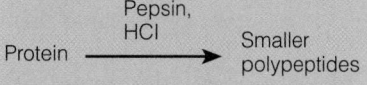

Mouth and salivary glands

Chewing and crushing moisten protein-rich foods and mix them with saliva to be swallowed

Stomach

Hydrochloric acid (HCl) uncoils protein strands and activates stomach enzymes:

Protein —(Pepsin, HCl)→ Smaller polypeptides

Small intestine and pancreas

Pancreatic and small intestinal enzymes split polypeptides further:

Polypeptides —(Pancreatic and intestinal proteases)→ Tripeptides, dipeptides, amino acids

Then enzymes on the surface of the small intestinal cells hydrolyze these peptides and the cells absorb them:

Peptides —(Intestinal tripeptidases and dipeptidases)→ Amino acids (absorbed)

HYDROCHLORIC ACID AND THE DIGESTIVE ENZYMES

In the stomach:

Hydrochloric acid (HCl)
- Denatures protein structure
- Activates pepsinogen to pepsin

Pepsin
- Cleaves proteins to smaller polypeptides and some free amino acids
- Inhibits pepsinogen synthesis

In the small intestine:

Enteropeptidase[a]
- Converts pancreatic trypsinogen to trypsin

Trypsin
- Inhibits trypsinogen synthesis
- Cleaves peptide bonds next to the amino acids lysine and arginine
- Converts pancreatic procarboxypeptidases to carboxypeptidases
- Converts pancreatic chymotrypsinogen to chymotrypsin

Chymotrypsin
- Cleaves peptide bonds next to the amino acids phenylalanine, tyrosine, tryptophan, methionine, asparagine, and histidine

Carboxypeptidases
- Cleave amino acids from the acid (carboxyl) ends of polypeptides

Elastase and collagenase
- Cleave polypeptides into smaller polypeptides and tripeptides

Intestinal tripeptidases
- Cleave tripeptides to dipeptides and amino acids

Intestinal dipeptidases
- Cleave dipeptides to amino acids

Intestinal aminopeptidases
- Cleave amino acids from the amino ends of small polypeptides (oligopeptides)

[a]Enteropeptidase was formerly known as *enterokinase.*

In the Stomach The major event in the stomach is the partial breakdown (hydrolysis) of proteins. Hydrochloric acid uncoils (denatures) each protein's tangled strands so that digestive enzymes can better attack the peptide bonds. The hydrochloric acid also converts the inactive form ♦ of the enzyme pepsinogen to its active form, **pepsin**. Pepsin initiates protein digestion by cleaving proteins—large polypeptides—into smaller polypeptides and some amino acids.

In the Small Intestine When polypeptides enter the small intestine, several pancreatic and intestinal proteases hydrolyze them further into short peptide

♦ The inactive form of an enzyme is called a **proenzyme** or a **zymogen** (ZYE-moh-jen).

pepsin: a gastric enzyme that hydrolyzes protein. Pepsin is secreted in an inactive form, **pepsinogen,** which is activated by hydrochloric acid in the stomach.

♦ A string of four to nine amino acids is an **oligopeptide** (OL-ee-go-PEP-tide).

- **oligo** = few

chains, ♦ tripeptides, dipeptides, and individual amino acids. Then **peptidase** enzymes on the membrane surfaces of the intestinal cells split most of the dipeptides and tripeptides into single amino acids. Only a few small peptides escape digestion and enter the blood intact. Figure 6-6 includes names of the digestive enzymes for protein and describes their actions.

Protein Absorption A number of specific carriers transport amino acids (and some dipeptides and tripeptides) into the intestinal cells. Once inside the intestinal cells, amino acids may be used for energy or to synthesize needed compounds. Amino acids that are not used by the intestinal cells are transported across the cell membrane into the surrounding fluid where they enter the capillaries on their way to the liver.

Consumers lacking nutrition knowledge may fail to realize that most proteins are broken down to amino acids before absorption. They may be misled by advertisements urging them to "Eat enzyme A. It will help you digest your food." Or "Don't eat food B. It contains enzyme C, which will digest cells in your body." In reality, though unless protected in some way, enzymes in foods are digested, just as all proteins are. Even the digestive enzymes—which function optimally at their specific pH—are denatured and digested when the pH of their environment changes. The enzyme pepsin, for example, which works best in the low pH of the stomach becomes inactive and digested when it enters the higher pH of the small intestine.

Another misconception is that eating predigested proteins (amino acid supplements) saves the body from having to digest proteins and keeps the digestive system from "overworking." Such a belief grossly underestimates the body's abilities. As a matter of fact, the digestive system handles whole proteins *better* than predigested ones because it dismantles and absorbs the amino acids at rates that are optimal for the body's use. (The last section of this chapter discusses amino acid supplements further.)

IN SUMMARY **Digestion is facilitated mostly by the stomach's acid and enzymes, which first denature dietary proteins, then cleave them into smaller polypeptides and some amino acids. Pancreatic and intestinal enzymes split these polypeptides further, to oligo-, tri-, and dipeptides, and then split most of these to single amino acids. Then carriers in the membranes of intestinal cells transport the amino acids into the cells, where they are released into the bloodstream.**

Proteins in the Body

The human body contains an estimated 30 000 different kinds of proteins, collectively known as **proteome**. Of these, about 3000 have been studied, ♦ although this number is growing rapidly with the recent surge in knowledge gained from sequencing the human genome. ♦ Only about 10 are described in this chapter—but these should be enough to illustrate the versatility, uniqueness, and importance of proteins. As you will see, each protein has a specific function, and that function is determined during protein synthesis.

♦ The study of the body's proteins is called **proteomics.**

♦ The **human genome** is the full set of chromosomes, including all of the genes and associated DNA.

Protein Synthesis Each human being is unique because of small differences in the body's proteins. These differences are determined by the amino acid sequences of proteins, which, in turn, are determined by genes. The following paragraphs describe in words the ways cells synthesize proteins; Figure 6-7 provides a pictorial description. Protein synthesis depends on a diet that provides adequate protein and essential amino acids.

The instructions for making every protein in a person's body are transmitted by way of the genetic information received at conception. This body of knowledge, which is filed in the DNA (deoxyribonucleic acid) within the nucleus of every cell, never leaves the nucleus.

peptidase: a digestive enzyme that hydrolyzes peptide bonds. *Tripeptidases* cleave tripeptides; *dipeptidases* cleave dipeptides. *Endopeptidases* cleave peptide bonds within the chain to create smaller fragments, whereas *exopeptidases* cleave bonds at the ends to release free amino acids.

- **tri** = three
- **di** = two
- **endo** = within
- **exo** = outside

proteome: all of the proteins synthesized by our cells.

FIGURE 6-7 Protein Synthesis

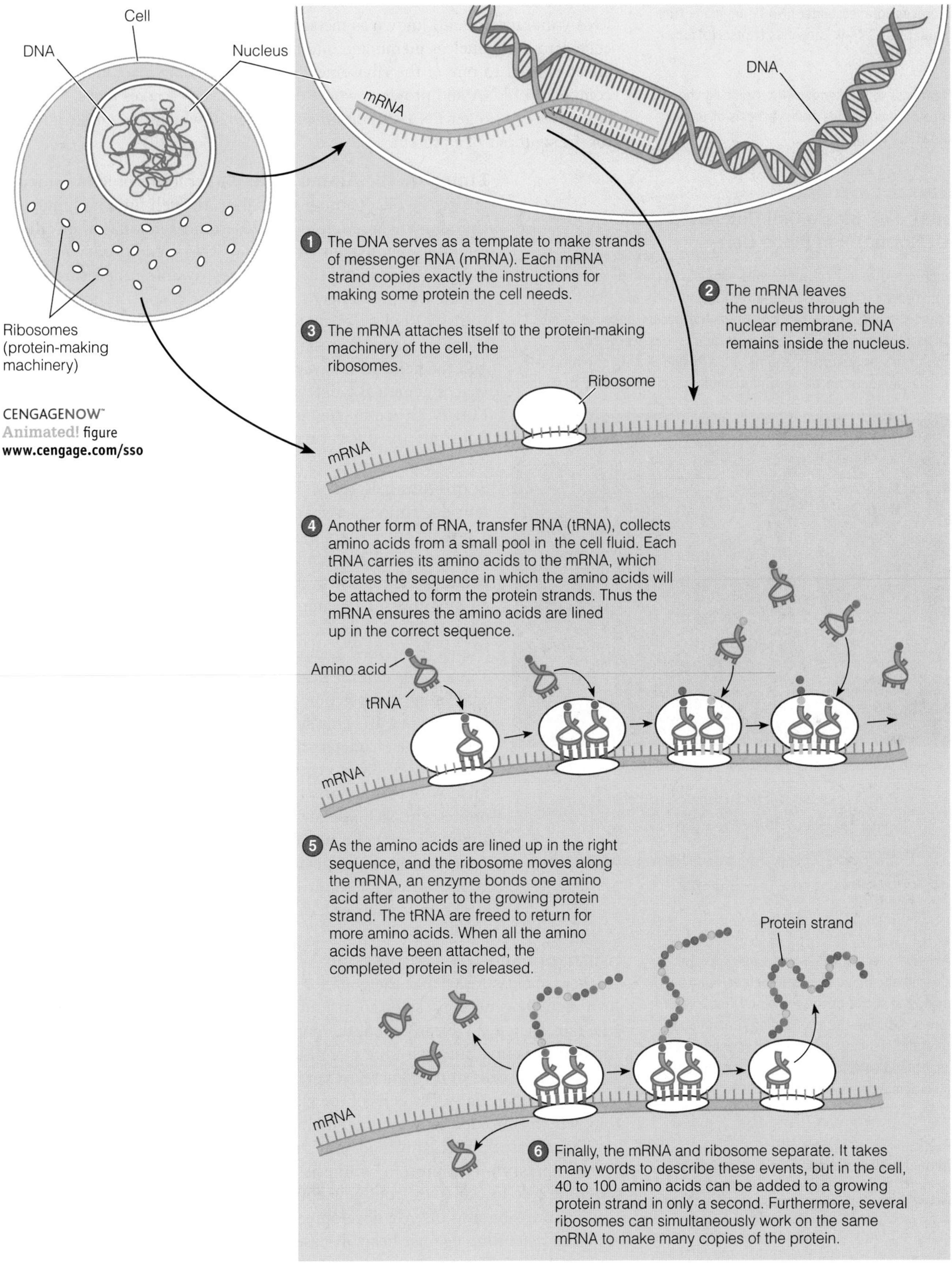
Cell
DNA
Nucleus
Ribosomes (protein-making machinery)
mRNA
DNA
1 The DNA serves as a template to make strands of messenger RNA (mRNA). Each mRNA strand copies exactly the instructions for making some protein the cell needs.
2 The mRNA leaves the nucleus through the nuclear membrane. DNA remains inside the nucleus.
3 The mRNA attaches itself to the protein-making machinery of the cell, the ribosomes.
Ribosome
mRNA
4 Another form of RNA, transfer RNA (tRNA), collects amino acids from a small pool in the cell fluid. Each tRNA carries its amino acids to the mRNA, which dictates the sequence in which the amino acids will be attached to form the protein strands. Thus the mRNA ensures the amino acids are lined up in the correct sequence.
Amino acid
tRNA
mRNA
5 As the amino acids are lined up in the right sequence, and the ribosome moves along the mRNA, an enzyme bonds one amino acid after another to the growing protein strand. The tRNA are freed to return for more amino acids. When all the amino acids have been attached, the completed protein is released.
Protein strand
mRNA
6 Finally, the mRNA and ribosome separate. It takes many words to describe these events, but in the cell, 40 to 100 amino acids can be added to a growing protein strand in only a second. Furthermore, several ribosomes can simultaneously work on the same mRNA to make many copies of the protein.

CENGAGENOW™
Animated! figure
www.cengage.com/sso

♦ This process of messenger RNA being made from a template of DNA is known as **transcription.**

♦ This process of messenger RNA directing the sequence of amino acids and synthesis of proteins is known as **translation.**

Delivering the Instructions Transforming the information in DNA into the appropriate sequence of amino acids needed to make a specific protein requires two major steps. In the first step, ♦ a stretch of DNA is used as a template to make a strand of RNA (ribonucleic acid) known as messenger RNA. Messenger RNA then carries the code across the nuclear membrane into the body of the cell. There it seeks out and attaches itself to one of the ribosomes (a protein-making machine, which is itself composed of RNA and protein), where the second step ♦ takes place. Situated on a ribosome, messenger RNA specifies the sequence in which the amino acids line up for the synthesis of a protein.

FIGURE 6-8 Sickle Cell Compared with Normal Red Blood Cell CENGAGENOW™ Animated! figure www.cengage.com/sso

Normally, red blood cells are disc-shaped, but in the inherited disorder sickle-cell anemia, red blood cells are sickle- or crescent-shaped. This alteration in shape occurs because valine replaces glutamic acid in the amino acid sequence of two of hemoglobin's polypeptide chains. As a result of this one alteration, the hemoglobin has a diminished capacity to carry oxygen.

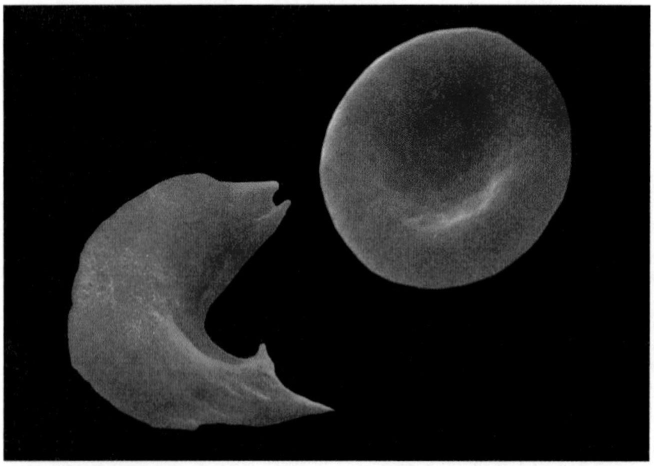

© Dr. Stanley Flegler/Visuals Unlimited

Sickle-shaped blood cell — Normal red blood cell

Amino acid sequence of normal hemoglobin:
Val–His–Leu–Thr–Pro–Glu–Glu

Amino acid sequence of sickle-cell hemoglobin:
Val–His–Leu–Thr–Pro–Val–Glu

Lining Up the Amino Acids Other forms of RNA, called transfer RNA, collect amino acids from the cell fluid and take them to the messenger. Each of the 20 amino acids has a specific transfer RNA. Thousands of transfer RNAs, each carrying its amino acid, cluster around the ribosomes, awaiting their turn to unload. When the messenger's list calls for a specific amino acid, the transfer RNA carrying that amino acid moves into position. Then the next loaded transfer RNA moves into place and then the next and the next. In this way, the amino acids line up in the sequence that is genetically determined, and enzymes bind them together. Finally, the completed protein strand is released, and the transfer RNAs are freed to return for other loads of amino acids.

Sequencing Errors The sequence of amino acids in each protein determines its shape, which supports a specific function. If a genetic error alters the amino acid sequence of a protein, or if a mistake is made in copying the sequence, an altered protein will result, sometimes with dramatic consequences. The protein hemoglobin offers one example of such a genetic variation. In a person with **sickle-cell anemia,** ♦ two of hemoglobin's four polypeptide chains (described earlier on p. 174) have the normal sequence of amino acids, but the other two chains do not—they have the amino acid valine in a position that is normally occupied by glutamic acid (see Figure 6-8). This single alteration in the amino acid sequence changes the characteristics and shape of hemoglobin so much that it loses its ability to carry oxygen effectively. The red blood cells filled with this abnormal hemoglobin stiffen into elongated sickle, or crescent, shapes instead of maintaining their normal pliable disc shape—hence the name, sickle-cell anemia. Sickle-cell anemia raises energy needs, causes many medical problems, and can be fatal.[1] Caring for children with sickle-cell anemia includes diligent attention to their water needs; dehydration can trigger a crisis.

♦ Anemia is a symptom of various diseases. In sickle-cell anemia, a defect in hemoglobin changes the shape of the red blood cells. Later chapters describe the anemias of vitamin and mineral deficiencies. In all cases of anemia, abnormal blood cells are unable to meet the body's oxygen demands.

Nutrients and Gene Expression When a cell makes a protein as described earlier, scientists say that the gene for that protein has been "expressed." Cells can regulate **gene expression** to make the type of protein, in the amounts and at the rate, they need. Nearly all of the body's cells possess the genes for making all human proteins, but each type of cell usually makes only the proteins it needs. For example, cells of the pancreas express the gene for insulin; in other cells, that gene is idle. Similarly, the cells of the pancreas do not make the protein hemoglobin, which is needed only by the red blood cells.

Recent research has unveiled some of the fascinating ways nutrients regulate gene expression and protein synthesis (see Highlight 6). Because diet plays an ongoing role in our lives from conception to death, it has a major influence on gene expression and disease development. The benefits of polyunsaturated fatty acids in defending against heart disease, for example, are partially explained by their role in influencing gene expression for lipid enzymes. Later chapters provide additional examples of relationships among nutrients, genes, and disease development.

sickle-cell anemia: a hereditary form of anemia characterized by abnormal sickle- or crescent-shaped red blood cells. Sickled cells interfere with oxygen transport and blood flow. Symptoms are precipitated by dehydration, exercise and insufficient oxygen (as may occur at high altitudes) and include hemolytic anemia (red blood cells burst), fever, and severe pain in the joints and abdomen.

gene expression: the process by which a cell converts the genetic code into RNA and protein.

IN SUMMARY **Cells synthesize proteins according to the genetic information provided by the DNA in the nucleus of each cell. This information dictates the sequence in which amino acids are linked together to form a given protein. Sequencing errors occasionally occur, sometimes with significant consequences.**

Roles of Proteins

Whenever the body is growing, repairing, or replacing tissue, proteins are involved. Sometimes their role is to facilitate or to regulate; other times it is to become part of a structure. Versatility is a key feature of proteins.

As Building Materials for Growth and Maintenance From the moment of conception, proteins form the building blocks of muscles, blood, and skin—in fact, of most body structures. For example, to build a bone or a tooth, cells first lay down a **matrix** of the protein **collagen** and then fill it with crystals of calcium, phosphorus, magnesium, fluoride, and other minerals.

Collagen also provides the material of ligaments and tendons and the strengthening "glue" between the cells of the artery walls that enables the arteries to withstand the pressure of the blood surging through them with each heartbeat. Also made of collagen are scars that knit the separated parts of torn tissues together.

Proteins are also needed for replacing dead or damaged cells. The life span of a skin cell is only about 30 days. As old skin cells are shed, new cells made largely of protein grow from underneath to replace them. Cells in the deeper skin layers synthesize new proteins to form hair and fingernails. Muscle cells make new proteins to grow larger and stronger in response to exercise.[2] Cells of the GI tract are replaced every few days. Both inside and outside, then, the body continuously deposits protein into the new cells that replace those that have been lost.

As Enzymes Some proteins act as **enzymes.** Digestive enzymes have appeared in every chapter since Chapter 3, but digestion is only one of the many processes facilitated by enzymes. Enzymes not only break down substances, but they also build substances (such as bone) ♦ and transform one substance into another (amino acids into glucose, for example). Figure 6-9 diagrams a synthesis reaction.

♦ Breaking down reactions are **catabolic,** whereas building up reactions are **anabolic.** (Chapter 7 provides more details.)

FIGURE 6-9 Enzyme Action

Each enzyme facilitates a specific chemical reaction. In this diagram, an enzyme enables two compounds to make a more complex structure, but the enzyme itself remains unchanged.

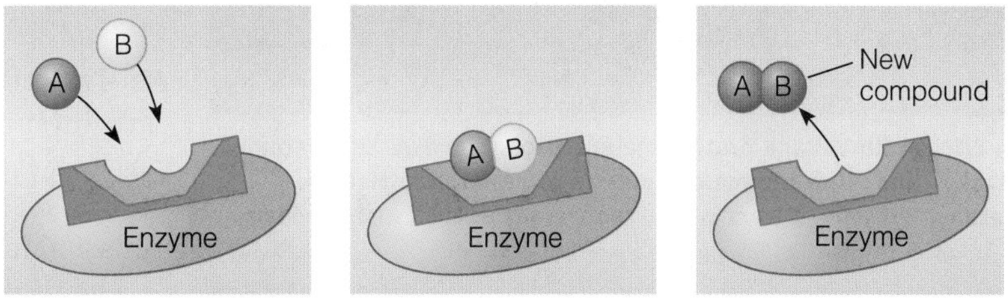
B
A
Enzyme
A B
Enzyme
A B
New compound
Enzyme

The separate compounds, A and B, are attracted to the enzyme's active site, making a reaction likely. | The enzyme forms a complex with A and B. | The enzyme is unchanged, but A and B have formed a new compound, AB.

An analogy may help to clarify the role of enzymes. Enzymes are comparable to the clergy and judges who make and dissolve marriages. When a minister marries two people, they become a couple, with a new bond between them. They are joined together—but the minister remains unchanged. The minister represents enzymes that synthesize large compounds from smaller ones. One minister can perform thousands of marriage ceremonies, just as one enzyme can perform billions of synthetic reactions.

Similarly, a judge who lets married couples separate may decree many divorces before retiring. The judge represents enzymes that hydrolyze larger compounds to smaller ones; for example, the digestive enzymes. The point is that, like the minister and the judge, enzymes themselves are not altered by the reactions they facilitate. They are catalysts, permitting reactions to occur more quickly and efficiently than if substances depended on chance encounters alone.

As Hormones The body's many hormones are messenger molecules, and *some* hormones are proteins. ♦ Various endocrine glands in the body release hormones in response to changes that challenge the body. The blood carries the hormones from these glands to their target tissues, where they elicit the appropriate responses to restore and maintain normal conditions.

♦ Some hormones, such as estrogen and testosterone, derive from the lipid cholesterol.

The hormone insulin provides a familiar example. After a meal, when blood glucose rises, the pancreas releases insulin. Insulin stimulates the translocation of glucose transporter molecules to the cell surface of muscle and adipose tissues, which then allow glucose into the cells much faster than during the

matrix (MAY-tricks): the basic substance that gives form to a developing structure; in the body, the formative cells from which teeth and bones grow.

collagen (KOL-ah-jen): the protein from which connective tissues such as scars, tendons, ligaments, and the foundations of bones and teeth are made.

enzymes: proteins that facilitate chemical reactions without being changed in the process; protein catalysts.

TABLE 6-2 Examples of Hormones and Their Actions

Hormones	Actions
Growth hormone	Promotes growth
Insulin and glucagon	Regulate blood glucose (see Chapter 4)
Thyroxin	Regulates the body's metabolic rate (see Chapter 8)
Calcitonin and parathyroid hormone	Regulate blood calcium (see Chapter 13)
Antidiuretic hormone	Regulates fluid and electrolyte balance (see Chapter 11)

NOTE: Hormones are chemical messengers that are secreted by endocrine glands in response to altered conditions in the body. Each travels to one or more specific target tissues or organs, where it elicits a specific response. For descriptions of many hormones important in nutrition, see APPENDIX A.

fasted state. After acting on the message, the cells either release or destroy insulin; released insulin is destroyed by the liver. As blood glucose falls back to normal, the pancreas slows its release of insulin. Many other proteins act as hormones, regulating a variety of actions in the body (see Table 6-2 for examples).

As Regulators of Fluid Balance Proteins help to maintain the body's **fluid balance.** Normally, proteins are found primarily within the cells and in the plasma (essentially blood without its red blood cells). Being large, proteins do not normally cross the walls of the blood vessels. During times of critical illness or protein malnutrition, however, plasma proteins leak out of the blood vessels into the tissues (between the cells). Because proteins attract water, fluid accumulates and causes swelling. Swelling due to an excess of fluid in the tissues is known as **edema.** The protein-related causes of edema include:

- Excessive protein losses caused by inflammation and critical illnesses
- Inadequate protein synthesis caused by liver disease
- Inadequate dietary intake of protein

Whatever the cause of edema, the result is the same: a diminished capacity to deliver nutrients and oxygen to the cells and to remove wastes from them. As a consequence, cells fail to function adequately.

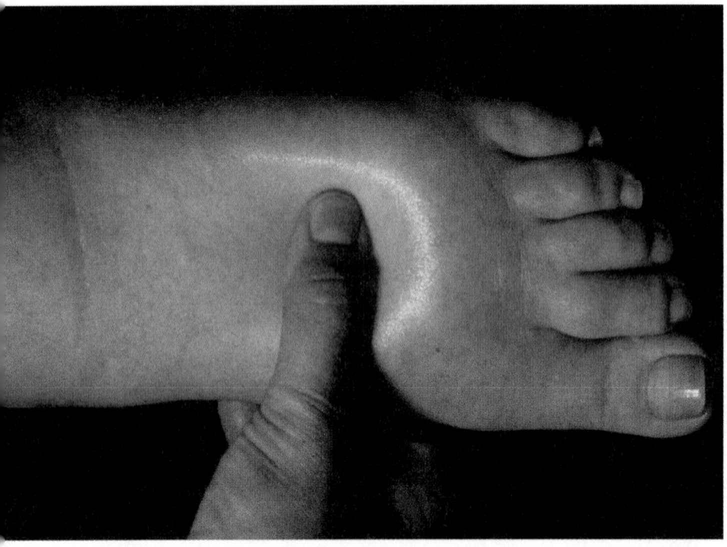

SPL/Photo Researchers, Inc.

In critical illness and protein malnutrition, blood vessels become "leaky" and allow plasma proteins to move into the tissues. Because proteins attract water, the tissues swell, causing edema.

As Acid–Base Regulators Proteins also help to maintain the balance between **acids** and **bases** within the body fluids. Normal body processes continually produce acids and bases, which the blood carries to the kidneys and lungs for excretion. The challenge is to do this without upsetting the blood's acid–base balance.

In an acid solution, hydrogen ions (H^+) abound; the more hydrogen ions, the more concentrated the acid. Proteins, which have negative charges on their surfaces, attract hydrogen ions, which have positive charges. By accepting and releasing hydrogen ions, ♦ proteins maintain the acid–base balance of the blood and body fluids.

The blood's acid–base balance is tightly controlled. The extremes of **acidosis** and **alkalosis** lead to coma and death, largely because they denature working proteins. Disturbing a protein's shape renders it useless. To give just one example, denatured hemoglobin loses its capacity to carry oxygen.

As Transporters Some proteins move about in the body fluids, carrying nutrients and other molecules. The protein hemoglobin carries oxygen from the lungs to the cells. The lipoproteins transport lipids around the body. Special transport proteins carry vitamins and minerals.

The transport of the mineral iron provides an especially good illustration of these proteins' specificity and precision. When iron is absorbed, it is captured in an intestinal cell by a protein. Before leaving the intestinal cell, iron is attached to another protein that carries it through the bloodstream to the cells. Once iron enters a cell, it is attached to a storage protein that will hold the iron until it is needed. When it is needed, iron is incorporated into proteins in the red blood cells and muscles that assist in oxygen transport and use. (Chapter 14 provides more details on how these protein carriers transport and store iron.)

Some transport proteins reside in cell membranes and act as "pumps," picking up compounds on one side of the membrane and releasing them on the other as needed. Each transport protein is specific for a certain compound or group of related compounds. Figure 6-10 illustrates how a membrane-bound transport protein helps to maintain the sodium and potassium concentrations in the fluids inside and outside cells. The balance of these two minerals is critical to nerve transmissions and muscle contractions; imbalances can cause irregular heartbeats, muscular weakness, kidney failure, and even death.

♦ Compounds that keep a solution's pH constant when acids or bases are added are called **buffers.**

fluid balance: maintenance of the proper types and amounts of fluid in each compartment of the body fluids (see also Chapter 11).

edema (eh-DEEM-uh): the swelling of body tissue caused by excessive amounts of fluid in the interstitial spaces; seen in protein deficiency (among other conditions).

acids: compounds that release hydrogen ions in a solution.

bases: compounds that accept hydrogen ions in a solution.

acidosis (assi-DOE-sis): higher-than-normal acidity in the blood and body fluids.

alkalosis (alka-LOE-sis): higher-than-normal alkalinity (base) in the blood and body fluids.

FIGURE 6-10 An Example of a Transport Protein

This transport protein resides within a cell membrane and acts as a two-door passageway. Molecules enter on one side of the membrane and exit on the other, but the protein doesn't leave the membrane. This example shows how the transport protein moves sodium and potassium in opposite directions across the membrane to maintain a high concentration of potassium and a low concentration of sodium within the cell. This active transport system requires energy.

CENGAGENOW™
Animated! figure
www.cengage.com/sso

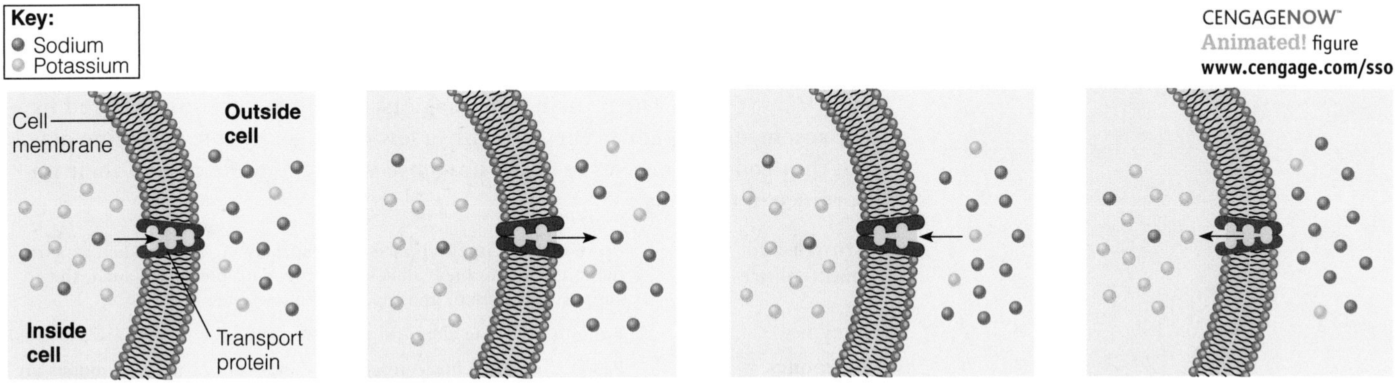
Key:
Sodium
Potassium
Cell membrane
Outside cell
Inside cell
Transport protein

The transport protein picks up sodium from inside the cell. The protein changes shape and releases sodium outside the cell. The transport protein picks up potassium from outside the cell. The protein changes shape and releases potassium inside the cell.

As Antibodies Proteins also defend the body against disease. A virus—whether it is one that causes flu, smallpox, measles, or the common cold—enters the cells and multiplies there. One virus may produce 100 replicas of itself within an hour or so. Each replica can then burst out and invade 100 different cells, soon yielding 10 000 viruses, which invade 10 000 cells. Left free to do their worst, they will soon overwhelm the body with disease.

Fortunately, when the body detects these invading **antigens**, it manufactures **antibodies**, giant protein molecules designed specifically to combat them. The antibodies work so swiftly and efficiently that in a normal, healthy individual, most diseases never have a chance to get started. Without sufficient protein, though, the body cannot maintain its army of antibodies to resist infectious diseases.

Each antibody is designed to destroy a specific antigen. Once the body has manufactured antibodies against a particular antigen (such as the measles virus), it "remembers" how to make them. Consequently, the next time the body encounters that same antigen, it produces antibodies even more quickly. In other words, the body develops a molecular memory, known as **immunity**. (Chapter 17 describes food allergies—the immune system's response to specific food proteins and food antigens). Note also that new food allergen labelling Regulations will come into effect on August 4, 2012.[3] These regulations are designed to enhance the labelling of foods that contain allergens (including mustard seeds), gluten, and added sulphites. In the meantime, the Canadian Food Inspection Agency is also encouraging food manufacturers to inform consumers that some cereal products made from oats or barley, for example, may also contain low levels of wheat. Where appropriate, such information would be helpful to those who may have severe wheat allergies. Health Canada has also informed consumers about the potential for low levels of wheat in some cereal grain-based foods.[4] Thus, it is important for those with allergies to wheat to look for precautionary labelling, for example, "may contain wheat" on cereal grain-based products.

As a Source of Energy and Glucose Without energy, cells die; without glucose, the brain and nervous system falter. Even though proteins are needed to do the work that only they can perform, they will be sacrificed to provide energy ♦ and glucose ♦ during times of starvation or insufficient carbohydrate or total energy intake. The body will break down its tissue proteins to make amino acids available for energy or glucose production. In this way, protein can maintain blood glucose levels, but at the expense of losing lean body tissue. Chapter 7 provides more details on energy metabolism.

♦ Protein provides 4 kcal/g. Return to p. 9 for a refresher on how to calculate the protein kcalories from foods.

♦ The making of glucose from noncarbohydrate sources such as amino acids is **gluconeogenesis.**

antigens: substances that elicit the formation of antibodies or an inflammation reaction from the immune system. A bacterium, a virus, a toxin, and a protein in food that causes allergy are all examples of antigens.

antibodies: large proteins of the blood and body fluids, produced by the immune system in response to the invasion of the body by foreign molecules (usually proteins called *antigens*). Antibodies combine with and inactivate the foreign invaders, thus protecting the body.

immunity: the body's ability to defend itself against diseases (see also Chapter 19).

Other Roles As mentioned earlier, proteins form integral parts of most body structures such as skin, muscles, and bones. They also participate in some of the body's most amazing activities such as blood clotting and vision. When a tissue is injured, a rapid chain of events leads to the production of fibrin, a stringy, insoluble mass of protein fibres that forms a solid clot from liquid blood. Later, more slowly, the protein collagen forms a scar to replace the clot and permanently heal the wound. The light-sensitive pigments in the cells of the eye's retina are molecules of the protein opsin. Opsin responds to light by changing its shape, thus initiating the nerve impulses that convey the sense of sight to the brain.

IN SUMMARY **The protein functions discussed here are summarized in the accompanying table. They are only a few of the many roles proteins play, but they convey some sense of the immense variety of proteins and their importance in the body.**

Growth and maintenance	Proteins form integral parts of most body structures such as skin, tendons, membranes, muscles, organs, and bones. As such, they support the growth and repair of body tissues.
Enzymes	Proteins facilitate chemical reactions (and all enzymes are proteins).
Hormones	Proteins regulate body processes. (Some, but not all, hormones are proteins.)
Fluid balance	Proteins help to maintain the volume and composition of body fluids.
Acid–base balance	Proteins help to maintain the acid–base balance of body fluids by acting as buffers.
Transportation	Proteins transport substances, such as lipids, vitamins, minerals, and oxygen, around the body.
Antibodies	Proteins inactivate foreign invaders, thus protecting the body against diseases.
Energy and glucose	Proteins provide some fuel, and glucose if needed, for the body's energy needs.

A Preview of Protein Metabolism

This section previews protein metabolism; Chapter 7 provides a full description. Cells have several metabolic options, depending on their protein and energy needs.

Protein Turnover and the Amino Acid Pool Within each cell, proteins are continually being made and broken down, a process known as **protein turnover.** When proteins break down, they free amino acids. ♦ These amino acids mix with amino acids from dietary protein to form a small "**amino acid pool**" within the cells and circulating blood. Note: Unlike glucose and fatty acids, amino acids are not stored for later use. The rate of protein degradation and the amount of protein intake may vary, but the pattern of amino acids within the pool remains fairly constant. Regardless of their source, any of these amino acids can be used to make body proteins or other nitrogen-containing compounds, or they can be stripped of their nitrogen, leaving a carbon backbone that can then be used for energy (either immediately or stored as fat for later use).

Nitrogen Balance Protein turnover and **nitrogen balance** go hand in hand. ♦ In healthy adults, protein synthesis balances with degradation, and protein intake from food balances with nitrogen excretion in the urine, feces, and sweat. When nitrogen intake equals nitrogen output, the person is in nitrogen equilibrium, or zero nitrogen balance (see Figure 6-11). Researchers use nitrogen balance studies to estimate protein requirements.

If the body synthesizes more than it degrades and adds protein, nitrogen status becomes positive. Nitrogen status is positive in growing infants, children, adolescents, pregnant women, individuals building muscle, and people recovering from protein deficiency or illness; their nitrogen intake exceeds their nitrogen output. They are retaining protein in new tissues as they add blood, bone, skin, and muscle cells to their bodies.

If the body degrades more than it synthesizes and loses protein, nitrogen status becomes negative. Nitrogen status is negative in people who become sedentary, are

♦ Amino acids (or proteins) that derive from within the body are **endogenous** (en-DODGE-eh-nus). In contrast, those that derive from foods are **exogenous** (eks-ODGE-eh-nus).

- **endo** = within
- **gen** = arising
- **exo** = outside (the body)

♦ Nitrogen balance:

- Nitrogen equilibrium (zero nitrogen balance): N in = N out
- Positive nitrogen: N in > N out
- Negative nitrogen: N in < N out

protein turnover: the degradation and synthesis of protein.

amino acid pool: the supply of amino acids derived from either food proteins or body proteins that collect in the cells and circulating blood and stand ready to be incorporated in proteins and other compounds or used for energy.

nitrogen balance: the amount of nitrogen consumed (N in) as compared with the amount of nitrogen excreted (N out) in a given period of time.*

*The genetic materials DNA and RNA contain nitrogen, but the quantity is insignificant compared with the amount in protein. Protein is 16 percent nitrogen. Said another way, the average protein weighs about 6.25 times as much as the nitrogen it contains, so scientists can estimate the amount of protein in a sample of food, body tissue, or other material by multiplying the weight of the nitrogen in it by 6.25.

FIGURE 6-11 Nitrogen Balance

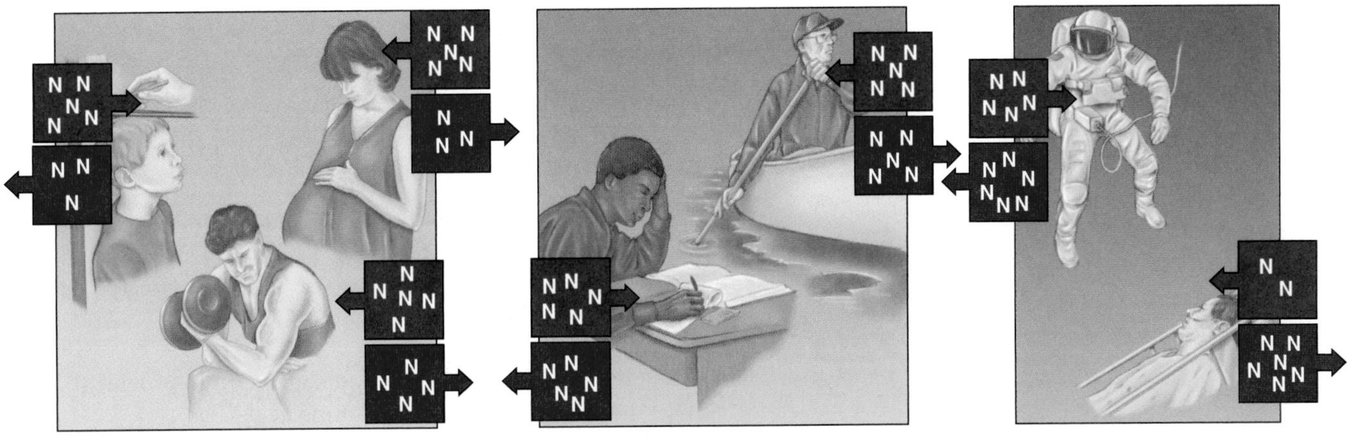

Positive Nitrogen Balance
These people, a growing child, a person building muscle, and a pregnant woman, are all retaining more nitrogen than they are excreting.

Nitrogen Equilibrium
These people, a healthy college student and a young retiree, are in nitrogen equilibrium.

Negative Nitrogen Balance
These people, an astronaut and a surgery patient, are losing more nitrogen than they are taking in.

© MBI/Alamy

starving, or suffering other severe stresses such as burns, injuries, infections, and fever; their nitrogen output exceeds their nitrogen intake. During these times, the body loses nitrogen as it breaks down muscle and other body proteins for energy.

Using Amino Acids to Make Other Compounds Cells can also use amino acids to make other compounds. For example, the amino acid tyrosine is used to make the **neurotransmitters** norepinephrine and epinephrine, which relay nervous system messages throughout the body. Tyrosine can also be made into the pigment melanin, which is responsible for brown hair, eye, and skin colour, or into the hormone thyroxin, which helps to regulate the metabolic rate. For another example, the amino acid tryptophan serves as a precursor for the vitamin niacin and for serotonin, a neurotransmitter important in sleep regulation, appetite control, and sensory perception.

Using Amino Acids for Energy and Glucose As mentioned earlier, when glucose or fatty acids are limited, cells are forced to use amino acids for energy and glucose. The body does not make a specialized storage form of protein as it does for carbohydrate and fat. Glucose is stored as glycogen in the liver and fat as triglycerides in adipose tissue, but protein in the body is available only from the working and structural components of the tissues. When the need arises, the body breaks down its tissue proteins and uses their amino acids for energy or glucose. Thus, over time, energy deprivation (starvation) always causes wasting of lean body tissue as well as fat loss. An adequate supply of carbohydrates and fats spares amino acids from being used for energy and allows them to perform their unique roles.

Using Amino Acids to Make Fat Amino acids may be used to make fat when energy and protein intakes exceed needs and carbohydrate intake is adequate. Note: Making fat from amino acids is energetically very expensive and unlikely to occur to any great extent under conditions where the diet is adequate but not overabundant in total energy. When protein is abundant, energy metabolism shifts to use more protein instead of fat. Excess amino acids can also be converted to fat which can then be stored for later use. Consequently, protein-rich foods that provide more energy than the body needs can contribute to weight gain.

Deaminating Amino Acids When amino acids are broken down (as occurs when they are used for energy or to make glucose or fat), they are first deaminated—stripped of their nitrogen-containing amino groups. Two products result from **deamination**: one is **ammonia** (NH_3); the other product is the carbon structure without its amino group—often a **keto acid.** Keto acids may enter a number of metabolic pathways—for example, they may be used for energy or for the production

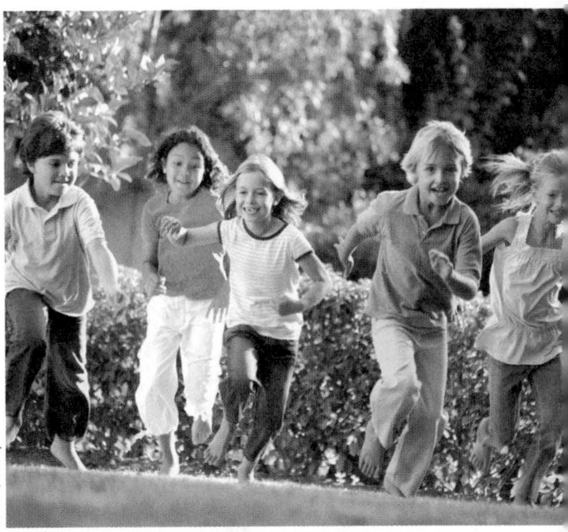

© MBI/Alamy

Growing children end each day with more bone, blood, muscle, and skin cells than they had at the beginning of the day.

neurotransmitters: chemicals that are released at the end of a nerve cell when a nerve impulse arrives there. They diffuse across the gap to the next cell and alter the membrane of that second cell to either inhibit or excite it.

deamination (dee-AM-ih-NAY-shun): removal of the amino (NH_2) group from a compound such as an amino acid.

ammonia: a compound with the chemical formula NH_3; produced during the deamination of amino acids.

keto (KEY-toe) **acid:** an organic acid that contains a carbonyl group (C=O).

FIGURE 6-12 Deamination and Synthesis of a Dispensable/Nonessential Amino Acid

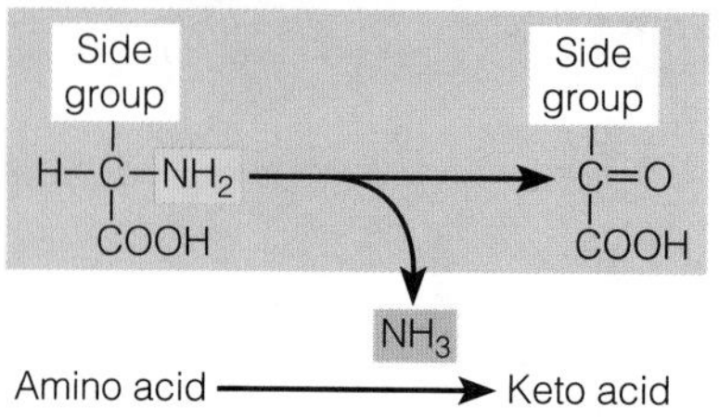
Side group
H–C–NH2
COOH
Side group
C=O
COOH
NH3
Amino acid
Keto acid

The deamination of an amino acid produces ammonia (NH_3) and a keto acid.

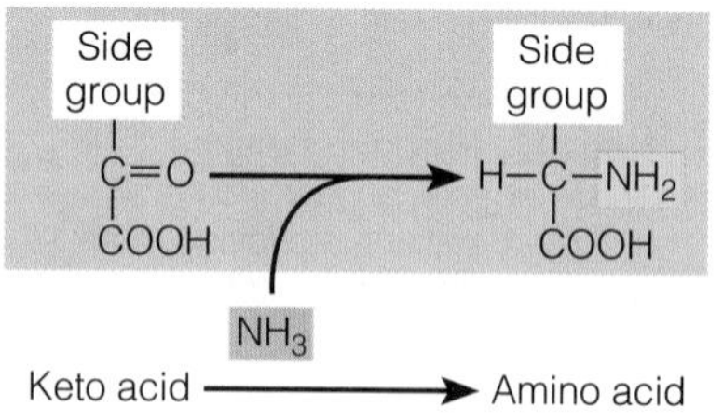
Side group
C=O
COOH
Side group
H–C–NH2
COOH
NH3
Keto acid
Amino acid

Given a source of NH_3, the body can make dispensable/nonessential amino acids from keto acids.

FIGURE 6-13 Transamination and Synthesis of a Dispensable/Nonessential Amino Acid

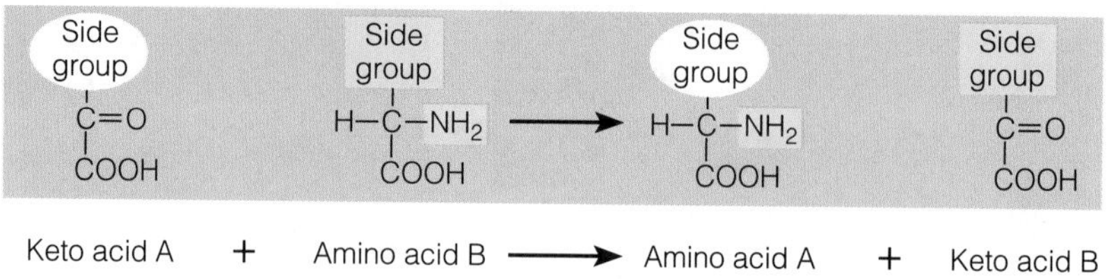
Side group
C=O
COOH
Side group
H–C–NH2
COOH
Side group
H–C–NH2
COOH
Side group
C=O
COOH
Keto acid A
+
Amino acid B
Amino acid A
+
Keto acid B

The body can transfer amino groups (NH_2) from an amino acid to a keto acid, forming a new *dispensable/nonessential* amino acid and a new keto acid. Transamination reactions require the vitamin B_6 coenzyme.

of glucose, ketones, cholesterol, or fat.* They may also be used to provide the carbon skeletons to make dispensable/nonessential amino acids.

Using Amino Acids to Make Proteins and Dispensable/Nonessential Amino Acids As mentioned, cells can assemble amino acids into the proteins they need to do their work. If an indispensable/essential amino acid is missing, the body may break down some available proteins to obtain it. If a particular dispensable/nonessential amino acid is not readily available, cells can make it from a keto acid—if a nitrogen source is available. Ammonia provides some of the nitrogen needed for the synthesis of dispensable/nonessential amino acids from keto acids (see Figure 6-12). Cells can also make a dispensable/nonessential amino acid by transferring an amino group from one amino acid to its corresponding keto acid, as shown in Figure 6-13. Through many such **transamination** reactions, involving many different keto acids, the liver cells can synthesize the dispensable/nonessential amino acids.

Converting Ammonia to Urea Ammonia is a toxic compound chemically identical to the strong-smelling ammonia in bottled cleaning solutions. Because ammonia is a base, the blood's critical acid–base balance becomes upset if the cells produce larger quantities than the liver can handle.

To prevent such a crisis, the liver combines ammonia with carbon dioxide to make **urea,** a much less toxic compound. Figure 6-14 provides a greatly oversimplified diagram of urea synthesis; details are shown in APPENDIX C. The production of urea increases as dietary protein increases, until production hits its maximum rate at intakes approaching 250 grams per day.

Excreting Urea Liver cells release urea into the blood, where it circulates until it passes through the kidneys (see Figure 6-15). The kidneys then filter urea out of the blood for excretion in the urine. Normally, the liver efficiently captures all the ammonia, makes urea from it, and releases the urea into the blood; then the kidneys clear all the urea from the blood. This division of labour allows easy diagnosis of diseases of both organs. In liver disease, blood ammonia will be high; in kidney disease, blood urea will be high.

Urea is the body's principal vehicle for excreting unused nitrogen, and the amount of urea produced increases with protein intake. To keep urea in solution, the body needs water. For this reason, a person who regularly consumes a high-protein diet (say, 100 grams a day or more) must drink plenty of water to dilute and excrete urea from the body. Without extra water, a person on a high-protein diet risks dehydration because the body uses its water to rid itself of urea. This explains some of the water loss that accompanies high-protein diets. Such losses may make high-protein diets *appear* to be effective, but water loss, of course, is of no value to the person who wants to lose body fat (as Highlight 8 explains).

FIGURE 6-14 Urea Synthesis

When amino acids are deaminated, ammonia is produced. The liver detoxifies ammonia before releasing it into the bloodstream by combining it with another waste product, carbon dioxide, to produce urea. See APPENDIX C for details.

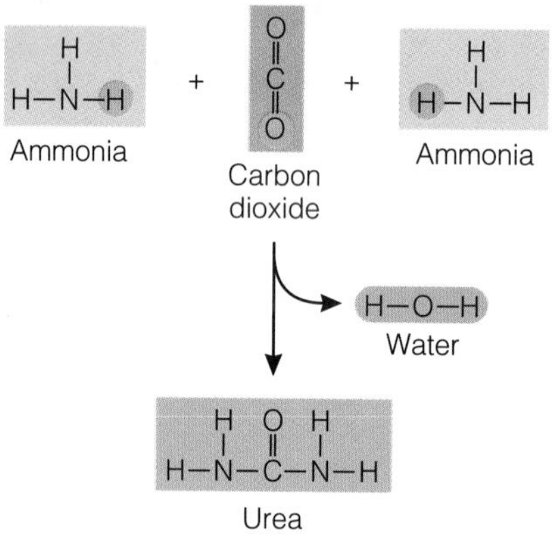
H–N–H
Ammonia
+
O=C=O
Carbon dioxide
+
H–N–H
Ammonia
H–O–H
Water
H–N–C–N–H
Urea

transamination (TRANS-am-ih-NAY-shun): the transfer of an amino group from one amino acid to a keto acid, producing a new dispensable/nonessential amino acid and a new keto acid.

urea (you-REE-uh): the principal nitrogen-excretion product of protein metabolism. Two ammonia fragments are combined with carbon dioxide to form urea.

*Chemists sometimes classify amino acids according to the destinations of their carbon fragments after deamination. If the fragment leads to the production of glucose, the amino acid is called *glucogenic;* if it leads to the formation of ketone bodies, fats, and sterols, the amino acid is called *ketogenic.* There is no sharp distinction between glucogenic and ketogenic amino acids, however. A few are both, most are considered glucogenic, only one (leucine) is clearly ketogenic.

IN SUMMARY Proteins are constantly being synthesized and broken down as needed. The body's assimilation of amino acids into proteins and its release of amino acids via protein degradation and excretion can be tracked by measuring nitrogen balance, which should be positive during growth and steady in adulthood. An energy deficit or an inadequate protein intake may force the body to use amino acids as fuel, creating a negative nitrogen balance. Protein eaten in excess of need is degraded and the remaining carbon backbones are converted to glucose or stored as body fat.

FIGURE 6-15 Urea Excretion

The liver and kidneys both play a role in disposing of excess nitrogen. Can you see why the person with liver disease has high blood ammonia, whereas the person with kidney disease has high blood urea? (Figure 12-2 provides details of how the kidneys work.)

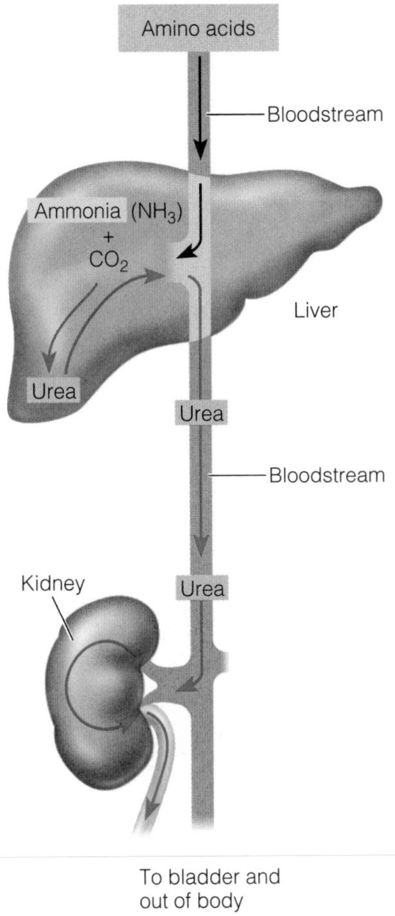
Amino acids
Bloodstream
Ammonia (NH_3)
+
CO_2
Liver
Urea
Urea
Bloodstream
Kidney
Urea
To bladder and
out of body

Protein in Foods

In Canada and the United States, where nutritious foods are abundant, most people eat protein in such large quantities that they receive all the amino acids they need. For example, while the RDA for young adult females and males is between 50 and 60 grams per day, CCHS 2.2 data reveal they consume an average of 73 and 107 grams per day, respectively. In countries where food is scarce and the people eat only marginal amounts of protein-rich foods, however, the *quality* of the protein becomes crucial.

Protein Quality

The protein quality of the diet determines, in large part, how well children grow and how well adults maintain their health. Put simply, **high-quality proteins** provide enough of all the essential amino acids needed to support the body's work, and low-quality proteins don't. Two factors influence protein quality—the protein's digestibility and its amino acid composition.

Digestibility As explained earlier, proteins must be digested before they can provide amino acids. **Protein digestibility** depends on such factors as the protein's source and the other foods eaten with it. The digestibility of most animal proteins is high (90 to 99 percent); plant proteins are less digestible (70 to 90 percent for most, but more than 90 percent for soy and legumes).

Amino Acid Composition To make proteins, a cell must have all the needed amino acids available simultaneously. The liver can make any dispensable/nonessential amino acid that may be in short supply so that the cells can continue linking amino acids into protein strands. If an indispensable/essential amino acid is missing, though, a cell must dismantle available proteins to obtain it. Therefore, to prevent protein breakdown in the body, dietary protein must supply at least the nine indispensable/essential amino acids plus enough nitrogen-containing amino groups and energy for the synthesis of the dispensable/nonessential ones. If the diet supplies too little of any essential amino acid, protein synthesis will be limited. The body makes whole proteins only; if one amino acid is missing, the others cannot form a "partial" protein. An essential amino acid supplied in less than the amount needed to support protein synthesis is called a **limiting amino acid.**

Reference Protein The quality of a food protein is determined by comparing its amino acid composition with the essential amino acid requirements of preschool-age children. Such a standard is called a **reference protein.** ♦ The rationale behind using the requirements of this age group is that if a protein will effectively support a young child's growth and development, then it will meet or exceed the requirements of older children and adults.

High-Quality Proteins As mentioned earlier, a high-quality protein contains all the indispensable/essential amino acids in relatively the same amounts and proportions that human beings require; it may or may not contain all the dispensable/nonessential amino acids. Proteins that are low in an indispensable/essential amino acid cannot, by themselves, support protein synthesis. Generally, foods derived from animals (meat, fish, poultry, cheese, eggs, yogurt, and milk) provide high-quality proteins, although gelatin is an exception. (It lacks tryptophan and cannot support growth and health as a diet's sole protein.) Proteins from plants

♦ In the past, egg protein was commonly used as the reference protein. Table D-1 in APPENDIX D presents the amino acid profile of egg. As the reference protein, egg was assigned the value of 100; Table D-3 includes scores of other food proteins for comparison.

high-quality proteins: dietary proteins containing all the indispensable/essential amino acids in relatively the same amounts that human beings require. They may also contain dispensable/nonessential amino acids.

protein digestibility: a measure of the amount of amino acids absorbed from a given protein intake.

limiting amino acid: the indispensable/essential amino acid found in the shortest supply relative to the amounts needed for protein synthesis in the body. Four amino acids are most likely to be limiting:

- Lysine
- Methionine
- Threonine
- Tryptophan

reference protein: a standard against which to measure the quality of other proteins.

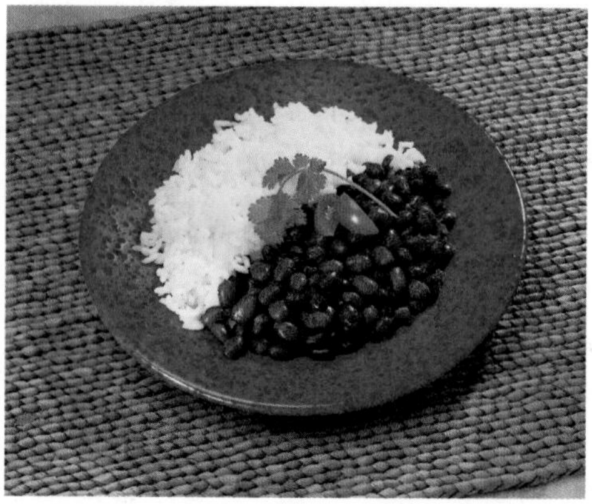

© Polara Studios, Inc.

Black beans and rice, a favourite Hispanic combination, together provide a balanced array of amino acids.

FIGURE 6-16 Complementary Proteins

In general, legumes provide plenty of isoleucine (Ile) and lysine (Lys) but fall short in methionine (Met) and tryptophan (Trp). Grains have the opposite strengths and weaknesses, making them a perfect match for legumes.

	Ile	Lys	Met	Trp
Legumes	✓	✓		
Grains			✓	✓
Together	✓	✓	✓	✓

(vegetables, nuts, seeds, grains, and legumes) have more diverse amino acid patterns and tend to be limiting in one or more indispensable/essential amino acids. Some plant proteins are notoriously low quality (e.g., corn protein). A few others are high quality (e.g., soy protein).

Researchers have developed several methods for evaluating the quality of food proteins and identifying high-quality proteins. APPENDIX D provides details.

Complementary Proteins In general, plant proteins are lower quality than animal proteins, and plants also offer less protein (per weight or measure of food). For this reason, many vegetarians improve the quality of proteins in their diets by combining plant-protein foods that have different but complementary amino acid patterns. This strategy yields **complementary proteins** that together contain all the essential amino acids in quantities sufficient to support health. The protein quality of the combination is greater than for either food alone (see Figure 6-16).

Many people have long believed that combining plant proteins at every meal is critical to protein nutrition. For most healthy vegetarians, though, it is *not* necessary to balance amino acids at each meal if the protein intake throughout the day is varied and energy intake is sufficient.[5] Vegetarians can receive all the amino acids they need over the course of a day by eating a variety of whole grains, legumes, seeds, nuts, and vegetables. Protein deficiency will develop, however, when fruits and certain vegetables make up the core of the diet, severely limiting both the *quantity* and *quality* of protein. Highlight 2 describes how to plan a nutritious vegetarian diet.

Measuring Protein Quality Researchers have developed many methods of evaluating the quality of food protein. Another important one is the **protein digestibility–corrected amino acid score (PDCAAS)**, which was used by the DRI committee to evaluate people's protein intakes. On the PDCAAS scale of 100 to 0, with 100 representing protein sources that are most readily digested and most perfectly balanced for meeting human needs, egg white, ground beef, chicken products, skim milk, and tuna all score 100. Soybean protein isn't far behind at 94, due in part, to a limited amount of certain amino acids (see Figure 6-16). Most legumes rank in the 60s and 50s. The wheat protein gluten, formed during bread making, ranks 25. Something interesting happens when pea flour (67) and whole-wheat flour (40) are combined: the score for the resulting flour is 82. Why? They are complementary proteins.

In trying to choose between peanut butter and chili in the grocery store, you may think you have no use for the PDCAAS. Although Canada does not presently have a value for %DV on our food labels, when you read the "% Daily Value" for protein listed on U.S. labels, you are using it indirectly. Manufacturers that list values for protein on food labels must use the PDCAAS to determine the protein quality of their products. Thus, protein values on labels reflect both the digestibility and the amino acid composition of the foods.

IN SUMMARY **A diet that supplies all of the indispensable/essential amino acids in adequate amounts ensures protein synthesis. The best guarantee of amino acid adequacy is to eat foods containing high-quality proteins or mixtures of foods containing complementary proteins that can each supply the amino acids missing in the other. In addition to its amino acid content, the quality of protein is measured by its digestibility and its ability to support growth. Such measures are of great importance in dealing with malnutrition worldwide, but in Canada and the United States, where protein deficiency is not common, protein quality of individual foods deserves little emphasis.**

Protein Regulations for Food Labels

All food labels must state the *quantity* of protein in grams. Food labels may also carry Nutrient Function and Nutrient Content Claims for protein provided the quantity and quality meet Health Canada's criteria that are set out in our Food and Drug Regulations.

complementary proteins: two or more dietary proteins whose amino acid assortments complement each other in such a way that the essential amino acids missing from one are supplied by the other.

protein digestibility–corrected amino acid score (PDCAAS): a measuring tool used to determine protein quality. The PDCAAS reflects a protein's digestibility as well as the proportions of amino acids that it provides.

Health Effects and Recommended Intakes of Protein and Amino Acids

As you know by now, protein is indispensable to life. It should come as no surprise that protein deficiency can have devastating effects on people's health. But, like the other nutrients, protein in excess can also be harmful. This section examines the health effects and recommended intakes of protein.

Protein-Energy Malnutrition

When people are deprived of protein, energy, or both, the result is **protein-energy malnutrition (PEM).** Although PEM touches many adult lives, it most often strikes early in childhood. It is one of the most prevalent and devastating forms of malnutrition in the world, afflicting one of every four children worldwide. Most of the 33 000 children who die each day are malnourished.[6]

Inadequate food intake leads to poor growth in children and to weight loss and wasting in adults. Children who are underweight for their height may be suffering from **acute PEM** (recent severe food deprivation), whereas children who are short for their age have experienced **chronic PEM** (long-term food deprivation). Poor growth due to PEM is easy to overlook because a small child may look quite normal, but it is the most common sign of malnutrition.

PEM is most prevalent in Africa, Central America, South America, and East and Southeast Asia. In North America, homeless people and those living in substandard housing in inner cities and rural areas have been diagnosed with PEM. In addition to those living in poverty, elderly people who live alone and adults who are addicted to drugs and alcohol are frequently victims of PEM. PEM can develop in young children when parents mistakenly provide "health-food beverages" ♦ that lack adequate energy or protein instead of milk, most commonly because of nutritional ignorance, perceived milk intolerance, or food faddism. Adult PEM is also seen in people hospitalized with infections such as AIDS or tuberculosis; these infections deplete body proteins, demand extra energy, induce nutrient losses, and alter metabolic pathways. Furthermore, poor nutrient intake during hospitalization worsens malnutrition and impairs recovery, whereas nutrition intervention often improves the body's response to other treatments and the chances of survival. PEM is also common in those suffering from the eating disorder anorexia nervosa (discussed in Highlight 8). Prevention emphasizes frequent, nutrient-dense, energy-dense meals and, equally important, resolution of the underlying causes of PEM—poverty, infections, and illness.

♦ Rice drinks are often sold as milk alternatives, but if they are not fortified they may fail to provide adequate protein, vitamins, and minerals.

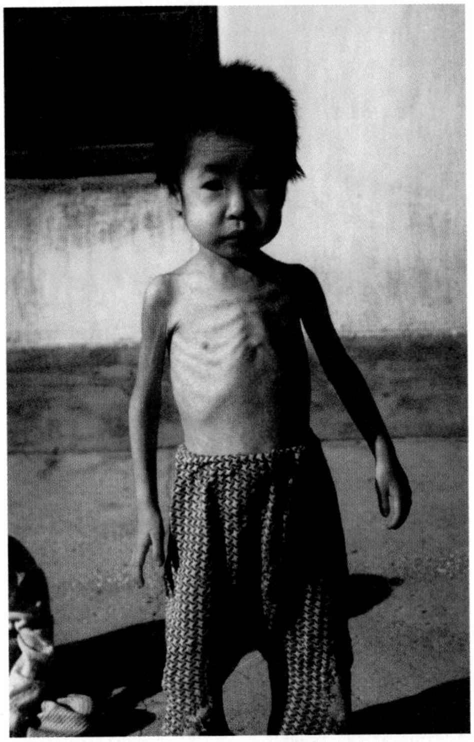

AP/Wide World Photos

The severe wasting characteristic of marasmus is apparent in this child's "matchstick" arms.

protein-energy malnutrition (PEM): a deficiency of protein, energy, or both, including kwashiorkor, marasmus, and instances in which they overlap; also called *protein-kcalorie malnutrition (PCM).*

acute PEM: protein-energy malnutrition caused by recent severe food restriction; characterized in children by underweight for height (wasting).

chronic PEM: protein-energy malnutrition caused by long-term food deprivation; characterized in children by short height for age (stunting).

TABLE 6-3 Features of Marasmus and Kwashiorkor in Children

Separating PEM into two classifications oversimplifies the condition, but at the extremes, marasmus and kwashiorkor exhibit marked differences. Marasmus-kwashiorkor mix presents symptoms common to both marasmus and kwashiorkor. In all cases, children are likely to develop diarrhea, infections, and multiple nutrient deficiencies.

Marasmus	Kwashiorkor
Infancy (less than 2 yr)	Older infants and young children (1 to 3 yr)
Severe deprivation, or impaired absorption, of protein, energy, vitamins, and minerals	Inadequate protein intake or, more commonly, infections
Develops slowly; chronic PEM	Rapid onset; acute PEM
Severe weight loss	Some weight loss
Severe muscle wasting, with no body fat	Some muscle wasting, with retention of some body fat
Growth: <60% weight-for-age	Growth: 60 to 80% weight-for-age
No detectable edema	Edema
No fatty liver	Enlarged fatty liver
Anxiety, apathy	Apathy, misery, irritability, sadness
Good appetite possible	Loss of appetite
Hair is sparse, thin, and dry; easily pulled out	Hair is dry and brittle; easily pulled out; changes colour; becomes straight
Skin is dry, thin, and easily wrinkles	Skin develops lesions

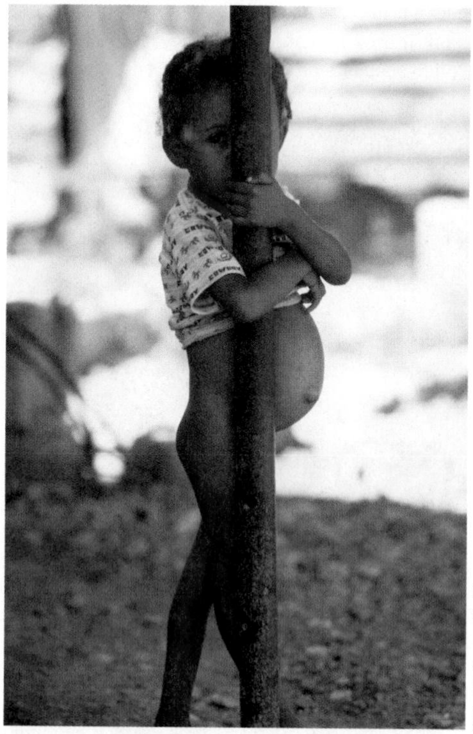

© Paul A. Souders/Corbis

The edema characteristic of kwashiorkor is apparent in this child's swollen belly. Malnourished children commonly have an enlarged abdomen from parasites as well.

Classifying PEM PEM occurs in two forms: marasmus and kwashiorkor, which differ in their clinical features (see Table 6-3 on p. 187). The following paragraphs present three clinical syndromes—marasmus, kwashiorkor, and the combination of the two.

Marasmus Appropriately named from the Greek word meaning "dying away," **marasmus** reflects a severe deprivation of food over a long time (chronic PEM). Put simply, the person is starving and suffering from an inadequate energy *and* protein intake (and inadequate essential fatty acids, vitamins, and minerals as well). Marasmus occurs most commonly in children from 6 to 18 months of age in all the overpopulated and impoverished areas of the world. Children living in poverty simply do not have enough to eat. They subsist on diluted cereal drinks that supply scant energy and protein of low quality; such food can barely sustain life, much less support growth. Consequently, marasmic children look like little old people—just "skin and bones."

Without adequate nutrition, muscles, including the heart, waste and weaken. Because the brain normally grows to almost its full adult size within the first two years of life, marasmus impairs brain development and learning ability. Reduced synthesis of key hormones slows metabolism and lowers body temperature. There is little or no fat under the skin to insulate against cold. Hospital workers find that children with marasmus need to be clothed, covered, and kept warm. Because these children often suffer delays in their mental and behavioural development, they also need loving care, a stimulating environment, and parental attention.

The starving child faces this threat to life by engaging in as little activity as possible—not even crying for food. The body musters all its forces to meet the crisis, so it cuts down on any expenditure of energy not needed for the functioning of the heart, lungs, and brain. Growth ceases; the child is no larger at age four than at age two. Enzymes are in short supply and the GI tract lining deteriorates. Consequently, what little food is eaten can't be properly digested and absorbed.

Kwashiorkor **Kwashiorkor** typically reflects a sudden and recent deprivation of food (acute PEM). *Kwashiorkor* is a Ghanaian word that refers to the birth position of a child and is used to describe the illness a child develops when the next child is born. When a mother who has been nursing her first child bears a second child, she weans the first child and puts the second one on the breast. The first child, suddenly switched from nutrient-dense, protein-rich breast milk to a starchy, protein-poor cereal, soon begins to sicken and die. Kwashiorkor typically sets in between 18 months and 2 years.

Kwashiorkor usually develops rapidly as a result of protein deficiency or, more commonly, is precipitated by an illness such as measles or other infection.[7] Other factors, such as aflatoxins (a contaminant sometimes found in mouldy grains), may also contribute to the development of, or symptoms that accompany, kwashiorkor.

The loss of weight and body fat is usually not as severe in kwashiorkor as in marasmus, but some muscle wasting may occur. Without adequate plasma proteins to maintain fluid balance, the child's limbs and abdomen become swollen with edema—a distinguishing feature of kwashiorkor. ♦ A fatty liver develops due to a lack of the protein carriers to transport lipids out of the liver. The fatty liver lacks enzymes to clear metabolic toxins from the body, so their harmful effects are prolonged. Inflammation in response to these toxins and to infections further contributes to the edema that accompanies kwashiorkor. Without sufficient tyrosine to make melanin, hair loses its colour, and inadequate protein synthesis leaves the skin patchy and scaly, often with sores that fail to heal. The lack of proteins to carry or store iron leaves iron free. Unbound iron is common in kwashiorkor and may contribute to illness and death by promoting bacterial growth and free-radical damage. (Free-radical damage is discussed fully in Highlight 12.)

♦ For this reason, kwashiorkor is sometimes referred to as "wet" PEM and marasmus as "dry" PEM.

Marasmus-Kwashiorkor Mix The combination of marasmus and kwashiorkor is characterized by the edema of kwashiorkor with the wasting of marasmus. Most often, the child suffers the effects of both malnutrition and infections.

Infections In PEM, antibodies to fight off invading bacteria are degraded to provide amino acids for other uses, leaving the malnourished child vulnerable to infections.

marasmus (ma-RAZ-mus): a form of PEM that results from a severe deprivation, or impaired absorption, of energy, protein, vitamins, and minerals.

kwashiorkor (kwash-ee-OR-core, kwash-ee-or-CORE): a form of PEM that results from inadequate protein intake and infections.

Blood proteins, including hemoglobin, are no longer synthesized, so the child becomes anemic and weak. **Dysentery**, an infection of the digestive tract, causes diarrhea, further depleting the body of nutrients and fluids. In the marasmic child, once infection sets in, kwashiorkor often follows, and the immune response weakens further.

The combination of infections, fever, fluid imbalances, and anemia often leads to heart failure and occasionally sudden death. Infections combined with malnutrition are responsible for two-thirds of the deaths of young children in developing countries. Measles, which might make a healthy child sick for a week or two, kills a child with PEM within two or three days.

Rehabilitation If caught in time, the life of a starving child may be saved with rehydration and nutrition intervention.[8] In severe cases, diarrhea will have incurred dramatic fluid and mineral losses that need to be replaced during the first 24 to 48 hours to help raise the blood pressure and strengthen the heartbeat. After that, protein and food energy may be given in *small* quantities several times a day, with intakes *gradually* increased as tolerated.[9] Severely malnourished people, especially those with edema, recover better with an initial diet that is relatively low in protein (10 percent of energy intake).

Experts assure us that we possess the knowledge, technology, and resources to end hunger. Programs that tailor interventions to the local people and involve them in the process of identifying problems and devising solutions have the most success. To win the war on hunger, those who have the food, technology, and resources must make fighting hunger a priority (see Chapter 21 for more on hunger).

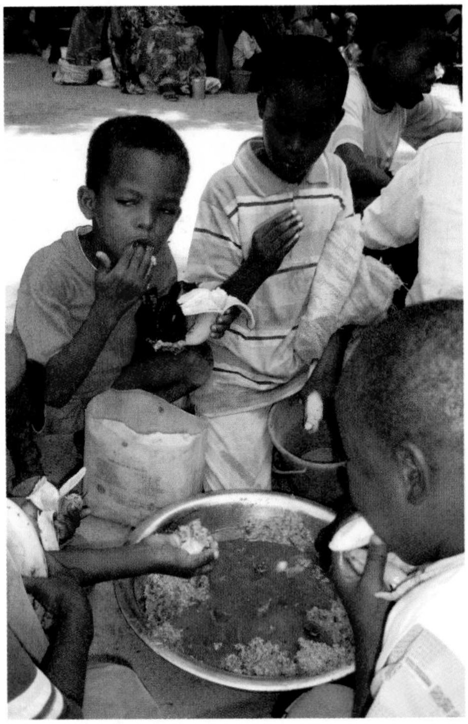

AP Photo/Mohamed Sheikh Nor/CP Images

Donated food saves some people from starvation, but it is usually insufficient to meet nutrient needs or even to defend against hunger.

Health Effects of Protein

While many of the world's people struggle to obtain enough food energy and protein, in developed countries both are so abundant that problems of excess are seen. Overconsumption of protein offers no benefits and may pose health risks. High-protein diets have been implicated in several chronic diseases, including heart disease, cancer, osteoporosis, obesity, and kidney stones, but evidence is insufficient to establish an Upper Level (UL).[10]

Researchers attempting to clarify the relationships between excess protein and chronic diseases face several obstacles. Population studies have difficulty determining whether diseases correlate with animal proteins or with their accompanying saturated fats, for example. Studies that rely on data from vegetarians must sort out the many lifestyle factors, in addition to a "no-meat diet," that might explain relationships between protein and health.

Heart Disease A high-protein diet may contribute to the progression of heart disease. As Chapter 5 mentions, foods rich in animal protein also tend to be rich in saturated fats. Consequently, it is not surprising to find a correlation between animal-protein intake (red meats and dairy products) and heart disease.[11] On the other hand, substituting vegetable protein for animal protein may improve blood lipids and decrease heart disease mortality.[12]

Research suggests that elevated levels of the amino acid homocysteine may be an independent risk factor for heart disease, heart attacks, and sudden death in patients with heart disease.[13] Researchers do not yet fully understand the many factors—including a diet high in saturated fatty acids—that can raise homocysteine in the blood or whether elevated levels are a cause or an effect of heart disease.[14] Elevated homocysteine is associated with increased oxidative stress and inflammation.[15] Until researchers can determine the exact role homocysteine plays in heart disease, they are following several leads in pursuit of the answers. Coffee's role in heart disease has been controversial, but research suggests it is among the most influential factors in raising homocysteine, which may explain some of the adverse health effects of heavy consumption.[16] Elevated homocysteine levels are among the many adverse health consequences of smoking cigarettes and drinking alcohol as well.[17] Homocysteine is also elevated with inadequate intakes of B vitamins and can usually be lowered with fortified foods or supplements of vitamin B_{12}, vitamin B_6, and folate.[18] Lowering homocysteine, however, may not help in preventing heart attacks.[19] Supplements of the B vitamins do not always benefit those with heart disease and, in fact, may actually increase the risks.[20]

dysentery (DISS-en-terry): an infection of the digestive tract that causes diarrhea.

In contrast to homocysteine, the amino acid arginine may help protect against heart disease by lowering blood pressure and homocysteine levels.[21] Additional research is needed to confirm the benefits of arginine. In the meantime, it is unwise for consumers to use supplements of arginine, or any other amino acid for that matter (as pp. 193–194 explain). Physicians may find it beneficial to add arginine supplements to their heart patients' treatment plan; however, Health Canada has advised that those who have had a heart attack should not consume arginine supplements because a recent study indicated there was a potential increased risk of death after such an event.[22]

♦ Processed meats include ham, bacon, pastrami, salami, sausage, bratwurst, and hot dogs; they have been preserved by smoking, curing, salting, or adding preservatives.

Cancer Protein does not seem to increase the risk of cancer, but some protein-rich foods do. For example, evidence suggests a strong correlation between high intakes of red meat and processed meats ♦ with cancer of the colon. Chapter 19 discusses dietary links with cancer, and Chapter 20 presents food-safety issues of processed meats.

Adult Bone Loss (Osteoporosis) Chapter 13 presents calcium metabolism, and Highlight 13 elaborates on the main factors that influence osteoporosis. This section briefly describes the relationships between protein intake and bone loss. When protein intake is high, calcium excretion increases. Whether excess protein depletes the bones of their chief mineral may depend upon the ratio of calcium intake to protein intake. After all, bones need both protein and calcium. An ideal ratio has not been determined, but a young woman whose intake meets recommendations for both nutrients has a calcium-to-protein ratio of more than 20 to 1 (milligrams to grams), which probably provides adequate protection for the bones. For most women in North America, however, average calcium intakes are lower and protein intakes are higher, yielding a 9-to-1 ratio, which may produce calcium losses significant enough to compromise bone health. In other words, the problem may reflect too little calcium, not too much protein. In establishing recommendations, the DRI Committee considered protein's effect on calcium metabolism and bone health, but it did not find sufficient evidence to warrant an adjustment for calcium or a UL for protein.[23]

Some (but not all) research suggests that animal protein may be more detrimental to calcium metabolism and bone health than vegetable protein.[24] Importantly, *inadequate* intakes of protein may compromise bone health. Osteoporosis is particularly common in elderly women and in adolescents with anorexia nervosa—groups who typically receive less protein than they need. For these people, increasing protein intake may be just what they need to protect their bones. It would also be prudent for these individuals to ensure adequate intakes of other important nutrients, including calcium and vitamin D.[25]

Weight Control Fad weight-loss diets that encourage a high-protein, low-carbohydrate diet may be effective, but only because they are low-kcalorie diets. Diets that provide adequate protein, moderate fat, and sufficient energy from carbohydrates can better support weight loss and good health. Including protein at each meal may help with weight loss by providing satiety.[26] Selecting too many protein-rich foods, such as meat and milk, may crowd out fruits, vegetables, and whole grains, making the diet inadequate in other nutrients and fibre.

Kidney Disease Excretion of the end products of protein metabolism depends, in part, on an adequate fluid intake and healthy kidneys. A high protein intake does not cause kidney disease, but it does increase the work of the kidneys and accelerate kidney deterioration in people with chronic kidney disease.[27] Restricting dietary protein may help to slow the progression of kidney disease in people who have this condition.[28]

IN SUMMARY **Protein deficiencies arise from both energy-poor and protein-poor diets and lead to the devastating diseases of marasmus and kwashiorkor. Together, these diseases are known as PEM (protein-energy malnutrition), a major form of malnutrition causing death in children worldwide. Excesses of protein offer no advantage; in fact, overconsumption of protein-rich foods may incur health problems as well.**

HOW TO Calculate Recommended Protein Intakes

To figure your protein RDA:

- Look up the healthy weight for a person of your height (inside back cover). If your present weight falls within that range, use it for the following calculations. If your present weight falls outside the range, use the midpoint of the healthy weight range as your reference weight.
- Convert pounds to kilograms, if necessary (pounds divided by 2.2 equals kilograms).
- Multiply kilograms by 0.8 to get your RDA in grams per day. (Teens 14 to 18 years old, multiply by 0.85.) Example:

$$\text{Weight} = 150 \text{ lb}$$

$$150 \text{ lb} \div 2.2 \text{ lb/kg} = 68 \text{ kg (rounded off)}$$

$$68 \text{ kg} \times 0.8 \text{ g/kg} = 54 \text{ g protein (rounded off)}$$

CENGAGENOW™
For additional practice log on to **www.cengage.com/sso**, go to Chapter 6, then to How to Calculate Recommended Protein Intakes.

TRY IT Calculate your protein RDA.

Recommended Intakes of Protein and Amino Acids

As mentioned earlier, the body continuously breaks down and loses some protein and cannot store amino acids. To replace protein, the body needs dietary protein for two reasons. First, dietary protein is the only source of the *indispensable/essential* amino acids, and second, it is a major source of *nitrogen* with which to build the dispensable/nonessential amino acids and other nitrogen-containing compounds the body needs.

Given recommendations that people's fat intakes should contribute 20 to 35 percent of total food energy and carbohydrate intakes should contribute 45 to 65 percent, that leaves 10 to 35 percent for protein. In a 2000-kcalorie diet, that represents 200 to 700 kcalories from protein, or 50 to 175 grams. Average intakes of young adults in Canada and the United States fall within this range.

Protein RDA The protein RDA ♦ for adults is 0.8 grams per kilogram of healthy body weight per day. For infants and children, the RDA is slightly higher. The table on the inside front cover lists the RDA for males and females at various ages in two ways—grams per day based on reference body weights and grams per kilogram body weight per day. Some evidence suggests that intakes greater than the protein RDA may be beneficial.[29]

♦ RDA for protein:
- 0.8 g/kg/day
- 10 to 35% of energy intake

The RDA covers the needs for replacing worn-out tissue, so it increases for larger people; it also covers the needs for building new tissue during growth, so it increases for infants, children, adolescents, and pregnant and lactating women. The protein RDA is the same for lightly active athletes as for others, even though more active athletes may need more protein and many fitness authorities recommend a higher range of protein intakes for athletes pursuing different activities ♦ (see Table 15-5 in Chapter 15 for details).[30] Even so, "higher" intakes still fall within the 10 to 35 percent Acceptable Macronutrient Distribution Range (AMDR).[31] The accompanying "How To" explains how to calculate your RDA for protein.

♦ Protein recommendations for athletes: 1.2–1.7 g/kg/day

In setting the RDA, the DRI Committee assumes that people are healthy and do not have unusual metabolic needs for protein, that the protein eaten will be of mixed quality (from both high- and low-quality sources), and that the body will use the protein efficiently. In addition, the committee assumes that the protein is consumed along with sufficient carbohydrate and fat to provide adequate energy and that other nutrients in the diet are also adequate.

Adequate Energy Note the qualification "adequate energy" in the preceding statement, and consider what happens if energy intake falls short of needs. An intake of 50 grams of protein provides 200 kcalories, which represents 10 percent of the total energy from protein, if the person receives 2000 kcalories a day. But

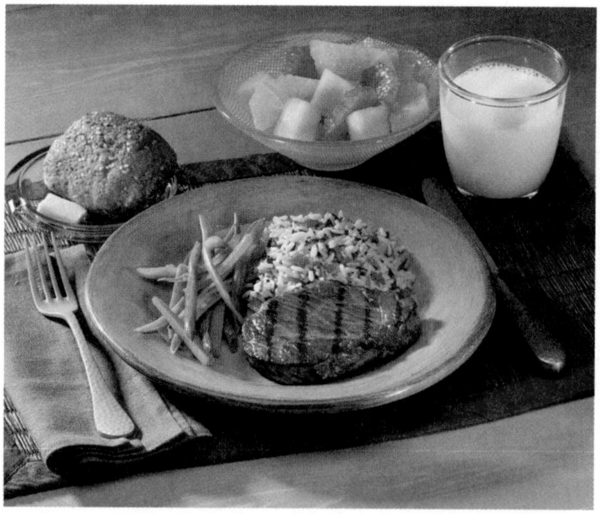
© Polara Studios, Inc.

For many people, this 150 gram steak provides almost all of the meat and much of the protein recommended for a day's intake.

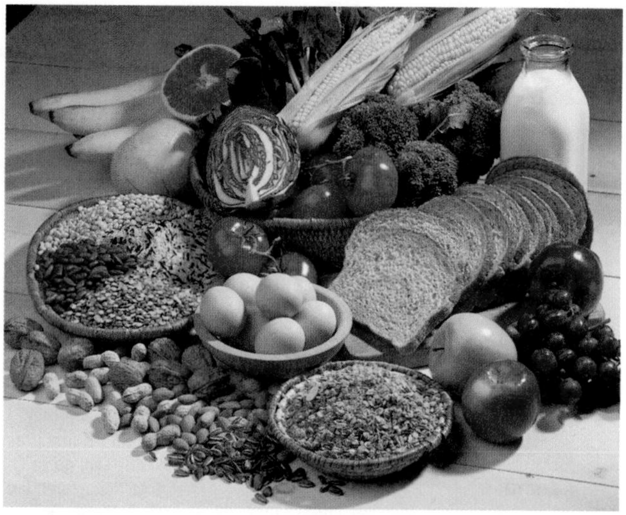
© Polara Studios, Inc.

Vegetarians obtain their protein from whole grains, legumes, nuts, vegetables, and, in some cases, eggs and milk products.

if the person cuts energy intake drastically—to, say, 800 kcalories a day—then an intake of 200 kcalories from protein is suddenly 25 percent of the total; yet it's still the same amount of protein (number of grams). The protein intake is reasonable, but the energy intake is not. The low energy intake forces the body to use the protein to meet energy needs rather than to replace lost body protein. Similarly, if the person's energy intake is high—say, 4000 kcalories—the 50 gram protein intake represents only 5 percent of the total; yet it *still* is a reasonable protein intake. Again, the energy intake is unreasonable for most people, but in this case, it permits the protein to be used to meet the body's needs.

Be careful when judging protein (or carbohydrate or fat) intake as a percentage of energy. Always consider the number of grams as well, and compare it with the RDA or another standard stated in grams. A recommendation stated as a percentage of energy intake is useful only if the energy intake is within reason.

Protein in Abundance Most people in Canada and the United States receive more protein than they need. Even athletes in training typically don't need to increase their protein intakes because the additional foods they eat to meet their high-energy needs deliver protein as well. (Chapter 15 provides full details on the energy and protein needs of athletes.) That protein intake is high is not surprising considering the abundance of food eaten and the central role meats hold in the North American diet. A 30 gram serving of meat (or 125 mL/½ cup legumes) delivers about 7 grams of protein, so a 240 gram portion of meat alone supply more than the RDA for an average-size person. Besides meat, well-fed people eat many other nutritious foods, many of which also provide protein. A cup of milk (250 mL) provides 8 grams of protein. Grains and vegetables provide small amounts of protein, but they can add up to significant quantities; fruits and fats provide no protein.

To illustrate how easy it is to overconsume protein, consider the amounts recommended by *Canada's Food Guide* for a 2000-kcalorie diet: 180 grams of grains provide about 18 grams of protein; 625 millilitres (2½ cups) of vegetables deliver about 10 grams; 750 millilitres (3 cups) of milk offer 24 grams; and 200 grams of meat supply 38 grams. This totals 90 grams of protein—higher than the protein RDA for most people and yet still lower than the average intake of most young adults in Canada.

People in Canada and the United States typically get more protein than they need. If they have an adequate *food* intake, they have a more-than-adequate protein intake. The key diet-planning principle to emphasize for protein is moderation. Even though most people receive plenty of protein, some feel compelled to take supplements as well, as the next section describes.

IN SUMMARY **The optimal diet is adequate in energy from carbohydrate and fat and delivers 0.8 grams of protein per kilogram of healthy body weight each day. Canadian and U.S. diets are typically more than adequate in this respect.**

Protein and Amino Acid Supplements Websites, health-food stores, and popular magazine articles advertise a wide variety of protein supplements, and people take these supplements for many different reasons. Athletes take protein powders to build muscle. Dieters take them to spare their bodies' protein while losing weight. Women take them to strengthen their fingernails. People take individual amino acids, too—to cure herpes, to make themselves sleep better, to lose weight, and to relieve pain and depression.* Like many other magic solutions to health problems, protein and amino acid supplements ♦ don't work these miracles. Furthermore, they may be harmful.

♦ Use of amino acids as dietary supplements is *inappropriate,* especially for:
- All women of childbearing age
- Pregnant or lactating women
- Infants, children, and adolescents
- Elderly people
- People with inborn errors of metabolism that affect their bodies' handling of amino acids
- Smokers
- People on low-protein diets
- People with chronic or acute mental or physical illnesses who take amino acids without medical supervision

Protein Powders Because the body builds muscle protein from amino acids, many athletes take protein powders with the false hope of stimulating muscle growth. Muscle work builds muscle; protein supplements do not, and athletes do not need them. Taking protein supplements does not improve athletic performance.[32] (Highlight 15 presents more information on other supplements athletes commonly use.) Protein powders can supply amino acids to the body, but nature's protein sources—lean meat, milk, eggs, and legumes—supply all these amino acids and more.

Whey and casein ♦ **protein** appear to be particularly popular among athletes hoping to achieve greater muscle gains. A waste product of cheese manufacturing, whey protein is a common ingredient in many low-cost protein powders. When combined with strength training, whey supplements may increase protein synthesis slightly, but they do not seem to enhance athletic performance. To build stronger muscles, athletes need to eat food with adequate energy and protein to support the weight-training work that does increase muscle mass. Those who still think they need more whey can drink a glass of milk; 250 millilitres (1 cup) provides 1.5 grams of whey.

♦ Casein Protein: Isolated casein protein is more slowly absorbed than isolated whey protein, however, manufacturers are now producing blends of both whey and casein. Also, those with allergies to milk protein need to be mindful of the fact that these proteins may be isolated from milk.

Purified protein preparations contain none of the other nutrients needed to support the building of muscle, and the protein they supply is not needed by athletes who eat food. It is excess protein, and the body dismantles it and uses it for energy or stores it as body fat. The deamination of excess amino acids places an extra burden on the liver as well as the kidneys to excrete unused nitrogen.

Amino Acid Supplements Single amino acids do not occur naturally in foods and offer no benefit to the body; in fact, they may be harmful. The body was not designed to handle the high concentrations and unusual combinations of amino acids found in supplements. Large doses of amino acids cause diarrhea.[33] An excess of one amino acid can create such a demand for a carrier that it limits the absorption of another amino acid, presenting the possibility of a deficiency. Those amino acids winning the competition enter in excess, creating the possibility of toxicity. Toxicity of single amino acids in animal studies raises concerns about their use in human beings. Anyone considering taking amino acid supplements should be cautious not to exceed levels normally found in foods.[34]

Most healthy athletes eating well-balanced diets do not need amino acid supplements. Advertisers point to research that identifies the **branched-chain amino acids** ♦ as the main ones used as fuel by exercising muscles. What the ads leave out is that compared to glucose and fatty acids, branched-chain amino acids provide very little fuel and that ordinary foods provide them in abundance anyway. Large doses of branched-chain amino acids can raise plasma ammonia concentrations, which can be toxic to the brain. Branched-chain amino acid supplements may be beneficial in conditions such as liver disease, but otherwise, they are not routinely recommended.[35]

♦ The branched-chain amino acids are leucine, isoleucine, and valine.

In two cases, recommendations for single amino acid supplements have led to widespread public use—lysine to prevent or relieve the infections that cause herpes cold sores on the mouth or genital organs, and tryptophan to relieve pain, depression, and insomnia. In both cases, enthusiastic popular reports preceded careful scientific experiments and health recommendations. Research is insufficient to determine whether lysine suppresses herpes infections, but it appears safe (up to 3 grams per day) when taken in divided doses with meals.[36]

whey protein: a by-product of cheese production; falsely promoted as increasing muscle mass. Whey is the watery part of milk that separates from the curds.

branched-chain amino acids: the essential amino acids leucine, isoleucine, and valine, which are present in large amounts in skeletal muscle tissue; falsely promoted as fuel for exercising muscles.

*Canada allows only single amino acid supplements to be sold as Natural Health Products or used as food additives.

Tryptophan may be effective with respect to pain and sleep, but its use for these purposes is experimental. About 20 years ago, more than 1500 people who elected to take tryptophan supplements developed a rare blood disorder known as eosinophilia-myalgia syndrome (EMS). EMS is characterized by severe muscle and joint pain, extremely high fever, and, in more than three dozen cases, death. Treatment for EMS usually involves physical therapy and low doses of corticosteroids to relieve symptoms temporarily. Both Health Canada and the U.S. Food and Drug Administration implicated impurities in the supplements, issued a recall of all products containing manufactured tryptophan, and warned that high-dose supplements of tryptophan might provoke symptoms of EMS even in the absence of impurities.[37]

IN SUMMARY **Normal, healthy people never need protein or amino acid supplements. It is safest to obtain lysine, tryptophan, arginine, and all other amino acids from protein-rich foods, eaten with abundant carbohydrate and some fat to facilitate their use in the body. With all that we know about science, it is hard to improve on nature.**

Nutrition Portfolio

Foods that derive from animals—meats, fish, poultry, eggs, and milk products—provide plenty of protein but are often accompanied by fat. Those that derive from plants—whole grains, vegetables, and legumes—may provide less protein but also less fat.

Go to Diet Analysis Plus and choose one of the days on which you have tracked your diet for the entire day. Go to the Intake Spreadsheet report. Scroll down until you see: protein (g).

- Which of your food choices provided you with the most protein on that day? Does that food also have a lot of fat? Refer to the fat (g) column for this information.
- Describe your dietary sources of proteins and whether you use mostly plant-based or animal-based protein foods in your diet.

Now take a look at the Intake vs. Goals report.

- How do your protein needs compare with your protein intake? Consider whether you receive enough, but not too much, protein daily. Remember, 100 percent means your intake is meeting your needs based on your intake and profile information.
- If your protein intake exceeds 100 percent, consider the possible negative consequences of a high protein intake over many years.
- Debate the risks and benefits of taking protein or amino acid supplements.

Diet Analysis PLUS **To complete this exercise, go to your Diet Analysis Plus at www.cengage.com/sso.**

Nutrition on the Net

CENGAGENOW™
For further study of topics covered in this chapter, log on to **www.cengage.com/sso.**

- Learn more from Health Canada about how well Canadians are doing in terms of protein intake: **www.hc-sc.gc.ca/fn-an/surveill/nutrition/commun/art-nutr-eng.php#a3**
- Learn more about sickle-cell anemia from the U.S. National Heart, Lung, and Blood Institute or the Sickle Cell Disease Association of America: **www.nhlbi.nih.gov** or **www.sicklecelldisease.org**
- Learn more about protein-energy malnutrition and world hunger from the World Health Organization Nutrition Programme or the U.S. National Institute of Child Health and Human Development: **www.who.int/nutrition/en** or **www.nichd.nih.gov**
- Chapter 21 offers many more websites on malnutrition and world hunger.

References

1. M. T. Gladwin and E. Vichinsky, Pulmonary complications of sickle cell disease, *New England Journal of Medicine* 359 (2008): 2254–2265; F. J. Kirkham, Therapy insight: Stroke risk and its management in patients with sickle cell disease, *Nature Clinical Practice. Neurology* 3 (2007): 264–278.
2. M. K. C. Hesselink, R. Minnaard, and P. Schrauwen, Eat the meat or feed the meat: Protein turnover in remodeling muscle, *Current Opinion in Clinical Nutrition and Metabolic Care* 9 (2006): 672–676.
3. Health Canada, Food and Nutrition, Food allergen labelling. www.hc-sc.gc.ca/fn-an/label-etiquet/allergen/index-eng.php, accessed September 1, 2011.
4. Canadian Food Inspection Agency, Allergen labelling information for manufacturers and importers of cereal grain-based products (May 20, 2011). www.inspection.gc.ca/english/fssa/labeti/allerg/20110520inde.shtml, accessed September 1, 2011.
5. Position of the American Dietetic Association, Vegetarian diets, *Journal of the American Dietetic Association* 109:7 (2009): 1266–1282.
6. Data from www.unicef.org, posted April 2005 and May 2006.
7. N. S. Scrimshaw, Fifty-five-year personal experience with human nutrition worldwide, *Annual Review of Nutrition* 27 (2007): 1–18.
8. J. F. Desjeux, Recent issues in energy-protein malnutrition in children, *Nestlé Nutrition Workshop Series: Pediatric Program* 58 (2006): 177–184.
9. D. R. Brewster, Critical appraisal of the management of severe malnutrition: 2. Dietary management, *Journal of Paediatrics and Child Health* 42 (2006): 575–582; A. A. Jackson, A. Ashworth, and S. Khanum, Improving child survival: Malnutrition Task Force and the paediatrician's responsibility, *Archives of Diseases in Childhood* 91 (2006): 706–710.
10. Committee on Dietary Reference Intakes, *Dietary Reference Intakes for Energy, Carbohydrate, Fiber, Fat, Fatty Acids, Cholesterol, Protein, and Amino Acids* (Washington, D.C.: National Academies Press, 2005), p. 694.
11. L. E. Kelemen and coauthors, Associations of dietary protein with disease and mortality in a prospective study of postmenopausal women, *American Journal of Epidemiology* 161 (2005): 239–249.
12. N. R. Matthan and coauthors, Effect of soy protein from differently processed products on cardiovascular disease risk factors and vascular endothelial function in hypercholesterolemic subjects, *American Journal of Clinical Nutrition* 85 (2007): 960–966; B. L. McVeigh and coauthors, Effect of soy protein varying in isoflavone content on serum lipids in healthy young men, *American Journal of Clinical Nutrition* 83 (2006): 244–251; Kelemen and coauthors, 2005.
13. M. Haim and coauthors, Serum homocysteine and long-term risk of myocardial infarction and sudden death in patients with coronary heart disease, *Cardiology* 107 (2006): 52–56; M. B. Kazemi and coauthors, Homocysteine level and coronary artery disease, *Angiology* 57 (2006): 9–14.
14. P. Berstad and coauthors, Dietary fat and plasma total homocysteine concentrations in 2 adult age groups: The Hordaland Homocysteine Study, *American Journal of Clinical Nutrition* 85 (2007): 1598–1605; J. Selhub, The many facets of hyperhomocysteinemia: Studies from the Framingham cohorts, *Journal of Nutrition* 136 (2006): 1726S–1730S.
15. C. Antoniades and coauthors, Asymmetrical dimethylarginine regulates endothelial function in methionine-induced but not in chronic homocystinemia in humans: Effect of oxidative stress and proinflammatory cytokines, *American Journal of Clinical Nutrition* 84 (2006): 781–788.
16. S. E. Chiuve and coauthors, Alcohol intake and methylenetetrahydrofolate reductase polymorphism modify the relation of folate intake to plasma homocysteine, *American Journal of Clinical Nutrition* 82 (2005): 155–162.
17. J. A. Troughton and coauthors, Homocysteine and coronary heart disease risk in the PRIME study, *Atherosclerosis* 191(2006): 90–97; Chiuve and coauthors, 2005.
18. T. J. Green and coauthors, Lowering homocysteine with B vitamins has no effect on biomarkers of bone turnover in older persons: A 2-y randomized controlled trial, *American Journal of Clinical Nutrition* 85 (2007): 460–464; D. Genser and coauthors, Homocysteine, folate and vitamin B_{12} in patients with coronary heart disease, *Annals of Nutrition & Metabolism* 50 (2006): 413–419; D. S. Wald and coauthors, Folic acid, homocysteine, and cardiovascular disease: Judging causality in the face of inconclusive trial evidence, *British Medical Journal* 333 (2006): 1114–1117.
19. B-Vitamin Treatment Trialists' Collaboration, Homocysteine-lowering trials for prevention of cardiovascular events: A review of the design and power of the large randomized trials, *American Heart Journal* 151 (2006): 282–287.
20. C. Baigent and R. Clarke, B Vitamins for the prevention of vascular diseases: Insufficient evidence to justify treatment, *Journal of the American Medical Association* 298 (2007): 1212–1214; R. L. Jamison and coauthors, Effect of homocysteine lowering on mortality and vascular disease in advanced chronic kidney disease and end-stage renal disease: A randomized controlled trial, *Journal of the American Medical Association* 298 (2007): 1163–1170; L. A. Bazzano and coauthors, Effect of folic acid supplementation on risk of cardiovascular diseases: A meta-analysis of randomized controlled trials, *Journal of the American Medical Association* 296 (2006): 2720–2726; K. H. Bonaa and coauthors, Homocysteine lowering and cardiovascular events after acute myocardial infarction, *New England Journal of Medicine* 354 (2006): 1578–1588; C. M. Carlsson, Homocysteine lowering with folic acid and vitamin B supplements: Effects on cardiovascular disease in older adults, *Drugs and Aging* 23 (2006): 491–502; E. Lonn and coauthors, Homocysteine lowering with folic acid and B vitamins in vascular disease, *New England Journal of Medicine* 354 (2006): 1567–1577.
21. S. G. West and coauthors, Oral L-arginine improves hemodynamic responses to stress and reduces plasma homocysteine in hypercholesterolemic men, *Journal of Nutrition* 135 (2005): 212–217.
22. B. S. Kendler, Supplemental conditionally essential nutrients in cardiovascular disease therapy, *Journal of Cardiovascular Nursing* 21 (2006): 9–16; Health Canada, Health Canada advises heart patients not to use products containing L-arginine. www.hc-sc.gc.ca/ahc-asc/media/advisories-avis/_2006/2006_30-eng.php, accessed June 17, 2011.
23. Committee on Dietary Reference Intakes, 2005, p. 841; Committee on Dietary Reference Intakes, *Dietary Reference Intakes for Calcium, Phosphorus, Magnesium, Vitamin D, and Fluoride* (Washington, D.C.: National Academies Press, 1997), pp. 75–76.
24. J. P. Bonjour, Dietary protein: An essential nutrient for bone health, *Journal of the American College of Nutrition* 24 (2005): 526S–536S; C. Weikert and coauthors, The relation between dietary protein, calcium and bone health in women: Results from the EPIC-Potsdam cohort, *Annals of Nutrition & Metabolism* 49 (2005): 312–318.
25. A. D. Conigrave, E. M. Brown, and R. Rizzoli, Dietary protein and bone health: Roles of amino acid-sensing receptors in the control of calcium metabolism and bone homeostasis, *Annual Review of Nutrition* 28 (2008): 131–155; A. Devine and coauthors, Protein consumption is an important predictor of lower limb bone mass in elderly women, *American Journal of Clinical Nutrition* 81 (2005): 1423–1428.
26. R. F. Kushner and B. Doerfler, Low-carbohydrate, high-protein diets revisited, *Current Opinion in Gastroenterology* 24 (2008): 198–203; A. Astrup, The satiating power of protein—A key to obesity prevention? *American Journal of Clinical Nutrition* 82 (2005): 1–2; D. S. Weigle and coauthors, A high-protein diet induces sustained reductions in appetite, ad libitum caloric intake, and body weight despite compensatory changes in diurnal plasma leptin and ghrelin concentrations, *American Journal of Clinical Nutrition* 82 (2005): 41–48.
27. A. M. Bernstein, L. Treyzon, and Z. Li, Are high-protein, vegetable-based diets safe for kidney function? A review of the literature, *Journal of the American Dietetic Association* 107 (2007): 644–650.
28. R. Pecoits-Filho, Dietary protein intake and kidney disease in Western diet, *Contributions to Nephrology* 155 (2007): 102–112; S. Mandayam and W. E. Mitch, Dietary protein restriction benefits patients with chronic kidney disease, *Nephrology* 11 (2006): 53–57.
29. R. R. Wolfe and S. L. Miller, The recommended dietary allowance of protein: A misunderstood concept, *Journal of the American Medical Association* 299 (2008): 2891–2893.
30. Position of the American Dietetic Association, Dietitians of Canada, and the American College of Sports Medicine, Nutrition and athletic performance, *Journal of the American Dietetic Association* 109 (2009): 509–527; S. M. Phillips, Dietary protein for athletes: From requirements to metabolic advantage, *Applied Physiology, Nutrition, and Metabolism* 31 (2006): 647–654.

31. S. M. Phillips, Dietary protein for athletes: From requirements to metabolic advantage, *Applied Physiology, Nutrition, and Metabolism* 31 (2006): 647–654.
32. L. L. Andersen and coauthors, The effect of resistance training combined with timed ingestion of protein on muscle fiber size and muscle strength, *Metabolism: Clinical and Experimental* 54 (2005): 151–156.
33. G. K. Grimble, Adverse gastrointestinal effects of arginine and related amino acids, *Journal of Nutrition* 137 (2007): 1693S–1701S.
34. *Dietary Reference Intakes—The Essential Guide to Nutrient Requirements* (Washington, D.C.: National Academies Press, 2006), p. 152.
35. S. Takeshita and coauthors, A snack enriched with oral branched-chain amino acids prevents a fall in albumin in patients with liver cirrhosis undergoing chemoembolization for hepatocellular carcinoma, *Nutrition Research* 29 (2009): 89–93; T. Kawaguchi and coauthors, Branched-chain amino acid–enriched supplementation improves insulin resistance in patients with chronic liver disease, *International Journal of Molecular Medicine* (2008): 105–112; S. Khanna and S. Gopalan, Role of branched-chain amino acids in liver disease: The evidence for and against, *Current Opinion in Clinical Nutrition and Metabolic Care* (2007): 297–303; M. Charlton, Branched-chain amino acid enriched supplements as therapy for liver disease, *Journal of Nutrition* 136 (2006): 295S–298S; Y. Shimomura and coauthors, Branched-chain amino acid catabolism in exercise and liver disease, *Journal of Nutrition* 136 (2006): 250S–253S.
36. M. M. Perfect and coauthors, Use of complementary and alternative medicine for the treatment of genital herpes, *Herpes* 12 (2005): 38–41.
37. Health Canada, Food and Nutrition, Frequently asked questions—Biotechnology and Genetically Modified Foods. www.hc-sc.gc.ca/fn-an/gmf-agm/fs-if/faq_4-eng.php#a11, accessed September 3, 2011; M. J. Smith and R. H. Garrett, A heretofore undisclosed crux of eosinophilia-myalgia syndrome: Compromised histamine degradation, *Inflammation Research* 54 (2005): 435–450.

HIGHLIGHT 6

Nutritional Genomics

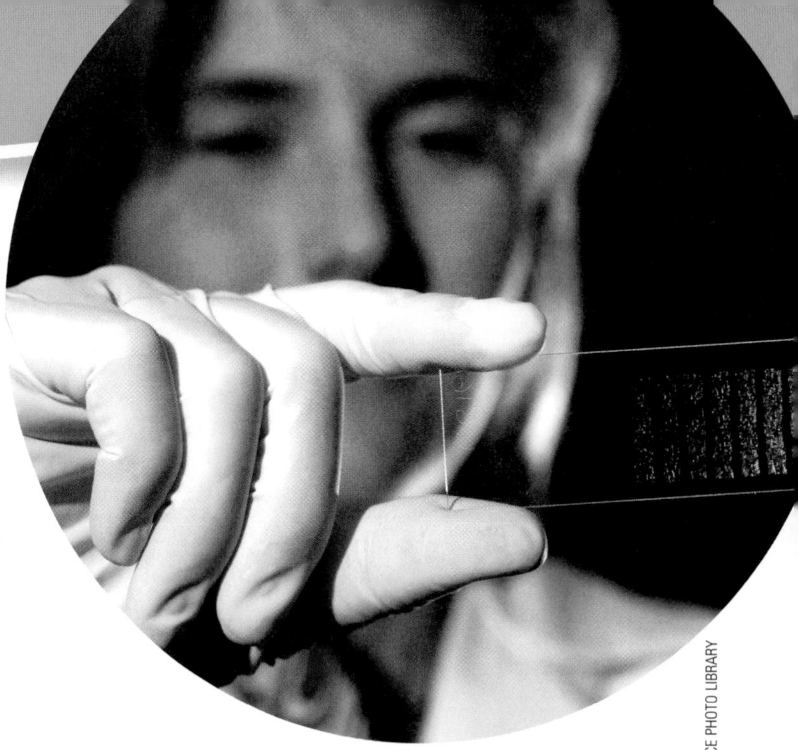
PATRICK DUMAS/EURELIOS/SCIENCE PHOTO LIBRARY

Imagine this scenario: A physician scrapes a sample of cells from inside your cheek and submits it to a **genomics** lab. The lab returns a report based on your genetic profile that reveals which diseases you are most likely to develop and makes recommendations for specific diet and lifestyle changes that can help you maintain good health. You may also be given a prescription for a dietary supplement that will best meet your personal nutrient requirements. Such a scenario may one day become reality as scientists uncover the relationships between **genetics,** diet, and disease. Until then, however, consumers need to know that current genetic test kits commonly available on the Internet are unproven and may create more problems than they resolve.[1]

Figure H6-1 (p. 198) introduces **nutritional genomics,** a new field of study that examines how nutrients influence gene activity (*nutrigenomics*) and how **genes** influence the activities of nutrients (*nutrigenetics*).[2] The accompanying glossary defines related terms.

Unlike sciences in the 20th century, nutritional genomics takes a comprehensive approach in analyzing information from several fields of study, providing an integrated understanding of the findings.[3] Consider how multiple disciplines contributed to our understanding of vitamin A over the past several decades, for example. Biochemistry revealed vitamin A's three chemical structures. Immunology identified the anti-infective properties of one of these structures while physiology focused on another structure and its role in vision. Epidemiology has reported improvements in the death rates and vision of malnourished children given vitamin A supplements, and biology has explored how such effects might be possible. A comprehensive understanding was slow to develop as researchers collected information on one gene, one action, and one nutrient at a time. Today's research in nutritional genomics involves all of the sciences, coordinating their multiple findings and explaining their interactions among several genes, actions, and nutrients in relatively little time. As a result, nutrition knowledge is growing at an incredibly fast pace.

The recent surge in genomics research grew from the Human Genome Project, an international effort by industry and government scientists to identify and describe all of the genes in the **human genome**—that is, all the genetic information contained within a person's cells. Completed in 2003, this project developed many of the research technologies needed to study genes and genetic variation. Scientists are now working to identify the individual proteins made by the genes (the proteome), the genes associated with aging and diseases, and the dietary and lifestyle choices that most influence the expression of those genes.[4] Such information will have major implications for society in general, and for health care in particular.[5]

GLOSSARY

chromosomes: structures within the nucleus of a cell made of DNA and associated proteins. Human beings have 46 chromosomes in 23 pairs. Each chromosome has many genes.

DNA (deoxyribonucleic acid): the double helix molecules of which genes are made.

epigenetics: the study of heritable changes in gene function that occur without a change in the DNA sequence.

gene expression: the process by which a cell converts the genetic code into RNA and protein.

genes: sections of chromosomes that contain the instructions needed to make one or more proteins.

genetics: the study of genes and inheritance.

genomics: the study of all the genes in an organism and their interactions with environmental factors.

human genome (GEE-nome): the full complement of genetic material in the chromosomes of a person's cells.

methylation: the addition of a methyl group (CH_3).

microarray technology: research tools that analyze the expression of thousands of genes simultaneously and search for particular gene changes associated with a disease. DNA microarrays are also called *DNA chips.*

mutations: permanent changes in the DNA that can be inherited.

nucleotide bases: the nitrogen-containing building blocks of DNA and RNA—cytosine (C), thymine (T), uracil (U), guanine (G), and adenine (A). In DNA, the base pairs are A–T and C–G and in RNA, the base pairs are A–U and C–G.

nucleotides: the subunits of DNA and RNA molecules, composed of a phosphate group, a 5-carbon sugar (deoxyribose for DNA and ribose for RNA), and a nitrogen-containing base.

nutritional genomics: the science of how nutrients affect the activities of genes (**nutrigenomics**) and how genes affect the interactions between diet and disease (**nutrigenetics**).

phenylketonuria (FEN-il-KEY-toe-NEW-ree-ah) or **PKU:** an inherited disorder characterized by failure to metabolize the amino acid phenylalanine to tyrosine.

RNA (ribonucleic acid): a compound similar to DNA, but RNA is a single strand with a ribose sugar instead of a deoxyribose sugar and uracil instead of thymine as one of its bases.

FIGURE H6-1 Nutritional Genomics

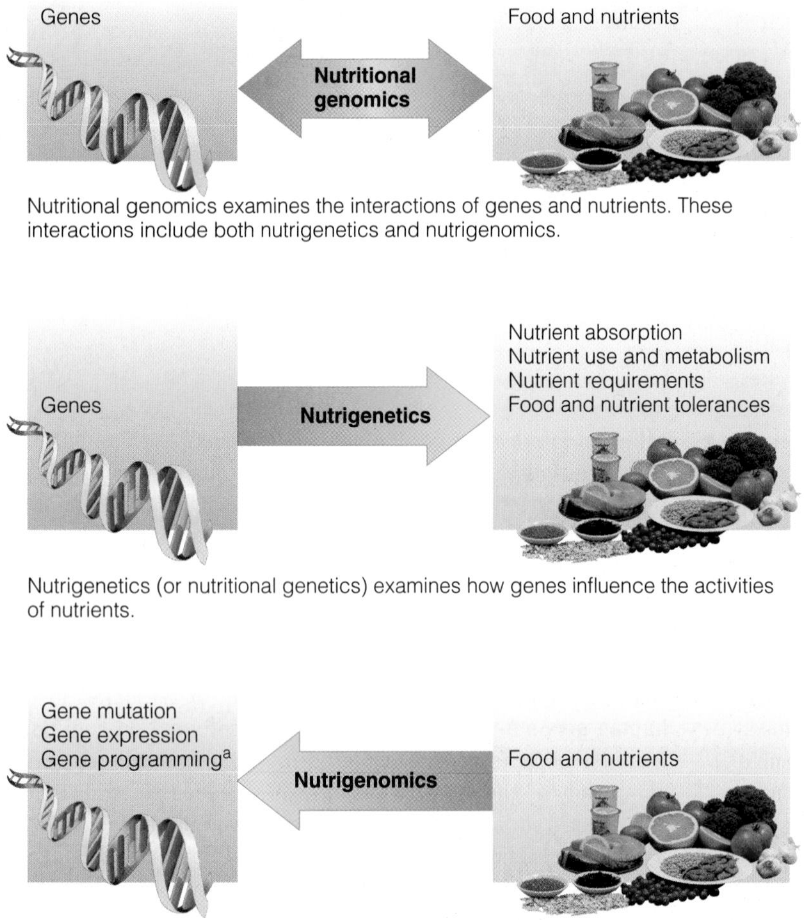
Genes
Nutritional genomics
Food and nutrients
Genes
Nutrigenetics
Nutrient absorption
Nutrient use and metabolism
Nutrient requirements
Food and nutrient tolerances
Gene mutation
Gene expression
Gene programming[a]
Nutrigenomics
Food and nutrients

Nutritional genomics examines the interactions of genes and nutrients. These interactions include both nutrigenetics and nutrigenomics.

Nutrigenetics (or nutritional genetics) examines how genes influence the activities of nutrients.

Nutrigenomics, which includes epigenetics, examines how nutrients influence the activities of genes.

[a]Chapter 18 introduces programming and describes how a mother's nutrition can permanently change gene expression in the fetus with consequences for future generations.

A Genomics Primer

Figure H6-2 shows the relationships among the materials that comprise the genome. As Chapter 6's discussion of protein synthesis points out, genetic information is encoded in DNA molecules within the nucleus of cells. The **DNA (deoxyribonucleic acid)** molecules and associated proteins are packed within 46 **chromosomes.** The genes are segments of a DNA strand that can eventually be translated into one or more proteins. The sequence of **nucleotide bases** within each gene determines the amino acid sequence of a particular protein. Scientists currently estimate that there are between 20 000 and 25 000 genes in the human genome.

As Figure 6-7 (p. 177) explains, when cells make proteins, a DNA sequence is used to make messenger **RNA (ribonucleic acid).** The **nucleotide** sequence in messenger RNA then determines the amino acid sequence to make a protein. This process—from genetic information to protein synthesis—is known as **gene expression.** Gene expression can be determined by measuring the amounts of messenger RNA in a tissue sample. **Microarray technology** (see photo on p. 197) allows researchers to detect messenger RNA and analyze the expression of thousands of genes simultaneously.

Simply having a certain gene does not determine that its associated trait will be expressed; the gene has to be activated. (Similarly, owning lamps does not ensure you will have light in your home unless you turn them on.) Nutrients are among many environmental factors that play key roles in either activating or silencing genes. Switching genes on and off does not change the DNA itself, but it can have dramatic consequences for a person's health.

The area of study that examines how environmental factors influence gene expression without changing the DNA is known as **epigenetics.**[6] To turn genes on, enzymes attach proteins near the beginning of a gene. If enzymes attach a methyl group (CH_3) instead, the protein is blocked from binding to the gene, and the gene remains switched off. Other factors influence gene expression as well, but methyl groups are currently the most well understood.[7] They also are known to have dietary connections.

The accompanying photo of two mice illustrates epigenetics and how diet can influence genetic traits such as hair colour and body weight. Both mice have a gene that tends to produce fat, yellow pups, but their mothers were given different diets during pregnancy. The mother of the mouse on the right was given a dietary supplement containing the B vitamins folate and vitamin B_{12}. These nutrients silenced the gene for "yellow and fat," resulting in brown pups with normal appetites. As Chapter 10 explains, one of the main roles of these B vitamins is to transfer methyl groups. In the case of the supplemented mice, methyl groups migrated onto DNA and silenced several genes, thus producing brown coats and protecting against the development of obesity and some related diseases. Keep in mind that these changes occurred epigenetically. In other words, the DNA sequence within the genes of the mice remained the same. Nutrition and other environmental factors can influence genes in a way that creates inheritable changes in the body's metabolism and susceptibility to disease.[8] In this way, the dietary habits of parents, and even grandparents, can influence future generations.

Many nutrients and phytochemicals regulate gene expression and influence health through their involvement in DNA **methylation.**[9] Some, such as folate, silence genes and protect against some cancers by providing methylation.[10] Others, such as phytochemicals found in green tea, activate genes and protect against some cancers by inhibiting methylation activity.[11] Whether silencing or activating a gene is beneficial or harmful depends on what the gene does. Silencing a gene that stimulates cancer growth, for example, would be beneficial, but silencing a gene

FIGURE H6-2 The Human Genome

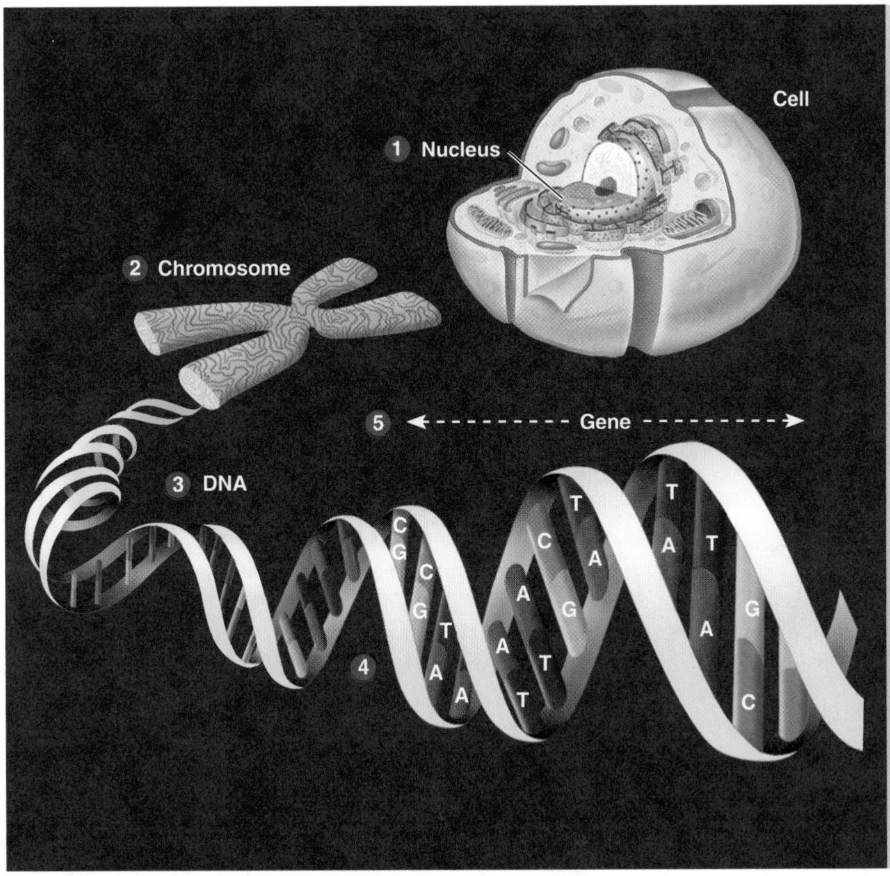
Cell
1 Nucleus
2 Chromosome
5 Gene
3 DNA
4
C G C G T A A T A C A G T A T A G C T T A T

1. The human genome is a complete set of genetic material organized into 46 chromosomes, located within the nucleus of a cell.
2. A chromosome is made of DNA and associated proteins.
3. The double helical structure of a DNA molecule is made up of two long chains of nucleotides. Each nucleotide is composed of a phosphate group, a 5-carbon sugar, and a base.
4. The sequence of nucleotide bases (C, G, A, T) determines the amino acid sequence of proteins. These bases are connected by hydrogen bonding to form base pairs—adenine (A) with thymine (T) and guanine (G) with cytosine (C).
5. A gene is a segment of DNA that includes the information needed to synthesize one or more proteins.

SOURCE: Adapted from "A Primer: From DNA to Life," Human Genome Project, U.S. Department of Energy Genome Programs; http://genomics.energy.gov.

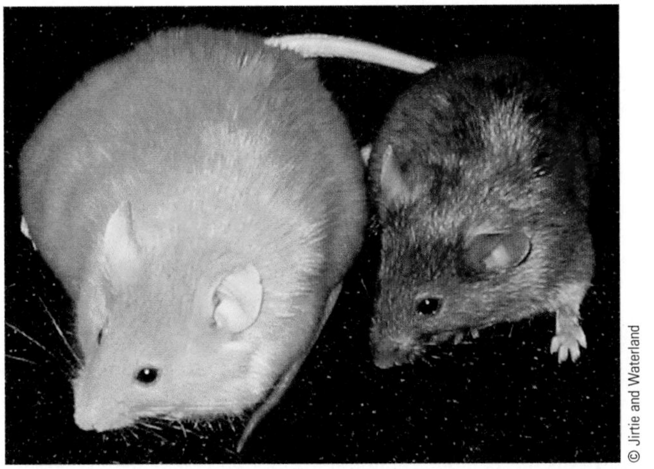
© Jirtie and Waterland

Both of these mice have the gene that tends to produce fat, yellow pups, but their mothers had different diets. The mother of the mouse on the right received a dietary supplement, which silenced the gene, resulting in brown pups with normal appetites.

that suppresses cancer growth would be harmful. Similarly, activating a gene that defends against obesity would be beneficial, but activating a gene that promotes obesity would be harmful.

Figure H6-3 (p. 200) illustrates how nutrient regulation of gene expression can influence a person's health. Much research is under way to determine which nutrients activate or silence which genes.

Genetic Variation and Disease

Except for identical twins, no two persons are genetically identical. Even then, over the years a particular gene may become active in one twin and silenced in the other because of epigenetic changes.

The variation in the genomes of any two persons is only about 0.1 percent, a difference of only one nucleotide base in every 1000. Yet it is this incredibly small difference that makes each of us unique and explains why, given the same environmental influences, some of us develop certain diseases and others do not. Similarly, genetic variation explains why some of us respond to interventions such as diet and others do not. For example, following a diet low in saturated fats will significantly lower LDL cholesterol for most people, but the degree of change varies dramatically among individuals, with some people having only a small decrease or even a slight increase.[12] In other words, dietary factors may be more helpful or more harmful depending on a person's particular genetic varia-

FIGURE H6-3 Nutrient Regulation of Gene Expression

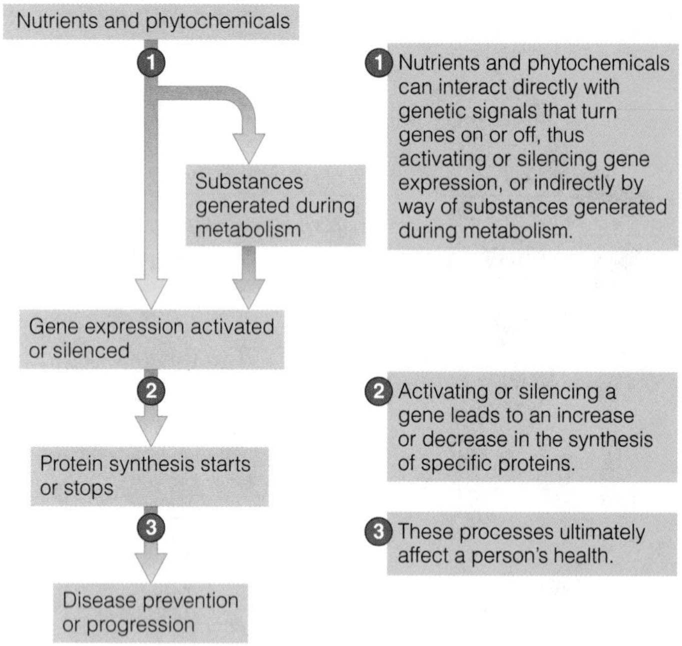
Nutrients and phytochemicals
1
Substances generated during metabolism
Gene expression activated or silenced
2
Protein synthesis starts or stops
3
Disease prevention or progression
1 Nutrients and phytochemicals can interact directly with genetic signals that turn genes on or off, thus activating or silencing gene expression, or indirectly by way of substances generated during metabolism.
2 Activating or silencing a gene leads to an increase or decrease in the synthesis of specific proteins.
3 These processes ultimately affect a person's health.

tions.[13] Such findings help to explain some of the conflicting results from research studies. The goal of nutritional genomics is to custom design *specific* recommendations that fit the needs of *each* individual. Such personalized recommendations are expected to provide more effective disease prevention and treatment solutions.

Diseases characterized by a single-gene disorder are genetically predetermined, usually exert their effects early in life, and greatly affect those touched by them; such diseases are relatively rare. The cause and effect of single-gene disorders is clear—those with the genetic defect get the disease and those without it don't. In contrast, the more common diseases, such as heart disease and cancer, are influenced by many genes and typically develop over several decades. These chronic diseases have multiple genetic components that *predispose* the prevention or development of a disease, depending on a variety of environmental factors (such as smoking, diet, and physical activity).[14] Both types are of interest to researchers studying nutritional genomics.

Single-Gene Disorders

Some disorders are caused by **mutations** in single genes that are inherited at birth. The consequences of a missing or malfunctioning protein can seriously disrupt metabolism and may require significant dietary or medical intervention. A classic example of a diet-related, single-gene disorder is **phenylketonuria,** or **PKU.**

Approximately one in every 15 000 infants in North America is born with PKU. PKU arises from mutations in the gene that codes for the enzyme that converts the essential amino acid phenylalanine to the amino acid tyrosine. Without this enzyme, phenylalanine and its metabolites accumulate and damage the nervous system, resulting in mental retardation, seizures, and behaviour abnormalities. At the same time, the body cannot make tyrosine or compounds made from it (such as the neurotransmitter epinephrine). Consequently, tyrosine becomes an essential amino acid: because the body cannot make it, the diet must supply it.

Although the most debilitating effect is on brain development, other symptoms of PKU become evident if the condition is left untreated. Infants with PKU may have poor appetites and grow slowly. They may be irritable or have tremors or seizures. Their bodies and urine may have a musty odour. Their skin colouring may be unusually pale, and they may develop skin rashes.

The effect of nutrition intervention in PKU is remarkable. In fact, the only current treatment for PKU is a diet that restricts phenylalanine and supplies tyrosine to maintain blood levels of these amino acids within safe ranges. Because all foods containing protein provide phenylalanine, the diet must depend on a special formula to supply a phenylalanine-free source of energy, protein, vitamins, and minerals. If the restricted diet is conscientiously followed, the symptoms can be prevented. Because phenylalanine is an essential amino acid, the diet cannot exclude it completely. Children with PKU need phenylalanine to grow, but they cannot handle excesses without detrimental effects. Therefore, their diets must provide enough phenylalanine to support normal growth and health but not enough to cause harm. The diet must also provide tyrosine. To ensure that blood concentrations of phenylalanine and tyrosine are close to normal, children and adults who have PKU must have blood tests periodically and adjust their diets as necessary, including the avoidance of food products and beverages containing aspartame, which contains phenylalanine.

Multigene Disorders

In multigene disorders, several genes can influence the progression of a disease, but no single gene causes the disease on its own. For this reason, genomics researchers must study the expression and interactions of *multiple* genes. Because multigene disorders are often sensitive to interactions with environmental influences, they are not as straightforward as single-gene disorders.

Heart disease provides an example of a chronic disease with multiple gene and environmental influences. Consider that major risk factors for heart disease include elevated blood cholesterol levels, obesity, diabetes, and hypertension, yet the underlying genetic and environmental causes of any of these individual risk factors is not completely understood. Genomic research can reveal details about each of these risk factors.[15] For example, tests could determine whether blood cholesterol levels are high due to increased cholesterol absorption or production or because of decreased cholesterol degradation. This information could then guide physicians and dietitians to prescribe the most appropriate medical and dietary interventions from among many possible solutions.[16] Today's dietary recommendations advise a low-fat diet, which helps people with a small type of LDL but not those with the large type. In fact, a low-fat diet is actually more harmful for people with the large type. Finding the best option for each person will be a challenge given the many possible interactions between genes and environmental factors and the millions of possible gene variations in the human genome that make each individual unique.[17]

The results of genomic research are helping to explain findings from previous nutrition research. Consider dietary fat and heart disease, for example. As Highlight 5 explains, epidemiological and clinical studies have found that a diet high in unsaturated fatty acids often helps to maintain a healthy blood lipid profile. Now genetic studies offer an underlying explanation of this relationship: diets rich in polyunsaturated fatty acids activate genes responsible for making enzymes (an epigenetic effect) that break down fats and silence genes responsible for making enzymes that synthesize fats.[18] Both actions change fat metabolism in the direction of lowering blood lipids.

To learn more about how individuals respond to diet, researchers examine the genetic differences between people. The most common genetic differences involve a change in a single nucleotide base located in a particular region of a DNA strand—thymine replacing cytosine, for example. Such variations are called single nucleotide polymorphisms (SNPs), and they commonly occur throughout the genome. Many SNPs (commonly pronounced "snips") have no effect on cell activity. In fact, SNPs are significant only if they affect the amino acid sequence of a protein in a way that alters its function *and* if that function is critical to the body's well-being. Research on a gene that plays a key role in lipid metabolism reveals differences in a person's response to diet depending on whether the gene has a common SNP. People with the SNP have lower LDL when eating a diet rich in polyunsaturated fatty acids—and higher LDL with a low intake—than those without the SNP.[19] These findings clearly show how diet (in this case, polyunsaturated fat) interacts with a gene (in this case, a fat metabolism gene with a SNP) to influence the development of a disease (changing blood lipids implicated in heart disease).

Clinical Concerns

Because multigene, chronic diseases are common, an understanding of the human genome will have widespread ramifications for health care.[20] This new understanding of the human genome is expected to change health care by:

- Providing knowledge of an individual's genetic predisposition to specific diseases.
- Allowing physicians to develop "designer" therapies—prescribing the most effective schedule of screening, behaviour changes (including diet), and medical interventions based on each individual's genetic profile.
- Enabling manufacturers to create new medications for each genetic variation so that physicians can prescribe the best medicine in the exact dose and frequency to enhance effectiveness and minimize the risks of side effects.[21]
- Providing a better understanding of the nongenetic factors that influence disease development.

Enthusiasm surrounding genomic research needs to be put into perspective, however, in terms of the present status of clinical medicine as well as people's willingness to make difficult lifestyle choices. Critics have questioned whether genetic markers for disease would be more useful than simple clinical measurements, which reflect both genetic *and* environmental influences. In other words, knowing that a person is genetically predisposed to diabetes is not necessarily more useful than knowing the person's actual risk factors.[22] Furthermore, if a disease has many genetic risk factors, each gene that contributes to susceptibility may have little influence on its own, so the benefits of identifying an individual genetic marker might be small. The long-range possibility is that many genetic markers will eventually be identified, and the hope is that the combined information will be a useful and accurate predictor of disease.

Having the knowledge to prevent disease and actually taking action do not always coincide. Despite the abundance of current dietary recommendations, many people are unwilling to make behaviour changes known to improve their health. For example, it has been estimated that heart disease and type 2 diabetes are 90 percent preventable when people adopt an appropriate diet, maintain a healthy body weight, and exercise regularly. Yet these two diseases remain among the leading causes of death. Given the difficulty that many people have with current recommendations, it may be unrealistic to expect that they will enthusiastically adopt an even more detailed list of lifestyle modifications. Then again, compliance may be better when it is supported by information based on a person's own genetic profile and the knowledge that the epigenetic profile can be changed.

The debate over nature versus nurture—whether genes or the environment are more influential—has quieted. The focus has shifted. Scientists acknowledge the important roles of each and understand the real answers lie within the myriad interactions. Current research is sorting through how nutrients and other dietary factors interact with genes to confer health benefits or risks. Answers from genomic research may not become apparent for years to come, but the opportunities and rewards may prove well worth the efforts.[23]

Nutrition on the Net

CENGAGENOW™
For further study of topics covered in this Highlight, log on to **www.cengage.com/sso**.

- Learn more about the inherited metabolic disease, Phenylketoneuria (PKU), including its prevalence in Canada, how to test for it, and how to treat it: **www.canpku.org/about-pku**
- Get information about human genomic discoveries and how they can be used to improve health from the Office of Public Health Genomics site of the U.S. Centers for Disease Control: **www.cdc.gov/genomics**

References

1. A. L. McGuire and W. Burke, An unwelcome side effect of direct-to-customer personal genome testing: Raiding the medical commons, *Journal of the American Medical Association* 300 (2008): 2669–2671.
2. P. J. Stover and M. A. Caudill, Genetic and epigenetic contributions to human nutrition and health: Managing genome-diet interactions, *Journal of the American Dietetic Association* 108 (2008): 1480–1487; J. Kaput, Nutrigenomics–2006 update, *Clinical Chemistry and Laboratory Medicine* 45 (2007): 279–287.
3. G. T. Keusch, What do *-omics* mean for the science and policy of the nutritional sciences? *American Journal of Clinical Nutrition* 83 (2006): 520S–522S.
4. G. W. Duff, Influence of genetics on disease susceptibility and progression, *Nutrition Reviews* 65 (2007): S177–S181; P. J. Gillies, Preemptive nutrition of pro-inflammatory states: A nutrigenomic model, *Nutrition Reviews* 65 (2007): S217–S220; T. A. Manolio, Study designs to enhance identification of genetic factors in healthy aging, *Nutrition Reviews* 65 (2007): S228–S233.
5. A. P. Feinberg, Epigenetics at the epicenter of modern medicine, *Journal of the American Medical Association* 299 (2008): 1345–1350.
6. G. P. Kauwell, Epigenetics: What it is and how it can affect dietetics practice, *Journal of the American Dietetic Association* 108 (2008): 1056–1059.
7. M. Esteller, Epigenetics in cancer, *New England Journal of Medicine* 358 (2008): 1148–1159; L. Cobiac, Epigenomics and nutrition, *Forum of Nutrition* 60 (2007): 31–41; T. M. Edwards and J. P. Myers, Environmental exposures and gene regulation in disease etiology, *Environmental Health Perspectives* 115 (2007): 1264–1270.
8. S. A. Ross and coauthors, Introduction: Diet, epigenetic events and cancer prevention, *Nutrition Reviews* 66 (2008): S1–S6; R. L. Jirtle and M. K. Skinner, Environmental epigenomics and disease susceptibility, *Nature Reviews: Genetics* 8 (2007): 253–262; R. A. Waterland and K. B. Michels, Epigenetic epidemiology of the developmental origins hypothesis, *Annual Review of Nutrition* 27 (2007): 363–388.
9. M. P. Lee and B. K. Dunn, Influence of genetic inheritance on global epigenetic states and cancer risk prediction with DNA methylation signature: Challenges in technology and data analysis, *Nutrition Reviews* 66 (2008): S69–S72.
10. C. M. Ulrich, M. C. Reed, and H. F. Nijhout, Modeling folate, one-carbon metabolism, and DNA methylation, *Nutrition Reviews* 66 (2008): S27–S30.
11. C. S. Yang and coauthors, Reverse of hypermethylation and reactivation of genes by dietary polyphenolic compounds, *Nutrition Reviews* 66 (2008): S18–S20.
12. D. Corella and J. M. Ordovas, Single nucleotide polymorphisms that influence lipid metabolism: Interaction with dietary factors, *Annual Review of Nutrition* 25 (2005): 341–390.
13. B. Fontaine-Bisson and coauthors, Genetic polymorphisms of tumor necrosis factor-α modify the association between dietary polyunsaturated fatty acids and fasting HDL-cholesterol and apo A-I concentrations, *American Journal of Clinical Nutrition* 86 (2007): 768–774; E. A. Ruiz-Narváez, P. Kraft, and H. Campos, Ala12 variant of the peroxisome proliferator-activated receptor-γ gene (*PPARG*) is associated with higher polyunsaturated fat in adipose tissue and attenuates the protective effect of polyunsaturated fat intake on the risk of myocardial infarction, *American Journal of Clinical Nutrition* 86 (2007): 1238–1242; E. Trujillo, C. Davis, and J. Milner, Nutrigenomics, proteomics, metabolomics, and the practice of dietetics, *Journal of the American Dietetic Association* 106 (2006): 403–413.
14. L. R. Ferguson and M. Philpott, Nutrition and mutagenesis, *Annual Review of Nutrition* 28 (2008): 313–329; J. Kaput and coauthors, The case for strategic international alliances to harness nutritional genomics for public and personal health, *British Journal of Nutrition* 94 (2005): 623–632.
15. J. H. Hardy and A. Singleton, Genomewide association studies and human disease, *New England Journal of Medicine* 360 (2009): 1759–1768.
16. R. M. DeBusk and coauthors, Nutritional genomics in practice: Where do we begin? *Journal of the American Dietetic Association* 105 (2005): 589–597.
17. J. M. Ordovas, Nutrigenetics, plasma lipids, and cardiovascular risk, *Journal of the American Dietetic Association* 106 (2006): 1074–1081.
18. H. Sampath and J. M. Ntambi, Polyunsaturated fatty acid regulation of genes of lipid metabolism, *Annual Review of Nutrition* 25 (2005): 317–340.
19. E. S. Tai and coauthors, Polyunsaturated fatty acids interact with PPARA–L162V polymorphism to affect plasma triglyceride apolipoprotein C-III concentrations in the Framingham Heart Study, *Journal of Nutrition* 135 (2005): 397–403.
20. M. M. Bergmann, U. Görman, and J. C. Mathers, Bioethical considerations for human nutrigenomics, *Annual Review of Nutrition* 28 (2008): 447–467; J. P. Evans, Health care in the age of genetic medicine, *Journal of the American Medical Association* 298 (2007): 2670–2672; S. Vakili and M. A. Caudill, Personalized nutrition: Nutritional genomics as a potential tool for targeted medical nutrition therapy, *Nutrition Reviews* 65 (2007): 301–315.
21. S. B. Shurin and E. G. Nabel, Pharmacogenomics—Ready for prime time? *New England Journal of Medicine* 358 (2008): 1061–1063.
22. J. B. Meigs and coauthors, Genotype score in addition to common risk factors for prediction of type 2 diabetes, *New England Journal of Medicine* 359 (2008): 2208–2219.
23. A. E. Guttmacher and F. S. Collins, Realizing the promise of genomics in biomedical research, *Journal of the American Medical Association* 294 (2005): 1399–1402.

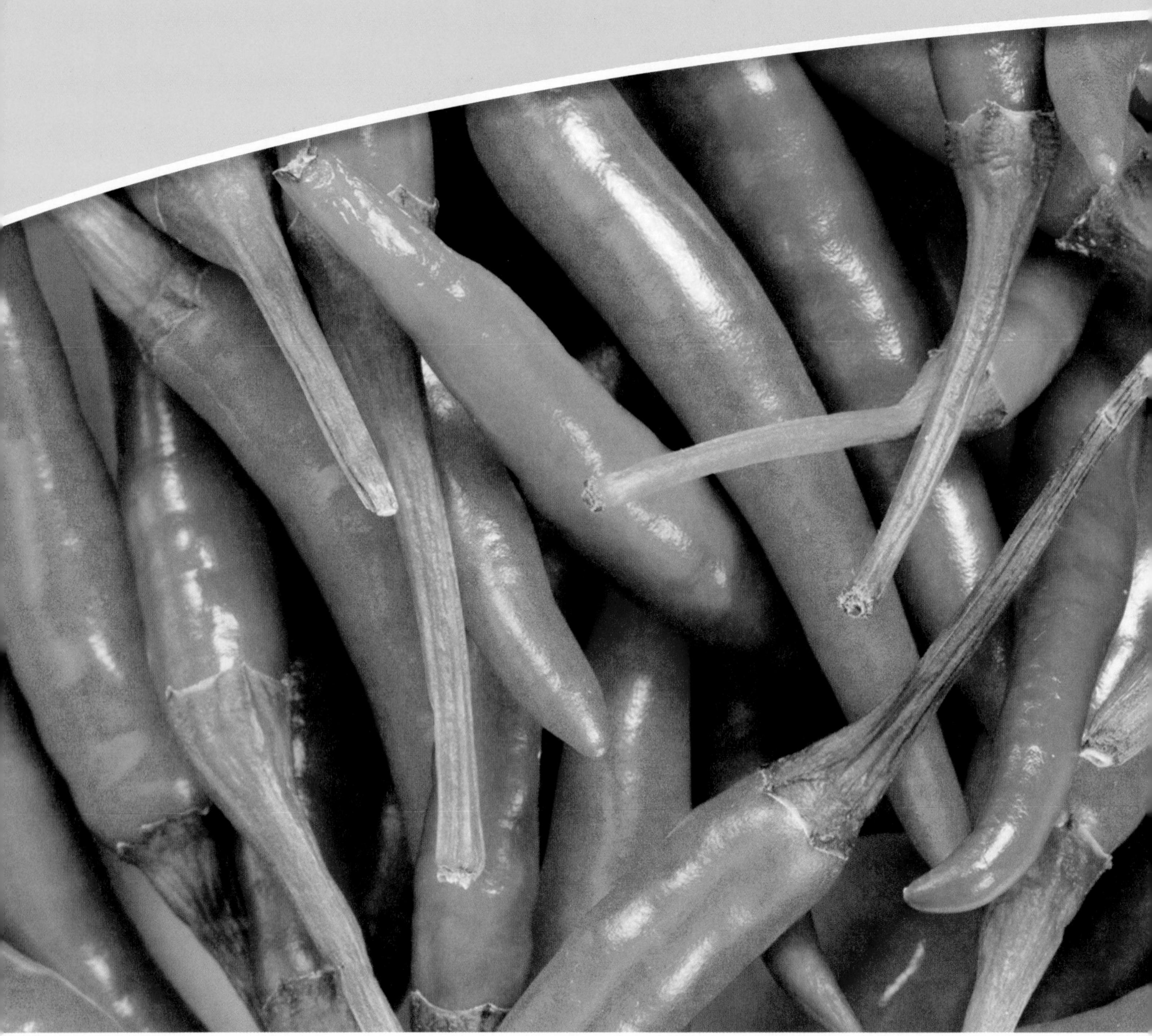

Elnur/shutterstock

Nutrition in Your Life

CENGAGENOW™

Throughout this chapter, the CengageNOW logo indicates an opportunity for online self-study, linking you to interactive tutorials, activities, and videos to increase your understanding of chapter concepts.
www.cengage.com/sso

You eat breakfast and hustle off to class. After lunch, you study for tomorrow's exam. Dinner is followed by an evening of dancing. Do you ever think about how the food you eat powers the activities of your life? What happens when you don't eat—or when you eat too much? Learn how the cells of your body transform carbohydrates, fats, and proteins into energy—and what happens when you give your cells too much or too little of any of these nutrients. Discover the metabolic pathways that lead to body fat and those that support physical activity. It's really quite fascinating.

CHAPTER 7

Metabolism: Transformations and Interactions

CHAPTER OUTLINE

Energy makes it possible for people to breathe, ride bicycles, compose music, and do everything else they do. As Chapter 1 explains, *energy* is the capacity to do work. Although every aspect of our lives depends on energy, the concept of energy can be difficult to grasp because it cannot be seen or touched, and it manifests in various forms, including heat, mechanical, electrical, and chemical energy. In the body, heat energy maintains a constant body temperature, mechanical energy moves muscles, and electrical energy sends nerve impulses. Energy is stored in foods and in the body as chemical energy. This chemical energy powers the myriad activities of all cells.

All the energy that sustains human life initially comes from the sun—the ultimate source of energy. During **photosynthesis,** plants make simple sugars from carbon dioxide and capture the sun's light energy in the chemical bonds of those sugars. Then human beings eat either the plants or animals that have eaten the plants. These foods provide energy, but how does the body obtain that energy from foods? This chapter answers that question by following the nutrients that provide the body with **fuel** through a series of reactions that release energy from their chemical bonds (e.g., breaking of C-C bonds). As these bonds break, they release energy in a controlled version of the same process by which wood burns in a fire. Both wood and food have the potential to provide energy. When wood burns in the presence of oxygen, it generates heat and light (energy), steam (water), and some carbon dioxide and ash (waste). Similarly, during **metabolism**, the body releases energy, water, and carbon dioxide (and other waste products).

By studying metabolism, you will understand how the body uses foods to meet its needs and why some foods meet those needs better than others. Readers who are interested in weight control will discover which foods contribute most to body fat and which to select when trying to gain or lose weight safely. Readers who are physically active will discover which foods best support endurance activities and which to select when trying to build lean body mass.

photosynthesis: the process by which green plants use the sun's energy to make carbohydrates from carbon dioxide and water.
- **photo** = light
- **synthesis** = put together (making)

fuel: compounds that cells can use for energy. The major fuels include glucose, fatty acids, and amino acids; other fuels include ketone bodies, lactate, glycerol, and alcohol.

metabolism: the sum total of all the chemical reactions that go on in living cells. Energy metabolism includes all the reactions by which the body obtains and expends the energy from food.
- **metaballein** = change

Chemical Reactions in the Body

Earlier chapters introduce some of the body's chemical reactions: the making and breaking of the bonds in carbohydrates, lipids, and proteins. Metabolism is the sum of these and all the other chemical reactions that go on in living cells; *energy metabolism* includes all the ways the body obtains and uses energy from food.

The Site of Metabolic Reactions—Cells The human body is made up of trillions of cells, and each cell busily conducts its metabolic work all the time. (APPENDIX A presents a brief summary of the structure and function of the cell.) Figure 7-1 depicts a typical cell and shows where the major reactions of energy metabolism take place. The type and extent of metabolic activities vary depending on the type of cell, but of all the body's cells, the liver cells are the most versatile and metabolically active. Table 7-1 offers insights into the liver's work.

The Building Reactions—Anabolism Earlier chapters describe how condensation reactions (that produce water as part of the reaction) combine the basic units of energy-yielding nutrients to build body compounds. Glucose molecules may be joined together to make glycogen chains. Glycerol and fatty acids may be assembled into triglycerides. Amino acids may be linked together to make proteins. Each of these reactions starts with small, simple compounds and uses them as building blocks to form larger, more complex structures. Because such reactions involve doing work, they require energy. The building up of body compounds is known as **anabolism.** Anabolic reactions are represented in this book, wherever possible, with "up" arrows in chemical diagrams (such as those shown at the top of Figure 7-2).

anabolism (an-AB-o-lism): reactions in which small molecules are put together to build larger ones. Anabolic reactions require energy.

- **ana** = (build) up

catabolism (ca-TAB-o-lism): reactions in which large molecules are broken down to smaller ones. Catabolic reactions release energy.

- **kata** = (break) down

The Breakdown Reactions—Catabolism The breaking down of body compounds is known as **catabolism;** catabolic reactions release energy and are represented, wherever possible, by "down" arrows in chemical diagrams (as in the bottom of Figure 7-2). Earlier chapters describe how hydrolysis reactions break

FIGURE 7-1 A Typical Cell (Simplified Diagram)

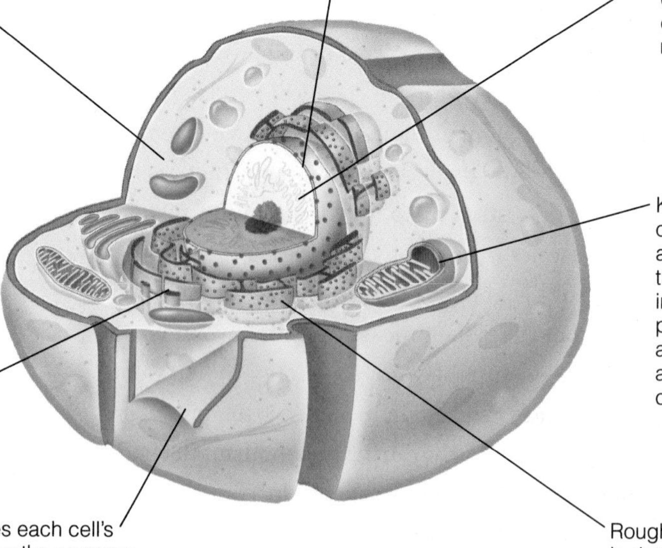
Inside the cell membrane lies the cytoplasm, a lattice-type structure that supports and controls the movement of the cell's structures. A protein-rich jelly-like fluid called cytosol fills the spaces within the lattice. The cytosol contains the enzymes involved in glycolysis.[a]
A separate inner membrane encloses the cell's nucleus.
Inside the nucleus are the chromosomes, which contain the genetic material DNA.
Known as the "powerhouses" of the cells, the mitochondria are intricately folded membranes that house all the enzymes involved in the conversion of pyruvate to acetyl CoA, fatty acid oxidation, the TCA cycle, and the electron transport chain.[b]
This network of membranes is known as smooth endoplasmic reticulum—the site of lipid synthesis.
A membrane encloses each cell's contents and regulates the passage of molecules in and out of the cell.
Rough endoplasmic reticulum is dotted with ribosomes—the site of protein synthesis.[c]

[a]Glycolysis is introduced on p. 211.
[b]The conversion of pyruvate to acetyl CoA, fatty acid oxidation, the TCA cycle, and the electron transport chain are described later in the chapter.
[c]Figure 6-7 on p. 177 describes protein synthesis.

TABLE 7-1 Metabolic Work of the Liver

The liver is the most active processing centre in the body. When nutrients enter the body from the digestive tract, the liver receives most of them first; then it metabolizes, packages, stores, or ships them out for use by other organs. When alcohol, drugs, or poisons enter the body, they are also sent directly to the liver; here they are detoxified and their by-products shipped out for excretion. An enthusiastic anatomy and physiology professor once remarked that given the many vital activities of the liver, we should express our feelings for others by saying, "I love you with all my liver" instead of "with all my heart." Granted, this declaration lacks romance, but it makes a valid point. Here are just some of the many jobs performed by the liver. To renew your appreciation for this remarkable organ, review Figure 3-12 (p. 78).

Carbohydrates

- Converts fructose and galactose to glucose
- Makes and stores glycogen
- Breaks down glycogen and releases glucose
- Breaks down glucose for energy when needed
- Makes glucose from some amino acids and glycerol when needed
- Converts excess glucose to fatty acids

Lipids

- Builds and breaks down triglycerides, phospholipids, and cholesterol as needed
- Breaks down fatty acids for energy when needed
- Packages extra lipids in lipoproteins for transport to other body organs
- Manufactures bile to send to the gallbladder for use in fat digestion
- Makes ketone bodies when necessary

Proteins

- Manufactures nonessential amino acids that are in short supply
- Removes from circulation amino acids that are present in excess of need and converts them to other amino acids or deaminates them and converts them to glucose or fatty acids
- Removes ammonia from the blood and converts it to urea to be sent to the kidneys for excretion
- Makes other nitrogen-containing compounds the body needs (such as bases used in DNA and RNA)
- Makes many transport and blood proteins

Other

- Detoxifies alcohol, other drugs, and poisons; prepares waste products for excretion
- Helps dismantle old red blood cells and captures the iron for recycling
- Stores most vitamins and many minerals
- Converts vitamin D into an intermediate metabolic form

FIGURE 7-2 Anabolic and Catabolic Reactions Compared

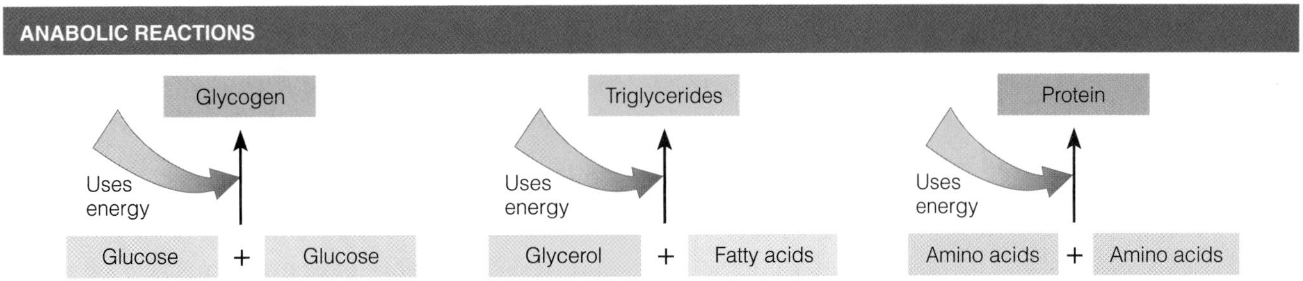
ANABOLIC REACTIONS
Glycogen
Uses energy
Glucose
+
Glucose
Triglycerides
Uses energy
Glycerol
+
Fatty acids
Protein
Uses energy
Amino acids
+
Amino acids

Anabolic reactions include the making of glycogen, triglycerides, and protein; these reactions require differing amounts of energy.

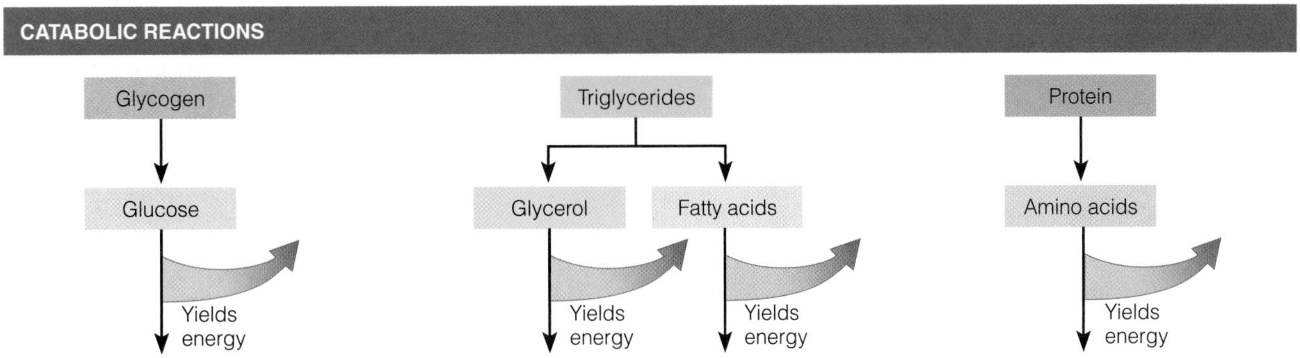
CATABOLIC REACTIONS
Glycogen
Glucose
Yields energy
Triglycerides
Glycerol
Fatty acids
Yields energy
Yields energy
Protein
Amino acids
Yields energy

Catabolic reactions include the breakdown of glycogen, triglycerides, and protein; the further catabolism of glucose, glycerol, fatty acids, and amino acids releases differing amounts of energy. Much of the energy released is captured in the high-energy bonds of adenosine triphosphate (ATP).

NOTE: You need not memorize a colour code to understand the figures in this chapter, but you may find it helpful to know that blue is used for carbohydrates, yellow for fats, and red for proteins.

FIGURE 7-3 ATP (Adenosine Triphosphate)

ATP is one of the body's high-energy molecules. Notice that the bonds connecting the three phosphate groups have been drawn as wavy lines, indicating a high-energy bond. When these bonds are broken, energy is released.

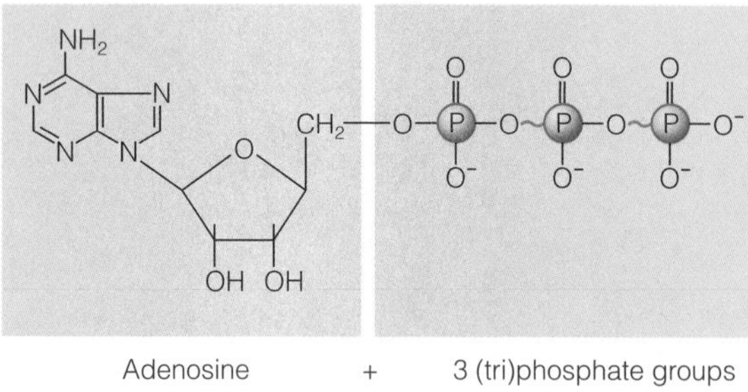
Adenosine
+
3 (tri)phosphate groups

down glycogen to glucose, triglycerides to fatty acids and glycerol, and proteins to amino acids. When the body needs energy, it breaks down any or all of these four basic units into even smaller units, as described later.

The Transfer of Energy in Reactions—ATP Some of the energy released during the breakdown of glucose, glycerol, fatty acids, and amino acids from foods is captured in the high-energy storage compound **ATP (adenosine triphosphate)**. ATP, as its name indicates, contains three phosphate groups (see Figure 7-3). ♦ The negative charges on the phosphate groups make ATP vulnerable to hydrolysis. When the bonds between the phosphate groups are hydrolyzed, they readily break, splitting off one or two phosphate groups and releasing energy. In this way, ATP provides the energy that powers all the activities of living cells. Figure 7-4 describes how the body captures and releases energy in the bonds of ATP.

Quite often, the hydrolysis of ATP occurs simultaneously with reactions that will use that energy—a metabolic duet known as **coupled reactions**. In essence, the body uses ATP to transfer the energy released during catabolic reactions to power its anabolic reactions. The body converts the chemical energy of food to the chemical energy of ATP with about 50 percent efficiency, radiating the rest as heat.[1] Some energy is lost as heat again when the body uses the chemical energy of ATP to do its work—moving muscles, synthesizing compounds, or transporting nutrients, for example.

♦ ATP = A—P~P~P.
Each ~ denotes a "high-energy" bond.

The Helpers in Metabolic Reactions—Enzymes and Coenzymes Metabolic reactions almost always require enzymes ♦ to facilitate their action. In many cases, the enzymes need assistants to help them. Enzyme helpers are called **coenzymes.** ♦

Coenzymes are complex organic molecules that associate closely with most enzymes but are not proteins themselves. The relationships between various coenzymes and their respective enzymes may differ in detail, but one thing is true of all: without its coenzyme, an enzyme cannot function. Some of the B vitamins serve as coenzymes that participate in the energy metabolism of glucose, glycerol, fatty acids, and amino acids. (Chapter 10 provides more details.)

♦ **Enzymes** are proteins that act as catalysts. **Catalysts** facilitate chemical reactions without being changed in the process.

♦ The general term for substances that facilitate enzyme action is **cofactors;** they include both organic coenzymes made from vitamins and inorganic substances such as minerals.

IN SUMMARY **During digestion the energy-yielding nutrients—carbohydrates, lipids, and proteins—are broken down to glucose (and other mono-**

FIGURE 7-4 The Capture and Release of Energy by ATP

It may help to think of the conversion of ADP to ATP as a rechargeable battery—capturing and releasing energy as it does the body's work.

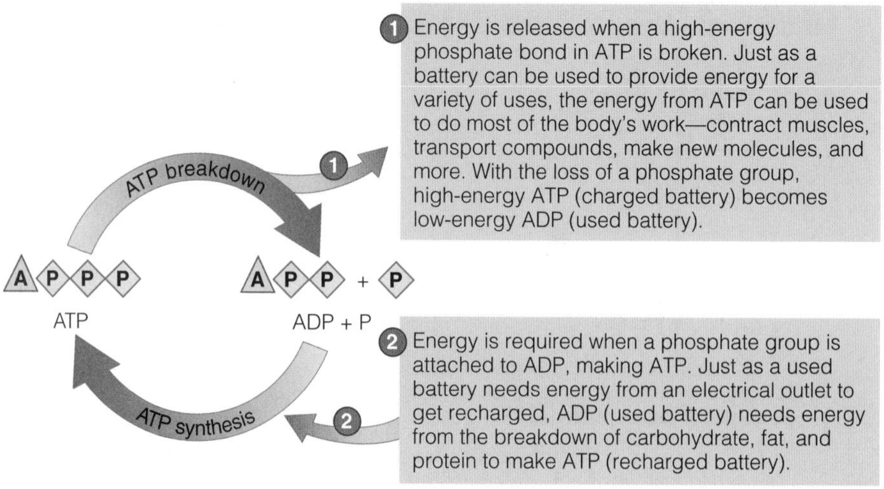
1 Energy is released when a high-energy phosphate bond in ATP is broken. Just as a battery can be used to provide energy for a variety of uses, the energy from ATP can be used to do most of the body's work—contract muscles, transport compounds, make new molecules, and more. With the loss of a phosphate group, high-energy ATP (charged battery) becomes low-energy ADP (used battery).
ATP breakdown
A P P P
ATP
A P P + P
ADP + P
ATP synthesis
2 Energy is required when a phosphate group is attached to ADP, making ATP. Just as a used battery needs energy from an electrical outlet to get recharged, ADP (used battery) needs energy from the breakdown of carbohydrate, fat, and protein to make ATP (recharged battery).

ATP or **adenosine** (ah-DEN-oh-seen) **triphosphate** (try-FOS-fate): a common high-energy compound composed of a purine (adenine), a sugar (ribose), and three phosphate groups.

coupled reactions: pairs of chemical reactions in which some of the energy released from the breakdown of one compound is used to create a bond in the formation of another compound.

coenzymes: complex organic molecules that work with enzymes to facilitate the enzymes' activity. Many coenzymes have B vitamins as part of their structures. (Figure 10-3 on p. 316 illustrates coenzyme action.)
- **co** = with

saccharides), glycerol, fatty acids, and amino acids. With the help of enzymes and coenzymes, the cells use these products of digestion to build more complex compounds (anabolism) or break them down further to release energy (catabolism). High-energy compounds such as ATP may capture the energy released during catabolism.

Breaking Down Nutrients for Energy

Chapters 4, 5, and 6 lay the groundwork for the study of metabolism; a brief review may be helpful. During digestion, the body breaks down the three energy-yielding nutrients—carbohydrates, lipids, and proteins—into four basic units that can be absorbed into the blood:

- From carbohydrates—glucose (and other monosaccharides)
- From fats (triglycerides)—glycerol and fatty acids
- From proteins—amino acids

The body uses carbohydrates and fats for most of its energy needs. Amino acids are used primarily as building blocks for proteins, but they also enter energy pathways, contributing about 10 to 15 percent of the day's energy use. Look for these four basic units—glucose, glycerol, fatty acids, and amino acids—to appear again and again in the metabolic reactions described in this chapter. Alcohol also enters many of the metabolic pathways; Highlight 7 focuses on how alcohol disrupts metabolism and how the body handles it.

Glucose, glycerol, fatty acids, and amino acids are the basic units derived from food, but, as described in earlier chapters, a molecule of each of these compounds is made of still smaller units, the atoms—carbons, nitrogens, oxygens, and hydrogens. During catabolism, the body separates these atoms from one another (i.e., breaks the bonds between them). To follow this action, recall how many carbons are in the "backbones" of these compounds:

- Glucose has 6 carbons:

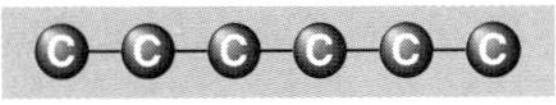

- Glycerol has 3 carbons:

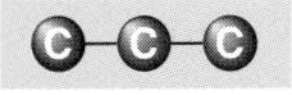

- A fatty acid usually has an even number of carbons, commonly 16 or 18 carbons:*

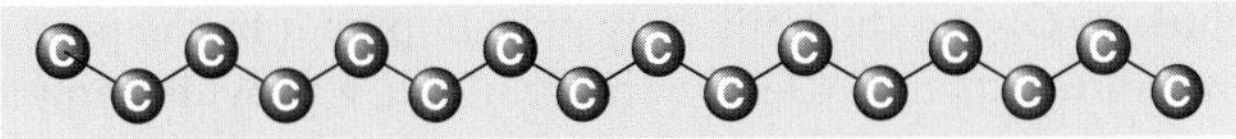

- An amino acid has 2, 3, or more carbons with a nitrogen attached:**

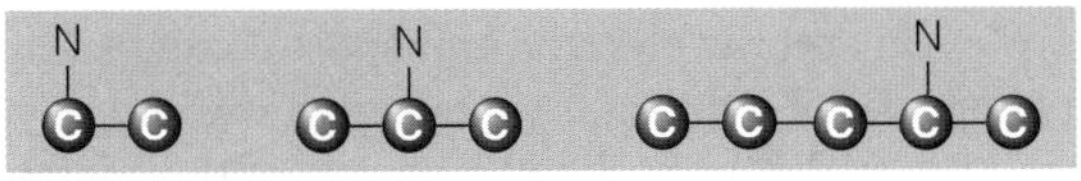
N
N
N

Full chemical structures and reactions appear both in the earlier chapters and in APPENDIX C; this chapter diagrams the reactions using just the compounds' carbon and nitrogen backbones.

As you will see, each of the compounds—glucose, glycerol, fatty acids, and amino acids—starts down a different path. Along the way, two new names appear—**pyruvate** (a 3-carbon structure) and **acetyl CoA** (a 2-carbon structure with a

pyruvate (PIE-roo-vate): a 3-carbon compound that plays a key role in energy metabolism.

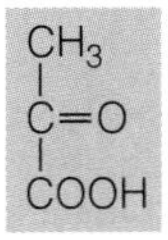
CH_3
C=O
COOH

acetyl CoA (ASS-eh-teel, or ah-SEET-il, coh-AY): a 2-carbon compound (*acetate,* or *acetic acid,* shown in Figure 5-1 on p. 130) to which a molecule of CoA is attached.

*The figures in this chapter show 16- or 18-carbon fatty acids. Fatty acids may have 4 to 22 or more carbons, with chain lengths of 16 and 18 carbons most prevalent.

**The figures in this chapter usually show amino acids as compounds of 2, 3, or 5 carbons arranged in a straight line, but in reality amino acids may contain other numbers of carbons and assume other structural shapes (see APPENDIX C).

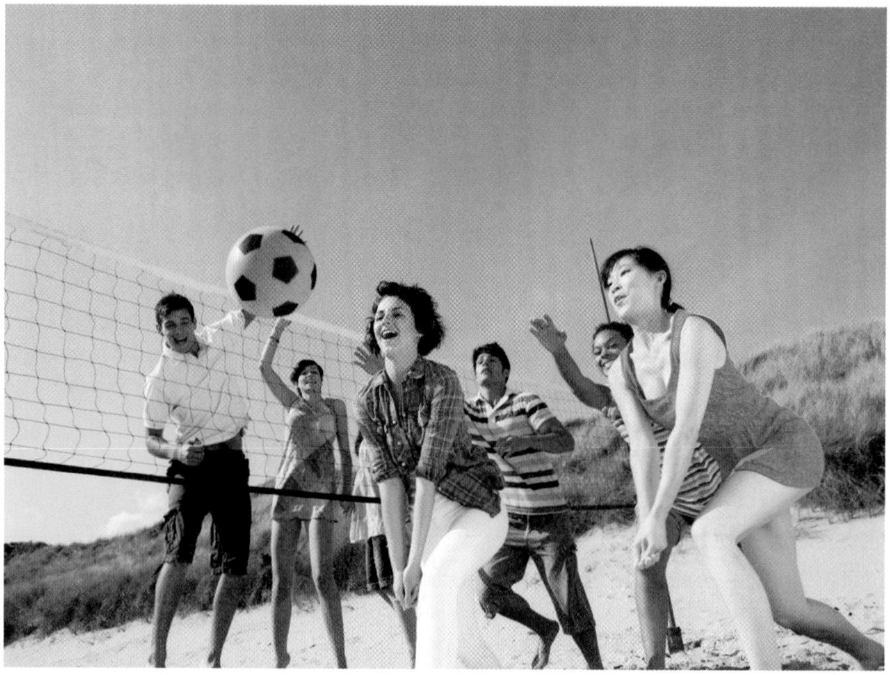

photos.com

All the energy used to keep the heart beating, the brain thinking, and the legs running comes from the carbohydrates, fats, and proteins in foods.

coenzyme, **CoA**, attached)—and the rest of the story falls into place around them.* Two major points to notice in the following discussion:

- Pyruvate can be used to make glucose.
- Acetyl CoA cannot be used to make glucose.

A key to understanding these metabolic pathways is learning which fuels can be converted to glucose and which cannot. The parts of protein and fat that can be converted to pyruvate *can* provide glucose for the body, whereas the parts that are converted to acetyl CoA *cannot* provide glucose but can readily provide energy or be used to make fat. The body must have glucose to fuel the activities of the central nervous system and red blood cells. Without glucose from food, the body will devour its own lean (protein-containing) tissue to get the amino acids needed to make glucose. Therefore, to keep this from happening, the body needs foods that can provide glucose—primarily carbohydrate. Giving the body only fat, which delivers mostly acetyl CoA, puts it in the position of having to break down protein tissue to make glucose. Giving the body only protein puts it in the position of having to convert protein to glucose. Clearly, the best diet ♦ provides ample carbohydrate, adequate protein, and some fat.

Eventually, all of the energy-yielding nutrients can enter the final energy pathways of the **TCA cycle** and the **electron transport chain.** ♦ (Similarly, people from three different cities can all enter an interstate highway and travel to the same destination.) Figure 7-5 provides a simplified overview of the energy-yielding pathways. The next sections of the text describe how each of the energy-yielding nutrients is broken down to acetyl CoA and other compounds in preparation for their entrance into the TCA cycle and electron transport chain. These final energy pathways have central roles in energy metabolism and receive full attention later in the chapter.

♦ A healthy diet provides:
- 45–65% kcalories from carbohydrate
- 10–35% kcalories from protein
- 20–35% kcalories from fat

♦ The TCA cycle is also called the **citric acid cycle** or the **Kreb's cycle.** The electron transport chain is also called the **respiratory chain.**

CoA (coh-AY): coenzyme A; the coenzyme derived from the B vitamin pantothenic acid and central to energy metabolism.

TCA cycle or **tricarboxylic** (try-car-box-ILL-ick) **acid cycle:** a series of metabolic reactions that break down molecules of acetyl CoA to carbon dioxide and hydrogen atoms; also called the *citric acid cycle* or the *Kreb's cycle* after the biochemist who elucidated its reactions.

electron transport chain: the final pathway in energy metabolism that transports electrons from hydrogen to oxygen and captures about half the energy released by breaking C-C bonds and storing it in the high-energy bonds of ATP.

Glucose

What happens to glucose, glycerol, fatty acids, and amino acids during energy metabolism can best be understood by starting with glucose. This discussion features glucose because of its central role in carbohydrate metabolism and because liver cells can convert the monosaccharides fructose and galactose to compounds that enter the same energy pathways.

*The term *pyruvate* means a salt of *pyruvic acid*. (Throughout this book, the ending *–ate* is used interchangeably with *–ic acid*; for our purposes they mean the same thing.)

FIGURE 7-5 **Simplified Overview of Energy-Yielding Pathways**

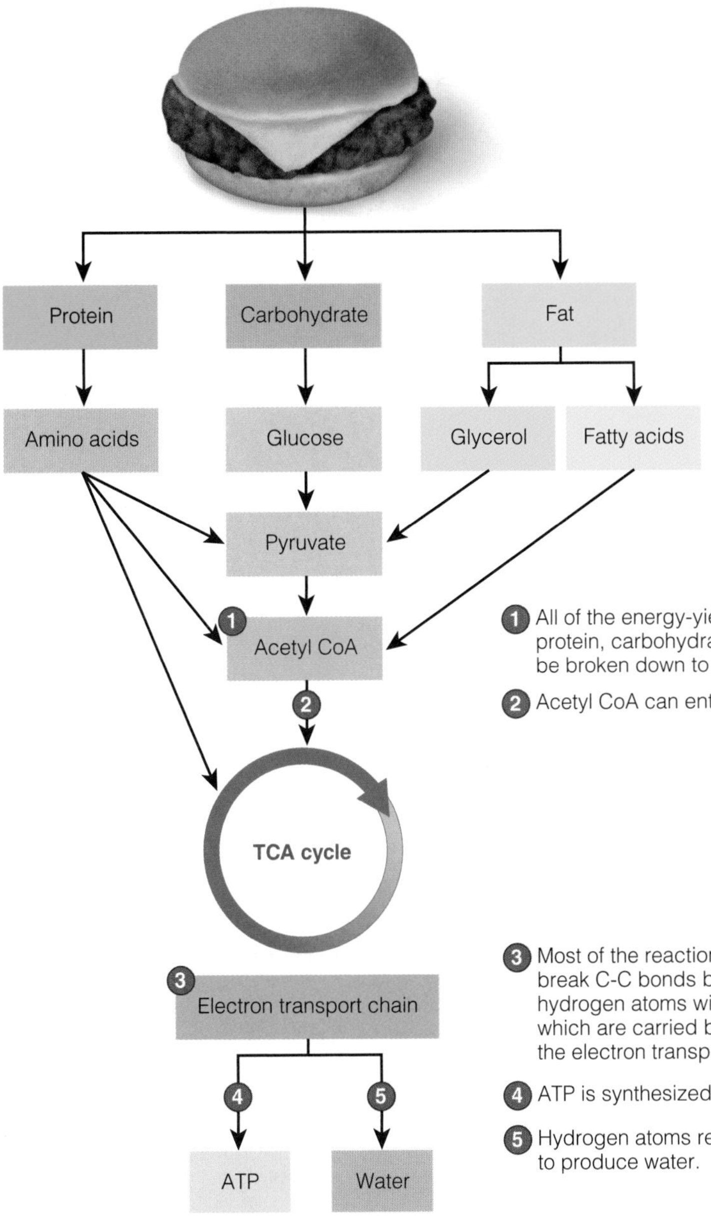
Protein
Carbohydrate
Fat
Amino acids
Glucose
Glycerol
Fatty acids
Pyruvate
1
Acetyl CoA
2
TCA cycle
3
Electron transport chain
4
5
ATP
Water

1 All of the energy-yielding nutrients—protein, carbohydrate, and fat—can be broken down to acetyl CoA.

2 Acetyl CoA can enter the TCA cycle.

3 Most of the reactions above not only break C-C bonds but also release hydrogen atoms with their electrons, which are carried by coenzymes to the electron transport chain.

4 ATP is synthesized.

5 Hydrogen atoms react with oxygen to produce water.

Glucose-to-Pyruvate The first pathway glucose takes on its way to yield energy is called **glycolysis** (glucose splitting).* Figure 7-6 (p. 212) shows a simplified drawing of glycolysis. (This pathway actually involves several steps and several enzymes, which are detailed in APPENDIX C.) In a series of reactions, the 6-carbon glucose is converted to similar 6-carbon compounds before being split in half (by breaking C-C bonds), forming two 3-carbon compounds. These 3-carbon compounds continue along the pathway until they are converted to pyruvate. Thus the net yield of one glucose molecule is two pyruvate molecules. The net yield of energy at this point is small; to start glycolysis, the cell uses a little energy and then produces only a little more than it had to invest initially.** In addition, as glucose breaks down to pyruvate, hydrogen atoms with their electrons are released and carried to the electron transport chain by coenzymes made from the B vitamins niacin and riboflavin. A later section of the chapter explains how oxygen

glycolysis (gly-COLL-ih-sis): the metabolic breakdown of glucose to pyruvate. Glycolysis can operate in both the presence (aerobic) or absence of oxygen (anaerobic).

- **glyco** = glucose
- **lysis** = breakdown

*Glycolysis takes place in the cytosol of the cell (see Figure 7-1, p. 206).

**The cell uses 2 ATP to begin the breakdown of glucose to pyruvate, but it then gains 4 ATP for a net gain of 2 ATP.

FIGURE 7-6 **Glycolysis: Glucose-to-Pyruvate**

This simplified overview of glycolysis illustrates the steps in the process of converting glucose to pyruvate. APPENDIX C provides more details.

CENGAGENOW™
Animated! figure
www.cengage.com/sso

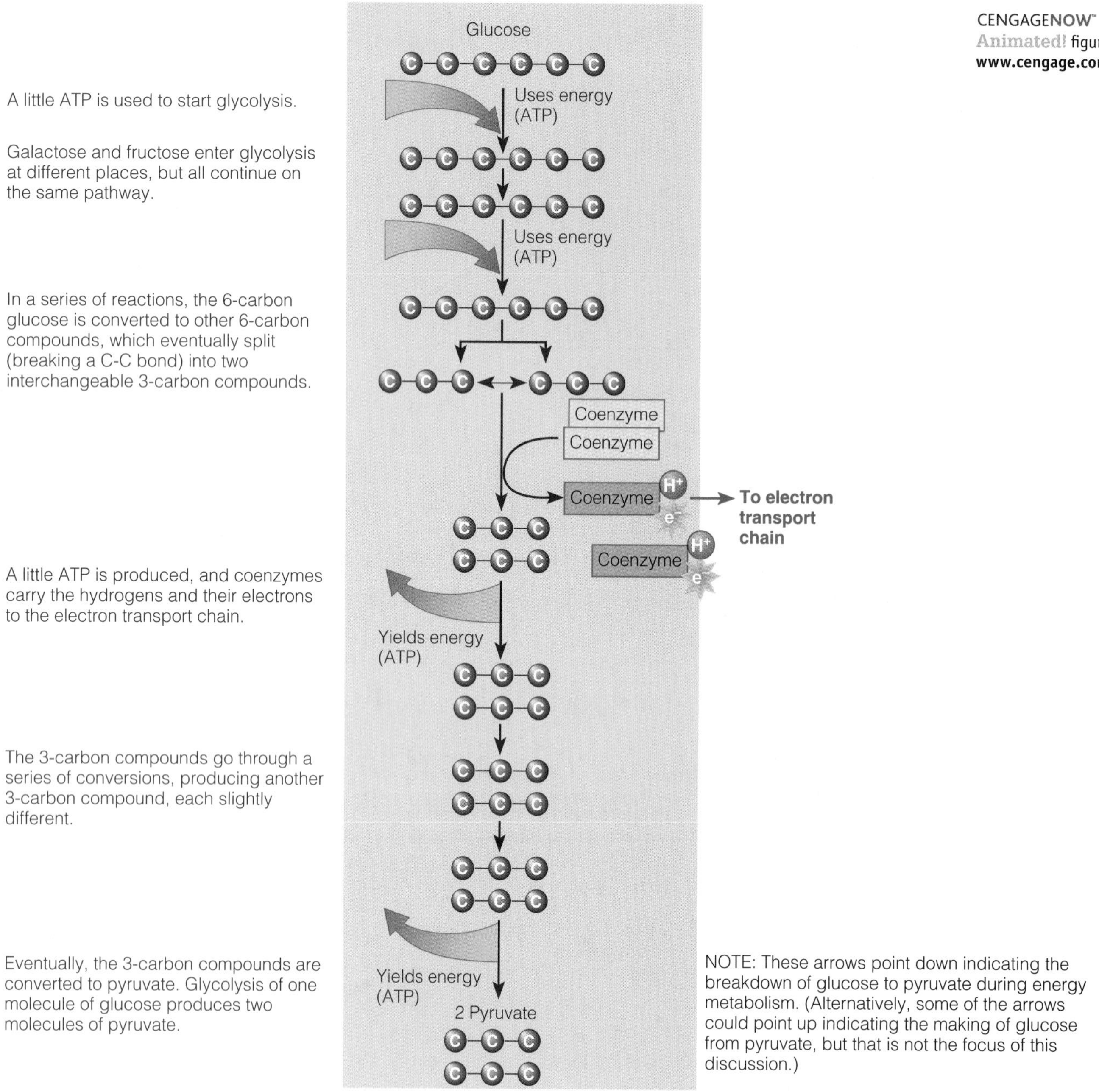
Glucose
A little ATP is used to start glycolysis.
Uses energy (ATP)
Galactose and fructose enter glycolysis at different places, but all continue on the same pathway.
Uses energy (ATP)
In a series of reactions, the 6-carbon glucose is converted to other 6-carbon compounds, which eventually split (breaking a C-C bond) into two interchangeable 3-carbon compounds.
Coenzyme
Coenzyme
Coenzyme
Coenzyme
H+
e−
To electron transport chain
A little ATP is produced, and coenzymes carry the hydrogens and their electrons to the electron transport chain.
Yields energy (ATP)
The 3-carbon compounds go through a series of conversions, producing another 3-carbon compound, each slightly different.
Eventually, the 3-carbon compounds are converted to pyruvate. Glycolysis of one molecule of glucose produces two molecules of pyruvate.
Yields energy (ATP)
2 Pyruvate
NOTE: These arrows point down indicating the breakdown of glucose to pyruvate during energy metabolism. (Alternatively, some of the arrows could point up indicating the making of glucose from pyruvate, but that is not the focus of this discussion.)

accepts the electrons and combines with the hydrogens to form water and how the process captures energy in the high-energy bonds of ATP.

This discussion focuses primarily on the breakdown of glucose for energy, but if needed, cells in the liver (and to some extent, the kidneys) can make glucose again from pyruvate in a process similar to the reversal of glycolysis. Making glucose requires energy, however, and a few different enzymes. Still, glucose can be made from pyruvate, so some of the arrows between glucose and pyruvate could point up as well as down. ♦

♦ Glucose may go "down" to make pyruvate, or pyruvate may go "up" to make glucose, depending on the cell's needs.

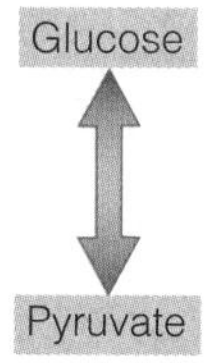
Glucose
Pyruvate

Pyruvate's Options—Anaerobic or Aerobic Whenever carbohydrates, fats, or proteins are broken down to provide energy, oxygen is always ultimately involved in the process. The role of oxygen in metabolism is worth noticing, for it helps our understanding of physiology and metabolic reactions. Chapter 15 describes the body's use of the energy nutrients to fuel physical activity, but the facts presented here offer a sneak preview.

When the body needs energy quickly—as occurs when you run 400 metres as fast as you can—pyruvate is converted to lactate. When the breakdown of glucose-to-pyruvate-to-lactate proceeds without oxygen, it is **anaerobic**. This anaerobic pathway yields energy quickly, but it cannot be sustained for long—a couple of minutes at most.

When energy expenditure proceeds at a slower pace—as occurs when you jog around the track for an hour—pyruvate breaks down to acetyl CoA in an **aerobic** pathway. Aerobic pathways produce energy more slowly, but because they can be sustained for a long time, their total energy yield is greater. The following paragraphs explain these pathways.

Pyruvate-to-Lactate (Aerobic and Anaerobic) As mentioned earlier, coenzymes carry the hydrogens from glucose breakdown to the electron transport chain. If the electron transport chain is unable to accept these hydrogens, as may occur when cells lack sufficient **mitochondria** (review Figure 7-1) or in the absence of sufficient oxygen, pyruvate can accept the hydrogens. As Figure 7-7 shows, by accepting the hydrogens, pyruvate becomes **lactate**, and the coenzymes are freed to return to glycolysis to pick up more hydrogens. In this way, glucose can continue providing a small amount of energy anaerobically for a while (see the left side of Figure 7-7).

The production of lactate occurs to a limited extent even at rest under aerobic conditions, especially in RBCs, since they lack the mitochondria needed for aerobic metabolism. During high-intensity exercise, however, the muscles rely heavily on anaerobic glycolysis to produce ATP quickly, and the concentration of lactate increases dramatically. The rapid rate of glycolysis produces abundant pyruvate and releases hydrogen-carrying coenzymes more rapidly than the mitochondria

anaerobic (AN-air-ROE-bic): not requiring oxygen.

- **an** = not

aerobic (air-ROE-bic): requiring oxygen.

mitochondria (my-toh-KON-dree-uh): the cellular organelles responsible for producing ATP aerobically; made of membranes (lipid and protein) with enzymes mounted on them. (The singular is *mitochondrion.*)

- **mitos** = thread (referring to their slender shape)
- **chondros** = cartilage (referring to their external appearance)

lactate: a 3-carbon compound produced from pyruvate during both aerobic and anaerobic metabolism.

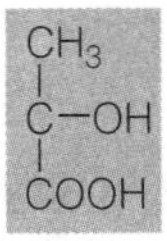
CH3
C—OH
COOH

FIGURE 7-7 Pyruvate-to-Lactate

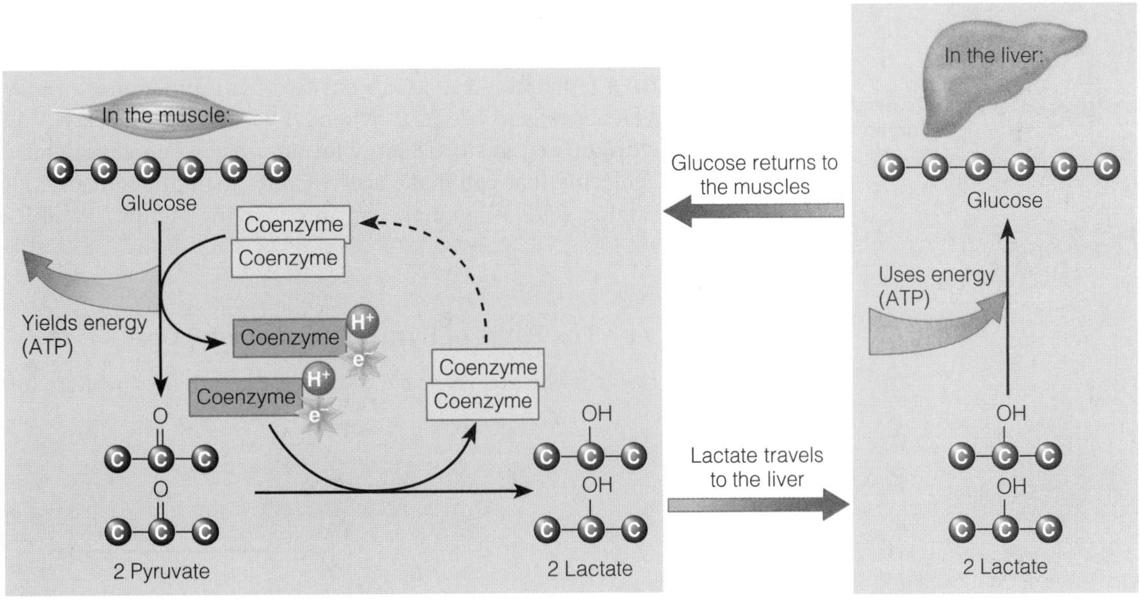
In the muscle:
Glucose
Coenzyme
Coenzyme
Yields energy (ATP)
Coenzyme
Coenzyme
Coenzyme
Coenzyme
O
O
2 Pyruvate
OH
OH
2 Lactate
Glucose returns to the muscles
Lactate travels to the liver
In the liver:
Glucose
Uses energy (ATP)
OH
OH
2 Lactate

Working muscles break down most of their glucose molecules anaerobically to pyruvate. If the cells lack sufficient mitochondria or in the absence of sufficient oxygen, pyruvate can accept the hydrogens from glucose breakdown and become lactate. This conversion frees the coenzymes so that glycolysis can continue.

NOTE: Other figures in this chapter focus narrowly on the carbons of pyruvate. Its oxygen group is included in this figure to more clearly illustrate this reaction. See definitions for the chemical structures of pyruvate and lactate.

Liver enzymes can convert lactate to glucose, but this reaction requires energy. The process of converting lactate from the muscles to glucose in the liver that can be returned to the muscles is known as the *Cori cycle.*

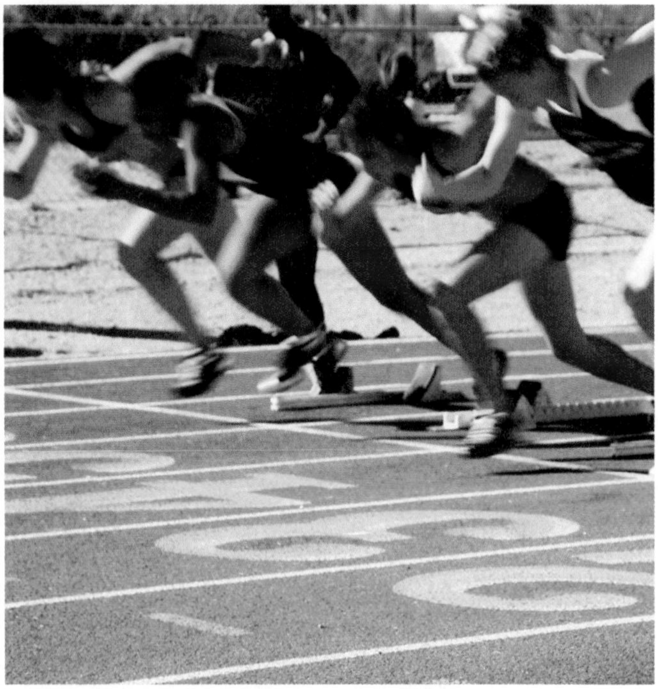
photos.com

The anaerobic breakdown of glucose-to-pyruvate-to-lactate is the major source of energy for short, intense exercise.

can handle them. To enable exercise to continue at this intensity, pyruvate is converted to lactate and coenzymes are released, which allows glycolysis to continue. The accumulation of lactate in the muscles coincides with—but does not seem to be the cause of—the subsequent drop in blood pH, burning pain, and fatigue that are commonly associated with intense exercise.[2] In fact, making lactate from pyruvate consumes two hydrogen ions, which actually diminishes acidity and improves the performance of tired muscles. A person performing the same exercise following endurance training actually experiences less discomfort—in part because the number of mitochondria in the muscle cells has increased. This adaptation improves the mitochondrias' ability to keep pace with the muscles' demand for energy.

One possible fate of lactate is to be transported from the muscles to the liver. There the liver can convert the lactate produced in muscles to glycogen or glucose, the latter of which can then be returned to the muscles. This recycling process is called the **Cori cycle** (see Figure 7-7). (Muscle cells cannot recycle lactate to glucose because they lack a necessary enzyme, but skeletal muscles, the heart, and the brain can all use lactate as an important source of energy.)

Pyruvate-to-Acetyl CoA (Aerobic) If the cell needs energy and oxygen is available, pyruvate molecules enter the mitochondria of the cell (review Figure 7-1, p. 206). There a carbon group (COOH) from the 3-carbon pyruvate is removed to produce a 2-carbon compound that bonds with a molecule of CoA, becoming acetyl CoA. The carbon group from pyruvate becomes carbon dioxide, which is released into the blood, circulated to the lungs, and breathed out. Figure 7-8 diagrams the pyruvate-to-acetyl CoA reaction.

The step from pyruvate to acetyl CoA is metabolically irreversible: a cell cannot retrieve the shed carbons from carbon dioxide to remake pyruvate and then glucose. It is a one-way step and is therefore shown with only a "down" arrow in Figure 7-9.

Acetyl CoA's Options Acetyl CoA has two main functions—it may be used to synthesize fats or to generate ATP. When ATP is abundant, acetyl CoA makes fat, the most efficient way to store energy for later use when energy may be needed. Thus any molecule that can make acetyl CoA—including glucose, glycerol, fatty acids, and amino acids—can make fat. In reviewing Figure 7-9, notice that acetyl

FIGURE 7-8 Pyruvate-to-Acetyl CoA

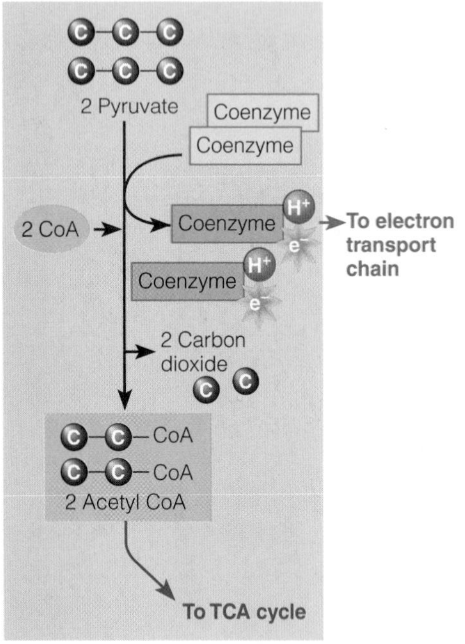
2 Pyruvate
Coenzyme
Coenzyme
2 CoA
Coenzyme
H+
e-
To electron transport chain
Coenzyme
H+
e-
2 Carbon dioxide
CoA
CoA
2 Acetyl CoA
To TCA cycle

Each pyruvate loses a carbon as carbon dioxide and picks up a molecule of CoA, becoming acetyl CoA. The arrow goes only one way (down) because the step is not reversible.

FIGURE 7-9 The Paths of Pyruvate and Acetyl CoA

Pyruvate may follow several reversible paths, but the path from pyruvate to acetyl CoA is irreversible.

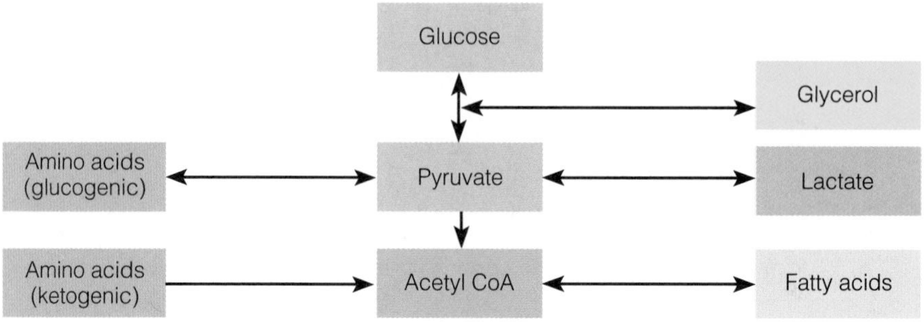
Glucose
Glycerol
Amino acids (glucogenic)
Pyruvate
Lactate
Amino acids (ketogenic)
Acetyl CoA
Fatty acids

NOTE: Amino acids that can be used to make glucose are called *glucogenic;* amino acids that are converted to acetyl CoA are called *ketogenic.*

Cori cycle: the path from muscle glycogen to glucose to pyruvate to lactate (which travels to the liver) to glucose (which can travel back to the muscle) to glycogen; named after the scientist who elucidated this pathway.

CoA can be used as a building block for fatty acids, but it cannot be used to make glucose or amino acids. When ATP is low and the cell needs energy, acetyl CoA may proceed through the TCA cycle, releasing energy in its C-C bonds and hydrogens, with their electrons, to the electron transport chain.

The story of acetyl CoA continues on p. 218 after a discussion of how fat and protein arrive at the same crossroads. For now, know that when acetyl CoA from the breakdown of glucose enters the aerobic pathways of the TCA cycle and electron transport chain, much more ATP is produced than during glycolysis. The role of glycolysis is to provide energy for short bursts of activity and to prepare glucose for the later energy pathways.

IN SUMMARY The breakdown of glucose to energy begins with glycolysis, a pathway that produces pyruvate. Keep in mind that glucose can be synthesized only from pyruvate or compounds earlier in the pathway. Pyruvate may be converted to lactate aerobically or anaerobically or to acetyl CoA aerobically. Once the commitment to acetyl CoA is made, glucose is not retrievable; acetyl CoA cannot go back to glucose. Figure 7-10 summarizes the breakdown of glucose.

FIGURE 7-10 Glucose Enters the Energy Pathway

This figure summarizes the breakdown of glucose-to-pyruvate-to-acetyl CoA. Details of the TCA cycle and the electron transport chain are given later and in APPENDIX C.

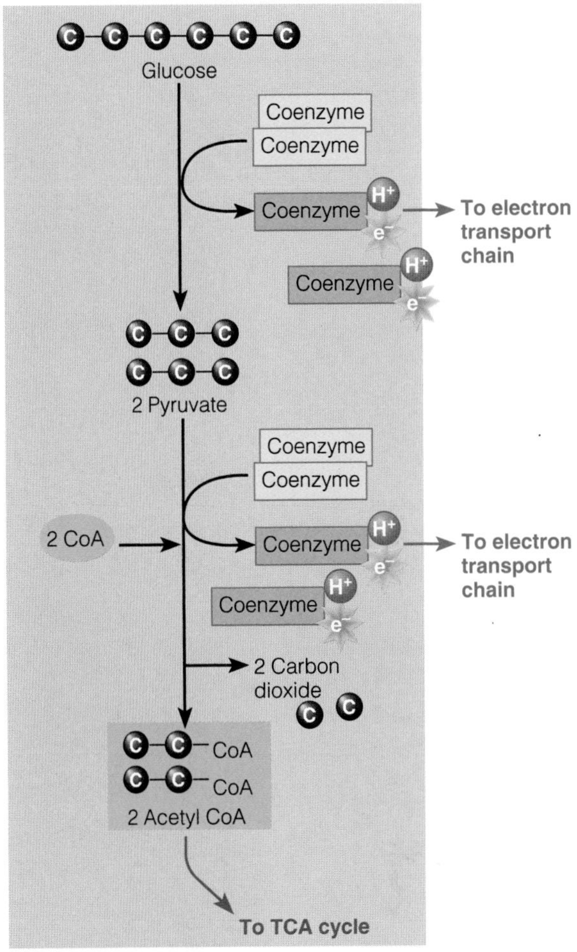
Glucose
Coenzyme
Coenzyme
Coenzyme
H+
e−
To electron transport chain
Coenzyme
2 Pyruvate
2 CoA
2 Carbon dioxide
CoA
CoA
2 Acetyl CoA
To TCA cycle

IN SUMMARY 1 glucose yields 2 pyruvate, which yield 2 acetyl CoA.

Glycerol and Fatty Acids

Once glucose breakdown is understood, fat and protein breakdown are easily learned, for all three eventually enter the same energy pathways. Recall that triglycerides can break down to glycerol and fatty acids.

Glycerol-to-Pyruvate Glycerol is a 3-carbon compound like pyruvate but with a different arrangement of H and OH on the C. As such, glycerol can easily be converted to another 3-carbon compound that can go either "up" the pathway to form glucose or "down" to form pyruvate and then acetyl CoA (review Figure 7-9 on p. 214).

Fatty Acids-to-Acetyl CoA Fatty acids are taken apart 2 carbons at a time in a series of reactions known as **fatty acid oxidation.*** Figure 7-11 (p. 216) illustrates fatty acid oxidation and shows that in the process, each 2-carbon fragment splits off and combines with a molecule of CoA to make acetyl CoA. As each 2-carbon fragment breaks off from a fatty acid during oxidation, hydrogens and their electrons are released and carried to the electron transport chain by coenzymes made from the B vitamins riboflavin and niacin. Figure 7-12 (p. 217) summarizes the breakdown of fats.

Fatty Acids Cannot Be Used to Synthesize Glucose Red blood cells and the brain and nervous system depend primarily on glucose as fuel. When carbohydrate is unavailable, the liver cells can make glucose from pyruvate and other 3-carbon compounds, such as glycerol. Importantly, cells cannot make glucose from the 2-carbon fragments of fatty acids. In chemical diagrams, the arrow between pyruvate and acetyl CoA always points only one way—down—and fatty acids enter the metabolic path below this arrow (review Figure7-9). The down arrow indicates that fatty acids cannot be used to make glucose.

Remember that almost all dietary fats are triglycerides and that triglycerides contain only one small molecule of glycerol with three fatty acids. The glycerol can yield glucose, ♦ but that represents only 3 of the 50 or so carbon atoms in a triglyceride—about 5 percent of its weight (see Figure 7-13 on p. 217). The other 95 percent cannot be converted to glucose.

♦ Making glucose from noncarbohydrate sources is called **gluconeogenesis.** The glycerol portion of a triglyceride and most amino acids can be used to make glucose (review Figure 7-9). The liver is the major site of gluconeogenesis, but the kidneys become increasingly involved under certain circumstances, such as starvation.

fatty acid oxidation: the metabolic breakdown of fatty acids to acetyl CoA; also called *beta oxidation.*

*Oxidation of fatty acids occurs in the mitochondria of the cells (review Figure 7-1, p. 206).

FIGURE 7-11 Fatty Acid-to-Acetyl CoA

Fatty acids are broken apart into 2-carbon fragments that combine with CoA to make acetyl CoA.

CENGAGENOW™
Animated! figure
www.cengage.com/sso

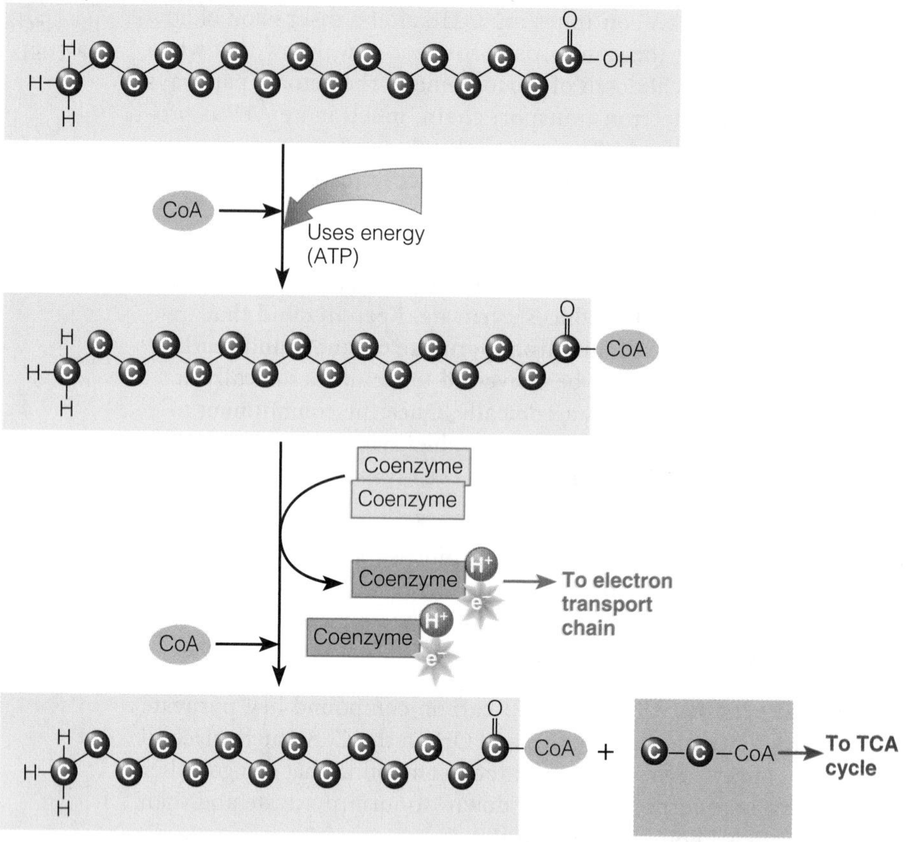
16-C fatty acid
H
H
H
C
O
OH
CoA
Uses energy
(ATP)
Coenzyme
Coenzyme
Coenzyme
H^+
e^-
To electron
transport
chain
CoA
To TCA
cycle

The fatty acid is first activated by coenzyme A.

As each carbon-carbon bond is cleaved, hydrogens and their electrons are released, and coenzymes pick them up.

Another CoA joins the chain, and the bond at the second carbon (the beta-carbon) weakens. Acetyl CoA splits off, leaving a fatty acid that is two carbons shorter.

The shorter fatty acid enters the pathway and the cycle repeats, releasing more hydrogens with their electrons and more acetyl CoA. The molecules of acetyl CoA enter the TCA cycle, and the coenzymes carry the hydrogens and their electrons to the electron transport chain.

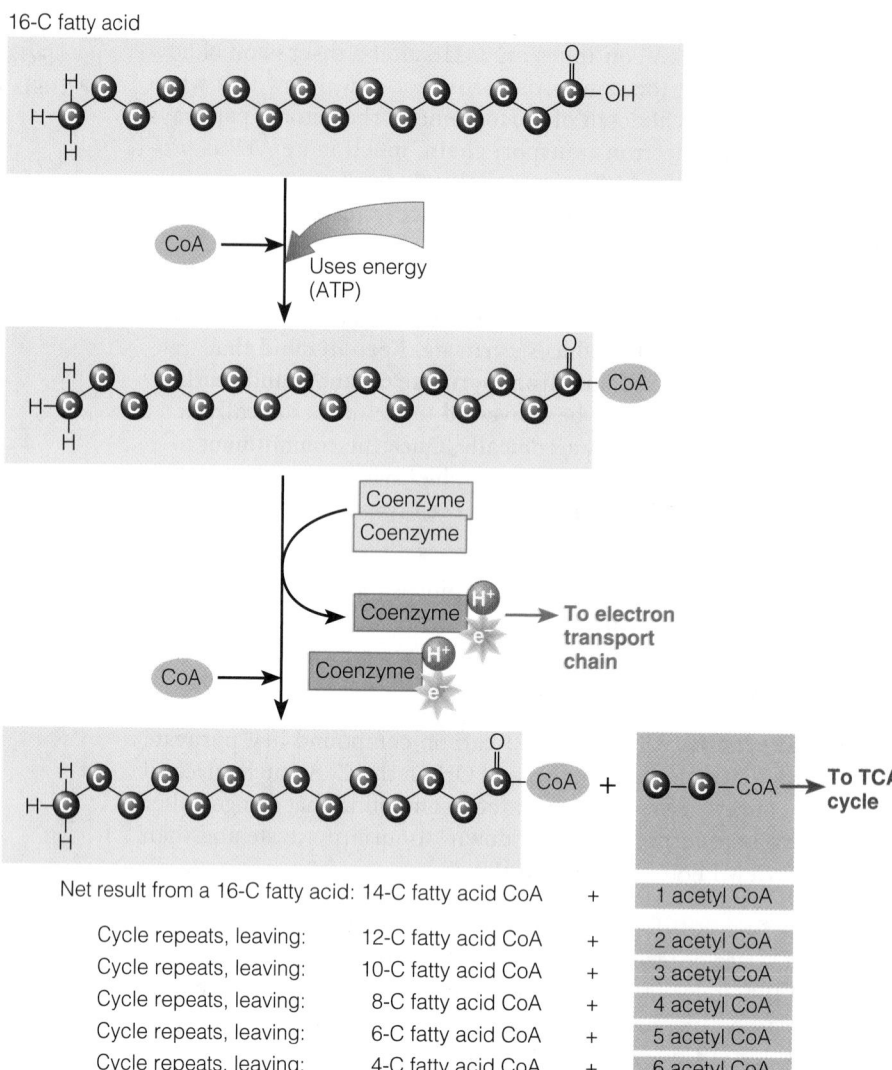

Net result from a 16-C fatty acid:	14-C fatty acid CoA	+	1 acetyl CoA
Cycle repeats, leaving:	12-C fatty acid CoA	+	2 acetyl CoA
Cycle repeats, leaving:	10-C fatty acid CoA	+	3 acetyl CoA
Cycle repeats, leaving:	8-C fatty acid CoA	+	4 acetyl CoA
Cycle repeats, leaving:	6-C fatty acid CoA	+	5 acetyl CoA
Cycle repeats, leaving:	4-C fatty acid CoA	+	6 acetyl CoA
Cycle repeats, leaving:	2-C fatty acid CoA*	+	7 acetyl CoA

*Notice that 2-C fatty acid CoA = acetyl CoA, so that the final yield from a 16-C fatty acid is 8 acetyl CoA.

IN SUMMARY **The body can convert the small glycerol portion of a triglyceride to either pyruvate (and then glucose) or acetyl CoA. The fatty acids of a triglyceride, on the other hand, cannot make glucose, but they can provide abundant acetyl CoA. Acetyl CoA may then enter the TCA cycle to release energy or combine with other molecules of acetyl CoA to make body fat.**

Amino Acids

The preceding two sections have described how the breakdown of carbohydrate and fat produces acetyl CoA, which can enter the pathways that provide energy for the body's use. One energy-yielding nutrient remains: protein or, rather, the amino acids of protein. Before entering the metabolic pathways, amino acids are deaminated (that is, they lose their nitrogen-containing amino group). Chapter 6 describes how deamination produces ammonia (NH_3), which provides the nitrogen needed to make dispensable/nonessential amino acids and other nitrogen-containing compounds. Any remaining ammonia is cleared from the body via urea synthesis in the liver and excretion by the kidneys.

FIGURE 7-12 Fats Enter the Energy Pathway

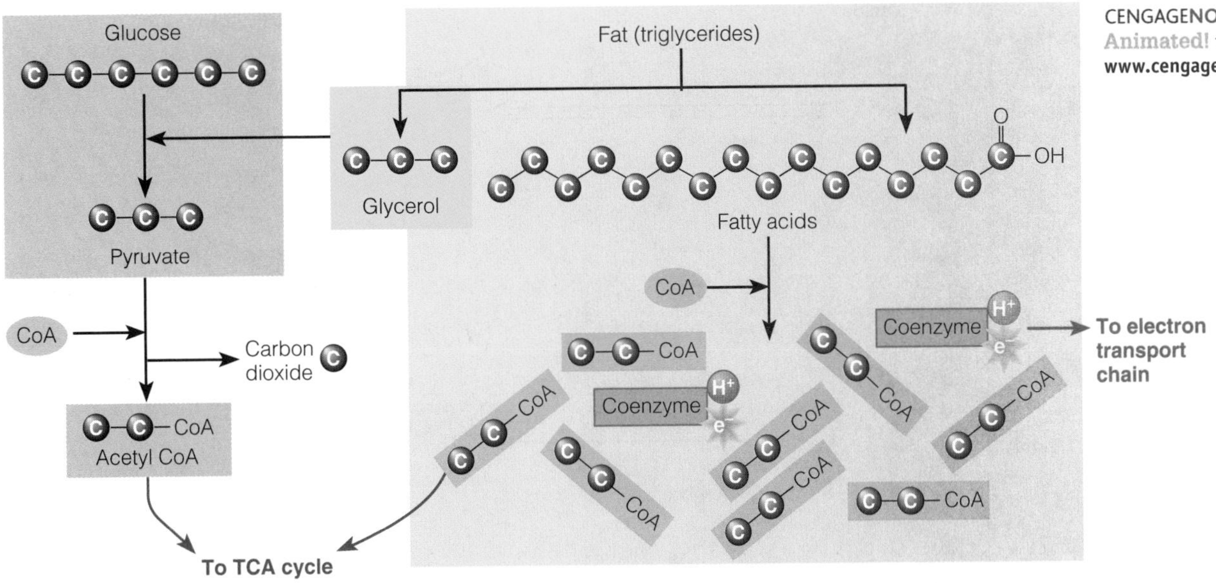
Glucose
Fat (triglycerides)
Glycerol
Fatty acids
Pyruvate
CoA
Carbon dioxide
Acetyl CoA
Coenzyme
To electron transport chain
To TCA cycle

CENGAGENOW™ Animated! figure www.cengage.com/sso

Glycerol enters the glycolysis pathway about midway between glucose and pyruvate. Fatty acids are broken down into 2-carbon fragments that combine with CoA to form acetyl CoA (shown in Figure 7-11).

IN SUMMARY A 16-carbon fatty acid yields 8 acetyl CoA.

Amino Acids-to-Energy Amino acids can enter the energy pathways in several ways. As Figure 7-14 (p. 218) illustrates, some amino acids can be converted to pyruvate, others are converted to acetyl CoA, and still others enter the TCA cycle directly as compounds other than acetyl CoA.

Amino Acids-to-Glucose As you might expect, amino acids that are used to make pyruvate can provide glucose, whereas those used to make acetyl CoA can provide additional energy or make body fat but cannot make glucose. ♦ Amino acids entering the TCA cycle directly can continue in the cycle and generate energy; alternatively, they can generate glucose.[3] Thus protein, unlike fat, is a fairly good source of glucose when carbohydrate is not available.

♦ Amino acids that can make glucose via either pyruvate or TCA cycle intermediates are **glucogenic;** amino acids that are degraded to acetyl CoA are **ketogenic.**

IN SUMMARY The body can use some amino acids to produce glucose, whereas others can be used either to provide energy or to make fat. Before an amino acid enters any of these metabolic pathways, its nitrogen-containing amino group must be removed through deamination.

FIGURE 7-13 The Carbons of a Typical Triglyceride

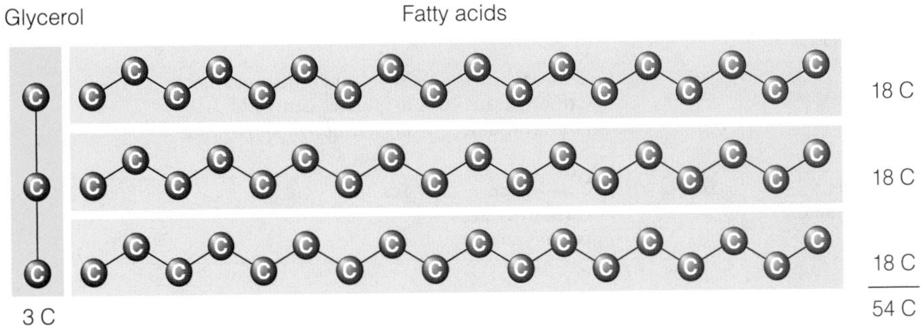
Glycerol
Fatty acids
18 C
18 C
18 C
54 C
3 C

A typical triglyceride contains only one small molecule of glycerol (3 C) but has three fatty acids (each commonly 16 C or 18 C, or about 48 C to 54 C in total). Only the glycerol portion of a triglyceride can yield glucose.

FIGURE 7-14 **Amino Acids Enter the Energy Pathway**

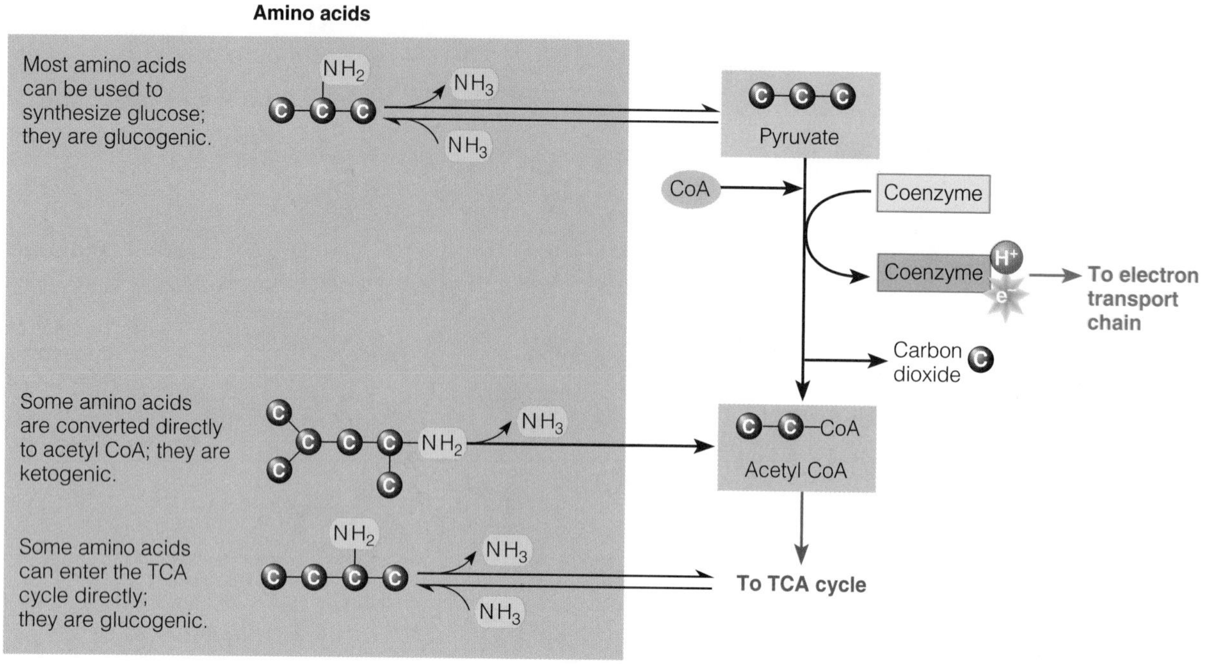
Amino acids
Most amino acids can be used to synthesize glucose; they are glucogenic.
NH2
NH3
NH3
C C C
Pyruvate
CoA
Coenzyme
Coenzyme
H+
e-
To electron transport chain
Carbon dioxide
Some amino acids are converted directly to acetyl CoA; they are ketogenic.
NH2
NH3
C C CoA
Acetyl CoA
Some amino acids can enter the TCA cycle directly; they are glucogenic.
NH2
NH3
NH3
To TCA cycle

NOTE: Deamination and the synthesis of urea are discussed and illustrated in Chapter 6, Figure 6-13 (p. 184). The arrows from pyruvate and the TCA cycle to amino acids are possible only for *dispensable/nonessential* amino acids; remember, the body cannot make essential amino acids.

Breaking Down Nutrients for Energy—In Summary To review the ways the body can use the energy-yielding nutrients, see the following summary table. To obtain energy, the body uses glucose and fatty acids as its primary fuels and amino acids to a lesser extent. To make glucose, the body can use all carbohydrates and most amino acids, but it can convert only 5 percent of fat (the glycerol portion of triglycerides) to glucose. Fatty acids cannot make glucose. To make proteins, the body needs amino acids. It can use glucose and glycerol to make some dispensable/nonessential amino acids when nitrogen is available; it cannot use fatty acids to make body proteins. Finally, when energy intake exceeds the body's needs, all three energy-yielding nutrients can contribute to body fat stores.

IN SUMMARY

Nutrient	Yields Energy?	Yields Glucose?	Yields Amino Acids and Body Proteins?	Yields Fat Stores?
Carbohydrates (glucose)	Yes	Yes	Yes—when nitrogen is available, can yield *dispensable/nonessential* amino acids	Yes
Lipids (fatty acids)	Yes	No	No	Yes
Lipids (glycerol)	Yes	Yes—when carbohydrate is unavailable	Yes—when nitrogen is available, can yield *dispensable/nonessential* amino acids	Yes
Proteins (amino acids)	Yes	Yes—when carbohydrate is unavailable	Yes	Yes

The Final Steps of Catabolism Thus far the discussion has followed each of the energy-yielding nutrients down three different pathways. All lead to the point where acetyl CoA enters the TCA cycle. The TCA cycle reactions take

FIGURE 7-15 A Mitochondrion

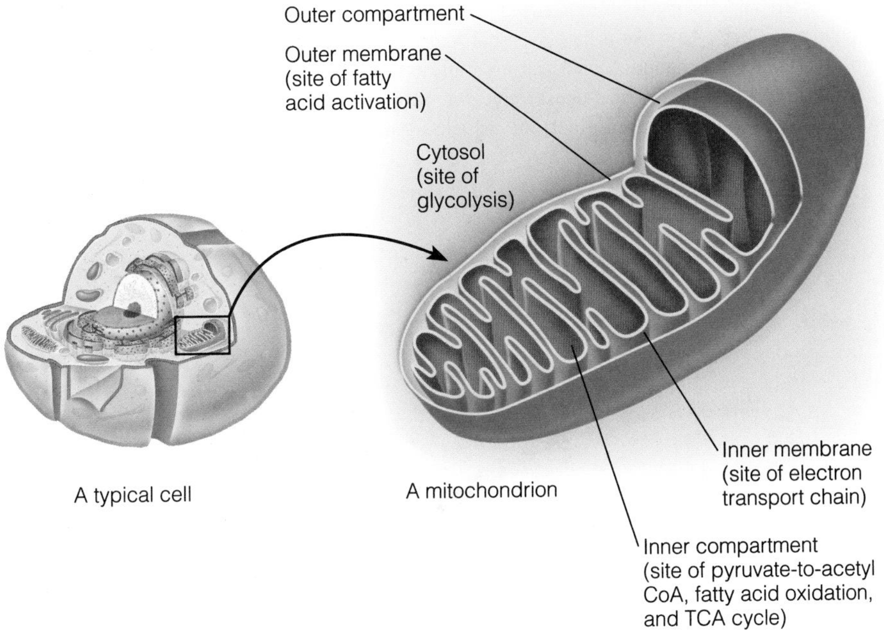
Outer compartment
Outer membrane (site of fatty acid activation)
Cytosol (site of glycolysis)
A typical cell
A mitochondrion
Inner membrane (site of electron transport chain)
Inner compartment (site of pyruvate-to-acetyl CoA, fatty acid oxidation, and TCA cycle)

place in the inner compartment of the mitochondria. Examine the structure of the mitochondria shown in Figure 7-15. The significance of its structure will become evident as details unfold.

The TCA Cycle Acetyl CoA enters the TCA cycle, a busy metabolic traffic centre. The TCA cycle is a circular path, but that doesn't mean it regenerates acetyl CoA. Acetyl CoA goes one way only—down to two carbon dioxide molecules and a coenzyme (CoA). The TCA cycle is a circular path because a 4-carbon compound known as **oxaloacetate** is needed in the first step and it is synthesized in the last step.

Oxaloacetate's role in replenishing the TCA cycle is critical. When oxaloacetate is insufficient, the TCA cycle slows down, and the cells face an energy crisis. Oxaloacetate is made primarily from pyruvate, although it can also be made from certain amino acids. Importantly, oxaloacetate cannot be made from fat. That oxaloacetate must be available for acetyl CoA to enter the TCA cycle underscores the importance of carbohydrates in the diet. A diet that provides ample carbohydrate ensures an adequate supply of oxaloacetate (because glucose produces pyruvate during glycolysis). (The chapter closes with more information on the consequences of low-carbohydrate diets.)

As Figure 7-16 (p. 220) shows, oxaloacetate is the first 4-carbon compound to enter the TCA cycle. Oxaloacetate picks up acetyl CoA (a 2-carbon compound), drops off one carbon (as carbon dioxide), then another carbon (as carbon dioxide), and returns to pick up another acetyl CoA. As for the acetyl CoA, its carbons go only one way—to carbon dioxide (see APPENDIX C for additional details).*

As acetyl CoA molecules break down to carbon dioxide, hydrogen atoms with their electrons are removed from the compounds in the cycle. Each turn of the TCA cycle releases a total of eight electrons. Coenzymes made from the B vitamins niacin and riboflavin receive the hydrogens and their electrons from the TCA cycle and transfer them to the electron transport chain—much like a taxi cab that picks up passengers in one location and drops them off in another.

*Actually, the carbons that enter the cycle in acetyl CoA may not be the exact ones that are given off as carbon dioxide. In one of the steps of the cycle, a 6-carbon compound of the cycle becomes symmetrical, both ends being identical. Thereafter it loses carbons to carbon dioxide at one end or the other. Thus only half of the carbons from acetyl CoA are given off as carbon dioxide in any one turn of the cycle; the other half become part of the compound that returns to pick up another acetyl CoA. It is true to say, though, that for each acetyl CoA that enters the TCA cycle, two carbons are given off as carbon dioxide. It is also true that with each turn of the cycle, the energy equivalent of one acetyl CoA is released.

oxaloacetate (OKS-ah-low-AS-eh-tate): a carbohydrate intermediate of the TCA cycle.

FIGURE 7-16 **The TCA Cycle**

Oxaloacetate, a compound made primarily from pyruvate, starts the TCA cycle. The 4-carbon oxaloacetate joins with the 2-carbon acetyl CoA to make a 6-carbon compound. This compound is changed a little to make a new 6-carbon compound, which releases carbons as carbon dioxide, becoming a 5- and then a 4-carbon compound. Each reaction changes the structure slightly until finally the original 4-carbon oxaloacetate forms again and picks up another acetyl CoA—from the breakdown of glucose, glycerol, fatty acids, and amino acids—and starts the cycle over again. The breakdown of acetyl CoA releases hydrogens with their electrons, which are carried by coenzymes made from B vitamins to the electron transport chain. (For more details, see APPENDIX C.)

CENGAGENOW™
Animated! figure
www.cengage.com/sso

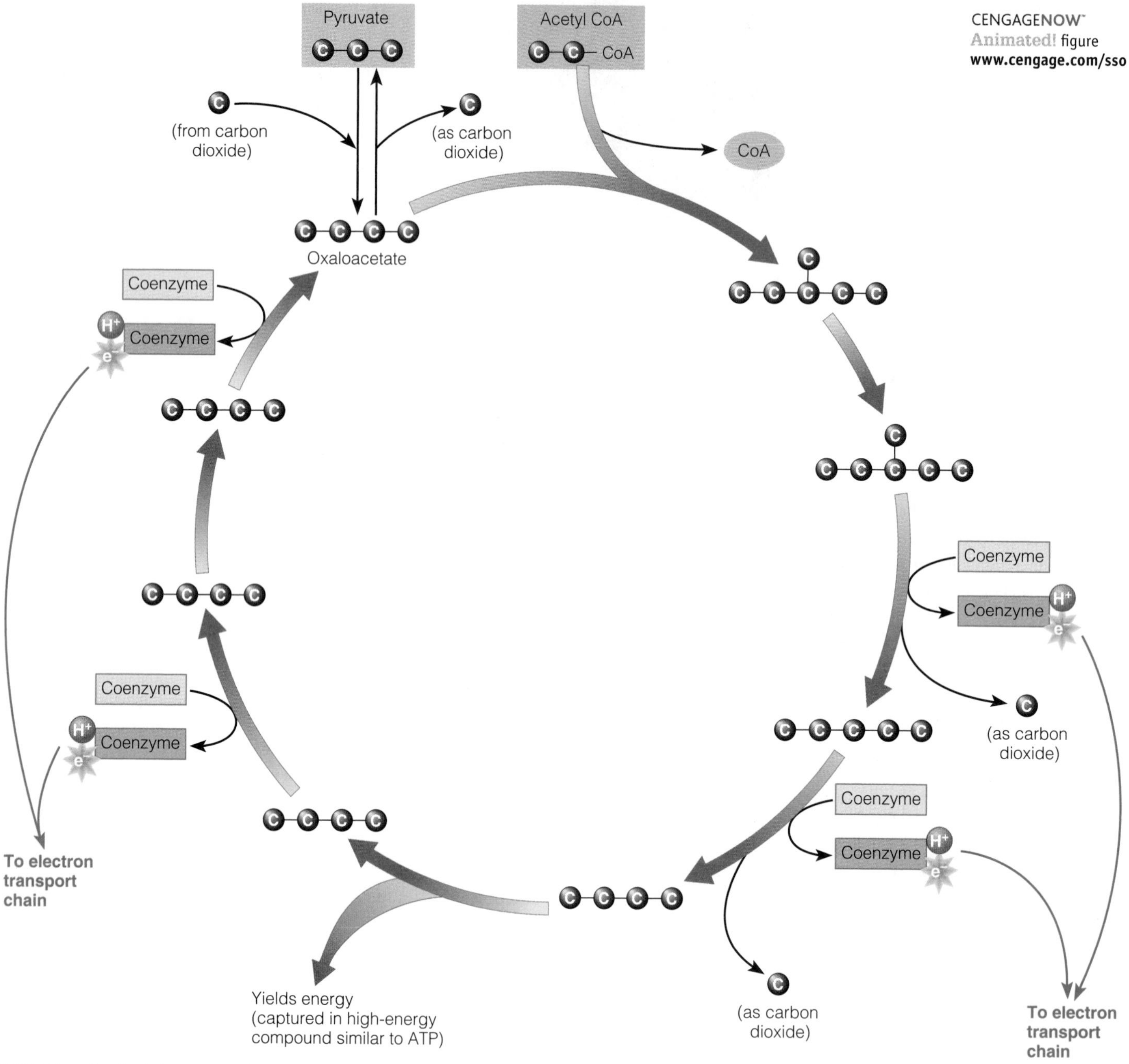
Pyruvate
Acetyl CoA
CoA
(from carbon dioxide)
(as carbon dioxide)
CoA
Oxaloacetate
Coenzyme
Coenzyme
Coenzyme
Coenzyme
Coenzyme
Coenzyme
Coenzyme
Coenzyme
(as carbon dioxide)
To electron transport chain
Yields energy (captured in high-energy compound similar to ATP)
(as carbon dioxide)
To electron transport chain

NOTE: Knowing that glucose produces pyruvate during glycolysis and that oxaloacetate must be available to start the TCA cycle, you can understand why the complete oxidation of fat requires carbohydrate.

The Electron Transport Chain In the final pathway, the electron transport chain, energy is captured in the high-energy bonds of ATP. The electron transport chain consists of a series of proteins that serve as electron "carriers." These carriers are mounted in sequence on the inner membrane of the mitochondria (review Figure 7-15). As the coenzymes deliver their electrons from the TCA cycle, glycolysis, and fatty acid oxidation to the electron transport chain, each carrier receives

FIGURE 7-17 Electron Transport Chain and ATP Synthesis

CENGAGENOW™
Animated! figure
www.cengage.com/sso

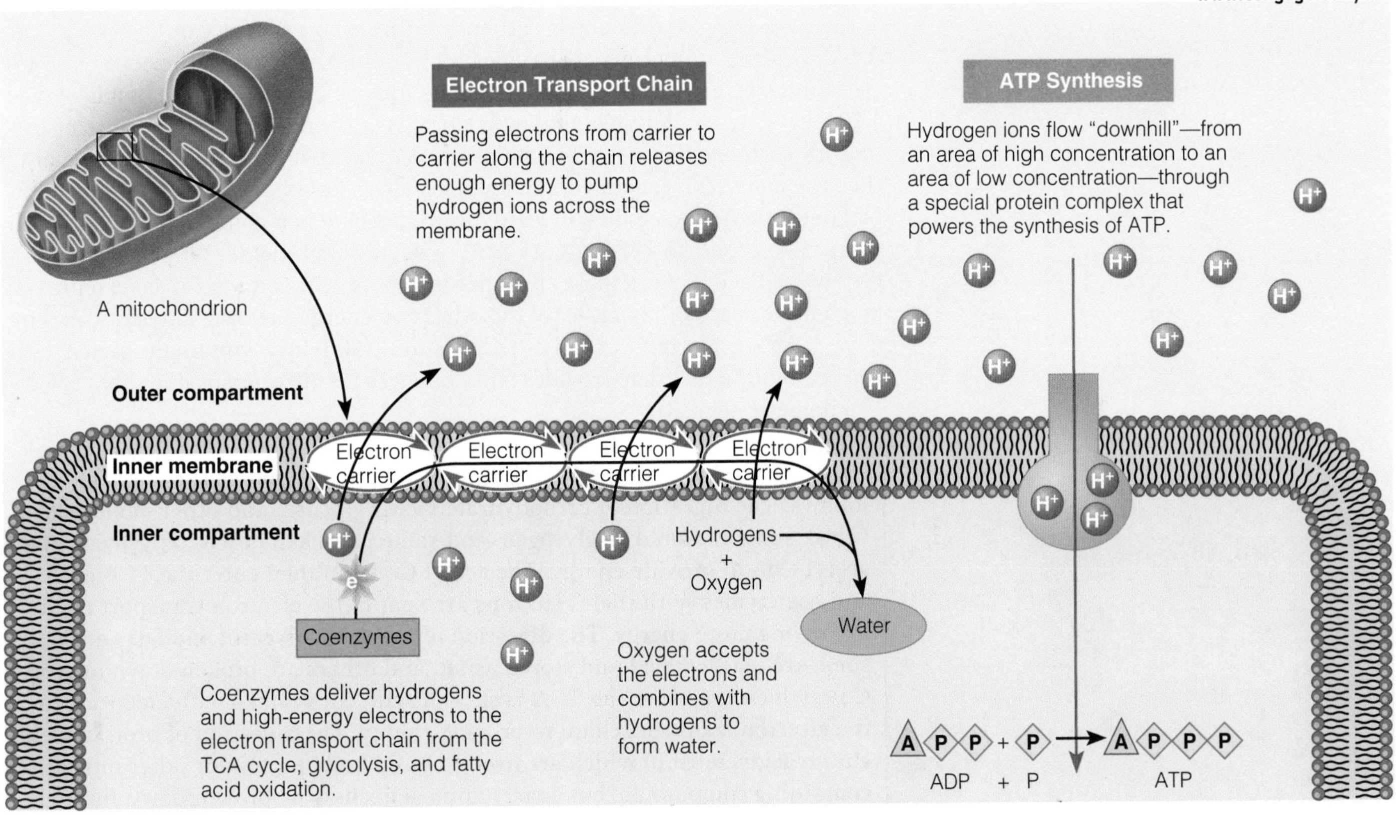
Electron Transport Chain
Passing electrons from carrier to carrier along the chain releases enough energy to pump hydrogen ions across the membrane.
ATP Synthesis
Hydrogen ions flow "downhill"—from an area of high concentration to an area of low concentration—through a special protein complex that powers the synthesis of ATP.
A mitochondrion
Outer compartment
Inner membrane
Inner compartment
Electron carrier
Electron carrier
Electron carrier
Electron carrier
H+
e-
Coenzymes
Hydrogens + Oxygen
Water
Coenzymes deliver hydrogens and high-energy electrons to the electron transport chain from the TCA cycle, glycolysis, and fatty acid oxidation.
Oxygen accepts the electrons and combines with hydrogens to form water.
A P P + P → A P P P
ADP + P
ATP

the electrons and passes them on to the next carrier. These electron carriers continue passing the electrons down until they reach oxygen at the end of the chain. Oxygen (O) accepts the electrons and combines with hydrogen atoms (H) to form water (H_2O). That oxygen must be available for energy metabolism explains why it is essential to life.

As electrons are passed from carrier to carrier, hydrogen ions are pumped across the membrane to the outer compartment of the mitochondria. The rush of hydrogen ions back into the inner compartment powers the synthesis of ATP. In this way, energy is captured in the bonds of ATP. The ATP leaves the mitochondria and enters the cytoplasm, where it can be used for energy. Figure 7-17 provides a simple diagram of the electron transport chain (see APPENDIX C for details).

The kCalories-per-Gram Secret Revealed Of the three energy-yielding nutrients, fat provides the most energy per gram. ♦ The reason may be apparent in Figure 7-18, which compares a fatty acid with a glucose molecule. Notice that nearly all the bonds in the fatty acid are between carbons and hydrogens. Oxygen can be added to all of them—forming carbon dioxide with the carbons and water with the hydrogens. As this happens, hydrogens are released to coenzymes heading for

♦ Fat = 9 kcal/g
Carbohydrate = 4 kcal/g
Protein = 4 kcal/g

FIGURE 7-18 Chemical Structures of a Fatty Acid and Glucose Compared

To ease comparison, the structure shown here for glucose is not the ring structure shown in Chapter 4, but an alternative way of drawing its chemical structure.

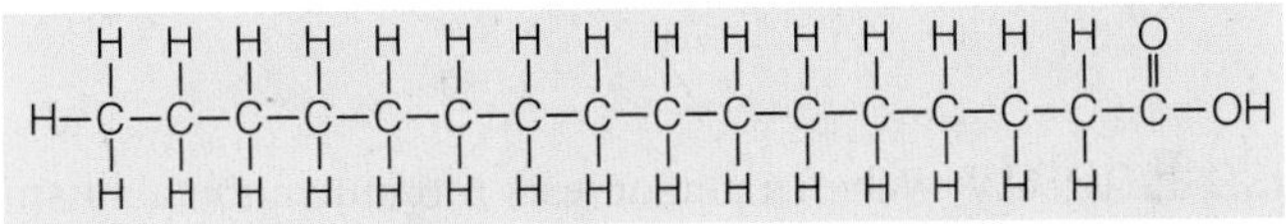

Fatty acid

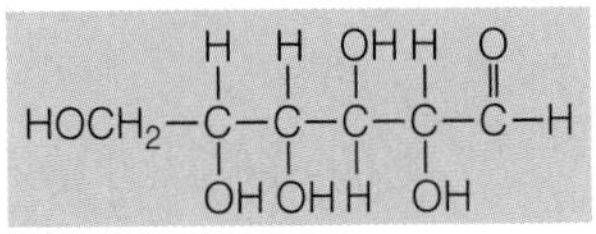

Glucose

the electron transport chain. In glucose, on the other hand, an oxygen is already bonded to each carbon. Thus there is less potential for oxidation, and fewer hydrogens are released when the remaining bonds are broken.

Because fat contains many carbon-hydrogen bonds that can be readily oxidized, it sends numerous coenzymes with their hydrogens and electrons to the electron transport chain where that energy can be captured in the bonds of ATP. This explains why fat yields more kcalories per gram than carbohydrate or protein. (Remember that each ATP holds energy and that kcalories measure energy; thus the more ATP generated, the more kcalories have been collected.) For example, one glucose molecule will yield 30 to 32 ATP when completely oxidized.[4] In comparison, one 16-carbon fatty acid molecule will yield 129 ATP when completely oxidized. Fat is a more efficient fuel source. Gram for gram, fat can provide much more energy than either of the other two energy-yielding nutrients, making it the body's preferred form of energy storage. (Similarly, you might prefer to fill your car with a fuel that provides 55 kilometres per litre versus one that provides 13 kilometres per litre.)

IN SUMMARY **After a balanced meal, the body handles the nutrients as follows. The digestion of carbohydrate yields glucose (and other monosaccharides); some is stored as glycogen, and some is broken down to pyruvate and acetyl CoA to provide energy. The acetyl CoA can then enter the TCA cycle and coenzymes with their electrons are sent to the electron transport chain to provide more energy. The digestion of fat yields glycerol and fatty acids; some are reassembled and stored as fat, and others are broken down to acetyl CoA, which can enter the TCA cycle and send coenzymes with electrons to the electron transport chain to provide energy. The digestion of protein yields amino acids, most of which are used to build body protein or other nitrogen-containing compounds, but some amino acids may be broken down through the same pathways as glucose to provide energy. Other amino acids enter directly into the TCA cycle, and these, too, can be broken down to yield energy.**

In summary, although carbohydrate, fat, and protein enter the TCA cycle by different routes, the final pathways are common to all energy-yielding nutrients. These pathways, which are shown as a simplified overview in Figure 7-5 (p. 211), are shown again in more detail in Figure 7-19. Instead of dismissing this figure as "too busy," take a few moments to appreciate the busyness of it all. Consider that this figure is merely an overview of energy metabolism, and then imagine how busy a cell really is during the metabolism of hundreds of compounds, each of which may be involved in several reactions, each requiring an enzyme. Now, if you really want a challenge, try to think about the entire process in reverse for each of the macronutrients—in other words, back to glucose or an amino acid or a fatty acid. Doing this will help you to better appreciate how the macronutrients in your diet "give you energy."

Energy Balance

Every day, a healthy diet delivers more than a thousand kcalories from foods, and the active body uses most of them to do its work. As a result, body weight changes little, if at all. Maintaining body weight reflects that the body's energy budget is balanced. Some people, however, eat too much or exercise too little and get fat; others eat too little or exercise too much and get thin. The metabolic details have already been described; the next sections review them from the perspective of the body fat gained or lost. The possible reasons why people gain or lose weight are explored in Chapter 8.

Feasting—Excess Energy

When a person eats too much, metabolism favours fat formation. Fat cells enlarge regardless of whether the excess in kcalo-

FIGURE 7-19 The Central Pathways of Energy Metabolism

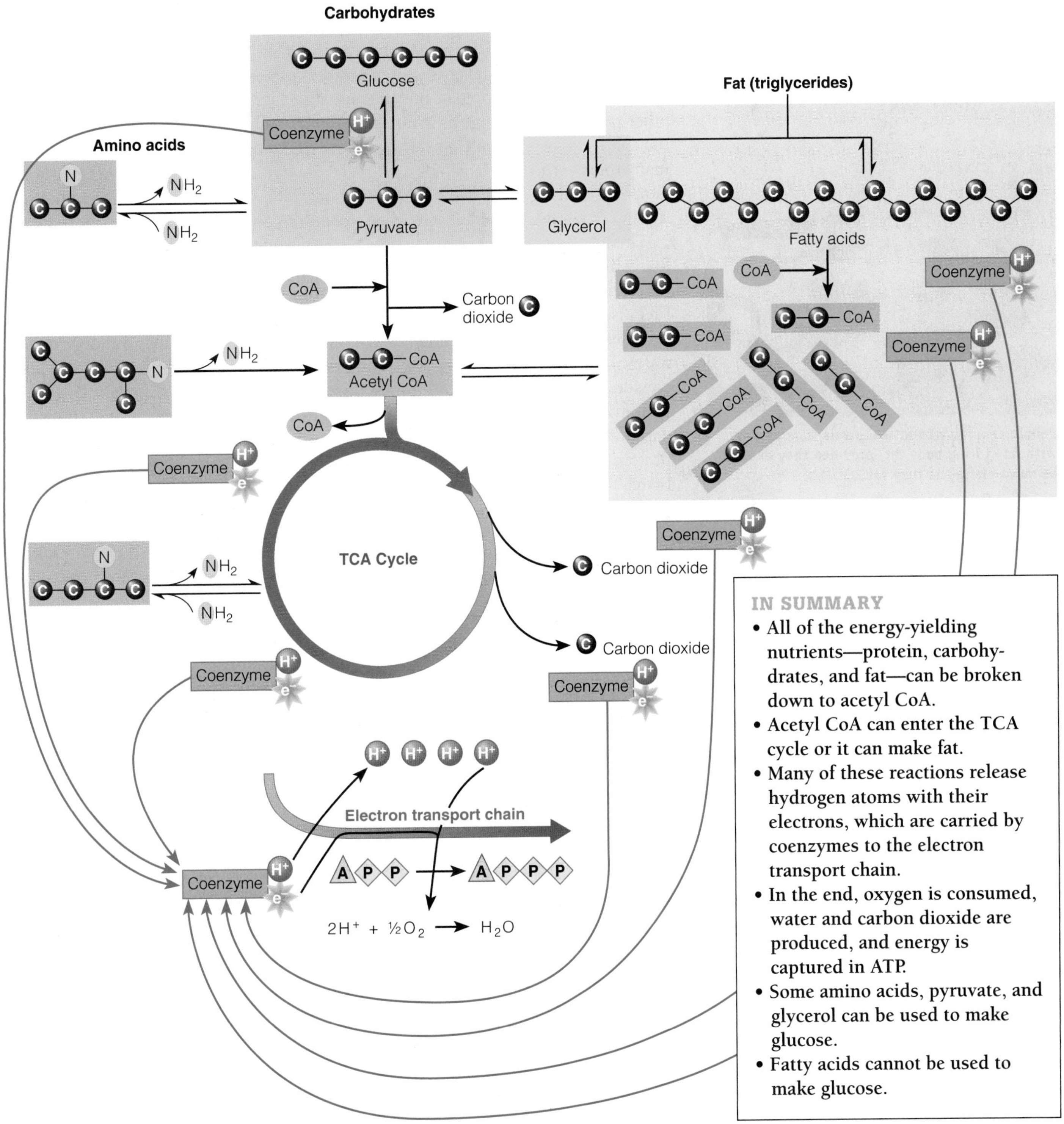
Carbohydrates
Glucose
Coenzyme
H^+
e
Amino acids
N
NH_2
NH_2
Pyruvate
Fat (triglycerides)
Glycerol
Fatty acids
CoA
Carbon dioxide
CoA
Acetyl CoA
CoA
TCA Cycle
Carbon dioxide
Carbon dioxide
Coenzyme
Electron transport chain
A P P
A P P P
$2H^+ + \frac{1}{2}O_2 \rightarrow H_2O$

IN SUMMARY

- All of the energy-yielding nutrients—protein, carbohydrates, and fat—can be broken down to acetyl CoA.
- Acetyl CoA can enter the TCA cycle or it can make fat.
- Many of these reactions release hydrogen atoms with their electrons, which are carried by coenzymes to the electron transport chain.
- In the end, oxygen is consumed, water and carbon dioxide are produced, and energy is captured in ATP.
- Some amino acids, pyruvate, and glycerol can be used to make glucose.
- Fatty acids cannot be used to make glucose.

ries derives from protein, carbohydrate, or fat. The pathway from dietary fat to body fat, however, is the most direct (requiring only a few metabolic steps) and the most efficient (costing only a few kcalories). Briefly, to convert a dietary triglyceride to a triglyceride in adipose tissue, the body removes two of the fatty acids from the glycerol backbone, absorbs the parts, and puts them (and others) together again. By comparison, to convert a molecule of sucrose, the body has to split glucose from fructose, absorb them, dismantle them to pyruvate and acetyl CoA, assemble many acetyl CoA molecules into fatty acid chains, and finally attach fatty acids to a glycerol backbone to make a triglyceride for storage in adipose

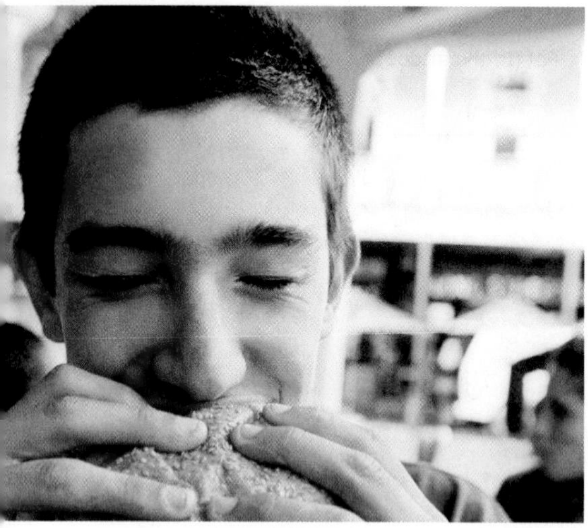
© Ocean/Corbis

People can enjoy bountiful meals such as this without storing body fat, provided they expend as much energy as they take in.

tissue. Quite simply, the body uses much less energy to convert dietary fat to body fat than it does to convert dietary carbohydrate to body fat. On average, storing excess energy from dietary fat as body fat uses only 5 percent of the ingested energy intake, but storing excess energy from dietary carbohydrate as body fat requires 25 percent of the ingested energy intake.

The pathways from excess protein and excess carbohydrate to body fat are not only indirect and inefficient, but they are also less preferred by the body (having other priorities for using these nutrients). Provided there is enough total energy in the diet from other sources, before entering fat storage, protein must first tend to its many roles in the body's lean tissues, and carbohydrate must fill the glycogen stores. Simply put, using these two nutrients to make fat is a low priority for the body. Still, if eaten in abundance, any of the energy-yielding nutrients can be made into fat.

This chapter has described each of the energy-yielding nutrients individually, but cells use a mixture of these fuels. How much of which nutrient is in the fuel mix depends, in part, on its availability from the diet.[5] (The proportion of each fuel also depends on physical activity, as Chapter 15 explains.) Dietary protein and dietary carbohydrate influence the mixture of fuel used during energy metabolism. Usually, protein's contribution to the fuel mix is relatively minor and fairly constant, but protein oxidation does increase when protein is eaten in excess. Similarly, carbohydrate eaten in excess significantly enhances carbohydrate oxidation. In contrast, fat oxidation does *not* respond to dietary fat intake. The more protein or carbohydrate in the fuel mix, the less fat contributes to the fuel mix. Instead of being oxidized, fat accumulates in storage. Details follow.

Excess Protein Recall from Chapter 6 that the body cannot store excess amino acids as such; it has to convert them to other compounds. Contrary to popular opinion, a person cannot grow muscle simply by overeating protein. Lean tissue such as muscle develops in response to a stimulus such as hormones or physical activity. When a person overeats protein, the body uses the surplus first by replacing normal daily losses and then by increasing protein oxidation. The body achieves protein balance this way, but any increase in protein oxidation displaces fat in the fuel mix. Any additional protein is then deaminated, and the remaining carbons are used to make fatty acids, which are stored as triglycerides in adipose tissue. Thus a person can grow fat by eating too much protein.

People who eat huge portions of meat and other protein-rich foods may wonder why they have weight problems. Not only does the fat in those foods lead to fat storage, but the protein can, too, when energy intake exceeds energy needs. Many fad weight-loss diets encourage high protein intakes based on the false assumption that protein builds only muscle, not fat.

Excess Carbohydrate Compared with protein, the proportion of carbohydrate in the fuel mix changes more dramatically when a person overeats. The body handles abundant carbohydrate by first storing it as glycogen, but glycogen storage areas are limited and fill quickly. Because maintaining glucose balance is critical, the body uses glucose frugally when the diet provides only small amounts and freely when supplies are abundant. In other words, glucose oxidation rapidly adjusts to the dietary intake of carbohydrate.

Excess glucose can also be converted to fat directly.[6] This pathway is relatively minor, however. As mentioned earlier, converting glucose to fat is energetically expensive and does not occur until after glycogen stores have been filled. Even then, only a little, if any, new fat is made from carbohydrate.

Nevertheless, excess dietary carbohydrate can displace fat in the fuel mix.[7] When this occurs, carbohydrate spares both dietary fat and body fat from oxidation—an effect that may be more pronounced in overweight people than in lean people. The net result: excess carbohydrate contributes to obesity or at least to the maintenance of an overweight body.

Excess Fat Unlike excess protein and carbohydrate, which both enhance their own oxidation, eating too much fat does not promote fat oxidation. Instead, excess dietary fat moves efficiently into the body's fat stores; almost all of the excess is stored.

IN SUMMARY If energy intake exceeds the body's energy needs, the result will be weight gain—regardless of whether the excess intake is from protein, carbohydrate, or fat. The difference is that the body is much more efficient at storing energy when the excess derives from dietary fat.

The Transition from Feasting to Fasting Figure 7-20 shows the metabolic pathways operating in the body as it shifts from feasting (part A) to

FIGURE 7-20 Feasting and Fasting

A When a person overeats (feasting): When a person eats in excess of energy needs, the body stores a small amount of glycogen and much larger quantities of fat.

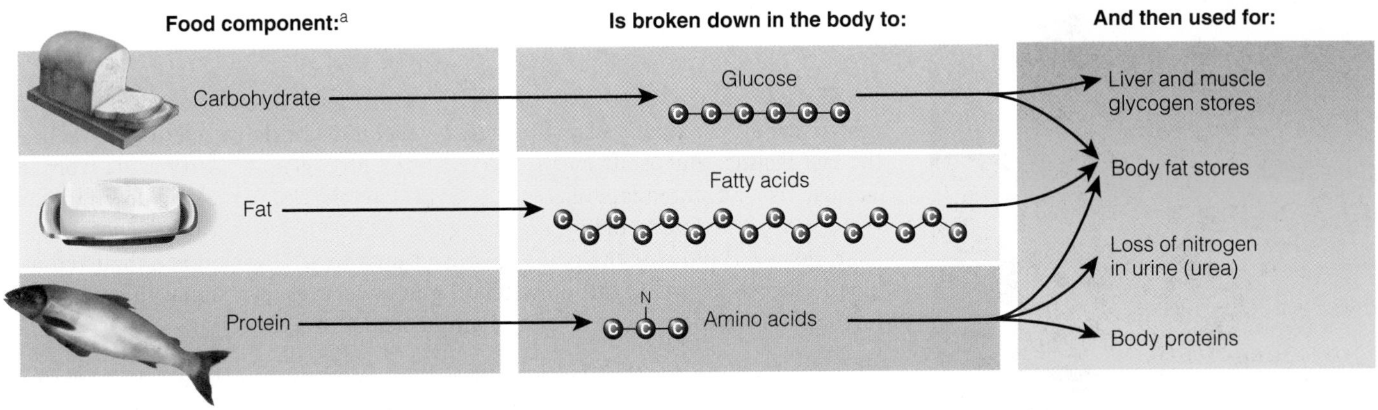
Food component:[a]
Is broken down in the body to:
And then used for:
Carbohydrate
Glucose
Liver and muscle glycogen stores
Fat
Fatty acids
Body fat stores
Loss of nitrogen in urine (urea)
Protein
N
Amino acids
Body proteins

B When a person draws on stores (fasting): When nutrients from a meal are no longer available to provide energy (about 2 to 3 hours after a meal), the body draws on its glycogen and fat stores for energy.

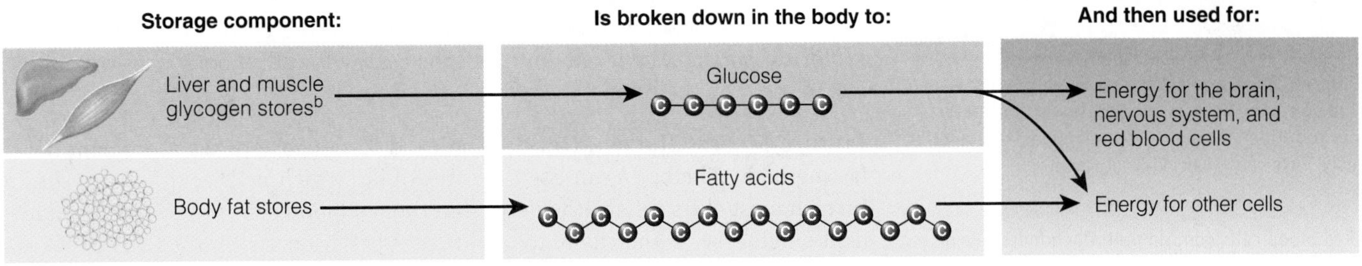
Storage component:
Is broken down in the body to:
And then used for:
Liver and muscle glycogen stores[b]
Glucose
Energy for the brain, nervous system, and red blood cells
Body fat stores
Fatty acids
Energy for other cells

C If the fast continues beyond glycogen depletion: As glycogen stores dwindle (after about 24 hours of starvation), the body begins to break down its protein (muscle and lean tissue) to amino acids to synthesize glucose needed for brain and nervous system energy. In addition, the liver converts fats to ketone bodies, which serve as an alternative energy source for the brain, thus slowing the breakdown of body protein.

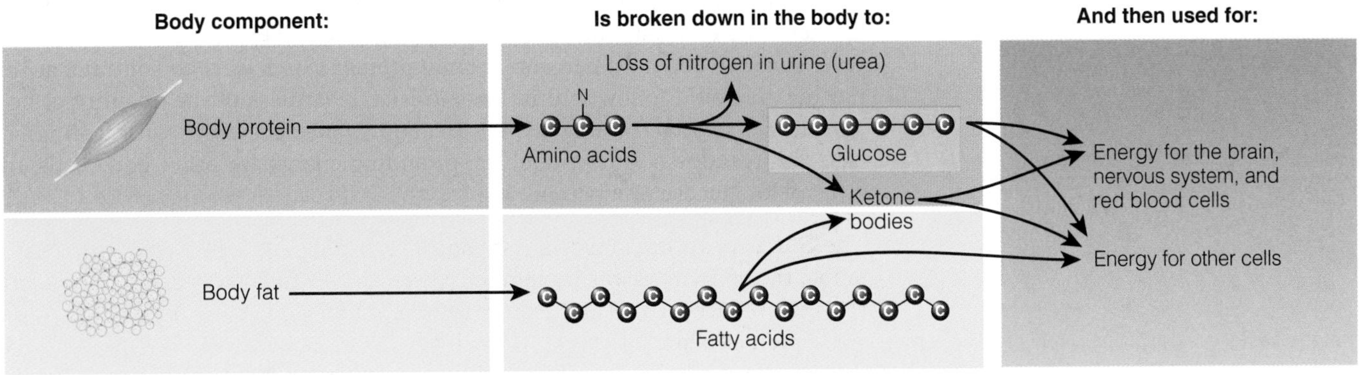
Body component:
Is broken down in the body to:
And then used for:
Loss of nitrogen in urine (urea)
Body protein
N
Amino acids
Glucose
Ketone bodies
Energy for the brain, nervous system, and red blood cells
Energy for other cells
Body fat
Fatty acids

[a]Alcohol is not included because it is a toxin and not a nutrient, but it does contribute energy to the body. After detoxifying the alcohol, the body uses the remaining two carbon fragments for energy (7 kcal/gram) or to build fatty acids and stores them as fat.

[b]The muscles' stored glycogen provides glucose only for the muscle in which the glycogen is stored.

fasting (parts B and C). After a meal, glucose, glycerol, and fatty acids from foods are used as needed and then stored. Later, as the body shifts from a fed state to a fasting one, it begins drawing on these stores. Glycogen and fat are released from storage to provide more glucose, glycerol, and fatty acids for energy.

Energy is needed all the time. Even when a person is asleep and totally relaxed, the cells of many organs are hard at work. In fact, this work—the cells' work that maintains all life processes ♦ without any conscious effort—represents about two-thirds of the total energy a person expends in a day. The small remainder is the work that a person's muscles perform voluntarily during waking hours.

♦ The cells' work that maintains all life processes refers to the body's **basal metabolism**, which is described in Chapter 8.

The body's top priority is to meet the cells' needs for energy, and it normally does this by periodic refuelling—that is, by eating several times a day. When food is not available, the body turns to its own tissues for other fuel sources. If people choose not to eat, we say they are fasting; if they have no choice, we say they are starving. The body makes no such distinction. In either case, the body is forced to draw on its reserves of carbohydrate and fat and, within a day or so, on its vital protein tissues as well.

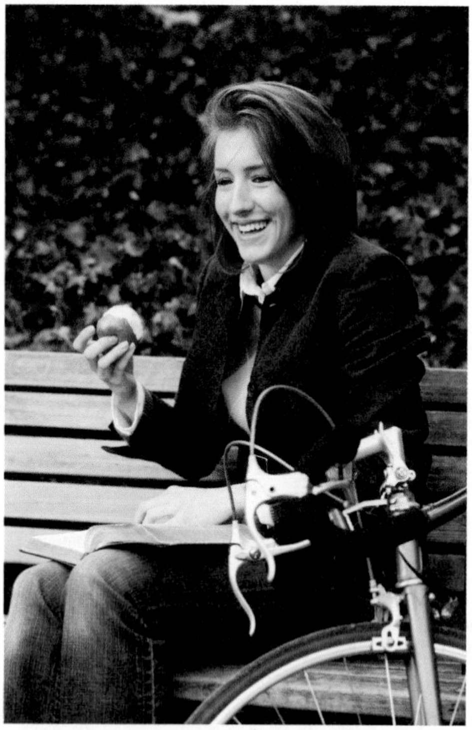
photos.com

The brain and nerve cells depend on glucose—either directly from carbohydrates or indirectly from proteins (through gluconeogenesis). Importantly, fats cannot provide glucose.

Fasting—Inadequate Energy

During fasting, carbohydrate, fat, and protein are all eventually used for energy—fuel must be delivered to every cell. As the fast begins, glucose from the liver's stored glycogen and fatty acids from the adipose tissue's stored fat are both flowing into cells, then breaking down to yield acetyl CoA, and finally delivering energy to power the cells' work. Several hours later, however, most of the glucose is used up—liver glycogen is exhausted and blood glucose begins to fall. Low blood glucose serves as a signal that promotes further fat breakdown and release of amino acids from muscles.

Glucose Needed for the Brain At this point, most of the cells are depending on fatty acids to continue providing their fuel. But, as mentioned earlier, red blood cells and the cells of the nervous system need glucose. Glucose is their primary energy fuel, and even when other energy fuels are available, glucose must be present to permit the energy-metabolizing machinery of the nervous system to work. Normally, the brain and nerve cells—which weigh only a little over 1 kilogram (3 pounds)—consume about half of the total *glucose* used each day (about 500 kcalories' worth). About one-fourth of the *energy* the adult body uses when it is at rest is spent by the brain.[8]

Protein Meets Glucose Needs The need for glucose poses a problem for the fasting body. The body can use its stores of fat, which may be quite generous, to furnish most of its cells with energy, but the red blood cells are completely dependent on glucose, ♦ and the brain and nerves prefer energy in the form of glucose. Amino acids that yield pyruvate can be used to make glucose. ♦ To obtain the amino acids, body proteins must be broken down. For this reason, body protein tissues such as muscle and liver always break down to some extent during fasting. The amino acids that can't be used to make glucose are used as an energy source for other body cells.

♦ Red blood cells contain no mitochondria. Review Figure 7-1, p. 206, to fully appreciate why red blood cells must depend on glucose for energy.

♦ 1 g protein can make ½ g glucose

The breakdown of body protein is an expensive way to obtain glucose. In the first few days of a fast, body protein provides about 90 percent of the needed glucose; glycerol, about 10 percent. If body protein losses were to continue at this rate, death would follow within three weeks, regardless of the quantity of fat a person had stored. Fortunately, fat breakdown also increases with fasting—in fact, fat breakdown almost doubles, providing energy for other body cells and glycerol for glucose production.

The Shift to Ketosis As the fast continues, the body finds a way to use its fat to fuel the brain. It adapts by combining acetyl CoA fragments derived from fatty acids to produce an alternate energy source, ketone bodies (see Figure 7-21). Normally produced and used only in small quantities, ketone bodies ♦ can efficiently provide fuel for brain cells.[9] Ketone body production rises until, after about ten days of fasting, it is meeting much of the nervous system's energy needs. Still,

♦ **Ketone bodies** are compounds produced during the incomplete breakdown of fat when glucose is not available.

many areas of the brain rely exclusively on glucose, and to produce it, the body continues to sacrifice protein—albeit at a slower rate than in the early days of fasting.

When ketone bodies contain an acid group (COOH), they are called **keto acids.** Small amounts of keto acids are a normal part of the blood chemistry, but when their concentration rises, the pH of the blood drops. This is ketosis, a sign that the body's chemistry is going awry. Acidic blood denatures proteins, leaving them unable to function. Elevated blood ketones (ketonemia) are excreted in the urine (ketonuria). A fruity odour on the breath (known as acetone breath) develops, reflecting the presence of the ketone acetone.

Suppression of Appetite Ketosis also induces a loss of appetite. As starvation continues, this loss of appetite becomes an advantage to a person without access to food because the search for food would be a waste of energy. When the person finds food and eats again, the body shifts out of ketosis, the hunger centre gets the message that food is again available, and the appetite returns.

FIGURE 7-21 Ketone Body Formation

1. The first step in the formation of ketone bodies is the condensation of two molecules of acetyl CoA and the removal of the CoA to form a compound that is converted to the first ketone body.
2. This ketone body may lose a molecule of carbon dioxide to become another ketone.
3. Or, the acetoacetate may add two hydrogens, becoming another ketone body (beta-hydroxybutyrate). See APPENDIX C for more details.

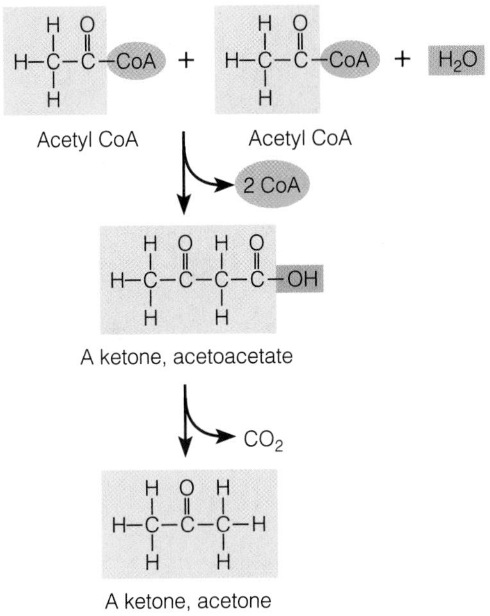
Acetyl CoA
Acetyl CoA
H_2O
2 CoA
A ketone, acetoacetate
CO_2
A ketone, acetone

Slowing of Metabolism In an effort to conserve body tissues for as long as possible, the hormones of fasting slow metabolism. As the body shifts to the use of ketone bodies, it simultaneously reduces its energy output and conserves both its fat and its lean tissue. Still the lean (protein-containing) tissues shrink and perform less metabolic work, reducing energy expenditures. As the muscles waste, they can do less work and so demand less energy, reducing expenditures further. Although fasting may promote dramatic *weight* loss, a low-kcalorie diet and physical activity better support *fat* loss while retaining lean tissue.

Symptoms of Starvation The adaptations just described—slowing of energy output and reduction in fat loss—occur in the starving child, the hungry homeless adult, the fasting religious person, the adolescent with anorexia nervosa, and the malnourished hospital patient. Such adaptations help to prolong their lives and explain the physical symptoms of starvation: wasting; slowed heart rate, respiration, and metabolism; lowered body temperature; impaired vision; organ failure; and reduced resistance to disease. Psychological effects of food deprivation include depression, anxiety, and food-related dreams.

The body's adaptations to fasting are sufficient to maintain life for a long time—up to two months. Mental alertness need not be diminished, and even some physical energy may remain unimpaired for a surprisingly long time. These remarkable adaptations, however, should not prevent anyone from recognizing the very real hazards that fasting presents.

IN SUMMARY **When fasting, the body makes a number of adaptations: increasing the breakdown of fat to provide energy for most of the cells, using glycerol and amino acids to make glucose for the red blood cells and central nervous system, producing ketones to fuel the brain, suppressing the appetite, and slowing metabolism. All of these measures conserve energy and minimize losses.**

Low-Carbohydrate Diets

When a person consumes a low-carbohydrate diet, a metabolism similar to that of fasting prevails. With little dietary carbohydrate coming in, the body uses its glycogen stores to provide glucose for the cells of the brain, nerves, and blood. Once the body depletes its glycogen reserves,

keto (KEY-toe) **acids:** organic acids that contain a carbonyl group (C=O).

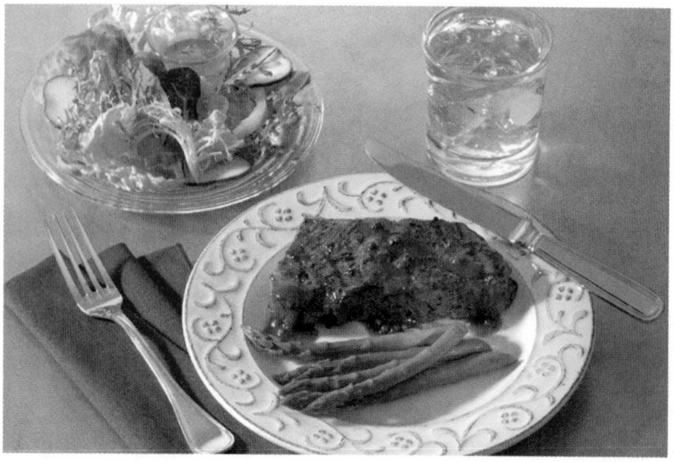
© Matthew Farruggio

Low-carbohydrate meals overemphasize meat, fish, poultry, eggs, and cheeses, and shun breads, pastas, fruits, and vegetables.

it begins making glucose from the amino acids of protein (gluconeogenesis). A low-carbohydrate diet may provide abundant protein from food, but the body still uses some protein from body tissues.

Dieters can know glycogen depletion has occurred and gluconeogenesis has begun by monitoring their urine. Whenever glycogen or protein is broken down, water is released and urine production increases. Low-carbohydrate diets also induce ketosis, and ketones can be detected in the urine. Ketones form whenever glucose is lacking and fat breakdown is incomplete.

Many fad diets regard ketosis as the key to losing weight, but studies comparing weight-loss diets find no relation between ketosis and weight loss.[10] People in ketosis may experience a loss of appetite and a dramatic weight loss within the first few days.[11] They should know that much of this weight loss reflects the loss of glycogen and protein together with large quantities of body fluids and important minerals. They need to appreciate the difference between loss of *fat* and loss of *weight*. Fat losses on ketogenic diets are no greater than on other diets providing the same number of kcalories. Once the dieter returns to well-balanced meals that provide adequate energy, carbohydrate, fat, protein, vitamins, and minerals, the body avidly retains these needed nutrients. The weight will return, quite often to a level higher than the starting point. Table 7-2 lists other consequences of a ketogenic diet.

TABLE 7-2 Adverse Side-effects of Low-Carbohydrate, Ketogenic Diets

- Nausea
- Fatigue (especially if physically active)
- Constipation
- Low blood pressure
- Elevated uric acid (which may exacerbate kidney disease and cause inflammation of the joints in those predisposed to gout)
- Stale, foul taste in the mouth (bad breath)
- In pregnant women, fetal harm and stillbirth

This chapter has probed the intricate details of metabolism at the level of the cells, exploring the transformations of nutrients to energy and to storage compounds. Several chapters and highlights build on this information. The highlight that follows this chapter shows how alcohol disrupts normal metabolism. Chapter 8 describes how a person's intake and expenditure of energy are reflected in body weight and body composition. Chapter 9 examines the consequences of unbalanced energy budgets—overweight and underweight. Chapter 10 shows the vital roles the B vitamins play as coenzymes assisting all the metabolic pathways described here. And Chapter 15 revisits metabolism to show how it supports the work of physically active people and how athletes can best apply that information in their choices of foods to eat.

Nutrition Portfolio

All day, every day, your cells dismantle carbohydrates, fats, and proteins, with the help of vitamins, minerals, and water, releasing energy to meet your body's immediate needs or storing it as fat for later use.

Go to Diet Analysis Plus and choose one of the days on which you have tracked your diet for the entire day. Go to the Intake vs. Goals report and answer the following questions. Keep in mind that in this report 100 percent means you are meeting your needs perfectly.

- How close were you to 100 percent for carbohydrates, fats, proteins, vitamins, minerals, and water? In general, which category was lowest? Which category was highest?
- Describe what types of foods best support aerobic and anaerobic activities.
- Consider whether you eat more protein, carbohydrate, or fat than your body needs.
- Explain how a low-carbohydrate diet forces your body into ketosis.

Diet Analysis PLUS

To complete this exercise, go to your Diet Analysis Plus at www.cengage.com/sso.

Nutrition on the Net

CENGAGENOW™
For further study of topics covered in this chapter, log on to **www.cengage.com/sso.**

- Learn more about how the body metabolizes/transforms omega-3 and omega-6 fatty acids in important biomolecules: **www.dhaomega3.org**
- Learn more about the metabolism of dispensable and indispensable amino acids into important biomolecules: **http://themedicalbiochemistrypage.org/amino-acid-metabolism.html**
- Learn more about the use of diets with different compositions of carbohydrate, fat, and protein for weight management: **www.nejm.org/doi/full/10.1056/NEJMoa0804748**

References

1. R. H. Garrett and C. M. Grisham, *Biochemistry* (Belmont, Calif.: Thomson Brooks/Cole, 2005), p. 73.
2. S. P. Cairns, Lactic acid and exercise performance: Culprit or friend? *Sports Medicine* 36 (2006): 279–291; J. P. Weir and coauthors, Is fatigue all in your head? A critical review of the central governor model, *British Journal of Sports Medicine* 40 (2006): 573–586; A. Philp, A. L. Macdonald, and P. W. Watt, Lactate: A signal coordinating cell and systemic function, *Journal of Experimental Biology* 208 (2005): 4561–4575.
3. S. S. Gropper, J. L. Smith, and J. L. Groff, *Advanced Nutrition and Human Metabolism* (Belmont, Calif.: Thomson Wadsworth, 2005), p. 198.
4. Garrett and Grisham, 2005, p. 669.
5. A. Wise, Transcriptional switches in the control of macronutrient metabolism, *Nutrition Reviews* 66 (2008): 321–325.
6. M. F. Chong and coauthors, Parallel activation of de novo lipogenesis and stearoyl-CoA desaturase activity after 3 d of high-carbohydrate feeding, *American Journal of Clinical Nutrition* 87 (2008): 817–823.
7. R. Roberts and coauthors, Reduced oxidation of dietary fat after a short term high-carbohydrate diet, *American Journal of Clinical Nutrition* 87 (2008): 824–831.
8. W. R. Leonard, J. J. Snodgrass, and M. L. Robertson, Effects of brain evolution on human nutrition and metabolism, *Annual Review of Nutrition* 27 (2007): 311–327.
9. G. F. Cahill, Fuel metabolism in starvation, *Annual Review of Nutrition* 26 (2006): 1–22.
10. M. D. Coleman and S. M. Nickols-Richardson, Urinary ketones reflect serum ketone concentration but do not relate weight loss in overweight premenopausal women following a low-carbohydrate/high-protein diet, *Journal of the American Dietetic Association* 105 (2005): 608–611.
11. A. M. Johnstone and coauthors, Effects of a high-protein ketogenic diet on hunger, appetite, and weight loss in obese men feeding ad libitum, *American Journal of Clinical Nutrition* 87 (2008): 44–55.

Alcohol and Nutrition

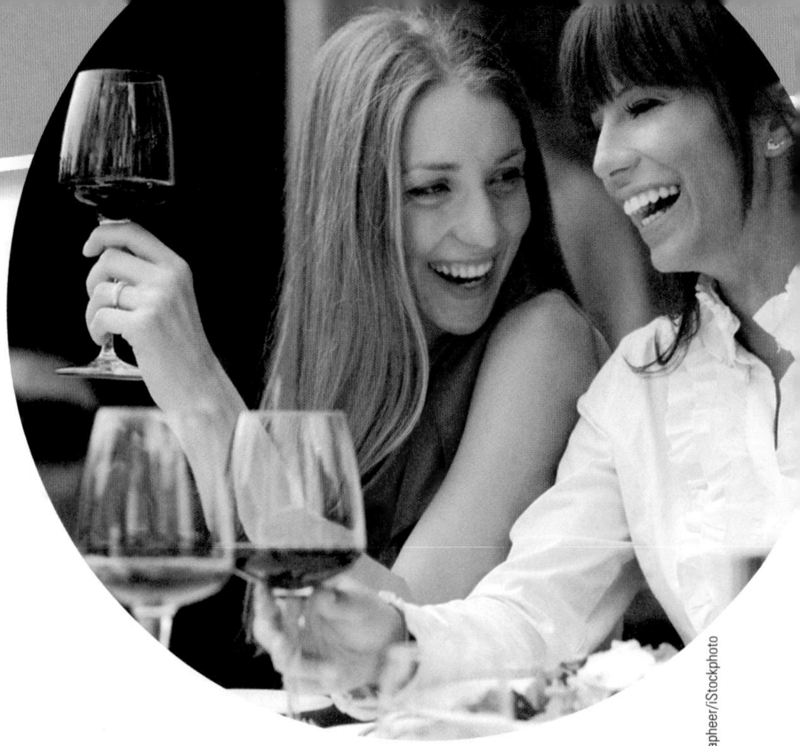

© webphotographeer/iStockphoto

With the understanding of metabolism gained from Chapter 7, you are in a position to understand how the body handles alcohol, how alcohol interferes with metabolism, and how alcohol impairs health and nutrition. Before examining alcohol's damaging effects, it may be appropriate to mention that drinking alcohol in *moderation* may have some health benefits, including reduced risks of heart attacks, strokes, dementia, diabetes, and osteoporosis.[1] Moderate alcohol consumption may lower mortality from all causes, but only in adults aged 35 and older.[2] No health benefits are evident before middle age.[3] Similarly, health benefits begin to disappear in older age, as metabolism changes and organs become more sensitive to toxic substances.[4] Importantly, any benefits of moderate alcohol use must be weighed against the many harmful effects of excessive alcohol use described in this highlight, as well as the possibility of alcohol abuse.

Alcohol in Beverages

To the chemist, **alcohol** refers to a class of organic compounds containing hydroxyl (OH) groups (the accompanying glossary defines alcohol and related terms). The glycerol to which fatty acids are attached in triglycerides is an example of an alcohol to a chemist. To most people, though, *alcohol* refers to the intoxicating

GLOSSARY

acetaldehyde (ass-et-AL-duh-hide): an intermediate in alcohol metabolism.

alcohol: a class of organic compounds containing hydroxyl (OH) groups.

alcohol abuse: a pattern of drinking that includes failure to fulfill work, school, or home responsibilities; drinking in situations that are physically dangerous (as in driving while intoxicated); recurring alcohol-related legal problems (as in aggravated assault charges); or continued drinking despite ongoing social problems that are caused by or worsened by alcohol.

alcohol dehydrogenase (dee-high-DROJ-eh-nayz): an enzyme active in the stomach and the liver that converts ethanol to acetaldehyde.

alcoholism: a pattern of drinking that includes a strong craving for alcohol, a loss of control and an inability to stop drinking once begun, withdrawal symptoms (nausea, sweating, shakiness, and anxiety) after heavy drinking, and the need for increasing amounts of alcohol to feel "high."

antidiuretic hormone (ADH): a hormone produced by the pituitary gland in response to dehydration (or a high sodium concentration in the blood). It stimulates the kidneys to reabsorb more water and therefore prevents water loss in urine (also called *vasopressin*). (This ADH should not be confused with the enzyme alcohol dehydrogenase, which is also sometimes abbreviated ADH.)

beer: an alcoholic beverage traditionally brewed by fermenting malted barley and adding hops for flavour.

binge drinking: four or more drinks for women and five or more drinks for men of alcohol in a row (within a couple of hours).

cirrhosis (seer-OH-sis): advanced liver disease in which liver cells turn orange, die, and harden, permanently losing their function; often associated with alcoholism.
- **cirrhos** = an orange

distilled liquor or **hard liquor:** an alcoholic beverage traditionally made by fermenting and distilling a carbohydrate source such as molasses, potatoes, rye, beets, barley, or corn; sometimes called *distilled spirits*.

drink: a dose of any alcoholic beverage that delivers 15 mL of pure ethanol:
- 150 mL of wine
- 300 mL of wine cooler
- 340 mL of beer
- 50 mL of hard liquor (80 proof whiskey, scotch, rum, or vodka)

drug: a substance that can modify one or more of the body's functions.

ethanol: a particular type of alcohol found in beer, wine, and distilled liquor; also called *ethyl alcohol* (see Figure H7-1). Ethanol is the most widely used—and abused—drug in our society. It is also the only legal, nonprescription drug that produces euphoria.

excessive drinking: heavy drinking, binge drinking, or both.

fatty liver: an early stage of liver deterioration seen in several diseases, including kwashiorkor and alcoholic liver disease. Fatty liver is characterized by an accumulation of fat in the liver cells.

fibrosis (fye-BROH-sis): an intermediate stage of liver deterioration seen in several diseases, including viral hepatitis and alcoholic liver disease. In fibrosis, the liver cells lose their function and assume the characteristics of connective tissue cells (fibres).

heavy drinking: more than one drink per day on average for women and more than two drinks per day on average for men.

MEOS or **microsomal** (my-krow-SO-mal) **ethanol-oxidizing system:** a system of enzymes in the liver that oxidize not only alcohol but also several classes of drugs.

moderation: in relation to alcohol consumption, not more than two drinks a day for the average-size man and not more than one drink a day for the average-size woman.

NAD (nicotinamide adenine dinucleotide): the main coenzyme form of the vitamin niacin. Its reduced form is NADH.

narcotic (nar-KOT-ic): a drug that dulls the senses, induces sleep, and becomes addictive with prolonged use.

proof: a way of stating the percentage of alcohol in distilled liquor. Liquor that is 100 proof is 50 percent alcohol; 90 proof is 45 percent, and so forth.

Wernicke-Korsakoff (VER-nee-key KORE-sah-kof) **syndrome:** a neurological disorder typically associated with chronic alcoholism and caused by a deficiency of the B vitamin thiamin; also called *alcohol-related dementia*.

wine: an alcoholic beverage traditionally made by fermenting a sugar source such as grape juice.

FIGURE H7-1 Two Alcohols: Glycerol and Ethanol

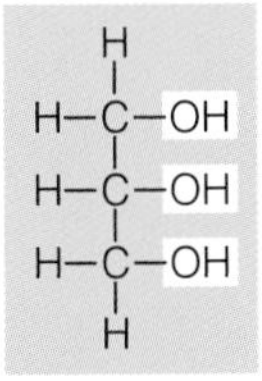

Glycerol is the alcohol used to make the carbon backbone to which 3 fatty acids become attached and form triglycerides.

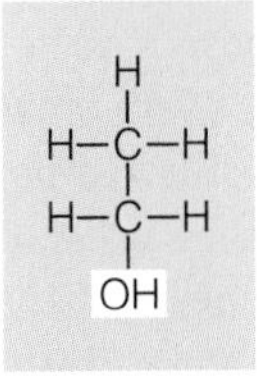

Ethanol is the alcohol in beer, wine, and distilled liquor.

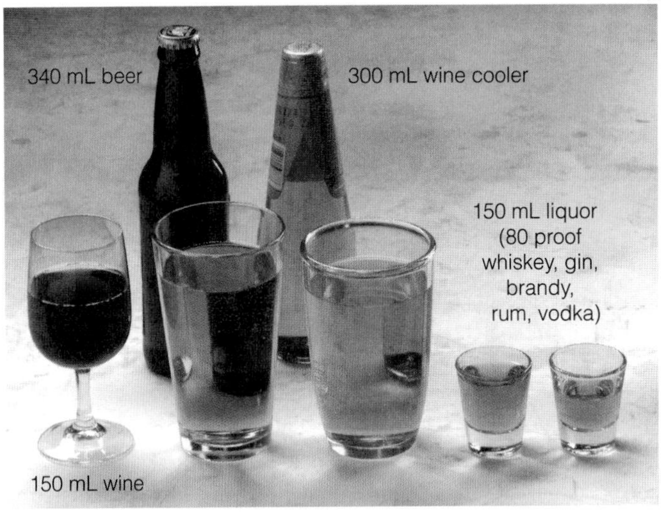
340 mL beer
300 mL wine cooler
150 mL liquor (80 proof whiskey, gin, brandy, rum, vodka)
150 mL wine

Each of these servings equals one drink.

ingredient in **beer, wine,** and **distilled liquor (hard liquor).** The chemist's name for this particular alcohol is *ethyl alcohol,* or **ethanol.** Glycerol has three carbons with three hydroxyl groups attached; ethanol has only two carbons and one hydroxyl group (see Figure H7-1). The remainder of this highlight talks about the particular alcohol ethanol but refers to it simply as *alcohol.*

Alcohols affect living things profoundly, partly because they act as lipid solvents. Their ability to dissolve lipids out of cell membranes allows alcohols to penetrate rapidly into cells, destroying cell structures and thereby killing the cells. For this reason, most alcohols are toxic in relatively small amounts; by the same token, because they kill microbial cells, they are useful as skin disinfectants.

Ethanol is less toxic than the other alcohols. Sufficiently diluted and taken in small enough doses, its action in the brain produces an effect that people seek—not with zero risk, but with a low enough risk (if the doses are low enough) to be tolerable. Used in this way, alcohol is a **drug**—that is, a substance that modifies body functions. Like all drugs, alcohol both offers benefits and poses hazards. The *Dietary Guidelines for Americans* (see APPENDIX I) advise "those who choose to drink alcoholic beverages to do so sensibly and in moderation."

Dietary Guidance for Canadians

- Those who choose to drink alcoholic beverages should do so sensibly and in moderation: up to one drink per day for women and two drinks per day for men.
- Alcoholic beverages should not be consumed by some individuals, including those who cannot restrict their alcohol intake, women of childbearing age who may become pregnant, pregnant and lactating women, children and adolescents, individuals taking medications that can interact with alcohol, and those with specific medical conditions.
- Alcoholic beverages should be avoided by individuals engaging in activities that require attention, skill, or coordination, such as driving or operating machinery.

The term **moderation** is important when describing alcohol use. How many drinks constitute moderate use, and how much is "a drink"? First, a **drink** is any alcoholic beverage that delivers 15 millilitres of *pure ethanol:*

- 150 mL of wine
- 300 mL of wine cooler
- 340 mL of beer
- 50 mL of distilled liquor (80 proof whiskey, scotch, rum, or vodka)

As a practical tip, prevent overpouring by measuring liquids and using tall, narrow glasses.[5]

Beer, wine, and liquor deliver different amounts of alcohol. The amount of alcohol in distilled liquor is stated as **proof:** 100 proof liquor is 50 percent alcohol, 80 proof is 40 percent alcohol, and so forth. Wine and beer have less alcohol than distilled liquor, although some fortified wines and beers have more alcohol than the regular varieties (see photo caption below).

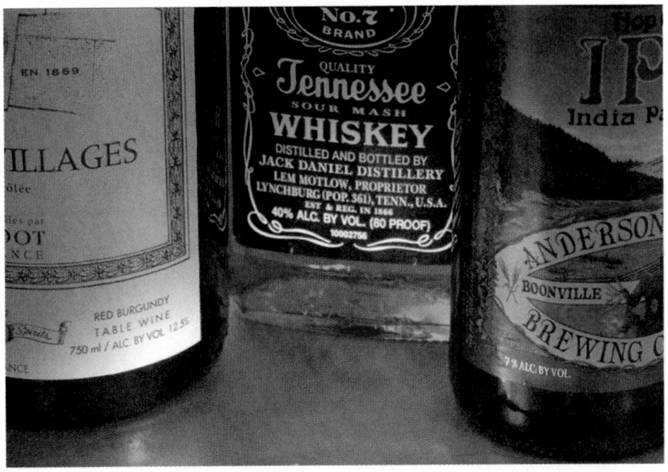
No.7
BRAND
QUALITY
Tennessee
SOUR MASH
WHISKEY
DISTILLED AND BOTTLED BY
JACK DANIEL DISTILLERY
LEM MOTLOW, PROPRIETOR
LYNCHBURG (POP. 361), TENN., U.S.A.
40% ALC. BY VOL. (80 PROOF)
ILLAGES
RED BURGUNDY
TABLE WINE
India Pa
ANDERSON
BOONVILLE
BREWING

Wines contain 7 to 24 percent alcohol by volume; those containing 14 percent or more must state their alcohol content on the label, whereas those with less than 14 percent may simply state "table wine" or "light wine." Beers typically contain less than 5 percent alcohol by volume and malt liquors, 5 to 8 percent.

Second, because people have different tolerances for alcohol, it is impossible to name an exact daily amount of alcohol that is appropriate for everyone. Authorities have attempted to identify amounts that are acceptable for most healthy people. An accepted definition of moderation is up to two drinks per day for men and up to one drink per day for women. (Pregnant women are advised to abstain from alcohol, as Highlight 16 explains.) Notice that this advice is stated as a maximum, not as an average; seven drinks one night a week would not be considered moderate, even though one a day would be. Doubtless, some people could consume slightly more; others could not handle nearly so much without risk. The amount a person can drink safely is highly individual, depending on genetics, health, gender, body composition, age, and family history.

Alcohol in the Body

From the moment an alcoholic beverage enters the body, alcohol is treated as if it has special privileges. Unlike foods, which require time for digestion, alcohol needs no digestion and is quickly absorbed across the walls of an empty stomach, reaching the brain within a few minutes. Consequently, a person can immediately feel euphoric when drinking, especially on an empty stomach.

When the stomach is full of food, alcohol has less chance of touching the walls and diffusing through, so its influence on the brain is slightly delayed. This information leads to another practical tip: eat snacks when drinking alcoholic beverages. Carbohydrate snacks slow alcohol absorption and high-fat snacks slow peristalsis, keeping the alcohol in the stomach longer. Salty snacks make a person thirsty; to quench thirst, drink water instead of more alcohol.

The stomach begins to break down alcohol with its **alcohol dehydrogenase** enzyme. Women produce less of this stomach enzyme than men; consequently, more alcohol reaches the intestine for absorption into the bloodstream. As a result, women absorb more alcohol than men of the same size who drink the same amount of alcohol. Consequently, they are more likely to become more intoxicated on less alcohol than men. Such differences between men and women help explain why women have a lower alcohol tolerance and a lower recommendation for moderate intake.

In the small intestine, alcohol is rapidly absorbed. From this point on, alcohol receives priority treatment: it gets absorbed and metabolized before most nutrients. Alcohol's priority status helps to ensure a speedy disposal and reflects two facts: alcohol cannot be stored in the body, and it is potentially toxic.

Alcohol Arrives in the Liver

As Chapter 3 explains, the capillaries of the digestive tract merge into veins that carry blood first to the liver. These veins branch and rebranch into capillaries that seemingly touch every liver cell. Consequently, liver cells are the first to receive alcohol-laden blood. Liver cells are also the only other cells in the body that can make enough of the alcohol dehydrogenase enzyme to oxidize alcohol at an appreciable rate. The routing of blood through the liver cells gives them the chance to dispose of some alcohol before it moves on.

Alcohol affects every organ of the body, but the most dramatic evidence of its disruptive behaviour appears in the liver. If liver cells could talk, they would describe alcohol as demanding, egocentric, and disruptive of the liver's efficient way of running its business. For example, liver cells normally prefer fatty acids as their fuel, and they like to package excess fatty acids into triglycerides and ship them out to other tissues. When alcohol is present, however, the liver cells are forced to metabolize alcohol and let the fatty acids accumulate, sometimes in huge stockpiles. Alcohol metabolism can also permanently change liver cell structure, impairing the liver's ability to metabolize fats. As a result, heavy drinkers develop fatty livers.

The liver is the primary site of alcohol metabolism.[6] It can process about 15 millilitres of *ethanol* per hour (the amount in a typical drink), depending on the person's body size, previous drinking experience, food intake, and general health. This maximum rate of alcohol breakdown is set by the amount of alcohol dehydrogenase available. If more alcohol arrives at the liver than the enzymes can handle, the extra alcohol travels to all parts of the body, circulating again and again until liver enzymes are finally available to process it. Another practical tip derives from this information: drink slowly enough to allow the liver to keep up—no more than one drink per hour.

The amount of alcohol dehydrogenase enzyme present in the liver varies with individuals, depending on the genes they have inherited and on how recently they have eaten. Fasting for as little as a day forces the body to degrade its proteins, including the alcohol-processing enzymes, and this can slow the rate of alcohol metabolism by half. Drinking after not eating all day thus causes the drinker to feel the effects more promptly for two reasons: rapid absorption and slowed breakdown. By maintaining higher blood alcohol concentrations for longer times, alcohol can anesthetize the brain more completely (as described later in this highlight).

The alcohol dehydrogenase enzyme breaks down alcohol by removing hydrogens in two steps. (Figure H7-2 provides a simplified diagram of alcohol metabolism; APPENDIX C provides the chemical details.) In the first step, alcohol dehydrogenase oxidizes alcohol to **acetaldehyde**—a highly reactive and toxic compound. High concentrations of acetaldehyde in the brain and other tissues are responsible for many of the damaging effects of **alcohol abuse.**

In the second step, a related enzyme, acetaldehyde dehydrogenase, converts acetaldehyde to acetate, which is then converted to either carbon dioxide (CO_2) or acetyl CoA—the "crossroads" compound introduced in Chapter 7. The reactions from alcohol to acetaldehyde to acetate produce hydrogens (H^+) and electrons. The B vitamin niacin, in its role as the coenzyme **NAD (nicotinamide adenine dinucleotide)**, helpfully picks up these hydrogens and electrons (becoming NADH) and escorts them through the electron transport chain. Thus, whenever the body breaks down alcohol, NAD diminishes and NADH accumulates. (Chapter 10 presents information on NAD and the other coenzyme roles of the B vitamins.)

FIGURE H7-2 **Alcohol Metabolism**

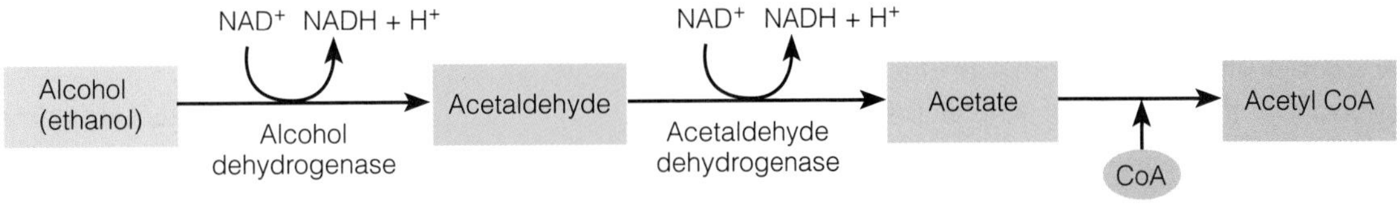
NAD+ NADH + H+
Alcohol (ethanol)
Alcohol dehydrogenase
Acetaldehyde
NAD+ NADH + H+
Acetaldehyde dehydrogenase
Acetate
CoA
Acetyl CoA

The conversion of alcohol to acetyl CoA requires the B vitamin niacin in its role as the coenzyme NAD. When the enzymes oxidize alcohol, they remove H atoms and attach them to NAD. Thus NAD is used up and NADH accumulates. NOTE: More accurately, NAD^+ is converted to NADH + H^+.

Alcohol Disrupts the Liver

During alcohol metabolism, the multitude of other metabolic processes for which NAD is required, including glycolysis, the TCA cycle, and the electron transport chain, falter. Its presence is sorely missed in these energy pathways because it is the chief carrier of the hydrogens that travel with their electrons along the electron transport chain. Without adequate NAD, these energy pathways cannot function. Traffic either backs up or an alternate route is taken. Such changes in the normal flow of energy pathways have striking physical consequences.

For one, the accumulation of hydrogen ions during alcohol metabolism shifts the body's acid–base balance toward acid. For another, the accumulation of NADH slows the TCA cycle, so pyruvate and acetyl CoA build up. Excess acetyl CoA then takes the route to fatty acid synthesis (as Figure H7-3 illustrates), and fat clogs the liver.

As you might expect, a liver overburdened with fat cannot function properly. Liver cells become less efficient at performing a number of tasks. Much of this inefficiency impairs a person's nutritional health in ways that cannot be corrected by diet alone. For example, the liver has difficulty activating vitamin D, as well as producing and releasing bile. To overcome such problems, a person needs to stop drinking alcohol.

The synthesis of fatty acids accelerates with exposure to alcohol. Fat accumulation can be seen in the liver after a single night of heavy drinking. **Fatty liver,** the first stage of liver deterioration seen in heavy drinkers, interferes with the distribution of nutrients and oxygen to the liver cells. Fatty liver is reversible with abstinence from alcohol. If fatty liver lasts long enough, however, the liver cells will die and form fibrous scar tissue. This second stage of liver deterioration is called **fibrosis.** Some liver cells can regenerate with good nutrition and abstinence from alcohol, but in the most advanced stage, **cirrhosis,** damage is the least reversible.

The fatty liver has difficulty making glucose from protein. Without gluconeogenesis, blood glucose can plummet, leading to irreversible damage to the central nervous system.

The lack of glucose together with the overabundance of acetyl CoA sets the stage for ketosis. The body uses excess acetyl CoA to make ketone bodies; their acidity pushes the acid–base balance further toward acid and suppresses nervous system activity.

Excess NADH also promotes the making of lactate from pyruvate. The conversion of pyruvate to lactate uses the hydrogens from NADH and restores some NAD, but a lactate build-up has serious

FIGURE H7-3 **Alternate Route for Acetyl CoA: To Fat**

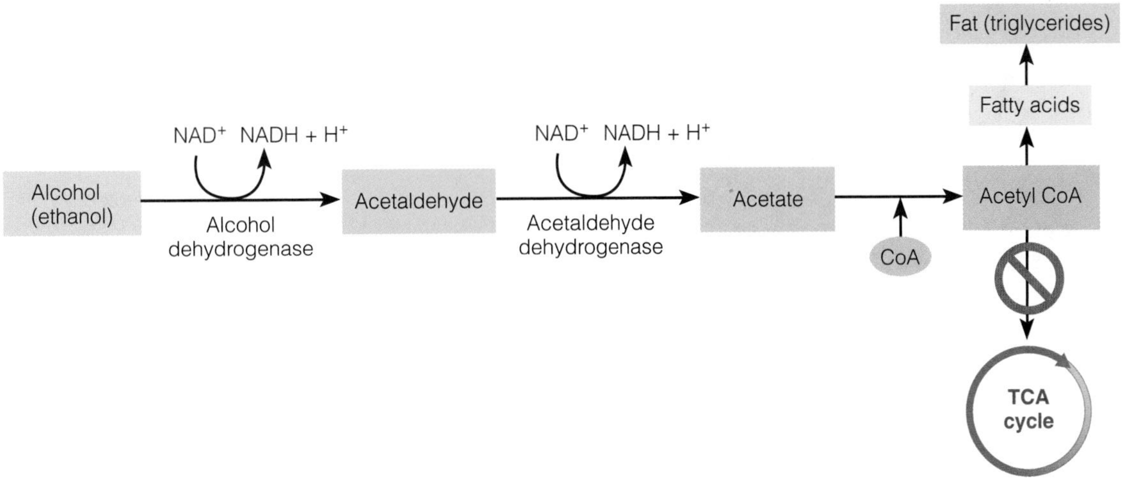
Fat (triglycerides)
Fatty acids
NAD+ NADH + H+
Alcohol (ethanol)
Alcohol dehydrogenase
Acetaldehyde
NAD+ NADH + H+
Acetaldehyde dehydrogenase
Acetate
CoA
Acetyl CoA
TCA cycle

Acetyl CoA molecules are blocked from getting into the TCA cycle by the low level of NAD. Instead of being used for energy, the acetyl CoA molecules become building blocks for fatty acids.

consequences of its own—it adds still further to the body's acid burden and interferes with the excretion of another acid, uric acid, causing inflammation of the joints.

Alcohol alters both amino acid and protein metabolism. Synthesis of proteins important in the immune system slows down, weakening the body's defences against infections. Evidence of protein deficiency becomes apparent, both from a diminished synthesis of proteins and from a poor diet. Normally, the cells would at least use the amino acids from the protein foods a person eats, but the drinker's liver deaminates the amino acids and uses the carbon fragments primarily to make fat or ketones. Eating well does not protect the drinker from protein depletion; a person has to stop drinking alcohol.

The liver's priority treatment of alcohol affects its handling of drugs as well as nutrients. In addition to the dehydrogenase enzyme already described, the liver possesses an enzyme system that metabolizes *both* alcohol and several other types of drugs. Called the **MEOS (microsomal ethanol-oxidizing system),** this system handles about one-fifth of the total alcohol a person consumes. At high blood concentrations or with repeated exposures, alcohol stimulates the synthesis of enzymes in the MEOS. The result is a more efficient metabolism of alcohol and tolerance to its effects.

As a person's blood alcohol rises, alcohol competes with—and wins out over—other drugs whose metabolism also relies on the MEOS. If a person drinks and uses another drug at the same time, the MEOS will dispose of alcohol first and metabolize the drug more slowly. While the drug waits to be handled later, the dose may build up so that its effects are greatly amplified—sometimes to the point of being fatal. Many drug labels provide warnings to avoid alcohol while taking the drug.

In contrast, once a heavy drinker stops drinking and alcohol is no longer competing with other drugs, the enhanced MEOS metabolizes drugs much faster than before. As a result, determining the correct dosages of medications can be challenging.

This discussion has emphasized the major way that the blood is cleared of alcohol—metabolism by the liver—but there is another way. About 10 percent of the alcohol leaves the body through the breath and in the urine. This is the basis for the breath and urine tests for drunkenness. The amounts of alcohol in the breath and in the urine are in proportion to the amount still in the bloodstream and brain. In nearly all provinces, legal drunkenness is set at 0.08 percent or less, reflecting the relationship between alcohol use and traffic and other accidents.

Alcohol Arrives in the Brain

Figure H7-4 describes alcohol's effects on the brain. Alcohol is a **narcotic.** People used it for centuries as an anesthetic because it can deaden pain. But alcohol was a poor anesthetic because one could never be sure how much a person would need and how much would be a fatal dose. Consequently, new, more predictable anesthetics have replaced alcohol. Nonetheless, alcohol continues to be used today as a kind of social anesthetic to help people relax or to

FIGURE H7-4 Alcohol's Effects on the Brain

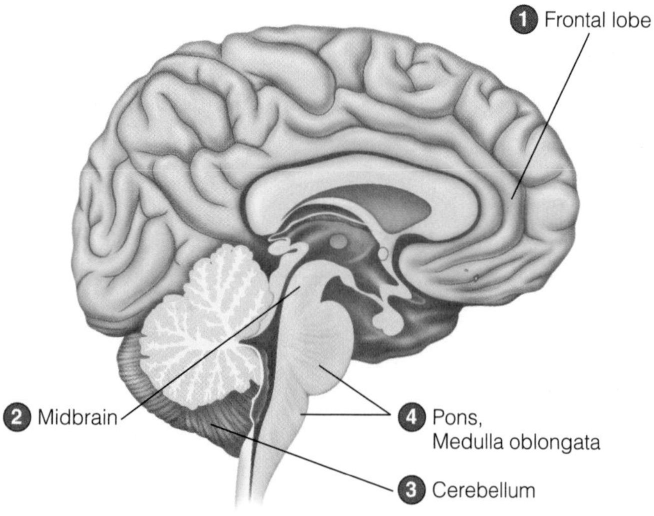

1 Frontal lobe
2 Midbrain
4 Pons, Medulla oblongata
3 Cerebellum

1. Judgment and reasoning centres are most sensitive to alcohol. When alcohol flows to the brain, it first sedates the frontal lobe, the centre of all conscious activity. As the alcohol molecules diffuse into the cells of these lobes, they interfere with reasoning and judgment.

2. Speech and vision centres in the midbrain are affected next. If the drinker drinks faster than the rate at which the liver can oxidize the alcohol, blood alcohol concentrations rise: the speech and vision centres of the brain become sedated.

3. Voluntary muscular control is then affected. At still higher concentrations, the cells in the cerebellum responsible for coordination of voluntary muscles are affected, including those used in speech, eye-hand coordination, and limb movements. At this point people under the influence stagger or weave when they try to walk, or they may slur their speech.

4. Respiration and heart action are the last to be affected. Finally, the conscious brain is completely subdued, and the person passes out. Now the person can drink no more; this is fortunate because higher doses would anesthetize the deepest brain centres that control breathing and heartbeat, causing death.

TABLE H7-1 Alcohol Doses and Approximate Blood Level Percentages for Men and Women

Drinks[a]	Body Weight in Pounds—Men								
	100	120	140	160	180	200	220	240	
	00	00	00	00	00	00	00	00	ONLY SAFE DRIVING LIMIT
1	.04	.03	.03	.02	.02	.02	.02	.02	IMPAIRMENT BEGINS
2	.08	.06	.05	.05	.04	.04	.03	.03	
3	.11	.09	.08	.07	.06	.06	.05	.05	DRIVING SKILLS SIGNIFICANTLY AFFECTED
4	.15	.12	.11	.09	.08	.08	.07	.06	
5	.19	.16	.13	.12	.11	.09	.09	.08	
6	.23	.19	.16	.14	.13	.11	.10	.09	
7	.26	.22	.19	.16	.15	.13	.12	.11	LEGALLY INTOXICATED
8	.30	.25	.21	.19	.17	.15	.14	.13	
9	.34	.28	.24	.21	.19	.17	.15	.14	
10	.38	.31	.27	.23	.21	.19	.17	.16	

Drinks[a]	Body Weight in Pounds—Women									
	90	100	120	140	160	180	200	220	240	
	00	00	00	00	00	00	00	00	00	ONLY SAFE DRIVING LIMIT
1	.05	.05	.04	.03	.03	.03	.02	.02	.02	IMPAIRMENT BEGINS
2	.10	.09	.08	.07	.06	.05	.05	.04	.04	DRIVING SKILLS SIGNIFICANTLY AFFECTED
3	.15	.14	.11	.10	.09	.08	.07	.06	.06	
4	.20	.18	.15	.13	.11	.10	.09	.08	.08	
5	.25	.23	.19	.16	.14	.13	.11	.10	.09	
6	.30	.27	.23	.19	.17	.15	.14	.12	.11	LEGALLY INTOXICATED
7	.35	.32	.27	.23	.20	.18	.16	.14	.13	
8	.40	.36	.30	.26	.23	.20	.18	.17	.15	
9	.45	.41	.34	.29	.26	.23	.20	.19	.17	
10	.51	.45	.38	.32	.28	.25	.23	.21	.19	

NOTE: Legal drinking age in Canada is 19 years old except in Alberta, Manitoba, and Quebec where it is 18 years old. The legal limit of blood alcohol content (BAC) is 0.08 (80 mg per 100 mL of blood); however, individual provinces or territories may impose sanctions on drivers with lower levels.

[a]Taken within an hour or so; each drink equivalent to 15 mL of pure ethanol.

SOURCE: National Clearinghouse for Alcohol and Drug Information; Susan Monroe, Legal drinking age in Canada, About.com Guide. http://canadaonline.about.com/od/canadianlaw/g/drinkingage.htm, accessed September 8, 2011; Canada Safety Council, Canada's blood alcohol laws among the strictest in the Western world (April 29, 2009). http://safety-council.org/news/archives/canada-s-blood-alcohol-laws-amongthe- strictest-in-the-western-world/, accessed September 8, 2011.

relieve anxiety. People think that alcohol is a stimulant because it seems to relieve inhibitions. Actually, though, it accomplishes this by sedating *inhibitory* nerves, which are more numerous than excitatory nerves. Ultimately, alcohol acts as a depressant and affects all the nerve cells.

It is lucky that the brain centres respond to a rising blood alcohol concentration in the order described in Figure H7-4 because a person usually passes out before managing to drink a lethal dose. It is possible, though, to drink so fast that the effects of alcohol continue to accelerate after the person has passed out. Occasionally, a person drinks so much as to stop breathing and die. Table H7-1 shows the blood alcohol levels that correspond to progressively greater intoxication, and Table H7-2 shows the brain responses that occur at these blood levels.

TABLE H7-2 Alcohol Blood Levels and Brain Responses

Blood Alcohol Concentration	Effect on Brain
0.05	Impaired judgment, relaxed inhibitions, altered mood, increased heart rate
0.10	Impaired coordination, delayed reaction time, exaggerated emotions, impaired peripheral vision, impaired ability to operate a vehicle
0.15	Slurred speech, blurred vision, staggered walk, seriously impaired coordination and judgment
0.20	Double vision, inability to walk
0.30	Uninhibited behaviour, stupor, confusion, inability to comprehend
0.40 to 0.60	Unconsciousness, shock, coma, death (cardiac or respiratory failure)

NOTE: Blood alcohol concentration depends on a number of factors, including alcohol in the beverage, the rate of consumption, the person's gender, and body weight. For example, a 45 kg female can become legally drunk (≥0.08 concentration) by drinking three beers in an hour, whereas a 100 kg male consuming that amount at the same rate would have a 0.05 blood alcohol concentration.

Like liver cells, brain cells die with excessive exposure to alcohol. Liver cells may be replaced, but not all brain cells can regenerate. Thus, some heavy drinkers suffer permanent brain damage. Whether alcohol impairs cognition in moderate drinkers is unclear.

People who drink alcoholic beverages may notice that they urinate more, but they may be unaware of the vicious cycle that results. Alcohol depresses production of **antidiuretic hormone (ADH),** a hormone produced by the pituitary gland that retains water—consequently, with less ADH, more water is lost. Loss of body water leads to thirst, and thirst leads to more drinking. Water will relieve dehydration, but the thirsty drinker may drink alcohol instead, which only worsens the problem. Such information provides another practical tip: drink water when thirsty and before each alcoholic drink. Drink an extra glass or two before going to bed. This strategy will help lessen the effects of a hangover.

Water loss is accompanied by the loss of important minerals. As Chapter 11 explains, these minerals are vital to the body's fluid balance and to many chemical reactions in the cells, including muscle action. Detoxification treatment includes restoration of mineral balance as quickly as possible.

Alcohol and Malnutrition

For many moderate drinkers, alcohol does not suppress food intake and may actually stimulate appetite. Moderate drinkers usually consume alcohol as *added* energy—on top of their normal food intake. In addition, alcohol in moderate doses is efficiently metabolized. Consequently, alcohol can contribute to body fat and weight gain—either by inhibiting oxidation or by being converted to fat.[7] Metabolically, alcohol is almost as efficient as fat in promoting obesity; each 30 grams of alcohol represents about a 15 millilitres of fat. Alcohol's contribution to body fat is most evident in the central obesity that commonly accompanies alcohol consumption, popularly—and appropriately—known as the "beer belly."[8] Alcohol in heavy doses, though, is not efficiently metabolized, generating more heat than fat. Heavy drinkers usually consume alcohol as *substituted* energy—instead of their normal food intake. They tend to eat poorly and suffer malnutrition.

Alcohol is rich in energy (7 kcalories per gram), but as with pure sugar or fat, the kcalories are empty of nutrients. The more alcohol people drink, the less likely that they will eat enough food to obtain adequate nutrients. The more kcalories used on alcohol, the fewer kcalories available to use on nutritious foods. Table H7-3 shows the kcalorie amounts of typical alcoholic beverages.

Chronic alcohol abuse not only displaces nutrients from the diet, but it also interferes with the body's metabolism of nutrients. Most dramatic is alcohol's effect on the B vitamin folate. The liver loses its ability to retain folate, and the kidneys increase their excretion of it. Alcohol abuse creates a folate deficiency that devastates digestive system function. The intestine normally releases and retrieves folate continuously, but it becomes damaged by folate deficiency and alcohol toxicity, so it fails to retrieve its own folate and misses any that may trickle in from food as well. Alcohol also interferes with the action of folate in converting the amino acid homocysteine to methionine. The result is an excess of homocysteine, which has been linked to heart disease, and an inadequate supply of methionine, which slows the production of new cells, especially the rapidly dividing cells of the intestine and the blood. The combination of poor folate status and alcohol consumption has also been implicated in promoting colorectal cancer.[9]

The inadequate food intake and impaired nutrient absorption that accompany chronic alcohol abuse frequently lead to a deficiency of another B vitamin—thiamin. In fact, the cluster of thiamin-deficiency symptoms commonly seen in chronic **alcoholism** has its own name—the **Wernicke-Korsakoff syndrome.**[10] This syndrome is characterized by paralysis of the eye muscles, poor muscle coordination, impaired memory, and damaged nerves; it and other alcohol-related memory problems may respond to thiamin supplements.

Acetaldehyde, an intermediate in alcohol metabolism (review Figure H7-2, p. 233), interferes with nutrient use, too. For example, acetaldehyde dislodges vitamin B_6 from its protective binding protein so that it is destroyed, causing a vitamin B_6 deficiency and, thereby, lowered production of red blood cells.

Malnutrition occurs not only because of lack of intake and altered metabolism but because of direct toxic effects as well. Alcohol causes stomach cells to oversecrete both gastric acid and histamine, an immune system agent that produces inflammation. Beer in particular stimulates gastric acid secretion, irritating the linings of the stomach and esophagus and making them vulnerable to ulcer formation.

Overall, nutrient deficiencies are virtually inevitable in alcohol abuse, not only because alcohol displaces food but also because alcohol directly interferes with the body's use of nutrients, making them ineffective even if they are present. Intestinal cells fail to absorb B vitamins, notably, thiamin, folate, and vitamin B_{12}. Liver cells lose efficiency in activating vitamin D. Cells in the retina of the eye, which normally process the alcohol form of vitamin A (retinol) to the aldehyde form needed in vision (retinal), find themselves processing ethanol to acetaldehyde instead. Likewise, the liver cannot convert the aldehyde form of vitamin A to its acid form (retinoic acid), which is needed to support the growth of its (and all) cells.

Regardless of dietary intake, excessive drinking over a lifetime creates deficits of all the nutrients mentioned in this discussion and more. No diet can compensate for the damage caused by heavy alcohol consumption.

TABLE H7-3 kCalories in Alcoholic Beverages and Mixers

Beverage	Amount (mL)	Energy (kcal)	Alcohol (g)
Beer			
Regular	340	153	14
Light	340	103	11
Nonalcoholic	340	32	0
Cocktails			
Daiquiri, canned	200	259	20
Daiquiri, from recipe	135	223	28
Piña colada, canned	200	526	20
Piña colada, from recipe	135	245	14
Tequila sunrise, canned	200	232	20
Whiskey sour, canned	200	249	20
Distilled liquor (gin, rum, vodka, whiskey)			
80 proof	45	97	14
86 proof	45	105	15
90 proof	45	110	16
94 proof	45	116	17
100 proof	45	124	18
Sake	45	58	7
Liqueurs			
Coffee and cream liqueur, 34 proof	45	154	7
Coffee liqueur, 53 proof	45	170	11
Coffee liqueur, 63 proof	45	160	14
Crème de menthe, 72 proof	45	186	15
Mixers			
Club soda	340	0	0
Cola	340	136	0
Cranberry juice cocktail	120	72	0
Ginger ale or tonic water	340	124	0
Grapefruit juice	120	48	0
Orange juice	120	56	0
Tomato or vegetable juice	120	21	0
Wine			
Champagne	150	105	13
Cooking	150	72	5
Dessert, dry	150	224	23
Dessert, sweet	150	236	23
Red or rosé	150	125	16
White	150	121	15
Wine cooler	300	150	11

How Much Alcohol Do Canadians Consume?

During 2010, just under 80 percent of Canadians over 15 years consumed alcohol, 44 percent of whom drink at least once a week.[11, 12] Beer comprises 80 percent of alcoholic beverages consumed by Canadians, which have risen to the level of just over 85 litres per person over the age of 15 years. In addition, almost 14 litres of wine are consumed annually by these individuals, as are 7.5 litres of spirits. Statistics Canada notes that these levels may be understated since they do not include homemade alcoholic beverages or those brewed on the premises, and so on. It should also be noted that over one in five (22.6 percent) drinkers exceeded the low-risk guidelines of less than 14 drinks per week for males and 9 drinks per week for females (i.e., engaged in **heavy drinking**), a behaviour more common among those 18 to 24 years of age.

Drinking habits span a wide spectrum: many adults drink no alcohol whatsoever, some take a glass of wine only with meals, others drink on social occasions, and others take in large quantities of alcohol daily because of a life-shattering situation.

Alcohol Consumption among Canadian University Students

According to a Canadian Institutes of Health Research (CIHR)–funded survey reported by Canada's Centre for Addiction and Mental Health (CAMH), a 2004 Canadian campus survey of over 6000 students from 40 universities revealed that 77 percent had consumed alcohol during the month prior to the study. Furthermore, 18.5 percent and 6.6 percent indicated that they consumed five or more or eight or more drinks (**binge drinking**), respectively, on a single occasion once every two weeks or more frequently.[13]

Also, almost one-third of students reported at least one indicator of dependent drinking (e.g., being unable to stop).Males reported drinking more and higher amounts than females (8.9 versus 4.5 drinks per week), as well as higher rates of **excessive drinking** and episodic drinking, most of which occurred on weekends and off-campus but in private premises. Social acceptance may make it difficult for binge drinkers to recognize themselves as problem drinkers. For this reason, interventions must focus both on educating individuals and on changing the campus social environment. The damage alcohol causes only becomes worse if the pattern is not broken. Alcohol abuse sets in much more quickly in young people than in adults. Those who start drinking at an early age more often suffer from alcoholism than people who start later on. Table H7-4 lists the key signs of alcoholism.

TABLE H7-4 Signs of Alcoholism

- Tolerance: the person needs higher and higher intakes of alcohol to achieve intoxication.
- Withdrawal: the person who stops drinking experiences anxiety, agitation, increased blood pressure, or seizures, or seeks alcohol to relieve these symptoms.
- Impaired control: the person intends to have 1 or 2 drinks, but has 9 or 10 instead, or the person tries to control or quit drinking, but fails.
- Disinterest: the person neglects important social, family, job, or school activities because of drinking.
- Time: the person spends a great deal of time obtaining and drinking alcohol or recovering from excessive drinking.
- Impaired ability: the person's intoxication or withdrawal symptoms interfere with work, school, or home.
- Problems: the person continues drinking despite physical hazards or medical, legal, psychological, family, employment, or school problems.

The presence of three or more of these conditions is required to make a diagnosis.

SOURCE: Adapted from *Diagnostic and Statistical Manual of Mental Disorders,* 4th ed [DSM-IV-TR]. (Arlington, VA American Psychiatric Association, 2000).

Alcohol's Long-Term Effects

The most devastating long-term effect of alcohol is the damage done to a child whose mother abused alcohol during pregnancy. The effects of alcohol on the unborn and the message that pregnant women should not drink alcohol are presented in Highlight 16.

For nonpregnant adults, a drink or two sets in motion many destructive processes in the body, but the next day's abstinence reverses them. As long as the doses are moderate, the time between them is ample, and nutrition is adequate, recovery is probably complete.

If the doses of alcohol are heavy and the time between them short, complete recovery cannot take place. Repeated onslaughts of alcohol gradually take a toll on all parts of the body (see Table H7-5 on p. 238). Compared with nondrinkers and moderate drinkers, heavy drinkers have significantly greater risks of dying from all causes.

Personal Strategies

One obvious option available to people attending social gatherings is to enjoy the conversation, eat the food, and drink nonalcoholic beverages. Several nonalcoholic beverages are available that mimic the look and taste of their alcoholic counterparts. For those who enjoy champagne or beer, sparkling ciders and beers without alcohol are available. Instead of drinking a cocktail, a person can sip tomato juice with a slice of lime and a stalk of celery or just a plain cola beverage. Any of these drinks can ease conversation.

The person who chooses to drink alcohol should sip each drink slowly with food while following Canada's 'new' Low-Risk Drinking Guidelines (e.g., 10 or less drinks a week for women; 15 or less drinks a week for men; include non-drinking days every week) found on the Centre for Addiction and Mental Health website.[14] The alcohol should arrive at the liver cells slowly enough that the enzymes can handle the load. It is best to space drinks, too, allowing about an hour or so to metabolize each drink.

If you want to help sober up a friend who has had too much to drink, don't bother walking arm in arm around the block. Walking muscles have to work harder, but muscle cells can't metabolize alcohol; only liver cells can. Remember that each person has a limited amount of the alcohol dehydrogenase enzyme that clears the blood at a steady rate. Time alone will do the job. Nor will it help to give your friend a cup of coffee. Caffeine is a stimulant, but it won't speed up alcohol metabolism. Table H7-6 (p. 238) presents other alcohol myths.

TABLE H7-5 Health Effects of Heavy Alcohol Consumption

Health Problem	Effects of Alcohol
Arthritis	Increases the risk of inflamed joints.
Cancer	Increases the risk of cancer of the liver, rectum, breast, mouth, pharynx, larynx, and esophagus.
Fetal alcohol syndrome	Causes physical and behavioural abnormalities in the fetus (see Highlight 16).
Heart disease	In heavy drinkers, raises blood pressure, blood lipids, and the risk of stroke and heart disease; when compared with those who abstain, heart disease risk is generally lower in light-to-moderate drinkers.
Hyperglycemia	Raises blood glucose.
Hypoglycemia	Lowers blood glucose, especially in people with diabetes.
Infertility	Increases the risks of menstrual disorders and spontaneous abortions (in women); suppresses luteinizing hormone (in women) and testosterone (in men).
Kidney disease	Enlarges the kidneys, alters hormone functions, and increases the risk of kidney failure.
Liver disease	Causes fatty liver, alcoholic hepatitis, and cirrhosis.
Malnutrition	Increases the risk of protein-energy malnutrition; low intakes of protein, calcium, iron, vitamin A, vitamin C, thiamin, vitamin B_6, and riboflavin; and impaired absorption of calcium, phosphorus, vitamin D, and zinc.
Nervous disorders	Causes neuropathy and dementia; impairs balance and memory.
Obesity	Increases energy intake, but is not a primary cause of obesity.
Psychological disturbances	Causes depression, anxiety, and insomnia.

NOTE: This list is by no means all-inclusive. Alcohol has direct toxic effects on all body systems.

People who have passed out from drinking need 24 hours to sober up completely. Let them sleep, but watch over them. Encourage them to lie on their sides, instead of their backs. That way, if they vomit, they won't choke.

Don't drive too soon after drinking. The lack of glucose for the brain to function and the length of time to clear the blood of alcohol make alcohol's adverse effects linger long after its blood concentration has fallen. Driving coordination is still impaired the morning *after* a night of drinking, even if the drinking was moderate. Responsible aircraft pilots know that they must allow 24 hours for their bodies to clear alcohol completely, and they do not fly any sooner. The U.S. Federal Aviation Administration and major airlines enforce this rule.

TABLE H7-6 Myths and Truths Concerning Alcohol

Myth:	Hard liquors such as rum, vodka, and tequila are more harmful than wine and beer.
Truth:	The damage caused by alcohol depends largely on the *amount* consumed. Compared with hard liquor, beer and wine have relatively low percentages of alcohol, but they are often consumed in larger quantities.
Myth:	Consuming alcohol with raw seafood diminishes the likelihood of getting hepatitis.
Truth:	People have eaten contaminated oysters while drinking alcoholic beverages and not gotten as sick as those who were not drinking. But do not be misled: hepatitis is too serious an illness for anyone to depend on alcohol for protection.
Myth:	Alcohol stimulates the appetite.
Truth:	For some people, alcohol may stimulate appetite, but it seems to have the opposite effect in heavy drinkers. Heavy drinkers tend to eat poorly and suffer malnutrition.
Myth:	Drinking alcohol is healthy.
Truth:	Moderate alcohol consumption is associated with a lower risk for heart disease. Higher intakes, however, raise the risks for high blood pressure, stroke, heart disease, some cancers, accidents, violence, suicide, birth defects, and deaths in general. Furthermore, excessive alcohol consumption damages the liver, pancreas, brain, and heart. No authority recommends that nondrinkers begin drinking alcoholic beverages to obtain health benefits.
Myth:	Wine increases the body's absorption of minerals.
Truth:	Wine may increase the body's absorption of potassium, calcium, phosphorus, magnesium, and zinc, but the alcohol in wine also promotes the body's excretion of these minerals, so no benefit is gained.
Myth:	Alcohol is legal and, therefore, not a drug.
Truth:	Alcohol is legal for adults 19 years old and older (18 in Alberta, Manitoba, and Quebec), but it is also a drug—a substance that alters one or more of the body's functions.
Myth:	A shot of alcohol warms you up.
Truth:	Alcohol diverts blood flow to the skin making you *feel* warmer, but it actually cools the body.
Myth:	Wine and beer are mild; they do not lead to alcoholism.
Truth:	Alcoholism is not related to the kind of beverage, but rather to the quantity and frequency of consumption.
Myth:	Mixing different types of drinks gives you a hangover.
Truth:	Too much alcohol in any form produces a hangover.
Myth:	Alcohol is a stimulant.
Truth:	People think alcohol is a stimulant because it seems to relieve inhibitions, but it does so by depressing the activity of the brain. Alcohol is medically defined as a depressant drug.
Myth:	Beer is a great source of carbohydrate, vitamins, minerals, and fluids.
Truth:	Beer does provide some carbohydrate, but most of its kcalories come from alcohol. The few vitamins and minerals in beer cannot compete with rich food sources. And the diuretic effect of alcohol causes the body to lose more fluid in urine than is provided by the beer.

Look again at the drawing of the brain in Figure H7-4 (p. 234), and note that when someone drinks, judgment fails first. Judgment might tell a person to limit alcohol consumption to two drinks at a party, but if the first drink takes judgment away, many more drinks may follow. The failure to stop drinking as planned, on repeated occasions, is a warning sign that the person should not drink at all.

The accompanying Nutrition on the Net provides websites for organizations that offer information about alcohol and alcohol abuse.

Ethanol interferes with a multitude of chemical and hormonal reactions in the body—many more than have been enumerated here. With heavy alcohol consumption, the potential for harm is great. If you drink alcoholic beverages, do so with care, and in moderation.

Nutrition on the Net

CENGAGENOW™
For further study of topics covered in this Highlight, log on to **www.cengage .com/sso**.

- Gather information on alcohol and drug abuse from the U.S. National Clearinghouse for Alcohol and Drug Information (NCADI): **ncadi.samhsa.gov**
- Learn more about alcoholism and drug dependence from the U.S. National Council on Alcoholism and Drug Dependence (NCADD): **www.ncadd.org**
- Visit the Centre for Addiction and Mental Health: **www.camh.net**
- Find help for a family alcohol problem from Alateen and Al-Anon Family support groups: **www.al-anon.alateen.org**
- Find help for an alcohol or drug problem from Alcoholics Anonymous (AA) or Narcotics Anonymous: **www.aa.org** or **www.na.org**

References

1. J. H. O'Keefe, K. A. Bybee, and C. J. Lavie, Alcohol and cardiovascular health: The razor-sharp double-edged sword, *Journal of the American College of Cardiology* 50 (2007): 1009–1014; D. J. Meyerhoff and coauthors, Health risks of chronic moderate and heavy alcohol consumption: How much is too much? *Alcoholism, Clinical and Experimental Research* 29 (2005): 1334–1340.
2. M. P. Ferreira and D. Willoughby, Alcohol consumption: The good, the bad, and the indifferent, *Applied Physiology, Nutrition, and Metabolism* 33 (2008): 12–20; V. Arndt and coauthors, Age, alcohol consumption, and all-cause mortality, *Annals of Epidemiology* 14 (2004): 750–753.
3. J. Connor and coauthors, The burden of death, disease, and disability due to alcohol in New Zealand, *New Zealand Medical Journal* 118 (2005): U1412.
4. P. Meier and H. K. Seitz, Age, alcohol metabolism and liver disease, *Current Opinion in Clinical Nutrition and Metabolic Care* 11 (2008): 21–26; H. K. Seitz and F. Stickel, Alcoholic liver disease in the elderly, *Clinics in Geriatric Medicine* 23 (2007): 905–921.
5. B. Wansink and K. van Ittersum, Shape of glass and amount of alcohol poured: Comparative study of effect of practice and concentration, *British Medicine Journal* 331 (2005): 1512–1514.
6. S. Zakhari, Overview: How is alcohol metabolized by the body? *Alcohol Research & Health* 29 (2006): 245–254.
7. R. A. Breslow and B. A. Smothers, Drinking patterns and body mass index in never smokers: National Health Interview Survey, 1997–2001, *American Journal of Epidemiology* 161 (2005): 368–376.
8. S. G. Wannamethee, A. G. Shaper, and P. H. Whincup, Alcohol and adiposity: Effects of quantity and type of drink and time relation with meals, *International Journal of Obesity and Related Metabolic Disorders* 29 (2005): 1436–1444.
9. M. Ryan-Harshman and W. Aldoori, Diet and colorectal cancer: Review of the evidence, *Canadian Family Physician* 53 (2007): 1913–1920.
10. A. D. Thomson and coauthors, Wernicke's encephalopathy: "Plus ça change, plus c'est la même chose," *Alcohol and Alcoholism* 43 (2008): 180–186.
11. Statistics Canada, Summary tables—Beverages (2006-2010). www40.statcan.gc.ca/l01/cst01/famil102c-eng.htm, accessed September 8, 2011.
12. Parliament of Canada, PRB 0620E, Substance abuse and public policy in Canada: V. Alcohol and related harms (June 28, 2006). www.parl.gc.ca/Content/LOP/researchpublications/prb0620-e.htm#aconsumption, accessed September 8, 2011.
13. E. M. Adlaf, A. Demers, and L. Gliksman (Eds.), Canadian Campus Survey 2004 (Toronto: Centre for Addiction and Mental Health, 2005). www.camh.net/Research/Areas_of_research/Population_Life_Course_Studies/ccs_2004_report.pdf, accessed September 8, 2011.
14. Centre for Addiction and Mental Health, Low-risk drinking guidelines. www.camh.net/About_Addiction_Mental_Health/Drug_and_Addiction_Information/low_risk_drinking_guidelines.html, accessed December 19, 2011.

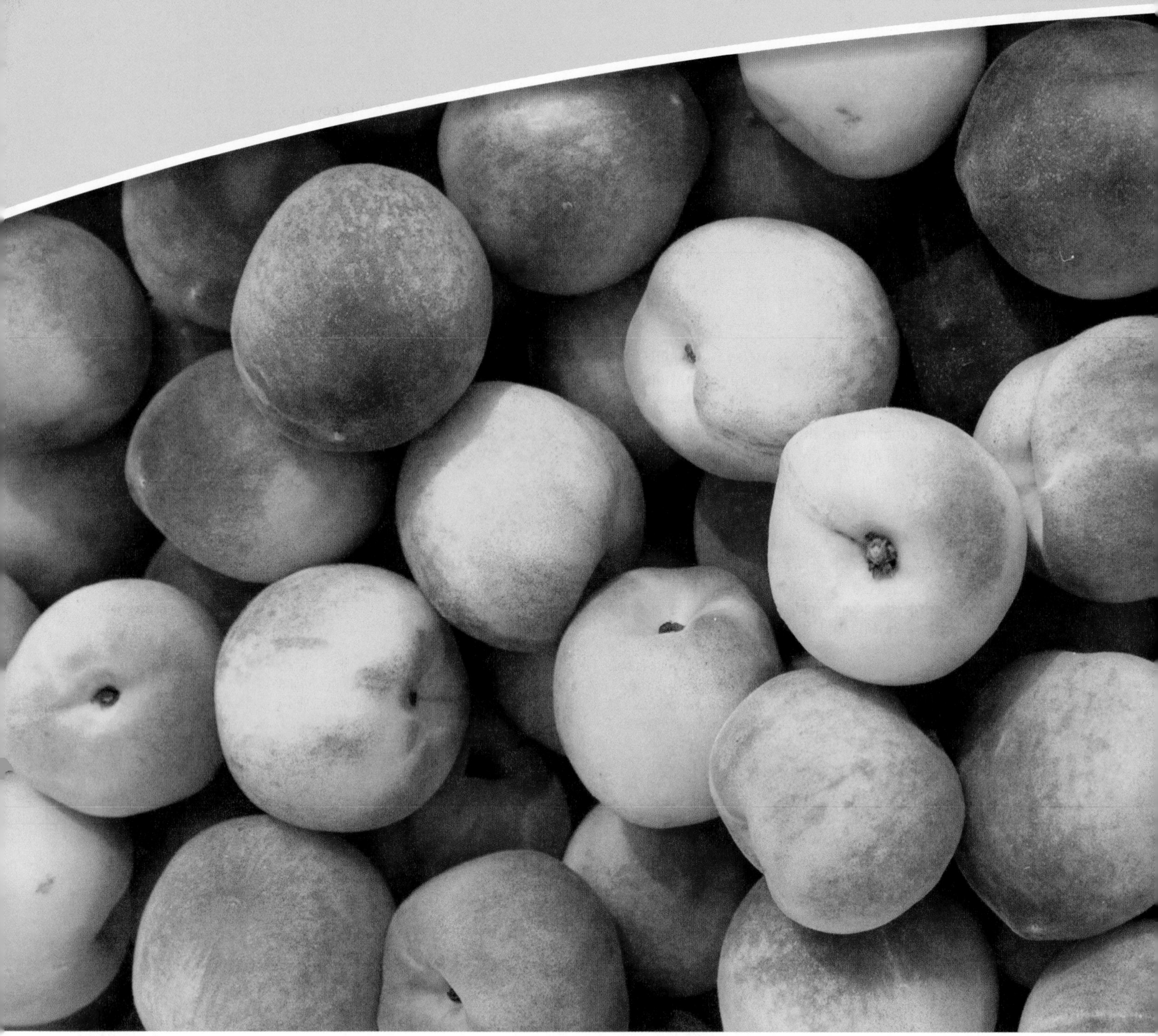

holbox/shutterstock

Nutrition in Your Life

CENGAGENOW™

Throughout this chapter, the CengageNOW logo indicates an opportunity for online self-study, linking you to interactive tutorials, activities, and videos to increase your understanding of chapter concepts.
www.cengage.com/sso

It's a simple equation: energy in + energy out = energy balance. The reality, of course, is much more complex. One day you may devour a dozen doughnuts at midnight and sleep through your morning workout—tipping the scales toward weight gain. Another day you may snack on veggies and train for a 10K race—shifting the balance toward weight loss. Your body weight—especially as it relates to your body fat—and your level of fitness have consequences for your health. So, how are you doing? Are you ready to see how your "energy in" and "energy out" balance and whether your body weight and fat measures are consistent with good health?

CHAPTER

8

Energy Balance and Body Composition

CHAPTER OUTLINE

The body's remarkable machinery can cope with many extremes of diet. As Chapter 7 explains, excess carbohydrate (glucose), excess protein (amino acids), and excess fat all can contribute to body fat. To some extent, amino acids can be used to make glucose. To a very limited extent, even fat (the glycerol portion) can be used to make glucose. But a grossly unbalanced diet imposes hardships on the body. If energy intake is too low or if too little carbohydrate or protein is supplied, the body must degrade its own lean tissue to meet its glucose and protein needs. If energy intake is too high, the body stores fat.

Both excessive and deficient body fat result from an energy imbalance. The simple picture is as follows. People who have consumed more food energy than they have expended bank the surplus as body fat. To reduce body fat, they need to expend more energy than they take in from food. In contrast, people who have consumed too little food energy to support their bodies' activities have relied on their bodies' fat stores and possibly some of their lean tissues as well. To gain weight, these people need to take in more food energy than they expend. As you will see, though, the details of the body's weight regulation are quite complex.[1] This chapter describes energy balance and body composition and examines the health problems associated with having too much or too little body fat. The next chapter presents strategies toward resolving these problems.

Energy Balance

People expend energy continuously and eat periodically to refuel. Ideally, their energy intakes cover their energy expenditures without too much excess. Excess energy is stored as fat, and stored fat is used for energy between meals. The amount of body fat a person deposits in, or withdraws from, storage on any given day depends on the energy balance for that day—the amount consumed (energy in) versus the amount expended (energy out). When a person is maintaining weight, energy in equals energy out. When the balance shifts, weight changes. For each 3500 kcalories eaten in excess, 454 grams (1 pound) of body fat is stored; similarly, 454 grams (1 pound) of fat is lost for each 3500 kcalories expended beyond those consumed. ♦ The fat

♦ 454 grams (1 lb) body fat = 3500 kcal
Body fat, or adipose tissue, is composed of a mixture of mostly fat, some protein, and water. Every 454 grams (1 pound) of body fat is approximately 87% fat, or (454 × 0.87) 395 g, and 395 g × 9 kcal/g = 3555 kcal.

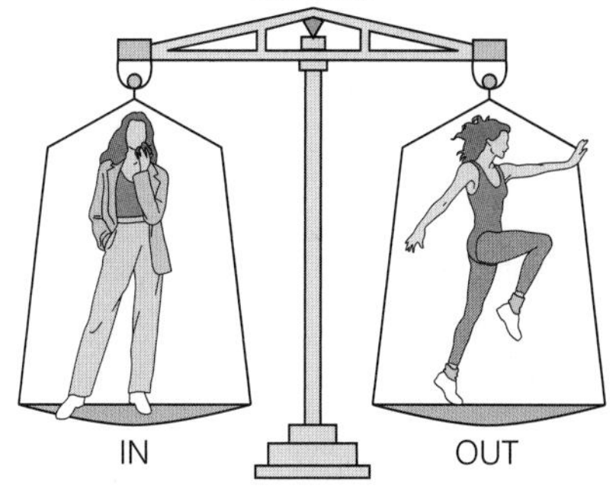
ENERGY
IN
OUT

When energy in balances with energy out and a person is in a stable hydration state, a person's body weight is stable.

stores of even a healthy-weight adult represent an ample reserve of energy—50 000 to 200 000 kcalories.

Dietary Guidance for Canadians

To maintain body weight in a healthy range, balance kcalories from foods and beverages with kcalories expended.

Quick changes in body weight are not simple changes in fat stores. Weight gained or lost rapidly includes some fat, large amounts of fluid, and some lean tissues such as muscle proteins and bone minerals. Because water constitutes about 60 percent of an adult's body weight, retention or loss of water can greatly influence body weight. Even over the long term, the composition of weight gained or lost is normally about 75 percent fat and 25 percent lean. During starvation, losses of fat and lean are about equal. (Recall from Chapter 7 that without adequate carbohydrate, protein-rich lean tissues break down to provide glucose.) Invariably, though, *fat* gains and losses are gradual. The next two sections examine the two sides of the energy-balance equation: energy in and energy out.

IN SUMMARY **When the energy consumed equals the energy expended, a person is in energy balance and body weight is stable. If more energy is taken in than is expended, a person gains weight. If more energy is expended than is taken in, a person loses weight.**

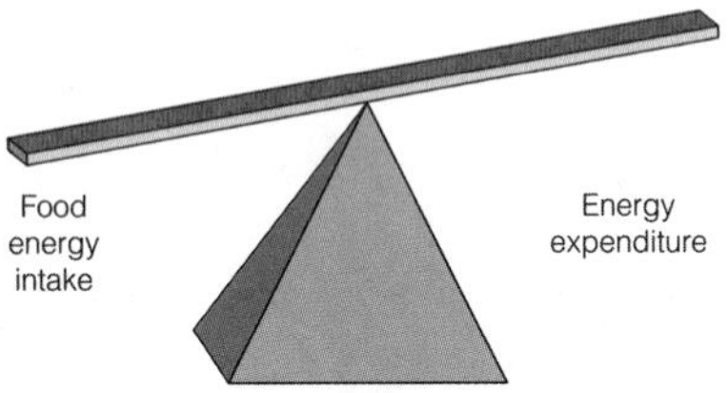
Food
energy
intake
Energy
expenditure

Weight loss occurs when energy expenditure exceeds energy intake.

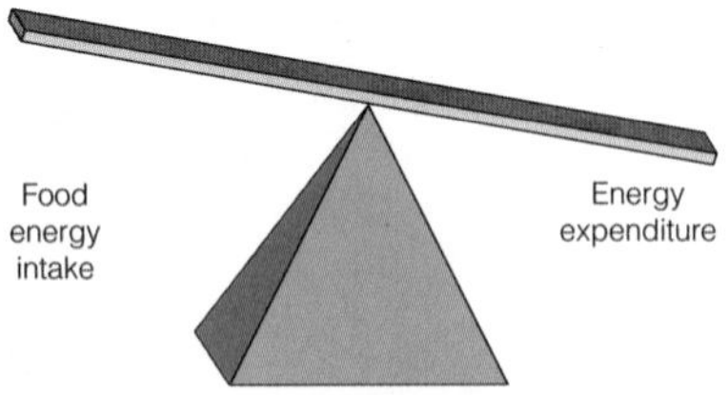
Food
energy
intake
Energy
expenditure

Weight gain occurs when energy intake exceeds energy expenditure.

Energy In: The kCalories Foods Provide

Foods and beverages provide the "energy in" part of the energy-balance equation. How much energy a person receives depends on the composition of the foods and beverages and on the amount the person eats and drinks.

Food Composition

To find out how many kcalories a food provides, a scientist can burn the food in a **bomb calorimeter** (see Figure 8-1). When the food burns, energy is released in the form of heat. The amount of heat given off provides a *direct* measure of the food's energy value (remember that kcalories are units of heat energy). In addition to releasing heat, these reactions generate carbon dioxide and water—just as the body's cells do when they metabolize the energy-yielding nutrients from foods. Details of the chemical reactions in a calorimeter and in the body differ, but the overall process is similar: when the food burns and the chemical bonds break, the carbons (C) and hydrogens (H) combine with oxygens (O) to form carbon dioxide (CO_2) and water (H_2O). The amount of oxygen consumed gives an *indirect* measure ♦ of the amount of energy released.

A bomb calorimeter measures the available energy in foods but overstates the amount of energy that the human body ♦ derives from foods. Why? Because the body is less efficient than a calorimeter and cannot metabolize all of the energy-yielding nutrients in a food completely. Researchers can correct for this discrepancy mathematically to create useful tables of the energy values of foods (such as APPENDIX H). These values provide reasonable estimates, but they do not reflect the *precise* amount of energy a person will derive from the foods consumed.

The energy values of foods can also be computed from the amounts of carbohydrate, fat, and protein (and alcohol, if present) in the foods.* For example, a food ♦ containing 12 grams of carbohydrate, 5 grams of fat, and 8 grams of protein will provide 48 carbohydrate kcalories, 45 fat kcalories, and 32 protein kcalories, for a total of 125 kcalories. (To review how to calculate the energy foods provide, turn to p. 9.)

*Some of the food energy values in the table of food composition in APPENDIX H were derived by bomb calorimetry, and many were calculated from their energy-yielding nutrient contents.

♦ Food energy values can be determined by:
- **Direct calorimetry,** which measures the amount of heat released.
- **Indirect calorimetry,** which measures the amount of oxygen consumed.

♦ The number of kcalories that the body derives from a food, in contrast to the number of kcalories determined by calorimetry, is the **physiological fuel value.**

♦
- 1 g carbohydrate = 4 kcal
- 1 g fat = 9 kcal
- 1 g protein = 4 kcal
- 1 g alcohol = 7 kcal

As Chapter 1 mentions, many scientists measure food energy in kilojoules instead. Conversion factors for these and other measures are in the Aids to Calculation section on the inside back cover of the book.

bomb calorimeter (KAL-oh-RIM-eh-ter): an instrument that measures the heat energy released when foods are burned, thus providing an estimate of the potential energy of the foods.
- **calor** = heat
- **metron** = measure

FIGURE 8-1 Bomb Calorimeter

When food is burned, energy is released in the form of heat. Heat energy is measured in kcalories.

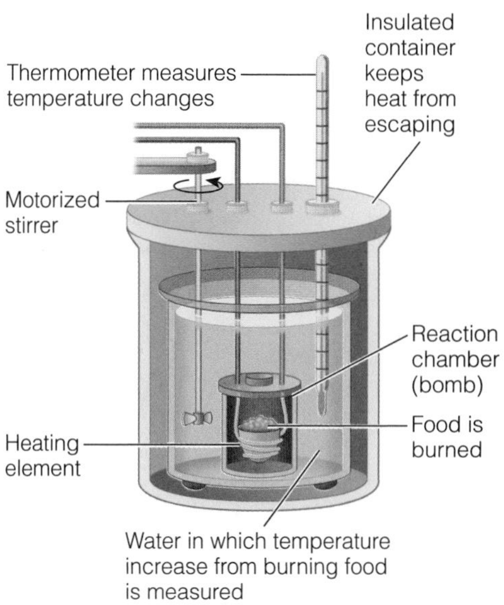
Insulated container keeps heat from escaping
Thermometer measures temperature changes
Motorized stirrer
Reaction chamber (bomb)
Food is burned
Heating element
Water in which temperature increase from burning food is measured

Food Intake

To achieve energy balance, the body must meet its needs without taking in too much or too little energy. **Appetite** prompts a person to eat—or not to eat.[2] Somehow the body decides how much and how often to eat—when to start eating and when to stop. As you will see, many signals—from both the environment and genetics—initiate or delay eating.[3]

Hunger People eat for a variety of reasons, most obviously (although not necessarily most commonly) because they are hungry. Most people recognize **hunger** as an irritating feeling that prompts thoughts of food and motivates them to start eating. In the body, hunger is the physiological response to a need for food triggered by nerve signals and chemical messengers originating and acting in the brain, primarily in the **hypothalamus.**[4] Hunger can be influenced by the presence or absence of nutrients in the bloodstream, the size and composition of the preceding meal, customary eating patterns, climate (heat reduces food intake; cold increases it), exercise, hormones, and physical and mental illnesses. Hunger determines what to eat, when to eat, and how much to eat.

The stomach is ideally designed to handle periodic batches of food, and people typically eat meals at roughly four-hour intervals. Four hours after a meal, most, if not all, of the food has left the stomach. Most people do not feel like eating again until the stomach is either empty or almost so. Even then, a person may not feel hungry for quite a while.

Satiation During the course of a meal, as food enters the GI tract and hunger diminishes, **satiation** develops. As receptors in the stomach stretch and hormones such as cholecystokinin become active, the person begins to feel full. The response: satiation occurs and the person stops eating.

Satiety After a meal, the feeling of **satiety** continues to suppress hunger and allows a person to not eat again for a while. Whereas *satiation* tells us to "stop eating," *satiety* reminds us to "not start eating again." Figure 8-2 (p. 244) summarizes the relationships among hunger, satiation, and satiety. Of course, people can override these signals, especially when presented with stressful situations or favourite foods.

Overriding Hunger and Satiety Not surprisingly, eating can be triggered by signals other than hunger, even when the body does not need food. Some people experience food cravings when they are bored or anxious. In fact, they may eat in response to any kind of stress, ♦ negative or positive. ("What do I do when I'm grieving? Eat. What do I do when I'm celebrating? Eat!") Not too surprisingly, repeatedly eating to relieve chronic stress can lead to overeating and weight gain.[5]

♦ Eating in response to arousal is called **stress eating.**

Many people respond to external cues such as the time of day ("It's time to eat") or the availability, sight, and taste of food ("I'd love a piece of chocolate even though I'm stuffed"). Environmental influences such as large portion sizes, favourite

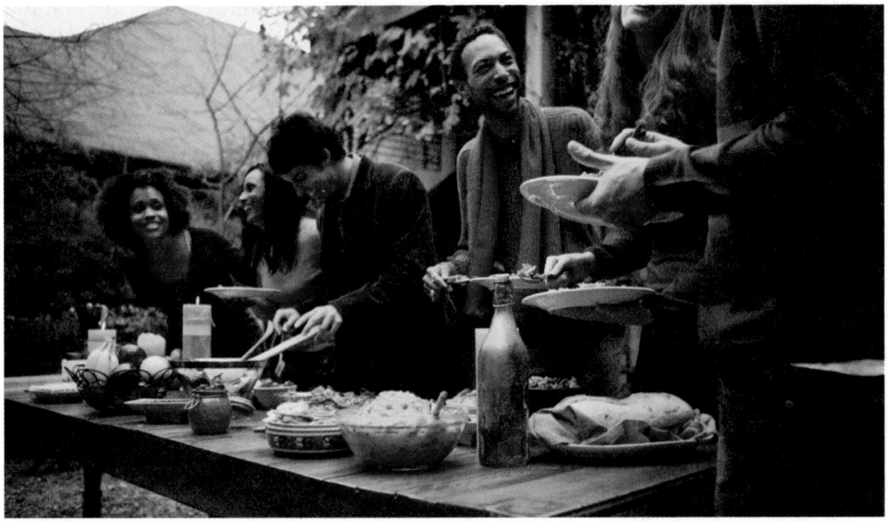
Jupiterimages/Getty Images

Regardless of hunger, people typically overeat when offered the abundance and variety of a buffet. To limit unhealthy weight gains, listen to hunger and satiety signals.

appetite: the integrated response to the sight, smell, thought, or taste of food that initiates or delays eating.

hunger: the painful sensation caused by a lack of food that initiates food-seeking behaviour.

hypothalamus (high-po-THAL-ah-mus): a brain centre that controls activities such as maintenance of water balance, regulation of body temperature, and control of appetite.

satiation (say-she-AY-shun): the feeling of satisfaction and fullness that occurs during a meal and halts eating. Satiation determines how much food is consumed during a meal.

satiety: the feeling of fullness and satisfaction that occurs after a meal and inhibits eating until the next meal. Satiety determines how much time passes between meals.

FIGURE 8-2 Hunger, Satiation, and Satiety

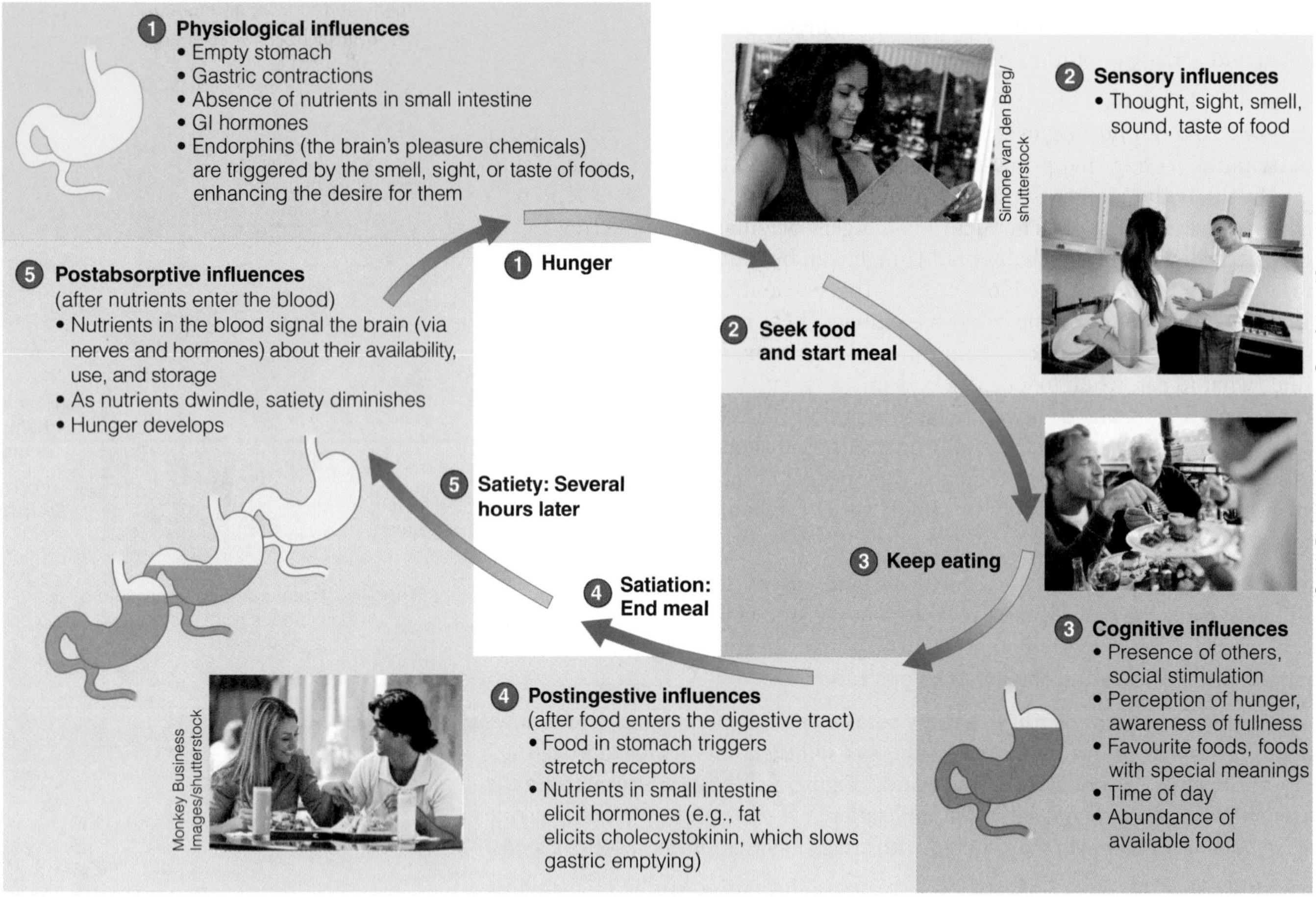
1 Physiological influences
• Empty stomach
• Gastric contractions
• Absence of nutrients in small intestine
• GI hormones
• Endorphins (the brain's pleasure chemicals) are triggered by the smell, sight, or taste of foods, enhancing the desire for them
2 Sensory influences
• Thought, sight, smell, sound, taste of food
Simone van den Berg/ shutterstock
© craftvision/iStockphoto
1 Hunger
2 Seek food and start meal
3 Keep eating
Corbis Photography
3 Cognitive influences
• Presence of others, social stimulation
• Perception of hunger, awareness of fullness
• Favourite foods, foods with special meanings
• Time of day
• Abundance of available food
4 Satiation: End meal
4 Postingestive influences
(after food enters the digestive tract)
• Food in stomach triggers stretch receptors
• Nutrients in small intestine elicit hormones (e.g., fat elicits cholecystokinin, which slows gastric emptying)
Monkey Business Images/shutterstock
5 Satiety: Several hours later
5 Postabsorptive influences
(after nutrients enter the blood)
• Nutrients in the blood signal the brain (via nerves and hormones) about their availability, use, and storage
• As nutrients dwindle, satiety diminishes
• Hunger develops

foods, or an abundance or variety of foods stimulate eating and increase energy intake. These cognitive influences ♦ can easily lead to weight gain.

♦ Cognitive influences include perceptions, memories, intellect, and social interactions.

Eating can also be suppressed by signals other than satiety, even when a person is hungry. People with the eating disorder anorexia nervosa, for example, use tremendous discipline to ignore the pangs of hunger. Some people simply cannot eat during times of stress, negative or positive. ("I'm too sad to eat." "I'm too excited to eat!") Why some people overeat in response to stress and others cannot eat at all remains a bit of a mystery, although researchers are beginning to understand the connections between stress hormones, brain activity, and "comfort foods." Factors that appear to be involved include how the person perceives the stress and whether usual eating behaviours are restrained. (Highlight 8 features anorexia nervosa and other eating disorders.)

Sustaining Satiation and Satiety The extent to which foods produce satiation and sustain satiety depends in part on the nutrient composition of a meal. Of the three energy-yielding nutrients, protein is considered the most **satiating.** In fact, too little protein in the diet can leave a person feeling hungry.[6]

Foods low in energy density ♦ are also more satiating. High-fibre foods effectively provide satiation by filling the stomach and delaying the absorption of nutrients. For this reason, eating a large salad as a first course helps a person eat less during the meal. In contrast, fat has a weak effect on satiation; consequently, eating high-fat foods may lead to passive overconsumption. High-fat foods are flavourful, which stimulates the appetite and entices people to eat more. High-fat foods are also energy dense; consequently, they deliver more kcalories per bite. (Chapter 1 introduces the concept of energy density, and Chapter 9 describes how considering a food's energy density can help with weight management.) Although

♦ Energy density is a measure of the energy a food provides relative to the amount of food (kcalories per gram). Foods with a low energy density provide fewer kcalories, and those with high energy density provide more kcalories, for the same amount of food.

satiating: having the power to suppress hunger and inhibit eating.

FIGURE 8-3 How Fat Influences Portion Sizes

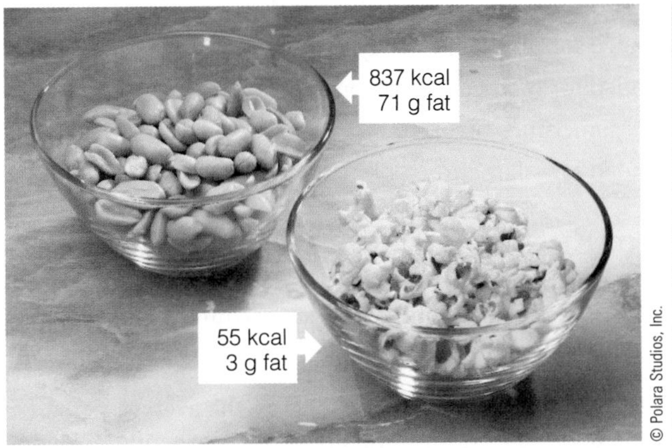
837 kcal
71 g fat
55 kcal
3 g fat
© Polara Studios, Inc.

For the same size portion, peanuts deliver more than 15 times the kcalories and 20 times the fat of popcorn.

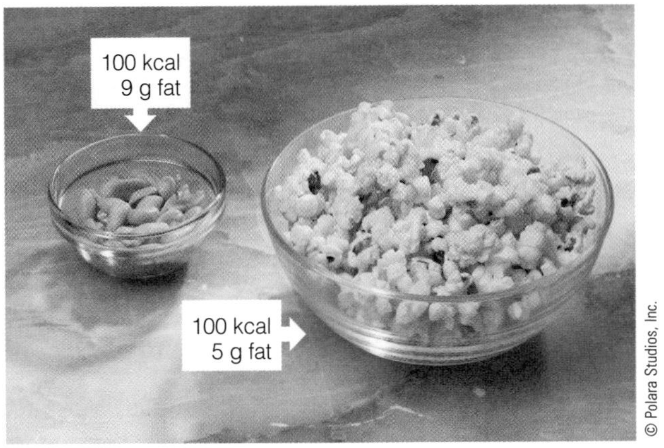
100 kcal
9 g fat
100 kcal
5 g fat
© Polara Studios, Inc.

For the same number of kcalories, a person can have a few high-fat peanuts or almost 2 cups of high-fibre popcorn. (This comparison used oil-based popcorn; using air-popped popcorn would double the amount of popcorn in this example.)

fat provides little satiation during a meal, it produces strong satiety signals once it enters the intestine. Fat in the intestine triggers the release of cholecystokinin—a hormone that signals satiety and inhibits food intake.

Eating high-fat foods while trying to limit energy intake requires small portion sizes, which can leave a person feeling unsatisfied. Portion size correlates directly with a food's satiety. Instead of eating small portions of high-fat foods and feeling deprived, a person can feel satisfied by eating large portions of low-fat, high-fibre, and low energy density foods. Figure 8-3 illustrates how fat influences portion size.

Message Central—The Hypothalamus As you can see, eating is a complex behaviour controlled by a variety of psychological, social, metabolic, and physiological factors. The hypothalamus appears to be the control centre, integrating messages about energy intake, expenditure, and storage from other parts of the brain and from the mouth, GI tract, and liver. Some of these messages influence satiation, which helps control the size of a meal; others influence satiety, which helps determine the frequency of meals.[7]

Dozens of gastrointestinal hormones ♦ influence appetite control and energy balance.[8] By understanding the action of these hormones, researchers may one day be able to develop anti-obesity treatments.[9] The greatest challenge now is to sort out the many actions of these brain chemicals. For example, one of these chemicals, **neuropeptide Y**, causes carbohydrate cravings, initiates eating, decreases energy expenditure, and increases fat storage—all factors favouring a positive energy balance and weight gain.

♦ Gastrointestinal hormones that regulate food intake:
- Amylin
- Cholecystokinin (CCK)
- Enterostatin
- Ghrelin
- Glucagon-like peptide-1 (GLP-1)
- Oxyntomodulin
- Pancreatic polypeptide (PP)
- Peptide YY (PYY)

IN SUMMARY A mixture of signals governs a person's eating behaviours. Hunger and appetite initiate eating, whereas satiation and satiety stop and delay eating, respectively. Each responds to messages from the nervous and hormonal systems. Superimposed on these signals are complex factors involving emotions, habits, and other aspects of human behaviour.

Energy Out: The kCalories the Body Expends

Chapter 7 explains that heat is released whenever the body breaks down carbohydrate, fat, or protein for energy and again when that energy is used to do work. The generation of heat, known as **thermogenesis**, can be measured to determine

neuropeptide Y: a chemical produced in the brain that stimulates appetite, diminishes energy expenditure, and increases fat storage.

thermogenesis: the generation of heat; used in physiology and nutrition studies as an index of how much energy the body is expending.

♦ Energy expenditure, like food energy, can be determined by:
- **Direct calorimetry,** which measures the amount of heat released.
- **Indirect calorimetry,** which measures the amount of oxygen consumed and carbon dioxide expelled.

the amount of energy expended. ♦ The total energy a body expends reflects three main categories of thermogenesis:

- Energy expended for basal metabolism
- Energy expended for physical activity
- Energy expended for food consumption

A fourth category is sometimes involved:

- Energy expended for adaptation

Components of Energy Expenditure

People expend energy when they are physically active, of course, but they also expend energy when they are resting quietly. In fact, quiet metabolic activities account for the lion's share of most people's energy expenditures, as Figure 8-4 shows.

Basal Metabolism About two-thirds of the energy the average person expends in a day supports the body's **basal metabolism.** Metabolic activities maintain the body temperature, keep the lungs inhaling and exhaling air, the bone marrow making new red blood cells, the heart beating 100 000 times a day, and the kidneys filtering wastes—in short, they support all the basic processes of life.

The **basal metabolic rate (BMR)** is the rate at which the body expends energy for these life-sustaining activities. ♦ The rate may vary from person to person and may vary for the same individual with a change in circumstance or physical condition. The rate is slowest when a person is sleeping undisturbed, but it is usually measured in a room with a comfortable temperature when the person is awake, but lying still, after a restful sleep and an overnight (12 to 14 hour) fast. A similar measure of energy output—called the **resting metabolic rate (RMR)**—is slightly higher than the BMR because its criteria for recent food intake and physical activity are not as strict. When energy needs cannot be measured, equations ♦ can provide reasonably accurate estimates.

♦ Quick and easy estimates for basal energy needs:
- Men: Slightly >1 kcal/min (1.1 to 1.3 kcal/min) or 24 kcal/kg/day
- Women: Slightly <1 kcal/min (0.8 to 1.0 kcal/min) or 23 kcal/kg/day

For perspective, a burning candle or a 75-watt light bulb releases about 1 kcal/min.

♦ BMR equations use actual weight in kilograms, height in centimetres, and age in years:
- Men: $(10 \times \text{wt}) + (6.25 \times \text{ht}) - (5 \times \text{age}) + 5$
- Women: $(10 \times \text{wt}) + (6.25 \times \text{ht}) - (5 \times \text{age}) - 161$

In general, the more a person weighs, the more *total* energy is expended on basal metabolism, but the amount of energy *per kilogram* of body weight may be lower. For example, an adult's BMR might be 1500 kcalories per day and an infant's only 500, but compared to body weight, the infant's BMR is more than twice as fast. Similarly, a normal-weight adult may have a metabolic rate one and a half times that of an obese adult when compared to body weight because lean tissue is metabolically more active than body fat.

Table 8-1 summarizes the factors that raise and lower the BMR. For the most part, the BMR is highest in people who are growing (children, adolescents, and pregnant women) and in those with considerable **lean body mass** (physically fit people and males). One way to increase the BMR then is to participate in endurance and strength-training activities regularly to maximize lean body mass. The BMR is also high in people with fever or under stress and in people with highly active thyroid glands. The BMR slows down with a loss of lean body mass and during fasting and malnutrition.

Physical Activity The second component of a person's energy output is physical activity: voluntary movement of the skeletal muscles and support systems. Physical activity is the most variable—and the most changeable—component of energy expenditure. Consequently, its influence on both weight gain and weight loss can be significant.

During physical activity, the muscles need extra energy to move, and the heart and lungs need extra energy to deliver nutrients and oxygen and dispose of wastes. The amount of energy needed for any activity, whether playing tennis or studying for an exam, depends on three factors: muscle mass, body weight, and activity. The larger the muscle mass and the heavier the weight of the body part being moved, the more energy is expended. Table 8-2 gives average energy expenditures for various activities in kcal/kg/min. The energy cost of physical activity can also be measured in units of metabolic equivalent tasks (METs), where 1 MET is equivalent to

basal metabolism: the energy needed to maintain life when a body is at complete digestive, physical, and emotional rest.

basal metabolic rate (BMR): the rate of energy use for metabolism under specified conditions: after a 12-hour fast and restful sleep, without any physical activity or emotional excitement, and in a comfortable setting. It is usually expressed as kcalories per kilogram body weight per hour.

resting metabolic rate (RMR): similar to the basal metabolic rate (BMR), a measure of the energy use of a person at rest in a comfortable setting, but with less stringent criteria for recent food intake and physical activity. Consequently, the RMR is slightly higher than the BMR.

lean body mass: the body minus its fat.

TABLE 8-1 Factors that Increase or Decrease the BMR and Energy Expenditure

Factors that Increase the BMR	
Height	In tall, thin people, the BMR is higher.[a]
Growth	In children, adolescents, and pregnant women, the BMR is higher.
Body composition (gender)	The more lean tissue, the higher the BMR (which is why males usually have a higher BMR than females). The more fat tissue, the lower the BMR.
Fever	Fever raises the BMR.[b]
Stresses	Stresses (including many diseases and certain drugs) raise the BMR.
Environmental temperature	Both heat and cold raise the BMR.
Hormones (gender)	The thyroid hormone thyroxin, for example, can speed up or slow down the BMR.[c] Premenstrual hormones slightly raise the BMR.
Smoking	Nicotine increases energy expenditure.
Caffeine	Caffeine increases energy expenditure.
Factors that Decrease the BMR	
Age	Lean body mass diminishes with age, slowing the BMR.[d]
Fasting/starvation	Fasting/starvation lowers the BMR.[e]
Malnutrition	Malnutrition lowers the BMR.
Sleep	BMR is lowest when sleeping.

[a]If two people weigh the same, the taller, thinner person will have the faster metabolic rate, reflecting the greater skin surface, through which heat is lost by radiation, in proportion to the body's volume (see the margin drawing on p. 249).
[b]Fever raises the BMR by 10 percent for each degree Celcius above 37 degrees and up to 40 degrees.
[c]The thyroid gland releases hormones that travel to the cells and influence cellular metabolism. Thyroid hormone activity can speed up or slow down the rate of metabolism by as much as 50 percent.
[d]The BMR begins to decrease an early adulthood (after growth and development cease) at a rate of about 2 percent/decade. A reduction in voluntary activity as well brings the total decline in energy expenditure to 5 percent/decade.
[e]Prolonged starvation reduces the total amount of metabolically active lean tissue in the body, although the decline occurs sooner and to a greater extent than body losses alone can explain. More likely, the neural and hormonal changes that accompany fasting are responsible for changes in the BMR.

FIGURE 8-4 Components of Energy Expenditure

The amount of energy spent in a day differs for each individual, but in general, basal metabolism is the largest component of energy expenditure and the thermic effect of food is the smallest. The amount spent in voluntary physical activities has the greatest variability, depending on a person's activity patterns. For a sedentary person, physical activities may account for less than half as much energy as basal metabolism, whereas an extremely active person may expend as much on activity as for basal metabolism.

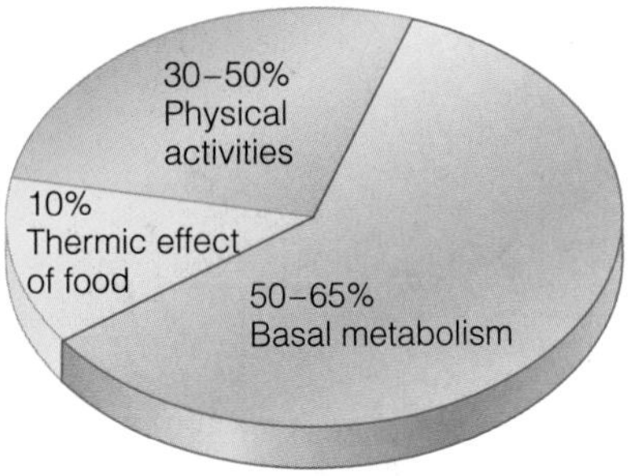
30–50%
Physical
activities
10%
Thermic effect
of food
50–65%
Basal metabolism

TABLE 8-2 Energy Expended on Various Activities

The values listed in this table reflect both the energy expended in physical activity *and* the amount used for BMR. To calculate kcalories spent per minute of activity for your own body weight, multiply kcal/kg/min (or kcal/lb/min) by your exact weight and then multiply that number by the number of minutes spent in the activity. For example, if you weigh 65 kilograms (142 pounds), and you want to know how many kcalories you spent doing 30 minutes of vigorous aerobic dance: $0.136 \times 65 = 8.8$ kcalories per minute; 8.8×30 minutes $= 264$ total kcalories spent.

Activity	kCal/kg min	kCal/lb min
Aerobic dance (vigorous)	.136	.062
Basketball (vigorous, full court)	.213	.097
Bicycling		
21 km/h	.099	.045
24 km/h	.108	.049
27 km/h	.125	.057
31 km/h	.167	.076
34 km/h	.198	.090
37 km/h	.240	.109
40 km/h	.306	.139
Canoeing, flat water, moderate pace	.099	.045
Cross-country skiing		
13 km/h	.229	.104
Gardening	.099	.045
Golf (carrying clubs)	.099	.045

Activity	kCal/kg min	kCal/lb min
Handball	.172	.078
Horseback riding (trot)	.114	.052
Rowing (vigorous)	.213	.097
Running		
8 km/h	.134	.061
10 km/h	.163	.074
12 km/h	.207	.094
14 km/h	.227	.103
16 km/h	.251	.114
18 km/h	.288	.131
Soccer (vigorous)	.213	.097
Studying	.024	.011
Swimming		
18 m/min	.070	.032
41 m/min	.128	.058
46 m/min	.154	.070

Activity	kCal/kg min	kCal/lb min
Table tennis (skilled)	.099	.045
Tennis (beginner)	.070	.032
Vacuuming and other household tasks	.066	.030
Walking (brisk pace)		
6 km/h	.077	.035
7 km/h	.106	.048
Weight lifting		
light-to-moderate effort	.053	.024
vigorous effort	.106	.048
Wheelchair basketball	.185	.084
Wheeling self in wheelchair	.066	.030
Wii games		
bowling	.046	.021
boxing	.047	.021
tennis	.048	.022

TABLE 8-3 Metabolic Equivalent Tasks (METs) of Selected Activities*

METs	Activity Type	Examples of Activities
≤1.0	Inactivity	Lying or sitting quietly, watching television; Reclining, reading, or talking on the phone; Meditating; Sleeping;
1.1–2.9	Light intensity	Standing quietly (e.g., in a line); Light office work (e.g., typing on computer); Spectator at sports event; Light effort household tasks (e.g., food preparation); Stretching, hatha yoga;
3.0–6.0	Moderate intensity	Walking 5 to 7 km/h; Golfing; Ice skating; Ballroom dancing; Mowing the lawn;
≥6.1	Vigorous intensity	Bicycling; Weight lifting, circuit training; Ball sports (e.g., soccer, basketball); Racquet sports (e.g., badminton, tennis, squash); Climbing hills with load;

*Example activities excerpted from B. E. Ainsworth and coauthors, Compendium of physical activities: An update of activity codes and MET intensities, *Medicine and Science in Sports and Exercise* 32 (2000): S498–S516; B. E. Ainsworth and coauthors, Compendium of physical activities: Classification of energy costs of human physical activities, *Medicine and Science in Sports and Exercise* 25 (1993): 71–80.

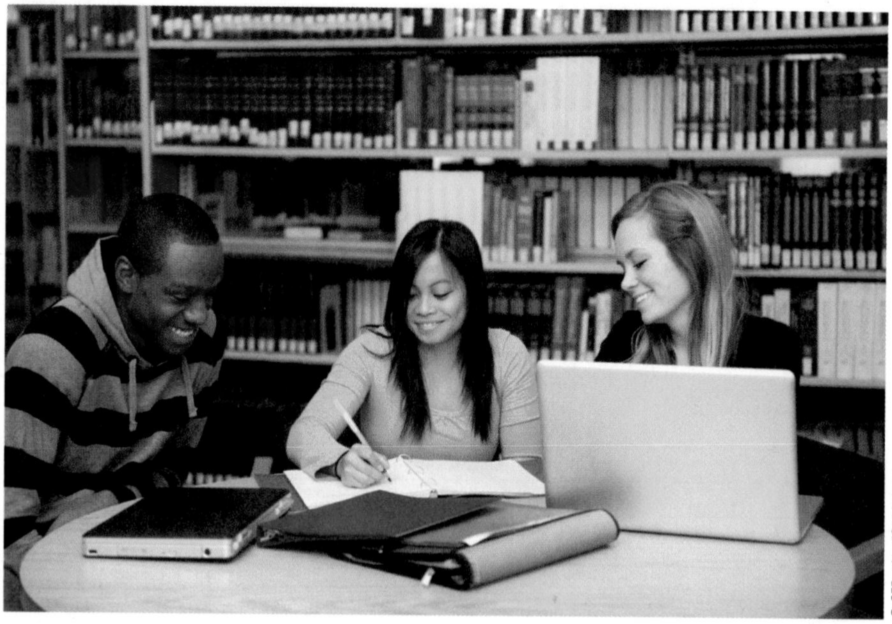
© CEFutcher/iStockphoto

It feels like work and it may make you tired, but studying requires only one or two kcalories per minute.

the amount of energy a person expends at rest—for example, lying quietly in bed awake and listening to music but not talking. Light intensity activities are assigned <3 METs, moderate intensity activities range between 3 and 6 METs, and vigorous intensity activities are greater than 6 METs.[10] Table 8-3 provides METs for a selected variety of activities. It is important to note that METs were not developed to estimate precise costs of energy in individuals; METs instead provide a classification system for determining the intensities of activities. Individual differences in body mass, body composition, age, sex, and other characteristics can affect the true energy costs to different people. The activity's duration, frequency, and intensity also influence energy expenditure: the longer, the more frequent, and the more intense the activity, the more kcalories expended. (Chapter 15 describes how an activity's duration, frequency, and intensity also influence the body's use of the energy-yielding nutrients.)

Thermic Effect of Food When a person eats, the GI tract muscles speed up their rhythmic contractions, the cells that manufacture and secrete digestive juices begin their tasks, and some nutrients are absorbed by active transport. This acceleration of activity requires energy and produces heat; it is known as the **thermic effect of food (TEF).**

The thermic effect of food is proportional to the food energy taken in and is usually estimated at 10 percent of energy intake. Thus a person who ingests 2000 kcalories probably expends about 200 kcalories on the thermic effect of food. The proportions vary for different foods, however, and are also influenced by factors such as meal size and frequency. In general, the thermic effect of food is greater for high-protein foods than for high-fat foods ♦ and for a meal eaten all at once rather than spread out over a couple of hours. For most purposes, however, the thermic effect of food can be ignored when estimating energy expenditure because its contribution to total energy output is smaller than the probable errors involved in estimating overall energy intake and output.

♦ Thermic effect of foods:
- Carbohydrate: 5–10%
- Fat: 0–5%
- Protein: 20–30%
- Alcohol: 15–20%

The percentages are calculated by dividing the energy expended during digestion and absorption (above basal) by the energy content of the food.

Adaptive Thermogenesis Some additional energy is spent when a person must adapt to dramatically changed circumstances (**adaptive thermogenesis**). When the body has to adapt to physical conditioning, extreme cold, overfeeding, starvation, trauma, or other types of stress, it has extra work to do, building the tissues and producing the enzymes and hormones necessary to cope with the demand. In some circumstances, this energy makes a considerable difference in the total energy expended. Because this component of energy expenditure is so variable and specific to individuals, it is not included when calculating energy requirements.

thermic effect of food (TEF): an estimation of the energy required to process food (digest, absorb, transport, metabolize, and store ingested nutrients); also called the *specific dynamic effect (SDE)* of food or the *specific dynamic activity (SDA)* of food. The sum of the TEF and any increase in the metabolic rate due to overeating is known as *diet-induced thermogenesis (DIT).*

adaptive thermogenesis: adjustments in energy expenditure related to changes in environment such as extreme cold and to physiological events such as overfeeding, trauma, and changes in hormone status.

Estimating Energy Requirements In estimating energy requirements, the DRI Committee developed equations based on research measuring total daily energy expenditure. These equations consider how the following factors influence energy expenditure: ♦

- *Gender.* In general, women have a lower BMR than men, in large part because men typically have more lean body mass. Two sets of energy equations—one for men and one for women—were developed to accommodate the influence of gender on energy expenditure.
- *Growth.* The BMR is high in people who are growing. For this reason, pregnant and lactating women, infants, children, and adolescents have their own sets of energy equations (provided in APPENDIX F).
- *Age.* The BMR declines during adulthood as lean body mass diminishes. This change in body composition occurs, in part, because some hormones that influence appetite, body weight, and metabolism become more, or less, active with age.[11] Physical activities tend to decline as well, bringing the average reduction in energy expenditure to about 5 percent per decade. The decline in BMR that occurs when a person becomes less active reflects the loss of lean body mass and may be minimized with ongoing physical activity. Because age influences energy expenditure, it is also factored into the energy equations.
- *Physical activity.* Using individual values for various physical activities (as in Table 8-2 on p. 247) is time-consuming and impractical for estimating the energy needs of a population. Instead, various activities are clustered according to the typical intensity of a day's efforts. Energy equations include a physical activity factor for various levels of intensity for each gender.
- *Body composition and body size.* The BMR is high in people who are tall and so have a large surface area. ♦ Similarly, the more a person weighs, the more energy is expended on basal metabolism. For these reasons, the energy equations include a factor for both height and weight.

As just explained, energy needs vary between individuals depending on such factors as gender, growth, age, physical activity, and body size and composition. Even when two people are similarly matched, however, their energy needs still differ because of genetic differences. Perhaps one day genetic research will reveal how to estimate requirements for each individual. For now, the "How To" on p. 250 provides instructions on calculating your estimated energy requirements using the DRI equations and physical activity factors. ♦

IN SUMMARY **A person in energy balance takes in energy from food and expends much of it on basal metabolic activities, some of it on physical activities, and a little on the thermic effect of food. Because energy requirements vary from person to person, such factors as gender, age, weight, and height as well as the intensity and duration of physical activity must be considered when estimating energy requirements.**

♦ Note that Table 8-1 (p. 247) lists these factors among those that influence BMR and consequently energy expenditure.

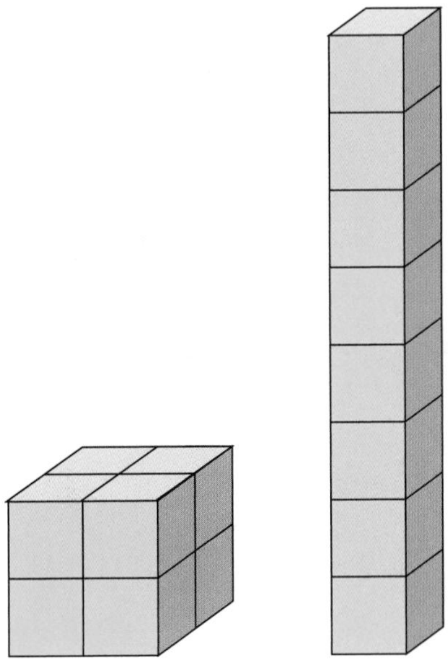

♦ Each of these structures is made of eight blocks. They weigh the same, but they are arranged differently. The short, wide structure has 24 sides exposed and the tall, thin one has 34. Because the tall, thin structure has a greater surface area, it will lose more heat (expend more energy) than the short, wide one. Similarly, two people of different heights might weigh the same, but the taller, thin one will have a higher BMR (expending more energy) because of the greater skin surface.

♦ APPENDIX F presents DRI tables that provide a shortcut to estimating total energy expenditure and instructions to help you determine the appropriate physical activity factor to use in the equation.

Body Weight, Body Composition, and Health

A person 1.78 metres tall who weighs 65 kilograms ♦ may carry only about 14 of those kilograms as fat. The rest is mostly water and lean tissues—muscles, organs such as the heart and liver, and the bones of the skeleton. Direct measures of **body composition** are impossible in living human beings; instead, researchers assess body composition indirectly based on the following assumption:

Body weight = fat + lean tissue (including water)

Weight gains and losses tell us nothing about how the body's composition may have changed, yet weight is the measure most people use to judge their "fatness."

♦ In Imperial terms, a person 5 feet 10 inches tall who weighs 150 pounds may carry only about 30 of those pounds as fat.

body composition: the proportions of muscle, bone, fat, and other tissue that make up a person's total body weight.

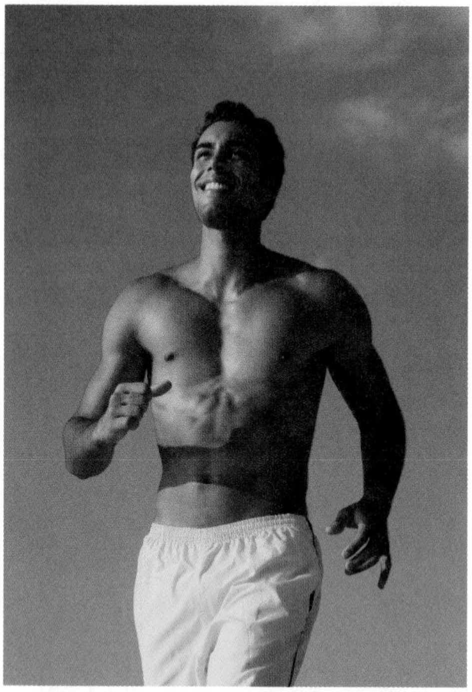

altrendo images/Getty Images

At 1.93 metres and 113 kilograms (6 feet 4 inches tall and 250 pounds), this runner would be considered over*weight* by most standards. Yet he is clearly not over*fat*.

For many people, overweight means overfat, but this is not always the case. Athletes with dense bones and well-developed muscles may be overweight by some standards but have little body fat. Conversely, inactive people may seem to have acceptable weights, when, in fact, they may have too much body fat.

Defining Healthy Body Weight How much should a person weigh? How can a person know if her weight is appropriate for her height? How can a person know if his weight is jeopardizing his health? Such questions seem so simple, yet the answers can be complex—and quite different depending on whom you ask.

HOW TO Estimate Energy Requirements

To determine your estimated energy requirement (EER), use the appropriate equation, inserting your age in years, weight (wt) in kilograms, height (ht) in metres, and physical activity (PA) factor from the accompanying table. (To convert pounds to kilograms, divide by 2.2; to convert inches to metres, divide by 39.37.)

- For men 19 years and older:
  $\text{EER} = [662 - (9.53 \times \text{age})] + \text{PA} \times [(15.91 \times \text{wt}) + (539.6 \times \text{ht})]$
- For women 19 years and older:
  $\text{EER} = [354 - (6.91 \times \text{age})] + \text{PA} \times [(9.36 \times \text{wt}) + (726 \times \text{ht})]$

For example, consider an active 30-year-old male who is 5 feet 11 inches tall and weighs 178 pounds. First, he converts his weight from pounds to kilograms and his height from inches to metres:

$$178 \text{ lb} \div 2.2 = 80.9 \text{ kg}$$
$$71 \text{ in} \div 39.37 = 1.8 \text{ m}$$

Next, he considers his level of daily physical activity and selects the appropriate PA factor from the accompanying table. (In this example, 1.25 for an active male.) Then, he inserts his age, PA factor, weight, and height into the appropriate equation:

$$\text{EER} = [662 - (9.53 \times 30)] + 1.25 \times [(15.91 \times 80.9) + (539.6 \times 1.8)]$$

(A reminder: Do calculations within the parentheses first.) He calculates:

$$\text{EER} = [662 - 286] + 1.25 \times [1287 + 971]$$

(Another reminder: Do calculations within the brackets next.)

$$\text{EER} = 376 + 1.25 \times 2258$$

(One more reminder: Do multiplication before addition.)

$$\text{EER} = 376 + 2823$$
$$\text{EER} = 3199$$

The estimated energy requirement for an active 30-year-old male who is 5 feet 11 inches tall and weighs 178 pounds is about 3200 kcalories/day. His actual requirement probably falls within a range ♦ of 200 kcalories above and below this estimate.

NOTE: APPENDIX F provides tables of energy expenditure for adults at various levels of activity and various heights and weights. It also includes EER equations for infants, children, adolescents, and pregnant women.

CENGAGENOW™
For additional practice log on to **www.cengage.com/sso**.

Physical Activity (PA) Factors for EER Equations

	Men	Women	Physical Activity
Sedentary	1.0	1.0	Typical daily living activities
Low active	1.11	1.12	Plus 30–60 min moderate activity
Active	1.25	1.27	Plus ≥ 60 min moderate activity
Very active	1.48	1.45	Plus ≥ 60 min moderate activity and 60 min vigorous or 120 min moderate activity

NOTE: Moderate activity is equivalent to walking at 5 to 7 km/h.

TRY IT Estimate your energy requirement based on your current age, weight, height, and activity level.

♦ For *most* people, the actual energy requirement falls within these ranges:
- For men, EER ± 200 kcal
- For women, EER ± 160 kcal

For *almost all* people, the actual energy requirement falls within these ranges:
- For men, EER ± 400 kcal
- For women, EER ± 320 kcal

The Criterion of Fashion In asking what is ideal, people often mistakenly turn to fashion for the answer and judge body weight by appearances. No doubt our society sets unrealistic ideals for body weight, especially for women. Magazines, movies, and television all convey the message that to be thin is to be beautiful and happy. As a result, the media have a great influence on the weight concerns and dieting patterns of people of all ages, but most tragically on young, impressionable children and adolescents.[12]

Importantly, perceived body image often has little to do with actual body weight or size. People of all shapes, sizes, and ages—including extremely thin fashion models with anorexia nervosa and fitness instructors with ideal body composition—have learned to be unhappy with their "overweight" bodies. Such dissatisfaction can lead to damaging behaviours, such as starvation diets, diet pill abuse, and health-care avoidance. The first step toward making healthy changes may be self-acceptance. Keep in mind that fashion is fickle; the body shapes valued by our society change with time. Furthermore, body shapes valued by our society differ from those of other societies. The standards defining "ideal" are subjective and frequently have little in common with health. Table 8-4 offers some tips for adopting health as an ideal, rather than society's misconceived image of beauty.

FIGURE 8-5 Distribution of Body Weights in Canadian Adults

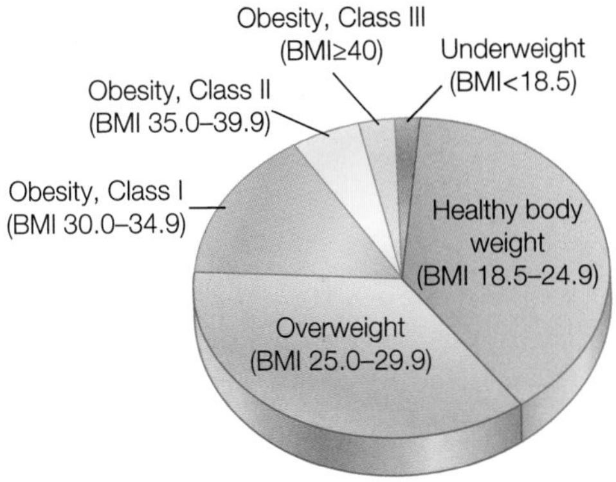
Obesity, Class III
(BMI≥40)
Underweight
(BMI<18.5)
Obesity, Class II
(BMI 35.0–39.9)
Obesity, Class I
(BMI 30.0–34.9)
Healthy body
weight
(BMI 18.5–24.9)
Overweight
(BMI 25.0–29.9)

SOURCE: Canadian Community Health Survey, 2004

The Criterion of Health Even if our society were to accept fat as beautiful, obesity would still be a major risk factor for several life-threatening diseases. For this reason, the most important criterion for determining how much a person should weigh and how much body fat a person needs is not appearance but good health and longevity. Ideally, a person has enough fat to meet basic needs ♦ but not so much as to incur health risks. This range of healthy body weights has been identified using a common measure of weight and height—the body mass index.

♦ Fat in the body:
- Provides energy
- Insulates against temperature extremes
- Protects against physical shock
- Forms cell membranes
- Makes compounds such as hormones, vitamin D, and bile

Body Mass Index The **body mass index (BMI)** describes relative weight for height: ♦

$$\text{BMI} = \frac{\text{weight (kg)}}{\text{height (m)}^2} \text{ or } \frac{\text{weight (lb)}}{\text{height (in)}^2} \times 703.$$

♦ To convert pounds to kilograms:
lb ÷ 2.2 lb/kg = kg
To convert inches to metres:
in ÷ 39.37 in/m = m

Weight classifications based on BMI are presented in Table 8-5 (p. 252). Notice that healthy weight falls between a BMI of 18.5 and 24.9, with **underweight** below 18.5, **overweight** 25.0 to 29.9, and **obese** 30.0 and above. Approximately six out of ten Canadian adults have a BMI 25.0 or greater, as Figure 8-5 shows.[13]

Obesity-related diseases become evident beyond a BMI of 25. For this reason, a BMI of 25 for adults represents a healthy goal for overweight people and an upper limit for others. The lower end of the healthy range may be a reasonable target for severely underweight people. BMI values slightly below the healthy range may be compatible with good health if food intake is adequate, but signs of illness, reduced work capacity, and poor reproductive function become apparent when BMI is below 17. For quick reference, the inside back cover presents weights and visual images associated with various BMI values. The accompanying "How To" (p. 253) describes how to determine your BMI and how to find a goal weight based on a desired BMI.

body mass index (BMI): an index of a person's weight in relation to height; determined by dividing the weight (in kilograms) by the square of the height (in metres).

underweight: body weight below some standard of acceptable weight that is usually defined in relation to height (such as BMI); BMI below 18.5.

overweight: body weight above some standard of acceptable weight that is usually defined in relation to height (such as BMI); BMI 25 to 29.9.

obese: overweight with adverse health effects;
- **Class I:** BMI 30 to 34.9
- **Class II:** BMI 35 to 39.9
- **Class III:** BMI 40 or higher.

TABLE 8-4 Tips for Accepting a Healthy Body Weight

- Value yourself and others for human attributes other than body weight. Realize that prejudging people by weight is as harmful as prejudging them by race, religion, or gender.
- Use positive, nonjudgmental descriptions of your body.
- Accept positive comments from others.
- Focus on your whole self including your intelligence, social grace, and professional and scholastic achievements.
- Accept that no magic diet exists.
- Stop dieting to lose weight. Adopt a lifestyle of healthy eating and physical activity permanently.
- Follow *Canada's Food Guide*. Never restrict food intake below the minimum levels that meet nutrient needs.
- Become physically active, not because it will help you get thin but because it will make you feel good and enhance your health.
- Seek support from loved ones. Tell them of your plan for a healthy life in the body you have been given.
- Seek professional counselling, *not* from a weight-loss counsellor, but from someone who can help you make gains in self-esteem without weight as a factor.
- Appreciate body weight for its influence on health, not appearance.

TABLE 8-5 Body Mass Index (BMI)

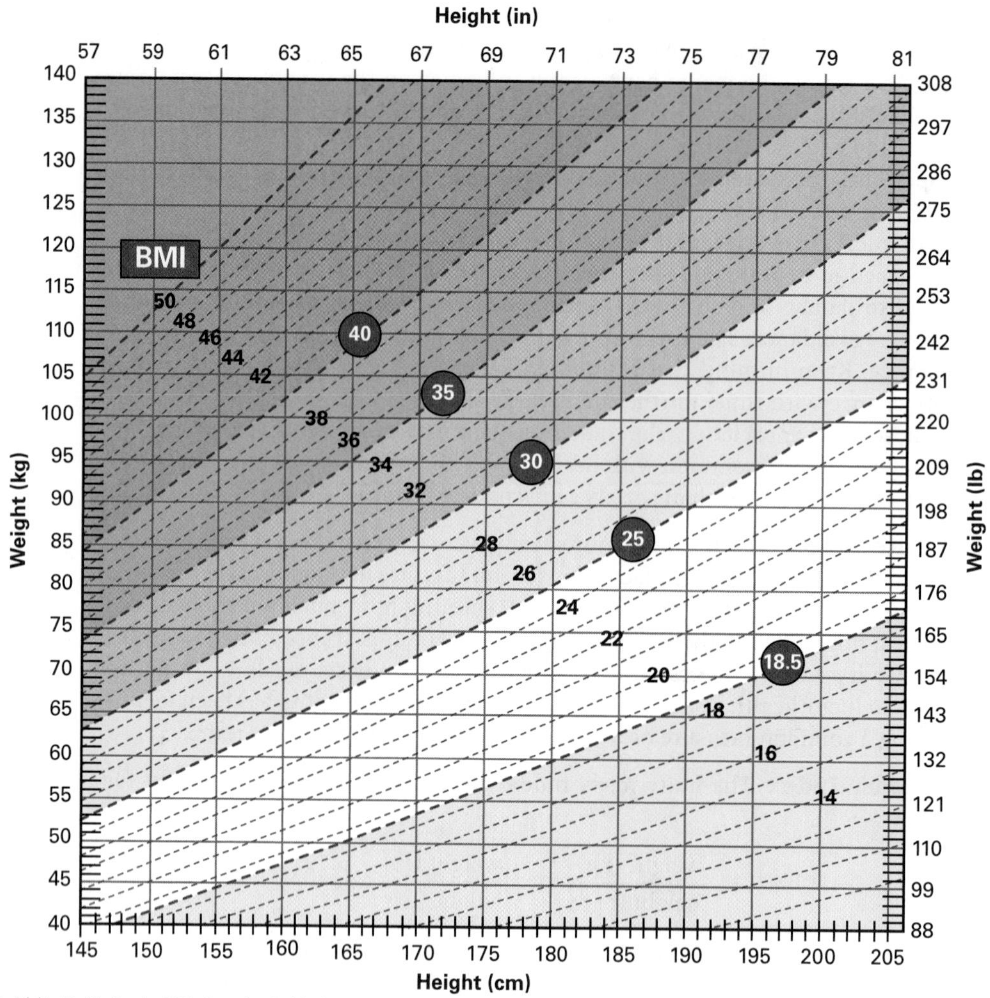
Height (in)
57 59 61 63 65 67 69 71 73 75 77 79 81
Weight (kg)
140 135 130 125 120 115 110 105 100 95 90 85 80 75 70 65 60 55 50 45 40
Weight (lb)
308 297 286 275 264 253 242 231 220 209 198 187 176 165 154 143 132 121 110 99 88
BMI
50 48 46 44 42 40 38 36 35 34 32 30 28 26 25 24 22 20 18.5 18 16 14
145 150 155 160 165 170 175 180 185 190 195 200 205
Height (cm)

SOURCE: Canadian Guidelines for Body Weight Classification in Adults. Health Canada, 2003. Reproduced with the permission of the Minister of Health, 2011. See also endnote 14 on page 259.

Keep in mind that BMI reflects height and weight measures and not body composition nor distribution of body fat. Consequently, muscular athletes may be classified as over*weight* by BMI standards and not be over*fat*.[15] At the peak of his bodybuilding career, Arnold Schwarzenegger won the Mr. Olympia competition with a BMI of 31; the runner on p. 250 also has a BMI greater than 30. Yet neither would be considered obese. Striking differences in body composition are also apparent among people of different ages and various ethnic and racial groups, making standard BMI guidelines inappropriate for some populations.[16] For example, black persons tend to have a greater bone density and protein content than white persons; consequently, using BMI as the standard may overestimate the prevalence of overweight and obesity among the black population.

IN SUMMARY **Current standards for body weight are based on a person's weight in relation to height, called the body mass index (BMI), and reflect disease risks. To its disadvantage, BMI does not reflect body fat, and it may misclassify very muscular people as overweight.**

Body Fat and Its Distribution

Although weight measures are inexpensive, easy to take, and highly accurate, they fail to reveal two valuable pieces of information in assessing disease risk: how much of the weight is fat and where the fat is located. The ideal amount of body fat depends partly on the person. A normal-weight man may have from 13 to 21 percent body fat; a woman, because of her greater quantity of essential fat, 23 to 31 percent. In general, health

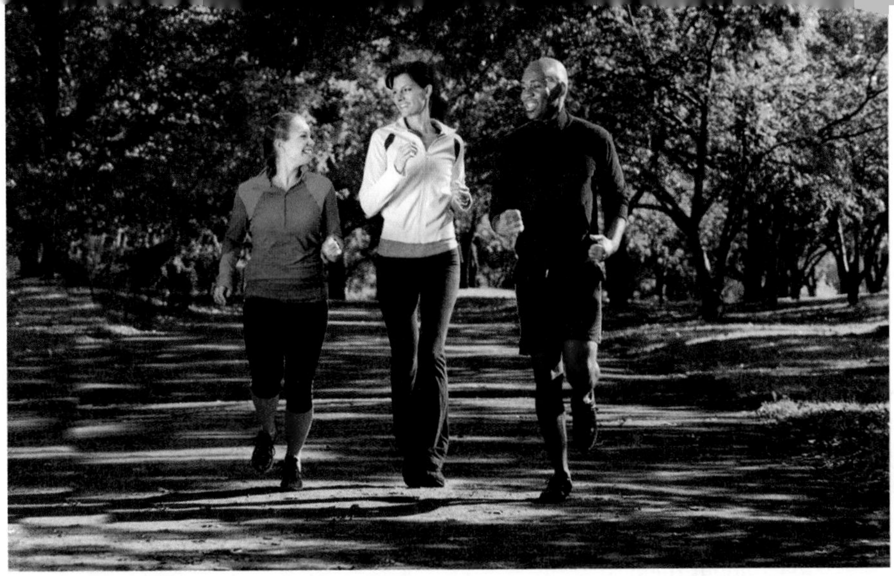
Tyler Olson/shutterstock

A healthy body contains enough lean tissue to support health and the right amount of fat to meet body needs.

problems typically develop when body fat exceeds 22 percent in young men, 25 percent in men older than age 40, 32 percent in young women, and 35 percent in women older than age 40. Body fat may contribute as much as 70 percent in excessively obese adults. Figure 8-6 (p. 254) compares the body composition of healthy-weight men and women.

Some People Need Less Body Fat For many athletes, a lower percentage of body fat may be ideal—just enough fat to provide fuel, insulate and protect the

HOW TO Determine BMI

To calculate your body mass index (BMI), use one of the following equations:

$$\text{BMI} = \frac{\text{weight (kg)}}{\text{height (m)}^2} \text{ or}$$

$$\text{BMI} = \frac{\text{weight (lb)}}{\text{height (in)}^2} \times 703$$

Consider, for example, a person who is 1.65 m (5'5") tall and weighs 79 kg (174 lb):

$$\text{BMI} = \frac{79 \text{ kg}}{1.65 \text{ m}^2} = 29 \text{ or}$$

$$\text{BMI} = \frac{174 \text{ lb}}{65 \text{ in}^2} \times 703 = 29$$

This person has a BMI of 29 and is considered overweight.

You could also use Table 8-5 to determine your BMI. Locate your height in the first column (in this example, 1.65 m). Then look across the row until you find the number that is closest to your weight (in this example, 79 kg). The number along the curve identifies your BMI (in this example, 29).

A reasonable initial target for most overweight people is a BMI 2 units below their current one. To determine a goal weight based on a desired BMI, locate your height in the first column and then look across the row until you reach the column with the desired BMI. In this example, to reach a BMI of 27, this person's goal weight is 74 kilograms, which represents a 5 kilogram weight loss. Such a determination can help a person set realistic weight goals using health risk as a guide.

CENGAGENOW™
For additional practice log on to **www.cengage.com/sso**.

TRY IT Calculate your BMI and determine whether you are underweight, healthy weight, overweight, or obese. If your BMI is less than 18.5 or 25.0 or greater, identify a weight that takes your BMI 2 units closer to the healthy weight range.

FIGURE 8-6 Male and Female Body Compositions Compared

The differences between male and female body compositions become apparent during adolescence. Lean body mass (primarily muscle) increases more in males than in females. Fat assumes a larger percentage of female body composition as essential body fat is deposited in the mammary glands and pelvic region in preparation for childbearing. Both men and women have essential fat associated with the bone marrow, the central nervous system, and the internal organs.

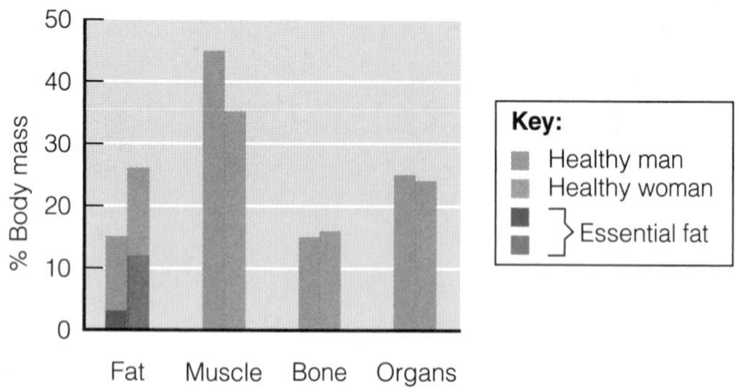
% Body mass
50
40
30
20
10
0
Fat
Muscle
Bone
Organs
Key:
Healthy man
Healthy woman
Essential fat

SOURCE: Advanced human nutrition by WILDMAN, ROBERT E. C. Copyright 2000. Reproduced with permission of TAYLOR & FRANCIS GROUP LLC - Print, other book, CD-DVD via Copyright Clearance Center.

body, assist in nerve impulse transmissions, and support normal hormone activity, but not so much as to burden the body with excess bulk. For some athletes, then, ideal body fat might be 5 to 10 percent for men and 15 to 20 percent for women. (Review the photo on p. 250 to appreciate what 8 percent body fat looks like.)

Some People Need More Body Fat For a Nunavut fisherman, a higher percentage of body fat is probably beneficial because fat provides an insulating blanket to prevent excessive loss of body heat in cold climates. A woman starting a pregnancy needs sufficient body fat to support conception and fetal growth. Below a certain threshold for body fat, hormone synthesis falters, and individuals may become infertile, develop depression, experience abnormal hunger regulation, or become unable to keep warm. These thresholds differ for each function and for each individual; much remains to be learned about them.

Fat Distribution The distribution of fat on the body may be more critical than the total amount of fat alone. **Visceral fat** that is stored around the organs of the abdomen is referred to as **central obesity** or upper-body fat (see Figure 8-7). Independently of BMI or total body fat, central obesity is associated with increased risks of heart disease, stroke, diabetes, insulin resistance, hypertension, gallstones, and some types of cancer.[17]

Visceral fat is most common in men and to a lesser extent in women past menopause. Even when total body fat is similar, men have more visceral fat than women. Regardless of gender, the risks of cardiovascular disease, diabetes, and mortality are increased for those with excessive visceral fat. Interestingly, smokers tend to have more visceral fat than nonsmokers even though they typically have lower BMI.[18]

Subcutaneous fat around the hips and thighs, sometimes referred to as lower-body fat, is most common in women during their reproductive years and seems relatively harmless. In fact, overweight people who have little visceral fat are less susceptible to health problems than overweight people with visceral fat. Figure 8-8 compares the body shapes of people with upper-body fat and lower-body fat.

Waist Circumference A person's **waist circumference** is a good indicator of fat distribution and central obesity.[19] In general, women with a waist circumference of equal to or greater than 88 centimetres (35 inches) and men with a waist circumference of equal to or greater than 102 centimetres (40 inches) have a high risk of central obesity–related health problems, such as diabetes and cardiovascular disease. As waist circumference increases, disease risks increase. Recent research suggests a need for ethnic-specific threshold measures for waist circumference, but generally as waist circumference increases, disease risks increase.[20] APPENDIX E includes instructions for measuring waist circumference and assessing abdominal fat.

Waist circumference is a better indicator of abdominal fat, but some researchers use the waist-to-hip ratio when studying disease risks. APPENDIX E explains a desirable waist-to-hip ratio for Canadian women is less than 0.8 and for men is less than 1.0. The ratio requires another step or two (measuring the hips and comparing that measure to the waist measure), but it does not provide any additional information. Therefore, waist circumference alone is the preferred method for assessing abdominal fat in a clinical setting.[21]

Other Measures of Body Composition Health-care professionals commonly use BMI and waist circumference measures because they are relatively easy and inexpensive. Together, these two measures prove most valuable in assessing a person's health risks and monitoring changes over time.[22] Researchers needing more precise measures of body composition may choose any of several other techniques to estimate body fat and its distribution (see Figure 8-9 on p. 256). Mastering these techniques requires proper instruction and practice to ensure

visceral fat: fat stored within the abdominal cavity in association with the internal abdominal organs; also called *intra-abdominal fat.*

central obesity: excess fat around the trunk of the body; also called *abdominal fat* or *upper-body fat.*

subcutaneous fat: fat stored directly under the skin.
- **sub** = beneath
- **cutaneous** = skin

waist circumference: an anthropometric measurement used to assess a person's abdominal fat.

FIGURE 8-7 Abdominal Fat

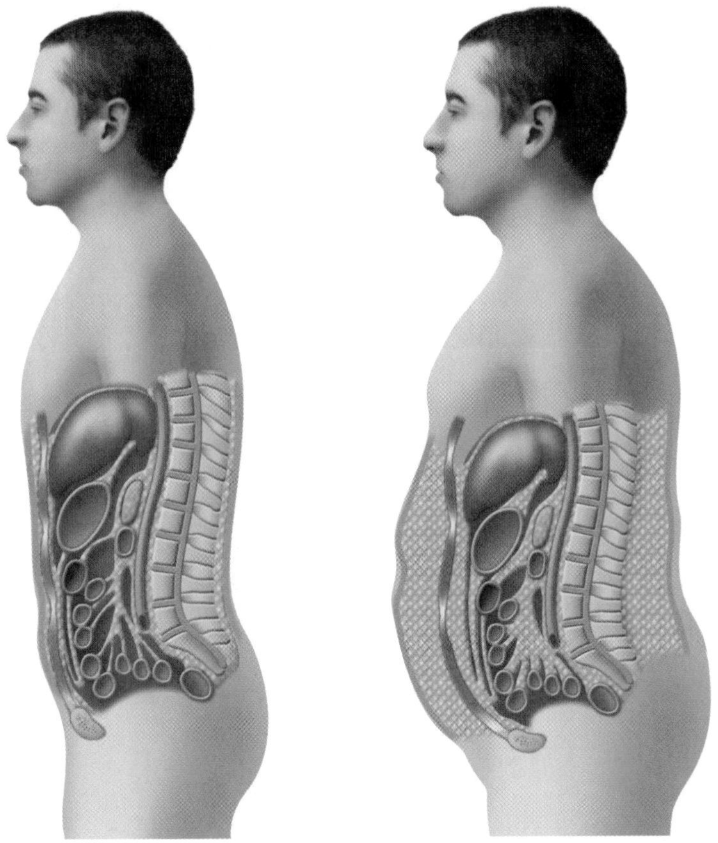

In healthy-weight people, some fat is stored around the organs of the abdomen.

In overweight people, excess abdominal fat increases the risks of diseases.

FIGURE 8-8 "Apple" and "Pear" Body Shapes Compared

Popular articles sometimes call bodies with upper-body fat "apples" and those with lower-body fat, "pears." Researchers sometimes refer to upper-body fat as "android" (manlike) obesity and to lower-body fat as "gynoid" (womanlike) obesity.

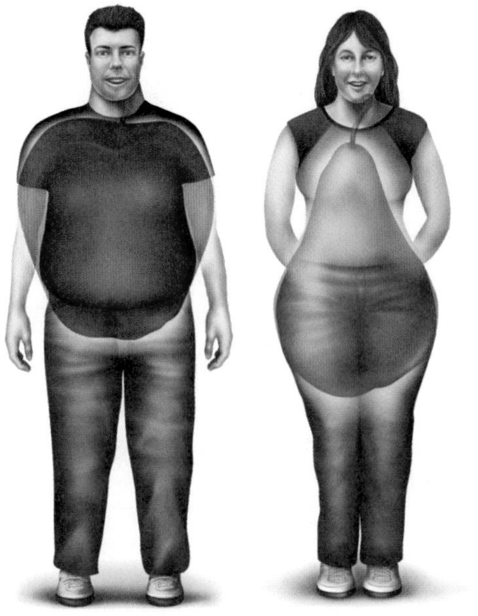

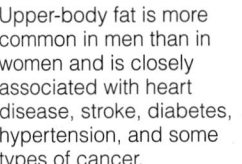

Upper-body fat is more common in men than in women and is closely associated with heart disease, stroke, diabetes, hypertension, and some types of cancer.

Lower-body fat is more common in women than in men and is not usually associated with chronic diseases.

reliability. In addition to the methods shown in Figure 8-9, researchers sometimes estimate body composition using these methods: total body water, dual energy X-ray absorptiometry, near-infrared spectrophotometry, ultrasound, computed tomography, and magnetic resonance imaging. Each method has advantages and disadvantages with respect to cost, technical difficulty, and precision of estimating body fat. APPENDIX E provides a comparison of the methods and includes many of the tables and charts routinely used in assessment procedures.

IN SUMMARY **The ideal amount of body fat varies from person to person, but researchers have found that body fat in excess of 22 percent for young men and 32 percent for young women (the levels rise slightly with age) poses health risks. Central obesity, in which excess abdominal fat is distributed around the trunk of the body, presents greater health risks than excess fat distributed on the lower body.**

Health Risks Associated with Body Weight and Body Fat

Insurance data indicate that body weight and fat distribution correlate with disease risks and life expectancy. The correlation suggests a greater *likelihood* of developing a chronic disease and shortening life expectancy. Not all overweight and underweight people will get sick and die before their time nor will all normal-weight people live long healthy lives. *Correlations* are not *causes*. For the most part, people with a BMI between 18.5 and 24.9 have relatively few weight-related health risks; risks increase as BMI falls below or rises above this

FIGURE 8-9 Methods Used to Assess Body Fat

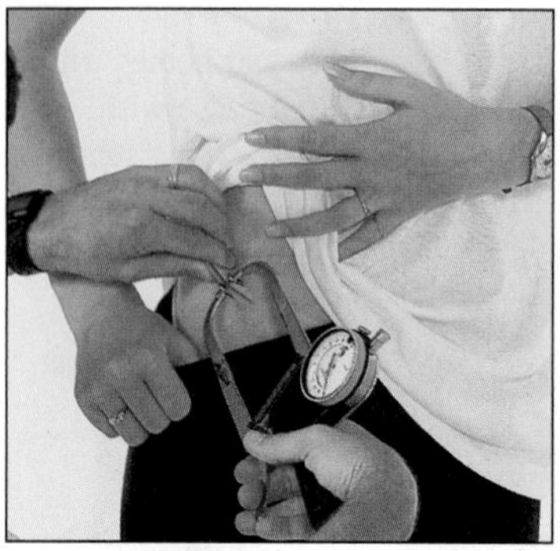

© Fitness & Wellness, Boise, Idaho

Skinfold measures estimate body fat by using a caliper to gauge the thickness of a fold of skin on the back of the arm (over the triceps), below the shoulder blade (subscapular), and in other places (including lower-body sites), and then comparing these measurements with standards.

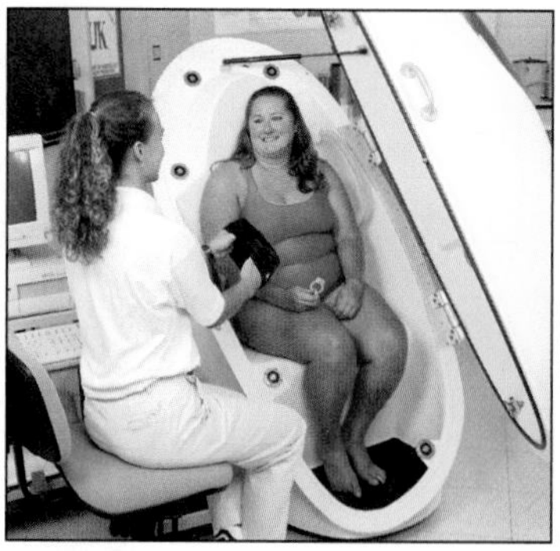

Photo courtesy of COSMED USA, Inc.

Air displacement plethysmography estimates body composition by having a person sit inside a chamber while computerized sensors determine the amount of air displaced by the person's body.

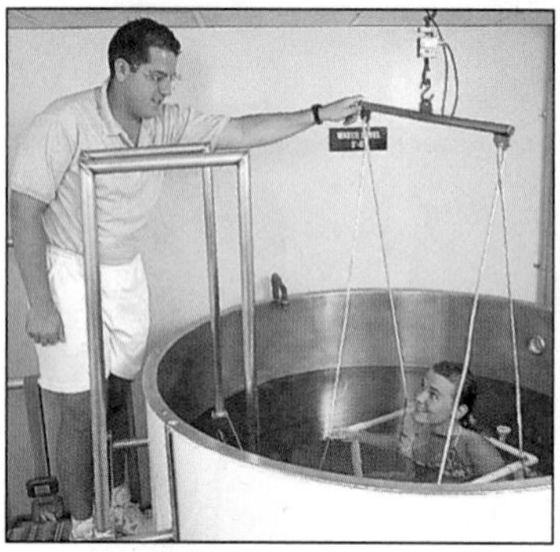

© David Young-Wolff/PhotoEdit

Hydrodensitometry measures body density by weighing the person first on land and then again while submerged in water. The difference between the person's actual weight and underwater weight provides a measure of the body's volume. A mathematical equation using the two measurements (volume and actual weight) determines body density, from which the percentage of body fat can be estimated.

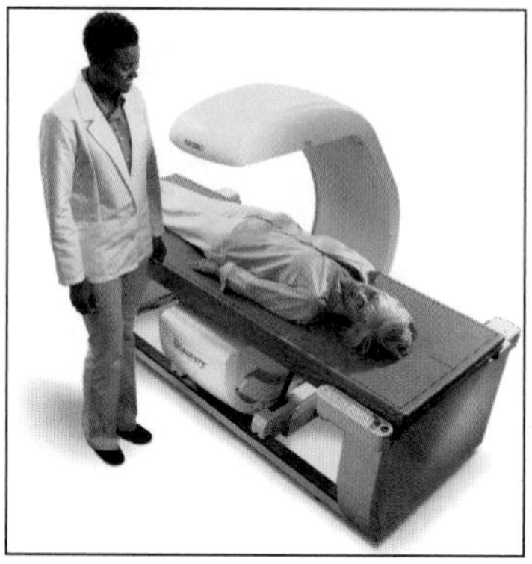

© Photo Courtesy of Hologic, Inc.

Dual energy X-ray absorptiometry (DEXA) uses two low-dose X-rays that differentiate among fat-free soft tissue (lean body mass), fat tissue, and bone tissue, providing a precise measurement of total fat and its distribution in all but extremely obese subjects.

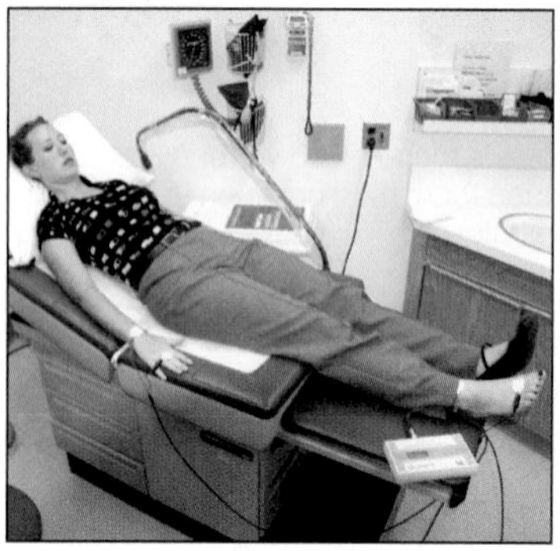

© Geri Engberg Photography

Bioelectrical impedance measures body fat by using a low-intensity electrical current. Because electrolyte-containing fluids, which readily conduct an electrical current, are found primarily in lean body tissues, the leaner the person, the less resistance to the current. The measurement of electrical resistance is then used in a mathematical equation to estimate the percentage of body fat.

range, indicating that both too little and too much body fat impair health.[23] Epidemiological data show a J- or U-shaped relationship between body weights and mortality (see Figure 8-10).[24] People who are extremely underweight or extremely obese carry higher risks of early deaths ♦ than those whose weights fall within the healthy, or even the slightly overweight, range.[25] These mortality risks decline with age.[26]

♦ BMI and mortality:
- BMI 22.5–24.9 = optimal survival
- BMI 30–34.9 = 3 years' loss of life
- BMI ≥40 = 10 years' loss of life (equivalent to lifetime of smoking)

Independently of BMI, factors such as smoking habits raise health risks, and physical fitness lowers them. A man with a BMI of 22 who smokes two packs of cigarettes a day is jeopardizing his health, whereas a woman with a BMI of 32 who walks briskly for an hour a day is improving her health.

Health Risks of Underweight Some underweight people enjoy an active, healthy life, but others are underweight because of malnutrition, smoking habits, substance abuse, or illnesses. Weight and fat measures alone would not reveal these underlying causes, but a complete assessment that includes a diet and medical history, physical examination, and biochemical analysis would.

An underweight person, especially an older adult, may be unable to preserve lean tissue during the fight against a wasting disease such as cancer or a digestive disorder, especially when the disease is accompanied by malnutrition. Without adequate nutrient and energy reserves, an underweight person will have a particularly tough battle against such medical stresses. Underweight women develop menstrual irregularities and become infertile. Those who do conceive may give birth to unhealthy infants. An underweight woman can improve her chances of having a healthy infant by gaining weight prior to conception, during pregnancy, or both. Underweight and significant weight loss are also associated with osteoporosis and bone fractures. For all these reasons, underweight people may benefit from enough of a weight gain to provide an energy reserve and protective amounts of all the nutrients that can be stored.

Health Risks of Overweight As for excessive body fat, the health risks are so many that it has been designated a disease—obesity. Among the health risks associated with obesity are diabetes, hypertension, cardiovascular disease, sleep apnea (abnormal ceasing of breathing during sleep), osteoarthritis, some cancers, gallbladder disease, kidney stones, respiratory problems (including Pickwickian syndrome, a breathing blockage linked with sudden death), infertility, and complications in pregnancy and surgery. Obese people are more likely to be disabled in their later years.[27]

The cost in terms of lives is also great. Mortality increases as excess weight increases.[28] People with a BMI of 35 or greater are about twice as likely to die of heart disease as others.[29] The risks associated with a high BMI appear to be greater for white persons than for black persons; in fact, the health risks associated with obesity do not become apparent in black women until a BMI of 37. In contrast, health risks appear to be greater for Asians than for Caucasians at the same BMI.[30]

Equally important, both central obesity and weight gains of more than 9 kilograms (20 pounds) between early and middle adulthood correlate with increased disease risks.[31] Fluctuations in body weight, as typically occur with "yo-yo" dieting, may also increase the risks of chronic diseases and premature death. In contrast, sustained weight loss improves physical well-being, reduces disease risks, and increases life expectancy.

Cardiovascular Disease The relationship between obesity and cardiovascular disease risk is strong, with links to both elevated blood cholesterol and hypertension. Central obesity may raise the risk of heart attack and stroke as much as the three leading risk factors (high LDL cholesterol, hypertension, and smoking) do. ♦ In addition to body fat and its distribution, weight gain also increases the risk of cardiovascular disease. Weight loss, on the other hand, can effectively lower both blood cholesterol and blood pressure in overweight and obese people. Of course, lean and normal-weight people may also have high blood cholesterol and blood pressure, and these factors are just as dangerous in lean people as in obese people.

Diabetes Most adults with type 2 diabetes are overweight or obese. Diabetes (type 2) is three times more likely to develop in an obese person than in a nonobese person. Furthermore, the person with type 2 diabetes often has central obesity. Central-body fat cells appear to be larger and more insulin-resistant than lower-body fat cells.[32] The association between **insulin resistance** and obesity is strong. Both are major risk factors for the development of type 2 diabetes.

Diabetes appears to be influenced by weight gains as well as by body weight. A weight gain of more than 4.5 kilograms (10 pounds) after the age of 18 doubles the risk of developing diabetes, even in women of average weight. In contrast, weight loss is effective in improving glucose tolerance and insulin resistance.[33]

Inflammation and the Metabolic Syndrome Chronic **inflammation** accompanies obesity, and inflammation contributes to chronic diseases.[34] As a person grows fatter, lipids first fill the adipose tissue and then migrate into other tissues such as the muscles and liver.[35] This accumulation of fat, especially in the abdominal

FIGURE 8-10 BMI and Mortality

This J-shaped curve describes the relationship between body mass index (BMI) and mortality and shows that both underweight and overweight present risks of a premature death.

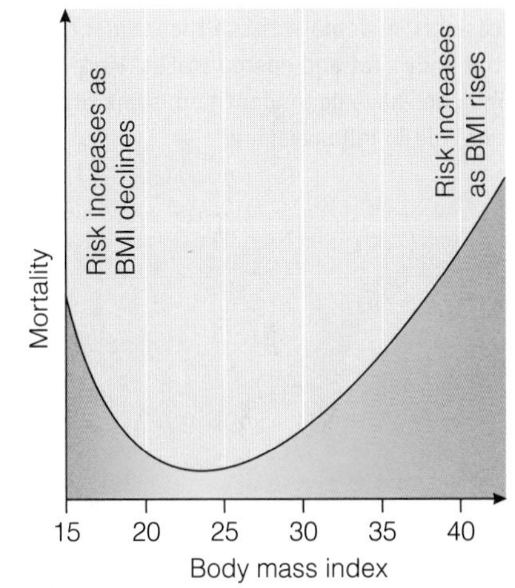
Risk increases as BMI declines
Risk increases as BMI rises
Mortality
15
20
25
30
35
40
Body mass index

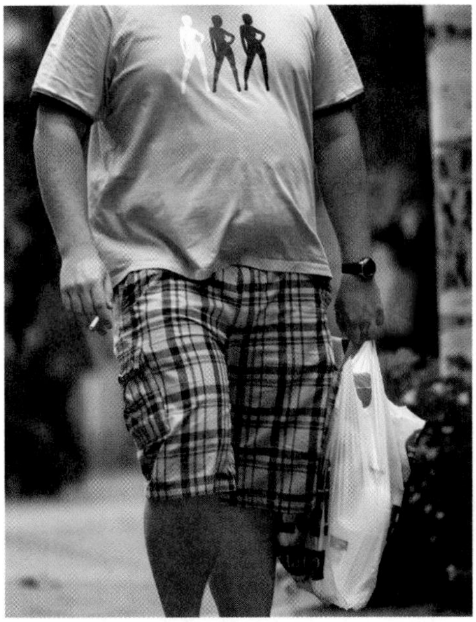

© Craig Stephen/Alamy

Smoking is the leading cause of preventable illnesses and early deaths. Obesity is a close second.

♦ Cardiovascular disease risk factors associated with obesity:
- High LDL cholesterol
- Low HDL cholesterol
- High blood pressure (hypertension)
- Diabetes

Chapter 19 provides many more details.

insulin resistance: the condition in which a normal amount of insulin produces a subnormal effect in muscle, adipose, and liver cells, resulting in an elevated fasting glucose; a metabolic consequence of obesity that precedes type 2 diabetes.

inflammation: an immunological response to cellular injury characterized by an increase in white blood cells.

♦ Metabolic syndrome is a cluster of at least three of the following risk factors:
- High blood pressure
- High blood glucose
- High blood triglycerides
- Low HDL cholesterol
- High waist circumference

♦ Chapter 5 introduced **adipokines**—proteins released from adipose tissue that signal changes in the body's fat and energy status. More than 50 adipokines have been identified, some of which play a role in inflammation.

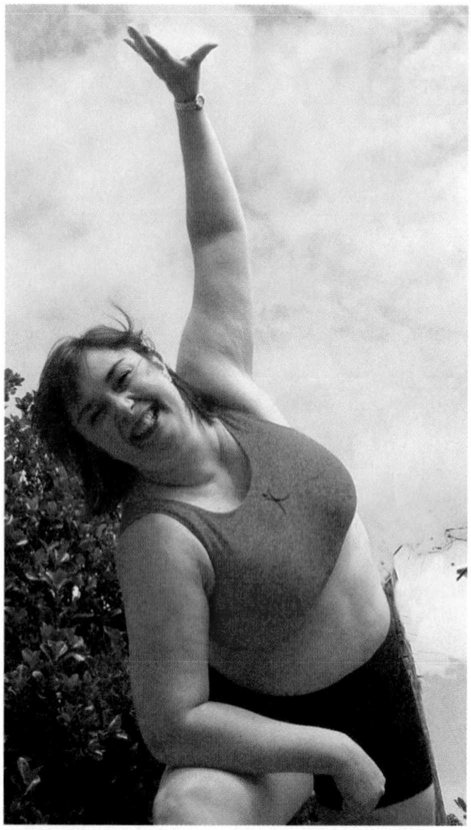

© Joe Libin

Being active—even if overweight—is healthier than being sedentary. With a BMI of 36, aerobics instructor Jennifer Portnick is considered obese, but her daily workout routine helps to keep her in good health.

region, changes the body's metabolism, resulting in insulin resistance, low HDL, high triglycerides, and high blood pressure.[36] This cluster of symptoms—collectively known as the metabolic syndrome—increases the risks for diabetes, hypertension, and atherosclerosis. ♦ Fat accumulation, especially in the abdominal region, activates genes that code for proteins ♦ involved in inflammation.[37] Furthermore, although relatively few immune cells are commonly found in adipose tissue, weight gain significantly increases their number and their role in inflammation.[38] Elevated blood lipids—whether due to obesity or to a high-fat diet—also promote inflammation.[39] Together, these factors help to explain why chronic inflammation accompanies obesity and how obesity contributes to the metabolic syndrome and the progression of chronic diseases.[40] Even in healthy youngsters, body fat correlates positively with chronic inflammation.[41] As might be expected, weight loss reduces the number of immune cells in adipose tissue and changes gene expression to reduce inflammation.[42]

Cancer The risk of some cancers increases with both body weight and weight gain, but researchers do not fully understand the relationships. One possible explanation may be that obese people have elevated levels of hormones that could influence cancer development. For example, adipose tissue is the major site of estrogen synthesis in women, obese women have elevated levels of estrogen, and estrogen has been implicated in the development of cancers of the female reproductive system—cancers that account for half of all cancers in women.

Fit and Fat versus Sedentary and Slim Importantly, BMI and weight gains and losses do not tell the whole story. Cardiorespiratory and muscular fitness play major roles in health and longevity, independently of body weight.[43] Normal-weight people who are fit have a lower risk of mortality than normal-weight people who are unfit. Furthermore, overweight but fit people have lower risks than normal-weight, unfit ones.[44] Fit people are also likely to gain less weight over the years.[45] Clearly, a healthy body weight is good, but it may not be good enough. Fitness, in and of itself, offers many health benefits, as Chapter 15 confirms. The next chapter explores weight management and the benefits of choosing nutritious foods and exercising regularly.

IN SUMMARY **The weight appropriate for an individual depends largely on factors specific to that individual, including body fat distribution, family health history, and current health status. At the extremes, both overweight and underweight carry clear risks to health.**

Nutrition Portfolio

When combined with fitness, a healthy body weight will help you to defend against chronic diseases.

Go to Diet Analysis Plus and choose one of the days on which you have tracked your diet for the entire day. Go to the Energy Balance report; use this report to help you answer the following questions:

- Describe how your daily food intake and physical activity balance with each other.
- What did the diet analysis program estimate as your daily energy requirement? What information was this based on?
- Describe any health risks that may be of concern for a person who continuously has very high "net kcalories" or very low "net kcalories" for many years? What would you do to achieve energy balance?

Diet Analysis PLUS

To complete this exercise, go to your Diet Analysis Plus at www.cengage.com/sso.

Nutrition on the Net

CENGAGENOW™
For further study of topics covered in this chapter, log on to **www.cengage.com/sso.**

- Obtain food composition data from the Canadian Nutrient File: **www.hc-sc.gc.ca/fn-an/nutrition/fiche-nutri-data/index-eng.php**
- Find physical activity guidelines for Canadians at the Canadian Society for Exercise Physiology website to: **www.csep.ca**
- Learn about the 10,000 Steps Program at Shape Up America: **www.shapeup.org**
- Visit the special web pages and interactive applications that Aim for a Healthy Weight: **www.nhlbi.nih.gov/health/public/heart/obesity/lose_wt**

References

1. G. A. Bray and C. M. Champagne, Beyond energy balance: There is more to obesity than kilocalories, *Journal of the American Dietetic Association* 105 (2005): S17–S23.
2. R. D. Mattes and coauthors, Appetite: Measurement and manipulation misgivings, *Journal of the American Dietetic Association* 105 (2005): S87–S97.
3. T. Rankinen and C. Bouchard, Genetics of food intake and eating behavior phenotypes in humans, *Annual Review of Nutrition* 26 (2006): 413–434.
4. C. D. Morrison and H. Berthoud, Neurobiology of nutrition and obesity, *Nutrition Reviews* 65 (2007): 517–534; M. J. Wolfgang and M. D. Lane, Control of energy homeostasis: Role of enzymes and intermediates of fatty acid metabolism in the central nervous system, *Annual Review of Nutrition* 26 (2006): 23–44.
5. T. C. Adam and E. S. Epel, Stress, eating and the reward system, *Physiology and Behavior* 91 (2007): 449–458; S. J. Torres and C. A. Nowson, Relationship between stress, eating behavior, and obesity, *Nutrition* 23 (2007): 887–894.
6. J. W. Apolzan and coauthors, Inadequate dietary protein increases hunger and desire to eat in young and older men, *Journal of Nutrition* 137 (2007): 1478–1482.
7. D. E. Cummings and J. Overduin, Gastrointestinal regulation of food intake, *Journal of Clinical Investigation* 117 (2007): 13–23.
8. E. Valassi, M. Scacchi, and F. Cavagnini, Neuroendocrine control of food intake, *Nutrition, Metabolism, and Cardiovascular Disease* 18 (2008): 158–168; Cummings and Overduin, 2007; K. G. Murphy, W. S. Dhillo, and S. R. Bloom, Gut peptides in the regulation of food intake and energy homeostasis, *Endocrine Reviews* 27 (2006): 719–727.
9. J. A. Harrold and J. C. Halford, The hypothalamus and obesity, *Recent Patents on CNS Drug Discovery* 1 (2006): 305–314.
10. B. E. Ainsworth and coauthors, Compendium of physical activities: An update of activity codes and MET intensities, *Medicine and Science in Sports and Exercise* 32 (2000): S498–S516; B. E. Ainsworth and coauthors, Compendium of physical activities: Classification of energy costs of human physical activities, *Medicine and Science in Sports and Exercise* 25 (1993): 71–80.
11. N. Meunier and coauthors, Basal metabolic rate and thyroid hormones of late-middle-aged and older human subjects: The ZENITH study, *European Journal of Clinical Nutrition* 59 (2005): S53–S57.
12. A. J. Hill, Motivation for eating behaviour in adolescent girls: The body beautiful, *Proceedings of the Nutrition Society* 65 (2006): 376–384.
13. M. Tjepkema, Adult obesity in Canada: Measured height and weight, Statistics Canada Cat. No. 82-620-MWE2005001. www.statcan.gc.ca/pub/82-620-m/2005001/article/adults-adultes/8060-eng.htm, accessed August 2010.
14. Public Health Agency of Canada, 2010. The Chronic Disease Infobase website. Retrieved October 30, 2010 from http://www.infobase.phac-aspc.gc.ca Mortality Data: The mortality data contained in these tables were provided to Health Canada from the Canadian Vital Statistics databases at Statistics Canada with the knowledge and consent of the provincial and territorial vital statistics registries which supply the data to Statistics Canada. Their cooperation is gratefully acknowledged. Incidence Data: The Source of the incidence data is the Canadian Council of Cancer Registries. Subsequent manipulation of data was performed by the Surveillance and Risk Assessment Division, CCDPC, Health Canada. Population estimates were provided by Statistics Canada. Data quality information was provided by the provincial and territorial cancer registries and the Health Statistics Division of Statistics Canada.
15. K. A. Witt and E. A. Bush, College athletes with an elevated body mass index often have a high upper arm muscle area, but not elevated triceps and subscapular skinfolds, *Journal of the American Dietetic Association* 105 (2005): 599–602.
16. R. Huxley and coauthors, Ethnic comparisons of the cross-sectional relationships between measures of body size with diabetes and hypertension, *Obesity Reviews* 9 (2008): 53–61.
17. K. F. Adams and coauthors, Body mass and colorectal cancer risk in the NIH-AARP cohort, *American Journal of Epidemiology* 166 (2007): 36–45; G. Hu and coauthors, Body mass index, waist circumference, and waist-hip ratio on the risk of total and type-specific stroke, *Archives of Internal Medicine* 167 (2007): 1420–1427; C. D. Lee and coauthors, Abdominal obesity and coronary artery calcification in young adults: The Coronary Artery Risk Development in Young Adults (CARDIA) Study, *American Journal of Clinical Nutrition* (2007): 48–54; S. B. Votruba and M. D. Jensen, Regional fat deposition as a factor in FFA metabolism, *Annual Review of Nutrition* 27 (2007): 149–163; G. R. Dagenais and coauthors, Prognostic impact of body weight and abdominal obesity in women and men with cardiovascular disease, *American Heart Journal* 149 (2005): 54–60; Y. Wang and coauthors, Comparison of abdominal adiposity and overall obesity in predicting risk of type 2 diabetes among men, *American Journal of Clinical Nutrition* 81 (2005): 555–563.
18. D. Canoy and coauthors, Cigarette smoking and fat distribution in 21,828 British men and women: A population-based study, *Obesity Research* 13 (2005): 1466–1475.
19. J. P. Després and coauthors, Abdominal obesity and the metabolic syndrome: Contribution to global cardiometabolic risk, *Arteriosclerosis, Thrombosis, and Vascular Biology* 28 (2008): 1039–1049; S. Klein and coauthors, Waist circumference and cardiometabolic risk: A consensus statement from Shaping America's Health: Association for Weight Management and Obesity Prevention; NAASO, The Obesity Society; The American Society for Nutrition; and the American Diabetes Association, *American Journal of Clinical Nutrition* 85 (2007): 1197–1202; Wang and coauthors, 2005.
20. P. T. Katzmarzyk and coauthors, Ethnic-specific BMI and waist circumference thresholds, *Obesity* (2011) doi:10.1038/oby.2010.319; S. M. Camhi and coauthors, The relationship of waist circumference and BMI to visceral, subcutaneous, and total body fat: Sex and race differences, *Obesity* 19 (2011): 402–408.
21. C. J. Dobbelsteyn, M. R. Joffres, D. R. MacLean, G. Flowerdew, and Canadian Heart Health Surveys Research Group. A comparative evaluation of waist circumference, waist-to-hip ratio and body mass index

as indicators of cardiovascular risk factors, the Canadian Heart Health Surveys, *International Journal of Obesity* 25 (2001): 652–661.

22. Position of the American Dietetic Association: Weight management, *Journal of the American Dietetic Association* 109 (2009): 330–346.
23. K. M. Flegal and B. I. Graubard, Estimates of excess deaths associated with body mass index and other anthropometric variables, *American Journal of Clinical Nutrition* 89 (2009): 1213–1219; D. M. Freedman and coauthors, Body mass index and all-cause mortality in a nationwide U.S. cohort, *International Journal of Obesity* 30 (2006): 822–829.
24. G. Whitlock and coauthors, Body-mass index and cause-specific mortality in 900000 adults: Collaborative analyses of 57 prospective studies, *Lancet* 373 (2009): 1083–1096; T. Pischon and coauthors, General and abdominal adiposity and risk of death in Europe, *New England Journal of Medicine* 359 (2008): 2105–2120.
25. K. M. Flegal and coauthors, Cause-specific excess deaths associated with underweight, overweight, and obesity, *Journal of the American Medical Association* 298 (2007): 2028–2037; C. L. Ogden and coauthors, The epidemiology of obesity, *Gastroenterology* 132 (2007): 2087–2102; G. M. Price and coauthors, Weight, shape, and mortality risk in older persons: Elevated waist-hip ratio, not high body mass index, is associated with a greater risk of death, *American Journal of Clinical Nutrition* 84 (2006): 449–460; K. M. Flegal and coauthors, Excess deaths associated with underweight, overweight, and obesity, *Journal of the American Medical Association* 293 (2005): 1861–1867; D. L. McGee, Body mass index and mortality: A meta-analysis based on person-level data from twenty-six observational studies, *Annals of Epidemiology* 15 (2005): 87–97.
26. Price and coauthors, 2006.
27. D. E. Alley and V. W. Chang, The changing relationship of obesity and disability, 1988–2004, *Journal of the American Medical Association* 298 (2007): 2020–2027.
28. R. P. Gelber and coauthors, Body mass index and mortality in men: Evaluating the shape of the association, *International Journal of Obesity* 31 (2007): 1240–1247.
29. A. Romero-Corral and coauthors, Association of bodyweight with total mortality and with cardiovascular events in coronary artery disease: A systematic review of cohort studies, *The Lancet* 368 (2006): 666–678; Flegal and coauthors, 2005.
30. Huxley and coauthors, 2008.
31. A. Scheinkiewitz and coauthors, Body mass index history and risk of type 2 diabetes: Results from the European Prospective Investigation into Cancer and Nutrition (EPIC)—Potsdam Study, *American Journal of Clinical Nutrition* 84 (2006): 427–433.
32. E. H. Livingston, Lower body subcutaneous fat accumulation and diabetes mellitus risk, *Surgery for Obesity and Related Diseases* 2 (2006): 362–368.
33. G. M. Reaven, The insulin resistance syndrome: Definition and dietary approaches to treatment, *Annual Review of Nutrition* 25 (2005): 391–406.
34. A. W. Fogarty and coauthors, A prospective study of weight change and systemic inflammation over 9 y, *American Journal of Clinical Nutrition* 87 (2008): 30–35; R. DeCaterina and coauthors, Nutritional mechanisms that influence cardiovascular disease, *American Journal of Clinical Nutrition* 83 (2006): 421S–426S.
35. E. N. Hansen, A. Torquati, and N. N. Abumrad, Results of bariatric surgery, *Annual Review of Nutrition* 26 (2006): 481–511.
36. S. L. Gray and A. J. Vidal-Puig, Adipose tissue expandability in the maintenance of metabolic homeostasis, *Nutrition Reviews* 65 (2007): S7–S12; C. S. Fox and coauthors, Abdominal visceral and subcutaneous adipose tissue compartments: Association with metabolic risk factors in the Framingham Heart Study, *Circulation* 116 (2007): 39–48; A. Pradhan, Obesity, metabolic syndrome, and type 2 diabetes: Inflammatory basis of glucose metabolic disorders, *Nutrition Reviews* 65 (2007): S152–S156; A. Tchernof, Visceral adipocytes and the metabolic syndrome, *Nutrition Reviews* 65 (2007): S24–S29; J. P. Despres, Is visceral obesity the cause of the metabolic syndrome, *Annals of Medicine* 38 (2006): 52–63.
37. P. Trayhurn, C. Bing, and I. S. Wood, Adipose tissue and adipokines—Energy regulation from the human perspective, *Journal of Nutrition* 136 (2006): 1935S–1939S.
38. A. H. Berg and P. E. Scherer, Adipose tissue, inflammation, and cardiovascular disease, *Circulation Research* 96 (2005): 939–968.
39. G. Boden, Fatty acid-induced inflammation and insulin resistance in skeletal muscle and liver, *Current Diabetes Reports* 6 (2006): 177–181.
40. P. Calabro and E. T. Yeh, Intra-abdominal adiposity, inflammation, and cardiovascular risk: New insight into global cardiometabolic risk, *Current Hypertension Reports* 10 (2008): 32–38; V. Z. Rocha and P. Libby, The multiple facets of the fat tissue, *Thyroid* 18 (2008): 175–183; D. C. W. Lau and coauthors, Adipokines: Molecular links between obesity and atherosclerosis, *American Journal of Physiology—Heart and Circulatory Physiology* 288 (2005): H2031–H2041.
41. A. Sbarbati and coauthors, Obesity and inflammation: Evidence for an elementary lesion, *Pediatrics* 117 (2006): 220–223; J. Warnberg and coauthors, Inflammatory proteins are related to total and abdominal adiposity in a healthy adolescent population: The AVENA Study, *American Journal of Clinical Nutrition* 84 (2006): 505–512.
42. J. P. Bastard and coauthors, Recent advances in the relationship between obesity, inflammation, and insulin resistance, *European Cytokine Network* 17 (2006): 4–12.
43. T. A. Lakka and D. E. Laaksonen, Physical activity in prevention and treatment of the metabolic syndrome, *Applied Physiology, Nutrition, and Metabolism* 32 (2007): 76–88; X. Sui and coauthors, Cardiorespiratory fitness and adiposity as mortality predictors in older adults, *Journal of the American Medical Association* 298 (2007): 2507–2516; R. D. Telford, Low physical activity and obesity: Causes of chronic disease or simply predictors? *Medicine & Science in Sports & Exercise* 39 (2007): 1233–1240.
44. R. P. Wildman and coauthors, The obese without cardiometabolic risk factor clustering and the normal weight with cardiometabolic risk factor clustering, *Archives of Internal Medicine* 168 (2008): 1617–1624.
45. C. Mason and coauthors, Musculoskeletal fitness and weight gain in Canada, *Medicine & Science in Sports & Exercise* 39 (2007): 38–43; P. T. Williams, Maintaining vigorous activity attenuates 7-yr weight gain in 8340 runners, *Medicine & Science in Sports & Exercise* 39 (2007): 801–809.

HIGHLIGHT 8

Eating Disorders

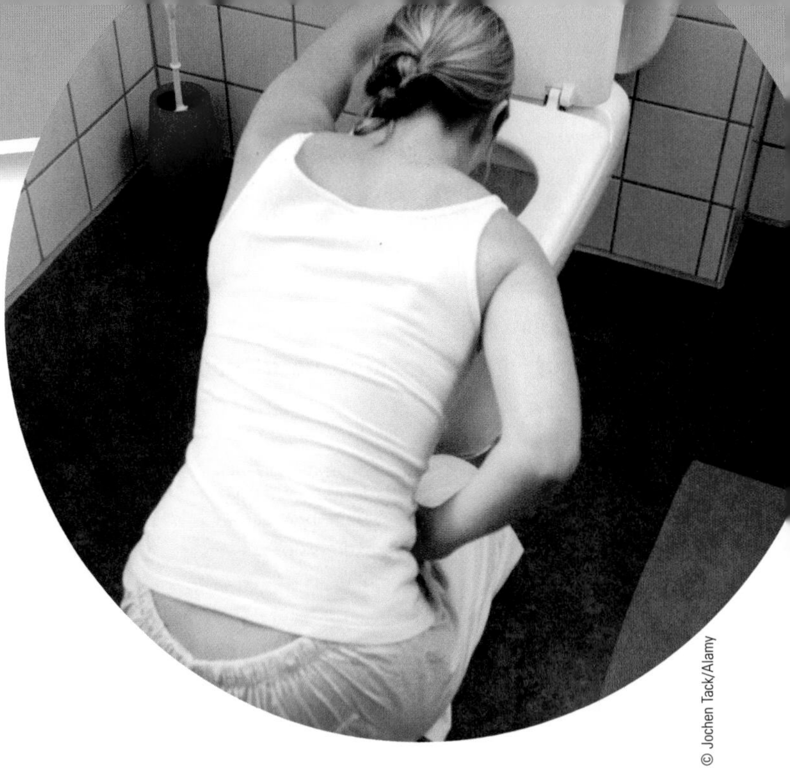

© Jochen Tack/Alamy

For some people, the struggle with body weight manifests itself as an **eating disorder.** (The accompanying glossary defines this and related terms.) Three eating disorders—anorexia nervosa, bulimia nervosa, and binge eating disorder—are relatively uncommon, but present real concerns because of their health consequences. It is estimated that 0.5 to 4 percent of women will suffer from anorexia nervosa at some time in their lives.[1] Prevalence of bulimia nervosa is slightly higher, with 1 to 4 percent of women affected. Binge eating disorder is found in about 2 percent of women. Many more suffer from other unspecified conditions that, even though they do not meet the strict criteria for an eating disorder, imperil a person's well-being.

Why do so many people in our society suffer from eating disorders? Most experts agree that the causes include multiple factors: sociocultural, psychological, and perhaps neurochemical. Excessive pressure to be thin is at least partly to blame. Comments and criticisms about body weight and shape from family and friends can have lasting effects.[2] Young people may have learned to identify discomforts such as anger, jealousy, or disappointment with "feeling fat." They often have other psychological issues such as depression, anxiety, or substance abuse. As weight issues become more of a focus, psychological problems worsen, and the likelihood of developing eating disorders intensifies. Unfortunately, few seek health care for eating disorders.[3] Athletes are among those most likely to develop eating disorders.

The Female Athlete Triad

At age 14, Suzanne was a top contender for a spot on the provincial gymnastics team. Each day her coach reminded team members that they must weigh no more than their assigned weights to qualify for competition. The coach chastized gymnasts who gained weight, and Suzanne was terrified of being singled out. Convinced that the less she weighed the better she would perform, Suzanne weighed herself several times a day to confirm that she had not exceeded her 36 kilogram limit. Driven to excel in her sport, Suzanne kept her weight down by eating very little and training very hard. Unlike many of her friends, Suzanne never began to menstruate. A few months before her fifteenth birthday, Suzanne's coach dropped her back to the second-level team. Suzanne blamed her poor performance on a slow-healing stress fracture. Mentally stressed and physically exhausted, she quit gymnastics and began overeating between periods of self-starvation. Suzanne had developed the dangerous combination of problems that characterize the **female athlete triad**—disordered eating, amenorrhea, and osteoporosis (see Figure H8-1 on p. 262).[4]

Disordered Eating

Part of the reason many athletes engage in **disordered eating** behaviours may be that they and their coaches have embraced unsuitable weight standards. An athlete's body must be heavier for a given height than a nonathlete's body because the athlete's body is dense, containing more healthy bone and muscle and less fat. When athletes rely only on the scales, they may mistakenly believe

GLOSSARY

amenorrhea (ay-MEN-oh-REE-ah): the absence of or cessation of menstruation. *Primary amenorrhea* is menarche delayed beyond 16 years of age. *Secondary amenorrhea* is the absence of three to six consecutive menstrual cycles.

anorexia (an-oh-RECK-see-ah) **nervosa:** an eating disorder characterized by a refusal to maintain a minimally normal body weight and a distortion in perception of body shape and weight.

- **an** = without
- **orex** = mouth
- **nervos** = of nervous origin

binge-eating disorder: an eating disorder with criteria similar to those of bulimia nervosa, excluding purging or other compensatory behaviours.

bulimia (byoo-LEEM-ee-ah) **nervosa:** an eating disorder characterized by repeated episodes of binge eating usually followed by self-induced vomiting, misuse of laxatives or diuretics, fasting, or excessive exercise.

- **buli** = ox

cathartic (ka-THAR-tik): a strong laxative.

disordered eating: eating behaviours that are neither normal nor healthy, including restrained eating, fasting, binge eating, and purging.

eating disorders: disturbances in eating behaviour that jeopardize a person's physical or psychological health.

emetic (em-ETT-ic): an agent that causes vomiting.

female athlete triad: a potentially fatal combination of three medical problems—disordered eating, amenorrhea, and osteoporosis.

muscle dysmorphia (dis-MORE-fee-ah): a psychiatric disorder characterized by a preoccupation with building body mass.

stress fractures: bone damage or breaks caused by stress on bone surfaces during exercise.

unspecified eating disorders: eating disorders that do not meet the defined criteria for specific eating disorders.

FIGURE H8-1 The Female Athlete Triad

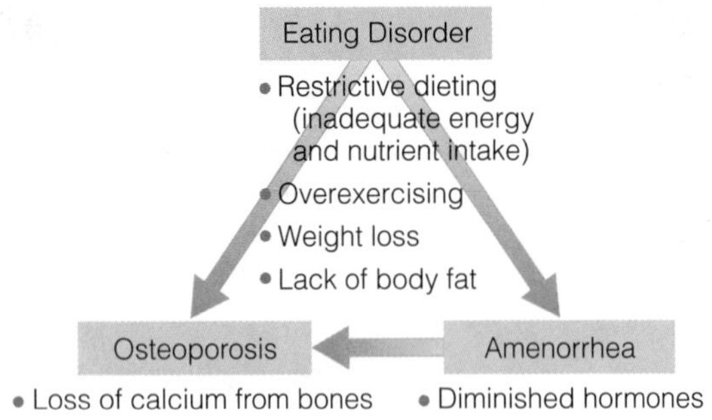
Eating Disorder
• Restrictive dieting (inadequate energy and nutrient intake)
• Overexercising
• Weight loss
• Lack of body fat
Osteoporosis
• Loss of calcium from bones
Amenorrhea
• Diminished hormones

they are too fat because weight standards, such as the BMI, do not provide adequate information about body composition.

Many young athletes severely restrict energy intakes to improve performance, enhance the aesthetic appeal of their performance, or meet the weight guidelines of their specific sports. They fail to realize that the loss of lean tissue that accompanies energy restriction actually impairs their physical performance. The increasing incidence of abnormal eating habits among athletes is cause for concern. Male athletes, especially wrestlers and gymnasts, are affected by these disorders as well, but females are most vulnerable. Risk factors for eating disorders among athletes include:

- Young age (adolescence)
- Pressure to excel at a chosen sport
- Focus on achieving or maintaining an "ideal" body weight or body fat percentage

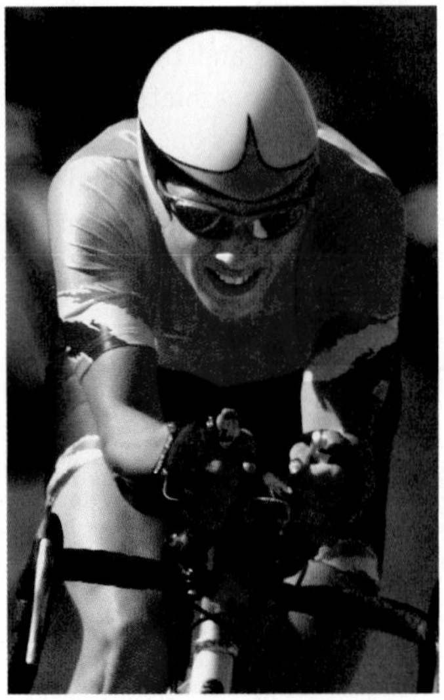

© Reuters NewMedia/Corbis

A few years ago, this Olympic gold medalist was weak and malnourished from anorexia nervosa. However, she recovered and set a world record in the cycling road race.

- Participation in sports or competitions that emphasize a lean appearance or judge performance on aesthetic appeal such as gymnastics, wrestling, figure skating, or dance[5]
- Weight-loss dieting at an early age
- Unsupervised dieting

Amenorrhea

The prevalence of **amenorrhea** among premenopausal women is about 2 to 5 percent overall, but among female athletes, it may be much higher. Contrary to previous notions, amenorrhea is *not* a normal adaptation to strenuous physical training: it is a symptom of something going wrong. Amenorrhea is characterized by low blood estrogen, infertility, and often bone mineral losses. Excessive training, depleted body fat, low body weight, and inadequate nutrition all contribute to amenorrhea. However amenorrhea evelops, it threatens the integrity of the bones. Bone losses remain significant even after recovery. (Women with bulimia frequently have menstrual irregularities, but because they rarely cease menstruating, they may be spared this loss of bone integrity.)

Osteoporosis

For most people, weight-bearing physical activity, dietary calcium, and (for women) the hormone estrogen protect against the bone loss of osteoporosis. For young women with disordered eating and amenorrhea, strenuous activity can impair bone health.[6] Vigorous training combined with inadequate food intake disrupts metabolic and hormonal balances. These disturbances compromise bone health, greatly increasing the risks of **stress fractures.**[7] Stress fractures, a serious form of bone injury, commonly occur among dancers and other competitive athletes with amenorrhea, low calcium intakes, and disordered eating. Many underweight young athletes have bones like those of postmenopausal women, and they may never recover their lost bone even after diagnosis and treatment—which makes prevention critical. Young athletes should be encouraged to consume 1300 milligrams of calcium each day, to eat nutrient-dense foods, and to obtain enough energy to support both weight gain and the energy expended in physical activity. Nutrition is critical to bone recovery.[8]

Other Dangerous Practices of Athletes

Only females face the threats of the female athlete triad, of course, but many male athletes face pressure to achieve a certain body weight and may develop eating disorders.[9] Each week throughout the season, David drastically restricts his food and fluid intake before a wrestling match in an effort to "make weight." Wrestlers and their coaches believe that competing in a lower weight class will give them a competitive advantage over smaller opponents. To that end, David practises in rubber suits, sits in saunas, and takes diuretics and laxatives to lose 2 to 3 kilograms (4 to 6 pounds). He hopes to replenish the lost fluids, glycogen, and lean tissue during the hours between his weigh-in and competition, but the body needs days to correct this metabolic mayhem. Reestablishing fluid and electrolyte balances may take a day or two, replenishing glycogen stores may take two to three days, and replacing lean tissue may take even longer.

Ironically, the combination of food deprivation and dehydration impairs physical performance by reducing muscle strength, decreasing anaerobic power, and reducing endurance capacity. For optimal performance, wrestlers need to first achieve their competitive weight during the off-season and then eat well-balanced meals and drink plenty of fluids during the competitive season.

Some athletes, usually males, go to extreme measures to bulk up and *gain* weight. People afflicted with **muscle dysmorphia** eat high-protein diets, take dietary supplements, weight train for hours at a time, and often abuse steroids in an attempt to increase muscle mass. Their bodies are large and muscular, yet they see themselves as puny 40 kilogram weaklings. They are preoccupied with the idea that their bodies are too small or inadequately muscular. Like others with distorted body images, people with muscle dysmorphia weigh themselves frequently and centre their lives on diet and exercise. Paying attention to diet and pumping iron for fitness is admirable, but obsessing over it can cause serious social, occupational, and physical problems.

Preventing Eating Disorders in Athletes

To prevent eating disorders in athletes and dancers, the performers, their coaches, and their parents must learn about inappropriate body weight ideals, improper weight-loss techniques, eating disorder development, proper nutrition, and safe weight-control methods. Young people naturally search for identity and will often follow the advice of a person in authority without question. Therefore, coaches and dance instructors should never encourage unhealthy weight loss to qualify for competition or to conform to distorted artistic ideals. Athletes who truly need to lose weight should try to do so during the off-season and under the supervision of a health-care professional. Frequent weigh-ins can push young people who are striving to lose weight into a cycle of starving to confront the scale, then bingeing uncontrollably afterward. The erosion of self-esteem that accompanies these events can interfere with normal psychological development and set the stage for serious problems later on.

Table H8-1 includes suggestions to help athletes and dancers protect themselves against developing eating disorders. The remaining sections describe eating disorders that anyone, athlete or nonathlete, may experience.

Anorexia Nervosa

Julie, 18 years old, is a superachiever in school. She watches her diet with great care, and she exercises daily, maintaining a rigorous schedule of self-discipline. She is thin, but she is determined to lose more weight. She is 1.68 metres tall and weighs 39 kilograms (roughly 5 feet 6 inches and 85 pounds). She has **anorexia nervosa.**

Characteristics of Anorexia Nervosa

Julie is unaware that she is undernourished, and she sees no need to obtain treatment. She developed amenorrhea several months ago and has become moody and chronically depressed. She views normal healthy body weight as too fat and insists that she needs to lose weight, although her eyes are sunk in deep hollows in her face. Julie denies that she is ever tired, although she is close to physical exhaustion and no longer sleeps easily. Her family is concerned, and though reluctant to push her, they have finally insisted that she see a psychiatrist. Julie's psychiatrist has diagnosed anorexia nervosa (see Table H8-2 on p. 264) and prescribed group therapy as a start. If she does not begin to gain weight soon, she may need to be hospitalized.

Central to the diagnosis of anorexia nervosa is a distorted body image that overestimates personal body fatness. When Julie looks at herself in the mirror, she sees a "fat" 39 kilogram body. The more Julie overestimates her body size, the more resistant she is to treatment, and the more unwilling to examine her faulty values and misconceptions. In fact, she finds value in her condition.[10] Malnutrition is known to affect brain functioning and judgment in this way, causing lethargy, confusion, and delirium.

Anorexia nervosa cannot be self-diagnosed. Many people in our society are engaged in the pursuit of thinness, and denial runs high among people with anorexia nervosa. Some women have all the attitudes and behaviours associated with the condition, but without the dramatic weight loss.

How can a person as thin as Julie continue to starve herself? Julie uses tremendous discipline against her hunger to strictly limit her portions of low-fat, high-fibre, low-kcalorie foods.[11] She

TABLE H8-1 Tips for Combating Eating Disorders

General Guidelines
• Never restrict food amounts to below those suggested for adequacy by *Canada's Food Guide* (see Table 2-2 on p. 39). • Eat frequently. Include healthy snacks between meals. The person who eats frequently never gets so hungry as to allow hunger to dictate food choices. • If not at a healthy weight, establish a reasonable weight goal based on a healthy body composition. • Allow a reasonable time to achieve the goal. A reasonable loss of excess fat can be achieved at the rate of about 10 percent of body weight in six months. • Establish a weight-maintenance support group with people who share interests.
Specific Guidelines for Athletes and Dancers
• Replace weight-based goals with performance-based goals. • Restrict weight-loss activities to the off-season. • Remember that eating disorders impair physical performance. Seek confidential help in obtaining treatment if needed. • Focus on proper nutrition as an important facet of your training, as important as proper technique.

TABLE H8-2 Criteria for Diagnosis of Anorexia Nervosa

A person with anorexia nervosa demonstrates the following:

A. Refusal to maintain body weight at or above a minimal normal weight for age and height (e.g., weight loss leading to maintenance of body weight less than 85 percent of that expected; or failure to make expected weight gain during period of growth, leading to body weight less than 85 percent of that expected).

B. Intense fear of gaining weight or becoming fat, even though underweight.

C. Disturbance in the way in which one's body weight or shape is experienced, undue influence of body weight or shape on self-evaluation, or denial of the seriousness of the current low body weight.

D. In females past puberty, amenorrhea—the absence of at least three consecutive menstrual cycles. (A woman is considered to have amenorrhea if her periods occur only following hormone, e.g., estrogen, administration.)

Two types:

- *Restricting type:* During the episode of anorexia nervosa, the person does not regularly engage in binge eating or purging behaviour (i.e., self-induced vomiting or the misuse of laxatives, diuretics, or enemas).
- *Binge eating/purging type:* During the episode of anorexia nervosa, the person regularly engages in binge eating or purging behaviour (i.e., self-induced vomiting or the misuse of laxatives, diuretics, or enemas).

SOURCE: Reprinted with permission from the Diagnostic and Statistical Manual of Mental Disorders, Fourth Edition, Text Revision, (Copyright © 2000). American Psychiatric Association.

will deny her hunger, and having adapted to so little food, she feels full after eating only a half-dozen carrot sticks. She knows the kcalorie intake of various foods and the kcalorie expenditure of different exercises. If she feels that she has gained only grams of weight, she runs or jumps rope until she is sure she has exercised it off. If she fears that the food she has eaten outweighs the exercise, she may take laxatives to hasten the passage of food from her system. She drinks water incessantly to fill her stomach, risking dangerous mineral imbalances. She is desperately hungry. In fact, she is starving, but she doesn't eat because her need for self-control dominates.

Many people, on learning of this disorder, say they wish they had "a touch" of it to get thin. They mistakenly think that people with anorexia nervosa feel no hunger. They also fail to recognize the pain of the associated psychological and physical trauma.

The starvation of anorexia nervosa damages the body just as the starvation of war and poverty does. In fact, after a few months, most people with anorexia nervosa have protein-energy malnutrition (PEM) that is similar to marasmus (described in Chapter 6). Their bodies have been depleted of both body fat and protein. Victims are dying to be thin—quite literally. In young people, growth ceases and normal development falters. They lose so much lean tissue that basal metabolic rate slows. In addition, the heart pumps inefficiently and irregularly, the heart muscle becomes weak and thin, the chambers diminish in size, and the blood pressure falls. Minerals that help to regulate heartbeat become unbalanced. Many deaths occur due to multiple organ system failure when the heart, kidneys, and liver cease to function.

Starvation brings other physical consequences as well, such as loss of brain tissue, impaired immune response, anemia, and a loss of digestive functions that worsens malnutrition. Peristalsis becomes sluggish, the stomach empties slowly, and the lining of the intestinal tract atrophies. The pancreas slows its production of digestive enzymes. The deteriorated GI tract fails to provide sufficient digestive enzymes and absorptive surfaces for handling any food that is eaten. The person may suffer from diarrhea, further worsening malnutrition.

Other effects of starvation include altered blood lipids, high blood vitamin A and vitamin E, low blood proteins, dry thin skin, abnormal nerve functioning, reduced bone density, low body temperature, low blood pressure, and the development of fine body hair (the body's attempt to keep warm). The electrical activity of the brain becomes abnormal, and insomnia is common. Both women and men lose their sex drives.

Women with anorexia nervosa develop amenorrhea. (It is one of the diagnostic criteria.) In young girls, the onset of menstruation is delayed. Menstrual periods typically resume with recovery, although some women never restart even after they have gained weight. Should an underweight woman with anorexia nervosa become pregnant, she is likely to give birth to an underweight baby—and low-birthweight babies face many health problems (as Chapter 16 explains). Mothers with anorexia nervosa may underfeed their children, who then fail to grow and may also suffer the other consequences of starvation.

Treatment of Anorexia Nervosa

Treatment of anorexia nervosa requires a multidisciplinary approach.[12] Teams of physicians, nurses, psychiatrists, family therapists, and dietitians work together to resolve two sets of issues and behaviours: those relating to food and weight and those involving relationships with oneself and others. The first dietary objective is to stop weight loss while establishing regular eating patterns. Appropriate diet is crucial to recovery and must be tailored to each individual's needs. Because body weight is low and fear of weight gain is high, initial food intake may be small—perhaps only 1200 kcalories per day.[13] A variety of foods and foods with a higher energy density help to ensure greater success.[14] As eating becomes more comfortable, clients should gradually increase energy intake. Initially, clients may be unwilling to eat for themselves. Those who do eat will have a good chance of recovering without additional interventions. Even after recovery, however, energy intakes and eating behaviours may not fully return to normal.[15] Furthermore, weight gains may be slow because energy needs may be slightly elevated due to anxiety, abdominal pain, and cigarette smoking.

Because anorexia nervosa is like starvation physically, health-care professionals classify clients based on indicators of PEM.* Low-risk clients need nutrition counselling. Intermediate-risk

*Indicators of protein-energy malnutrition: a low percentage of body fat, low serum albumin, low serum transferrin, and impaired immune reactions.

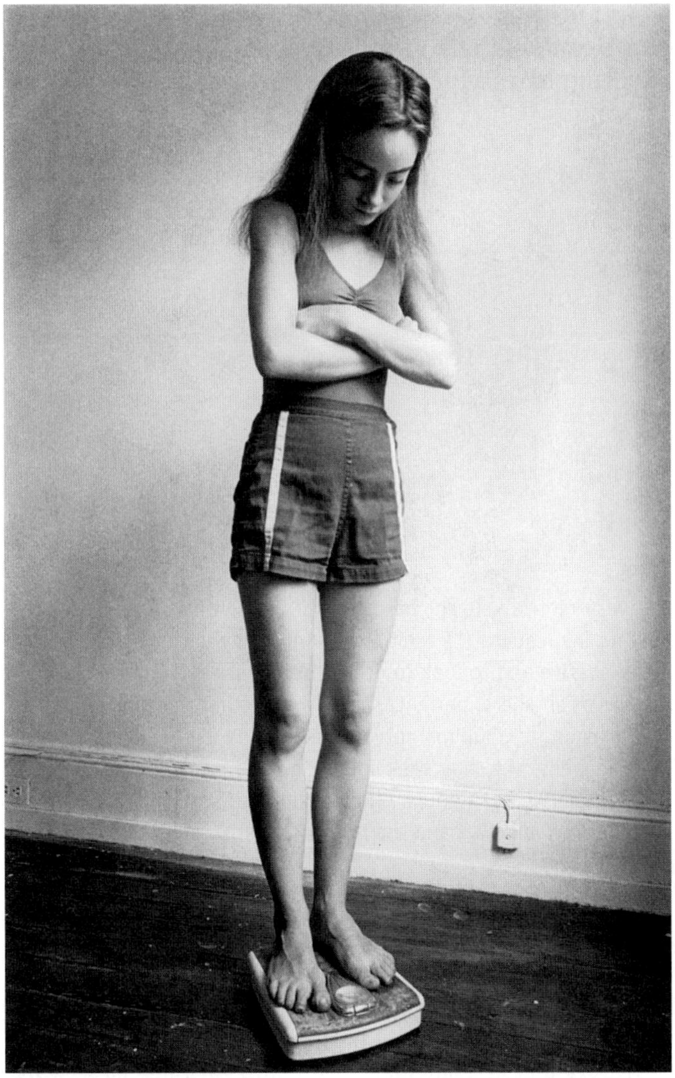

Susan Rosenberg/Photo Researchers, Inc

People with anorexia nervosa see themselves as fat, even when they are dangerously underweight.

clients may need supplements such as high-kcalorie, high-protein formulas in addition to regular meals. High-risk clients may require hospitalization and may need to be fed by tube at first to prevent death.[16] This step may cause psychological trauma. Although drugs are commonly prescribed, they play a limited role in treatment.

Denial runs high among those with anorexia nervosa. Few seek treatment on their own. About half of the women who are treated can maintain their body weight at 85 percent or more of a healthy weight, and at that weight, many of them may begin menstruating again. The other half have poor to fair treatment outcomes, relapse into abnormal eating behaviours, or die. Anorexia nervosa has one of the highest mortality rates among psychiatric disorders—most commonly from cardiac complications or by suicide.[17]

Before drawing conclusions about someone who is extremely thin or who eats very little, remember that diagnosis requires professional assessment. Several national organizations offer information for people who are seeking help with anorexia nervosa, either for themselves or for others.*

*Internet sites are listed at the end of this highlight.

Bulimia Nervosa

Kelly is a charming, intelligent, 30-year-old flight attendant of normal weight who thinks constantly about food. She alternates between starving herself and secretly bingeing, and when she has eaten too much, she makes herself vomit. Most readers recognize these symptoms as those of **bulimia nervosa.**

Characteristics of Bulimia Nervosa

Bulimia nervosa is distinct from anorexia nervosa and is more prevalent, although the true incidence is difficult to establish because bulimia nervosa is not as physically apparent. More men suffer from bulimia nervosa than from anorexia nervosa, but bulimia nervosa is still more common in women than in men. The secretive nature of bulimic behaviours makes recognition of the problem difficult, but once it is recognized, diagnosis is based on the criteria listed in Table H8-3.

Like the typical person with bulimia nervosa, Kelly is single, female, and white. She is well educated and close to her ideal body weight, although her weight fluctuates over a range of 4 to 5 kilograms (or so) every few weeks. She prefers to weigh less than the weight that her body maintains naturally.

Kelly seldom lets her eating disorder interfere with work or other activities, although a third of all bulimics do. From early childhood, she has been a high achiever and emotionally dependent on her parents. As a young teen, Kelly frequently followed severely

TABLE H8-3 Criteria for Diagnosis of Bulimia Nervosa

A person with bulimia nervosa demonstrates the following:

A. Recurrent episodes of binge eating. An episode of binge eating is characterized by both of the following:
   1. Eating, in a discrete period of time (e.g., within any two-hour period), an amount of food that is definitely larger than most people would eat during a similar period of time and under similar circumstances.
   2. A sense of lack of control over eating during the episode (e.g., a feeling that one cannot stop eating or control what or how much one is eating).

B. Recurrent inappropriate compensatory behaviour to prevent weight gain, such as self-induced vomiting; misuse of laxatives, diuretics, enemas, or other medications; fasting; or excessive exercise.

C. Binge eating and inappropriate compensatory behaviours both occur, on average, at least twice a week for three months.

D. Self-evaluation unduly influenced by body shape and weight.

E. The disturbance does not occur exclusively during episodes of anorexia nervosa.

Two types:

- *Purging type:* The person regularly engages in self-induced vomiting or the misuse of laxatives, diuretics, or enemas.
- *Nonpurging type:* The person uses other inappropriate compensatory behaviours, such as fasting or excessive exercise, but does not regularly engage in self-induced vomiting or the misuse of laxatives, diuretics, or enemas.

SOURCE: Reprinted with permission from the Diagnostic and Statistical Manual of Mental Disorders, Fourth Edition, Text Revision, (Copyright © 2000). American Psychiatric Association.

restricted diets but could never maintain the weight loss. Kelly feels anxious at social events and cannot easily establish close personal relationships. She is usually depressed, is often impulsive, and has low self-esteem. When crisis hits, Kelly responds by replaying events, worrying excessively, and blaming herself but never asking for help—behaviours that interfere with effective coping.

Like the person with anorexia nervosa, the person with bulimia nervosa spends much time thinking about body weight and food. The preoccupation with food manifests itself in secret binge-eating episodes, which usually progress through several emotional stages: anticipation and planning, anxiety, urgency to begin, rapid and uncontrollable consumption of food, relief and relaxation, disappointment, and finally shame or disgust.

A bulimic binge is characterized by a sense of lacking control over eating. During a binge, the person consumes food for its emotional comfort and cannot stop eating or control what or how much is eaten. A typical binge occurs periodically, in secret, usually at night, and lasts an hour or more. Because a binge frequently follows a period of rigid dieting, eating is accelerated by intense hunger. Energy restriction followed by bingeing can set in motion a pattern of weight cycling, which may make weight loss and maintenance more difficult over time.

During a binge, Kelly consumes thousands of kcalories of easy-to-eat, low-fibre, high-fat, and, especially, high-carbohydrate foods. Typically, she chooses cookies, cakes, and ice cream—and she eats the entire bag of cookies, the whole cake, and every last spoonful in a carton of ice cream. After the binge, Kelly pays the price with swollen hands and feet, bloating, fatigue, headache, nausea, and pain.

To purge the food from her body, Kelly may use a **cathartic**—a strong laxative that can injure the lower intestinal tract. Or she may induce vomiting, with or without the use of an **emetic**—a drug intended as first aid for poisoning. These purging behaviours are often accompanied by feelings of shame or guilt. Hence a vicious cycle develops: negative self-perceptions followed by dieting, bingeing, and purging, which in turn lead to negative self-perceptions (see Figure H8-2).

On first glance, purging seems to offer a quick and easy solution to the problems of unwanted kcalories and body weight. Many people perceive such behaviour as neutral or even positive, when, in fact, binge eating and purging have serious physical consequences. Signs of subclinical malnutrition are evident in a compromised immune system. Fluid and mineral imbalances caused by vomiting or diarrhea can lead to abnormal heart rhythms and injury to the kidneys. Urinary tract infections can lead to kidney failure. Vomiting causes irritation and infection of the pharynx, esophagus, and salivary glands; erosion of the teeth; and dental caries. The esophagus may rupture or tear, as may the stomach. Sometimes the eyes become red from pressure during vomiting. The hands may be calloused or cut by the teeth while inducing vomiting. Overuse of emetics depletes potassium concentrations and can lead to death by heart failure.

Unlike Julie, Kelly is aware that her behaviour is abnormal, and she is deeply ashamed of it. She wants to recover, and this makes recovery more likely for her than for Julie, who clings to denial. Feeling inadequate ("I can't even control my eating"), Kelly tends to be passive and to look to others for confirmation of her sense of worth. When she experiences rejection, either in reality or in her imagination, her bulimia nervosa becomes worse. If Kelly's depression deepens, she may seek solace in drug or alcohol abuse or in other addictive behaviours. Clinical depression is common in people with bulimia nervosa, and the rates of substance abuse are high.

FIGURE H8-2 The Vicious Cycle of Restrictive Dieting and Binge Eating

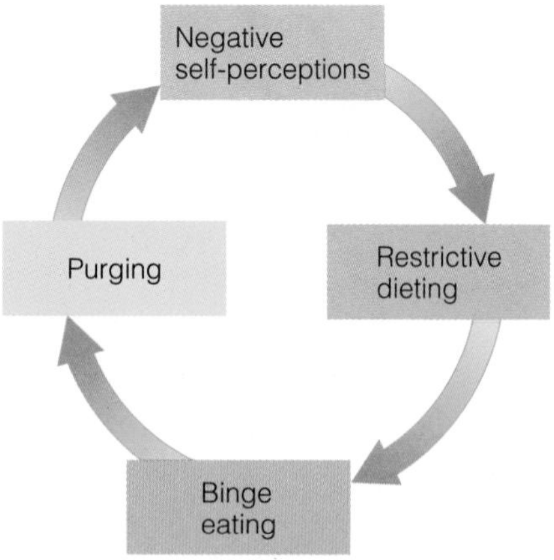
Negative self-perceptions
Restrictive dieting
Binge eating
Purging

Treatment of Bulimia Nervosa

Kelly needs to establish regular eating patterns. She may also benefit from a regular exercise program. Weight maintenance, rather than cyclic weight gains and losses, is the treatment goal. Major steps toward recovery include discontinuing purging and restrictive dieting habits and learning to eat three meals a day plus snacks. Initially, energy intake should provide enough food to satisfy hunger and maintain body weight. Table H8-4 offers diet strategies to correct the eating problems of bulimia nervosa. Most women diagnosed with bulimia nervosa recover within five to ten years, with or without treatment, but treatment probably speeds the recovery process.

A mental health professional should be on the treatment team to help clients with their depression and addictive behaviours. Some physicians prescribe the antidepressant drug fluoxetine in the treatment of bulimia nervosa.* Another drug that may be useful in the management of bulimia nervosa is naloxone, an opiate antagonist that suppresses the consumption of sweet and high-fat foods in binge eaters.

Anorexia nervosa and bulimia nervosa are distinct eating disorders, yet they sometimes overlap in important ways. Anorexia victims may purge, and victims of both disorders may be overly concerned with body weight and have a tendency to drastically undereat. Many perceive foods as "forbidden" and "give in" to an eating binge. The two disorders can also appear in the same

*Fluoxetine is marketed under the trade name Prozac.

TABLE H8-4 Diet Strategies for Combating Bulimia Nervosa

Planning Principles

- Plan meals and snacks; record plans in a food diary prior to eating.
- Plan meals and snacks that require eating at the table and using utensils.
- Refrain from finger foods.
- Refrain from "dieting" or skipping meals.

Nutrition Principles

- Eat a well-balanced diet and regularly timed meals consisting of a variety of foods.
- Include raw vegetables, salad, or raw fruit at meals to prolong eating times.
- Choose whole-grain, high-fibre breads, pasta, rice, and cereals to increase bulk.
- Consume adequate fluid, particularly water.

Other Tips

- Choose foods that provide protein and fat for satiety and bulky, fibre-rich carbohydrates for immediate feelings of fullness.
- Try including soups and other water-rich foods for satiety.
- Choose portions that meet the definition of "a serving" according to *Canada's Food Guide* (pp. 38–42).
- For convenience (and to reduce temptation) select foods that naturally divide into portions. Select one potato, rather than rice or pasta that can be overloaded onto the plate; purchase yogurt and cottage cheese in individual containers; look for small packages of precut steak or chicken; choose frozen dinners with measured portions.
- Engage in moderate physical activity every day—exercise may be an important tool in defeating bulimia.

person, or one can lead to the other. Treatment is challenging and relapses are not unusual. Other people have **unspecified eating disorders** that fall short of the criteria for anorexia nervosa or bulimia nervosa but share some of their features, for example, females who meet all the criteria for anorexia nervosa except that they have regular menstrual cycles or except that they have had recent substantial weight loss but their current body weight is in the normal range. Without a doubt, eating disorders of any type are complex problems that involve biological, psychological, and social causes. Just as research suggests genetic factors may increase risk for eating disorders, the emphasis society places on body thinness may also contribute to increased risk.[18] Another example of unspecified eating disorders is binge-eating disorder.

TABLE H8-5 Unspecified Eating Disorders, Including Binge-Eating Disorder

Criteria for Diagnosis of Unspecified Eating Disorders, in General

Many people have eating disorders but do not meet all the criteria to be classified as having anorexia nervosa or bulimia nervosa. Some examples include those who:

A. Meet all of the criteria for anorexia nervosa, except irregular menses.
B. Meet all of the criteria for anorexia nervosa, except that their current weights fall within the normal ranges.
C. Meet all of the criteria for bulimia nervosa, except that binges occur less frequently than stated in the criteria.
D. Are of normal body weight and who compensate inappropriately for eating small amounts of food (example: self-induced vomiting after eating two cookies).
E. Repeatedly chew food but spit it out without swallowing.
F. Have recurrent episodes of binge eating but do not compensate as do those with bulimia nervosa.

Criteria for Diagnosis of Binge-Eating Disorder, Specifically

A person with a binge-eating disorder demonstrates the following:

A. Recurrent episodes of binge eating. An episode of binge eating is characterized by both of the following:
   1. Eating, in a discrete period of time (e.g., within any two-hour period) an amount of food that is definitely larger than most people would eat in a similar period of time under similar circumstances.
   2. A sense of lack of control over eating during the episode (e.g., a feeling that one cannot stop eating or control what or how much one is eating).
B. Binge-eating episodes are associated with at least three of the following:
   1. Eating much more rapidly than normal.
   2. Eating until feeling uncomfortably full.
   3. Eating large amounts of food when not feeling physically hungry.
   4. Eating alone because of being embarrassed by how much one is eating.
   5. Feeling disgusted with oneself, depressed, or very guilty after overeating.
C. The binge eating causes marked distress.
D. The binge eating occurs, on average, at least twice a week for six months.
E. The binge eating is not associated with the regular use of inappropriate compensatory behaviours (e.g., purging, fasting, excessive exercise) and does not occur exclusively during the course of anorexia nervosa or bulimia nervosa.

SOURCE: Reprinted with permission from the Diagnostic and Statistical Manual of Mental Disorders, Fourth Edition, Text Revision, (Copyright © 2000). American Psychiatric Association.

Binge-Eating Disorder

Charlie is a 40-year-old schoolteacher who has been overweight all his life. His friends and family are forever encouraging him to lose weight, and he has come to believe that if he only had more willpower, dieting would work. He periodically gives dieting his best shot—restricting energy intake for a day or two only to succumb to uncontrollable cravings, especially for high-fat foods. Like Charlie, up to half of the obese people who try to lose weight periodically binge; unlike people with bulimia nervosa, however, they typically do not purge. Such an eating disorder does not meet the criteria for either anorexia nervosa or bulimia nervosa—yet such compulsive overeating is a problem and occurs in people of normal weight as well as those who are severely overweight. Table H8-5 lists criteria for unspecified eating disorders, including binge eating. Obesity alone is not an eating disorder.

Clinicians note differences between people with bulimia nervosa and those with binge-eating disorder. People with **binge-eating disorder** consume less during a binge, rarely purge, and exert less restraint during times of dieting. Similarities also exist, including feeling out of control, disgusted, depressed, embarrassed, guilty, or distressed because of their self-perceived gluttony.

There are also differences between obese binge eaters and obese people who do not binge. Those with the binge-eating disorder report higher rates of self-loathing, disgust about body size, depression, and anxiety. Their eating habits differ as well. Obese binge eaters tend to consume more kcalories and more dessert and snack-type foods during regular meals and binges than obese people who do not binge.

Binge eating is a behavioural disorder that can be resolved with treatment. Even a simple Internet-based treatment program can help.[19] Reducing binge eating makes participation in weight-control programs easier. It also improves physical health, mental health, and the chances of success in breaking the cycle of rapid weight losses and gains.

Eating Disorders in Society

Society plays a central role in eating disorders. Adolescent girls who read magazine articles on dieting and weight loss are likely to engage in unhealthy eating habits.[20] Further proof of society's influence is found in the demographic distribution of eating disorders—they are known only in developed nations, and they become more prevalent as wealth increases and food becomes plentiful. Some people point to the vomitoriums of ancient times and claim that bulimia nervosa is not new, but the two are actually distinct. Ancient people were eating for pleasure, without guilt, and in the company of others; they vomited so that they could rejoin the feast. Bulimia nervosa is a disorder of isolation and is often accompanied by low self-esteem.

Chapter 8 describes how our society sets unrealistic ideals for body weight, especially in women, and devalues those who do not conform to them. Anorexia nervosa and bulimia nervosa are not a form of rebellion against these unreasonable expectations, but rather an exaggerated acceptance of them. In fact, body dissatisfaction is a primary factor in the development of eating disorders. Not everyone who is dissatisfied will develop an eating disorder, but everyone with an eating disorder is dissatisfied.

Characteristics of disordered eating such as restrained eating, fasting, binge eating, purging, fear of fatness, and distortion of body image are extraordinarily common among young girls. Most are "on diets," and many are poorly nourished. Some eat too little food to support normal growth; thus they miss out on their adolescent growth spurts and may never catch up. Many eat so little that hunger propels them into binge-purge cycles.

Perhaps a person's best defence against these disorders is to learn to appreciate his or her own uniqueness. When people discover and honour their body's real physical needs, they become unwilling to sacrifice health for conformity. To respect and value oneself may be lifesaving.

Nutrition on the Net

CENGAGENOW™
For further study of topics covered in this Highlight, log on to **www.cengage.com/sso**.

- Learn more about eating disorders from the National Eating Disorder Information Centre: **www.nedic.ca**
- Find resources and referrals from the National Association of Anorexia Nervosa and Associated Disorders: **www.anad.org**
- Get facts about eating disorders from the U.S. National Institute of Mental Health: **www.nimh.nih.gov/health/topics/eating-disorders/index.shtml**
- The U.S. National Eating Disorders Association offers general and audience-specific information for individuals and families affected by eating disorders: **nationaleatingdisorders.org**
- Take the Eating Attitudes Test to determine if you might need to seek medical advice regarding an eating disorder: **psychcentral.com/quizzes/eat.htm**

Be aware that some websites encourage disordered eating behaviours and may have a negative impact.

References

1. Public Health Association of Canada, A report on mental illnesses in Canada, Ottawa (2002). www.phac-aspc.gc.ca/publicat/miic-mmac/index-eng.php, accessed August 2010.
2. C. B. Taylor and coauthors, The adverse effect of negative comments about weight and shape from family and siblings on women at high risk for eating disorders, *Pediatrics* 118 (2006): 731–738.
3. H. W. Hoek, Incidence, prevalence and mortality of anorexia nervosa and other eating disorders, *Current Opinion in Psychiatry* 19 (2006): 389–394.
4. American College of Sports Medicine, Position stand: The female athlete triad, *Medicine & Science in Sports & Exercise* 39 (2007): 1867–1882; C. M. Lebrun, The female athlete triad: What's a doctor to do? *Current Sports Medicine Reports* 6 (2007): 397–404.
5. M. F. Reinking and L. E. Alexander, Prevalence of disordered-eating behaviors in undergraduate female collegiate athletes and nonathletes, *Journal of Athletic Training* 40 (2005): 47–51; M. K. Torstveit and J. Sundgot-Borgen, The female athlete triad: Are elite athletes at increased risk? *Medicine & Science in Sports & Exercise* 37 (2005): 184–193.
6. M. T. Barrack and coauthors, Dietary restraint and low bone mass in female adolescent endurance runners, *American Journal of Clinical Nutrition* 87 (2008): 36–43.

7. J. L. Kelsey and coauthors, Risk factors for stress fracture among young female cross-country runners, *Medicine and Science in Sports and Exercise* 39 (2007): 1457–1463.
8. J. Dominguez and coauthors, Treatment of anorexia nervosa is associated with increases in bone mineral density, and recovery is a biphasic process involving both nutrition and return of menses, *American Journal of Clinical Nutrition* 86 (2007): 92–99.
9. M. Vertalino and coauthors, Participation in weight-related sports is associated with higher use of unhealthful weight-control behaviors and steroid use, *Journal of the American Dietetic Association* 107 (2007): 434–440.
10. R. H. S. Nordbø and coauthors, The meaning of self-starvation: Qualitative study of patients' perception of anorexia nervosa, *International Journal of Eating Disorders* 39 (2006): 556–564.
11. M. Misra and coauthors, Nutrient intake in community-dwelling adolescent girls with anorexia nervosa and in healthy adolescents, *American Journal of Clinical Nutrition* 84 (2006): 698–706.
12. Position of the American Dietetic Association: Nutrition intervention in the treatment of anorexia nervosa, bulimia nervosa, and other eating disorders, *Journal of the American Dietetic Association* 106 (2006): 2073–2082.
13. J. Yager and A. E. Andersen, Anorexia nervosa, *New England Journal of Medicine* 353 (2005): 1481–1488.
14. J. E. Schebendach and coauthors, Dietary energy density and diet variety as predictors of outcome in anorexia nervosa, *American Journal of Clinical Nutrition* 87 (2008): 810–816.
15. R. Sysko and coauthors, Eating behavior among women with anorexia nervosa, *American Journal of Clinical Nutrition* 82 (2005): 296–301.
16. E. Attia and B. T. Walsh, Behavioral management for anorexia nervosa, *New England Journal of Medicine* 360 (2009): 500–506.
17. J. M. Holm-Denoma and coauthors, Deaths by suicide among individuals with anorexia as arbiters between competing explanations of the anorexia-suicide link, *Journal of Affective Disorders* 107 (2008): 231–236; G. Murialdo and coauthors, Alterations in the autonomic control of heart rate variability in patients with anorexia or bulimia nervosa: Correlations between sympathovagal activity, clinical features, and leptin levels, *Journal of Endocrinological Investigation* 30 (2007): 356–362; D. Casiero and W. H. Frishman, Cardiovascular complications of eating disorders, *Cardiology in Review* 14 (2006): 227–231; M. Pompili and coauthors, Suicide and attempted suicide in eating disorders, obesity and weight-image concern, *Eating Behaviors* 7 (2006): 384–394.
18. M. P. Levine and S. K. Murnen, "Everybody knows that mass media are/are not [pick one] a cause of eating disorders": A critical review of evidence for a causal link between media, negative body image, and disordered eating in females, *Journal of Social and Clinical Psychology* 28 (2009): 9–42; J. Yager and A. E. Andersen, Anorexia nervosa, *New England Journal of Medicine* 353 (2005): 1481–1488.
19. M. Jones and coauthors, Randomized, controlled trial of an Internet-facilitated intervention for reducing binge eating and overweight in adolescents, *Pediatrics* 121 (2008): 453–462.
20. P. Van den Berg and coauthors, Is dieting advice from magazines helpful or harmful? Five-year associations with weight-control behaviors and psychological outcomes in adolescents, *Pediatrics* 119 (2007): e30–e37.

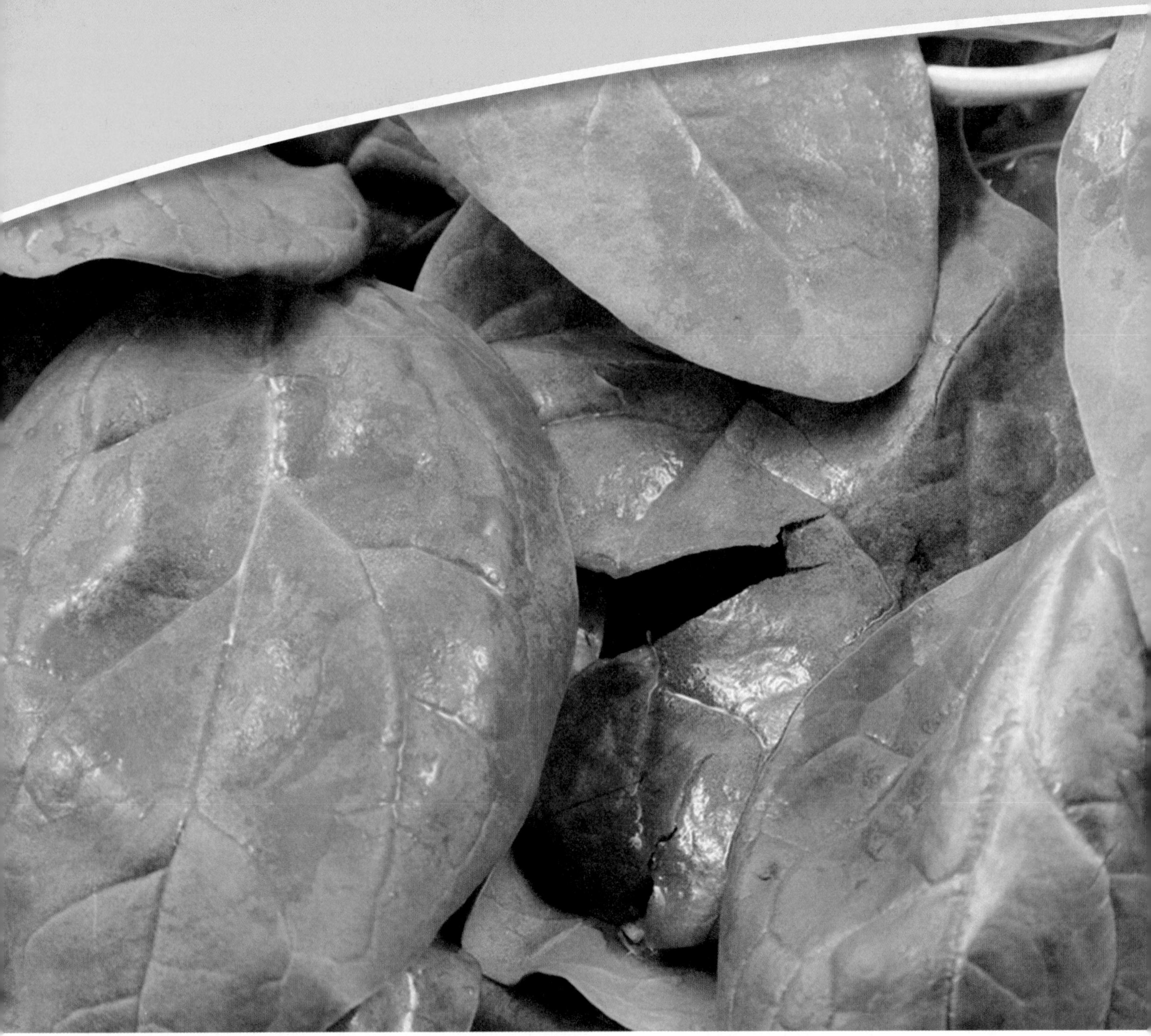

photos.com

Nutrition in Your Life

CENGAGENOW™

Throughout this chapter, the CengageNOW logo indicates an opportunity for online self-study, linking you to interactive tutorials, activities, and videos to increase your understanding of chapter concepts.
www.cengage.com/sso

Are you pleased with your body weight? If so, you are a rare individual. Most people in our society think they should weigh more or less (mostly less) than they do. Usually, their primary concern is appearance, but they often understand that physical health is also somehow related to body weight. One does not necessarily cause the other—that is, an ideal body weight does not ensure good health. Instead, both depend on diet and physical activity. A well-balanced diet and active lifestyle support good health—and help maintain body weight within a reasonable range.

CHAPTER

9

Weight Management: Overweight, Obesity, and Underweight

CHAPTER OUTLINE

The previous chapter described how body weight is stable when energy in equals energy out. Weight gains occur when energy intake exceeds energy expended, and conversely, weight losses occur when energy expended exceeds energy intake. At the extremes, both overweight and underweight present health risks. **Weight management** is a key component of good health.

This chapter emphasizes overweight and obesity, partly because they have been more intensively studied and partly because they represent a major health problem in Canada and a growing concern worldwide. Information on underweight is presented at the end of the chapter. The highlight that follows this chapter examines fad diet plans.

Overweight and Obesity

Despite our preoccupation with body image and weight loss, the prevalence of overweight and obesity in Canada continues to rise dramatically.[1] In the past two decades, obesity increased in many provinces in both genders, and across all ages, races, and educational levels (see Figure 9-1 on p. 272). A majority of Canadian adults—almost 60 percent—are now considered overweight or obese, as defined by a BMI of 25 or greater.[2] ♦ It was estimated that in 2006 the direct costs of obesity and overweight were $6 billion in Canada.[3]

The prevalence of overweight among children in Canada has also risen at an alarming rate. An estimated 26 percent of children and adolescents aged 2 to 17 years are either overweight or obese.[4] Chapter and Highlight 17 present information on overweight during childhood and adolescence.

♦ BMI:
- Underweight: <18.5
- Healthy weight: 18.5–24.9
- Overweight: 25.0–29.9
- Obese:
  Class I: 30.0–34.9
  Class II: 35.0–39.9
  Class III: ≥40.0

weight management: maintaining body weight in a healthy range by preventing gradual weight gain over time and losing weight if overweight.

FIGURE 9-1 Increasing Prevalence of Self-reported Obesity (BMI ≥ 30) among Canadian Adults

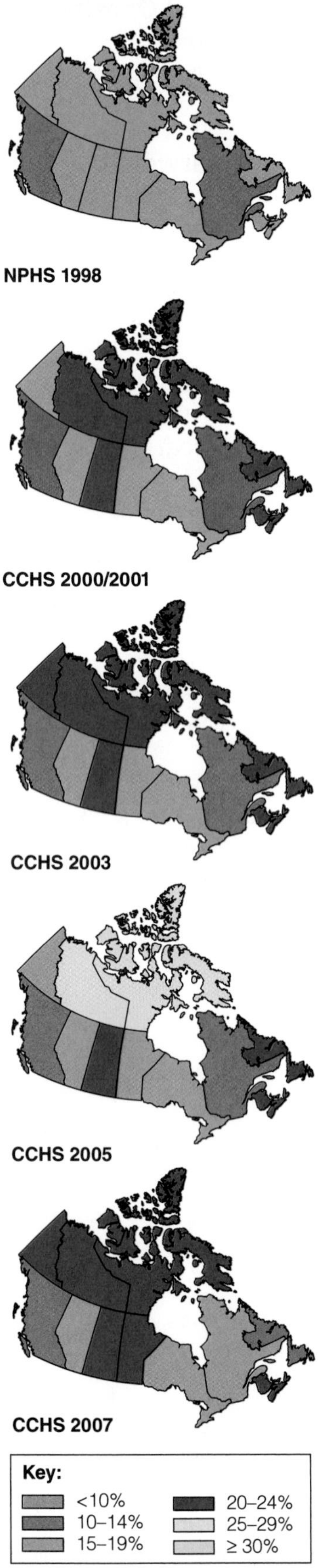
NPHS 1998
CCHS 2000/2001
CCHS 2003
CCHS 2005
CCHS 2007
Key:
<10%
10–14%
15–19%
20–24%
25–29%
≥ 30%

SOURCE: Public Health Agency of Canada, 2010. The Chronic Disease Infobase website (www.infobase.phac-aspc.gc.ca). Retrieved October 30, 2010.

Obesity in Canada is widespread. This **epidemic** of obesity has spread worldwide, affecting more than 300 million adults and 155 million children.[5] Contrary to popular opinion, obesity is not limited to industrialized nations; more than 115 million people in developing countries suffer from obesity-related problems. Before examining the suspected causes of obesity and the various strategies used to treat it, it is helpful to understand the development and metabolism of body fat.

Fat Cell Development

When "energy in" exceeds "energy out," much of the excess energy is stored in the fat cells of adipose tissue. The amount of fat in a person's body reflects both the *number* and the *size* of the fat cells. The number of fat cells increases most rapidly during the growing years of late childhood and early puberty. After growth ceases, fat cell number may continue to increase whenever energy balance is positive. Obese people have more fat cells than healthy-weight people; their fat cells are also larger.

As fat cells accumulate triglycerides, they expand in size (review Figure 5-20 on p. 144). When the cells enlarge, they stimulate cell proliferation so that their numbers increase again. Thus obesity develops ♦ when a person's fat cells increase in number, in size, or quite often both. Figure 9-2 illustrates fat cell development.

When "energy out" exceeds "energy in," the size of fat cells dwindles, but not their number. People with extra fat cells tend to regain lost weight rapidly; with weight gain, their many fat cells readily fill. In contrast, people with an average number of enlarged fat cells may be more successful in maintaining weight losses; when their cells shrink, both cell size and number are normal. Prevention of obesity is most critical, then, during the growing years of childhood and adolescence when fat cells increase in number.[6] Researchers are exploring ways to induce fat cell death—which would decrease the number.[7] ♦

As mentioned, excess fat first fills the body's natural storage site—adipose tissue. Then it becomes necessary to deposit excess fat in organs such as the heart or liver, which plays a key role in the development of diseases such as heart failure or fatty liver.[8] ♦ Metabolic changes such as insulin resistance become apparent, and chronic inflammation develops as adipose tissue produces its adipokines.[9]

Fat Cell Metabolism

The enzyme lipoprotein lipase (LPL) ♦ removes triglycerides from the blood for storage in both adipose tissue and muscle cells. Obese people generally have much more LPL activity in their adipose cells than lean people do (their muscle cell LPL activity is similar, though). This high LPL activity makes fat storage especially efficient. Consequently, even modest excesses in energy intake have a more dramatic impact on obese people than on lean people.

The activity of LPL in different regions of the body is partially influenced by gender.[10] In women, fat cells in the breasts, hips, and thighs produce abundant LPL, putting fat away in those body sites; in men, fat cells in the abdomen produce abundant LPL. This enzyme activity explains why men tend to develop central obesity around the abdomen (apple-shaped) whereas women more readily develop lower-body fat around the hips and thighs (pear-shaped).

Gender differences are also apparent in the activity of the enzymes ♦ controlling the release and breakdown of fat in various parts of the body. The release of lower-body fat is less active in women than in men, whereas the release of upper-body fat is similar. Furthermore, the rate of fat breakdown is lower in women than in men. Consequently, women may have a more difficult time losing fat in general, and from the hips and thighs in particular.

Enzyme activity may also explain why some people who lose weight regain it so easily. After weight loss, adipose LPL activity increases.[11] Apparently, weight loss serves as a signal to the gene that produces the LPL enzyme, saying, "Make more of the enzyme that stores fat." People easily regain weight after having lost it because they are battling against enzymes that want to store fat. Not only is fat storage efficient, but fat oxidation is not. Dietary fat oxidation correlates negatively with body fatness: obese people have the least activity.[12] The activities of these and other proteins provide an explanation for the observation that some inner mechanism seems to set a person's weight or body composition at a fixed point; the body will adjust to restore that **set point** if the person tries to change it.

FIGURE 9-2 Fat Cell Development

Fat cells are capable of increasing their size by 20-fold and their number by several thousandfold.

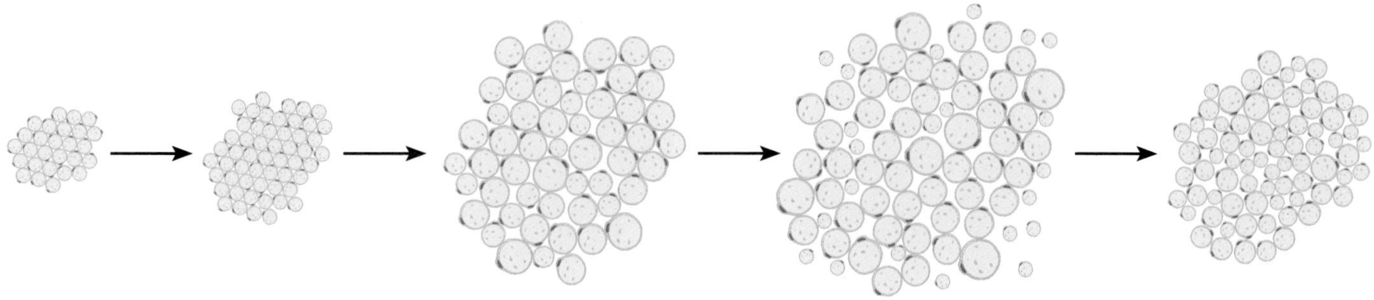
During growth, fat cells increase in number.
When energy intake exceeds expenditure, fat cells increase in size.
When fat cells have enlarged and energy intake continues to exceed energy expenditure, fat cells increase in number again.
With fat loss, the size of the fat cells shrinks but not the number.

Set-Point Theory

Many internal physiological variables, such as blood glucose, blood pH, and body temperature, remain fairly stable under a variety of conditions. The hypothalamus and other regulatory centres constantly monitor and delicately adjust conditions to maintain homeostasis. The stability of such complex systems may depend on set-point regulators that maintain variables within specified limits.

Researchers have confirmed that after weight gains or losses, the body adjusts its metabolism to restore the original weight. Energy expenditure increases after weight gain and decreases after weight loss. These changes in energy expenditure differ from those that would be expected based on body composition alone, and they help to explain why it is so difficult for an underweight person to maintain weight gains and an overweight person to maintain weight losses.[13]

Thrifty Gene Theory

How much energy we need to get through the day is influenced by our ability to use energy efficiently. The thrifty gene theory suggests a different perspective on energy use. The theory proposes that people who use energy sparingly will store fat more readily, putting them at greater risk for weight gain. While having the ability to efficiently store energy would have been important in days gone by when food supplies were unpredictable and scarce, in today's world of food abundance it may be a contributing factor to unwanted weight gain. Recent advances in identifying interactions between obesity-related genes, behaviours, and environmental factors have broadened our understanding of the complex network of factors that affect body weight.[14]

IN SUMMARY **Fat cells develop by increasing in number and size. Prevention of excess weight gain depends on maintaining a reasonable number of fat cells. With weight gains or losses, the body adjusts in an attempt to return to its previous status.**

- Obesity due to an increase in the *number* of fat cells is **hyperplastic obesity.** Obesity due to an increase in the *size* of fat cells is **hypertrophic obesity.**
- Cell death is known as **apoptosis.**
- The adverse effects of fat in nonadipose tissues are known as **lipotoxicity.**
- **Lipoprotein lipase (LPL)** is an enzyme that hydrolyzes triglycerides passing by in the bloodstream and directs their parts into the cells, where they can be metabolized or reassembled for storage.
- Enzymes involved in the breakdown of fat include **hormone-sensitive lipase** and **adipose tissue lipase.**

Causes of Overweight and Obesity

Why do people accumulate excess body fat? The obvious answer is that they take in more food energy than they expend. But that answer falls short of explaining why they do this. Is it genetic? Environmental? Cultural? Behavioural? Socioeconomic? Psychological? Metabolic? All of these? Most likely, obesity has many interrelated causes. Why an imbalance between energy intake and energy expenditure occurs remains a bit of a mystery; the next sections summarize possible explanations.

epidemic (ep-ih-DEM-ick): the appearance of a disease (usually infectious) or condition that attacks many people at the same time in the same region.
- **epi** = upon
- **demos** = people

set point: the point at which controls are set (e.g., on a thermostat). The set-point theory that relates to body weight proposes that the body tends to maintain a certain weight by means of its own internal controls.

♦ Environmental factors include diet and physical activity.

Genetics and Epigenetics Genetics plays a true causative role in relatively few cases of obesity, for example, in Prader-Willi syndrome—a genetic disorder characterized by excessive appetite, massive obesity, short stature, and often mental retardation. Most cases of obesity, however, do not stem from a single gene, yet genetic influences do seem to be involved. Highlight 6 describes epigenetics—the influence of environmental factors ♦ on gene expression. Obesity provides a classic example.[15]

Researchers have found that adopted children tend to be more similar in weight to their biological parents than to their adoptive parents. Studies of twins yield similar findings: compared with fraternal twins, identical twins are twice as likely to weigh the same.[16] These findings suggest an important role for genetics in determining a person's *predisposition* to obesity.[17] In other words, genes interact with the diet and activity patterns that lead to obesity and the metabolic pathways that influence satiety and energy balance.[18] Even identical twins with identical genes become different over the years as epigenetic changes accumulate. This raises an important point: you cannot change the genome you inherit, but you can influence the epigenome. Vigorous exercise, for example, can minimize the genetic influences on BMI.[19]

Clearly, something genetic makes a person more or less likely to gain or lose weight when overeating or undereating.[20] Some people gain more weight than others on comparable energy intakes. Given an extra 1000 kcalories a day for 100 days, some pairs of identical twins gain less than 4.5 kilograms while others gain up to 14 kilograms. Within each pair, the amounts of weight gained, percentages of body fat, and locations of fat deposits are similar. Similarly, some people lose more weight than others following comparable exercise routines.

Researchers have been examining the human genome in search of genetic and epigenetic answers to obesity questions.[21] As the section on protein synthesis in Chapter 6 describes, each cell expresses only the genes for the proteins it needs, and each protein performs a unique function. The following paragraphs describe some recent research involving proteins that might help explain appetite control, energy regulation, and obesity development.

Leptin Researchers have identified an obesity gene, called *ob,* that is expressed primarily in the adipose tissue and codes for the protein **leptin.** Leptin acts as a hormone, primarily in the hypothalamus. Research suggests that leptin from adipose tissue signals sufficient energy stores and promotes a negative energy balance by suppressing appetite and increasing energy expenditure.[22] Changes in energy expenditure primarily reflect changes in basal metabolism but may also include changes in physical activity patterns. Leptin is also released from stomach cells in response to the presence of food, suggesting a role for both short-term and long-term regulation of food intake and energy storage.[23]

Mice with a defective *ob* gene do not produce leptin and can weigh up to three times as much as normal mice and have five times as much body fat (see Figure 9-3). When injected with a synthetic form of leptin, the mice rapidly lose body fat. (Because leptin is a protein, it would be destroyed during digestion if given orally; consequently, it must be given by injection.) The fat cells not only lose fat, but they self-destruct (reducing cell number), which may explain why weight gains are delayed when the mice are fed again.

Although extremely rare, a genetic deficiency of leptin or genetic mutation of its receptor has been identified in human beings as well.[24] Extremely obese children with barely detectable blood levels of leptin have little appetite control; they are constantly hungry and eat considerably more than their siblings or peers. Given daily injections of leptin, these children lose a substantial amount of weight, confirming leptin's role in regulating appetite and body weight.

Not too surprisingly, leptin injections are effective in suppressing appetite and supporting weight loss only when overeating and obesity are the result of a leptin deficiency. Very few obese people have a leptin deficiency, however. In fact, leptin levels increase as BMI increases.[25] Leptin rises but fails to suppress appetite or enhance energy expenditure—a condition researchers describe as leptin

leptin: a protein produced by fat cells under direction of the *ob* gene that decreases appetite and increases energy expenditure.

- **leptos** = thin

FIGURE 9-3 Mice with and without Leptin Compared

Both of these mice have a defective *ob* gene. Consequently, they do not produce leptin. They both became obese, but the one on the right received daily injections of leptin, which suppressed food intake and increased energy expenditure, resulting in weight loss.

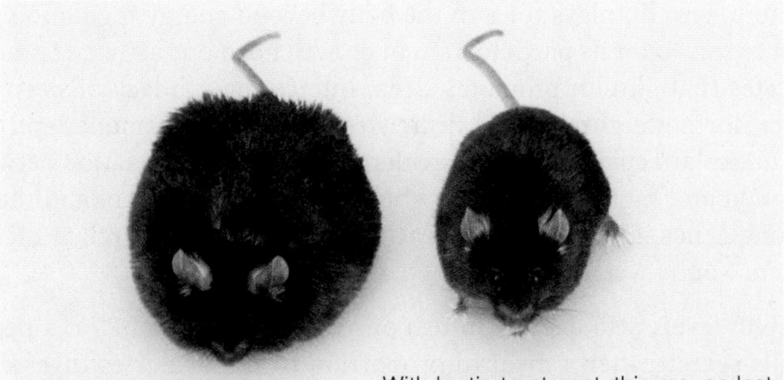

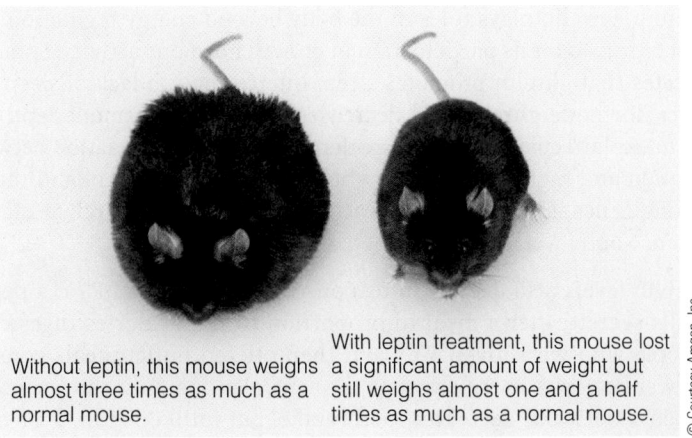

Without leptin, this mouse weighs almost three times as much as a normal mouse.

With leptin treatment, this mouse lost a significant amount of weight but still weighs almost one and a half times as much as a normal mouse.

resistance.[26] Interestingly, excessive fructose consumption seems to induce leptin resistance and accelerate fat storage.[27]

Some researchers have re-examined the evidence on leptin from another point of view—one of undernutrition. Instead of focusing on leptin's role as a satiety signal that might help prevent obesity by diminishing appetite, they view leptin as a starvation hormone that signals energy deficits. When energy intake is low, leptin levels decline, and metabolism slows in an effort to reduce energy demands. Clearly, leptin plays a major role in energy regulation, but additional research is needed to clarify its actions when intake is either excessive or deficient.

In addition to its involvement in energy regulation, leptin plays several other roles in the body. For example, leptin may inform the female reproductive system about body fat reserves; stimulate growth of new blood vessels, especially in the cornea of the eye; enhance the maturation of bone marrow cells; promote formation of red blood cells; and help support a normal immune response. Elevated leptin levels may be partially responsible for the early maturation that commonly occurs in obese children.

Adiponectin In addition to leptin, adipose tissue secretes another protein known as **adiponectin.** Unlike leptin, however, adiponectin correlates inversely with body fat: lean people have higher amounts than obese people—which helps to explain some of the relationships between obesity and diseases.[28] Adiponectin seems to have the beneficial effects of inhibiting inflammation and protecting against insulin resistance, type 2 diabetes, and cardiovascular disease.[29] Researchers are hopeful that if they can find ways to raise adiponectin levels or enhance its activity, they will be able to reduce the disease risks associated with obesity.[30]

Ghrelin Another protein, known as **ghrelin,** also acts as a hormone primarily in the hypothalamus.[31] In contrast to leptin or adiponectin, ghrelin is secreted primarily by the stomach cells and promotes a positive energy balance by stimulating appetite and promoting efficient energy storage.[32] The role ghrelin plays in regulating food intake and body weight is currently the subject of intensive research.[33]

Ghrelin triggers the desire to eat. Blood levels of ghrelin typically rise before and fall after a meal in proportion to the kcalories ingested—reflecting the hunger and satiety that precede and follow eating. In general, fasting blood levels correlate inversely with body weight: lean people have high ghrelin levels and obese people have low levels.[34]

Ghrelin fights to maintain a stable body weight. In fact, some researchers speculate that its role is to maximize fat stores during times of famine.[35] On average,

adiponectin: a protein produced by the fat cells that inhibits inflammation and protects against insulin resistance, type 2 diabetes, and cardiovascular disease.

ghrelin (GRELL-in): a protein produced by the stomach cells that enhances appetite and decreases energy expenditure.

- **ghre** = growth

ghrelin levels are high whenever the body is in negative energy balance, as occurs during low-kcalorie diets, for example. This response may help explain why weight loss is so difficult to maintain. Weight loss is more successful with exercise and after gastric bypass surgery, in part because ghrelin levels are relatively low.[36] Ghrelin levels decline again whenever the body is in positive energy balance, as occurs with weight gains.

Like leptin, ghrelin plays roles in the body beyond energy regulation. In fact, it was first recognized for its participation in growth hormone activity. Some research also indicates that ghrelin promotes sleep. Interestingly, a lack of sleep increases the hunger hormone ghrelin and decreases the satiety hormone leptin—which may help to explain epidemiological evidence finding an association between short sleep duration and high BMI.[37] Researchers are trying to understand the relationships among genes, sleep disorders, eating habits, and other related factors that may influence body weight and weight gain.[38]

PYY Ghrelin levels also decline in response to high levels of PYY, a peptide that the GI cells secrete after a meal in proportion to the kcalories ingested. In one study, people who were given PYY and then offered buffet meals consumed 30 percent fewer kcalories in the day than the control group. Like the hormone leptin, PYY signals satiety and decreases food intake, but unlike leptin, PYY may be an effective treatment for obesity. An ideal diet would maintain the satiating hormones (leptin, PYY, and cholecystokinin) and minimize the appetite-stimulating hormone (ghrelin); fortunately, the diet that seems to do that best is one that is low in fat and rich in fibre.[39]

Table 9-1 summarizes the actions of the proteins just described. It also includes a few more to illustrate the many complex factors involved in the regulation of food intake and energy homeostasis.

Uncoupling Proteins Genes also code for proteins involved in energy metabolism. These proteins may influence the storing or expending of energy with different efficiencies or in different types of fat. The body has two types of fat: white and **brown adipose tissue.**[40] White adipose tissue stores fat for other cells to use for energy; brown adipose tissue releases stored energy as heat. Recall from Chapter 7 that when fat is oxidized, some of the energy is released in heat and some is captured in ATP. In brown adipose tissue, oxidation is uncoupled ♦ from ATP formation, producing heat only.[41] By radiating energy away as heat, the body expends, rather than stores, energy. In contrast, efficient coupling leads to fat storage.[42] In

♦ In **coupled reactions,** the energy released from the breakdown of one compound is used to create a bond in the formation of another compound. In **uncoupled reactions,** the energy is released as heat.

brown adipose tissue: masses of specialized fat cells packed with pigmented mitochondria that produce heat instead of ATP.

TABLE 9-1 Proteins Involved in Regulation of Food Intake and Energy Homeostasis

Protein	Concentration	Secreted from	Action
Adiponectin	Lower in obesity	Adipose tissue	Increases insulin sensitivity
Ghrelin	Increases with fasting Decreases after a meal	Stomach	Stimulates appetite
Leptin	Higher in obesity	Adipose tissue	Suppresses appetite Increases energy expenditure
Oxyntomodulin	Increases after a meal	Central nervous system GI tract	Suppresses appetite
Pancreatic peptide (PP)	Increases after a meal	Pancreas	Suppresses appetite
PYY	Lower in obesity Increases after a meal	Small intestine	Suppresses appetite
Resistin	Higher in obesity	Adipose tissue, bone marrow, and immune system cells	Provides short-term satiety Opposes insulin
Visfatin	Higher in obesity	Adipose tissue (specifically visceral)	Mimics glucose-lowering effects of insulin

SOURCES: Adapted from S. S. Gropper, J. L. Smith, and J. L. Groff, Advanced Nutrition and Human Metabolism, 5th ed. (Belmont, Calif.: Thomson Cengage, 2009) p. 299; M. H. Rokling-Andersen and coauthors, Effects of long-term exercise and diet intervention on plasma adipokine concentrations, American Journal of Clinical Nutrition 86 (2007): 1293–1301; H. Xie and coauthors, Insulin-like effects of visfatin on human osteoblasts, Calcifi ed Tissue International 80 (2007): 201–210; M. E. Shills and coauthors, Modern Nutrition in Health and Disease, 10th ed. (Philadelphia: Lippincott Williams and Wilkins, 2006); S. Tovar and coauthors, Central administration of resistin promotes short-term satiety in rats: A review, European Journal of Endocrinology 153 (2005): R1–R5; J. Berndt and coauthors, Plasma visfatin concentrations and fat depot-specific mRNA expression in humans, Diabetes 54 (2005): 2911–2916.

other words, weight gains or losses may depend on whether the body dissipates the energy from an ice cream sundae as heat or stores it in body fat.

Brown fat and heat production is particularly important in newborns and in animals exposed to cold weather, especially those that hibernate.[43] They have plenty of brown adipose tissue. In contrast, most human adults have little brown fat—less than 1 percent of all fat cells and interspersed among the white fat cells.[44] Brown fat activity is most apparent during exposure to cold.[45] Importantly, brown fat quantity is inversely related with BMI; overweight and obese individuals have less brown fat activity than others.[46] The role of brown fat in body weight regulation is not yet understood, but such an understanding may prove most useful in developing obesity treatments.[47]

Uncoupling proteins are active not only in brown fat, but also in white fat and many other tissues. Their actions seem to influence the basal metabolic rate (BMR) and oppose the development of obesity. Animals with abundant amounts of these uncoupling proteins resist weight gain, whereas those with minimal amounts gain weight easily. Similarly, people with a genetic variant of an uncoupling protein have lower metabolic rates and are more overweight than others.

Environment With obesity rates rising and the **gene pool** remaining relatively unchanged, environment must also play a role in obesity. Obesity reflects the interactions between genes and the environment.[48] The *environment* includes all of the circumstances that we encounter daily that push us toward fatness or thinness. Over the past four decades, the demand for physical activity has decreased as the abundance of food has increased.[49]

Keep in mind that genetic and environmental factors are not mutually exclusive; in fact, their *interactions* create the epigenetics that provide a greater understanding of obesity and related diseases.[50] Genes can influence eating behaviours, for example, and food and activity behaviours influence the genes that regulate body weight. Interestingly, even social relationships can influence the development of obesity.[51] The likelihood that a person will become obese increases when a friend, sibling, or spouse becomes obese.

Overeating One explanation for obesity is that overweight people overeat, although diet histories may not always reflect high intakes. Diet histories are not always accurate records of actual intakes; both normal-weight and obese people commonly misreport their dietary intakes.[52] Most importantly, current dietary intakes may not reflect the eating habits that led to obesity. Obese people who had a positive energy balance for years and accumulated excess body fat may not currently have a positive energy balance. This reality highlights an important point: the energy-balance equation must consider time. Both present *and* past eating and activity patterns influence current body weight.

We live in an environment that exposes us to an abundance of high-kcalorie, high-fat foods that are readily available, relatively inexpensive, heavily advertised, ♦ and reasonably tasty. Food is available everywhere, all the time—thanks largely to fast food. Our highways are lined with fast-food restaurants, and convenience stores and service stations offer fast food as well. Fast food is available in our schools, malls, and airports. It's convenient and it's available morning, noon, and night—and all times in between.

♦ The food industry spends billions of dollars a year on advertising. The message? "Eat more."

Most alarming are the extraordinarily large serving sizes and ready-to-go meals that offer supersize ♦ combinations. People buy the large sizes and combinations, perceiving them to be a good value, but then they eat more than they need—a bad deal. In fact, one U.S. research study calculated that for the 67 cents extra to upsize a meal, consumers receive an extra 400 kcalories, an extra 36 grams of body fat, and an extra $1 to $7 in health-care costs.[53]

♦ "Want fries with that?" A supersize portion delivers more than 600 kcalories.

Large package or portion sizes can increase consumption—even when the food is not particularly appealing. Moviegoers given stale popcorn ate more when eating from a huge container than from a large container (both sizes were greater than anyone could finish).[54] Simply put, large portion sizes deliver more kcalories. And portion sizes of virtually all foods and beverages have increased

gene pool: all the genetic information of a population at a given time.

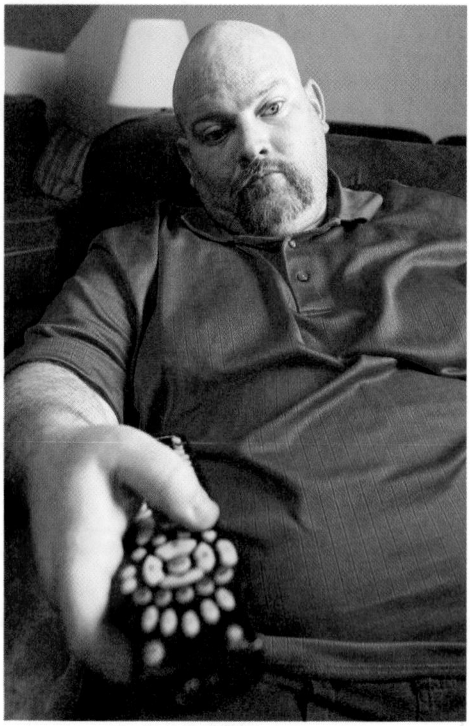
© Terry J Alcorn/iStockphoto LP

Lack of physical activity fosters obesity.

markedly in the past several decades, most notably at fast-food restaurants. Not only have portion sizes increased over time, but they are now two to eight times larger than standard serving sizes. The trend toward large portion sizes parallels the increasing prevalence of overweight and obesity in Canada, beginning in the 1970s, increasing sharply in the 1980s, and continuing today.

Restaurant food, especially fast food, contributes significantly to the development of obesity. Fast food is often energy-dense food, which increases energy intake, BMI, and body fatness.[55] The combination of large portions and energy-dense foods is a double whammy.[56] Reducing portion sizes is somewhat helpful, but the real kcalorie savings come from lowering the energy density. After all, large portions of foods with low energy density such as lean meats, vegetables, and fruits can help with weight loss. Unfortunately, low-energy-dense foods tend to be more expensive and less convenient than energy-dense foods.[57] The financial interests of the food industry do not always align with consumer health goals.[58] Consumers' health would benefit from restaurants providing appropriate portion sizes and offering more vegetables, fruits, legumes, and whole grains. Restaurant portion size decisions, however, are based on the chefs' plate presentations, food costs, and customer expectations—not customer health needs.[59]

Physical Inactivity Our environment fosters physical inactivity as well.[60] Life requires little exertion—escalators carry us up stairs, automobiles take us across town, buttons roll down windows, and remote controls change television channels from a distance. Modern technology has replaced physical activity at home, at work, and in transportation. Inactivity contributes to weight gain and poor health. In turn, watching television, playing video games, and using the computer may contribute most to physical inactivity. The more time people spend in these sedentary activities, the more likely they are to be overweight.

Sedentary activities contribute to weight gain in several ways. First, they require little energy beyond the resting metabolic rate. Second, they replace time spent in more vigorous activities. Third, watching television influences food purchases and correlates with between-meal snacking on the high-kcalorie, high-fat foods most heavily advertised.

Some obese people are so extraordinarily inactive that even when they eat less than lean people, they still have an energy surplus. Reducing their food intake further would incur nutrient deficiencies and jeopardize health. Physical activity is a necessary component of nutritional health. People must be physically active if they are to eat enough food to deliver all the nutrients they need without unhealthy weight gain. In fact, *to prevent weight gain,* the DRI ♦ suggests an accumulation of 60 minutes of moderately intense physical activities every day in addition to the less intense activities of daily living. Recommendations *to lose weight* encourage even greater duration, intensity, or frequency of physical activity (as a later section of the chapter discusses). For adults who want to gain health benefits from being active, the Canadian Society for Exercise Physiology in conjunction with the Public Health Agency of Canada recently released physical activity guidelines that recommend adults between the ages of 18 to 64 years include at least 150 minutes of moderate-to-vigorous activity every week, in bouts of 10 minutes or more.[61]

♦ DRI for physical activity: 60 min/day (moderate intensity)

People may be obese, therefore, not because they eat too much, but because they move too little—both in purposeful exercise and in the activities of daily life. Studies report that the differences in the time obese and lean people spent lying, sitting, standing, and moving account for about 350 kcalories a day.[62] In general, lean people tend to be more spontaneously active in their occupations and their leisure time.[63] The energy expended ♦ in these everyday spontaneous activities plays a pivotal role in energy balance and weight management.[64]

♦ The energy expenditure associated with everyday spontaneous activities is called **nonexercise activity thermogenesis (NEAT).**

IN SUMMARY **Obesity has many causes and different combinations of causes in different people. Some causes, such as overeating and physical inactivity, may be within a person's control, and some, such as genetics, may be beyond it.**

Problems of Overweight and Obesity

An estimated 44 percent of Canadian adults are trying to lose weight at any given time, which is comparatively lower than 50 percent of U.S. adults.[65] Some of these people do not even need to lose weight. Others may benefit from weight loss, but they are not successful. Relatively few people succeed in losing weight, and even fewer succeed permanently. Whether a person needs to lose weight is a question of health.

Health Risks

Chapter 8 describes some of the health problems that commonly accompany obesity. In evaluating the risks to health from obesity, health-care professionals use three indicators:[66]

- Body mass index ♦ (BMI, as Chapter 8 describes)
- Waist circumference ♦ (as Chapter 8 describes)
- Disease risk profile

Importantly, the disease risk profile takes into account life-threatening diseases, family history, and common risk factors for chronic diseases (such as blood lipid profile).[67] The higher the BMI, the greater the waist circumference, and the more risk factors—the greater the urgency to treat obesity.

People can best decide whether weight loss might be beneficial by considering their health status and motivation. People who are overweight by BMI standards, but otherwise in good health, might not benefit from losing weight; they might focus on preventing further weight gains instead. In contrast, those who are obese and suffering from a life-threatening disease such as diabetes might improve their health substantially by adopting a diet and exercise plan that supports weight loss. Motivation is a key component; to lose weight, a person needs to be ready and willing to make lifestyle changes for a lifetime.

Overweight in Good Health Often a person's motivations for weight loss have nothing to do with health. A healthy young woman with a BMI of 26 ♦ might want to lose a few pounds for spring break, but doing so might not improve her health. In fact, if she opts for a starvation diet or diet pills, she would be healthier *not* trying to lose weight.

Obese or Overweight with Risk Factors Weight loss is recommended for people who are obese and those who are overweight (or who have a high waist circumference) with two or more risk factors for chronic diseases. ♦ A 50-year-old man with a BMI of 28 ♦ who has high blood pressure and a family history of heart disease can improve his health by adopting a diet low in saturated fat and a regular exercise plan.

Obese or Overweight with Life-Threatening Condition Weight loss is also recommended for a person who is either obese or overweight and suffering from a life-threatening condition such as heart disease, diabetes, or sleep apnea. ♦ The health benefits of weight loss are clear. For example, a 30-year-old man with a BMI of 40 ♦ might be able to prevent or control diabetes by losing 34 kilograms (75 pounds). Although the effort required to do so may be great, it may be no greater than the effort and consequences of living with diabetes.

Perceptions and Prejudices

Many people assume that every obese person can achieve slenderness and should pursue that goal. First consider that most obese people do not—for whatever reason—successfully lose weight and maintain their losses. Then consider the prejudice involved in that assumption. People come with varying weight tendencies, just as they come with varying potentials for height and degrees of health, yet we do not expect tall people to shrink or healthy people to get sick in an effort to become "normal."

♦ BMI 25.0–29.9 = overweight
BMI ≥30 = obese

♦ Men: ≥102 cm (40 in)
Women: ≥88 cm (35 in)

♦ For reference, a woman with a BMI of 26 might be:
- 1.60 m, 66.2 kg (5 ft 3 in, 146 lb)
- 1.65 m, 70.8 kg (5 ft 5 in, 156 lb)
- 1.70 m, 75.3 kg (5 ft 7 in, 166 lb)

♦ Obese people and overweight people with two or more of these risk factors require aggressive treatment:
- Hypertension
- Cigarette smoking
- High LDL
- Low HDL
- Impaired glucose tolerance
- Family history of heart disease
- Men ≥45 yr; women ≥55 yr

♦ For reference, a man with a BMI of 28 might be:
- 1.73 m, 83.5 kg (5 ft 8 in, 184 lb)
- 1.78 m, 88.5 kg (5 ft 10 in, 195 lb)
- 1.83 m, 93.4 kg (6 ft, 206 lb)

♦ Obese people and overweight people with any of these diseases require aggressive treatment:
- Heart disease
- Diabetes (type 2)
- Sleep apnea (a disturbance of breathing during sleep, including temporarily stopping)

♦ For reference, a man with a BMI of 40 might be:
- 1.73 m, 120.2 kg (5 ft 8 in, 265 lb)
- 1.78 m, 127 kg (5 ft 10 in, 280 lb)
- 1.83 m, 133.8 kg (6 ft, 295 lb)

FIGURE 9-4 The Psychology of Weight Cycling

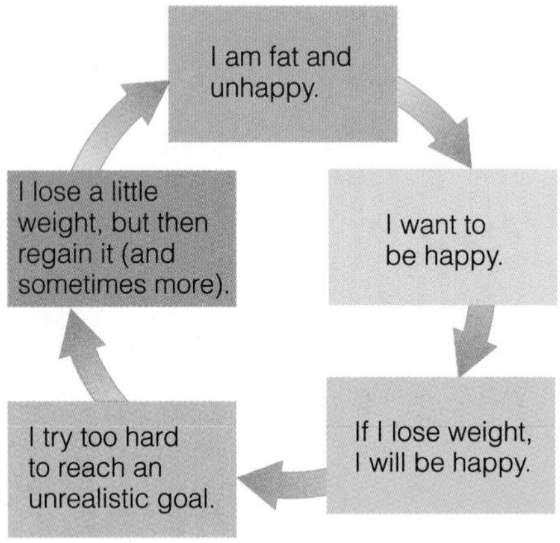
I am fat and unhappy.
I want to be happy.
If I lose weight, I will be happy.
I try too hard to reach an unrealistic goal.
I lose a little weight, but then regain it (and sometimes more).

Social Consequences Large segments of our society place such enormous value on thinness that obese people face prejudice and discrimination on the job, at school, and in social situations: they are judged on their appearance more than on their character. Socially, obese people are stereotyped as lazy and lacking in self-control. Such a critical view of overweight is not prevalent in many other cultures, including segments of our own society. Instead, overweight is simply accepted or even embraced as a sign of robust health and beauty. Many overweight people today are tired of the focus on weight control and simply want to be accepted as they are. To free society of its obsession with body weight and prejudice against obesity, people must first learn to judge others for who they are and not for what they weigh.

Psychological Problems Psychologically, obese people may suffer embarrassment when others treat them with hostility and contempt, and some have even come to view their own bodies as grotesque and loathsome. Feelings of rejection, shame, or depression are common among obese people.

Most weight-loss programs assume that the problem can be solved simply by applying willpower and hard work. If determination were the only factor involved, though, the success rate would be far greater than it is. Overweight people may readily assume blame for failure to lose weight and maintain the losses when, in fact, it is the programs that have failed. Ineffective treatment and its associated sense of failure add to a person's psychological burden. Figure 9-4 illustrates how the devastating psychological effects of obesity and dieting perpetuate themselves.

Dangerous Interventions

Some people attach so many dreams of happiness to weight loss that they willingly risk huge sums of money for the slightest chance of success. As a result, weight-loss schemes flourish. Of the tens of thousands of claims, treatments, and theories for losing weight, few are effective—and many are downright dangerous. The negative effects must be carefully considered before embarking on any weight-loss program. Some interventions ♦ entail greater dangers than the risk of being overweight. Physical problems may arise from fad diets, "yo-yo" dieting, and drug use, and psychological problems may emerge from repeated "failures."

♦ Scrutinize fad diets, magic potions, and wonder gizmos with a healthy dose of skepticism.

Some of the nation's most popular diet books and weight-loss programs have misled consumers with unsubstantiated claims and deceptive testimonials. Furthermore, they fail to provide an assessment of the short- and long-term results of their treatment plans, even though such evaluations are possible and would permit consumers to make informed decisions. Of course, some weight-loss programs are better than others in terms of cost, approach, and customer satisfaction, but few are particularly successful in helping people keep off lost weight. Clients can expect reputable programs to abide by a consumer bill of rights that explains the risks associated with weight-loss programs and provides honest predictions of success (see Table 9-2).

Fad Diets **Fad diets** often sound good, but they typically fall short of delivering on their promises. They espouse exaggerated or false theories of weight loss and advise consumers to follow inadequate diets. Some fad diets are hazardous to health as Highlight 9 explains. Adverse reactions can be as minor as headaches, nausea, and dizziness or as serious as death. Table H9-3 (p. 307) offers guidelines for identifying unsound weight-loss schemes and fad diets.

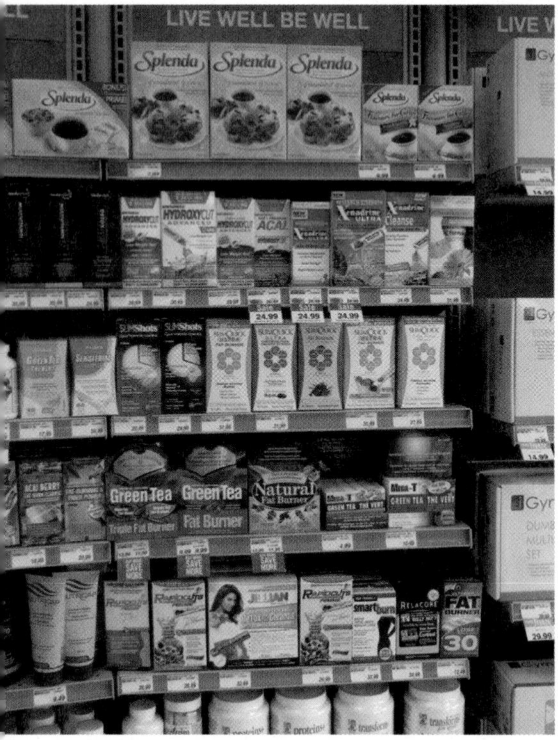
LIVE WELL BE WELL
Splenda
Green Tea
Fat Burner

Dick Hemingway

So many promises, so little success.

Weight-Loss Products Many people in Canada use nonprescription weight-loss products. Most of them are women, especially young overweight women, but almost 10 percent are of normal weight.

In their search for weight-loss magic, some consumers turn to "natural" herbal products and dietary supplements, even though few have proved to be effective.[68] St. John's wort, for example, contains substances that inhibit the uptake of **serotonin** and thus suppress appetite. In addition to the many cautions that accompany the use of all herbal remedies, consumers should be aware that St. John's wort is often prepared in combination with the herbal stimulant ephedrine. ♦ Ephedrine-containing

♦ Ephedrine is an amphetamine-like substance extracted from the Chinese ephedra herb *ma huang*.

fad diets: popular eating plans that promise quick weight loss. Most fad diets severely limit certain foods or overemphasize others (for example, never eat potatoes or pasta or eat cabbage soup daily).

serotonin (ser-oh-TONE-in): a neurotransmitter important in sleep regulation, appetite control, and sensory perception, among other roles. Serotonin is synthesized in the body from the amino acid tryptophan with the help of vitamin B_6.

TABLE 9-2 Weight-Loss Consumer Bill of Rights (An Example)

1. *Warning:* Rapid weight loss may cause serious health problems. Rapid weight loss is weight loss of more than 0.7 to 0.9 kilograms (1½ to 2 pounds) per week or weight loss of more than 1 percent of body weight per week after the second week of participation in a weight-loss program.
2. Consult your personal physician before starting any weight-loss program.
3. Only permanent lifestyle changes, such as making healthful food choices and increasing physical activity, promote long-term weight loss and successful maintenance.
4. Qualifications of this provider are available upon request.
5. *You have a right to:*
   - Ask questions about the potential health risks of this program and its nutritional content, psychological support, and educational components.
   - Receive an itemized statement of the actual or estimated price of the weight-loss program, including extra products, services, supplements, examinations, and laboratory tests.
   - Know the actual or estimated duration of the program.
   - Know the name, address, and qualifications of the dietitian or nutritionist who has reviewed and approved the weight-loss program.

supplements promote modest short-term weight loss (about 1 kilogram a month), but the associated risks are high. These supplements have been implicated in several cases of heart attacks and seizures and have been linked to about 100 deaths. For this reason, Health Canada allows the sale of ephedrine in nasal decongestants and homeopathic medicines only to a maximum of 8 milligrams per dose or 32 milligrams per day. Table 9-3 presents the claims and the dangers behind ephedrine and several other dietary supplements commonly used for weight loss.[69]

TABLE 9-3 Selected Herbal and Other Dietary Supplements Marketed for Weight Loss

Product	Claims	Research Findings	Risks
Bitter orange[a] (*Citrus aurantium,* a natural flavouring that contains synephrine, a compound structurally similar to epinephrine)	Stimulates weight loss; provides an alternative to ephedra	Little evidence available	May increase blood pressure; may interact with drugs
Chitosan[b] (pronounced KITE-oh-san; derived from chitin, the substance that forms the hard shells of lobsters, crabs, and other crustaceans)	Binds to dietary fat, preventing digestion and absorption	Ineffective	Impaired absorption of fat-soluble vitamins
Chromium (trace mineral)	Eliminates body fat	Ineffective; weight gain reported when not accompanied by exercise	Headaches, sleep disturbances, and mood swings; hexavalent form is toxic and carcinogenic
Conjugated linoleic acid (CLA; a group of fatty acids related to linoleic acid, but with different *cis-* and *trans-*configurations)	Reduces body fat and suppresses appetite	Some evidence in animal studies, modest fat loss in human studies	None known
Ephedrine[c] (amphetamine-like substance derived from the Chinese ephedra herb *ma huang*)	Speeds body's metabolism	Short-term weight loss and dangerous side-effects	Insomnia, tremors, heart attacks, strokes, and death; Health Canada has placed a partial ban on the sale of these products
Fucoxanthin[d] (derived from seaweed)	Speeds metabolism; burns fat	No evidence available	None known
Hoodia (derived from cactus)	Suppresses appetite	Little evidence available	None known
Hydroxycitric acid[e] (active ingredient derived from the rind of the tropical fruit *garcinia cambogia*)	Inhibits the enzyme that converts citric acid to fat; suppresses appetite	Ineffective	Toxicity symptoms reported in animal studies; headaches, respiratory, and gastrointestinal distress in humans
Pyruvate[f] (3-carbon compound produced during glycolysis)	Speeds body's metabolism	Modest weight loss with high doses	GI distress
Yohimbine (derived from the bark of a West African tree)	Promotes weight loss	Ineffective	Nervousness, insomnia, anxiety, dizziness, tremors, headaches, nausea, vomiting, hypertension

[a] Marketed under the trade names Xenadrine EFX, Metabolife Ultra, NOW Diet Support.
[b] Marketed under the trade names Chitorich, Exofat, Fat Breaker, Fat Blocker, Fat Magnet, Fat Trapper, and Fatsorb.
[c] Marketed under the trade names Diet Fuel, Metabolife, and Nature's Nutrition Formula One.
[d] Marketed under the trade name FucoThin.
[e] Marketed under the trade names Ultra Burn, Citralean, CitriMax, Citrin, Slim Life, Brindleslim, Medislim, and Beer Belly Busters.
[f] Marketed under the trade names Exercise in a Bottle, Pyruvate Punch, Pyruvate-c, and Provate.
NOTE: Health Canada has not approved the use of most of these products; many products are used in conjunction with a 1000- to 1800-kcalorie diet.

Herbal laxatives containing senna, aloe, rhubarb root, cascara, castor oil, and buckthorn (or various combinations) are commonly sold as "dieter's tea." Such concoctions commonly cause nausea, vomiting, diarrhea, cramping, and fainting and may have contributed to the deaths of four women who had drastically reduced their food intakes. Consumers mistakenly believe that laxatives will diminish nutrient absorption and reduce kcalorie intake, but remember that absorption occurs primarily in the small intestine and laxatives act on the large intestine. Highlight 19 explores the possible benefits and potential dangers of herbal products and other alternative therapies. As it explains, current laws do not require manufacturers of dietary supplements to test the safety or effectiveness of any product. Consumers cannot assume that an herb or dietary supplement of any kind is safe or effective just because it is available on the market. More than 70 tainted dietary supplements that contain undeclared active pharmaceutical ingredients that can have serious consequences such as seizures and heart attacks have been identified. In addition, many weight-loss supplements do not contain the amounts of active ingredients listed on the labels. Anyone using dietary supplements for weight loss should first consult with a physician.

Other Gimmicks Other gimmicks don't help with weight loss either. Hot baths do not speed up metabolism so that kilograms can be lost in hours. Steam and sauna baths do not melt the fat off the body, although they may dehydrate people so that they lose water weight. Brushes, sponges, wraps, creams, and massages intended to move, burn, or break up "**cellulite**" do nothing of the kind because there is no such thing as cellulite.

IN SUMMARY **The question of whether a person should lose weight depends on many factors: among them are the extent of overweight, age, health, and genetic makeup. Not all obesity will cause disease or shorten life expectancy. Just as there are unhealthy, normal-weight people, there are healthy, obese people. Some people may risk more in the process of losing weight than in remaining overweight. Fad diets and weight-loss supplements can be as physically and psychologically damaging as excess body weight.**

Aggressive Treatments for Obesity

The appropriate strategies for weight reduction depend on the degree of obesity and the risk of disease. An overweight person in good health may need only to improve eating habits and increase physical activity, but someone with **clinically severe obesity** may need more aggressive treatment ♦ options—drugs or surgery. Drugs appear to be modestly effective and safe, at least in the short term; surgery appears to be dramatically effective but can have severe complications, at least for some people.

Drugs

Based on new understandings of obesity's genetic basis and its classification as a chronic disease, much research effort has focused on drug treatments for obesity. Experts reason that if obesity is a chronic disease, it should be treated as such—and the treatment of most chronic diseases includes drugs. The challenge, then, is to develop an effective drug—or more likely, a combination of drugs—that can be used over time without adverse side-effects or the potential for abuse.[70]

Several drugs for weight loss have been tried over the years. When used as part of a long-term, comprehensive weight-loss program, drugs ♦ can help with modest weight loss.[71] Because weight regain commonly occurs with the discontinuation of drug therapy, treatment must be long term. Yet the long-term use of drugs poses risks. We don't yet know whether a person would be harmed more from maintaining a 50 kilogram excess or from taking a drug for a decade to keep the 50 kilograms off. Physicians must prescribe drugs appropriately, inform consumers of the potential risks, and monitor side-effects carefully. Health Canada has approved three prescription drugs to treat obesity.[72]

♦ The field of medicine that specializes in treating obesity is called **bariatrics.**
- **bar** = weight

♦ Drugs may be an option for people with all of the following conditions:
- Unable to achieve adequate weight loss with diet and exercise
- BMI $\geq$30 or BMI $\geq$27 with weight-related health problems
- No medical contraindications

cellulite (SELL-you-light or SELL-you-leet): supposedly, a lumpy form of fat; actually, a fraud. Fatty areas of the body may appear lumpy when the strands of connective tissue that attach the skin to underlying muscles pull tight where the fat is thick. The fat itself is the same as fat anywhere else in the body. If the fat in these areas is lost, the lumpy appearance disappears.

clinically severe obesity: a BMI of 40 or greater or a BMI of 35 or greater with additional medical problems. A less preferred term used to describe the same condition is *morbid obesity.*

Orlistat **Orlistat** takes a different approach to weight control.* It inhibits pancreatic lipase activity in the GI tract, thus blocking dietary fat digestion and absorption by about 30 percent. The drug is taken with meals and is most effective when accompanied by a reduced-kcalorie, low-fat diet. Side-effects include gas, frequent bowel movements, and reduced absorption of fat-soluble vitamins.

Phentermine and Diethylproprion Phentermine and diethylproprion enhance the release of the neurotransmitter norepinephrine, which tends to reduce food intake.** Weight reduction is modest. Side-effects include increased blood pressure and insomnia.

Other Drugs Some physicians prescribe drugs that have not been approved for weight loss, a practice known as "off-label" use. These drugs have been approved for other conditions (such as seizures) and incidentally cause modest weight loss.[73] Physicians using off-label drugs must be well-informed of the drugs' use and effects and monitor their patients' responses closely.

Surgery

Surgery ♦ as an approach to weight loss is justified in some specific cases of clinically severe obesity.[74] As Figure 9-5 shows, surgical procedures effectively limit food intake by reducing the capacity of the stomach. In addition, they suppress hunger by reducing production of the hormone ghrelin.[75] The results are significant: depending on the type of surgery, initial weight loss is 20 to 32 percent of body weight and 14 to 25 percent after ten years.[76] Importantly, most people experience dramatic improvements in their diabetes, blood lipids, and blood

*Orlistat is marketed under the trade name Xenical.
**Phentermine is marketed under the trade names Fastin and Ionamin. Diethylproprion is marketed under the trade name Tenuate.

♦ Surgery may be an option for people with all of the following conditions:
- Unable to achieve adequate weight loss with diet and exercise
- BMI ≥40 or BMI ≥35 with weight-related health problems (such as diabetes or hypertension)
- No medical or psychological contraindications
- Understanding of risks and strong motivation to comply with post-surgery treatment plan

FIGURE 9-5 Gastric Surgery Used in the Treatment of Severe Obesity

Both of these surgical procedures limit the amount of food that can be comfortably eaten.

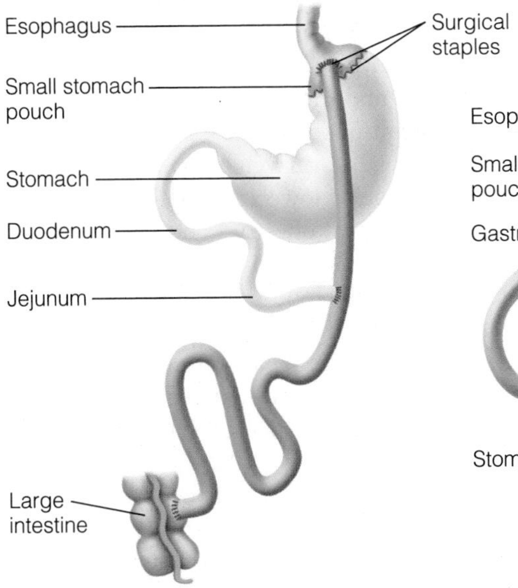
Esophagus
Surgical staples
Small stomach pouch
Stomach
Duodenum
Jejunum
Large intestine

In gastric bypass, the surgeon constructs a small stomach pouch and creates an outlet directly to the small intestine, bypassing most of the stomach, the entire duodenum, and some of the jejunum. (Dark areas highlight the flow of food through the GI tract; pale areas indicate bypassed sections.)

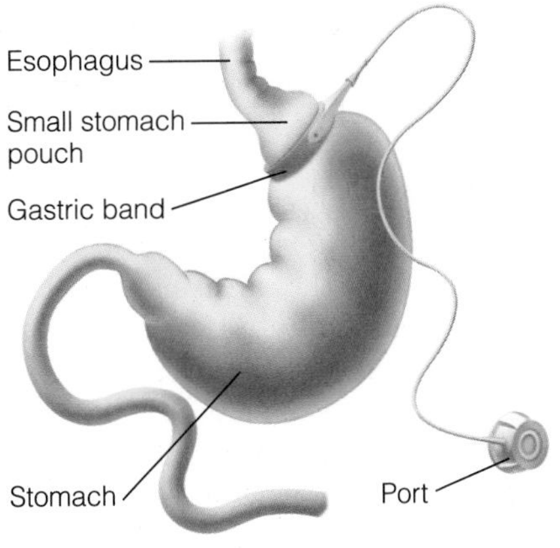
Esophagus
Small stomach pouch
Gastric band
Stomach
Port

In gastric banding, the surgeon uses a gastric band to reduce the opening from the esophagus to the stomach. The size of the opening can be adjusted by inflating or deflating the band by way of a port placed in the abdomen just beneath the skin.

orlistat (OR-leh-stat): a drug used in the treatment of obesity that inhibits the absorption of fat in the GI tract, thus limiting kcaloric intake.

pressure.[77] Whether surgery is a reasonable option for obese teens is the subject of much debate among pediatricians and bariatric surgeons (see Chapter 17).

The long-term safety and effectiveness of gastric surgery depend, in large part, on compliance with dietary instructions. Common immediate post-surgical complications include infections, nausea, vomiting, and dehydration. In the long term, vitamin and mineral deficiencies are common.[78] Weight regain and psychological problems may also occur. Lifelong medical supervision is necessary for those who choose the surgical route, but in suitable candidates, the possible health benefits of weight loss—improved blood lipid profile, blood pressure, and insulin sensitivity—may balance the risks.[79] Overall mortality is lower for obese people after surgery than for other obese people.[80]

Another surgical procedure is used, not to treat obesity, but to remove some of the evidence. Plastic surgeons can extract some fat deposits by suction lipectomy, or "liposuction." This cosmetic procedure has little effect on body weight (less than 5 kilograms), but can alter body shape slightly in specific areas. Liposuction is a popular procedure in part because of its perceived safety, but, in fact, serious complications can occasionally result in death. Furthermore, removing adipose tissue by way of liposuction does not provide the health benefits that typically accompany weight loss.[81] In other words, liposuction does not improve blood pressure, inflammation, blood lipid profile, or insulin sensitivity. Furthermore, as with other weight-loss attempts, fat deposits will return when dietary intake exceeds needs.

IN SUMMARY **Obese people with high risks of medical problems may need aggressive treatment, including drugs or surgery. Others may benefit most from improving eating and exercise habits.**

Weight-Loss Strategies

Successful weight-loss strategies embrace small changes, moderate losses, and reasonable goals.[82] People who lose 5 to 10 kilograms (10 to 20 pounds) in a year by consistently choosing nutrient-dense foods and engaging in regular physical activity are much more likely to maintain the loss and reap health benefits than if they were to lose more weight in less time by adopting a radical fad diet. In keeping with this philosophy, Health Canada and the Public Health Agency of Canada promote and support healthy eating and regular physical activity through advice given in *Eating Well with Canada's Food Guide* and the *Canadian Physical Activity Guidelines*. Even modest weight loss brings health benefits.

Modest weight loss, even when a person is still overweight, can improve glucose control and reduce the risks of heart disease by lowering blood pressure and blood cholesterol, especially for those with central obesity.[83] Improvements in physical capabilities and bodily pain become evident with even a 2–3 kilogram weight loss. For these reasons, parameters such as blood pressure, blood cholesterol, or even vitality are more useful than body weight in marking success. People less concerned with disease risks may prefer to set goals for personal fitness, such as being able to play with children or climb stairs without becoming short of breath. Importantly, they can enjoy living a healthy life instead of focusing on the elusive goal of losing weight.

Whether the goal is health or fitness, expectations need to be reasonable. Unreachable targets ensure frustration and failure. When realistic, yet moderately challenging, goals are achieved or exceeded, people enjoy rewards instead of finding disappointment.

Research findings highlight the great disparity between lofty expectations and reasonable success.[84] Before beginning a weight-loss program, obese women identified the weights they would describe as "dream," "happy," "acceptable," and "disappointing" (see Figure 9-6). All of these weights were below their starting weight. Their goal weights far exceeded the 5 to 10 percent recommended by experts, or even the 15 percent reported by the most successful

FIGURE 9-6 Reasonable Weight Goals and Expectations Compared

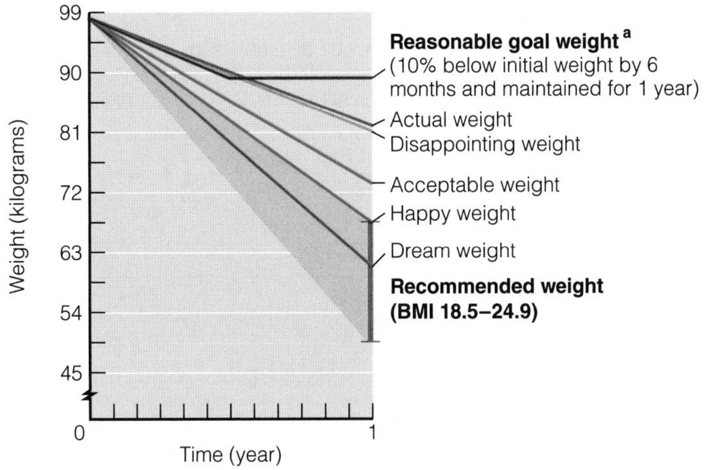
Weight (kilograms)
99
90
81
72
63
54
45
0
Time (year)
1
Reasonable goal weight a
(10% below initial weight by 6 months and maintained for 1 year)
Actual weight
Disappointing weight
Acceptable weight
Happy weight
Dream weight
Recommended weight
(BMI 18.5–24.9)

[a]Reasonable goal weights reflect kilograms lost over time. Given more time, reasonable goals may eventually fall within the recommended weight range.

SOURCE: Copyright © 1997 by the American Psychological Association. Adapted with permission. Adapted from G. D. Foster and coauthors, What is a reasonable weight loss? Patients' expectations and evaluations of obesity treatment outcomes, Journal of Consulting and Clinical Psychology 65 (1997): 79–85. The use of APA information does not imply endorsement by APA.

weight-loss studies. Even their "disappointing" weights exceeded recommended goals. Close to a year later, and after an average loss of 16 kilograms, almost half of the women did not achieve even their "disappointing" weights. They did, however, experience more physical, social, and psychological benefits than they had predicted for that weight. Still, in a culture that overvalues thinness, these women were not satisfied with a 16 percent reduction in weight—not because their efforts were unsuccessful, but because their expectations were unrealistic.

Depending on initial body weight, a reasonable rate of weight loss for overweight people is ¼ to 1 kilogram (½ to 2 pounds) a week, ♦ or 10 percent of body weight over six months.[85] For a person weighing 110 kilograms (250 pounds), a 10 percent loss is 11 kilograms (25 pounds), or about 0.5 kilogram (1 pound) a week for six months. Such gradual weight losses are more likely to be maintained than rapid losses. Keep in mind that pursuing good health is a lifelong journey. Most adults are keenly aware of their body weights and shapes and realize that what they eat and what they do can make a difference to some extent. Those who are most successful at weight management seem to have fully incorporated healthful eating and physical activity into their daily lives. Such advice—to reduce energy intake and increase physical activity—would hardly surprise anyone, yet relatively few people trying to control their weight follow these recommendations.

♦ Safe rate for weight loss:
- 0.25 to 1.0 kg (½ to 2 lb/week)
- 10% body weight/6 months

Eating Plans

Contrary to the claims of fad diets, no single food plan is magical, and no specific food must be included or avoided in a weight-management program. In designing a plan, people need only consider foods that they like or can learn to like, that are available, and that are within their means. *Eating Well with Canada's Food Guide* provides a useful framework for choosing an adequate, varied, and balanced diet that fits into a healthy weight-loss plan.

Be Realistic about Energy Intake The main characteristic of a weight-loss diet is that it provides less energy than the person needs to maintain present body weight. If food energy is restricted too severely, dieters may not receive sufficient nutrients and may lose lean tissue. Rapid weight loss usually means excessive loss of lean tissue, a lower BMR, and a rapid weight gain to follow. In addition, restrictive eating may set in motion the unhealthy behaviours of eating disorders as described in Highlight 8.

Table 9-4 (p. 286) outlines the recommendations of a weight-loss diet. Energy intake should provide nutritional adequacy without excess—that is, somewhere

TABLE 9-4 Recommendations for a Weight-Loss Diet

Nutrient	Recommended Intake
kCalories	
For people with BMI ≥35	Approximately 500 to 1000 kcalories per day reduction from usual intake
For people with BMI between 27 and 35	Approximately 300 to 500 kcalories per day reduction from usual intake
Total fat	30% or less of total kcalories
Saturated fatty acids[a]	8 to 10% of total kcalories
Monounsaturated fatty acids	Up to 15% of total kcalories
Polyunsaturated fatty acids	Up to 10% of total kcalories
Cholesterol[a]	300 mg or less per day
Protein[b]	Approximately 15% of total kcalories
Carbohydrate[c]	55% or more of total kcalories
Sodium chloride	No more than 2400 mg of sodium or approximately 6 g of sodium chloride (salt) per day
Calcium	1000 to 1500 mg per day
Fibre[c]	20 to 30 g per day

[a]People with high blood cholesterol should aim for less than 7 percent kcalories from saturated fat and 200 milligrams of cholesterol per day.
[b]Protein should be derived from plant sources and lean sources of animal protein.
[c]Carbohydrates and fibre should be derived from vegetables, fruits, and whole grains.
SOURCE: National Institutes of Health Obesity Education Initiative, The Practical Guide: Identification, Evaluation, and Treatment of Overweight and Obesity in Adults (Washington, D.C.: U.S. Department of Health and Human Services, 2000), p. 27.

between deprivation and complete freedom to eat whatever, whenever. A reasonable suggestion is that an adult needs to increase activity and reduce food intake enough to create a deficit of 500 to 1000 kcalories per day. Such a deficit produces a weight loss of ½ to 1 kilogram (1 to 2 pounds) per week—a rate that supports the loss of fat efficiently while retaining lean tissue.[86] In general, weight-loss diets provide about 1200 kcalories per day for women and 1600 kcalories a day for men.[87]

Some people skip meals, typically breakfast, in an effort to reduce energy intake, but research suggests such a strategy may be counterproductive. Breakfast frequency is inversely associated with obesity—that is, people who frequently eat breakfast have lower BMI than those who tend to skip breakfast.[88] Furthermore, when people eat breakfast, overall diet quality is better and daily energy density is lower—two factors that support healthy body weight.[89]

Emphasize Nutritional Adequacy Nutritional adequacy is difficult to achieve on fewer than 1200 kcalories a day, and most healthy adults need never consume any less. A plan that provides an adequate intake supports a healthier and more successful weight loss than a restrictive plan that creates feelings of starvation and deprivation, which can lead to an irresistible urge to binge.

Keep in mind that well-balanced diets that emphasize vegetables, fruits, whole grains, low-fat milk or milk alternatives, and lean meats or meat alternatives offer many health rewards even when they don't result in weight loss.[90] A dietary supplement providing vitamins and minerals at or below 100 percent of the Daily Values can help people following low-kcalorie diets to achieve nutrient adequacy.[91]

Eat Small Portions As mentioned earlier, portion sizes at markets, at restaurants, and even at home have increased dramatically over the years. We have come to expect large portions, and we have learned to clean our plates. Many of us pay more attention to these external cues defining how much to eat than to our internal cues of hunger and satiety. For health's sake, we may need to learn to eat less food at each meal—one piece of chicken for dinner instead of two, 5 millilitres (a teaspoon) of butter on vegetables instead of 15 millilitres (a tablespoon), and one cookie for dessert instead of six. The goal is to eat enough food for adequate energy, abundant vitamins and minerals, and some pleasure, but not more. This amount should leave a person feeling satisfied—not stuffed.

Keep in mind that even fat-free and low-fat foods can deliver a lot of kcalories when a person eats large quantities. A low-fat cookie or two can be a sweet treat even on a weight-loss diet, but larger portions defeat the savings.

People who have difficulty making low-kcalorie selections or controlling portion sizes may find it easier to use structured meal replacement plans. Meal replacements that provide low-kcalorie, nutritious meals or snacks can support weight loss while easing the task of diet planning.[92] Ideally, those using a meal replacement plan will seek advice from a registered dietitian to learn how to select appropriately from conventional food choices as well.

Lower Energy Density Most people take their cues about how much to eat based on portion sizes, and the larger the portion size, the more they eat—even when the food is not particularly tasty.[93] To lower energy intake, a person can either reduce the portion size or reduce the energy density.[94] Reducing energy density while maintaining food quantity, especially by including vegetables and fruits, seems to be a successful strategy to control hunger and lose weight.[95] Figure 9-7 illustrates how water, fibre, and fat influence energy density, and the "How To" feature on p. 288 compares foods based on their energy density. Foods containing water, those rich in fibre, and those low in fat help to lower energy density, providing more satiety for fewer kcalories.[96] Because a low-energy-density diet is a low-fat, high-fibre diet rich in many vitamins and minerals, it supports good health in addition to weight loss.[97] Unfortunately, low-energy-density foods tend to be relatively expensive.[98]

Remember Water Water helps with weight management in several ways. For one, foods with high water content (such as broth-based soups) increase fullness, reduce hunger, and consequently reduce energy intake.[99] For another, drinking a large glass of water before a meal may ease hunger, fill the stomach, and reduce energy intake.[100] Importantly, water adds no kcalories. Consuming large portions of kcaloric beverages increases energy intake.[101] Simply replacing nutrient-poor, energy-dense beverages with water could save a person up to 7 kilograms (15 pounds) a year.[102] Water also helps the GI tract adapt to a high-fibre diet.

Focus on Fibre Healthy meals and snacks centre on high-fibre foods. Fresh vegetables, fruits, legumes, and whole grains offer abundant vitamins, minerals, and fibre but little fat. Consequently, diets rich in fibre tend to be relatively low in energy and high in nutrients.

High-fibre foods also require effort to eat—an added bonus. Eating fibre-rich vegetables and fruits reduces energy density, lowers kcalorie intake, and promotes satiety. A person who slows down and savours each bite eats less before the satiety signal reaches the brain. Consequently, energy intake is lower when meals are

FIGURE 9-7 Energy Density

Decreasing the energy density (kcal/g) of foods allows a person to eat satisfying portions while still reducing energy intake. To lower energy density, select foods high in water or fibre and low in fat.

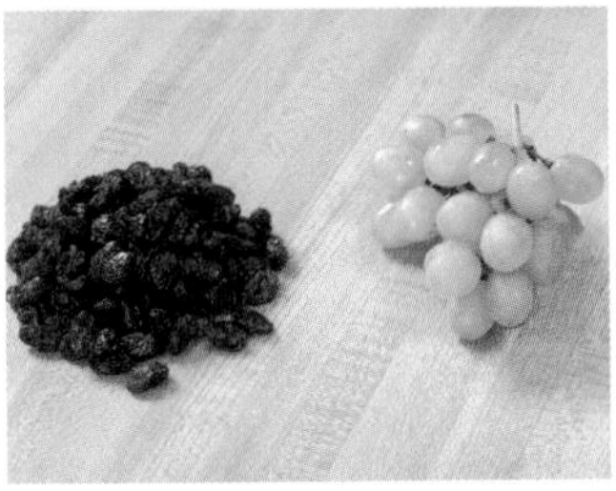
© Matthew Farruggio
Selecting grapes with their high water content instead of raisins increases the volume and cuts the energy intake in half.

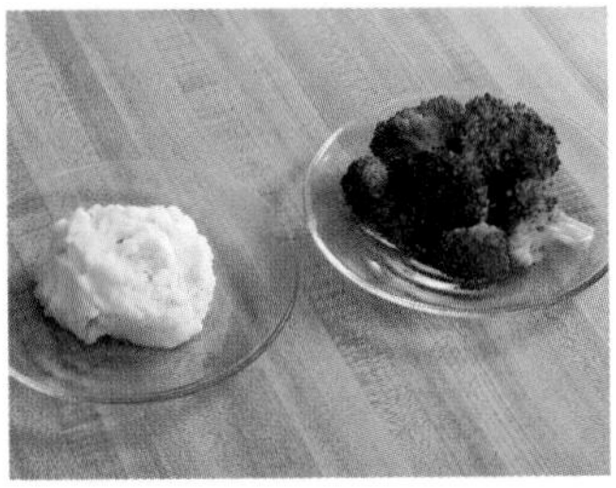
© Matthew Farruggio
Even at the same weight and similar serving sizes, the fibre-rich broccoli delivers twice the fibre of the potatoes for about one-fourth the energy.

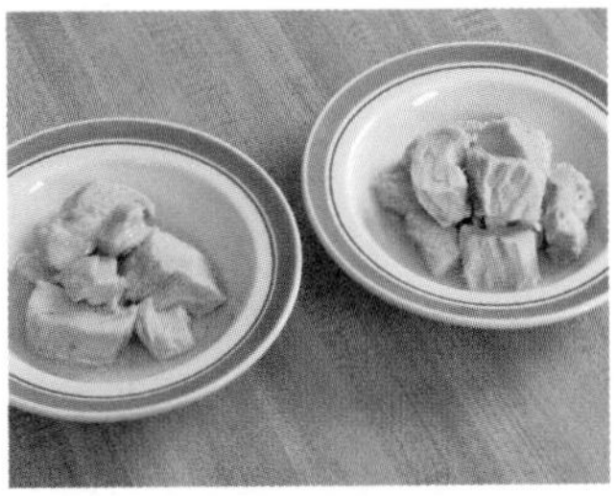
© Matthew Farruggio
By selecting the water-packed tuna (on the right) instead of the oil-packed tuna (on the left), a person can enjoy the same amount for fewer kcalories.

HOW TO Compare Foods Based on Energy Density

Chapter 2 describes how to evaluate foods based on their nutrient density—their nutrient contribution per kcalorie. Another way to evaluate foods is to consider their energy density—their energy contribution per gram. This example compares carrot sticks with french fries. The conclusion is no surprise, but understanding the mathematics may offer valuable insight into the concept of energy density. A carrot weighing 72 grams delivers 31 kcalories. To calculate the energy density, divide kcalories by grams:

$$\frac{31 \text{ kcal}}{72 \text{ g}} = 0.43 \text{ kcal/g}$$

Do the same for french fries weighing 50 grams and contributing 167 kcalories:

$$\frac{167 \text{ kcal}}{50 \text{ g}} = 3.34 \text{ kcal/g}$$

The more kcalories per gram, the greater the energy density. French fries are more energy dense than carrots. They provide more energy per gram—and per bite. Considering a food's energy density is especially useful in planning diets for weight management. Foods with a high energy density help with weight gain, whereas foods with a low energy density help with weight loss.

CENGAGENOW™
For additional practice log on to **www.cengage.com/sso.**

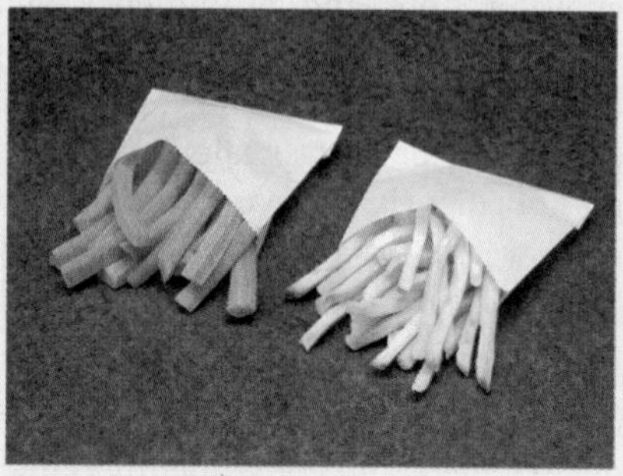

© Matthew Farruggio

TRY IT Compare the energy density of a hard-boiled egg (50 grams and 78 kcalories) with light tuna canned in water (57 grams and 66 kcalories).

eaten slowly.[103] Savouring each bite also activates the pleasure centres of the brain. Some research suggests that people may overeat when the brain doesn't sense enough gratification from food.[104] Faster eating correlates with higher weights.[105]

Choose Fats Sensibly Ideally, a weight-loss diet is both high in fibre and low in fat. Lowering the fat content of a food lowers its energy density—for example, selecting skim milk instead of whole milk. That way, a person can consume the usual amount (say, a 250 mL glass of milk) at a lower energy intake (85 instead of 150 kcalories).

Fat has a weak satiating effect, and satiation plays a key role in determining food intake during a meal. Consequently, a person eating a high-fat meal raises energy intake by adding more food and more fat kcalories. For these reasons, measure fat with extra caution. (Review pp. 152–154 for strategies to lower fat in the diet.) Be careful not to take this advice to extremes, however; too little fat in the diet or in the body carries health risks as well, as Chapter 5 explains.

Whether a low-fat diet is the best option for weight loss is the subject of some controversy and much debate. An important point to notice in any discussion on weight-loss diets is total energy intake. *Low fat* simply means the energy derived from fat is relatively low compared with the total energy intake; it does not mean total energy intake is low. And reducing energy intake to less than expended is essential for weight loss. One way to lower energy intake is to lower fat intake. In these cases, adopting a low-fat diet can help with weight loss.

Select Carbohydrates Carefully Another currently popular way to lower energy intake is to lower carbohydrate intake. Highlight 4's discussion of carbohydrate-restricted and carbohydrate-modified diets reached the same conclusions as the previous paragraph on low-fat diets: they only work when kcalorie intake is less than kcalorie output.

People trying to control weight often use foods and beverages sweetened with artificial sweeteners. Using artificial sweeteners instead of sugar lowers the energy density of foods and beverages. Most studies find no difference in hunger and no compensation in food intakes when diet soft drinks replace regular ones.[106] In this way, people who eat or drink artificially sweetened products can lower their energy intakes and expect modest weight losses.[107]

To what extent artificial sweeteners can help someone lose weight depends in part on the person's motivations and actions. For example, one person might drink an artificially sweetened beverage now so as to be able to eat a high-kcalorie food later. This person's energy intake might stay the same or increase. A person trying to control food energy intake might drink an artificially sweetened beverage now and choose a low-kcalorie food later. This plan would help reduce the person's total energy intake. Using artificial sweeteners will not automatically lower energy intake. To control energy intake successfully, a person needs to make informed diet and activity decisions throughout the day.

Watch for Other Empty kCalories A person trying to achieve or maintain a healthy weight needs to pay attention not only to fat, but to sugar and alcohol, too. Using sugar or alcohol for pleasure on occasion is compatible with health as long as most daily choices are of nutrient-dense foods. Not only does alcohol add kcalories, but accompanying mixers can also add both kcalories and fat, especially in creamy drinks such as piña coladas (review Table H7-3 on p. 236). Furthermore, drinking alcohol reduces a person's inhibitions, which can sabotage weight-control efforts—at least temporarily.

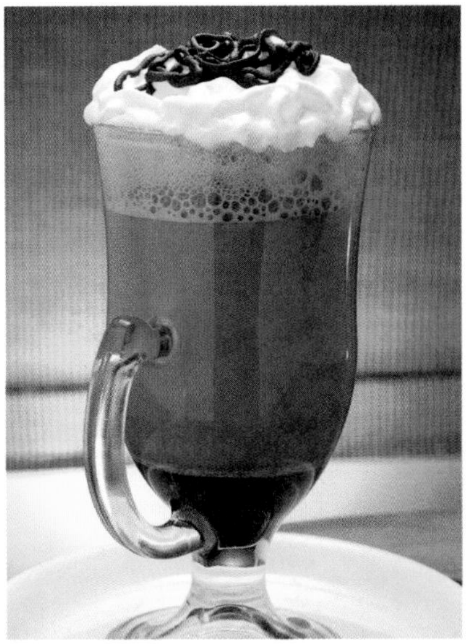

Santiago Cornejo/shutterstock

If you want to lose weight, steer clear of the empty kcalories in fancy coffee drinks. A 500 millilitre (16-ounce) café mocha delivers 400 kcalories—half of them from fat.

IN SUMMARY **A person who adopts a lifelong "eating plan for good health" rather than a "diet for weight loss" will be more likely to keep the lost weight off. Table 9-5 (p. 290) provides several tips for successful weight management.**

Physical Activity

The best approach to weight management includes physical activity.[108] The *Canadian Physical Activity Guidelines* help Canadians of all ages find ways to incorporate exercise into their daily lives.[109] The greater the energy used in exercise, the greater the body fat loss.[110] Yet among people trying to lose weight, fewer than half are physically active and only half of the active group meet minimal recommendations.[111] To prevent weight gains and support weight losses, current DRI recommendations advise 60 minutes of moderately intense physical activity a day in addition to activities of daily life.[112] People who combine diet and exercise typically lose more fat, retain more muscle, and regain less weight than those who only follow a weight-loss diet. Even when people who include physical activity in their weight-management program do not lose more weight, they seem to follow their diet plans more closely and maintain their losses better than those who do not exercise. Consequently, they benefit from taking in a little less energy as well as from expending a little more energy in physical activity. Importantly, those who exercise reduce abdominal obesity and improve their blood pressure, insulin resistance, and cardiorespiratory fitness, regardless of weight loss.[113] Chapter 15 presents the many health benefits of physical activity; the focus here is on its role in weight management.

Dietary Guidance for Canadians

To help manage body weight and prevent gradual, unhealthy body weight gain in adulthood, engage in regular bouts of moderate- to vigorous-intensity activity on most days of the week while not exceeding kcaloric intake requirements.

Activity and Energy Expenditure Table 8-2 (p. 247) shows how much energy each of several activities uses. Physical activities of lower intensity and longer duration (e.g., brisk walking) typically use less carbohydrate and more fat as fuel. The total number of kcalories spent in an activity depends on body weight, intensity, and duration. For example, a person who weighs 65 kilograms (150 pounds)

TABLE 9-5 Weight-Management Strategies

In General
• Focus on healthy eating and activity habits, not on weight losses or gains. • Adopt reasonable expectations about health and fitness goals and about how long it will take to achieve them. • Make nutritional adequacy a high priority. • Learn, practise, and follow a healthful eating plan for the rest of your life. • Participate in some form of physical activity regularly. • Adopt permanent lifestyle changes to achieve and maintain a healthy weight.
For Weight Loss
• Energy out should exceed energy in by about 500 kcalories/day. Increase your physical activity enough to spend more energy than you consume from foods. • Emphasize foods with a low energy density and a high nutrient density. • Eat small portions. Share a restaurant meal with a friend or take home half for lunch tomorrow. • Eat slowly. • Limit high-fat foods. Make legumes, whole grains, vegetables, and fruits central to your diet plan. • Limit low-fat treats to the serving size on the label. • Limit concentrated sweets and alcoholic beverages. • Drink a glass of water before you begin to eat and another while you eat. Drink plenty of water throughout the day. • Keep a record of diet and exercise habits; it reveals problem areas, the first step toward improving behaviours. • Learn alternative ways to deal with emotions and stresses. • Attend support groups regularly or develop supportive relationships with others.
For Weight Gain
• Energy in should exceed energy out by at least 500 kcalories/day. Increase your food intake enough to store more energy than you expend in exercise. Exercise and eat to build muscles. • Expect weight gain to take time (1 pound per month would be reasonable). • Emphasize energy-dense foods. • Eat at least three meals a day. • Eat large portions of foods and expect to feel full. • Eat snacks between meals. • Drink plenty of juice and milk.

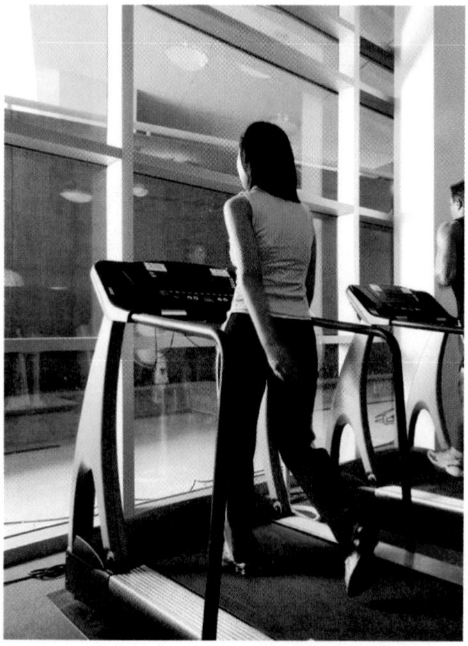

© Corbis Super RF/Alamy

The key to good health is to combine sensible eating with regular exercise.

and walks 6 kilometres (3½ miles) in 60 minutes expends about 300 kcalories. That same person running 5 kilometres (3 miles) in 30 minutes uses a similar amount. By comparison, a 90 kilogram (200-pound) person running 5 kilometres (3 miles) in 30 minutes expends an additional 140 kcalories or so. The goal is to expend as much energy as your time allows. The greater the energy deficit created by exercise, the greater the fat loss. And be careful not to compensate for the energy expended in exercise by eating more food. Otherwise, energy balance won't shift and fat loss will be less significant.

Activity and Discretionary kCalories Discretionary kcalories refer to the difference in kcalories needed to supply nutrients and those needed to maintain energy balance. Because exercise expends energy, the energy allowance to maintain weight increases with increased physical activity—yet the energy needed to deliver needed nutrients remains about the same. In this way, physical activity increases the number of discretionary kcalories (see Figure 9-8). Having a larger discretionary kcalorie allowance puts a little more wiggle room in a weight-loss diet for such options as second helpings, sweet treats, or alcoholic beverages on occasion. Of course, selecting nutrient-dense foods and *not* using discretionary kcalories will maximize weight loss.

Activity and Metabolism Activity also contributes to energy expenditure in an indirect way—by speeding up metabolism. It does this both immediately and over the long term. On any given day, metabolism remains slightly elevated for several hours after intense and prolonged exercise.[114] ♦ Over the long term, a person who

♦ This postexercise effect may raise the energy expenditure of exercise up to 15 percent.

FIGURE 9-8 Influence of Physical Activity on Discretionary kCalories

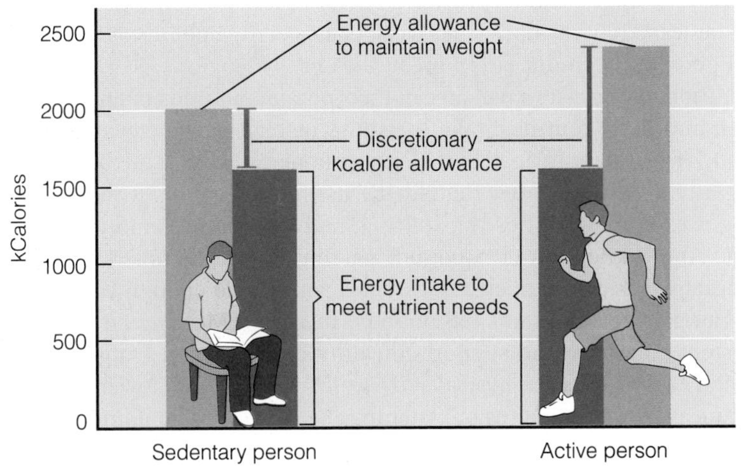
kCalories
2500
2000
1500
1000
500
0
Energy allowance to maintain weight
Discretionary kcalorie allowance
Energy intake to meet nutrient needs
Sedentary person
Active person

CENGAGENOW™ Animated! figure www.cengage.com/sso

engages in daily vigorous activity gradually develops more lean tissue. Metabolic rate rises accordingly, and this supports continued weight loss or maintenance.

Activity and Body Composition Physically active people have less body fat than sedentary people do—even if they have the same BMI. Physical activity, even without weight loss, changes body composition: body fat decreases and lean body mass increases. Furthermore, strength training exercises specifically prevent increases in body fat and abdominal fat.[115]

Activity and Appetite Control Many people think that exercising will make them eat more, but this is not entirely true. Active people do have healthy appetites, but *immediately* after an intense workout, most people do not feel like eating. They may be thirsty and want to shower, but they are not hungry.[116] The body has released fuels from storage to support the exercise, so glucose and fatty acids are abundant in the blood. At the same time, the body has suppressed its digestive functions. Hard physical work and eating are not compatible. A person must calm down, put energy fuels back in storage, and relax before eating. At that time, a physically active person may eat more than a sedentary person, but not so much as to fully compensate for the kcalories expended in exercise.

Exercise may help curb the inappropriate appetite that accompanies boredom, anxiety, or depression. Weight-management programs encourage people who feel the urge to eat when not hungry to go out and exercise instead. The activity passes time, relieves anxiety, and prevents inappropriate eating.

Activity and Psychological Benefits Activity also helps reduce stress. Because stress itself cues inappropriate eating for many people, activity can help here, too. In addition, the fit person looks and feels healthy and, as a result, gains self-esteem. High self-esteem motivates a person to persist in seeking good health and fitness, which keeps the beneficial ♦ cycle going.

Choosing Activities Clearly, physical activity is a plus in a weight-management program. What kind of physical activity is best? People should choose activities that they enjoy and are willing to do regularly. ♦ What schedule of physical activity is best? It doesn't matter; whether a person chooses several short bouts of exercise or one continuous workout, the fitness and weight-loss benefits are the same—and any activity is better than being sedentary.

Health-care professionals frequently advise people to engage in activities of low-to-moderate intensity for a long duration, such as an hour-long, fast-paced walk. The reasoning behind such advice is that people exercising at low-to-moderate intensity are more likely to stick with their activity for longer times and are less

♦ Benefits of physical activity in a weight-management program:
- Short-term increase in energy expenditure (from exercise and from a slight rise in metabolism)
- Long-term increase in BMR (from an increase in lean tissue)
- Improved body composition
- Appetite control
- Stress reduction and control of stress eating
- Physical, and therefore psychological, well-being
- Improved self-esteem

Chapter 15 presents additional benefits of physical activity.

♦ For an active life, limit sedentary activities, engage in strength and flexibility activities, enjoy leisure activities often, engage in moderately intense to vigorous activities regularly, and be as active as possible every day (see the *Canadian Physical Activity Guidelines* in Chapter 15).

♦ Estimated energy expended when walking at a moderate pace = 1 kcal/1.6 km/kg body weight.

likely to injure themselves. A person who stays with an activity routine long enough to enjoy the rewards will be less inclined to give it up and will, over the long term, reap many health benefits. Activity of low-to-moderate intensity ♦ that expends at least 2000 kcalories per week is especially helpful for weight management. Higher levels produce even greater losses.

In addition to exercise, a person can incorporate hundreds of energy-expending activities into daily routines: take the stairs instead of the elevator, walk to the neighbour's apartment instead of making a phone call, and rake the leaves instead of using a blower. Remember that sitting uses more kcalories than lying down, standing uses more kcalories than sitting, and moving uses more kcalories than standing. An 80 kilogram (175-pound) person who replaces a 30-minute television program with a 3 kilometre walk a day can expend enough energy to lose (or at least not gain) 8 kilograms (18 pounds) in a year. Meeting an activity goal of 10 000 steps a day helps to support a healthy BMI.[117] By wearing a pedometer, a person can easily increase physical activity, lose weight, and lower blood pressure without measuring kilometres or watching the clock.[118] The point is to be active. Walk. Run. Swim. Dance. Cycle. Climb. Skip. Do whatever you enjoy doing—and do it often.

Spot Reducing People sometimes ask about "spot reducing." Unfortunately, muscles do not "own" the fat that surrounds them. Fat cells all over the body release fat in response to the demand of physical activity for use by whatever muscles are active. Specific exercises—whether moderate or intense—do not influence the site of adipose tissue loss.[119]

Exercise can help with trouble spots in another way, though. The "trouble spot" for most men is the abdomen, their primary site of fat storage. During aerobic exercise, abdominal fat readily releases its stores, providing fuel to the physically active body. With regular exercise and weight loss, men will deplete these abdominal fat stores before those in the lower body. Women may also deplete abdominal fat with exercise, but their "trouble spots" are more likely to be their hips and thighs.

In addition to aerobic activity, strength training can help to improve the tone of muscles in a trouble area, and stretching to gain flexibility can help with associated posture problems. A combination of aerobic, strength, and flexibility workouts best improves fitness and physical appearance.

> **IN SUMMARY** **Physical activity should be an integral part of a weight-control program. Physical activity can increase energy expenditure, improve body composition, help control appetite, reduce stress and stress eating, and enhance physical and psychological well-being.**

Environmental Influences

Chapter 8 describes how hormones regulate hunger, satiety, and satiation, but people don't always pay close attention to such internal signals. Instead, their eating behaviours are often dictated by environmental factors. Environmental factors include those surrounding the eating experience as well as those pertaining to the food itself. Changing any of these factors can influence how much a person eats.

Atmosphere The environment surrounding a meal or snack influences its duration. When the lighting, décor, aromas, and sounds of an environment are pleasant and comfortable, people tend to spend more time eating and thus eat more. A person needn't eat under neon lights with offensive music to eat less, of course. Instead, after completing a meal, remove food from the table and enjoy the ambience—without the presence of visual cues to stimulate additional eating.

Accessibility Among the strongest influences on how much we eat are the accessibility, ease, and convenience of obtaining food. In general, the less effort needed to obtain food, the more likely food will be eaten. Are you more likely to eat if half a leftover pizza is in your refrigerator or if you have to drive to the grocery store, buy a frozen pizza, and bake it for 45 minutes? Having food nearby and visible encourages eating. In one study, secretaries ate more chocolates when the candy was on their desks than when they had to walk two metres.[120] Interestingly, the secretaries underestimated the amount of chocolates they had eaten when the candy was on their desk and overestimated when it was a short distance away. The message is clear for people wanting to eat less candy (or any other tempting item)—keep it out of sight and in an inconvenient place (or don't even buy it).

Socializing People tend to eat more when socializing with others. Pleasant conversations extend the duration of a meal, allowing a person more time to eat more, and research confirms that the longer the meal, the greater the consumption.[121] In addition, by taking a visual cue from companions, a person might eat more when others at the table clean their plates or go to the buffet line for seconds. One way to eat less is to pace yourself with the person who seems to be eating the least and slowest.

Social interactions also distract a person from paying attention to how much has been eaten. In some cases, socializing with friends during a meal may provide comfort and lower a person's motivation to limit consumption. In other cases, socializing with unfamiliar people during a meal—during a job interview or blind date, for example—may create stress and reduce food consumption. To eat less while socializing, pay attention to portion size.

Distractions Distractions influence food intake by initiating eating, interfering with internal controls to stop eating, and extending the duration of eating. Some people start eating dinner when a favourite television program comes on, regardless of hunger. Other people continue eating breakfast until they finish reading the newspaper. Such mindless eating can easily become overeating. Distractions also interfere with a person's ability to monitor and regulate how much is consumed.[122] If distractions are a part of the eating experience, extra care is needed to control portion sizes.

Presence The mere sight (or smell, or even thought) of a food can prompt a person to start eating—regardless of hunger. The chocolates in the clear candy dishes on the secretaries' desks were eaten much faster than those in opaque containers.[123]

Multiple Choices When offered a large assortment of foods, or several flavours of the same food, people tend to eat more. Interestingly, they tend to eat more even when the number of choices is only *perceived*. Given six flavours of jelly beans, people will eat more when offered an assorted mixture than when presented with the exact same flavours and quantities sorted in a sectioned container.

Having multiple choices is both pleasing and distracting—two factors that slow the eating experience and delay satiation.[124] To limit intake, then, focus on a limited number of foods per meal. Be careful not to misunderstand and abandon variety in diet planning. Eating a variety of nutrient-dense foods from each of the food groups is still a healthy plan.

Package and Portion Sizes As noted earlier, the sizes of packages in grocery stores and portion sizes at restaurants and at home have increased dramatically in recent decades, contributing to the increase in obesity in Canada. Put simply, we tend to clean our plates and finish the package. The larger the bag of potato chips, the greater the intake. To keep from overeating, repackage snacks into smaller containers or eat them from a plate, not directly from the package.

Serving Containers We often use plates, utensils, and glasses as visual cues to guide our decisions on how much to eat and drink.[125] If you plan to eat a bowl of ice cream, it matters whether the bowl you select holds 250 millilitres or 750 millilitres. Even the size of the serving container matters. Students took more—and ate more—snacks when serving from two large bowls instead of from four medium bowls.[126]

Large dinner plates and wide glasses create illusions and misperceptions about quantities consumed. A scoop of mashed potatoes on a small

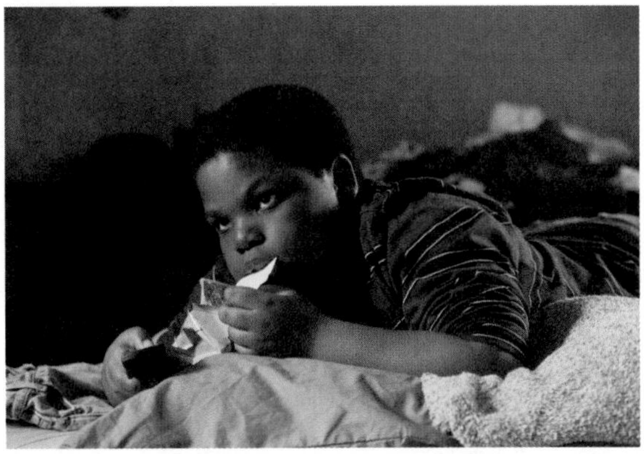

Photodisc/Getty Images

Eating from the package while distracted by television is a weight-gaining combination.

plate looks larger than the same-size scoop on a large plate, leading a person to underestimate the amount of food eaten.[127] To control portion sizes, use small bowls and plates, small serving spoons, and tall, narrow glasses.[128] Of course, using a small plate will not result in less food eaten if multiple servings are taken.[129]

Behaviour and Attitude

Changes in behaviour and attitude can be very effective in supporting efforts to achieve and maintain appropriate body weight and composition.[130] **Behaviour modification** focuses on how to change behaviours to increase energy expenditure and decrease energy intake.[131] A person must commit to taking action.

Adopting a positive, matter-of-fact attitude helps to ensure success. Healthy eating and activity choices are an essential part of healthy living and should simply be incorporated into the day—much like brushing one's teeth or wearing a seat belt.

Become Aware of Behaviours To solve a problem, a person must first identify all the behaviours that created the problem. Keeping a record ♦ will help to identify eating and exercise behaviours that may need changing (see Figure 9-9). It will also establish a baseline against which to measure future progress.

Change Behaviours Behaviour modification strategies ♦ focus on learning desired eating and exercise behaviours and eliminating unwanted behaviours. With so many possible behaviour changes, a person can feel overwhelmed. Start with small time-specific goals for each behaviour—for example, "I'm going to take a 30 minute walk after dinner every evening" instead of "I'm going to run in a marathon someday." Practise desired behaviours until they become routine. Addressing multiple behaviours that focus on a common goal simultaneously may better support changes than taking on one at a time.[132] Using a reward system also seems to effectively support weight-loss efforts.[133]

Cognitive Skills Successful behaviour changes depend in part on two cognitive skills—problem solving and cognitive restructuring.[134] Problem solving requires a person to identify the problem, generate potential solutions, list the pros and cons and the risks and benefits of each, implement the most feasible solution, and evaluate to determine whether behaviours should be continued or abandoned.

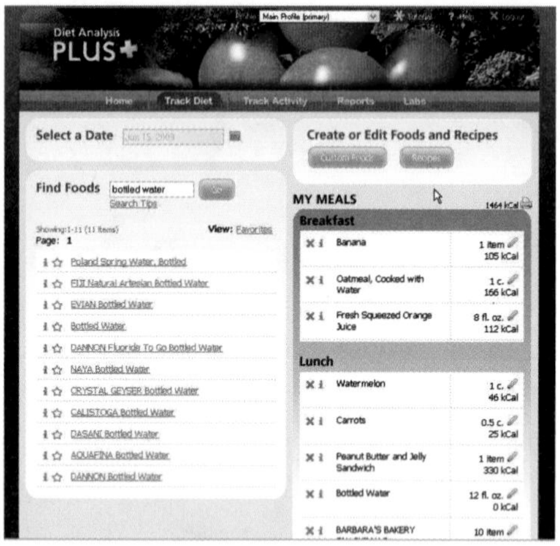
Diet Analysis
PLUS+
Select a Date
Create or Edit Foods and Recipes
Find Foods
MY MEALS
Breakfast
Lunch

Diet analysis programs help people identify high-kcalorie foods and monitor their eating habits.

♦ Visit myfoodguide.ca to find menu planning and diet assessment resources.

♦ Examples of behavioural strategies to support weight change:
- Do not grocery shop when hungry.
- Eat slowly (pause during meals, chew thoroughly, put down utensils between bites).
- Exercise when watching television.

behaviour modification: the changing of behaviour by the manipulation of antecedents (cues or environmental factors that trigger behaviour), the behaviour itself, and consequences (the penalties or rewards attached to behaviour).

FIGURE 9-9 Food Record

The entries in a food record should include the times and places of meals and snacks, the types and amounts of foods eaten, and a description of the individual's feelings when eating. The diary should also record physical activities: the kind, the intensity level, the duration, and the person's feelings about them.

Time	Place	Activity or food eaten	People present	Mood
10:30–10:40	School vending machine	6 peanut butter crackers and 12 oz. cola	by myself	starved
12:15–12:30	Restaurant	Sub sandwich and 12 oz. cola	friends	relaxed & friendly
3:00–3:45	Gym	Weight training	work out partner	tired
4:00–4:10	Snack bar	Small frozen yogurt	by myself	OK

Cognitive restructuring requires a person to replace negative thoughts that derail success with positive thoughts that support behaviour change.

Personal Attitude For many people, overeating and being overweight have become an integral part of their identity. Those who fully understand their personal relationships with food are best prepared to make healthful changes in eating and exercise behaviours.

Sometimes habitual behaviours that are hazardous to health, such as smoking or drinking alcohol, contribute positively by helping people adapt to stressful situations. Similarly, many people overeat to cope with the stresses of life. To break out of that pattern, they must first identify the particular stressors that trigger the urge to overeat. Then, when faced with these situations, they must learn and practise problem-solving skills that will help them to respond appropriately.

All this is not to imply that psychological therapy holds the magic answer to a weight problem. Still, efforts to improve one's general well-being may result in healthy eating and activity habits even when weight loss is not the primary goal. When the problems that trigger the urge to overeat are resolved in alternative ways, people may find they eat less. They may begin to respond appropriately to internal cues of hunger rather than inappropriately to external cues of stress. Sound emotional health supports a person's ability to take care of physical health in all ways—including nutrition, weight management, and fitness.

Support Groups Group support can prove helpful when making life changes. Some people find it useful to join a group such as Take Off Pounds Sensibly (TOPS), Weight Watchers (WW), Overeaters Anonymous (OA), or others. Some dieters prefer to form their own self-help groups or find support online. The Internet offers numerous opportunities for weight-loss education and counselling that may be effective alternatives to face-to-face programs.[135] As always, consumers need to choose wisely and avoid rip-offs.

IN SUMMARY **A surefire remedy for obesity has yet to be found, although many people find a combination of the approaches just described to be most effective. Diet and exercise shift energy balance so that more energy is being expended than is taken in. Physical activity increases energy expenditure, builds lean tissue, and improves health. Energy intake should be reduced by 500 to 1000 kcalories per day, depending on starting body weight and usual food intake. Behaviour modification and cognitive restructuring retrain habits to support a healthy eating and exercise plan. This treatment package requires time, individualization, and sometimes the assistance of a registered dietitian or support group.**

Weight Maintenance

People who are successful often experience much of their weight loss within half a year and then reach a plateau. This slowdown can be disappointing, but it should be recognized as an opportunity for the body to adjust to its new weight. Reaching a plateau provides a little relief from the distraction of weight-loss dieting. An appropriate goal at this point is to continue the eating and activity behaviours that will maintain weight. Attempting to lose additional weight at this point would require major effort and would almost certainly meet with failure.

The prevalence of **successful weight-loss maintenance** is difficult to determine, in part because researchers have used different criteria. Some look at success after one year and others after five years; some quantify success as 5 or more kilograms lost and others as 5 or 10 percent of initial body weight lost. Furthermore, most research studies examine the success of one episode of weight loss in a structured program, but this scenario does not necessarily reflect the experiences of the general population. In reality, most people have lost weight several times in their lifetimes and did so on their own, not in a formal program. Almost 50 percent of people who intentionally lost weight have successfully maintained the loss for at least a year.[136]

Those who are successful in maintaining their weight loss have established moderately intense to vigorous exercise regimens and careful eating patterns, taking in

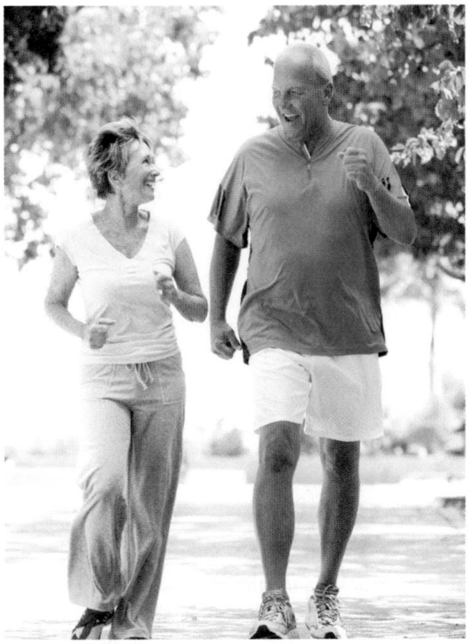

Monkey Business Images/shutterstock

Maintaining a healthy body weight requires maintaining the moderately intense to vigorous physical activities and careful eating habits that supported weight loss.

successful weight-loss maintenance: achieving a weight loss of at least 10 percent of initial body weight and maintaining the loss for at least one year.

less energy and a lower percentage of kcalories from fat than the national average. Because these people are more efficient at storing fat, they do not have the same flexibility in their food and activity habits as their friends who have never been overweight. With weight loss, metabolism shifts downward so that formerly overweight people require less energy than might be expected given their current body weight and body composition. This decrease in energy expenditure persists over time.[137] Consequently, to keep weight off, they must either eat less or exercise more than people the same size who have never been obese. Put simply, it takes more to prevent weight *regain* than to prevent weight gain.[138]

Physical activity plays a key role in maintaining weight loss. Those who engage in moderately intense or vigorous physical activities are far more successful than those who are inactive. Weight maintenance may require a person to expend at least 2500 kcalories in physical activity per week.[139] To accomplish this, a person might exercise either moderately (such as brisk walking at 6 kilometres [4 miles] per hour) for 60 minutes a day or vigorously (such as fast bicycling at 30 kilometres [18 miles] per hour) for 30 minutes a day, for example. Being ac-tive during both work hours and leisure time also helps a person to maintain weight loss.[140]

Dietary Guidance for Canadians

To sustain weight loss and minimize functional decline in adulthood, some people may need to engage in more than 150 minutes of moderate- to vigorous-intensity activity per week and strengthening activities more than twice a week while not exceeding their kcaloric intake requirements. It is advisable to consult with a health-care provider before participating in this level of activity.

In addition to limiting energy intake and exercising regularly, one other strategy helps with weight maintenance: frequent self-monitoring.[141] People who weigh themselves periodically and monitor their eating and exercise habits regularly can detect weight gains in the early stages and promptly initiate changes to prevent relapse.[142]

Losing weight and maintaining the loss may not be easy, but it is possible. Strategies of those who have been successful may differ in the details, but in general, most do the following:

- Eat a low-kcalorie diet (usually small portions four to five times a day).
- Eat a consistent diet day to day (simplicity helps to keep the focus).
- Eat breakfast (curbs hunger).
- Be very physically active (at least 60 minutes of moderate activity daily).
- Weigh frequently (take prompt action with small gains).
- Watch only a limited amount of television (less than 10 hours a week).
- Don't allow small weight gains to become large ones.

Importantly, people who are successful losing weight find that it gets easier with time—the changes in diet and activity patterns become permanent.[143]

Prevention Given the information presented up to this point in the chapter, the adage "An ounce of prevention is worth a pound of cure" seems particularly apropos. Preventing weight gain would benefit almost everybody.[144] Obesity is a major risk factor for numerous diseases, and losing weight is challenging and often temporary. Strategies for preventing weight gain ♦ are very similar to those for losing weight, with one exception: they begin early. Over the years, they become an integral part of a person's life. It is much easier for a person to resist doughnuts for breakfast if he rarely eats them. Similarly, a person will have little trouble walking each morning if she has always been active.

♦ To prevent weight gain:
- Eat regular meals and limit snacking.
- Drink water instead of high-kcalorie beverages.
- Select sensible portion sizes and limit daily energy intake to no more than energy expended.
- Become physically active and limit sedentary activities.

Dietary Guidance for Canadians

To prevent gradual weight gain over time, make small decreases in food and beverage kcalories and increase physical activity.

Public Health Programs Has anyone in the North America *not* heard the message that obesity raises the risks of chronic diseases and that overweight people should aim for a healthy weight by eating sensibly and becoming physically active? Not likely. Yet implementing such advice is difficult in an environment of abundant food and physical inactivity. To successfully treat obesity, we may have to change the environment in which we live through public health law.[145] Table 9-6 provides examples of public health strategies that have been suggested to improve the nutrition environment in the United States, many of which also apply in Canada.[146] Some of these strategies may seem radical, but dramatic measures may be needed if we are to curb the obesity epidemic that is sweeping across North America. Whether changes in public policy—such as a tax on sugared beverages and snack foods—will influence diet habits or simply generate revenues remains to be seen.[147] Clearly, effective strategies will need to reach beyond individuals to address social networks, community institutions, and government policies.[148]

IN SUMMARY **Preventing weight gains and maintaining weight losses require vigilant attention to diet and physical activity. Taking care of oneself is a lifelong responsibility.**

Underweight

Underweight ♦ is a far less prevalent problem than overweight, affecting no more than 2 percent of Canadian adults (review Figure 8-5 on p. 252). Whether the underweight person needs to gain weight is a question of health and, like weight loss, a highly individual matter. People who are healthy at their present weight may stay there; there are no compelling reasons to try to gain weight. Those who are thin because of malnourishment or illness, however, might benefit from a diet that supports weight gain. Medical advice can help make the distinction.

♦ **Underweight** is a body weight so low as to have adverse health effects; it is generally defined as BMI <18.5.

Thin people may find gaining weight difficult. Those who wish to gain weight for appearance's sake or to improve their athletic performance need to be aware that healthful weight gains can be achieved only by physical conditioning combined with high energy intakes. On a high-kcalorie diet alone, a person may gain weight, but it will be mostly fat. Even if the gain improves appearance, it can be detrimental to health and might impair athletic performance. Therefore, in weight gain, as in weight loss, physical activity and energy intake are essential components of a sound plan.

Problems of Underweight The causes of underweight may be as diverse as those of overweight—genetic tendencies, hunger, appetite, and satiety irregularities;

TABLE 9-6 Suggested Public Health Strategies

Strategies	Examples of Suggested Nutritional Strategies	Examples of Successful Nonnutritional Strategies
Impose safety standards to reduce the potential for harm.	• Regulate the energy or fat density of foods. • Regulate the size of packages of high-fat foods.	• Mandate safety glass in automobiles. • Regulate the lead content of paint.
Control commercial advertising to limit the influence of harmful products.	• Improve nutrition labelling and product packaging. • Restrict the promotion of high-fat foods (especially when directed at children).	• Restrict cigarette advertising (especially when directed at children). • Add health warnings to alcoholic beverages.
Control the conditions under which products are sold to limit exposure to hazardous substances.	• Remove high-fat, low-nutrient density foods from school vending machines. • Restrict the number of vendors licensed to sell high-fat foods.	• Mandate minimum-age laws for the use of tobacco, alcohol, and automobiles. • Restrict the number of vendors licensed to sell alcohol.
Control prices to reduce consumption.	• Tax soft drinks and other foods high in kcalories, fat, or sugar.	• Tax alcohol and tobacco.

SOURCES: Adapted from L. O. Gostin, Law as a tool to facilitate healthier lifestyles and prevent obesity, *Journal of the American Medical Association* 297 (2007): 87–90; M. Nestle and M. F. Jacobson, Halting the obesity epidemic: A public health policy approach, *Public Health Reports* 115 (2000): 12–24.

psychological traits; and metabolic factors. Habits learned early in childhood, especially food aversions, may perpetuate themselves.

The demand for energy to support physical activity and growth often contributes to underweight. An active, growing boy may need more than 4000 kcalories a day to maintain his weight and may be too busy to take time to eat adequately. Underweight people find it hard to gain weight due, in part, to their expenditure of energy in adaptive thermogenesis. So much energy may be expended adapting to a higher food intake that at first as many as 750 to 800 extra kcalories a day may be needed to gain a half a kilogram a week. Like those who want to lose weight, people who want to gain must learn new habits and learn to like new foods. They are also similarly vulnerable to potentially harmful schemes and would be wise to review the consumer bill of rights on p. 281, using "weight gain" instead of "weight loss" where appropriate.

As described in Highlight 8, the underweight condition anorexia nervosa sometimes develops in people who employ self-denial to control their weight. They go to such extremes that they become severely undernourished, achieving final body weights of 30 kilograms (70 pounds) or even less. One difference between a person with anorexia nervosa and other underweight people is that starvation is intentional. Another difference is the levels of hormones such as leptin and ghrelin.[149] (See Highlight 8 for a review of anorexia nervosa and other eating disorders.)

Weight-Gain Strategies

Adequacy and balance are the key diet-planning strategies for weight gain. Meals focus on energy-dense foods to provide many kcalories in a small volume and exercise to build muscle.

Energy-Dense Foods Energy-dense foods (the very ones eliminated from a successful weight-loss diet) hold the key to weight gain. Pick the highest-kcalorie items from each food group—that is, milk shakes instead of skim milk, salmon instead of snapper, avocados instead of cucumbers, a glass of grape juice instead of a small apple, and whole-wheat muffins instead of whole-wheat bread. Because fat provides more than twice as many kcalories per 5 millilitres as sugar does, fat adds kcalories without adding much bulk.

Although eating high-kcalorie, high-fat foods is not healthy for most people, it may be essential for an underweight individual who needs to gain weight. An underweight person who is physically active and eating a nutritionally adequate diet can afford a few extra kcalories from fat. For health's sake, it is wise to select foods with monounsaturated and polyunsaturated fats instead of those with saturated or *trans* fats: for example, sautéing vegetables in canola oil instead of butter or hydrogenated margarine.

Regular Meals Daily People who are underweight need to make meals a priority and take the time to plan, prepare, and eat each meal. They should eat at least three healthy meals every day. Another suggestion is to eat meaty appetizers or the main course first and leave the soup or salad until later.

Large Portions Underweight people need to learn to eat more food at each meal. For example, they can add extra slices of ham and cheese on a sandwich for lunch, drink milk from a larger glass, and eat cereal from a larger bowl.

The person should expect to feel full. Most underweight individuals are accustomed to small quantities of food. When they begin eating significantly more, they feel uncomfortable. This is normal and passes over time.

Extra Snacks Because a substantially higher energy intake is needed each day, in addition to eating more food at each meal, it is necessary to eat more frequently. Between-meal snacks do not interfere with later meals; they can readily lead to weight gains. For example, a student might make three sandwiches in the morning and eat them between classes in addition to the day's three regular meals. Snacking on dried fruit, nuts, and seeds is also an easy way to add kcalories.

Juice and Milk Beverages provide an easy way to increase energy intake. Consider that 1500 millilitres (6 cups) of cranberry juice add almost 1000 kcalories to the day's intake. kCalories can be added to milk by mixing in powdered milk or packets of instant breakfast.

For people who are underweight due to illness, concentrated liquid formulas are often recommended because a weak person can swallow them easily. A physician or registered dietitian can recommend high-protein, high-kcalorie formulas to help an underweight person maintain or gain weight. Used in addition to regular meals, these supplements can help considerably.

Exercising to Build Muscles To gain weight, use strength training primarily, and increase energy intake to support that exercise. Eating extra food will then support a gain of both muscle and fat. An additional 500 to 1000 kcalories a day above normal energy needs is enough to support the exercise as well as the building of muscle.[150]

IN SUMMARY **Both the incidence of underweight and the health problems associated with it are less prevalent than overweight and its associated problems. To gain weight, a person must train physically and increase energy intake by selecting energy-dense foods, eating regular meals, taking larger portions, and consuming extra snacks and beverages. Table 9-5 (p. 290) includes a summary of weight-gain strategies.**

Nutrition Portfolio

To enjoy good health and maintain a reasonable body weight, combine sensible eating habits and regular physical activity.

Go to Diet Analysis Plus and choose one of the days on which you have tracked your diet for the entire day. Go to the Energy Balance and Intake vs. Goals reports.

- Calculate your BMI and consider whether you need to lose or gain weight for the sake of good health. If you do need to gain or lose weight, do the Diet Analysis reports give you insight into why you may be overweight or underweight?
- Reflect on your weight over the past year or so and explain any weight gains or losses. Using the Intake vs. Goals report, can you identify areas in which you need to adjust your food intake, perhaps eating more or less?
- Describe the potential risks and possible benefits of fad diets and over-the-counter weight-loss drugs or herbal supplements.

Diet Analysis PLUS

To complete this exercise, go to your Diet Analysis Plus at www.cengage.com/sso.

Nutrition on the Net

CENGAGENOW™
For further study of topics covered in this chapter, log on to **www.cengage.com/sso.**

- Review the 2006 Canadian Clinical Practice Guidelines on the Management and Prevention of Obesity in Adults and Children: **www.cmaj.ca/cgi/content/full/176/8/S1/DC1**
- Use *Eating Well with Canada's Food Guide* and the *Canadian Physical Activity Guidelines* to help you achieve and maintain a healthy body weight. **www.hc-sc.gc.ca/fn-an/food-guide-aliment/index-eng.php and www.csep.ca**
- Visit weight-loss support groups, such as Take Off Pounds Sensibly (TOPS), Overeaters Anonymous (OA), and Weight Watchers: **www.tops.org, www.oa.org,** and **www.weightwatchers.ca**
- Learn about Canadian initiatives in obesity research at the Canadian Obesity Network: **www.obesitynetwork.ca**
- Learn about the 10,000 Steps Program from Shape Up America!: **www.shapeup.org**
- Find helpful information on achieving and maintaining a healthy weight from the Calorie Control Council: **www.caloriecontrol.org**

- Learn how to end size discrimination from the U.S. National Association to Advance Fat Acceptance: **www.naafa.org**
- Explore the Weight Management section of the U.S. government site: **www.nutrition.gov**
- Learn about weight control and the Weight-control Information Network (WIN) program: **www.win.niddk.nih.gov**

References

1. M. Tjepkema, Adult obesity in Canada: Measured height and weight, Statistics Canada Cat. No. 82-620-MWE2005001. www.statcan.gc.ca/pub/82-620-m/2005001/article/adults-adultes/8060-eng.htm, accessed August 18, 2010.
2. Public Health Agency of Canada, Obesity in Canada–Snapshot, 2009. www.phac-aspc.gc.ca/publicat/2009/oc/index-eng.php#tot, accessed August 18, 2010.
3. A. H. Anis and coauthors, Obesity and overweight in Canada: An updated cost-of-illness study, *Obesity Reviews* 11 (2010): 31–40.
4. M. Shields, Overweight Canadian children and adolescents, 2006. www.statcan.gc.ca/pub/82-620-m/2005001/article/child-enfant/8061-eng.htm, accessed August 18, 2010.
5. P. Hossain, B. Kawar, and M. El Nahas, Obesity and diabetes in the developing world—A growing challenge, *New England Journal of Medicine* 356 (2007): 213–215.
6. A. McCarthy and coauthors, Birth weight; postnatal, infant, and childhood growth; and obesity in young adulthood: Evidence from the Barry Caerphilly Growth Study, *American Journal of Clinical Nutrition* 86 (2007): 907–913.
7. C. Nelson-Dooley and coauthors, Novel treatments for obesity and osteoporosis: Targeting apoptotic pathways in adipocytes, *Current Medicinal Chemistry* 12 (2005): 2215–2225.
8. P. Angulo, Obesity and nonalcoholic fatty liver disease, *Nutrition Reviews* 65 (2007): S57–S63; E. Yan and coauthors, Nonalcoholic fatty liver disease: Pathogenesis, identification, progression, and management, *Nutrition Reviews* 65 (2007): 376–384.
9. W. L. Holland and coauthors, Lipid mediators of insulin resistance, *Nutrition Reviews* 65 (2007): S39–S46; R. Weiss, Fat distribution and storage: How much, where, and how? *European Journal of Endocrinology* 157 (2007): S39–S45.
10. S. B. Votruba and M. D. Jensen, Sex differences in abdominal, gluteal, and thigh LPL activity, *American Journal of Physiology: Endocrinology and Metabolism* 292 (2007): E1823–E1828.
11. M. Patalay and coauthors, The lowering of plasma lipids following a weight reduction program is related to increased expression of the LDL receptor and lipoprotein lipase, *Journal of Nutrition* 135 (2007): 735–739.
12. K. R. Westerterp and coauthors, Dietary fat oxidation as a function of body fat, *American Journal of Clinical Nutrition* 87 (2008): 132–135.
13. G. C. Major and coauthors, Clinical significance of adaptive thermogenesis, *International Journal of Obesity* 31 (2007): 204–212.
14. T. Agurs-Collins and C. Bouchard, Gene-nutrition and gene-physical activity interactions in the etiology of obesity, *Obesity* 16 (2008): S2–S4.
15. R. A. Waterland, Epigenetic epidemiology of obesity: Application of epigenomic technology, *Nutrition Reviews* 66 (2008): S21–S23.
16. J. Wardle and coauthors, Evidence for a strong genetic influence on childhood adiposity despite the force of the obesogenic environment, *American Journal of Clinical Nutrition* 87 (2008): 398–404.
17. C. M. Lindgren and M. I. McCarthy, Mechanisms of disease: Genetic insights into the etiology of type 2 diabetes and obesity, *Nature Clinical Practice. Endocrinology & Metabolism* 4 (2008): 156–163.
18. A. Newell and coauthors, Addressing the obesity epidemic: A genomics perspective, *Preventing Chronic Disease* 4 (2007): 1–6; R. J. F. Loos and T. Rankinen, Gene-diet interactions on body weight changes, *Journal of the American Dietetic Association* 105 (2005): S29–S34; S. Tholin and coauthors, Genetic and environmental influences on eating behavior: The Swedish Young Male Twins Study, *American Journal of Clinical Nutrition* 81 (2005): 564–569.
19. J. M. McCaffery and coauthors, Gene x environment interaction of vigorous exercise and body mass index among male Vietnam-era twins, *American Journal of Clinical Nutrition* 89 (2009): 1011–1018.
20. T. Rankinen and C. Bouchard, Genetics of food intake and eating behavior phenotypes in humans, *Annual Review of Nutrition* 26 (2006): 413–434; H. N. Lyon and J. N. Hirschhorn, Genetics of common forms of obesity: A brief overview, *American Journal of Clinical Nutrition* 82 (2005): 215S–217S.
21. R. J. Loos and C. Bouchard, FTO: The first gene contributing to common forms of human obesity, *Obesity Reviews* 9 (2008): 246–250; N. J. Timpson and coauthors, The fat mass- and obesity-associated locus and dietary intake in children, *American Journal of Clinical Nutrition* 88 (2008): 971–978; A. Körner and coauthors, Polygenic contribution to obesity: Genome-wide strategies reveal new targets, *Frontiers of Hormone Research* 36 (2008): 12–36; R. L. Leibel, Energy in, energy out, and the effects of obesity-related genes, *New England Journal of Medicine* (2008): 2603–2604; C. L. Saunders and coauthors, Meta-analysis of genome-wide linkage studies in BMI and obesity, *Obesity* (2007): 2263–2275.
22. M. Rosenbaum and coauthors, Leptin reverses weight loss—Induced changes in regional neural activity responses to visual food stimuli, *Journal of Clinical Investigation* 118 (2008): 2583–2591; I. S. Farooqi and coauthors, Leptin regulates striatal regions and human eating behavior, *Science* 317 (2007): 1355.
23. P. G. Cammisotto and M. Bendayan, Leptin secretion by white adipose tissue and gastric mucosa, *Histology and Histopathology* 22 (2007): 199–210.
24. I. S. Farooqi and coauthors, Clinical and molecular genetic spectrum of congenital deficiency of the leptin receptor, *New England Journal of Medicine* 356 (2007): 237–247.
25. C. E. Ruhl and coauthors, Body mass index and serum leptin concentration independently estimate percentage body fat in older adults, *American Journal of Clinical Nutrition* 85 (2007): 1121–1126; V. Monti and coauthors, Relationship of ghrelin and leptin hormones with body mass index and waist circumference in a random sample of adults, *Journal of the American Dietetic Association* 106 (2006): 822–828.
26. M. G. Myers, M. A. Cowley, and H. Münzberg, Mechanisms of leptin action and leptin resistance, *Annual Review of Physiology* 70 (2008): 537–556; P. J. Enriori and coauthors, Leptin resistance and obesity, *Obesity* (2006): 254S–258S.
27. A. Shapiro and coauthors, Fructose-induced leptin resistance exacerbates weight gain in response to subsequent high fat feeding, *American Journal of Physiology. Regulatory, Integrative and Comparative Physiology* 295 (2008): R1370–R1375.
28. J. Beltowski, A. Jamroz-Wisniewska, and S. Widomska, Adiponectin and its role in cardiovascular disease, *Cardiovascular & Hematological Disorders Drug Targets* 8 (2008): 7–46.
29. G. Wolf, New insights into thiol-mediated regulation of adiponectin secretion, *Nutrition Reviews* 66 (2008): 642–645; M. Garaulet and coauthors, Adiponectin, the controversial hormone, *Public Health Nutrition* 10 (2007): 1145–1150; Y. Takemura, K. Walsh, and N. Ouchi, Adiponectin and cardiovascular inflammatory responses, *Current Atherosclerosis Report* 9 (2007): 238–243.
30. M. Guerre-Millo, Adiponectin: An update, *Diabetes & Metabolism* 34 (2008): 12–18.
31. V. Popovic and L. H. Duntas, Brain somatic cross-talk: Ghrelin, leptin, and ultimate challengers of obesity, *Nutritional Neuroscience* 8 (2005): 1–5.

32. D. E. Cummings, K. E. Foster-Schubert, and J. Overduin, Ghrelin and energy balance: Focus on current controversies, *Current Drug Targets* 6 (2005): 153–169.
33. Cummings, Foster-Schubert, and Overduin, 2005.
34. Monti and coauthors, 2006.
35. Cummings, Foster-Schubert, and Overduin, 2005.
36. D. R. Broom and coauthors, Exercise induced suppression of acylated ghrelin in humans, *Journal of Applied Physiology* 102 (2007): 2165–2171; Cummings, Foster-Schubert, and Overduin, 2005.
37. N. D. Kohatsu and coauthors, Sleep duration and body mass index in rural population, *Archives of Internal Medicine* 166 (2006): 1701–1705; S. R. Patel and coauthors, Association between reduced sleep and weight gain in women, *American Journal of Epidemiology* 164 (2006): 947–954; R. D. Verona and coauthors, Overweight and obese patients in a primary care population report less sleep than patients with a normal body mass index, *Archives of Internal Medicine* 165 (2005): 25–34.
38. P. Hamet and J. Tremblay, Genetics of sleep-wake cycles and its disorders, *Metabolism* 55 (2006): S7–S12.
39. J. Orr and B. Davy, Dietary influences on peripheral hormones regulating energy intake: Potential applications for weight management, *Journal of the American Dietetic Association* 105 (2005): 1115–1124.
40. S. Enerbäck, The origins of brown adipose tissue, *New England Journal of Medicine* 360 (2009): 2021–2023; A. S. Avram, M. M. Avram, and W. D. James, Subcutaneous fat in normal and diseased states: 2. Anatomy and physiology of white and brown adipose tissue, *Journal of the American Academy of Dermatology* 53 (2005): 671–673
41. J. S. Kim-Han and L. L. Dugan, Mitochondrial uncoupling proteins in the central nervous system, *Antioxidants and Redox Signaling* 7 (2005): 1173–1181; R. J. F. Roos and T. Rankinen, Gene-diet interactions on body weight changes, *Journal of the American Dietetic Association* 105 (2005): S29–S34; P. Trayhurn, The biology of obesity, *Proceedings of the Nutrition Society* 64 (2005): 31–38.
42. M. Harper, K. Green, and M. D. Brand, The efficiency of cellular energy transduction and its implications for obesity, *Annual Review of Nutrition* 28 (2008): 13–33.
43. P. Laurberg, S. Andersen, and J. Karmisholt, Cold adaptation and thyroid hormone metabolism, *Hormone and Metabolic Research* 37 (2005): 545–549.
44. Avram, Avram, and James, 2005.
45. W. D. van Marken Lichtenbelt and coauthors, Cold-activated brown adipose tissue in healthy men, *New England Journal of Medicine* 360 (2009): 1500–1508.
46. A. M. Cypess and coauthors, Identification and importance of brown adipose tissue in adult humans, *New England Journal of Medicine* 360 (2009): 1509–1517.
47. K. A. Virtanen and coauthors, Functional brown adipose tissue in healthy adults, *New England Journal of Medicine* 360 (2009): 1518–1525.
48. L. Qi and Y. A. Cho, Gene-environment interaction and obesity, *Nutrition Reviews* 66 (2008): 684–694.
49. W. P. James, The fundamental drivers of the obesity epidemic, *Obesity Reviews* 9 (2008): S6–S13.
50. I. Romao and J. Roth, Genetic and environmental interactions in obesity and type 2 diabetes, *Journal of the American Dietetic Association* 108 (2008): S24–S28.
51. N. A. Christakis and J. H. Fowler, The spread of obesity in a large social network over 32 years, *New England Journal of Medicine* 357 (2007): 370–379.
52. J. M. Abbot and coauthors, Psychosocial and behavioral profile and predictors of self-reported energy underreporting in obese middle-aged women, *Journal of the American Dietetic Association* 108 (2008): 114–119; A. Amend and coauthors, Validation of dietary intake data in black women with type 2 diabetes, *Journal of the American Dietetic Association* 107 (2007): 112–117; R. L. Bailey and coauthors, Assessing the effect of underreporting energy intake on dietary patterns and weight status, *Journal of the American Dietetic Association* 107 (2007): 64–71; S. Hendrickson and R. Mattes, Financial incentive for diet recall accuracy does not affect reported energy intake or number of underreporters in a sample of overweight females, *Journal of the American Dietetic Association* 107 (2007): 118–121; J. Maurer and coauthors, The psychological and behavioral characteristics related to energy misreporting, *Nutrition Reviews* 64 (2006): 53–66.
53. R. N. Close and D. A. Schoeller, The financial reality of overeating, *Journal of the American College of Nutrition* 25 (2006): 203–209.
54. B. Wansink and J. Kim, Bad popcorn in big buckets: Portion size can influence intake as much as taste, *Journal of Nutrition Education and Behavior* 37 (2005): 242–245.
55. L. Johnson and coauthors, Energy-dense, low-fiber, high-fat dietary pattern is associated with increased fatness in childhood, *American Journal of Clinical Nutrition* 87 (2008): 846–854; N. C. Howarth and coauthors, Dietary energy density is associated with overweight status among 5 ethnic groups in the Multiethnic Cohort Study, *Journal of Nutrition* 136 (2006): 2243–2248.
56. B. J. Rolls, L. S. Roe, and J. S. Meengs, Reductions in portion size and energy density of foods are additive and lead to sustained decreases in energy intake, *American Journal of Clinical Nutrition* 83 (2006): 11–17.
57. L. H. Epstein and coauthors, Price and maternal obesity influence purchasing of low- and high-energy-dense foods, *American Journal of Clinical Nutrition* 86 (2007): 914–922; P. Monsivais and A. Drewnowski, The rising cost of low-energy-density foods, *Journal of the American Dietetic Association* 107 (2007): 2071–2076; A. Drewnowski and N. Darmon, The economics of obesity: Dietary energy density and energy cost, *American Journal of Clinical Nutrition* 82 (2005): 265S–273S.
58. D. S. Ludwig and M. Nestle, Can the food industry play a constructive role in the obesity epidemic? *Journal of the American Medical Association* 300 (2008): 1808–1811.
59. M. Condrasky and coauthors, Chefs' opinions of restaurant portion sizes, *Obesity* (2007): 2086–2094.
60. J. L. Black and J. Macinko, Neighborhoods and obesity, *Nutrition Reviews* 66 (2008): 2–20; M. C. Nelson and coauthors, Built and social environments: Associations with adolescent overweight and activity, *American Journal of Prevention Medicine* 31 (2006): 109–117; K. M. Booth, M. M. Pinkston, and W.S.C. Poston, Obesity and the built environment, *Journal of the American Dietetic Association* 105 (2005): S110–S117.
61. D. E. R. Warburton and coauthors, Evidence-informed physical activity guidelines for Canadian adults, *Applied Physiology, Nutrition, and Metabolism* 32 (2007): S16–S68.
62. J. A. Levine and coauthors, Non-exercise activity thermogenesis: The Crouching Tiger Hidden Dragon of society weight gain, *Arteriosclerosis, Thrombosis, and Vascular Biology* 26 (2006): 729–736; J. A. Levine and coauthors, Interindividual variation in posture allocation: Possible role in human obesity, *Science* 307 (2005): 584–586.
63. J. A. Teske, C. J. Billington, and C. M. Kotz, Neuropeptidergic mediators of spontaneous physical activity and non-exercise activity thermogenesis, *Neuroendocrinology* 87 (2008): 71–90.
64. J. A. Levine, Nonexercise activity thermogenesis—Liberating the life-force, *Journal of Internal Medicine* 262 (2007): 273–287; M. Marra and coauthors, BMR variability in women of different weight, *Clinical Nutrition* 26 (2007): 567–572.
65. Nielsen Global Online Survey, Diet and healthy eating: A Canadian perspective (2009). http://ca.nielsen.com/content/dam/nielsen/en_ca/documents/pdf/reports/DietandHealthyEating_English.pdf, accessed September 8, 2011; American on the move: Steps to a healthier way of life, press release, September 10, 2007.
66. R. F. Kushner and D. J. Blatner, Risk assessment of the overweight and obese patient, *Journal of the American Dietetic Association* 105 (2005): S53–S62; National Institutes of Health Obesity Education Initiative, *The Practical Guide: Identification, Evaluation, and Treatment of Overweight and Obesity in Adults,* NIH publication no. 00-4084 (Washington, D.C.: U.S. Department of Health and Human Services, 2000).
67. National Institutes of Health Obesity Education Initiative, 2000.
68. Ethics opinion: Weight loss products and medications, *Journal of the American Dietetic Association* 108 (2008): 2109–2113; H. M. Blanck and coauthors, Use of nonprescription dietary supplements for weight loss is common among Americans, *Journal of the American Dietetic Association* 107 (2007): 441–447.
69. J. T. Dwyer, D. B. Allison, and P. M. Coates, Dietary supplements in weight reduction, *Journal of the American Dietetic Association* 105 (2005): S80–S86.
70. R. F. Kushner, Anti-obesity drugs, *Expert Opinion on Pharmacotherapy* 9 (2008): 1339–1350.

71. D. Rucker and coauthors, Long-term pharmacotherapy for obesity and overweight: Updated meta-analysis, *British Medical Journal* 335 (2007): 1194–1199.
72. R. H. Eckel, Nonsurgical management of obesity in adults, *New England Journal of Medicine* 358 (2008): 1941–1950.
73. S. B. Moyers, Medications as adjunct therapy for weight loss: Approved and off-label agents in use, *Journal of the American Dietetic Association* 105 (2005): 948–959.
74. E. J. DeMaria, Bariatric surgery for morbid obesity, *New England Journal of Medicine* 356 (2007): 2176–2183.
75. Cummings, Foster-Schubert, and Overduin, 2005.
76. L. Sjöström and coauthors, Effects of bariatric surgery on mortality in Swedish obese subjects, *New England Journal of Medicine* 357 (2007): 741–752; G. L. Blackburn, Solutions in weight control: Lessons from gastric surgery, *American Journal of Clinical Nutrition* 82 (2005): 248S–252S.
77. J. B. Dixon and coauthors, Adjustable gastric banding and conventional therapy for type 2 diabetes: A randomized controlled trial, *Journal of the American Medical Association* 299 (2008): 316–323; E. N. Hansen, A. Torquati, and N. N. Abumrad, Results of bariatric surgery, *Annual Review of Nutrition* 26 (2006): 481–511.
78. S. Singh and A. Kumar, Wernicke encephalopathy after obesity surgery, *Neurology* 68 (2007): 807–811; M. Shah, V. Simha, and A. Garg, Long-term impact of bariatric surgery on body weight, co-morbidities, and nutritional status: A review, *Journal of Clinical Endocrinology and Metabolism* 91 (2006): 4223–4231.
79. J. A. Vogel and coauthors, Reduction in predicted coronary heart disease risk after substantial weight reduction after bariatric surgery, *American Journal of Cardiology* 99 (2007): 222–226; Hansen, Torquati, and Abumrad, 2006.
80. T. D. Adams and coauthors, Long-term mortality after gastric bypass surgery, *New England Journal of Medicine* 357 (2007): 753–761; Sjöström and coauthors, 2007.
81. Hansen, Torquati, and Abumrad, 2006.
82. C. A. Nonas and G. D. Foster, Setting achievable goals for weight loss, *Journal of the American Dietetic Association* 105 (2005): S118–S123.
83. D. R. Jacobs and coauthors, Association of 1-y changes in diet pattern with cardiovascular disease risk factors and adipokines: Results from the 1-y randomized Oslo Diet and Exercise Study, *American Journal of Clinical Nutrition* 89 (2009): 509–517; M. L. Fernandez, The metabolic syndrome, *Nutrition Reviews* 65 (2007): S30–S34; C. Galani and H. Schneider, Prevention and treatment of obesity with lifestyle interventions: Review and meta-analysis, *International Journal of Public Health* 52 (2007): 348–359.
84. G. D. Foster and coauthors, Obese patients' perceptions of treatment outcomes and the factors that influence them, *Archives of Internal Medicine* 161 (2001): 2133–2139.
85. National Institutes of Health Obesity Education Initiative, 2000, p. 2.
86. Position of the American Dietetic Association: Weight management, *Journal of the American Dietetic Association* 109 (2009): 330–346.
87. National Institutes of Health Obesity Education Initiative, 2000, pp. 26–27.
88. M. T. Timlin and coauthors, Breakfast eating and weight change in a 5-year prospective analysis of adolescents: Project EAT (Eating Among Teens), *Pediatrics* 121 (2008): e638; M. T. Timlin and M. A. Pereira, Breakfast frequency and quality in the etiology of adult obesity and chronic diseases, *Nutrition Reviews* 65 (2007): 268–281.
89. A. K. Kant and coauthors, Association of breakfast energy density with diet quality and body mass index in American adults: National Health and Nutrition Examination Surveys, 1999–2004, *American Journal of Clinical Nutrition* 88 (2008): 1396–1404.
90. M. Bulló and coauthors, Inflammation, obesity and comorbidities: The role of diet, *Public Health Nutrition* 10 (2007): 1164–1172.
91. J. T. Dwyer, D. B. Allison, and P. M. Coates, Dietary supplements in weight reduction, *Journal of the American Dietetic Association* 105 (2005): S80–S86.
92. Position of the American Dietetic Association, 2009.
93. B. J. Rolls, L. S. Roe, and J. S. Meengs, The effect of large portion sizes on energy intake is sustained for 11 days, *Obesity* 15 (2007): 1535–1543; Wansink and Kim, 2005.
94. M. P. Mattson, Energy intake, meal frequency, and health: A neurobiological perspective, *Annual Review of Nutrition* 25 (2005): 237–260.
95. K. E. Leahy, L. L. Birch, and B. J. Rolls, Reducing the energy density of multiple meals decreases the energy intake of preschool-age children, *American Journal of Clinical Nutrition* 88 (2008): 1459–1468; J. A. Ello-Martin and coauthors, Dietary energy density in the treatment of obesity: A year-long trial comparing 2 weight-loss diets, *American Journal of Clinical Nutrition* 85 (2007): 1465–1477; M. J. Franz and coauthors, Weight-loss outcomes: A systematic review and meta-analysis of weight-loss clinical trials with a minimum 1-year follow-up, *Journal of the American Dietetic Association* 107 (2007): 1755–1767; J. H. Ledikwe, J. A. Ello-Martin, and B. J. Rolls, Portion sizes and the obesity epidemic, *Journal of Nutrition* 135 (2005): 905–909; J. A. Ello-Martin, J. H. Ledikwe, and B. J. Rolls, The influence of food portion size and energy density on energy intake: Implications for weight management, *American Journal of Clinical Nutrition* 82 (2005): 236S–241S.
96. B. J. Rolls, A. Drewnowski, and J. H. Ledikwe, Changing the energy density of the diet as a strategy for weight management, *Journal of the American Dietetic Association* 105 (2005): S98–S103.
97. J. H. Ledikwe and coauthors, Reductions in dietary energy density are associated with weight loss in overweight and obese participants in the PREMIER trial, *American Journal of Clinical Nutrition* 85 (2007): 1212–1221; J. H. Ledikwe and coauthors, Low-energy-density diets are associated with high diet quality in adults in the United States, *Journal of the American Dietetic Association* 106 (2006): 1172–1180.
98. P. Monsivais and A. Drewnowski, The rising cost of low-energy-density foods, *Journal of the American Dietetic Association* 107 (2007): 2071–2076.
99. J. E. Flood and B. J. Rolls, Soup preloads in a variety of forms reduce meal energy intake, *Appetite* 49 (2007): 626–634.
100. B. M. Davy and coauthors, Water consumption reduces energy intake at a breakfast meal in obese older adults, *Journal of the American Dietetic Association* 108 (2008): 1236–1239; E. L. Van Walleghen and coauthors, Pre-meal water consumption reduces meal energy intake in older but not younger subjects, *Obesity* 15 (2007): 93–99.
101. J. E. Flood and coauthors, The effect of increased beverage portion size on energy intake at a meal, *Journal of the American Dietetic Association* 106 (2006): 1984–1990.
102. B. M. Popkin and coauthors, A new proposed guidance system for beverage consumption in the United States, *American Journal of Clinical Nutrition* 83 (2006): 529–542.
103. A. M. Andrade and coauthors, Eating slowly led to decreases in energy intake within meals in healthy women, *Journal of the American Dietetic Association* 108 (2008): 1186–1191.
104. E. Stice and coauthors, Relation between obesity and blunted striatal response to food is moderated by *TaqIA* A1 allele, *Science* 322 (2008): 449–452.
105. C. H. Llewellyn and coauthors, Eating rate is a heritable phenotype related to weight in children, *American Journal of Clinical Nutrition* 88 (2008): 1560–1566.
106. F. Bellisle and A. Drewnowski, Intense sweeteners, energy intake and the control of body weight, *European Journal of Clinical Nutrition* 61 (2007): 691–700; P. Monsivais, M. M. Perrigue, and A. Drewnowski, Sugars and satiety: Does the type of sweetener make a difference? *American Journal of Clinical Nutrition* 86 (2007): 116–123.
107. Bellisle and Drewnowski, 2007.
108. J. M. Jakicic and A. D. Otto, Treatment and prevention of obesity: What is the role of exercise? *Nutrition Reviews* 64 (2006): S57–S61.
109. Canadian Society for Exercise Physiology, *Canadian Physical Activity Guidelines for Adults 18 to 64 years* (2010). www.csep.ca/english/view.asp?x=804, accessed September 8, 2011.
110. S. J. Elder and S. B. Roberts, The effects of exercise on food intake and body fatness: A summary of published studies, *Nutrition Reviews* 65 (2007): 1–19.
111. J. Kruger, M. M. Yore, and H. W. Kohl, III, Leisure-time physical activity patterns by weight control status: 1999-2002 NHANES, *Medicine & Science in Sports & Exercise* 39 (2007): 788–795.
112. Committee on Dietary Reference Intakes, *Dietary Reference Intakes for Energy, Carbohydrate, Fiber, Fat, Fatty Acids, Cholesterol, Pro-tein, and Amino Acids* (Washington, D.C.: National Academies Press, 2005).
113. L. L. Frank and coauthors, Effects of exercise on metabolic risk variables in overweight postmenopausal women: A randomized clinical trial, *Obesity Research* 13 (2005): 615–625.

114. K. Ohkawara and coauthors, Twenty-four-hour analysis of elevated energy expenditure after physical activity in a metabolic chamber: Models of daily total energy expenditure, *American Journal of Clinical Nutrition* 87 (2008): 1268–1276.
115. K. H. Schmitz and coauthors, Strength training and adiposity in premenopausal women: Strong, Healthy, and Empowered study, *American Journal of Clinical Nutrition* 86 (2007): 566–572.
116. S. J. Elder and S. B. Roberts, The effects of exercise on food intake and body fatness: A summary of published studies, *Nutrition Reviews* 65 (2007): 1–19.
117. H. R. Wyatt and coauthors, A Colorado statewide survey of walking and its relation to excessive weight, *Medicine and Science in Sports and Exercise* 37 (2005): 724–730.
118. D. M. Bravata and coauthors, Using pedometers to increase physical activity and improve health: A systematic review, *Journal of the American Medical Association* 298 (2007): 2296–2304.
119. B. J. Nicklas and coauthors, Effect of exercise intensity on abdominal fat loss during calorie restriction in overweight and obese postmenopausal women: A randomized, controlled trial, *American Journal of Clinical Nutrition* 89 (2009): 1043–1052.
120. B. Wansink, J. E. Painter, and Y. K. Lee, The office candy dish: Proximity's influence on estimated and actual consumption, *International Journal of Obesity* 30 (2006): 871–875.
121. P. Pliner and coauthors, Meal duration mediates the effect of "social facilitation" on eating in humans, *Appetite* 46 (2006): 189–198.
122. J. M. Poothullil, Recognition of oral sensory satisfaction and regulation of the volume of intake in humans, *Nutritional Neuroscience* 8 (2005): 245–250.
123. Wansink, Painter, and Lee, 2006.
124. M. M. Hetherington and coauthors, Understanding variety: Tasting different foods delays satiation, *Physiology and Behavior* 87 (2006): 263–271.
125. B. Wansink, J. E. Painter, and J. North, Bottomless bowls: Why visual cues of portion size may influence intake, *Obesity Research* 13 (2005): 93–100.
126. B. Wansink and M. M. Cheney, Super bowls: Serving bowl size and food consumption, *Journal of the American Medical Association* 293 (2005): 1727–1728.
127. B. Wansink, K. van Ittersum, and J. E. Painter, Ice cream illusions bowls, spoons, and self-served portion sizes, *American Journal of Preventive Medicine* 31 (2006): 240–243.
128. B. Wansink and K. van Ittersum, Shape of glass and amount of alcohol poured: Comparative study of effect of practice and concentration, *British Medical Journal* 331 (2005): 1512–1514.
129. B. J. Rolls and coauthors, Using a smaller plate did not reduce energy intake at meals, *Appetite* 49 (2007): 652–660.
130. J. W. Anderson, S. B. Conley, and A. S. Nicholas, One hundred-pound weight losses with an intensive behavioral program: Changes in risk factors in 118 patients with long-term follow-up, *American Journal of Clinical Nutrition* 86 (2007): 301–307.
131. L. A. Berkel and coauthors, Behavioral interventions for obesity, *Journal of the American Dietetic Association* 105 (2005): S35–S43; G. D. Foster, A. P. Makris, and B. A. Bailer, Behavioral treatment of obesity, *American Journal of Clinical Nutrition* 82 (2005): 230S–235S.
132. D. J. Hyman and coauthors, Simultaneous vs sequential counseling for multiple behavior change, *Archives of Internal Medicine* 167 (2007): 1152–1158.
133. K. G. Volpp and coauthors, Financial incentive-based approaches for weight loss: A randomized trial, *Journal of the American Medical Association* 300 (2008): 2631–2637.
134. A. N. Fabricatore, Behavior therapy and cognitive-behavioral therapy of obesity: Is there a difference? *Journal of the American Dietetic Association* 107 (2007): 92–99.
135. L. P. Svetkey and coauthors, Comparison of strategies for sustaining weight loss: The weight loss maintenance randomized controlled trial, *Journal of the American Medical Association* 299 (2008): 1139–1148.
136. G. L. Blackburn, and B. A. Waltman, Expanding the limits of treatment: New strategic initiatives, *Journal of the American Dietetic Association* 105 (2005): S131–S135.
137. M. Rosenbaum and coauthors, Long-term persistence of adaptive thermogenesis in subjects who have maintained a reduced body weight, *American Journal of Clinical Nutrition* 88 (2008): 906–912.
138. S. Phelan and coauthors, Empirical evaluation of physical activity recommendations for weight control in women, *Medicine & Science in Sports & Exercise* 39 (2007): 1832–1836.
139. V. A. Catenacci and coauthors, Physical activity patterns in the National Weight Control Registry, *Obesity* 16 (2008): 153–161; D. F. Tate and coauthors, Long-term weight losses associated with prescription of higher physical activity goals. Are higher levels of physical activity protective against weight regain? *American Journal of Clinical Nutrition* 85 (2007): 954–959.
140. E. C. Weiss and coauthors, Weight regain in U.S. adults who experienced substantial weight loss, 1999–2002, *American Journal of Preventive Medicine* 33 (2007): 34–40; D. A. Raynor and coauthors, Television viewing and long-term weight maintenance: Results from the National Weight Control Registry, *Obesity* 14 (2006): 1816–1824.
141. D. L. Helsel, J. M. Jakicic, and A. D. Otto, Comparison of techniques for self-monitoring eating and exercise behaviors on weight loss in a correspondence-based intervention, *Journal of the American Diet Association* 107 (2007): 1807–1810; L. F. Tinker and coauthors, Predictors of dietary change and maintenance in the Women's Health Initiative Dietary Modification Trial, *Journal of the American Dietetic Association* 107 (2007): 1155–1165.
142. R. R. Wing and coauthors, A self-regulation program for maintenance of weight loss, *New England Journal of Medicine* 355 (2006): 1563–1571.
143. R. R. Wing and S. Phelan, Long-term weight loss maintenance, *American Journal of Clinical Nutrition* 82 (2005): 222S–225S.
144. J. O. Hill, H. Thompson, and H. Wyatt, Weight maintenance: What's missing? *Journal of the American Dietetic Association* 105 (2005): S63–S66.
145. W. P. James, The epidemiology of obesity: The size of the problem, *Journal of Internal Medicine* 263 (2008): 336–352; L. O. Gostin, Law as a tool to facilitate healthier lifestyles and prevent obesity, *Journal of the American Medical Association* 297 (2007): 87–90; M. M. Mello, D. M. Studdert, and T. A. Brennan, Obesity: The new frontier of public health law, *New England Journal of Medicine* 354 (2006): 2601–2610.
146. Gostin, 2007.
147. K. D. Brownell and T. R. Frieden, Ounces of prevention—The public policy case for taxes on sugared beverages, *New England Journal of Medicine* 360 (2009): 1805–1808; F. Kuchler, A. Tegene, and J. M. Harris, Taxing snack foods: What to expect for diet and tax revenues, *Current Issues in Economics of Food Markets,* Agriculture Information Bulletin No. 747–08, August 2004.
148. T. T. Huang and T. A. Glass, Transforming research strategies for understanding and preventing obesity, *Journal of the American Medical Association* 300 (2008): 1811–1813.
149. N. Germain and coauthors, Constitutional thinness and lean anorexia nervosa display opposite concentrations of peptide YY, glucagon-like peptide 1, ghrelin, and leptin, *American Journal of Clinical Nutrition* 85 (2007): 967–971.
150. Position Paper: Nutrition and athletic performance: Position of the American Dietetic Association, Dietitians of Canada, and the American College of Sports Medicine, *Journal of the American Dietetic Association* 100 (2000): 1543–1556.

The Latest and Greatest Weight-Loss Diet—Again

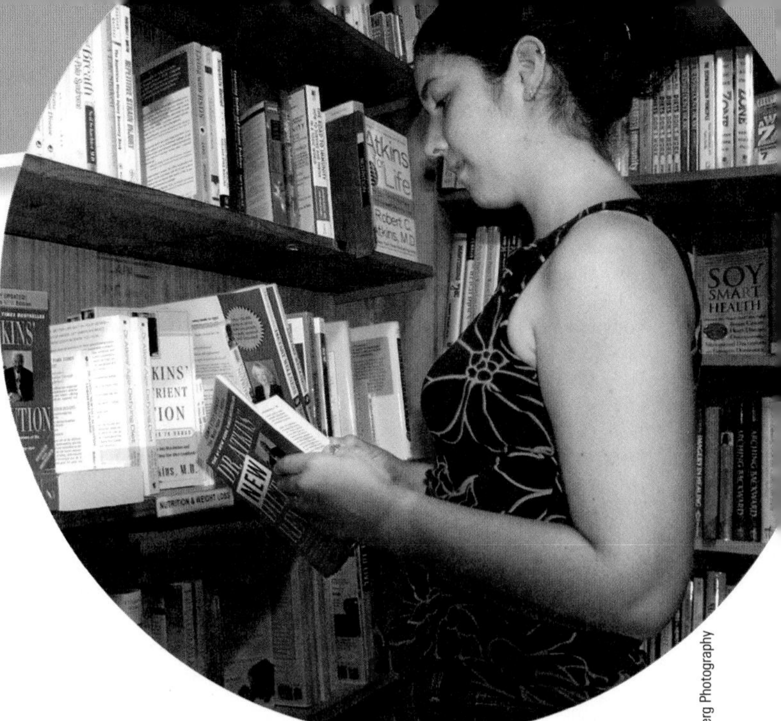
Atkins
SOY SMART HEALTH
© Geri Engberg Photography

To paraphrase William Shakespeare, "a fad diet by any other name would still be a fad diet." And the names are legion: the Atkins Diet, the Calories Don't Count Diet, the Cheater's Diet, the South Beach Diet, the Zone Diet.* Year after year, "new and improved" diets appear on bookstore shelves and circulate among friends. People of all sizes eagerly try the best diet on the market ever, hoping that this one will really work. Sometimes these diets seem to work for a while, but more often than not, their success is short-lived. Then another diet takes the spotlight. Here's how Dr. K. Brownell, an obesity researcher at Yale University, describes this phenomenon: "When I get calls about the latest diet fad, I imagine a trick birthday cake candle that keeps lighting up and we have to keep blowing it out."

Realizing that fad diets do not offer a safe and effective long-term plan for weight loss, health professionals speak out, but they never get the candle blown out permanently. New fad diets can keep making outrageous claims because no one requires their advocates to prove what they say. Fad diet gurus do not have to conduct credible research on the benefits or dangers of their diets. They can simply make recommendations and then later, if questioned, search for bits and pieces of research that support the conclusions they have already reached. That's backward. Diet and health recommendations should *follow* years of sound scientific research *before* being offered to the public.

Because anyone can publish anything—in books or on the Internet—peddlers of fad diets can make unsubstantiated statements that fall far short of the truth but sound impressive to the uninformed. They often offer distorted bits of legitimate research. They may start with one or more actual facts but then leap from one erroneous conclusion to the next. Anyone who wants to believe these claims has to wonder how the thousands of scientists working on obesity research over the past century could possibly have missed such obvious connections. Table H9-1 presents some of the claims and truths of fad diets.

*The following sources offer comparisons and evaluations of various fad diets for your review: New diet winners, *Consumer Reports,* June 2007, pp. 12–17; Battle of the diet books II, *Nutrition Action Healthletter,* July/August 2006, pp. 10–11; B. Liebman, Weighing the diet books, *Nutrition Action Healthletter,* January/February 2004, pp. 1–8; S. T. St. Jeor and coauthors, Dietary protein and weight reduction: A statement for healthcare professionals from the nutrition committee of the Council on Nutrition, Physical Activity, and Metabolism of the American Heart Association, *Circulation* 104 (2001): 1869–1874.

Fad diets come in almost as many shapes and sizes as the people who search them out. Some restrict fats or carbohydrates, some limit portion sizes, some focus on food combinations, and some claim that a person's genetic type or blood type determines the foods best suited to manage weight and prevent disease. Table H9-2 (p. 306) compares some of today's more popular diets. Table H9-3 (p. 307) offers guidelines for identifying fad diets and other weight-loss scams; it includes the hallmarks of a reasonable weight-loss program as well.

Fad Diets' Appeal

With more than half of our nation's adults overweight and many more concerned about their weight, the market for a weight-loss book, product, or program is huge (no pun intended). In a recent survey commissioned by the Heart and Stroke Foundation, 20- to 39-year-old Canadians spent the greatest dollars on weight-loss efforts (e.g., club or gym fees, diet foods, supplements).[1] Even a plan that offers only minimal weight-loss success easily attracts a following.

Perhaps the greatest appeal of fad diets is that they tend to ignore dietary recommendations. Foods such as meats and milk products that need to be selected carefully to limit saturated fat can be eaten with abandon. Whole grains, legumes, vegetables, and fruits that should be eaten in abundance can now be bypassed. For some people, this is a dream come true: steaks without the potatoes, ribs without the coleslaw, and meatballs without the pasta. Who can resist the promise of weight loss while eating freely from a list of favourite foods?

Dieters are also lured into fad diets by sophisticated—yet often erroneous—explanations of the metabolic consequences of eating certain foods. Terms such as *eicosanoids* and *de novo lipogenesis* are scattered about, often intimidating readers into believing that the authors must be right given their brilliance in understanding the body.

If fad diets were as successful as some people claim, then consumers who tried them would lose weight, and their obesity problems would be solved. But this is not the case. Similarly, if fad diets were as worthless as others claim, then consumers would eventually stop pursuing them. Clearly, this is not happening either. Most fad diets have enough going for them that they work for some people at least for a short time, but they fail to produce long-lasting results for most people.

Don't Count kCalories

Who wants to count kcalories? Even experienced dieters find counting kcalories burdensome, not to mention timeworn. They want a new, easy way to lose weight, and fad diet plans seem to offer this boon. But, though fad diets often claim to disregard kcalories, their design typically ensures a low energy intake. Most of the sample menu plans, especially in the early stages, are designed to deliver an average of 1200 kcalories a day.

Even when counting kcalories is truly not necessary, total kcalories tend to be low simply because food intake is so limited. Diets that omit hundreds of foods and several food groups limit a person's options and lack variety. Chapter 2 praises variety as a valuable way to ensure an adequate intake of nutrients, but variety also entices people to eat more food and gain more weight. Without variety, some people lose interest in eating, which further reduces energy intake. Even if the allowed foods are favourites, eating the same foods week after week can become monotonous.

Without its refried beans, tortilla wrapping, and chopped vegetables, a burrito is reduced to a pile of ground beef. Without the baked potato, there's no need for butter and sour cream. Weight loss occurs because of the low energy intake. This is an important point. Any diet can produce weight loss, at least temporarily, if intake is restricted. The real value of a diet is determined by its ability to maintain weight loss and support good health over the long term. The goal is not simply weight loss, but health gains—and most fad diets cannot support optimal health over time.

When food choices are limited, nutrient intakes may be inadequate. To help shore up some of these inadequacies, fad diets often recommend a dietary supplement. Conveniently, many of the companies selling fad diets also peddle these supplements. But as Highlights 10 and 12 explain, foods offer many more health benefits than any supplement can provide. Quite simply, if the diet is inadequate, it needs to be improved, not supplemented.

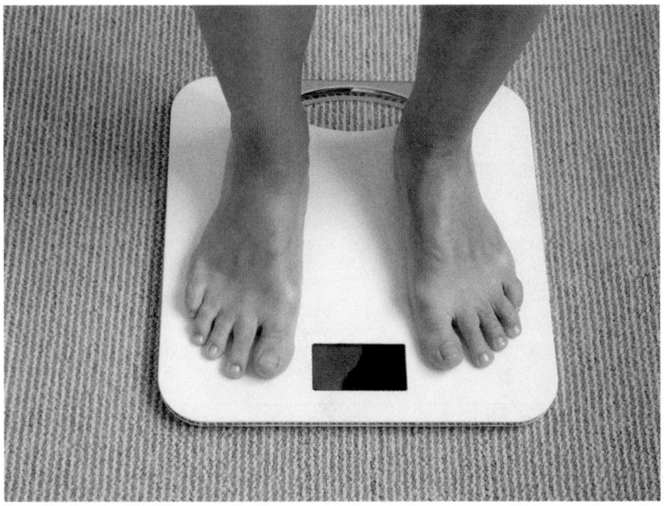

Philip Lange/shutterstock

The wise consumer seeks a diet that supports not only weight loss, but health gains.

TABLE H9-1 The Claims and Truths of Fad Diets

The Claim:	You can lose weight "easily."
The Truth:	Most fad diet plans have complicated rules that require you to calculate protein requirements, count carbohydrate grams, combine certain foods, time meal intervals, purchase special products, plan daily menus, and measure serving sizes.
The Claim:	You can lose weight by eating a specific ratio of carbohydrate, protein, and fat.
The Truth:	Weight loss depends on expending more energy than you take in, not on the proportion of energy nutrients.
The Claim:	This "revolutionary diet" can "reset your genetic code."
The Truth:	You inherited your genes and cannot alter your genetic code.
The Claim:	High-protein diets are popular, selling millions of books, because they work.
The Truth:	Weight-loss books are popular because people grasp for quick fixes and simple solutions to their weight problems. If book sales were an indication of weight-loss success, we would be a lean nation—but they're not, and neither are we.
The Claim:	People gain weight on low-fat diets.
The Truth:	People can gain weight on low-fat diets if they overindulge in carbohydrates and proteins while cutting fat; low-fat diets are not necessarily low-kcalorie diets. But people can also lose weight on low-fat diets if they cut kcalories as well as fat.
The Claim:	High-protein diets energize the brain.
The Truth:	The brain depends on glucose for its energy; the primary dietary source of glucose is carbohydrate, not protein.
The Claim:	Thousands of people have been successful with this plan.
The Truth:	Authors of fad diets have not published their research findings in scientific journals. Success stories are anecdotal and failures are not reported.
The Claim:	Carbohydrates raise blood glucose levels, triggering insulin production and fat storage.
The Truth:	Insulin promotes fat storage when energy intake exceeds energy needs. Furthermore, insulin is only one hormone involved in the complex processes of maintaining the body's energy balance and health.
The Claim:	Eat protein and lose weight.
The Truth:	For every complicated problem, there is a simple—and wrong—solution.

TABLE H9-2 Popular Diets Compared

Diet	Major Premise Promoted	Strong Point(s)	Weak Point(s)
Atkins Diet	• People are overweight or obese because they have metabolic imbalances caused by eating too many carbohydrates; by restricting carbohydrates, these imbalances can be corrected. • You can lose weight without lowering kcalorie intake.	• Quick, short-term weight loss is achieved.	• Restricts carbohydrates to a level that induces ketosis. • Ketosis can cause nausea, light-headedness, and fatigue. • Ketosis can worsen existing medical problems such as kidney disease. • A diet high in fat such as Atkins can increase the risk of heart disease and some cancers.
Cheater's Diet	• Successful weight loss depends on eliminating boredom and allowing indulgences. • Cheating on weekends "stokes your metabolism."	• Meals are proportioned one-half fruit or vegetables, one-fourth lean protein, and one-fourth whole grains. • Encourages as much exercise as possible.	• No scientific data on cheating boosting metabolism or supporting weight loss.
Eat Right 4 Your Type	• Your blood type determines which foods you should eat or not eat.	None	• Food groups or individual foods are excluded, depending on blood type. • No scientific data on the relationship between blood type and food choices.
Glucose Revolution	• Low glycemic index foods satisfy hunger, control blood glucose, and promote weight loss.	• Emphasizes fibre-rich vegetables, legumes, fruits, and whole grains. • Minimizes saturated fat intake.	• Difficult to know the glycemic index of some foods.
Ornish Diet	• By strictly limiting fat (both animal and vegetable), you eat fewer kcalories without eating less food.	• High-fibre, low-fat foods in this plan can lower blood cholesterol and blood pressure.	• So little fat that essential fatty acids may be lacking. • Limits fish, nuts, and olive oil, which may protect against heart disease.
Pritikin Program	• By eating low-fat, mainly plant-based foods, you can eat more food and still feel satisfied.	• No food group is completely eliminated in this high-fibre, low-fat diet program. • Some use of foods rich in omega-3 fatty acids is encouraged.	• For some people, very low-fat diets may be unsatisfying and therefore difficult to adhere to.
Sonoma Diet	• Enjoying portion-controlled Mediterranean-style foods supports weight loss and promotes good health.	• Emphasizes nutrient-dense foods.	• Initial phase restricts fruits and limits milk products.
South Beach Diet	• Eating "good carbohdrates" such as vegetables, whole-wheat pastas, and brown rice will maintain satiety and resist cravings for "bad carbohydrates" such as white rice and potatoes.	• Encourages consumption of vegetables, lean meats, and fish, and the use of unsaturated oils when cooking. • Restricts fatty meats and cheeses as well as sweets.	• Starchy carbohydrates and all fruits are completely excluded during the first two weeks.
Ultimate Weight Solution Diet	• Foods that require great effort to prepare and eat are nutrient-dense; eating these kinds of foods (raw vegetables, vegetable soups, whole grains, beans, meats, poultry, and fish) will lead to weight loss. • Foods that take little effort to prepare and eat provide excess kcalories relative to nutrients; eating these kinds of foods (fast foods, puddings, high-kcalorie convenience foods, processed foods) leads to uncontrolled eating and weight gain.	• Encourages consumption of lean meats and fish; whole grains; vegetables; fruit; and low-fat milk, yogurt, and cheese. • Restricts fatty meats and cheeses as well as sweets. • Encourages exercise.	• Confusing as to exactly what to eat or how much.
Zone Diet	• Eating the correct proportions of carbohydrates, fat, and protein leads to hormonal balance, weight loss, disease prevention, and increased vitality.	• Promotes weight loss because it is a low-kcalorie diet.	• The diet is rigid, restrictive, and complicated, making it difficult for most people to follow accurately. • The overblown health claims of the diet's proponents are based on misinterpreted science and remain unsubstantiated.

TABLE H9-3 Guidelines for Identifying Fad Diets and Other Weight-Loss Scams

Fad Diets and Weight-Loss Scams	Healthy Diet Guidelines
1. They promise dramatic, rapid weight loss.	1. Weight loss should be gradual and not exceed 1 kilogram per week.
2. They promote diets that are nutritionally unbalanced or extremely low in kcalories.	2. Diets should provide: • A reasonable number of kcalories (not fewer than 1000 kcalories per day for women and 1200 kcalories per day for men) • Enough, but not too much, protein (between the RDA and twice the RDA) • Enough, but not too much, fat (between 20 and 35% of daily energy intake from fat) • Enough carbohydrates to spare protein and prevent ketosis (at least 100 grams per day) and 20 to 30 grams of fibre from food sources • A balanced assortment of vitamins and minerals from a variety of foods from each of the food groups • At least 1 litre (about 1 quart) of water daily or 1 millilitre per kcalorie daily—whichever is more
3. They use liquid formulas rather than foods.	3. Foods should accommodate a person's ethnic background, taste preferences, and financial means.
4. They attempt to make clients dependent upon special foods or devices.	4. Programs should teach clients how to make good choices from the conventional food supply.
5. They fail to encourage permanent, realistic lifestyle changes.	5. Programs should teach physical activity plans that involve expending at least 300 kcalories a day and behaviour-modification strategies that help to correct poor eating habits.
6. They misrepresent salespeople as "counsellors" supposedly qualified to give guidance in nutrition and/or general health.	6. Even if adequately trained, such "counsellors" would still be objectionable because of the obvious conflict of interest that exists when providers profit directly from products they recommend and sell.
7. They collect large sums of money at the start or require that clients sign contracts for expensive, long-term programs.	7. Programs should be reasonably priced and run on a pay-as-you-go basis.
8. They fail to inform clients of the risks associated with weight loss in general or the specific program being promoted.	8. They should provide information about dropout rates, the long-term success of their clients, and possible diet side-effects.
9. They promote unproven or spurious weight-loss aids such as human chorionic gonadotropin hormone (HCG), starch blockers, diuretics, sauna belts, body wraps, passive exercise, ear stapling, acupuncture, electric muscle-stimulating (EMS) devices, spirulina, amino acid supplements (e.g., arginine, ornithine), glucomannan, methylcellulose (a "bulking agent"), "unique" ingredients, and so forth.	9. They should focus on nutrient-rich foods and regular exercise.
10. They fail to provide for weight maintenance after the program ends.	10. They should provide a plan for weight maintenance after successful weight loss.

SOURCES: Adapted from American College of Sports Medicine, *ACSM's Guidelines for Exercise Testing and Prescription* (Baltimore: Williams & Wilkins, 1995), pp. 218–219; J. T. Dwyer, Treatment of obesity: Conventional programs and fad diets, in *Obesity*, ed. P. Björntorp and B. N. Brodoff (Philadelphia: J.B. Lippincott, 1992), p. 668; *National Council against Health Fraud Newsletter,* March/April 1987, National Council against Health Fraud, Inc.

Follow a Plan

Most people need specific instructions and examples to make dietary changes. Popular diets offer dieters a plan. The user doesn't have to decide what foods to eat, how to prepare them, or how much to eat. Unfortunately, these instructions serve only short-term weight-loss needs. They do not provide for long-term changes in lifestyle that will support weight maintenance or health goals.

The success of any weight-loss diet depends on the person adopting the plan and sticking with it.[2] People who prefer a high-protein, low-carbohydrate diet over a high-carbohydrate, low-fat diet, for example, may have more success at sticking with it. Keep in mind, though, that weight loss occurs because of the duration of a low-kcalorie plan—not the proportion of energy nutrients.

The Real Deal

Fad diets attribute magical powers to their weight-loss plans, but in reality, the magic is in tipping the energy balance so that activities expend more kcalories than foods bring in. Because new diets emerge in the market regularly, it can be challenging to sort the fad diets from the healthy options. Furthermore, it can be difficult determining a diet's overall quality rates and how it compares with others. One study used the Healthy Eating Index tool to compare popular weight-loss plans—based on a healthful approach, not on weight loss.[3] Of the eight popular plans examined, Ornish ranked highest and Atkins ranked lowest.

Keep in mind that healthy weight loss requires long-term lifestyle changes in eating and activity habits—not quick, short-term fixes. A healthy plan may not be quick but it allows for flexibility and a variety of foods, including some favourite treats on occasion.

Fad diets may not harm healthy people if used for only a little while, but they cannot support optimal health for long. Chapter 9 includes reasonable approaches to weight management and concludes that the ideal diet is one you can live with for the rest of your life. Keep that criterion in mind when you evaluate the next "latest and greatest weight-loss diet" that comes along.

Nutrition on the Net

CENGAGENOW™
For further study of topics covered in this Highlight, log on to **www.cengage.com/sso**.

- Find tips for getting active on the Public Health Agency of Canada's website: **www.phac-aspc.gc.ca/hp-ps/hl-mvs/pa-ap/04paap-eng.php**
- Get quick facts and statistics about the physical activity levels of Canadians at the ParticipACTION website: **www.participaction.com/en-us/Get-Informed/Facts-And-Stats.aspx**
- Try out the Heart and Stroke Foundation's interactive My Healthy Weight Action Plan to find ways to achieve and maintain a healthy body weight: **ww1.heartandstroke.ca/hwplan.asp?media=hw_HSF1**

References

1. Heart and Stroke Foundation, Canadians trapped on weight-loss rollercoaster, press release. www.heartandstroke.com/site, accessed August 21, 2010.
2. M. L. Dansinger and coauthors, Comparison of the Atkins, Ornish, Weight Watchers, and Zone Diets for weight loss and heart disease risk reduction: A randomized trial, *Journal of the American Medical Association* 293 (2005): 43–53.
3. Y. Ma and coauthors, A dietary quality comparison of popular weight-loss plans, *Journal of the American Dietetic Association* 107 (2007): 1786–1791.

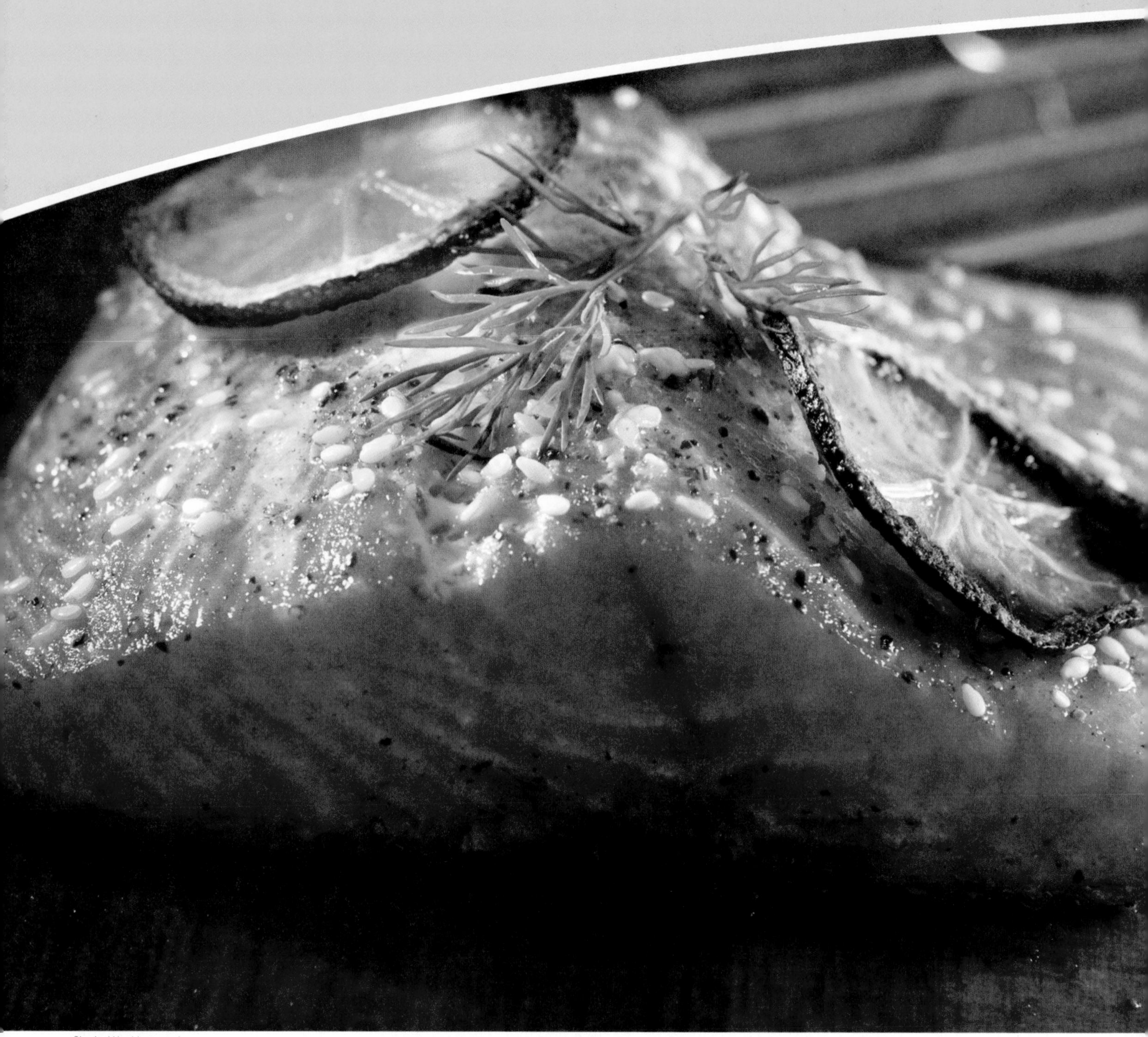

Olga Lyubkina/shutterstock

CENGAGENOW™

Throughout this chapter, the CengageNOW logo indicates an opportunity for online self-study, linking you to interactive tutorials, activities, and videos to increase your understanding of chapter concepts.
www.cengage.com/sso

Nutrition in Your Life

Do you have the energy you need to get through the day? If not, then maybe you lack the nutrients needed for energy metabolism. Many people do not realize how the B vitamins work in concert with each other and how some of the trace minerals support the generation of cellular energy from the carbohydrates, fats, and proteins in the foods that we eat. Treat your body well: eat a balanced and varied diet of nutrient-dense foods to provide you with the vitamins and minerals that will help you generate enough energy to get you through the day.

CHAPTER 10

Nutrients for Energy Metabolism

CHAPTER OUTLINE

Earlier chapters focused attention on the energy-yielding nutrients—carbohydrates, fats, and proteins. This and the following four chapters feature the vitamins and minerals—nutrients that have many important roles, including how they assist in generating energy from the macronutrients, maintain fluid and electrolyte balance, act as antioxidants, keep bones strong, and contribute to blood health.

This chapter starts with an overview of the vitamins and minerals that presents their chemical nature and bioavailability from foods, their treatment by the body, and their common nutrient interactions. Once introduced, attention is then drawn to the topic of this chapter, the vitamins and minerals used in energy metabolism. Following a brief introduction to the micronutrients that support energy production, the spotlight is turned on the B vitamins. A discussion of the synergistic interactions between the B vitamins gives rise to an in-depth focus on each B vitamin individually: specifically the roles, recommendations, deficiencies and toxicities, and food sources for the eight B vitamins. The focus on B vitamins concludes with a look at their collective power. Finally, to close Chapter 10 attention shifts from the vitamins to the minerals that are involved in energy metabolism: sulphur, iodine, manganese, and chromium.

The Vitamins and Minerals—An Overview

Researchers first recognized that foods contain substances that are "vital to life" in the early 1900s. Since then, the world of vitamins has opened up dramatically. Our understanding of the roles of minerals has also increased dramatically during recent times because advancing technologies have been able to detect smaller and smaller amounts of minerals in different body tissues. The **vitamins** and **minerals** ♦ are powerful substances, as their *absence* attests. Vitamin A deficiency can cause blindness; a lack of the B vitamin niacin can cause dementia; an inadequate intake of iron can lead to anemia; and a lack of calcium can slow bone growth. The consequences of deficiencies are so dire, and the effects of restoring the needed

♦ The **vitamins** are organic, essential nutrients required in tiny amounts to perform specific functions that promote growth, reproduction, or the maintenance of health and life.
- **vita** = life
- **amine** = containing nitrogen (the first vitamins discovered contained nitrogen)

The **minerals** are inorganic, essential nutrients required in varying amounts that function primarily as structural components or regulators of body processes.

vitamins and minerals so dramatic, that people spend billions of dollars every year in the belief that vitamin and mineral pills will cure a host of ailments (see Highlight 10). Vitamins and minerals certainly support sound nutritional health, but they do not cure all ills. Furthermore, vitamin and mineral supplements do not offer the many benefits that come from eating micronutrient-rich foods.

The *presence* of vitamins and minerals also attests to their power. The B vitamin folate helps to prevent birth defects and calcium and vitamin K allow blood to clot. As you will see, the roles of vitamins and minerals in supporting optimal health extend far beyond preventing deficiency diseases. In fact, some of the credit given to low-fat diets in preventing disease actually belongs to the vitamins found in vegetables, fruits, and whole grains (see Highlight 12 for more on vitamins and minerals in disease prevention).

The vitamins and minerals differ from carbohydrates, fats, and proteins in the following ways:

- *Structure.* Vitamins are individual units; they are not linked together (as are molecules of glucose or amino acids). APPENDIX C presents the chemical structure for each of the vitamins. Minerals are inorganic elements that always retain their chemical identity, from the time they are ingested to when they are excreted from the body.
- *Function.* Vitamins do not yield usable energy when broken down; many assist the enzymes that release energy from carbohydrates, fats, and proteins. Minerals, like vitamins, do not yield usable energy but do assist enzymes that release energy from the macronutrients. Unlike vitamins, minerals cannot be degraded.
- *Food contents.* The amounts of vitamins people ingest daily from foods and the amounts they require are measured in *micrograms* (µg) or *milligrams* (mg), whereas the amounts of minerals consumed daily varies more widely ranging from micrograms (µg) to *grams* (g). ♦

♦ For perspective, a five dollar bill weighs about 1 g.
1 g = 1000 mg
1 mg = 1000 µg
The Aids to Calculation section at the back of this book explains how to convert a measurement from one unit of measure to another.

The vitamins are similar to the energy-yielding nutrients, though, in that they are vital to life, organic, and available from foods. While minerals are also vital to life and available from foods, a few characteristics distinguish them from the vitamins, most notably their inorganic chemical nature and retention of chemical identity. Some minerals share similarities with vitamins—for example, potassium is easily absorbed into the blood, transported freely, and readily excreted by the kidneys, much like the water-soluble vitamins. Other minerals, such as calcium, are more like fat-soluble vitamins in that they must have carriers to be absorbed and transported. And, like some of the fat-soluble vitamins, minerals taken in excess can be toxic.

Bioavailability The amount of vitamins and minerals available from foods depends not only on the quantity provided by a food but also on the amount absorbed and used by the body—referred to as **bioavailability.** The vitamins and minerals differ in the amounts the body can absorb and the extent to which they must be specially handled. The quantity of vitamins and minerals in a food can be determined relatively easily. Researchers analyze foods to determine their content and publish the results in tables of food composition such as in APPENDIX H. Determining the bioavailability of a vitamin or mineral is a more complex task because it depends on many factors, including:

- Efficiency of digestion and time of transit through the GI tract
- Previous nutrient intake and nutrition status
- Method of food preparation (raw, cooked, or processed)
- Source of the nutrient (synthetic, fortified, or naturally occurring)
- Other foods consumed at the same time
- Naturally occurring **binders** found in foods, such as phytates present in legumes and whole grains and oxalates found in some vegetables, chemically combine with minerals preventing their absorption
- Fibres present in foods can reduce mineral absorption by trapping them and carrying them out of the body

bioavailability: the rate at and the extent to which a nutrient is absorbed and used.

binders: chemical compounds in foods that combine with nutrients (especially minerals) to form complexes the body cannot absorb. Examples include *phytates* (FYE-tates) and *oxalates* (OCK-sa-lates)

Chapters 10 to 14 describe factors that inhibit or enhance the absorption of individual vitamins and minerals. Experts consider these factors when estimating recommended intakes.

Precursors Some of the vitamins are available from foods in inactive forms known as **precursors**, or provitamins. Once inside the body, the precursor is converted to an active form of the vitamin. Thus, in measuring a person's vitamin intake, it is important to count both the amount of the active vitamin and the potential amount available from its precursors. The discussions and summary tables throughout this and the following four chapters indicate which vitamins have precursors. Minerals ♦ are often found in a usable salt form rather than a precursor form in foods.

Chemical Nature Being organic, ♦ vitamins can be destroyed and left unable to function. Therefore, they must be handled with care during storage and in cooking. Prolonged heating may destroy much of the thiamin in food. Because riboflavin can be destroyed by the ultraviolet rays of the sun or by fluorescent light, foods stored in transparent glass containers are most likely to lose riboflavin. Oxygen destroys vitamin C, so losses occur when foods are cut, processed, and stored; these losses may be enough to reduce its action in the body.[1] Table 10-1 summarizes ways to minimize vitamin losses in the kitchen, and Chapter 20 provides more details. Being inorganic, minerals do not change chemical identity in foods or when absorbed and used in the body. Iron, for example, may temporarily combine with other charged elements in salts, but it is always iron. Neither can minerals be destroyed by heat, air, acid, or mixing. Consequently, little care is needed to preserve minerals during food preparation. In fact, the ash that remains when a food is completely combusted in a bomb calorimeter contains all of the minerals that were in the food originally. Minerals can be lost from food only when they leach into cooking water that is then poured down the drain.

Solubility As you may recall, carbohydrates and proteins are hydrophilic and lipids are hydrophobic. The vitamins divide along the same lines—the hydrophilic, water-soluble ones ♦ are the eight B vitamins and vitamin C; the hydrophobic, fat-soluble ones are vitamins A, D, E, and K. As each vitamin was discovered, it was given a name and sometimes a letter and number as well. Many of the water-soluble vitamins have multiple names, which has led to some confusion. The margin lists the standard names, and summary tables throughout this and the following four chapters provide the common alternative names.

Solubility is apparent in the food sources of the different vitamins, and it affects their absorption, transport, storage, and excretion by the body. The water-soluble vitamins are found in the watery compartments of foods; the fat-soluble vitamins usually occur together in the fats and oils of foods. On being absorbed, the water-soluble vitamins move directly into the blood. Like fats, however, the fat-soluble vitamins must first enter the lymph, then the blood. Once in the blood, many of the water-soluble vitamins travel freely, whereas many of the fat-soluble vitamins require transport proteins. Upon reaching the cells, water-soluble vitamins freely circulate in the water-filled compartments of the body, but fat-soluble vitamins are held in fatty tissues and the liver until needed. The kidneys, monitoring the blood that flows through them, detect and remove small excesses of water-soluble vitamins; large excesses, however, may overwhelm the system, creating adverse effects.

TABLE 10-1 Minimizing Vitamin Losses

- To slow the degradation of vitamins, refrigerate (most) fruits and vegetables.
- To minimize the oxidation of vitamins, store fruits and vegetables that have been cut in airtight wrappers, and store juices that have been opened in closed containers (and refrigerate them).
- To prevent losses during washing, rinse fruits and vegetables before cutting (not after).
- To minimize losses during cooking, use a microwave oven or steam vegetables in a small amount of water. Add vegetables after water has come to a boil. Use the cooking water in mixed dishes such as casseroles and soups. Avoid high temperatures and long cooking times.

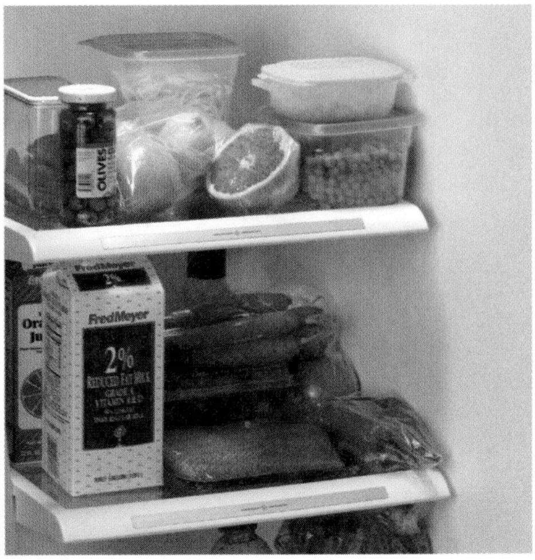
OLIVES
FredMeyer
2%
REDUCED FAT MILK

To minimize vitamin losses, wrap cut fruits and vegetables or store them in airtight containers.

♦ **Major minerals:**
- Sodium
- Potassium
- Chloride
- Phosphorus
- Calcium
- Magnesium
- Sulphur

Trace minerals:
- Selenium
- Fluoride
- Iodine
- Chromium
- Manganese
- Iron
- Zinc
- Copper

♦ **Water-soluble vitamins:**
- B vitamins:
  Thiamin
  Riboflavin
  Niacin
  Biotin
  Pantothenic acid
  Vitamin B_6
  Folate
  Vitamin B_{12}
- Vitamin C

Fat-soluble vitamins:
- Vitamin A
- Vitamin D
- Vitamin E
- Vitamin K

♦ Organic nutrients contain carbon.

precursors: substances that precede others; with regard to vitamins, compounds that can be converted into active vitamins; also known as *provitamins.*

Fat-soluble vitamins tend to remain in fat-storage sites in the body rather than being excreted, and so are more likely to reach toxic levels when consumed in excess.

Because the body stores fat-soluble vitamins, they can be eaten in large amounts once in a while and still meet the body's needs over time. Water-soluble vitamins are retained for varying lengths of time in the body. Although a single day's omission from the diet does not bring on a deficiency, the water-soluble vitamins must still be eaten more regularly than the fat-soluble vitamins. Minerals on the other hand, have varying solubility, which affects their absorption. For example, calcium citrate has greater solubility and is better absorbed than calcium carbonate. Iron has a higher solubility and is better absorbed when it is consumed with acidic foods. Vitamin C is an organic acid found in foods that helps with the absorption of iron. Acid entering the upper part of the small intestine from the stomach causes a localized low pH aiding the absorption of minerals such as iron and zinc.

Nutrient Interactions Chapters 10 to 14 describe how the presence or absence of one vitamin or mineral can affect another's absorption, metabolism, and excretion. For example, Figure 10-11 (page 329) shows how folate and vitamin B_{12} interact to mutually enhance absorption and perform metabolic roles. The interactions between sodium and calcium cause both to be excreted when sodium intakes are high. Another mineral–mineral interaction is observed when phosphorus binds with magnesium in the GI tract, so magnesium absorption is limited when phosphorus intakes are high. Discussions in this and the following four chapters point out additional problems that arise from such interactions. As you read through these chapters, notice how often they reflect an excess of one nutrient creating an inadequacy of another and how supplements—not foods—are most often to blame.

Toxicity Knowledge about some of the amazing roles of vitamins and minerals has prompted many people to assume that "more is better" and take vitamin and mineral supplements. Just as an inadequate intake can cause harm, so can an excessive intake. Even some of the water-soluble micronutrients have adverse effects when taken in large doses.

That a vitamin or mineral can be both essential and harmful may seem surprising, but the same is true of most nutrients. The effects of every substance depend on its dose, and this is one reason consumers should not self-prescribe supplements for their ailments. Figure 10-1 shows three possible relationships between dose levels and effects. The third diagram represents the situation with nutrients—more is better up to a point, but beyond that point, still more can be harmful.

The Committee on Dietary Reference Intakes (DRI) addresses the possibility of adverse effects from high doses of nutrients by establishing Tolerable Upper Intake Levels (UL). The UL defines the highest amount of a nutrient that is likely not to cause harm for most healthy people when consumed daily. The risk of harm

FIGURE 10-1 Dose Levels and Effects

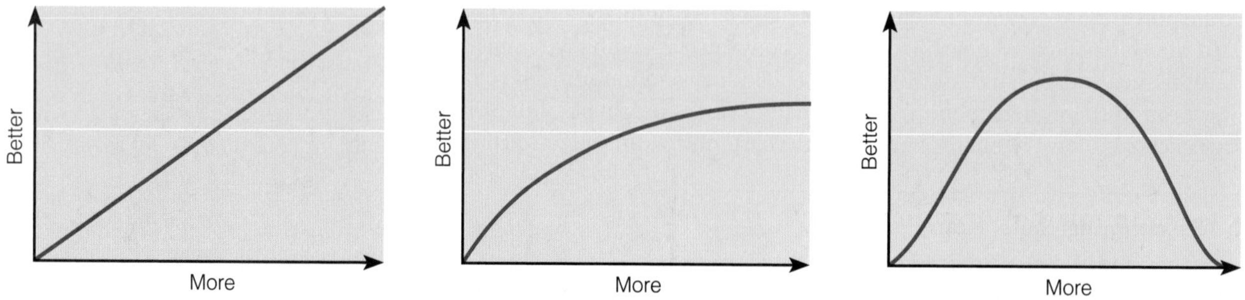
Better
More
Better
More
Better
More

As you progress in the direction of more, the effect gets better and better, with no end in sight (real life is seldom, if ever, like this).

As you progress in the direction of more, the effect reaches a maximum and then a plateau, becoming no better with higher doses.

As you progress in the direction of more, the effect reaches an optimum at some intermediate dose and then declines, showing that more is better up to a point and then harmful. That too much can be as harmful as too little represents the situation with most nutrients.

increases as intakes rise above the UL. Of the nutrients discussed in this chapter, niacin, vitamin B_6, folate, choline, iodine, and manganese have UL, as shown in the summary table (page 343). Insufficient data exist to establish UL for the remaining vitamins and minerals discussed in this chapter: thiamin, riboflavin, biotin, pantothenic acid, vitamin B_{12}, sulphur, and chromium, but this does not mean that excessively high intakes would be without risk. (The inside front cover pages present UL for the vitamins and minerals.)

Figure 10-2 shows the amounts of the **major minerals** found in the body and, for comparison, some of the **trace minerals.** The distinction between the major and trace minerals does not mean that one group is more important than the other—all minerals are vital to life. The major minerals are so named because they are present, and needed, in larger amounts in the body. They are shown at the top of the figure and the trace minerals are shown at the bottom. Major and trace minerals are discussed in this and the following four chapters.

IN SUMMARY **The vitamins are essential nutrients needed in tiny amounts in the diet both to prevent deficiency diseases and to support optimal health. The water-soluble vitamins are the B vitamins and vitamin C; the fat-soluble vitamins are vitamins A, D, E, and K. The minerals are essential, water-soluble nutrients needed in varying amounts in the diet, and used mainly for structural functions and regulatory processes. The major minerals are sodium, potassium, chloride, phosphorus, calcium, magnesium, and sulphur; the trace minerals include selenium, fluoride, iodine, chromium, manganese, iron, zinc, and copper. The accompanying table focuses on differences between the water-soluble and fat-soluble vitamins.**

	Water-Soluble Vitamins: B Vitamins and Vitamin C	Fat-Soluble Vitamins: Vitamins A, D, E, and K
Absorption	Directly into the blood	First into the lymph, then the blood
Transport	Travel freely	Many require transport proteins
Storage	Circulate freely in water-filled parts of the body	Stored in the cells associated with fat
Excretion	Kidneys detect and remove excess in urine	Less readily excreted; tend to remain in fat-storage sites
Toxicity	Possible to reach toxic levels when consumed from supplements	Likely to reach toxic levels when consumed from supplements
Requirements	Needed in frequent doses (perhaps 1 to 3 days)	Needed in periodic doses (perhaps weeks or even months)

NOTE: Exceptions occur, but these differences between the water-soluble and fat-soluble vitamins are valid generalizations.

major minerals: essential mineral nutrients the human body requires in relatively large amounts (greater than 100 milligrams per day); sometimes called *macrominerals*.

trace minerals: essential mineral nutrients the human body requires in relatively small amounts (less than 100 milligrams per day); sometimes called *microminerals*.

As we move away from the overview of vitamins and minerals toward taking a more in-depth look at the vitamins and minerals used for energy metabolism, it is important to underscore many of their interrelationships. The remainder of this chapter introduces the micronutrients used in energy production and notes some of their common interactions. These interconnections illustrate the consequences of having too little or too much of a nutrient in the body and allow the focus to shift to examining the B vitamins individually. However, it is important not to lose sight of how the B vitamins work together in impressive ways, so a view of how they work in concert concludes the exploration of the B vitamins. The final section of chapter 10 explores specific minerals that assist in generating energy from the carbohydrates, fats, and proteins.

FIGURE 10-2 **Minerals in a 60-kilogram (132-pound) Human Body**

Not only are the major minerals needed by the body in larger amounts, but they are also present in the body in larger amounts than the trace minerals.

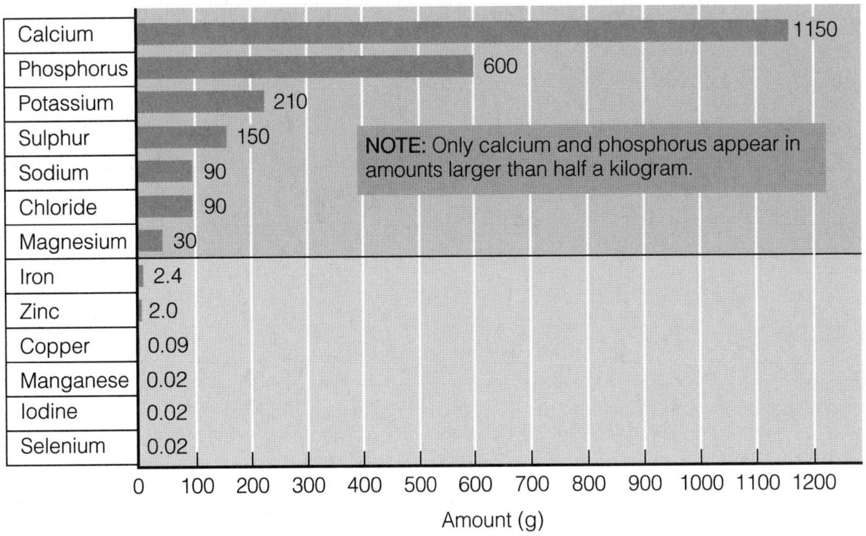
Calcium 1150
Phosphorus 600
Potassium 210
Sulphur 150
Sodium 90
Chloride 90
Magnesium 30
Iron 2.4
Zinc 2.0
Copper 0.09
Manganese 0.02
Iodine 0.02
Selenium 0.02
NOTE: Only calcium and phosphorus appear in amounts larger than half a kilogram.
0 100 200 300 400 500 600 700 800 900 1000 1100 1200
Amount (g)

Nutrients for Energy Metabolism

Despite supplement advertisements that claim otherwise, the vitamins and minerals do not provide the body with fuel for energy. It is true, though, that without B vitamins the body would lack energy. In Chapters 4 through 6, you learned that the energy-yielding nutrients—carbohydrate, fat, and protein—are sources of fuel; in this chapter you will learn how the B vitamins help the body use that fuel. Several of the B vitamins—*thiamin, riboflavin, niacin, pantothenic acid,* and *biotin*—form part of the coenzymes ♦ that assist enzymes in yielding energy from carbohydrate, fat, and protein. The vitamin portion of a coenzyme allows a chemical reaction to occur; the remaining portion of the coenzyme binds to the enzyme. Without its coenzyme, an enzyme cannot function. Thus symptoms of B vitamin deficiencies directly reflect the disturbances of metabolism caused by a lack of coenzymes. Figure 10-3 illustrates the action of the B vitamin coenzymes. The remaining three B vitamins also form coenzymes and play other indispensable roles in metabolism. *Vitamin* B_6 assists enzymes that metabolize amino acids. *Folate and vitamin* B_{12} help cells to multiply, including red blood cells and the cells lining the GI tract—cells that deliver energy to all the others.

♦ A **coenzyme** is a small organic molecule that associates closely with certain enzymes; many B vitamins form an integral part of coenzymes.

The vitamin-like compound *choline* is often clustered with the B vitamins because of common roles such as metabolizing fats, cholesterol, and homocysteine. *Sulphur* is a major mineral found as a component of thiamin and biotin and in the sulphur-containing amino acids. In these different roles, sulphur exerts an energy-generating effect.

The trace minerals used in energy metabolism are required in miniscule amounts, but once they enter the body they take on big jobs to sustain your energy. Insulin can't deliver glucose without *chromium*, the thyroid hormones require *iodide* for activation, and *manganese* facilitates the action of many metalloenzymes. Each trace mineral is involved in a vital role that only it can perform. Eating a varied and balanced diet supplies the B vitamins and trace minerals needed for energy metabolism.

Introducing the B Vitamins

The B vitamins work together in impressive ways: the presence or absence of one affects another's absorption, metabolism, and excretion. Riboflavin and vitamin B_6 provide an example of this interdependence. One of the riboflavin coenzymes, flavin mononucleotide, assists the enzyme that converts vitamin B_6 to its

FIGURE 10-3 Coenzyme Action

Some vitamins form part of the coenzymes that enable enzymes either to synthesize compounds (as illustrated by the lower enzymes in this figure) or to dismantle compounds (as illustrated by the upper enzymes).

CENGAGENOW™ Animated! figure www.cengage.com/sso

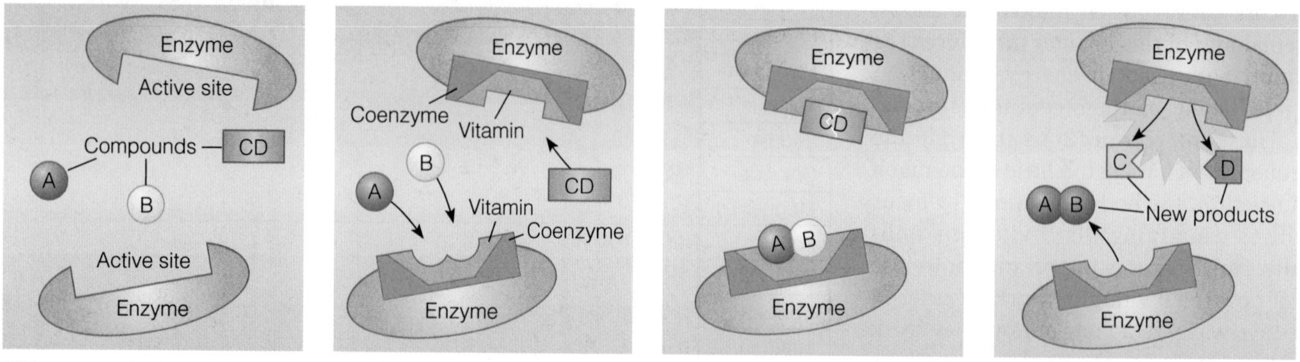
Enzyme
Active site
Compounds
CD
A
B
Active site
Enzyme
Enzyme
Coenzyme
Vitamin
B
A
CD
Vitamin
Coenzyme
Enzyme
Enzyme
CD
A B
Enzyme
Enzyme
C
D
A B
New products
Enzyme

Without coenzymes, compounds A, B, and CD don't respond to their enzymes.

With the coenzymes in place, compounds are attracted to their sites on the enzymes . . .

. . . and the reactions proceed instantaneously. The coenzymes often donate or accept electrons, atoms, or groups of atoms.

The reactions are completed with either the formation of a new product, AB, or the breaking apart of a compound into two new products, C and D, and the release of energy.

HOW TO Evaluate Foods for Their Nutrient Contributions

Figure 10-5 (p. 319) is the first of a series of figures in this and the next four chapters that present the vitamins and minerals in foods. Each figure presents the same 24 foods, which were selected based on their frequency of consumption and to ensure a variety of choices representative of each of the food groups in *Eating Well with Canada's Food Guide*. For example, a dark green and an orange vegetable were chosen from the vegetables and fruit group. Commonly consumed fruits were chosen. The suggestion to make at least half of your grain products whole grains was also considered: whole-wheat bread and pasta and high-fibre cereal, among other grain products. Foods were selected for the milk and alternatives and meat and alternatives groups in a similar way. In addition to the 24 foods that appear in all of the figures, three different foods were selected for each of the nutrients to add variety and often reflect excellent, and sometimes unusual, sources.

Notice that the figures list the food, the serving size, and the food energy (kcalories) on the left. The amount of the nutrient per serving is presented in the graph on the right along with the RDA (or AI) for adults, so you can see how many servings would be needed to meet recommendations.

The coloured bars show at a glance which food groups best provide a nutrient: green for Vegetables and Fruit; yellow for Grain Products; white for Milk and Alternatives; and red for Meat and Alternatives.

Notice how the bar graphs shift in the various figures. Careful study of all of the figures taken together will confirm that variety is the key to nutrient adequacy.

Another way to evaluate foods for their nutrient contributions is to consider their nutrient density (their thiamin *per 100 kcalories,* for example). Quite often, vegetables rank higher on a nutrient-per-kcalorie list than they do on a nutrient-per-serving list (see p. 37 to review how to evaluate foods based on nutrient density). The left column in the figure highlights between two and six of the 24 commonly consumed foods that offer the best nutrient density. Notice how many of them are vegetables.

Realistically, people cannot eat for single nutrients. Fortunately, most foods deliver more than one nutrient, allowing people to combine foods into nourishing meals.

CENGAGENOW™
For additional practice log on to **www.cengage.com/sso.**

TRY IT Calculate which food provides more riboflavin per 30 gram serving—a pork chop (90 g, 291 kcal, 0.25 mg riboflavin) or cheddar cheese (50 g, 165 kcal, 0.11 mg riboflavin). Which food is more nutrient dense with respect to riboflavin?

coenzyme form pyridoxal phosphate. Consequently, a severe riboflavin deficiency can impair vitamin B_6 activity illustrating how a deficiency of one nutrient may alter the action of another. Additionally, a deficiency of one nutrient may create a deficiency of another. For example, both riboflavin and vitamin B_6 (and the mineral iron) are required for the conversion of tryptophan to niacin. Consequently, an inadequate intake of either riboflavin or vitamin B_6 can diminish the body's niacin supply. These interdependent relationships are evident in many of the metabolic roles that B vitamins play in the body.

Metabolism is the body's work, and the B vitamin coenzymes are indispensable to every step. The pathways used to break down glucose to pyruvate, interconvert amino acids in preparation for break down, and oxidize fatty acids to form two-carbon molecules depend on a steady adequate supply of the B vitamin coenzymes. Low dietary intakes of the B vitamins will affect energy-producing pathways. Deficiencies of single B vitamins are rare in North America, but when people consume nutritionally poor diets, deficiencies of multiple B vitamins can appear. Because B vitamins are water-soluble, our bodies do not typically store them in quantity, which makes it important to eat foods rich in these nutrients every day. Accordingly, B vitamin toxicities from food intake are unknown, but they can occur when people overuse supplements. Foods provide a package of nutrients (and nonnutrients) in amounts that benefit health; supplements can overwhelm cells with large doses of nutrients and disrupt normal metabolic processes. The following sections describe individual B vitamins and note many coenzyme and metabolic pathways. Keep in mind that a later discussion assembles these pieces of information into a whole picture. The following sections also present the deficiencies, toxicities, recommendations, and food sources of each nutrient. For thiamin, riboflavin, niacin, vitamin B_6, folate, and vitamin B_{12}, sufficient data were available to establish an RDA; for biotin, pantothenic acid, and choline, an Adequate Intake (AI) was set; and only niacin, vitamin B_6, and choline have Tolerable Upper Intake Levels (UL).[2] These values appear in the summary tables and figures that follow and on the pages of the inside front cover.

The B Vitamins—As Individuals

Thiamin

Thiamin is the vitamin part of the coenzyme TPP (thiamin pyrophosphate), which assists in energy metabolism. The TPP coenzyme participates in the conversion of pyruvate to acetyl CoA (described in Chapter 7). The reaction removes one carbon from the 3-carbon pyruvate to make the 2-carbon acetyl CoA and carbon dioxide (CO_2). In a similar step in the TCA cycle, TPP helps convert a 5-carbon compound to a 4-carbon compound. Besides playing these pivotal roles in energy metabolism, thiamin occupies a special site on the membranes of nerve cells. Consequently, nerve activity and muscle activity in response to nerves depend heavily on thiamin.

Thiamin Recommendations Dietary recommendations are based primarily on thiamin's role in enzyme activity. Generally, thiamin needs will be met if a person eats enough food to meet energy needs—if that energy comes from nutritious foods. The average thiamin intake in Canada and the United States meets or exceeds recommendations.

Thiamin Deficiency and Toxicity People who fail to eat enough food to meet energy needs risk nutrient deficiencies, including thiamin deficiency. Inadequate thiamin intakes have been reported among the nation's malnourished and homeless people. Similarly, people who derive most of their energy from empty-kcalorie foods and beverages risk thiamin deficiency. Alcohol is a good example. ♦ It contributes energy but provides few, if any, nutrients and often displaces food. In addition, alcohol impairs thiamin absorption and enhances thiamin excretion in the urine, doubling the risk of deficiency. An estimated four out of five alcoholics are thiamin deficient.

♦ Severe thiamin deficiency in alcohol abusers is called the **Wernicke-Korsakoff** (VER-nee-key KORE-sah-kof) **syndrome.** Symptoms include disorientation, loss of short-term memory, jerky eye movements, and staggering gait.

Prolonged thiamin deficiency can result in the disease **beriberi**, which was first observed in Indonesia when the custom of polishing rice became widespread.[3] Rice provided 80 percent of the energy intake of the people of that area, and the germ and bran of the rice grain had been their principal source of thiamin. When the germ and bran were removed in the preparation of white rice, beriberi became rampant.

thiamin (THIGH-ah-min): a B vitamin. The coenzyme form is **TPP (thiamin pyrophosphate).**

beriberi: the thiamin-deficiency disease.

- **beri** = weakness
- **beriberi** = "I can't, I can't"

Beriberi is often described as "dry" or "wet." Dry beriberi reflects damage to the nervous system and is characterized by muscle weakness in the arms and legs. Wet beriberi reflects damage to the cardiovascular system and is characterized by dilated blood vessels, which cause the heart to work harder and the kidneys to retain salt and water, resulting in edema. Typically, both types of beriberi appear together, with one set of symptoms predominating. Figure 10-4 presents the edema of beriberi. No adverse effects have been associated with excesses of thiamin and no UL has been determined.

FIGURE 10-4 Thiamin-Deficiency Symptom—The Edema of Beriberi

Physical examination confirms that this person has wet beriberi. Notice how the impression of the physician's thumb remains on the leg.

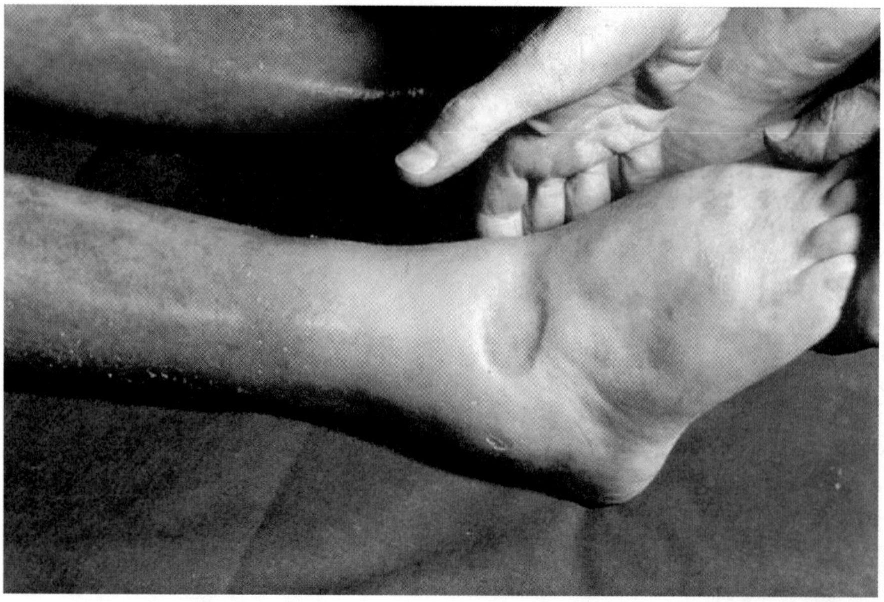

© NMSB/Custom Medical Stock Photo

Thiamin Food Sources Before examining Figure 10-5, you may want to read the "How To" on page 317, which describes the many features found in this and similar figures in this chapter and the next four chapters. When you look at Figure 10-5, notice that thiamin occurs in small quantities in many nutritious foods. The longer red bars near the bottom of the figure show that fortified meat analogues like soy burgers and meats in the pork family are exceptionally rich in thiamin. Yellow bars confirm that enriched grains are a reliable source of thiamin.

FIGURE 10-5 Thiamin in Selected Foods

See the "How To" section on p. 317 for more information on using this figure.

Food	Serving size (kcalories)
Broccoli, boiled	125 mL (29 kcal)
Carrots, boiled	125 mL (29 kcal)
Tomato, fresh	1 medium (22 kcal)
Apple, fresh	1 medium (72 kcal)
Banana	1 medium (105 kcal)
Blueberries, fresh	125 mL (44 kcal)
Bread, whole wheat	1 slice, 35 g (86 kcal)
Pasta, whole grain, cooked	125 mL (92 kcal)
Rice, white, cooked	125 mL (89 kcal)
Oatmeal, cooked	175 mL (144 kcal)
Pita, white	½ pita, 35 g (96 kcal)
Cereal, high fibre	30 g (78 kcal)
Milk, 2%	250 mL (129 kcal)
Cheddar cheese	50 g (202 kcal)
Yogurt, 2% plain	175 g (110 kcal)
Soy beverage, fortified	250 mL (110 kcal)
Kefir	175 g (104 kcal)
Ice cream, strawberry	125 mL (134 kcal)
Chicken breast, roasted	75 g (220 kcal)
Ground beef, lean, baked	75 g (191 kcal)
Egg, poached	1 large (72 kcal)
Tuna, canned in water	75 g (87 kcal)
Tofu, made with a calcium salt	150 g (114 kcal)
Peanut butter	30 mL (184 kcal)
Excellent, and sometimes unusual, sources:	
Vegetarian/soy burger	150 g (266 kcal)
Pork chop, lean, fried	75 g (174 kcal)
Acorn squash, baked	125 mL (61 kcal)

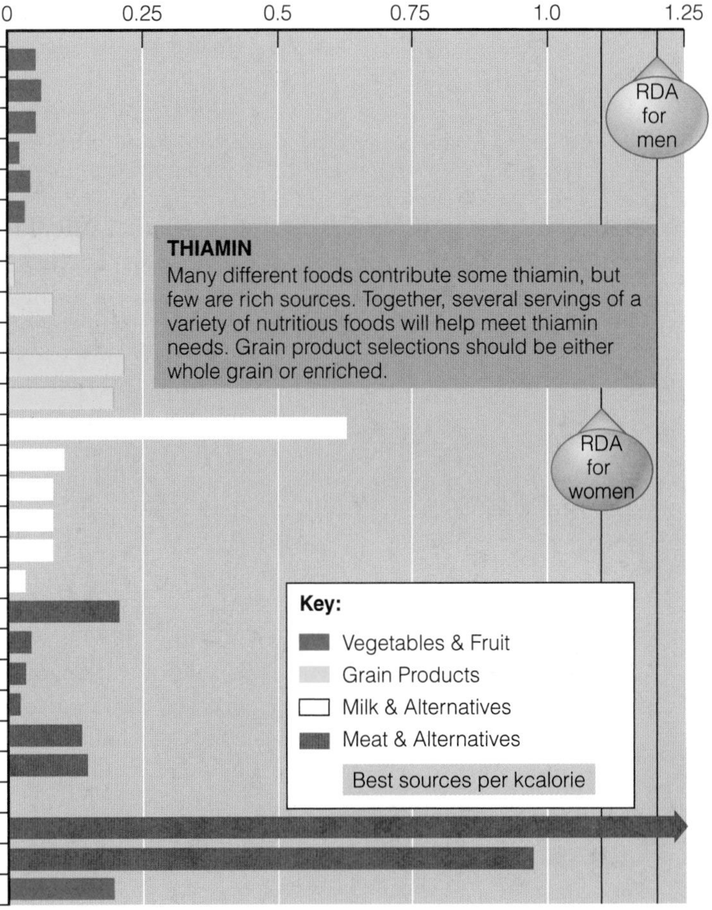
0
0.25
0.5
0.75
1.0
1.25
RDA for men
THIAMIN
Many different foods contribute some thiamin, but few are rich sources. Together, several servings of a variety of nutritious foods will help meet thiamin needs. Grain product selections should be either whole grain or enriched.
RDA for women
Key:
Vegetables & Fruit
Grain Products
Milk & Alternatives
Meat & Alternatives
Best sources per kcalorie

SOURCE: Canadian Nutrient File. Health Canada, 2008. Reproduced with the permission of the Minister of Health, 2011.

As mentioned earlier, prolonged cooking can destroy thiamin. Also, like other water-soluble vitamins, thiamin leaches into water when foods are boiled or blanched. Cooking methods that require little or no water such as steaming and microwave heating conserve thiamin and other water-soluble vitamins. The accompanying table provides a summary of thiamin.

IN SUMMARY Thiamin

Other Names

Vitamin B_1

Recommended Dietary Allowance (RDA)

Men: 1.2 mg/day

Women: 1.1 mg/day

Chief Functions in the Body

Part of coenzyme TPP (thiamin pyrophosphate) used in energy metabolism

Significant Sources

Whole-grain, fortified, or enriched grain products; moderate amounts in all nutritious food; pork

Easily destroyed by heat

Deficiency Disease

Beriberi (wet, with edema; dry, with muscle wasting)

Deficiency Symptoms[a]

Enlarged heart, cardiac failure; muscular weakness; apathy, poor short-term memory, confusion, irritability; anorexia, weight loss

Toxicity Symptoms

None reported

[a]Severe thiamin deficiency is often related to heavy alcohol consumption with limited food consumption (Wernicke-Korsakoff syndrome).

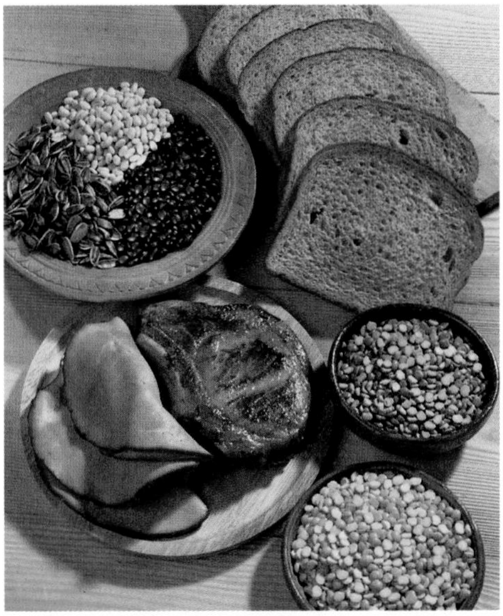

Pork is a rich source of thiamin, but enriched or whole-grain products typically make the greatest contribution to a day's intake because of the quantities consumed. Legumes such as split peas are also valuable sources of thiamin.

Riboflavin Like thiamin, **riboflavin** serves as a coenzyme in many reactions, most notably in energy metabolism. The coenzyme forms of riboflavin are FMN (flavin mononucleotide) and FAD (flavin adenine dinucleotide); both can accept and then donate two hydrogens (see Figure 10-6). During energy metabolism, FAD picks up two hydrogens (with their electrons) from the TCA cycle and delivers them to the electron transport chain (described in Chapter 7).

Riboflavin Recommendations Like thiamin's RDA, riboflavin's RDA is based primarily on its role in enzyme activity. Most people in Canada meet or exceed riboflavin recommendations.

Riboflavin Deficiency and Toxicity Riboflavin deficiency ♦ most often accompanies other nutrient deficiencies. Lack of the vitamin causes inflammation of the membranes of the mouth, skin, eyes, and GI tract. Excesses of riboflavin appear to cause no harm and no UL has been established.

♦ Riboflavin deficiency is called **ariboflavinosis** (ay-RYE-boh-FLAY-vin-oh-sis).
- **a** = not
- **osis** = condition

Riboflavin Food Sources The greatest contributions of riboflavin come from milk and alternatives (see Figure 10-7). Whole-grain or enriched bread and cereal products are also valuable sources because of the quantities typically consumed. When riboflavin sources are ranked by nutrient density (per kcalorie), ♦ many dark green, leafy vegetables (such as broccoli, turnip greens, asparagus, and spinach) appear high on the list. Vegans and others who don't use milk must rely on ample servings of dark greens and enriched grains for riboflavin. Nutritional yeast is another good source.

♦ Turn to p. 37 for a review of how to evaluate foods based on nutrient density (per kcalorie).

Ultraviolet light and irradiation destroy riboflavin. For these reasons, milk is sold in cardboard or opaque plastic containers, instead of clear glass bottles. Precautions are also taken when vitamin D is added to milk by irradiation.* In contrast, riboflavin is stable to heat, so cooking does not destroy it. The accompanying table provides a summary of riboflavin.

*Vitamin D can be added to milk by feeding cows irradiated yeast or by irradiating the milk itself.

FIGURE 10-6 Riboflavin Coenzyme, Accepting and Donating Hydrogens

This figure shows the chemical structure of the riboflavin portion of the coenzyme only; the remainder of the coenzyme structure is represented by dotted lines (see APPENDIX C for the complete chemical structures of FAD and FMN). The reactive sites that accept and donate hydrogens are highlighted in white.

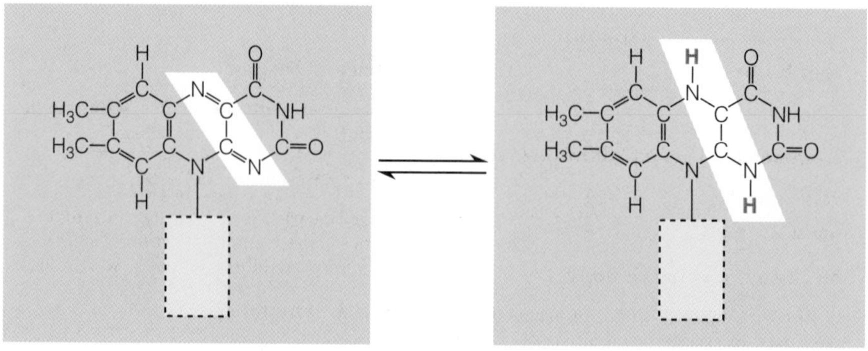

FAD ⇌ $FADH_2$

During the TCA cycle, compounds release hydrogens, and the riboflavin coenzyme FAD picks up two of them. As it accepts two hydrogens, FAD becomes $FADH_2$.

$FADH_2$ carries the hydrogens to the electron transport chain. At the end of the electron transport chain, the hydrogens are accepted by oxygen, creating water, and $FADH_2$ becomes FAD again. For every $FADH_2$ that passes through the electron transport chain, two ATP are generated.

riboflavin (RYE-boh-flay-vin): a B vitamin. The coenzyme forms are **FMN (flavin mononucleotide)** and **FAD (flavin adenine dinucleotide).**

FIGURE 10-7 Riboflavin in Selected Foods

See the "How To" section on p. 317 for more information on using this figure.

Food	Serving size (kcalories)
Broccoli, boiled	125 mL (29 kcal)
Carrots, boiled	125 mL (29 kcal)
Tomato, fresh	1 medium (22 kcal)
Apple, fresh	1 medium (72 kcal)
Banana	1 medium (105 kcal)
Blueberries, fresh	125 mL (44 kcal)
Bread, whole wheat	1 slice, 35 g (86 kcal)
Pasta, whole grain, cooked	125 mL (92 kcal)
Rice, white, cooked	125 mL (89 kcal)
Oatmeal, cooked	175 mL (144 kcal)
Pita, white	½ pita, 35 g (96 kcal)
Cereal, high fibre	30 g (78 kcal)
Milk, 2%	250 mL (129 kcal)
Cheddar cheese	50 g (202 kcal)
Yogurt, 2% plain	175 g (110 kcal)
Soy beverage, fortified	250 mL (110 kcal)
Kefir	175 g (104 kcal)
Ice cream, strawberry	125 mL (134 kcal)
Chicken breast, roasted	75 g (220 kcal)
Ground beef, lean, baked	75 g (191 kcal)
Egg, poached	1 large (72 kcal)
Tuna, canned in water	75 g (87 kcal)
Tofu, made with a calcium salt	150 g (114 kcal)
Peanut butter	30 mL (184 kcal)
Excellent, and sometimes unusual, sources:	
Beef liver, fried	75 g (178 kcal)
Mushrooms, white, stir-fried	125 mL (15 kcal)
Oysters, steamed	75 g (122 kcal)

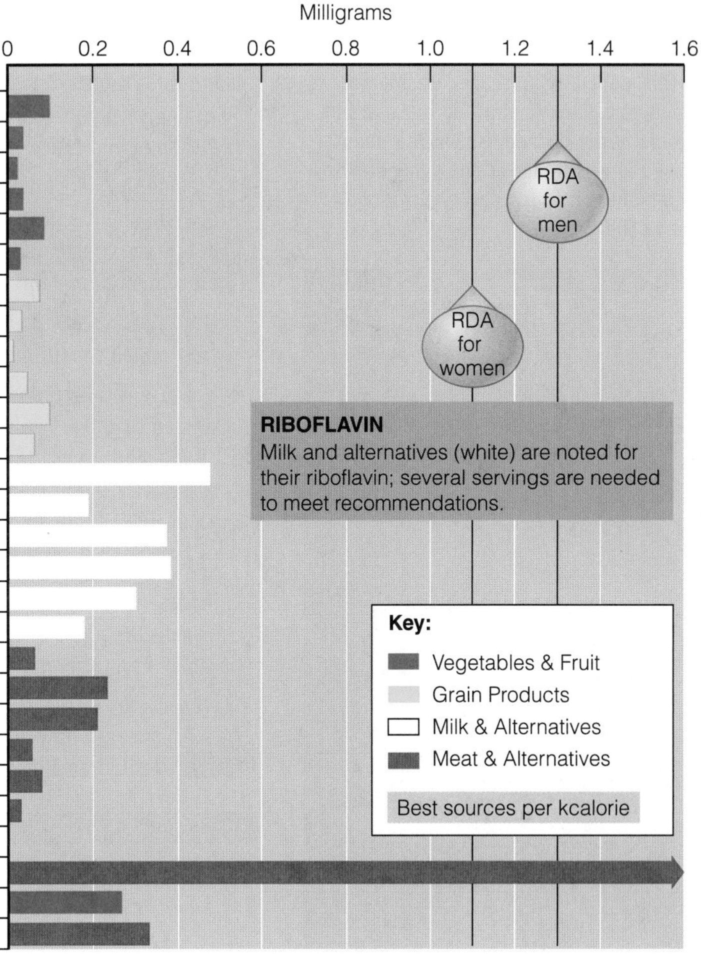
Milligrams
0
0.2
0.4
0.6
0.8
1.0
1.2
1.4
1.6
RDA for men
RDA for women
RIBOFLAVIN
Milk and alternatives (white) are noted for their riboflavin; several servings are needed to meet recommendations.
Key:
Vegetables & Fruit
Grain Products
Milk & Alternatives
Meat & Alternatives
Best sources per kcalorie

SOURCE: Canadian Nutrient File. Health Canada, 2008. Reproduced with the permission of the Minister of Health, 2011.

IN SUMMARY Riboflavin

Other Names

Vitamin B_2

RDA

Men: 1.3 mg/day

Women: 1.1 mg/day

Chief Functions in the Body

Part of coenzymes FMN (flavin mononucleotide) and FAD (flavin adenine dinucleotide) used in energy metabolism

Significant Sources

Milk products (yogurt, cheese); whole-grain, fortified, or enriched grain products; liver

Easily destroyed by ultraviolet light and irradiation

Deficiency Disease

Ariboflavinosis (ay-RYE-boh-FLAY-vin-oh-sis)

Deficiency Symptoms

Sore throat; cracks and redness at corners of mouth;[a] painful, smooth, purplish red tongue;[b] inflammation characterized by skin lesions covered with greasy scales

Toxicity Symptoms

None reported

[a]Cracks at the corners of the mouth are called *angular stomatitis* or *cheilosis* (kye-LOH-sis or kee-LOH-sis).

[b]Smoothness of the tongue is caused by loss of its surface structures and is termed *glossitis* (gloss-EYE-tis).

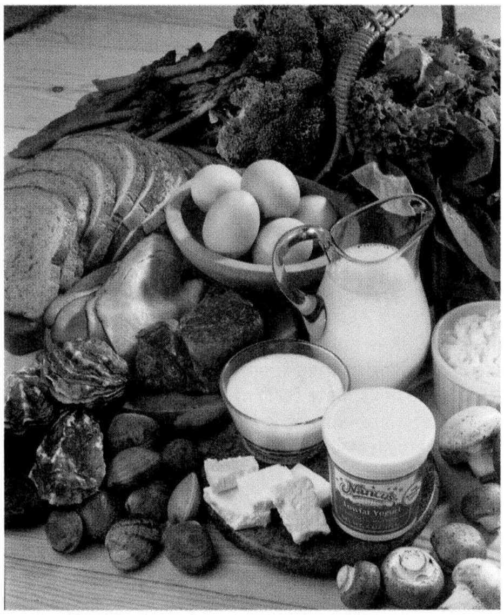

All of these foods are rich in riboflavin, but milk and alternatives provide much of the riboflavin in the diets of many people.

Niacin

The name **niacin** describes two chemical structures: nicotinic acid and nicotinamide (also known as niacinamide). The body can easily convert nicotinic acid to nicotinamide, which is the major form of niacin in the blood.

The two coenzyme forms of niacin, NAD (nicotinamide adenine dinucleotide) and NADP (the phosphate form), participate in numerous metabolic reactions.

FIGURE 10-8 Niacin-Deficiency Symptom—The Dermatitis of Pellagra

In the dermatitis of pellagra, the skin darkens and flakes away as if it were sunburned. The protein-deficiency disease kwashiorkor also produces a "flaky paint" dermatitis, but the two are easily distinguished. The dermatitis of pellagra is bilateral and symmetrical and occurs only on those parts of the body exposed to the sun.

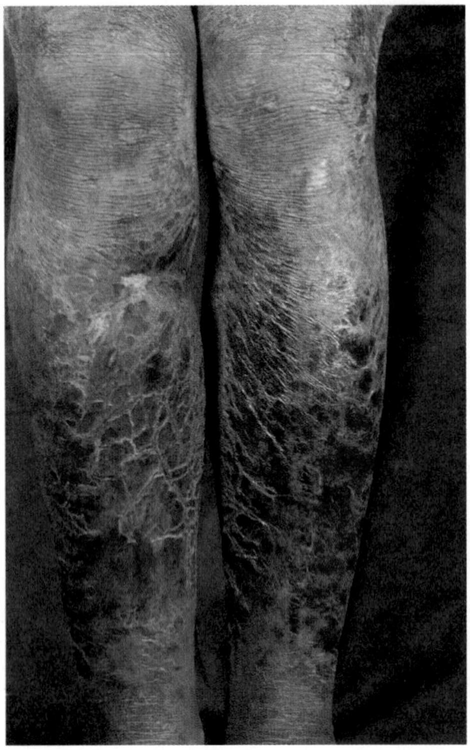

Dr. M.A. Ansary/Photo Researchers, Inc

HOW TO Estimate Niacin Equivalents

Niacin recommendations are expressed as niacin equivalents (NE), but diet analysis programs and food composition tables report only preformed niacin. To estimate niacin equivalents from the tryptophan in dietary protein:

- Assume that most dietary proteins contain about 1 percent tryptophan. To determine the amount of tryptophan in protein, divide grams of protein by 100.
- Multiply by 1000 to convert grams of tryptophan to milligrams.
- Because it takes 60 milligrams of tryptophan to make 1 milligram of niacin, divide milligrams of tryptophan by 60 to get niacin equivalents.
- Add the amount of preformed niacin obtained in the diet.

Consider, for example, a person who consumes 80 grams of protein and 5 milligrams of preformed niacin.

- Estimate the amount of tryptophan in 80 grams of protein and convert to milligrams:

$$80 \text{ g protein} \div 100 = 0.8 \text{ g tryptophan}$$
$$0.8 \text{ g tryptophan} \times 1000 = 800 \text{ mg tryptophan}$$

- Convert milligrams of tryptophan to niacin equivalents:

$$800 \text{ mg tryptophan} \div 60 = 13 \text{ mg NE}$$

To determine the total amount of niacin available from the diet, add the amount available from tryptophan to the amount preformed in the diet.

$$13 \text{ mg NE} + 5 \text{ mg preformed niacin} = 18 \text{ mg NE}$$

CENGAGENOW™
For additional practice log on to **www.cengage.com/sso.**

TRY IT Calculate how many niacin equivalents a person receives from a diet that delivers 60 grams protein and 6 milligrams niacin.

They are central in energy-transfer reactions, especially the metabolism of glucose, fat, and alcohol. NAD is similar to the riboflavin coenzymes in that it carries hydrogens (and their electrons) during metabolic reactions, including the pathway from the TCA cycle to the electron transport chain. NAD also protects against neurological degeneration.[4]

Niacin Recommendations Niacin is unique among the B vitamins in that the body can make it from the amino acid tryptophan. This use of tryptophan occurs only after protein synthesis needs have been met.[5] Approximately 60 milligrams of dietary tryptophan is needed to make 1 milligram of niacin. For this reason, recommended intakes are stated in **niacin equivalents** (NE). ♦ A food containing 1 milligram of niacin and 60 milligrams of tryptophan provides the equivalent of 2 milligrams of niacin, or 2 niacin equivalents. The RDA for niacin allows for this conversion and is stated in niacin equivalents; average niacin intakes in Canada exceed recommendations. The accompanying "How To" feature shows how to estimate niacin equivalents from both tryptophan and preformed niacin in the diet.

♦ 1 NE = 1 mg niacin or 60 mg tryptophan

Niacin Deficiency The niacin-deficiency disease, **pellagra**, produces the symptoms of diarrhea, dermatitis, dementia, and eventually death (often called "the four Ds"). Figure 10-8 illustrates the dermatitis of pellagra.

In the early 1900s, pellagra caused widespread misery and some 87 000 deaths in the U.S. South, where many people subsisted on a low-protein diet centred on corn. This diet supplied neither enough niacin nor enough tryptophan. At least 70 percent of the niacin in corn is bound to complex carbohydrates and small peptides, making it unavailable for absorption. Furthermore, corn is high in the

niacin (NIGH-a-sin): a B vitamin. The coenzyme forms are **NAD (nicotinamide adenine dinucleotide)** and **NADP (the phosphate form of NAD).** Niacin can be eaten preformed or made in the body from its precursor, tryptophan, an essential amino acid.

niacin equivalents (NE): the amount of niacin present in food, including the niacin that can theoretically be made from its precursor, tryptophan, present in the food.

pellagra (pell-AY-gra): the niacin-deficiency disease.
- **pellis** = skin
- **agra** = rough

amino acid leucine, which interferes with the tryptophan-to-niacin conversion, thus further contributing to the development of pellagra.

Pellagra was originally believed to be caused by an infection. Medical researchers spent many years and much effort searching for infectious microbes until they realized that the problem was not what was *present* in the food but what was *absent* from it. That a disease such as pellagra could be caused by diet—and not by pathogens—was a groundbreaking discovery. It contradicted commonly held medical opinions that diseases were caused only by infectious agents. By carefully following the scientific method (as described in Chapter 1), researchers advanced the science of nutrition dramatically.

Niacin Toxicity Naturally occurring niacin from foods ♦ causes no harm, but large doses from supplements or drugs produce a variety of adverse effects, most notably "**niacin flush.**" Niacin flush occurs when nicotinic acid is taken in doses only three to four times the RDA. It dilates the capillaries and causes a tingling sensation that can be painful. The nicotinamide form does not produce this effect.

♦ When a normal dose of a nutrient (levels commonly found in foods) provides a normal blood concentration, the nutrient is having a **physiological** effect. When a large dose (levels commonly available only from supplements) overwhelms some body system and acts like a drug, the nutrient is having a **pharmacological** effect.
- **physio** = natural
- **pharma** = drug

Large doses of nicotinic acid have been used to lower LDL cholesterol, raise HDL cholesterol, and increase adiponectin levels—all factors that help to protect against heart disease.[6] Such therapy must be closely monitored. People with the following conditions may be particularly susceptible to the toxic effects of niacin: liver disease, diabetes, peptic ulcers, gout, irregular heartbeats, inflammatory bowel disease, migraine headaches, and alcoholism. The nicotinamide form does not improve blood cholesterol levels.

Niacin Food Sources Tables of food composition typically list preformed niacin only, but as mentioned, niacin can also be made in the body from the amino acid tryptophan. Dietary tryptophan could meet about half the daily niacin need for most people, but the average diet easily supplies enough preformed niacin.

Figure 10-9 (p. 324) presents niacin in selected foods. Meat, poultry, legumes, and enriched and whole grains contribute about half the niacin people consume. Mushrooms, potatoes, and tomatoes are among the richest vegetable sources, and they can provide abundant niacin when eaten in generous amounts.

Niacin is less vulnerable to losses during food preparation and storage than other water-soluble vitamins. Being fairly heat resistant, niacin can withstand reasonable cooking times, but like other water-soluble vitamins, it will leach into cooking water. The accompanying table provides a summary of niacin.

niacin flush: a temporary burning, tingling, and itching sensation that occurs when a person takes a large dose of nicotinic acid; often accompanied by a headache and reddened face, arms, and chest.

biotin (BY-oh-tin): a B vitamin that functions as a coenzyme in metabolism.

IN SUMMARY Niacin

Other Names	Significant Sources
Nicotinic acid, nicotinamide, niacinamide, vitamin B_3; precursor is dietary tryptophan (an amino acid)	Milk, eggs, meat, poultry, fish; whole-grain, fortified, and enriched grain products; nuts and all protein-containing foods
RDA	**Deficiency Disease**
Men: 16 mg NE/day Women: 14 mg NE/day	Pellagra
Upper Level	**Deficiency Symptoms**
Adults: 35 mg/day	Diarrhea, abdominal pain, vomiting; inflamed, swollen, smooth, bright red tongue;[a] depression, apathy, fatigue, loss of memory, headache; bilateral symmetrical rash on areas exposed to sunlight
Chief Functions in the Body	**Toxicity Symptoms**
Part of coenzymes NAD (nicotinamide adenine dinucleotide) and NADP (its phosphate form) used in energy metabolism	Painful flush, hives, and rash ("niacin flush"); nausea and vomiting; liver damage, impaired glucose tolerance

[a]Smoothness of the tongue is caused by loss of its surface structures and is termed *glossitis* (gloss-EYE-tis).

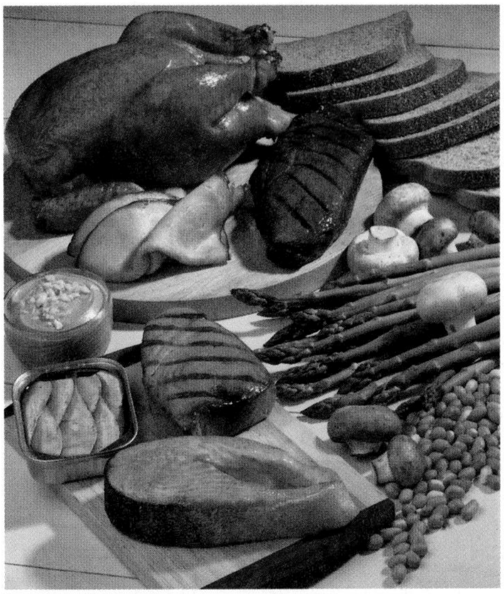

© Polara Studios, Inc.

Protein-rich foods such as meat, fish, poultry, and peanut butter contribute much of the niacin in people's diets. Enriched breads and cereals and a few vegetables are also rich in niacin.

Biotin

Biotin plays an important role in metabolism as a coenzyme that carries activated carbon dioxide. This role is critical in the TCA cycle: biotin delivers a

FIGURE 10-9 Niacin in Selected Foods

See the "How To" section on p. 317 for more information on using this figure.

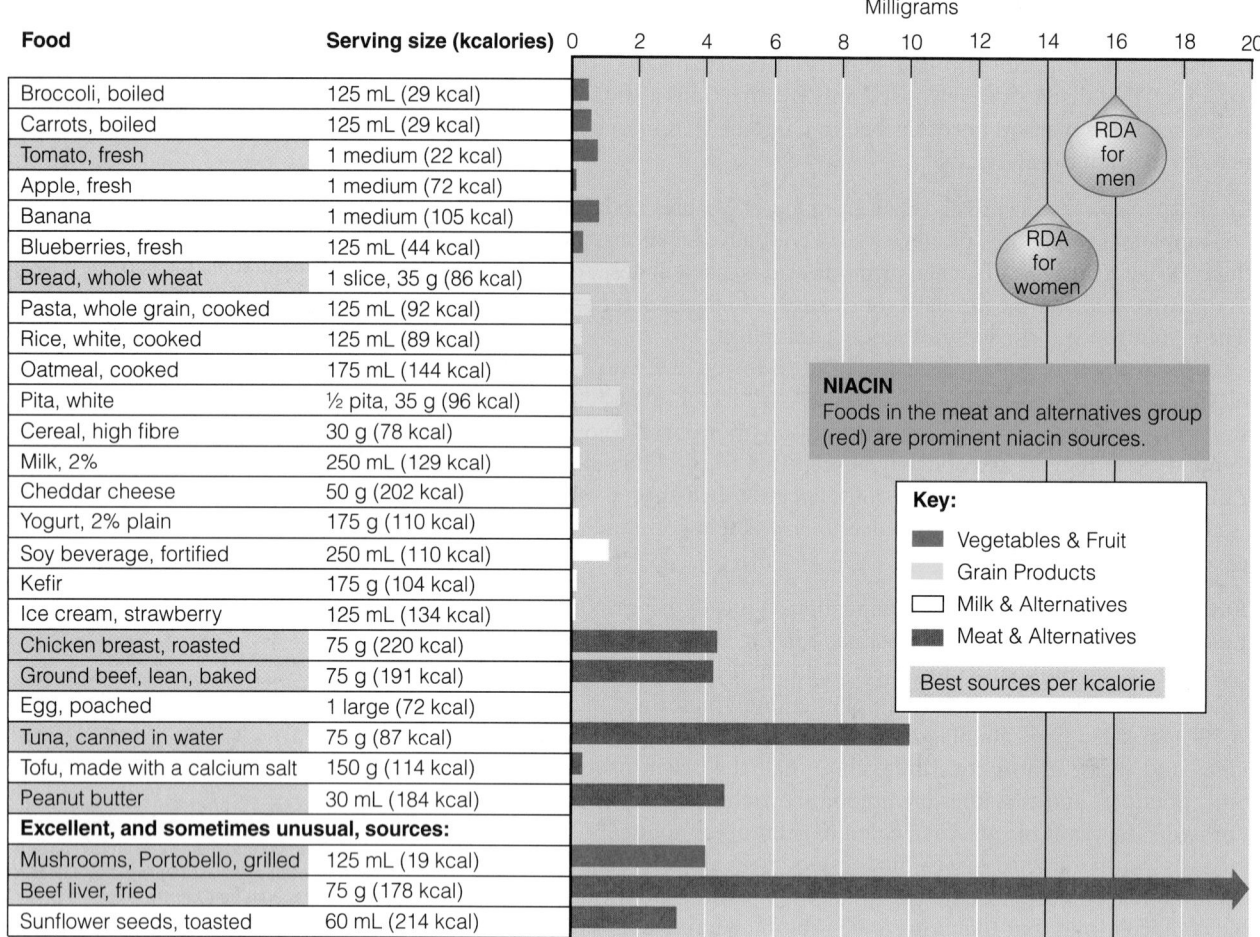

Food	Serving size (kcalories)
Broccoli, boiled	125 mL (29 kcal)
Carrots, boiled	125 mL (29 kcal)
Tomato, fresh	1 medium (22 kcal)
Apple, fresh	1 medium (72 kcal)
Banana	1 medium (105 kcal)
Blueberries, fresh	125 mL (44 kcal)
Bread, whole wheat	1 slice, 35 g (86 kcal)
Pasta, whole grain, cooked	125 mL (92 kcal)
Rice, white, cooked	125 mL (89 kcal)
Oatmeal, cooked	175 mL (144 kcal)
Pita, white	½ pita, 35 g (96 kcal)
Cereal, high fibre	30 g (78 kcal)
Milk, 2%	250 mL (129 kcal)
Cheddar cheese	50 g (202 kcal)
Yogurt, 2% plain	175 g (110 kcal)
Soy beverage, fortified	250 mL (110 kcal)
Kefir	175 g (104 kcal)
Ice cream, strawberry	125 mL (134 kcal)
Chicken breast, roasted	75 g (220 kcal)
Ground beef, lean, baked	75 g (191 kcal)
Egg, poached	1 large (72 kcal)
Tuna, canned in water	75 g (87 kcal)
Tofu, made with a calcium salt	150 g (114 kcal)
Peanut butter	30 mL (184 kcal)
Excellent, and sometimes unusual, sources:	
Mushrooms, Portobello, grilled	125 mL (19 kcal)
Beef liver, fried	75 g (178 kcal)
Sunflower seeds, toasted	60 mL (214 kcal)

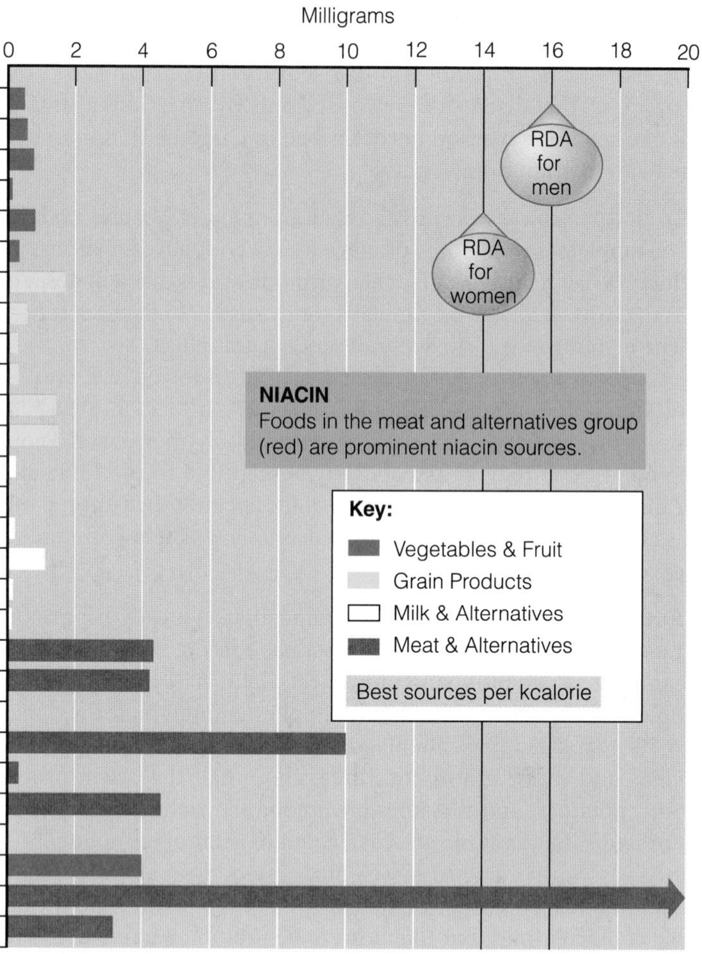
Milligrams
0 2 4 6 8 10 12 14 16 18 20
RDA for men
RDA for women
NIACIN
Foods in the meat and alternatives group (red) are prominent niacin sources.
Key:
Vegetables & Fruit
Grain Products
Milk & Alternatives
Meat & Alternatives
Best sources per kcalorie

♦ **Gluconeogenesis** is the synthesis of glucose from noncarbohydrate sources such as amino acids or glycerol.

♦ The protein **avidin** (AV-eh-din) in egg whites binds biotin.
- **avid** = greedy

carbon to 3-carbon pyruvate, thus replenishing oxaloacetate, the 4-carbon compound needed to combine with acetyl CoA to keep the TCA cycle turning (review Figure 7-16 on p. 220). The biotin coenzyme also participates in gluconeogenesis, ♦ fatty acid synthesis, and the breakdown of certain fatty acids and amino acids.

Biotin Recommendations Biotin is needed in very small amounts. Because there is insufficient research on biotin requirements, an Adequate Intake (AI) has been determined, instead of an RDA.

Biotin Deficiency and Toxicity Biotin deficiencies rarely occur. Researchers can induce a biotin deficiency in animals or human beings by feeding them raw egg whites, which contain a protein ♦ that binds biotin and thus prevents its absorption. Biotin-deficiency symptoms include skin rash, hair loss, and neurological impairment. More than two dozen raw egg whites must be consumed daily for several months to produce these effects; cooking eggs denatures the binding protein. No adverse effects from high biotin intakes have been reported. Biotin does not have a UL.

Biotin Food Sources Biotin is widespread in foods (including egg yolks), so eating a variety of foods protects against deficiencies. Some biotin is also synthesized by GI tract bacteria, but this amount may not contribute much to the biotin absorbed. The accompanying table provides a summary of biotin.

IN SUMMARY Biotin

Adequate Intake (AI)	Deficiency Symptoms
Adults: 30 μg/day	Depression, lethargy, hallucinations, numb or tingling sensation in the arms and legs; red, scaly rash around the eyes, nose, and mouth; hair loss
Chief Functions in the Body	**Toxicity Symptoms**
Part of a coenzyme used in energy metabolism, fat synthesis, amino acid metabolism, and glycogen synthesis	None reported
Significant Sources	
Widespread in foods; liver, egg yolks, soybeans, fish, whole grains; also produced by GI bacteria	

Pantothenic Acid

Pantothenic acid is part of the chemical structure of coenzyme A—the same CoA that forms acetyl CoA, the "crossroads" compound in several metabolic pathways, including the TCA cycle. (APPENDIX C presents the chemical structures of these two molecules and shows that coenzyme A is made up in part of pantothenic acid.) As such, it is involved in more than 100 different steps in the synthesis of lipids, neurotransmitters, steroid hormones, and hemoglobin.

Pantothenic Acid Recommendations An Adequate Intake (AI) for pantothenic acid has been set. It reflects the amount needed to replace daily losses.

Pantothenic Acid Deficiency and Toxicity Pantothenic acid deficiency is rare. Its symptoms involve a general failure of all the body's systems and include fatigue, GI distress, and neurological disturbances. The "burning feet" syndrome that affected prisoners of war in Asia during World War II is thought to have been caused by pantothenic acid deficiency. No toxic effects have been reported, and no UL has been established.

Pantothenic Acid Food Sources Pantothenic acid is widespread in foods, and typical diets seem to provide adequate intakes. Beef, poultry, whole grains, potatoes, tomatoes, and broccoli are particularly good sources. Losses of pantothenic acid during food production can be substantial because it is readily destroyed by the freezing, canning, and refining processes. The accompanying table provides a summary of pantothenic acid.

IN SUMMARY Pantothenic Acid

AI	Deficiency Symptoms
Adults: 5 mg/day	Vomiting, nausea, stomach cramps; insomnia, fatigue, depression, irritability, restlessness, apathy; hypoglycemia, increased sensitivity to insulin; numbness, muscle cramps, inability to walk
Chief Functions in the Body	**Toxicity Symptoms**
Part of coenzyme A, used in energy metabolism	None reported
Significant Sources	
Widespread in foods; chicken, beef, potatoes, oats, tomatoes, liver, egg yolk, broccoli, whole grains	
Easily destroyed by food processing	

Vitamin B_6

Vitamin B_6 occurs in three forms—pyridoxal, pyridoxine, and pyridoxamine. All three can be converted to the coenzyme PLP (pyridoxal phosphate), which is active in amino acid metabolism. Because PLP can transfer amino groups (NH_2) from an amino acid to a keto acid, the body can make dispensable/nonessential amino acids (review Figure 6-12 on p. 184). The ability to add and remove amino groups makes PLP valuable in protein and urea metabolism as well. The conversions of the amino acid tryptophan to niacin or to the neurotransmitter serotonin ♦ also depend on PLP. In addition, PLP participates in the synthesis of heme (the nonprotein portion of hemoglobin), nucleic acids (such as DNA and RNA), and lecithin (a phospholipid).

♦ **Serotonin** is a neurotransmitter important in appetite control, sleep regulation, and sensory perception, among other roles; it is synthesized in the body from the amino acid tryptophan with the help of vitamin B_6.

pantothenic (PAN-toe-THEN-ick) **acid:** a B vitamin. The principal active form is part of coenzyme A, called "CoA" throughout Chapter 7.

- **pantos** = everywhere

vitamin B_6: a family of compounds—pyridoxal, pyridoxine, and pyridoxamine. The primary active coenzyme form is **PLP (pyridoxal phosphate).**

A surge of research in the last decade has revealed that vitamin B_6 influences cognitive performance, immune function, and steroid hormone activity. Unlike other water-soluble vitamins, vitamin B_6 is stored extensively in muscle tissue.

Vitamin B_6 Recommendations Because vitamin B_6 coenzymes participate in amino acid metabolism, previous RDA were expressed in terms of protein intakes; the current RDA for vitamin B_6, however, is not. Research does not support claims that large doses of vitamin B_6 enhance muscle strength or physical endurance. As Highlight 15 explains, dietary supplements cannot compete with a nutritious diet and physical training.

Vitamin B_6 Deficiency Without adequate vitamin B_6, synthesis of key neurotransmitters diminishes, and abnormal compounds produced during tryptophan metabolism accumulate in the brain. Early symptoms of vitamin B_6 deficiency include depression and confusion; advanced symptoms include abnormal brain wave patterns and convulsions.

Alcohol contributes to the destruction and loss of vitamin B_6 from the body. As Highlight 7 describes, when the body breaks down alcohol, it produces acetaldehyde. If allowed to accumulate, acetaldehyde dislodges the PLP coenzyme from its enzymes; once loose, PLP breaks down and is excreted.

Another drug that acts as a vitamin B_6 **antagonist** is isoniazid, a medication that inhibits the growth of the tuberculosis bacterium.* This drug has saved countless lives, but because isoniazid binds and inactivates vitamin B_6, it can induce a deficiency. Whenever isoniazid is used to treat tuberculosis, vitamin B_6 supplements must be given to protect against deficiency.

Vitamin B_6 Toxicity The first major report of vitamin B_6 toxicity appeared in the early 1980s. Until that time, most researchers and dietitians believed that, like the other water-soluble vitamins, vitamin B_6 could not reach toxic concentrations in the body. The report described neurological damage in people who had been taking more than 2 *grams* of vitamin B_6 daily (20 times the current UL of 100 *milligrams* per day) for two months or more.

Some people have taken vitamin B_6 supplements in an attempt to cure **carpal tunnel syndrome** even though such treatment appears to be ineffective.[7] Self-prescribing is ill advised because large doses of vitamin B_6 may cause irreversible nerve degeneration.

Vitamin B_6 Food Sources As you can see from the colours in Figure 10-10, meats, fish, and poultry (red bars) and some vegetables and fruit (green bars) offer vitamin B_6. As is true of most of the other vitamins, vegetables and fruits rank considerably higher when foods are judged by nutrient density (vitamin B_6 per kcalorie). Several servings of vitamin B_6–rich foods are needed to meet recommended intakes.

Foods lose vitamin B_6 when heated. Information is limited, but vitamin B_6 bioavailability from plant-derived foods seems to be lower than from animal-derived foods. Fibre does not appear to interfere with vitamin B_6 absorption. The accompanying table provides a summary of vitamin B_6.

Folate

Folate, also known as folacin or folic acid, has a chemical name that would fit a flying dinosaur: pteroylglutamic acid (PGA for short). Its primary coenzyme form, THF (tetrahydrofolate), serves as part of an enzyme complex that transfers 1-carbon compounds that arise during metabolism. This action converts vitamin B_{12} to one of its coenzyme forms, synthesizes the DNA required for all rapidly growing cells, and regenerates the amino acid methionine from homocysteine.

antagonist: a competing factor that counteracts the action of another factor. When a drug displaces a vitamin from its site of action, the drug renders the vitamin ineffective and thus acts as a vitamin antagonist.

carpal tunnel syndrome: a pinched nerve at the wrist, causing pain or numbness in the hand. It is often caused by repetitive motion of the wrist.

folate (FOLE-ate): a B vitamin; also known as folic acid, folacin, or pteroylglutamic (tare-o-EEL-glue-TAM-ick) acid (PGA). The coenzyme forms are **DHF (dihydrofolate)** and **THF (tetrahydrofolate).**

*Isoniazid (eye-so-NYE-uh-zid) is also known as INH (isonicotinic acid hydrazide).

FIGURE 10-10 Vitamin B_6 in Selected Foods

See the "How To" section on p. 317 for more information on using this figure.

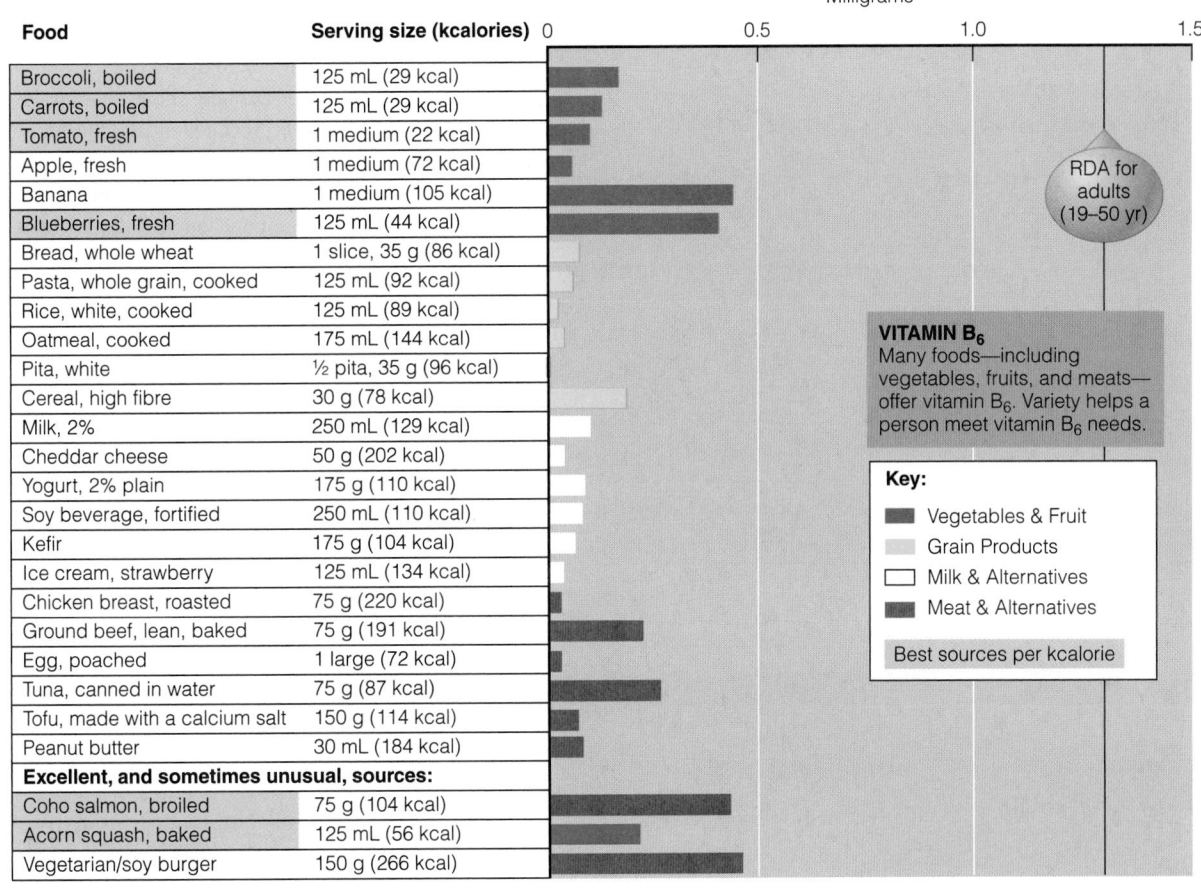

Food	Serving size (kcalories)
Broccoli, boiled	125 mL (29 kcal)
Carrots, boiled	125 mL (29 kcal)
Tomato, fresh	1 medium (22 kcal)
Apple, fresh	1 medium (72 kcal)
Banana	1 medium (105 kcal)
Blueberries, fresh	125 mL (44 kcal)
Bread, whole wheat	1 slice, 35 g (86 kcal)
Pasta, whole grain, cooked	125 mL (92 kcal)
Rice, white, cooked	125 mL (89 kcal)
Oatmeal, cooked	175 mL (144 kcal)
Pita, white	½ pita, 35 g (96 kcal)
Cereal, high fibre	30 g (78 kcal)
Milk, 2%	250 mL (129 kcal)
Cheddar cheese	50 g (202 kcal)
Yogurt, 2% plain	175 g (110 kcal)
Soy beverage, fortified	250 mL (110 kcal)
Kefir	175 g (104 kcal)
Ice cream, strawberry	125 mL (134 kcal)
Chicken breast, roasted	75 g (220 kcal)
Ground beef, lean, baked	75 g (191 kcal)
Egg, poached	1 large (72 kcal)
Tuna, canned in water	75 g (87 kcal)
Tofu, made with a calcium salt	150 g (114 kcal)
Peanut butter	30 mL (184 kcal)
Excellent, and sometimes unusual, sources:	
Coho salmon, broiled	75 g (104 kcal)
Acorn squash, baked	125 mL (56 kcal)
Vegetarian/soy burger	150 g (266 kcal)

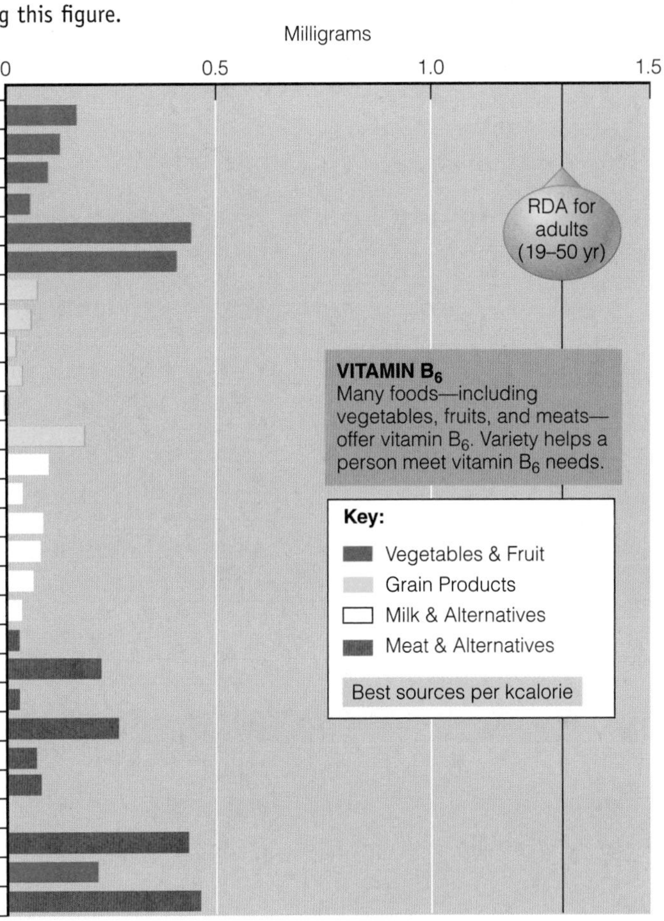

Milligrams
0
0.5
1.0
1.5
RDA for adults (19–50 yr)
VITAMIN B6
Many foods—including vegetables, fruits, and meats—offer vitamin B6. Variety helps a person meet vitamin B6 needs.
Key:
Vegetables & Fruit
Grain Products
Milk & Alternatives
Meat & Alternatives
Best sources per kcalorie

SOURCE: Canadian Nutrient File. Health Canada, 2008. Reproduced with the permission of the Minister of Health, 2011.

IN SUMMARY Vitamin B_6

Other Names

Pyridoxine, pyridoxal, pyridoxamine

RDA

Adults (19–50 yr): 1.3 mg/day

Upper Level

Adults: 100 mg/day

Chief Functions in the Body

Part of coenzymes PLP (pyridoxal phosphate) and PMP (pyridoxamine phosphate) used in amino acid and fatty acid metabolism; helps to convert tryptophan to niacin and to serotonin; helps to make red blood cells

Significant Sources

Meats, fish, poultry, potatoes and other starchy vegetables, legumes, noncitrus fruits, fortified cereals, liver, fortified soy products

Easily destroyed by heat

Deficiency Symptoms

Scaly dermatitis; anemia (small-cell type);[a] depression, confusion, convulsions

Toxicity Symptoms

Depression, fatigue, irritability, headaches, nerve damage causing numbness and muscle weakness leading to an inability to walk and convulsions; skin lesions

[a]Small-cell-type anemia is called *microcytic anemia*.

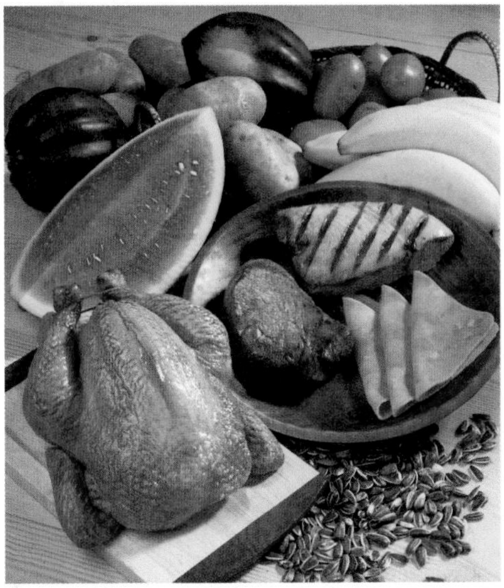

Most protein-rich foods such as meat, fish, and poultry provide ample vitamin B_6; some vegetables and fruits are good sources, too.

HOW TO Estimate Dietary Folate Equivalents

Folate is expressed in terms of DFE (dietary folate equivalents) because synthetic folate from supplements and fortified foods is absorbed at almost twice (1.7 times) the rate of naturally occurring folate from other foods. Use the following equation to calculate:

$$\text{DFE} = \mu\text{g food folate} + (1.7 \times \mu\text{g synthetic folate})$$

Consider, for example, a pregnant woman who takes a supplement and eats a bowl of fortified cornflakes, 2 slices of fortified bread, and a cup of fortified pasta. From the supplement and fortified foods, she obtains synthetic folate:

Supplement	100 μg folate
Fortified cornflakes	100 μg folate
Fortified bread	40 μg folate
Fortified pasta	60 μg folate
	300 μg folate

To calculate the DFE, multiply the amount of synthetic folate by 1.7:

$$300\ \mu\text{g} \times 1.7 = 510\ \mu\text{g DFE}$$

Now add the naturally occurring folate from the other foods in her diet—in this example, another 90 μg of folate.

$$510\ \mu\text{g DFE} + 90\ \mu\text{g} = 600\ \mu\text{g DFE}$$

Notice that if we had not converted synthetic folate from supplements and fortified foods to DFE, then this woman's intake would appear to fall short of the 600 μg recommendation for pregnancy (300 μg + 90 μg = 390 μg) in the DRI for folate. But as our example shows, her intake does meet the DRI recommendation. However, *Eating Well with Canada's Food Guide* recommends women of childbearing years who are capable of becoming pregnant take a multivitamin supplement containing 400 μg of folic acid every day, in addition to meeting the DRI-RDA recommendation. At this time, supplement and fortified food labels list folate in μg only, not μg DFE, making such calculations necessary.

CENGAGENOW™
For additional practice log on to **www.cengage.com/sso.**

TRY IT Calculate how many dietary folate equivalents a person receives from 200 μg folate from a supplement, 75 μg folate from fortified cereal, and 120 μg folate from other foods.

Figure 10-11 summarizes folate's absorption, activation, and relationship with vitamin B_{12}. It explains that foods deliver folate mostly in the "bound" form—that is, combined with a string of amino acids (all glutamate), known as polyglutamate. (See APPENDIX C for the chemical structure.) Enzymes on the intestinal cell surfaces hydrolyze the polyglutamate to monoglutamate—folate with only one glutamate attached—and several glutamates. The monoglutamate is then attached to a methyl group (CH_3) and delivered to the liver and other body cells. To activate folate, the methyl group must be removed by an enzyme that requires the help of vitamin B_{12}. Without that help, folate becomes trapped inside cells in its methyl form, unavailable to support DNA synthesis and cell growth.

To dispose of excess folate, the liver secretes most of it into bile that is sent to the gallbladder. Thus folate returns to the intestine in an enterohepatic circulation route like that of bile itself (review Figure 5-16 on p. 140).

This complicated system for handling folate is vulnerable to GI tract injuries. Because folate is actively secreted back into the GI tract with bile, it can be reabsorbed repeatedly. If the GI tract cells are damaged, then folate is lost. Such is the case in alcohol abuse; folate deficiency rapidly develops and, ironically, further damages the GI tract. Remember, folate is active in cell multiplication—and the cells lining the GI tract are among the most rapidly replaced cells in the body. When unable to make new cells, the GI tract deteriorates and not only loses folate, but fails to absorb other nutrients as well.

♦ To calculate DFE:
DFE = μg food folate + (1.7 × μg synthetic folate)
Using the example in the text:

	100 μg food
+	170 μg supplement (1.7 × 100 μg)
	270 μg DFE

dietary folate equivalents (DFE): the amount of folate available to the body from naturally occurring sources, fortified foods, and supplements, accounting for differences in the bioavailability from each source.

Folate Recommendations The bioavailability of folate ranges from 50 percent for foods to 100 percent for supplements taken on an empty stomach. These differences in bioavailability were considered when establishing the folate RDA. Naturally occurring folate from foods is given full credit. Synthetic folate (folic acid) from fortified foods and supplements is given extra credit because, on average, it is 1.7 times more available than naturally occurring food folate. Thus a person consuming 100 micrograms of folate from foods and 100 micrograms of folic acid in a supplement receives 270 **dietary folate equivalents (DFE)**. ♦ (The "How To" describes how to estimate dietary folate equivalents.) The need for folate rises considerably during pregnancy and whenever cells are multiplying, so the recommendations for pregnant women are considerably higher than for other adults.

FIGURE 10-11 Folate's Absorption and Activation

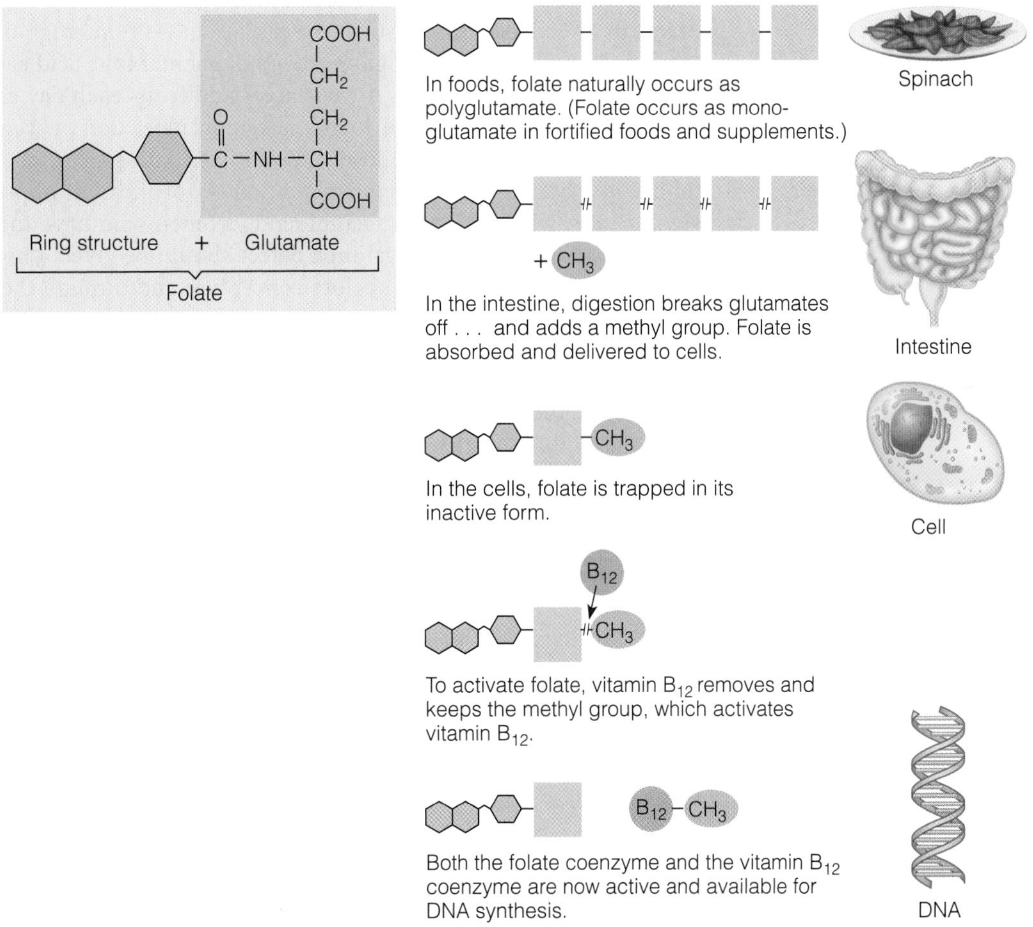
COOH
CH_2
O
CH_2
C − NH − CH
COOH
Ring structure + Glutamate
Folate
In foods, folate naturally occurs as polyglutamate. (Folate occurs as monoglutamate in fortified foods and supplements.)
Spinach
+ CH_3
In the intestine, digestion breaks glutamates off . . . and adds a methyl group. Folate is absorbed and delivered to cells.
Intestine
CH_3
In the cells, folate is trapped in its inactive form.
Cell
B_{12}
CH_3
To activate folate, vitamin B_{12} removes and keeps the methyl group, which activates vitamin B_{12}.
B_{12} − CH_3
Both the folate coenzyme and the vitamin B_{12} coenzyme are now active and available for DNA synthesis.
DNA

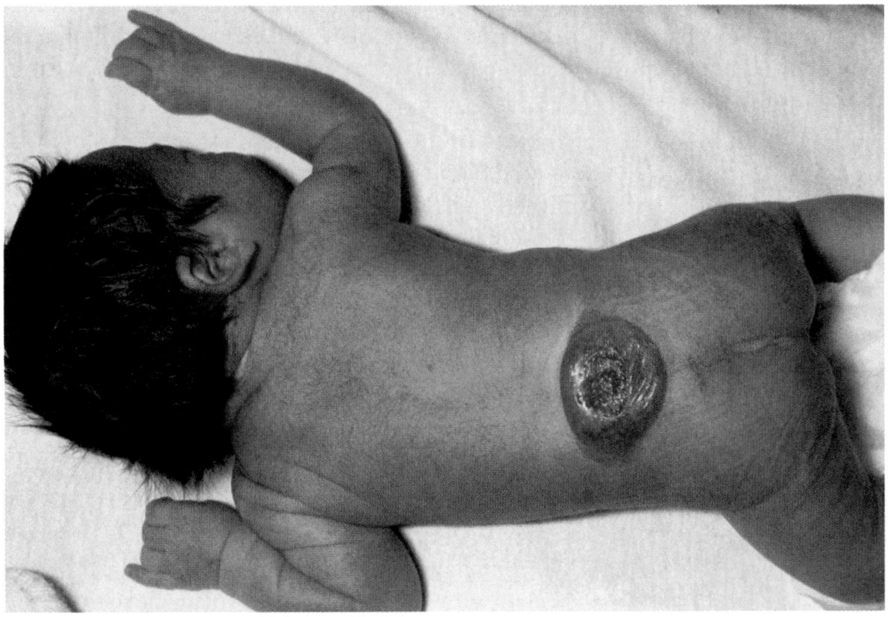

Folate helps to protect against spina bifida, a neural tube defect characterized by the incomplete closure of the spinal cord and its bony encasement.

Folate and Neural Tube Defects The brain and spinal cord develop from the **neural tube**, and defects in its orderly formation during the early weeks of pregnancy may result in various central nervous system disorders and death. (Chapter 16 includes photos of neural tube development and an illustration of a neural tube defect.)

neural tube: the embryonic tissue that forms the brain and spinal cord.

♦ The two main types of neural tube defects are **spina bifida** (literally, "split spine") and **anencephaly** ("no brain").

♦ Women of childbearing age (15 to 45 yr) should:
- Eat folate-rich foods
- Eat folate-fortified foods
- Take a multivitamin daily (most provide 400 μg folate)

♦ A milligram (mg) is one-thousandth of a gram. A microgram (μg) is one-thousandth of a milligram (or one-millionth of a gram).
- 0.4 mg = 400 μg

Folic acid supplements taken one month before conception and continued throughout the first trimester of pregnancy can help prevent **neural tube defects.** ♦ For this reason, all women of childbearing age ♦ who are capable of becoming pregnant are advised to consume 0.4 milligram (400 micrograms) of folate from foods and another 400 micrograms of supplemental folic acid each day. ♦ Women who eat at least five servings of vegetables and fruits each day can meet the daily folate recommendation from foods, although most don't eat enough servings.[8] Furthermore, the bioavailability of food folate is less than that of supplemental folic acid.[9] Consequently, supplementation or fortification improves folate status significantly. Health Canada recommends women who have increased risk for a pregnancy affected by a neural tube defect should be given a higher dose of folic acid daily (4 to 5 milligrams) before conception and through the first trimester of pregnancy.

Because half of the pregnancies each year are unplanned and because neural tube defects occur early in development before most women realize they are pregnant, Health Canada has mandated that certain grain products be fortified to deliver folic acid to the Canadian population.* Fortification has improved folate status in women of childbearing age and lowered the number of neural tube defects that occur each year, as Figure 10-12 shows. In the four years after mandatory fortification came into effect in 1998, the prevalence of neural tube defects fell 46 percent and geographical differences disappeared across Canada.[10]

Some research suggests that folate may also prevent other congenital birth defects, such as cleft lip and palate.[11] Such findings strengthen recommendations for pregnant women to pay attention to their folate needs.

Folic acid fortification raises safety concerns as well. Because high intakes of folate can mask a vitamin B_{12} deficiency, folate consumption should not exceed 1 milligram daily without close medical supervision.[12] The risks and benefits of folate fortification continue to be a topic of current debate.[13]

Folate and Heart Disease Health Canada's decision to fortify grain products with folic acid was strengthened by research suggesting a role for folate in protecting against heart disease.[14] One of folate's key roles in the body is to break down the amino acid homocysteine. Without folate, homocysteine accumulates, which seems to enhance formation of blood clots and atherosclerotic lesions. Fortified foods and folic acid supplements raise blood folate and reduce blood homocysteine, but do not seem to reduce the risk of heart attacks, strokes, or death from cardiovascular causes.[15]

neural tube defects: malformations of the brain, spinal cord, or both during embryonic development that often result in lifelong disability or death.

FIGURE 10-12 Reduction in Neural-Tube Defects after Folic Acid Fortification in Canada

Neural tube defects have declined since folate fortification began in 1998.

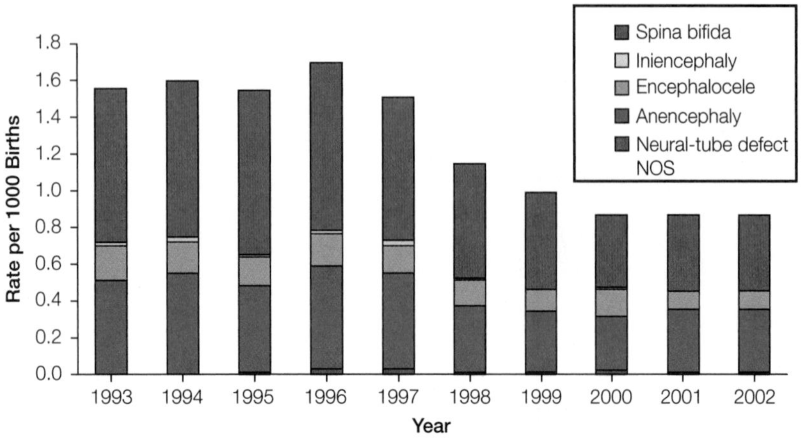
Spina bifida
Iniencephaly
Encephalocele
Anencephaly
Neural-tube defect NOS
1.8
1.6
1.4
1.2
1.0
0.8
0.6
0.4
0.2
0.0
Rate per 1000 Births
1993
1994
1995
1996
1997
1998
1999
2000
2001
2002
Year

SOURCE: P. De Wals et al., "Reduction in neural-tube defects after folic acid fortification in Canada", New England Journal of Medicine 357(2). Copyright 2007 Massachusetts Medical Society.

Folate and Cancer Because the synthesis of DNA and the transfer of methyl groups depend on folate, its relationships with cancer are complex, depending on the type of cancer and the timing of folate supplementation. Sufficient folate may protect against the initiation of cancer, but it may enhance progression once cancer has begun.[16] In general, foods containing folate probably reduce the risk of pancreatic cancer.[17] Some evidence suggests folate may also reduce the risk of colorectal cancer, but may increase risk of postmenopausal breast cancer in women carrying a particular genetic marker.[18]

Folate Deficiency Folate deficiency impairs cell division and protein synthesis—processes critical to growing tissues. In a folate deficiency, the

*White flour and enriched pasta and corn meal must be fortified to a level of 0.15 to 0.20 milligrams per 100 grams of product. For perspective, 100 grams is roughly 3 slices of bread; 250 mL (1 cup) of flour; 125 mL (1/2 cup) of cornmeal, farina, or 185 mL (3/4 cup) of macaroni or noodles.

replacement of red blood cells and GI tract cells falters. Not surprisingly, then, two of the first symptoms of a folate deficiency are **anemia** and GI tract deterioration.

The anemia of folate deficiency is characterized by large, ♦ immature red blood cells. Without folate, DNA damage destroys many of the red blood cells as they attempt to divide and mature. The result is fewer, but larger, red blood cells that cannot carry oxygen or travel through the capillaries as efficiently as normal red blood cells.

Primary folate deficiencies may develop from inadequate intake and have been reported in infants who were fed goat's milk, which is notoriously low in folate. Secondary folate deficiencies may result from impaired absorption or an unusual metabolic need for the vitamin. Metabolic needs increase in situations where cell multiplication must speed up, such as pregnancies involving twins and triplets; cancer; skin-destroying diseases such as chicken pox and measles; and burns, blood loss, GI tract damage, and the like.

Of all the vitamins, folate appears to be most vulnerable to interactions with drugs, which can also lead to a secondary deficiency. Some medications, notably anticancer drugs, have a chemical structure similar to folate's structure and can displace the vitamin from enzymes and interfere with normal metabolism. Like all cells, cancer cells need the real vitamin to multiply—without it, they die. Unfortunately, anticancer drugs affect both cancerous cells and healthy cells, creating a folate deficiency for all cells. (Highlight 18 discusses nutrient–drug interactions and includes a figure illustrating the similarities between the vitamin folate and the anticancer drug methotrexate.)

Aspirin and antacids also interfere with the body's folate status: aspirin inhibits the action of folate-requiring enzymes, and antacids limit the absorption of folate. Healthy adults who use these drugs to relieve an occasional headache or upset stomach need not be concerned, but people who rely heavily on aspirin or antacids should be aware of the nutrition consequences. Oral contraceptives may also impair folate status, as may smoking.[19]

Folate Toxicity Naturally occurring folate from foods alone appears to cause no harm. Excess folate from fortified foods or supplements, however, can reach levels that are high enough to obscure a vitamin B_{12} deficiency and delay diagnosis of neurological damage. For this reason, a UL has been established for folate from fortified foods or supplements (see the inside front cover).

Folate Food Sources Figure 10-13 (p. 332) shows that folate is especially abundant in legumes, fruits, and vegetables. The vitamin's name suggests the word *foliage,* and indeed, leafy green vegetables are outstanding sources. With fortification, grain products also contribute folate. See Table 10-2 for the folate fortification level in grain products that is required by Canada's Food and Drug Regulations. The small red and white bars in Figure 10-13 indicate that meats and milk products are poor folate sources. Heat and oxidation during cooking and storage can destroy as much as half of the folate in foods. The accompanying table provides a summary of folate.

IN SUMMARY Folate

Other Names	Significant Sources
Folic acid, folacin, pteroylglutamic acid (PGA)	Fortified grains, leafy green vegetables, legumes, seeds, liver
	Easily destroyed by heat and oxygen
RDA	**Deficiency Symptoms**
Adults: 400 µg/day	Anemia (large-cell type);[a] smooth, red tongue;[b] mental confusion, weakness, fatigue, irritability, headache; shortness of breath; elevated homocysteine
Upper Level	
Adults: 1000 µg/day	
Chief Functions in the Body	**Toxicity Symptoms**
Part of coenzymes THF (tetrahydrofolate) and DHF (dihydrofolate) used in DNA synthesis and therefore important in new cell formation	Masks vitamin B_{12}–deficiency symptoms

[a]Large-cell-type anemia is known as either *macrocytic* or *megaloblastic anemia.*

[b]Smoothness of the tongue is caused by loss of its surface structures and is termed *glossitis* (gloss-EYE-tis).

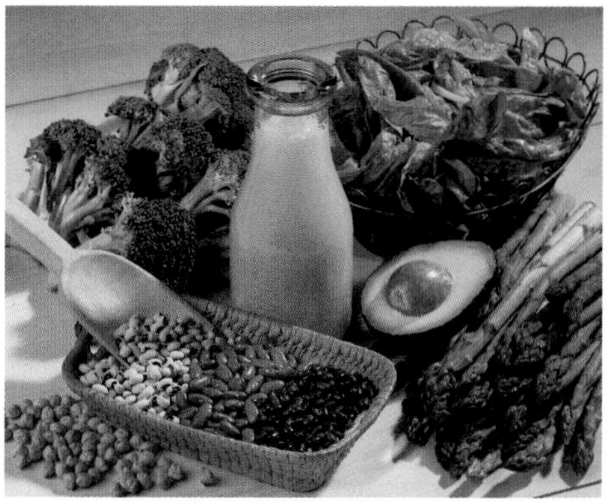

© Polara Studios, Inc.

Leafy dark green vegetables (such as spinach and broccoli), legumes (such as black beans, kidney beans, and black-eyed peas), liver, and some fruits (notably citrus fruits and juices) are naturally rich in folate.

♦ Large-cell anemia is known as **macrocytic** or **megaloblastic** anemia.
- **macro** = large
- **cyte** = cell
- **mega** = large

TABLE 10-2 Mandatory Fortification of Grain Products in Canada

Current levels in 100 grams of flour, white flour, enriched flour, or enriched white flour

Nutrient	Level
Thiamin (mg)	0.64
Riboflavin (mg)	0.40
Niacin (mg)	5.30
Folic acid (mg)	0.15
Iron (mg)	4.4

SOURCE: Justice Canada, Food and Drug Regulations, Part B, Division 13, 13.001.[S], Grain and bakery products.

anemia (ah-NEE-me-ah): literally, "too little blood." Anemia is any condition in which too few red blood cells are present, or the red blood cells are immature (and therefore large) or too small or contain too little hemoglobin to carry the normal amount of oxygen to the tissues. It is not a disease itself but can be a consequence of many different disease conditions, including many nutrient deficiencies, bleeding, excessive red blood cell destruction, and defective red blood cell formation.
- **an** = without
- **emia** = blood

FIGURE 10-13 **Folate in Selected Foods**

See the "How To" section on p. 317 for more information on using this figure.

Food	Serving size (kcalories)
Broccoli, boiled	125 mL (29 kcal)
Carrots, boiled	125 mL (29 kcal)
Tomato, fresh	1 medium (22 kcal)
Apple, fresh	1 medium (72 kcal)
Banana	1 medium (105 kcal)
Blueberries, fresh	125 mL (44 kcal)
Bread, whole wheat	1 slice, 35 g (86 kcal)
Pasta, whole grain, cooked	125 mL (92 kcal)
Rice, white, cooked	125 mL (89 kcal)
Oatmeal, cooked	175 mL (144 kcal)
Pita, white	½ pita, 35 g (96 kcal)
Cereal, high fibre	30 g (78 kcal)
Milk, 2%	250 mL (129 kcal)
Cheddar cheese	50 g (202 kcal)
Yogurt, 2% plain	175 g (110 kcal)
Soy beverage, fortified	250 mL (110 kcal)
Kefir	175 g (104 kcal)
Ice cream, strawberry	125 mL (134 kcal)
Chicken breast, roasted	75 g (220 kcal)
Ground beef, lean, baked	75 g (191 kcal)
Egg, poached	1 large (72 kcal)
Tuna, canned in water	75 g (87 kcal)
Tofu, made with a calcium salt	150 g (114 kcal)
Peanut butter	30 mL (184 kcal)
Excellent, and sometimes unusual, sources:	
Asparagus, boiled	125 mL (21 kcal)
Lentils, boiled	175 mL (170 kcal)
Orange juice, from concentrate	125 mL (59 kcal)

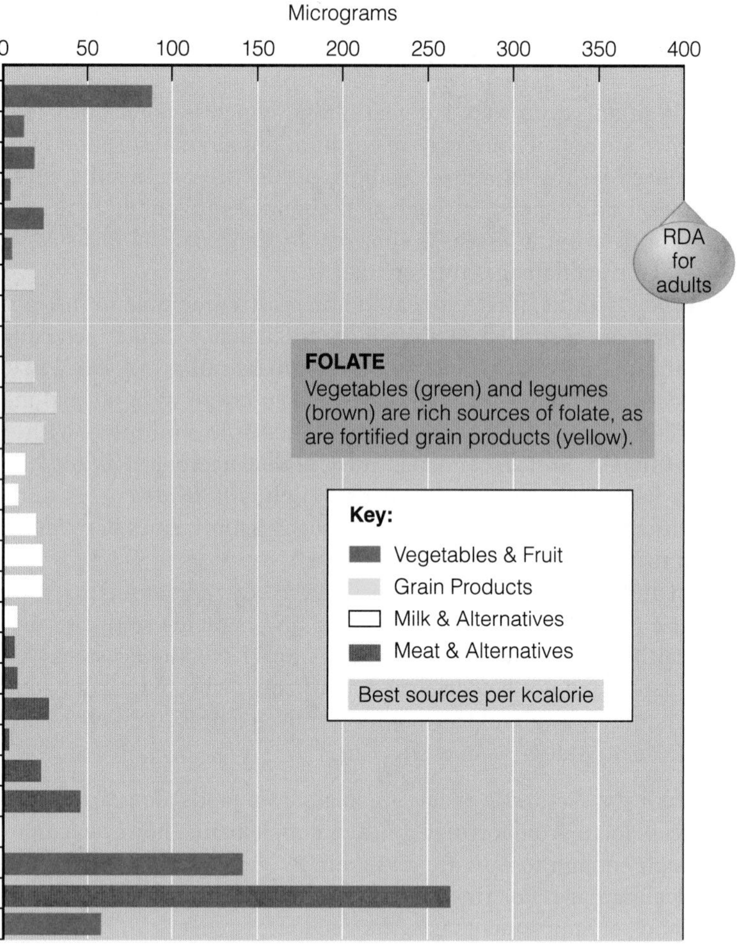
Micrograms
0
50
100
150
200
250
300
350
400
RDA for adults
FOLATE
Vegetables (green) and legumes (brown) are rich sources of folate, as are fortified grain products (yellow).
Key:
Vegetables & Fruit
Grain Products
Milk & Alternatives
Meat & Alternatives
Best sources per kcalorie

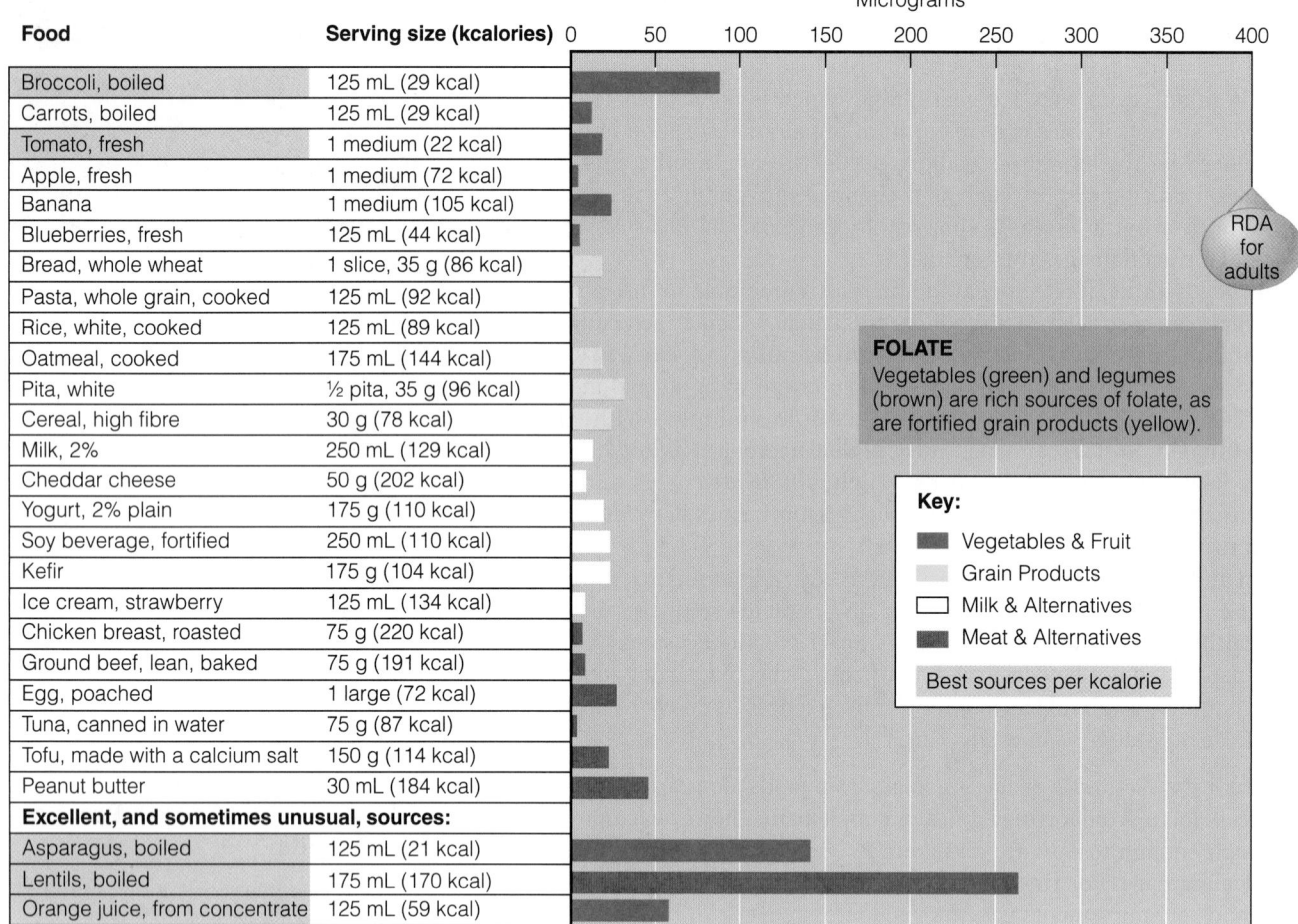

SOURCE: Canadian Nutrient File. Health Canada, 2008. Reproduced with the permission of the Minister of Health, 2011.

Vitamin B_{12}

Vitamin B_{12} and folate are closely related: each depends on the other for activation. Recall that vitamin B_{12} removes a methyl group to activate the folate coenzyme. When folate gives up its methyl group, the vitamin B_{12} coenzyme becomes activated (review Figure 10-11 on p. 329).

The regeneration of the amino acid methionine and the synthesis of DNA and RNA depend on both folate and vitamin B_{12}.* In addition, without any help from folate, vitamin B_{12} maintains the sheath that surrounds and protects nerve fibres and promotes their normal growth. Bone cell activity and metabolism also depend on vitamin B_{12}.

Vitamin B_{12} is a large molecule with a cobalt centre (see Figure 10-14). Because of its physical and chemical characteristics, the digestion and absorption of vitamin B_{12} depend on several steps. In the stomach, hydrochloric acid and the digestive enzyme pepsin release vitamin B_{12} from the proteins to which it is attached in foods. Then as vitamin B_{12} passes from the stomach to the small intestine, it binds with a stomach secretion called **intrinsic factor.** Bound together, intrinsic factor and vitamin B_{12} travel to the end of the small intestine, where receptors recognize the complex. Importantly, the receptors do not recognize vitamin B_{12} without intrinsic factor. The vitamin is gradually absorbed into the bloodstream as the intrinsic factor is degraded. Transport of vitamin B_{12} in the blood depends on specific binding proteins.

Like folate, vitamin B_{12} enters the enterohepatic circulation—continually being secreted into bile and delivered to the intestine where it is reabsorbed. Because

vitamin B_{12}: a B vitamin characterized by the presence of cobalt. The active forms of coenzyme B_{12} are methylcobalamin and deoxyadenosylcobalamin.

intrinsic factor: a glycoprotein (a protein with short polysaccharide chains attached) secreted by the stomach cells that binds with vitamin B_{12} in the small intestine to aid in the absorption of vitamin B_{12}.
- **intrinsic** = on the inside

atrophic (a-TRO-fik) **gastritis** (gas-TRY-tis): chronic inflammation of the stomach accompanied by a diminished size and functioning of the mucous membrane and glands.
- **atrophy** = wasting
- **gastro** = stomach
- **itis** = inflammation

*In the body, methionine serves as a methyl (CH_3) donor. In doing so, methionine can be converted to other amino acids. Some of these amino acids can regenerate methionine, but methionine is still considered an essential amino acid that is needed in the diet.

most vitamin B_{12} is reabsorbed, healthy people rarely develop a deficiency even when their intake is minimal.

Vitamin B_{12} Recommendations The RDA for adults is only 2.4 micrograms of vitamin B_{12} a day—just over two-millionths of a gram. The ink in the period at the end of this sentence may weigh about 2.4 micrograms. As tiny as this amount appears to the human eye, it contains billions of molecules of vitamin B_{12}, enough to provide coenzymes for all the enzymes that need its help.

Vitamin B_{12} Deficiency and Toxicity Most vitamin B_{12} deficiencies reflect inadequate absorption, not poor intake. Inadequate absorption typically occurs for one of two reasons: a lack of hydrochloric acid or a lack of intrinsic factor. Without hydrochloric acid, the vitamin is not released from the dietary proteins and so is not available for binding with the intrinsic factor. Without the intrinsic factor, the vitamin cannot be absorbed.

Vitamin B_{12} deficiency is common among the elderly.[20] Many people, especially those older than 50, develop **atrophic gastritis**, a condition that damages the cells of the stomach. Atrophic gastritis may also develop in response to iron deficiency or infection with *Helicobacter pylori*, the bacterium implicated in ulcer formation. Without healthy stomach cells, production of hydrochloric acid and intrinsic factor diminishes. Even with an adequate intake from foods, vitamin B_{12} status suffers. The vitamin B_{12} deficiency caused by atrophic gastritis and a lack of intrinsic factor is known as **pernicious anemia.**

Some people inherit a defective gene for the intrinsic factor. In such cases, or when the stomach has been injured and cannot produce enough of the intrinsic factor, vitamin B_{12} must be injected to bypass the need for intestinal absorption. Alternatively, the vitamin may be delivered by nasal spray; absorption is rapid, high, and well tolerated.

A prolonged inadequate intake, as can occur with a vegan diet, ♦ may also create a vitamin B_{12} deficiency. People who stop eating animal-derived foods containing vitamin B_{12} may take several years to develop deficiency symptoms because the body recycles much of its vitamin B_{12}, reabsorbing it over and over again. Even when the body fails to absorb vitamin B_{12}, deficiency may take up to three years to develop because the body conserves its supply. Neurological degeneration, a sign of vitamin B_{12} deficiency, appears more rapidly in infants born to mothers with unsupplemented vegan diets or untreated pernicious anemia.[21]

Because vitamin B_{12} is required to convert folate to its active form, one of the most obvious vitamin B_{12}–deficiency symptoms is the anemia of folate deficiency. This anemia is characterized by large, immature red blood cells, which indicate slow DNA synthesis and an inability to divide (see Figure 10-15). When folate is trapped in its inactive (methyl folate) form due to vitamin B_{12} deficiency or is unavailable due to folate deficiency itself, DNA synthesis slows.

First to be affected in a vitamin B_{12} or folate deficiency are the rapidly growing blood cells. Either vitamin B_{12} or folate will clear up the anemia, but if folate is given when vitamin B_{12} is needed, the result is disastrous: devastating neurological symptoms. Remember that vitamin B_{12}, but not folate, maintains the sheath that surrounds and protects nerve fibres and promotes their normal growth. Folate "cures" the *blood*

FIGURE 10-14 Cobalt in Vitamin B_{12}

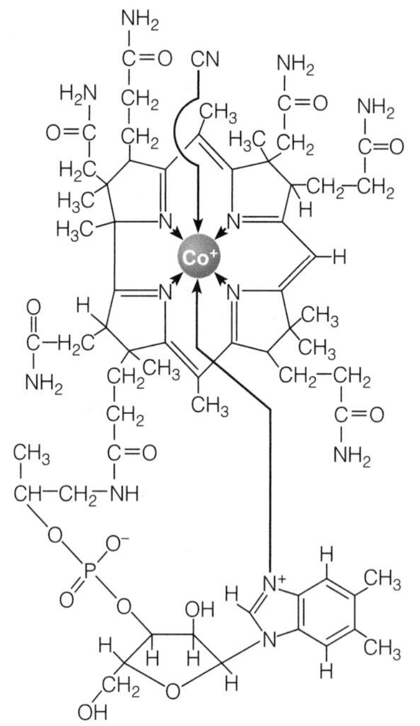

The intricate vitamin B_{12} molecule contains one atom of the mineral cobalt. The alternative name for vitamin B_{12}, cobalamin, reflects the presence of cobalt in its structure.

♦ Vitamin B_{12} is found primarily in foods derived from animals.

pernicious (per-NISH-us) **anemia:** a blood disorder that reflects a vitamin B_{12} deficiency caused by lack of intrinsic factor and characterized by abnormally large and immature red blood cells. Other symptoms include muscle weakness and irreversible neurological damage.
- **pernicious** = destructive

FIGURE 10-15 Normal and Anemic Blood Cells

The anemia of folate deficiency is indistinguishable from that of vitamin B_{12} deficiency. APPENDIX E describes the biochemical tests used to differentiate the two conditions.

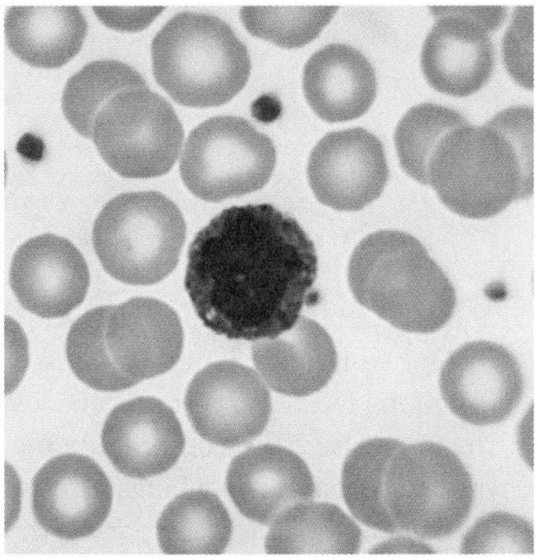

© Carolina Biological/Visuals Unlimited

Normal blood cells. The size, shape, and colour of these red blood cells show that they are normal.

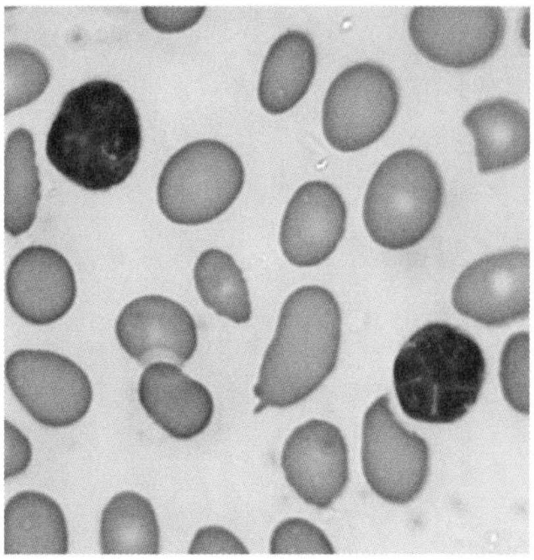

© Carolina Biological/Visuals Unlimited

Blood cells in pernicious anemia (megaloblastic). These megaloblastic blood cells are slightly larger (macrocytic) than normal red blood cells, and their shapes are irregular.

symptoms of a vitamin B_{12} deficiency, but cannot stop the *nerve* symptoms from progressing.[22] By doing so, folate "masks" a vitamin B_{12} deficiency.

Marginal vitamin B_{12} deficiency impairs cognition.[23] Advanced neurological symptoms include a creeping paralysis that begins at the extremities and works inward and up the spine. Early detection and correction are necessary to prevent permanent nerve damage and paralysis. With sufficient folate in the diet, the neurological symptoms of vitamin B_{12} deficiency can develop without evidence of anemia. Such interactions between folate and vitamin B_{12} highlight some of the safety issues surrounding the use of supplements and the fortification of foods.[24] No adverse effects have been reported for excess vitamin B_{12}, and no UL has been set.

Vitamin B_{12} Food Sources Vitamin B_{12} is unique among the vitamins in being found almost exclusively in foods derived from animals. Its bioavailability is greatest from milk and fish.[25] Anyone who eats reasonable amounts of animal-derived foods is most likely to have an adequate intake, including vegetarians who use milk products or eggs. Vegans, who restrict all foods derived from animals, need a reliable source, such as vitamin B_{12}–fortified soy beverage or vitamin B_{12} supplements. Yeast grown on a vitamin B_{12}–enriched medium and mixed with that medium provides some vitamin B_{12}, but yeast itself does not contain active vitamin B_{12}. Fermented soy products such as miso (a soybean paste) and sea algae such as spirulina also do *not* provide active vitamin B_{12}. Extensive research shows that the amounts listed on the labels of these plant products are inaccurate and misleading because the vitamin B_{12} is in an inactive, unavailable form.

As mentioned earlier, the water-soluble vitamins are particularly vulnerable to losses in cooking. For most of these nutrients, microwave heating minimizes losses as well as, or better than, traditional cooking methods. Such is not the case for vitamin B_{12}, however. Microwave heating inactivates vitamin B_{12}. To preserve this vitamin, use the oven or stovetop instead of a microwave to cook meats and milk products (major sources of vitamin B_{12}). The accompanying table provides a summary of vitamin B_{12}.

IN SUMMARY Vitamin B_{12}

Other Names

Cobalamin (and related forms)

RDA

Adults: 2.4 μg/day

Chief Functions in the Body

Part of coenzymes methylcobalamin and deoxyadenosylcobalamin used in new cell synthesis; helps to maintain nerve cells; reforms folate coenzyme; helps to break down some fatty acids and amino acids

Significant Sources

Foods of animal origin (meat, fish, poultry, shellfish, milk, cheese, eggs)

Easily destroyed by microwave cooking

Deficiency Disease

Pernicious anemia[a]

Deficiency Symptoms

Anemia (large-cell type);[b] fatigue, degeneration of peripheral nerves progressing to paralysis; sore tongue, loss of appetite, constipation

Toxicity Symptoms

None reported

[a]The name *pernicious anemia* refers to the vitamin B_{12} deficiency caused by atrophic gastritis and a lack of intrinsic factor, but not to that caused by inadequate dietary intake.

[b]Large-cell-type anemia is known as either *macrocytic* or *megaloblastic anemia*.

Vitamin-Like Compounds

Nutrition scientists debate whether other dietary compounds might also be considered vitamins. These compounds may have functions in the body, but to be a vitamin, a compound must be dietarily essential. In some cases, the compounds may be conditionally essential—that is, needed by the body from foods when synthesis becomes insufficient to support normal growth and metabolism. In other cases, the compounds may simply not be needed from the diet under any circumstances.

Choline Determining whether the nitrogen-containing compound choline is an essential nutrient has been blurry for decades, in part because the body can make choline from the amino acid methionine. Furthermore, choline is commonly found in foods such as milk, eggs, and peanuts and as part of lecithin, a food additive commonly used as an emulsifying agent (review Figure 5-9 on p. 136). Consequently, choline deficiencies are rare. Without any dietary choline, however, synthesis alone appears to be insufficient to meet the body's needs, making choline a conditionally essential nutrient. For this reason, the DRI Committee established an Adequate Intake (AI) for choline. The body uses choline to make the neurotransmitter acetylcholine and the phospholipid lecithin. During fetal development, choline supports the structure and function of the brain and spinal cord, by supporting neural tube closure and enhancing learning performance.[26] The UL for choline is based on its critical effect in lowering blood pressure. The accompanying table provides a summary of choline.

IN SUMMARY Choline

AI	Deficiency Symptoms
Men: 550 mg/day	Liver damage
Women: 425 mg/day	**Toxicity Symptoms**
Upper Level	Body odour, sweating, salivation, reduced growth rate, low blood pressure, liver damage
Adults: 3500 mg/day	**Significant Sources**
Chief Functions in the Body	Milk, liver, eggs, peanuts
Needed for the synthesis of the neurotransmitter acetylcholine and the phospholipid lecithin	

Inositol and Carnitine **Inositol** is a part of cell membrane structures, and **carnitine** transports long-chain fatty acids from the cytosol to the mitochondria for oxidation. Like choline, these two substances can be made by the body, but unlike choline, no recommendations have been established. Researchers continue to explore the possibility that these substances may be essential. Even if they are essential, though, supplements are unnecessary because these compounds are widespread in foods.

Some vitamin companies include choline, inositol, and carnitine in their formulations to make their vitamin pills look more "complete" than others, but this strategy offers no real advantage. For a rational way to compare vitamin-mineral supplements, read Highlight 10.

Nonvitamins Other substances have been mistaken for essential nutrients for human beings because they are needed for growth by bacteria or other forms of life. Among them are PABA (para-aminobenzoic acid, a component of folate's chemical structure), the bioflavonoids (vitamin P or hesperidin), pyrroloquinoline quinone (methoxatin), orotic acid, lipoic acid, and ubiquinone (coenzyme Q_{10}). Other names erroneously associated with vitamins are "vitamin O" (oxygenated saltwater), "vitamin B_5" (another name for pantothenic acid), "vitamin B_{15}" (also called "pangamic acid," a hoax), and "vitamin B_{17}" (laetrile, an alleged "cancer cure" and not a vitamin or a cure by any stretch of the imagination—in fact, laetrile is a potentially dangerous substance).

IN SUMMARY **The B vitamins serve as coenzymes that facilitate the work of every cell. They are active in carbohydrate, fat, and protein metabolism and in the making of DNA and thus new cells. Historically famous B vitamin–deficiency diseases are beriberi (thiamin), pellagra (niacin), and pernicious anemia (vitamin B_{12}). Pellagra can be prevented by adequate protein because the amino acid tryptophan can be converted to niacin in the body. A high intake of folate can mask the blood symptoms of a vitamin B_{12} deficiency, but it will not prevent the associated nerve damage. Vitamin B_6 participates in amino acid metabolism and can be harmful in excess. Biotin and pantothenic acid serve important roles in energy metabolism and are common in a variety of foods. Many substances that people claim as B vitamins are not.**

inositol (in-OSS-ih-tall): a nonessential nutrient that can be made in the body from glucose. Inositol is a part of cell membrane structures.

carnitine (CAR-neh-teen): a nonessential, nonprotein amino acid made in the body from lysine that helps transport fatty acids across the mitochondrial membrane.

The B Vitamins—In Concert

This chapter has described some of the remarkable ways that vitamins work individually, as if their many actions in the body could easily be disentangled. In fact, it is often difficult to tell which vitamin is truly responsible for a given effect because the nutrients are interdependent. You have already seen this interdependence with vitamin B_{12} and folate. The consequences of a deficiency of vitamin B_{12} limit the activation of the folate coenzyme THF, resulting in macrocytic anemia. You've also seen how an inadequate intake of either riboflavin or vitamin B_6 can compromise your niacin status. Evidence of interdependent roles for the B vitamins exists in many of the body's tissues.

B Vitamin Roles Figure 10-16 summarizes the metabolic pathways introduced in Chapter 7 and conveys an *impression* of the many ways B vitamins assist in metabolic pathways. Metabolism is the body's work, and the B vitamin coenzymes are indispensable to every step. In scanning the pathways of metabolism depicted in the figure, note the many abbreviations for the coenzymes that keep the processes going.

Look at the now-familiar pathway of glucose breakdown. To break down glucose to pyruvate, the cells must have certain enzymes. For the enzymes to work, they must have the niacin coenzyme NAD. Cells can make NAD, but only if they have enough niacin (or enough of the amino acid tryptophan to make niacin).

The next step is the breakdown of pyruvate to acetyl CoA. The enzymes involved in this step require both NAD and the thiamin and riboflavin coenzymes TPP and FAD, respectively. The cells can manufacture the enzymes they need from the vitamins, if the vitamins are in the diet.

Another coenzyme needed for this step is CoA. Predictably, the cells can make CoA except for an essential part that must be obtained in the diet—pantothenic acid. Another coenzyme requiring biotin serves the enzyme complex involved in converting pyruvate to oxaloacetate, the compound that combines with acetyl CoA to start the TCA cycle.

These and other coenzymes participate throughout all the metabolic pathways. Vitamin B_6 is an indispensable part of PLP—a coenzyme required for many amino acid conversions, for a crucial step in the making of the iron-containing portion of hemoglobin for red blood cells, and for many other reactions. Folate becomes THF—the coenzyme required for the synthesis of new genetic material and therefore new cells. The vitamin B_{12} coenzyme, in turn, regenerates THF to its active form; thus vitamin B_{12} is also necessary for the formation of new cells.

Thus each of the B vitamin coenzymes is involved, directly or indirectly, in energy metabolism. Some facilitate the energy-releasing reactions themselves; others help build new cells to deliver the oxygen and nutrients that allow the energy reactions to occur.

B Vitamin Deficiencies Now suppose the body's cells lack one of these B vitamins—niacin, for example. Without niacin, the cells cannot make NAD. Without NAD, the enzymes involved in every step of the glucose-to-energy pathway cannot function. Then, because all the body's activities require energy, literally everything begins to grind to a halt. This is no exaggeration. The deadly disease pellagra, caused by niacin deficiency, produces the "devastating four *Ds*": dermatitis, which reflects a failure of the skin; dementia, a failure of the nervous system; diarrhea, a failure of digestion and absorption; and eventually, as would be the case for any severe nutrient deficiency, death. These symptoms are the obvious ones, but a niacin deficiency affects all other organs, too, because all are dependent on the energy pathways.

All the vitamins are as essential as niacin. With any B vitamin deficiency, many body systems become deranged, and similar symptoms may appear. A lack of any of them can have disastrous and far-reaching effects.

FIGURE 10-16 Metabolic Pathways Involving B Vitamins

These metabolic pathways are introduced in Chapter 7 and are presented here to highlight the many coenzymes that facilitate the reactions. These coenzymes depend on the following vitamins:

- NAD and NADP: niacin
- TPP: thiamin
- CoA: pantothenic acid
- B_{12}: vitamin B_{12}
- FMN and FAD: riboflavin
- THF: folate
- PLP: vitamin B_6
- Biotin

Pathways leading toward acetyl CoA and the TCA cycle are catabolic, and those leading toward amino acids, glycogen, and fat are anabolic. For further details, see APPENDIX C.

CENGAGENOW™ Animated! figure www.cengage.com/sso

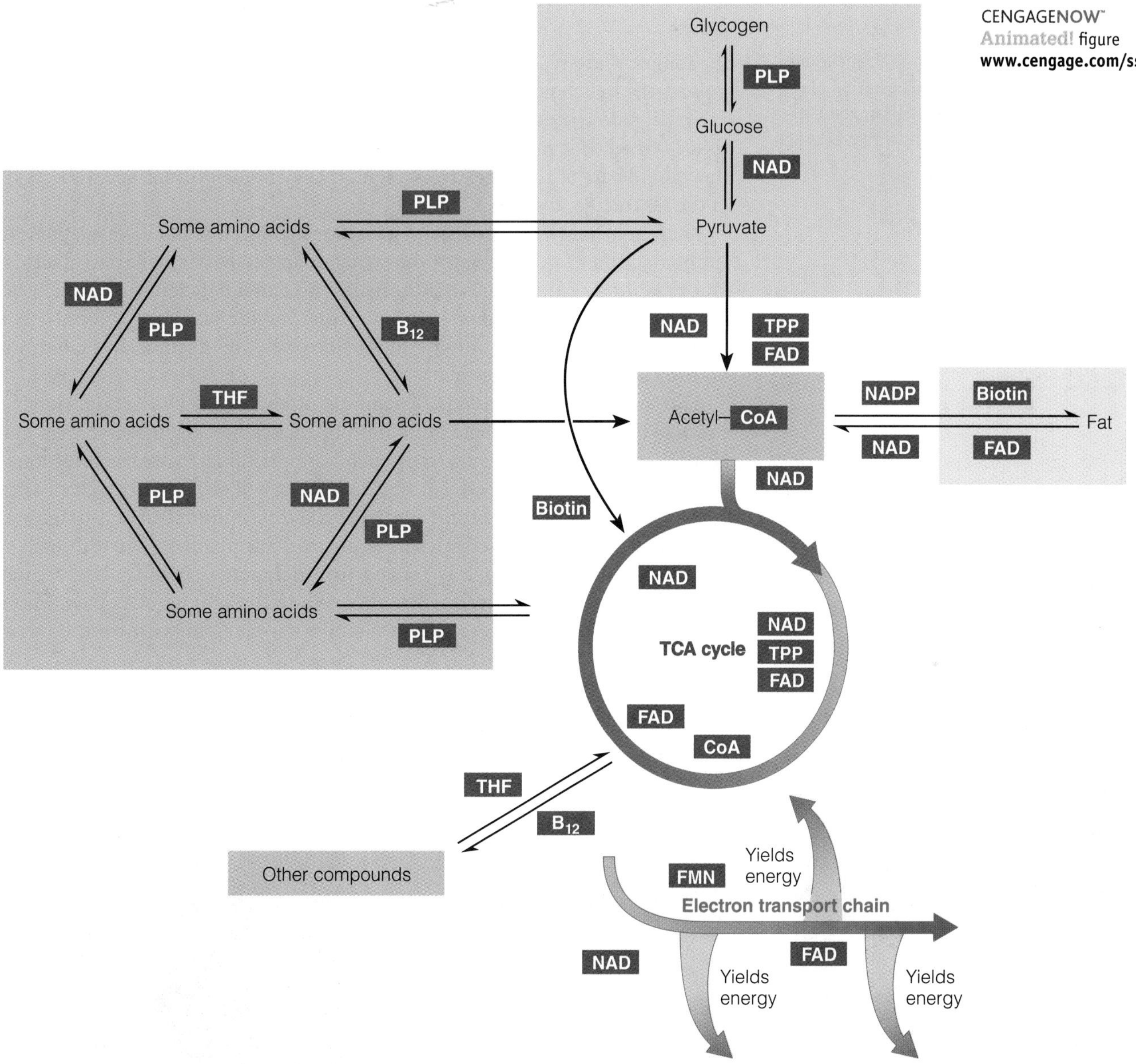
Glycogen
PLP
Glucose
NAD
Pyruvate
PLP
Some amino acids
NAD
PLP
B12
THF
Some amino acids
Some amino acids
PLP
NAD
PLP
Some amino acids
PLP
NAD
TPP
FAD
Acetyl–CoA
NADP
Biotin
Fat
NAD
FAD
NAD
Biotin
NAD
TCA cycle
NAD
TPP
FAD
FAD
CoA
THF
B12
Other compounds
Yields energy
FMN
Electron transport chain
NAD
FAD
Yields energy
Yields energy

Deficiencies of single B vitamins seldom show up in isolation, however. After all, people do not eat nutrients singly; they eat foods, which contain mixtures of nutrients. Only in two cases described earlier—beriberi and pellagra—have dietary deficiencies associated with single B vitamins been observed on a large scale in human populations. Even in these cases, several vitamins were lacking even though one vitamin stood out above the rest. When foods containing the vitamin known to be needed were provided, the other vitamins that were in short supply came as part of the package.

♦ Two common signs of B vitamin deficiencies are **glossitis** (gloss-EYE-tis), an inflammation of the tongue, and **cheilosis** (kye-LOH-sis or kee-LOH-sis), a condition of reddened lips with cracks at the corners of the mouth.

- **glossa** = tongue
- **cheilos** = lip

Major deficiency diseases of epidemic proportions such as pellagra and beriberi are no longer seen in Canada, but lesser deficiencies of nutrients, including the B vitamins, sometimes occur in people whose food choices are poor because of poverty, ignorance, illness, or poor health habits like alcohol abuse. (Review Highlight 7 to fully appreciate how alcohol induces vitamin deficiencies and interferes with energy metabolism.) Remember from Chapter 1 that deficiencies can arise not only from deficient intakes (primary causes), but also for other (secondary) reasons.

In identifying nutrient deficiencies, it is important to realize that a particular sign or symptom may not always have the same cause. The skin and the tongue (shown in Figure 10-17) appear to be especially sensitive to B vitamin deficiencies, but focusing on these body parts gives them undue emphasis. Both the skin and the tongue ♦ are readily visible in a physical examination. The physician sees and reports the deficiency's outward signs, but the full impact of a vitamin deficiency occurs inside the cells of the body. If the skin develops a rash or lesions, other tissues beneath it may be degenerating, too. Similarly, the mouth and tongue are the visible part of the digestive system; if they are abnormal, most likely the rest of the GI tract is, too.

Keep in mind that the cause of a sign or symptom is not always apparent. The summary tables in this chapter show that deficiencies of riboflavin, niacin, biotin, and vitamin B_6 can all cause skin rashes. So can a deficiency of protein, linoleic acid, or vitamin A. Because skin is on the outside and easy to see, it is a useful indicator of "things going wrong inside cells." By itself, a skin condition says nothing about its possible cause.

The same is true of anemia. Anemia is often caused by iron deficiency, but it can also be caused by a folate or vitamin B_{12} deficiency; by digestive tract failure to absorb any of these nutrients; or by such nonnutritional causes as infections, parasites, cancer, or loss of blood. No single nutrient will always cure a given symptom.

A person who feels chronically tired may be tempted to self-diagnose iron-deficiency anemia and self-prescribe an iron supplement. But this will relieve tiredness only if the cause is indeed iron-deficiency anemia. If the cause is a folate deficiency, taking iron will only prolong the fatigue. A person who is better informed may decide to take a vitamin supplement with iron, covering the

FIGURE 10-17 B Vitamin–Deficiency Symptoms—The Smooth Tongue of Glossitis and the Skin Lesions of Cheilosis

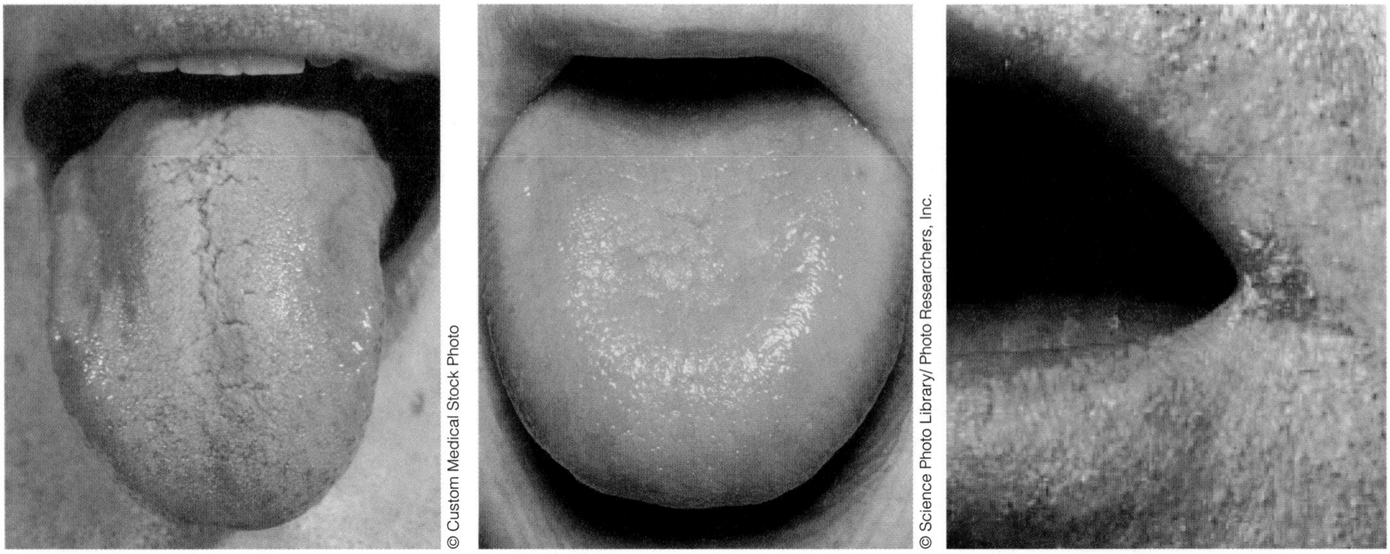

A healthy tongue has a rough and somewhat bumpy surface.

In a B vitamin deficiency, the tongue becomes smooth and swollen due to atrophy of the tissue (glossitis).

In a B vitamin deficiency, the corners of the mouth become irritated and inflamed (cheilosis).

possibility of a vitamin deficiency. But the symptom may have a nonnutritional cause. If the cause of the tiredness is actually hidden blood loss due to cancer, the postponement of a diagnosis may be fatal. When fatigue is caused by a lack of sleep, of course, no nutrient or combination of nutrients can replace a good night's rest. A person who is chronically tired should see a physician rather than self-prescribe. If the condition is nutrition related, a registered dietitian should be consulted as well.

B Vitamin Toxicities Toxicities of the B vitamins from foods alone are unknown, but they can occur when people overuse dietary supplements. With supplements, the quantities can quickly overwhelm the cells. Consider that one small capsule can easily deliver 2 milligrams of vitamin B_6, but it would take more than 3000 bananas, 6600 cups of rice, or 3600 chicken breasts to supply an equivalent amount. When the cells become oversaturated with a vitamin, they must work to eliminate the excess. The cells dispatch water-soluble vitamins to the urine for excretion, but sometimes they cannot keep pace with the onslaught. Homeostasis becomes disturbed and symptoms of toxicity develop.

B Vitamin Food Sources Significantly, deficiency diseases, such as beriberi and pellagra, were eliminated by supplying foods—not pills. Vitamin pill advertisements make much of the fact that vitamins are indispensable to life, but human beings obtained their nourishment from foods for centuries before vitamin pills existed. If the diet lacks a vitamin, the first solution is to adjust food intake to obtain that vitamin.

The bar graphs of selected foods in this chapter, taken together, sing the praises of a balanced diet. The Vegetables and Fruit group is an excellent source of folate. The Grain Products deliver thiamin riboflavin, niacin, and folate. The Milk and Alternatives group stands out for riboflavin and vitamin B_{12}. The Meat and Alternatives group serves thiamin, niacin, vitamin B_6, and vitamin B_{12} well. A diet that offers a variety of foods from each group, prepared with reasonable care, serves up ample B vitamins.

IN SUMMARY **The B vitamin coenzymes work together in energy metabolism. Some facilitate the energy-releasing reactions themselves; others help build cells to deliver the oxygen and nutrients that permit the energy pathways to run. These vitamins depend on one another to function optimally; a deficiency of any of them creates multiple problems. Fortunately, a variety of foods from each of the food groups provides an adequate supply of all of the B vitamins.**

Minerals for Energy Metabolism

Sulphur **Sulphate** is the oxidized form of the mineral **sulphur**, as it exists in food and water. The body's need for sulphate is easily met by a variety of foods and beverages. In addition, the body receives sulphate from the amino acids methionine and cysteine, which are found in dietary proteins. These sulphur-containing amino acids help determine the contour of protein molecules. The sulphur-containing side chains in cysteine molecules can link to each other via disulphide bridges, which stabilize the protein structure. (See the drawing of insulin with its disulphide bridges on p. 173.) Skin, hair, and nails contain some of the body's more rigid proteins, which have a high sulphur content.

Because the body's sulphate needs are easily met with normal protein intakes, there is no recommended intake for sulphate. Deficiencies do not occur when diets contain protein. Only when people lack protein to the point of severe deficiency will they lack the sulphur-containing amino acids.

sulphate: a salt produced from the oxidation of sulphur.

sulphur: a mineral present in the body as part of some proteins.

FIGURE 10-18 Iodine-Deficiency Symptom—The Enlarged Thyroid of Goiter

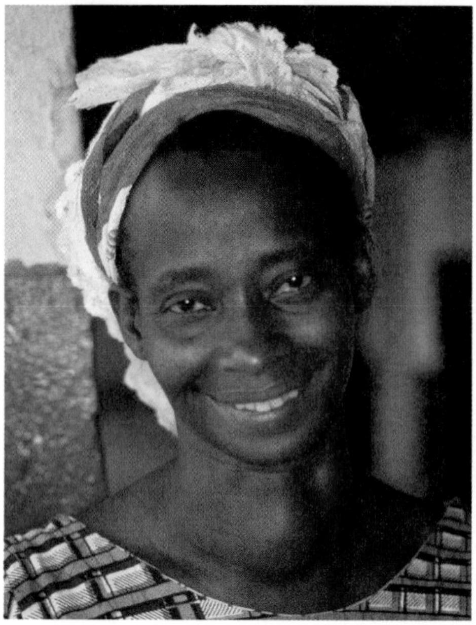

Scott Camazine/Photo Researchers, Inc.

In iodine deficiency, the thyroid gland enlarges—a condition known as simple goiter. Iodine toxicity also enlarges the thyroid gland, creating a similar-looking goiter.

♦ The ion form of iodine is called **iodide.**

♦ The thyroid gland releases tetraiodothyronine (T_4), commonly known as *thyroxine* (thigh-ROCKS-in), to its target tissues. Upon reaching the cells, T_4 is deiodinated to triiodothyronine (T_3), which is the active form of the hormone.

♦ Thyroid-stimulating hormone is also called **thyrotropin.**

♦ Examples of goitrogen-containing foods:
- Cabbage, spinach, radishes, rutabagas
- Soybeans, peanuts
- Peaches, strawberries

♦ The underactivity of the thyroid gland is known as **hypothyroidism** and may be caused by iodine deficiency or any number of other causes. Without treatment, an infant with **congenital hypothyroidism** will develop the physical and mental retardation of **cretinism.**

goiter (GOY-ter): an enlargement of the thyroid gland due to an iodine deficiency, malfunction of the gland, or overconsumption of a goitrogen. Goiter caused by iodine deficiency is sometimes called *simple goiter.*

goitrogen (GOY-troh-jen): a substance that enlarges the thyroid gland and causes *toxic goiter.* Goitrogens occur naturally in such foods as cabbage, kale, Brussels sprouts, cauliflower, broccoli, and kohlrabi.

cretinism (CREE-tin-ism): a congenital disease characterized by mental and physical retardation and commonly caused by maternal iodine deficiency during pregnancy.

Iodine

Traces of the iodine ion (called iodide) ♦ are indispensable to life. In the GI tract, iodine from foods becomes iodide. This chapter uses the term *iodine* when referring to the nutrient in foods and *iodide* when referring to it in the body. Iodide occurs in the body in minuscule amounts, but its principal role in the body and its requirement are well established.

Iodide Roles in the Body Iodide is an integral part of the thyroid hormones ♦ that regulate body temperature, metabolic rate, reproduction, growth, blood cell production, nerve and muscle function, and more. By controlling the rate at which the cells use oxygen, these hormones influence the amount of energy released during basal metabolism.

Iodine Deficiency The hypothalamus regulates thyroid hormone production by controlling the release of the pituitary's thyroid-stimulating hormone (TSH). ♦ With iodine deficiency, thyroid hormone production declines, and the body responds by secreting more TSH in a futile attempt to accelerate iodide uptake by the thyroid gland. If a deficiency persists, the cells of the thyroid gland enlarge to trap as much iodide as possible. Sometimes the gland enlarges until it makes a visible lump in the neck, a **goiter** (shown in Figure 10-18).

Goiter afflicts about 200 million people the world over, many of them in South America, Asia, and Africa. In all but 4 percent of these cases, the cause is iodine deficiency. As for the 4 percent (8 million), most have goiter because they regularly eat excessive amounts of foods ♦ that contain an antithyroid substance **(goitrogen)** whose effect is not counteracted by dietary iodine. The goitrogens present in plants remind us that even natural components of foods can cause harm when eaten in excess.

Goiter may be the earliest and most obvious sign of iodine deficiency, but the most tragic and prevalent damage occurs in the brain. Iodine deficiency is the most common cause of *preventable* mental retardation and brain damage in the world. Children with even a mild iodine deficiency typically have goiters and perform poorly in school. With sustained treatment, however, mental performance in the classroom as well as thyroid function improves.

A severe iodine deficiency during pregnancy causes the extreme and irreversible mental and physical retardation known as **cretinism.** ♦ Cretinism affects approximately six million people worldwide and can be averted by the early diagnosis and treatment of maternal iodine deficiency. A worldwide effort to provide iodized salt to people living in iodine-deficient areas has been dramatically successful. Because iron deficiency is common among people with iodine deficiency and because iron deficiency reduces the effectiveness of iodized salt, dual fortification with both iron and iodine may be most beneficial.[27]

Iodine Toxicity Excessive intakes of iodine can interfere with thyroid function and enlarge the gland, just as deficiency can.[28] During pregnancy, exposure to excessive iodine from foods, prenatal supplements, or medications is especially damaging to the developing infant. An infant exposed to toxic amounts of iodine during gestation may develop a goiter so severe as to block the airways and cause suffocation. The UL is 1100 micrograms ♦ per day for an adult—several times higher than average intakes.

Iodine Recommendations and Sources The ocean is the world's major source of iodine. In coastal areas, kelp, seafood, water, and even iodine-containing sea mist are dependable iodine sources. Further inland, the amount of iodine in foods is variable and generally reflects the amount present in the soil in which plants are grown or on which animals graze. Landmasses that were once under the ocean have soils rich in iodine; those in flood-prone areas where water leaches iodine from the soil are poor in iodine. In Canada and the United States, the iodization of salt ♦ has eliminated the widespread misery caused by iodine deficiency during the 1930s, but iodized salt is not available in many parts of the world.

Some countries add iodine to bread, fish paste, or drinking water instead. Families that do not use iodized foods have a higher prevalence of child malnutrition and mortality.[29]

Although average consumption of iodine in the United States exceeds recommendations, it falls below toxic levels. Current levels of iodine intake for Canada are not available, but they are likely similar to that in the United States. The recent Canadian Health Measures Survey tested urinary iodine as a marker of the iodine nutritional status of Canadians. Results will be released soon. Some of the excess iodine in the U.S. diet stems from fast foods, which use iodized salt liberally. Also, iodine comes from bakery products and from milk. The baking industry uses iodates (iodine salts) as dough conditioners, and most dairies feed cows iodine-containing medications and use iodine to disinfect milking equipment. Now that these sources have been identified, food industries have reduced their use of these compounds, but the sudden emergence of this problem points to a need for continued surveillance of the food supply. Processed foods in Canada can contain iodized or noniodized salt.

The recommended intake of iodine for adults is a minuscule amount. The need for iodine is easily met by consuming seafood, vegetables grown in iodine-rich soil, and iodized salt. ♦ In Canada, all table salt is iodized but specialized salts often are not. Canadian labelling laws do not require food processors to indicate on a food label if the salt used as an ingredient in a food is iodized or not. In the United States, labels indicate whether salt is iodized.

♦ For perspective, most foods provide 3 to 75 μg iodine per serving.

♦ Iodized salt contains about 60 μg iodine per gram salt.

♦ On average, 2 mL (½ tsp) iodized salt provides the RDA for iodine.

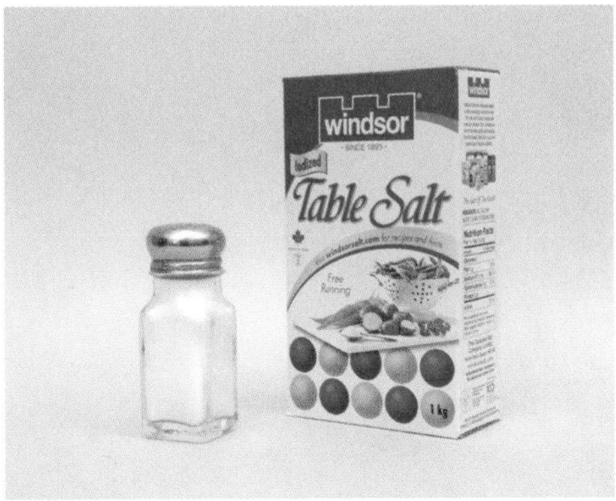
windsor
Iodized
Table Salt
1 kg

Dick Hemingway

Only "iodized salt" has had iodine added.

IN SUMMARY **Iodide, the ion of the mineral iodine, is an essential component of the thyroid hormone. An iodine deficiency can lead to simple goiter (enlargement of the thyroid gland) and can impair fetal development, causing cretinism. Iodization of salt has largely eliminated iodine deficiency in Canada and the United States. The accompanying table provides a summary of iodine.**

Iodine

RDA	**Deficiency Disease**
Adults: 150 μg/day	Simple goiter, cretinism
Upper Level	**Deficiency Symptoms**
1100 μg/day	Underactive thyroid gland, goiter, mental and physical retardation in infants (cretinism)
Chief Functions in the Body	**Toxicity Symptoms**
A component of two thyroid hormones that help to regulate growth, development, and metabolic rate	Underactive thyroid gland, elevated TSH, goiter
Significant Sources	
Iodized salt, seafood, bread, dairy products, plants grown in iodine-rich soil and animals fed those plants	

Manganese

The human body contains a tiny 20 milligrams of manganese. Most of it can be found in the bones and metabolically active organs such as the liver, kidneys, and pancreas.

Manganese Roles in the Body

Manganese acts as a cofactor for many enzymes that facilitate the metabolism of carbohydrate, lipids, and amino acids. In addition, manganese-containing metalloenzymes assist in bone formation and the conversion of pyruvate to a TCA cycle compound.

Manganese Deficiency and Toxicity

Manganese requirements are low, and many plant foods contain significant amounts of this trace mineral, so deficiencies are rare. As is true of other trace minerals, however, dietary factors such as phytates inhibit its absorption. In addition, high intakes of iron and calcium limit manganese absorption, so people who use supplements of those minerals regularly may impair their manganese status.

Toxicity is more likely to occur from an environment contaminated with manganese than from dietary intake. Miners who inhale large quantities of manganese dust on the job over prolonged periods show symptoms of a brain disease, along with abnormalities in appearance and behaviour. Still, a UL has been established based on intakes from food, water, and supplements.

Manganese Recommendations and Sources Grain products make the greatest contribution of manganese to the diet. With insufficient information to establish an RDA, an AI was set based on average intakes.

IN SUMMARY **Manganese-dependent enzymes are involved in bone formation and various metabolic processes. Because manganese is widespread in plant foods, deficiencies are rare, although regular use of calcium and iron supplements may limit manganese absorption. The accompanying table provides a summary of manganese.**

Manganese

AI	Significant Sources
Men: 2.3 mg/day	Nuts, whole grains, leafy vegetables, tea
Women: 1.8 mg/day	**Deficiency Symptoms**
Upper Level	Rare
Adults: 11 mg/day	**Toxicity Symptoms**
Chief Functions in the Body	Nervous system disorders
Cofactor for several enzymes; bone formation	

Chromium

Chromium is an essential mineral that participates in carbohydrate and lipid metabolism. Like iron, chromium assumes different charges. In chromium, the Cr^{+++} ion is the most stable and most commonly found in foods.

Chromium Roles in the Body Chromium helps maintain glucose homeostasis by enhancing the activity of the hormone insulin. ♦ When chromium is lacking, a diabetes-like condition may develop with elevated blood glucose and impaired glucose tolerance, insulin response, and glucagon response. Some research findings suggest that chromium supplements improve glucose or insulin responses in diabetes, but other studies have found no improvements.[30]

♦ Small organic compounds that enhance insulin's action are called **glucose tolerance factors (GTF).** Some glucose tolerance factors contain chromium.

Chromium Recommendations and Sources Chromium is present in a variety of foods. The best sources are unrefined foods, particularly liver, brewer's yeast, and whole grains. The more refined foods people eat, the less chromium they ingest.

Chromium Supplements Supplement advertisements have succeeded in convincing consumers that they can lose fat and build muscle by taking chromium picolinate. Whether chromium supplements (either picolinate or plain) reduce body fat or improve muscle strength remains controversial. (Highlight 15 revisits chromium picolinate and other supplements athletes use in the hopes of improving their performance.)

IN SUMMARY **Chromium enhances insulin's action. A deficiency can result in a diabetes-like condition. Chromium is widely available in unrefined foods including brewer's yeast, whole grains, and liver. The accompanying table provides a summary of chromium.**

Chromium

AI	
Men: 35 μg/day	
Women: 25 μg/day	

Chief Functions in the Body

Enhances insulin action and may improve glucose tolerance

Significant Sources

Meats (especially liver), whole grains, brewer's yeast

Deficiency Symptoms

Diabetes-like condition

Toxicity Symptoms

None reported

Although vitamins and minerals are not direct sources of energy, they play critical support roles in generating cellular energy from the macronutrients. The interrelated roles of the B vitamins and various minerals in energy-yielding pathways emphasize the importance of regularly consuming adequate amounts of all of these nutrients. Without B vitamin coenzymes and the trace minerals, you would not be able to metabolize carbohydrates, fats, and proteins into energy that allows you to perform your daily activities and sustain life. The accompanying summary table condenses the information provided in this chapter for a quick review.

IN SUMMARY Nutrients for Energy Metabolism

Nutrient and Chief Functions	Deficiency Symptoms	Toxicity Symptoms	Food Sources
Thiamin Part of coenzyme TPP in energy metabolism	Beriberi (edema or muscle wasting), anorexia and weight loss, neurological disturbances, muscular weakness, heart enlargement and failure	None reported	Enriched, fortified, or whole-grain products; pork
Riboflavin Part of coenzymes FAD and FMN in energy metabolism	Inflammation of the mouth, skin, and eyelids	None reported	Milk products; enriched, fortified, or whole-grain products; liver
Niacin Part of coenzymes NAD and NADP in energy metabolism	Pellagra (diarrhea, dermatitis, and dementia)	Niacin flush, liver damage, impaired glucose tolerance	Protein-rich foods
Biotin Part of coenzyme in energy metabolism	Skin rash, hair loss, neurological disturbances	None reported	Widespread in foods; GI bacteria synthesis
Pantothenic acid Part of coenzyme A in energy metabolism	Digestive and neurological disturbances	None reported	Widespread in foods
Vitamin B_6 Part of coenzymes used in amino acid and fatty acid metabolism	Scaly dermatitis, depression, confusion, convulsions, anemia	Nerve degeneration, skin lesions	Protein-rich foods
Folate Activates vitamin B_{12}; helps synthesize DNA for new cell growth	Anemia, glossitis, neurological disturbances, elevated homocysteine	Masks vitamin B_{12} deficiency	Legumes, vegetables, fortified grain products
Vitamin B_{12} Activates folate; helps synthesize DNA for new cell growth; protects nerve cells	Anemia; nerve damage and paralysis	None reported	Foods derived from animals
Sulphur As part of proteins, stabilizes their shape by forming disulphide bridges; part of the vitamins biotin and thiamin and the hormone insulin	None known; protein deficiency would occur first	Toxicity would occur only if sulphur-containing amino acids were eaten; in excess this (in animals) suppresses growth	All protein-containing foods (meats, fish, poultry, eggs, milk, legumes, nuts)
Iodine A component of the thyroid hormones that help to regulate-growth, development, and metabolic rate	Underactive thyroid gland, goiter, mental and physical retardation (cretinism)	Elevated TSH, goiter	Iodized salt; seafood; plants grown in iodine-rich soil and animals fed those plants
Manganese Cofactor for several enzymes; bone formation	Rare	Nervous symptom disorders	Nuts, whole grains, leafy vegetables, tea
Chromium Enhances insulin action, may improve glucose intolerance	Diabetes-like condition	None reported	Meats (liver), whole grains, brewer's yeast

Nutrition Portfolio

To obtain the vitamins and minerals that you need daily for energy metabolism, be sure to select a variety of foods from all of the four food groups.

Go to Diet Analysis Plus and choose one of the days on which you tracked your diet. Select the Intake vs. Goals report and then consider the following questions. Remember that scoring 100 percent on this report means you met your daily nutrient goal.

- On your Intake vs. Goals report, check your intake for three B vitamins: riboflavin, folate and vitamin B_{12}. How was your intake of these nutrients? How could you improve your intake? Why is this important?
- If you are a woman of childbearing age, calculate the dietary folate equivalents you received from folate-rich foods, fortified foods, and supplements, then compare that to your RDA.

Now click on the Intake Spreadsheet report and consider the following questions:

- Check your intake of Grain Products. Determine the proportion of your thiamin, riboflavin, and niacin intakes that come from these foods. What are your other key sources of these B vitamins?
- Examine the variety in your food intake, taking particular notice of how often you include foods from the Vegetables and Fruit and Milk and Alternatives groups in your daily diet. These foods can be substantial sources of folate and riboflavin, respectively. How could you improve your intake of these foods?
- Describe the advantages of using iodized versus non-iodized salt.

Diet Analysis PLUS

To complete this exercise, go to your Diet Analysis Plus at www.cengage.com/sso.

Nutrition on the Net

CENGAGENOW™
For further study of topics covered in this chapter, log on to **www.cengage.com/sso.**

- Search for "vitamins" and "minerals" at the Dietitians of Canada's website: **www.dietitians.ca**
- Learn more about neural tube defects from Health Canada: **www.hc-sc.gc.ca/hl-vs/iyh-vsv/med/folic-folique-eng.php**
- Become more knowledgeable about iodine and thyroid disease from the Thyroid Foundation of Canada: **www.thyroid.ca**
- Read about Health Canada's food fortification policy on their website: **www.hc-sc.gc.ca/fn-an/nutrition/vitamin/index-eng.php**

References

1. C. S. Johnston and J. C. Hale, Oxidation of ascorbic acid in stored orange juice is associated with reduced plasma vitamin C concentrations and elevated lipid peroxides, *Journal of the American Dietetic Association* 105 (2005): 106–109.
2. Committee on Dietary Reference Intakes, *Dietary Reference Intakes for Vitamin C, Vitamin E, Selenium, and Carotenoids* (Washington, D.C.: National Academies Press, 2000); Committee on Dietary Reference Intakes, *Dietary Reference Intakes for Thiamin, Riboflavin, Niacin, Vitamin B_6, Folate, Vitamin B_{12}, Pantothenic Acid, Biotin, and Choline* (Washington, D.C.: National Academies Press, 1998).
3. K. J. Carpenter, *Beriberi, White Rice, and Vitamin B: A Disease, a Cause, and a Cure* (Berkeley: University of California Press, 2000).
4. K. L. Bogan and C. Brenner, Nicotinic acid, nicotinamide, and nicotinamide riboside: A molecular evaluation of NAD+ precursor vitamins in human nutrition, *Annual Review of Nutrition* 28 (2008): 115–130.
5. Committee on Dietary Reference Intakes, 1998, pp. 128–129.
6. L. Zhang and coauthors, Niacin inhibits surface expression of ATP synthase β chain in HepG2 cells: Implications for raising HDL, *Journal of Lipid Research* 49 (2008): 1195–1201; P. L. Canner, C. D. Furberg, and M. E. McGovern, Benefits of niacin in patients with versus without the metabolic syndrome and healed myocardial infarction (from the Coronary Drug Project), *American Journal of Cardiology* 97 (2006): 477–479; S. Westphal and coauthors, Adipokines and treatment with niacin, *Metabolism* 55 (2006): 1283–1285.
7. D. B. Piazzini and coauthors, A systematic review of conservative treatment of carpal tunnel syndrome, *Clinical Rehabilitation* 21 (2007): 299–314.
8. P. De Wals and coauthors, Reduction in neural-tube defects after folic acid fortification in Canada, *New England Journal of Medicine* 357 (2007): 135-142; Q. Yang and coauthors, Race-ethnicity differences in folic acid intake in women of childbearing age in the United States after folic acid fortification: Findings from the National Health and

Nutrition Examination Survey, 2001–2002, *American Journal of Clinical Nutrition* 85 (2007): 1409–1416; Use of dietary supplements containing folic acid among women of childbearing age: United States, 2005, *Morbidity and Mortality Weekly Report* 54 (2005): 955–957.

9. R. M. Winkels and coauthors, Bioavailability of food folates is 80% of that of folic acid, *American Journal of Clinical Nutrition* 85 (2007): 465–473.
10. P. D. Wals and coauthors, Reduction in neural-tube defects after folic acid fortification in Canada, *New England Journal of Medicine* 357 (2007): 135–142; T.G.K. Bentley and coauthors, Population-level changes in folate intake by age, gender, and race/ethnicity after folic acid fortification, *American Journal of Public Health* 96 (2006): 2040–2047; T. Tamura and M. F. Picciano, Folate and human reproduction, *American Journal of Clinical Nutrition* 83 (2006): 993–1016; A. M. Shuaibi and coauthors, Folate status of young Canadian women after folic acid fortification of grain products *Journal of the American Dietetic Association* 108 (2008): 2090–2094.
11. A. J. Wilcox and coauthors, Folic acid supplements and risk of facial clefts: National population-based case-control study, *British Medical Journal* 334 (2007): 464–469; Y. I. Goh and coauthors, Prenatal multivitamin supplementation and rates of congenital anomalies: A meta-analysis, *Journal of Obstetrics and Gynaecology Canada* 28 (2006): 680–689.
12. Committee on Dietary Reference Intakes, 1998.
13. O. Dary, Nutritional interpretation of folic acid interventions, *Nutrition Reviews* 67 (2009): 235–244; A. D. Smith, Y. I. Kim, and H. Refsum, Is folic acid good for everyone? *American Journal of Clinical Nutrition* 87 (2008): 517–533; Y. Kim, Folic acid fortification and supplementation: Good for some but not so good for others, *Nutrition Reviews* 65 (2007): 504–511; I. H. Rosenberg, Folic acid fortification, *Nutrition Reviews* 65 (2007): 503; N. W. Solomons, Food fortification with folic acid: Has the other shoe dropped? *Nutrition Reviews* 65 (2007): 512–515; R. L. Brent and G. P. Oakley, The folate debate, *Pediatrics* 117 (2006): 1418–1419; J. I. Rader and B. O. Schneeman, Prevalence of neural tube defects, folate status, and folate fortification of enriched cereal-grain products in the United States, *Pediatrics* 117 (2006): 1394–1399.
14. A. de Bree, L. A. van Mierlo, and R. Draijer, Folic acid improves vascular reactivity in humans: A meta-analysis of randomized controlled trials, *American Journal of Clinical Nutrition* 86 (2007): 610–617; D. S. Wald and coauthors, Folic acid, homocysteine, and cardiovascular disease: Judging causality in the face of inconclusive trial evidence, *British Journal of Medicine* 333 (2006): 1114–1117.
15. C. M. Albert and coauthors, Effect of folic acid and B vitamins on risk of cardiovascular events and total mortality among women at high risk for cardiovascular disease: A randomized trial, *Journal of the American Medical Association* 299 (2008): 2027–2036; M. Ebbing and coauthors, Mortality and cardiovascular events in patients treated with homocysteine-lowering B vitamins after coronary angiography, *Journal of the American Medical Association* 300 (2008): 795–801; E. Lonn, Homocysteine-lowering B vitamin therapy in cardiovascular prevention—Wrong again? *Journal of the American Medical Association* 299 (2008): 2086–2087; C. Baigent and R. Clarke, B Vitamins for the prevention of vascular disease: Insufficient evidence to justify treatment, *Journal of the American Medical Association* 298 (2007): 1212–1214; R. L. Jamison and coauthors, Effect of homocysteine lowering on mortality and vascular disease in advanced chronic kidney disease and end-stage renal disease: A randomized trial, *Journal of the American Medical Association* 298 (2007): 1163–1170; L. A. Bazzano and coauthors, Effect of folic acid supplementation on risk of cardiovascular diseases—A meta-analysis of randomized controlled trials, *Journal of the American Medical Association* 296 (2006): 2720–2726; C. M. Carlsson, Homocysteine lowering with folic acid and vitamin B supplements: Effects on cardiovascular disease in older adults, *Drugs and Aging* 23 (2006): 491–502; The Heart Outcomes Prevention Evaluation (HOPE) 2 Investigators, Homocysteine lowering with folic acid and B vitamins in vascular disease, *New England Journal of Medicine* 354 (2006): 1567–1577.
16. J. B. Mason, Folate, cancer risk, and the Greek god, Proteus: A tale of two chameleons, *Nutrition Reviews* 67 (2009): 206–212; Smith, Kim, and Refsum, 2008; C. M. Ulrich, Folate and cancer prevention: A closer look at a complex picture, *American Journal of Clinical Nutrition* 86 (2007): 271–273.
17. A. R. Hart, H. Kennedy, and I. Harvey, Pancreatic cancer: A review of the evidence on causation, *Clinical Gastroenterology Hepatology* 6 (2008): 275–282; World Cancer Research Fund and American Institute for Cancer Research, *Food, Nutrition, Physical Activity, and the Prevention of Cancer: A Global Perspective* (Washington, D.C.: AICR, 2007), pp. 106–107.
18. U. C. Ericson, M. I. L. Ivarsson, E. Sonestedt, B. Gullberg, J. Carlson, H. Olsson, and E. Wirfält, Increased breast cancer risk at high plasma folate concentrations among women with the MTHFR 677T allele, *American Journal of Clinical Nutrition* 90 (2009): 1380–1389; A. D. Smith, Y. Kim, and H. Refsum, Is folic acid good for everyone? *American Journal of Clinical Nutrition* 87 (2008): 517–533; C. M. Ulrich and J. D. Potter, Folate supplementation: Too much of a good thing? *Cancer Epidemiology, Biomarkers & Prevention* 15 (2006): 189–193; M. A. Sanjoaquin, A. N. Couto, A. W. Roddam, and T. J. Key, Folate intake and colorectal cancer risk: a meta-analytical approach, *International Journal of Cancer* 113 (2005): 825–828.
19. K. D. Stark and coauthors, Status of plasma folate after folic acid fortification of the food supply in pregnant African American women and the influences of diet, smoking, and alcohol consumption, *American Journal of Clinical Nutrition* 81 (2005): 669–671.
20. L. H. Allen, How common is vitamin B-12 deficiency? *American Journal of Clinical Nutrition* 89 (2009): 693S–696S; S. P. Stabler and coauthors, Elevated serum S-adenosylhomocysteine in cobalamin-deficient elderly and response to treatment, *American Journal of Clinical Nutrition* 84 (2006): 1422–1429.
21. D. K. Dror and L. H. Allen, Effect of vitamin B_{12} deficiency on neurodevelopment in infants: Current knowledge and possible mechanisms, *Nutrition Reviews* 66 (2008): 250–255.
22. K. F. Wykoff and V. Ganji, Proportion of individuals with low serum vitamin B-12-concentrations without macrocytosis is higher in the post-folic acid fortification period than in the pre-folic acid fortification period, *American Journal of Clinical Nutrition* 86 (2007): 1187–1192.
23. R. Clarke and coauthors, Low vitamin B-12; status and risk of cognitive decline in older adults, *American Journal of Clinical Nutrition* 86 (2007): 1384–1391; C. McCracken and coauthors, Methylmalonic acid and cognitive function in the Medical Research Council Cognitive Function and Ageing Study, *American Journal of Clinical Nutrition* 84 (2006): 1406–1411.
24. M. A. Johnson, If high folic acid aggravates vitamin B_{12} deficiency what should be done about it? *Nutrition Reviews* 65 (2007): 451–458.
25. A. Vogiatzoglou and coauthors, Dietary sources of vitamin B-12 and their association with plasma vitamin B-12 concentrations in the general population: The Hordaland Homocysteine Study, *American Journal of Clinical Nutrition* 89 (2009): 1078–1087.
26. L. M. Sanders and S. H. Zeisel, Choline: Dietary requirements and role in brain development, *Nutrition Today* 42 (2007): 181–186; S. H. Zeisel, Choline: Critical role during fetal development and dietary requirements in adults, *Annual Review of Nutrition* 26 (2006): 229–250.
27. M. B. Zimmerman, The influence of iron status on iodine utilization and thyroid function, *Annual Review of Nutrition* 26 (2006): 367–389.
28. W. Teng and coauthors, Effect of iodine intake on thyroid diseases in China, *New England Journal of Medicine* 354 (2006): 2783–2793.
29. R. D. Semba and coauthors, Child malnutrition and mortality among families not utilizing adequately iodized salt in Indonesia, *American Journal of Clinical Nutrition* 87 (2008): 438–444.
30. E. M. Balk and coauthors, Effect of chromium supplementation on glucose metabolism and lipids: A systematic review of randomized controlled trials, *Diabetes Care* 30 (2007): 2154–2163; C. L. Broadhurst and P. Domenico, Clinical studies on chromium picolinate supplementation in diabetes mellitus—A review, *Diabetes Technology and Therapeutics* 8 (2006): 677–687; P. R. Trumbo and K. C. Ellwood, Chromium picolinate intake and risk of type 2 diabetes: An evidence-based review by the United States Food and Drug Administration, *Nutrition Reviews* 64 (2006): 357–363; M. L. Diaz, B. A. Watkins, Y. Li, R. A. Anderson, and W. W. Campbell, Chromium picolinate and conjugated linoleic acid do not synergistically influence diet- and exercise-induced changes in body composition and health indexes in overweight women, *The Journal of Nutritional Biochemistry* 19 (2008): 61–68.

HIGHLIGHT 10

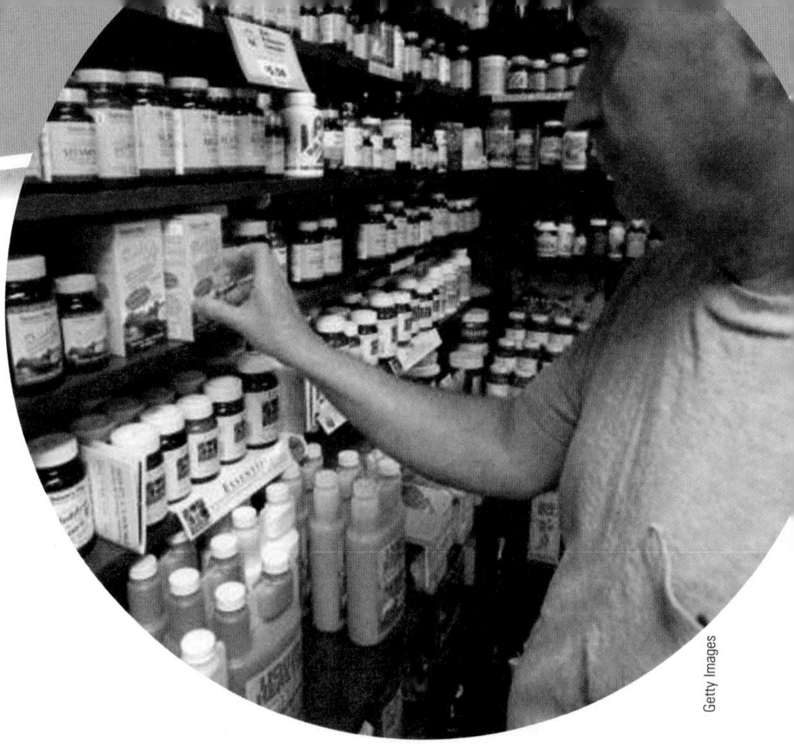
Getty Images

Vitamin and Mineral Supplements

An estimated 75 000 supplements are currently on the market. More than half of the adults in Canada take a **dietary supplement** regularly.[1] Many people take supplements as dietary insurance—in case they are not meeting their nutrient needs from foods alone. Others take supplements as health insurance—to protect against certain diseases.[2]

Multinutrient supplements are most frequently used, but many people take large doses of single nutrients, most commonly, vitamin C, vitamin E, beta-carotene, iron, and calcium. In many cases, taking supplements is a costly but harmless practice; sometimes, it is both costly and harmful to health.

For the most part, people self-prescribe supplements, taking them on the advice of friends, advertisements, websites, or books that may or may not be reliable. Sometimes, they take supplements on the recommendation of a physician. When such advice follows a valid nutrition assessment, supplementation may be warranted, but even then the preferred course of action is to improve food choices and eating habits.[3] Without an assessment, the advice to take supplements may be inappropriate. A registered dietitian can help with the decision.

When people think of dietary supplements, they often think of vitamins, but a diet that lacks vitamins probably lacks several minerals as well. This highlight asks several questions related to vitamin-mineral supplements. (The accompanying glossary defines dietary supplements and related terms.) What are the arguments *for* taking supplements? What are the arguments *against* taking them? Finally, if people do take supplements, how can they choose the appropriate ones? (Amino acid supplements and herbal supplements are discussed in Chapter 6 and Highlight 19, respectively.)

Arguments for Supplements

Vitamin-mineral supplements may be appropriate in some circumstances. In some cases, they can prevent or correct deficiencies; in others, they can reduce the risk of diseases. Consumers should discuss supplement use with their health-care professionals who can help monitor for adverse effects or nutrient–drug interactions.[4]

Correct Overt Deficiencies

In Canada, adults rarely suffer nutrient deficiency diseases such as scurvy, pellagra, and beriberi, but nutrient deficiencies do still occur. To correct an overt deficiency disease, a physician may prescribe therapeutic doses two to ten times the RDA (or AI) of a nutrient. At such high doses, the supplement is acting as a drug.

Support Increased Nutrient Needs

As Chapters 16 through 18 explain, nutrient needs increase during certain stages of life, making it difficult to meet some of those needs without supplementation. For example, women who lose a lot of blood and therefore a lot of iron during menstruation each month may need an iron supplement. Women of childbearing age need folate supplements to reduce the risks of neural tube defects. Similarly, pregnant women and women who are breastfeeding their infants have exceptionally high nutrient needs and so usually need special supplements. Newborns routinely receive a single dose of vitamin K at birth to prevent abnormal bleeding. Infants may need other supplements as well, depending on whether they are breastfed or receiving formula, and on whether their water contains fluoride.

GLOSSARY

dietary supplement: any pill, capsule, tablet, liquid, or powder that contains vitamins, minerals, herbs, or amino acids; intended to increase dietary intake of these substances.

Health Canada, Natural Health Products Directorate: authority that ensures Canadians have access to safe, high quality, and effective natural health products, which include vitamins and minerals, herbal remedies, homeopathic medicines, traditional medicines such as traditional Chinese medicines, probiotics, and other products such as amino acids and essential fatty acids.

high potency: 100 percent or more of the Daily Value for the nutrient in a single supplement and for at least two-thirds of the nutrients in a multinutrient supplement.

Improve Nutrition Status

In contrast to the classical deficiencies, which present a multitude of symptoms and are relatively easy to recognize, subclinical deficiencies are subtle and easy to overlook—and they are also more likely to occur. People who do not eat enough food to deliver the needed amounts of nutrients, such as habitual dieters and the elderly, risk developing subclinical deficiencies.[5] Similarly, vegetarians who restrict their use of entire food groups without appropriate substitutions may fail to fully meet their nutrient needs. If there is no way for these people to eat enough nutritious foods to meet their needs, then vitamin-mineral supplements may be appropriate to help prevent nutrient deficiencies.

Improve the Body's Defenses

Health-care professionals may provide special supplementation to people being treated for addictions to alcohol or other drugs and to people with prolonged illnesses, extensive injuries, or other severe stresses such as surgery. Illnesses that interfere with appetite, eating, or nutrient absorption impair nutrition status. For example, the stomach condition atrophic gastritis often creates a vitamin B_{12} deficiency. In addition, nutrient needs are often heightened by diseases or medications. In all these cases, supplements are appropriate.

Reduce Disease Risks

Few people consume the optimal amounts of all the vitamins and minerals by diet alone. Inadequate intakes have been linked to chronic diseases such as heart disease, some cancers, and osteoporosis. For this reason, some physicians recommend that all adults take vitamin-mineral supplements. Such regular supplementation would provide an optimum intake to enhance metabolic harmony and prevent disease at relatively little cost. Others recognize the lack of conclusive evidence and the potential harm of supplementation and advise against such a recommendation.[6] The most recent statement from the U.S. National Institutes of Health acknowledges that evidence is insufficient to recommend either for or against the use of supplements to prevent chronic diseases.[7]

Highlight 12 reviews the relationships between supplement use and disease prevention. It describes some of the accumulating evidence suggesting that intakes of certain nutrients at levels much higher than can be attained from foods alone may be beneficial in reducing disease risks. It also presents research confirming the associated risks.[8] Clearly, consumers must be cautious in taking supplements to prevent disease.

Who Needs Supplements?

In summary, the following list acknowledges that in these specific conditions, these people may need to take supplements:

- People with specific nutrient deficiencies need specific nutrient supplements.
- People whose energy intakes are particularly low (fewer than 1600 kcalories per day) need multivitamin-mineral supplements.
- Vegetarians who eat all-plant diets (vegans) and older adults with atrophic gastritis need vitamin B_{12}.
- People who have lactose intolerance or milk allergies or who otherwise do not consume enough milk products to forestall extensive bone loss need calcium.
- People in certain stages of the life cycle who have increased nutrient requirements need specific nutrient supplements. For example, infants need iron and fluoride, women of childbearing age and pregnant women need folate and iron, and the elderly need vitamin B_{12} and vitamin D.
- People who have inadequate milk intakes, limited sun exposure, or heavily pigmented skin need vitamin D.
- People who have diseases, infections, or injuries or who have undergone surgery that interferes with the intake, absorption, metabolism, or excretion of nutrients may need specific nutrient supplements.
- People taking medications that interfere with the body's use of specific nutrients may need specific nutrient supplements.

Except for people in these circumstances, most adults can normally get all the nutrients they need by eating a varied diet of nutrient-dense foods. Even athletes can meet their nutrient needs without the help of supplements, as Chapter 15 explains.

Arguments against Supplements

Foods rarely cause nutrient imbalances or toxicities, but supplements can. The higher the dose, the greater the risk of harm. People's tolerances for high doses of nutrients vary, just as their risks of deficiencies do. Amounts that some can tolerate may be harmful for others, and no one knows who falls where along the spectrum. It is difficult to determine just how much of a nutrient is enough—or too much. The Tolerable Upper Intake Levels of the DRI answer the question "How much is too much?" by defining the highest amount that appears safe for most healthy people. Table H10-1 (p. 348) presents the Upper Levels and Daily Values for selected vitamins and minerals and the quantities typically found in supplements.

Toxicity

Supplement users are more likely to have excessive intakes of certain nutrients—notably iron, zinc, vitamin A, and niacin.[9] The extent and severity of supplement toxicity remain unclear. Only a few alert health-care professionals can recognize toxicity, even when it is acute. When it is chronic, with the effects developing subtly and progressing slowly, it often goes unrecognized. In view of the potential hazards, some authorities believe supplements should bear warning labels, advising consumers that large doses may be toxic.

Toxic overdoses of vitamins and minerals in children are more readily recognized and, unfortunately, fairly common. Fruit-flavoured, chewable vitamins shaped like cartoon characters entice young children to eat them like candy in amounts that can cause poisoning. Iron supplements (30 milligrams of iron or more per tablet) are especially toxic and are the leading cause of accidental ingestion fatalities among children. Even mild overdoses cause GI distress, nausea, and black diarrhea, which reflects gastric bleeding. Severe overdoses result in bloody diarrhea, shock, liver damage, coma, and death.

Life-Threatening Misinformation

Another problem arises when people who are ill come to believe that high doses of vitamins or minerals can be therapeutic. Not only can high doses be toxic, but the person may take them instead of seeking medical help. Furthermore, there are no guarantees that the supplements will be effective. Taking B vitamin

TABLE H10-1 Vitamin and Mineral Intakes for Adults

Nutrient	Tolerable Upper Intake Levels[a]	Daily Values[e]	Typical Multivitamin-Mineral Supplement	Average Single-Nutrient Supplement
Vitamins				
Vitamin A	3000 μg (10 000 IU)	3300 IU	5000 IU	8000 to 10 000 IU
Vitamin D	50 μg (2000 IU)	200 IU	400 IU	400 IU
Vitamin E	1000 mg (1500 to 2200 IU)[b]	15 IU	30 IU	100 to 1000 IU
Vitamin K	—[c]	80 μg	40 μg	—[f]
Thiamin	—[c]	1.3 mg	1.5 mg	50 mg
Riboflavin	—[c]	1.6 mg	1.7 mg	25 mg
Niacin (as niacinamide)	35 mg[b]	23 mg	20 mg	100 to 500 mg
Vitamin B_6	100 mg	1.8 mg	2 mg	100 to 200 mg
Folate	1000 μg[b]	220 μg	400 μg	400 μg
Vitamin B_{12}	—[c]	2 μg	6 μg	100 to 1000 μg
Pantothenic acid	—[c]	7 mg	10 mg	100 to 500 mg
Biotin	—[c]	300 μg	30 μg	300 to 600 μg
Vitamin C	2000 mg	60 mg	10 mg	500 to 2000 mg
Choline	3500 mg	—	10 mg	250 mg
Minerals				
Calcium	2500 mg	1000 mg	160 mg	250 to 600 mg
Phosphorus	4000 mg	1000 mg	110 mg	—[f]
Magnesium	350 mg[d]	400 mg	100 mg	250 mg
Iron	45 mg	18 mg	18 mg	18 to 30 mg
Zinc	40 mg	15 mg	15 mg	10 to 100 mg
Iodine	1100 μg	150 μg	150 μg	—[f]
Selenium	400 μg	70 μg	10 μg	50 to 200 μg
Fluoride	10 mg	—	—	—[f]
Copper	10 mg	2 mg	0.5 mg	—[f]
Manganese	11 mg	2 mg	5 mg	—[f]
Chromium	—[c]	120 μg	25 μg	200 to 400 μg

[a]Unless otherwise noted, Upper Levels represent total intakes from food, water, and supplements.
[b]Upper Levels represent intakes from supplements, fortified foods, or both.
[c]These nutrients have been evaluated by the DRI Committee for Tolerable Upper Intake Levels, but none were established because of insufficient data. No adverse effects have been reported with intakes of these nutrients at levels typical of supplements, but caution is still advised, given the potential for harm that accompanies excessive intakes.
[d]Upper Levels represent intakes from supplements only.
[e]Table 6.5, Recommended Daily Intake for Vitamins and Mineral Nutrients, Guide to Food Labelling and Advertising.
[f]Available as a single nutrient supplement by prescription.

supplements instead of medication may sound appealing, but they do not protect against the progression of atherosclerosis.[10] Marketing materials for supplements often make health statements that are required to be "truthful and not misleading," but they often fall far short of both. Highlight 19 revisits this topic and includes a discussion of herbal preparations and other alternative therapies.

Unknown Needs

Another argument against the use of supplements is that no one knows exactly how to formulate the "ideal" supplement. What nutrients should be included? Which, if any, of the phytochemicals should be included? How much of each? On whose needs should the choices be based? Surveys have repeatedly shown little relationship between the supplements people take and the nutrients they actually need.

False Sense of Security

Another argument against supplement use is that it may lull people into a false sense of security. A person might eat irresponsibly, thinking, "My supplement will cover my needs." Or, experiencing a warning symptom of a disease, a person might postpone seeking a diagnosis, thinking, "I probably just need a supplement to make this go away." Such self-diagnosis is potentially dangerous.

Other Invalid Reasons

Other invalid reasons people might use for taking supplements include:

- The belief that the food supply or soil contains inadequate nutrients
- The belief that supplements can provide energy
- The belief that supplements can enhance athletic performance or build lean body tissues without physical work or faster than work alone (see Highlight 15)
- The belief that supplements will help a person cope with stress
- The belief that supplements can prevent, treat, or cure conditions ranging from the common cold to cancer

Ironically, people with health problems are more likely to take supplements than other people, yet today's health problems are more likely to be due to overnutrition and poor lifestyle choices than to nutrient deficiencies. The truth—that most people would benefit from improving their eating and exercise habits—is harder to swallow than a supplement pill.

Bioavailability and Antagonistic Actions

In general, the body absorbs nutrients best from foods in which the nutrients are diluted and dispersed among other substances that may facilitate their absorption. Taken in pure, concentrated form, nutrients are likely to interfere with one another's absorption or with the absorption of nutrients in foods eaten at the same time. Documentation of these effects is particularly extensive for minerals: zinc hinders copper and calcium absorption, iron hinders zinc absorption, calcium hinders magnesium and iron absorption, and magnesium hinders the absorption of calcium and iron. Similarly, binding agents in supplements limit mineral absorption.

Although minerals provide the most-familiar and best-documented examples, interference among vitamins is now being seen as supplement use increases. The vitamin A precursor beta-carotene, long thought to be nontoxic, interferes with vitamin E metabolism when taken over the long term as a dietary supplement. Vitamin E, on the other hand, antagonizes vitamin K activity and so should not be used by people being treated for blood-clotting disorders. Consumers who want the benefits of optimal absorption of nutrients should eat ordinary foods, selected for nutrient density and variety.

Whenever the diet is inadequate, the person should first attempt to improve it so as to obtain the needed nutrients from foods. If that is truly impossible, then the person needs a multivitamin-mineral supplement that supplies between 50 and 150 percent of the Daily Value for each of the nutrients. These amounts reflect the ranges commonly found in foods and therefore are compatible with the body's normal handling of nutrients (its physiologic tolerance). The next section provides some pointers to assist in the selection of an appropriate supplement.

Selection of Supplements

Whenever a physician or registered dietitian recommends a supplement, follow the directions carefully. When selecting a supplement yourself, look for a single, balanced vitamin-mineral supplement. Supplements with an 8-digit Natural Products Number (NPN) have been assessed for safety, quality, and efficacy by Health Canada.

If you decide to take a vitamin-mineral supplement, ignore the eye-catching art and meaningless claims. Pay attention to the form the supplements are in, the list of ingredients, and the price. Here's where the truth lies, and from it you can make a rational decision based on facts. You have two basic questions to answer.

Form

The first question: What form do you want—chewable, liquid, or pills? If you'd rather drink your supplements than chew them, fine. If you choose a chewable form, though, be aware that chewable vitamin C can dissolve tooth enamel. If you choose pills, look for statements about the disintegration time. The Natural Health Products (NHP) regulations state that supplements should completely disintegrate within 45 to 60 minutes. Obviously, supplements that don't dissolve have little chance of entering the bloodstream, so look for a brand that claims to meet NHP regulatory disintegration standards.

Contents

The second question: What vitamins and minerals do *you* need? Generally, an appropriate supplement provides vitamins and minerals in amounts that do not exceed recommended intakes. Avoid supplements that, in a daily dose, provide more than the Tolerable Upper Intake Level for *any* nutrient. Avoid preparations with more than 10 milligrams of iron per dose, except as prescribed by a physician. Iron is hard to get rid of once it's in the body, and an excess of iron can cause problems, just as a deficiency can (see Chapter 14).

Misleading Claims

Manufacturers of *organic* or natural vitamins boast that their pills are purified from real foods rather than synthesized in a laboratory. These supplements are no more effective than others and often cost more. The word *synthetic* may sound like "fake," but to synthesize just means to put together. Think back on the course of human evolution; it is not natural to take any kind of pill. In reality, the finest, most natural vitamin "supplements" available are vegetables, fruits, whole grains, milk and alternatives, and meat, fish, poultry, eggs, legumes, nuts, and seeds.

Avoid products that make **"high potency"** claims. More is not better (review Figure 10-1 on p. 314). Remember that foods are also providing these nutrients. Nutrients can build up and cause unexpected problems. For example, a man who takes vitamins and begins to lose his hair may think his hair loss means he needs *more* vitamins, when in fact it may be the early sign of a vitamin A overdose. (Of course, it may be completely unrelated to nutrition as well.)

Be aware that fake vitamins and preparations that contain items not needed in human nutrition, such as carnitine and inositol, reflect a marketing strategy aimed at your pocket, not at your health. The manufacturer wants you to believe that its pills contain the latest "new" nutrient that other brands omit, but in reality, these substances are not known to be needed by human beings.

Realize that the claim that supplements "relieve stress" is another marketing ploy. If you give even passing thought to what people mean by "stress," you'll realize manufacturers could never design a supplement to meet everyone's needs. Is it stressful to take an exam? Well, yes. Is it stressful to survive a major car wreck with third-degree burns and multiple bone fractures? Definitely, yes. The body's responses to these stresses are different. The body does use vitamins and minerals in mounting a stress response, but a body fed a well-balanced diet can meet the needs of most minor stresses. For the major ones, medical intervention is needed. In any case, taking a dietary supplement won't make life any less stressful.

Other marketing tricks to sidestep are "green" pills that contain dehydrated, crushed parsley, alfalfa, and other fruit and vegetable extracts. The nutrients and phytochemicals advertised can be obtained from a serving of vegetables more easily and for less money. Such pills may also provide enzymes, but enzymes are inactivated in the stomach during protein digestion.

Recognize the latest nutrition buzzwords. Manufacturers were marketing "antioxidant" supplements before the print had time to dry on the first scientific reports of antioxidant vitamins' action in preventing cancer and cardiovascular disease. Remember, too, that high doses can alter a nutrient's action in the body. An antioxidant in physiological quantities may be beneficial, but in pharmacological quantities, it may act as a prooxidant and produce harmful by-products. Highlight 12 explores antioxidants and supplement use in more detail.

Finally, be aware that advertising on the Internet is cheap and not closely regulated. Promotional e-mails can be sent to millions of people in an instant. Internet messages can easily cite references and provide links to other sites, implying an endorsement when in fact none has been given. Be cautious when examining unsolicited information and search for a balanced perspective.

Cost

When shopping for supplements, remember that local or store brands may be just as good as nationally advertised brands. If they are less expensive, it may be because the price does not have to cover the cost of national advertising.

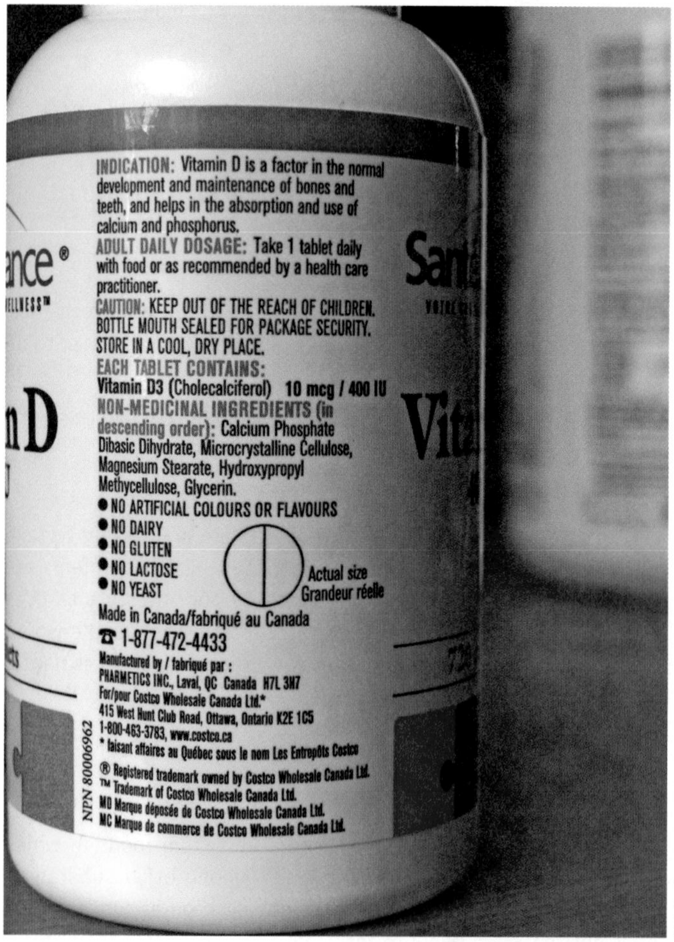
INDICATION: Vitamin D is a factor in the normal development and maintenance of bones and teeth, and helps in the absorption and use of calcium and phosphorus.
ADULT DAILY DOSAGE: Take 1 tablet daily with food or as recommended by a health care practitioner.
CAUTION: KEEP OUT OF THE REACH OF CHILDREN.
BOTTLE MOUTH SEALED FOR PACKAGE SECURITY.
STORE IN A COOL, DRY PLACE.
EACH TABLET CONTAINS:
Vitamin D3 (Cholecalciferol) 10 mcg / 400 IU
NON-MEDICINAL INGREDIENTS (in descending order): Calcium Phosphate Dibasic Dihydrate, Microcrystalline Cellulose, Magnesium Stearate, Hydroxypropyl Methycellulose, Glycerin.
NO ARTIFICIAL COLOURS OR FLAVOURS
NO DAIRY
NO GLUTEN
NO LACTOSE
NO YEAST
Actual size
Grandeur réelle
Made in Canada/fabriqué au Canada
1-877-472-4433
Manufactured by / fabriqué par :
PHARMETICS INC., Laval, QC Canada H7L 3H7
For/pour Costco Wholesale Canada Ltd.*
415 West Hunt Club Road, Ottawa, Ontario K2E 1C5
1-800-463-3783, www.costco.ca
* faisant affaires au Québec sous le nom Les Entrepôts Costco
® Registered trademark owned by Costco Wholesale Canada Ltd.
™ Trademark of Costco Wholesale Canada Ltd.
MD Marque déposée de Costco Wholesale Canada Ltd.
MC Marque de commerce de Costco Wholesale Canada Ltd.
NPN 80006962
Dick Hemingway

This supplement container shows a nutrient function claim that meets specific criteria set by Health Canada.

Regulation of Supplements

In Canada, over-the-counter vitamin and mineral supplements are regulated as natural health products, which are governed by **Health Canada, Natural Health Products Directorate,** and must comply with the NHP regulations. Vitamin and mineral supplements requiring a prescription are regulated under the Food and Drug Regulations. NHP labels must comply with the NHP regulations, which enable consumers to make informed choices about nutrient supplements (see Figure H10-1). Consumers can expect to find the following information on vitamin and mineral supplement labels:

- *Brand name:* must appear on the label as the identifiable name of the product
- *Product number:* all non-prescription vitamin and mineral supplements must be identified by the prefix NHP followed by the 8-digit product number
- *Dosage form:* tablet, packet, or other form of supplement must be provided
- *Sterile products:* for these products, the word "sterile" must be specified on the principal display panel
- *Net amount:* refers to the total number of dosage units in the container, given by weight, measure, or number
- *Medicinal ingredients:* the medicinal ingredients are often listed by proper name followed by a common name; for example, Medicinal ingredient: Echinacea angustifolia (Echinacea)
- *Description of source material of each medicinal ingredient:* the source (e.g., leaf, flower, root) is required; for example, Medicinal ingredient: Echinacea angustifolia (Echinacea) (root)
- *Quantity (and potency, if any) of each medicinal ingredient per dosage unit:* medicinal ingredients should be listed in descending order of quantity, and the quantity of dosage unit must be associated with each name
- *Recommended use or purpose:* a health claim that links the product to a disease or health-related condition is required and must comply with Section 3 of the Food and Drugs Act as they apply to NHP
- *Recommended route of administration, dose, and duration of use (if any):* the recommended route of administration, the number and frequency of dosage units, and the duration of use is required
- *Risk information:* cautions, warnings, known adverse reactions, and contraindications must be identical to the information approved by the NHP Directorate
- *Recommended storage conditions, if any:* must be listed (e.g., dry, well-ventilated premises at 15–25°C or "Must be refrigerated.")
- *Lot number:* must be displayed and remain legible through the useful life of the product
- *Expiry date:* must meet one the following two requirements: (1) the date (year and month), up to and including which a NHP maintains its purity and physical characteristics and its medicinal ingredients maintain their quantity per dosage unit and their potency, and (2) the date (year and month), after which the manufacturer recommends that the NHP should not be used
- *Non-medicinal ingredients:* must be identified as non-medicinal ingredients, and can be listed in any order

The multi-billion-dollar-a-year supplement industry spends much money and effort influencing these regulations. Should a problem arise, the burden falls to Health Canada to prove the supplement poses a risk of illness or injury and remove it from the market. When asked, most Canadians express support for greater regulation of dietary supplements. In fact, Health Canada relies on consumers and health-care professionals to report any adverse reactions or side effects to health products. The MedEffect™ Canada website offers an online reporting system; consumers can also complete a report at a local pharmacy. It's important that Health Canada receive these reports as it allows them to identify previously unknown rare or serious adverse reactions; make changes in product safety information; contribute to international data on the benefits, risks, or effectiveness of health products; issue public warnings and advisories; and remove unsafe products from the Canadian market.

If all the nutrients we need can come from food, why not just eat food? Foods have so much more to offer than supplements do. Nutrients in foods come in an infinite variety of combinations with a multitude of different carriers and absorption enhancers. They come with water, fibre, and an array of beneficial phytochemicals. Foods stimulate the GI tract to keep it healthy. They provide energy, and as long as you need energy each day, why not have nutritious foods deliver it? Foods offer pleasure, satiety, and opportunities for socializing while eating. Quite simply, foods meet human health needs far better than dietary supplements. For further proof, read Highlight 12.

FIGURE H10-1 An Example of a Supplement Label

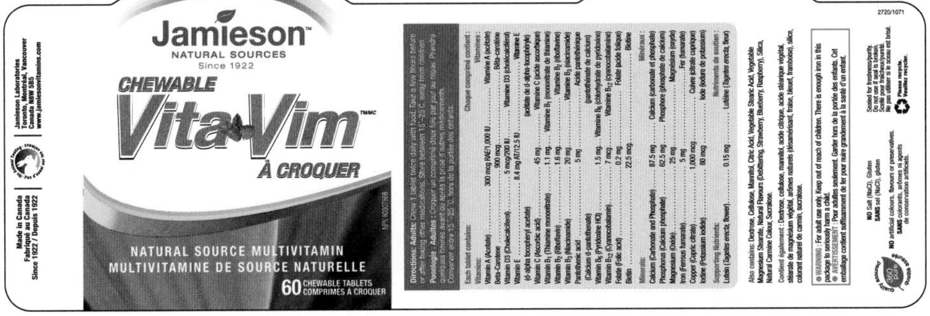
Jamieson
NATURAL SOURCES
Since 1922
CHEWABLE
Vita-Vim
À CROQUER
NATURAL SOURCE MULTIVITAMIN
MULTIVITAMINE DE SOURCE NATURELLE
60 CHEWABLE TABLETS
COMPRIMÉS À CROQUER

Nutrition on the Net

CENGAGENOW™
For further study of topics covered in this Highlight, log on to **www.cengage.com/sso**.

- Gather information from Health Canada: **www.hc-sc.gc.ca**
- Learn more about vitamin and mineral supplements as natural health products from the Natural Health Products Directorate: **www.hc-sc.gc.ca/dhp-mps/prodnatur/index-eng.php**
- Report adverse reactions associated with dietary supplements to Health Canada's MedEffect™ program: **www.hc-sc.gc.ca/dhp-mps/medeff/index-eng.php**
- Search for "supplements" at the Dietitians of Canada's website: **www.dietitians.ca**
- Learn more about supplements from the U.S. FDA Center for Food Safety and Applied Nutrition: **www.fda.gov/Food/DietarySupplements**
- Obtain consumer information on dietary supplements from the U.S. Pharmacopeia: **www.usp.org**
- Review the Federal Trade Commission policies for dietary supplement advertising: **www.ftc.gov/bcp**
- Gather information from the U.S. Office of Dietary Supplements: **http://ods.od.nih.gov**

References

1. H. Vatanparast, J. L. Adolphe, and S. J. Whiting, Socio-economic status and vitamin/mineral supplement use in Canada, *Health Reports* 21 (2010): 1–7; X. Guo, N. Willows, S. Kuhle, G. Jhangri, and P. J. Veugelers, Use of vitamin and mineral supplements among Canadian adults, *Canadian Journal of Public Health* 100 (2009): 357–360.
2. E. Sloan, Why people use vitamin and mineral supplements, *Nutrition Today* 42 (2007): 55–61.
3. Dietitians of Canada: Do I need a vitamin or mineral supplement? www.dietitians.ca/Nutrition-Resources-A-Z/Fact-Sheet-Pages%28HTML%29/Miscellaneous/Do-I-Need-a-Supplement-.aspx, accessed September 9, 2011.
4. E. A. Yetley, Multivitamin and multimineral dietary supplements: Definitions, characterization, bioavailability, and drug interactions, *American Journal of Clinical Nutrition* 85 (2007): 269S–276S; B. B. Timbo and coauthors, Dietary supplements in a National Survey: Prevalence of use and reports of adverse events, *Journal of the American Dietetic Association* 106 (2006): 1966–1974.
5. R. S. Sebastian and coauthors, Older adults who use vitamin/mineral supplements differ from nonusers in nutrient intake adequacy and dietary attitudes, *Journal of the American Dietetic Association* 107 (2007): 1322–1332.
6. H. Huang and coauthors, The efficacy and safety of multivitamin and mineral supplement use to prevent cancer and chronic disease in adults: A systematic review for a National Institutes of Health State-of-the-Science Conference, *Annals of Internal Medicine* 145 (2006): 372–385.
7. National Institutes of Health, 2006.
8. G. Bjelakovic and coauthors, Mortality in randomized trials of antioxidant supplements for primary and secondary prevention, *Journal of the American Medical Association* 297 (2007): 842–857; K. A. Lawson and coauthors, Multivitamin use and risk of prostate cancer in the National Institutes of Health-AARP Diet and Health Study, *Journal of the National Cancer Institute* 99 (2007): 754–764.
9. S. P. Murphy and coauthors, Multivitamin-multimineral supplements' effect on total nutrient intake, *American Journal of Clinical Nutrition* 85 (2007): 280S–284S.
10. J. Bleys and coauthors, Vitamin-mineral supplementation and the progression of atherosclerosis: A meta-analysis of randomized controlled trials, *American Journal of Clinical Nutrition* 84 (2006): 880–887; D. B. McCormick, The dubious use of vitamin-mineral supplements in relation to cardiovascular disease, *American Journal of Clinical and Nutrition* 84 (2006): 680–681.

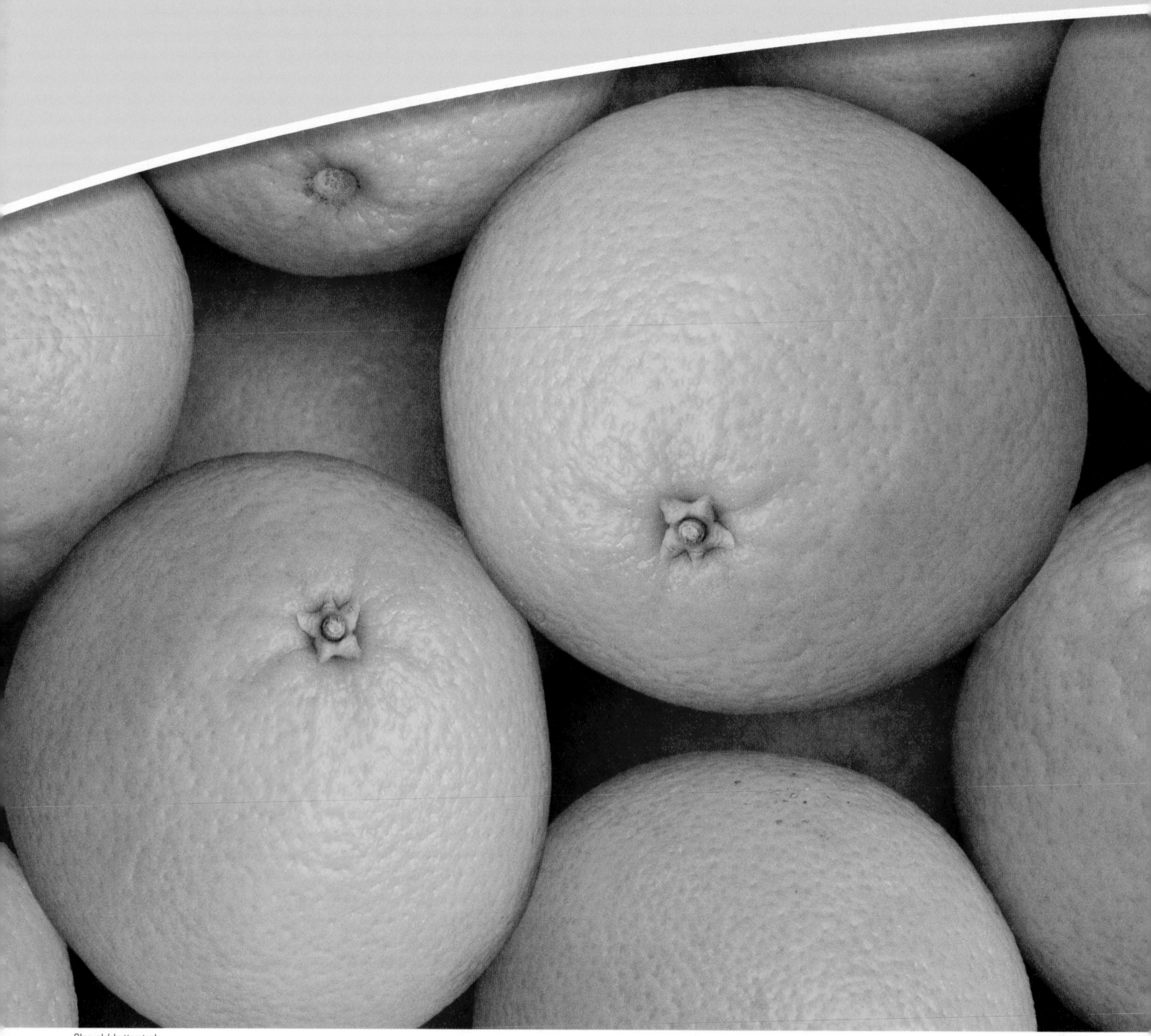

Olegusk/shutterstock

Nutrition in Your Life

CENGAGENOW™

Throughout this chapter, the CengageNOW logo indicates an opportunity for online self-study, linking you to interactive tutorials, activities, and videos to increase your understanding of chapter concepts.
www.cengage.com/sso

What's your beverage of choice? If you said water, then congratulate yourself for recognizing its important role in maintaining your body's fluid balance. Without water, you would realize within days how vital it is to your survival. Water and the major minerals sodium, chloride, potassium, and phosphorus support fluid balance throughout the body. Before getting too comfortable reading this chapter, pour yourself a glass of water. Your body will thank you.

CHAPTER 11

Water and the Electrolytes

CHAPTER OUTLINE

Water is an essential nutrient, more important to life than any of the others. The body needs more water each day than any other nutrient. Furthermore, you can survive only a few days without water, whereas a deficiency of the other nutrients may take weeks, months, or even years to develop.

The first nutrient profiled in this chapter is water. The body maintains an appropriate balance and distribution of fluids with the help of water and another class of nutrients—the minerals. Sodium, chloride, potassium, and phosphorus are the notable electrolytes. This chapter describes how water and these minerals help to regulate the distribution of body fluids and perform other important functions in the body. Chapter 20 revisits water as a beverage and addresses consumer concerns about its safety.

Water and the Body Fluids

Water constitutes about 60 percent of an adult's body weight and a higher percentage of a child's (see Figure 1-1, p. 6). Because water makes up about three-fourths of the weight of lean tissue and less than one-fourth of the weight of fat, a person's body composition influences how much of the body's weight is water. The proportion of water is generally smaller in females, obese people, and the elderly because of their smaller proportion of lean tissue.

In the body, water is the fluid in which all life processes occur. The water in the body fluids:

- Carries nutrients and waste products throughout the body
- Maintains the structure of large molecules such as proteins and glycogen
- Participates in metabolic reactions
- Serves as the solvent for minerals, vitamins, amino acids, glucose, and many other small molecules so that they can participate in metabolic activities
- Acts as a lubricant and cushion around joints and inside the eyes, the spinal cord, and, in pregnancy, the amniotic sac surrounding the fetus in the womb
- Aids in the regulation of normal body temperature, as the evaporation of sweat from the skin removes excess heat from the body
- Maintains blood volume

To support these and other vital functions, the body actively maintains an appropriate **water balance.** ♦

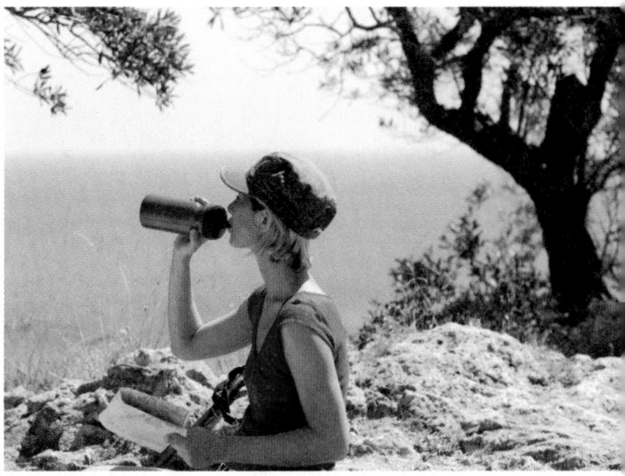

Diego Cervo/shutterstock

Water is the most indispensable nutrient.

♦ Water balance: intake = output

water balance: the balance between water intake and output (losses).

Water Balance and Recommended Intakes

Water Balance and Recommended Intakes Every cell contains fluid of the exact composition that is best for that cell. Fluid inside cells is called **intracellular fluid**, whereas fluid outside cells is called **extracellular fluid.** ♦ The extracellular fluid that surrounds each cell is called **interstitial fluid.** Figure 11-1 illustrates a cell and its associated fluids. The composition of intercellular and extracellular fluids differ from one another. They continually lose and replace their components, yet the composition in each compartment remains remarkably constant under normal conditions. Because imbalances can be devastating, the body quickly responds by adjusting both water intake and excretion as needed. Consequently, the entire system of cells and fluids remains in a delicate, but controlled, state of homeostasis.

♦ Fluids in the body:
- Intracellular (inside cells)
- Extracellular (outside cells)
  - Interstitial (between cells)
  - Intravascular (inside blood vessels)

Water Intake **Thirst** and satiety influence water intake, apparently in response to changes sensed by the mouth, hypothalamus, ♦ and nerves.[1] When water intake is inadequate, the blood becomes concentrated (having lost water but not the dissolved substances within it), the mouth becomes dry, and the hypothalamus initiates drinking behaviour. When water intake is excessive, the stomach expands and stretch receptors send signals to stop drinking. Similar signals are sent from receptors in the heart as blood volume increases.

♦ The **hypothalamus** is a brain centre that controls activities such as maintenance of water balance, regulation of body temperature, and control of appetite.

Thirst drives a person to seek water, but it lags behind the body's need. When too much water is lost from the body and not replaced, **dehydration** develops. A first sign of dehydration is thirst, the signal that the body has already lost some of its fluid. If a person is unable to obtain fluid or, as in many elderly people, fails to perceive the thirst message, the symptoms of dehydration may progress rapidly from thirst to weakness, exhaustion, and delirium—and end in death if not corrected. Highlight 11 more closely examines the effects of progressive states of dehydration. Dehydration may easily develop with either water deprivation or excessive water losses. (Chapter 15 revisits dehydration and the fluid needs of athletes.)

Water intoxication, on the other hand, is rare but can occur with excessive water ingestion and kidney disorders that reduce urine production. The symptoms may include confusion, convulsions, and even death in extreme cases. Excessive water ingestion (10 to 20 litres) within a few hours dilutes the sodium concentration of the blood and contributes to a dangerous condition known as **hyponatremia.** For this reason, guidelines suggest limiting fluid intake during times of heavy sweating to between 1 and 1.5 litres per hour. (Chapter 15 revisits hyponatremia as sometimes seen in endurance athletes.)

♦ Water generated during metabolism is called **metabolic water.**

Water Sources The obvious dietary sources of water are water itself and other beverages, but nearly all foods also contain water. Most fruits and vegetables contain up to 90 percent water, and many meats and cheeses contain at least 50 percent. See Table 11-1 for selected foods and APPENDIX H for many more. Also, water is produced as an end-product ♦ of condensation reactions and during the oxidation of energy-yielding nutrients. Recall from Chapter 7 that when the energy-yielding nutrients break down, their carbons and hydrogens combine with oxygen to yield carbon dioxide (CO_2) and water (H_2O). As Table 11-2 shows, the water derived daily from these three sources averages about 2½ litres (roughly 10½ cups).

♦ The amount of water the body has to excrete each day to dispose of its wastes is the **obligatory** (ah-BLIG-ah-TORE-ee) **water excretion**—about 500 mL (2 cups).

Water Losses The body must excrete a minimum of about 500 millilitres (2 cups) of water each day ♦ as urine—enough to carry away the waste products generated by a day's metabolic activities. Above this amount, excretion adjusts to balance intake. If a person drinks more water, the kidneys excrete more urine, and the urine becomes more dilute. In addition to urine, water is lost from the lungs as vapour and from the skin as sweat; some is also lost in feces.* The amount of fluid lost from each source varies, depending on the environment (such as heat or humidity) and physical conditions (such as exercise or fever). On average, daily losses total about 2.5 litres. Table 11-2 shows how daily water losses and intakes balance; maintaining this balance requires healthy kidneys and an adequate intake of fluids.

FIGURE 11-1 One Cell and Its Associated Fluids

Fluids are found within the cells (intracellular) or outside the cells (extracellular). Extracellular fluids include plasma (the fluid portion of blood in the intravascular spaces of blood vessels) and interstitial fluids (the tissue fluid that fills the intercellular spaces between the cells).

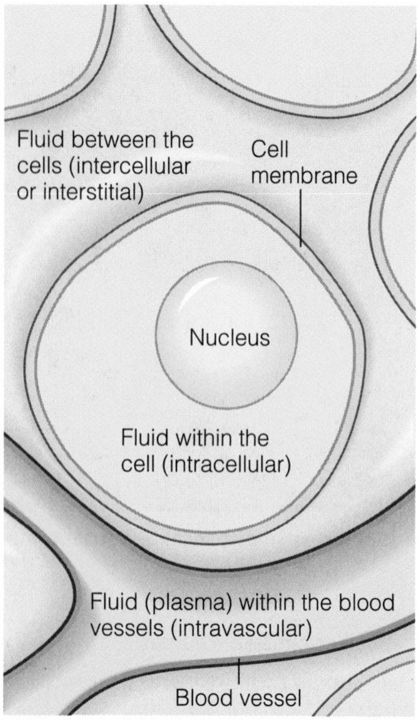
Fluid between the cells (intercellular or interstitial)
Cell membrane
Nucleus
Fluid within the cell (intracellular)
Fluid (plasma) within the blood vessels (intravascular)
Blood vessel

Water Recommendations Because water needs vary depending on diet, activity, environmental temperature, and humidity, a general water requirement is difficult

*Water lost from the lungs and skin accounts for almost one-half of the daily losses even when a person is not visibly perspiring; these losses are commonly referred to as *insensible water losses.*

TABLE 11-1 Percentage of Water in Selected Foods

100%	Water
90–99%	Skim milk, strawberries, watermelon, lettuce, cabbage, celery, spinach, broccoli
80–89%	Fruit juice, yogurt, apples, grapes, oranges, carrots
70–79%	Shrimp, bananas, corn, potatoes, avocados, cottage cheese, ricotta cheese
60–69%	Pasta, legumes, salmon, ice cream, chicken breast
50–59%	Ground beef, hot dogs, feta cheese
40–49%	Pizza
30–39%	Cheddar cheese, bagels, bread
20–29%	Pepperoni, sausage, cake, biscuits
10–19%	Butter, margarine, raisins
1–9%	Crackers, cereals, pretzels, taco shells, peanut butter, nuts
0%	Oils, sugars

to establish. Recommendations ♦ are sometimes expressed in proportion to the amount of energy expended under average environmental conditions.[2] The recommended water intake for a person who expends 2000 kcalories a day, for example, is 2 to 3 litres of water (about 8 to 12 cups). This recommendation is in line with the Adequate Intake (AI) for *total* water set by the DRI Committee. ♦ Total water includes not only drinking water, but water in other beverages and in foods as well.

Because a wide range of water intakes will prevent dehydration and its harmful consequences, the AI is based on average intakes. People who are physically active or who live in hot environments may need more.[3]

Which beverages are best? Any beverage can readily meet the body's fluid needs, but those with few or no kcalories do so without contributing to weight gain. Given that obesity is a major health problem and that beverages represent about 15 to 20 percent of Canadians' total energy intake, water is the best choice for most people.[4] Other choices include tea, coffee, skim and 1% milk, fortified soy beverage, artificially sweetened beverages, fruit and vegetable juices, sports drinks, and lastly, sweetened nutrient-poor beverages.

Some research indicates that people who drink caffeinated beverages lose a little more fluid than when drinking water because caffeine acts as a diuretic. The DRI Committee considered such findings in their recommendations for water intake and concluded: "Caffeinated beverages contribute to the daily total water intake similar to that contributed by non-caffeinated beverages."[5] In other words, it doesn't seem to matter whether people rely on caffeine-containing beverages or other beverages to meet their fluid needs.

As Highlight 7 explains, alcohol acts as a diuretic and can impair a person's health. Alcohol should not be used to meet fluid needs.

Health Effects of Water In addition to meeting the body's fluid needs, drinking plenty of water may protect against urinary stones and constipation.[6] Even mild dehydration seems to interfere with daily tasks involving concentration, alertness, and short-term memory.[7]

TABLE 11-2 Water Balance

Water Sources	Amount (mL)	Water Losses	Amount (mL)
Liquids	550 to 1500	Kidneys (urine)	500 to 1400
Foods	700 to 1000	Skin (sweat)	450 to 900
Metabolic water	200 to 300	Lungs (breath)	350
Total	1450 to 2800	GI tract (feces)	150
		Total	1450 to 2800

NOTE: For perspective, 100 millilitres is a little less than ½ cup and 1000 millilitres is a little more than 1 quart.

*For those using kilojoules: 4.2 to 6.3 mL/kJ expended.

♦ Water recommendation:
- 1.0 to 1.5 mL/kcal expended (adults)*
- 1.5 mL/kcal expended (infants and athletes)

Conversion factors:
- 125 mL ≈ ½ c

Easy estimation: ½ c per 100 kcal expended

♦ AI for *total* water:
- Men: 3.7 L/day
- Women: 2.7 L/day

Conversion factors:
- 1 L ≈ 4 c

intracellular fluid: fluid within the cells, usually high in potassium and phosphate. Intracellular fluid accounts for approximately two-thirds of the body's water.
- **intra** = within

extracellular fluid: fluid outside the cells. Extracellular fluid includes two main components—the interstitial fluid between cells and the intravascular fluid of plasma. Extracellular fluid accounts for approximately one-third of the body's water.
- **extra** = outside

interstitial (IN-ter-STISH-al) **fluid:** fluid between the cells (intercellular), usually high in sodium and chloride. Interstitial fluid is a large component of extracellular fluid.
- **inter** = in the midst, between

thirst: a conscious desire to drink.

dehydration: the condition in which body water output exceeds water input. Symptoms include thirst, dry skin and mucous membranes, rapid heartbeat, low blood pressure, and weakness.

water intoxication: the rare condition in which body water contents are too high in all body fluid compartments.

hyponatremia (HIGH-po-na-TREE-me-ah): a decreased concentration of sodium in the blood.

FIGURE 11-2 How Hard is Your Water?

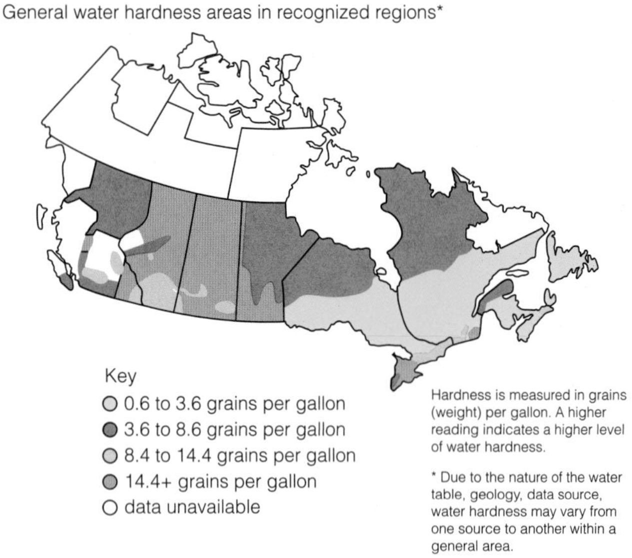
General water hardness areas in recognized regions*
Key
0.6 to 3.6 grains per gallon
3.6 to 8.6 grains per gallon
8.4 to 14.4 grains per gallon
14.4+ grains per gallon
data unavailable
Hardness is measured in grains (weight) per gallon. A higher reading indicates a higher level of water hardness.
* Due to the nature of the water table, geology, data source, water hardness may vary from one source to another within a general area.

SOURCE: Canadian Water Quality Association (CWQA). Reprinted with permission.

The kind of water a person drinks may also make a difference to health. Water is usually either hard or soft. **Hard water** has high concentrations of calcium and magnesium; sodium or potassium is the principal mineral of **soft water.** (See the accompanying glossary for these and other common terms used to describe water.) Figure 11-2 shows the distribution of hard and soft water in different regions of Canada. In practical terms, soft water makes more bubbles with less soap; hard water leaves a ring on the tub, a crust of rocklike crystals in the teakettle, and a grey residue in the laundry.

Soft water may seem more desirable around the house, and some homeowners purchase water softeners that replace magnesium and calcium with sodium. In the body, however, soft water with sodium may aggravate hypertension and heart disease. In contrast, the minerals in hard water may benefit these conditions.

Soft water also more easily dissolves certain contaminant minerals, such as cadmium and lead, from old plumbing pipes. As Chapter 14 explains, these contaminant minerals harm the body by displacing the nutrient minerals from their normal sites of action. People who live in buildings with old plumbing should run the cold water tap a minute or two to flush out harmful minerals whenever the water faucet has been off for more than six hours.[8]

Many people select **bottled water**, believing it to be safer than tap water and therefore worth its substantial cost. Chapter 20 offers a discussion of bottled water safety and regulations.

IN SUMMARY **Water makes up about 60 percent of the adult body's weight. To maintain water balance, intake from liquids, foods, and metabolism must equal losses from the kidneys, skin, lungs, and GI tract. The amount and type of water a person drinks may have positive or negative health effects.**

Water

Adequate Intake (AI)

Adults: 2.7 litres/day (women)
3.7 litres/day (men)

Chief Functions in the Body

Maintains normal blood volume and pressure, fluid balance, and acid-base balance, transports nutrients to cells and waste products from cells, participates in chemical reactions, acts as a solvent, serves as a shock absorber, and regulates body temperature

Deficiency Symptoms

Thirst, concentrated urine

Toxicity Symptoms

Confusion, convulsions, death in extreme cases

Significant Sources

Water, beverages, and foods, especially fruits and vegetables

GLOSSARY OF TYPES OF WATER

artesian water: water drawn from a well that taps a confined aquifer in which the water is under pressure.

bottled water: drinking water sold in bottles.

carbonated water: water that contains carbon dioxide gas, either naturally occurring or added, that causes bubbles to form in it; also called *bubbling* or *sparkling water.* Seltzer, soda, and tonic waters are legally soft drinks and are not regulated as water.

distilled water: water that has been vapourized and recondensed, leaving it free of dissolved minerals.

filtered water: water treated by filtration, usually through *activated carbon filters* that reduce the lead in tap water, or by *reverse osmosis* units that force pressurized water across a membrane removing lead, arsenic, and some microorganisms from tap water.

hard water: water with a high calcium and magnesium content.

mineral water: water from a spring or well that naturally contains dissolved minerals. Minerals give water a distinctive flavour. Many mineral waters are high in sodium.

natural water: water obtained from a spring or well that is certified to be safe and sanitary. The mineral content may not be changed, but the water may be treated in other ways such as with ozone or by filtration.

public water: water from a municipal water system that has been treated and disinfected.

purified water: water that has been treated by distillation or other physical or chemical processes that remove dissolved solids. Because purified water contains no minerals or contaminants, it is useful for medical and research purposes.

soft water: water with a high sodium or potassium content.

spring water: water originating from an underground spring or well. It may be bubbly (carbonated), or "flat" or "still," meaning not carbonated. Brand names such as "Spring Pure" do not necessarily mean that the water comes from a spring.

well water: water drawn from groundwater by tapping into an aquifer.

Blood Volume and Blood Pressure Fluids maintain the blood volume, which in turn influences blood pressure. The kidneys are central to the regulation of blood volume and blood pressure.[9] All day, every day, the kidneys reabsorb needed substances and water and excrete wastes with some water in the urine (see Figure 11-3). The kidneys meticulously adjust the volume and the concentration of the urine to accommodate changes in the body, including variations in the day's food and beverage intakes. Instructions on whether to retain or release substances or water come from ADH, renin, angiotensin, and aldosterone.

ADH Whenever blood volume or blood pressure falls too low, or whenever the extracellular fluid becomes too concentrated, the hypothalamus signals the pituitary gland to release antidiuretic hormone (ADH). ♦ ADH is a water-conserving hormone ♦ that stimulates the kidneys to reabsorb water. Consequently, the more water you need, the less your kidneys excrete. These events also trigger thirst. Drinking water and retaining fluids raise the blood volume and dilute the concentrated fluids, thus helping to restore homeostasis.

Renin Cells in the kidneys respond to low blood pressure by releasing an enzyme called **renin**. Through a complex series of events, renin causes the kidneys to reabsorb sodium. Sodium reabsorption, in turn, is always accompanied by water retention, which helps to restore blood volume and blood pressure.

Angiotensin In addition to its role in sodium retention, renin hydrolyzes a protein from the liver called angiotensinogen to **angiotensin I**. Angiotensin I is inactive until another enzyme converts it to its active form—**angiotensin II**. Angiotensin II is a powerful **vasoconstrictor** that narrows the diameters of blood vessels, thereby raising the blood pressure.

♦ **Antidiuretic hormone (ADH)** is a hormone produced by the pituitary gland in response to dehydration (or a high sodium concentration in the blood). It stimulates the kidneys to reabsorb more water and therefore to excrete less.

♦ Recall from Highlight 7 that alcohol depresses ADH activity, thus promoting fluid losses and dehydration. In addition to its antidiuretic effect, ADH elevates blood pressure and so is also called **vasopressin** (VAS-oh-PRES-in).
- **vaso** = vessel
- **press** = pressure

renin (REN-in): an enzyme from the kidneys that hydrolyzes the protein angiotensinogen to angiotensin I.

angiotensin I (AN-gee-oh-TEN-sin): an inactive precursor that is converted by an enzyme to yield active angiotensin II.

angiotensin II: a hormone involved in blood pressure regulation.

vasoconstrictor (VAS-oh-kon-STRIK-tor): a substance that constricts or narrows the blood vessels.

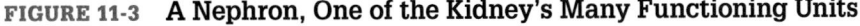

FIGURE 11-3 A Nephron, One of the Kidney's Many Functioning Units

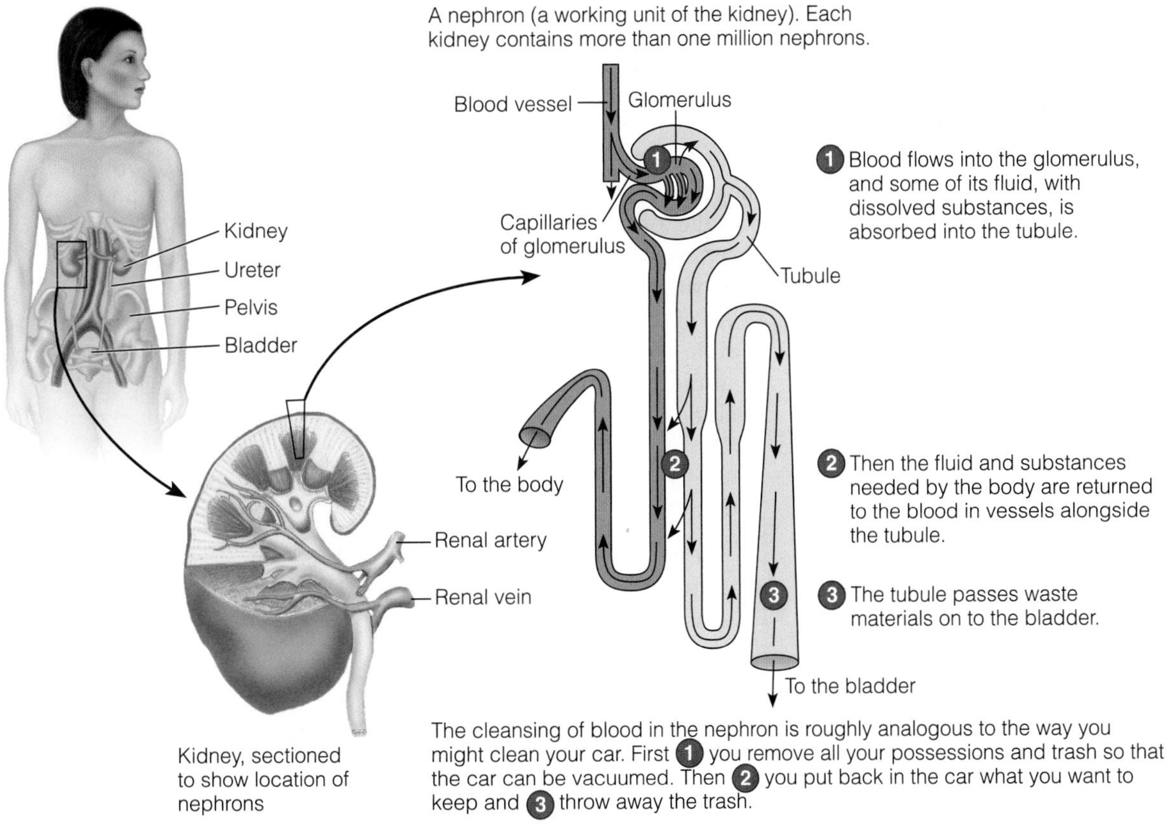
A nephron (a working unit of the kidney). Each kidney contains more than one million nephrons.
Blood vessel
Glomerulus
Capillaries of glomerulus
Tubule
1 Blood flows into the glomerulus, and some of its fluid, with dissolved substances, is absorbed into the tubule.
Kidney
Ureter
Pelvis
Bladder
To the body
Renal artery
Renal vein
2 Then the fluid and substances needed by the body are returned to the blood in vessels alongside the tubule.
3 The tubule passes waste materials on to the bladder.
To the bladder
Kidney, sectioned to show location of nephrons
The cleansing of blood in the nephron is roughly analogous to the way you might clean your car. First 1 you remove all your possessions and trash so that the car can be vacuumed. Then 2 you put back in the car what you want to keep and 3 throw away the trash.

FIGURE 11-4 How the Body Regulates Blood Volume

The renin-angiotensin-aldosterone system helps regulate blood volume and therefore blood pressure.

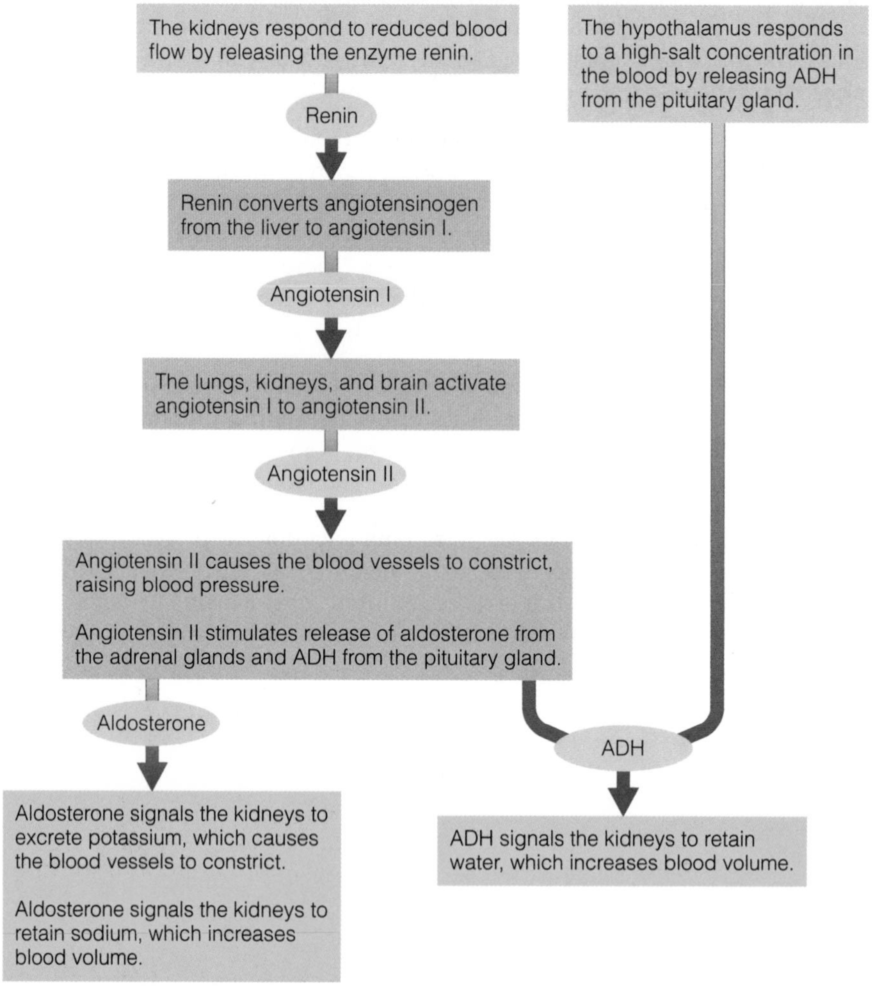
The kidneys respond to reduced blood flow by releasing the enzyme renin.
The hypothalamus responds to a high-salt concentration in the blood by releasing ADH from the pituitary gland.
Renin
Renin converts angiotensinogen from the liver to angiotensin I.
Angiotensin I
The lungs, kidneys, and brain activate angiotensin I to angiotensin II.
Angiotensin II
Angiotensin II causes the blood vessels to constrict, raising blood pressure.
Angiotensin II stimulates release of aldosterone from the adrenal glands and ADH from the pituitary gland.
Aldosterone
ADH
Aldosterone signals the kidneys to excrete potassium, which causes the blood vessels to constrict.
Aldosterone signals the kidneys to retain sodium, which increases blood volume.
ADH signals the kidneys to retain water, which increases blood volume.

Aldosterone In addition to acting as a vasoconstrictor, angiotensin II stimulates the release of the hormone **aldosterone** from the **adrenal glands.** Aldosterone signals the kidneys to excrete potassium and to retain more sodium, and therefore water, because when sodium moves, water follows. Again, the effect is that when more water is needed, less is excreted.

All of these actions are presented in Figure 11-4 and help to explain why high-sodium diets aggravate conditions such as hypertension or edema. Too much sodium causes water retention and an accompanying rise in blood pressure or swelling in the interstitial spaces. Chapter 19 discusses hypertension in detail.

IN SUMMARY **The body responds to low blood volume, low blood pressure, or highly concentrated body fluids by producing:**

- **ADH, which stimulates the kidneys to reabsorb water.**
- **Renin, which initiates the pathway that leads to the production of angiotensin II.**
- **Angiotensin II, which constricts blood vessels and stimulates the release of aldosterone and ADH.**
- **Aldosterone, which regulates potassium and sodium levels.**

All these actions combine to effectively restore homeostasis. Water balance can be maintained only if a person drinks enough water.

aldosterone (al-DOS-ter-own): a hormone secreted by the adrenal glands that regulates blood pressure by increasing the reabsorption of sodium by the kidneys. Aldosterone also regulates chloride and potassium concentrations.

adrenal glands: glands adjacent to, and just above, each kidney.

Fluid and Electrolyte Balance Maintaining a balance of about two-thirds of the body fluids inside the cells and one-third outside is vital to the life of the cells. If too much water were to enter the cells, they might rupture; if too much water were to leave, they would collapse. To control the movement of water, the cells direct the movement of the major minerals. ♦

Dissociation of Salt in Water When a mineral **salt** such as sodium chloride (NaCl) dissolves in water, it separates **(dissociates)** into **ions**—positively and negatively charged particles (Na^+ and Cl^-). The positive ions are **cations**; the negative ones are **anions.** ♦ Unlike pure water, which conducts electricity poorly, ions dissolved in water carry electrical current. For this reason, salts that dissociate into ions are called **electrolytes,** and fluids that contain them are **electrolyte solutions.**

In all electrolyte solutions, anion and cation concentrations are balanced (the number of negative and positive charges are equal). If a fluid contains 1000 negative charges, it must contain 1000 positive charges, too. If an anion enters the fluid, a cation must accompany it or another anion must leave so that electrical neutrality will be maintained. Thus, whenever sodium (Na^+) ions leave a cell, potassium (K^+) ions enter, for example. In fact, it's a good bet that whenever Na^+ and K^+ ions are moving, they are going in opposite directions.

Table 11-3 shows that, indeed, the positive and negative charges inside and outside cells are perfectly balanced even though the numbers of each kind of ion differ over a wide range. Inside the cells, the positive charges total 202 and the negative charges balance these perfectly. Outside the cells, the amounts and proportions of the ions differ from those inside, but again the positive and negative charges balance. Scientists count these charges in milliequivalents, mEq. ♦

Electrolytes Attract Water Electrolytes attract water. Each water molecule has a net charge of zero, ♦ but the oxygen side of the molecule has a slight negative charge, and the hydrogens have a slight positive charge. Figure 11-5 (p. 362) shows the result in an electrolyte solution: both positive and negative ions attract clusters of water molecules around them. This attraction dissolves salts in water and enables the body to move fluids into appropriate compartments.

♦ The major minerals:
- Sodium
- Chloride
- Potassium
- Calcium
- Phosphorus
- Magnesium
- Sulphur

♦ To remember the difference between cations and anions, think of the "t" in cations as a "plus" (+) sign and the "n" in anions as a "negative."

♦ The concentration of electrolytes in a volume of solution is expressed as **milliequivalents per litre (mEq/L).** Milliequivalents are a useful measure when considering ions because the number of charges reveals characteristics about the solution that are not evident when the concentration is expressed in terms of weight.

♦ A neutral molecule, such as water, that has opposite charges spatially separated within the molecule is **polar.** See APPENDIX B for more details.

TABLE 11-3 Important Body Electrolytes

Electrolytes	Intracellular (inside cells) Concentration (mEq/L)	Extracellular (outside cells) Concentration (mEq/L)
Cations (positively charged ions)		
Sodium (Na^+)	10	142
Potassium (K^+)	150	5
Calcium (Ca^{++})	2	5
Magnesium (Mg^{++})	40	3
	202	155
Anions (negatively charged ions)		
Chloride (Cl^-)	2	103
Bicarbonate (HCO_3^-)	10	27
Phosphate ($HPO_4^=$)	103	2
Sulphate ($SO_4^=$)	20	1
Organic acids (lactate, pyruvate)	10	6
Proteins	57	16
	202	155

NOTE: The numbers of positive and negative charges in a given fluid are the same. For example, in extracellular fluid, the cations and anions both equal 155 milliequivalents per litre (mEq/L). Of the cations, sodium ions make up 142 mEq/L; and potassium, calcium, and magnesium ions make up the remainder. Of the anions, chloride ions number 103 mEq/L; bicarbonate ions number 27; and the rest are provided by phosphate ions, sulphate ions, organic acids, and protein.

salt: a compound composed of a positive ion other than H^+ and a negative ion other than OH^-. An example is sodium chloride ($Na^+ Cl^-$).
- **Na** = sodium
- **Cl** = chloride

dissociates (dis-SO-see-aites): physically separates.

ions (EYE-uns): atoms or molecules that have gained or lost electrons and therefore have electrical charges. Examples include the positively charged sodium ion (Na^+) and the negatively charged chloride ion (Cl^-). For a closer look at ions, see APPENDIX B.

cations (CAT-eye-uns): positively charged ions.

anions (AN-eye-uns): negatively charged ions.

electrolytes: salts that dissolve in water and dissociate into charged particles called ions.

electrolyte solutions: solutions that can conduct electricity.

FIGURE 11-5 Water Dissolves Salts and Follows Electrolytes

The structural arrangement of the two hydrogen atoms and one oxygen atom enables water to dissolve salts. Water's role as a solvent is one of its most valuable characteristics.

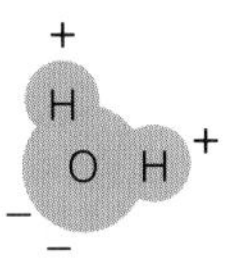
+
H
O H
+
–
–

The negatively charged electrons that bond the hydrogens to the oxygen spend most of their time near the oxygen atom. As a result, the oxygen is slightly negative, and the hydrogens are slightly positive (see APPENDIX B).

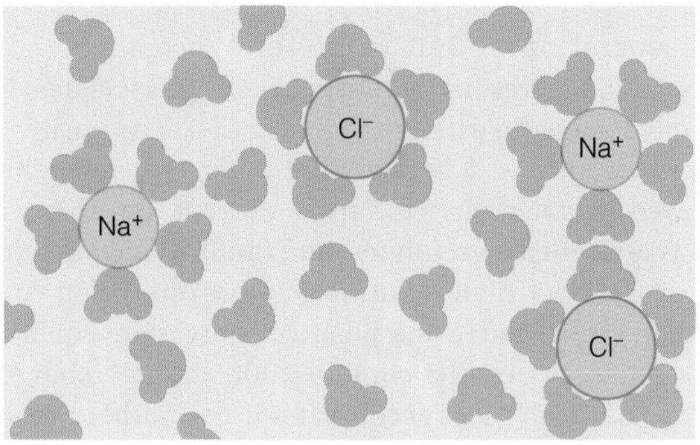
Cl⁻
Na⁺
Na⁺
Cl⁻

In an electrolyte solution, water molecules are attracted to both anions and cations. Notice that the negative oxygen atoms of the water molecules are drawn to the sodium cation (Na^+), whereas the positive hydrogen atoms of the water molecules are drawn to the chloride ions (Cl^-).

Water Follows Electrolytes As Figure 11-6 shows, some electrolytes reside primarily outside the cells (notably, sodium and chloride), whereas others reside predominantly inside the cells (notably, potassium, magnesium, phosphate, and sulphate). Cell membranes are *selectively permeable,* meaning that they allow the passage of some molecules, but not others. Whenever electrolytes move across the membrane, water follows.

solutes (SOLL-yutes): the substances that are dissolved in a solution. The number of molecules in a given volume of fluid is the *solute concentration.*

osmosis: the movement of water across a membrane *toward* the side where the solutes are more concentrated.

osmotic pressure: the amount of pressure needed to prevent the movement of water across a membrane.

The movement of water across a membrane toward the more concentrated **solutes** is called **osmosis.** The amount of pressure needed to prevent the movement of water across a membrane is called the **osmotic pressure.** Figure 11-7 presents osmosis, and the photos of salted eggplant and rehydrated raisins provide familiar food examples.

FIGURE 11-6 A Cell and Its Electrolytes

All of these electrolytes are found both inside and outside the cells, but each can be found mostly on one side or the other of the cell membrane.

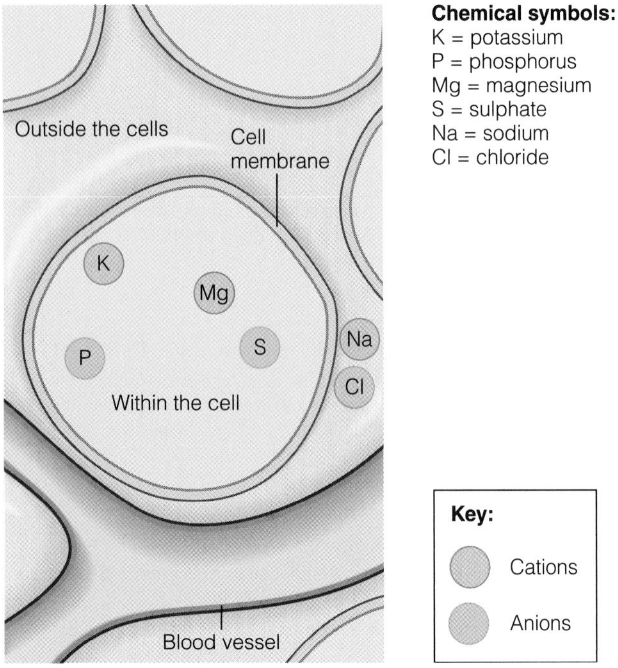
Outside the cells
Cell membrane
K
Mg
P
S
Na
Cl
Within the cell
Blood vessel
Chemical symbols:
K = potassium
P = phosphorus
Mg = magnesium
S = sulphate
Na = sodium
Cl = chloride
Key:
Cations
Anions

Proteins Regulate Flow of Fluids and Ions Chapter 6 describes how proteins attract water and help to regulate fluid movement. In addition, transport proteins in the cell membranes regulate the passage of positive ions and other substances from one side of the membrane to the other. Negative ions follow positive ions, and water flows toward the more concentrated solution.

A protein that regulates the flow of fluids and ions in and out of cells is the sodium-potassium pump. The pump actively exchanges sodium for potassium across the cell membrane, using ATP as an energy source. Figure 6-10 on p. 181 illustrates this action.

Regulation of Fluid and Electrolyte Balance The amounts of various minerals in the body must remain nearly constant. Regulation occurs chiefly at two sites: the GI tract and the kidneys.

The digestive juices of the GI tract contain minerals. These minerals and those from foods are reabsorbed in the large intestine as needed. Each day, 8 litres of fluids and associated minerals are recycled this way, providing ample opportunity for the regulation of electrolyte balance.

The kidneys' control of the body's *water* content by way of the hormone ADH has already been described (see p. 359). The kidneys regulate the *electrolyte* contents by responding to the hormone aldosterone (explained on p. 360). If the body's sodium is low, aldosterone stimulates sodium reabsorption from the kidneys. As sodium is reabsorbed, potassium (another positive ion) is excreted in accordance with the rule that total positive charges must remain in balance with total negative charges.

FIGURE 11-7 Osmosis

Water flows in the direction of the more highly concentrated solution.

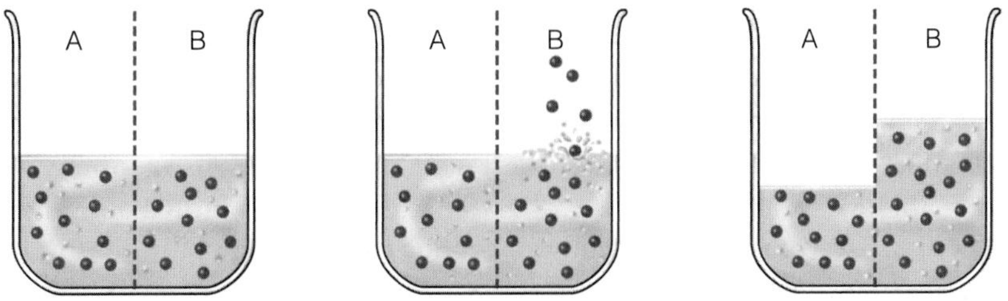
A
B
A
B
A
B

1. With equal numbers of solute particles on both sides of the semipermeable membrane, the concentrations are equal, and the tendency of water to move in either direction is about the same.
2. Now additional solute is added to side B. Solute cannot flow across the divider (in the case of a cell, its membrane).
3. Water can flow both ways across the divider, but has a greater tendency to move from side A to side B, where there is a greater concentration of solute. The volume of water becomes greater on side B, and the concentrations on side A and B become equal.

Fluid and Electrolyte Imbalance Normally, the body defends itself successfully against fluid and electrolyte imbalances. Certain situations and some medications, however, may overwhelm the body's ability to compensate. Severe, prolonged vomiting and diarrhea as well as heavy sweating, burns, and traumatic wounds may incur such great fluid and electrolyte losses as to precipitate a medical emergency.

Different Solutes Lost by Different Routes Different solutes are lost depending on why fluid is lost. If fluid is lost by vomiting or diarrhea, sodium is lost indiscriminately. If the adrenal glands oversecrete aldosterone, as may occur when they develop a tumour, the kidneys may excrete too much potassium. Also, the person with uncontrolled diabetes may lose glucose, a solute not normally excreted, and large amounts of fluid with it. Each situation results in dehydration, but drinking water alone cannot restore electrolyte balance. Medical intervention is required.

Replacing Lost Fluids and Electrolytes In many cases, people can replace the fluids and minerals lost in sweat or in a temporary bout of diarrhea by drinking plain cool water and eating regular foods. Some cases, however, demand rapid replacement of fluids and electrolytes—for example, when diarrhea threatens the life of a malnourished child. Caregivers around the world have learned to use simple formulas ♦ to treat mild-to-moderate cases of diarrhea. These lifesaving formulas do not require hospitalization and can be prepared from ingredients

♦ Health-care workers use **oral rehydration therapy (ORT)**—a simple solution of sugar, salt, and water, taken by mouth—to treat dehydration caused by diarrhea. A simple ORT recipe (cool before giving):

- ½ L boiling water
- A small handful of sugar (20 mL/4 tsp)
- 3 pinches of salt (2 mL/½ tsp)

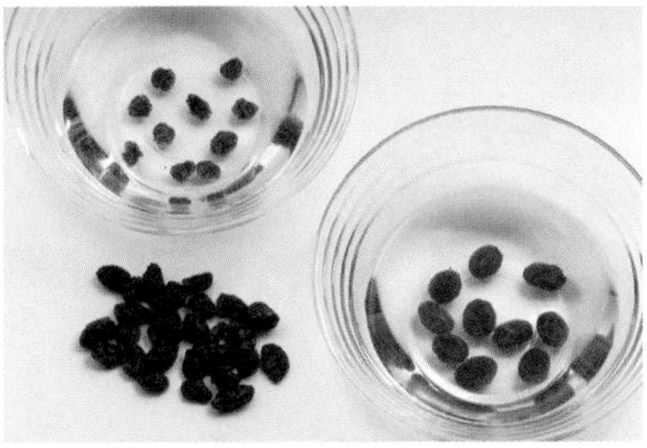

© Craig M. Moore

When immersed in water, raisins become plump because water moves toward the higher concentration of sugar inside the raisins.

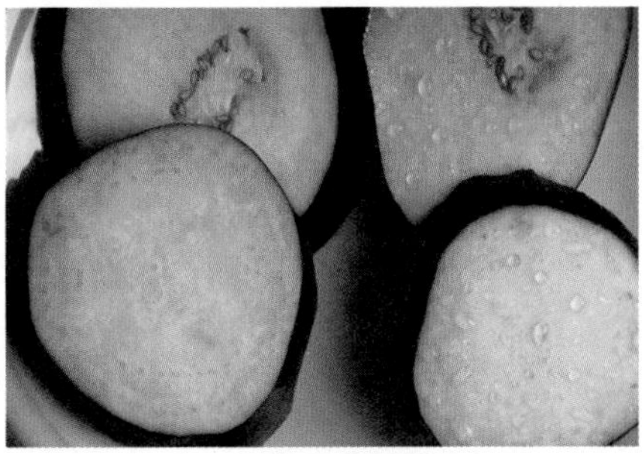

© Craig M. Moore

When sprinkled with salt, vegetables "sweat" because water moves toward the higher concentration of salt outside the eggplant.

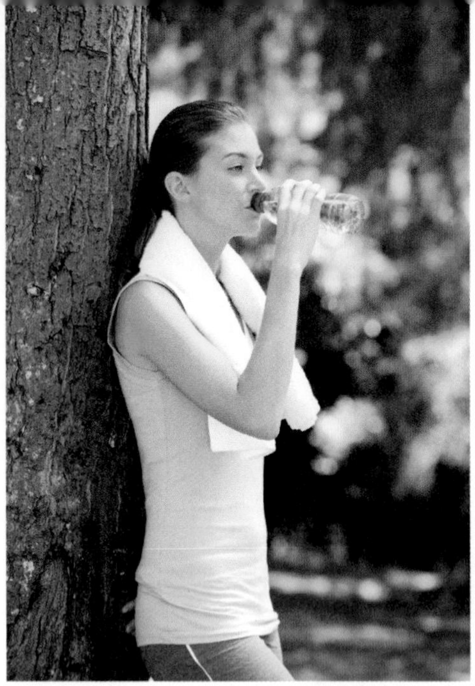

dean bertoncelj/shutterstock

Physically active people must remember to replace their body fluids.

♦ **pH** is the unit of measure expressing a substance's acidity or alkalinity.

♦ The lower the pH, the higher the H^+ ion concentration and the stronger the acid. A pH above 7 is alkaline, or base—a solution in which OH^- ions predominate.

♦ **Bicarbonate** is an alkaline compound with the formula HCO_3. It is produced in all cell fluids from the dissociation of carbonic acid to help maintain the body's acid–base balance. (Bicarbonate is also secreted from the pancreas during digestion as part of the pancreatic juice.)

carbonic acid: a compound with the formula H_2CO_3 that results from the combination of carbon dioxide (CO_2) and water (H_2O); of particular importance in maintaining the body's acid–base balance.

available locally. Caregivers need only learn to measure ingredients carefully and use sanitary water. Once rehydrated, a person can begin eating foods. (Chapter 15 presents a discussion of sport drinks.)

Acid–Base Balance

The body uses its ions not only to help maintain fluid and electrolyte balance, but also to regulate the acidity (pH) ♦ of its fluids. The pH scale introduced in Chapter 3 is repeated here, in Figure 11-8, with the normal and abnormal pH ranges of the blood added. As you can see, the body must maintain the pH within a narrow range to avoid life-threatening consequences. Slight deviations in either direction can denature proteins, rendering them useless. Enzymes couldn't catalyze reactions and hemoglobin couldn't carry oxygen—to name just two examples.

The acidity of the body's fluids is determined by the concentration of hydrogen ions (H^+). ♦ A high concentration of hydrogen ions is very acidic. Normal energy metabolism generates hydrogen ions, as well as many other acids, that must be neutralized. Three systems defend the body against fluctuations in pH—buffers in the blood, respiration in the lungs, and excretion in the kidneys.

Regulation by the Buffers Bicarbonate ♦ (a base) and **carbonic acid** (an acid) in the body fluids, as well as some proteins, protect the body against changes in acidity by acting as buffers—substances that can neutralize acids or bases. Carbon dioxide, which is formed all the time during energy metabolism, dissolves in water to form carbonic acid in the blood. Carbonic acid, in turn, dissociates to form hydrogen ions and bicarbonate ions. The appropriate balance between carbonic acid and bicarbonate is essential to maintaining optimal blood pH. Figure 11-9

FIGURE 11-8 The pH Scale

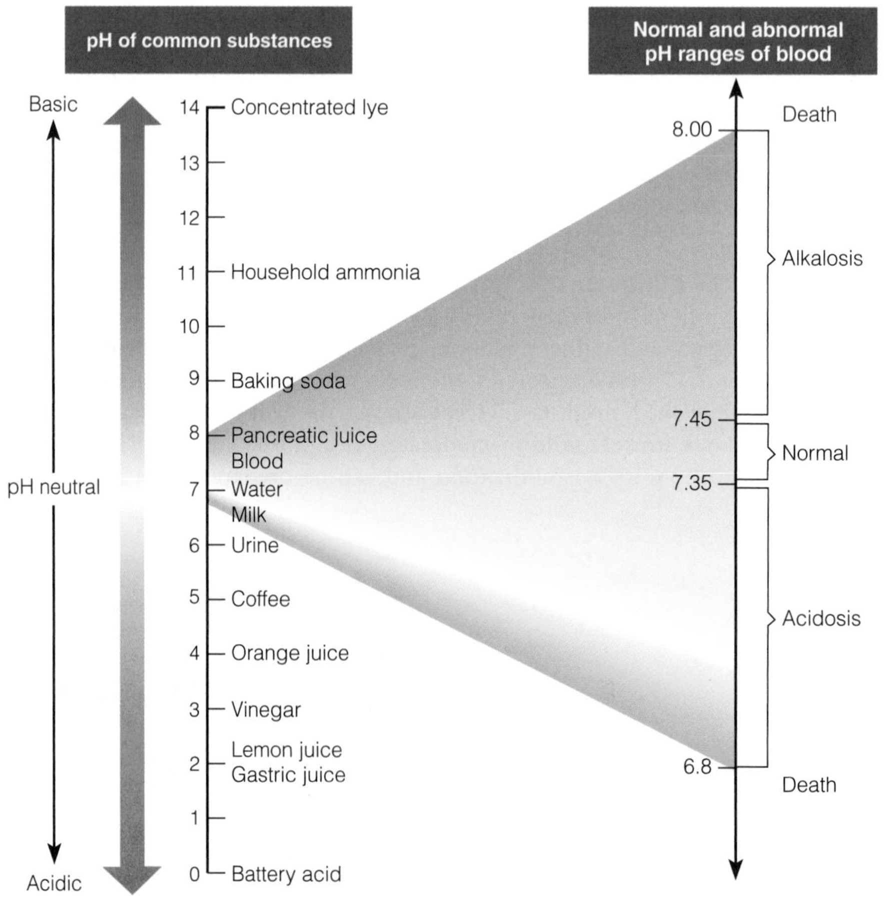

pH of common substances
Normal and abnormal pH ranges of blood
Basic
pH neutral
Acidic
14 Concentrated lye
13
12
11 Household ammonia
10
9 Baking soda
8 Pancreatic juice
Blood
7 Water
Milk
6 Urine
5 Coffee
4 Orange juice
3 Vinegar
2 Lemon juice
Gastric juice
1
0 Battery acid
Death
8.00
Alkalosis
7.45
Normal
7.35
Acidosis
6.8
Death

NOTE: Each step is ten times as concentrated in base (1/10 as much acid, or H^+) as the one below it.

presents the chemical reactions of this buffer system, which is primarily under the control of the lungs and kidneys.

Regulation in the Lungs The lungs control the concentration of carbonic acid by raising or slowing the respiration rate, depending on whether the pH needs to be increased or decreased. If too much carbonic acid builds up, the respiration rate speeds up; this hyperventilation increases the amount of carbon dioxide exhaled, thereby lowering the carbonic acid concentration and restoring homeostasis. Conversely, if bicarbonate builds up, the respiration rate slows; carbon dioxide is retained and forms more carbonic acid. Again, homeostasis is restored.

Regulation in the Kidneys The kidneys control the concentration of bicarbonate by either reabsorbing or excreting it, depending on whether the pH needs to be increased or decreased, respectively. Their work is complex, but the net effect is easy to sum up. The *body's* total acid burden remains nearly constant; the acidity of the *urine* fluctuates to accommodate that balance.

FIGURE 11-9 Bicarbonate–Carbonic Acid Buffer System

The reversible reactions of the bicarbonate–carbonic acid buffer system help to regulate the body's pH. Recall from Chapter 7 that carbon dioxide and water are formed during energy metabolism.

Carbon dioxide (CO_2) is a volatile gas that quickly dissolves in water (H_2O), forming carbonic acid (H_2CO_3):

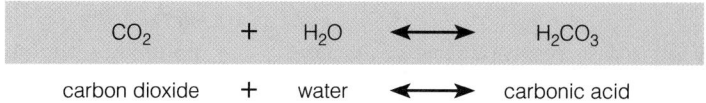

$$CO_2 + H_2O \longleftrightarrow H_2CO_3$$

carbon dioxide + water ⟷ carbonic acid

Carbonic acid readily dissociates to a hydrogen ion (H^+) and a bicarbonate ion (HCO_3^-):

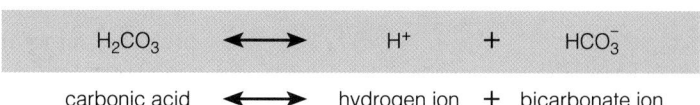

$$H_2CO_3 \longleftrightarrow H^+ + HCO_3^-$$

carbonic acid ⟷ hydrogen ion + bicarbonate ion

IN SUMMARY **Electrolytes (charged minerals) in the fluids help distribute the fluids inside and outside the cells, thus ensuring the appropriate water balance and acid–base balance to support all life processes. Excessive losses of fluids and electrolytes upset these balances, and the kidneys play a key role in restoring homeostasis.**

♦ AI for sodium:
- 1500 mg/day (19–50 yr)
- 1300 mg/day (51–70 yr)
- 1200 mg/day (>70 yr)

Sodium

sodium: the principal cation in the extracellular fluids of the body; critical to the maintenance of fluid balance, nerve impulse transmissions, and muscle contractions.

People have held salt (sodium chloride) in high regard throughout recorded history. We describe someone we admire as "the salt of the earth" and people we consider worthless as "not worth their salt." Even the word *salary* comes from the Latin word for salt.

Cultures vary in their use of salt, but most people find its taste innately appealing. Salt brings its own tangy taste and enhances other flavours, most likely by suppressing the bitter flavours. You can taste this effect for yourself: tonic water with its bitter quinine tastes sweeter with a little salt added.

Sodium Roles in the Body

Important to maintaining the body's fluid balance, **sodium** is the principal cation of the extracellular fluid and the primary regulator of its volume. Sodium also helps maintain acid–base balance and is essential to nerve impulse transmission and muscle contraction.*

Sodium is readily absorbed by the intestinal tract and travels freely in the blood until it reaches the kidneys, which filter all the sodium out of the blood. Then, with great precision, the kidneys return to the bloodstream the exact amount of sodium the body needs. Normally, the amount excreted is approximately equal to the amount ingested on a given day. When blood sodium rises, as when a person eats salted foods, thirst signals the person to drink until the appropriate sodium-to-water concentration is restored. Then the kidneys excrete both the excess water and the excess sodium together.

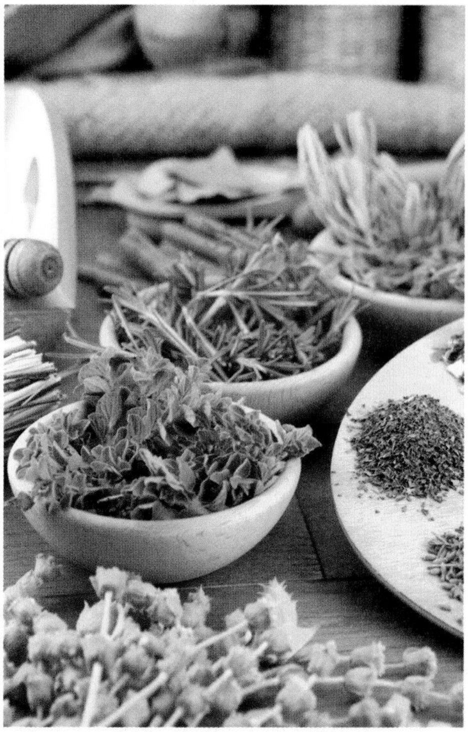

Gts/shutterstock

Fresh herbs add flavour to a recipe without adding salt.

Sodium Recommendations

Diets rarely lack sodium, and even when intakes are low, the body adapts by reducing sodium losses in urine and sweat, thus making deficiencies unlikely. Sodium recommendations ♦ are set low enough

*One of the ways the kidneys regulate acid–base balance is by excreting hydrogen ions (H^+) in exchange for sodium ions (Na^+).

to protect against high blood pressure, but high enough to allow an adequate intake of other nutrients with a typical diet. Because high sodium intakes correlate with high blood pressure, the Upper Level (UL) for adults is set at 2300 milligrams per day, slightly lower than the Daily Value used on food labels (2400 milligrams). The average sodium intake for adults in Canada is about 3400 mg per day, which exceeds the UL.[10]

Sodium and Hypertension

For years, a high *sodium* intake was considered the primary factor responsible for high blood pressure. Then research pointed to *salt* (sodium chloride) ♦ as the dietary culprit. Salt has a greater effect on blood pressure than either sodium or chloride alone or in combination with other ions.

♦ Salt (sodium chloride) is about 40% sodium.
1 g salt contributes about 400 mg sodium
6 g salt = 5 mL (1 tsp)
5 mL (1 tsp) salt contributes about 2300 mg sodium

For some individuals—most notably, those with hypertension and people older than 40 years of age—blood pressure increases in response to excesses in salt intake.[11] **Salt sensitivity** is apparent in about 25 percent of those with normal blood pressure and in about 50 percent of those with high blood pressure.[12] For them, a high salt intake correlates strongly with heart disease, and salt restriction (to no more than 1500 milligrams of sodium per day) helps to lower blood pressure.

In fact, a salt-restricted diet lowers blood pressure in people without hypertension as well. Because reducing salt intake causes no harm and diminishes the risk of hypertension and heart disease, in 2007, Health Canada convened the Sodium Working Group to develop a nationwide strategy to reduce the sodium intake of Canadians. Stakeholders in the group represented Health Canada, the health professional and scientific communities, health-focused and consumer nongovernmental organizations, food manufacturing and food service industries, and other federal government officials. In 2010, the working group released the *Sodium Reduction Strategy for Canada* that recommends an interim sodium intake goal of 2300 mg per day (about 5 mL or 1 tsp of salt) be achieved by 2016, and lower intakes to follow in subsequent years.[13] Specific recommendations were also developed for food manufacturers and food service establishments, consumer awareness and education, sodium-related research, monitoring the implementation of the strategy and evaluating short, intermediate, and long-term outcomes. Higher intakes seem to be well tolerated in most healthy people, however. The "How To" on p. 367 offers strategies for cutting salt (and therefore sodium) intake.

Dietary Guidance for Canadians

Consume less than 2300 milligrams (approximately 5 mL or 1 tsp of salt) of sodium per day.

One diet plan, known as the DASH (Dietary Approaches to Stop Hypertension) diet, may also lower blood pressure. The DASH approach emphasizes fruits, vegetables, and low-fat milk products; includes whole grains, nuts, poultry, and fish; and calls for reduced intakes of red meat, butter, and other high-fat foods. The DASH diet in combination with a reduced sodium intake is even more effective in lowering blood pressure than either strategy alone. Chapter 19 offers a complete discussion of hypertension and the dietary recommendations for its prevention and treatment.

Sodium and Bone Loss (Osteoporosis)

A high salt intake is also associated with increased calcium excretion, but its influence on bone loss is less clear. In addition, potassium may prevent the calcium excretion caused by a high-salt diet. For these reasons, dietary advice to prevent bone loss parallels that suggested for hypertension—a DASH diet that is low in sodium and abundant in potassium-rich vegetables and fruits and calcium-rich skim or 1% milk.

Sodium in Foods

In general, processed foods have the most sodium, whereas unprocessed foods such as fresh fruits, vegetables, milk, and meats have the least. In fact, as much as 75 percent of the sodium in people's diets comes from salt added to foods by manufacturers; about 15 percent comes from salt added

salt sensitivity: a characteristic of individuals who respond to a high salt intake with an increase in blood pressure or to a low salt intake with a decrease in blood pressure.

HOW TO Cut Salt (and Sodium) Intake

Most people eat more salt (and therefore sodium) than they need. Some people can lower their blood pressure by avoiding highly salted foods and removing the salt shaker from the table. Foods eaten without salt may seem less tasty at first, but with repetition, people can learn to enjoy the natural flavours of many unsalted foods. Strategies to cut salt intake include:

- Select fresh, unprocessed foods.
- Cook with little or no added salt.
- Prepare foods with sodium-free spices such as basil, bay leaves, curry, garlic, ginger, mint, oregano, pepper, rosemary, and thyme; lemon juice; vinegar; or wine.
- Add little or no salt at the table; taste foods before adding salt.
- Read labels with an eye open for sodium. (See the glossary on p. 53 for terms used to describe the sodium content of foods on labels.)
- Select low-salt or salt-free products when available.

Use these foods sparingly:

- Foods prepared in brine, such as pickles, olives, and sauerkraut
- Salty or smoked meats, such as bologna, corned or chipped beef, bacon, hot dogs, ham, lunchmeats, salt pork, sausage, and smoked tongue
- Salty or smoked fish, such as anchovies, caviar, salted and dried cod, herring, sardines, and smoked salmon
- Snack items such as potato chips, pretzels, salted popcorn, salted nuts, and crackers
- Condiments such as bouillon cubes; seasoned salts; MSG; soy, teriyaki, Worcestershire, and barbeque sauces; prepared horseradish, ketchup, and mustard
- Cheeses, especially processed types
- Canned and instant soups

CENGAGENOW™
For additional practice log on to **www.cengage.com/sso**.

TRY IT Compare the sodium contents of 30 grams of the following foods: a plain bagel, potato chips, and animal crackers.

during cooking and at the table; and only 10 percent comes from the natural content in foods. To help consumers limit their intake, public health organizations and policymakers in the *Sodium Reduction Strategy for Canada* have called on food manufacturers and food suppliers in food service establishments to reduce sodium in the nation's food supply.

Because processed foods may contain sodium without chloride, as in additives such as sodium bicarbonate or sodium saccharin, they do not always taste salty. Most people are surprised to learn that 30 grams of some cereals contains more sodium than 30 grams of salted peanuts—and that 125 millilitres (½ cup) of instant chocolate pudding contains still more. The peanuts taste saltier because the salt is all on the surface, where the tongue's taste receptors immediately pick it up.

Figure 11-10 (p. 368) shows that processed foods not only contain more sodium than their less-processed counterparts but also have less potassium. Low potassium may be as significant as high sodium when it comes to blood pressure regulation, so processed foods have two strikes against them.[14]

Dietary Guidance for Canadians
Choose and prepare foods with little salt. At the same time, consume potassium-rich foods, such as fruits and vegetables.

Sodium Deficiency

If blood sodium drops, as may occur with vomiting, diarrhea, or heavy sweating, both sodium and water must be replenished. Under normal conditions of sweating due to physical activity, salt losses can easily be replaced later in the day with ordinary foods. Salt tablets are not recommended because too much salt, especially if taken with too little water, can induce dehydration. During intense activities, such as ultra-endurance events, athletes can lose so much sodium and drink so much water that they develop hyponatremia—the dangerous condition ♦ of having too little sodium in the blood. Chapter 15 offers details about hyponatremia and guidelines for ultra-endurance athletes.

♦ Symptoms of hyponatremia:
- Headache, confusion, stupor
- Seizures, coma

FIGURE 11-10 What Processing Does to the Sodium and Potassium Contents of Foods

People who eat foods high in salt often happen to be eating fewer potassium-containing foods at the same time. Notice how potassium is lost and sodium is gained as foods become more processed, causing the potassium-to-sodium ratio to fall dramatically. Even when potassium isn't lost, the addition of sodium still lowers the potassium-to-sodium ratio. Limiting sodium intake may help in two ways, then—by lowering blood pressure in salt-sensitive individuals and by indirectly raising potassium intakes in all individuals.

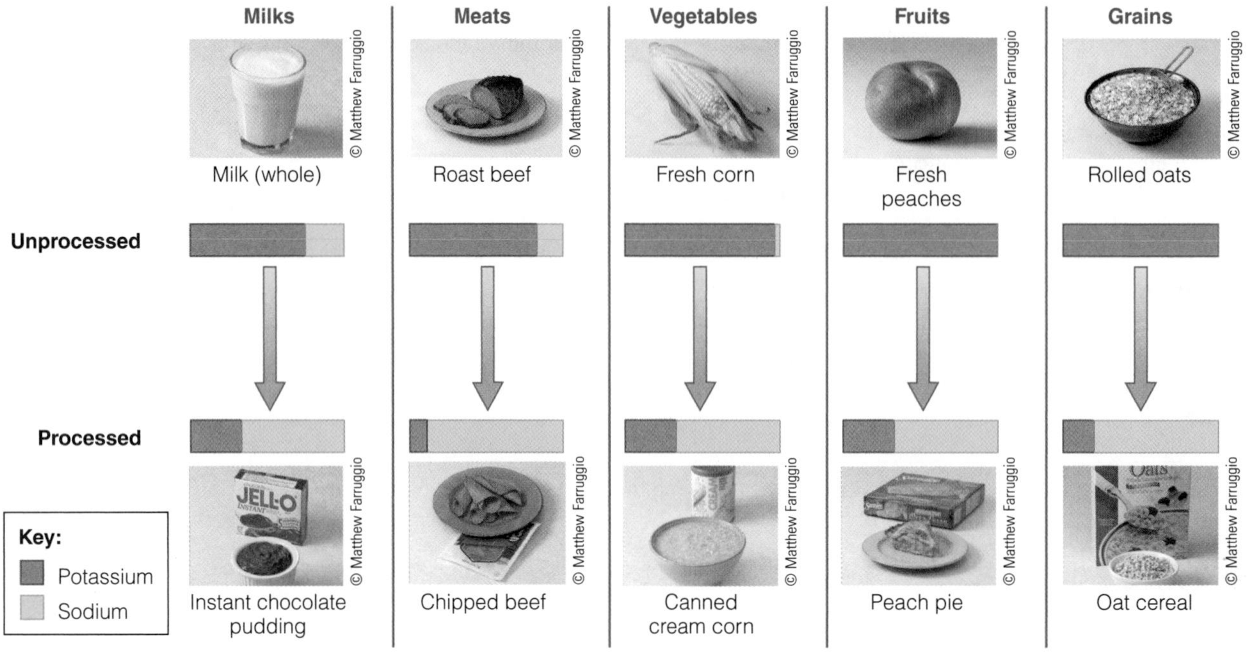
Milks
Meats
Vegetables
Fruits
Grains
Milk (whole)
Roast beef
Fresh corn
Fresh peaches
Rolled oats
Unprocessed
Processed
Key:
Potassium
Sodium
Instant chocolate pudding
Chipped beef
Canned cream corn
Peach pie
Oat cereal
© Matthew Farruggio

Sodium Toxicity and Excessive Intakes

The immediate symptoms of acute sodium toxicity are edema and high blood pressure. Prolonged excessive sodium intake ♦ may contribute to hypertension in some people, as explained earlier.

♦ UL for sodium: 2300 mg/day

IN SUMMARY **Sodium is the main cation outside cells and one of the primary electrolytes responsible for maintaining fluid balance. Dietary deficiency is rare, and excesses may aggravate hypertension in some people. For this reason, health professionals advise a diet moderate in salt and sodium. The accompanying table provides a summary of sodium.**

Sodium

Adequate Intake (AI)
Adults: 1500 mg/day (19–50 yr) 1300 mg/day (51–70 yr) 1200 mg/day (>70 yr)

Upper Level
Adults: 2300 mg/day

Chief Functions in the Body
Maintains normal fluid and electrolyte balance; assists in nerve impulse transmission and muscle contraction

Deficiency Symptoms
Muscle cramps, mental apathy, loss of appetite

Toxicity Symptoms
Edema, acute hypertension

Significant Sources
Table salt, soy sauce; moderate amounts in meats, milks, breads, and vegetables; large amounts in processed foods

Chloride

The element *chlorine* (Cl_2) is a poisonous gas. When chlorine reacts with sodium or hydrogen, however, it forms the negative chloride ion (Cl^-). *Chloride,* an essential nutrient, is required in the diet.

Chloride Roles in the Body

Like sodium, potassium, and phosphorus, chloride helps to maintain fluid and electrolyte balance. **Chloride** is the major anion of the extracellular fluids (outside the cells), where it occurs mostly in association with sodium. Chloride moves passively across membranes through channels and so also associates with potassium inside cells.

In the stomach, the chloride ion is part of hydrochloric acid, which maintains the strong acidity of the gastric juice. One of the most serious consequences of vomiting is the loss of this acid ♦ from the stomach, which upsets the acid–base balance.* Such imbalances are commonly seen in bulimia nervosa, as described in Highlight 8.

♦ The loss of acid can lead to **alkalosis,** an above-normal alkalinity in the blood and body fluids.

Chloride Recommendations and Intakes

Chloride is abundant in foods (especially processed foods) as part of sodium chloride and other salts. Chloride recommendations are slightly higher than, but still equivalent to, those of sodium. In other words, 4 millilitres (¾ tsp) of salt ♦ will deliver some sodium, more chloride, and still meet the AI for both.

♦ Salt (sodium chloride) is about 60% chloride.
1 g salt contributes about 600 mg chloride
6 g salt = 5 mL (1 tsp)
5 mL (1 tsp) salt contributes about 3700 mg chloride

Chloride Deficiency and Toxicity

Diets rarely lack chloride. Chloride losses may occur in conditions such as heavy sweating, chronic diarrhea, and vomiting. The only known cause of high blood chloride concentrations is dehydration due to water deficiency. In both cases, consuming ordinary foods and beverages can restore chloride balance.

IN SUMMARY **Chloride is the major anion outside cells, and it associates closely with sodium. In addition to its role in fluid balance, chloride is part of the stomach's hydrochloric acid. The accompanying table provides a summary of chloride.**

Chloride

AI	**Deficiency Symptoms**
Adults: 2300 mg/day (19–50 yr) 2000 mg/day (51–70 yr) 1800 mg/day (>70 yr)	Do not occur under normal circumstances
Upper Level	**Toxicity Symptoms**
Adults: 3600 mg/day	Vomiting
Chief Functions in the Body	**Significant Sources**
Maintains normal fluid and electrolyte balance; part of hydrochloric acid found in the stomach, necessary for proper digestion	Table salt, soy sauce; moderate amounts in meats, milks, eggs; large amounts in processed foods

Potassium

Like sodium, **potassium** is a positively charged ion. In contrast to sodium, potassium is the body's principal intracellular cation, *inside* the body cells.

chloride (KLO-ride): the major anion in the extracellular fluids of the body. Chloride is the ionic form of chlorine, Cl^-. See APPENDIX B for a description of the chlorine-to-chloride conversion.

potassium: the principal cation within the body's cells; critical to the maintenance of fluid balance, nerve impulse transmissions, and muscle contractions.

*Hydrochloric acid secretion into the stomach involves the addition of bicarbonate ions (base) to the plasma. These bicarbonate ions (HCO_3^-) are neutralized by hydrogen ions (H^+) from the gastric secretions that are reabsorbed into the plasma. When hydrochloric acid is lost during vomiting, these hydrogen ions are no longer available for reabsorption, and so, in effect, the concentrations of bicarbonate ions in the plasma are increased. In this way, excessive vomiting of acidic gastric juices leads to *metabolic alkalosis.*

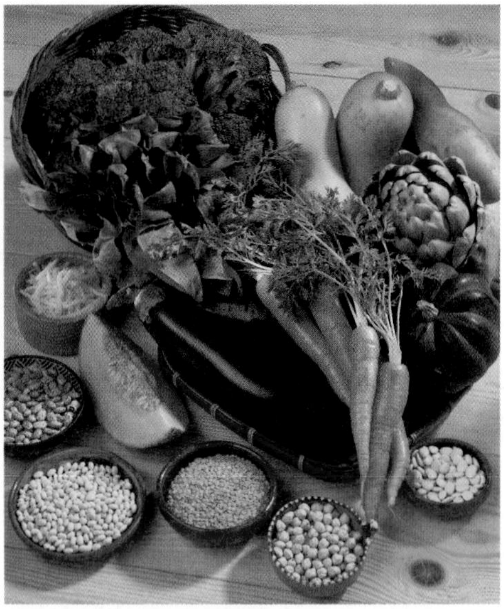

Fresh foods, especially fruits and vegetables, provide potassium in abundance.

♦ The DASH diet, used to lower blood pressure, emphasizes potassium-rich foods such as fruits and vegetables.

Potassium Roles in the Body Potassium plays a major role in maintaining fluid and electrolyte balance and cell integrity. During nerve impulse transmission and muscle contraction, potassium and sodium briefly trade places across the cell membrane. The cell then quickly pumps them back into place. Controlling potassium distribution is a high priority for the body because it affects many aspects of homeostasis, including a steady heartbeat.

Potassium Recommendations and Intakes Potassium is abundant in all living cells. Because cells remain intact unless foods are processed, the richest sources of potassium are *fresh* foods—as Figure 11-11 shows. In contrast, most processed foods such as canned vegetables, ready-to-eat cereals, and luncheon meats contain less potassium—and more sodium (recall Figure 11-10 on p. 368). To meet the AI for potassium, most people need to increase their intake of vegetables and fruits to five to nine servings daily.

Potassium and Hypertension Diets low in potassium seem to play an important role in the development of high blood pressure. Low potassium intakes, especially when combined with high sodium intakes, raise blood pressure and increase the risk of death from heart disease.[15] In contrast, high potassium intakes, especially when combined with low sodium intakes, appear to both prevent and correct hypertension. ♦ Potassium-rich fruits and vegetables also appear to reduce the risk of stroke—more so than can be explained by the reduction in blood pressure alone.

FIGURE 11-11 Potassium in Selected Foods

See the "How To" section on p. 317 for more information on using this figure.

Food	Serving size (kcalories)
Broccoli, boiled	125 mL (29 kcal)
Carrots, boiled	125 mL (29 kcal)
Tomato, fresh	1 medium (22 kcal)
Apple, fresh	1 medium (72 kcal)
Banana	1 medium (105 kcal)
Blueberries, fresh	125 mL (44 kcal)
Bread, whole wheat	1 slice, 35 g (86 kcal)
Pasta, whole grain, cooked	125 mL (92 kcal)
Rice, white, cooked	125 mL (89 kcal)
Oatmeal, cooked	175 mL (144 kcal)
Pita, white	½ pita, 35 g (96 kcal)
Cereal, high fibre	30 g (78 kcal)
Milk, 2%	250 mL (129 kcal)
Cheddar cheese	50 g (202 kcal)
Yogurt, 2% plain	175 g (110 kcal)
Soy beverage, fortified	250 mL (110 kcal)
Kefir	175 g (104 kcal)
Ice cream, strawberry	125 mL (134 kcal)
Chicken breast, roasted	75 g (220 kcal)
Ground beef, lean, baked	75 g (191 kcal)
Egg, poached	1 large (72 kcal)
Tuna, canned in water	75 g (87 kcal)
Tofu, made with a calcium salt	150 g (114 kcal)
Peanut butter	30 mL (184 kcal)
Excellent, and sometimes unusual, sources:	
Dried apricots	75 mL (99 kcal)
Lima beans, boiled	175 mL (160 kcal)
Potato: small, baked	138 g (128 kcal)

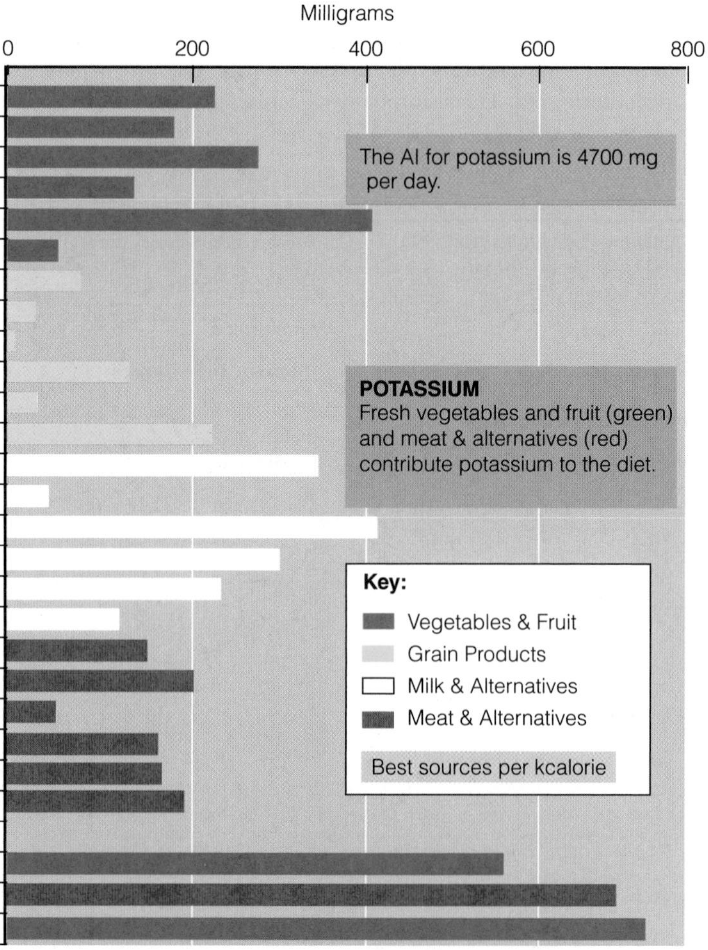
Milligrams
0
200
400
600
800
The AI for potassium is 4700 mg per day.
POTASSIUM
Fresh vegetables and fruit (green) and meat & alternatives (red) contribute potassium to the diet.
Key:
Vegetables & Fruit
Grain Products
Milk & Alternatives
Meat & Alternatives
Best sources per kcalorie

SOURCE: Canadian Nutrient File. Health Canada, 2008. Reproduced with the permission of the Minister of Health, 2011.

Potassium Deficiency Potassium deficiency is characterized by an increase in blood pressure, salt sensitivity, kidney stones, and bone turnover. As deficiency progresses, symptoms include irregular heartbeats, muscle weakness, and glucose intolerance.

Potassium Toxicity Potassium toxicity does not result from overeating foods high in potassium; therefore a UL has not been set. It can result from overconsumption of potassium salts or supplements (including some "energy fitness shakes") and from certain diseases or treatments. Given more potassium than the body needs, the kidneys accelerate their excretion. If the GI tract is bypassed, however, and potassium is injected directly into a vein, it can stop the heart.

IN SUMMARY **Potassium, like sodium and chloride, is an electrolyte that plays an important role in maintaining fluid balance. Potassium is the primary cation inside cells; fresh foods, notably fruits and vegetables, are its best sources. The accompanying table provides a summary of potassium.**

Potassium

AI	Toxicity Symptoms
Adults: 4700 mg/day	Muscular weakness; vomiting; if given into a vein, can stop the heart
Chief Functions in the Body	**Significant Sources**
Maintains normal fluid and electrolyte balance; facilitates many reactions; supports cell integrity; assists in nerve impulse transmission and muscle contractions	All whole foods: meats, milks, vegetables, fruits, grains, legumes
Deficiency Symptoms[a]	
Irregular heartbeat, muscular weakness, glucose intolerance	

[a]Deficiency accompanies dehydration.

Phosphorus

Phosphorus is the second most abundant mineral in the body. Although about 85 percent of it is found combined with calcium in the hydroxyapatite crystals of bones and teeth (see Chapter 13) it has other important roles in the body.

Phosphorus Roles in the Body Phosphorus, predominately as a phosphorus salt (phosphate, PO_4^{3-}), is the major negatively charged electrolyte found inside cells. It works with potassium, the major positively charged electrolyte inside cells, to maintain electrical neutrality. In fact, phosphorus is found in all body cells and acts as part of a major buffer system (phosphoric acid and its salts). Phosphorus is also part of DNA and RNA and is therefore necessary for all growth. The phospholipid bilayer that forms cell membranes and the phospholipids found in lipoproteins (see Chapter 5) also contain phosphorus. As a component in adenosine triphosphate (ATP), phosphorus has a critical role in transferring cellular energy from metabolic fuels. And lastly, phosphorus is often used to activate enzymes that catalyze reactions in the body.

Phosphorus Recommendations and Intakes For all adults, the RDA for phosphorus is 700 milligrams per day and the UL is set at 4000 milligrams per day. Figure 11-12 (p. 372) shows foods rich in proteins are the best sources of phosphorus. Milk and cheese contribute about one-fourth of the phosphorus in the North American diet.

Phosphorus Deficiency and Toxicity Because phosphorus is commonly found in almost all foods, dietary deficiencies are unlikely and adverse effects of high dietary phosphorus intakes have not been reported.

phosphorus: a major mineral found mostly in the body's bones and teeth.

FIGURE 11-12 Phosphorus in Selected Foods

See the "How To" section on p. 317 for more information on using this figure.

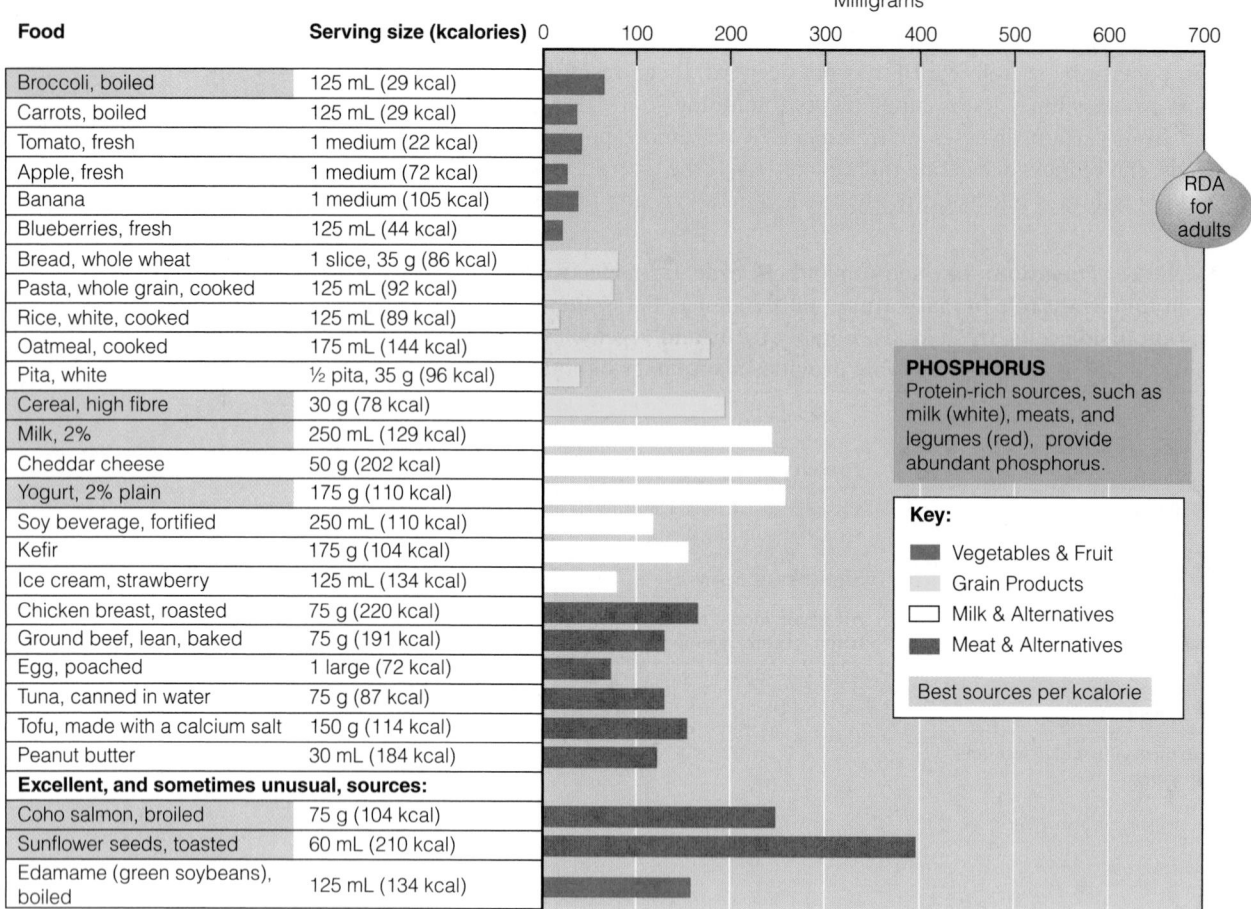

Food	Serving size (kcalories)
Broccoli, boiled	125 mL (29 kcal)
Carrots, boiled	125 mL (29 kcal)
Tomato, fresh	1 medium (22 kcal)
Apple, fresh	1 medium (72 kcal)
Banana	1 medium (105 kcal)
Blueberries, fresh	125 mL (44 kcal)
Bread, whole wheat	1 slice, 35 g (86 kcal)
Pasta, whole grain, cooked	125 mL (92 kcal)
Rice, white, cooked	125 mL (89 kcal)
Oatmeal, cooked	175 mL (144 kcal)
Pita, white	½ pita, 35 g (96 kcal)
Cereal, high fibre	30 g (78 kcal)
Milk, 2%	250 mL (129 kcal)
Cheddar cheese	50 g (202 kcal)
Yogurt, 2% plain	175 g (110 kcal)
Soy beverage, fortified	250 mL (110 kcal)
Kefir	175 g (104 kcal)
Ice cream, strawberry	125 mL (134 kcal)
Chicken breast, roasted	75 g (220 kcal)
Ground beef, lean, baked	75 g (191 kcal)
Egg, poached	1 large (72 kcal)
Tuna, canned in water	75 g (87 kcal)
Tofu, made with a calcium salt	150 g (114 kcal)
Peanut butter	30 mL (184 kcal)
Excellent, and sometimes unusual, sources:	
Coho salmon, broiled	75 g (104 kcal)
Sunflower seeds, toasted	60 mL (210 kcal)
Edamame (green soybeans), boiled	125 mL (134 kcal)

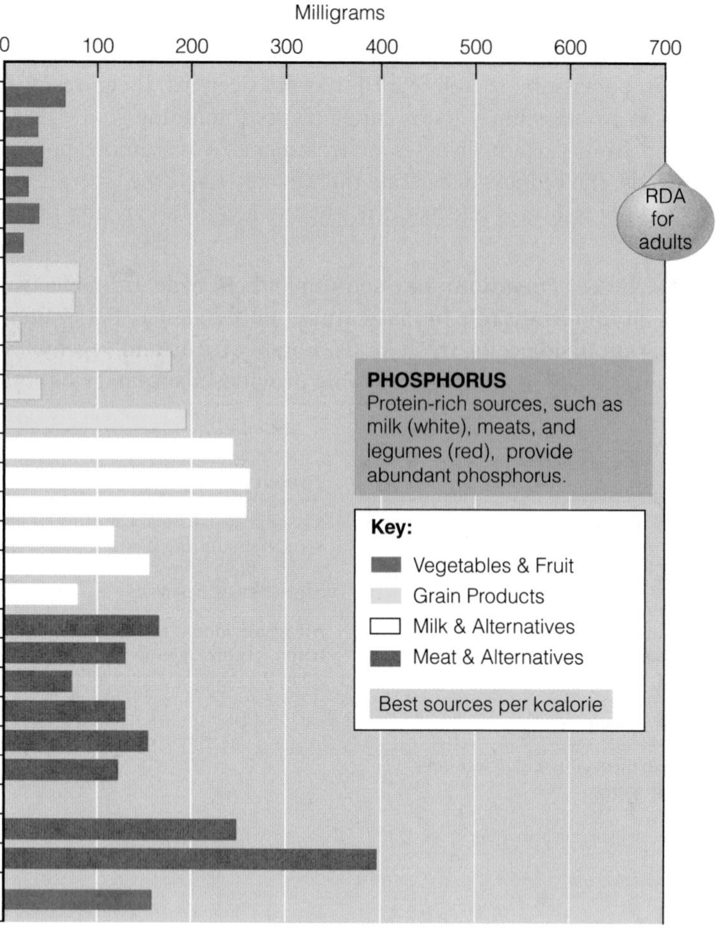
Milligrams
0
100
200
300
400
500
600
700
RDA for adults
PHOSPHORUS
Protein-rich sources, such as milk (white), meats, and legumes (red), provide abundant phosphorus.
Key:
Vegetables & Fruit
Grain Products
Milk & Alternatives
Meat & Alternatives
Best sources per kcalorie

SOURCE: Canadian Nutrient File. Health Canada, 2008. Reproduced with the permission of the Minister of Health, 2011.

IN SUMMARY Phosphorus has many roles beyond its role in fluid balance. It teams up with calcium to provide strength to bones, is important in energy metabolism, is part of phospholipids and lipoproteins, and is a necessary component of the genetic materials DNA and RNA.

Phosphorus

Recommended Dietary Allowance (RDA)

Adults: 700 mg/day

Upper Level

Adults (19–70 yr): 4000 mg/day

Chief Functions in the Body

Mineralization of bones and teeth; part of every cell; important in genetic material, part of phospholipids, used in energy transfer and in buffer systems that maintain acid–base balance

Deficiency Symptoms

Muscular weakness, bone pain[a]

Toxicity Symptoms

Calcification of nonskeletal tissues, particularly the kidneys

Significant Sources

All animal tissues (meat, fish, poultry, eggs, milk)

[a]Dietary deficiency rarely occurs, but some drugs can bind with phosphorus, making it unavailable and resulting in bone loss that is characterized by weakness and pain.

IN SUMMARY Water, quite simply, keeps us alive. It liquefies food during the process of digestion to allow for the absorption of nutrients into the body. Water is essential to transport nutrients to the cells, used in metabolic reactions within cells, and removes waste products from cells for excretion from the body.

Like the other nutrients, minerals' actions are coordinated to get the body's work done. The major minerals, especially sodium, chloride, potassium, and phosphorus, influence the body's fluid balance; whenever an anion moves, a cation moves—always maintaining homeostasis. They are also the primary nutrients involved in regulating blood pressure. Sodium, chloride, and potassium are key members of the team of nutrients that direct nerve impulse transmission and muscle contraction. The accompanying table provides a summary of water and the major minerals that act as electrolytes.

Water and the Electrolytes

Nutrient Chief Functions	Deficiency Symptoms	Toxicity Symptoms	Significant Sources
Water Transports nutrients to and waste products from cells; participates in chemical reactions; acts as a solvent and shock absorber; helps to regulate body temperature	Thirst, concentrated urine, dehydration	Confusion, convulsions, death in certain circumstances	Water, beverages, foods, particularly vegetables and fruits
Sodium Maintains normal fluid and electrolyte balance; assists in nerve impulse transmission and muscle contraction	Muscle cramps, mental apathy, loss of appetite	Edema, acute hypertension	Table salt, soy sauce; moderate amounts in meats, milks, breads, and vegetables; large amounts in processed foods
Chloride Maintains normal fluid and electrolyte balance; part of hydrochloric acid found in the stomach, necessary for proper digestion	Do not occur under normal circumstances	Vomiting	Table salt, soy sauce; moderate amounts in meats, milks, eggs; large amounts in processed foods
Potassium Maintains normal fluid and electrolyte balance; facilitates many reactions; supports cell integrity; assists in nerve impulse transmission and muscle contractions	Irregular heartbeat, muscular weakness, glucose intolerance	Muscular weakness; vomiting; if given into a vein, can stop the heart	All whole foods; meats, milks, fruits, vegetables, grains, legumes
Phosphorus Mineralization of bones and teeth; part of every cell; important in genetic material, part of phospholipids, used in energy transfer and in buffer systems that maintain acid–base balance	Muscular weakness, bone pain[a]	Calcification of nonskeletal tissues, particularly the kidneys	All animal tissues (meat, fish, poultry, eggs, milk)

[a]Dietary deficiency rarely occurs, but some drugs can bind with phosphorus, making it unavailable and resulting in bone loss that is characterized by weakness and pain.

The tasks that these minerals perform are of great importance to many life processes. Consuming enough of each of them every day is easy when choosing a variety of foods from each of the food groups. For an adequate intake of all the nutrients, including the minerals that act primarily as electrolytes, choose different foods from each of the four food groups. And . . . drink plenty of water.

TABLE 11-4 Adult Canadians' Average Daily Nutrient Intakes from Food* Compared to the Dietary Reference Intakes

	Intake Men	Women	RDA[a]/AI[b] Men	Women
Water (g/d)	2974	2624	3700[b]	2700[b]
Sodium (mg/d)	3587	2658	1500[b,c]	1500[b,c]
Potassium (mg/d)	3460	2798	4700[b]	4700[b]
Phosphorus (mg/d)	1515	1181	700[a]	700[a]

*Canadian Community Healthy Survey, Cycle 2.2, Nutrition (2004) Nutrient intakes from food.
[a]Represents RDA values; RDA refers to Recommended Dietary Allowance.
[b]Represents AI values; AI refers to Adequate Intake.
[c]19–50 Years; 51–70 years: 1300 mg/d; 70+ years: 1200 mg/d.

After learning about the importance of water for many body functions and the roles of electrolytes in maintaining fluid balance, you may be interested to see how Canadians' intakes of these nutrients compare with current recommendations. Table 11-4 (p. 373) shows the average daily intake of the nutrients discussed in this chapter for adults 19 years and older. These intakes suggest that most Canadians could adjust their water, sodium, and potassium intakes to bring them closer to the recommended intakes.

Nutrition Portfolio

Many people may miss the mark when it comes to drinking enough water to keep their bodies well hydrated; in contrast, sodium intakes often exceed those recommended for health.

Go to Diet Analysis Plus and choose one of the days on which you tracked your diet. Select the Intake vs. Goals report and then consider the following questions. Remember that scoring 100 percent on this report means you met your daily nutrient goal.

Were you above, below, or at your goal for water intake? Was that a typical day for you? Describe your strategy for ensuring that you drink plenty of water—about eight glasses—every day.

- Take a look at your sodium intake in this report. Most people in Canada exceed the UL. Did you? Explain the importance of selecting and preparing foods with less salt. Make a plan to lower your sodium intake. Which foods would you consume more and which foods would you consume less to help bring your sodium intake closer to the recommendation?
- How was your intake of potassium for that day? If you are not getting enough potassium, then list at least three foods you would be willing to eat that would improve your intake.

Diet Analysis PLUS **To complete this exercise, go to your Diet Analysis Plus at www.cengage.com/sso.**

Nutrition on the Net

CENGAGENOW™
For further study of topics covered in this chapter, log on to **www.cengage.com/sso.**

- Search for "electrolytes" at Dietitians of Canada: **www.dietitians.ca**
- Learn how vegetables and fruit support a healthy diet low in sodium and chloride and rich in potassium from the Mix it up! program: **www.5to10aday.com**
- Search for the "DASH diet" at the Heart and Stroke Foundation: **www.heartandstroke.com**
- Learn about the Sodium Reduction Strategy for Canada from Health Canada: **www.hc-sc.gc.ca/fn-an/nutrition/sodium/strateg/index-eng.php**
- Find out more about the safety of drinking water by searching for "Drinking Water and Your Health" at Health Canada: **www.hc-sc.gc.ca**
- Read more about regional differences in water hardness across Canada: **www.cwqa.com**

References

1. A. K. Johnson, The sensory psychobiology of thirst and salt appetite, *Medicine & Science in Sports & Exercise* 39 (2007): 1388–1400.
2. F. Manz and A. Wentz, Hydration status in the United States and Germany, *Nutrition Reviews* 63 (2005): S55–S62.
3. M. N. Sawka, S. N. Cheuvront, and R. Carter III, Human water needs, *Nutrition Reviews* 63 (2005): S30–S39.1.
4. D. Garriguet, Beverage consumption of Canadian adults, Statistics Canada, *Health Reports* 19 (2008): 23–29; D. Garriguet, Beverage consumption of children and teens, Statistics Canada, *Health Reports* 19 (2008): 1–6.
5. Committee on Dietary Reference Intakes, *Dietary Reference Intakes for Water, Potassium, Sodium, Chloride, and Sulfate* (Washington, D.C.: National Academies Press, 2004), p. 67.
6. F. Manz and A. Wentz, The importance of good hydration for the prevention of chronic diseases, *Nutrition Reviews* 63 (2005): S2–S5.
7. P. Ritz and G. Berrut, The importance of good hydration for day-to-day health, *Nutrition Reviews* 63 (2005): S6–S13.
8. Actions You Can Take to Reduce Lead in Drinking Water, www.epa.gov/ogwdw/lead/lead1.html, updated April 2008.

9. K. M. O'Shaughnessy and F. E. Karet, Salt handling and hypertension, *Annual Review of Nutrition* 26 (2006): 343–365.
10. Health Canada, Statistics Canada, Canadian Community Health Survey, Cycle 2.2, Nutrition (2004)—Nutrient intakes from food, Provincial, Regional and National Summary Data Tables, Volume 1 (2007).
11. Centers for Disease Control and Prevention, Application of lower sodium intake recommendations to adults: United States, 1999–2006, *Morbidity and Mortality Weekly Report* 58 (2009): 281–283.
12. B. Rodriguez-Iturbe and N. D. Vaziri, Salt-sensitive hyptertension—Update on novel findings, *Nephrology, Dialysis, Transplantation: Official Publication of the European Dialysis and Transplant Association* 22 (2007): 992–995.
13. Health Canada, *Sodium Reduction Strategy for Canada* (Ottawa, ON.: Nutrition Evaluation Division, Health Canada, 2010).
14. H. J. Adrogué and N. E. Madias, Sodium and potassium in the pathogenesis of hypertension, *New England Journal of Medicine* 356 (2007): 1966–1978.
15. M. Umesawa and coauthors, Relations between dietary sodium and potassium intakes and mortality from cardiovascular disease: The Japan Collaborative Cohort Study for Evaluation of Cancer Risks, *American Journal of Clinical Nutrition* 88 (2008): 195–202; Adrogué and Madias, 2007.

Fluid Balance

To appreciate the importance of water, consider just a few of our many needs for water throughout the body: water is essential to enable the smooth movement of joints, a normal blood volume, transporting nutrients to cells, removing waste products from the body, participating in reactions, allowing cells to live or die, and stabilizing body temperature. When we consume just the right amount, too little, or too much water, our bodies rely on electrolytes to help equilibrate a balance of water in the various fluid compartments. Highlighted earlier in Chapter 11 were the important interrelationships between water and electrolytes. Maintaining fluid homeostasis would not be possible without adequate electrolytes and adequate water intake to replenish losses. To sustain life, an appropriate water distribution in the body's fluid compartments is required.

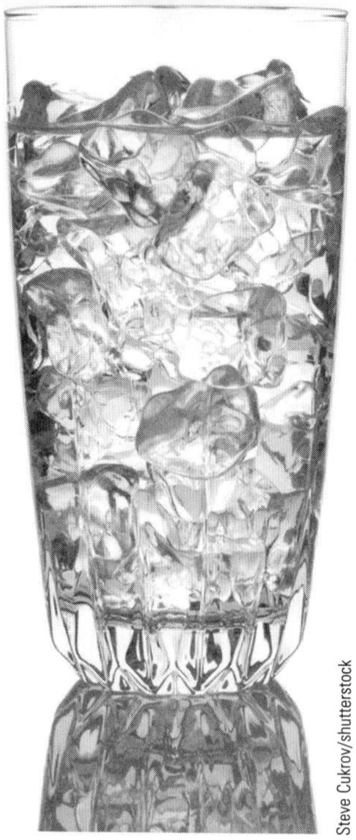

Steve Cukrov/shutterstock

Regulation of Fluid Balance

The regulation of fluid balance is composed of two factors: the control of electrolyte balance and the control of water balance. Sodium is the primary electrolyte regulator of extracellular fluid volume, of which interstitial fluid and blood are parts. The kidneys are the primary organ regulator of the salt load in the blood, constantly adjusting sodium output in the urine to account for input from the diet and losses through the skin. An important impact of regulating salt balance is the long-term regulation of extracellular fluid volume, which in turn helps to maintain normal blood pressure. For example, during times of low blood volume, water can move freely from the intracellular and interstitial compartments into the bloodstream. Conversely, at times of high blood volume, water can move out of the bloodstream into and around cells. The process of osmosis directs water flow to the fluid compartment with the greatest concentration of electrolytes causing cells to expand or collapse. Some of the symptoms observed in later stages of dehydration and heat illness are due to brain neurons not functioning normally because of a fluid imbalance.[1]

In conjunction with the kidneys' role in establishing a salt balance between sodium input and output, they are the primary organ regulator of water balance. The amount of water excreted in the urine compensates for variable water intake and water losses through breathing, sweating, and fecal waste removal. When overall water intake, physical exertion, and environmental conditions are moderate, the body is exceptionally capable of maintaining fluid homeostasis. It is when moderate conditions develop into abnormal situations that life can become threatened and actions are necessary to re-establish fluid balance in the body.

Although people's water intake is more often too little than too much, fluid balance covers a wide range of fluid distribution in the body. Too little as well as too much water in the body can have detrimental effects on body metabolism and survival. This highlight starts by focusing on some of the common causes of dehydration followed by the effects of sequentially decreasing amounts of water in the body. It concludes with a look at the relatively rare condition of water intoxication.

Dehydration

There are many causes of dehydration, all of which lead to a higher amount of water lost from the body relative to the amount of water entering the body. Let's begin with some of the common causes of dehydration, including diarrhea, vomiting, fever, unmanaged diabetes, and abuse of diuretics and laxatives.

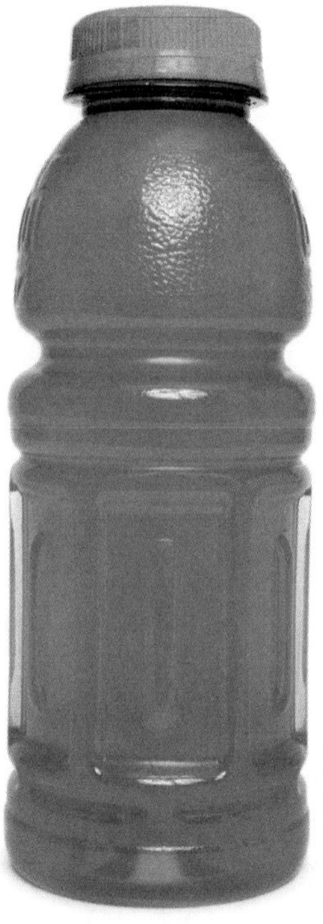

Filaphoto/shutterstock

Sports beverages become an increasingly important source of energy, electrolytes, and water for people who participate in higher intensity activities that extend beyond 60 minutes.

Diarrhea is characterized by the expulsion of frequent, watery, and loose stools. Quick movement of dietary content through the intestines limits the normal absorption of water from foods and beverages. Viruses, bacteria, parasites, food components including undigested lactose and sugar alcohols, medications, and disorders of the gastrointestinal tract such as irritable bowel syndrome, colitis, and celiac disease can hasten the movement of intestinal content. Treatment of diarrhea will depend on the cause, but all treatments will aim to restore the large amounts of electrolytes and water that leave the body. Prompt treatment is especially important for children and the elderly because the effects of dehydration are more pronounced and immediate during these life stages.

Often associated with nausea, vomiting is the expulsion of stomach content up through the esophagus and the mouth. A common symptom of many conditions, treatment for vomiting depends on the cause. Most mild cases can be managed by taking rest and drinking small amounts of fluid as tolerated. Intense or frequent episodes of vomiting can result in large losses of fluids and sodium, placing a person at risk for dehydration. Ascertaining the underlying cause will determine the appropriate treatment protocol.

High fevers accompanied by heavy sweating can jeopardize a person's hydration state due to fluid and electrolytes lost through the skin. Losses need to be replaced to restore water and salt balance in the body.

Increased thirst and urination resulting from uncontrolled diabetes can lead to dehydration. When blood glucose levels are high, the brain detects an increased blood concentration. This stimulates the thirst mechanism, causing people to drink more water. However, with high levels of blood glucose, some is lost in the urine. When glucose leaves the blood and enters the urine, water follows the glucose, resulting in more frequent urination and a higher potential for dehydration.

Diuretics and laxatives are common over-the-counter purchases and when taken as instructed are effective in relieving symptoms of water retention and constipation, respectively. Because diuretics and laxatives can cause large losses of fluids, excessive use of these products should be avoided. If problems persist, consult with your health-care provider to determine the cause of your symptoms and an appropriate treatment plan.

Now that you are aware of some of the causes of dehydration, let's now turn our attention to the damaging effects of increasing levels of dehydration in the body.

Thirst

When your blood becomes more concentrated than normal due to restricted water intake or increased water loss, your brain detects the change and initiates your thirst mechanism. Responding to thirst is important to re-establish normal fluid balance; however, thirst signals are often ignored due to a variety of reasons, such as being preoccupied with current activities and not having ready access to beverages. Even though a loss of 1 to 2 percent of total body weight as water stimulates a neural response, thirst is not a reliable signal of dehydration because it lags behind the body's need for water. It is therefore important to be proactive and regularly drink water throughout the day to minimize bouts of thirst. Table H11-1 shows typical symptoms of dehydration with varying amounts of body water loss.

TABLE H11-1 Signs of Dehydration

Body Weight Lost (%)	Symptoms
1–2	Thirst, fatigue, weakness, vague discomfort, loss of appetite
3–4	Impaired physical performance, dry mouth, reduction in urine, flushed skin, impatience, apathy
5–6	Difficulty concentrating, headache, irritability, sleepiness, impaired temperature regulation, increased respiratory rate
7–10	Dizziness, spastic muscles, loss of balance, delirium, exhaustion, collapse

NOTE: The onset and severity of symptoms at various percentages of body weight lost depend on the activity, fitness level, degree of acclimation, temperature, and humidity. If not corrected, dehydration can lead to death.

Ignoring Your Thirst

When you ignore your thirst, the body starts to conserve water. The earlier section on blood volume and blood pressure (pages 359–360) explained how enzymes, hormones, and proteins that act mostly at the level of the kidneys are used to re-establish fluid balance and normal blood volume. Despite actions taken to reduce water loss through the kidneys, we continue to lose water in our breathing, sweating, and feces. These insensible losses must be accounted for by increasing water intake through foods and beverages. Likewise, water losses experienced through vomiting and diarrhea must be replenished. As Table H11-1 shows, water conservation mechanisms are initiated when there is a 3 to 4 percent loss of body weight as water. Strong evidence indicates sweating beyond 2 percent of body weight in temperate and warm-hot environments can affect thermoregulation and blood circulation and impair performance in endurance activities.[2]

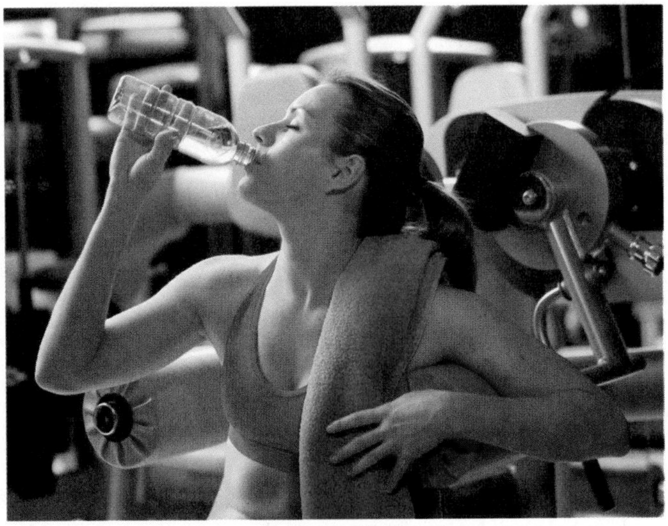

wavebreakmedia ltd/shutterstock

When being active, water is always a good companion.

Thirst and water conservation are early stages of dehydration. When left unmanaged, dehydration can become a serious medical condition. A lower-than-normal total body water content can increase core temperature and lead to physiological heat stress.[3] This is particularly true during bouts of extended physical activity or outdoor work in hot environments. Ignoring signals experienced under these conditions during the early stages of dehydration can lead to increasingly severe forms of heat-related illnesses: heat cramps, heat exhaustion, and heat stroke.[4]

Heat Illnesses

Heat Cramps

Heat-related illnesses occur along a continuum from heat cramps to heat stroke as a result of the body being unable to properly cool. Risk for heat illness is directly related to environmental conditions, hydration, and electrolyte status.[5] People who sweat a lot because they work outside or engage in intense activities in hot weather can experience painful heat cramps during or after activity. Symptoms may first appear as subtle twitches or spasms usually in muscles of the arms, legs, or abdomen, but can quickly become widespread debilitating and painful muscle spasms. Heat cramps are caused by excessive loss of water and sodium from the muscles usually occurring due to strenuous activity in hot environments.

When experiencing muscle cramps it is important to stop all activity, seek a cool place, and sit quietly. Call for immediate medical attention if you have heart problems or are on a low-sodium diet; otherwise drink juice, a sports beverage, or simply water, preferably with a pinch of salt. If the cramps remain after an hour, seek medical assistance. Avoid returning to the activity for a few hours after the cramps subside as this exertion could lead to heat exhaustion or heat stroke.[6]

Heat Exhaustion

Exertional activities—for example, during heavy labour or sports competitions in hot environments—increase the risk for heat exhaustion.[7] When possible, restrict strenuous activities to cooler times in the day. At times of excessive loss of water and sodium the body sweats profusely in an attempt to cool down. The skin is often cool and wet. Other signs of heat exhaustion include headache, nausea, vertigo, weakness, rapid breathing, and thirst.[8] With heat exhaustion, there is increased body heat production and less body water to stabilize body temperature. In extreme situations, a person experiencing heat exhaustion may lose consciousness and suffer heat collapse. In these cases, blood can pool in the extremities reducing the movement of heat from the core of the body to the skin for the release of heat from the surface to cool the body.[9]

People experiencing symptoms of heat exhaustion should be moved to a cool place and given a cool, hydrating drink such as a chilled sports beverage.[10] Remove gear such as a helmet or equipment and loosen clothing to allow the body to cool. Fan the body to evaporate the sweat from the skin. A cool shower, bath, or water sprayed over the body or a cold pack placed in areas that respond to quick cooling—for example, around the neck, under the arms, or in the groin area—can also help reduce the body's temperature. A person experiencing heat exhaustion should be treated and not left alone since heat exhaustion can lead to the life-threatening condition of heat stroke.

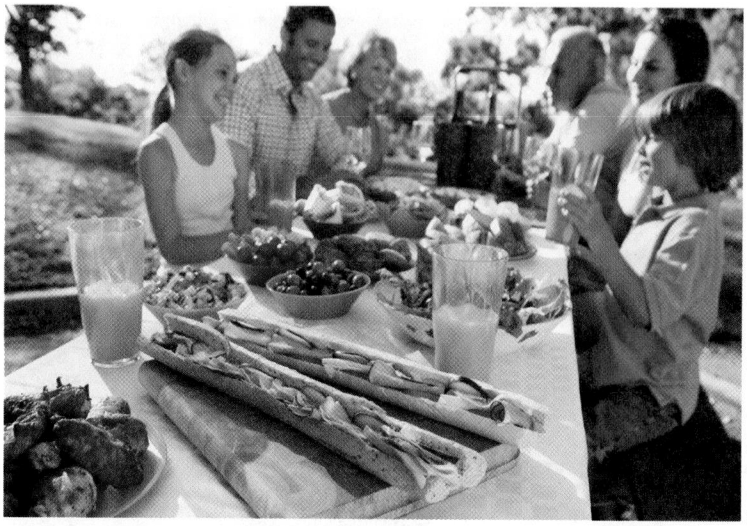
Monkey Business Images/shutterstock

Drinking hydrating beverages proactively throughout the day will reduce your risk of experiencing dehydration.

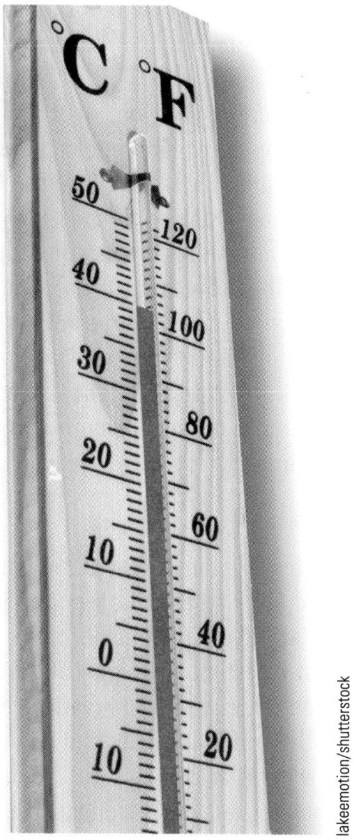
°C °F
50
40
30
20
10
0
10
120
100
80
60
40
20
lakeemotion/shutterstock

When the temperature rises, take precautions not to overexert yourself.

Heat Stroke

Heat stroke is a serious medical condition that occurs when the body cannot regulate its temperature. It requires immediate emergency assistance. Body water reserves are so low that sweating stops, the core temperature rises rapidly sometimes up to over 40°C in a matter of minutes, and the body cannot cool down. The heart works harder to pump blood from the body core to the extremities. People can feel weak and nauseous; hyperventilate; experience a rapid pulse and headaches; have red, hot, and dry skin; and be confused, disoriented, or act strangely. In later stages, a person may lose consciousness or have convulsions.[11] Overexertion during strenuous outdoor work or physical activity in hot humid conditions along with low body water and electrolyte imbalance causes heat stroke, which can lead to death if not treated immediately.

To treat a person with heat stroke, call 9-1-1 immediately and follow their instructions. You will likely be asked to move the person to a shady or cool place and use cold packs, towels, or a water hose to spray the body while awaiting medical attention. If muscle spasms occur as a result of heat stroke, prevent the person from self-inflicted injury; if vomiting occurs, keep their air passage open by laying the person on his or her side.

Just as too little body water can threaten life, so can too much. Let's now turn our attention to the relatively uncommon condition of water intoxication.

Water Intoxication

When water intake exceeds the kidneys ability to excrete the excess, sodium becomes diluted in the blood. The condition of hyponatremia can produce serious side-effects, such as headaches, cramps, convulsions, blurred vision, and death in extreme cases.[12] Drinking too much water without adequate sodium replacement during or after prolonged activities such as marathons and triathlons can increase the risk for hyponatremia in endurance athletes.[13] Current guidance suggests athletes "drink according to thirst" and not over consume water during these types of events.[14] For most healthy Canadians, drinking too much water is not a nutritional issue, which lies in contrast to many who do not drink enough water. The side-effects of rapid ingestion of large quantities of water have been observed when the kidneys' maximal water excretion rate of approximately 1 litre per hour is surpassed.[15]

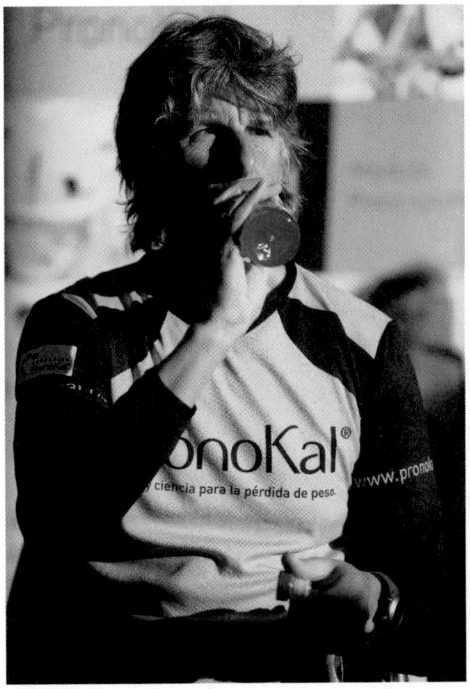

onoKal®
ciencia para la pérdida de peso
www.prono

JOSEP LAGO/AFP/Getty Images

During endurance activities, sports beverages may be a better choice than water alone.

References

1. L. E. Armstrong, and coauthors, American College of Sports Medicine position stand, Exertional heat illness during training and competition, *Medicine and Science in Sports and Exercise* 39 (2007): 556–572.
2. T. L. Merry and coauthors, Effects of aerobic fitness on hypohydration-induced physiological strain and exercise impairment, *Acta Physiologica* 198 (2010): 179–190; M. N. Sawka, Does dehydration impair exercise performance? *Medicine and Science in Sports and Exercise* 39 (2007): 1209–1217.
3. M. N. Sawka, Physiological consequences of hypohydration: Exercise performance and thermoregulation, *Medicine and Science in Sports and Exercise* 24 (1992): 657–670.
4. L. E. Armstrong, and coauthors, American College of Sports Medicine position stand, 2007.
5. M. F. Bergeron, Heat cramps: Fluid and electrolyte challenges during tennis in the heat, *Journal of Science and Medicine in Sport* 6 (2003): 19–27.
6. Centres for Disease Control and Prevention, Extreme heat: A prevention guide to promote your personal health and safety (2009). www.bt.cdc.gov/disasters/extremeheat/heat_guide.asp, accessed September 10, 2011.
7. L. E. Armstrong, and coauthors, American College of Sports Medicine position stand, 2007.
8. P. Bray and coauthors, Heat-related illnesses: Opportunities for prevention, *Journal of Occupational and Environmental Medicine* 52 (2010): 844–845.
9. L. E. Armstrong, and coauthors, American College of Sports Medicine position stand, 2007.
10. Centres for Disease Control and Prevention, Extreme heat: A prevention guide to promote your personal health and safety, (2009). www.bt.cdc.gov/disasters/extremeheat/heat_guide.asp, accessed September 10, 2011.
11. Ontario Ministry of Labour, Occupational Health and Safety Branch, Heat stress health and safety guideline, (2011). www.labour.gov.on.ca/english/hs/pdf/gl_heat.pdf, accessed September 10, 2011.
12. D. J. Farrell and L. Bower, Fatal water intoxication, *Journal of Clinical Pathology* 56 (2003): 803-804.
13. M. H. Rosner and J. Kirven, Exercise-associated hyponatremia, *Clinical Journal of the American Society of Nephrology* 2 (2007): 151–161.
14. S. Malik and coauthors, The collapsed athlete, in C. E. Lawless (Ed.) Sports Cardiology Essentials: Evaluation, Management and Case Studies (New York: Springer, 2011).
15. Food and Nutrition Board, Dietary Reference Intakes for Water, Potassium, Sodium, Chloride, and Sulfate (2005): Washington DC, The National Academies Press. http://books.nap.edu/openbook.php?record_id=10925&page=R1, accessed September 10, 2011.

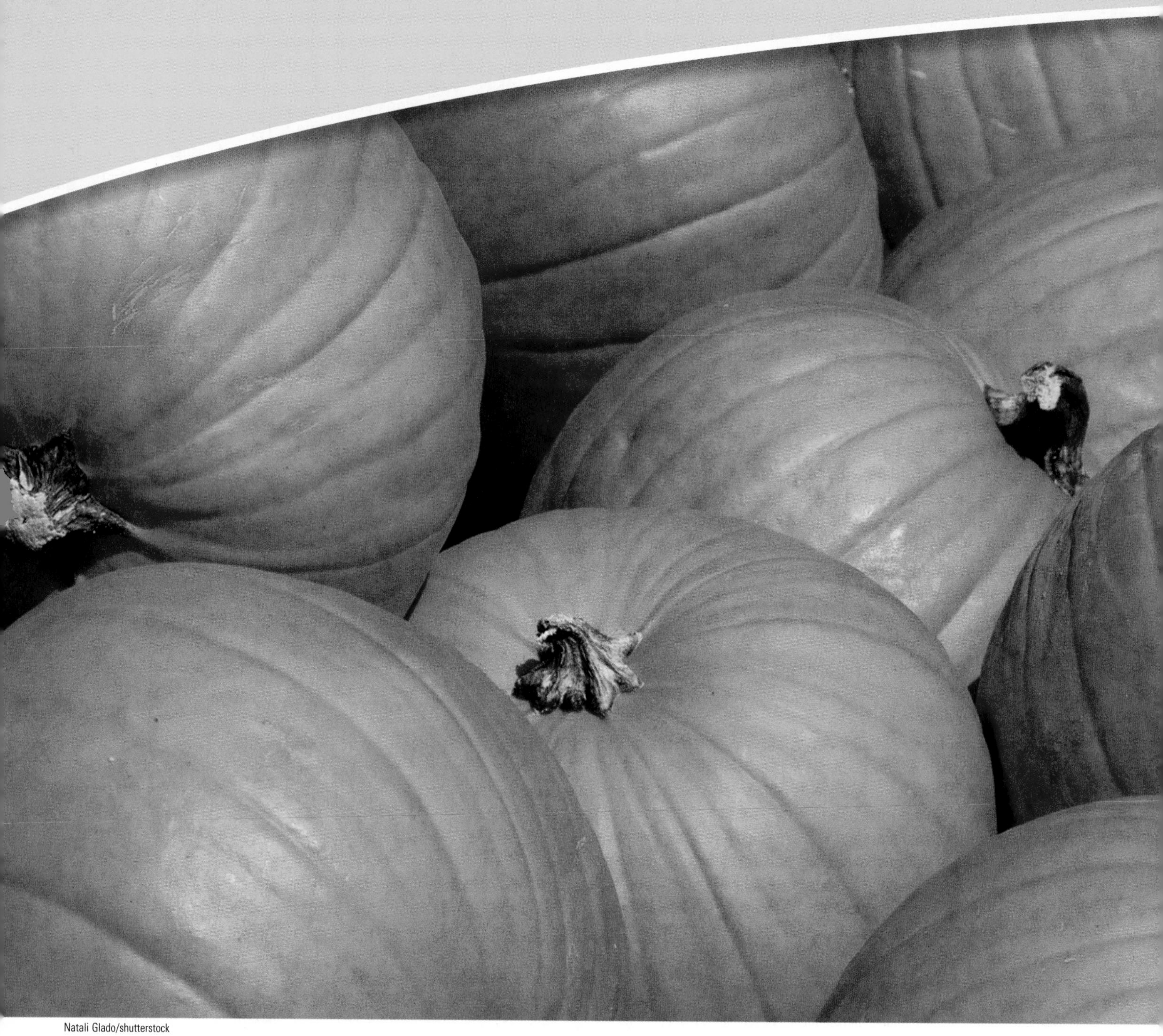

Natali Glado/shutterstock

CENGAGENOW™

Throughout this chapter, the CengageNOW logo indicates an opportunity for online self-study, linking you to interactive tutorials, activities, and videos to increase your understanding of chapter concepts.
www.cengage.com/sso

Nutrition in Your Life

Realizing that vitamin A from vegetables participates in vision, a mom encourages her children to "eat your carrots" because "they're good for your eyes." A dad gives his children oranges because the vitamin C can help reduce damage caused by free radicals. A physician recommends that a patient use vitamin E to slow the progression of heart disease. These common daily occurrences highlight some of the heroic work of the nutrients associated with having antioxidant roles in the body.

CHAPTER

12

The Antioxidant Nutrients

CHAPTER OUTLINE

The Antioxidant Nutrients—An Overview

The nutrients that act as antioxidants to protect our cells from oxidative damage are the fat-soluble vitamins A (including beta-carotene) and E, the water-soluble vitamin C, and the trace mineral selenium. Distinctive in their roles, the vitamin antioxidants donate electrons to quench free radicals that cause damage and can lead to cancer and heart disease, whereas trace mineral antioxidants are cofactors required by enzyme systems that exert protective effects. Also important to protecting against oxidative damage are enzymes that require the trace minerals manganese, iron, zinc, and copper. While only mentioned here, they are later presented in Chapters 13 and 14 where their roles in energy metabolism and blood health are highlighted. In addition to the nutrient antioxidants, foods offer many phytochemicals that protect our cells from oxidative damage. With more than half of Canadian adults consuming fewer than the minimum recommended number of daily servings of vegetables and fruit[1]—a food group that provides a rich supply of antioxidants and phytochemicals—we need to remind ourselves to regularly consume adequate amounts of these foods in our diets. Before we profile each antioxidant nutrient, let's take a brief look at why we need antioxidants to protect against diseases caused by free radicals.

Oxidation occurs as a part of normal metabolism. Chapter 7 describes how oxygen is used in metabolism to produce cellular energy. During metabolic reactions when atoms lose electrons, oxidation occurs, and when atoms gain electrons, reduction occurs. Most often, when molecules are broken down, bonds break and re-form with a redistribution of atoms and a rearrangement of bonds to form new, stable compounds (see APPENDIX B for a review of basic chemistry concepts). Sometimes an atom loses an electron that is not paired up with another electron, leaving a highly unstable atom. An atom with an unpaired electron in its outer orbital is called a **free radical**. Free radicals cause damage by attacking lipids in cell membranes and lipoproteins, our DNA and RNA, and body proteins resulting in widespread damage and increasing our risk for disease. Antioxidants donate one

free radical: unstable and highly reactive atom or molecule that has one or more unpaired electrons in the outer orbital.

of their own electrons to pair up with the unpaired electron in the outer orbital of free radicals, thus neutralizing the damaging effects. A key feature of antioxidants is their stability in both oxidized and reduced forms, so they do not create new free radicals. Highlight 12 describes free radicals in more detail and how antioxidants can stabilize free radicals to help slow the progression of disease. Now let's turn our attention to the antioxidant nutrients, starting with vitamin A and beta-carotene.

Vitamin A and Beta-Carotene

Vitamin A was the first fat-soluble vitamin to be recognized. A century later, vitamin A and its precursor, **beta-carotene**, ♦ continue to intrigue researchers with their diverse roles and profound effects on health.

Three different forms of vitamin A are active in the body: retinol, retinal, and retinoic acid. Collectively, these compounds are known as **retinoids.** Foods derived from animals provide compounds (retinyl esters) that are readily digested and absorbed as retinol in the intestine.[2] Foods derived from plants provide **carotenoids,** ♦ a class of phytochemicals. The most studied of the carotenoids is beta-carotene, which can be split to form retinol in the intestine and liver. Beta-carotene's absorption and conversion are significantly less efficient than those of the retinoids. Figure 12-1 illustrates the structural similarities and differences of these vitamin A compounds and the cleavage of beta-carotene.

Alpha-carotene and beta-cryptoxanthin are two other carotenoids with pro-vitamin A properties—that is, like beta-carotene they can be converted into retinol, the most active form of vitamin A. Common carotenoids with no **vitamin A activity** include lycopene, lutein, and zeaxanthin. Although not considered essential nutrients, they have shown positive health effects. A focus of research for lycopene has been on its role in reducing risk for cancer—in particular, prostate cancer—whereas research into the roles of lutein and zeaxanthin in eye health has indicated these carotenoids may be involved in preventing age-related macular degeneration.[3] Even though over 600 carotenoids exist in nature, about 50 are found in the foods humans eat. Past and emerging research strongly suggests an adequate daily intake of vegetables and fruit offers the potential to yield substantial health benefits.

The cells can convert retinol and retinal to the other active forms of vitamin A as needed. The conversion of retinol to retinal is reversible, but the further conversion of retinal to retinoic acid is irreversible (see Figure 12-2). This irreversibility is significant because each form of vitamin A performs a function that the others cannot.

♦ A compound that can be converted into an active vitamin is called a **precursor.**

♦ Carotenoids are among the best-known phytochemicals.

vitamin A: all naturally occurring compounds with the biological activity of **retinol** (RET-ih-nol), the alcohol form of vitamin A.

beta-carotene (BAY-tah KARE-oh-teen): one of the carotenoids; an orange pigment and vitamin A precursor found in plants.

retinoids (RET-ih-noyds): chemically related compounds with biological activity similar to that of retinol; metabolites of retinol.

carotenoids (kah-ROT-eh-noyds): pigments commonly found in plants and animals, some of which have vitamin A activity. The carotenoid with the greatest vitamin A activity is beta-carotene.

vitamin A activity: a term referring to both the active forms of vitamin A and the precursor forms in foods without distinguishing between them.

FIGURE 12-1 Forms of Vitamin A

In this diagram, corners represent carbon atoms, as in all previous diagrams in this book. A further simplification here is that methyl groups (CH_3) are understood to be at the ends of the lines extending from corners. (See APPENDIX C for complete structures.)

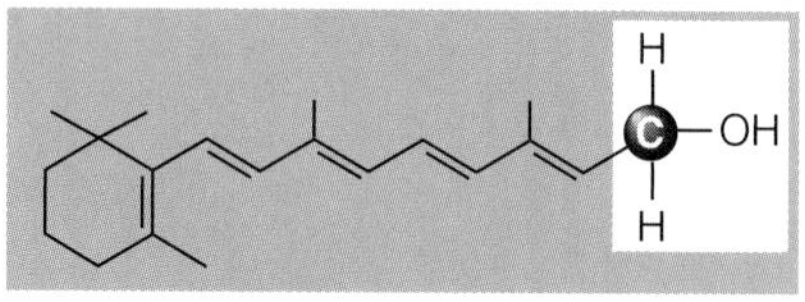
H
C
OH
H

Retinol, the alcohol form

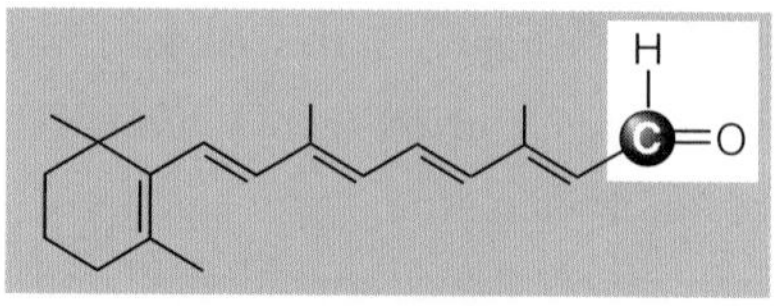
H
C
O

Retinal, the aldehyde form

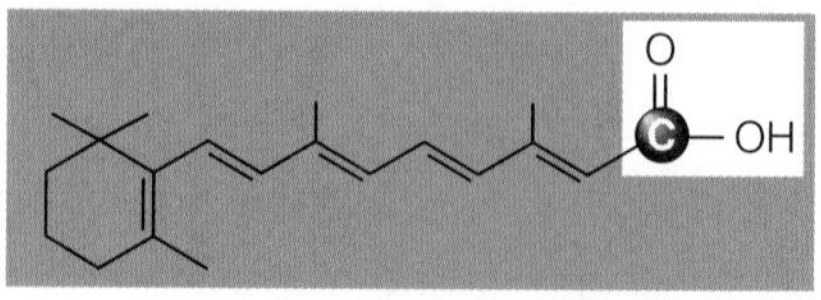
O
C
OH

Retinoic acid, the acid form

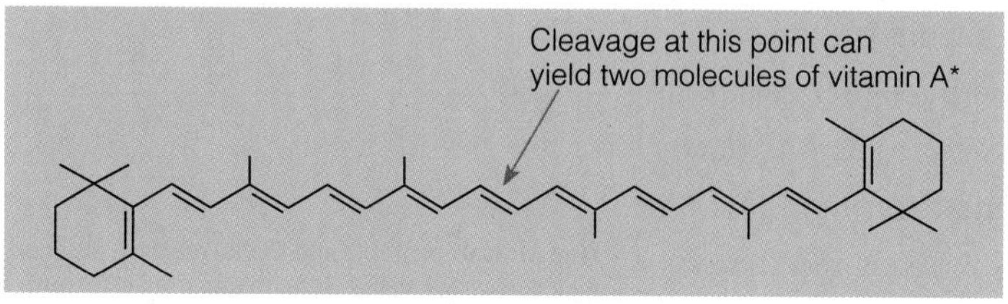
Cleavage at this point can yield two molecules of vitamin A*

Beta-carotene, a precursor

*Sometimes cleavage occurs at other points as well, so that one molecule of beta-carotene may yield only one molecule of vitamin A. Furthermore, not all beta-carotene is converted to vitamin A, and absorption of beta-carotene is not as efficient as that of vitamin A. For these reasons, 12 µg of beta-carotene are equivalent to 1 µg of vitamin A. Conversion of other carotenoids to vitamin A is even less efficient.

Several proteins participate in the digestion and absorption of vitamin A.[4] After absorption via the lymph system, vitamin A eventually arrives at the liver, where it is stored. There, a special transport protein, **retinol-binding protein (RBP)**, picks up vitamin A from the liver and carries it in the blood. Cells that use vitamin A have special protein receptors for it, and its action within each cell may differ depending on the receptor.[5] For example, retinoic acid can stimulate cell growth in the skin and inhibit cell growth in tumours.[6]

FIGURE 12-2 Conversion of Vitamin A Compounds

Notice that the conversion from retinol to retinal is reversible, whereas the pathway from retinal to retinoic acid is not.

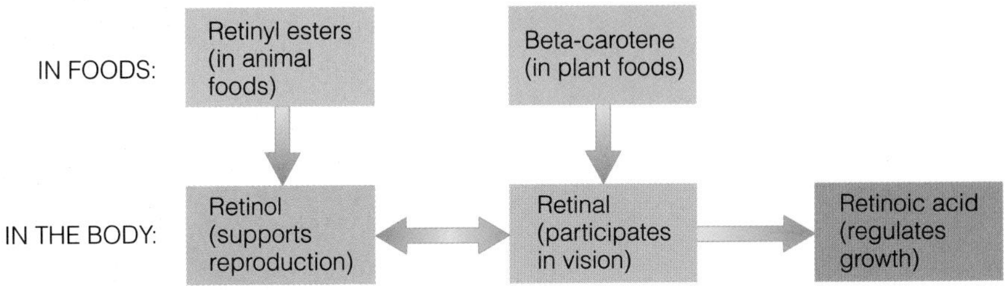
IN FOODS:
Retinyl esters (in animal foods)
Beta-carotene (in plant foods)
IN THE BODY:
Retinol (supports reproduction)
Retinal (participates in vision)
Retinoic acid (regulates growth)

Vitamin A Roles in the Body

Vitamin A is a versatile vitamin, known to regulate the expression of several hundred genes.[7] Its major roles include:

- Promoting vision
- Participating in protein synthesis and cell differentiation, thereby maintaining the health of epithelial tissues and skin
- Supporting reproduction and growth

As mentioned, each form of vitamin A performs specific tasks. Retinol supports reproduction and is the major transport and storage form of the vitamin. Retinal is active in vision and is also an intermediate in the conversion of retinol to retinoic acid (review Figure 12-2). Retinoic acid acts like a hormone, regulating cell differentiation, growth, and embryonic development. Animals raised on retinoic acid as their sole source of vitamin A can grow normally, but they become blind because retinoic acid cannot be converted to retinal.

Vitamin A in Vision Vitamin A plays two indispensable roles in the eye: it helps maintain a crystal-clear outer window, the **cornea**, and it participates in the conversion of light energy into nerve impulses at the **retina** (see Figure 12-3 for details). Some of the photosensitive cells ♦ of the retina contain **pigment** molecules called **rhodopsin**; each rhodopsin molecule is composed of a protein called **opsin** bonded to a molecule of retinal. ♦ When light passes through the cornea of the eye and strikes the retina, rhodopsin responds by changing shape and becoming bleached. As it does, the retinal shifts from a *cis* to a *trans* configuration, just as fatty acids do during hydrogenation (see p. 134–135). The bleached *trans*-retinal cannot remain bonded to opsin. When retinal is released, opsin changes shape, thereby disturbing the membrane of the cell and generating an electrical impulse

♦ Photosensitive cells of the retina:
- Rods contain the rhodopsin pigment and respond to faint light.
- Cones contain the iodopsin pigment and function in colour vision.

♦ More than 100 million cells reside in the retina, and each contains about 30 million molecules of vitamin A–containing visual pigments.

retinol-binding protein (RBP): the specific protein responsible for transporting retinol.

cornea (KOR-nee-uh): the transparent membrane covering the outside of the eye.

retina (RET-in-uh): the innermost membrane of the eye, composed of several layers including one that contains the rods and cones.

pigment: a molecule capable of absorbing certain wavelengths of light so that it reflects only those that we perceive as a certain colour.

rhodopsin (ro-DOP-sin): a light-sensitive pigment of the retina; contains the retinal form of vitamin A and the protein opsin.
- **hod** = red (pigment)
- **opsin** = visual protein

opsin (OP-sin): the protein portion of the visual pigment molecule.

FIGURE 12-3 Vitamin A's Role in Vision

The retina receives the image formed by the lens and converts light energy into chemical energy and nerve signals that reach the brain via the optic nerve.

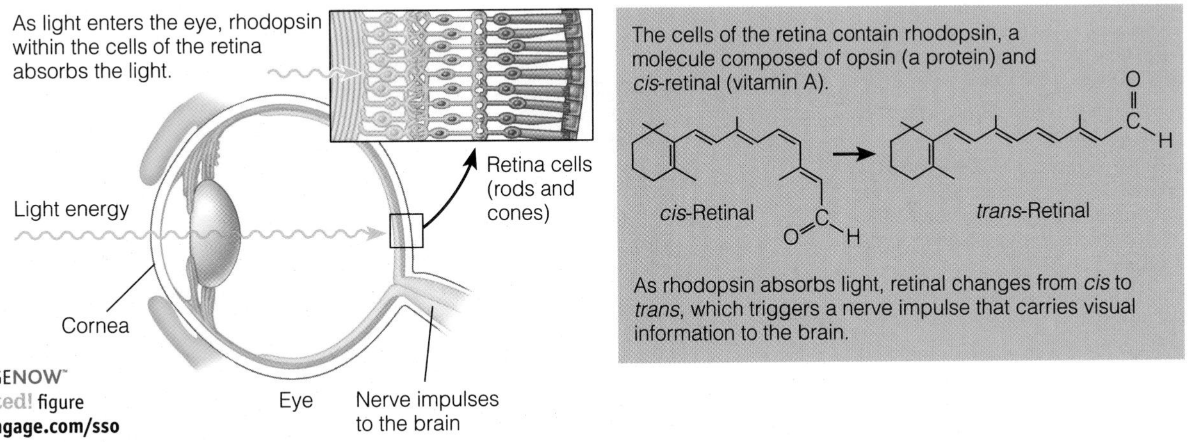
As light enters the eye, rhodopsin within the cells of the retina absorbs the light.
Light energy
Retina cells (rods and cones)
Cornea
Eye
Nerve impulses to the brain
The cells of the retina contain rhodopsin, a molecule composed of opsin (a protein) and cis-retinal (vitamin A).
cis-Retinal
trans-Retinal
As rhodopsin absorbs light, retinal changes from cis to trans, which triggers a nerve impulse that carries visual information to the brain.

CENGAGENOW™ Animated! figure **www.cengage.com/sso**

that travels along the cell's length. At the other end of the cell, the impulse is transmitted to a nerve cell, which conveys the message to the brain. Much of the retinal is then converted back to its active *cis* form and combined with the opsin protein to regenerate the pigment rhodopsin. Some retinal, however, may be oxidized to retinoic acid, a biochemical dead end for the visual process. Visual activity leads to repeated small losses of retinal, necessitating its constant replenishment either directly from foods or indirectly from retinol stores.

Vitamin A in Protein Synthesis and Cell Differentiation Despite its important role in vision, only one-thousandth of the body's vitamin A is in the retina. Much more is in the cells lining the body's surfaces. There, the vitamin participates in protein synthesis and **cell differentiation,** a process by which each type of cell develops to perform a specific function.

All body surfaces, both inside and out, are covered by layers of cells known as **epithelial cells.** The **epithelial tissue** on the outside of the body is, of course, the skin—and vitamin A helps to protect against skin damage from sunlight. The epithelial tissues that line the inside of the body are the **mucous membranes**: the linings of the mouth, stomach, and intestines; the linings of the lungs and the passages leading to them; the linings of the urinary bladder and urethra; the linings of the uterus and vagina; and the linings of the eyelids and sinus passageways. Within the body, the mucous membranes of the GI tract alone line an area larger than a quarter of a football field, and vitamin A helps to maintain their integrity (see Figure 12-4).

Vitamin A promotes differentiation of epithelial cells and goblet cells, one-celled glands that synthesize and secrete mucus. Mucus coats and protects the epithelial cells from invasive microorganisms and other potentially damaging substances, such as gastric juices.

Vitamin A in Reproduction and Growth As mentioned, vitamin A also supports reproduction and growth. In men, retinol participates in sperm development, and in women, vitamin A supports normal fetal development during pregnancy. Children lacking vitamin A fail to grow. When given vitamin A supplements, these children gain weight and grow taller.

The growth of bones illustrates that growth is a complex phenomenon of **remodelling.** To convert a small bone into a large bone, the bone-remodelling cells must "undo" some parts of the bone as they go, ♦ and vitamin A participates in the dismantling. The cells that break down bone contain sacs of degradative enzymes. ♦ With the help of vitamin A, these enzymes eat away at selected sites in the bone, removing the parts that are not needed.

Beta-Carotene as an Antioxidant In the body, beta-carotene serves primarily as a vitamin A precursor.[8] Not all dietary beta-carotene is converted to active vitamin A, however. Some beta-carotene may act as an antioxidant ♦ capable of protecting the body against disease. (See Highlight 12 for details.) In fact, a diet rich in vegetables and fruits containing beta-carotene and other carotenoids helps to defend against some cancers.

♦ The cells that destroy bone during growth are **osteoclasts;** those that build bone are **osteoblasts.**
- **osteo** = bone
- **clast** = break
- **blast** = build

♦ The sacs of degradative enzymes are **lysosomes** (LYE-so-zomes).

♦ Key antioxidant nutrients:
- Vitamin C, vitamin E, beta-carotene
- Selenium

cell differentiation (DIF-er-EN-she-AY-shun): the process by which immature cells develop specific functions different from those of the original that are characteristic of their mature cell type.

epithelial (ep-i-THEE-lee-ul) **cells:** cells on the surface of the skin and mucous membranes.

epithelial tissue: the layer of the body that serves as a selective barrier between the body's interior and the environment. (Examples are the cornea of the eyes, the skin, the respiratory lining of the lungs, and the lining of the digestive tract.)

mucous (MYOO-kus) **membranes:** the membranes, composed of mucus-secreting cells, that line the surfaces of body tissues.

remodelling: the dismantling and re-formation of a structure.

FIGURE 12-4 Mucous Membrane Integrity

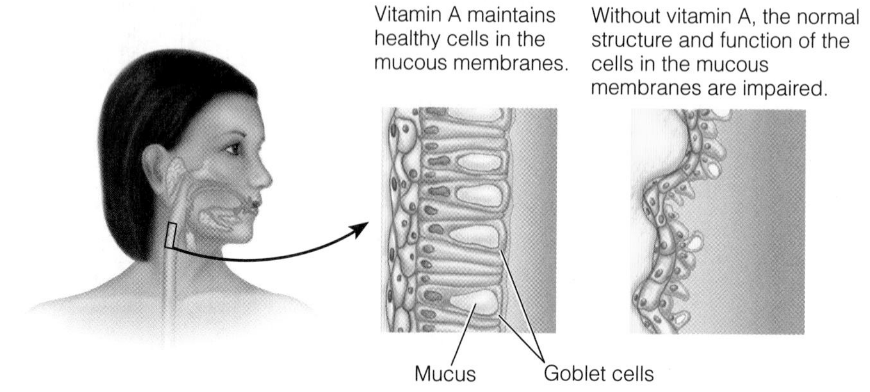
Vitamin A maintains healthy cells in the mucous membranes.
Without vitamin A, the normal structure and function of the cells in the mucous membranes are impaired.
Mucus
Goblet cells

Vitamin A Deficiency

Vitamin A status depends mostly on the adequacy of vitamin A stores, 90 percent of which are in the liver. Vitamin A status also depends on a person's protein status because retinol-binding protein serves as the vitamin's transport carrier inside the body.

If a person were to stop eating vitamin A–containing foods, deficiency symptoms would not begin to appear until after stores were depleted—one to two years for a healthy adult but much sooner for a growing child. Then the consequences would be profound and severe.[9] Vitamin A deficiency is uncommon in North America, but it is a major nutrition problem in many developing countries. An estimated 250 million children worldwide have some degree of vitamin A deficiency and thus are vulnerable to infectious diseases and blindness. About 1 to 2 percent of them become blind every year, half of them dying within a year of losing their sight. Routine vitamin A supplementation and food fortification can be a lifesaving intervention.[10]

Infectious Diseases In developing countries around the world, measles is a devastating infectious disease, killing more than 500 children each day.[11] The severity of the illness often correlates with the degree of vitamin A deficiency; deaths are usually due to related infections such as pneumonia and severe diarrhea. Providing large doses of vitamin A reduces the risk of dying from these infections.

The World Health Organization (WHO) and UNICEF (the United Nations International Children's Emergency Fund) have made the control of vitamin A deficiency a major goal in their quest to improve child health and survival throughout the developing world. They recommend routine vitamin A supplementation for all children with measles in areas where vitamin A deficiency is a problem or where the measles death rate is high. Vitamin A supplementation also protects against the complications of other life-threatening infections, including malaria, lung diseases, and HIV (human immunodeficiency virus, the virus that causes AIDS).

Night Blindness **Night blindness** is one of the first detectable signs of vitamin A deficiency and permits early diagnosis. In night blindness, the retina does not receive enough retinal to regenerate the visual pigments bleached by light. The person loses the ability to recover promptly from the temporary blinding that follows a flash of bright light at night or to see after the lights go out. In many parts of the world, after the sun goes down, vitamin A–deficient people become night-blind. They often cling to others or sit still, afraid that they may trip and fall or lose their way if they try to walk alone. Figure 12-5 shows the eyes' slow recovery in response to a flash of bright light in night blindness.

Blindness (Xerophthalmia) Beyond night blindness is total blindness—failure to see at all. Night blindness is caused by a lack of vitamin A at the back of the

night blindness: slow recovery of vision after flashes of bright light at night or an inability to see in dim light; an early symptom of vitamin A deficiency.

FIGURE 12-5 Vitamin A–Deficiency Symptom—Night Blindness

These photographs illustrate the eyes' slow recovery in response to a flash of bright light at night. In animal research studies, the response rate is measured with electrodes.

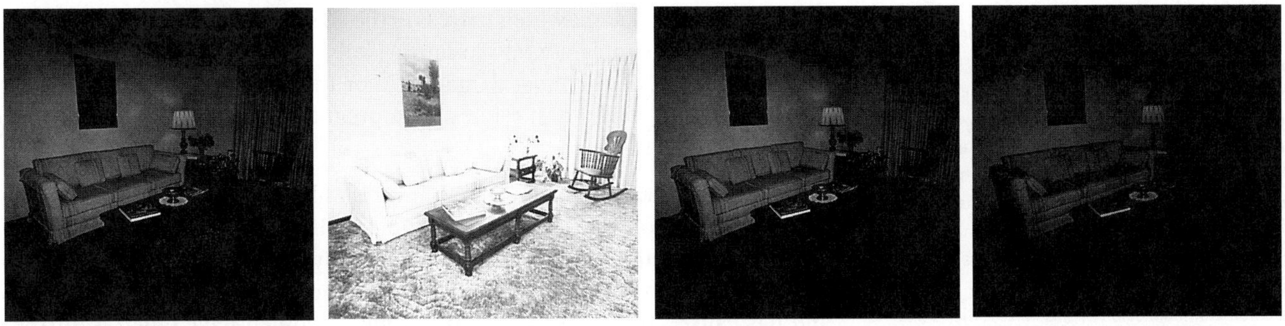

In dim light, you can make out the details in this room. You are using your rods for vision.

A flash of bright light momentarily blinds you as the pigment in the rods is bleached.

You quickly recover and can see the details again in a few seconds.

With inadequate vitamin A, you do not recover but remain blinded for many seconds.

Photos by Deavid J. Farr/ImageSmythe

FIGURE 12-6 Vitamin A–Deficiency Symptom—The Rough Skin of Keratinization

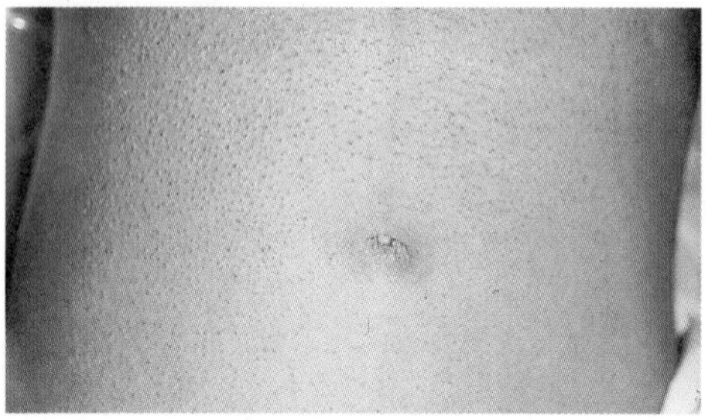

Ken Greer/Visuals Unlimited

In vitamin A deficiency, the epithelial cells secrete the protein keratin in a process known as *keratinization*. (Keratinization doesn't occur in the GI tract, but mucus-producing cells dwindle and mucus production declines.) The extreme of this condition is *hyperkeratinization* or *hyperkeratosis*. When keratin accumulates around hair follicles, the condition is known as *follicular hyperkeratosis*.

eye, the retina; total blindness is caused by a lack at the front of the eye, the cornea. Severe vitamin A deficiency is the major cause of childhood blindness in the world, causing more than half a million preschool children to lose their sight each year. Blindness due to vitamin A deficiency, known as **xerophthalmia**, develops in stages. At first, the cornea becomes dry and hard because of inadequate mucus production—a condition known as **xerosis.** Then, corneal xerosis can quickly progress to **keratomalacia**, the softening of the cornea that leads to irreversible blindness.

Keratinization Elsewhere in the body, vitamin A deficiency affects other surfaces. On the body's outer surface, the epithelial cells change shape and begin to secrete the protein **keratin**—the hard, inflexible protein of hair and nails. As Figure 12-6 shows, the skin becomes dry, rough, and scaly as lumps of keratin accumulate (**keratinization**). Without vitamin A, the goblet cells in the GI tract diminish in number and activity, limiting the secretion of mucus. With less mucus, normal digestion and absorption of nutrients falter, and this, in turn, worsens malnutrition by limiting the absorption of whatever nutrients the diet may deliver. Similar changes in the cells of other epithelial tissues weaken defenses, making infections of the respiratory tract, the GI tract, the urinary tract, the vagina, and inner ear likely.

Vitamin A Toxicity

Just as a deficiency of vitamin A affects all body systems, so does a toxicity. Symptoms of toxicity begin to develop when all the binding proteins are swamped, and free vitamin A damages the cells. Such effects are unlikely when a person depends on a balanced diet for nutrients, but toxicity is a real possibility when concentrated amounts of **preformed vitamin A** in foods derived from animals, fortified foods, or supplements is consumed.[12] Children are most vulnerable to toxicity because they need less vitamin A and are more sensitive to overdoses. An Upper Level (UL) has been set for preformed vitamin A (see inside front cover).

Beta-carotene, which is found in a wide variety of vegetables and fruits, is not converted efficiently enough in the body to cause vitamin A toxicity; instead, it is stored in the fat just under the skin. Although overconsumption of beta-carotene from foods may turn the skin yellow, this is not harmful (see Figure 12-7). In contrast, overconsumption of beta-carotene from supplements may be quite harmful. In excess, this antioxidant may act as a prooxidant, promoting cell division and destroying vitamin A. Furthermore, the adverse effects of beta-carotene supplements are most evident in people who drink alcohol and smoke cigarettes.

Bone Defects Excessive intake of vitamin A over the years may weaken the bones and contribute to fractures and osteoporosis.[13] Vitamin A suppresses bone-building activity, stimulates bone-dismantling activity, and interferes with vitamin D's ability to maintain normal blood calcium.[14] Research findings suggest that most people should not take vitamin A supplements.[15] Even multivitamin supplements ♦ provide more vitamin A than most people need.

Birth Defects Excessive vitamin A during pregnancy leads to abnormal cell death in the spinal cord, which increases the risk of birth defects.[16] ♦ High intakes (10 000 IU ♦ of supplemental vitamin A daily) before the seventh week of pregnancy appear to be the most damaging. For this reason, vitamin A is not given as a supplement in the first trimester of pregnancy without specific evidence of deficiency, which is rare.

Not for Acne Adolescents need to know that massive doses of vitamin A have no beneficial effect on **acne**. The prescription medicine Accutane is made from vitamin A but is chemically different.* Taken orally, Accutane is effective against the deep lesions of cystic acne. It is highly toxic, however, especially during growth, and has caused birth defects in infants when women have taken it during their

*The generic name for Accutane is isotretinoin.

♦ Multivitamin supplements typically provide:
- 750 µg (2500 IU)
- 1500 µg (5000 IU)

For perspective, the RDA for vitamin A is 700 µg for women and 900 µg for men.

♦ A substance that causes abnormal fetal development and birth defects is called a **teratogen** (ter-AT-oh-jen).
- **terato** = monster
- **gen** = to produce

♦ For perspective, 10 000 IU ≈ 3000 µg vitamin A, roughly four times the RDA for women.

xerophthalmia (zer-off-THAL-mee-uh): progressive blindness caused by inadequate tear production due to severe vitamin A deficiency.
- **xero** = dry
- **ophthalm** = eye

xerosis (zee-ROW-sis): abnormal drying of the skin and mucous membranes; a sign of vitamin A deficiency.

keratomalacia (KARE-ah-toe-ma-LAY-shuh): softening of the cornea that leads to irreversible blindness; seen in severe vitamin A deficiency.

keratin (KARE-uh-tin): a water-insoluble protein; the normal protein of hair and nails.

keratinization: accumulation of keratin in a tissue; a sign of vitamin A deficiency.

preformed vitamin A: dietary vitamin A in its active form.

acne: a chronic inflammation of the skin's follicles and oil-producing glands, which leads to an accumulation of oils inside the ducts that surround hairs; usually associated with the maturation of young adults.

pregnancies. For this reason, women taking Accutane must begin using effective forms of contraception at least one month before taking the drug and continue using contraception at least one month after discontinuing its use. They should also refrain from taking any supplements containing vitamin A to avoid additive toxic effects.

Another vitamin A relative, Retin-A, fights acne, the wrinkles of aging, and other skin disorders.* Applied topically, this ointment smooths and softens skin; it also lightens skin that has become darkly pigmented after inflammation. During treatment, the skin becomes red and tender and peels.

Vitamin A Recommendations Because the body can derive vitamin A from various retinoids and carotenoids, its content in foods and its recommendations are expressed as **retinol activity equivalents (RAE).** One microgram of retinol counts as 1 RAE, ♦ as does 12 micrograms of dietary beta-carotene. Most food and supplement labels report their vitamin A contents using International Units (IU), ♦ a measure of vitamin activity used before direct chemical analysis was possible. The accompanying "How To" feature (p. 389) explains how to convert IU to a weight measurement.

Vitamin A in Foods The richest sources of the retinoids are foods derived from animals—liver, fish liver oils, milk and milk products, butter, and eggs. Because vitamin A is fat soluble, it is lost when milk is skimmed. To compensate, 2%, 1%, and skim milks are often fortified so as to supply 6 to 10 percent of the Daily Value per cup.** In Canada, margarine is fortified to provide about the same amount of vitamin A as butter.

Plants contain no retinoids, but many vegetables and some fruits contain vitamin A precursors—the carotenoids, red and yellow pigments of plants. Only a few carotenoids have vitamin A activity; the carotenoid with the greatest vitamin A activity is beta-carotene. The bioavailability of carotenoids depends in part on fat accompanying the meal.[17] More carotenoids are absorbed when salads have regular dressing than when reduced-fat dressing is used, and essentially no carotenoid absorption occurs when fat-free dressing is used.

The Colours of Vitamin A Foods Dark leafy greens (like spinach—not celery or cabbage) and rich yellow or deep orange vegetables and fruits (such as winter squash, cantaloupe, carrots, and sweet potatoes—not corn or bananas) help people meet their vitamin A needs (see Figure 12-8 on p. 388). A diet including several servings of such carotene-rich sources helps to ensure a sufficient intake.

An attractive meal that includes foods of different colours most likely supplies vitamin A as well. Most foods with vitamin A activity are brightly coloured—green, yellow, orange, and red. Any plant-derived food with significant vitamin A activity must have some colour because beta-carotene is a rich, deep yellow, almost orange compound. The beta-carotene in dark green, leafy vegetables is abundant but masked by large amounts of the green pigment **chlorophyll.**

Bright colour is not always a sign of vitamin A activity, however. Beets and corn, for example, derive their colours from the red and yellow **xanthophylls,** which have no vitamin A activity. As for white plant foods such as potatoes, cauliflower, pasta, and rice, they also offer little or no vitamin A. Similarly, fast foods often lack vitamin A. Anyone who dines frequently on hamburgers, french fries, and colas is wise to emphasize colourful vegetables and fruits at other meals.

Vitamin A–Rich Liver People sometimes wonder if eating liver too frequently can cause vitamin A toxicity. Liver is a rich source because vitamin A is stored in the livers of animals, just as in humans.*** Arctic explorers who have eaten large quantities of polar bear liver have become ill with symptoms suggesting vitamin

*The generic name for Retin-A is tretinoin topical.
**Typically vitamin A fortification of fat-reduced milks in Canada is to a level higher than is naturally found in whole milk (about 1600 IU per litre).
***The liver is not the only organ that stores vitamin A. The kidneys, adrenal glands, and other organs do, too, but the liver stores the most and is the most commonly eaten organ meat.

FIGURE 12-7 Symptom of Beta-Carotene Excess—Discoloration of the Skin

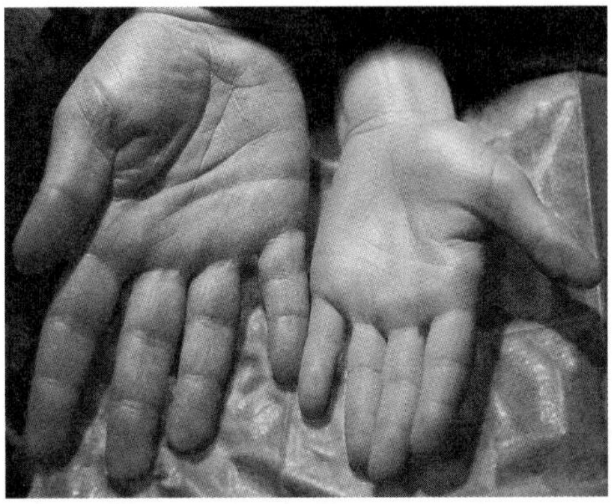

The hand on the right shows the skin discoloration that occurs when blood levels of beta-carotene rise in response to a low-kcalorie diet that features carrots, pumpkins, and orange juice. (The hand on the left belongs to someone else and is shown here for comparison.)

♦ 1 μg RAE = 1 μg retinol
= 2 μg beta-carotene (supplement)
= 12 μg beta-carotene (dietary)
= 24 μg of other vitamin A precursor carotenoids

♦ 1 IU retinol = 0.3 μg retinol or 0.3 μg RAE
1 IU beta-carotene (supplement) = 0.5 IU retinol or 0.15 μg RAE
1 IU beta-carotene (dietary) = 0.165 IU retinol or 0.05 μg RAE
1 IU other vitamin A precursor carotenoids = 0.025 μg RAE

retinol activity equivalents (RAE): a measure of vitamin A activity; the amount of retinol that the body will derive from a food containing preformed retinol or its precursor beta-carotene.

chlorophyll (KLO-row-fil): the green pigment of plants, which absorbs light and transfers the energy to other molecules, thereby initiating photosynthesis.

xanthophylls (ZAN-tho-fills): pigments found in plants; responsible for the colour changes seen in autumn leaves.

FIGURE 12-8 Vitamin A in Selected Foods

See the "How To" section on p. 317 for more information on using this figure.

Food	Serving size (kcalories)
Broccoli, boiled	125 mL (29 kcal)
Carrots, boiled	125 mL (29 kcal)
Tomato, fresh	1 medium (22 kcal)
Apple, fresh	1 medium (72 kcal)
Banana	1 medium (105 kcal)
Blueberries, fresh	125 mL (44 kcal)
Bread, whole wheat	1 slice, 35 g (86 kcal)
Pasta, whole grain, cooked	125 mL (92 kcal)
Rice, white, cooked	125 mL (89 kcal)
Oatmeal, cooked	175 mL (144 kcal)
Pita, white	½ pita, 35 g (96 kcal)
Cereal, high fibre	30 g (78 kcal)
Milk, 2%	250 mL (129 kcal)
Cheddar cheese	50 g (202 kcal)
Yogurt, 2% plain	175 g (110 kcal)
Soy beverage, fortified	250 mL (110 kcal)
Kefir	175 g (104 kcal)
Ice cream, strawberry	125 mL (134 kcal)
Chicken breast, roasted	75 g (220 kcal)
Ground beef, lean, baked	75 g (191 kcal)
Egg, poached	1 large (72 kcal)
Tuna, canned in water	75 g (87 kcal)
Tofu, made with a calcium salt	150 g (114 kcal)
Peanut butter	30 mL (184 kcal)
Excellent, and sometimes unusual, sources:	
Beef liver, fried	75 g (178 kcal)
Yams, baked, no skin	125 mL (95 kcal)
Papaya, fresh	150 g (59 kcal)

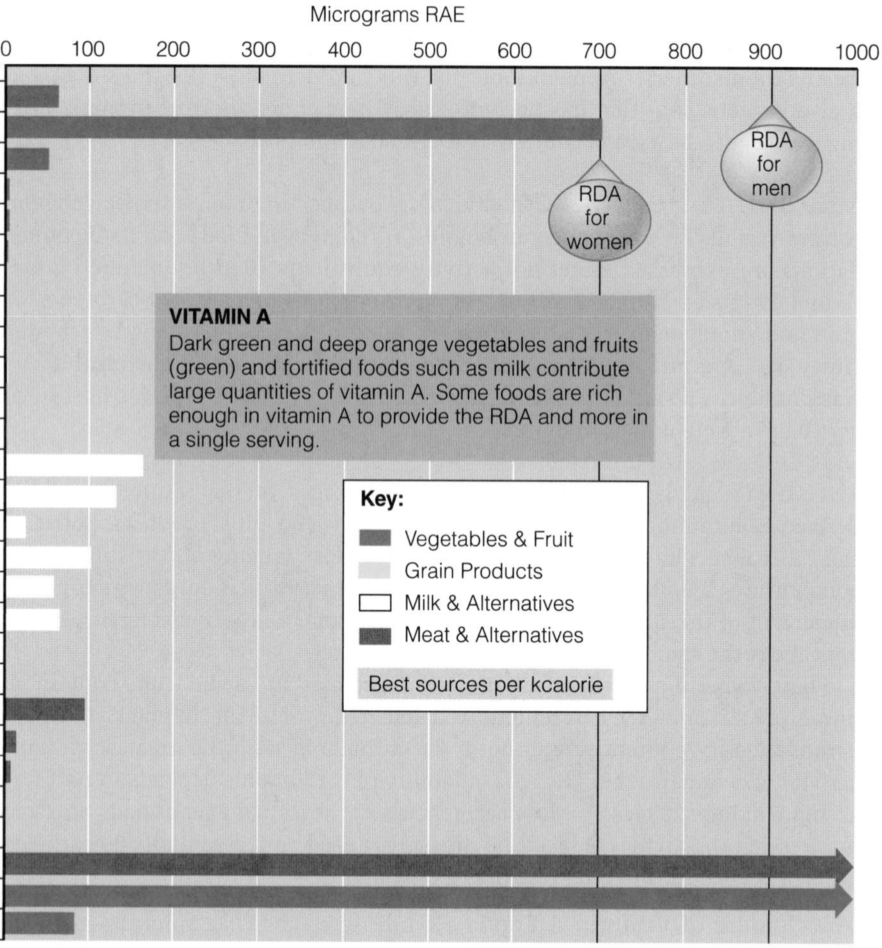
Micrograms RAE
0
100
200
300
400
500
600
700
800
900
1000
RDA for women
RDA for men
VITAMIN A
Dark green and deep orange vegetables and fruits (green) and fortified foods such as milk contribute large quantities of vitamin A. Some foods are rich enough in vitamin A to provide the RDA and more in a single serving.
Key:
Vegetables & Fruit
Grain Products
Milk & Alternatives
Meat & Alternatives
Best sources per kcalorie

SOURCE: Canadian Nutrient File. Health Canada, 2008. Reproduced with the permission of the Minister of Health, 2011.

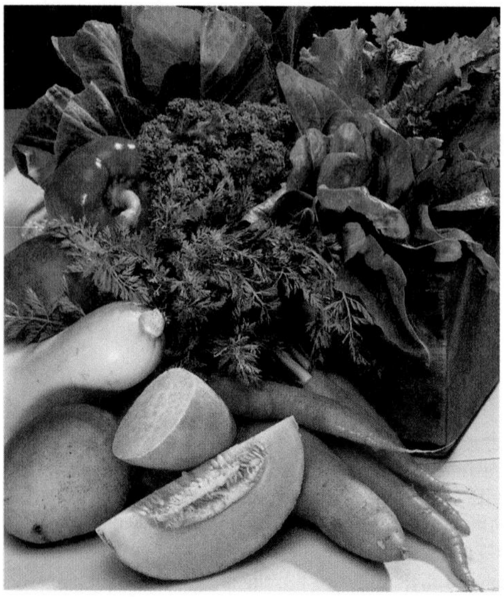

© Polara Studios Inc.

The carotenoids in foods bring colours to meals; the retinoids in our eyes allow us to see them.

A toxicity, as have young children who regularly ate a chicken liver spread that provided three times their daily recommended intake. Liver offers many nutrients, and eating it periodically may improve a person's nutrition status. But caution is warranted not to eat too much too often, especially for pregnant women. With 30 grams of beef liver providing more than three times the RDA for vitamin A, intakes can rise quickly.

IN SUMMARY Vitamin A is found in the body in three forms: retinol, retinal, and retinoic acid. Together, they are essential to vision, healthy epithelial tissues, and growth. Vitamin A deficiency is a major health problem worldwide, leading to infections, blindness, and keratinization. Toxicity can also cause problems and is most often associated with supplement abuse. Animal-derived foods such as liver and whole or fortified milk provide retinoids, whereas brightly coloured plant-derived foods such as spinach, carrots, and pumpkins provide beta-carotene and other carotenoids. In addition to serving as a precursor for vitamin A, beta-carotene may act as an antioxidant in the body. The accompanying table provides a summary of vitamin A.

Vitamin A

Other Names	Deficiency Disease
Retinol, retinal, retinoic acid; precursors are carotenoids such as beta-carotene	Hypovitaminosis A

Other Names
Retinol, retinal, retinoic acid; precursors are carotenoids such as beta-carotene

Recommended Dietary Allowance (RDA)
Men: 900 µg RAE/day
Women: 700 µg RAE/day

Upper Level
Adults: 3000 µg/day

Chief Functions in the Body
Vision; maintenance of cornea, epithelial cells, mucous membranes, skin; bone and tooth growth; reproduction; immunity

Significant Sources
Retinol: fortified milk, cheese, cream, butter, fortified margarine, eggs, liver
Beta-carotene: spinach and other dark leafy greens; broccoli, deep orange fruits (apricots, cantaloupe) and vegetables (squash, carrots, sweet potatoes, pumpkin)

Deficiency Disease
Hypovitaminosis A

Deficiency Symptoms
Night blindness, corneal drying (xerosis), triangular gray spots on eye (Bitot's spots), softening of the cornea (keratomalacia), and corneal degeneration and blindness (xerophthalmia); impaired immunity (infectious diseases); plugging of hair follicles with keratin, forming white lumps (hyperkeratosis)

Toxicity Disease
Hypervitaminosis A[a]

Chronic Toxicity Symptoms
Increased activity of osteoclasts[b] causing reduced bone density; liver abnormalities; birth defects

Acute Toxicity Symptoms
Blurred vision, nausea, vomiting, vertigo; increase of pressure inside skull, mimicking brain tumour; headaches; muscle incoordination

[a]A related condition, *hypercarotenemia,* is caused by the accumulation of too much of the vitamin A precursor beta-carotene in the blood, which turns the skin noticeably yellow. Hypercarotenemia is not, strictly speaking, a toxicity symptom.

[b]*Osteoclasts* are the cells that destroy bone during its growth. Those that build bone are *osteoblasts*.

HOW TO Convert International Units (IU) to Weight Measurements

Supplement labels often list the amount of fat-soluble vitamins in International Units (IU), a universally accepted measure of a vitamin's biological effect. Such a measure allows scientists to compare the potency of substances and was most useful decades ago before chemicals could be purified and weighed accurately.

Because IU measures biological activity and not weight, the conversion factors differ for each fat-soluble vitamin:

For vitamin A (retinol):

- 1 IU = 0.3 µg
- 1 µg = 3.33 IU

For vitamin D (cholecalciferol):

- 1 IU = 0.025 µg
- 1 µg = 40 IU

For vitamin E (natural α-tocopherol):

- 1 IU = 0.67 mg
- 1 mg = 1.49 IU

To convert from IU to a weight measurement, multiply IU by the appropriate equivalent. For example, for a supplement listing 5000 IU vitamin A, 400 IU vitamin D, and 30 IU vitamin E:

5000 IU × 0.3 µg/IU = 1500 µg retinol
400 IU × 0.025 µg/IU = 10 µg cholecalciferol
30 IU × 0.67 mg/IU = 20 mg α-tocopherol

CENGAGENOW™
For additional practice log on to **www.cengage.com/sso.**

TRY IT Convert these values on a supplement label from IU to weight measurements: 4000 IU vitamin A, 600 IU vitamin D, and 12 IU vitamin E.

Vitamin E

Researchers discovered a component of vegetable oils necessary for reproduction in rats and named this antisterility factor **tocopherol**, which means "to bring forth offspring." When chemists isolated four different tocopherol compounds, they designated them by the first four letters of the Greek alphabet: alpha, beta, gamma, and delta. The tocopherols consist of a complex ring structure and a long saturated side chain. (APPENDIX C provides the chemical structures.) The positions of methyl groups (CH_3) on the side chain and their chemical rotations distinguish one tocopherol from another. **Alpha-tocopherol** is the only one with vitamin E activity in the human body.[18] The other tocopherols are not readily converted to alpha-tocopherol in the body, nor do they perform the same roles. Whether these other tocopherols might be beneficial in other ways is the subject of current research.[19]

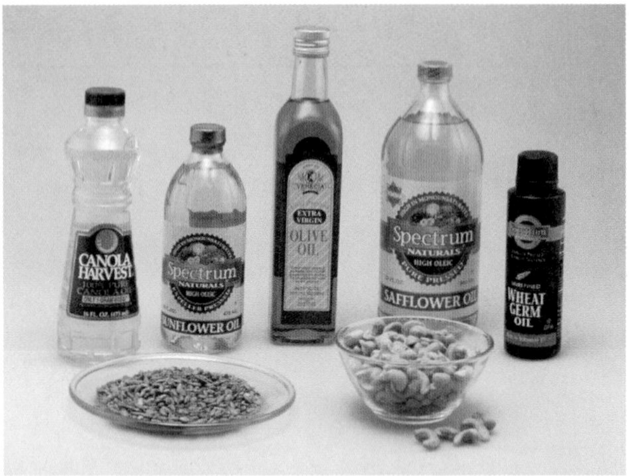
CANOLA HARVEST
Spectrum
OLIVE OIL
Spectrum
SAFFLOWER OIL
WHEAT GERM OIL

Fat-soluble vitamin E is found predominantly in vegetable oils, seeds, and nuts.

Vitamin E Role as an Antioxidant

Vitamin E is a fat-soluble antioxidant and one of the body's primary defenders against the adverse effects of free radicals. Its main action is to stop the chain reaction of free radicals producing more free radicals (see Highlight 12). In doing so, vitamin E protects the vulnerable components of the cells and their membranes from destruction. Most notably, vitamin E prevents the oxidation of the polyunsaturated fatty acids, but it protects other lipids and related compounds (e.g., vitamin A) as well.

Accumulating evidence suggests that vitamin E may reduce the risk of heart disease by protecting low-density lipoproteins (LDL) against oxidation and reducing inflammation.[20] The oxidation of LDL and inflammation have been implicated as key factors in the development of heart disease. Highlight 12 explains how vitamin E and other antioxidants might protect against chronic diseases, such as heart disease and cancer, and explores whether foods or supplements might be most helpful—or harmful.

Vitamin E Deficiency

A primary deficiency of vitamin E (from poor dietary intake) is rare; deficiency is usually associated with diseases of fat malabsorption such as cystic fibrosis. Without vitamin E, the red blood cells break open and spill their contents, probably due to oxidation of the polyunsaturated fatty acids in their membranes. This classic sign of vitamin E deficiency, known as **erythrocyte hemolysis**, is seen in premature infants, born before the transfer of vitamin E from the mother to the infant that takes place in the last weeks of pregnancy. Vitamin E treatment corrects **hemolytic anemia.**

Prolonged vitamin E deficiency also causes neuromuscular dysfunction involving the spinal cord and retina of the eye. Common symptoms include loss of muscle coordination and reflexes and impaired vision and speech. Vitamin E treatment corrects these neurological symptoms of vitamin E deficiency.

Two other conditions seem to respond to vitamin E treatment, although results are inconsistent. One is **fibrocystic breast disease**, a nonmalignant breast disease. The other is **intermittent claudication**, an abnormality of blood flow that causes cramping in the legs.

Vitamin E Toxicity

Vitamin E supplement use has risen in recent years as its protective actions against chronic diseases have been recognized. Fortunately, the liver carefully regulates vitamin E concentrations.[21] Toxicity is rare, and vitamin E appears safe across a broad range of intakes.[22] The UL for vitamin E (1000 milligrams) is more than 65 times greater than the recommended intake for adults (15 milligrams). Extremely high doses of vitamin E may interfere with the blood-clotting action of vitamin K and enhance the effects of drugs used to oppose blood clotting, causing hemorrhage. Additional research is needed to determine whether vitamin E supplements increase the risk of hemorrhagic stroke.[23]

tocopherol (tuh-KOFF-er-ol): a general term for several chemically related compounds, one of which has vitamin E activity. (See APPENDIX C for chemical structures.)

alpha-tocopherol: the active vitamin E compound.

erythrocyte (eh-RITH-ro-cite) **hemolysis** (he-MOLL-uh-sis): the breaking open of red blood cells (erythrocytes); a symptom of vitamin E–deficiency disease in human beings.

- **erythro** = red
- **cyte** = cell
- **hemo** = blood
- **lysis** = breaking

hemolytic (HE-moh-LIT-ick) **anemia:** the condition of having too few red blood cells as a result of erythrocyte hemolysis.

fibrocystic (FYE-bro-SIS-tik) **breast disease:** a harmless condition in which the breasts develop lumps, sometimes associated with caffeine consumption. In some, it responds to abstinence from caffeine; in others, it can be treated with vitamin E.

- **fibro** = fibrous tissue
- **cyst** = closed sac

intermittent claudication (klaw-dih-KAY-shun): severe calf pain caused by inadequate blood supply. It occurs when walking and subsides during rest.

- **intermittent** = at intervals
- **claudicare** = to limp

Vitamin E Recommendations The current RDA for vitamin E is based on the alpha-tocopherol form only. As mentioned earlier, the other tocopherols cannot be converted to alpha-tocopherol, nor can they perform the same metabolic roles in the body. A person who consumes large quantities of polyunsaturated fatty acids needs more vitamin E. Fortunately, vitamin E and polyunsaturated fatty acids tend to occur together in the same foods. Current research suggests that most adults in the United States fall short of recommended intakes for vitamin E and that smokers may have a higher requirement.[24] No reports of vitamin E intakes for Canadians exist, but intakes are likely similar to reports for Americans.

Vitamin E in Foods Vitamin E is widespread in foods. Much of the vitamin E in the diet comes from vegetable oils and products made from them, such as margarine and salad dressings. Wheat germ oil is especially rich in vitamin E.

Because vitamin E is readily destroyed by heat processing (such as deep-fat frying) and oxidation, fresh or lightly processed foods are preferable sources. Most processed and convenience foods do not contribute enough vitamin E to ensure an adequate intake.

Prior to 2000, values of the vitamin E in foods reflected all of the tocopherols and were expressed in "milligrams of tocopherol equivalents." ♦ These measures overestimated the amount of alpha-tocopherol. To estimate the alpha-tocopherol content of foods stated in tocopherol equivalents, multiply by 0.8.[25]

♦ APPENDIX H accurately presents vitamin E data in milligrams of alpha-tocopherol.

IN SUMMARY **Vitamin E acts as an antioxidant, defending lipids and other components of the cells against oxidative damage. Deficiencies are rare, but they do occur in premature infants, the primary symptom being erythrocyte hemolysis. Vitamin E is found predominantly in vegetable oils and appears to be one of the least toxic of the fat-soluble vitamins. The accompanying table provides a summary of vitamin E.**

Vitamin E

Other Names	**Significant Sources**
Alpha-tocopherol	Polyunsaturated plant oils, margarine, salad dressings, leafy green vegetables (spinach, turnip greens, collard greens, broccoli), wheat germ, whole grains, liver, egg yolks, nuts, seeds
RDA	Easily destroyed by heat and oxygen
Adults: 15 mg/day	**Deficiency Symptoms**
Upper Level	Red blood cell breakage,[a] nerve damage
Adults: 1000 mg/day	**Toxicity Symptoms**
Chief Functions in the Body	Augments the effects of anticlotting medication
Antioxidant (stabilization of cell membranes, regulation of oxidation reactions, protection of polyunsaturated fatty acids [PUFA] and vitamin A)	

[a]The breaking of red blood cells is called *erythrocyte hemolysis*.

Vitamin C

Two hundred and sixty years ago, any man who joined the crew of a seagoing ship knew he had at best a 50–50 chance of returning alive—not because he might be slain by pirates or die in a storm, but because he might contract **scurvy**. As many as two-thirds of a ship's crew could die of scurvy during a long voyage. Only men on short voyages, especially around the Mediterranean Sea, were free of scurvy. No one knew the reason: that on long ocean voyages, the ship's cook used up the fresh fruits and vegetables early and then served only cereals and meats until the return to port.

scurvy: the vitamin C–deficiency disease.

The first nutrition experiment ever performed on human beings was devised in the mid-1700s to find a cure for scurvy. James Lind, a British physician, divided 12 sailors with scurvy into 6 pairs. Each pair received a different supplemental ration: cider, vinegar, sulphuric acid, seawater, oranges and lemons, or a strong laxative mixed with spices. Those receiving the citrus fruits quickly recovered, but sadly, it was 50 years before the British navy required all vessels to provide every sailor ♦ with lime juice daily.

The antiscurvy "something" in limes and other foods was dubbed the **antiscorbutic factor.** Nearly 200 years later, the factor was isolated and found to be a 6-carbon compound similar to glucose; it was named **ascorbic acid.**

♦ The tradition of providing British sailors with citrus juice daily to prevent scurvy gave them the nickname "limeys."

Vitamin C Roles in the Body

Vitamin C parts company with the B vitamins in its mode of action. In some settings, vitamin C serves as a cofactor ♦ helping a specific enzyme perform its job, but in others, it acts as an antioxidant participating in more general ways.

♦ A **cofactor** is a small, inorganic or organic substance that facilitates the action of an enzyme.

As an Antioxidant Vitamin C loses electrons easily, a characteristic that allows it to perform as an **antioxidant.** In the body, antioxidants defend against **free radicals.** (Free radicals are discussed fully in Highlight 12.) As mentioned previously, a free radical is a molecule with one or more unpaired electrons, which makes it unstable and highly reactive. By donating an electron or two, antioxidants neutralize free radicals and protect other substances from their damage. Figure 12-9 illustrates how vitamin C can give up electrons to stop free-radical damage and then accept them again to become reactivated. This recycling of vitamin C is key to limiting losses and maintaining a reserve of antioxidants in the body. Transporting and concentrating vitamin C in the cells enhances its role as an antioxidant.[26]

Vitamin C is like a bodyguard for water-soluble substances; it stands ready to sacrifice its own life to save theirs. In the cells and body fluids, vitamin C protects tissues from **oxidative stress** and thus may play an important role in preventing diseases. In the intestines, vitamin C enhances iron absorption by protecting iron from oxidation. (Chapter 14 provides more details about the relationship between vitamin C and iron.)

As a Cofactor in Collagen Formation Vitamin C helps to form the fibrous structural protein of connective tissues known as collagen. ♦ Collagen serves as the matrix on which bones and teeth are formed. When a person is wounded, collagen glues the separated tissues together, forming scars. Cells are held together largely by collagen; this is especially important in the walls of the blood vessels, which must withstand the pressure of blood surging with each beat of the heart.

♦ **Collagen** is the structural protein from which connective tissues such as scars, tendons, ligaments, and the foundations of bones and teeth are made.

antiscorbutic (AN-tee-skor-BUE-tik) **factor:** the original name for vitamin C.
- **anti** = against
- **scorbutic** = causing scurvy

ascorbic acid: one of the two active forms of vitamin C (see Figure 12-9). Many people refer to vitamin C by this name.
- **a** = without
- **scorbic** = having scurvy

antioxidant: a substance in foods that significantly decreases the adverse effects of free radicals on normal physiological functions in the human body.

free radicals: unstable molecules with one or more unpaired electrons.

oxidative stress: a condition in which the production of oxidants and free radicals exceeds the body's ability to handle them and prevent damage.

Chapter 6 describes how the body makes proteins by stringing together chains of amino acids. During the synthesis of collagen, each time a proline or lysine is added to the growing protein chain, an enzyme hydroxylates it (adds an OH group to it), making the amino acid hydroxyproline or hydroxylysine, respectively. These two special amino acids facilitate the binding together of collagen fibres to make strong, ropelike structures. The conversion of proline to hydroxyproline requires both vitamin C and iron. Iron works as a cofactor in the reaction, and vitamin C protects iron from oxidation, thereby allowing iron to perform its duty. Without vitamin C and iron, the hydroxylation step does not occur.

FIGURE 12-9 Active Forms of Vitamin C

The two hydrogens highlighted in yellow give vitamin C its acidity and its ability to act as an antioxidant.

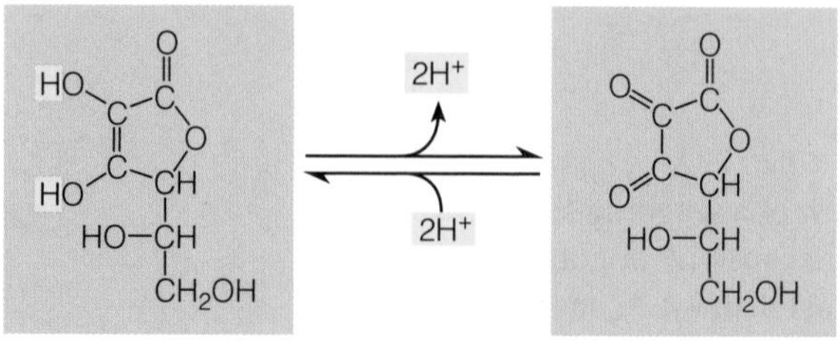
HO
HO
HO—CH
CH₂OH
2H⁺
2H⁺
HO—CH
CH₂OH

Ascorbic acid protects against oxidative damage by donating its two hydrogens with their electrons to free radicals (molecules with unpaired electrons). In doing so, ascorbic acid becomes dehydroascorbic acid.

Dehydroascorbic acid can readily accept hydrogens to become ascorbic acid. The reversibility of this reaction is key to vitamin C's role as an antioxidant.

As a Cofactor in Other Reactions Vitamin C also serves as a cofactor in the synthesis of several other compounds. As in collagen formation, vitamin C helps in the hydroxylation of carnitine, a compound that transports fatty acids, especially long-chain fatty acids, across the inner membrane of mitochondria in cells. It participates in the conversions of the amino acids tryptophan and tyrosine to the neurotransmitters serotonin and norepinephrine, respectively. Vitamin C also assists in the making of hormones, including thyroxin, which regulates the metabolic rate; when metabolism speeds up in times of extreme physical stress, the body's use of vitamin C increases.

In Stress The adrenal glands contain more vitamin C than any other organ in the body. ♦ During stress, the adrenal glands release vitamin C, together with hormones, into the blood.[27] The vitamin's exact role in the stress reaction remains unclear, but physical stresses raise vitamin C needs. Among the stresses known to increase vitamin C needs are infections; burns; extremely high or low temperatures; intakes of toxic heavy metals such as lead, mercury, and cadmium; the chronic use of certain medications, including aspirin, barbiturates, and oral contraceptives; and cigarette smoking.

When immune system cells are called into action, they use a great deal of oxygen and produce free radicals. In this case, free radicals are helpful. They act as ammunition in an "oxidative burst" that demolishes the offending viruses and bacteria and destroys the damaged cells. Vitamin C steps in as an antioxidant to control this oxidative activity.

♦ Vitamin C is found in:
- Adrenal glands, pituitary glands
- Liver, spleen, heart, kidneys, lungs, pancreas, white blood cells
- Muscles, red blood cells

In the Prevention and Treatment of the Common Cold Vitamin C has been a popular option for the prevention and treatment of the common cold for decades, but research supporting such claims has been conflicting and controversial. Some studies find no relationship between vitamin C and the occurrence of the common cold, whereas others report modest benefits—fewer colds, fewer days, and shorter duration of severe symptoms, especially for those exposed to physical and environmental stresses.[28] A review of the research on vitamin C in the treatment and prevention of the common cold reveals a slight, but consistent reduction (of 8 percent) in the duration of the common cold in favour of those taking a daily dose of at least 200 milligrams of vitamin C.[29] The question for consumers to consider is, "Is this enough to warrant routine daily supplementation?" Findings from one study show that consumers want their colds to be at least 25 percent less severe to justify the costs of taking vitamin C supplements regularly.[30]

Discoveries about how vitamin C works in the body provide possible links between the vitamin and the common cold. Anyone who has ever had a cold knows the discomfort of a runny or stuffed-up nose. Nasal congestion develops in response to elevated blood **histamine**, and people commonly take antihistamines for relief. Like an antihistamine, vitamin C comes to the rescue and deactivates histamine.

In Disease Prevention Whether vitamin C may help in preventing or treating cancer, heart disease, cataract, and other diseases is still being studied, and findings are presented in Highlight 12's discussion on antioxidants. Conducting research in Canada and the United States can be difficult, however, because diets typically contribute enough vitamin C to provide optimal health benefits.

Vitamin C Recommendations

For decades, vitamin C ranked at the top of dietary supplement sales. How much vitamin C does a person need? As is true of all the vitamins, recommendations are set generously above the minimum requirement to prevent deficiency disease and well below the toxicity level (see Figure 12-10 on page 394).[31]

The requirement—the amount needed to prevent the overt symptoms of scurvy—is only 10 milligrams daily. However, 10 milligrams a day does not saturate all the body tissues; higher intakes will increase the body's total vitamin C. At about 100 milligrams ♦ per day, 95 percent of the population probably reaches tissue saturation. Recommendations are slightly lower, ♦ based on the amounts needed to provide antioxidant protection. At about 200 milligrams, absorption reaches a maximum, and there is little, if any, increase in blood concentrations at higher doses. Excess vitamin C is readily excreted.

As mentioned earlier, cigarette smoking increases the need for vitamin C. Cigarette smoke contains oxidants, which greedily deplete this potent antioxidant.

♦ For perspective, 250 mL (1 cup) orange juice provides >100 mg vitamin C.

♦ Vitamin C RDA
- Men: 90 mg/day
- Women: 75 mg/day

histamine (HISS-tah-mean or HISS-tah-men): a substance produced by cells of the immune system as part of a local immune reaction to an antigen; participates in causing inflammation.

FIGURE 12-10 Vitamin C Intake (mg/day)

Recommendations for vitamin C are set generously above the minimum requirement and well below the toxicity level.

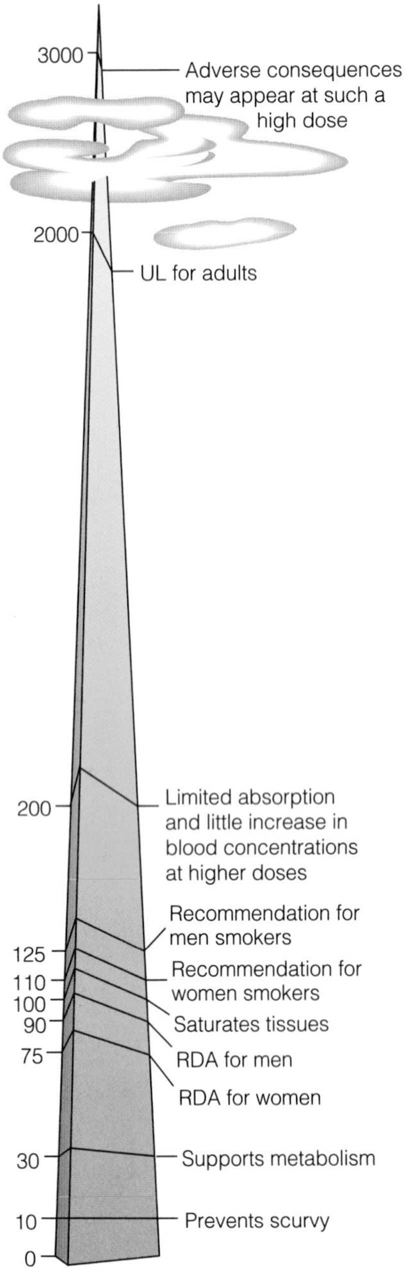
3000
Adverse consequences may appear at such a high dose
2000
UL for adults
200
Limited absorption and little increase in blood concentrations at higher doses
Recommendation for men smokers
125
110
100
90
Recommendation for women smokers
Saturates tissues
75
RDA for men
RDA for women
30
Supports metabolism
10
Prevents scurvy
0

♦ **Gout** is a metabolic disease in which uric acid crystals precipitate in the joints.

false positive: a test result indicating that a condition is present (positive) when in fact it is not present (therefore false).

false negative: a test result indicating that a condition is not present (negative) when in fact it is present (therefore false).

Exposure to cigarette smoke, especially when accompanied by low dietary intakes of vitamin C, depletes the body's vitamin C in both active and passive smokers. People who chew tobacco also have low levels of vitamin C. Because people who smoke cigarettes regularly suffer significant oxidative stress, their requirement for vitamin C is increased an additional 35 milligrams; nonsmokers regularly exposed to cigarette smoke should also be sure to meet their RDA for vitamin C.

Vitamin C Deficiency

Two of the most notable signs of a vitamin C deficiency reflect its role in maintaining the integrity of blood vessels. The gums bleed easily around the teeth, and capillaries under the skin break spontaneously, producing pinpoint hemorrhages (see Figure 12-11).

When vitamin C concentrations fall to about a fifth of optimal levels (this may take more than a month on a diet lacking vitamin C), scurvy symptoms begin to appear. Inadequate collagen synthesis causes further hemorrhaging. Muscles, including the heart muscle, degenerate. The skin becomes rough, brown, scaly, and dry. Wounds fail to heal because scar tissue will not form. Bone rebuilding falters; the ends of the long bones become softened, malformed, and painful, and fractures develop. The teeth become loose as the cartilage around them weakens. Anemia and infections are common. There are also characteristic psychological signs, including hysteria and depression. Sudden death is likely, caused by massive internal bleeding.

Once diagnosed, scurvy is readily resolved by vitamin C. Moderate doses in the neighbourhood of 100 milligrams per day are sufficient, curing the scurvy within about five days. Such an intake is easily achieved by including vitamin C–rich foods in the diet.

Vitamin C Toxicity

The availability of vitamin C supplements and the publication of books recommending vitamin C to prevent colds and cancer have led thousands of people to take large doses of vitamin C. Not surprisingly, side effects of vitamin C supplementation such as gastrointestinal distress and diarrhea have been reported. The UL for vitamin C was established based on these symptoms.

Several instances of interference with medical regimens are also known. Large amounts of vitamin C excreted in the urine obscure the results of tests used to detect glucose or ketones in the diagnosis of diabetes. In some instances, excess vitamin C gives a **false positive** result; in others, a **false negative.** People taking anticlotting medications may unwittingly counteract the effect if they also take massive doses of vitamin C. Those with kidney disease, a tendency toward gout, ♦ or a genetic abnormality that alters vitamin C's breakdown to its excretion products are prone to forming kidney stones if they take large doses of vitamin C.* Vitamin C supplements may adversely affect people with iron overload. As Chapter 14

*Vitamin C is inactivated and degraded by several routes, and sometimes oxalate, which can form kidney stones, is produced along the way. People may also develop oxalate crystals in their kidneys regardless of vitamin C status.

FIGURE 12-11 Vitamin C–Deficiency Symptoms—Scorbutic Gums and Pinpoint Hemorrhages

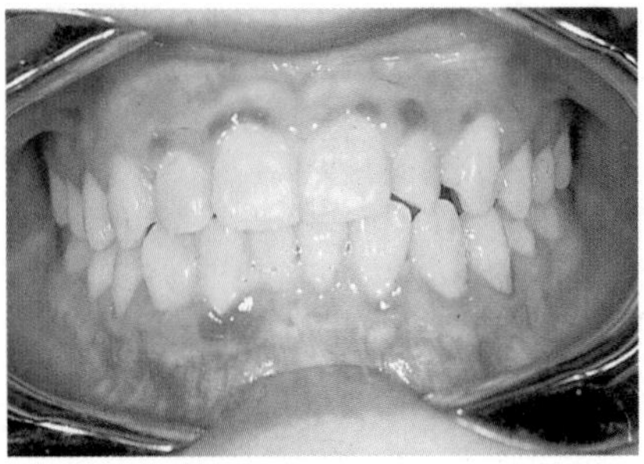

© L. V. Bergman & Associates, Inc.

Scorbutic gums. Unlike other lesions of the mouth, scurvy presents a symmetrical appearance without infection.

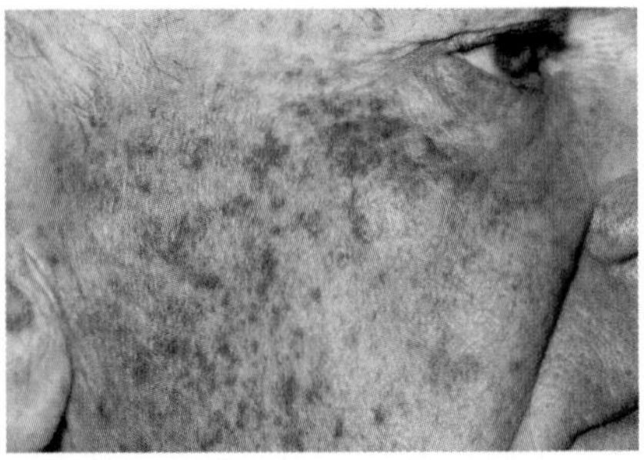

Dr. P. Marazzi/Photo Researchers, Inc

Pinpoint hemorrhages. Small red spots appear in the skin, indicating spontaneous bleeding internally.

explains, vitamin C enhances iron absorption and releases iron from body stores; too much free iron causes the kind of cellular damage typical of free radicals. These adverse consequences of vitamin C's effects on iron have not been seen in clinical studies, but they illustrate how vitamin C can act as a *pro*oxidant when quantities exceed the body's needs.[32]

Vitamin C Food Sources Fruits and vegetables can easily provide a generous amount of vitamin C. A cup of orange juice at breakfast, a salad for lunch, and a stalk of broccoli and a potato for dinner alone provide more than 300 milligrams. ♦ Clearly, a person making such food choices does not need vitamin C supplements.

♦ For perspective, review Figure 12-10.

Figure 12-12 shows the amounts of vitamin C in various common foods. The overwhelming abundance of green bars reveals not only that the citrus fruits are justly famous for being rich in vitamin C, but that other fruits and vegetables are in the same league. A half cup or 125 millilitres of broccoli, bell pepper, or strawberries provides more than 50 milligrams of the vitamin (and an array of other nutrients). Because vitamin C is vulnerable to heat, raw fruits and vegetables usually have a higher nutrient density than their cooked counterparts. Similarly, because vitamin C is readily destroyed by oxygen, foods and juices should be stored properly and consumed within a week of opening.

The potato is an important source of vitamin C, not because one potato by itself meets the daily need, but because potatoes are such a common staple that they make significant contributions. In fact, scurvy was unknown in Ireland until

FIGURE 12-12 Vitamin C in Selected Foods

See the "How To" section on p. 317 for more information on using this figure.

Food	Serving size (kcalories)
Broccoli, boiled	125 mL (29 kcal)
Carrots, boiled	125 mL (29 kcal)
Tomato, fresh	1 medium (22 kcal)
Apple, fresh	1 medium (72 kcal)
Banana	1 medium (105 kcal)
Blueberries, fresh	125 mL (44 kcal)
Bread, whole wheat	1 slice, 35 g (86 kcal)
Pasta, whole grain, cooked	125 mL (92 kcal)
Rice, white, cooked	125 mL (89 kcal)
Oatmeal, cooked	175 mL (144 kcal)
Pita, white	½ pita, 35 g (96 kcal)
Cereal, high fibre	30 g (78 kcal)
Milk, 2%	250 mL (129 kcal)
Cheddar cheese	50 g (202 kcal)
Yogurt, 2% plain	175 g (110 kcal)
Soy beverage, fortified	250 mL (110 kcal)
Kefir	175 g (104 kcal)
Ice cream, strawberry	125 mL (134 kcal)
Chicken breast, roasted	75 g (220 kcal)
Ground beef, lean, baked	75 g (191 kcal)
Egg, poached	1 large (72 kcal)
Tuna, canned in water	75 g (87 kcal)
Tofu, made with a calcium salt	150 g (114 kcal)
Peanut butter	30 mL (184 kcal)
Excellent, and sometimes unusual, sources:	
Red bell pepper, raw	125 mL (24 kcal)
Guava, fresh	125 mL (59 kcal)
Kiwi, fresh	1 large (56 kcal)

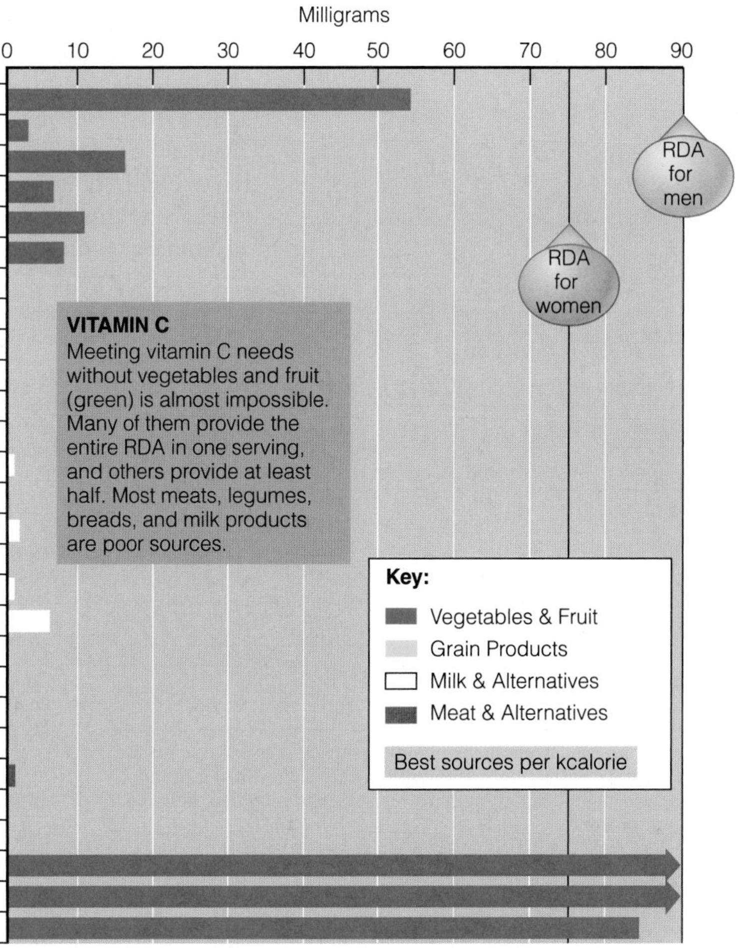
Milligrams
0
10
20
30
40
50
60
70
80
90
RDA for men
RDA for women
VITAMIN C
Meeting vitamin C needs without vegetables and fruit (green) is almost impossible. Many of them provide the entire RDA in one serving, and others provide at least half. Most meats, legumes, breads, and milk products are poor sources.
Key:
Vegetables & Fruit
Grain Products
Milk & Alternatives
Meat & Alternatives
Best sources per kcalorie

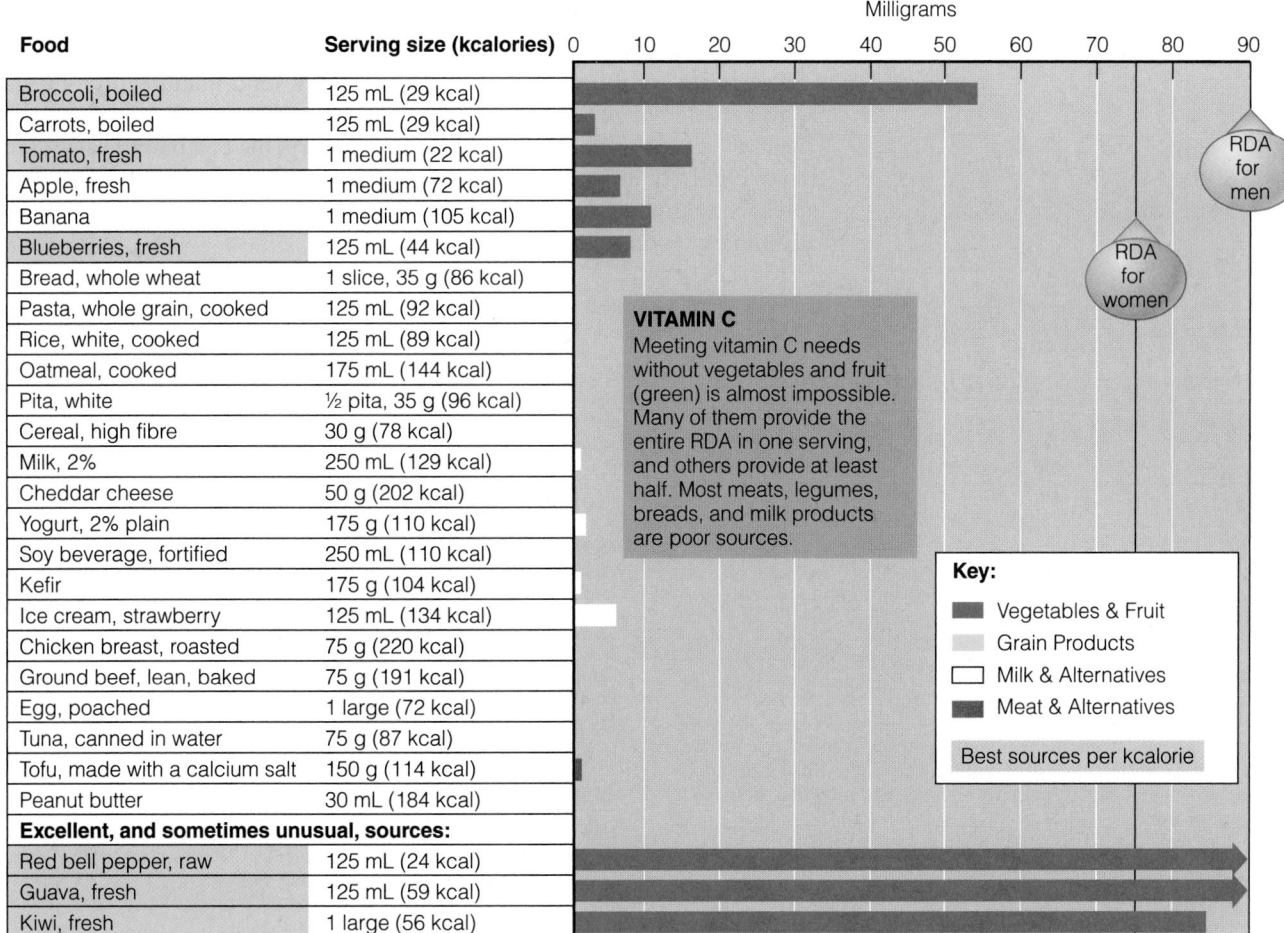

SOURCE: Canadian Nutrient File. Health Canada, 2008. Reproduced with the permission of the Minister of Health, 2011

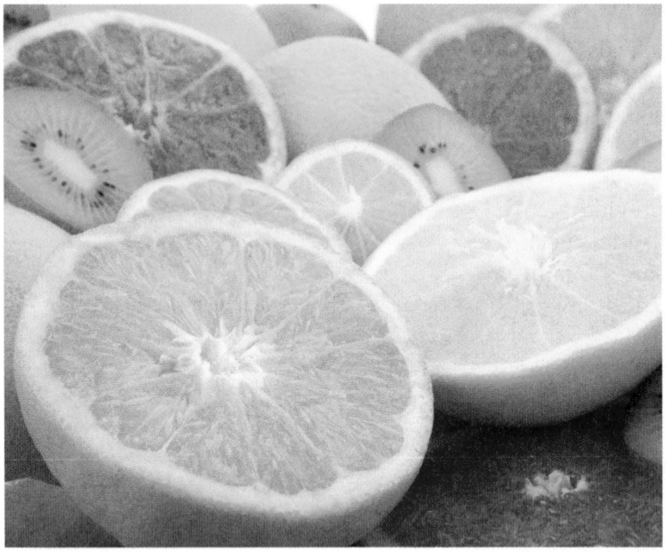

photos.com

When dietitians say "vitamin C," people think "citrus fruits" . . .

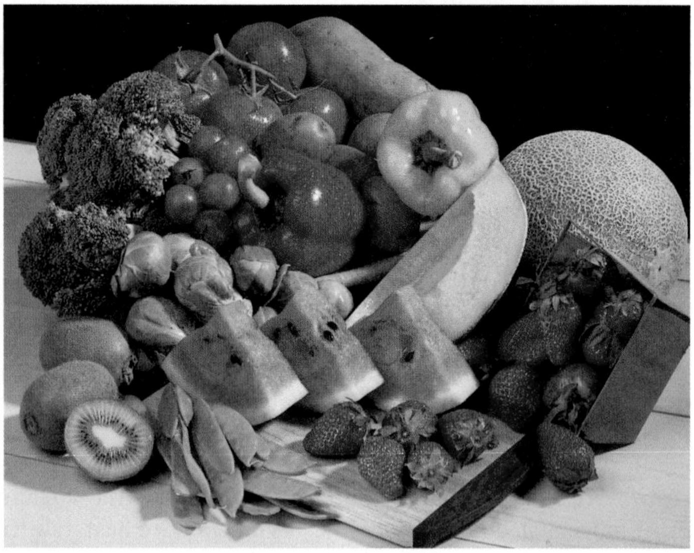

© Polara Studios Inc.

. . . but these foods are also rich in vitamin C.

the potato blight of the mid-1840s when some two million people died of malnutrition and infection.

The lack of yellow, white, and red bars in Figure 12-12 confirms that grain products, milk and alternatives, and meat and alternatives are notoriously poor sources of vitamin C. Organ meats (liver, kidneys, and others) and raw meats contain some vitamin C, but most people don't eat large quantities of these foods. Raw meats and fish contribute enough vitamin C to be significant sources in parts of Canada, Alaska, and Japan, but elsewhere vegetables and fruits are necessary to supply sufficient vitamin C.

Because of vitamin C's antioxidant property, food manufacturers sometimes add a variation of vitamin C to some beverages and most cured meats, such as luncheon meats, to prevent oxidation and spoilage. This compound safely preserves these foods, but it does not have vitamin C activity in the body. Simply put, "ham and bacon cannot replace fruits and vegetables." The accompanying table provides a summary of vitamin C.

IN SUMMARY Vitamin C

Other Names

Ascorbic acid

RDA

Men: 90 mg/day

Women: 75 mg/day

Smokers: +35 mg/day

Upper Level

Adults: 2000 mg/day

Chief Functions in the Body

Collagen synthesis (strengthens blood vessel walls, forms scar tissue, provides matrix for bone growth), antioxidant, thyroxin synthesis, amino acid metabolism, strengthens resistance to infection, helps in absorption of iron

Significant Sources

Citrus fruits, cabbage-type vegetables (such as Brussels sprouts and cauliflower), dark green vegetables (such as bell peppers and broccoli), cantaloupe, strawberries, lettuce, tomatoes, potatoes, papayas, mangoes

Easily destroyed by heat and oxygen

Deficiency Disease

Scurvy

Deficiency Symptoms

Anemia (small-cell type),[a] atherosclerotic plaques, pinpoint hemorrhages; bone fragility, joint pain; poor wound healing, frequent infections; bleeding gums, loosened teeth; muscle degeneration, pain, hysteria, depression; rough skin, blotchy bruises

Toxicity Symptoms

Nausea, abdominal cramps, diarrhea; headache, fatigue, insomnia; hot flashes; rashes; interference with medical tests, aggravation of gout symptoms, urinary tract problems, kidney stones[b]

[a]Small-cell-type anemia is *microcytic anemia*.

[b]People with kidney disease, a tendency toward gout, or a genetic abnormality that alters the breakdown of vitamin C are prone to forming kidney stones. Vitamin C is inactivated and degraded by several routes, sometimes producing oxalate, which can form stones in the kidneys.

Selenium

The essential mineral **selenium** shares some of the chemical characteristics of the mineral sulphur. This similarity allows selenium to substitute for sulphur in the amino acids methionine, cysteine, and cystine.

Selenium Roles in the Body

Selenium is one of the body's antioxidant nutrients, working primarily as a part of proteins—most notably, the enzyme glutathione peroxidase.[33] Glutathione peroxidase and vitamin E work in tandem. Glutathione peroxidase prevents free-radical formation, thus blocking the chain reaction before it begins; if free radicals do form and a chain reaction starts, vitamin E stops it. (Highlight 12 describes free-radical formation, chain reactions, and antioxidant action in detail.) Another enzyme that converts the thyroid hormone to its active form also contains selenium.

Selenium Deficiency

Selenium deficiency is associated with a heart disease ♦ that is prevalent in regions of China where the soil and foods lack selenium. Although the primary cause of this heart disease is probably a virus, selenium deficiency appears to predispose people to it, and adequate selenium seems to prevent it.

♦ The heart disease associated with selenium deficiency is named **Keshan** (KESH-an or ka-SHAWN) **disease** for one of the provinces of China where it was first studied. Keshan disease is characterized by heart enlargement and insufficiency; fibrous tissue replaces the muscle tissue that normally composes the middle layer of the walls of the heart.

Selenium and Cancer

Some research suggests that selenium may protect against some types of cancers. Given the potential for harm and the lack of conclusive evidence, however, recommendations to take selenium supplements would be premature—and perhaps ineffective as well. Selenium from foods appears to be more effective in inhibiting cancer growth than selenium from supplements. Such a finding reinforces a theme that has been repeated throughout this text—foods offer many more health benefits than supplements.

Selenium Recommendations and Sources

Selenium is found in the soil, and therefore in the crops grown for consumption.[34] Soil levels of selenium vary across Canada, but in the major grain- and legume-producing provinces of Alberta, Saskatchewan, and Manitoba, the average selenium content in soil is higher than many other regions in the world.[35] Figure 12-13 shows average selenium distribution in Prairie soils. People living in regions with selenium-poor soil may still get enough selenium, partly because they eat vegetables and grains transported from other regions and partly because they eat meats, milk, and eggs, which are reliable sources of selenium. Eating as few as two Brazil nuts a day effectively improves selenium status.[36] Average intakes in Canada and the United States are above the RDA, which is based on the amount needed to maximize glutathione peroxidase activity.

FIGURE 12-13 Average Selenium Distribution in Canadian Prairie Soils

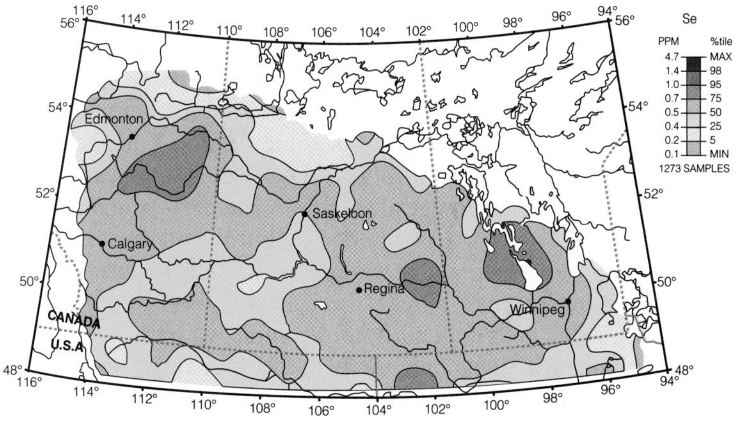
Se
PPM %tile
4.7 MAX
1.4 98
1.0 95
0.7 75
0.5 50
0.4 25
0.2 5
0.1 MIN
1273 SAMPLES
Edmonton
Calgary
Saskatoon
Regina
Winnipeg
CANADA
U.S.A.

selenium (se-LEEN-ee-um): a trace element.

Selenium Toxicity Because high doses of selenium are toxic, a UL has been set. Selenium toxicity causes loss and brittleness of hair and nails, garlic breath odour, and nervous system abnormalities.

IN SUMMARY **Selenium is an antioxidant nutrient that works closely with the glutathione peroxidase enzyme and vitamin E. Selenium is found in association with protein in foods. Deficiencies are associated with a predisposition to a type of heart abnormality known as Keshan disease. The accompanying table provides a summary of selenium.**

Selenium

RDA	Deficiency Symptoms
Adults: 55 µg/day	Predisposition to heart disease characterized by cardiac tissue becoming fibrous (Keshan disease)
Upper Level	**Toxicity Symptoms**
Adults: 400 µg/day	Loss and brittleness of hair and nails; skin rash, fatigue, irritability, and nervous system disorders; garlic breath odour
Chief Functions in the Body	
Defends against oxidation; regulates thyroid hormone	
Significant Sources	
Seafood, meat, whole grains, vegetables and fruits (depending on soil content)	

As mentioned earlier (page 381) the trace minerals manganese, iron, zinc, and copper also have antioxidant properties. More specifically, manganese, zinc, and copper are cofactors for superoxide dismutase that catalyzes the conversion of superoxide atoms to a less toxic hydrogen peroxide form; and iron activates catalase, an enzyme that converts hydrogen peroxide to water and oxygen gas. Chapter 10 describes the importance of manganese and Chapter 14 discusses iron, zinc, and copper. Consuming diets that include ample vegetables and fruits in the context of well-balanced and varied food choices provide us not only with antioxidant nutrients but also with many health benefits.

The Antioxidant Nutrients—In Summary

The fat-soluble vitamins A (including beta-carotene) and E, the water-soluble vitamin C, and the trace mineral selenium function as antioxidants in our bodies. Their presence affects the health of cell membranes, low-density lipoproteins, our DNA and RNA, and proteins that have important functional roles in the body. Deficiencies of the antioxidant nutrients compromise our defences against free-radical damage. Toxicities, usually caused by people using supplements, also pose possible ill health effects since high intakes of the nutrient antioxidants may act as pro-oxidants by stimulating the generation of free radicals.

The interactions between antioxidant nutrients serve to illustrate the importance of consuming all of them in adequate amounts. For example, selenium works synergistically with vitamin E: as a cofactor in glutathione peroxidase, selenium quenches free radicals and spares the use of some vitamin E for non-antioxidant roles. Vitamin E protects vitamin A from oxidation and in the case of vitamin E deficiency, the absorption and storage of vitamin A and beta-carotene are impaired. The ability of vitamin C to donate or accept an electron and remain stable in both its oxidized and reduced forms can regenerate the antioxidant activity of vitamin E once it has donated an electron to a free radical. The antioxidant nutrients also play important roles in other body functions: for example, vitamin A for bone growth and remodelling, vitamin E for proper immune function and growth and development, vitamin C for the synthesis of collagen and increasing the absorption of iron, and selenium for regulating the production of thyroid hormones.

Eating a wide variety of nourishing foods daily can ensure an appropriate intake of antioxidants, not too little and not too much. The accompanying table provides a summary of the antioxidant nutrients.

IN SUMMARY The Antioxidant Nutrients

Nutrient and Chief Functions	Deficiency Symptoms	Toxicity Symptoms	Significant Sources
Vitamin A and Beta-Carotene Vision; maintenance of cornea, epithelial cells, mucous membranes, skin; bone and tooth growth; reproduction; immunity	Infectious diseases, night blindness, blindness (xerophthalmia), keratinization	Reduced bone mineral density, liver abnormalities, birth defects	Retinol: milk and milk products Beta-carotene: dark green leafy and deep orange vegetables
Vitamin E Antioxidant (stabilization of cell membranes, regulation of oxidation reactions, protection of polyunsaturated fatty acids [PUFA] and vitamin A)	Erythrocyte hemolysis, nerve damage	Hemorrhagic effects	Vegetable oils, nuts, and seeds
Vitamin C Antioxidant; synthesis of collagen, carnitine, hormones, neurotransmitters	Scurvy (bleeding gums, pinpoint hemorrhages, abnormal bone growth, and joint pain)	Diarrhea, GI distress	Vegetables and fruit, especially citrus and berries
Selenium Part of an enzyme that defends against oxidation; regulates thyroid hormones	Associated with Keshan disease	Nail and hair brittleness and loss; fatigue, irritability, and nervous system disorders; skin rash; garlic breath odour	Seafoods, organ meats, other meats, whole grains, vegetables, and fruits

Nutrition Portfolio

Consuming a well-balanced diet that contains a mix of colourful vegetables and fruits, fortified milk or soy products, and vegetable oils can provide ample antioxidant nutrients. Using supplements of antioxidant nutrients should be done cautiously, if at all. Go to Diet Analysis Plus and choose one of the days on which you tracked your diet for an entire day. Select the MyPlate report and then consider the following questions:

- How was your overall intake in the Vegetables and Fruit group? Do you need improvement in this area? What are some changes you could make that would align your choices with the types recommended in the *Food Guide*?

Now look at the report titled Intake Spreadsheet to answer the following questions:

- Examine your choice of vegetables and evaluate whether you meet the daily recommendation for at least one dark green and one orange vegetable.
- Describe the vegetable oils you use when you cook and their vitamin contributions. What, if any, effect does heat have on the vitamin content of your oils?
- Which of your foods provided vitamin C? How could you bring your vitamin C intake closer to the recommended amount?

Diet Analysis PLUS

To complete this exercise, go to your Diet Analysis Plus at www.cengage.com/sso.

Nutrition on the Net

CENGAGENOW™
For further study of topics covered in this chapter, log on to **www.cengage.com/sso.**

- Search for "antioxidants" at the Dietitians of Canada's website: **www.dietitians.ca**
- Review the Dietary Reference Intakes for vitamin C, vitamin E, selenium, and the carotenoids by searching for "DRI Antioxidants": **www.nap.edu**
- Visit the World Health Organization to learn about "antioxidant" initiatives around the world: **www.who.int**
- Search for "antioxidants" at Health Canada's website: **www.hc-sc.gc.ca**
- Learn about the health effects of consuming vegetables and fruits from the Mix it up! program: **www.5to10aday.com**

References

1. D. Garriguet, Canadians' eating habits. *Health Reports* 18 (2007): 17–32.
2. E. H. Harrison, Mechanisms of digestion and absorption of dietary vitamin A, *Annual Review of Nutrition* 25 (2005): 87–103.
3. B. Burton-Freeman and K. Reimers, Tomato consumption and health: Emerging benefits, *American Journal of Lifestyle Medicine* 5 (2011): 182–191; L. Ma and X. Lin, Effects of lutein and zeaxanthin on aspects of eye health, *Journal of the Science of Food and Agriculture* 90 (2010): 2–12; R. L. Roberts and coauthors, Lutein and zeaxanthin in eye and skin health, *Clinics in Dermatology* 27 (2009): 195–201.
4. Harrison, 2005.
5. G. Wolf, Identification of a membrane receptor for retinol-binding protein functioning in the cellular uptake of retinol, *Nutrition Reviews* 65 (2007): 385–388.
6. G. Wolf, Retinoic acid as cause of cell proliferation or cell growth inhibition depending on activation of one of two different nuclear receptors, *Nutrition Reviews* 66 (2008): 55–59.
7. R. Blomhoff and H. K. Blomhoff, Overview of retinoid metabolism and function, *Journal of Neurobiology* 66 (2006): 606–630.
8. Committee on Dietary Reference Intakes, *Dietary Reference Intakes for Vitamin C, Vitamin E, Selenium, and Carotenoids* (Washington, D.C.: National Academies Press, 2000).
9. A. Sommer, Vitamin A deficiency and clinical disease: An historical overview, *Journal of Nutrition* 138 (2008): 1835–1839.
10. S. A. Abrams and D. C. Hilmers, Postnatal vitamin A supplementation in developing countries: An intervention whose time has come? *Pediatrics* 122 (2008): 180–181; K. Kraemer and coauthors, Are low tolerable upper intake levels for vitamin A undermining effective food fortification efforts? *Nutrition Reviews* 66 (2008): 517–525.
11. www.who.int/mediacentre/factsheets, f286, revised December 2008.
12. A. Sheth, R. Khurana, and V. Khurana, Potential liver damage associated with over-the-counter vitamin supplements, *Journal of the American Dietetic Association* 108 (2008): 1536–1537; K. L. Penniston and S. A. Tanumihardjo, The acute and chronic toxic effects of vitamin A, *American Journal of Clinical Nutrition* 83 (2006): 191–201.
13. J. D. Ribaya-Mercado and J. B. Blumberg, Vitamin A: Is it a risk factor for osteoporosis and bone fracture? *Nutrition Reviews* 65 (2007): 425–438; M. Kneissel and coauthors, Retinoid-induced bone thinning is caused by subperiosteal osteoclast activity in adult rodents, *Bone* 36 (2005): 202–214.
14. P. S. Genaro and L. A. Martini, Vitamin A supplementation and risk of skeletal fracture, *Nutrition Reviews* 62 (2004): 65–72.
15. H. A. Jackson and A. H. Sheehan, Effect of vitamin A on fracture risk, *The Annals of Pharmacotherapy* 39 (2005): 2086–2090.
16. J. Zhao and coauthors, Retinoic acid downregulates microRNAs to induce abnormal development of spinal cord in spina bifida rat model, *Child's Nervous System* 24 (2008): 485–492; S. Reijntjes and coauthors, The control of morphogen signaling: Regulation of the synthesis and catabolism of retinoic acid in the developing embryo, *Developmental Biology* 285 (2005): 224–237.
17. J. D. Ribaya-Mercado and coauthors, Carotene-rich plant foods ingested with minimal dietary fat enhance the total-body vitamin A pool size in Filipino schoolchildren as assessed by stable-isotopedilution methodology, *American Journal of Clinical Nutrition* 85 (2007): 1041–1049.
18. Committee on Dietary Reference Intakes, 2000.
19. S. Devaraj and I. Jialal, Failure of vitamin E in clinical trials: Is gammatocopherol the answer? *Nutrition Reviews* 63 (2005): 290–293; M. C. Morris and coauthors, Relation of the tocopherol forms to incident Alzheimer disease and to cognitive change, *American Journal of Clinical Nutrition* 81 (2005): 508–514.
20. D. L. Rainwater and coauthors, Vitamin E dietary supplementation significantly affects multiple risk factors for cardiovascular disease in baboons, *American Journal of Clinical Nutrition* 86 (2007): 597–603; U. Singh, S. Devaraj, and I. Jialal, Vitamin E, oxidative stress, and inflammation, *Annual Review of Nutrition* 25 (2005): 151–174.
21. M. G. Traber, Vitamin E regulatory mechanisms, *Annual Review of Nutrition* 27 (2007): 347–362.
22. J. N. Hathcock and coauthors, Vitamins E and C are safe across a broad range of intakes, *American Journal of Clinical Nutrition* 81 (2005): 736–745.
23. Committee on Dietary Reference Intakes, 2000, p. 252.
24. R. S. Bruno and coauthors, α-Tocopherol disappearance is faster in cigarette smokers and is inversely related to their ascorbic acid status, *American Journal of Clinical Nutrition* 81 (2005): 95–103.
25. Committee on Dietary Reference Intakes, 2000.
26. J. X. Wilson, Regulation of vitamin C transport, *Annual Review of Nutrition* 25 (2005): 105–125.
27. S. J. Padayatty and coauthors, Human adrenal glands secrete vitamin C in response to adrenocorticotrophic hormone, *American Journal of Clinical Nutrition* 86 (2007): 145–149.
28. M. Simasek and D. A. Blandino, Treatment of the common cold, *American Family Physician* 75 (2007): 515–520; S. Sasazuki and coauthors, Effect of vitamin C on common cold: Randomized controlled trial, *European Journal of Clinical Nutrition* 60 (2006): 9–17; B. Arroll, Nonantibiotic treatments for upper-respiratory tract infections (common cold), *Respiratory Medicine* 99 (2005): 1477–1484.
29. R. M. Douglas and coauthors, Vitamin C for preventing and treating the common cold, *Cochrane Database of Systematic Reviews* 3 (2007): CD000980; E. S. Wintergerst, S. Maggini, and D. H. Hornig, Immuneenhancing role of vitamin C and zinc and effect on clinical conditions, *Annals of Nutrition and Metabolism* 50 (2006): 85–94.
30. B. Barrett and coauthors, Sufficiently important difference for common cold: Severity reduction, *Annals of Family Medicine* 5 (2007): 216–223.
31. Committee on Dietary Reference Intakes, 2000.
32. Q. Chen, M. G. Espey, A. Y. Sun, C. Pooput, K. L. Kirk, M. C. Krishna, D. B. Khosh, J. Drisko, and M. Levine, Pharmacologic doses of ascorbate act as a prooxidant and decrease growth of aggressive tumor xenografts in mice, *Proceedings of the National Academy of Sciences* 105 (2008): 11105–11109; J. N. Hathcock and coauthors, Vitamins E and C are safe across a broad range of intakes, *American Journal of Clinical Nutrition* 81 (2005): 736–745.
33. X. G. Lei, W. Cheng, and J. P. McClung, Metabolic regulation and function of glutathione peroxidase-1, *Annual Review of Nutrition* 27 (2007): 41–61; R. F. Burk and K. E. Hill, Selenoprotein P: An extracellular protein with unique physical characteristics and a role in selenium homeostasis, *Annual Review of Nutrition* 25 (2005): 215–235.
34. J. W. Finley, Selenium accumulation in plant foods, *Nutrition Reviews* 63 (2005): 196–202.
35. R. G. Garrett, Selenium, a bioessential element and its abundance in Prairie agricultural soils, Applied Geochemistry and Mineralogy Subdivision, Geological Survey of Canada, Natural Resources Canada, Ottawa (2003).
36. C. D. Thomson and coauthors, Brazil nuts: An effective way to improve selenium status, *American Journal of Clinical Nutrition* 87 (2008): 379–384.

HIGHLIGHT 12

Antioxidant Nutrients in Disease Prevention

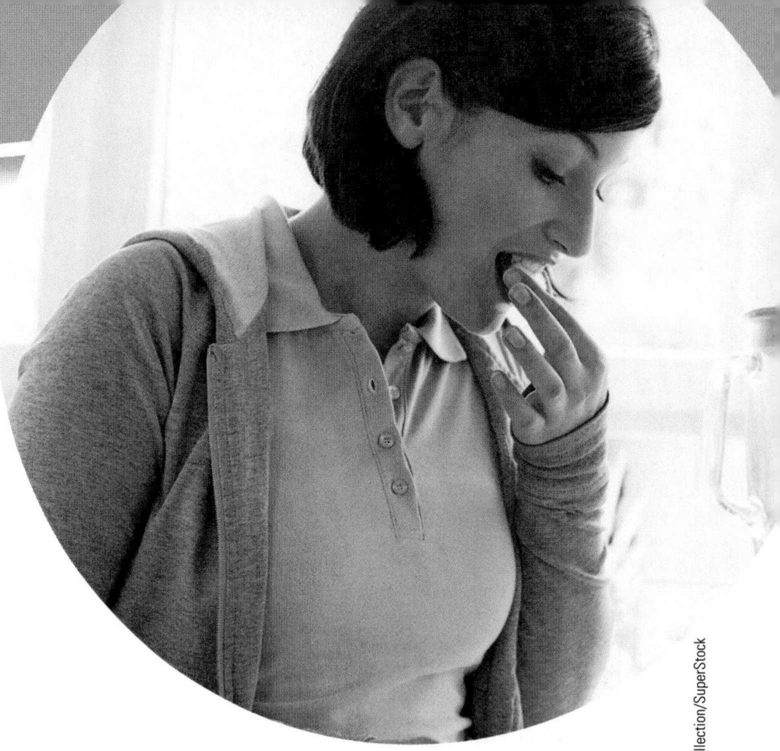

© Fancy Collection/SuperStock

Count on supplement manufacturers to exploit the day's hot topics in nutrition. The moment bits of research news surface, new supplements appear—and terms like *antioxidants* and *lycopene* become household words. Friendly faces in TV commercials try to persuade us that these supplements hold the magic in the fight against aging and disease. New supplements hit the market and cash registers ring. Vitamin C, for years the leading single nutrient supplement, gains new popularity, and sales of lutein, beta-carotene, and vitamin E supplements soar as well.

In the meantime, scientists and medical experts around the world continue their work to clarify and confirm the roles of antioxidants in preventing chronic diseases. This highlight summarizes some of the accumulating evidence. It also revisits the advantages of foods over supplements. But first it is important to introduce the troublemakers—the **free radicals.** (The accompanying glossary defines free radicals and related terms.)

Free Radicals and Disease

Chapter 7 describes how the body's cells use oxygen in metabolic reactions. In the process, oxygen sometimes reacts with body compounds and produces highly unstable molecules known as free radicals. In addition to normal body processes, environmental factors such as ultraviolet radiation, air pollution, and tobacco smoke generate free radicals.

A free radical is a molecule with one or more unpaired electrons.* An electron without a partner is unstable and highly reactive. To regain its stability, the free radical quickly finds a stable but vulnerable compound from which to steal an electron.

With the loss of an electron, the formerly stable molecule becomes a free radical itself and steals an electron from another nearby molecule. Thus, an electron-snatching chain reaction is under way with free radicals producing more free radicals. **Antioxidants** neutralize free radicals by donating one of their own electrons, thus ending the chain reaction. When they lose electrons, antioxidants do not become free radicals because they are stable in either form. (Review Figure 12-9 on p. 392 to see how ascorbic acid can give up two hydrogens with their electrons and become dehydroascorbic acid.)

Once formed, free radicals attack. Occasionally, these free-radical attacks are helpful. For example, cells of the immune system use free radicals as ammunition in an "oxidative burst" that demolishes disease-causing viruses and bacteria. Most often, however, free-radical attacks cause widespread damage. They commonly damage the polyunsaturated fatty acids in lipoproteins and in cell membranes, disrupting the transport of substances into and out of cells. Free radicals also alter DNA, RNA, and proteins, creating excesses and deficiencies of specific proteins, impairing cell functions, and eliciting an inflammatory response. All of these actions contribute to cell damage, disease progression, and aging (see Figure H12-1 on page 402).

The body's natural defences and repair systems try to control the destruction caused by free radicals, but these systems are not 100 percent effective. In fact, they become less effective with age, and the unrepaired damage accumulates. To some extent, dietary antioxidants defend the body against **oxidative stress,** but if antioxidants are unavailable or if free-radical production becomes excessive, health problems may develop.[1] Oxygen-derived free radicals may cause diseases, not only by indiscriminately destroying the valuable components of cells, but also by serving as signals for specific activities within the cells. Scientists have identified oxidative stress as a causative factor and antioxidants as a protective factor in cognitive performance and the aging process as well as in the development of diseases such as cancer, arthritis, cataracts, diabetes, and heart disease.

*Many free radicals exist, but oxygen-derived free radicals are most common in the human body. Examples of oxygen-derived free radicals include superoxide radical ($O_2{\cdot}^-$), hydroxyl radical ($OH\cdot$), and nitric oxide ($NO\cdot$). (The dots in the symbols represent the unpaired electrons.) Technically, hydrogen peroxide (H_2O_2) and singlet oxygen are not free radicals because they contain paired electrons, but the unstable conformation of their electrons makes radical-producing reactions likely. Scientists sometimes use the term *reactive oxygen species (ROS)* to describe all of these compounds.

HIGHLIGHT 12

GLOSSARY

antioxidants: substances typically found in foods that significantly decrease the adverse effects of free radicals on normal functions in the body.

free radicals: unstable and highly reactive atoms or molecules that have one or more unpaired electrons in the outer orbital. (See APPENDIX B for a review of basic chemistry concepts.)

oxidants (OKS-ih-dants): compounds (such as oxygen itself) that oxidize other compounds. Compounds that prevent oxidation are called *antioxidants,* whereas those that promote it are called *pro-oxidants.*

- **anti** = against
- **pro** = for

oxidative stress: a condition in which the production of oxidants and free radicals exceeds the body's ability to handle them and prevent damage.

phytochemicals: nonnutrient compounds found in plant-derived foods that have biological activity in the body.

pro-oxidants: substances that significantly induce oxidative stress.

Defending against Free Radicals

The body maintains a couple lines of defence against free-radical damage. A system of enzymes disarms the most harmful **oxidants.*** The action of these enzymes depends on the minerals selenium, copper, manganese, and zinc. If the diet fails to provide adequate supplies of these minerals, this line of defense weakens. The body also uses the antioxidant vitamins—vitamin E, beta-carotene, and vitamin C. Vitamin E defends the body's lipids (cell membranes and lipoproteins, for example) by efficiently stopping the free-radical chain reaction. Beta-carotene also acts as an antioxidant in lipid membranes. Vitamin C protects other tissues, such as the skin and fluid of the blood, against free-radical attacks.[2] Vitamin C seems especially adept at neutralizing free radicals from polluted air and cigarette smoke; it also restores oxidized vitamin E to its active state.

*These enzymes include glutathione peroxidase, thioredoxin reductase, superoxide dismutase, and catalase.

FIGURE H12-1 Free-Radical Damage

Free radicals are highly reactive. They might attack the polyunsaturated fatty acids in a cell membrane, which generates lipid radicals that damage cells and accelerate disease progression. Free radicals might also attack and damage DNA, RNA, and proteins, which interferes with the body's ability to maintain normal cell function, causing disease and premature aging.

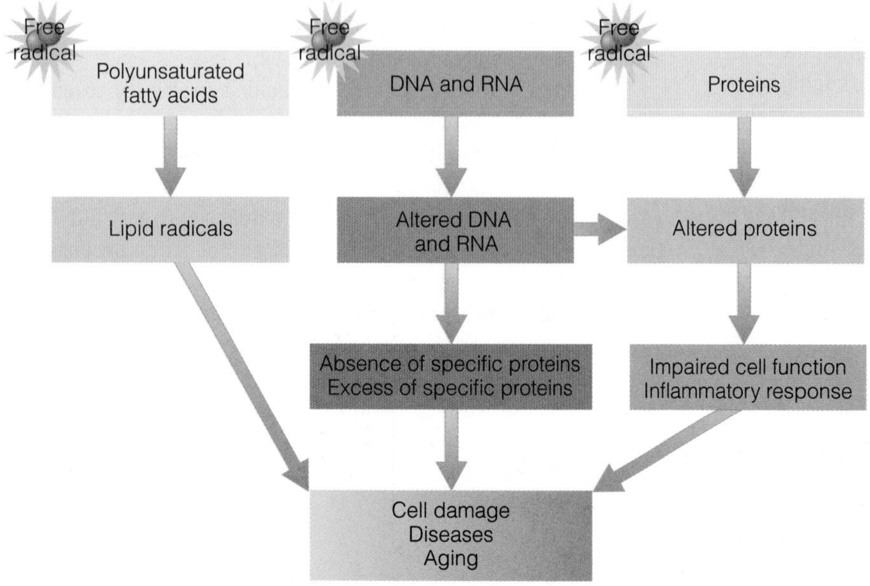
Free radical
Polyunsaturated fatty acids
Free radical
DNA and RNA
Free radical
Proteins
Lipid radicals
Altered DNA and RNA
Altered proteins
Absence of specific proteins
Excess of specific proteins
Impaired cell function
Inflammatory response
Cell damage
Diseases
Aging

Dietary antioxidants may also include some of the **phytochemicals** (featured in Highlight 14). Together, nutrients and phytochemicals with antioxidant activity minimize damage in the following ways:

- Limiting free-radical formation
- Destroying free radicals or their precursors
- Stimulating antioxidant enzyme activity
- Repairing oxidative damage
  - Stimulating repair enzyme activity
  - Supporting a healthy immune system[3]

These actions play key roles in defending the body against chronic diseases such as cancer and heart disease.

Defending against Cancer

Cancers arise when cellular DNA is damaged—sometimes by free-radical attacks. Antioxidants may reduce cancer risks by protecting DNA from this damage. Many researchers have reported low rates of cancer in people whose diets include abundant vegetables and fruits, rich in antioxidants.[4] Preliminary reports suggest an inverse relationship between DNA damage and vegetable intake and a positive relationship with beef and pork intake. Laboratory studies with animals and with cells in tissue culture also seem to support such findings.

Foods rich in vitamin C seem to protect against certain types of cancers, especially those of the esophagus. Such a correlation may reflect the benefits of a diet rich in fruits and vegetables and low in fat; it does not necessarily support taking vitamin C supplements to treat or prevent cancer. At high doses vitamin C acts as a **pro-oxidant,** generating free radicals. Limited research suggests this action may be useful in destroying cancer cells.[5]

Researchers hypothesize that vitamin E might inhibit cancer formation by attacking free radicals that damage DNA. Evidence that vitamin E helps guard against cancer, however, is contradictory and inconclusive.[6]

Several studies report a cancer-preventing benefit of vegetables and fruits rich in beta-carotene and the other carotenoids as well. Carotenoids seem to protect against oxidative damage to DNA.[7] High concentrations of beta-carotene are associated with a lower mortality from all causes and lower rates of some cancers.[8] These benefits may simply reflect a healthy diet abundant in fruits and vegetables.[9]

Research suggests the trace mineral selenium may be another important nutrient in the arsenal of nutritional cancer prevention. The anti-carcinogenic property of selenium is thought to be mediated primarily through the activity of selenoproteins, such as the enzyme glutathione peroxidase.[10] Yet, despite showing promise in some cancer studies, results from other studies have not confirmed antitumour activity. Until we understand the underlying mechanisms of selenium's action, it is not prudent to use selenium supplements for the purpose of cancer prevention.[11]

Defending against Heart Disease

High blood cholesterol carried in LDL is a major risk factor for cardiovascular disease, but how do LDL exert their damage? One scenario is that free radicals within the arterial walls oxidize LDL, changing their structure and function. The oxidized LDL then accelerate the formation of artery-clogging plaques. These free radicals also oxidize the polyunsaturated fatty acids of the cell membranes, sparking additional changes in the arterial walls, which impede the flow of blood. Susceptibility to such oxidative damage within the arterial walls is heightened by a diet high in saturated fat or cigarette smoke. In contrast, diets that include plenty of fruits and vegetables, especially when combined with little saturated fat, strengthen antioxidant defences against LDL oxidation.

Antioxidants, especially vitamin E, may protect against cardiovascular disease. Epidemiological studies suggest that people who eat foods rich in vitamin E have relatively few atherosclerotic plaques and low rates of death from heart disease. Similarly, large doses of vitamin E supplements may slow the progression of heart disease.[12] Among its many protective roles, vitamin E defends against LDL oxidation, inflammation, arterial injuries, and blood clotting.[13]

Vitamin C supplements may reduce the risk of heart disease. Some studies suggest that vitamin C protects against LDL oxidation, raises HDL, lowers total cholesterol, and improves blood pressure. Vitamin C may also minimize inflammation and the free-radical action within the arterial wall.[14]

Antioxidant nutrients taken as supplements seem to slow the early progression of atherosclerosis. Less clear is whether antioxidant supplements benefit people who already have heart disease or multiple risk factors for it. Antioxidant supplements may not be beneficial and, in fact, may even be harmful for these people.[15]

Numerous studies have shown high blood selenium levels are associated with adverse blood lipids and increased risk for heart disease.[16] At present, the mechanisms are unclear. On the other hand, a recent British study suggested a modest improvement in blood lipids for people who had low blood selenium levels at the start of the supplementation trial.[17] Conflicting results are not unusual in scientific investigations and push researchers to conduct well-designed investigations. Clearly, further research is required to determine the optimal selenium activity levels that can benefit cardiovascular health.

Foods, Supplements, or Both?

In the process of scavenging and quenching free radicals, antioxidants themselves become oxidized. To some extent, they can be regenerated, but losses still occur and free radicals attack continuously. To maintain defences, a person must replenish dietary antioxidants regularly. But should antioxidants be replenished from foods or from supplements?

Foods—especially fruits and vegetables—offer not only antioxidants, but an array of other valuable vitamins and minerals as well. Importantly, deficiencies of these nutrients can damage DNA as readily as free radicals can. Eating vegetables and fruits in abundance protects against both deficiencies and diseases—and is associated with reduced mortality.[18] A major review of the evidence gathered from metabolic studies, epidemiologic studies, and dietary intervention trials identified three dietary strategies most effective in preventing heart disease:

- Use unsaturated fats (that have not been hydrogenated) instead of saturated or *trans* fats (see Highlight 5).
- Select foods rich in omega-3 fatty acids (see Chapter 5).
- Consume a diet high in vegetables, fruits, nuts, seeds, and whole grains and low in refined grain products.

Such a diet combined with exercise, weight control, and not smoking serves as the best prescription for health. Notably, taking supplements is not among these disease-prevention recommendations.

Some research suggests a protective effect from as little as a daily glass of orange juice or carrot juice (rich sources of vitamin C and beta-carotene, respectively). Other intervention studies, however, have used levels of nutrients that far exceed current recommendations and can be achieved only by taking supplements. In making their recommendations for the antioxidant nutrients, members of the DRI Committee considered whether these studies support substantially higher intakes to help protect against chronic diseases. They did raise the recommendations for vitamins C and E, but they do not support taking vitamin pills over eating a healthy diet. Based on the 2004 Canadian Community Health Survey,[19] as a whole the Canadian population gets 32 percent of its vitamin C from fruit juices and another 11 percent from fruit drinks. Citrus fruits follow in third place representing 7 percent of vitamin C intake from foods. Collectively, these three foods provide about half of the vitamin C intake of Canadians. Overall, about 17 percent of the population does not meet the recommended intake for vitamin C. For the 31 percent of Canadians who take vitamin C supplements, an inadequate intake of vitamin C is virtually eliminated. Despite ensuring adequate vitamin C intakes for many people, the use of supplements cannot replace the synergistic effects found among the multiple nutrients and phytochemicals provided by foods.

While awaiting additional research, should people anticipate the "go-ahead" and start taking antioxidant supplements now? Most scientists agree that the evidence is insufficient for such a recommendation.[20] Those finding sufficient evidence discourage supplement use.[21] Though fruits and vegetables containing many antioxidant nutrients and phytochemicals have been associated with a diminished risk of many cancers, supplements have not always proved beneficial. In fact, sometimes the benefits are more apparent when the vitamins come from foods rather than from supplements. In other words, the antioxidant actions of fruits and vegetables are greater than their nutrients alone can explain. Without data to confirm the benefits of supplements, we cannot accept the potential risks.[22] And the risks are real.

Consider the findings from a meta-analysis of the relationships between supplements of vitamin A, vitamin E, beta-carotene, or combinations and total mortality. Researchers concluded that supplements either had *no benefit* or *increased* mortality and should

TABLE H12-1 Vitamin Antioxidants and Chronic Disease Risk

Antioxidant	Disease	Risk from Foods	Risk from Supplements
Vitamin C	Coronary heart disease	Inconsistent results	Inconsistent results
	Breast cancer	Inconsistent results	—
	Colorectal cancer	Inconsistent results	—
	Gastrointestinal cancer	—	Not known
	Lung cancer	No effect	Not known
Vitamin E	Coronary heart disease	Inconsistent results	No effect or possible increased risk
	Breast cancer	—	No effect
	Colorectal cancer	Inconsistent results	—
	Gastrointestinal cancer	—	No effect
	Lung cancer	No effect	No effect
	Prostate cancer	Decreased risk	Decreased risk in smokers
Beta-carotene	Coronary heart disease	Decreased risk	No effect in nonsmokers, increased risk in smokers
	Lung cancer	Inconsistent results	No effect in nonsmokers, increased risk in smokers
	Colorectal cancer	Decreased risk	—
	Gastrointestinal cancer	—	No effect
	Prostate cancer	No effect	—
Other carotenoids	Lung cancer	Decreased risk for beta-cryptoxanthin	—
	Colorectal cancer	Decreased risk	—
	Prostate cancer	Decreased risk for lycopene	—
Vegetables and fruit	Coronary heart disease	Decreased risk	
	Breast cancer	No effect	
	Colorectal cancer	Inconsistent results	
	Gastric and esophageal cancer	Decreased risk	
	Lung cancer	Decreased risk for fruits, no effect for vegetables	
	Prostate cancer	No effect	
Supplement containing a combination of antioxidants	Coronary heart disease		Possibly increased risk
	Gastroinestinal cancer		Possibly increased risk
	Lung cancer		No effect in nonsmokers, increased risk in smokers

SOURCE: Verhagen, et al., "The State of Antioxidant Affairs", Nutrition Today (41), 2006, pp. 244–249. Reprinted by permission.

be avoided.[23] In fact, beta-carotene *enhances* the risk of lung cancer in smokers by increasing the formation of free radicals.[24]

Similarly, studies using mineral antioxidant supplements (e.g., selenium) have provided inconclusive evidence of reducing risk of chronic diseases. The Selenium and Vitamin E Cancer Prevention Trial was stopped early after five years due to no evidence of the supplements preventing prostate cancer. In fact, there was a nonsignificant but slight increased rate of prostate cancer in the men who were supplemented with vitamin E and a nonsignificant but slightly increased rate of diabetes in the men who were taking the selenium supplements.[25]

Even if research clearly proves that a particular nutrient is the ultimate protective ingredient in foods, supplements would not be the answer because their contents are limited. Vitamin E supplements, for example, usually contain alpha-tocopherol, but foods provide an assortment of tocopherols among other nutrients, many of which provide valuable protection against free-radical damage. In addition to a full array of nutrients, foods provide phytochemicals that also fight against many diseases. Supplements shortchange users. Furthermore, supplements should be used only as an adjunct to other measures such as smoking cessation, weight control, physical activity, and medication as needed.

Clearly, much more research is needed to define optimal and dangerous levels of intake. This much we know: antioxidants behave differently under various conditions. At physiological levels typical of a healthy diet, they act as antioxidants, but at pharmacological doses typical of supplements, they may act as prooxidants, stimulating the production of free radicals and altering metabolism in a way that may promote disease. A high intake of vitamin C from supplements, for example, may *increase* the risk of heart disease in women with diabetes. Until the optimum intake of antioxidant nutrients can be determined, the risks of supplement use remain unclear. Table H12-1 presents a summary of the relationships between vitamin antioxidants and chronic diseases—sorted by foods or supplements.[26] As you can see, many studies report either no effect or inconsistent results. Any decrease in risk is attributed to foods 9 out of 10 times. Any increase in risk is always from supplements, and often in smokers. Clearly, the best way to add antioxidants to the diet is to eat generous servings of vegetables and fruits daily.

It should be clear by now that we cannot know the identity and action of every chemical in every food. Even if we did, why create a supplement to replicate a food? Why not eat foods and enjoy the pleasure, nourishment, and health benefits they provide? The beneficial constituents in foods are widespread among plants. Among the fruits, pomegranates, berries, and citrus rank high in antioxidants; top antioxidant vegetables include kale, spinach, and Brussels sprouts; millet and oats contain the most antioxidants among the grains; pinto beans and soybeans are the outstanding legumes; and walnuts outshine the other nuts. But don't try to single out one particular food for its "magical" nutrient, antioxidant, or phytochemical. Instead, eat a wide variety of vegetables, fruits, grains, legumes, nuts, and seeds every day—and get *all* the benefits these foods have to offer.

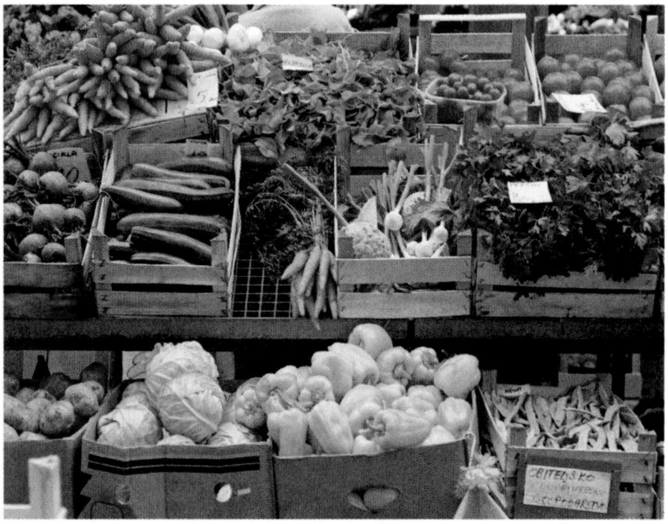

Baloncici/shutterstock

Many cancer-fighting products are available now at your local produce counter.

References

1. H. Verhagen and coauthors, The state of antioxidant affairs, *Nutrition Today* 41 (2006): 244–250; A. J. McEligot, S. Yang, and F. L. Meyskens, Redox regulation by intrinsic species and extrinsic nutrients in normal and cancer cells, *Annual Review of Nutrition* 25 (2005): 261–295.
2. M. V. Catani and coauthors, Biological role of vitamin C in keratinocytes, *Nutrition Reviews* 63 (2005): 81–90.
3. A. L. Webb and E. Villamor, Update: Effects of antioxidant and non-antioxidant vitamin supplementation on immune function, *Nutrition Reviews* 65 (2007): 181–217.
4. D. P. Hayes, The protective role of fruits and vegetables against radiation-induced cancer, *Nutrition Reviews* 63 (2005): 303–311.
5. Q. Chen and coauthors, Pharmacologic doses of ascorbate act as a prooxidant and decrease growth of aggressive tumor xenografts in mice, *Proceedings of the National Academy of Sciences* 105 (2008): 11105–11109.
6. D. Q. Pham and R. Plakogiannis, Vitamin E supplementation in cardiovascular disease and cancer prevention: Part 1, *Annals of Pharmacotherapy* 39 (2005): 1870–1878.
7. X. Zhao and coauthors, Modification of lymphocyte DNA damage by carotenoid supplementation in postmenopausal women, *American Journal of Clinical Nutrition* 83 (2006): 163–169.
8. S. C. Larsson and coauthors, Vitamin A, retinol, and carotenoids and the risk of gastric cancer: A prospective cohort study, *American Journal of Clinical Nutrition* 85 (2007): 497–503; B. Buijsse and coauthors, Plasma carotene and α-tocopherol in relation to 10-y all-cause and cause-specific mortality in European elderly: The Survey in Europe on Nutrition and the Elderly, a Concerted Action (SENECA), *American Journal of Clinical Nutrition* 82 (2005): 879–886.
9. L. Gallicchio and coauthors, Carotenoids and the risk of developing lung cancer: A systematic review, *American Journal of Clinical Nutrition* 88 (2008): 372–383.
10. I. Zwolak and H. Zaporowska, Selenium interactions and toxicity: A review, *Cell Biology and Toxicology* 27 (2011): doi: 10.1007/s10565-011-9203-9.

11. M. I. Jackson and G. F. Combs Jr, Selenium and anticarcinogenesis: Underlying mechanisms, *Current Opinion in Clinical Nutrition and Metabolic Care* 11 (2008): 718–726; L. Novotny, P. Rauko, S. B. Kombian, and I. O. Edafiogho, Selenium as a chemoprotective anti-cancer agent: Reality or wishful thinking? *Neoplasma* 57 (2010): 383–391.
12. J. Zingg, A. Azzi, and M. Meydani, Genetic polymorphisms as determinants for disease-preventive effects of vitamin E, *Nutrition Reviews* 66 (2008): 406–414; S. Devaraj and coauthors, Effect of high-dose α-tocopherol supplementation on biomarkers of oxidative stress and inflammation and carotid atherosclerosis in patients with coronary artery disease, *American Journal of Clinical Nutrition* 86 (2007): 1392–1398.
13. U. Singh, S. Devaraj, and I. Jialal, Vitamin E, oxidative stress, and inflammation, *Annual Review of Nutrition* 25 (2005): 151–174.
14. S. G. Wannamethee and coauthors, Associations of vitamin C status, fruit and vegetable intakes, and markers of inflammation and hemostasis, *American Journal of Clinical Nutrition* 83 (2006): 567–574.
15. N. R. Cook and coauthors, A randomized factorial trial of vitamins C and E and beta carotene in the secondary prevention of cardiovascular events in women: Results from the Women's Antioxidant Cardiovascular Study, *Archives of Internal Medicine* 167 (2007): 1610–1618; The HOPE and HOPE-TOO Investigators, Effects of long-term vitamin E supplementation on cardiovascular events and cancer: A randomized controlled trial, *Journal of the American Medical Association* 293 (2005): 1338–1347.
16. S. Stranges and coauthors, Associations of selenium status with cardiometabolic risk factors: An 8-year follow-up analysis of the Olivetti Heart Study, *Atherosclerosis* 217 (2011): 274–278; S. Stranges and coauthors, Higher selenium status is associated with adverse blood lipid profile in British adults, *Journal of Nutrition* 140 (2010): 81–87; M. Laclaustra and coauthors, Serum selenium and serum lipids in US adults: National Health and Nutrition Examination Survey (NHANES) 2003–2004, *Atherosclerosis* 210 (2010): 643–648.
17. M. Rayman and coauthors, Effect of supplementation with high-selenium yeast on plasma lipids: A randomized trial, *Annals of Internal Medicine* 154 (2011): 656–665.
18. A. Agudo and coauthors, Fruit and vegetable intakes, dietary antioxidant nutrients, and total mortality in Spanish adults: Findings from the Spanish cohort of the European Prospective Investigation into Cancer and Nutrition (EPIC-Spain), *American Journal of Clinical Nutrition* 85 (2007): 1634–1642.
19. D. Garriguet, The effect of supplement use on vitamin C intake, *Health Reports* 21 (2010): 1–6.
20. H. Y. Huang and coauthors, The efficacy and safety of multivitamin and mineral supplement use to prevent cancer and chronic disease in adults: A systematic review for a National Institutes of Health state-of-the-science conference, *Annals of Internal Medicine* 145 (2006): 372–385.
21. D. Q. Pham and R. Plakogiannis, Vitamin E supplementation in cardiovascular disease and cancer prevention: Part 1, *Annals of Pharmacotherapy* 39 (2005): 1870–1878.
22. S. Hercberg, The history of β-Carotene and cancers: From observational to intervention studies. What lessons can be drawn for future research on polyphenols? *American Journal of Clinical Nutrition* 81 (2005): 218S–222S.
23. G. Bjelakovic and coauthors, Mortality in randomized trials of antioxidant supplements for primary and secondary prevention: Systematic review and meta-analysis, *Journal of the American Medical Association* 297 (2007): 842–857; I. Lee and coauthors, Vitamin E in the primary prevention of cardiovascular disease and cancer: The Women's Health Study: A randomized controlled trial, *Journal of the American Medical Association* 294 (2005): 56–65; E. R. Miller and coauthors, Meta-analysis: High-dosage vitamin E supplementation may increase all-cause mortality, *Annals of Internal Medicine* 142 (2005): 37–46.
24. Y. G. J. van Helden and coauthors, β-Carotene metabolites enhance inflammation-induced oxidative DNA damage in lung epithelial cells, *Free Radical Biology and Medicine* 46 (2009): 299–304.
25. S. M. Lippman and coauthors, Effect of selenium and vitamin E on risk of prostate cancer and other cancers: The Selenium and Vitamin E Cancer Prevention Trial (SELECT), *Journal of the American Medical Association* 301 (2009): 39–51.
26. Verhagen and coauthors, 2006.

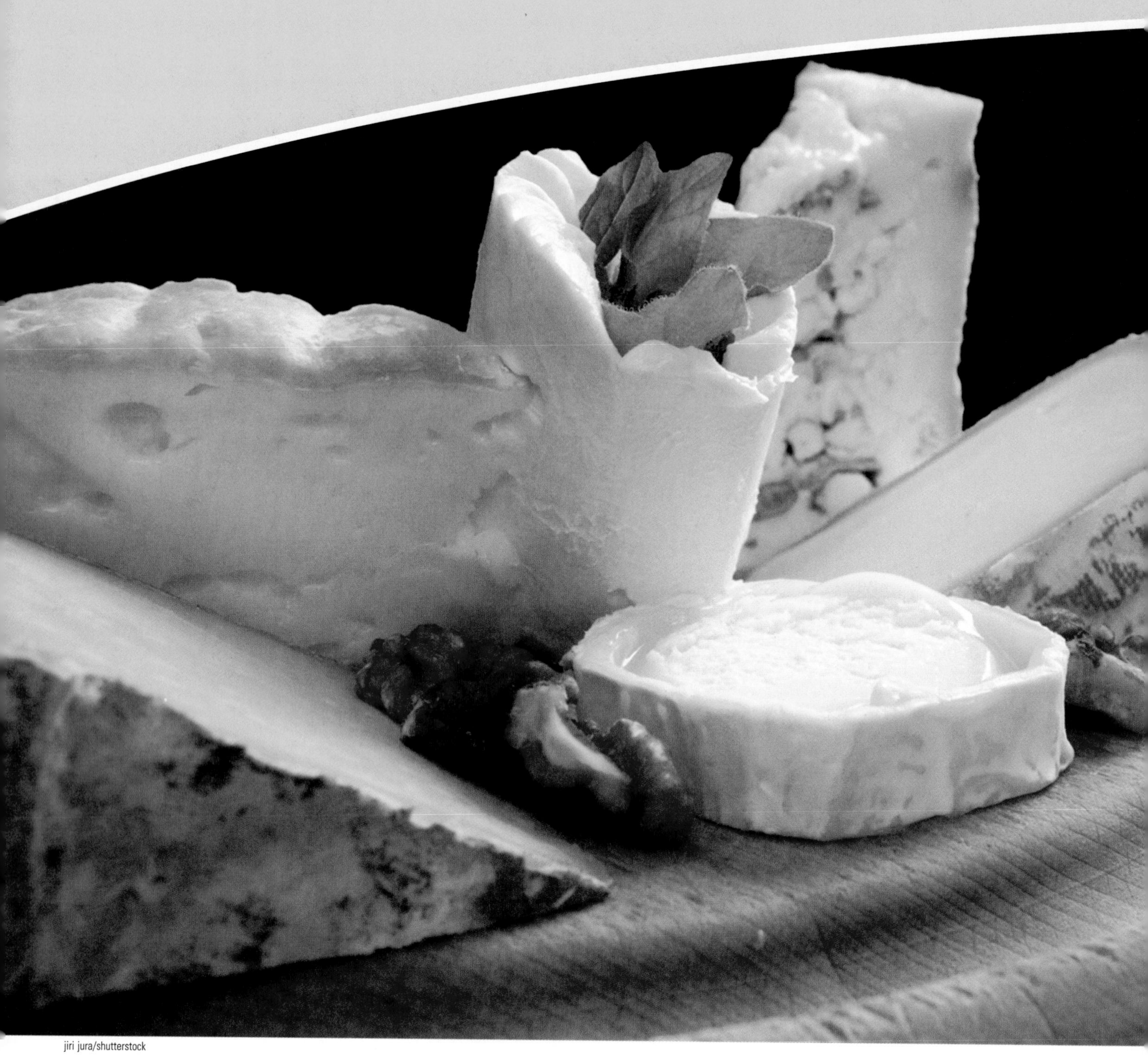

jiri jura/shutterstock

CENGAGENOW™

Throughout this chapter, the CengageNOW logo indicates an opportunity for online self-study, linking you to interactive tutorials, activities, and videos to increase your understanding of chapter concepts.
www.cengage.com/sso

Nutrition in Your Life

What's your beverage of choice? If you said water, then congratulate yourself for recognizing its importance in hydrating your body. If you answered milk, then pat yourself on the back for taking good care of your bones while hydrating your body. Milk is naturally rich in calcium and phosphorus, and vitamin D is added to all milks sold in Canada. The consequences of a lack of calcium-rich foods can have dramatic effects on your bones that may not become apparent for decades. Your bone health depends on the minerals calcium, phosphorus, magnesium, and fluoride and the fat-soluble vitamins A, D, and K. Before getting too comfortable reading this chapter, pour yourself a tall glass of nourishing milk. Your bones will thank you!

CHAPTER 13

Nutrients for Bone Health

CHAPTER OUTLINE

About Bones

What have you done for your bones today? Perhaps you poured yourself a tall glass of milk, had yogurt at breakfast, or participated in a weight-training class during your lunch hour. Or, perhaps you had canned salmon in your sandwich or took a brisk walk across campus to get to class. Many dietary, exercise, and other lifestyle choices are important to bone health. Regardless of your age, it's up to you to make choices that will benefit your bones.

If you make healthy choices that maximize your bone mineral density while you are young, you can reduce your risk for developing the bone-deficiency disease, osteoporosis, when you are older. Although calcium is the nutrient most commonly associated with bone health, the minerals phosphorus, magnesium, and fluoride are also important. And not only minerals—vitamins A, D, and K have important roles in the development and maintenance of your skeletal system. Chapter 12 described vitamin A and its role in the bone remodelling process. In this chapter, you will learn that calcium, phosphorus, magnesium, and fluoride are used to form mineral crystals that give bone its strength; vitamin D is required for the activation of transporter proteins that enhance the absorption of calcium, phosphorus, and magnesium; and vitamin K is required for the activation of a protein that binds to the minerals during the formation of bone. But before we study the roles of nutrients in bone health, let's take a brief look at bone composition, growth, and shaping; the general importance of bones; and what we can do to benefit our bone health.

What Makes Up My Bones? Bones are composed of about 65 percent inorganic matter in the form of mineral crystals that are deposited onto a protein (collagen) matrix, which accounts for the remaining 35 percent of bone matter. The inorganic mineral composition of bone provides *strength* and structural support to keep us upright and protects our internal organs. The organic collagen portion of bone allows *flexibility*, which is important during times of applied stress such as when jumping or walking. **Bone mineral density** is the term used to describe how tightly the mineral crystals are packed into your protein matrix, and is used to indicate bone strength. In effect, it is a ratio of your bone mineral content to your bone size. Dual energy X-ray absorptiometry accurately measures your bone mineral density and is often used to determine your risk for osteoporosis.

bone mineral density: a measure of bone strength. When minerals fill the bone matrix (making it dense), they give it strength.

Bone consists of two tissue types: **cortical bone** and **trabecular bone**. Detailed in Highlight 13, but in brief here, cortical bone is a very dense and ivory-like tissue that provides strength along the outer wall of larger bones and constitutes the main tissue of smaller bones. Trabecular bone is more susceptible to changes in circulating hormone levels and more readily releases minerals from its lacy, less-dense architecture. Over the life span, an excessive loss of bone can lead to osteoporosis, a disease most often associated with calcium deficiency. Osteoporosis and calcium are the focus of Highlight 13.

In What Ways Are My Bones Metabolically Active? Contrary to what most people think, your skeleton is a metabolically active organ system that is constantly being broken down and rebuilt. In fact, when you go to sleep, you lose bone overnight and when you get up, nourish your body, and move about, you rebuild your overnight losses. When we look at the processes taking place in bone, it is not surprising to see why bones are so metabolically active.

When you think of red blood cells, do you think of your bones? Perhaps not, but the bone marrow deep within your long bones is the site for synthesizing red blood cells that are needed to transport oxygen from our lungs to our cells to generate energy. Have you ever thought that nerves and blood vessels run through your bones? Indeed, nerves and blood vessels are integral components that support bone activity and help to maintain bone health. These are a few of the processes that happen in bones.

How Do My Bones Grow? Your bones are genetically programmed to grow in length from the time you are conceived into your teen years. Bone mineral density also accrues during these years and can extend into young adulthood. The process of bone lengthening tends to stop earlier for girls who commonly reach their adult height around 14 years of age than for boys who typically reach adult height a little later, around 17 years of age. Concurrent with periods of bone *growth*, the ongoing process of bone *modelling* determines the shape of our bones. In this process, enzymes in the **osteoclasts** of bone degrade parts of bone that are then filled in with new bone by enzymes found in the **osteoblasts**. Once bones have reached their adult size and shape, the process of *remodelling* occurs throughout the remainder of life. Remodelling helps to repair microdamage that happens to bone and strengthens areas of bone that receive physical force, such as when playing sports. Over our adult lives, osteoblast cells gradually lose their activity while osteoclast cells remain active, resulting in a natural process of bone loss. The rate at which we lose bone will depend on genetic factors that we can't control and other factors that we can control.

What Can I Do for My Bones? It is never too late to start taking care of your bones! Whether you are in your teens, twenties, or older, you can make dietary, exercise, and lifestyle choices that will benefit your bones. When you choose a varied and well-balanced diet containing all of the bone-health nutrients, pay particular attention to consuming adequate intakes of calcium and vitamin D. When your calcium and vitamin D intakes are inadequate, use a supplement until your dietary intake meets your recommended intake level. Make some of your exercise choices weight-bearing types of activities, such as walking, jogging, jumping, ball sports, and racquet sports, to name a few. Try to minimize alcohol consumption and smoking, as both are toxic to bone. Choose alcohol in moderation, if at all, and quit the habit if you smoke. Other lifestyle factors that benefit your bones include getting adequate sleep, reducing your stress level, and achieving a healthy body weight. The time to start taking care of your bones is today. So, get a good night's sleep, grab a yogurt, and get off the bus one or two stops early.

Calcium

Calcium is the most abundant mineral in the body. It receives much emphasis in this chapter and in the highlight that follows because an adequate intake helps grow a healthy skeleton in early life and minimize bone loss in later life.

cortical bone: the very dense bone tissue that forms the outer shell surrounding trabecular bone and comprises the shaft of a long bone.

trabecular bone: the lacy inner structure of calcium crystals that supports the bone's structure and provides a calcium storage bank.

osteoclasts: cells that destroy bone during growth.

osteoblasts: cells that build bone during growth.

calcium: the most abundant mineral in the body; found primarily in the body's bones and teeth.

Calcium Roles in the Body Ninety-nine percent of the body's calcium is in the bones (and teeth), where it plays two roles. First, it is an integral part of bone structure, providing a rigid frame that holds the body upright and serves as attachment points for muscles, making motion possible. Second, it serves as a calcium bank, offering a readily available source of the mineral to the body fluids should a drop in blood calcium occur. The remaining 1 percent of the body's calcium is in the body fluids.

Calcium in Bones As bones begin to form, calcium salts form crystals, called **hydroxyapatite**, on a matrix of the protein collagen. During **mineralization**, as the crystals become denser, they give strength and rigidity to the maturing bones. As a result, the long leg bones of children can support their weight by the time they have learned to walk.

Many people have the idea that once a bone is built, it is inert like a rock. Actually, the bones are gaining and losing minerals continuously in an ongoing process of remodelling. Growing children gain more bone than they lose, and healthy adults maintain a reasonable balance. When withdrawals substantially exceed deposits, problems such as osteoporosis develop (as described in Highlight 13).

The formation of teeth follows a pattern similar to that of bones. The turnover of minerals in teeth is not as rapid as in bone, however; fluoride hardens and stabilizes the crystals of teeth, opposing the withdrawal of minerals from them.

Calcium in Body Fluids Although only 1 percent of the body's calcium circulates in the extracellular and intracellular fluids, its presence there is vital to life. Cells throughout the body can detect calcium in the extracellular fluids and respond accordingly. Many of calcium's actions help to maintain normal blood pressure, perhaps by stabilizing the smooth muscle cells of the blood vessels or by releasing relaxing factors from the blood vessel cell walls.[1] Extracellular calcium also participates in blood clotting.

The calcium in intracellular fluids binds to proteins within the cells and activates them. ♦ These proteins participate in the regulation of muscle contractions, the transmission of nerve impulses, the secretion of hormones, and the activation of some enzyme reactions.

Calcium and Disease Prevention Calcium may protect against hypertension, although research results are inconsistent and inconclusive.[2] Considering the success of the Dietary Approaches to Stop Hypertension (DASH) diet in lowering blood pressure, restricting sodium to treat hypertension may be narrow advice. The DASH diet is not particularly low in sodium, but it is rich in calcium, as well as in magnesium and potassium. As mentioned earlier, the DASH diet, together with a reduced sodium intake, is more effective in lowering blood pressure than either strategy alone. Some research also suggests

♦ An example of a protein that calcium binds with and activates is **calmodulin** (cal-MOD-you-lin). One of calmodulin's roles is to activate the enzymes involved in breaking down glycogen, which releases energy for muscle contractions.

hydroxyapatite (high-drox-ee-APP-ah-tite): crystals made of calcium and phosphorus.

mineralization: the process in which calcium, phosphorus, and other minerals crystallize on the collagen matrix of a growing bone, hardening the bone.

FIGURE 13-1 Calcium Balance

CENGAGENOW™ Animated! figure www.cengage.com/sso

Blood calcium is regulated in part by vitamin D and two hormones—calcitonin and parathyroid hormone. Bone serves as a reservoir when blood calcium is high and as a source of calcium when blood calcium is low. Osteoclasts break down bone and release calcium into the blood; osteoblasts build new bone using calcium from the blood.

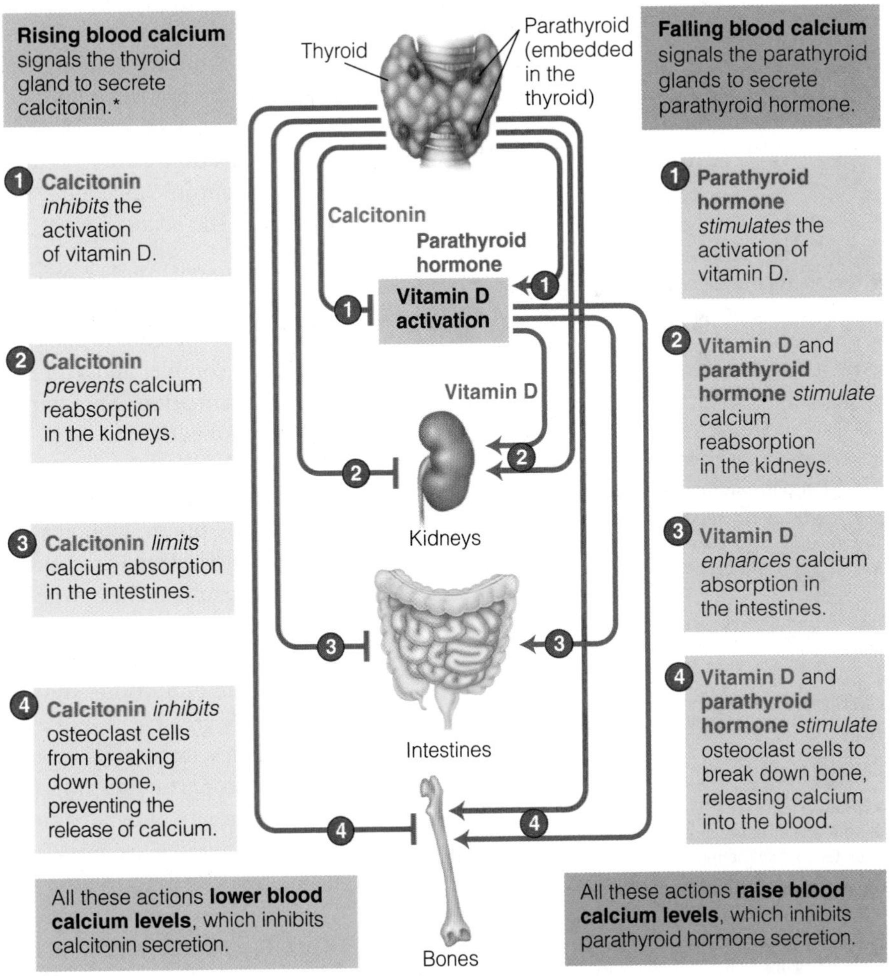
Rising blood calcium signals the thyroid gland to secrete calcitonin.*
Thyroid
Parathyroid (embedded in the thyroid)
Falling blood calcium signals the parathyroid glands to secrete parathyroid hormone.
1 Calcitonin inhibits the activation of vitamin D.
Calcitonin
Parathyroid hormone
Vitamin D activation
1 Parathyroid hormone stimulates the activation of vitamin D.
2 Calcitonin prevents calcium reabsorption in the kidneys.
Vitamin D
Kidneys
2 Vitamin D and parathyroid hormone stimulate calcium reabsorption in the kidneys.
3 Calcitonin limits calcium absorption in the intestines.
3 Vitamin D enhances calcium absorption in the intestines.
Intestines
4 Calcitonin inhibits osteoclast cells from breaking down bone, preventing the release of calcium.
4 Vitamin D and parathyroid hormone stimulate osteoclast cells to break down bone, releasing calcium into the blood.
All these actions lower blood calcium levels, which inhibits calcitonin secretion.
Bones
All these actions raise blood calcium levels, which inhibits parathyroid hormone secretion.

*Calcitonin plays a major role in defending infants and young children against the dangers of rising blood calcium that can occur when regular feedings of milk deliver large quantities of calcium to a small body. In contrast, calcitonin plays a relatively minor role in adults because their absorption of calcium is less efficient and their bodies are larger, making elevated blood calcium unlikely.

FIGURE 13-2 Maintaining Blood Calcium from the Diet and from the Bones

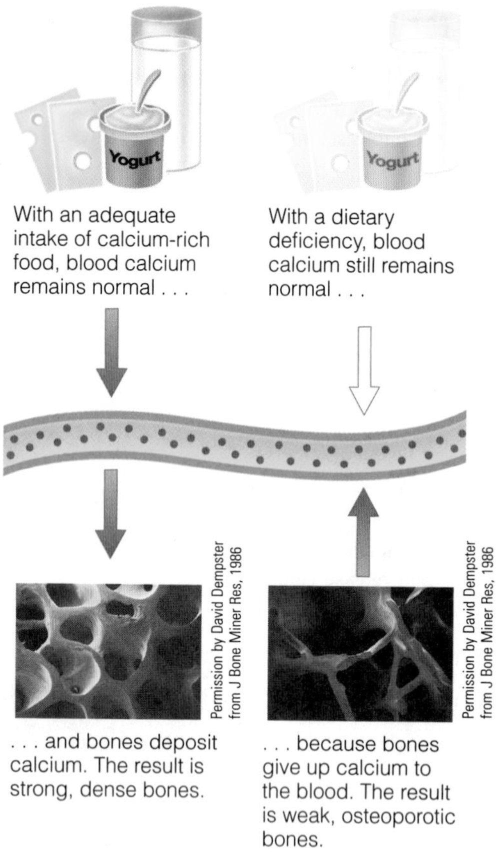
Yogurt
Yogurt
With an adequate intake of calcium-rich food, blood calcium remains normal . . .
With a dietary deficiency, blood calcium still remains normal . . .
Permission by David Dempster from J Bone Miner Res, 1986
Permission by David Dempster from J Bone Miner Res, 1986
. . . and bones deposit calcium. The result is strong, dense bones.
. . . because bones give up calcium to the blood. The result is weak, osteoporotic bones.

protective relationships between dietary calcium and blood cholesterol, diabetes, and colon cancer.[3] Highlight 13 explores calcium's role in preventing osteoporosis.

Calcium and Body Weight Calcium may also play a role in maintaining a healthy body weight.[4] Epidemiological studies suggest an inverse relationship between calcium intake and body weight: the higher the calcium intake, the lower the prevalence of overweight. In particular, calcium from dairy foods, but *not* from supplements, seems to influence body weight.[5] An adequate dietary calcium intake may help prevent excessive fat accumulation by stimulating hormonal action that targets the breakdown of stored fat. Not all research suggests that consumption of calcium or dairy foods alters fat metabolism or energy expenditure or improves body weight or composition.[6] Large, well-designed clinical studies are needed to clarify the effects of dietary calcium intake on body weight.

Calcium Balance Calcium homeostasis involves a system of hormones and vitamin D.[7] Whenever blood calcium falls too low or rises too high, three organ systems respond: the intestines, bones, and kidneys. Figure 13-1 (p. 411) illustrates how vitamin D and two hormones—**parathyroid hormone** and **calcitonin**—return blood calcium to normal.

The calcium in bone provides a nearly inexhaustible bank of calcium for the blood. The blood borrows and returns calcium as needed so that even with a dietary deficiency, *blood* calcium remains normal—even as *bone* calcium diminishes (see Figure 13-2). Blood calcium changes only in response to abnormal regulatory control, not to diet. A person can have an inadequate calcium intake for years and suffer no noticeable symptoms. Only later in life does it become apparent that bone integrity has been compromised.

Blood calcium above normal results in **calcium rigour**: the muscles contract and cannot relax. Similarly, blood calcium below normal causes **calcium tetany**—also characterized by uncontrolled muscle contraction. These conditions do *not* reflect a *dietary* excess or lack of calcium; they are caused by a lack of vitamin D or by abnormal secretion of the regulatory hormones. A chronic *dietary* deficiency of calcium, or a chronic deficiency due to poor absorption over the years, depletes the bones. Again: the *bones*, not the blood, are robbed by a calcium deficiency.

Calcium Absorption Because many factors affect calcium absorption, the most effective way to ensure adequacy is to increase calcium intake.[8] On average, adults absorb about 30 percent of the calcium they ingest. The stomach's acidity helps to keep calcium soluble, and vitamin D helps to make the **calcium-binding protein** needed for absorption. This explains why calcium-rich milk is the best food for vitamin D fortification.

Whenever calcium is needed, the body increases its production of the calcium-binding protein to improve calcium absorption. The result is obvious in the case of a pregnant woman, who absorbs 50 percent of the calcium from the milk she drinks. Similarly, growing children and teens absorb 50 to 60 percent of the calcium they consume. Then, when bone growth slows or stops, absorption falls to the adult level of about 30 percent. In addition, absorption becomes more efficient during times of inadequate intakes.

Many of the conditions that enhance calcium absorption inhibit its absorption when they are absent. For example, sufficient vitamin D supports absorption, and a deficiency impairs it. In addition, fibre, in general, and the binders phytate and oxalate, in particular, interfere with calcium absorption, but their effects are relatively minor in typical Canadian diets. Vegetables with oxalates and whole grains with phytates are nutritious foods, of course, but they are not useful calcium sources. The margin note ♦ presents factors that influence calcium balance.

♦ Factors that *enhance* calcium absorption:

- Stomach acid
- Vitamin D
- Lactose (in infants only)

Factors that *inhibit* calcium absorption:

- Lack of stomach acid
- Vitamin D deficiency
- High phosphorus intake
- Phytates (in seeds, nuts, grains)
- Oxalates (in beet greens, rhubarb, spinach, sweet potatoes)

Calcium Deficiency

A low calcium intake during the growing years limits the bones' ability to reach their optimal mass and density. Most people achieve a peak bone mass by their late 20s, and dense bones best protect against age-related bone loss and fractures (see Figure 13-3). All adults lose bone as they grow older, beginning between the ages of 30 and 40. When bone losses reach the point

parathyroid hormone: a hormone from the parathyroid glands that regulates blood calcium by raising it when levels fall too low; also known as *parathormone* (PAIR-ah-THOR-moan).

calcitonin (KAL-seh-TOE-nin): a hormone secreted by the thyroid gland that regulates blood calcium by lowering it when levels rise too high.

calcium rigour: hardness or stiffness of the muscles caused by high blood calcium concentrations.

calcium tetany (TET-ah-nee): intermittent spasm of the extremities due to nervous and muscular excitability caused by low blood calcium concentrations.

calcium-binding protein: a protein in the intestinal cells, made with the help of vitamin D, that facilitates calcium absorption.

FIGURE 13-3 Phases of Bone Development throughout Life

The active growth phase occurs from birth to approximately age 20. The next phase of peak bone mass development occurs between the ages of 12 and 30. The final phase, when bone resorption exceeds formation, begins between the ages of 30 and 40 and continues through the remainder of life.

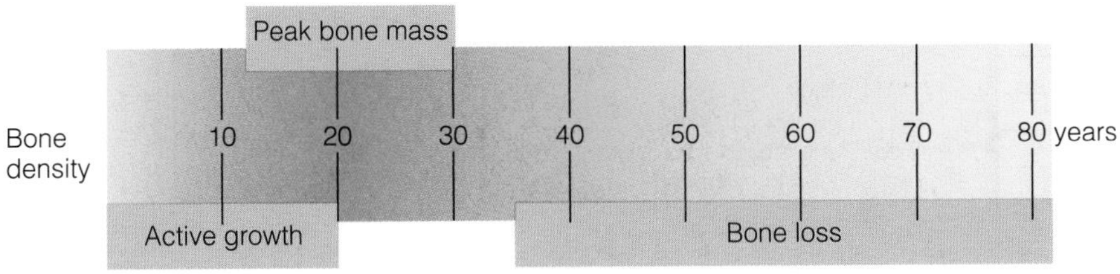
Peak bone mass
Bone density
10
20
30
40
50
60
70
80 years
Active growth
Bone loss

of causing fractures under common, everyday stresses, the condition is known as **osteoporosis**. Almost two million Canadians—about one in four women (mostly older women) and at least one in eight men over the age of 50—are living with osteoporosis.[9]

Unlike many diseases that make themselves known through symptoms such as pain, shortness of breath, skin lesions, tiredness, and the like, osteoporosis is silent. The body sends no signals saying bones are losing their calcium and, as a result, their integrity. Blood samples offer no clues because blood calcium remains normal regardless of bone content, and measures of bone density may not be routinely taken until later in life. Highlight 13 suggests strategies to protect against bone loss, of which eating calcium-rich foods is only one.

Calcium Recommendations and Sources

Calcium is unlike most other nutrients in that hormones maintain its *blood* concentration regardless of dietary intake. As Figure 13-2 shows, when calcium intake is high, the *bones* benefit; when intake is low, the *bones* suffer. Calcium recommendations are therefore based on the amount needed to retain the most calcium in bones. By retaining the most calcium possible, the bones can develop to their fullest potential in size and density—their **peak bone mass**—within genetic limits.

Calcium Recommendations Calcium recommendations have been set high enough to accommodate a 30 percent absorption rate. Because obtaining enough calcium during growth helps to ensure that the skeleton will be strong and dense, the recommendation for adolescents up to the age of 18 years is 1300 milligrams daily. Between the ages of 19 and 50 for all adults, and males between the ages of 51 and 70 years, recommendations are lowered to 1000 milligrams a day; for females between the ages of 51 and 70 years, and all adults 71 years or older, recommendations are raised again to 1200 milligrams a day to minimize the bone loss that tends to occur later in life. Some authorities advocate as much as 1500 milligrams a day for women older than 50. Although males fare better than females, many adult Canadians have calcium intakes below current recommendations.[10] High intakes of calcium from supplements may have adverse effects such as kidney stone formation.[11] For this reason, a UL has been established. ♦

♦ UL for calcium: 2500 mg/day

High intakes of both dietary protein and sodium increase calcium losses, but whether these losses impair bone development remains unclear. In the case of protein, high intakes of either animal or plant proteins may be problematic, but the effects are minimized by the beneficial effects of other nutrients in the food and diet—for example, by the potassium in legumes and the calcium in milk. In establishing a Recommended Dietary Allowance (RDA) for calcium, the DRI Committee considered these nutrient interactions and did not adjust dietary recommendations based on this information.

Calcium in Milk Products Figure 13-4 (p. 414) shows that calcium is found most abundantly in a single class of foods—milk. ♦ The person who doesn't like to

♦ Suggested daily *Food Guide* servings of Milk and Alternatives:

- Young children (2 to 8 yr): 2 servings each day
- Older children and teenagers: (9 to 18 yr): 3–4 servings each day
- Adults (19 to 50 yr): 2 servings each day
- Adults (51+ yr): 3 servings each day

osteoporosis (OS-tee-oh-pore-OH-sis): a disease in which the bones become porous and fragile due to a loss of minerals; also called *adult bone loss.*

- **osteo** = bone
- **porosis** = porous

peak bone mass: the highest attainable bone density for an individual, developed during the first three decades of life.

FIGURE 13-4 **Calcium in Selected Foods**

See the "How To" section on p. 317 for more information on using this figure.

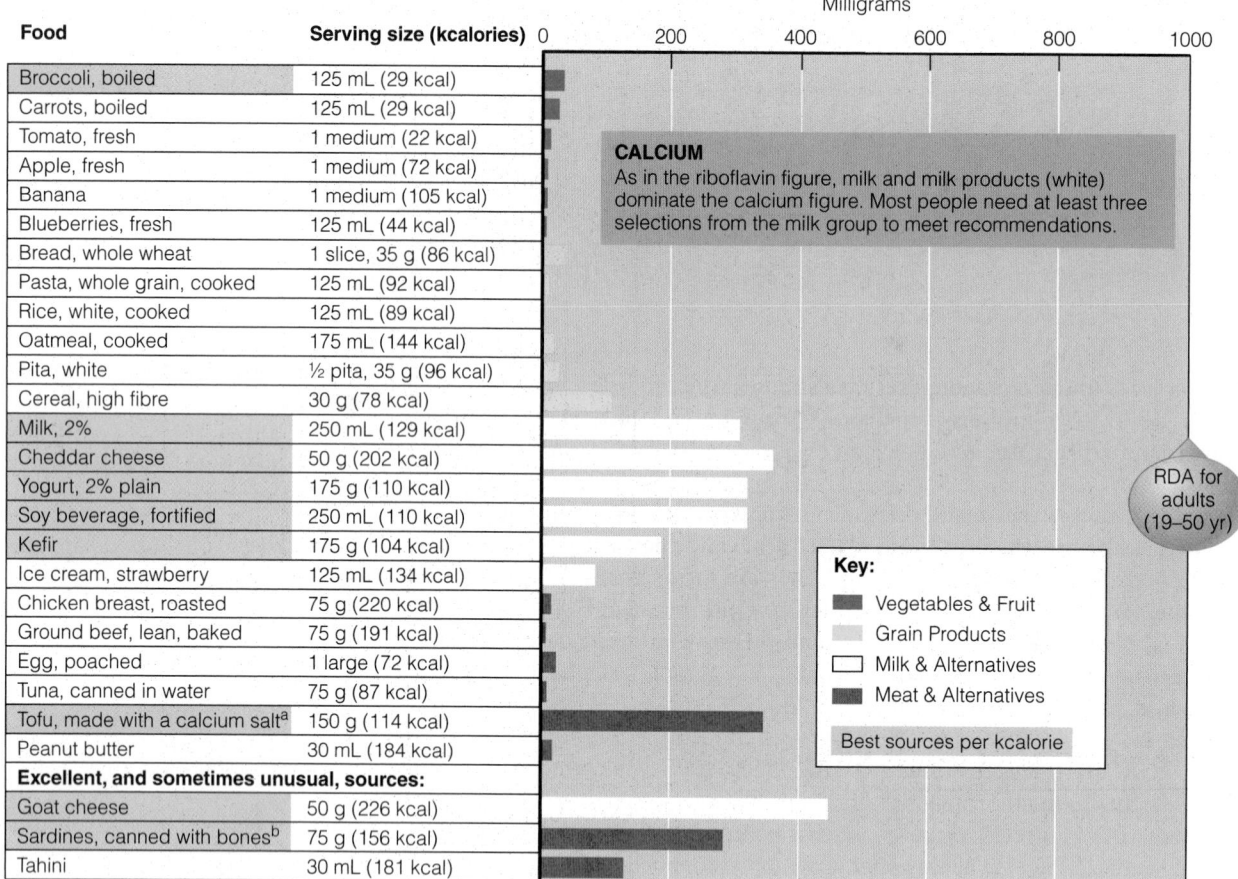

Food	Serving size (kcalories)
Broccoli, boiled	125 mL (29 kcal)
Carrots, boiled	125 mL (29 kcal)
Tomato, fresh	1 medium (22 kcal)
Apple, fresh	1 medium (72 kcal)
Banana	1 medium (105 kcal)
Blueberries, fresh	125 mL (44 kcal)
Bread, whole wheat	1 slice, 35 g (86 kcal)
Pasta, whole grain, cooked	125 mL (92 kcal)
Rice, white, cooked	125 mL (89 kcal)
Oatmeal, cooked	175 mL (144 kcal)
Pita, white	½ pita, 35 g (96 kcal)
Cereal, high fibre	30 g (78 kcal)
Milk, 2%	250 mL (129 kcal)
Cheddar cheese	50 g (202 kcal)
Yogurt, 2% plain	175 g (110 kcal)
Soy beverage, fortified	250 mL (110 kcal)
Kefir	175 g (104 kcal)
Ice cream, strawberry	125 mL (134 kcal)
Chicken breast, roasted	75 g (220 kcal)
Ground beef, lean, baked	75 g (191 kcal)
Egg, poached	1 large (72 kcal)
Tuna, canned in water	75 g (87 kcal)
Tofu, made with a calcium salt[a]	150 g (114 kcal)
Peanut butter	30 mL (184 kcal)
Excellent, and sometimes unusual, sources:	
Goat cheese	50 g (226 kcal)
Sardines, canned with bones[b]	75 g (156 kcal)
Tahini	30 mL (181 kcal)

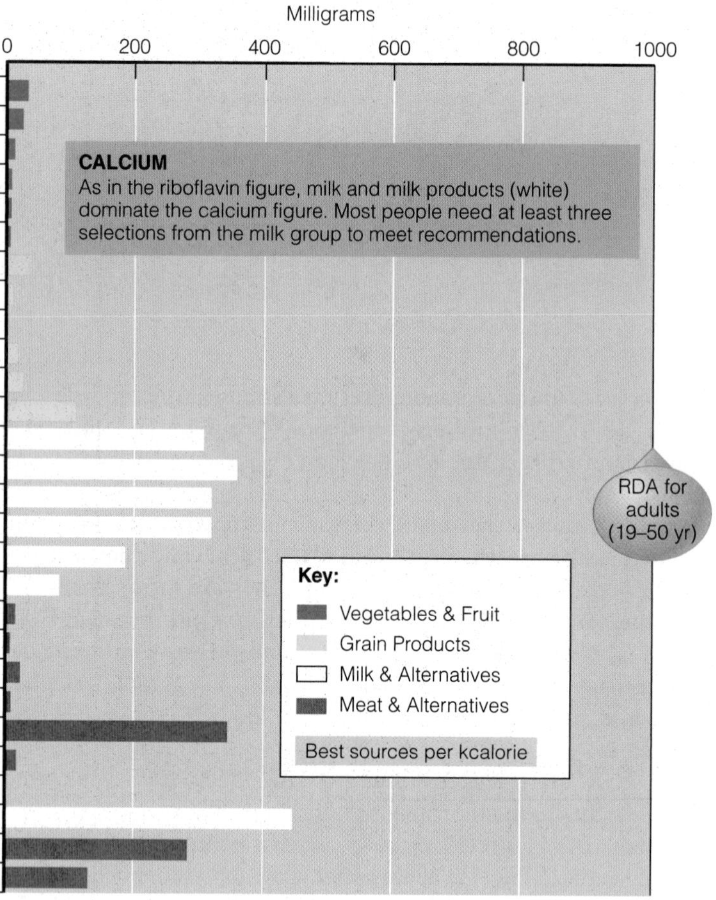
Milligrams
0
200
400
600
800
1000
CALCIUM
As in the riboflavin figure, milk and milk products (white) dominate the calcium figure. Most people need at least three selections from the milk group to meet recommendations.
RDA for adults (19–50 yr)
Key:
Vegetables & Fruit
Grain Products
Milk & Alternatives
Meat & Alternatives
Best sources per kcalorie

SOURCE: Canadian Nutrient File. Health Canada, 2008. Reproduced with the permission of the Minister of Health, 2011.
[a]Values based on products containing added calcium salts; the calcium in ½ c soybeans is about ⅔ as much as in ½ c tofu.
[b]If bones are discarded, calcium declines dramatically.

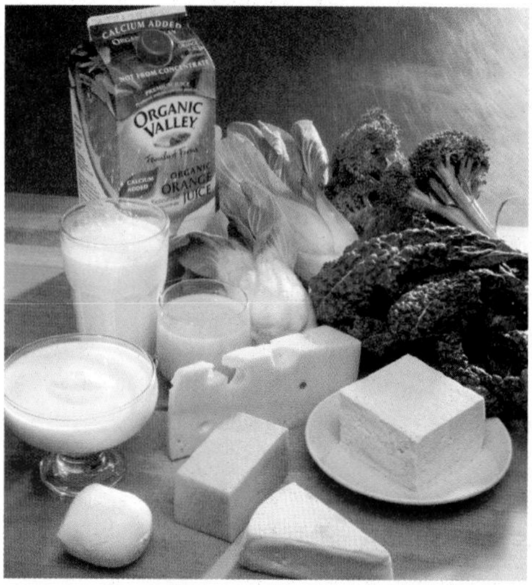
ORGANIC VALLEY

© Matthew Farruggio

Milk and milk products are well known for their calcium, but calcium-set tofu, fortified soy beverage, bok choy, kale, calcium-fortified orange juice, and broccoli also provide some calcium.

♦ People with lactose intolerance may be able to consume small quantities of milk, as Chapter 4 explains.

drink milk may prefer to eat cheese or yogurt. Alternatively, milk and milk products can be concealed in foods. Powdered skim milk can be added to casseroles, soups, and other mixed dishes during preparation; 25 grams (5 heaping tablespoons) offer the equivalent of 250 millilitres (1 cup) of milk. This simple step is an excellent way for older women not only to obtain extra calcium, but more protein, vitamins, and minerals as well.

It is especially difficult for children who don't drink milk to meet their calcium needs.[12] Children who don't drink milk have lower calcium intakes and poorer bone health than those who drink milk regularly. The consequences of drinking too little milk during childhood and adolescence persist into adulthood. Women who seldom drank milk as children or teenagers have lower bone density and greater risk of fractures than those who drank milk regularly.[13] It is possible for people who do not drink milk to obtain adequate calcium, but only if they carefully select other calcium-rich foods.

Calcium in Other Foods Many people, for a variety of reasons, cannot or do not drink milk. Some cultures do not use milk in their cuisines; some vegetarians exclude milk as well as meat; and some people are allergic to milk protein or are lactose intolerant. ♦ Others simply do not enjoy the taste of milk. These people need to find nonmilk sources of calcium to help meet their calcium needs. Some brands of tofu, some nuts (such as almonds), and some seeds (such as sesame seeds) can supply calcium for the person who doesn't use milk products. A slice of most breads contains only about 5 to 10 percent of the calcium found in milk, but it can be a major source for people who eat many slices because the calcium is well absorbed. Oysters are also a rich source of calcium, as are small fish eaten with their bones, such as canned sardines or canned salmon.

Among the vegetables, mustard and turnip greens, bok choy, kale, parsley, watercress, and broccoli are good sources of available calcium. So are some seaweeds such as the nori popular in Japanese cooking. Some dark green, leafy vegetables—notably spinach and Swiss chard—appear to be calcium-rich but actually provide little, if any, calcium to the body because of the binders they contain. It would take 200 millilitres (8 cups) of spinach—containing six times as much calcium as 250 millilitres (1 cup) of milk—to deliver the equivalent in *absorbable* calcium.

With the exception of foods such as spinach that contain calcium binders, however, the calcium content of foods is usually more important than bioavailability. Consequently, recognizing that people eat a variety of foods containing calcium, the DRI Committee did not consider calcium bioavailability when setting recommendations. Figure 13-5 ranks selected foods according to their calcium bioavailability.

Some mineral waters provide as much as 500 milligrams of calcium per litre, offering a convenient way to meet both calcium and water needs.[14] Similarly, calcium-fortified orange juice and other fruit and vegetable juices allow a person to obtain both calcium and vitamins easily. High-calcium milk (milk with extra calcium added) is another example of a calcium-fortified food. Fortified juices and foods help consumers increase calcium intakes, but depending on the calcium sources, the bioavailability may be significantly less than quantities listed on food labels.[15] The accompanying "How To" describes a shortcut method for estimating your calcium intake. Highlight 13 discusses calcium supplements.

A generalization that has been gaining strength throughout this book is supported by the information given here about calcium. A balanced diet that supplies a variety of foods is the best plan to ensure adequacy for all essential nutrients. All food groups should be included, and none should be overemphasized. In our culture, calcium intake is usually inadequate wherever milk is lacking in the diet—whether through ignorance, poverty, simple dislike, fad dieting, lactose intolerance, or allergy. By contrast, iron is usually lacking whenever milk is overemphasized, as Chapter 14 explains.

FIGURE 13-5 Bioavailability of Calcium from Selected Foods

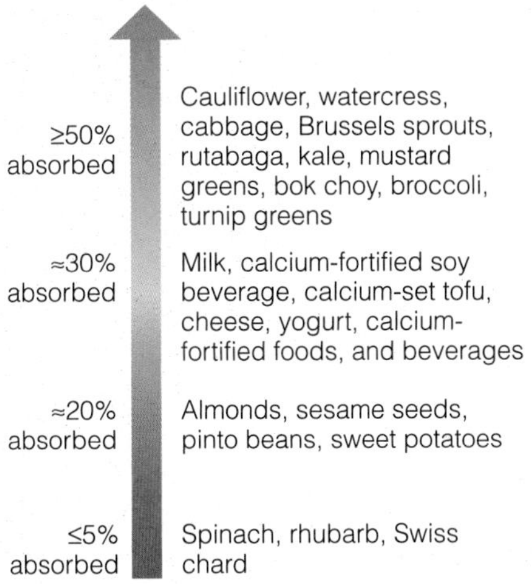
≥50% absorbed
Cauliflower, watercress, cabbage, Brussels sprouts, rutabaga, kale, mustard greens, bok choy, broccoli, turnip greens
≈30% absorbed
Milk, calcium-fortified soy beverage, calcium-set tofu, cheese, yogurt, calcium-fortified foods, and beverages
≈20% absorbed
Almonds, sesame seeds, pinto beans, sweet potatoes
≤5% absorbed
Spinach, rhubarb, Swiss chard

IN SUMMARY **Most of the body's calcium is in the bones where it provides a rigid structure and a reservoir of calcium for the blood. Blood calcium participates in muscle contraction, blood clotting, and nerve impulses, and it is closely regulated by a system of hormones and vitamin D. Calcium is found predominantly in milk, milk products, and milk alternatives, but some other foods including certain vegetables and calcium-set tofu also provide calcium. Even when calcium intake is inadequate, blood calcium remains normal, but at the expense of bone loss, which can lead to osteoporosis. The following table provides a summary of calcium.**

Calcium

Recommended Dietary Allowance (RDA)

All adults: (19–50 yr) 1000 mg/day
Male adults: (51–70 yr) 1000 mg/day
Female adults: (51–70 yr) 1200 mg/day
All adults: (>70 yr) 1200 mg/day

Upper Level

Adults: 2500 mg/day (19–50 yr)
2000 mg/day (>50 yr)

Chief Functions in the Body

Mineralization of bones and teeth; also involved in muscle contraction and relaxation, nerve functioning, blood clotting, blood pressure

Deficiency Symptoms

Stunted growth in children; bone loss (osteoporosis) in adults

Toxicity Symptoms

Constipation; increased risk of urinary stone formation and kidney dysfunction; interference with absorption of other minerals

Significant Sources

Milk, milk products, and milk alternatives, canned fish (with bones), calcium-set tofu (bean curd), greens (bok choy, broccoli, chard, kale), legumes

HOW TO Estimate Your Calcium Intake

Most dietitians have developed useful shortcuts to help them estimate nutrient intakes and "see" inadequacies in the diet. They can tell at a glance whether a day's meals fall short of calcium recommendations, for example.

To estimate calcium intakes, keep two bits of information in mind:

- 250 millilitres (1 cup) of milk provides about 300 milligrams of calcium.
- Adults need between 1000 and 1200 milligrams of calcium per day, which represents 800 to 1000 millilitres (3 to 4 cups) of milk—or the equivalent:

$$1000 \text{ mg} \div 300 \text{ mg/250 mL} = 833 \text{ mL}$$
$$1200 \text{ mg} \div 300 \text{ mg/250 mL} = 1000 \text{ mL}$$

If a person drinks 800 to 1000 millilitres (3 to 4 cups) of milk a day, it's easy to see that calcium needs are being met. If not, it takes some detective work to identify the other sources and estimate total calcium intake.

To estimate a person's daily calcium intake, use this shortcut, which compares the calcium in calcium-rich foods to the calcium content of milk. The calcium in a cup of milk is assigned 1 point, and the goal is to attain 3 to 4 points per day. Foods are given points as follows:

- 250 mL (1 c) milk, yogurt, or fortified soy beverage or 50 g cheese = 1 point
- 90 g canned fish with bones (sardines) = 1 point
- 250 mL (1 c) ice cream, cottage cheese, or calcium-rich vegetable (see the text) = ½ point

Then, because other foods also contribute small amounts of calcium, together they are given a point.

- Well-balanced diet containing a variety of foods = 1 point

Now consider a day's meals with calcium in mind. Cereal with 250 mL (1 cup) of milk for breakfast (1 point for milk), a ham and cheese sub sandwich for lunch (1 point for cheese), and 250 mL (1 cup) of broccoli and lasagne for dinner (½ point for calcium-rich vegetable and 1 point for cheese in lasagne)—plus 1 point for all other foods eaten that day—adds up to 4½ points. This shortcut estimate indicates that calcium recommendations have been met, and a diet analysis of these few foods reveals a calcium intake of more than 1000 milligrams. By knowing the best sources of each nutrient, you can learn to scan the day's meals and quickly see if you are meeting your daily goals.

CENGAGENOW™
For additional practice log on to **www.cengage.com/sso.**

TRY IT Compare the calcium contents of 125 millilitres (½ cup) of the following foods: almonds, broccoli, and yogurt.

Phosphorus

Second in quantity only to calcium, **phosphorus** is a mineral found in abundance in the human body. About 85 percent of our body's phosphorus as phosphate (PO_4^{3-}) is combined with calcium in the hydroxyapatite crystals ♦ of bones and teeth. The other 15 percent is distributed in soft tissues, including muscle and the kidneys.

♦ Hydroxyapatite, the major mineral crystal found in bone
$Ca^{2+}{}_{10}(PO_4^{3-})_6(OH^-)_2$
Bone consists of mineral crystals of different sizes and shapes. In hydroxyapatite:
Mg^{2+}, Sr^{2+}, Na^+, or K^+ can replace Ca^{2+}
CO_3^{2-} or HPO_4^{2-} can replace PO_4^{3-}
CO_3^{2-} or F^- can replace OH^-

Phosphorus Role in Bone Health Hydroxyapatite is the major mineral crystal found in our skeleton and teeth. Our skeleton protects our vital organs, allows us to stand upright, and interacts with muscles and tendons, allowing us to move. Our teeth help us to chew solid foods, a critical step in the process of digesting foods. The nonbone health roles for phosphorus are presented in Chapter 11.

Phosphorus Deficiency and Toxicity Dietary deficiencies of phosphorus are unlikely because it is found in many foods. No adverse effects of high dietary phosphorus intakes have been reported.

phosphorus: a major mineral found mostly in the body's bones and teeth.

Phosphorus Recommendations and Sources For all adults, the RDA for phosphorus is 700 milligrams per day and the UL is 4000 milligrams per day. Phosphorus is widespread in the food supply; however, protein-rich foods tend to provide higher amounts (see Figure 11-12 on page 372). Of notable importance to bone health, milk and cheese contribute about one-fourth of the phosphorus in the North American diet. For some people, the phosphorus added to soft drinks in the form of phosphoric acid can significantly contribute to their daily intake. In cases where calcium intake is already low, a high ratio of dietary phosphorus-to-calcium can be detrimental to bones[16] and teeth. Recently a team of researchers at McGill University reported calcium loss from teeth exposed to diet and regular cola-type soft drinks.[17]

IN SUMMARY **Phosphorus is critical to bone health, most notably as a component of the hydroxyapatite mineral crystal that provides strength to bone. As outlined in Chapter 11, phosphorus is also critical to fluid balance, energy metabolism, phospholipids and lipoproteins, and DNA and RNA.**

Vitamin D

Vitamin D (calciferol) ♦ is different from all the other nutrients in that the body can synthesize it, with the help of sunlight, from a precursor that the body makes from cholesterol. Therefore, vitamin D is not an essential nutrient; given enough time in the sun, people need no vitamin D from foods.

Figure 13-6 diagrams the pathway for making and activating vitamin D in the body. Ultraviolet rays from the sun hit the precursor in the skin and convert it to previtamin D_3. This compound diffuses from the skin into the blood and is converted to its active form with the help of the body's heat. The biological activity of the active vitamin is 500- to 1000-fold greater than that of its precursor.

Regardless of whether the body manufactures vitamin D or obtains it directly from foods, two hydroxylation reactions must occur before the vitamin becomes fully active.[18] First, the liver adds an OH group, and then the kidneys add another OH group to produce the active vitamin. ♦ A review of Figure 13-6 reveals how diseases affecting either the liver or the kidneys can interfere with the activation of vitamin D and produce symptoms of deficiency.

Vitamin D Roles in the Body

Though called a vitamin, the active form of vitamin D is actually a hormone—a compound manufactured by one part of the body that travels through the blood and causes another body part to respond.[19] Like vitamin A, vitamin D has a binding protein that carries it to the target organs—most notably, the intestines, the kidneys, and the bones. All respond to vitamin D by making the minerals needed for bone growth and maintenance available.

Vitamin D in Bone Growth Vitamin D is a member of a large and cooperative bone-making and maintenance team ♦ composed of nutrients and other compounds, including vitamins A and K; the hormones parathyroid hormone and calcitonin; the protein collagen; and the minerals calcium, phosphorus, magnesium, and fluoride. Vitamin D's special role in bone health is to assist in the absorption of calcium and phosphorus, thus helping to maintain blood concentrations of these minerals.[20] The bones grow denser and stronger as they absorb and deposit these minerals. Details of how vitamin D affects calcium balance in the GI tract, bone, and kidneys appear in Figure 13-1 (page 411).

Vitamin D raises blood concentrations of bone minerals in three ways. When the diet is sufficient, vitamin D enhances their absorption from the GI tract. When the diet is insufficient, vitamin D provides the needed minerals from other sources: reabsorption by the kidneys and mobilization from the bones into the

FIGURE 13-6 Vitamin D Synthesis and Activation

The precursor of vitamin D is made in the liver from cholesterol (see Figure 5-11 on p. 138 and APPENDIX C). The activation of vitamin D is closely regulated by parathyroid hormone. The final product, active vitamin D, is also known as 1,25-dihydroxycholecalciferol (or calcitriol).

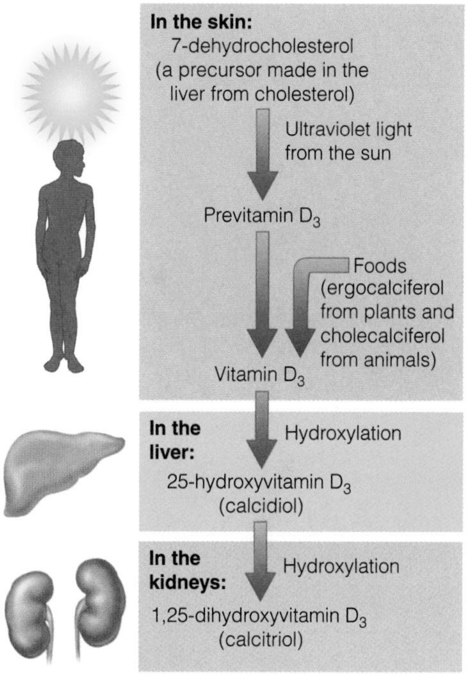
In the skin:
7-dehydrocholesterol
(a precursor made in the liver from cholesterol)
Ultraviolet light from the sun
Previtamin D3
Foods (ergocalciferol from plants and cholecalciferol from animals)
Vitamin D3
In the liver:
Hydroxylation
25-hydroxyvitamin D3 (calcidiol)
In the kidneys:
Hydroxylation
1,25-dihydroxyvitamin D3 (calcitriol)

CENGAGENOW™
Animated! figure
www.cengage.com/sso

♦ Vitamin D comes in many forms, but the two most important in the diet are a plant version called **vitamin D_2** or **ergocalciferol** (ER-go-kal-SIF-er-ol) and an animal version called **vitamin D_3** or **cholecalciferol** (KO-lee-kal-SIF-er-ol).

♦ Before hydroxylation, vitamin D in the blood is known as **calciol;** after hydroxylation in the liver, vitamin D is known as **calcidiol** (or **25-hydroxyvitamin D**); and after hydroxylation in the kidneys, **active vitamin D** is known as **calcitriol** (or **1,25-dihydroxyvitamin D**).

♦ Key bone nutrients:
- Vitamin D, vitamin K, vitamin A
- Calcium, phosphorus, magnesium, fluoride

blood.[21] The vitamin may work alone, as it does in the GI tract, or in combination with parathyroid hormone, as it does in the bones and kidneys.[22]

Vitamin D in Other Roles Scientists have discovered many other tissues that respond to vitamin D, including cells of the immune system, brain and nervous system, pancreas, skin, muscles and cartilage, and reproductive organs.[23] In many cases, vitamin D enhances or suppresses the activity of genes that regulate cell growth.[24] As such, it may be valuable in treating a number of diseases.[25] Despite studies that show benefit, a recent systematic review of evidence commissioned by Health Canada, the Public Health Agency of Canada, and several U.S. government agencies concludes considerable uncertainty of benefits due to inconsistent findings. Further research is warranted to substantiate the extent of vitamin D protection against tuberculosis, inflammation, multiple sclerosis, hypertension, some cancers, and other diseases.[26]

Vitamin D Deficiency

Overt signs of vitamin D deficiency are relatively rare, but vitamin D insufficiency is remarkably common.[27] Factors that contribute to vitamin D deficiency include dark skin, breastfeeding without supplementation, lack of sunlight, and not using fortified milk. In vitamin D deficiency, production of a protein that binds calcium ♦ in the intestinal cells slows. Thus, even when calcium in the diet is adequate, it passes through the GI tract unabsorbed, leaving the bones undersupplied. Consequently, a vitamin D deficiency creates a calcium deficiency and increases the risks of several chronic diseases.[28] Vitamin D–deficient adolescents may not reach their peak bone mass.[29] Low blood calcium due to a vitamin D deficiency can also trigger seizures.[30]

♦ Synthesis of **calbindin,** a calcium-binding transport protein, requires vitamin D.

Rickets Worldwide, the prevalence of the vitamin D–deficiency disease **rickets** is extremely high, affecting more than half of the children in countries such as Mongolia, Tibet, and the Netherlands.[31] In Canada, rickets is persistent especially among children living in the northern territories and darker-skinned infants who are breastfed without appropriate vitamin D supplementation.[32] To prevent rickets, recommendations from Health Canada and the Canadian Paediatric Society state that infants and children receive 10 micrograms (400 IU) of vitamin D each day through diet or supplementation.[33] ♦ In rickets, the bones fail to calcify normally, causing growth retardation and skeletal abnormalities. The bones become so weak that they bend when they have to support the body's weight (see Figure 13-7). A child with rickets who is old enough to walk characteristically develops bowed legs, often the most obvious sign of the disease. Another sign is the beaded ribs ♦ that result from the poorly formed attachments of the bones to the cartilage.

♦ For perspective, 250 ml (1 cup) of fortified milk provides about 100 IU vitamin D.

♦ Because the poorly formed rib attachments resemble rosary beads, this symptom is commonly known as **rachitic** (ra-KIT-ik) **rosary** ("the rosary of rickets").

Osteomalacia In adults, the poor mineralization of bone results in the painful bone disease **osteomalacia.**[34] The bones become increasingly soft, flexible, brittle, and deformed.

Osteoporosis Any failure to synthesize adequate vitamin D or obtain enough from foods sets the stage for a loss of calcium from the bones, which can result in fractures. Highlight 13 describes the many factors that lead to osteoporosis, a condition of reduced bone density.

The Elderly Vitamin D deficiency is especially likely in older adults for several reasons. For one, the skin, liver, and kidneys lose their capacity to make and activate vitamin D with advancing age. For another, older adults typically drink little or no milk—the main dietary source of vitamin D. And finally, older adults typically spend much of the day indoors, and when they do venture outside, many of them cautiously wear protective clothing or apply sunscreen to all sun-exposed areas of their skin. Dark-skinned people living in northern regions are particularly vulnerable. All of these factors increase the likelihood of vitamin D deficiency and its consequences: bone losses and fractures. Health Canada recommends all adults 51 years of age and older

rickets: the vitamin D–deficiency disease in children characterized by inadequate mineralization of bone (manifested in bowed legs or knock-knees, outward-bowed chest, and knobs on ribs). A rare type of rickets, not caused by vitamin D deficiency, is known as *vitamin D–refractory rickets.*

osteomalacia (OS-tee-oh-ma-LAY-shuh): a bone disease characterized by softening of the bones. Symptoms include bending of the spine and bowing of the legs. The disease occurs most often in adult women.

- **osteo** = bone
- **malacia** = softening

FIGURE 13-7 Vitamin D–Deficiency Symptoms—Bowed Legs and Beaded Ribs of Rickets

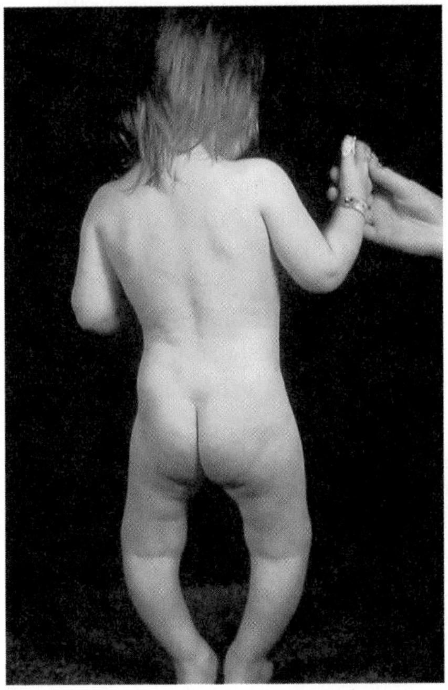

Biophoto Associates/Photo Researchers, Inc.

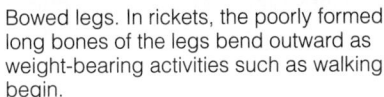

Bowed legs. In rickets, the poorly formed long bones of the legs bend outward as weight-bearing activities such as walking begin.

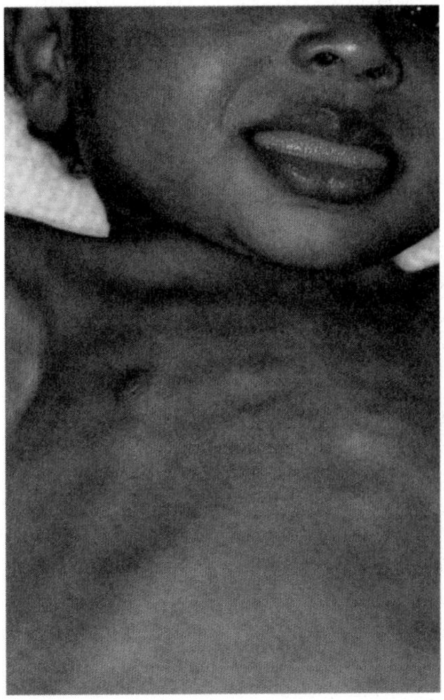

Photo Courtesy of Dr. Norman Carvalho at Children's Healthcare of Atlanta

Beaded ribs. In rickets, a series of "beads" develop where the cartilages and bones attach.

take 400 IU (10 micrograms) of vitamin D in supplement form each day, in addition to their dietary intake, to help raise blood levels, reduce bone loss, improve muscle performance, and lower the risks of falls and fractures, especially in elderly persons.[35]

Vitamin D Toxicity Vitamin D clearly illustrates how nutrients in optimal amounts support health, but both inadequacies and excesses cause trouble. Vitamin D is the most likely of the vitamins to have toxic effects when consumed in excessive amounts. The amounts of vitamin D made by the skin and found in foods are well within the safe limits set by the UL, but supplements containing the vitamin in concentrated form should be kept out of the reach of children and used cautiously by adults.

Excess vitamin D raises the concentration of blood calcium.[36] ♦ Excess blood calcium tends to precipitate in the soft tissue, forming stones, especially in the kidneys where calcium is concentrated in an effort to excrete it. Calcification may also harden the blood vessels and is especially dangerous in the major arteries of the brain, heart, and lungs, where it can cause death.

♦ High blood calcium is known as **hypercalcemia** and may develop from a variety of disorders, including vitamin D toxicity. It does *not* develop from a high calcium intake.

Vitamin D Recommendations and Sources Only a few foods—notably oily fish and egg yolks—contain vitamin D naturally. Fortunately, the body can make vitamin D with the help of a little sunshine. In setting the 2011 Recommended Dietary Allowance (RDA), however, the expert scientific committee assumed no vitamin D synthesis was available from skin exposure to the sun. The new RDA were increased for all Canadians from the previous 1997 levels, reflecting research that has shown bone health benefits and safety at the newly established levels.[37] The 2011 daily recommendation for children, adolescents, and adults up to the age of 70 years is 600 IU, and 800 IU for adults 71 years of age and older. Although some research suggests even higher vitamin D intakes benefit broader aspects of health,[38] the committee did not find consistent evidence to support these claims. Prior to release of the new recommendations, ♦ 90

♦ Current recommendations: 15 to 20 μg/day

percent of Canadians had vitamin D blood levels considered adequate for bone health, and 30 percent had higher levels thought to benefit overall health and help in disease prevention.[39] Canadians' reliance on diet and supplements rather than solar-induced synthesis of vitamin D is important due to our northern latitude. Exposure to the sun is the most important risk factor for skin cancer prompting the Canadian Cancer Society to recommend reliance on diet and supplements for vitamin D throughout the year.[40]

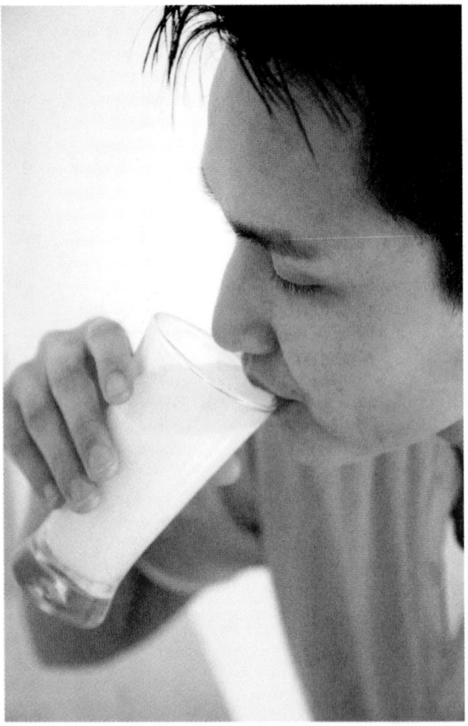

A cold glass of milk refreshes as it replenishes vitamin D and other bone-building nutrients.

Vitamin D in Foods Most adults, especially in sunny regions, need not make special efforts to obtain vitamin D from food. People who are not outdoors much or who live in northern or predominantly cloudy or smoggy areas are advised to drink at least 500 millilitres (2 cups) of vitamin D–fortified milk a day. The fortification of milk with vitamin D is the best guarantee that people will meet their needs and underscores the importance of milk in a well-balanced diet.* Despite vitamin D fortification, the average intake in Canada falls short of recommendations. Oily fish such as salmon, mackerel, and sardines are the best natural sources of vitamin D.

Meeting vitamin D needs is difficult without adequate sunshine, fortification, or supplementation.[41] Vegetarians who do not include milk in their diets may use vitamin D–fortified soy "milk" and cereals. Importantly, feeding infants and young children nonfortified "health beverages" instead of milk or infant formula can create severe nutrient deficiencies, including rickets.

Vitamin D from the Sun Most of the world's population relies on natural exposure to sunlight to maintain adequate vitamin D nutrition. The sun imposes no risk of vitamin D toxicity; prolonged exposure to sunlight degrades the vitamin D precursor in the skin, preventing its conversion to the active vitamin. Even lifeguards on southern beaches are safe from vitamin D toxicity from the sun.

Prolonged exposure to sunlight can, however, prematurely wrinkle the skin and cause skin cancer. Sunscreens help reduce these risks, but sunscreens with a sun protection factor (SPF) of 8 and higher can also reduce vitamin D synthesis. Still, even with an SPF 15–30 sunscreen, sufficient vitamin D synthesis can be obtained in 10 to 20 minutes of sun exposure.[42] Alternatively, a person could apply sunscreen after enough time has elapsed to provide sufficient vitamin D synthesis. For most people, exposing hands, face, and arms on a clear summer day for 5 to 10 minutes two or three times a week should be sufficient to maintain vitamin D nutrition.

The pigments of dark skin provide some protection from the sun's damage, but they also reduce vitamin D synthesis. Dark-skinned people require longer sunlight exposure than light-skinned people: heavily pigmented skin achieves the same amount of vitamin D synthesis in three hours as fair skin in a half hour. Latitude, season, and time of day ♦ also have dramatic effects on vitamin D synthesis and status (see Figure 13-8).[43] Heavy clouds, smoke, or smog block the ultraviolet (UV) rays of the sun that promote vitamin D synthesis. Differences in latitude may account for the finding that Canadians living in the Yukon, Northwest, and Nunavut territories are more likely than other Canadians to be vitamin D deficient and develop rickets. Vitamin D deficiency is especially prevalent in the winter.[44] To ensure an adequate vitamin D status, supplements may be needed.[45] The body's vitamin D supplies from summer synthesis alone are insufficient to meet winter needs.

♦ Factors that may limit sun exposure and, therefore, vitamin D synthesis:
- Geographic location
- Season of the year
- Time of day
- Air pollution
- Clothing
- Tall buildings
- Indoor living
- Sunscreens

Dietary Guidance for Canadians

People with dark skin and those with insufficient exposure to sunlight should consume extra vitamin D from vitamin D–fortified foods and/or supplements. *Eating Well with Canada's Food Guide* recommends adults over the age of 50 years take a daily supplement containing 400 IU (10 micrograms) of vitamin D in addition to their food intake.

*Vitamin D fortification of milk in Canada is 9 to 12 micrograms (350 to 470 IU) per litre.

FIGURE 13-8 Vitamin D Synthesis and Latitude

Above 40° north latitude (and below 40° south latitude in the southern hemisphere), vitamin D synthesis essentially ceases for the four months of winter. Synthesis increases as spring approaches, peaks in summer, and declines again in the fall. People living in regions of extreme northern (or extreme southern) latitudes may miss as much as six months of vitamin D production.

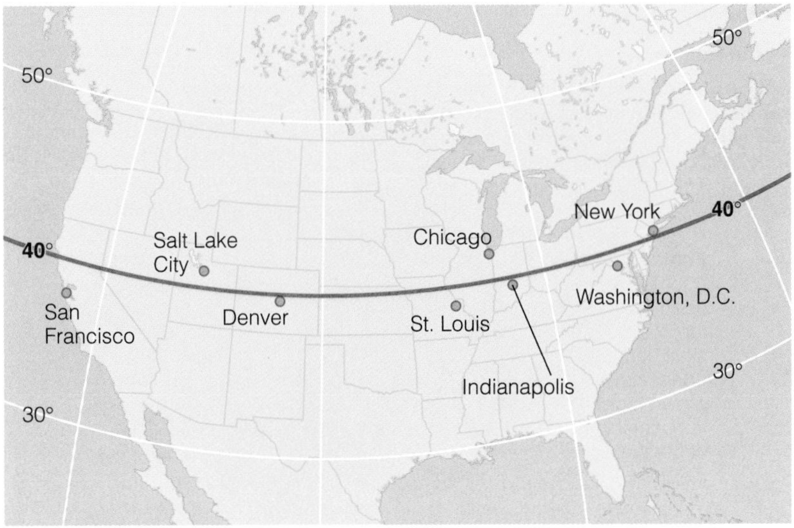
50°
50°
40°
40°
Salt Lake City
Chicago
New York
San Francisco
Denver
St. Louis
Washington, D.C.
Indianapolis
30°
30°

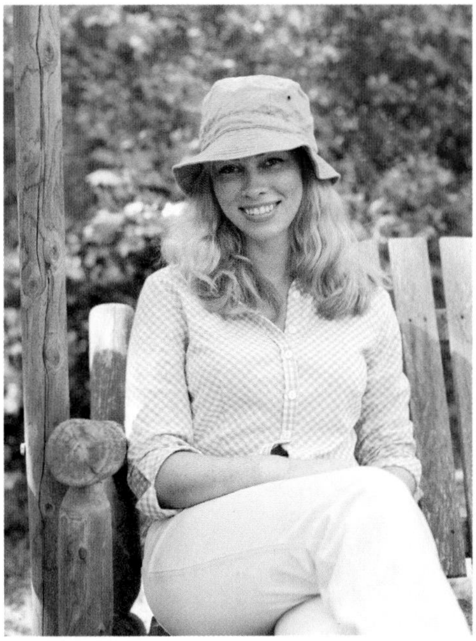
photos.com

The sunshine vitamin—vitamin D.

Depending on the radiation used, the UV rays from tanning lamps and tanning beds may also stimulate vitamin D synthesis and increase bone density. The potential hazards of skin damage, however, may outweigh any possible benefits.* Health Canada warns that if the lamps are not properly filtered, people using tanning booths risk burns, damage to the eyes and blood vessels, and skin cancer.

IN SUMMARY **Vitamin D can be synthesized in the body with the help of sunlight or obtained from fortified milk. It sends signals to three primary target sites: the GI tract to absorb more calcium and phosphorus, the bones to release more, and the kidneys to retain more. These actions maintain blood calcium concentrations and support bone formation. A deficiency causes rickets in childhood and osteomalacia in later life. The accompanying table provides a summary of vitamin D.**

Vitamin D

Other Names

ergocalciferol (vitamin D_2): vitamin D derived from plants in the diet and made from the yeast and plant sterol ergosterol.

cholecalciferol (vitamin D_3 or calciol): vitamin D derived from animals in the diet or made in the skin from 7-dehydrocholesterol, a precursor of cholesterol, with the help of sunlight.

calcidiol (25-hydroxyvitamin D): vitamin D found in the blood that is made from the hydroxylation of cholecalciferol in the liver.

calcitriol (1,25-dihydroxyvitamin D): vitamin D that is made from the hydroxylation of calcidiol in the kidneys; the biologically active hormone, sometimes called **active vitamin D.**

RDA

Adults: 600 IU/day or 15 μg/day (19–70 yr)
800 IU/day or 20 μg/day (>70 yr)

Upper Level

Adults: 4000 IU/day or 100 μg/day

Chief Functions in the Body

Mineralization of bones (raises blood calcium and phosphorus by increasing absorption from digestive tract, withdrawing calcium from bones, stimulating retention by kidneys)

*The best wavelengths for vitamin D synthesis are UV-B rays between 290 and 310 nanometres. Some tanning parlours advertise "UV-A rays only, for a tan without the burn," but UV-A rays can damage the skin.

Significant Sources	
Synthesized in the body with the help of sunlight; fortified milk, margarine, and some juices; veal, beef, egg yolks, liver, fatty fish (herring, salmon, sardines) and their oils	
Deficiency Diseases	
Rickets, osteomalacia	
Deficiency Symptoms	
Rickets in children	
Inadequate calcification, resulting in misshapen bones (bowing of legs); enlargement of ends of long bones (knees, wrists); deformities of ribs (bowed, with beads or knobs);[a] delayed closing of fontanel, resulting in rapid enlargement of head (see figure below); lax muscles resulting in protrusion of abdomen; muscle spasms	
Osteomalacia or Osteoporosis in adults	
Loss of calcium, resulting in soft, flexible, brittle, and deformed bones; progressive weakness; pain in pelvis, lower back, and legs	
Toxicity Disease	
Hypervitaminosis D	
Toxicity Symptoms	
Elevated blood calcium; calcification of soft tissues (blood vessels, kidneys, heart, lungs, tissues around joints)	

Fontanel
A fontanel is an open space in the top of a baby's skull before the bones have grown together. In rickets, closing of the fontanel is delayed.

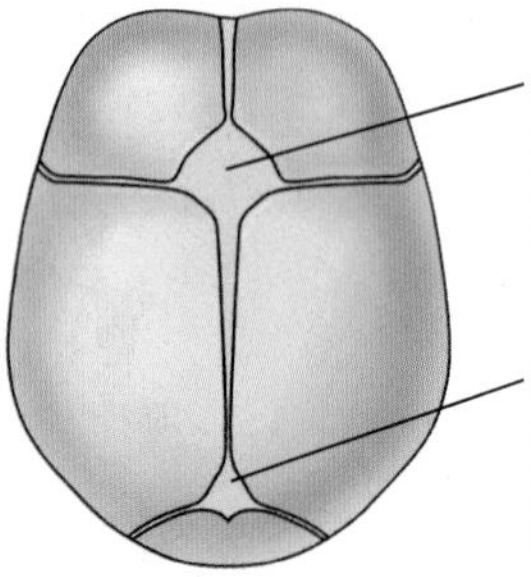
Anterior fontanel normally closes by the end of the second year.
Posterior fontanel normally closes by the end of the first year.

[a]Bowing of the ribs causes the symptoms known as *pigeon breast*. The beads that form on the ribs resemble rosary beads; thus this symptom is known as *rachitic* (ra-KIT-ik) *rosary* ("the rosary of rickets").

Magnesium

Only about 30 grams of **magnesium** is present in the body of a 60 kilogram (130-pound) person. More than half of the body's magnesium is in the bones. Much of the rest is in the muscles and soft tissues, with only 1 percent in the extracellular fluid. As with calcium, bone magnesium may serve as a reservoir to ensure normal blood concentrations.

Magnesium Roles in the Body In addition to maintaining bone health, magnesium acts in all the cells of the soft tissues, where it forms part of the protein-making machinery and is necessary for energy metabolism. It participates in hundreds of enzyme systems. A major role of magnesium is as a catalyst ♦ in the reaction that adds the last phosphate to the high-energy compound ATP, making it essential to the body's use of glucose; the synthesis of protein, fat, and nucleic acids; and the cells' membrane transport systems. Together with calcium, magnesium is involved in muscle contraction and blood clotting: calcium promotes the processes, whereas magnesium inhibits them. This dynamic interaction between the two minerals helps regulate blood pressure and lung function. Like many other nutrients, magnesium supports the normal functioning of the immune system.

♦ A **catalyst** is a compound that facilitates chemical reactions without itself being changed in the process.

Magnesium Deficiency Even with average magnesium intakes below recommendations, deficiency symptoms rarely appear except with diseases. Magnesium deficiency may develop in cases of alcohol abuse, protein malnutrition, kidney disorders, and prolonged vomiting or diarrhea. People using diuretics may also show symptoms. A severe magnesium deficiency causes a tetany similar to the calcium tetany described earlier. Magnesium deficiencies also impair central nervous system activity and may be responsible for the hallucinations experienced during alcohol withdrawal.

Magnesium and Hypertension Magnesium is critical to heart function and seems to protect against hypertension and heart disease. Interestingly, people living in areas with hard water, which contains high concentrations of

magnesium: a cation within the body's cells, active in many enzyme systems.

FIGURE 13-9 Magnesium in Selected Foods

See the "How To" section on p. 317 for more information on using this figure.

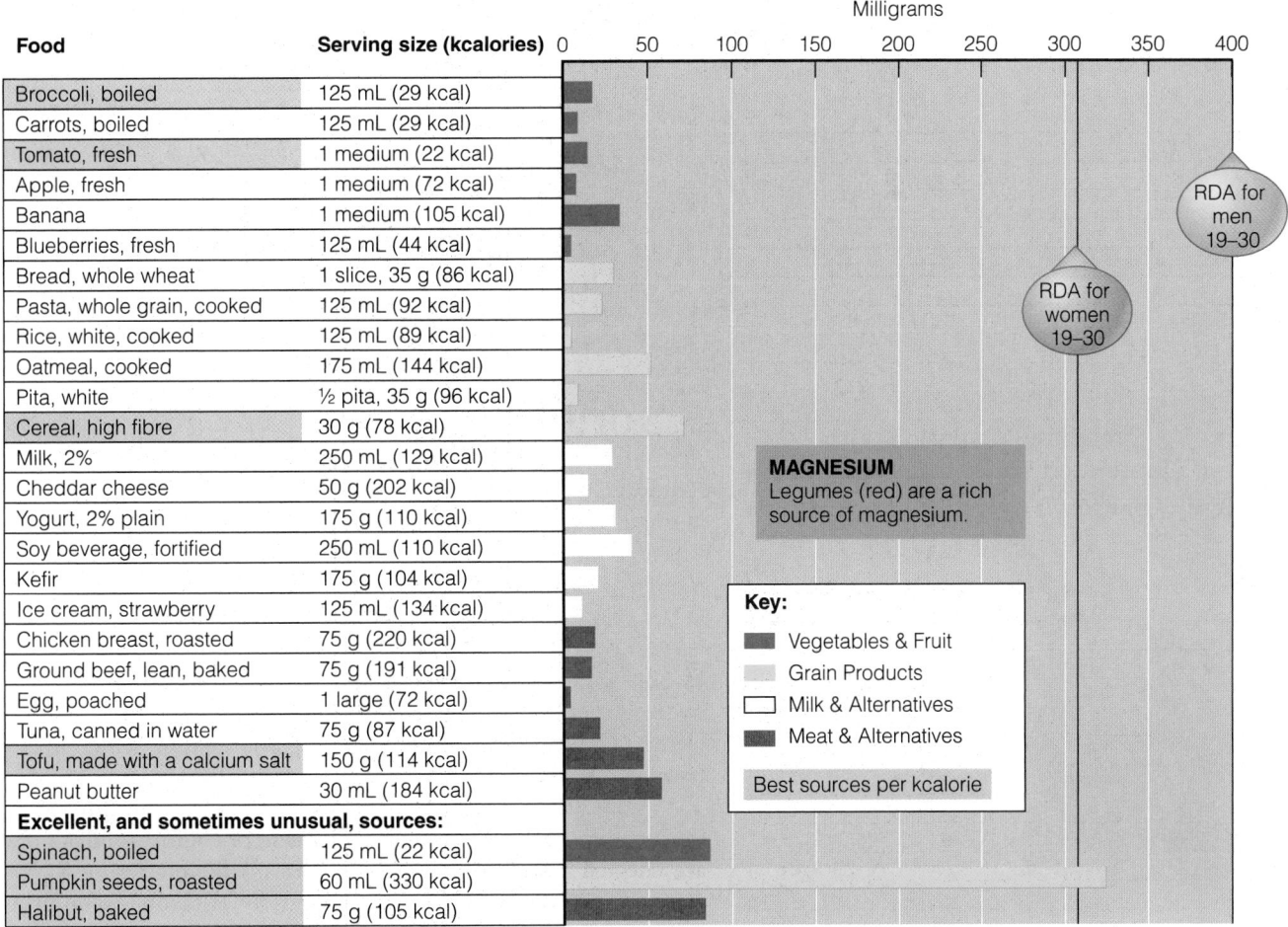

Food	Serving size (kcalories)
Broccoli, boiled	125 mL (29 kcal)
Carrots, boiled	125 mL (29 kcal)
Tomato, fresh	1 medium (22 kcal)
Apple, fresh	1 medium (72 kcal)
Banana	1 medium (105 kcal)
Blueberries, fresh	125 mL (44 kcal)
Bread, whole wheat	1 slice, 35 g (86 kcal)
Pasta, whole grain, cooked	125 mL (92 kcal)
Rice, white, cooked	125 mL (89 kcal)
Oatmeal, cooked	175 mL (144 kcal)
Pita, white	½ pita, 35 g (96 kcal)
Cereal, high fibre	30 g (78 kcal)
Milk, 2%	250 mL (129 kcal)
Cheddar cheese	50 g (202 kcal)
Yogurt, 2% plain	175 g (110 kcal)
Soy beverage, fortified	250 mL (110 kcal)
Kefir	175 g (104 kcal)
Ice cream, strawberry	125 mL (134 kcal)
Chicken breast, roasted	75 g (220 kcal)
Ground beef, lean, baked	75 g (191 kcal)
Egg, poached	1 large (72 kcal)
Tuna, canned in water	75 g (87 kcal)
Tofu, made with a calcium salt	150 g (114 kcal)
Peanut butter	30 mL (184 kcal)
Excellent, and sometimes unusual, sources:	
Spinach, boiled	125 mL (22 kcal)
Pumpkin seeds, roasted	60 mL (330 kcal)
Halibut, baked	75 g (105 kcal)

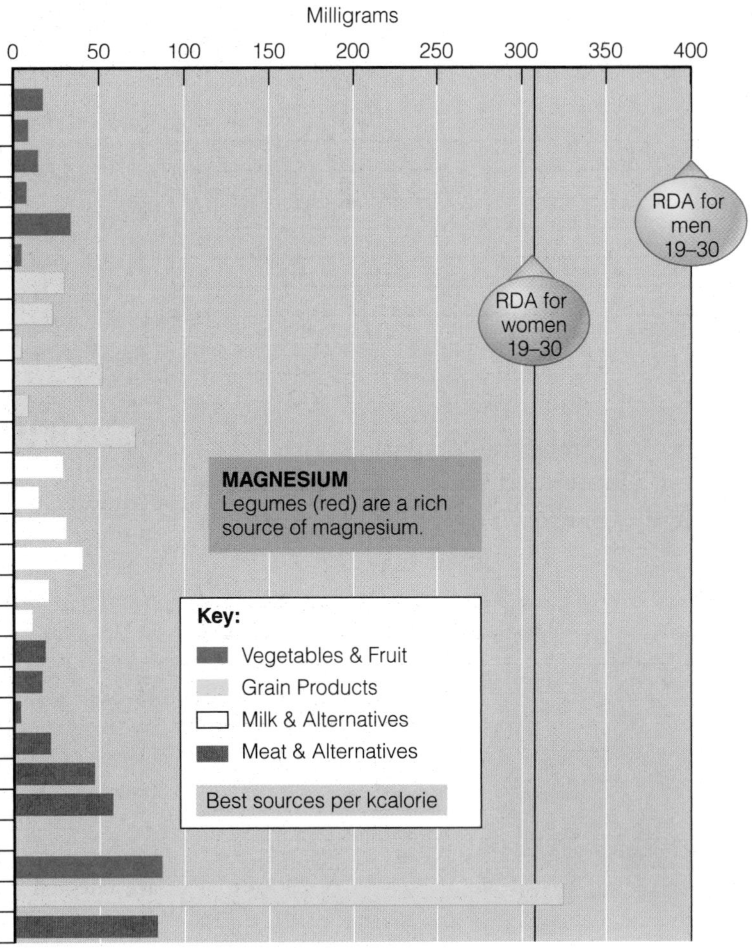
Milligrams
0
50
100
150
200
250
300
350
400
RDA for men 19–30
RDA for women 19–30
MAGNESIUM
Legumes (red) are a rich source of magnesium.
Key:
Vegetables & Fruit
Grain Products
Milk & Alternatives
Meat & Alternatives
Best sources per kcalorie

SOURCE: Canadian Nutrient File. Health Canada, 2008. Reproduced with the permission of the Minister of Health, 2011.

calcium and magnesium, tend to have low rates of heart disease.[46] With magnesium deficiency, the walls of the arteries and capillaries tend to constrict—a possible explanation for the hypertensive effect.

Magnesium Toxicity Magnesium toxicity is rare, but it can be fatal. The UL for magnesium applies only to nonfood sources such as supplements or magnesium salts.

Magnesium Intakes and Sources Average dietary magnesium intakes of Canadian adults fall below recommendations.[47] Dietary intake data, however, do not include the contribution made by water. In areas with hard water, the water contributes both calcium and magnesium to daily intakes. Mineral waters noted earlier for their calcium content may also be magnesium-rich and can be important sources of this mineral for those who drink them. Bioavailability of magnesium from mineral water is about 50 percent, but it improves when the water is consumed with a meal.

The foods in Figure 13-9 show that legumes make significant magnesium contributions. Magnesium is part of the chlorophyll molecule, so leafy green vegetables are also good sources.

IN SUMMARY **Like calcium and phosphorus, magnesium supports bone mineralization. Magnesium is also involved in numerous enzyme systems and in heart function. It is found abundantly in legumes and leafy green vegetables and, in some areas, in water. The accompanying table provides a summary of magnesium.**

Magnesium

RDA	Deficiency Symptoms
Men (19–30 yr): 400 mg/day Women (19–30 yr): 310 mg/day	Weakness; confusion; if extreme, convulsions, bizarre muscle movements (especially of eye and face muscles), hallucinations, and difficulty in swallowing; in children, growth failure[a]
Upper Level	**Toxicity Symptoms**
Adults: 350 mg nonfood magnesium/day	From nonfood sources only; diarrhea, alkalosis, dehydration
Chief Functions in the Body	**Significant Sources**
Bone mineralization, building of protein, enzyme action, normal muscle contraction, nerve impulse transmission, maintenance of teeth, and functioning of immune system	Nuts, legumes, whole grains, dark green vegetables, seafood, chocolate, cocoa

[a]A still more severe deficiency causes tetany, an extreme, prolonged contraction of the muscles similar to that caused by low blood calcium.

FIGURE 13-10 Canadian Population with Access to Fluoridated Water through Public Water Systems, 2007

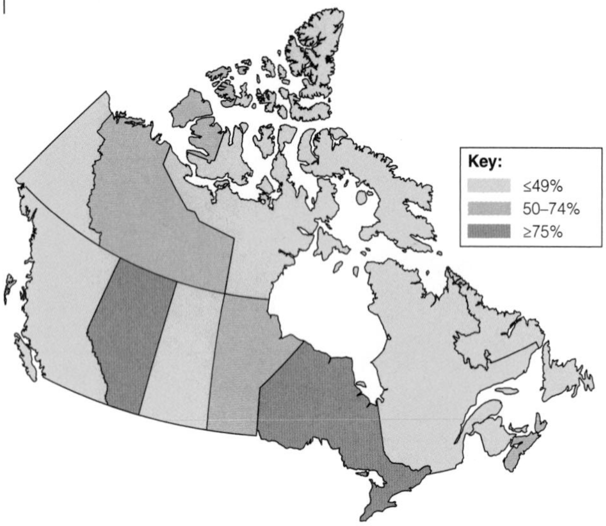
Key:
≤49%
50–74%
≥75%

SOURCE: Danielle Rabb-Waytowich, MLIS, "Water Fluoridation in Canada: Past and Present", *Journal of the Canadian Dental Association* 75(6), 2009

♦ For perspective, 1 part per million (1 ppm) is approximately 1 mg per litre.

♦ To prevent fluorosis:
- Monitor the fluoride content of the local water supply.
- Supervise toddlers when they brush their teeth—using only a little toothpaste (pea-size amount).
- Use fluoride supplements only as prescribed by a physician.

fluorapatite (floor-APP-uh-tite): the stabilized form of bone and tooth crystal, in which fluoride has replaced the hydroxyl groups of hydroxyapatite.

fluorosis (floor-OH-sis): discolouration and pitting of tooth enamel caused by excess fluoride during tooth development.

Fluoride

Fluoride is present in virtually all soils, water supplies, plants, and animals. Only a trace of fluoride occurs in the human body, but with this amount, the crystalline deposits in bones and teeth are larger and more perfectly formed.

Fluoride Roles in the Body

During the mineralization of bones and teeth, calcium and phosphorus form crystals called hydroxyapatite. Then fluoride replaces the hydroxyl (OH) portions of the hydroxyapatite crystal, forming **fluorapatite**, which makes the bones stronger and the teeth more resistant to decay.

Dental caries ranks as the nation's most widespread chronic disease in Canadian children: close to 60 percent of children and adolescents are affected by one or more dental caries.[48] By interfering with a person's ability to chew and eat a wide variety of foods, dental problems can quickly lead to a multitude of nutrition problems. Where fluoride is lacking, dental decay is common.

Drinking water offers a reliable source of fluoride; however, only 45 percent of Canadians are served by fluoridated public water systems (see Figure 13-10).[49] (Most bottled waters lack fluoride.) Fluoridation of drinking water (to raise the concentration to 1 part fluoride per 1 million ♦ parts water) offers good protection against dental caries at virtually no risk of toxicity.[50] By fluoridating the drinking water, a community offers its residents, particularly the children, a safe, economical, practical, and effective way to defend against dental caries.

Fluoride Toxicity

Too much fluoride can damage the teeth, causing **fluorosis**.[51] For this reason, a UL has been established. In mild cases, the teeth develop small white specks; in severe cases, the enamel becomes pitted and permanently stained (as shown in Figure 13-11). Fluorosis occurs only during tooth development and cannot be reversed, making its prevention ♦ a high priority. To limit fluoride ingestion, take care not to swallow fluoride-containing dental products such as toothpaste and mouthwash.

Fluoride Recommendations and Sources

As mentioned earlier, almost half of the Canadian population has access to fluoridated water. Fish and most teas contain appreciable amounts of natural fluoride.

IN SUMMARY **Fluoride makes bones stronger and teeth more resistant to decay. Fluoridation of public water supplies can significantly reduce the incidence of dental caries, but excess fluoride during tooth development can cause fluorosis—discoloured and pitted tooth enamel. The accompanying table provides a summary of fluoride.**

Fluoride

Adequate Intake (AI)	Significant Sources
Men: 4 mg/day Women: 3 mg/day	Drinking water (if fluoride containing or fluoridated), tea, seafood
Upper Level	**Deficiency Symptoms**
Adults: 10 mg/day	Susceptibility to tooth decay
Chief Functions in the Body	**Toxicity Symptoms**
Maintains health of bones and teeth; helps to make teeth resistant to decay	Fluorosis (pitting and discolouration of teeth)

FIGURE 13-11 Fluoride-Toxicity Symptom—The Mottled Teeth of Fluorosis

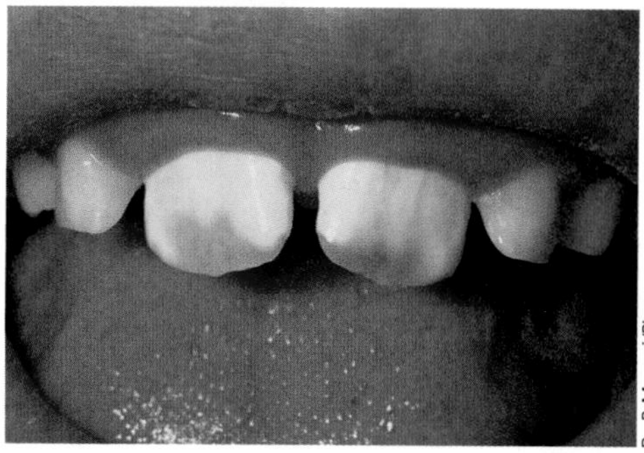

Dr. P. Marazzi/Photo Researchers, Inc

Vitamin K

Vitamin K is historically known for its role in blood clotting, but the health of bone proteins also depends on this fat-soluble vitamin.

Vitamin K Role in Bone Health Vitamin K participates in the metabolism of the bone protein **osteocalcin**. More specifically, vitamin K is needed to activate a carboxylase enzyme. When vitamin K is inadequate, osteocalcin is undercarboxylated and therefore less effective in binding calcium to form bone, resulting in low bone density.[52] An adequate intake of vitamin K helps to decrease bone turnover and protect against fractures,[53] although the effectiveness of vitamin K supplements on bone health is inconclusive.[54]

Vitamin K Deficiency and Toxicity Although rare, vitamin K deficiency profoundly affects our ability to clot blood; however, the long-term effects of vitamin K deficiency on bone health require further study. Similar to a low risk of deficiency, vitamin K toxicity is also rare. No adverse effects have been reported with high intakes of vitamin K and consequently a UL has not been set.

Vitamin K Recommendations and Sources The billions of bacteria found in the GI tract represent one source of vitamin K. Once synthesized, vitamin K is absorbed and stored in the liver. Bacterial synthesis of vitamin K provides only about half of a person's needs. Vitamin K–rich foods such as green vegetables and vegetable oils can easily supply the rest. The absorption of vitamin K from foods ranges between 40 and 70 percent.

IN SUMMARY **Aside from its role in blood clotting, certain proteins in bone require vitamin K. Bacteria in the GI tract synthesize about half of the human requirement for vitamin K, and the other half can be obtained from foods such as green vegetables and vegetable oils. The accompanying table provides a summary of vitamin K.**

Vitamin K

Other Names	Significant Sources
Phylloquinone, menaquinone, menadione, naphthoquinone	Bacterial synthesis in the digestive tract;[a] liver; leafy green vegetables, cabbage-type vegetables; milk
AI	**Deficiency Symptoms**
Men: 120 μg/day Women: 90 μg/day	Hemorrhaging
Chief Functions in the Body	**Toxicity Symptoms**
Synthesis of bone proteins and blood-clotting proteins	None known

osteocalcin (os-teo-KAL-sen): a calcium-binding protein in bones, essential for normal mineralization.

Nutrients for Bone Health—In Summary

After learning about the ways in which the minerals and vitamins—calcium, phosphorus, vitamin D, magnesium, fluoride, and vitamin K—support the development and maintenance of your bones and teeth, you may think to grab a glass of milk with your next meal or make a sandwich from canned salmon for lunch. Although these nutrients are closely associated with bone health, consuming foods rich in these nutrients also affect other important aspects of health. For example, calcium is required for muscle contraction and the regulation of blood pressure, and phosphorus and magnesium is essential to reactions involving glucose, fatty acids, amino acids, and vitamins. After familiarizing yourself with the various roles of these vitamins and minerals, by now you are likely realizing the importance of eating a wide variety of nutrient-dense foods each day to maintain a healthy body for life.

IN SUMMARY Nutrients for Bone Health

Bone Health Nutrients and Chief Functions	Deficiency Symptoms	Toxicity Symptoms	Significant Sources
Calcium			
Mineralization of bones and teeth; also involved in muscle contraction and relaxation, nerve functioning, blood clotting, and blood pressure	Stunted growth in children; bone loss (osteoporosis) in adults	Constipation; increased risk of urinary stone formation and kidney dysfunction; interference with absorption of other minerals	Milk, milk products, and milk alternatives, canned fish (with bones), calcium-set tofu, greens (bok choy, broccoli, chard), legumes
Phosphorus			
Mineralization of bones and teeth; part of every cell; important in genetic material; part of phospholipids; used in energy transfer and in buffer systems that maintain acid–base balance	Muscular weakness, bone pain[a]	Calcification of nonskeletal tissues, particularly the kidneys	All animal tissues (meat, fish, poultry, eggs, milk)
Vitamin D			
Mineralization of bones (raises blood calcium and phosphorus by increasing absorption from digestive tract, withdrawing calcium from bones, stimulating retention by kidneys)	Rickets, osteomalacia	Calcium imbalance (calcification of soft tissues and formation of stones)	Synthesized in the body with the help of sunshine, fortified milk
Magnesium			
Bone mineralization; building of protein; enzyme action; normal muscle contraction; nerve impulse transmission; maintenance of teeth; functioning of immune system	Weakness; confusion; if extreme, convulsions, bizarre muscle movements (especially of eye and face muscles), hallucinations, and difficulty in swallowing; in children, growth failure[b]	From nonfood sources only; diarrhea, alkalosis, dehydration	Nuts, legumes, whole grains, dark green vegetables, seafood, chocolate, cocoa
Fluoride			
Maintains health of bones and teeth; confers decay resistance on teeth	Susceptibility to tooth decay	Fluorosis (pitting and discolouration) of teeth	Drinking water (if fluoridated), tea, seafood
Vitamin K			
Synthesis of bone proteins and blood-clotting proteins	Hemorrhage	None known	Synthesized in the body by GI bacteria, green leafy vegetables

[a]Dietary deficiency rarely occurs, but some drugs can bind with phosphorus, making it unavailable and resulting in bone loss that is characterized by weakness and pain.
[b]A severe deficiency causes tetany, an extreme, prolonged contraction of the muscles similar to that caused by low blood calcium.

TABLE 13-1 Adult Canadians' Average Daily Nutrient Intakes from Food* Compared to the Dietary Reference Intakes

	Intake Men	Intake Women	RDA Men	RDA Women
Calcium (mg/d)	931	793	1000[a]	1000[a]
Phosphorus (mg/d)	1515	1181	700	700
Vitamin D (μg/d)	6.2	5.0	15[b]	15[b]
Magnesium (mg/d)	364	296	400[c]	310[c]

*Canadian Community Healthy Survey, Cycle 2.2, Nutrition (2004) Nutrient intakes from food. No published intake data exist for fluoride and vitamin K.
[a]19–50 years; 51–70 years: males 1000 mg/d and females 1200 mg/d; 71+ years: 1200 mg/d
[b]0–70 years; 71+ years: 20 μg/d
[c]19–30 years; 31+ years: males 420 mg/d and females 320 mg/d

Despite the need for a strong skeleton to carry us upright and healthy teeth to mechanically process food, you may be surprised by the average daily intake of the nutrients discussed in this chapter. How do adult Canadians' intakes of the bone health nutrients stack up against the current recommendations? Table 13-1 points out inadequate intakes of calcium, vitamin D, and magnesium. With low intakes of these nutrients, it is not surprising that osteoporosis is a public health issue in Canada, and it will become an even greater issue as the population ages. It is never too late to take care of your bones. Get the nutrients you need in amounts that you need and be physically active to maintain your bones.

Nutrition Portfolio

To obtain all the vitamins and minerals that your bones need each day, be sure to select a variety of foods from each of the four food groups.

Go to Diet Analysis Plus and choose one of the days on which you tracked your diet. Go to the Intake vs. Goals report. Near the bottom of this report, you will see all of the vitamins grouped together and all of the minerals grouped together; using this section of the report for reference, answer the following questions:

- How was your vitamin intake overall? Did you consume too much or too little of any vitamin? Which vitamins concerned you most? How was your vitamin D intake?
- Now, ask yourself about your mineral intake overall. Did you consume too much or too little of any mineral? How was your calcium intake?

Next go to the Intake Spreadsheet report, and looking at each of the vitamins, answer the following questions:

- Which of your foods provided high intakes of vitamins and minerals important to bone health?
- Which of your foods provided little or no calcium, phosphorus, magnesium, vitamin D, or vitamin K?
- Examine your daily choices of whole or enriched grains, dark green leafy and orange vegetables, citrus fruits, legumes, 1% milk products, and lean meats, then evaluate their contributions to your vitamin intakes.
- Compare any vitamin and mineral intakes you obtained from supplements with their respective UL.

Diet Analysis PLUS

To complete this exercise, go to your Diet Analysis Plus at www.cengage.com/sso.

Nutrition on the Net

CENGAGENOW™
For further study of topics covered in this chapter, log on to **www.cengage.com/sso.**

- Search for "osteoporosis" at the Dietitians of Canada's website: **www.dietitians.ca**
- Learn about our national facts and statistics on osteoporosis at Osteoporosis Canada: **www.osteoporosis.ca**
- Learn more about the new DRI calcium and vitamin D recommendations: **www.hc-sc.gc.ca/fn-an/nutrition/vitamin/vita-d-eng.php**
- Learn more about the DASH diet: **www.nhlbi.nih.gov/health/public/heart/hbp/dash/new_dash.pdf**
- Learn about the benefits of calcium and find tips and recipes for including more milk in your diet: **www.dairygoodness.ca**

References

1. P. R. Trumbo and K. C. Ellwood, Supplemental calcium and risk reduction of hypertension, pregnancy-induced hypertension, and preeclampsia: An evidence-based review by the US Food and Drug Administration, *Nutrition Reviews* 65 (2007): 78–87.
2. Trumbo and Ellwood, 2007.
3. J. Ishihara and coauthors, Dietary calcium, vitamin D, and the risk of colorectal cancer, *American Journal of Clinical Nutrition* 88 (2008): 1576–1583; C. S. Guerreiro and coauthors, The *D1822V APC* polymorphism interacts with fat, calcium, and fiber intakes in modulating the risk of colorectal cancer in Portuguese persons, *American Journal of Clinical Nutrition* 85 (2007): 1592–1597; M. E. Martínez and E. T. Jacobs, Calcium supplementation and prevention of colorectal neoplasia: Lessons from clinical trials, *Journal of the National Cancer Institute* 99 (2007): 99–100; S. C. Larsson and coauthors, Calcium and dairy food intakes are inversely associated with colorectal cancer risk in the Cohort of Swedish Men, *American Journal of Clinical Nutrition* 83 (2006): 667–673; A. Flood and coauthors, Calcium from diet and supplements is associated with reduced risk of colorectal cancer in a prospective cohort of women, *Cancer Epidemiology, Biomarkers, and Prevention* 14 (2005): 126–132.
4. R. P. Heaney and K. Rafferty, Preponderance of the evidence: An example from the issue of calcium intake and body composition, *Nutrition Reviews* 67 (2009): 32–39; G. C. Major and coauthors, Recent developments in calcium-related obesity research, *Obesity Reviews* 9 (2008): 428–445; G. Barba and P. Russo, Dairy foods, dietary calcium and obesity: A short review of the evidence, *Nutrition, Metabolism, and Cardiovascular Diseases* 16 (2006): 445–451; S. Schrager, Dietary calcium intake and obesity, *Journal of the American Board of Family Practice* 18 (2005): 205–210.
5. J. K. Lorenzen and coauthors, Calcium supplementation for 1 y does not reduce body weight or fat mass in young girls, *American Journal of Clinical Nutrition* 83 (2006): 18–23.
6. M. Bortolotti and coauthors, Dairy calcium supplementation in overweight or obese persons: Its effect on markers of fat metabolism, *American Journal of Clinical Nutrition* 88 (2008): 877–885; S. N. Rajpathak and coauthors, Calcium and dairy intakes in relation to long-term weight gain in US men, *American Journal of Clinical Nutrition* 83 (2006): 559–566; C. W. Gunther and coauthors, Dairy products do not lead to alterations in body weight or fat mass in young women in a 1-y intervention, *American Journal of Clinical Nutrition* 81 (2005): 751–756.
7. R. C. Khanal and I. Nemere, Regulation of intestinal calcium transport, *Annual Review of Nutrition* 28 (2008): 179–196.
8. F. Bronner, Recent developments in intestinal calcium absorption, *Nutrition Reviews* 67 (2009): 109–113.
9. Osteoporosis Canada, Breaking barriers not bones, 2008–2009 annual review. www.osteoporosis.ca, accessed December 2010; E. J. Waugh, M. A. Lam, G. A. Hawker, J. McGowan, A. Papaioannou, A. M. Cheung, A. B. Hodsman, W. D. Leslie, K. Siminoski, and S. A. Jamal, Risk factors for low bone mass in healthy 40–60 year old women: A systematic review of the literature, *Osteoporosis International* 20 (2009): 1–21.
10. H. Vatanaparast, J. H. Dolega-Cieszkowski, and S. J. Whiting, Many adult Canadians are not meeting current calcium recommendations from food and supplement intake, *Applied Physiology, Nutrition, and Metabolism* 34 (2009): 191–196.
11. R. D. Jackson and coauthors, Calcium plus vitamin D supplementation and the risk of fractures, *New England Journal of Medicine* 354 (2006): 669–683.
12. X. Gao and coauthors, Meeting adequate intake for dietary calcium without dairy foods in adolescents aged 9 to 18 years (National Health and Nutrition Examination Survey 2001–2002), *Journal of the American Dietetic Association* 106 (2006): 1759–1765.
13. F. R. Greer, N. F. Krebs, and the Committee on Nutrition, Optimizing bone health and calcium intakes of infants, children, and adolescents, *Pediatrics* 117 (2006): 578–585.
14. R. P. Heaney, Absorbability and utility of calcium in mineral waters, *American Journal of Clinical Nutrition* 84 (2006): 371–374.
15. R. P. Heaney and coauthors, Calcium fortification systems differ in bioavailability, *Journal of the American Dietetic Association* 105 (2005): 807–809.
16. K. Tucker and coauthors, Colas, but not other carbonated beverages, are associated with low bone mineral density in older women: The Framingham Osteoporosis Study, *American Journal of Clinical Nutrition* 84 (2006): 936–942; R. P. Heaney and K. Rafferty, Carbonated beverages and urinary calcium excretion, *American Journal of Clinical Nutrition* 74 (2001): 343–347; S. J. Whiting and coauthors, Relationship between carbonated and other low nutrient dense beverages and bone mineral content of adolescents, *Nutrition Research* 21 (2001): 1107–1115.
17. A. Borjian and coauthors. Pop-cola acids and tooth erosion: An in vitro, in vivo, electron-microscopic, and clinical report, *International Journal of Dentistry* (2010): doi:10.1155/2010/957842
18. P. Lips, Vitamin D physiology, *Progress in Biophysics and Molecular Biology* 92 (2006): 4–8.
19. H. F. Deluca, Evolution of our understanding of vitamin D, *Nutrition Reviews* 66 (2008): S73–S87; A. W. Norman, From vitamin D to hormone D: Fundamentals of the vitamin D endocrine system essential for good health, *American Journal of Clinical Nutrition* 88 (2008): 491S–499S.
20. R. P. Heaney, Vitamin D and calcium interactions: Functional outcomes, *American Journal of Clinical Nutrition* 88 (2008): 541S–544S.
21. Deluca, 2008; M. R. Haussler and coauthors, Vitamin D receptor: Molecular signaling and actions of nutritional ligands in disease prevention, *Nutrition Reviews* 66 (2008): S98–S112.
22. R. C. Khanal and I. Nemere, Regulation of intestinal calcium transport, *Annual Review of Nutrition* 28 (2008): 179–196.
23. A. W. Norman, Minireview: Vitamin D receptor—new assignments for an already busy receptor, *Endocrinology* 147 (2006): 5542–5548.
24. S. Samual and M. D. Sitrin, Vitamin D's role in cell proliferation and differentiation, *Nutrition Reviews* 66 (2008): S116–S124.
25. E. van Etten and coauthors, Regulation of vitamin D homeostasis: Implications for the immune system, *Nutrition Reviews* 66 (2008): S125–S134.
26. M. Chung and coauthors, Vitamin D and calcium: A systematic review of health outcomes, AHRQ Publication No. 09-E015 Agency for Healthcare Research and Quality, Rockville, MD (2009). Available at www.ahrq.gov/clinic/tp/vitadcaltp.htm; M. T. Cantorna, Vitamin D and multiple sclerosis: An update, *Nutrition Reviews* 66 (2008): S135–S138; M. F. Holick, Vitamin D: A d-lightful health perspective, *Nutrition Reviews* 66 (2008): S182–S194; S. E. Judd and coauthors, Optimal vitamin D status attenuates the age-associated increase in systolic blood pressure in white Americans: Results from the third National Health and Nutrition Examination Survey, *American Journal of Clinical Nutrition* 87 (2008): 136–141; G. E. Mullin and A. Dobs, Vitamin D and its role in cancer and immunity: A prescription for sunlight, *Nutrition in Clinical Practice* 22 (2007): 305–322; Y. Cui and T. E. Rohan, Vitamin D, calcium, and breast cancer risk: A review, *Cancer*

Epidemiological, Biomarkers and Prevention 15 (2006): 1427–1437; A. F. Gombart, Q. T. Luong, and H. P. Koeffler, Vitamin D compounds: Activity against microbes and cancer, *Anticancer Research* 26 (2006): 2531–2542; P. T. Liu and coauthors, Toll-like receptor triggering of a vitamin D–mediated human antimicrobial response, *Science* 311 (2006): 1770–1773; L. A. Martini and R. J. Wood, Vitamin D status and the metabolic syndrome, *Nutrition Reviews* 64 (2006): 479–486; K. L. Munger and coauthors, Serum 25-hydroxyvitamin D levels and risk of multiple sclerosis, *Journal of the American Medical Association* 296 (2006): 2832–2838; S. S. Schleithoff and coauthors, Vitamin D supplementation improves cytokine profiles in patients with congestive heart failure: A double-blind, randomized, placebo-controlled trial, *American Journal of Clinical Nutrition* 83 (2006): 754–759; T. Dietrich and coauthors, Association between serum concentrations of 25-hydroxyvitamin D and gingival inflammation, *American Journal of Clinical Nutrition* 82 (2005): 575–580.

27. L. S. Greene-Finestone, C. Berger, M. de Groh, D. A. Hanley, N. Hidiroglou, K. Sarafin, S. Poliquin, J. Krieger, J. B. Richards, D. Goltzman, and CaMos Research Group, 25-Hydroxyvitamin D in Canadian adults: Biological, environmental, and behavioral correlates, *Osteoporosis International* 21, doi: 10.1007/s00198-010-1362-7; S. A. Bowden and coauthors, Prevalence of vitamin D deficiency and insufficiency in children with osteopenia or osteoporosis referred to a pediatric metabolic bone clinic, *Pediatrics* 121 (2008): e1585–e1590; M. L. Neuhouser and coauthors, Vitamin D insufficiency in a multiethnic cohort of breast cancer survivors, *American Journal of Clinical Nutrition* 88 (2008): 133–139.
28. L. A. Martini and R. J. Wood, Vitamin D and blood pressure connection: Update on epidemiologic, clinical, and mechanistic evidence, *Nutrition Reviews* 66 (2008): 291–297; T. J. Wang and coauthors, Vitamin D deficiency and risk of cardiovascular disease, *Circulation* 117 (2008): 503–511; M. F. Holick, Vitamin D deficiency, *New England Journal of Medicine* 357 (2007): 266–281.
29. K. D. Cashman and coauthors, Low vitamin D status adversely affects bone health parameters in adolescents, *American Journal of Clinical Nutrition* 87 (2008): 1039–1044.
30. D. Schnadower and coauthors, Hypocalcemic seizures and secondary bilateral femoral fractures in an adolescent with primary vitamin D deficiency, *Pediatrics* 118 (2006): 2226–2230.
31. A. Prentice, Vitamin D deficiency: A global perspective, *Nutrition Reviews* 66 (2008): S153–S164.
32. L. M. Ward, I. Gaboury, M. Ladhani, and S. Zlotkin, Vitamin D–deficiency rickets among children in Canada, *Canadian Medical Association Journal* 177 (2007): 161–166.
33. Canadian Paediatric Surveillance Program, Rickets: A re-emerging public health problem in Canada? *Paediatric Child Health* 13 (2008): 73.
34. M. F. Holick, High prevalence of vitamin D inadequacy and implications for health, *Mayo Clinic Proceedings* 81 (2006): 353–373.
35. B. Dawson-Hughes, Serum 25-hydroxyvitamin D and functional outcomes in the elderly, *American Journal of Clinical Nutrition* 88 (2008): 537S–540S; S. A. Talwar and coauthors, Dose response to vitamin D supplementation among postmenopausal African American women, *American Journal of Clinical Nutrition* 86 (2007): 1657–1662; H. A. Bischoff-Ferrari and coauthors, Fracture prevention with vitamin D supplementation: A meta-analysis of randomized controlled trials, *Journal of the American Medical Association* 293 (2005): 2257–2264.
36. G. Jones, Pharmacokinetics of vitamin D toxicity, *American Journal of Clinical Nutrition* 88 (2008): 582S–586S.
37. A. C. Ross, C. L. Taylor, A. L. Yaktine, and H. B. Del Valle, Dietary Reference Intakes for calcium and vitamin D (Washington, D.C.: National Academies Press, 2011); R. P. Heaney, Vitamin D: Criteria for safety and eficacy, *Nutrition Reviews* 66 (2008): S178–S181; L. Mosekilde, Vitamin D requirement and setting recommendation levels: Long-term perspectives, *Nutrition Reviews* 66 (2008): S170–S177; R. Vieth and coauthors, The urgent need to recommend an intake of vitamin D that is effective, *American Journal of Clinical Nutrition* 85 (2007): 649–650; H. A. Bischoff-Ferrari and coauthors, Estimation of optimal serum concentrations of 25-hydroxyvitamin D for multiple health outcomes, *American Journal of Clinical Nutrition* 84 (2006): 18–28.
38. K. D. Cashman and coauthors, Estimation of the dietary requirement for vitamin D in healthy adults, *American Journal of Clinical Nutrition* 88 (2008): 1535–1542; J. F. Aloia and coauthors, Vitamin D intake to attain a desired serum 25-hydroxyvitamin D concentration, *American Journal of Clinical Nutrition* 87 (2008): 1952–1958.
39. K. Langlois and coauthors, Vitamin D status of Canadians as measured in the 2007 to 2009 Canadian Health Measures Survey, *Health Reports* 21 (2010): 47–55.
40. Canadian Cancer Society, Vitamin D (2011). www.cancer.ca/Canada-wide/Prevention/Vitamin D.aspx?sc_lang=en, accessed September 15, 2011.
41. A. Burgaz and coauthors, Associations of diet, supplement use, and ultraviolet B radiation exposure with vitamin D status in Swedish women during winter, *American Journal of Clinical Nutrition* 86 (2007): 1399–1404; R. M. van Dam and coauthors, Potentially modifiable determinants of vitamin D status in an older population in the Netherlands: The Hoorn Study, *American Journal of Clinical Nutrition* 85 (2007): 755–761.
42. B. A. Gilchrest, Sun exposure and vitamin D sufficiency, *American Journal of Clinical Nutrition* 88 (2008): 570S–577S.
43. M. J. Bolland and coauthors, The effects of seasonal variation of 25-hydroxyvitamin D and fat mass on a diagnosis of vitamin D sufficiency, *American Journal of Clinical Nutrition* 86 (2007): 959–964.
44. E. Hyppönen and C. Power, Hypovitaminosis D in British adults at age 45 y: Nationwide cohort study of dietary and lifestyle predictors, *American Journal of Clinical Nutrition* 85 (2007): 860–868; F. L. Weng and coauthors, Risk factors for low serum 25-hydroxyvitamin D concentrations in otherwise healthy children and adolescents, *American Journal of Clinical Nutrition* 86 (2007): 150–158.
45. L. Steingrimsdottir and coauthors, Relationship between serum parathyroid hormone levels, vitamin D sufficiency, and calcium intake, *Journal of the American Medical Association* 294 (2005): 2336–2341.
46. B. L. Tamboli, D. P. Singh, and K. Sharma, Role of waterborne magnesium in preventing chronic diseases, *International Journal of Collaborative Research* on *Internal Medicine & Public Health* 3 (2011): 78–87.
47. Health Canada and Statistics Canada, *Canadian Community Health Survey,* Cycle 2.2 Nutrition (2004) Nutrient intakes from food: Provincial, regional, and national summary data tables, Volume 2. www.hc-sc.gc.ca/fn-an/surveill/nutrition/commun/index-eng.php, accessed September 15, 2011.
48. The Canadian Dental Association: Dental Statistics (2010). www.cda-adc.ca/en/cda/media_room/health_month, accessed September 19, 2011.
49. Health Canada, It's Your Health: Fluoride and Human Health (2010), www.hc-sc.gc.ca/hl-vs/iyh-vsv/environ/fluor-eng.php, accessed September 15, 2011; Health Canada Office of the Chief Dental Officer, Provincial and territorial estimates for community water fluoridation coverage in 2007 (2007). www.hc-sc.gc.ca/ahc-asc/branch-dirgen/fnihb-dgspni/ocdo-bdc/project-eng.php, accessed September 15, 2011.
50. Position of the American Dietetic Association: The impact of fluoride on health, *Journal of the American Dietetic Association* 105 (2005): 1620–1628.
51. Surveillance for dental caries, dental sealants, tooth retention, edentulism, and enamel fluorosis: United States, 1988–1994 and 1999–2002, *Morbidity and Mortality Weekly Report* 54 (2005): 1–44.
52. H. M. Macdonald and coauthors, Vitamin K1 intake is associated with higher bone mineral density and reduced bone resorption in early postmenopausal Scottish women: No evidence of gene-nutrient interaction with apolipoprotein E polymorphisms, *American Journal of Clinical Nutrition* 87 (2008): 1513–1520; K. L. Berkner, The vitamin K-dependent carboxylase, *Annual Review of Nutrition* 25 (2005): 127–149.
53. S. Cockayne and coauthors, Vitamin K and the prevention of fractures: Systematic review and meta-analysis of randomized controlled trials, *Archives of Internal Medicine* 166 (2006): 1256–1261; J. Iwamoto, T. Takeda, and Y. Sato, Menatetrenone (vitamin K2) and bone quality in the treatment of postmenopausal osteoporosis, *Nutrition Reviews* 64 (2006): 509–517; K. D. Cashman, Vitamin K status may be an important determinant of childhood bone health, *Nutrition Reviews* 63 (2005): 284–293.
54. K. D. Cashman and E. O'Connor, Does high vitamin K1 intake protect against bone loss in later life? *Nutrition Reviews* 66 (2008): 532–538; M. K. Shea and S. L. Booth, Update on the role of vitamin K in skeletal health, *Nutrition Reviews* 66 (2008): 549–557.

HIGHLIGHT 13

Osteoporosis and Calcium

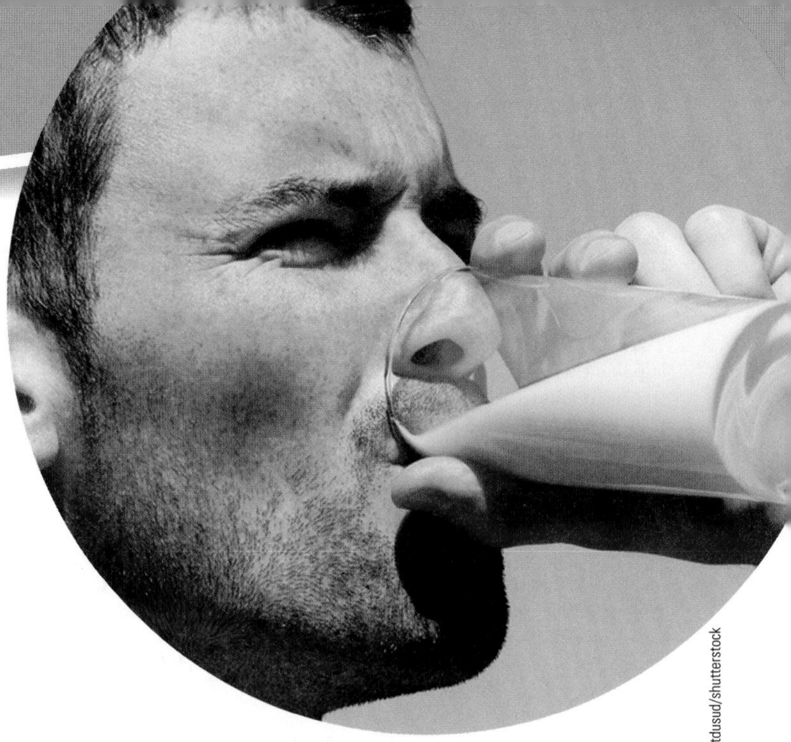

ventdusud/shutterstock

Osteoporosis most often becomes apparent during the later years, but it develops much earlier—and without warning. Few people are aware that their bones are being robbed of their strength. The problem often first becomes evident when someone's hip suddenly gives way. People say, "She fell and broke her hip," but in fact the hip may have been so fragile that it broke *before* she fell. Even bumping into a table may be enough to shatter a porous bone into fragments so numerous and scattered that they cannot be reassembled. Removing them and replacing them with an artificial joint requires major surgery. In Canada, at age 50, women and men have a lifetime risk of fracture of 12.1 percent and 5.2 percent, respectively.[1] The majority of hip fractures are related to osteoporosis and falls. In 2005–2006, over 28 000 Canadians were hospitalized for hip fracture.[2] These hospital visits last more than 10 days, placing an economic burden on the Canadian health-care system. The annual cost for treating people with hip and other fractures caused by osteoporosis is estimated at 1.9 billion dollars.[3] But more than having an economic impact, fractures affect people's quality of life. People with fractures frequently experience increased pain, limited mobility, and reduced ability for self-care.[4] Only 44 percent of hospitalized patients are able to return home, and 25 percent will die of complications within one year. Although these data are striking in magnitude, there is a downward trend in age-adjusted hip fracture rates in Canada, mostly due to better diagnosis and treatment protocols.[5] Given the burden of living with fracture, government has set prevention and proper diagnosis and treatment of osteoporosis as a priority public health issue.

This highlight examines osteoporosis, one of the most prevalent diseases of aging, affecting almost 2 million people in Canada—most of them women older than 50 years.[6] It reviews the many factors that contribute to breaks in the bones of the hips, vertebrae, wrists, arms, and ankles that happen each year. It also presents strategies to reduce the risks, paying special attention to the role of dietary calcium.

Bone Development and Disintegration

Bone has two compartments: the outer, hard shell of **cortical bone** and the inner, lacy matrix of **trabecular bone.** (The glossary defines these and other bone-related terms.) Both can lose minerals, but in different ways and at different rates. The photograph on p. 431 shows a human leg bone sliced lengthwise, exposing the lacy, calcium-containing crystals of trabecular bone. These crystals give up calcium to the blood when the diet runs short, and they take up calcium again when the supply is plentiful (review Figure 13-2 on p. 412). For people who have eaten calcium-rich foods throughout the bone-forming years of their youth, these deposits make bones dense and provide a rich reservoir of calcium.

Surrounding and protecting the trabecular bone is a dense, ivory-like exterior shell—the cortical bone. Cortical bone composes the shafts of the long bones, and a thin cortical shell caps the end of the bone, too. Both compartments confer strength on

GLOSSARY

antacids: medications used to relieve indigestion by neutralizing acid in the stomach. Calcium-containing preparations (such as Tums) contain available calcium. Antacids with aluminum or magnesium hydroxides (such as Rolaids) can accelerate calcium losses.

bone meal or **powdered bone:** crushed or ground bone preparations intended to supply calcium to the diet. Calcium from bone is not well absorbed and is often contaminated with toxic minerals such as arsenic, mercury, lead, and cadmium.

bone mineral density: a measure of bone strength. When minerals fill the bone matrix (making it dense), they give it strength.

coral: the skeleton of marine polyps, comprised mostly of calcium carbonate.

cortical bone: the very dense bone tissue that forms the outer shell surrounding trabecular bone and comprises the shaft of a long bone.

dolomite: a compound of minerals (calcium magnesium carbonate) found in limestone and marble. Dolomite is powdered and is sold as a calcium-magnesium supplement. However, it may be contaminated with toxic minerals, is not well absorbed, and interacts adversely with absorption of other esssential minerals.

osteoporosis: a disease characterized by porous and fragile bones.

oyster shell: a product made from the powdered shells of oysters that is sold as a calcium supplement, but it is not well absorbed by the digestive system.

trabecular (tra-BECK-you-lar) **bone:** the lacy inner structure of calcium crystals that supports the bone's structure and provides a calcium storage bank.

type I osteoporosis: osteoporosis characterized by rapid bone losses, primarily of trabecular bone.

type II osteoporosis: osteoporosis characterized by gradual losses of both trabecular and cortical bone.

bone: cortical bone provides the sturdy outer wall, and trabecular bone provides support along the lines of stress.

The two types of bone play different roles in calcium balance and osteoporosis. Supplied with blood vessels and metabolically active, trabecular bone is sensitive to hormones that govern day-to-day deposits and withdrawals of calcium. It readily gives up minerals whenever blood calcium needs replenishing. Losses of trabecular bone start becoming significant for men and women in their 30s, although losses can occur whenever calcium withdrawals exceed deposits.

Cortical bone also gives up calcium, but slowly and at a steady pace. Cortical bone losses typically begin at about age 40 and continue slowly but surely thereafter.

Losses of trabecular and cortical bone reflect two types of osteoporosis, which cause two types of bone breaks. **Type I osteoporosis** involves losses of trabecular bone (see Figure H13-1). These losses sometimes exceed three times the expected rate, and bone breaks may occur suddenly. Trabecular bone becomes so fragile that even the body's own weight can overburden the spine—vertebrae may suddenly disintegrate and crush down, painfully pinching major nerves.[7] Wrists may break as bone ends weaken, and teeth may loosen or fall out as the trabecular bone of the jaw recedes. Women are most often the victims of this type of osteoporosis, outnumbering men six to one.

In **type II osteoporosis,** the calcium of both cortical and trabecular bone is drawn out of storage, but slowly over the years. As old age approaches, the vertebrae may compress into wedge shapes, forming what is often called a "dowager's hump," the posture many older people assume as they "grow shorter." Figure H13-2 (p. 432) shows the effect of compressed spinal bone on a woman's height and posture. Because both the cortical shell and the trabecular interior weaken, breaks most often occur in the hip, as mentioned in the introductory paragraph. A woman is twice as likely as a man to suffer type II osteoporosis.

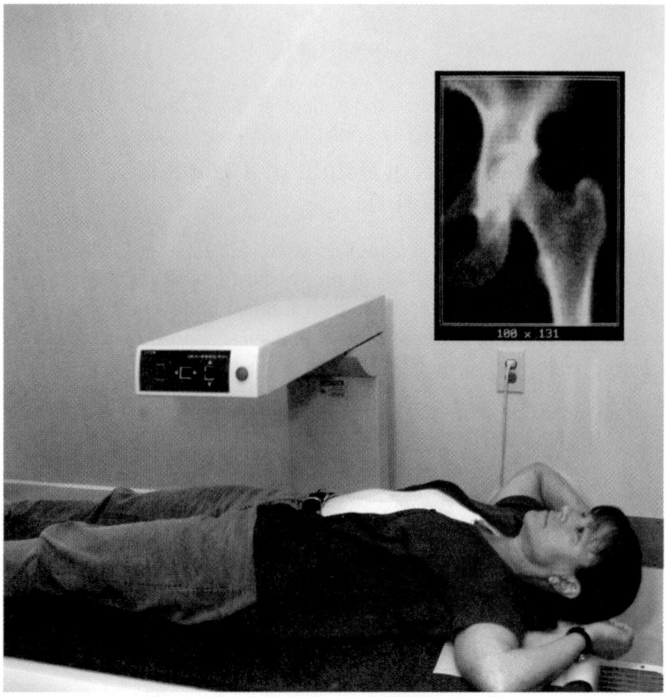
100 x 131
© David Young Wolff/PhotoEdit

Using a DEXA (dual-energy X-ray absorpiometry) test to measure bone mineral density identifies osteoporosis, determines risks for fractures, and tracks responses to treatment.

FIGURE H13-1 Healthy and Osteoporotic Trabecular Bones

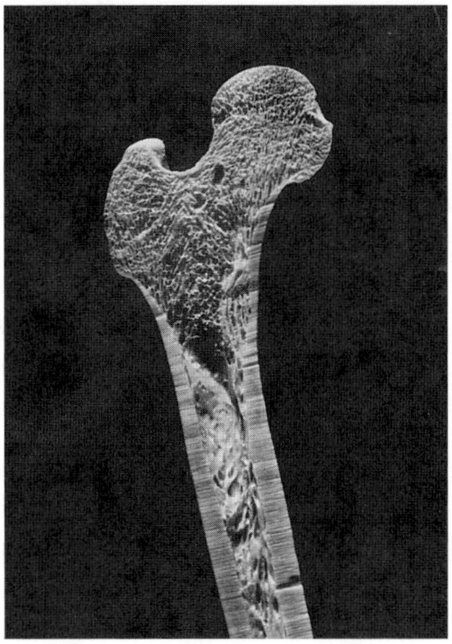
Courtesy of Gjon Mili

Trabecular bone is the lacy network of calcium-containing crystals that fills the interior. Cortical bone is the dense, ivorylike bone that forms the exterior shell.

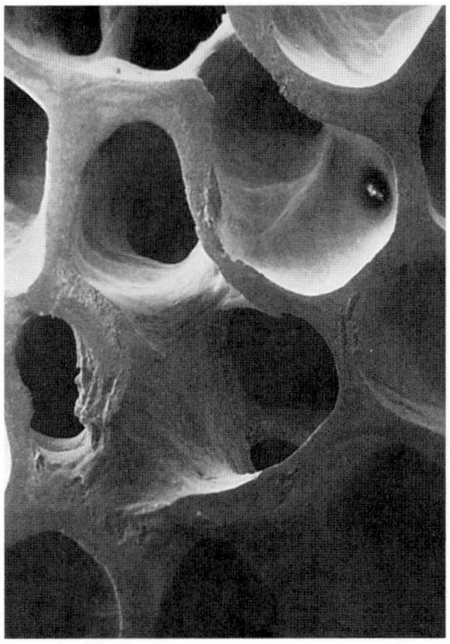
Permission by David Dempster from J Bone Miner Res, 1986

Electron micrograph of healthy trabecular bone.

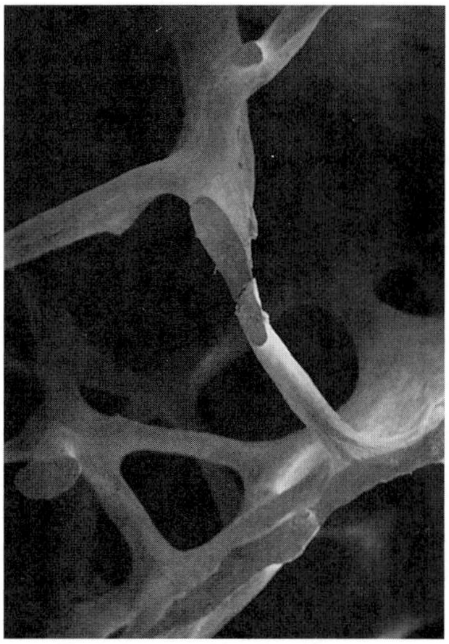
Permission by David Dempster from J Bone Miner Res, 1986

Electron micrograph of trabecular bone affected by osteoporosis.

FIGURE H13-2 Loss of Height in a Woman Caused by Osteoporosis

The woman on the left is about 50 years old. On the right, she is 80 years old. Her legs have not grown shorter. Instead, her back has lost length due to collapse of her spinal bones (vertebrae). Collapsed vertebrae cannot protect the spinal nerves from pressure that causes excruciating pain.

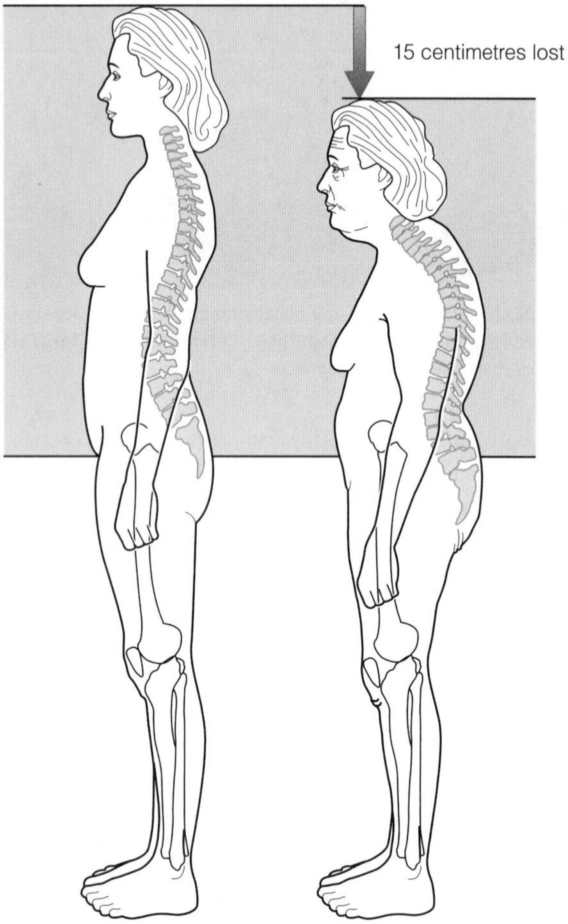
15 centimetres lost
50 years old
80 years old

TABLE H13-1 Types of Osteoporosis Compared

	Type I	Type II
Other name	Postmenopausal osteoporosis	Senile osteoporosis
Age of onset	50 to 70 years old	70 years and older
Bone loss	Trabecular bone	Both trabecular and cortical bone
Fracture sites	Wrist and spine	Hip
Gender incidence	6 women to 1 man	2 women to 1 man
Primary causes	Rapid loss of estrogen in women following menopause; loss of testosterone in men with advancing age	Reduced calcium absorption, increased bone mineral loss, increased propensity to fall

TABLE H13-2 Risk Factors and Protective Factors for Osteoporosis

Risk Factors	Protective Factors
• Older age	• Younger age
• Low BMI	• High BMI
• Caucasian, Asian, or Hispanic heritage	
• Cigarette smoking	• No smoking
• Alcohol consumption in excess	• Alcohol consumption in moderation
• Sedentary lifestyle	• Regular weight-bearing exercise
• Use of glucocorticoids or anticonvulsants	
• Female gender	• Male gender
• Maternal history of osteoporosis fracture or personal history of fracture	• Bone density assessment and treatment (if necessary)
• Estrogen deficiency in women (amenorrhea or menopause, especially early or surgically induced); testosterone deficiency in men	• Use of estrogen therapy
• Lifetime diet inadequate in calcium and vitamin D	• Lifetime diet rich in calcium and vitamin D

Table H13-1 summarizes the differences between the two types of osteoporosis. Physicians can diagnose osteoporosis and assess the risk of bone fractures by measuring **bone mineral density** using dual-energy X-ray absorptiometry (DEXA scan) or ultrasound. They also consider risk factors that predict bone fractures, including age, personal and family history of fracture, BMI, and physical inactivity.[8] The 2010 clinical practice guidelines for the diagnosis and management of osteoporosis in Canada outline recommendations for risk assessment and strategies for fracture prevention.[9] Table H13-2 summarizes the major risk factors and protective factors for osteoporosis. The more risk factors that apply to a person, the greater the chances of bone loss. Notice that several risk factors that are influential in the development of osteoporosis—such as age, gender, and genetics—cannot be changed. Other risk factors—such as diet, physical activity, body weight, smoking, and alcohol use—are personal behaviours that can be changed. By eating a calcium-rich, well-balanced diet, being physically active, abstaining from smoking, and drinking alcohol in moderation (if at all), people can defend themselves against osteoporosis. These decisions are particularly important for those with other risk factors that cannot be changed.

Whether a person develops osteoporosis seems to depend on the interactions of several factors, including nutrition. Age is the strongest predictor of bone density: osteoporosis is responsible for at least 80 percent of the hip fractures in people older than the age of 60.[10]

Age and Bone Calcium

Two major stages of life are critical in the development of osteoporosis. The first is the bone-acquiring stage of childhood and adolescence. The second is the bone-losing decades of late adulthood, especially in women after menopause. The bones gain strength and density all through the growing years and into young adulthood. As people age, the cells that build bone gradually become less active, but those that dismantle bone continue working. The result is that bone loss exceeds bone formation. Some bone loss is inevitable, but losses can be curtailed by maximizing bone mass.

Maximizing Bone Mass

To maximize bone mass, the diet must deliver an adequate supply of calcium during the first three decades of life. Children and teens who get enough calcium and vitamin D have denser bones than those with inadequate intakes.[11] With little or no calcium from the diet, the body must depend on bone to supply calcium to the blood—bone mass diminishes, and bones lose their density and strength. When people reach the bone-losing years of middle age, those who formed dense bones during their youth have the advantage. They simply have more bone starting out and can lose more before suffering ill effects. Figure H13-3 demonstrates this effect.

FIGURE H13-3 Bone Losses over Time Compared

Peak bone mass is achieved by age 30. Women gradually lose bone mass until menopause, when losses accelerate dramatically and then gradually taper off.

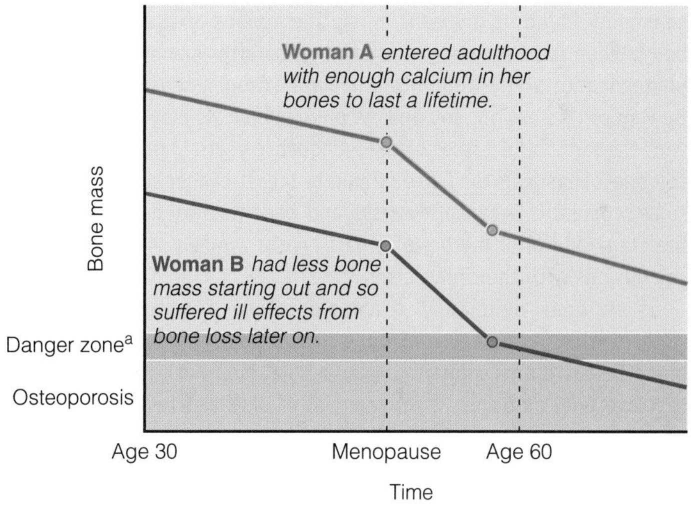

Woman A entered adulthood with enough calcium in her bones to last a lifetime.
Woman B had less bone mass starting out and so suffered ill effects from bone loss later on.
Bone mass
Danger zone[a]
Osteoporosis
Age 30
Menopause
Age 60
Time

[a]People with a moderate degree of bone mass reduction are said to have *osteopenia* and are at increased risk of fractures.

SOURCE: Data from Committee on Dietary Reference Intakes, *Dietary Reference Intakes for Calcium, Phosphorus, Magnesium, Vitamin D, and Fluoride* (Washington, D.C.: National Academy Press, 1997), pp. 71–145.

Minimizing Bone Loss

Not only does dietary calcium build strong bones in youth, but it remains important in protecting against losses in the later years. Unfortunately, calcium intakes of older adults are typically low, and calcium absorption declines after menopause. The kidneys do not activate vitamin D as well as they did earlier (recall that active vitamin D enhances calcium absorption). Also, sunlight is needed to form vitamin D, and many older people spend little or no time outdoors in the sunshine. For these reasons, and because intakes of vitamin D are typically low anyway, blood vitamin D declines.

Some of the hormones that regulate bone and calcium metabolism—parathyroid hormone, calcitonin, and estrogen—also change with age and accelerate bone mineral withdrawal. Together, these age-related factors contribute to bone loss: inefficient bone remodelling, reduced calcium intakes, impaired calcium absorption, poor vitamin D status, and hormonal changes that favour bone mineral withdrawal.

Gender and Hormones

After age, gender is the next strongest predictor of osteoporosis. Men have greater bone density than women at maturity, and women have greater losses than men in later life. Consequently, men develop bone problems about 10 years later than women, and women account for four out of five cases of osteoporosis. Menopause imperils women's bones. Bone dwindles rapidly when the hormone estrogen diminishes and menstruation ceases. The lack of estrogen contributes to the release of cytokines that produce inflammation and accelerate bone loss.[12] Women may lose up to 20 percent of their bone mass during the six to eight years following menopause. Eventually, losses taper off so that women again lose bone at the same rate as men their age. Losses of bone minerals continue throughout the remainder of a woman's lifetime, but not at the free-fall pace of the menopause years (review Figure H13-3).

Rapid bone losses also occur when *young* women's ovaries fail to produce enough estrogen, causing menstruation to cease. In some cases, diseased ovaries are to blame and must be removed; in others, the ovaries fail to produce sufficient estrogen because the women suffer from anorexia nervosa and have unreasonably restricted their body weight (see Highlight 8). The amenorrhea and low body weights explain much of the bone loss seen in these young women, even years after diagnosis and treatment. Estrogen therapy can help nonmenstruating women prevent further bone loss and reduce the incidence of fractures. Because estrogen therapy may increase the risks for breast cancer, women must carefully weigh any potential benefits against the possible dangers.

The two main classes of drugs used to prevent or treat osteoporosis are antiresorptive agents that block bone resorption by inhibiting osteoclast activity (examples include raloxifene, alendronate, risedronate, and calcitonin) and anabolic agents that stimulate bone formation by acting on osteoblasts (an example is parathyroid hormone).*[13] A combination of these drugs or of hormone replacement and a drug may be most beneficial.[14]

*Raloxifene (rah-LOX-ih-feen) is a selective estrogen-receptor modulator (SERM), marketed as Evista; alendronate (a-LEN-droe-nate) is a bisphosphonate, marketed as Fosamax; risedronate (rih-SEH-droe-nate) is a bisphosphonate, marketed as Actonel; and calcitonin is a hormone, marketed as Calcimar and Miacalcin.

Some women who choose not to use estrogen therapy turn to soy as an alternative treatment. Interestingly, the phytochemicals commonly found in soybeans mimic the actions of estrogen in the body. When natural estrogen is lacking, as after menopause, these phytochemicals may step in to stimulate estrogen-sensitive tissues. By way of this action, soy and its phytochemicals may help to prevent the rapid bone losses of the menopause years.[15] Unfortunately, soy photochemicals may also stimulate breast cancer cell growth in some women.[16] Because the risks and benefits vary depending on life stage and prior history of breast cancer, women should discuss soy options with their physicians.[17]

If estrogen deficiency is a major cause of osteoporosis in women, what is the cause of bone loss in men? The male sex hormone testosterone appears to play a role. Men with low levels of testosterone, as occurs after removal of diseased testes or when testes lose function with aging, suffer more fractures. Other common causes of osteoporosis in men include corticosteroid use and alcohol abuse.[18] Treatment for men with osteoporosis includes testosterone replacement therapy. Thus both male and female sex hormones participate in the development and treatment of osteoporosis.

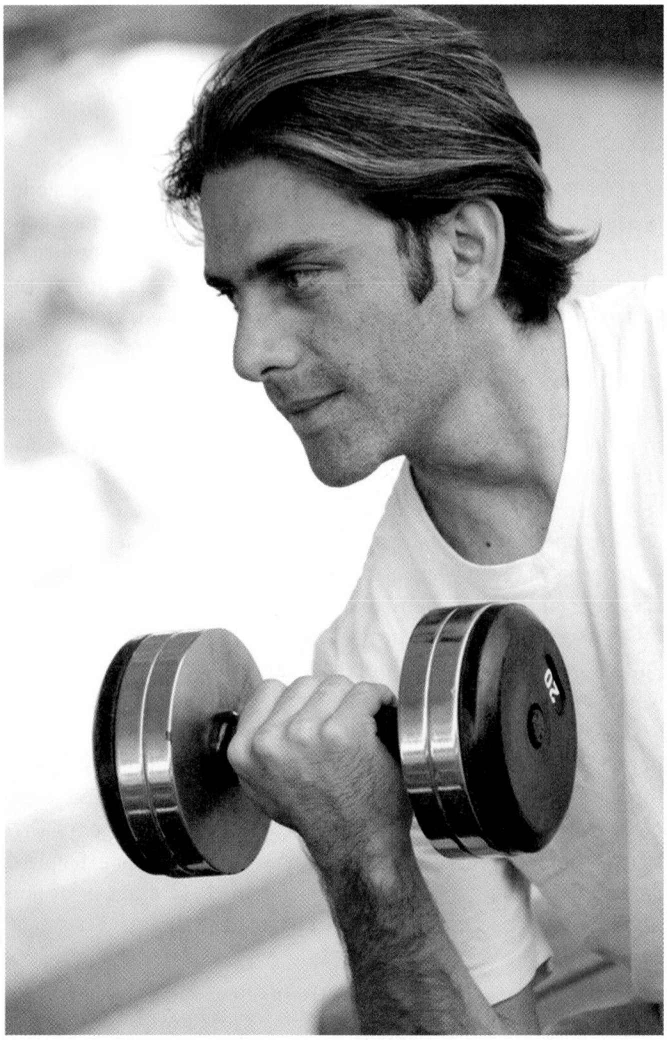
20

Paul Burns/Getty Images

Strength training helps to build strong bones.

Genetics and Ethnicity

Osteoporosis may, in part, be hereditary, and family history of osteoporosis or fracture is a risk factor.[19] The exact role of genetics is unclear, but it most likely influences both the peak bone mass achieved during growth and the bone loss incurred during the later years. The extent to which a given genetic potential is realized, however, depends on many outside factors. Diet and physical activity, for example, can maximize peak bone density during growth, whereas alcohol and tobacco abuse can accelerate bone losses later in life.

Risks of osteoporosis appear to run along racial lines and reflect genetic differences in bone development. Those of African descent, for example, seem to use and retain calcium more efficiently than Caucasians.[20] Consequently, even though their calcium intakes are typically lower, black people have denser bones than white people do. Greater bone density expresses itself in less bone loss, fewer fractures, and a lower rate of osteoporosis among black people.[21] Fractures, for example, are about twice as likely in white women age 65 or older as in black women.

Other ethnic groups have a high risk of osteoporosis. Asians from China and Japan, Hispanic people from Central and South America, and Inuit people from St. Lawrence Island typically have lower bone density than Caucasians. One might expect that these groups would suffer more bone fractures, but this is not always the case. Again, genetic differences may explain why. Asians, for example, generally have small, compact hips, which makes them less susceptible to fractures.

Findings from around the world demonstrate that although a person's genes may lay the groundwork for bone health, environmental factors influence the genes' ultimate expression. Diet, in general, and calcium, in particular, are among those environmental factors. Others include physical activity, body weight, smoking, and alcohol. Importantly, all of these factors are within a person's control.

Physical Activity and Body Weight

Physical activity may be the single most important factor supporting bone growth during adolescence.[22] Furthermore, physical activity during the adolescent years of bone growth appears to have lasting benefits for older women.[23] Muscle strength and bone strength go together. When muscles work, they pull on the bones, stimulating them to develop more trabeculae and grow denser. The hormones that promote new muscle growth also favour the building of bone. As a result, active bones are denser and stronger than sedentary bones.[24]

To keep bones healthy, a person should engage in weight training or weight-bearing endurance activities (such as tennis and jogging or vigorous walking) regularly.[25] Regular physical activity combined with an adequate calcium intake helps to maximize bone density in adolescence.[26] Adults can also maximize and maintain bone density with a regular program of weight training. Even past menopause, when most women are losing bone, weight training improves bone density.

Heavier body weights and weight gains place a similar stress on the bones and promote their density. In fact, being overweight may protect bones against the negative effects of a low-calcium diet.[27] Interestingly, leptin may play a key role in the relationship between body weight and bone mass.[28] Obese mice that are deficient in leptin show increases in bone formation. In contrast, weight losses reduce bone density and increase the risk of fractures—in part because energy restriction diminishes calcium absorption and compromises calcium balance. When calcium intake meets recommendations, however, calcium absorption is sufficient to maintain bone density during weight loss.[29] As mentioned in Highlight 8, the combination of underweight, severely restricted energy intake, extreme daily exercise, and amenorrhea reliably predicts bone loss.

Smoking and Alcohol

Add bone damage to the list of ill consequences associated with smoking. The bones of smokers are less dense than those of nonsmokers—even after controlling for differences in age, body weight, and physical activity habits.[30] Fortunately, the damaging effects can be reversed with smoking cessation. Blood indicators of beneficial bone activity are apparent six weeks after a person stops smoking. In time, bone density is similar for former smokers and nonsmokers.

People who abuse alcohol often suffer from osteoporosis and experience more bone breaks than others. Several factors appear to be involved. Alcohol enhances fluid excretion, leading to excessive calcium losses in the urine; upsets the hormonal balance required for healthy bones; slows bone formation, leading to lower bone density; stimulates bone breakdown; and increases the risk of falling. Limited research suggests that *moderate* alcohol consumption increases bone mineral density.[31]

Dietary Calcium

For older adults, an adequate calcium intake alone cannot protect against bone fractures.[32] Bone strength later in life depends most on how well the bones were built during childhood and adolescence. Adequate calcium nutrition during the growing years is essential to achieving optimal peak bone mass. Simply put, growing children who do not get enough calcium do not have strong bones. Neither do adults who did not get enough calcium during their childhood and adolescence. To that end, the DRI Committee recommends 1300 milligrams of calcium per day for everyone 9 through 18 years of age. Unfortunately, few girls meet the recommendations for calcium during these bone-forming years. (Boys generally obtain intakes close to those recommended because they eat more food.) Consequently, most girls start their adult years with less-than-optimal bone density. As adults, women rarely meet their recommended intakes of 1000 to 1200 milligrams from food. Some authorities suggest 1500 milligrams of calcium for postmenopausal women who are not receiving estrogen, but they warn that intakes exceeding 2500 milligrams a day could cause health problems.

Other Nutrients

Much research has focused on calcium, but other nutrients support bone health, too.[33] Adequate protein protects bones and reduces the likelihood of hip fractures.[34] As mentioned earlier, vitamin D is needed to maintain calcium metabolism and optimal bone health.[35] Supplementation with vitamin D reduces bone loss and the risk of fractures.[36] Vitamin K decreases bone turnover and protects against hip fractures. Vitamin C may slow bone losses.[37] The minerals magnesium and potassium also help to maintain bone mineral density. Vitamin A is needed in the bone-remodelling process, but too much vitamin A may be associated with osteoporosis.[38] Omega-3 fatty acids may help preserve bone integrity.[39] Additional research points to the bone benefits not of a specific nutrient, but of a diet rich in vegetables and fruits such as the DASH diet.[40] Phytochemicals such as lycopene reduce oxidative stress, which may help to defend against osteoporosis.[41] In contrast, diets containing too much salt are associated with bone losses. Similarly, diets containing too many colas or commercially baked snack and fried foods are associated with low bone mineral density.[42] Clearly, a well-balanced diet that depends on all the food groups to supply a full array of nutrients is central to bone health.

A Perspective on Supplements

Bone health depends, in part, on calcium. People who do not consume milk products or other calcium-rich foods in amounts that provide even half the recommended calcium should consider consulting a registered dietitian who can assess the diet and suggest food choices to correct any inadequacies. Calcium from foods may support bone health better than calcium from supplements.[43] For those who are unable to consume enough calcium-rich foods, however, taking calcium supplements—especially in combination with vitamin D—may help to enhance bone density and protect against bone loss and fractures.[44] Because calcium supplements may increase the risk of heart attacks, women should consult their physicians when making this decision.[45]

Selecting a calcium supplement requires a little investigative work to sort through the many options. Before examining calcium supplements, recognize that multivitamin-mineral pills contain little or no calcium. The label may list a few milligrams of calcium, but remember that the recommended intake is a gram or more for adults.

Calcium supplements are typically sold as compounds of calcium carbonate (common in **antacids** and fortified chocolate candies), citrate, gluconate, lactate, malate, or phosphate. These supplements often include magnesium, vitamin D, or both. In addition, some calcium supplements are made from **bone meal, oyster shell, coral,** or **dolomite** (limestone). Many calcium supplements, especially those derived from these natural products, contain lead—which impairs health in numerous ways, as Chapter 13 points out. Fortunately, calcium interferes with the absorption and action of lead in the body.

The first question to ask is how much calcium the supplement provides. Most calcium supplements provide between 250 and 1000 milligrams of calcium. To be safe, total calcium intake from both foods and supplements should not exceed 2500 milligrams a day. Read the label to find out how much a dose supplies. Unless the label states otherwise, supplements of calcium carbonate are 40 percent calcium; those of calcium citrate are 21 percent; lactate, 13 percent; and gluconate, 9 percent. Select a low-dose supplement and take it several times a day rather than taking a large-dose supplement all at once. Taking supplements in doses of 500 milligrams or less improves absorption. Small doses also help ease the GI distress (constipation, intestinal bloating, and excessive gas) that sometimes accompanies calcium supplement use.

The next question to ask is how well the body absorbs and uses the calcium from various supplements. Most healthy people absorb calcium equally well (and as well as from milk) from any of these supplements: calcium carbonate, citrate, or phosphate. More important than supplement solubility is tablet disintegration. When manufacturers compress large quantities of calcium into small pills, the stomach acid has difficulty penetrating the pill. To test a supplement's ability to dissolve, drop it into 175 millilitres (6 ounces) of vinegar, and stir occasionally. A high-quality formulation will dissolve within half an hour.

Finally, people who choose supplements must take them regularly. Furthermore, consideration should be given to the best time to take the supplements. To circumvent adverse nutrient interactions, take calcium supplements between, not with, meals. (Importantly, do not take calcium supplements with iron supplements or iron-rich meals; calcium inhibits iron absorption.) To enhance calcium absorption, take supplements with meals. If such contradictory advice drives you crazy, reconsider the benefits of food sources of calcium. Most experts agree that foods are the best source of most nutrients.

Some Closing Thoughts

Unfortunately, many of the strongest risk factors for osteoporosis are beyond people's control: age, gender, and genetics. But several strategies are still effective for prevention. First, ensure an optimal peak bone mass during childhood and adolescence by eating a balanced diet rich in calcium and engaging in regular physical activity. Then, maintain that bone mass by continuing those healthy diet and activity habits, abstaining from cigarette smoking, and using alcohol moderately, if at all. Finally, minimize bone loss by maintaining an adequate nutrition and exercise regimen, and, for women, consult a physician about calcium supplements or other drug therapies that may be effective both in preventing bone loss and in restoring lost bone. Also, minimize risk of falling to reduce the most common type of fall injury, hip fracture. The reward is the best possible chance of preserving bone health throughout life.

Nutrition on the Net

CENGAGENOW™
For furthur study of topics covered in this Highlight, log on to **www.cengage.com/sso.**

- Obtain additional information from Osteoporosis Canada: **www.osteoporosis.ca**
- Visit the Public Health Agency of Canada's Aging and Seniors website: **www.publichealth.gc.ca/seniors**
- Visit the U.S. National Institutes of Health Osteoporosis and Related Bone Diseases' National Resource Center: **www.niams.nih.gov/Health_Info/Bone**
- Learn more about osteoporosis from the National Osteoporosis Foundation: **www.nof.org**
- Review the U.S. Surgeon General's Report on Bone Health and Osteoporosis: **http://surgeongeneral.gov/library/bonehealth/content.html**
- Search for "falls and fractures" at the U.S. National Institute on Aging: **www.nia.nih.gov**
- Search for "vitamin D recommendations" at the Canadian Cancer Society's website: **www.cancer.ca**

References

1. R. B. Hopkins and coauthors, Estimation of the lifetime risk of hip fracture for women and men in Canada, *Osteoporosis International* (2011), doi: 10.1007/s00198-011-1652-8.
2. Canadian Institute for Health Information, Health Indicators 2007 (Ottawa: CIHI, 2007).
3. Osteoporosis Canada, Facts and statistics (2011). www.osteoporosis.ca/index.php/ci_id/8867/la_id/1.htm, accessed September 15, 2011.
4. A. Papaioannou and coauthors, The impact of incident fractures on health-related quality of life: 5 years of data from the Canadian Multicentre Osteoporosis Study, *Osteoporosis International* 20 (2009): 703–714.
5. W. D. Leslie and coauthors, Trends in hip fracture rates in Canada, *Journal of the American Medical Association* 30 (2009): 883–889.
6. Osteoporosis Canada, Facts and Statistics (2011); Public Health Agency of Canada, Fast Facts from the *2009 Canadian Community Health Survey-Osteoporosis Rapid Response* (2010). www.phac-aspc.gc.ca/cd-mc/osteoporosis-osteoporose/index-eng.php, accessed September 15, 2011; L. A. Fraser and coauthors, Fragility fractures and the osteoporosis care gap in women: The Canadian Multicentre Osteoporosis Study, *Osteoporosis International* 22 (2011): 789–796.
7. A. M. Cheung and A. S. Detsky, Osteoporosis and fractures: Missing the bridge? *Journal of the American Medical Association* 299 (2008): 1468–1470.
8. L. G. Raisz, Screening for osteoporosis, *New England Journal of Medicine* 353 (2005): 164–171.
9. A. Papaioannou and coauthors, 2010 clinical practice guidelines for the diagnosis and management of osteoporosis in Canada: Summary, *Canadian Medical Association Journal* 182 (2010): 1864–1873.
10. Osteoporosis Canada, Facts and statistics, 2011.
11. F. R. Greer, N. F. Krebs, and the Committee on Nutrition, Optimizing bone health and calcium intakes of infants, children, and adolescents, *Pediatrics* 117 (2006): 578–585.
12. G. R. Mundy, Osteoporosis and inflammation, *Nutrition Reviews* 65 (2007): S147–S151.
13. C. J. Rosen, Postmenopausal osteoporosis, *New England Journal of Medicine* 353 (2005): 595–603.
14. R. P. Heaney and R. R. Recker, Combination and sequential therapy of osteoporosis, *New England Journal of Medicine* 353 (2005): 624–625.
15. A. Atmaca and coauthors, Soy isoflavones in the management of postmenopausal osteoporosis, *Menopause* 15 (2008): 748–757; R. C. Poulsen and M. C. Kruger, Soy phytoestrogens: Impact on postmenopausal bone loss and mechanisms of action, *Nutrition Reviews* 66 (2008): 359–374.
16. W. G. Helferich, J. E. Andrade, and M. S. Hoagland, Phytoestrogens and breast cancer: A complex story, *Inflammopharmacology* 16 (2008): 219–226; Y. Zhang and coauthors, Soy isoflavones and their bone protective effect, *Inflammopharmacology* 16 (2008): 213–215.
17. S. Reinwald and C. M. Weaver, Soy isoflavones and bone health: A double-edged sword? *Journal of Natural Products* 69 (2006): 450–459.
18. P. R. Ebeling, Osteoporosis in men, *New England Journal of Medicine* 358 (2008): 1474–1482.
19. S. H. Ralston and B. de Crombrugghe, Genetic regulation of bone mass and susceptibility to osteoporosis, *Genes Development* 20 (2006): 2492–2506.
20. M. Braun and coauthors, Racial differences in skeletal calcium retention in adolescent girls with varied controlled calcium intakes, *American Journal of Clinical Nutrition* 85 (2007): 1657–1663; K. Wigertz and coauthors, Racial differences in calcium retention in response to dietary salt in adolescent girls, *American Journal of Clinical Nutrition* 81 (2005): 845–850.
21. J. A. Cauley and coauthors, Longitudinal study of changes in hip bone mineral density in Caucasian and African-American women, *Journal of the American Geriatrics Society* 53 (2005): 183–189; J. A. Cauley and coauthors, Bone mineral density and the risk of incident nonspinal fractures in black and white women, *Journal of the American Medical Association* 293 (2005): 2102–2108.
22. A. J. Lanou, S. E. Berkow, and N. D. Barnard, Calcium, dairy products, and bone health in children and young adults: A reevaluation of the evidence, *Pediatrics* 115 (2005): 736–743.
23. C. Rideout, H. McKay, and S. Barr, Self-reported lifetime physical activity and areal bone mineral density in healthy postmenopausal women: The importance of teenage activity, *Calcified Tissue International* 79 (2006): 214–222.
24. K. T. Borer, Physical activity in the prevention and amelioration of osteoporosis in women: Interaction of mechanical, hormonal and dietary factors, *Sports Medicine* 35 (2005): 779–830; F. R. Greer, Bone health: It's more than calcium intake, *Pediatrics* 115 (2005): 792–794.
25. American College of Sports Medicine Position Stand, Physical activity and bone health, *Medicine & Science in Sports & Exercise* 36 (2004): 1985–1996.
26. J. M. Welch and C. M. Weaver, Calcium and exercise affect the growing skeleton, *Nutrition Reviews* 63 (2005): 361–373.
27. M. Varenna and coauthors, Effects of dietary calcium intake on body weight and prevalence of osteoporosis in early postmenopausal women, *American Journal of Clinical Nutrition* 86 (2007): 639–644.
28. G. Wolf, Energy regulation by the skeleton, *Nutrition Reviews* 66 (2008): 229–233.
29. C. S. Riedt and coauthors, Premenopausal overweight women do not lose bone during moderate weight loss with adequate or higher calcium intake, *American Journal of Clinical Nutrition* 85 (2007): 972–980.
30. M. Lorentzon and coauthors, Smoking is associated with lower bone mineral density and reduced cortical thickness in young men, *Journal of Clinical Endocrinology and Metabolism* 92 (2007): 497–503.
31. R. Jugdaohsingh and coauthors, Moderate alcohol consumption and increased bone mineral density: Potential ethanol and non-ethanol mechanisms, *Proceedings of the Nutrition Society* 65 (2006): 291–310.
32. H. A. Bischoff-Ferrari and coauthors, Calcium intake and hip fracture risk in men and women: A meta-analysis of prospective cohort studies and randomized controlled trials, *American Journal of Clinical Nutrition* 86 (2007): 1780–1790.
33. C. Palacios, The role of nutrients in bone health, from A to Z, *Critical Reviews of Food Science and Nutrition* 46 (2006): 621–628; J. W. Nieves, Osteoporosis: The role of micronutrients, *American Journal of Clinical Nutrition* 81 (2005): 1232S–1239S.
34. A. D. Conigrave, E. M. Brown, and R. Rizzoli, Dietary protein and bone health: Roles of amino acid–sensing receptors in the control of calcium metabolism and bone homeostasis, *Annual Review of Nutrition* 28 (2008): 131–155.
35. K. D. Cashman and coauthors, Low vitamin D status adversely affects bone health parameters in adolescents, *American Journal of Clinical Nutrition* 87 (2008): 1039–1044; L. Steingrimsdottir and coauthors, Relationship between serum parathyroid hormone levels, vitamin D sufficiency, and calcium intake, *Journal of the American Medical Association* 294 (2005): 2336–2341.
36. H. A. Bischoff-Ferrari and coauthors, Fracture prevention with vitamin D supplementation: A meta-analysis of randomized controlled trials, *Journal of the American Medical Association* 293 (2005): 2257–2264.
37. S. Sahni and coauthors, High vitamin C intake is associated with lower 4-year bone loss in elderly men, *Journal of Nutrition* 138 (2008): 1931–1938.
38. J. D. Ribaya-Mercado and J. B. Blumberg, Vitamin A: Is it a risk factor for osteoporosis and bone fracture? *Nutrition Reviews* 65 (2007): 425–438; K. L. Penniston and coauthors, Serum retinyl esters are not elevated in postmenopausal women with and without osteoporosis whose preformed vitamin A intakes are high, *American Journal of Clinical Nutrition* 84 (2006): 1350–1356.
39. A. E. Griel and coauthors, An increase in dietary n-3 fatty acids decreases a marker of bone resorption in humans, *Nutrition Journal* 6 (2007): 2; M.

Högström, P. Nordström, and A. Nordström, n-3 Fatty acids are positively associated with peak bone mineral density and bone accrual in healthy men: The NO_2 Study, *American Journal of Clinical Nutrition* 85 (2007): 803–807; L. A. Weiss, E. Barrett-Connor, and D. von Mühlen, Ratio of n-6 to n-3 fatty acids and bone mineral density in older adults: The Rancho Bernardo Study, *American Journal of Clinical Nutrition* 81 (2005): 934–938.
40. H. Vatanparast and coauthors, Positive effects of vegetable and fruit consumption and calcium intake on bone mineral accrual in boys during growth from childhood to adolescence: The University of Saskatchewan Pediatric Bone Mineral Accrual Study, *American Journal of Clinical Nutrition* 82 (2005): 700–706.
41. L. G. Rao and coauthors, Lycopene consumption decreases oxidative stress and bone resorption markers in postmenopausal women, *Osteoporosis International* 18 (2007): 109–115.
42. L. M. Troy and coauthors, Dihydrophylloquinone intake is associated with low bone mineral density in men and women, *American Journal of Clinical Nutrition* 86 (2007): 504–508; K. L. Tucker and coauthors, Colas, but not other carbonated beverages, are associated with low bone mineral density in older women: The Framingham Osteoporosis Study, *American Journal of Clinical Nutrition* 84 (2006): 936–942.
43. Y. Manios and coauthors, Changes in biochemical indexes of bone metabolism and bone mineral density after a 12-mo dietary intervention program: The Postmenopausal Health Study, *American Journal of Clinical Nutrition* 86 (2007): 781–789; N. Napoli and coauthors, Effects of dietary calcium compared with calcium supplements on estrogen metabolism and bone mineral density, *American Journal of Clinical Nutrition* 85 (2007): 1428–1433.
44. H. A. Bischoff-Ferrari and coauthors, Effect of calcium supplementation on fracture risk: A double-blind randomized controlled trial, *American Journal of Clinical Nutrition* 87 (2008): 1945–1951; R. M. Daly and coauthors, The skeletal benefits of calcium- and vitamin D_3-fortified milk are sustained in older men after withdrawal of supplementation: An 18-mo follow-up study, *American Journal of Clinical Nutrition* 87 (2008): 771–777; M. F. Hitz, J. B. Jensen, and P. C. Eskildsen, Bone mineral density and bone markers in patients with a recent low-energy fracture: Effect of 1 y of treatment with calcium and vitamin D, *American Journal of Clinical Nutrition* 86 (2007): 251–259; B. M. P. Tang and coauthors, Use of calcium or calcium in combination with vitamin D supplementation to prevent fractures and bone loss in people aged 50 years and older: A meta-analysis, *Lancet* 370 (2007): 657–666; V. Matkovic and coauthors, Calcium supplementation and bone mineral density in females from childhood to young adulthood: A randomized controlled trial, *American Journal of Clinical Nutrition* 81 (2005): 175–188; R. P. Dodiuk-Gad and coauthors, Sustained effect of short-term calcium supplementation on bone mass in adolescent girls with low calcium intake, *American Journal of Clinical Nutrition* 81 (2005): 168–174.
45. M. J. Bolland and coauthors, Vascular events in healthy older women receiving calcium supplementation: Randomised controlled trial, *British Medical Journal* 336 (2008): 262–266.

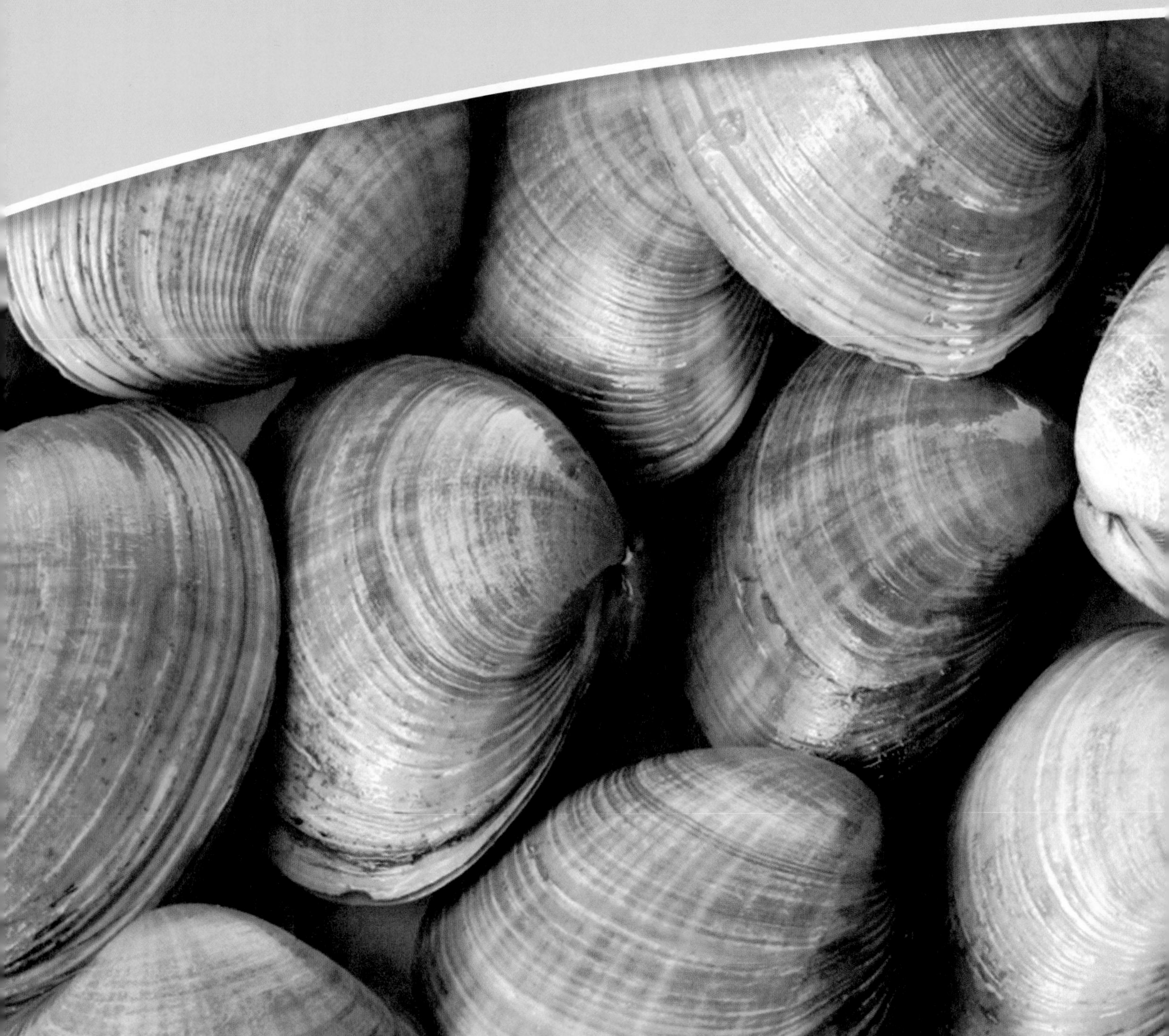

JIANG HONGYAN/shutterstock

CENGAGENOW™

Throughout this chapter, the CengageNOW logo indicates an opportunity for online self-study, linking you to interactive tutorials, activities, and videos to increase your understanding of chapter concepts.
www.cengage.com/sso

Nutrition in Your Life

Do you ever feel so endlessly tired that it prevents you from participating in the things that you want to do? Do you have trouble keeping warm? Do you run out of energy much sooner than your fellow ball players? If so, these may be signs that you have low body iron. A simple blood test will determine if your iron stores are low and need replenishing. With appropriate treatment, you will soon be able to resume your favourite activities and keep up with your friends. Reminding yourself to make iron-rich food choices throughout the day helps to maintain the health of your blood.

CHAPTER

14

Nutrients for Blood Health

CHAPTER OUTLINE

About Blood

Blood is in continual movement as it flows through your body, delivering a constant supply of oxygen and nutrients to different tissues. One key nutrient in blood is water. In Chapter 11, you learned about the role of water in blood and its effect on blood pressure. Remarkably, about 5 litres of blood in women and 5.5 litres in men accomplish the delivery task as well as the removal of metabolic waste products for exit from the body. It takes only about one minute to circulate blood from the heart, around the body, and back to the heart. In this time, the constituents in blood sustain life through many actions, including buffering blood pH, maintaining electrolyte balance, suspending assorted substances, and stabilizing body temperature. While Chapter 11 addressed water and the effects of the quantity of your blood, the nutrients profiled in this chapter focus on the effects of the quality of your blood.

Maintaining healthy blood is critical to life. Blood is the only fluid tissue in our body, giving it unique characteristics that differ from other tissues. Healthy blood depends on key micronutrients to perform its many roles, importantly carrying nutrients and oxygen to the cells and removing waste from the cells. Iron, as a working part of hemoglobin in red blood cells, is essential for transporting oxygen from the lungs to the rest of the body; zinc assists metalloenzymes that are involved in widespread metabolic processes including the production of hemoglobin; and the action of copper allows iron to bind to transferrin for transport to the bone marrow and then incorporation into hemoglobin. Without adequate vitamin K, we would hemorrhage. Our bodies rely on these and other micronutrients to heal wounds and maintain a healthy quality of blood that can carry nutrients from one site to another.

When whole blood is centrifuged, about 55 percent of the volume is plasma, 45 percent is red blood cells, and the remaining less than 1 percent is platelets and white blood cells (see Figure 14-1 on page 442). Our ability to fight infection, feel energetic, clot blood, or have normal blood pressure relies on the quality and quantity of our blood. Chapter 13 profiled the importance of vitamin K in bone health. In this chapter, we will explore the vital role of vitamin K in blood clotting and the ways in which iron, zinc, and copper assist in maintaining healthy blood and other body functions.

Vitamin K

Vitamin K is well-known for its role in activating proteins involved in the blood-clotting process (see Figure 14-2 on page 442).

FIGURE 14-1 Blood Components

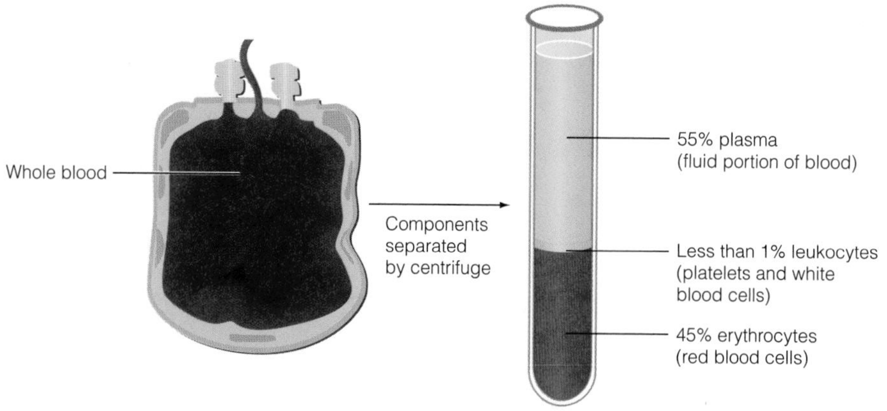
Whole blood
Components separated by centrifuge
55% plasma (fluid portion of blood)
Less than 1% leukocytes (platelets and white blood cells)
45% erythrocytes (red blood cells)

FIGURE 14-2 Blood-Clotting Process

When blood is exposed to air, foreign substances, or secretions from injured tissues, platelets (small, cell-like structures in the blood) release a phospholipid known as thromboplastin. Thromboplastin catalyzes the conversion of the inactive protein prothrombin to the active enzyme thrombin. Thrombin then catalyzes the conversion of the precursor protein fibrinogen to the active protein fibrin that forms the clot.

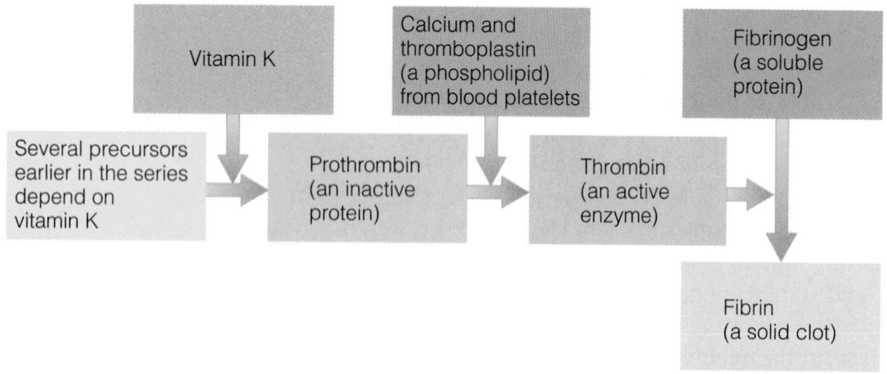
Vitamin K
Calcium and thromboplastin (a phospholipid) from blood platelets
Fibrinogen (a soluble protein)
Several precursors earlier in the series depend on vitamin K
Prothrombin (an inactive protein)
Thrombin (an active enzyme)
Fibrin (a solid clot)

Vitamin K Role in Blood Health

Danish scientists were the first to discover a blood-clotting role for vitamin K and named the vitamin "K" after *koagulation*, the Danish word for coagulation. Clotting is important for repairing damage to blood vessels and other tissues and involves numerous proteins in the multistep process. Vitamin K, specifically, is required to convert prothrombin to thrombin, which in turn, changes fibrinogen to active fibrin, causing a clot to form.

Vitamin K Deficiency and Toxicity

Without adequate vitamin K, blood clotting is compromised and may not occur at all. Under these conditions, wounds take a longer time to heal or do not heal at all, and internal or external hemorrhaging can continue unabated. The risk for a deficiency or toxicity of vitamin K is rare.

Vitamin K Recommendations and Sources

The AI for vitamin K is 120 μg/day for men and 90 μg/day for women. No adverse effects have been reported with high intakes of vitamin K; consequently, a UL has not been set. Bacteria in the GI tract produce vitamin K but not enough to meet all of our needs, so dietary recommendations have been established. Vitamin K represents a family of fat-soluble compounds that are found in plant and animal foods such as green vegetables, plant oils, and fish oils.

IN SUMMARY **Vitamin K has an important role in blood clotting. Bacteria in the GI tract synthesize about half of the human requirement for fat-soluble vitamin K and the other half can be obtained from foods such as green leafy vegetables, plant oils, and fish oils. The accompanying table provides a summary of vitamin K.**

Vitamin K

Other Names	**Significant Sources**
Phylloquinone, menaquinone, menadione, naphthoquinone	Bacterial synthesis in the digestive tract;[a] liver; leafy green vegetables, cabbage-type vegetables; milk, canola oil
Adequate Intake (AI)	**Deficiency Symptoms**
Men: 120 μg/day Women: 90 μg/day	Hemorrhaging
Chief Functions in the Body	**Toxicity Symptoms**
Synthesis of blood-clotting and bone proteins	None known

[a]Vitamin K needs cannot be met from bacterial synthesis alone; however, it is a potentially important source in the small intestine, where absorption efficiency ranges from 40 to 70 percent.

Iron

Iron is an essential nutrient, vital to many of the cells' activities, but it poses a problem for millions of people. Some people simply don't eat enough iron-containing foods to support their health optimally, whereas others absorb so much iron that it threatens their health. Iron exemplifies the principle that both too little and too much of a nutrient in the body can be harmful. In its wisdom, the body has several ways to achieve iron homeostasis, protecting against both deficiency and overload.

Iron Roles in the Body

Iron has the knack of switching back and forth between two ionic states. ♦ In the reduced state, iron has lost two electrons and therefore has a net positive charge of two; it is known as *ferrous iron*. In the oxidized state, iron has lost a third electron, has a net positive charge of three, and is known as *ferric iron*. Ferrous iron can be oxidized to ferric iron, and ferric iron can be reduced to ferrous iron. Thus iron can serve as a cofactor ♦ to enzymes involved in oxidation-reduction reactions—reactions so widespread in metabolism that they occur in all cells. Enzymes involved in making amino acids, collagen, hormones, and neurotransmitters all require iron. (For details about ions, oxidation, and reduction, see APPENDIX B.)

Iron forms a part of the electron carriers that participate in the electron transport chain (discussed in Chapter 7).* In this pathway, these carriers transfer hydrogens and electrons to oxygen, forming water, and in the process, make ATP for the cells' energy use.

Most of the body's iron is found in two proteins: hemoglobin ♦ in the red blood cells and **myoglobin** in the muscle cells. In both, iron helps accept, carry, and then release oxygen.

♦ Iron's two ionic states:
- Ferrous iron (reduced): Fe^{++}
- Ferric iron (oxidized): Fe^{+++}

♦ A **cofactor** is a substance that works with an enzyme to facilitate a chemical reaction.

♦ **Hemoglobin** is the oxygen-carrying protein of the red blood cells that transports oxygen from the lungs to tissues throughout the body; hemoglobin accounts for 80% of the body's iron.

Iron Absorption and Metabolism

The body conserves iron. Because it is difficult to excrete iron once it is in the body, balance is maintained primarily through absorption. More iron is absorbed when stores are empty and less is absorbed when stores are full.[1]

Iron Absorption Special proteins help the body absorb iron from food (see Figure 14-3). The iron-storage protein **ferritin** captures iron from food and stores it in the cells of the small intestine. When the body needs iron, ferritin releases some iron to an iron transport protein called **transferrin.** If the body does not

myoglobin: the oxygen-holding protein of the muscle cells.
- **myo** = muscle

ferritin (FAIR-ih-tin): the iron-storage protein.

transferrin (trans-FAIR-in): the iron transport protein.

*The iron-containing electron carriers of the electron transport chain are known as *cytochromes*. See APPENDIX C for details of this pathway.

FIGURE 14-3 Iron Absorption

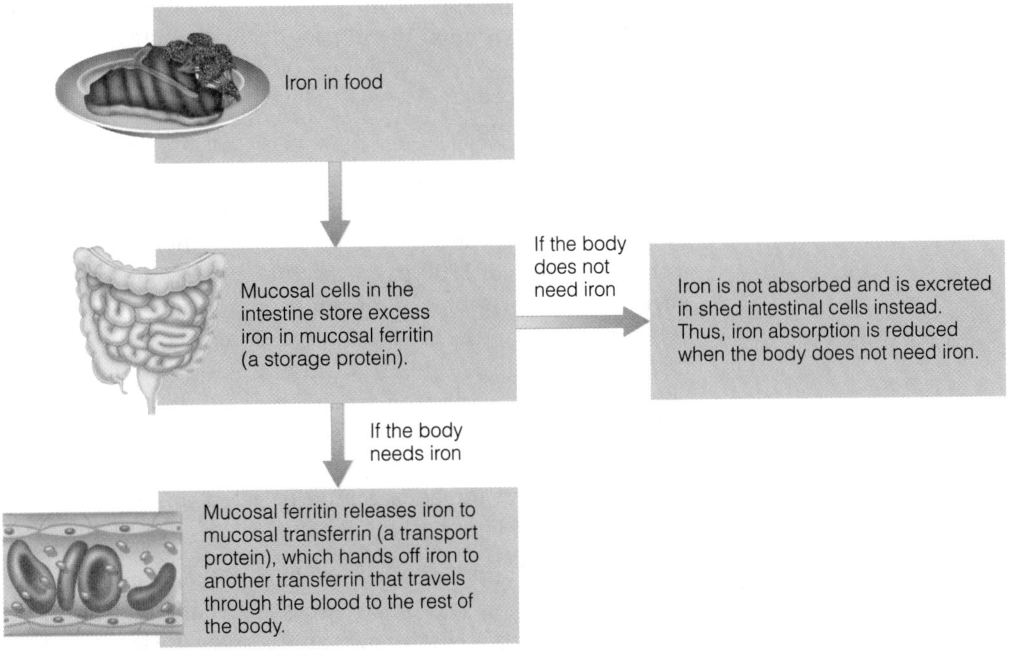
Iron in food
Mucosal cells in the intestine store excess iron in mucosal ferritin (a storage protein).
If the body does not need iron
Iron is not absorbed and is excreted in shed intestinal cells instead. Thus, iron absorption is reduced when the body does not need iron.
If the body needs iron
Mucosal ferritin releases iron to mucosal transferrin (a transport protein), which hands off iron to another transferrin that travels through the blood to the rest of the body.

FIGURE 14-4 Heme and Nonheme Iron in Foods

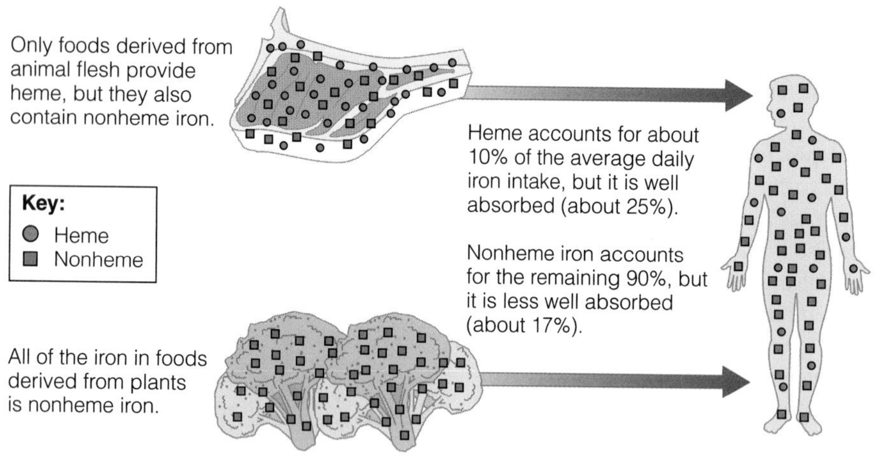
Only foods derived from animal flesh provide heme, but they also contain nonheme iron.
Key:
Heme
Nonheme
All of the iron in foods derived from plants is nonheme iron.
Heme accounts for about 10% of the average daily iron intake, but it is well absorbed (about 25%).
Nonheme iron accounts for the remaining 90%, but it is less well absorbed (about 17%).

need iron, it is carried out when the intestinal cells are shed and excreted in the feces; intestinal cells are replaced about every three to five days. By holding iron temporarily, these cells control iron absorption by either delivering iron when the day's intake falls short or disposing of it when intakes exceed needs.

Heme and Nonheme Iron Iron absorption depends in part on its dietary source. Iron occurs in two forms in foods: as **heme iron**, which is found only in foods derived from the flesh of animals, such as meats, poultry, eggs, and fish, and as **nonheme iron**, which is found in both plant-derived and animal-derived foods (see Figure 14-4). ♦ On average, heme iron represents about 10 percent of the iron a person consumes in a day. Even though heme iron accounts for only a small proportion of the intake, it is so well absorbed that it contributes significant iron. About 25 percent of heme iron and 17 percent of nonheme iron is absorbed, depending on dietary factors and the body's iron stores.[2] In iron deficiency, absorption increases.[3] In iron overload, absorption declines. Researchers disagree as to whether heme iron absorption responds to iron stores as sensitively as nonheme iron absorption does.

♦ About 40% of the iron in meat, fish, poultry, and eggs is bound into heme; the other 60% is nonheme iron. All of the iron in plant foods is nonheme iron.

Absorption-Enhancing Factors Meat, fish, and poultry contain not only the well-absorbed heme iron, but also a peptide (called the **MFP factor**) that promotes the absorption of nonheme iron ♦ from other foods eaten at the same meal.[4] Vitamin C also enhances nonheme iron absorption from foods eaten in the same meal by capturing the iron and keeping it in the reduced ferrous form, ready for absorption. Some acids and sugars also enhance nonheme iron absorption.

♦ Factors that *enhance* nonheme iron absorption:
- MFP factor
- Vitamin C (ascorbic acid)

Absorption-Inhibiting Factors Some dietary factors bind with nonheme iron, inhibiting absorption. ♦ These factors include the phytates in legumes, whole grains, and rice; the vegetable proteins in soybeans, other legumes, and nuts; the calcium in milk; and the polyphenols (such as tannic acid) in tea, coffee, grain products, oregano, and red wine.

♦ Factors that *inhibit* nonheme iron absorption:
- Phytates (legumes, grains, and rice)
- Vegetable proteins (soybeans, legumes, nuts)
- Calcium (milk)
- Tannic acid (and other polyphenols in tea and coffee)

Dietary Factors Combined The many dietary enhancers, inhibitors, and their combined effects make it difficult to estimate iron absorption.[5] Most of these factors exert a strong influence individually, but not when combined with the others in a meal. Furthermore, the impact of the combined effects diminishes when a diet is evaluated over several days. When multiple meals are analyzed together, three factors appear to be most relevant: MFP and vitamin C as enhancers and phytates as inhibitors.

Individual Variation Overall, about 18 percent of dietary iron is absorbed from mixed diets and only about 10 percent from vegetarian diets.[6] As you might expect, vegetarian diets do not have the benefit of easy-to-absorb heme iron or the help of MFP in enhancing absorption. In addition to dietary influences, iron absorption also depends on an individual's health, stage in the life cycle, and iron status. Absorption can be as low as 2 percent in a person with GI disease or as high as 35 percent in a rapidly growing, healthy child. The body adapts to absorb more iron when a person's iron stores fall short or when the need increases for any reason (such as pregnancy). The body makes more ferritin to absorb more iron from the small intestine and more transferrin to carry more iron around the body. Similarly, when iron stores are sufficient, the body adapts to absorb less iron.

Iron Transport and Storage The blood transport protein transferrin delivers iron to the bone marrow and other tissues. The bone marrow uses large quantities to make new red blood cells, whereas other tissues use less. Surplus iron is stored in the

heme (HEEM) **iron:** the iron in foods that is bound to the hemoglobin and myoglobin proteins; found only in meat, fish, poultry, and eggs.

nonheme iron: the iron in foods that is not bound to proteins; found in both plant-derived and animal-derived foods.

MFP factor: a peptide released during the digestion of **m**eat, **f**ish, and **p**oultry that enhances nonheme iron absorption.

FIGURE 14-5 Iron Recycled in the Body

Once iron enters the body, most of it is recycled. Some is lost with body tissues and must be replaced by eating iron-containing food.

CENGAGENOW™
Animated! figure
www.cengage.com/sso

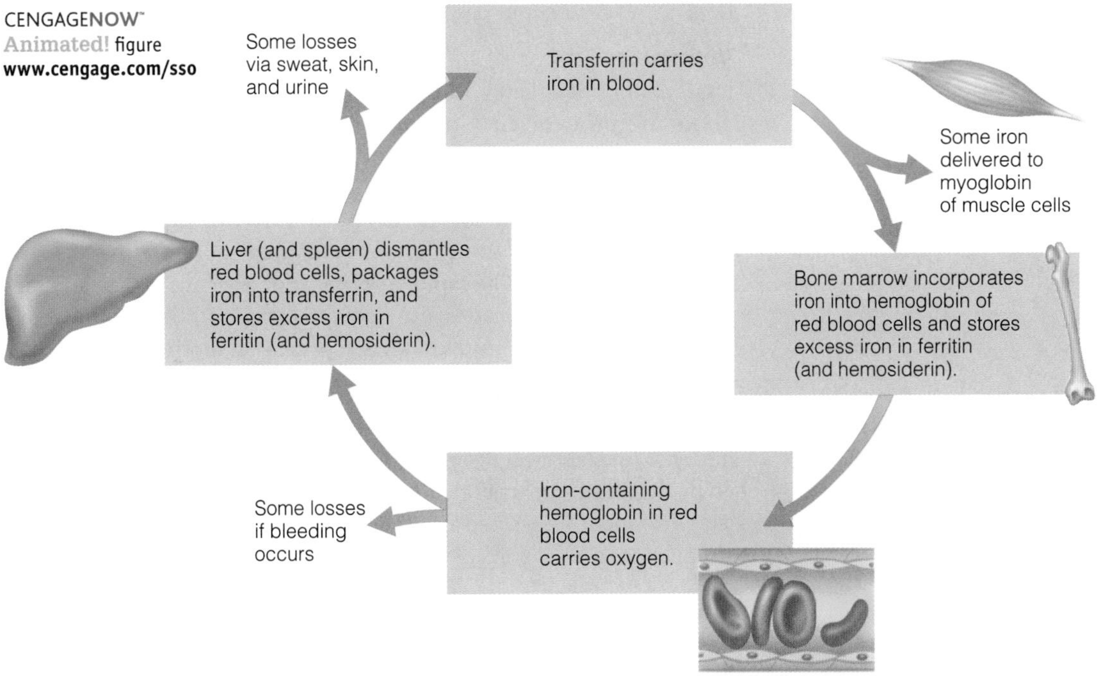
Some losses via sweat, skin, and urine
Transferrin carries iron in blood.
Some iron delivered to myoglobin of muscle cells
Liver (and spleen) dismantles red blood cells, packages iron into transferrin, and stores excess iron in ferritin (and hemosiderin).
Bone marrow incorporates iron into hemoglobin of red blood cells and stores excess iron in ferritin (and hemosiderin).
Some losses if bleeding occurs
Iron-containing hemoglobin in red blood cells carries oxygen.

protein ferritin, primarily in the liver, but also in the bone marrow and spleen. When dietary iron has been plentiful, ferritin is constantly and rapidly made and broken down, providing an ever-ready supply of iron. When iron concentrations become abnormally high, the liver converts some ferritin into another storage protein called **hemosiderin.** Hemosiderin releases iron more slowly than ferritin does. Storing excess iron in hemosiderin protects the body against the damage that free iron can cause. Free iron acts as a free radical, attacking cell lipids, DNA, and protein. (See Highlight 12 for more information on free radicals and the damage they can cause.)

Iron Recycling The average red blood cell lives about four months; then the spleen and liver cells remove it from the blood, take it apart, and prepare the degradation products for excretion or recycling. The iron is salvaged: the liver attaches it to transferrin, which transports it back to the bone marrow to be reused in making new red blood cells. Thus, although red blood cells live for only about four months, the iron recycles through each new generation of cells (see Figure 14-5). The body loses some iron daily via the GI tract and, if bleeding occurs, in blood. Only tiny amounts of iron are lost in urine, sweat, and shed skin.*

Iron Balance Maintaining iron balance depends on the careful regulation of iron absorption, transport, storage, recycling, and losses. The hormone **hepcidin** is central to the regulation of iron balance.[7] Produced by the liver, hepcidin helps to maintain blood iron within the normal range by limiting absorption from the small intestine and controlling release from the liver, spleen, and bone marrow.

Iron Deficiency

Worldwide, **iron deficiency** is the most common nutrient deficiency, with **iron-deficiency anemia** affecting more than 1.6 billion people—almost half of preschool children and pregnant women.[8] In Canada and the United States, iron deficiency is less prevalent, but it still affects 10 percent of toddlers, adolescent girls, and women of childbearing age. Iron deficiency is also relatively

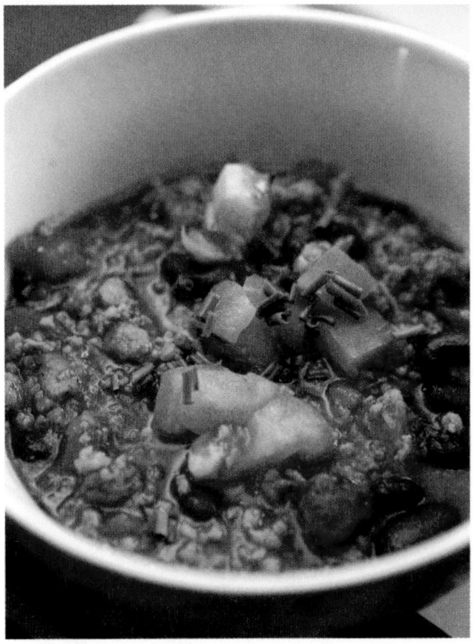
haak78/shutterstock

This chili dinner provides several factors that may enhance iron absorption: heme and nonheme iron and MFP from meat, nonheme iron from legumes, and vitamin C from tomatoes.

hemosiderin (heem-oh-SID-er-in): an iron-storage protein primarily made in times of iron overload.

hepcidin: a hormone produced by the liver that regulates iron balance.

iron deficiency: the state of having depleted iron stores.

iron-deficiency anemia: severe depletion of iron stores that results in low hemoglobin and small, pale red blood cells. Anemias that impair hemoglobin synthesis are *microcytic* (small cell).

- **micro** = small
- **cytic** = cell

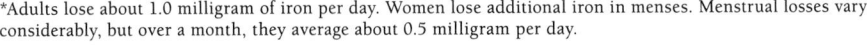

*Adults lose about 1.0 milligram of iron per day. Women lose additional iron in menses. Menstrual losses vary considerably, but over a month, they average about 0.5 milligram per day.

common among overweight children and adolescents compared with those who are normal weight.[9] The association between iron deficiency and obesity has yet to be explained, but researchers are currently examining the relationships between the inflammation that develops with excess body fat and reduced iron absorption.[10] Preventing and correcting iron deficiency are high priorities.

♦ High risk for iron deficiency:
- Women in their reproductive years
- Pregnant women
- Infants and young children
- Teenagers

Vulnerable Stages of Life Some stages of life ♦ demand more iron but provide less, making deficiency likely. Women in their reproductive years are especially prone to iron deficiency because of repeated blood losses during menstruation. Pregnancy demands additional iron to support the added blood volume, growth of the fetus, and blood loss during childbirth. Infants and young children receive little iron from high-milk diets, yet need extra iron to support their rapid growth and brain development.[11] Iron deficiency among toddlers in Canada and the United States is common.[12] The rapid growth of adolescence, especially for males, and the menstrual losses of females also demand extra iron that a typical teen diet may not provide. An adequate iron intake is especially important during these stages of life.

♦ The iron content of blood is about 0.5 mg/100 mL blood. A person donating a pint of blood (approximately 500 mL) loses about 2.5 mg of iron.

Blood Losses Bleeding ♦ from any site incurs iron losses. In some cases, such as an active ulcer, the bleeding may not be obvious, but even small chronic blood losses significantly deplete iron reserves. In developing countries, blood loss is often brought on by malaria and parasitic infections of the GI tract. People who donate blood regularly also incur losses and may benefit from iron supplements. As mentioned, menstrual losses can be considerable as they tap women's iron stores regularly.

♦ Stages of iron deficiency:
- Iron stores diminish
- Transport iron decreases
- Hemoglobin production declines

Assessment of Iron Deficiency Iron deficiency develops in stages. ♦ This section provides a brief overview of how to detect these stages, and APPENDIX E provides more details. In the first stage of iron deficiency, iron stores diminish. Measures of serum ferritin (in the blood) reflect iron stores and are most valuable in assessing iron status at this earliest stage.[13]

The second stage of iron deficiency is characterized by a decrease in transport iron: serum iron falls, and the iron-carrying protein transferrin *increases* (an adaptation that enhances iron absorption). Together, measurements of serum iron and transferrin can determine the severity of the deficiency—the more transferrin and the less iron in the blood, the more advanced the deficiency is. Transferrin saturation—the percentage of transferrin that is saturated with iron—decreases as iron stores decline.

The third stage of iron deficiency occurs when the lack of iron limits hemoglobin production. Now the hemoglobin precursor, **erythrocyte protoporphyrin,** begins to accumulate as hemoglobin and **hematocrit** values decline.

Hemoglobin and hematocrit tests are easy, quick, and inexpensive, so they are the tests most commonly used in evaluating iron status. Their usefulness in detecting iron deficiency is limited, however, because they are late indicators. Furthermore, other nutrient deficiencies and medical conditions can influence their values.

♦ Iron-deficiency anemia is a **microcytic** (my-cro-SIT-ic) **hypochromic** (high-po-KROME-ic) **anemia.**
- **micro** = small
- **cytic** = cell
- **hypo** = too little
- **chrom** = colour

Iron Deficiency and Anemia Notice that iron deficiency and iron-deficiency anemia are not the same: people may be iron deficient without being anemic. The term *iron deficiency* refers to depleted body iron stores without regard to the degree of depletion or to the presence of anemia. The term *iron-deficiency anemia* refers to the severe depletion of iron stores that results in a low hemoglobin concentration. In iron-deficiency anemia, hemoglobin synthesis decreases, resulting in red blood cells that are pale (hypochromic) and small (microcytic), ♦ as shown in Figure 14-6. These cells can't carry enough oxygen from the lungs to the tissues. Without adequate iron, energy metabolism in the cells falters. The result is fatigue, weakness, headaches, apathy, pallor, and poor resistance to cold temperatures. Because hemoglobin is the bright red pigment of the blood, the skin of a fair person who is anemic may become noticeably pale. In a dark-skinned person, the tongue and eye lining, normally pink, is very pale.

The fatigue that accompanies iron-deficiency anemia differs from the tiredness a person experiences from a simple lack of sleep. People with anemia feel fatigue only when they exert themselves. Iron supplementation can relieve the fatigue and improve the body's response to physical activity. (The iron needs of physically active people and the special iron deficiency known as sports anemia are discussed in Chapter 15.)

erythrocyte protoporphyrin (PRO-toe-PORE-fe-rin): a precursor to hemoglobin.

hematocrit (hee-MAT-oh-krit): measurement of the volume of the red blood cells packed by centrifuge in a given volume of blood.

FIGURE 14-6 Normal and Anemic Blood Cells

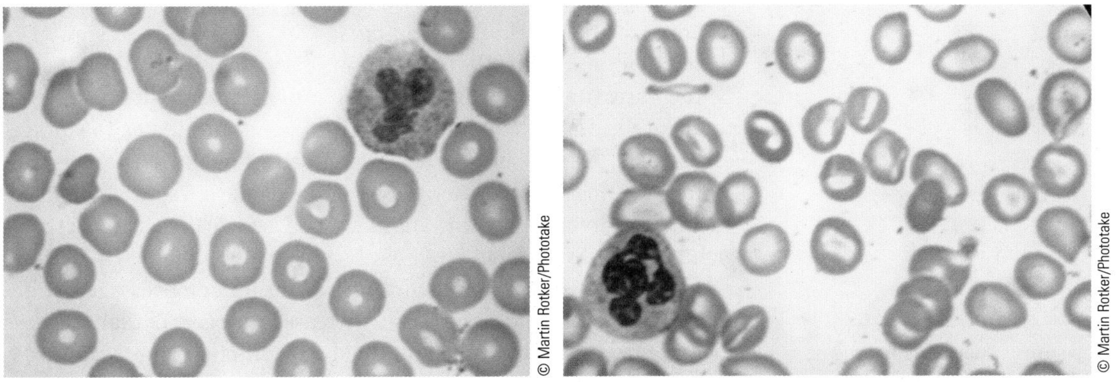
© Martin Rotker/Phototake
© Martin Rotker/Phototake

Both size and colour are normal in these blood cells.

Blood cells in iron-deficiency anemia are small (microcytic) and pale (hypochromic) because they contain less hemoglobin.

Iron Deficiency and Behaviour Long before the red blood cells are affected and anemia is diagnosed, a developing iron deficiency affects behaviour.[14] Even at slightly lowered iron levels, energy metabolism is impaired and neurotransmitter synthesis is altered, reducing physical work capacity and mental productivity. Without the physical energy and mental alertness to work, plan, think, play, sing, or learn, people simply do these things less. They have no obvious deficiency symptoms; they just appear unmotivated, apathetic, and less physically fit. Work productivity and voluntary activities decline.

Many of the symptoms associated with iron deficiency are easily mistaken for behavioural or motivational problems. A restless child who fails to pay attention in class might be thought contrary. An apathetic homemaker who has let housework pile up might be thought lazy. No responsible dietitian would ever claim that all behavioural problems are caused by nutrient deficiencies, but poor nutrition is always a possible contributor to problems like these. When investigating a behavioural problem, check the adequacy of the diet and seek a routine physical examination before undertaking more expensive, and possibly more harmful, treatment options. Treatment with long-term, low-dose iron supplements may improve cognitive skills and physical development.[15] The effects of iron deficiency on children's behaviour are discussed further in Chapter 17.

Iron Deficiency and Pica A curious behaviour seen in some iron-deficient people, especially in women and children of low-income groups, is **pica**—the craving and consumption of ice, chalk, starch, and other nonfood substances. ♦ These substances contain no iron and cannot remedy a deficiency; in fact, clay actually inhibits iron absorption, which may explain the iron deficiency that accompanies such behaviour. Pica is poorly understood. Its cause is unknown, but researchers hypothesize that it may be motivated by hunger, nutrient deficiencies, or an attempt to protect against toxins or microbes.[16] The consequence of pica is anemia.

♦ Pica is known as *geophagia* (gee-oh-FAY-gee-uh) when referring to eating clay, baby powder, chalk, ash, ceramics, paper, paint chips, or charcoal; *pagophagia* (pag-oh-FAY-gee-uh) when referring to eating large quantities of ice; and *amylophagia* (AM-ee-low-FAY-gee-ah) when referring to eating uncooked starch (flour, laundry starch, or raw rice).

Iron Toxicity

In general, even a diet that includes fortified foods poses no special risk for iron toxicity. The body normally absorbs less iron when its stores are full, but some individuals are poorly defended against excess iron. Once considered rare, **iron overload** has emerged as an important disorder of iron metabolism and regulation.

Iron Overload The iron overload disorder known as **hemochromatosis** is usually caused by a genetic failure to prevent unneeded iron in the diet from being absorbed.[17] Recent research suggests that just as insulin supports normal glucose homeostasis and its absence or ineffectiveness causes diabetes, the hormone hepcidin supports iron homeostasis and its absence or ineffectiveness causes hemochromatosis.

Hereditary hemochromatosis is the most common genetic disorder in Canada and the United States. Other causes of iron overload include repeated blood transfusions (which bypass the intestinal defence), massive doses of supplementary

pica (PIE-ka): a craving for and consumption of nonfood substances.

iron overload: toxicity from excess iron.

hemochromatosis (HE-moh-KRO-ma-toe-sis): a genetically determined failure to prevent absorption of unneeded dietary iron that is characterized by iron overload and tissue damage.

iron (which overwhelm the intestinal defence), and other rare metabolic disorders. Excess iron may cause **hemosiderosis**, a condition characterized by deposits of the iron-storage protein hemosiderin in the liver, heart, joints, and other tissues.

Some of the signs and symptoms of iron overload are similar to those of iron deficiency: apathy, lethargy, and fatigue. Therefore, taking iron supplements before assessing iron status is clearly unwise; hemoglobin tests alone would fail to make the distinction because excess iron accumulates in storage. Iron overload assessment tests measure transferrin saturation and serum ferritin.

Iron overload is characterized by tissue damage, especially in iron-storing organs such as the liver. Infections are likely because viruses and bacteria thrive on iron-rich blood.[18] Symptoms are most severe in alcohol abusers because alcohol damages the small intestine, further impairing its defenses against absorbing excess iron. Untreated hemochromatosis increases the risks of diabetes, liver cancer, heart disease, and arthritis. Treatment involves iron-chelation therapy.[19] ♦

♦ Chelation therapy uses a compound to sequester a toxic substance, rendering it inactive or less harmful.

Iron overload is much more common in men than in women and is twice as prevalent among men as iron deficiency.[20] The widespread fortification of foods with iron makes it difficult for people with hemochromatosis to follow a low-iron diet, and greater dangers lie in the indiscriminate use of iron and vitamin C supplements. Vitamin C not only enhances iron absorption, but also releases iron from ferritin, allowing free iron to wreak the damage typical of free radicals. Thus vitamin C acts as a *pro*oxidant when taken in high doses. (See Highlight 12 for a discussion of free radicals and their effects on disease development.)

Iron and Heart Disease Some research suggests a link between heart disease and excess iron, especially when accompanied by alcohol consumption.[21] As mentioned, free radicals can attack ferritin, causing it to release iron from storage. Free iron, in turn, acts as an oxidant that can generate more free radicals. Reducing iron stores, however, does not appear to reduce the risks of heart attack, stroke, or mortality.[22]

Iron and Cancer There may be an association between iron and some cancers.[23] Explanations for how iron might be involved in causing cancer focus on its free-radical activity, which can damage DNA (see Highlight 12). One of the benefits of a high-fibre diet may be that the accompanying phytates bind iron, making it less available for such reactions.

Iron Poisoning Large doses of iron supplements cause GI distress, including constipation, nausea, vomiting, and diarrhea. These effects may not be as serious as other consequences of iron toxicity, but they are consistent enough to establish a UL of 45 milligrams per day for adults.

Ingestion of iron-containing supplements remains a leading cause of accidental poisoning in young children.[24] Symptoms of toxicity include nausea, vomiting, diarrhea, a rapid heartbeat, a weak pulse, dizziness, shock, and confusion. As few as five iron tablets containing as little as 200 milligrams of iron have caused the deaths of dozens of young children. The exact cause of these deaths is uncertain, but excessive free-radical damage is thought to play a role in heart failure and respiratory distress. Autopsy reports reveal iron deposits and cell death in the stomach, small intestine, liver, and blood vessels (which can cause internal bleeding). As with medicines and other potentially toxic substances, keep iron-containing tablets out of the reach of children. If you suspect iron poisoning, call 9-1-1 immediately.

Iron Recommendations and Sources

To obtain enough iron, people must first select iron-rich foods—both naturally occurring and enriched or fortified—and then take advantage of factors that maximize iron absorption. This discussion begins by identifying iron-rich foods and then reviews the factors affecting absorption.

Recommended Iron Intakes The usual diet in Canada provides about 6 to 7 milligrams of iron per 1000 kcalories.[25] The recommended daily intake for men is 8 milligrams, and because most men eat more than 2000 kcalories a day, they can meet their iron needs with little effort. Women in their reproductive years, however, need 18 milligrams a day. The "How To" on p. 449 explains how to calculate the recommended intake.

hemosiderosis (HE-moh-sid-er-OH-sis): a condition characterized by the deposition of hemosiderin in the liver and other tissues.

HOW TO Estimate the Recommended Daily Intake for Iron

To calculate the recommended daily iron intake, the DRI Committee considers a number of factors. For example, for a woman of childbearing age (19 to 50):

- Losses from feces, urine, sweat, and shed skin: 1.0 milligram
- Losses through menstruation: 0.5 milligram (about 14 milligrams total averaged over 28 days)

These losses reflect an average daily need (total) of 1.5 milligrams of *absorbed* iron.

An estimated average requirement is determined based on the daily need and the assumption that an average of 18 percent of ingested iron is absorbed:

1.5 mg iron (needed)
÷ 0.18 (percent iron absorbed)
= 8 mg iron (estimated average requirement)

Then, a margin of safety is added to cover the needs of essentially all women of childbearing age, and the RDA is set at 18 milligrams.

CENGAGENOW™
For additional practice log on to **www.cengage.com/sso.**

TRY IT Calculate how many slices of whole-wheat bread, millilitres of broccoli, grams of hamburger meat, and millilitres of milk it takes to provide 18 milligrams of iron.

Vegetarians need 1.8 times as much iron ♦ to make up for the low bioavailability typical of their diets.[26] To maximize iron absorption, vegetarians should incorporate iron-rich foods into a diet that is low in inhibitors (foods such as leavened breads and fermented soy products such as miso and tempeh) and high in enhancers (foods rich in vitamin C and the organic acids found in fruits and vegetables). Good vegetarian sources of iron include soy foods (such as soybeans and tofu), legumes (such as lentils and kidney beans), nuts (such as cashews and almonds), seeds (such as pumpkin seeds and sunflower seeds), cereals (such as cream of wheat and oatmeal), dried fruit (such as apricots and raisins), vegetables (such as mushrooms and potatoes), and blackstrap molasses.

♦ To calculate the RDA for vegetarians, multiply by 1.8:
- 8 mg × 1.8 = 14 mg/day (vegetarian men)
- 18 mg × 1.8 = 32 mg/day (vegetarian women, 19 to 50 yr)

Because women have higher iron needs and lower energy needs, they sometimes have trouble obtaining enough iron. On average, women receive only 12 to 13 milligrams of iron per day, which is not enough iron for women until after menopause. To meet their iron needs from foods, premenopausal women need to select iron-rich foods at every meal.

Dietary Guidance for Canadians

Women of childbearing age who may become pregnant should eat foods high in heme iron and/or consume iron-rich plant foods or iron-fortified foods along with an enhancer of iron absorption, such as vitamin C–rich foods.

Iron in Foods Figure 14-7 (p. 450) shows the amounts of iron in selected foods. Meats, fish, and poultry contribute the most iron per serving; other protein-rich foods such as legumes and eggs are also good sources. Although an indispensable part of the diet, foods in the Milk and Milk Alternatives group are notoriously poor in iron. Grain products vary, with whole-grain, enriched, and fortified breads and cereals contributing significantly to iron intakes. Finally, dark green vegetables (such as broccoli) and dried fruits (such as raisins) contribute some iron.

Iron-Enriched Foods The Food and Drug Regulations (FDR) in Canada mandate the iron fortification of flour and "enriched" corn meal.* One serving of enriched bread or cereal provides only a little iron, but because people eat many servings of these foods, the contribution can be significant. Iron added to foods is nonheme iron, which is

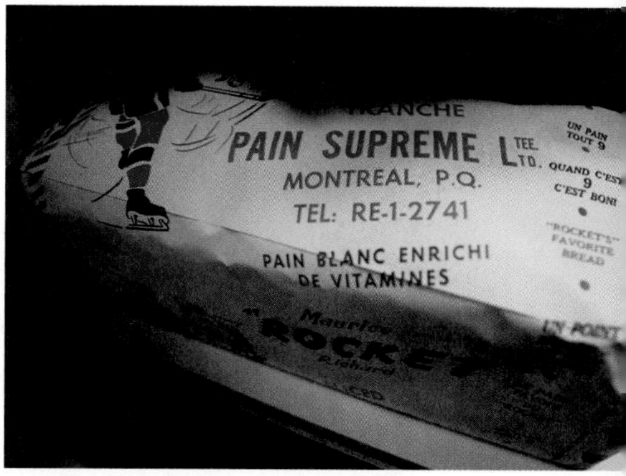
PAIN SUPREME LTÉE. LTD.
MONTREAL, P.Q.
TEL: RE-1-2741
PAIN BLANC ENRICHI DE VITAMINES

THE CANADIAN PRESS/Paul Chiasson

When the label on a grain product says "enriched," it means iron and several B vitamins have been added to meet FDR standards.

*The FDR standards require 4.4 milligrams of iron per 100 grams of flour.

FIGURE 14-7 Iron in Selected Foods

See the "How To" section on p. 317 for more information on using this figure.

Food	Serving size (kcalories)
Broccoli, boiled	125 mL (29 kcal)
Carrots, boiled	125 mL (29 kcal)
Tomato, fresh	1 medium (22 kcal)
Apple, fresh	1 medium (72 kcal)
Banana	1 medium (105 kcal)
Blueberries, fresh	125 mL (44 kcal)
Bread, whole wheat	1 slice, 35 g (86 kcal)
Pasta, whole grain, cooked	125 mL (92 kcal)
Rice, white, cooked	125 mL (89 kcal)
Oatmeal, cooked	175 mL (144 kcal)
Pita, white	½ pita, 35 g (96 kcal)
Cereal, high fibre	30 g (78 kcal)
Milk, 2%	250 mL (129 kcal)
Cheddar cheese	50 g (202 kcal)
Yogurt, 2% plain	175 g (110 kcal)
Soy beverage, fortified	250 mL (110 kcal)
Kefir	175 g (104 kcal)
Ice cream, strawberry	125 mL (134 kcal)
Chicken breast, roasted	75 g (220 kcal)
Ground beef, lean, baked	75 g (191 kcal)
Egg, poached	1 large (72 kcal)
Tuna, canned in water	75 g (87 kcal)
Tofu, made with a calcium salt	150 g (114 kcal)
Peanut butter	30 mL (184 kcal)
Excellent, and sometimes unusual, sources:	
Clams, boiled	75 g (111 kcal)
Parsley, fresh	125 mL (12 kcal)
Beef liver, fried	75 g (178 kcal)

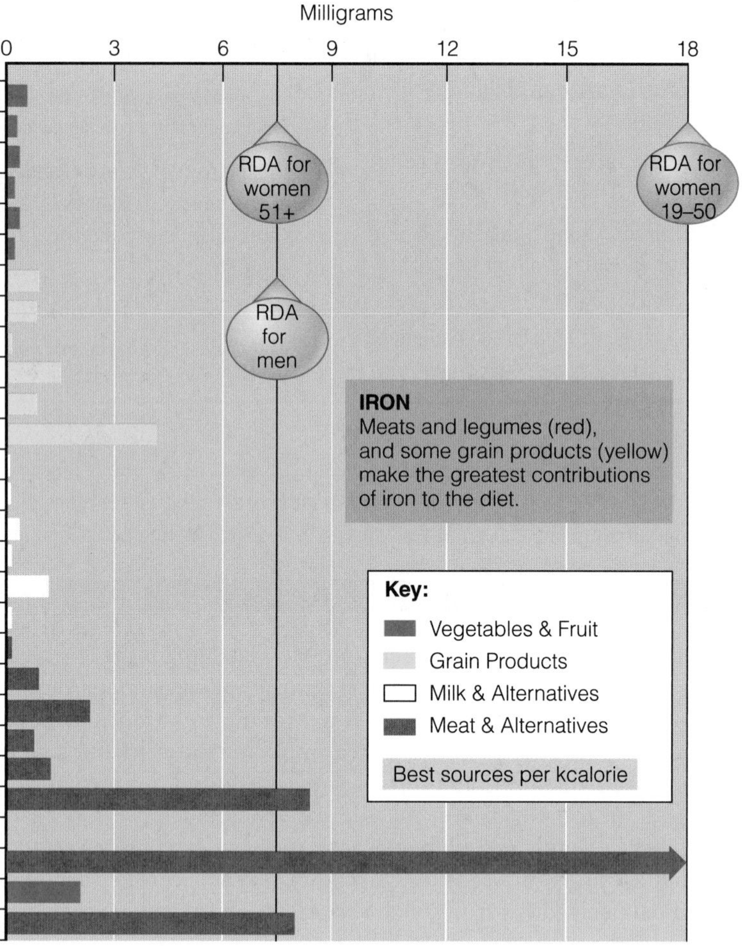
Milligrams
0
3
6
9
12
15
18
RDA for women 51+
RDA for men
RDA for women 19–50
IRON
Meats and legumes (red), and some grain products (yellow) make the greatest contributions of iron to the diet.
Key:
Vegetables & Fruit
Grain Products
Milk & Alternatives
Meat & Alternatives
Best sources per kcalorie

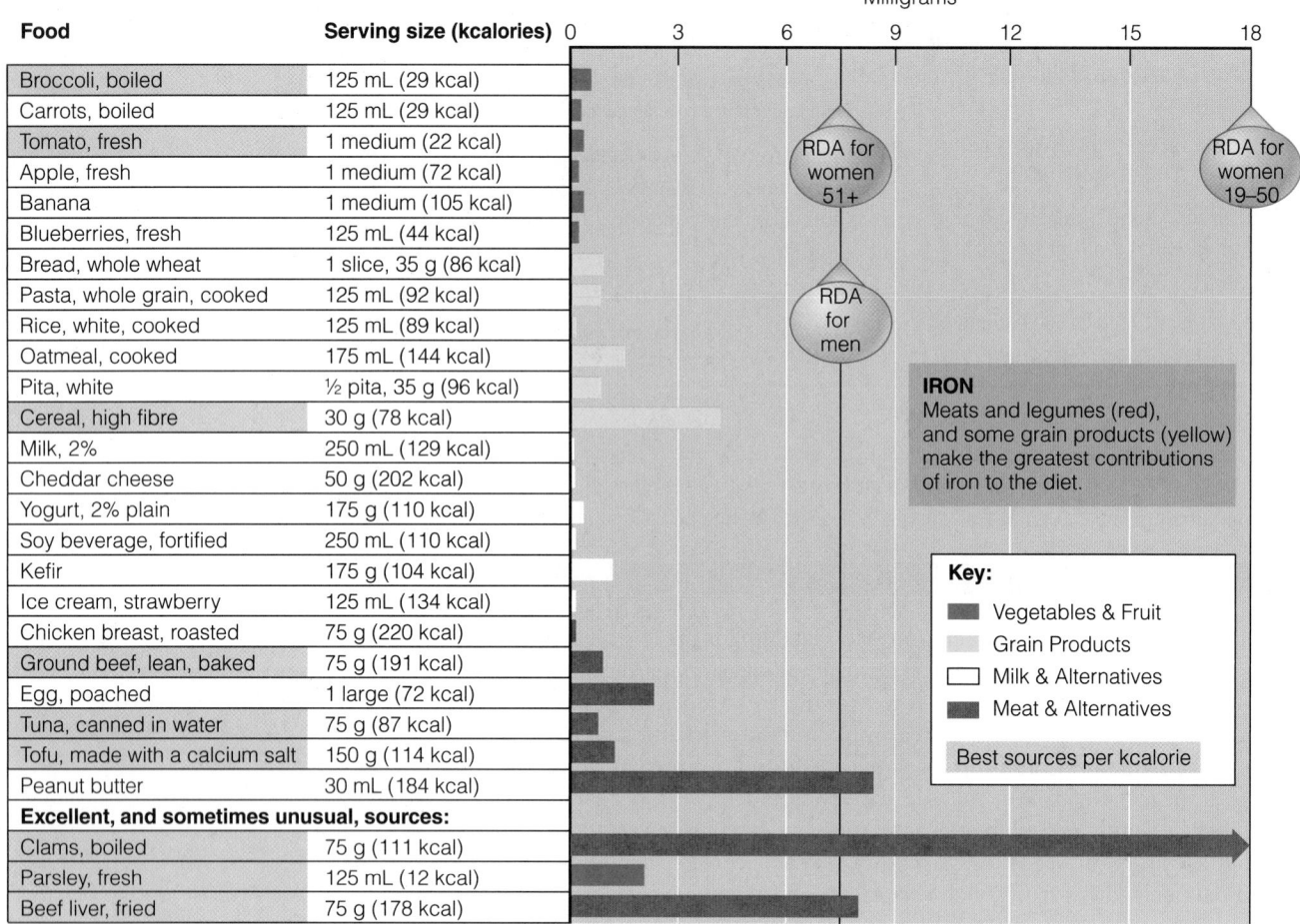

SOURCE: Canadian Nutrient File. Health Canada, 2008. Reproduced with the permission of the Minister of Health, 2011.

not absorbed as well as heme iron, but when eaten with absorption-enhancing foods, enrichment iron can increase iron stores and reduce iron deficiency.[27] In cases of iron overload, enrichment may exacerbate the problem.

Maximizing Iron Absorption In general, the bioavailability of iron is high in meats, fish, and poultry, intermediate in grains and legumes, and low in most vegetables, especially those containing oxalates such as spinach. As mentioned earlier, the amount of iron ultimately absorbed from a meal depends on the combined effects of several enhancing and inhibiting factors. For maximum absorption of nonheme iron, eat meat for MFP and fruits or vegetables for vitamin C. The iron of baked beans, for example, will be enhanced by the MFP in a piece of ham served with them. The iron of bread will be enhanced by the vitamin C in a slice of tomato on a sandwich.

♦ Increase in iron content (mg) for selected foods (90 g) after cooking in iron skillet:

Beef stew	0.66 → 3.40
Chili	0.96 → 6.27
Cornbread	0.67 → 0.86
Hamburger	1.49 → 2.29
Pancake	0.63 → 1.31
Rice	0.67 → 1.97
Scrambled egg	1.49 → 4.76
Spaghetti sauce	0.61 → 5.77

Iron Contamination and Supplementation

In addition to the iron from foods, **contamination iron** from nonfood sources of inorganic iron salts can contribute to the day's intakes. People can also get iron from supplements.

Contamination Iron Foods cooked in iron cookware take up iron salts. The more acidic the food and the longer it is cooked in iron cookware, the higher the iron content. ♦ The iron content of eggs can triple in the time it takes to scramble them in an iron pan. Admittedly, the absorption of this iron may be poor (perhaps only 1 to 2 percent), but every little bit helps a person who is trying to increase iron intake.

contamination iron: iron found in foods as the result of contamination by inorganic iron salts from iron cookware, iron-containing soils, and the like.

Iron Supplements People who are iron deficient may need supplements as well as an iron-rich, absorption-enhancing diet. Many physicians routinely recommend iron supplements to pregnant women, infants, and young children. Iron from supplements is less well absorbed than that from food, so the doses must be high. The absorption of iron taken as ferrous sulphate or as an iron **chelate** is better than that from other iron supplements. Absorption also improves when supplements are taken between meals, at bedtime on an empty stomach, and with liquids (other than milk, tea, or coffee, which inhibit absorption). Taking iron supplements in a single dose instead of several doses per day is equally effective and may improve a person's willingness to take it regularly.

There is no benefit to taking iron supplements with orange juice because vitamin C does not enhance absorption from supplements as it does from foods. Vitamin C enhances iron absorption by converting insoluble ferric iron in foods to the more soluble ferrous iron, and supplemental iron is already in the ferrous form. Constipation is a common side effect of iron supplementation; drinking plenty of water may help to relieve this problem. The best strategy to ensure compliance is to individualize the dose, formulation, and schedule.[28] Most importantly, iron supplements should be taken only when prescribed by a physician who has assessed an iron deficiency.

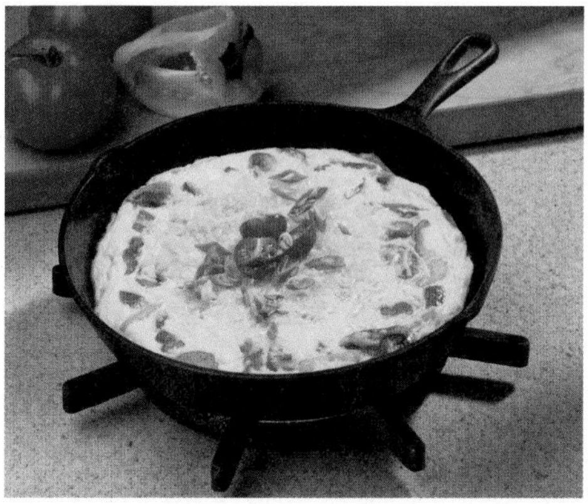

© Polara Studios, Inc.

An old-fashioned iron skillet adds iron to foods.

IN SUMMARY **Most of the body's iron is in hemoglobin and myoglobin where it carries oxygen for use in energy metabolism; some iron is also required for enzymes involved in a variety of reactions. Special proteins assist with iron absorption, transport, and storage—all helping to maintain an appropriate balance, because both too little and too much iron can be damaging. Iron deficiency is most common among infants and young children, teenagers, women of childbearing age, and pregnant women. Symptoms include fatigue and anemia. Iron overload is most common in men. Heme iron, which is found only in meat, fish, poultry, and eggs, is better absorbed than nonheme iron, which occurs in most foods. Nonheme iron absorption is improved by eating iron-containing foods with foods containing the MFP factor and vitamin C; absorption is limited by phytates and oxalates. The accompanying table provides a summary of iron.**

Iron

Recommended Dietary Allowance (RDA)
Men: 8 mg/day
Women: 18 mg/day (19–50 yr) 8 mg/day (51+)

Upper Level
Adults: 45 mg/day

Chief Functions in the Body
Part of the protein hemoglobin, which carries oxygen in the blood; part of the protein myoglobin in muscles, which makes oxygen available for muscle contraction; necessary for the utilization of energy as part of the cells' metabolic machinery

Significant Sources
Red meats, fish, poultry, shellfish, eggs, legumes, dried fruits

Deficiency Symptoms
Anemia: weakness, fatigue, headaches; impaired work performance and cognitive function; impaired immunity; pale skin, nail beds, mucous membranes, and palm creases; concave nails; inability to regulate body temperature; pica

Toxicity Symptoms
GI distress
Iron overload: infections, fatigue, joint pain, skin pigmentation, organ damage

Zinc

Zinc is a versatile trace element required as a cofactor by more than 100 enzymes. Virtually all cells contain zinc, but the highest concentrations are found in muscle and bone.[29]

Zinc Roles in the Body

Zinc supports the work of numerous proteins in the body, such as the **metalloenzymes**, ♦ which are involved in a variety of metabolic processes, including the regulation of gene expression.* In addition, zinc stabilizes

*Among the metalloenzymes requiring zinc are carbonic anhydrase, deoxythymidine kinase, DNA and RNA polymerase, and alkaline phosphatase.

♦ Metalloenzymes that require zinc:
- Help make parts of the genetic materials DNA and RNA
- Manufacture heme for hemoglobin
- Participate in essential fatty acid metabolism
- Release vitamin A from liver stores
- Metabolize carbohydrates
- Synthesize proteins
- Metabolize alcohol in the liver
- Dispose of damaging free radicals

chelate (KEY-late): a substance that can grasp the positive ions of a mineral.

chele = claw

metalloenzymes (meh-tal-oh-EN-zimes): enzymes that contain one or more minerals as part of their structures.

cell membranes, helping to strengthen their defence against free-radical attacks. Zinc also assists in immune function and in growth and development. Zinc participates in the synthesis, storage, and release of the hormone insulin in the pancreas, although it does not appear to play a direct role in insulin's action. Zinc interacts with platelets in blood clotting, affects thyroid hormone function, and influences behaviour and learning performance. It is needed to produce the active form of vitamin A (retinal) in visual pigments and the retinol-binding protein that transports vitamin A. It is essential to normal taste perception, wound healing, sperm production, and fetal development. A zinc deficiency impairs all these and other functions, underlining the vast importance of zinc in supporting the body's proteins.

Zinc Absorption and Metabolism

The body's handling of zinc resembles that of iron in some ways and differs in others. A key difference is the circular passage of zinc from the small intestine to the body and back again.

Zinc Absorption The rate of zinc absorption varies from about 15 to 40 percent, depending on a person's zinc status—if more is needed, more is absorbed. Also, dietary factors influence zinc absorption. For example, phytates bind zinc, thus limiting its bioavailability.[30]

Upon absorption into an intestinal cell, zinc has two options. Zinc may participate in the metabolic functions of the intestinal cell itself, or it may be retained within the intestinal cells by **metallothionein** until the body needs zinc.

Zinc Recycling Some zinc eventually reaches the pancreas, where it is incorporated into many of the digestive enzymes that the pancreas releases into the small intestine at mealtimes. The small intestine thus receives two doses of zinc with each meal—one from foods and the other from the zinc-rich pancreatic secretions. The recycling of zinc in the body from the pancreas to the small intestine and back to the pancreas is referred to as the **enteropancreatic circulation** of zinc. Each time zinc circulates through the small intestine, it may be excreted in shed intestinal cells or reabsorbed into the body (see Figure 14-8). The body loses zinc primarily in feces. Smaller losses occur in urine, shed skin, hair, sweat, menstrual fluids, and semen.

metallothionein (meh-TAL-oh-THIGH-oh-neen): a sulphur-rich protein that avidly binds with and transports metals such as zinc.
- **metallo** = containing a metal
- **thio** = containing sulphur
- **ein** = a protein

enteropancreatic (EN-ter-oh-PAN-kree-AT-ik) **circulation:** the circulatory route from the pancreas to the small intestine and back to the pancreas.

Zinc Transport Zinc's main transport vehicle in the blood is the protein albumin. Some zinc also binds to transferrin—the same transferrin that carries iron in the

FIGURE 14-8 Enteropancreatic Circulation of Zinc

Some zinc from food is absorbed by the small intestine and sent to the pancreas to be incorporated into digestive enzymes that return to the small intestine. This cycle is called the enteropancreatic circulation of zinc.

CENGAGENOW™
Animated! figure
www.cengage.com/sso

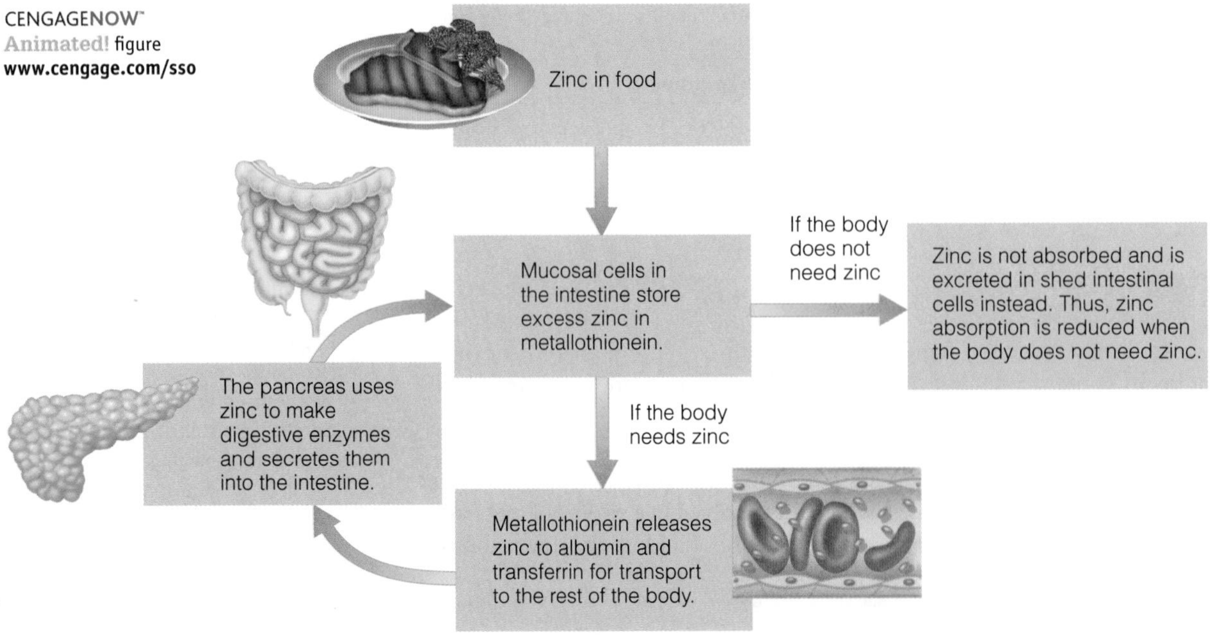
Zinc in food
Mucosal cells in the intestine store excess zinc in metallothionein.
If the body does not need zinc
Zinc is not absorbed and is excreted in shed intestinal cells instead. Thus, zinc absorption is reduced when the body does not need zinc.
If the body needs zinc
Metallothionein releases zinc to albumin and transferrin for transport to the rest of the body.
The pancreas uses zinc to make digestive enzymes and secretes them into the intestine.

blood. In healthy individuals, transferrin is usually less than 50 percent saturated with iron, but in iron overload, it is more saturated. Diets that deliver more than twice as much iron as zinc leave too few transferrin sites available for zinc. The result is poor zinc absorption. The converse is also true: large doses of zinc inhibit iron absorption.

Large doses of zinc create a similar problem with another essential mineral, copper. These nutrient interactions highlight one of the many reasons why people should use supplements conservatively, if at all: supplementation can easily create imbalances.

Zinc Deficiency Severe zinc deficiencies are not widespread in developed countries, but they do occur in vulnerable groups—pregnant women, young children, the elderly, and the poor.[31] Human zinc deficiency was first reported in the 1960s in children and adolescent boys in Egypt, Iran, and Turkey. Children have especially high zinc needs because they are growing rapidly and synthesizing many zinc-containing proteins, and the native diets among those populations were not meeting these needs. Middle Eastern diets are typically low in the richest zinc source, meats. Furthermore, the staple foods in these diets are legumes, unleavened breads, and other whole-grain foods—all high in fibre and phytates, which inhibit zinc absorption.*

Figure 14-9 shows the severe growth retardation and mentions the immature sexual development characteristic of zinc deficiency. In addition, zinc deficiency hinders digestion and absorption, causing diarrhea, which worsens malnutrition not only for zinc, but for all nutrients. It also impairs the immune response, making infections likely—among them, GI tract infections, which worsen malnutrition, including zinc malnutrition (a classic downward spiral of events). Chronic zinc deficiency damages the central nervous system and brain and may lead to poor motor development and cognitive performance. Because zinc deficiency directly impairs vitamin A metabolism, vitamin A–deficiency symptoms often appear. Zinc deficiency also disturbs thyroid function and the metabolic rate. It alters taste, causes loss of appetite, and slows wound healing—in fact, its symptoms are so pervasive that generalized malnutrition and sickness are more likely to be the diagnosis than simple zinc deficiency.

FIGURE 14-9 Zinc-Deficiency Symptom—The Stunted Growth of Dwarfism

The growth retardation, known as dwarfism, is rightly ascribed to zinc deficiency because it is partially reversible when zinc is restored to the diet.

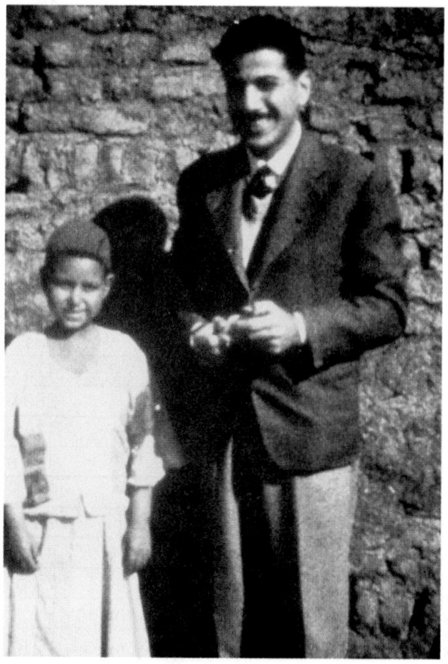

© H. Sandstead

The Egyptian man on the right is an adult of average height. The Egyptian boy on the left is 17 years old but is only 122 centimetres (4 feet) tall, like a 7-year-old in Canada. His genitalia are like those of a 6-year-old.

Zinc Toxicity High doses (more than 50 milligrams) of zinc may cause vomiting, diarrhea, headaches, exhaustion, and other symptoms. The UL for adults was set at 40 milligrams based on zinc's interference in copper metabolism—an effect that, in animals, leads to degeneration of the heart muscle.

Zinc Recommendations and Sources Figure 14-10 (p. 454) shows zinc amounts in foods per serving. Zinc is highest in protein-rich foods such as shellfish (especially oysters), meats, poultry, milk, and cheese. Legumes and whole-grain products are good sources of zinc if eaten in large quantities; in typical Canadian diets, the phytate content of grains is not high enough to impair zinc absorption. Vegetables vary in zinc content depending on the soil in which they are grown. Average intakes in Canada meet current recommendations, ranging between 5 and 6 milligrams of zinc per 1000 kcalories.[32]

Zinc Supplementation In developed countries, most people obtain enough zinc from the diet without resorting to supplements. In developing countries, zinc supplementation plays a major role in the treatment of childhood infectious diseases.[33] Zinc supplements effectively reduce the incidence of disease and death associated with diarrhea in children.[34] Similarly, zinc supplements reduce the incidence of pneumonia and associated deaths in older adults.[35]

The use of zinc lozenges to treat the common cold has been controversial and inconclusive, with some studies finding them effective and others not.[36] The different study results may reflect the effectiveness of various zinc compounds. Some studies using zinc gluconate report shorter duration of cold symptoms, whereas most studies using other combinations of zinc report no effect. Common side effects of zinc lozenges include nausea and bad taste reactions.

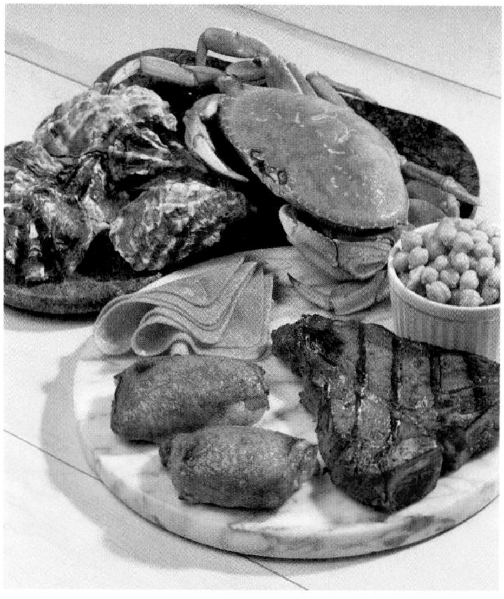

© Polara Studios, Inc.

Zinc is highest in protein-rich foods such as oysters, beef, poultry, legumes, and nuts.

*Unleavened bread contains no yeast, which normally breaks down phytates during fermentation.

FIGURE 14-10 Zinc in Selected Foods

See the "How To" section on p. 317 for more information on using this figure.

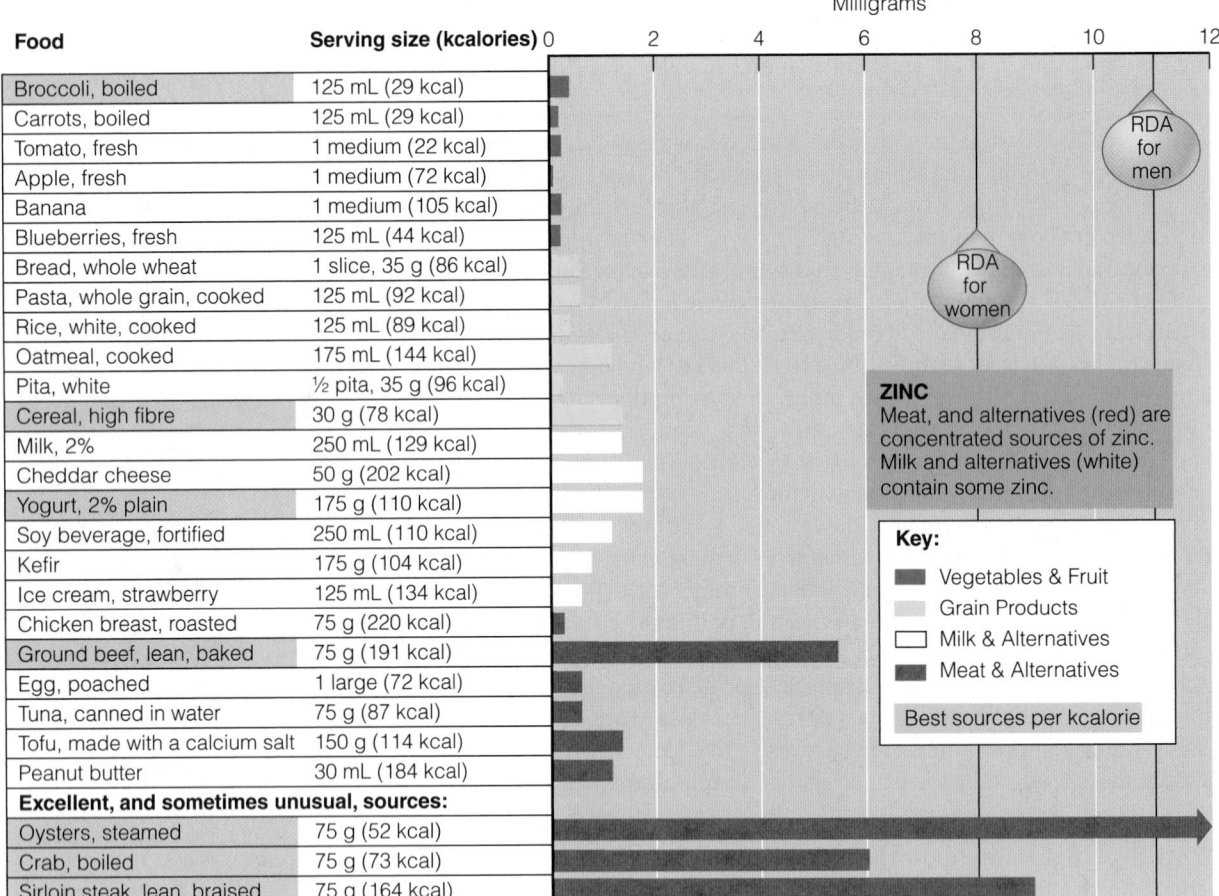

Food	Serving size (kcalories)
Broccoli, boiled	125 mL (29 kcal)
Carrots, boiled	125 mL (29 kcal)
Tomato, fresh	1 medium (22 kcal)
Apple, fresh	1 medium (72 kcal)
Banana	1 medium (105 kcal)
Blueberries, fresh	125 mL (44 kcal)
Bread, whole wheat	1 slice, 35 g (86 kcal)
Pasta, whole grain, cooked	125 mL (92 kcal)
Rice, white, cooked	125 mL (89 kcal)
Oatmeal, cooked	175 mL (144 kcal)
Pita, white	½ pita, 35 g (96 kcal)
Cereal, high fibre	30 g (78 kcal)
Milk, 2%	250 mL (129 kcal)
Cheddar cheese	50 g (202 kcal)
Yogurt, 2% plain	175 g (110 kcal)
Soy beverage, fortified	250 mL (110 kcal)
Kefir	175 g (104 kcal)
Ice cream, strawberry	125 mL (134 kcal)
Chicken breast, roasted	75 g (220 kcal)
Ground beef, lean, baked	75 g (191 kcal)
Egg, poached	1 large (72 kcal)
Tuna, canned in water	75 g (87 kcal)
Tofu, made with a calcium salt	150 g (114 kcal)
Peanut butter	30 mL (184 kcal)
Excellent, and sometimes unusual, sources:	
Oysters, steamed	75 g (52 kcal)
Crab, boiled	75 g (73 kcal)
Sirloin steak, lean, braised	75 g (164 kcal)

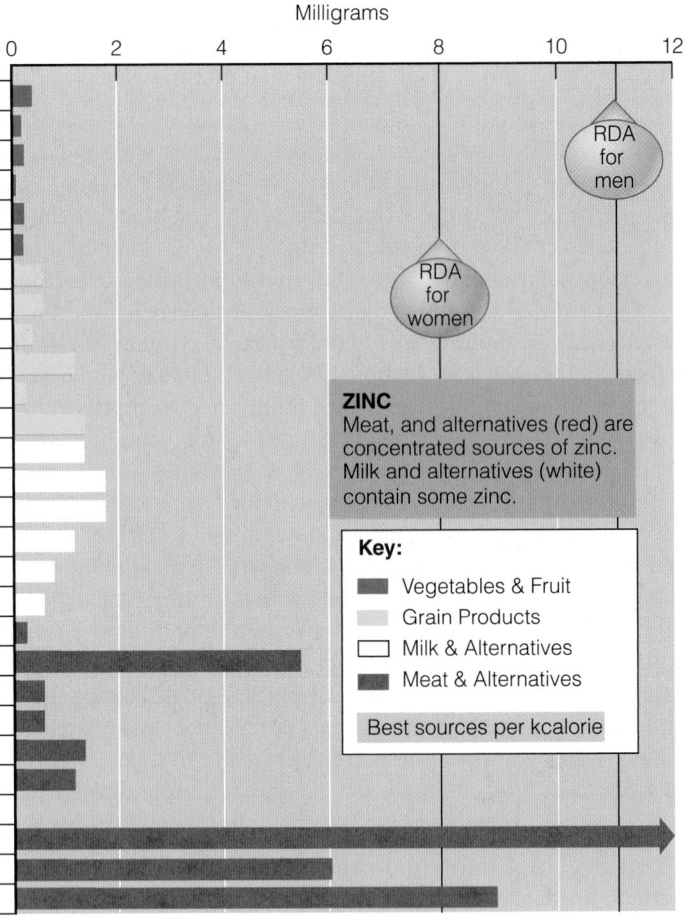
Milligrams
0
2
4
6
8
10
12
RDA for men
RDA for women
ZINC
Meat, and alternatives (red) are concentrated sources of zinc. Milk and alternatives (white) contain some zinc.
Key:
Vegetables & Fruit
Grain Products
Milk & Alternatives
Meat & Alternatives
Best sources per kcalorie

SOURCE: Canadian Nutrient File. Health Canada, 2008. Reproduced with the permission of the Minister of Health, 2011.

IN SUMMARY Zinc-requiring enzymes participate in a multitude of reactions affecting growth, vitamin A activity, and pancreatic digestive enzyme synthesis, among others. Both dietary zinc and zinc in pancreatic secretions (via enteropancreatic circulation) are available for absorption. Absorption is monitored by a special binding protein (metallothionein) in the small intestine. Protein-rich foods derived from animals are the best sources of bioavailable zinc. Fibre and phytates in cereals bind zinc, limiting absorption. Growth retardation and sexual immaturity are hallmark symptoms of zinc deficiency. The following table provides a summary of zinc.

Zinc

RDA

Men: 11 mg/day

Women: 8 mg/day

Upper Level

Adults: 40 mg/day

Chief Functions in the Body

Part of many enzymes; associated with the hormone insulin; involved in making genetic material and proteins, immune reactions, transport of vitamin A, taste perception, wound healing, the making of sperm, and the normal development of the fetus

Significant Sources

Protein-containing foods: red meats, shellfish, whole grains; some fortified cereals

Deficiency Symptoms[a]

Growth retardation, delayed sexual maturation, impaired immune function, hair loss, eye and skin lesions, loss of appetite

Toxicity Symptoms

Loss of appetite, impaired immunity, low HDL, copper and iron deficiencies

[a]A rare inherited disease of zinc malabsorption, *acrodermatitis* (AK-roh-der-ma-TIE-tis) *enteropathica* (EN-ter-oh-PATH-ick-ah), causes additional and more severe symptoms.

Copper

The body contains about 100 milligrams of copper in a variety of cells and tissues. Copper balance and transport depend on a system of proteins.[37]

Copper Roles in the Body Copper serves as a constituent of several enzymes. The copper-containing enzymes have diverse metabolic roles with one common characteristic: all involve reactions that consume oxygen or oxygen radicals. For example, copper-containing enzymes catalyze the oxidation of ferrous iron to ferric iron, which allows iron to bind to transferrin. Copper's role in iron metabolism makes it a key factor in hemoglobin synthesis. Copper- and zinc-containing enzymes participate in the body's natural defence against the oxidative damage of free radicals. Still other copper enzymes help to manufacture collagen, inactivate histamine, and degrade serotonin. Copper, like iron, is needed in many of the metabolic reactions related to the release of energy.

Copper Deficiency and Toxicity Typical North American diets provide adequate amounts of copper and deficiency is rare. In animals, copper deficiency raises blood cholesterol and damages blood vessels, raising questions about whether low dietary copper might contribute to cardiovascular disease in humans.

Some genetic disorders create a copper toxicity, but excessive intakes from foods are unlikely. Excessive intakes from supplements may cause liver damage, and therefore a UL has been set.

Two rare genetic disorders affect copper status in opposite directions. In Menkes disease, the intestinal cells absorb copper, but cannot release it into circulation, causing a life-threatening deficiency. Treatment involves giving copper intravenously. In Wilson's disease, copper accumulates in the liver and brain, creating a life-threatening toxicity. Wilson's disease can be controlled by reducing copper intake, using chelating agents such as penicillamine, and taking zinc supplements, which interfere with copper absorption.

Copper Recommendations and Sources The richest food sources of copper are legumes, whole grains, nuts, shellfish, and seeds. More than half of the copper from foods is absorbed, and the major route of elimination appears to be bile. Water may also provide copper, depending on the type of plumbing pipe and the hardness of the water.

IN SUMMARY **Copper is a component of several enzymes, all of which are involved in some way with oxygen or oxidation. Some act as antioxidants; others are essential to iron metabolism. Legumes, whole grains, and shellfish are good sources of copper. The accompanying table provides a summary of copper.**

Copper

RDA	**Significant Sources**
Adults: 900 µg/day	Seafood, nuts, whole grains, seeds, legumes
Upper Level	**Deficiency Symptoms**
Adults: 10 000 µg/day (10 mg/day)	Anemia, bone abnormalities
Chief Functions in the Body	**Toxicity Symptoms**
Necessary for the absorption and use of iron in the formation of hemoglobin; part of several enzymes	Liver damage

The health of your blood affects many metabolic processes, including the amount of energy that you generate each day. Although minute in need, the trace minerals tackle big jobs in forming and maintaining your blood. For example, at low intakes of iron, you produce less hemoglobin. Now think about the lack of energy you would have with insufficient hemoglobin to transport the oxygen from your lungs to your cells. Or, consider how an inadequate intake of copper can compromise the movement of iron out of the liver for transport in the blood and later incorporation into hemoglobin. From what you have learned in this chapter, you can now realize the importance of keeping your blood healthy by choosing nourishing foods that are rich in micronutrients, especially vitamin K and the minerals iron, zinc, and copper.

Other Trace Minerals

Research to determine whether other trace minerals are essential is difficult because their quantities in the body are so small and also because human deficiencies are unknown. Guessing their functions in the body can be particularly problematic. Much of the available knowledge comes from research using animals.

Nickel may serve as a cofactor for certain enzymes. Silicon is involved in the formation of bones and collagen. Vanadium, too, is necessary for growth and bone development and for normal reproduction. As described earlier in Chapter 10 (pp. 332–333), cobalt is a key mineral in the large vitamin B_{12} molecule, but it is not an essential nutrient and no recommendation has been established. Boron may play a key role in bone health, brain activities, and immune response.[38]

In the future, we may discover that many other trace minerals play key nutritional roles. Even arsenic—famous as a poison used by murderers and known to be a carcinogen—may turn out to be essential for human beings in tiny quantities. It has already proved useful in the treatment of some types of leukemia.[39]

heavy metals: mineral ions such as mercury and lead, so called because they are of relatively high atomic weight. Many heavy metals are poisonous.

Contaminant Minerals

Chapters 10 to 14 explain the many ways minerals serve the body—maintaining fluid and electrolyte balance, supporting antioxidant enzyme systems, providing structural support to the bones, transporting oxygen, and assisting enzymes. In contrast to the minerals that the body requires, contaminant minerals impair the body's growth, work capacity, and general health. Contaminant minerals include the **heavy metals** lead, mercury, and cadmium that enter the food supply by way of soil, water, and air pollution. This section focuses on lead poisoning because it is a serious environmental threat to young children and because reducing blood lead levels in children is a goal of Health Canada.[40] Much of the information on lead applies to the other contaminant minerals as well—they all disrupt body processes and impair nutrition status similarly.

Like other minerals, lead is indestructible and the body cannot change its chemistry. Chemically similar to nutrient minerals like iron, calcium, and zinc (cations with two positive charges), lead displaces them from some of the metabolic sites they normally occupy but is then unable to perform their roles. For example, lead competes with iron in heme, but it cannot carry oxygen. Similarly, lead competes with calcium in the brain, but it cannot signal messages from nerve cells. Excess lead in the blood also deranges the structure of red blood cell membranes, making them leaky and fragile. Lead interacts with white blood cells, too, impairing their ability to fight infection, and it binds to antibodies, thwarting their effort to resist disease. Chapter 17 examines the damaging effects of lead toxicity on a child's growth and development.

Lead typifies the ways all heavy metals behave in the body: they interfere with nutrients that are trying to do their jobs. The "good guy" nutrients are shoved aside by the "bad guy" contaminants. Then, when the contaminants cannot perform the roles of the nutrients, health diminishes. To safeguard our health, we must defend ourselves against contamination by eating nutrient-rich foods and preserving a clean environment.

Closing Thoughts on the Nutrients

This chapter completes the introductory lessons on the nutrients. Each nutrient, from the amino acids to zinc, has been described thoroughly—its chemistry, roles in the body, sources in the diet, symptoms of deficiency and toxicity, and influences on health and disease. Such a detailed examination is informative, but it can also be misleading. It is important to step back from the detailed study of the individual nutrients to look at them as a whole. After all, people eat foods, not nutrients, and most foods deliver dozens of nutrients. Furthermore, nutrients work cooperatively with one another in the body; their actions are most often *inter*actions. This chapter alone mentioned how iron depends on vitamin C to keep it in its active form and copper to incorporate it into hemoglobin, and how zinc is needed to activate and transport vitamin A. The following table provides a summary of the nutrients involved in blood health.

IN SUMMARY Nutrients for Blood Health

Vitamin or Nutrient and Chief Functions	Deficiency Symptoms	Toxicity Symptoms[a]	Significant Sources
Vitamin K Synthesis of blood-clotting proteins and bone proteins	Hemorrhage	None known	Synthesized in the body by GI bacteria; green leafy vegetables, oils
Iron Part of the protein hemoglobin, which carries oxygen in the blood; part of the protein myoglobin in muscles, which makes oxygen available for muscle contraction; necessary for energy metabolism	Anemia: weakness, fatigue, headaches; impaired work performance; impaired immunity; pale skin, nail beds, mucous membranes, and palm creases; concave nails; inability to regulate body temperature; pica	GI distress; iron overload: infections, fatigue, joint pain, skin pigmentation, organ damage	Red meats, fish, poultry, shellfish, eggs, legumes, dried fruits
Zinc Part of insulin and many enzymes; involved in making genetic material and proteins, immune reactions, transport of vitamin A, taste perception, wound healing, the making of sperm, and normal fetal development	Growth retardation, delayed sexual maturation, impaired immune function, hair loss, eye and skin lesions, loss of appetite	Loss of appetite, impaired immunity, low HDL, copper and iron deficiencies	Protein-containing foods: red meats, fish, shellfish, poultry, whole grains; fortified cereals
Copper Helps form hemoglobin; part of several enzymes	Anemia, bone abnormalities	Liver damage	Seafood, nuts, legumes, whole grains, seeds

[a]Acute toxicities of many minerals cause abdominal pain, nausea, vomiting, and diarrhea.

How much of each particular nutrient does the body need? Estimates fall somewhere between intakes that are inadequate and cause illness and intakes that are excessive and cause illness. A wide range of intakes that support health, to varying degrees, lies between deficiency and toxicity. In the past, nutrient needs were determined by how much was needed to prevent deficiency symptoms. If lack of a nutrient caused illness, it was defined as essential. Today, nutrient needs are based on how much is needed to support optimal health. The amount of vitamin C needed to prevent scurvy is much less than the amount correlated with reducing the risk of cancer, for example. Furthermore, nutrients are being examined within the context of the whole diet. Health benefits are not credited to vitamin C alone, but also to the vitamin C–rich fruits and vegetables that provide many other nutrients—and nonnutrients (phytochemicals)—important to health. Highlight 14 presents current perspectives on phytochemicals and their interactions with human health.

People can also improve their health with physical activity. Energy expenditure is unlike money expenditure: it is desirable to *spend* energy, not to save it (within reason, of course). The more energy people spend, the more food they can afford to eat—food that delivers both nutrients and pleasure. The next chapter presents details on nutrition and physical activity.

Nutrition Portfolio

To obtain the trace minerals that keep your blood healthy, be sure to select a variety of foods from all of the four food groups each day. Animal foods provide especially rich sources of bioavailable iron, zinc, and copper.

Go to Diet Analysis Plus and choose one of the days on which you tracked your diet. Select the Intake vs. Goals report and then consider the following questions. Remember that scoring 100 percent on this report means you met your daily nutrient goal.

- Your Intake vs. Goals report may only display your intake for two of the trace minerals: iron and zinc. How was your intake for these two trace minerals? How could you improve your intake of these nutrients?

Now click on the Intake Spreadsheet report and consider the following questions:

- Examine the variety in your food intake, taking particular notice of how often you include meats, seafood, poultry, legumes, and enriched or fortified grain products. These foods contain iron, zinc, and other trace minerals. How could you improve your intake of these foods?
- Estimate your relative intake of heme versus nonheme iron by examining your iron sources from animal and plant foods. Remember about 40 percent of the iron found in animal foods is heme iron and the other 60 percent of iron in animal foods and all of the iron in plant foods is nonheme.

Diet Analysis PLUS **To complete this exercise, go to your Diet Analysis Plus at www.cengage.com/sso.**

Nutrition on the Net

CENGAGENOW™
For further study of topics covered in this chapter, log on to **www.cengage.com/sso.**

- Read about Canada's Lead Risk Reduction Strategy from Health Canada: **www.hc-sc.gc.ca/ahc-asc/media/nr-cp/_2010/2010_203fsb-eng.php**
- Learn more about iron overload from the Canadian Hemochromatosis Society: **www.cdnhemochromatosis.ca**
- Search for "vitamins" and "minerals" at the Dietitians of Canada's website: **www.dietitians.ca**

References

1. R. E. Fleming and B. R. Bacon, Orchestration of iron homeostasis, *New England Journal of Medicine* 352 (2005): 1741–1744.
2. Committee on Dietary Reference Intakes, *Dietary Reference Intakes for Vitamin A, Vitamin K, Arsenic, Boron, Chromium, Copper, Iodine, Iron, Manganese, Molybdenum, Nickel, Silicon, Vanadium, and Zinc* (Washington, D.C.: National Academies Press, 2001), p. 315.
3. P. Thankachan and coauthors, Iron absorption in young Indian women: The interaction of iron status with the influence of tea and ascorbic acid, *American Journal of Clinical Nutrition* 87 (2008): 881–886.
4. R. F. Hurrell and coauthors, Meat protein fractions enhance nonheme iron absorption in humans, *Journal of Nutrition* 136 (2006): 2808–2812.
5. R. E. Conway, J. J. Powell, and C. A. Geissler, A food-group based algorithm to predict non-heme iron absorption, *International Journal of Food Sciences and Nutrition* 58 (2007): 29–41.
6. Committee on Dietary Reference Intakes, 2001, p. 351.
7. M. D. Knutson, Into the matrix: Regulation of the iron regulatory hormone hepcidin by matriptase-2, *Nutrition Reviews* 67 (2009): 284–288; M. F. Young and coauthors, Serum hepcidin is significantly associated with iron absorption from food and supplemental sources in healthy young women, *American Journal of Clinical Nutrition* 89 (2009): 533–538; M. U. Muckenthaler, B. Galy, and M. W. Hentze, Systemic iron homeostasis and the iron-responsive element/iron-regulatory protein (IRE/IRP) regulatory network, *Annual Review of Nutrition* 28 (2008): 197–213; E. Nemeth and T. Ganz, Regulation of iron metabolism by hepcidin, *Annual Review of Nutrition* 26 (2006): 323–342.
8. Worldwide prevalence of anaemia 1993–2005: WHO Global Database on Anaemia, published 2008, available at www.who.org.
9. L. M. Tussing-Humphreys and coauthors, Excess adiposity, inflammation, and iron-deficiency in female adolescents, *Journal of the American Dietetic Association* 109 (2009): 297–302.
10. J. P. McClung and J. P. Karl, Iron deficiency and obesity: The contribution of inflammation and diminished iron absorption, *Nutrition Reviews* 67 (2008): 100–104.
11. J. L. Beard, Why iron deficiency is important in infant development, *Journal of Nutrition* 138 (2008): 2534–2536.
12. K. C. White, Anemia is a poor predictor of iron deficiency among toddlers in the United States: For heme the bell tolls, *Pediatrics* 115 (2005): 315–320.
13. Z. Yang and coauthors, Comparison of plasma ferritin concentration with the ratio of plasma transferrin receptor to ferritin in estimating body iron stores: Results of 4 intervention trials, *American Journal of Clinical Nutrition* 87 (2008): 1892–1898.
14. J. C. McCann and B. N. Ames, An overview of evidence for a causal relation between iron deficiency during development and deficits in cognitive or behavioral function, *American Journal of Clinical Nutrition* 85 (2007): 931–945.

15. L. L. Iannotti and coauthors, Iron supplementation in early childhood: Health benefits and risks, *American Journal of Clinical Nutrition* 84 (2006): 1261–1276.
16. S. L. Young and coauthors, Toward a comprehensive approach to the collection and analysis of pica substances, with emphasis on geophagic materials, *PLoS ONE* 3 (2008): e3147.
17. A. Pietrangelo, Hereditary hemochromatosis, *Annual Review of Nutrition* 26 (2006): 251–270.
18. H. Drakesmith and A. Prentice, Viral infection and iron metabolism, *Nature Reviews. Microbiology* 6 (2008): 541–552; A. M. Prentice, Iron metabolism, malaria, and other infections: What is all the fuss about? *Journal of Nutrition* 138 (2008): 2537–2541; C. Ratledge, Iron metabolism and infection, *Food and Nutrition Bulletin* 28 (2007): S515–S523.
19. F. Dreyfus, The deleterious effects of iron overload in patients with myelodysplastic syndromes, *Blood Reviews* 22 (2008): S29–S34.
20. K. J. Allen and coauthors, Iron-overload: Related disease in *HFE* hereditary hemochromatosis, *New England Journal of Medicine* 358 (2008): 221–230.
21. F. B. Hu, The iron-heart hypothesis: Search for the ironclad evidence, *Journal of the American Medical Association* 297 (2007): 639–641; D. Lee, A. R. Folsom, and D. R. Jacobs, Iron, zinc, and alcohol consumption and mortality from cardiovascular diseases: The Iowa Women's Health Study, *American Journal of Clinical Nutrition* 81 (2005): 787–791.
22. L. R. Zacharski and coauthors, Reduction of iron stores and cardiovascular outcomes in patients with peripheral arterial disease: A randomized controlled trial, *Journal of the American Medical Association* 297 (2007): 603–610.
23. A. G. Mainous and coauthors, Iron, lipids, and risk of cancer in the Framingham Offspring Cohort, *American Journal of Epidemiology* 160 (2005): 1115–1122.
24. A. S. Manoguerra and coauthors, Iron ingestion: An evidence-based consensus guideline for out-of-hospital management, *Clinical Toxicology* 43 (2005): 553–570.
25. Health Canada, Statistics Canada, Canadian Community Health Survey, Cycle 2.2, Nutrition (2004)—Nutrient intakes from food, Provincial, Regional and National Summary Data Tables, Volumes 1 and 2 (Revised 2009).
26. Committee on Dietary Reference Intakes, 2001, p. 351.
27. D. Moretti and coauthors, Extruded rice fortified with micronized ground ferric pyrophosphate reduces iron deficiency in Indian schoolchildren: A double-blind randomized controlled trial, *American Journal of Clinical Nutrition* 84 (2006): 822–829; F. Pizarro and coauthors, Ascorbyl palmitate enhances iron bioavailability in iron-fortified bread, *American Journal of Clinical Nutrition* 84 (2006): 830–834.
28. M. Alleyne, M. K. Horne, and J. L. Miller, Individualized treatment for iron-deficiency anemia in adults, *American Journal of Medicine* 121 (2008): 943–948.
29. H. Tapiero and K. D. Tew, Trace elements in human physiology and pathology: Zinc and metallothioneins, *Biomedicine and Pharmacotherapy* 57 (2003): 399–411.
30. J. R. Hunt, J. M. Beiseigel, and L. K. Johnson, Adaptation in human zinc absorption as influenced by dietary zinc and bioavailability, *American Journal of Clinical Nutrition* 87 (2008): 1336–1345.
31. S. N. Meydani and coauthors, Serum zinc and pneumonia in nursing home elderly, *American Journal of Clinical Nutrition* 86 (2007): 1167–1173; J. M. Schneider and coauthors, The prevalence of low serum zinc and copper levels and dietary habits associated with serum zinc and copper in 12- to 36-month-old children from low-income families at risk for iron deficiency, *Journal of the American Dietetic Association* 107 (2007): 1924–1929.
32. Health Canada, Statistics Canada, Canadian Community Health Survey, Cycle 2.2, Nutrition (2004)—Nutrient intakes from food, Provincial, Regional and National Summary Data Tables, Volumes 1 and 2 (Revised 2009).
33. D. E. Roth and coauthors, Acute lower respiratory infections in childhood: Opportunities for reducing the global burden through nutritional interventions, *Bulletin of the World Health Organization* 86 (2008): 321–416.
34. M. Lukacik, R. L. Thomas, and J. V. Aranda, A meta-analysis of the effects of oral zinc in the treatment of acute and persistent diarrhea, *Pediatrics* 121 (2008): 326–336; S. E. Wuehler, F. Sempértegui, and K. H. Brown, Dose-response trial of prophylactic zinc supplements, with or without copper, in young Ecuadorian children at risk of zinc deficiency, *American Journal of Clinical Nutrition* 87 (2008): 723–733; R. Aggarwal, J. Sentz, and M. A. Miller, Role of zinc administration in prevention of childhood diarrhea and respiratory illnesses: A meta-analysis, *Pediatrics* 119 (2007): 1120–1130; J.M.M. Gardner and coauthors, Zinc supplementation and psychosocial stimulation: Effects on the development of undernourished Jamaican children, *American Journal of Clinical Nutrition* 82 (2005): 399–405.
35. Meydani and coauthors, 2007.
36. G. A. Eby and W. W. Halcomb, Ineffectiveness of zinc gluconate nasal spray and zinc orotate lozenges in common-cold treatment: A double-blind placebo-controlled clinical trial, *Alternative Therapies in Health and Medicine* 12 (2006): 34–48; B. Arroll, Non-antibiotic treatments for upper-respiratory tract infections (common cold), *Respiratory Medicine* 99 (2005): 1477–1484.
37. J. R. Prohaska, Role of copper transporters in copper homeostasis, *American Journal of Clinical Nutrition* 88 (2008): 826S–829S.
38. F. H. Nielsen, Is boron nutritionally relevant? *Nutrition Reviews* 66 (2008): 183–191.
39. M. S. Tallman, What is the role of arsenic in newly diagnosed APL? *Best Practice and Research Clinical Haematology* 21 (2008): 659–666.
40. Committee on Environmental Health, Lead exposure in children: Prevention, detection, and management, *Pediatrics* 116 (2005): 1036–1046; Blood lead levels: United States, 1999–2002, *Morbidity and Mortality Weekly Report* 54 (2005): 513–527.

HIGHLIGHT 14

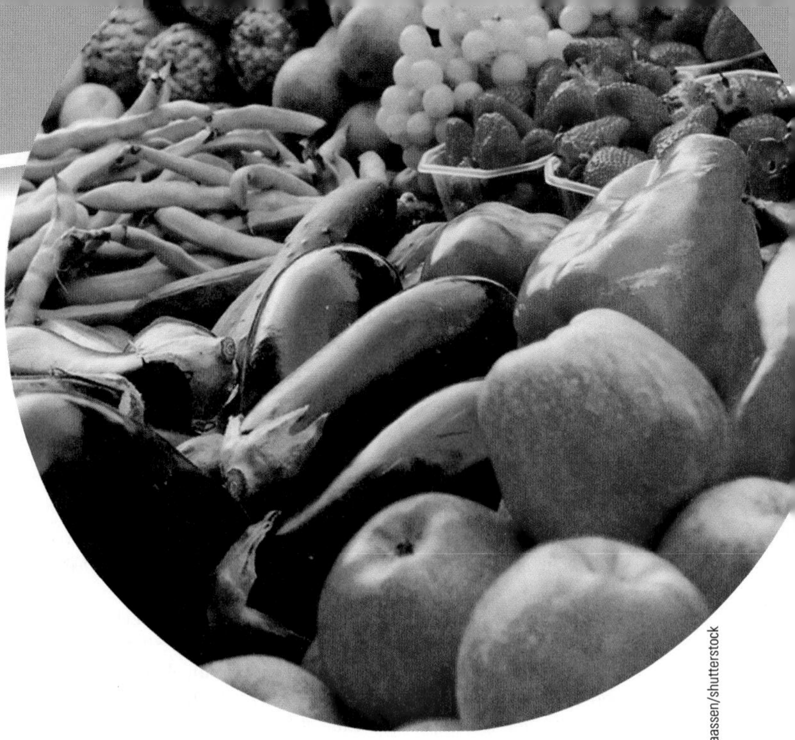
Regien Paassen/shutterstock

Phytochemicals and Functional Foods

This chapter completes the introductory discussions on the six classes of nutrients—carbohydrates, lipids, proteins, vitamins, minerals, and water. In addition to these nutrients, foods contain thousands of nonnutrient compounds, including the **phytochemicals.** Chapter 1 introduces the phytochemicals as compounds found in plant-derived foods (*phyto* means plant) that have biological activity in the body. Research on phytochemicals is unfolding daily, adding to our knowledge of their roles in human health, but there are still many questions and only tentative answers. Just a few of the tens of thousands of phytochemicals have been researched at all, and only a sampling are mentioned in this highlight—enough to illustrate their wide variety of food sources and roles in supporting health.

The concept that foods provide health benefits beyond those of the nutrients emerged from numerous epidemiological studies showing the protective effects of plant-based diets on cancer and heart disease. People have been using foods to maintain health and prevent disease for years, but now these foods have been given a name—they are called **functional foods.**[1] (The accompanying glossary defines this and other terms.) As Chapter 1 explains, functional foods include all foods (whole, fortified, or modified foods) that have a potentially beneficial effect on health.[2] Much of this text touts the benefits of nature's functional foods—whole grains rich in dietary fibres, oily fish rich in omega-3 fatty acids, and fresh fruits rich in phytochemicals, for example. This highlight begins with a look at some of these familiar functional foods, the phytochemicals they contain, and their roles in disease prevention. Then the discussion turns to examine the most controversial of functional foods—novel foods to which phytochemicals have been added to promote health. How these foods fit into a healthy diet is still unclear.

The Phytochemicals

In foods, phytochemicals impart tastes, aromas, colours, and other characteristics. They give hot peppers their burning sensation, garlic its pungent flavour, and tomatoes their dark red colour. In the body, phytochemicals can have profound physiological effects—acting as antioxidants, mimicking hormones, stimulating enzymes, interfering with DNA replication, destroying bacteria, and binding physically to cell walls. Any of these actions may suppress the development of diseases. They might also have adverse effects when consumed in excess.[3] Table H14-1 (p. 461) presents the names, possible effects, and food sources of some of the better-known phytochemicals.

Defending against Cancer

A variety of phytochemicals from a variety of foods appear to protect against DNA damage and defend the body against cancer. A few examples follow.

Soybeans and products made from them correlate with low rates of breast and prostate cancers.[4] Soybeans—as well as other legumes, **flaxseeds,** whole grains, vegetables, and fruits—are a

GLOSSARY

flavonoids (FLAY-von-oyds): yellow pigments in foods; phytochemicals that may exert physiological effects on the body.

flaxseeds: the small brown seeds of the flax plant; valued as a source of linseed oil, fibre, and omega-3 fatty acids.

functional foods: foods that contain physiologically active compounds that provide health benefits beyond basic nutrition.

lignans: phytochemicals present in flaxseed, but not in flax oil, that are converted to phytosterols by intestinal bacteria and are under study as possible anticancer agents.

lutein (LOO-teen): a plant pigment of yellow hue; a phytochemical believed to play roles in eye functioning and health.

lycopene (LYE-koh-peen): a pigment responsible for the red colour of tomatoes and other red-hued vegetables; a phytochemical that may act as an antioxidant in the body.

phytochemicals: nonnutrient compounds found in plant-derived foods that have biological activity in the body.

phytoestrogens: plant-derived compounds that have structural and functional similarities to human estrogen. Phytoestrogens include the isoflavones genistein, daidzein, and glycitein.

phytosterols: plant-derived compounds that have structural similarities to cholesterol and lower blood cholesterol by competing with cholesterol for absorption. Phytosterols include sterol esters and stanol esters.

TABLE H14-1 Phytochemicals—Their Food Sources and Actions

Name	Possible Effects	Food Sources
Alkylresorcinols (phenolic lipids)	May contribute to the protective effect of grains in reducing the risks of diabetes, heart disease, and some cancers	Whole-grain wheat and rye
Allicin (organosulphur compound)	Antimicrobial that may reduce ulcers; may lower blood cholesterol	Chives, garlic, leeks, onions
Capsaicin	Modulates blood clotting, possibly reducing the risk of fatal clots in heart and artery disease	Hot peppers
Carotenoids (include beta-carotene, lycopene, lutein, and hundreds of related compounds)	Act as antioxidants, possibly reducing risks of cancer and other diseases	Deeply pigmented vegetables and fruit (apricots, broccoli, cantaloupe, carrots, pumpkin, spinach, sweet potatoes, tomatoes)
Curcumin	Acts as an antioxidant and anti-inflammatory agent; may reduce blood clot formation; may inhibit enzymes that activate carcinogens	Turmeric, a yellow-coloured spice
Flavonoids (include flavones, flavonols, isoflavones, catechins, and others)	Act as antioxidants; scavenge carcinogens; bind to nitrates in the stomach, preventing conversion to nitrosamines; inhibit cell proliferation	Berries, black tea, celery, citrus fruits, green tea, olives, onions, oregano, purple grapes, purple grape juice, soybeans and soy products, vegetables, whole wheat, wine
Genistein and daidzein (isoflavones)	Phytoestrogens that inhibit cell replication in GI tract; may reduce risk of breast, colon, ovarian, prostate, and other estrogen-sensitive cancers; may reduce cancer cell survival; may reduce risk of osteoporosis	Soybeans, soy flour, soy-based beverages, tofu, textured vegetable protein, other legume products
Indoles (organosulphur compound)	May trigger production of enzymes that block DNA damage from carcinogens; may inhibit estrogen action	Cruciferous vegetables such as broccoli, Brussels sprouts, cabbage, cauliflower; horseradish, mustard greens, kale
Isothiocyanates (organosulphur compounds that include sulphoraphane)	Act as antioxidants; inhibit enzymes that activate carcinogens; activate enzymes that detoxify carcinogens; may reduce risk of breast cancer, prostate cancer	Cruciferous vegetables such as broccoli, Brussels sprouts, cabbage, cauliflower; horseradish, mustard greens, kale
Lignans	Phytoestrogens that block estrogen activity in cells possibly reducing the risk of cancer of the breast, colon, ovaries, and prostate	Flaxseed and its oil, whole grains
Monoterpenes (including limonene)	May trigger enzyme production to detoxify carcinogens; inhibit cancer promotion and cell proliferation	Citrus fruit peels and oils
Phenolic acids	May trigger enzyme production to make carcinogens water soluble, facilitating excretion	Coffee beans, fruits (apples, blueberries, cherries, grapes, oranges, pears, prunes), oats, potatoes, soybeans
Phytic acid	Binds to minerals, preventing free-radical formation, possibly reducing cancer risk	Whole grains
Resveratrol	Acts as antioxidant; may inhibit cancer growth; reduce inflammation, LDL oxidation, and blood clot formation	Red wine, peanuts, grapes, raspberries
Saponins (glucosides)	May interfere with DNA replication, preventing cancer cells from multiplying; stimulate immune response	Alfalfa sprouts, other sprouts, green vegetables, potatoes, tomatoes
Tannins	Act as antioxidants; may inhibit carcinogen activation and cancer promotion	Black-eyed peas, grapes, lentils, red and white wine, tea

rich source of an array of phytochemicals, among them the **phytoestrogens.** Because the chemical structure of these phytochemicals is similar to the steroid hormone estrogen, they can weakly mimic or modulate the effects of estrogen in the body. They also have antioxidant activity that appears to slow the growth of some cancers.[5] However, the use of phytoestrogen supplements is ill-advised as they may stimulate the growth of estrogen-dependent cancers (such as breast cancer).[6] Soy foods may be most effective when consumed in moderation throughout life. The role of soy foods for breast cancer survivors is less certain. The Canadian Cancer Society recommends breast cancer survivors should consult with their health-care team about eating soy-based foods. Until more research is done to determine the role of soy in breast cancer, it is prudent for breast cancer survivors to avoid high doses of soy and soy isoflavones.[7]

Limited evidence suggests that tomatoes may offer protection against some cancers.[8] Among the phytochemicals thought to be responsible for this effect is **lycopene,** one of beta-carotene's many carotenoid relatives.[9] Lycopene is the pigment that gives apricots, guava, papaya, pink grapefruits, and watermelon their red colour—and it is especially abundant in tomatoes and cooked tomato products. Lycopene is a powerful antioxidant that seems to inhibit the growth of cancer cells.[10] Importantly, the benefits of lycopene are not consistently evident.[11] When benefits have been seen, it has been from people having eaten *foods* containing lycopene.[12]

Soybeans and tomatoes are only two of the many foods credited with providing anticancer activity. Strong and convincing evidence shows that the risk of many cancers, and perhaps of cancer in general, decreases when diets include an abundance of vegetables and fruits.[13] To that end, current recommendations urge consumers to eat seven to ten servings of vegetables and fruits a day.

Defending against Heart Disease

Diets based primarily on unprocessed foods appear to support heart health better than those founded on highly refined foods—perhaps because of the abundance of nutrients, fibres, or phytochemicals such as the **flavonoids.** Flavonoids, a large group of phytochemicals known for their health-promoting qualities, are found in whole grains, legumes, soy, vegetables, fruits, herbs, spices, teas, chocolate, nuts, olive oil, and red wines. Flavonoids are powerful antioxidants that may help to protect LDL cholesterol against oxidation, minimize inflammation, and reduce blood platelet stickiness, thereby slowing the progression of atherosclerosis and making blood clots less likely.[14] Whereas an abundance of flavonoid-containing *foods* in the diet may lower the risks of chronic diseases, no claims can be made for flavonoids themselves as the protective factor, particularly when they are extracted from foods and sold as supplements. In fact, some research suggests that the antioxidant activity of flavonoid-rich foods is *not* because of the flavonoids themselves.[15]

In addition to flavonoids, fruits and vegetables are rich in carotenoids such as beta-carotene and **lutein.** Studies suggest that a diet rich in carotenoids is also associated with a lower risk of heart disease.[16]

The **phytosterols** of soybeans and the **lignans** of flaxseed may also protect against heart disease.[17] These cholesterol-like molecules are naturally found in all plants and inhibit cholesterol absorption in the body.[18] As a result, LDL cholesterol in the blood declines and HDL blood cholesterol remains relatively stable.[19] These phytochemicals also seem to protect against heart disease by reducing inflammation and lowering blood pressure.[20]

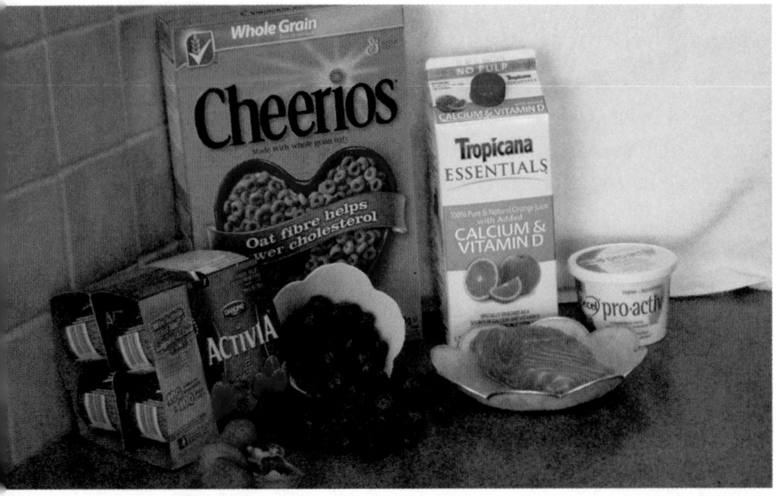
Whole Grain
Cheerios
Oat fibre helps
wer cholesterol
NO PULP
Tropicana
ESSENTIALS
CALCIUM &
VITAMIN D
pro·activ
ACTIVIA

© Craig M. Moore

Nature offers a variety of functional foods that provide us with many health benefits.

In 2010, Health Canada approved the addition of plant sterols to spreads, mayonnaise, margarines, salad dressings, yogurts, and vegetable and fruit juices. Health claims are permitted on labels of functional foods with added phytosterols. A primary statement of "[Serving size from Nutrition Facts table in metric and common household measures] of [the product's name] provides X% of the daily amount* of plant sterols shown to help reduce/lower cholesterol in adults." may be accompanied by a secondary statement: "Plant sterols help reduce [or help lower] cholesterol." The daily amount for adults is 2 grams per day.[21] Following a recent safety assessment, Health Canada advises plant sterols up to 3 grams a day for adults and 1 gram a day for children pose no health threat. Caution should be taken against consuming higher levels through foods or supplements. When plant sterols are added to food products intended for normal consumption as part of a healthy diet, they are considered foods. When added to the diet in supplemental form, they are considered natural health products.

The Phytochemicals in Perspective

Because foods deliver thousands of phytochemicals in addition to dozens of nutrients, researchers must be careful in giving credit for particular health benefits to any one compound. Diets rich in whole grains, legumes, vegetables, fruits, and nuts seem to protect against heart disease and cancer, but identifying *the* specific foods or components of foods that are responsible is difficult. Each food possesses a unique array of phytochemicals—citrus fruits provide monoterpenes; grapes, resveratrol; and flaxseed, lignans. (Review Table H14-1 for the possible effects and other food sources of these phytochemicals.) Broccoli may contain as many as 10 000 different phytochemicals—each with the potential to influence some action in the body. Beverages such as wine, spices such as oregano, and oils such as olive oil (especially virgin olive oil) contain many phytochemicals that may explain, in part, why people who live in the Mediterranean region have reduced risks of heart disease and cancer.[22] Phytochemicals might also explain why the DASH diet is so effective in lowering blood pressure and blood lipids. Even identifying all of the phytochemicals and their effects doesn't answer all the questions because the actions of phytochemicals may be complementary or overlapping—which reinforces the principle of variety in diet planning. For an appreciation of the array of phytochemicals offered by a variety of foods, see Figure H14-1 (p. 463).

Functional Foods

Because foods naturally contain thousands of phytochemicals that are biologically active in the body, virtually all of them have some special value in supporting health. In other words, even simple, whole foods, in reality, are functional foods. Cranberries may

*This mycoprotein product is marketed in the United States under the trade name Quorn (pronounced KWORN). It is not available in Canada.

help prevent urinary tract infections; garlic may lower blood cholesterol; and green tea may inhibit ulcer infections, just to name a few examples.[23] But that hasn't stopped food manufacturers from trying to create functional foods as well. The creation of more functional foods has become the fastest-growing trend and the greatest influence transforming the global food supply.[24]

Many processed foods become functional foods when they are fortified with nutrients or enhanced with phytochemicals or herbs (calcium-fortified orange juice, for example). Less frequently, an entirely new food is created, as in the case of a meat substitute made of mycoprotein—a protein derived from a fungus.* This functional food not only provides dietary fibre, polyunsaturated fats, and high-quality protein, but it lowers LDL cholesterol, raises HDL cholesterol, improves glucose response, and prolongs satiety after a meal. Such a novel functional food raises the question—is it a food or a drug?

Foods as Pharmacy

Not too long ago, most of us could agree on what was a food and what was a drug. Today, functional foods blur the distinctions.[25] They have characteristics similar to both foods and drugs, but do not fit neatly into either category. Consider margarine, for example.

Eating nonhydrogenated margarine sparingly instead of butter generously may lower blood cholesterol slightly over several months and clearly falls into the food category. Taking a statin drug, on the other hand, lowers blood cholesterol significantly within weeks and

FIGURE H14-1 **An Array of Phytochemicals in a Variety of Fruits and Vegetables**

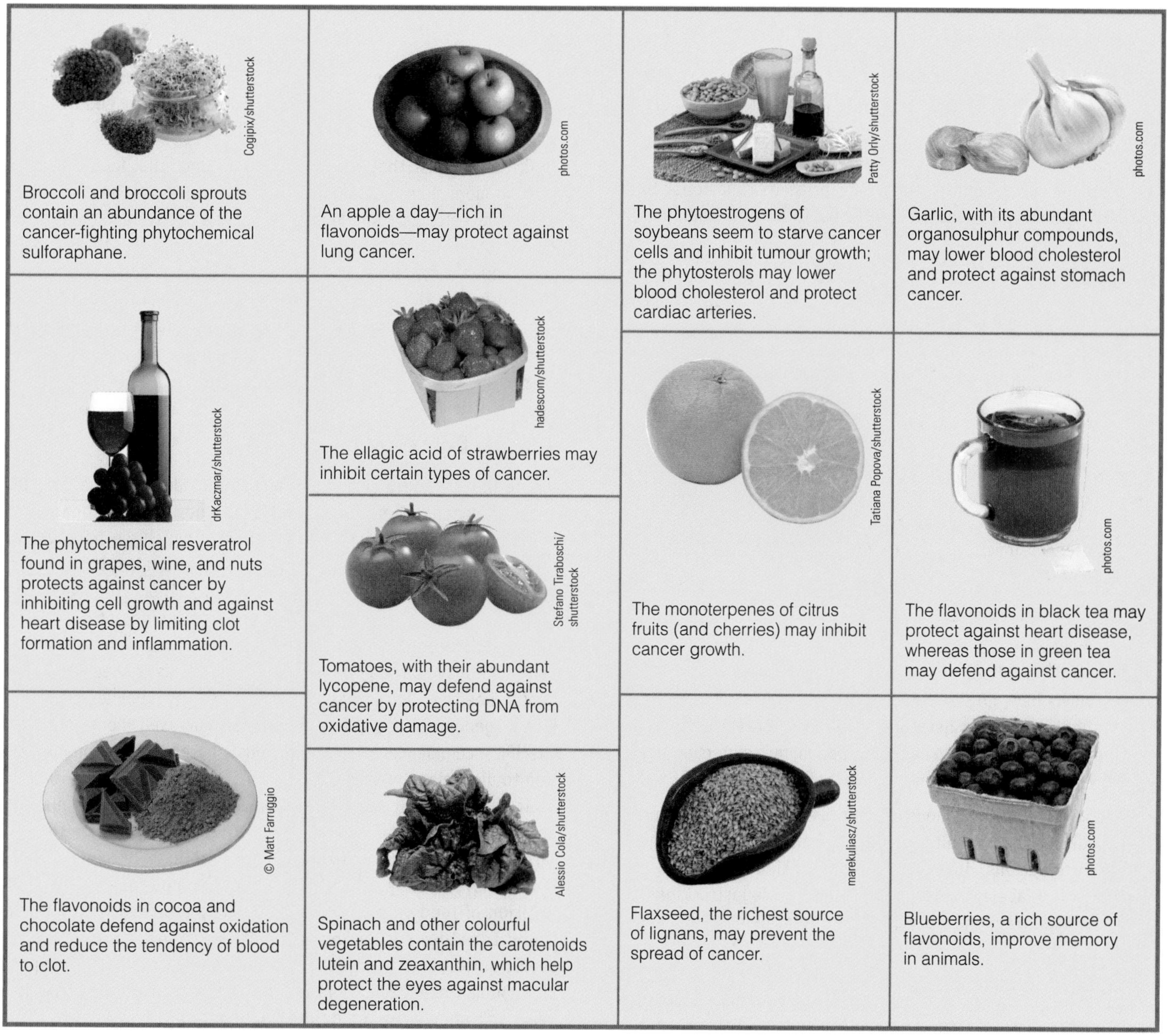
Cogipix/shutterstock
photos.com
Patty Orly/shutterstock
photos.com
drKaczmar/shutterstock
hadescom/shutterstock
Tatiana Popova/shutterstock
photos.com
Stefano Tiraboschi/shutterstock
© Matt Farruggio
Alessio Cola/shutterstock
marekuliasz/shutterstock
photos.com

Broccoli and broccoli sprouts contain an abundance of the cancer-fighting phytochemical sulforaphane.

An apple a day—rich in flavonoids—may protect against lung cancer.

The phytoestrogens of soybeans seem to starve cancer cells and inhibit tumour growth; the phytosterols may lower blood cholesterol and protect cardiac arteries.

Garlic, with its abundant organosulphur compounds, may lower blood cholesterol and protect against stomach cancer.

The phytochemical resveratrol found in grapes, wine, and nuts protects against cancer by inhibiting cell growth and against heart disease by limiting clot formation and inflammation.

The ellagic acid of strawberries may inhibit certain types of cancer.

The monoterpenes of citrus fruits (and cherries) may inhibit cancer growth.

The flavonoids in black tea may protect against heart disease, whereas those in green tea may defend against cancer.

Tomatoes, with their abundant lycopene, may defend against cancer by protecting DNA from oxidative damage.

The flavonoids in cocoa and chocolate defend against oxidation and reduce the tendency of blood to clot.

Spinach and other colourful vegetables contain the carotenoids lutein and zeaxanthin, which help protect the eyes against macular degeneration.

Flaxseed, the richest source of lignans, may prevent the spread of cancer.

Blueberries, a rich source of flavonoids, improve memory in animals.

clearly falls into the drug category. But margarine enhanced with a phytosterol that lowers blood cholesterol is in a grey area between the two. The margarine looks and tastes like a food, but it acts like a drug.

The use of functional foods as drugs creates a whole new set of diet-planning challenges. Not only must foods provide an adequate intake of all the nutrients to support good health, but they must also deliver drug-like ingredients to protect against disease. Like drugs used to treat chronic diseases, functional foods may need to be eaten several times a day for several months or years to have a beneficial effect. Sporadic users may be disappointed in the results. Margarine enriched with 2 to 3 grams of phytosterols may reduce cholesterol by up to 15 percent, much more than regular margarine does, but not nearly as much as the more than 30 percent reduction seen with cholesterol-lowering drugs.[26] For this reason, functional foods may be more useful for prevention and mild cases of disease than for intervention and more severe cases.

Foods and drugs differ dramatically in cost as well. Functional foods such as vegetables and fruits incur no added costs, of course, but foods that have been manufactured with added phytochemicals can be expensive, costing up to six times as much as their conventional counterparts. The price of functional foods typically falls between that of traditional foods and medicines.

Unanswered Questions

To achieve a desired health effect, which is the better choice: to eat a food designed to affect some body function or simply to adjust the diet? Does it make more sense to use a margarine enhanced with a phytosterol that lowers blood cholesterol or simply to limit the amount of butter eaten?* Is it smarter to eat eggs enriched with omega-3 fatty acids or to restrict egg consumption? Might functional foods offer a sensible solution for improving our nation's health—if done correctly? Perhaps so, but research determining the safety and effectiveness of these substances is still in progress. Until this work is complete, consumers may be asking the following questions:

- *Does it work?* Research is generally lacking and findings are often inconclusive.
- *How much does it contain?* Food labels are not required to list the quantities of added phytochemicals. Even if they were, consumers have no standard for comparison and cannot deduce whether the amounts listed are a little or a lot. Most importantly, until research is complete, food manufacturers do not know what amounts (if any) are most effective—or most toxic.
- *Is it safe?* Functional foods can act like drugs. They contain ingredients that can alter body functions and cause allergies, drug interactions, drowsiness, and other side effects. Yet, unlike drug labels, food labels do not provide instructions for the dosage, frequency, or duration of treatment.

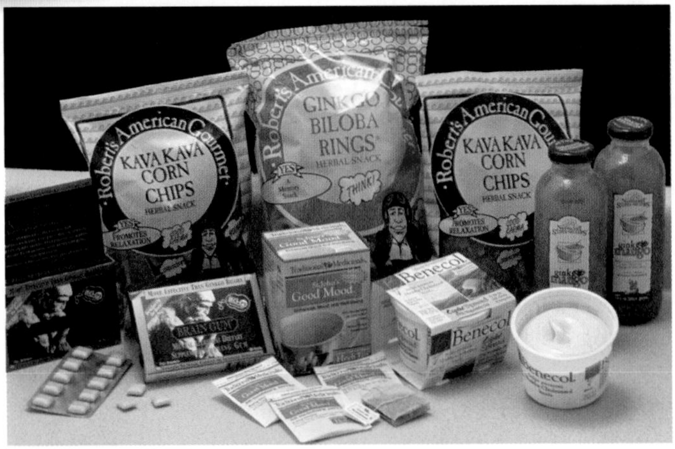
Robert's American Gourmet
KAVA KAVA CORN CHIPS
GINKGO BILOBA RINGS
Benecol
© Craig M. Moore

Functional foods currently on the market promise to "enhance mood," "promote relaxation and good karma," "increase alertness," and "improve memory," among other claims.

- *Is it healthy?* Adding phytochemicals to a food does not magically make it a healthy choice. A chocolate bar may be fortified with phytochemicals, but it is still made mostly of sugar and fat.

Critics suggest that the designation "functional foods" may be nothing more than a marketing tool. After all, even the most experienced researchers cannot yet identify the perfect combination of nutrients and phytochemicals to support optimal health. Yet manufacturers are freely experimenting with various concoctions as if they possessed that knowledge. Is it okay for them to sprinkle phytochemicals on fried snack foods or caramel candies and label them "functional," thus implying health benefits?

Future Foods

Nature has elegantly designed foods to provide us with a complex array of dozens of nutrients and thousands of additional compounds that may benefit health—most of which we have yet to identify or understand. Over the years, we have taken those foods, deconstructed them, and then reconstructed them in an effort to "improve" them. With new scientific understandings of how nutrients—and the myriad other compounds in foods—interact with genes, we may someday be able to design foods to meet the *exact* health needs of *each* individual. Indeed, our knowledge of the human genome and of human nutrition may well merge to allow specific recommendations for individuals based on their predisposition to diet-related diseases.

If the present trend continues, someday physicians may be able to prescribe the perfect foods to enhance your health, and farmers will be able to grow them. As Highlight 20 explains, scientists have already developed gene technology to alter the composition of food crops. They can grow rice enriched with vitamin A and tomatoes containing a hepatitis vaccine, for example. It seems quite likely that foods can be created to meet every possible human need. But then, in a sense, that was largely true 100 years ago when we relied on the bounty of nature.

*Margarine products that lower blood cholesterol contain either sterol esters from vegetable oils, soybeans, and corn or stanol esters from wood pulp.

Nutrition on the Net

CENGAGENOW™
For furthur study of topics covered in this Highlight, log on to **www.cengage.com/sso.**

- Search for "functional foods" at the International Food Information Council: **www.foodinsight.org**
- Read more about health claims for functional foods from Health Canada: **www.hc-sc.gc.ca/fn-an/label-etiquet/claims-reclam/nutra-funct_foods-nutra-fonct_aliment-eng.php**
- Find out if a "food recall alert" has been issued at the Canadian Food Inspection Agency's website: **www.inspection.gc.ca**

References

1. W. A. Walker and coauthors, Functional foods for health promotion: Microbes and health extended abstracts from the 11th Annual Conference on Functional Foods for Health Promotion, April 2008, *Nutrition Reviews* 67 (2009): 40–48.
2. Position of the American Dietetic Association: Functional foods, *Journal of the American Dietetic Association* 104 (2004): 814–826.
3. J. D. Lambert, S. Sang, and C. S. Yang, Possible controversy over dietary polyphenols: Benefits vs risks, *Chemical Research in Toxicology* 20 (2007): 583–585.
4. E. Cheung and coauthors, Diet and prostate cancer risk reduction, *Expert Review of Anticancer Therapy* 8 (2008): 43–50; E. Linos, and W. C. Willett, Diet and breast cancer risk reduction, *Journal of the National Comprehensive Cancer Network* 5 (2007): 711–718; M. B. Schabath and coauthors, Dietary phytoestrogens and lung cancer risk, *Journal of the American Medical Association* 294 (2005): 1493–1504.
5. T. A. Ryan-Borchers and coauthors, Soy isoflavones modulate immune function in healthy postmenopausal women, *American Journal of Clinical Nutrition* 83 (2006): 1118–1125.
6. M. Messina, W. McCaskill-Stevens, and J. W. Lampe, Addressing the soy and breast cancer relationship: Review, commentary, and workshop proceedings, *Journal of the National Cancer Institute* 98 (2006): 1275–1284.
7. Canadian Cancer Society, Nutrition concerns when you have breast cancer: Phytoestrogens. www.cancer.ca, accessed December 2010; G. Maskarinec, Soy foods for breast cancer survivors and women at high risk for breast cancer? *Journal of the American Dietetic Association* 105 (2005): 1524–1528.
8. C. J. Kavanaugh, P. R. Trumbo, and K. C. Ellwood, The U.S. Food and Drug Administration's evidence-based review for qualified health claims: Tomatoes, lycopene, and cancer, *Journal of the National Cancer Institute* 99 (2007): 1074–1085.
9. J. R. Mein, F. Lian, and X. Wang, Biological activity of lycopene metabolites: Implications for cancer prevention, *Nutrition Reviews* 66 (2008): 667–683; A. Vrieling and coauthors, Lycopene supplementation elevates circulating insulin-like growth factor-binding protein-1 and -2 concentrations in persons at greater risk of colorectal cancer, *American Journal of Clinical Nutrition* 86 (2007): 1456–1462.
10. N. Khan, F. Afaq, and H. Mukhtar, Cancer chemoprevention through dietary antioxidants: Progress and promise, *Antioxidants and Redox Signaling* 10 (2008): 475–510.
11. U. Peters and coauthors, Serum lycopene, other carotenoids, and prostate cancer risk: A nested case-control study in the Prostate, Lung, Colorectal, and Ovarian Cancer Screening Trial, *Cancer Epidemiology, Biomarkers, and Prevention* 16 (2007): 962–968.
12. S. Ellinger, J. Ellinger, and P. Stehle, Tomatoes, tomato products and lycopene in the prevention and treatment of prostate cancer: Do we have the evidence from intervention studies? *Current Opinion in Clinical Nutrition and Metabolic Care* 9 (2006): 722–727.
13. C. A. Gonzalez, Nutrition and cancer: The current epidemiological evidence, *British Journal of Nutrition* 96 (2006): S42–S45; H. Vainio and E. Weiderpass, Fruit and vegetables in cancer prevention, *Nutrition and Cancer* 54 (2006): 111–142.
14. R. di Giuseppe and coauthors, Regular consumption of dark chocolate is associated with low serum concentrations of C-reactive protein in a healthy Italian population, *Journal of Nutrition* 138 (2008): 1939–1945; I. Erlund and coauthors, Favorable effects of berry consumption on platelet function, blood pressure, and HDL cholesterol, *American Journal of Clinical Nutrition* 87 (2008): 323–331; L. Hooper and coauthors, Flavonoids, flavonoid-rich foods, and cardiovascular risk: A meta-analysis of randomized controlled trials, *American Journal of Clinical Nutrition* 88 (2008): 38–50; W. M. Loke and coauthors, Pure dietary flavonoids quercetin and (–)-epicatechin augment nitric oxide products and reduce endothelin-1 acutely in healthy men, *American Journal of Clinical Nutrition* 88 (2008): 1018–1025; S. Baba and coauthors, Continuous intake of polyphenolic compounds containing cocoa powder reduces LDL oxidative susceptibility and has beneficial effects on plasma HDL-cholesterol concentrations in humans, *American Journal of Clinical Nutrition* 85 (2007): 709–717; A. Basu and E. A. Lucas, Mechanisms and effects of green tea on cardiovascular health, *Nutrition Reviews* 65 (2007): 361–375; D. R. Jacobs, L. F. Andersen, and R. Blomhoff, Whole-grain consumption is associated with a reduced risk of noncardiovascular, noncancer death attributed to inflammatory diseases in the Iowa Women's Health Study, *American Journal of Clinical Nutrition* 85 (2007): 1606–1614; D. L. McKay and J. B. Blumberg, Cranberries *(Vaccinium macrocarpon)* and cardiovascular disease risk factors, *Nutrition Reviews* 65 (2007): 490–502; K. Taku and coauthors, Soy isoflavones lower serum total and LDL cholesterol in humans: A meta-analysis of 11 randomized controlled trials, *American Journal and Clinical Nutrition* 85 (2007): 1148–1156; S. S. Wijeratne, M. M. Abou-Zaid, and F. Shahidi, Antioxidant polyphenols in almond and its coproducts, *Journal of Agricultural and Food Chemistry* 54 (2006): 312–318.
15. S. B. Lotito and B. Frei, Consumption of flavonoid-rich foods and increased plasma antioxidant capacity in humans: Cause, consequence, or epiphenomenon? *Free Radical Biology and Medicine* 41 (2006): 1727–1746.
16. S. Voutilainen and coauthors, Carotenoids and cardiovascular health, *American Journal of Clinical Nutrition* 83 (2006): 1265–1271.
17. N. Lee, Phytoestrogens as bioactive ingredients in functional foods: Canadian regulatory update, *Journal of the AOAC International* 89 (2006): 1135–1137.
18. R. E. Ostlund, Jr., Phytosterols, cholesterol absorption and healthy diets, *Lipids* 42 (2007): 41–45.
19. B. Hansel and coauthors, Effect of low-fat, fermented milk enriched with plant sterols on serum lipid profile and oxidative stress in moderate hypercholesterolemia, *American Journal of Clinical Nutrition* 86 (2007): 790–796; L. H. Ellegård and coauthors, Dietary plant sterols and cholesterol metabolism, *Nutrition Reviews* 65 (2007): 39–45; V. W. Y. Lau, M. Journoud, and P. J. H. Jones, Plant sterols are efficacious in lowering plasma LDL and non-HDL cholesterol in hypercholesterolemic type 2 diabetic and nondiabetic persons, *American Journal of Clinical Nutrition* 81 (2005): 1351–1358; S. Zhan and S. C. Ho, Meta-analysis of the effects

of soy protein containing isoflavones on the lipid profile, *American Journal of Clinical Nutrition* 81 (2005): 397–408.
20. D. Fuchs and coauthors, Proteomic biomarkers of peripheral blood mononuclear cells obtained from postmenopausal women undergoing an intervention with soy isoflavones, *American Journal of Clinical Nutrition* 86 (2007): 1369–1375; S. Devaraj, B. C. Autret, and I. Jialal, Reduced-calorie orange juice beverage with plant sterols lowers C-reactive protein concentrations and improves the lipid profile in human volunteers, *American Journal of Clinical Nutrition* 84 (2006): 756–761.
21. Health Canada, Plant sterols and blood cholesterol lowering (2010). www.hc-sc.gc.ca/fn-an/label-etiquet/claims-reclam/assess-evalu/phytosterols-eng.php, accessed September 18, 2011.
22. D. M. Minich and J. S. Bland, Dietary management of the metabolic syndrome beyond macronutrients, *Nutrition Reviews* 66 (2008): 429–444; M. I. Covas and coauthors, The effect of polyphenols in olive oil on heart disease risk factors: A randomized trial, *Annals of Internal Medicine* 145 (2006): 333–341.
23. S. Y. Lee, Y. W. Shin, and K. B. Hahm, Phytoceuticals: Mighty but ignored weapons against *Helicobacter pylori* infection, *Journal of Digestive Diseases* 9 (2008): 129–139; Y. Liu and coauthors, Cranberry changes the physicochemical surface properties of *E. coli* and adhesion with uroepithelial cells, *Colloids and Surfaces. B, Biointerfaces* 65 (2008): 35–42; S. Gorinstein and coauthors, The atherosclerotic heart disease and protecting properties of garlic: Contemporary data, *Molecular Nutrition and Food Research* 51 (2007): 1365–1381; A. B. Howell, Bioactive compounds in cranberries and their role in prevention of urinary tract infections, *Molecular Nutrition and Food Research* 51 (2007): 732–737.
24. I. Siró and coauthors, Functional food. Product development, marketing and consumer acceptance—A review, *Appetite* 51 (2008): 456–467.
25. P. J. Jones and K. A. Varady, Are functional foods redefining nutritional requirements? *Applied Physiology, Nutrition, and Metabolism* 33 (2008): 118–123.
26. C. S. Patch, L. C. Tapsell, and P. G. Williams, Plant sterol/stanol prescription is an effective treatment strategy for managing hypercholesterolemia in outpatient clinical practice, *Journal of the American Dietetic Association* 105 (2005): 46–52.

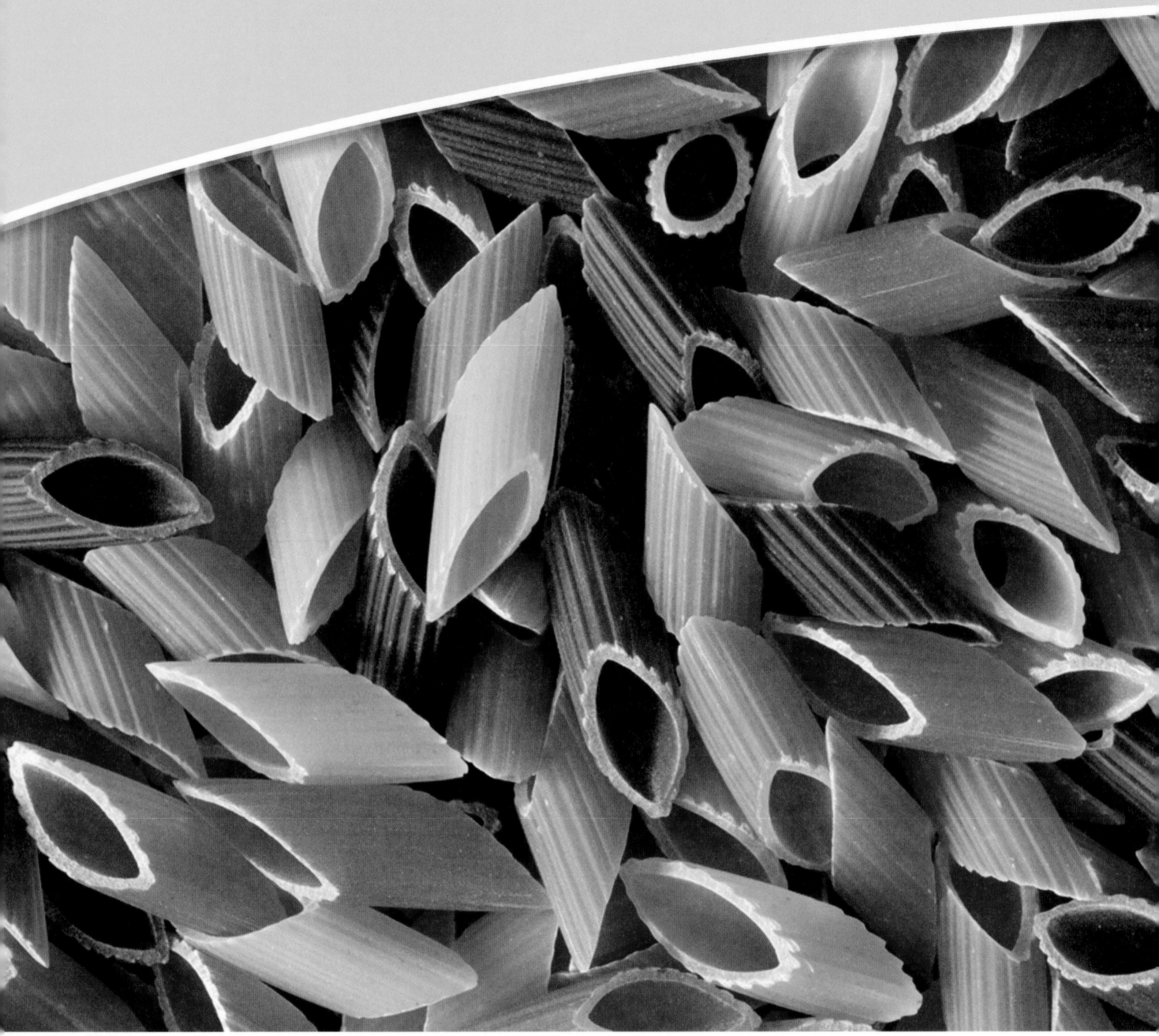

ajt/shutterstock

Nutrition in Your Life

CENGAGENOW™

Throughout this chapter, the CengageNOW logo indicates an opportunity for online self-study, linking you to interactive tutorials, activities, and videos to increase your understanding of chapter concepts.
www.cengage.com/sso

You choose to be physically active or inactive, and your choice can make a huge difference in how well you feel and how long you live. Today's world makes it easy to be inactive—too easy in fact—but the many health rewards of being physically active make it well worth the effort. You may even discover how much fun it is to be active, and with a little perseverance, you may become physically fit as well. As you become more active, you will find that the foods you eat can make a difference in how fast you run, how far you swim, or how much weight you lift. It's up to you. The choice is yours.

CHAPTER
15
Fitness: Physical Activity, Nutrients, and Body Adaptations

CHAPTER OUTLINE

Are you physically fit? If so, the following description applies to you. Your joints are flexible, your muscles are strong, and your body is lean with enough, but not too much, fat. You have the endurance to engage in daily physical activities with enough reserve energy to handle added challenges. Carrying heavy suitcases, opening a stuck window, or climbing four flights of stairs, which might strain an unfit person, is easy for you. What's more, you are prepared to meet mental and emotional challenges, too. All these characteristics of **fitness** describe the same wonderful condition of a healthy body.

Or perhaps you are leading a **sedentary** life. Today's world encourages inactivity, and people who go through life exerting minimal physical effort become weak and unfit and may begin to feel unwell. In fact, a sedentary lifestyle fosters the development of several chronic diseases.[1]

Regardless of your level of fitness, this chapter is written for "you," whoever you are and whatever your goals—whether you want to improve your health, lose weight, hone your athletic skills, ensure your position on a sports team, or simply adopt an active lifestyle. This chapter begins by discussing fitness and its benefits, and then goes on to explain how the body uses energy nutrients to fuel physical activity. Finally, it describes diets to support fitness.

Fitness

Fitness depends on a certain minimum amount of **physical activity** or **exercise**. Both physical activity and exercise involve body movement, muscle contraction, and enhanced energy expenditure, but a distinction is made between the two terms. Exercise is often considered to be vigorous, structured, and planned physical activity. This chapter focuses on how the active body uses energy nutrients—whether that body is pedalling a bike across campus or pedalling a stationary bike in a gym. Thus, for our purposes, the terms *physical activity* and *exercise* are used interchangeably.

fitness: the characteristics that enable the body to perform physical activity; more broadly, the ability to meet routine physical demands with enough reserve energy to rise to a physical challenge; or the body's ability to withstand stress of all kinds.

sedentary: physically inactive (literally, "sitting down a lot").

physical activity: bodily movement produced by muscle contractions that substantially increase energy expenditure.

exercise: planned, structured, and repetitive body movements that promote or maintain physical fitness.

♦ Each comparison influences the risks associated with chronic disease and death similarly:

- Vigorous exercise vs. minimal exercise
- Healthy weight vs. 20% overweight
- Nonsmoking vs. smoking (one pack a day)

Benefits of Fitness Extensive evidence confirms that regular physical activity promotes physical fitness, ♦ a factor that reduces the risk of developing a number of diseases and premature death.[2] Still, despite an increasing awareness of the health benefits that physical activity confers, data from the 2007/2008 Canadian Community Health Survey indicate about 25 percent of Canadian adults are moderately active, 23 percent are active, and over half of Canadians are inactive.[3] For some taking a pill to achieve the benefits of physical activity might be appealing. In fact, preliminary research on mice suggests that skeletal muscles respond to some drugs similarly to the way they do to exercise.[4] Regular physical activity, however, has beneficial effects far beyond those of muscles—many more than a pill can offer. Consider that physical inactivity is linked to the major degenerative diseases—heart disease, cancer, stroke, diabetes, and hypertension—the primary killers of adults in developed countries.[5] The *Canadian Physical Activity Guidelines* emphasize the importance of being physically active to promote health and reduce the risk of disease.[6]

Physical Activity Guidance for Canadians

All adults should avoid inactivity. Some physical activity is better than none, and adults who participate in any amount of physical activity gain some health benefits.

As a person becomes physically fit, the health of the entire body improves. In general, physically fit people enjoy:

- *Restful sleep.* Rest and sleep occur naturally after periods of physical activity. During rest, the body repairs injuries, disposes of wastes generated during activity, and builds new physical structures.
- *Nutritional health.* Physical activity expends energy and thus allows people to eat more food. If they choose wisely, active people will consume more nutrients and be less likely to develop nutrient deficiencies.
- *Optimal body composition.* A balanced program of physical activity limits body fat and increases or maintains lean tissue. Thus physically active people have relatively less body fat than sedentary people at the same body weight.[7]
- *Optimal bone density.* Weight-bearing physical activity builds bone strength and protects against osteoporosis.[8]
- *Resistance to colds and other infectious diseases.* Fitness enhances immunity.[*9]
- *Low risks of some types of cancers.* Lifelong physical activity may help to protect against colon cancer, breast cancer, and some other cancers.[10]
- *Strong circulation and lung function.* Physical activity that challenges the heart and lungs strengthens the circulatory system.
- *Low risk of cardiovascular disease.* Physical activity lowers blood pressure, slows resting pulse rate, and lowers blood cholesterol, thus reducing the risks of heart attacks and strokes.[11] Some research suggests that physical activity may reduce the risk of cardiovascular disease in another way as well—by reducing intra-abdominal fat stores.[12]
- *Low risk of type 2 diabetes.* Physical activity normalizes glucose tolerance.[13] Regular physical activity reduces the risk of developing type 2 diabetes and benefits those who already have the condition.
- *Reduced risk of gallbladder disease.* Regular physical activity reduces the risk of gallbladder disease—perhaps by facilitating weight control and lowering blood lipid levels.[14]
- *Low incidence and severity of anxiety and depression.* Physical activity may improve mood and enhance the quality of life by reducing depression and anxiety.[15]
- *Strong self-image.* The sense of achievement that comes from meeting physical challenges promotes self-confidence.
- *Long life and high quality of life in the later years.* Active people live longer, healthier lives than sedentary people do.[16] Even a 3 kilometre walk daily

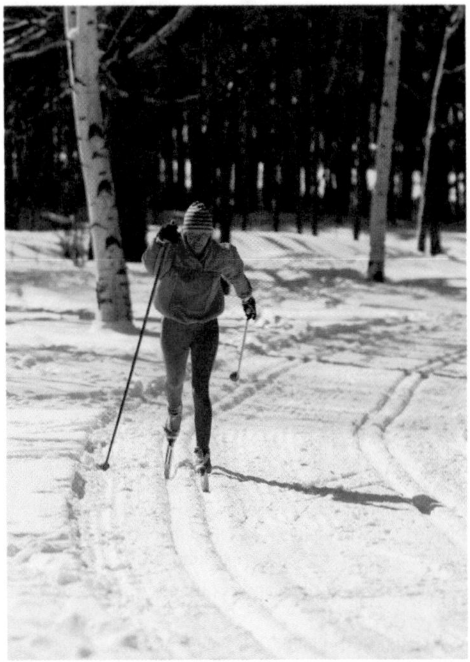

photos.com

Physical activity, or lack of it, exerts a significant and pervasive influence on everyone's nutrition and overall health.

*Moderate physical activity can stimulate immune function. Intense, vigorous, prolonged activity such as marathon running, however, may compromise immune function.

TABLE 15-1 Levels of Physical Activity Intensity Compared

Level of Intensity	Breathing and/or Heart Rate	Perceived Exertion (on a Scale of 0 to 10)	Talk Test	Energy Expenditure	Walking Pace
Light	Little to no increase	<5	Able to sing	<3.5 kcal/min	<5 km/h (<3 mph)
Moderate	Some increase	5 or 6	Able to have a conversation	3.5 to 7 kcal/min	5 to 7 km/h (3 to 4.5 mph)
Vigorous	Large increase	7 or 8	Conversation is difficult or "broken"	>7 kcal/min	>7 km/h (>4.5 mph)

SOURCE: Centers for Disease Control and Prevention, www.cdc.gov/physicalactivity/everyone; accessed August 21, 2010.

can add years to a person's life. In addition to extending longevity, physical activity supports independence and mobility in later life by reducing the risk of falls and minimizing the risk of injury should a fall occur.[17]

What does a person have to do to reap the health rewards of physical activity? The *Canadian Physical Activity Guidelines* recommend healthy adults accumulate at least 150 minutes of **aerobic physical activity** each week (**moderate-intensity physical activity** to **vigorous-intensity physical activity**), in bouts of 10 minutes or more, to achieve substantial health benefits. To gain greater health benefits, we should engage in more varied and intense physical activity over a longer duration and/or more frequently. Canadians are also encouraged to add muscle and bone strengthening activities at least two days a week (see Figure 15-1).[18] Table 15-1 compares intensity levels. The *Canadian Physical Activity Guidelines*, the Canadian

FIGURE 15-1 *Canadian Physical Activity Guidelines* for Adults

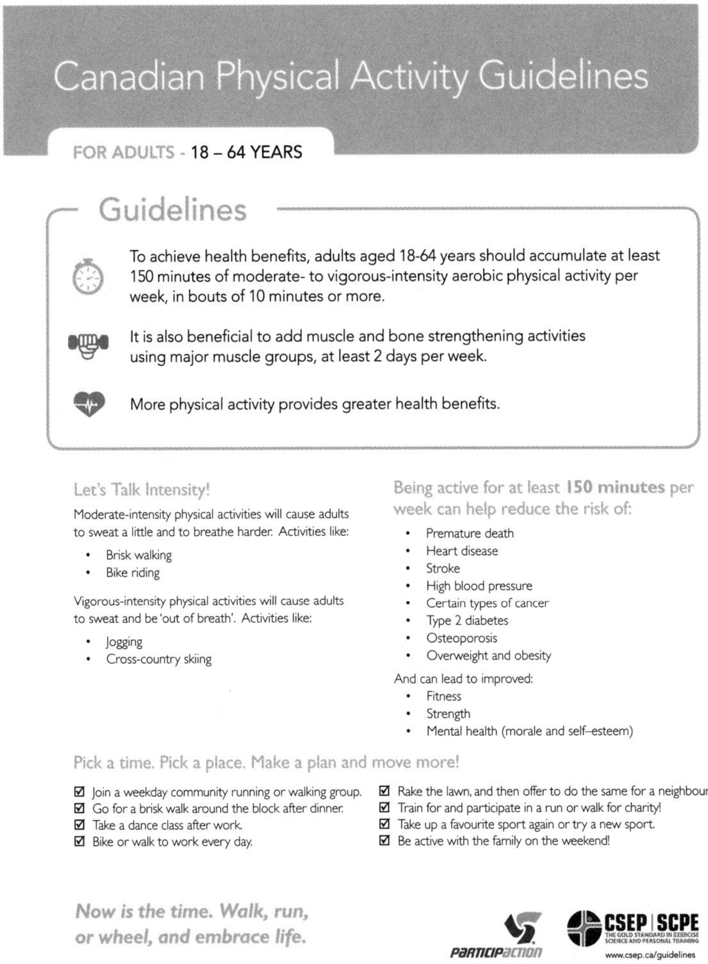
Canadian Physical Activity Guidelines
FOR ADULTS - 18 – 64 YEARS
Guidelines
To achieve health benefits, adults aged 18-64 years should accumulate at least 150 minutes of moderate- to vigorous-intensity aerobic physical activity per week, in bouts of 10 minutes or more.
It is also beneficial to add muscle and bone strengthening activities using major muscle groups, at least 2 days per week.
More physical activity provides greater health benefits.
Let's Talk Intensity!
Moderate-intensity physical activities will cause adults to sweat a little and to breathe harder. Activities like:
• Brisk walking
• Bike riding
Vigorous-intensity physical activities will cause adults to sweat and be 'out of breath'. Activities like:
• Jogging
• Cross-country skiing
Being active for at least 150 minutes per week can help reduce the risk of:
• Premature death
• Heart disease
• Stroke
• High blood pressure
• Certain types of cancer
• Type 2 diabetes
• Osteoporosis
• Overweight and obesity
And can lead to improved:
• Fitness
• Strength
• Mental health (morale and self-esteem)
Pick a time. Pick a place. Make a plan and move more!
☑ Join a weekday community running or walking group.
☑ Go for a brisk walk around the block after dinner.
☑ Take a dance class after work.
☑ Bike or walk to work every day.
☑ Rake the lawn, and then offer to do the same for a neighbour.
☑ Train for and participate in a run or walk for charity!
☑ Take up a favourite sport again or try a new sport.
☑ Be active with the family on the weekend!
Now is the time. Walk, run, or wheel, and embrace life.
PARTICIPACTION
CSEP | SCPE
www.csep.ca/guidelines

SOURCE: Canadian Physical Activity Guidelines, © 2011. Used with permission from the Canadian Society for Exercise Physiology, www.csep.ca/guidelines.

aerobic physical activity: activity in which the body's large muscles move in a rhythmic manner for a sustained period of time. Aerobic activity, also called *endurance activity,* improves cardiorespiratory fitness. Brisk walking, running, swimming, and bicycling are examples.

moderate-intensity physical activity: physical activity that requires some increase in breathing and/or heart rate and expends 3.5 to 7 kcalories per minute. Walking at a speed of 5 to 7 kilometres (3 to 4.5 miles) per hour (about 8 to 12 minutes to walk 1 kilometre is an example.

vigorous-intensity physical activity: physical activity that requires a large increase in breathing and/or heart rate and expends more than 7 kcalories per minute. Walking at a very brisk pace, >7 kilometres (4.5 miles) per hour, or running at a pace of at least 8 kilometres (5 miles) per hour are examples.

Society for Exercise Physiology, ParticipACTION, the Public Health Agency of Canada, and the DRI Committee, however, all advise that greater aerobic physical activity brings more extensive health benefits such as maintaining a healthy body weight (BMI of 18.5 to 24.9) and further reducing the risk of chronic diseases.

Physical Activity Guidance for Canadians

- For substantial health benefits, adults should do at least 150 minutes (2 hours and 30 minutes) a week of moderate- to vigorous-intensity aerobic physical activity. Aerobic activity should be performed in episodes of at least 10 minutes and should be spread throughout the week.
- For additional and more extensive health benefits, adults should increase their aerobic physical activity and strengthen their muscles and bones by engaging in resistance activities at least two days a week.

To develop and maintain *fitness*, the Public Health Agency of Canada, the Canadian Society for Exercise Physiology, and ParticipACTION recommend endurance and strengthening types of physical activities (see Table 15-2).[19] Following these guidelines will help adults improve their cardiorespiratory endurance, body composition, ♦ and strength. At this level of fitness, a person can reap still greater health benefits (substantially lower risk of premature death compared with those who are inactive, improved cardiorespiratory fitness, and improved body composition, for example).[20]

♦ **Body composition** refers to the proportions of muscle, bone, fat, and other tissue that make up a person's total body weight.

The bottom line is that any physical activity, even moderate activity, provides some health benefits, and these benefits follow a dose-response relationship. Therefore, some activity is better than none, and more activity is better still—up to a point. (Pursued in excess, intense physical activity, especially when combined with poor eating habits, can undermine health, as Highlight 8 on Eating Disorders explains.)

Developing Fitness To be physically fit, a person must develop enough flexibility, muscle strength and endurance, and cardiorespiratory endurance to

TABLE 15-2 Guidelines for Physical Fitness

	Cardiorespiratory Endurance	Resistance Training
	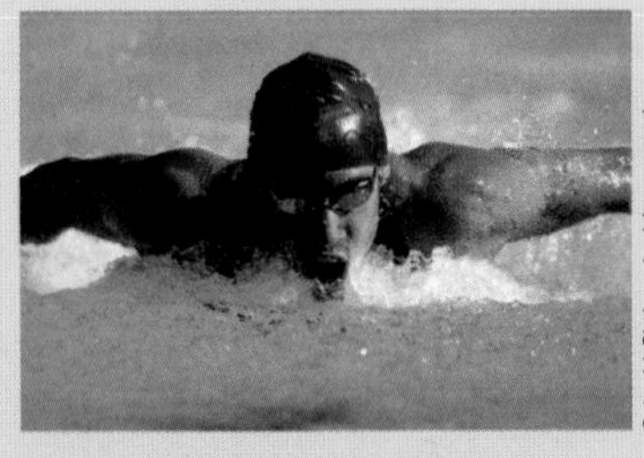 Schmid Christophe/shutterstock	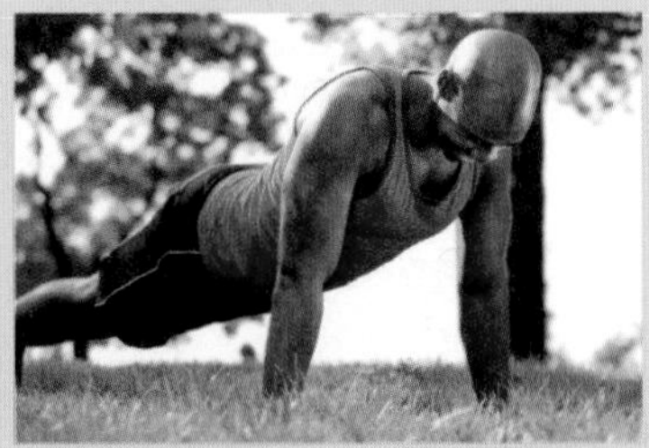 Tyler Olson/shutterstock
Type of Activity	Aerobic activity that uses large-muscle groups and can be maintained continuously	Resistance activity that is performed at a controlled speed and through a full range of motion
Frequency	At least 150 minutes per week	At least 2 days per week
Intensity	Moderate to vigorous[a]	Enough to enhance muscle strength and improve body composition
Duration	In bouts of at least 10 minutes	8 to 12 repetitions of 8 to 10 different exercises
Examples	Running, cycling, swimming, inline skating, rowing, power walking, cross-country skiing, kickboxing, jumping rope; sports activities such as basketball, soccer, racquetball, tennis, volleyball	Pull-ups, push-ups, weight lifting, pilates

[a]Moderate-intensity physical activities will cause adults to breathe harder and sweat more than usual such as walking at a brisk pace and riding a bike. During vigorous-intensity physical activity, adults will sweat and be "out of breath," such as when jogging or cross-country skiing.

SOURCE: Canadian Society for Exercise Physiology, *Canadian Physical Activity Guidelines*, www.csep.ca/guidelines, accessed September 12, 2011.

meet the everyday demands of life with some to spare and to achieve a reasonable body weight and body composition. **Flexibility** allows the joints to move freely, reducing the risk of injury. **Muscle strength** and **muscle endurance** enable muscles to work harder and longer without fatigue. **Cardiorespiratory endurance** supports the ongoing activity of the heart and lungs. Physical activity supports lean body tissues and reduces excess body fat. A person who practises a physical activity *adapts* by becoming better able to perform that activity after each session—with more flexibility, more strength, and more endurance.

The principles of **conditioning** apply to each component of fitness—flexibility, strength, and endurance. During conditioning, the body adapts microscopically to perform the work it is asked to do. The way to achieve conditioning is by **training**, primarily by applying the **progressive overload principle**—that is, by asking a little more of the body in each training session.

The Overload Principle You can apply the progressive overload principle in several different ways. You can perform the activity more often—that is, increase its **frequency.** You can perform it more strenuously—that is, increase its **intensity.** Or you can do it for longer time periods—that is, increase its **duration.** All three strategies, individually or in combination, work well. The rate of progression depends on individual characteristics such as fitness level, health status, age, and preference. If you enjoy your workout, do it more often. If you do not have much time, increase intensity. If you dislike hard work, take it easy, and do it for longer time periods. If you want continuous improvements, remember to overload progressively as you reach higher levels of fitness.

When increasing the frequency, intensity, or duration of a workout, however, exercise to a point that only *slightly* exceeds the comfortable capacity to work. It is better to progress slowly than to risk injury by overexertion.

The Body's Response to Physical Activity Fitness develops in response to demand and wanes when demand ceases. Muscles gain size and strength after being made to work repeatedly, a response called **hypertrophy.** Conversely, without activity, muscles diminish in size and lose strength, a response called **atrophy.**

Hypertrophy and atrophy are adaptive responses to the muscles' greater and lesser work demands, respectively. Thus cyclists often have strong, well-developed legs but less arm and chest strength; a tennis player may have one superbly strong arm, while the other is just average. A variety of physical activities produces the best overall fitness, and to this end, people need to work different muscle groups from day to day. This strategy provides a day or two of rest for different muscle groups, giving them time to replenish nutrients and to repair any minor damage incurred by the activity.

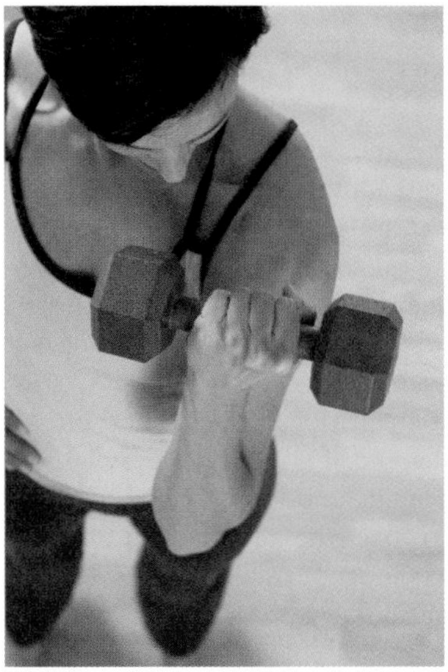

photos.com

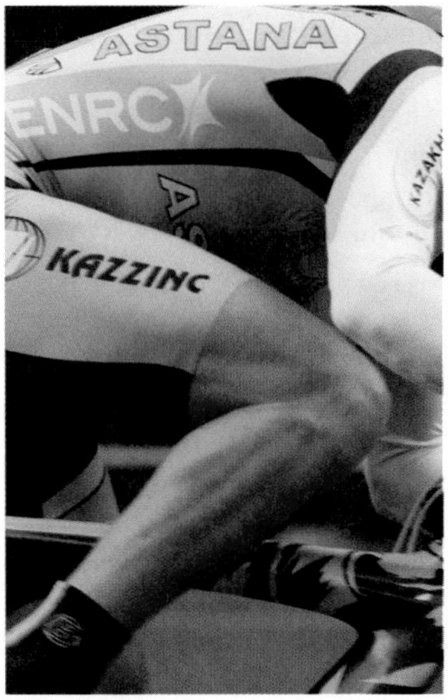
ASTANA
ENRC
KAZZINC

© Kanwarjit Singh Boparai/Alamy

People's bodies are shaped by the activities they perform.

flexibility: the capacity of the joints to move through a full range of motion; the ability to bend and recover without injury.

muscle strength: the ability of muscles to work against resistance.

muscle endurance: the ability of a muscle to contract repeatedly without becoming exhausted.

cardiorespiratory endurance: the ability to perform large-muscle, dynamic exercise of moderate to high intensity for prolonged periods.

conditioning: the physical effect of training; improved flexibility, strength, and endurance.

training: practising an activity regularly, which leads to conditioning. (Training is what you do; conditioning is what you get.)

progressive overload principle: the training principle that a body system, in order to improve, must be worked at frequencies, durations, or intensities that gradually increase physical demands.

frequency: the number of occurrences per unit of time (e.g., the number of activity sessions per week).

intensity: the degree of exertion while exercising (e.g., the amount of weight lifted or the speed of running).

duration: length of time (e.g., the time spent in each activity session).

hypertrophy (high-PER-tro-fee): growing larger; with regard to muscles, an increase in size (and strength) in response to use.

atrophy (AT-ro-fee): becoming smaller; with regard to muscles, a decrease in size (and strength) because of disuse, undernutrition, or wasting diseases.

Other tips for building fitness and minimizing the risk of overuse injuries are:

- Be active all week, not just on the weekends.
- Use proper equipment and attire.
- Perform exercises using proper form.
- Include **warm-up** and **cool-down** activities in each session. Warming up helps to prepare muscles, ligaments, and tendons for the upcoming activity and mobilizes fuels to support strength and endurance activities. Cooling down reduces muscle cramping and allows the heart rate to slow gradually.
- Train hard enough to challenge your strength or endurance a few times each week rather than every time you work out. Between challenges, do moderate workouts and include at least one day of rest each week.
- Pay attention to body signals. Symptoms such as abnormal heartbeat, dizziness, lightheadedness, cold sweat, confusion, or pain or pressure in the middle of the chest, teeth, jaw, neck, or arm demand immediate medical attention.
- Work out wisely. Do not start with activities so demanding that pain stops you within a day or two. Learn to enjoy small steps toward improvement. Fitness builds slowly.

Cautions on Starting a Fitness Program Before beginning a fitness program, make sure it is safe for you to do so. Most apparently healthy people can begin a moderate exercise program such as walking or increasing daily activities without a medical examination, but people with any of the risk factors listed in the margin ♦ may need medical advice. For healthy people who have been inactive, start by gradually increasing the duration, intensity, and frequency of activity in a stepwise progression to meet the guidelines.[21]

♦ Major coronary risk factors:
- Family history of heart disease
- Cigarette smoking
- Hypertension
- Serum cholesterol >200 mg/dL or HDL <40 mg/dL, or taking lipid-lowering medication
- Diabetes
- Sedentary lifestyle
- Obesity (BMI ≥30)

Cardiorespiratory Endurance

The length of time a person can remain active with an elevated heart rate—that is, the ability of the heart, lungs, and blood to sustain a given demand—defines a person's cardiorespiratory endurance. Cardiorespiratory endurance training improves a person's ability to sustain vigorous activities such as running, brisk walking, or swimming. Such training enhances the capacity of the heart, lungs, and blood to deliver oxygen to, and remove waste from, the body's cells. Cardiorespiratory endurance training, therefore, is *aerobic*. ♦ As the cardiorespiratory system gradually adapts to the demands of aerobic activity, the body delivers oxygen more efficiently. In fact, the accepted measure of a person's cardiorespiratory fitness is maximal oxygen uptake (**VO_2max**). The benefits of cardiorespiratory training are not just physical, though, because all of the body's cells, including the brain cells, require oxygen to function. When the cells receive more oxygen more readily, both the body and the mind benefit.

♦ Recall from Chapter 7 that **aerobic** means requiring oxygen.

Cardiorespiratory Conditioning **Cardiorespiratory conditioning** ♦ occurs as aerobic workouts improve heart and lung activities. **Cardiac output** increases, thus enhancing oxygen delivery. The heart becomes stronger, and each beat pumps more blood. Because the heart pumps more blood with each beat, fewer beats are necessary, and the resting heart rate slows down. The average resting pulse rate for adults is around 70 beats per minute, but people who achieve cardiorespiratory conditioning may have resting pulse rates of 50 or even lower. The muscles that work the lungs become stronger, too, so breathing becomes more efficient. Circulation through the arteries and veins improves. Blood moves easily, and blood pressure falls.[22]

♦ Cardiorespiratory conditioning:
- Increases cardiac output and oxygen delivery
- Increases blood volume per heartbeat (stroke volume)
- Slows resting pulse
- Increases breathing efficiency
- Improves circulation
- Reduces blood pressure

Cardiorespiratory endurance reflects the health of the heart and circulatory system, on which all other body systems depend. Figure 15-2 shows the major relationships among the heart, circulatory system, and lungs.

To improve your cardiorespiratory endurance, the activity you choose must be sustained for 20 minutes or longer and use most of the large-muscle groups of the body (legs, buttocks, and abdomen). You must also train at an intensity that elevates your heart rate.

warm-up: 5 to 10 minutes of light activity, such as easy jogging or cycling, prior to a workout to prepare the body for more vigorous activity.

cool-down: 5 to 10 minutes of light activity, such as walking or stretching, following a vigorous workout to gradually return the body's core to near-normal temperature.

VO_2max: the maximum rate of oxygen consumption by an individual at sea level.

cardiorespiratory conditioning: improvements in heart and lung function and increased blood volume, brought about by aerobic training.

cardiac output: the volume of blood discharged by the heart each minute; determined by multiplying the stroke volume by the heart rate. The stroke volume is the amount of oxygenated blood the heart ejects toward the tissues at each beat. Cardiac output (volume/minute) = stroke volume (volume/beat) × heart rate (beats/minute)

FIGURE 15-2 Delivery of Oxygen by the Heart and Lungs to the Muscles

The cardiorespiratory system responds to the muscles' demand for oxygen by building up its capacity to deliver oxygen. Researchers can measure cardiorespiratory fitness by measuring the maximum amount of oxygen a person consumes per minute while working out, a measure called VO_2max.

CENGAGENOW™ Animated! figure www.cengage.com/sso

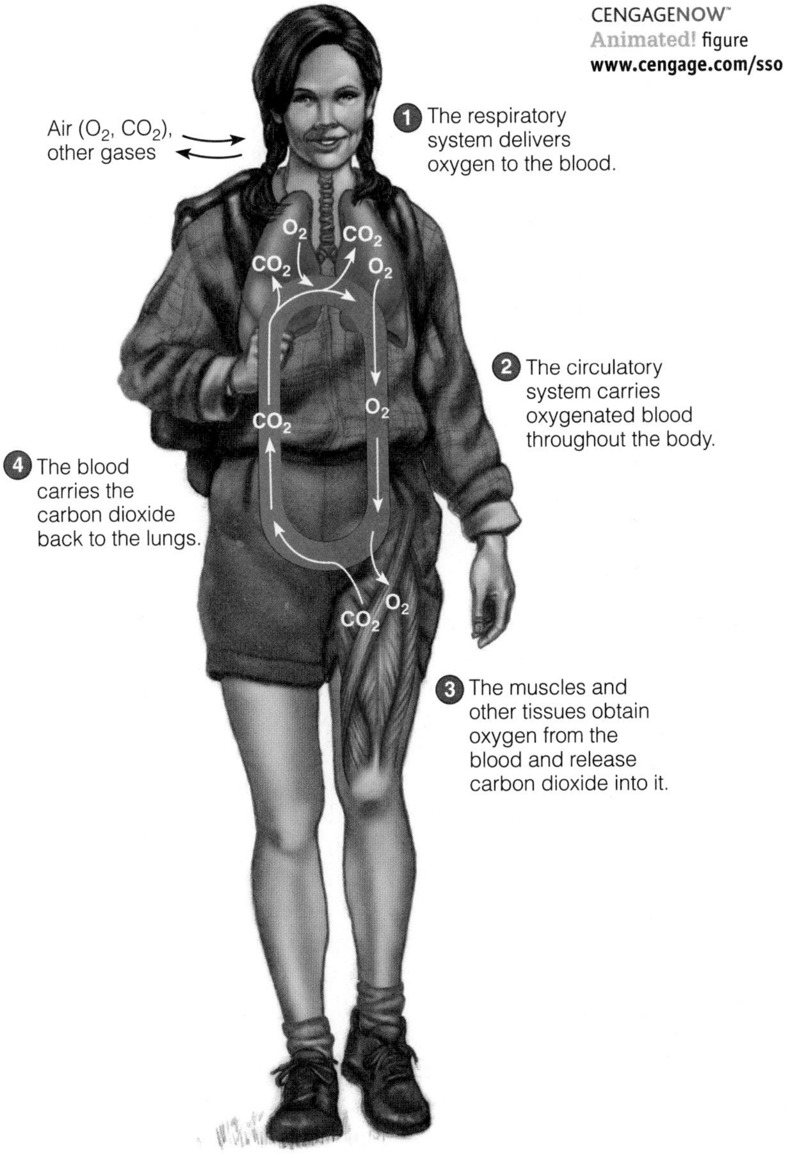
Air (O_2, CO_2), other gases
1 The respiratory system delivers oxygen to the blood.
O_2
CO_2
CO_2
O_2
2 The circulatory system carries oxygenated blood throughout the body.
CO_2
O_2
4 The blood carries the carbon dioxide back to the lungs.
CO_2
O_2
3 The muscles and other tissues obtain oxygen from the blood and release carbon dioxide into it.

A person's own perceived effort is usually a reliable indicator of the intensity of an activity. In general, when you're working out, do so at an intensity that raises your heart rate but still leaves you able to talk comfortably. If you are more competitive and want to work to your limit on some days, a treadmill test can reveal your maximum heart rate. You can work out safely at up to 90 percent of that rate.

Muscle Conditioning One of the benefits of cardiorespiratory training is that fit muscles use oxygen efficiently, reducing the heart's workload. An added bonus is that muscles that use oxygen efficiently can burn fat longer—a plus for body composition and weight control.

A Balanced Fitness Program The intensity and type of physical activities that are best for one person may not be good for another. A person who has been

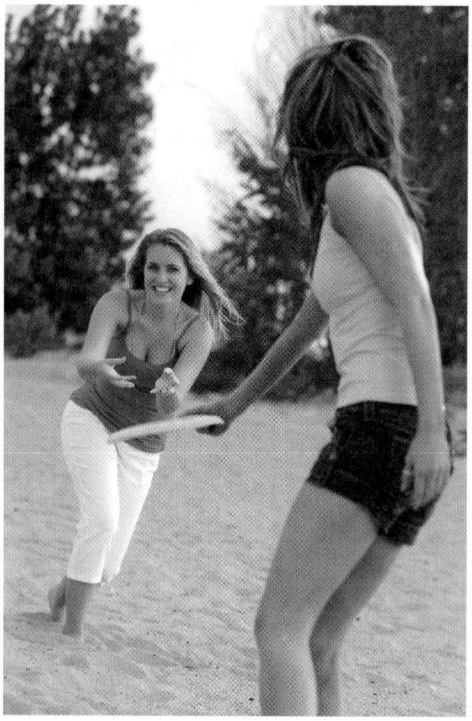

© Jim Jurica/iStockphoto

The key to regular physical activity is finding an activity you enjoy.

sedentary will initially perform at a dramatically different level of intensity than a fit person.

The type of physical activity that is best for you depends, too, on what you want to achieve and what you enjoy doing. Some people love walking, whereas others prefer to dance or ride a bike. If you want to be stronger and firmer, lift weights. And remember, muscle is more metabolically active than body fat, so the more muscle you have, the more energy you'll burn.

In a balanced fitness program, aerobic activity improves cardiorespiratory fitness, stretching enhances flexibility, and resistance training develops muscle strength, **muscle power**, and muscle endurance. Table 15-3 provides an example of a balanced fitness program.

TABLE 15-3 A Sample Balanced Fitness Program

Monday, Wednesday, Friday:
• 5 minutes of warm-up activity • 45 minutes of aerobic activity • 10 minutes of cool-down activity and stretching
Thursday, Saturday:
• 5 minutes of warm-up activity • 30 minutes of resistance training • 10 minutes of cool-down activity and stretching
Saturday and/or Sunday:
• Sports, walking, hiking, biking, or swimming

Resistance Training

Resistance training has long been recognized as a means to build muscle mass and develop and maintain muscle strength, muscle power, and muscle endurance. Resistance training can also help to maximize and maintain bone mass.[23] Even in women past menopause (when most women are losing bone), resistance training can improve bone density, especially in combination with adequate dietary calcium and vitamin D intake.[24] Additional benefits of resistance training have also emerged. Progressive resistance training helps prevent and manage several chronic diseases, including cardiovascular disease, and enhances psychological well-being.[25]

Physical Activity Guidance for Canadians

Adults should also do muscle- and bone-strengthening activities that involve all major muscle groups at least two days a week, as these activities provide additional health benefits.

By promoting strong muscles in the back and abdomen, resistance training can improve posture and reduce the risk of back injury. Resistance training can also help prevent the decline in physical mobility that often accompanies aging.[26] Older adults, even those in their eighties, who participate in resistance training programs not only gain muscle strength but also improve their muscle endurance, which enables them to walk longer before exhaustion. Leg strength and walking endurance are powerful indicators of an older adult's physical abilities.

Resistance training builds muscle strength, muscle power, and muscle endurance. To emphasize muscle strength, combine high resistance (heavy weight) with a low number (8 to 12) of repetitions.[27] To emphasize muscle power, combine moderate resistance (light to medium weight) with high velocity (as fast as safely possible). To emphasize muscle endurance, combine less resistance (lighter weight) with more (10 to 15) repetitions. Resistance training enhances performance in other sports, too. Swimmers can develop a more efficient stroke and tennis players, a more powerful serve, when they train with weights.

IN SUMMARY **Physical activity brings positive rewards: good health and long life. To develop fitness—whose components are flexibility, muscle strength and endurance, and cardiorespiratory endurance—a person must condition the body, through training, to adapt to the activity performed.**

Energy Systems and Fuels to Support Activity

Nutrition and physical activity go hand in hand. Activity demands carbohydrate and fat as fuel, protein to build and maintain lean tissues, vitamins and minerals to support both energy metabolism and tissue building, and water to help distribute the fuels and to dissipate the resulting heat and wastes. This section describes how nutrition supports a person who decides to get up and go.

muscle power: the product of force generation (strength) and movement velocity (speed); the speed at which a given amount of exertion is completed.

resistance training: the use of free weights or weight machines to provide resistance for developing muscle strength, power, and endurance; also called *weight training.* A person's own body weight may also be used to provide resistance as when a person does push-ups, pull-ups, or abdominal crunches.

The Energy Systems of Physical Activity—ATP and CP

Muscles contract fast. When called upon, they respond quickly without taking time to metabolize fat or carbohydrate for energy. In the first fractions of a second, muscles starting to move depend on their supplies of quick-energy compounds to power their movements. Exercise physiologists know these compounds by their abbreviations, ATP and CP.

ATP As Chapter 7 describes, all of the energy-yielding nutrients—carbohydrate, fat, and protein—can enter metabolic pathways that make the high-energy compound ATP (adenosine triphosphate). ATP is present in small amounts in all body tissues all the time, and it can deliver energy instantly. In the muscles, ATP provides the chemical driving force for contraction. When an ATP molecule is split, its energy is released, and the muscle cells channel some of that energy into mechanical movement and most of it into heat.

CP Immediately after the onset of a demand, before muscle ATP pools dwindle, a muscle enzyme begins to break down another high-energy compound that is stored in the muscle, **CP**, or **creatine phosphate.** ♦ CP is made from creatine, a compound commonly found in muscles, with a phosphate group attached. CP can split (anaerobically) ♦ to release phosphate and replenish ATP supplies. Supplies of CP in a muscle last for only about 10 seconds, producing enough quick energy, without oxygen, for a 100 metre dash.

When activity ceases and the muscles are resting, ATP gives up one of its phosphate groups to creatine. Thus CP is produced during rest by reversing the process that occurs during muscular activity. ♦ (Highlight 15 includes creatine supplements in its discussion of substances commonly used in the pursuit of fitness.)

♦ Creatine phosphate is also called **phosphocreatine (PC).**

♦ Recall from Chapter 7 that **anaerobic** means not requiring oxygen.

♦ During rest: ATP + creatine → CP
During activity: CP → ATP + creatine

The Energy-Yielding Nutrients To meet the more prolonged demands of sustained activity, the muscles generate ATP from the more abundant fuels: carbohydrate, fat, and protein. The breakdown of these nutrients generates ATP all day every day, and so maintains the supply. Muscles always use a mixture of fuels—never just one.

During rest, the body derives more than half of its ATP from fatty acids and most of the rest from glucose, along with a small percentage from amino acids. During physical activity, the body adjusts its mixture of fuels. How much of which fuel ♦ the muscles use during physical activity depends on an interplay among the fuels available from the diet, the intensity and duration of the activity, and the degree to which the body is conditioned to perform that activity. The next sections explain these relationships by examining each of the energy-yielding nutrients individually, but keep in mind that although one fuel may predominate at a given time, the other two will still be involved. Table 15-4 shows how fuel use changes according to the intensity and duration of the activity.

♦ Fuel mixture during activity depends on:
- Diet
- Intensity and duration of activity
- Training

As you read about each of the energy-yielding nutrients, notice how its contribution to the fuel mixture shifts depending on whether the activity is anaerobic or aerobic. Anaerobic activities are associated with strength, agility, and split-second surges of power. The jump of the basketball player, the slam of the tennis serve, the heave of a bodybuilder lifting weights, and the blast of the fullback through the opposing line all involve anaerobic work. Such high-intensity, short-duration activities depend mostly on glucose as the chief energy fuel.

CP, creatine phosphate (also called **phosphocreatine**): a high-energy compound in muscle cells that acts as a reservoir of energy that can maintain a steady supply of ATP. CP provides the energy for short bursts of activity.

TABLE 15-4 Fuels Used for Activities of Different Intensities and Durations

Activity Intensity	Activity Duration	Preferred Fuel Source	Oxygen Needed?	Activity Example
Extreme[a]	8 to 10 sec	ATP-CP (immediate availability)	No (anaerobic)	100 metre dash, shot put
Very high	20 sec to 3 min	ATP from carbohydrate (lactate)	No (anaerobic)	400 metre run at maximal speed
High	3 min to 20 min	ATP from carbohydrate	Yes (aerobic)	Cycling, swimming, or running
Moderate	More than 20 min	ATP from fat	Yes (aerobic)	Hiking

[a]All levels of activity intensity use the ATP-CP system initially; extremely intense short-term activities rely solely on the ATP-CP system.

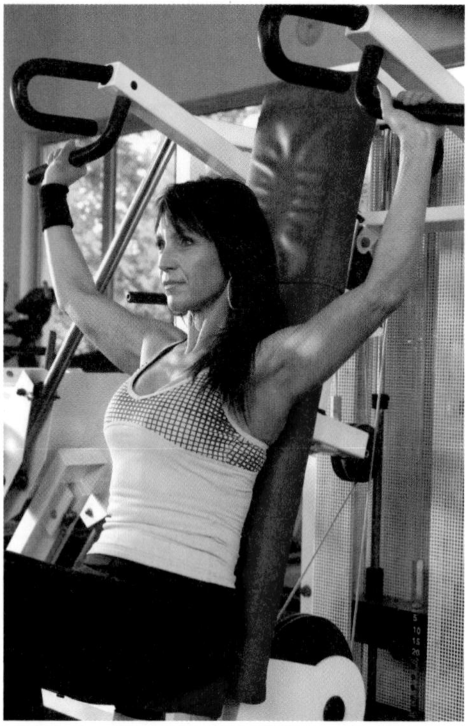

Photoline/shutterstock

Split-second surges of power as in the heave of a barbell or jump of a basketball player involve *anaerobic* work.

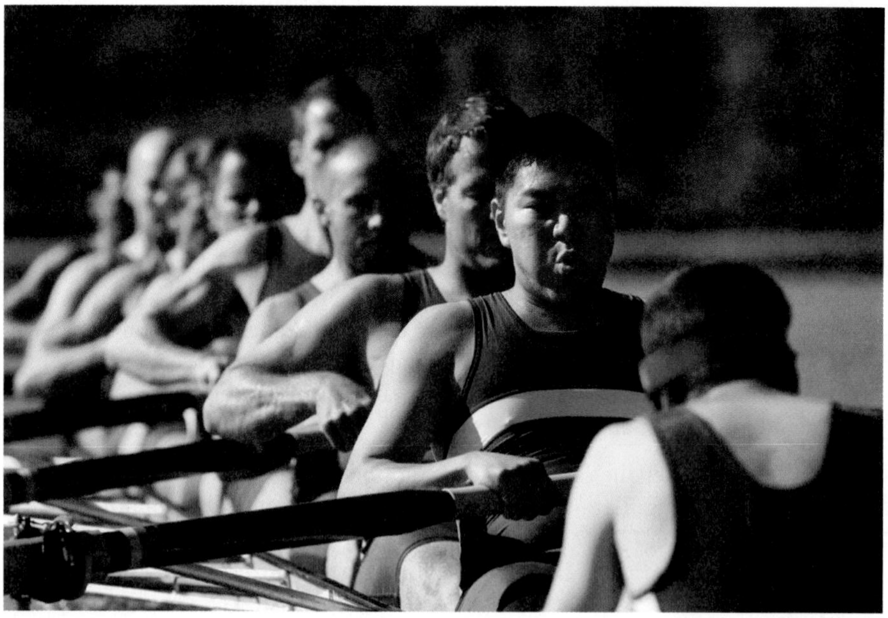

© Corbis Super RF/Alamy

Sustained muscular efforts as in a long-distance rowing event or a cross-country run involve *aerobic* work.

Endurance activities of low to moderate intensity and long duration depend more on fat to provide energy aerobically. The ability to continue swimming to the shore, to keep on hiking to the top of the mountain, or to continue pedalling all the way home reflects aerobic capacity. As mentioned earlier, aerobic capacity is also crucial to maintaining a healthy heart and circulatory system. The relationships among fuels and physical activity bear heavily on what foods best support your chosen activities.

Glucose Use during Physical Activity Glucose, stored in the liver and muscles as glycogen, is vital to physical activity. During exertion, the liver breaks down its glycogen and releases the glucose into the bloodstream. The muscles use this glucose as well as their own private glycogen stores to fuel their work. Glycogen supplies can easily support everyday activities but are limited to less than 2000 kcalories of energy, enough for about 30 kilometres of running.[28] The more glycogen the muscles store, the longer the glycogen will last during physical activity, which in turn influences performance. When glycogen is depleted, the muscles become fatigued.

Diet Affects Glycogen Storage and Use How much carbohydrate a person eats influences how much glycogen is stored. ♦ A classic study compared fuel use during activity among three groups of runners on different diets.[29] For several days before testing, one group consumed a normal mixed diet, a second group consumed a high-carbohydrate diet, and the third group consumed a no-carbohydrate diet (fat and protein diet). As Figure 15-3 shows, the high-carbohydrate diet allowed the runners to keep going longer before exhaustion. This study and many others that followed have confirmed that high-carbohydrate diets enhance endurance by ensuring ample glycogen stores.

♦ To fill glycogen stores, eat plenty of carbohydrate-rich foods.

Intensity of Activity Affects Glycogen Use How long an exercising person's glycogen will last depends not only on diet, but also on the intensity of the activity. Moderate activities such as jogging, during which breathing is steady and easy, use glycogen slowly. The lungs and circulatory system have no trouble keeping up with the muscles' need for oxygen. The individual breathes easily, and the heart beats steadily—the activity is aerobic. The muscles derive their energy from both glucose and fatty acids. By depending partly on fatty acids, moderate aerobic activity conserves glycogen.

FIGURE 15-3 The Effect of Diet on Physical Endurance

A high-carbohydrate diet can increase an athlete's endurance. In this study, the fat and protein diet provided 94 percent of kcalories from fat and 6 percent from protein; the normal mixed diet provided 55 percent of kcalories from carbohydrate; and the high-carbohydrate diet provided 83 percent of kcalories from carbohydrate.

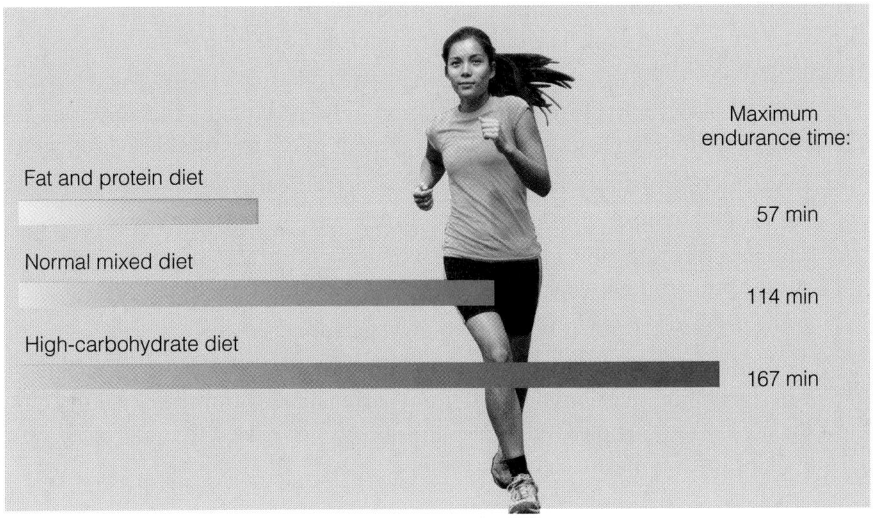
Maximum endurance time:
Fat and protein diet
57 min
Normal mixed diet
114 min
High-carbohydrate diet
167 min
Maridav/shutterstock

Intense activities—the kind that make it difficult "to catch your breath," such as a 400 metre race—use glycogen quickly. In such activities, the muscles break down glucose to pyruvate anaerobically, producing ATP quickly.

Lactate When the rate of glycolysis exceeds the capacity of the mitochondria to accept hydrogens with their electrons for the electron transport chain, the accumulating pyruvate molecules are converted to lactate. ♦ At low intensities, lactate is readily cleared from the blood, but at higher intensities, lactate accumulates. When the rate of lactate production exceeds the rate of clearance, intense activity can be maintained for only one to three minutes (as in a 400 to 800 metre race or a boxing match). Lactate has long been blamed for muscle fatigue, but recent research disputes this idea. Working muscles may produce lactate and experience fatigue, but the lactate does not cause the fatigue.[30]

♦ **Lactate** is the product of anaerobic glycolysis.

Lactate quickly leaves the muscles and travels in the blood to the liver. There, liver enzymes convert the lactate back into glucose. Glucose can then return to the muscles to fuel additional activity. (The recycling process that regenerates glucose from lactate is known as the *Cori cycle,* as shown in Figure 7-7 on p. 213.)

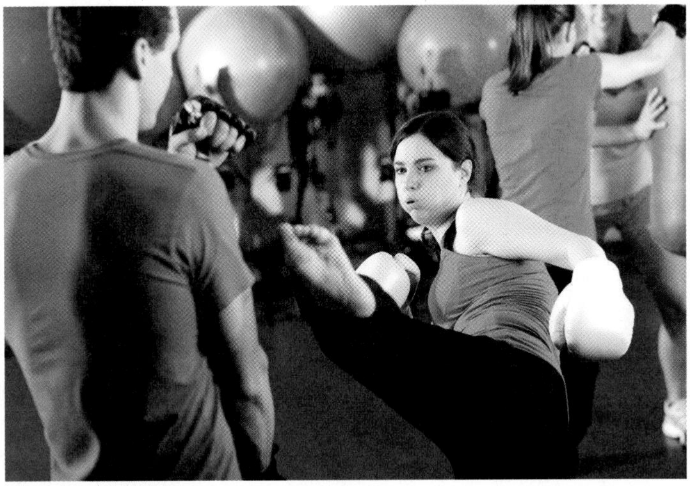
Kzenon/shutterstock

Moderate- to high-intensity aerobic exercises that can be sustained for only a short time (less than 20 minutes) use some fat, but more glucose for fuel.

Duration of Activity Affects Glycogen Use Glycogen use depends not only on the intensity of an activity, but also on its duration. Within the first 20 minutes or so of moderate activity, a person uses mostly glycogen for fuel—about one-fifth of the available glycogen. As the muscles devour their own glycogen, they become ravenous for more glucose, and the liver responds by emptying out its glycogen stores.

After 20 minutes, a person who continues exercising moderately (mostly aerobically) begins to use less and less glycogen and more and more fat for fuel (review Table 15-4 on p. 477). Still, glycogen use continues, and if the activity lasts long enough and is intense enough, blood glucose declines and muscle and liver glycogen stores are depleted. Physical activity can continue for a short time thereafter only because the liver scrambles to produce, from lactate and certain amino acids, the minimum amount of glucose needed to briefly forestall total depletion.

Glucose Depletion After a couple of hours of strenuous activity, glucose stores are depleted. When depletion occurs, it brings nervous system function to a near halt, making continued exertion at the same intensity almost impossible. Marathon runners refer to this point of glucose exhaustion as "hitting the wall."

To avoid such debilitation, endurance athletes try to maintain their blood glucose for as long as they can. The following guidelines will help endurance athletes maximize glucose supply:

- Eat a high-carbohydrate diet (approximately 8 grams of carbohydrate per kilogram of body weight or about 70 percent of energy intake) regularly.*
- Take glucose (usually in sports drinks) periodically during activities that last for one hour or more.
- Eat carbohydrate-rich foods (approximately 60 grams of carbohydrate) ♦ immediately following activity.
- Train the muscles to store as much glycogen as possible.

♦ For perspective, snack ideas providing 60 g carbohydrate:
- 175 mL sports drink and a small bagel
- 500 mL milk and 4 oatmeal cookies
- 250 mL pineapple juice and a granola bar

The last section of this chapter, "Diets for Physically Active People," discusses how to design a high-carbohydrate diet for performance, and the accompanying "How To" describes **carbohydrate loading**—a technique used to maximize glycogen stores for long endurance competitions.

Glucose during Activity Muscles can obtain the glucose they need not only from glycogen stores, but also from foods and beverages consumed during activity. Consuming carbohydrate is especially useful during exhausting endurance activities (lasting more than one hour) and during games such as soccer or hockey, which last for hours and demand repeated bursts of intense activity.[31]

Endurance athletes often run short of glucose by the end of competitive events. To ensure optimal carbohydrate intake, sports nutrition experts recommend 30 to 60 grams of carbohydrate per hour during prolonged events.[32] Carbohydrate-based sports drinks offer a convenient way to meet this recommendation and also help replace water and electrolyte losses. ♦ Thus, to ensure optimal hydration and carbohydrate intake, endurance athletes are advised to drink one-half to one litre of a 4 to 8 percent carbohydrate-based sports drink per hour, in small, frequent doses during activity.[33] During the last stages of an endurance competition, when glycogen is running low, glucose consumed during the event can slowly make its way from the digestive tract to the muscles and augment the body's supply of glucose enough to forestall exhaustion.

♦ A later section discusses fluid and electrolyte balance during activity.

Some researchers have questioned whether adding protein to carbohydrate-containing sports beverages would offer a performance advantage to endurance athletes.[34] Evidence so far suggests that when carbohydrate intake is optimal, protein provides no additional performance benefit.[35]

Glucose after Activity Eating high-carbohydrate foods *after* physical activity also enlarges glycogen stores. A high-carbohydrate meal eaten within 15 minutes after physical activity accelerates the rate of glycogen storage by 300 percent. After two hours, the rate of glycogen storage declines by almost half. Despite this slower rate of glycogen restoration, muscles continue to accumulate glycogen as long as athletes eat carbohydrate-rich foods within two hours following activity.[36] This is particularly important to athletes who train hard more than once a day.

Chapter 4 introduces the glycemic response and discusses the possible health benefits of eating a *low* glycemic diet. For athletes wishing to maximize muscle glycogen synthesis after strenuous training, however, eating foods with a *high*

carbohydrate loading: a regimen of moderate exercise followed by the consumption of a high-carbohydrate diet that enables muscles to store glycogen beyond their normal capacities; also called *glycogen loading* or *glycogen super compensation.*

*Percentage of energy intake is meaningful only when total energy intake is known. Consider that at high energy intakes (say, 5000 kcalories/day), even a moderate carbohydrate diet (50 percent of energy intake) supplies 625 grams of carbohydrate—enough for a 75 kilogram (165-pound) athlete in heavy training. By comparison, at a moderate energy intake (2000 kcalories/day), a high carbohydrate intake (70 percent of energy intake) supplies 350 grams—plenty of carbohydrate for most people, but not enough for athletes in heavy training.

HOW TO Maximize Glycogen Stores: Carbohydrate Loading

Some athletes use a technique called *carbohydrate loading* to maximize their muscle glycogen stores before a competition. Carbohydrate loading can nearly double muscle glycogen concentrations. In general, the athlete tapers training during the week before the competition and then eats a high-carbohydrate diet during the three days just prior to the event.[a] Specifically, the athlete follows the plan in the accompanying table.

[a]E. Coleman, Carbohydrate and exercise, in *Sports Nutrition: A Practical Manual for Professionals,* 4th ed., ed. M. Dunford (Chicago: American Dietetic Association, 2006), pp. 14–32.

Extra glycogen gained through carbohydrate loading can benefit an athlete who must keep going for 90 minutes or longer. Those who exercise for shorter times simply need a regular high-carbohydrate diet. In a hot climate, extra glycogen confers an additional advantage: as glycogen breaks down, it releases water, which helps to meet the athlete's fluid needs.

CENGAGENOW™
For additional practice log on to **www.cengage.com/sso.**

Before the Event	Training Intensity	Training Duration	Dietary Carbohydrate
6 days	Moderate (70% VO_2max)	90 min	Normal (5 g/kg body weight)
4–5 days	Moderate (70% VO_2max)	40 min	Normal (5 g/kg body weight)
2–3 days	Moderate (70% VO_2max)	20 min	High-carbohydrate (10 g/kg body weight)
1 day	Rest	—	High-carbohydrate (10 g/kg body weight)

TRY IT Estimate the carbohydrate needs of a 70 kilogram (154-pound) athlete during the week before an event.

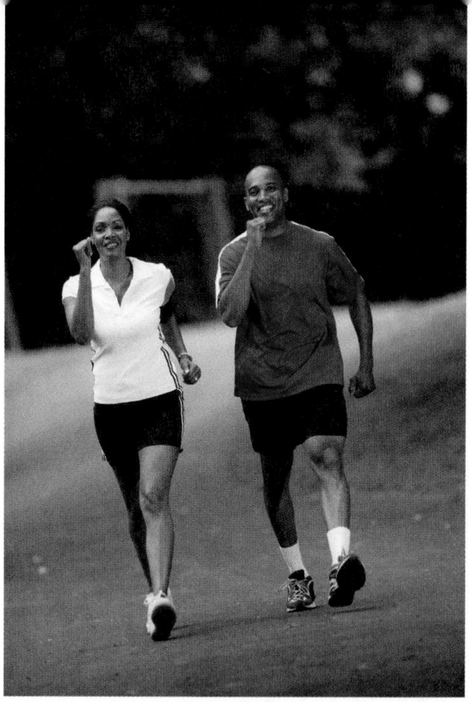

© Ocean/Corbis

Low- to moderate-intensity aerobic exercises that can be sustained for a long time (more than 20 minutes) use some glucose, but more fat for fuel.

glycemic index may be more beneficial (see Figure 4-13 on p. 107).[37] ♦ Foods with a high glycemic index elicit greater rates of glycogen synthesis compared to foods with a low glycemic index.[38] ♦

Training Affects Glycogen Use Training, too, affects how much glycogen muscles will store. Muscle cells that repeatedly deplete their glycogen through hard work adapt to store greater amounts of glycogen to support that work.

Conditioned muscles also rely less on glycogen and more on fat for energy, so glycogen breakdown and glucose use occur more slowly in trained than in untrained individuals at a given work intensity. A person attempting an activity for the first time uses much more glucose than an athlete who is trained to perform it. Oxygen delivery to the muscles by the heart and lungs plays a role, but equally importantly, trained muscles are better equipped to use the oxygen because their cells contain more mitochondria. ♦ Untrained muscles depend more heavily on anaerobic glucose breakdown, even when physical activity is just moderate.

Fat Use during Physical Activity

As Figure 15-3 (p. 479) shows, researchers have long recognized the importance of a high-carbohydrate diet for endurance performance. When endurance athletes "fat load" by consuming high-fat, low-carbohydrate diets for one to three days, their performance is impaired because their small glycogen stores are depleted quickly.[39] Endurance athletes who adhere to a high-fat, low-carbohydrate diet for more than a week, however, adapt by relying more on fat to fuel activity. Even with fat adaptation, however, performance benefits are not consistently evident.[40] In some cases, athletes on high-fat diets experience greater fatigue and perceive the activity to be more strenuous than athletes on high-carbohydrate diets.

♦ Chapter 4 (pp. 106–108) explains that the glycemic index is a method of classifying foods according to their potential to raise blood glucose. Processed foods made from refined flour such as snack foods, breads, and ready-to-eat cereals have a high glycemic index.

♦ In popular magazine articles and on the Internet, foods with a high glycemic index are sometimes called "high impact carbs," and foods with a low glycemic index are sometimes called "low impact carbs."

♦ The **mitochondria** are the structures within a cell responsible for producing ATP (see Figure 7-15 on p. 219).

Diets high in saturated fat carry risks of heart disease, too. Physical activity offers some protection against cardiovascular disease, but athletes, like everyone else, can suffer heart attacks and strokes. Most nutrition experts agree that the potential for adverse health effects of prolonged high-fat diets outweighs any possible benefit to performance.

Sports nutrition experts recommend that endurance athletes consume 20 to 35 percent of their energy from fat to meet nutrient and energy needs.[41] Athletes who restrict fat below 20 percent of total energy intake may fail to consume adequate energy and nutrients.

In contrast to *dietary* fat, *body* fat stores are extremely important during physical activity, as long as the activity is not too intense. Unlike glycogen stores, the body's fat stores can usually provide more than 70 000 kcalories and fuel hours of activity without running out.

The fat used in physical activity is liberated as fatty acids from the internal fat stores and from the fat under the skin. Areas that have the most fat to spare donate the greatest amounts (although they may not be the areas that appear fattiest). Thus "spot reducing" doesn't work because muscles do not "own" the fat that surrounds them. Fat cells release fatty acids into the blood, not into the underlying muscles. Then the blood gives to each muscle the amount of fat that it needs. Proof of this is found in a tennis player's arms—the skinfold measures of fat are the same in both arms, even though the muscles of one arm work much harder and may be larger than those of the other. A balanced fitness program that includes strength training, however, will tighten muscles underneath the fat, improving the overall appearance. Keep in mind that some body fat is essential to good health. ♦

♦ Chapter 8 (pp. 256–257) discusses the health risks of too little body fat.

Duration of Activity Affects Fat Use Early in an activity, as the muscles draw on fatty acids, blood levels fall. If the activity continues for more than a few minutes, the hormone epinephrine signals the fat cells to begin breaking down their stored triglycerides and liberating fatty acids into the blood. After about 20 minutes of physical activity, the blood fatty acid concentration surpasses the normal resting concentration. Thereafter, sustained, moderate activity uses body fat stores as its major fuel.

Intensity of Activity Affects Fat Use The intensity of physical activity also affects fat use. As the intensity of activity increases, fat makes less and less of a contribution to the fuel mixture. Remember that fat can be broken down for energy only by aerobic metabolism. For fat to fuel activity, then, oxygen must be abundantly available. If a person is breathing easily during activity, the muscles are getting all the oxygen they need and are able to use more fat in the fuel mixture.

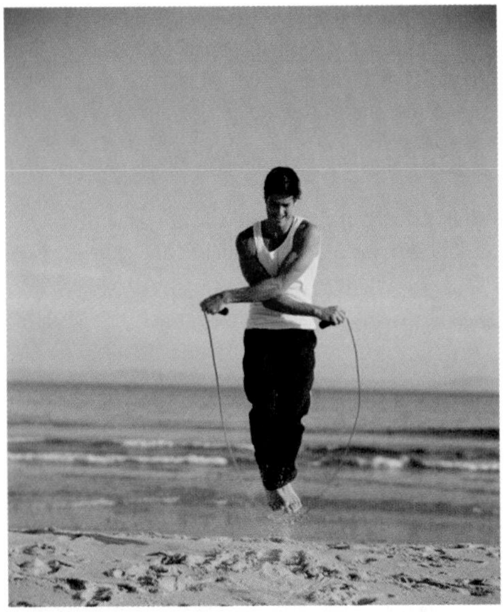
Paul Viant/Getty Images

Abundant energy from the breakdown of fat can come only from aerobic metabolism.

Training Affects Fat Use Training—repeated aerobic activity—produces the adaptations that permit the body to draw more heavily on fat for fuel. Training stimulates the muscle cells to manufacture more and larger mitochondria, the "powerhouse" structures of the cells that produce ATP for energy. Another adaptation: the heart and lungs become stronger and better able to deliver oxygen to muscles at high activity intensities. Still another: hormones in the body of a trained person slow glucose release from the liver and speed up the use of fat instead. These adaptations reward not only trained athletes but all active people; a person who trains by way of aerobic activities such as distance running or cycling becomes well suited to the activity.

Protein Use during Physical Activity—and between Times

Table 15-4 on p. 477 summarizes the fuel uses discussed so far, but does not include the third energy-yielding nutrient, protein, because protein is not a major fuel for physical activity. Nevertheless, physically active people use protein just as other people do—to build muscle and other lean tissues and, to some extent, to fuel activity. The body does, however, handle protein differently during activity than during rest.

Protein Used in Muscle Building Synthesis of body proteins is suppressed during activity. In the hours of recovery following activity, though, protein synthesis accelerates beyond normal resting levels. As noted earlier, eating high-carbohydrate foods immediately after exercise accelerates muscle glycogen storage. Similarly, research shows that eating high-quality protein, either by itself or together with carbohydrate, enhances muscle protein synthesis.[42] Remember that the body adapts and builds the molecules, cells, and tissues it needs for the next period of activity. Whenever the body remodels a part of itself, it also tears down old structures to make way for new ones. Repeated activity, with just a slight overload, triggers the protein-dismantling and protein-synthesizing equipment of each muscle cell to make needed changes—that is, to adapt.

The physical work of each muscle cell acts as a signal to its DNA and RNA to begin producing the kinds of proteins that will best support that work. Take running, for example. In the first difficult sessions, the body is not yet equipped to perform aerobic work easily, but with each session, the cells' genetic material gets the message that an overhaul is needed. In the hours that follow the session, the genes send molecular messages to the protein-building equipment that tell it what old structures to break down and what new structures to build. Within the limits of its genetic potential, the body responds. Running (or any aerobic activity) stimulates synthesis of mitochondrial protein to facilitate efficient aerobic metabolism. Over time, the body adapts and running becomes easier.

The body of a weight lifter responds to training, as well, but the response differs from that of aerobic training. Weight lifting stimulates synthesis of muscle fibre protein to enhance muscle mass and strength—with little change in mitochondrial protein. An athlete may add between between 7 and 28 grams (¼ ounce and 1 ounce) of protein to muscle mass each day during active muscle-building phases of training.

Protein Used as Fuel Not only do athletes retain more protein in their muscles, but they also use more protein as fuel. Muscles speed up their use of amino acids for energy during physical activity, just as they speed up their use of fat and carbohydrate. Still, protein contributes up to only about 10 percent of the total fuel used, both during activity and during rest. The most active people of all, endurance athletes, use up large amounts of all energy fuels, including protein, during performance, but such athletes also eat more food and therefore usually consume enough protein.

Diet Affects Protein Use during Activity The factors that affect how much protein is used during activity seem to be the same three that influence the use of fat and carbohydrate—one factor is diet. People who consume diets adequate in energy and rich in *carbohydrate* ♦ use less protein than those who eat protein- and fat-rich diets. Recall that carbohydrates spare proteins from being broken down to make glucose when needed. Because physical activity requires glucose, a diet lacking in carbohydrate necessitates the conversion of amino acids to glucose. The same is true for a diet high in fat because fatty acids can never provide glucose.

♦ To conserve protein, eat a diet adequate in energy and rich in carbohydrate.

Intensity and Duration of Activity Affect Protein Use during Activity A second factor, the intensity and duration of activity, also modifies protein use. Endurance athletes who train for more than an hour a day, engaging in aerobic activity of moderate intensity and long duration, may deplete their glycogen stores by the end of their workouts and become somewhat more dependent on body protein for energy.

In contrast, anaerobic strength training does not use more protein for energy, but it does demand more protein to build muscle. Thus the protein needs of both endurance and strength athletes are higher than those of sedentary people, but certainly not as high as the protein intakes many athletes consume.

Training Affects Protein Use A third factor that influences a person's use of protein during physical activity is the extent of training. Particularly in strength athletes such as bodybuilders, the higher the degree of training, the less protein a person uses during an activity.

TABLE 15-5 Recommended Protein Intakes for Athletes

	Recommendations (g/kg/day)	Protein Intakes (g/day)	
		Males	*Females*
RDA for adults	0.8	56	44
Recommended intake for power (strength or speed) athletes	1.2–1.7	84–119	66–94
Recommended intake for endurance athletes	1.2–1.4	84–98	66–77
Canadian average intake from food		99	73

NOTE: Daily protein intakes are based on a 70 kilogram (154-pound) man and 55 kilogram (121-pound) woman.
SOURCES: Health Canada and Statistics Canada, Canadian Community Health Survey, Cycle 2.2, Nutrition (2004), Nutrient Intakes from Food, Provincial, Regional and National Summary Data Tables, Volume 3. www.hc-sc.gc.ca/fn-an/surveill/nutrition/commun/cchs_focus-volet_escc-eng.php, accessed September 12, 2011; Committee on Dietary Reference Intakes, *Dietary Reference Intakes for Energy, Carbohydrate, Fiber, Fat, Fatty Acids, Cholesterol, Protein and Amino Acids* (Washington, D.C.: National Academies Press, 2005), pp. 660–661; Position of the American Dietetic Association, Dietitians of Canada, and the American College of Sports Medicine: Nutrition and athletic performance, *Journal of the American Dietetic Association* 109 (2009): 509–527.

Protein Recommendations for Active People As mentioned, all active people, and especially athletes in training, probably need more protein than sedentary people do.[43] Endurance athletes, such as long-distance runners and cyclists, use more protein for fuel than strength or power athletes do, and they retain some, especially in the muscles used for their sport. Strength athletes, such as weight lifters, and power athletes, such as football players, use less protein for fuel, but they still use some and retain much more. Therefore, *all* athletes in training should attend to protein needs, but they should first meet their energy needs with adequate carbohydrate intakes. Without adequate protein intake, athletes will burn off as fuel the very protein that they wish to retain in muscle.

How much protein, then, should an active person consume? Although the DRI Committee does not recommend greater than normal protein intakes for athletes, other authorities do.[44] These recommendations specify different protein intakes for athletes pursuing different activities (see Table 15-5).[45] A later section translates protein recommendations into a diet plan and shows that no one needs protein supplements, or even large servings of meat, to obtain the highest recommended protein intakes. (Chapter 6 concludes that most people receive more than enough protein without supplements and reviews the potential dangers of using protein and amino acid supplements.)

IN SUMMARY **The mixture of fuels the muscles use during physical activity depends on diet, the intensity and duration of the activity, and training. During intense activity, the fuel mix is mostly glucose, whereas during less intense, moderate activity, fat makes a greater contribution. With endurance training, muscle cells adapt to store more glycogen and to rely less on glucose and more on fat for energy. Athletes in training may need more protein than sedentary people do, but they typically eat more food as well and therefore obtain enough protein.**

Vitamins and Minerals to Support Activity

Many of the vitamins and minerals assist in releasing energy from fuels and in transporting oxygen. This knowledge has led many people to believe, mistakenly, that vitamin and mineral *supplements* offer physically active people both health benefits and athletic advantages. (Review Highlight 10 for a discussion of vitamin and mineral supplements, and see Highlight 15, which explores supplements and other products people use in the hope of enhancing athletic performance.)

Supplements Nutrient supplements do not enhance the performance of well-nourished people. Deficiencies of vitamins and minerals, however, do impede performance. As a reminder, supplements are intended to supplement dietary intake, not substitute for making unhealthy food choices. In general, active people who eat enough nutrient-dense foods to meet energy needs also meet their vitamin and mineral needs. After all, active people eat more food; it stands to reason that with the right choices, they'll get more nutrients.

Athletes who lose weight to meet low body-weight requirements, however, may eat so little food that they fail to obtain all the nutrients they need.[46] The practice of "making weight" is opposed by many health and fitness organizations, but for athletes who choose this course of action, a single daily multivitamin-mineral supplement that provides no more than the DRI recommendations for nutrients may be beneficial.

Some athletes believe that taking vitamin or mineral supplements directly before competition will enhance performance. These beliefs are contrary to scientific reality. Most vitamins and minerals function as small parts of larger working units. After entering the blood, they have to wait for the cells to combine them with their appropriate other parts so that they can do their work. This takes time—hours or days. Vitamins or minerals taken right before an event are useless for improving performance, even if the person is actually suffering deficiencies of them.

Nutrients of Concern In general, then, most active people who eat well-balanced meals do not need vitamin or mineral supplements. Two nutrients, vitamin E and iron, do merit special mention here, however, each for a different reason. Vitamin E is discussed because so many athletes take vitamin E supplements. ♦ Iron is discussed because some athletes may be unaware that they need iron supplements. The B vitamins, calcium, and vitamin D also warrant mention because of their respective roles in energy metabolism, muscle contraction, and bone health.

♦ The Tolerable Upper Intake Level (UL) for vitamin E is 1000 mg per day.

Vitamin E During prolonged, high-intensity physical activity, the muscles' consumption of oxygen increases tenfold or more, which increases the production of free radicals in the body.[47] As Highlight 12 states, vitamin E is a potent antioxidant that vigorously defends cell membranes against the oxidative damage of free radicals.

Does vitamin E supplementation protect against exercise-induced oxidative stress? Some studies find that it does; others show no effect, and still others report enhanced oxidative stress.[48] Recent research may offer some insight into these inconsistencies. Although free radicals are usually damaging, during repeated episodes of endurance activities, they may actually be beneficial. Free radicals activate powerful antioxidant enzymes, which may enhance the athlete's tolerance to such oxidative stresses.[49] Researchers speculate that antioxidant supplements such as vitamin E interfere with this adaptive response. This may explain why, in some studies, athletes taking vitamin E show signs of increased oxidative stress. The supplements interfere with protective adaptations. Clearly, more research is needed on supplements, but in the meantime, active people can benefit by using vitamin E–rich vegetable oils and eating generous servings of antioxidant-rich vegetables and fruits regularly.

Iron Deficiency Physically active young women, especially those who engage in endurance activities such as distance running, are prone to iron deficiency.[50] Habitually low intakes of iron-rich foods, high iron losses through menstruation, and the high demands of muscles for the iron-containing electron carriers of the mitochondria and the muscle protein myoglobin can cause iron deficiency in physically active young women.[51]

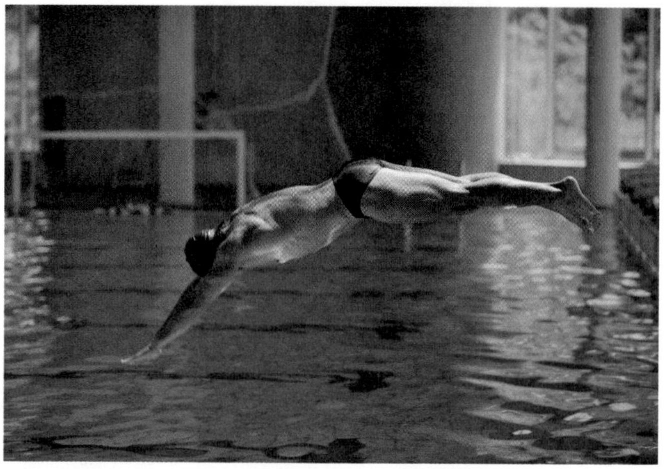
Benis Arapovic/shutterstock

For perfect functioning, every nutrient is needed.

Adolescent female athletes who eat vegetarian diets may be particularly vulnerable to iron deficiency. As Chapter 14 explains, the bioavailability of iron is often poor in vegetarian diets.[52] To protect against iron deficiency, vegetarian athletes need to select good dietary sources of iron (fortified cereals, legumes, nuts, and seeds) and include vitamin C–rich foods with each meal. As long as vegetarian athletes, like all athletes, consume enough nutrient-dense foods, they can perform as well as anyone.

Iron-Deficiency Anemia Iron-deficiency anemia impairs physical performance because the hemoglobin in red blood cells is needed to deliver oxygen to the cells for energy metabolism. ♦ Without adequate oxygen, an active person cannot perform aerobic activities and tires easily. Whether iron deficiency without clinical signs of anemia impairs physical performance is less clear.[53]

♦ Iron is an essential component of hemoglobin, the protein that transports oxygen throughout the body.

Sports Anemia Early in training, athletes may develop low blood hemoglobin for a while. This condition, sometimes called "**sports anemia**," is not a true iron-deficiency condition. Strenuous aerobic activity promotes destruction of the more fragile, older red blood cells, and the resulting cleanup work reduces the blood's iron content temporarily. Strenuous activity also expands the blood's plasma volume, thereby reducing the red blood cell count per unit of blood. However, the red blood cells do not diminish in size or number as in anemia, so their oxygen-carrying capacity is not hindered. Most researchers view sports anemia as an *adaptive,* temporary response to endurance training. Iron-deficiency anemia requires iron supplementation, but sports anemia does not.

Iron Recommendations for Athletes The best strategy for maintaining adequate iron nutrition depends on the individual. Menstruating women may border on iron deficiency even without the iron losses incurred by physical activity. Active teens of both genders have high iron needs because they are growing. Especially for women and teens, then, prescribed supplements may be needed to correct iron deficiencies. Physicians use the results of blood tests to determine whether such supplementation is needed. (Review Chapter 14 for many more details about iron, and see APPENDIX E for a description of the tests used in assessing its status.)

sports anemia: a transient condition of low hemoglobin in the blood, associated with the early stages of sports training or other strenuous activity.

B Vitamins As described in Chapter 10, the B vitamins play critical support roles in generating energy from the carbohydrates, fats, and proteins. The need for B vitamins is the same or slightly higher for active versus sedentary people, but because active people tend to consume more energy overall, when they choose a nutritious, varied, and balanced diet they have adequate intakes of the B vitamins. One notable exception is vegan athletes, who may be at risk for low vitamin B_{12} intakes. Examples of foods supplemented with vitamin B_{12} include meat analogues and fortified plant-based beverages.

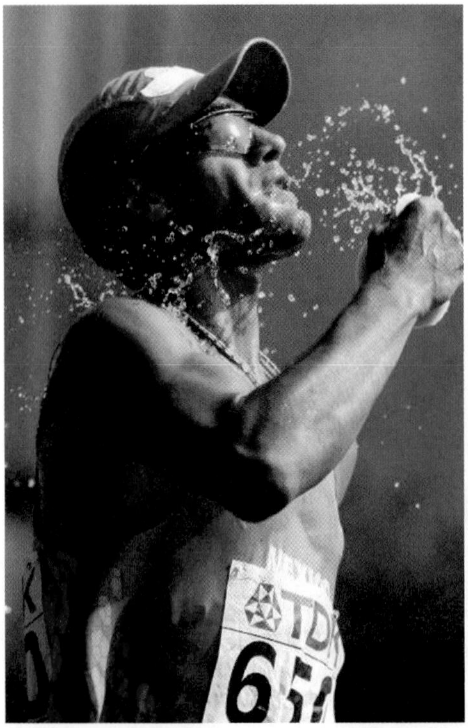
Getty Images

To prevent dehydration and the fatigue that accompanies it, drink liquids before, during, and after physical activity.

Calcium and Vitamin D Restricting foods found in the Milk and Alternatives food group compromises calcium and vitamin D intake, two nutrients important to bone health. This is especially important for women who tend to consume less food overall than men and shun milk and milk products because they consider them to be high-fat foods. Currently, Canadian women do not meet recommended intakes for both of these nutrients. As described in Chapter 13, vitamin D aids calcium absorption and calcium has important roles in bone health and muscle contraction. During times of increased intense activity the risk for stress fractures can increase. Moreover, some women who engage in extreme levels of activity can also experience amenorrhea, a loss of regular menstrual cycles for a period of three months or more without pregnancy; this is a condition that needs to be treated by a physician. When amenorrhea is combined with restricted eating it can lead to bone loss, otherwise referred to as the female-athlete triad: a combination of amenorrhea, disordered eating, and osteoporosis. Highlight 8 examines the female athlete triad. An adequate intake of calcium and vitamin D may not help restore menstrual regularity, but an inadequate intake can intensify bone loss.

IN SUMMARY With the possible exception of iron, well-nourished active people and athletes do not need nutrient supplements. Female athletes need to pay special attention to their iron needs.

Fluids and Electrolytes to Support Activity

The need for water far surpasses the need for any other nutrient. The body relies on watery fluids as the medium for all of its life-supporting activities, and if it loses too much water, its well-being will be compromised.

Obviously, the body loses water via sweat. Breathing uses water, too, exhaled as vapour. During physical activity, water losses from both routes are significant, and dehydration becomes a threat. Dehydration's first symptom is fatigue: a water loss of greater than 2 percent of body weight can reduce a person's capacity to do muscular work.[54] With a water loss of about 7 percent, a person is likely to collapse.

Temperature Regulation

As Chapter 7 discusses, working muscles produce heat as a by-product of energy metabolism. During intense activity, muscle heat production can be 15 to 20 times greater than at rest. The body cools itself by sweating. Each litre of sweat dissipates almost 600 kcalories of heat, preventing a rise in body temperature of almost 10 degrees ♦ on the Celsius scale. The body routes its blood supply through the capillaries just under the skin, and the skin secretes sweat to evaporate and cool the skin and the underlying blood. The blood then flows back to cool the deeper body chambers.

♦ Note: 10° on the Celsius scale is about 50° on the Fahrenheit scale.

Hyperthermia In hot, humid weather, sweat doesn't evaporate well because the surrounding air is already laden with water. In **hyperthermia**, body heat builds up and triggers maximum sweating, but without sweat evaporation, little cooling takes place. In such conditions, active people must take precautions to prevent **heat stroke.** To reduce the risk of heat stroke, drink enough fluid before and during the activity, rest in the shade when tired, and wear lightweight clothing that allows sweat to evaporate.[55] (Hence the danger of rubber or heavy suits that supposedly promote weight loss during physical activity—they promote profuse sweating, prevent sweat evaporation, and invite heat stroke.) If you ever experience any of the symptoms of heat stroke listed in the margin, ♦ stop your activity, sip fluids, seek shade, and ask for help. Heat stroke can be fatal, young people often die of it, and these symptoms demand attention.

♦ Symptoms of dehydration and heat stroke:
- Headache
- Nausea
- Dizziness
- Clumsiness
- Stumbling
- Sudden cessation of sweating (hot, dry skin)
- Confusion or other mental changes

Hypothermia In cold weather, **hypothermia,** or low body temperature, can be as serious as heat stroke is in hot weather. Inexperienced, slow runners participating in long races on cold or wet, chilly days are especially vulnerable to hypothermia. Slow runners who produce little heat can become too cold if clothing is inadequate. Early symptoms of hypothermia include shivering and euphoria. As body temperature continues to fall, shivering may stop, and weakness, disorientation, and apathy may occur. Each of these symptoms can impair a person's ability to act against a further drop in body temperature. Even in cold weather, however, the active body still sweats and still needs fluids. The fluids should be warm or at room temperature to help protect against hypothermia.

Fluid Replacement via Hydration Endurance athletes can easily lose 1.5 litres or more of fluid during *each hour* of activity. To prepare for fluid losses, a person must hydrate before activity. To replace fluid losses, the person must rehydrate during and after activity. (Table 15-6 on page 488 presents one schedule of hydration for physical activity.) Even then, in hot weather, the GI tract may not be able to absorb enough water fast enough to keep up with sweat losses, and some degree of dehydration may be inevitable. Athletes who know their body's **hourly sweat rate** can strive to replace the total amount of fluid lost during activity to prevent dehydration.[56]

hyperthermia: an above-normal body temperature.

heat stroke: a dangerous accumulation of body heat with accompanying loss of body fluid.

hypothermia: a below-normal body temperature.

hourly sweat rate: the amount of weight lost plus fluid consumed during exercise per hour.

TABLE 15-6 Hydration Schedule for Physical Activity

When to Drink	Amount of Fluid
2 to 3 hr before activity	500 to 750 mL (2 to 3 c)
15 min before activity	250 to 500 mL (1 to 2 c)
Every 15 min during activity	125 to 250 mL (1/2 to 1 c) (Drink enough to minimize loss of body weight, but don't overdrink.)
After activity	500 mL (2 c) for each half kilogram of body weight lost[a]

[a]Drinking 500 mL of fluid every 20 to 30 minutes after exercise until the total amount required is consumed is more effective for rehydration than drinking the needed amount all at once. Rapid fluid replacement after exercise stimulates urine production and results in less body water retention.

SOURCES: Adapted from American College of Sports Medicine, Position stand, Exercise and fluid replacement, *Medicine & Science in Sports & Exercise* 39 (2007): 377–390; C. K. Seto, D. Way, and N. O'Connor, Environmental illness in athletes, *Clinics in Sports Medicine* 24 (2005): 695–718; R. Murray, Fluid, electrolytes, and exercise in *Sports Nutrition: A Practice Manual for Professionals*. 4th ed., ed. M. Dunford (Chicago: American Dietetic Association, 2006), pp. 94–115; D. J. Casa, P. M. Clarkson, and W. O. Roberts, American College of Sports Medicine Roundtable on Hydration and Physical Activity: Consensus statements, *Current Sports Medicine Reports* 4 (2005): 115–127.

Athletes who are preparing for competition are often advised to drink extra fluids in the *days* immediately before the event, especially if they are still training. The extra water is not stored in the body, but drinking extra water ensures maximum hydration at the start of the event. Full hydration is imperative for every athlete both in training and in competition. The athlete who arrives at an event even slightly dehydrated begins with a disadvantage.

What is the best fluid for an exercising body? For noncompetitive, everyday active people, plain, cool water is recommended, especially in warm weather, for two reasons: (1) water rapidly leaves the digestive tract to enter the tissues where it is needed, and (2) it cools the body from the inside out. For endurance athletes, carbohydrate-containing beverages may be appropriate. Fluid ingestion during the event has the dual purposes of replenishing water lost through sweating and providing a source of carbohydrate to supplement the body's limited glycogen stores. Carbohydrate depletion brings on fatigue in the athlete, but as already mentioned, fluid loss and the accompanying build-up of body heat can be life-threatening. Thus the first priority for endurance athletes should be to replace fluids. Many good-tasting drinks are marketed for active people; a later section compares them with water.

hyponatremia (HIGH-poe-na-TREE-mee-ah): a decreased concentration of sodium in the blood.

- **hypo** = below
- **natrium** = sodium (Na)
- **emia** = blood

Electrolyte Losses and Replacement When a person sweats, small amounts of electrolytes—the electrically charged minerals sodium, potassium, chloride, and magnesium—are lost from the body along with water. Losses are greatest in beginners; training improves electrolyte retention.

To replenish lost electrolytes, a person ordinarily needs only to eat a regular diet that meets energy and nutrient needs. In events lasting more than one hour, sports drinks may be needed to replace fluids and electrolytes. Salt tablets can worsen dehydration and impair performance; they increase potassium losses, irritate the stomach, and cause vomiting.

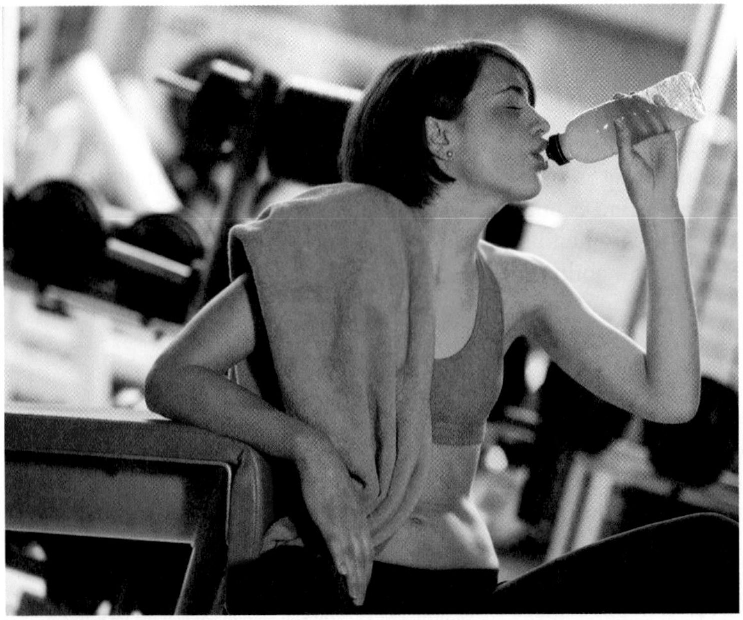

dean bertoncelj/shutterstock

Water is the best fluid for most physically active people, but some consumers prefer the flavours of sports drinks.

Hyponatremia When athletes compete in endurance sports replenishing electrolytes is crucial.[57] If athletes sweat profusely over a long period of time and do not replace lost sodium, a dangerous condition known as **hyponatremia** may result. Research shows that some athletes who sweat profusely may also lose more sodium in their sweat than others—and are prone to debilitating heat cramps.[58] These athletes lose twice as much sodium in sweat as athletes who don't cramp. Depending on individual variation, exercise intensity, and changes in ambient temperature and humidity, sweat rates for these athletes can exceed 2 litres per hour.[59]

Hyponatremia may also occur when endurance athletes drink such large amounts of water over the course of a long event that they overhydrate, diluting the body's fluids to such an extent that the sodium concentration becomes extremely low. During long competitions, when athletes lose sodium through heavy sweating *and* consume excessive amounts of liquids, especially water, hyponatremia becomes likely.

Some athletes may still be vulnerable to hyponatremia even when they drink sports drinks during an event. Sports drinks do contain sodium, but as a later section points out, the sodium content of sports drinks is low and, in some cases, too low to replace sweat losses. Still, sports drinks do offer more sodium than plain water.

To prevent hyponatremia, athletes need to replace sodium during prolonged events. They should favour sports drinks over water and eat pretzels in the last half of a long race. Some athletes may need beverages with higher sodium concentrations than commercial sports drinks. In the days before the event, especially an event in the heat, athletes should not restrict salt in their diets. The symptoms of hyponatremia are similar to, but not the same as, those of dehydration (see the margin). ♦

♦ Symptoms of hyponatremia:
- Severe headache
- Vomiting
- Bloating, puffiness from water retention (shoes tight, rings tight)
- Confusion
- Seizure

Sports Drinks Hydration is critical to optimal performance. As stated earlier, water best meets the fluid needs of most people, yet manufacturers market many good-tasting sports drinks that deliver both fluid and carbohydrate for active people. The term *sports drink* generally refers to beverages that contain carbohydrates and electrolytes in specific concentrations, and they are the focus of this discussion. Table 15-7 compares popular sports drinks.

Many sports drinks compete for their share of the more than $1 billion market in North America. What do sports drinks have to offer?

Fluid Sports drinks offer fluids to help offset the loss of fluids during physical activity, but plain water can do this, too. Alternatively, diluted fruit juices or flavoured water can be used if preferred to plain water.

Glucose Sports drinks offer simple sugars or **glucose polymers** that help maintain hydration and blood glucose and enhance performance as effectively as, or in some circumstances, even better than, water. Such measures are especially beneficial for strenuous endurance activities lasting longer than one hour, during

glucose polymers: compounds that supply glucose, not as single molecules, but linked in chains somewhat like starch. The objective is to attract less water from the body into the digestive tract (osmotic attraction depends on the number, not the size, of particles).

TABLE 15-7 Selected Sports Drinks Compared

Beverage	Serving Size	Energy (kCal)	Na[a] (mg)	K[a] (mg)	Mg[a] (mg)	Carb (g)	Fat (g)	Protein (g)	Carbohydrate Source	Carb (%)	Lactic Acid Buffer
Accelerade	355 mL	120	190	65	120	21	1	5	Sucrose, trehalose, fructose, maltodextrin	6	None
CarbBoom	250 mL	70	160	50	15	17	0	0	Maltodextrin, sucrose, glucose, fructose	7	None
Cytomax	500 mL	90	120	60	14	22	0	0	Amylopectin, maltodextrin, fructose, dextrose	5	Alpha-L-PolyLactate
eLoad	500 mL	109	370	97	13	27	0	0	Dextrose, sucrose	6	MultiCitrate
Gatorade	250 mL	50	110	30	0	14	0	0	Glucose, sucrose, fructose	6	None
GU20	500 mL	100	240	40	0	26	0	0	Maltodextrin, fructose	6	None
Hammer Nutrition Heed	500 mL	100	39	16	16	25	0	0	Maltodextrin	6	L-carnosine
Powerade	250 mL	56	52	32	0	15	0	0	High-fructose corn syrup	7	None
Ultima	250 mL	10	38	75	12	3	0	0	Maltodextrin	1	None

[a]Na = sodium; K = potassium; Mg = magnesium

NOTE: Except for Powerade, which is available only in liquid form, values reflect sports drink powders prepared with water according to package directions.

intense activities, or during prolonged competitive games that demand repeated intermittent activity.[60] Sports drinks are also suitable for events lasting less than one hour, although plain water is appropriate as well. Fluid transport to the tissues from beverages containing up to 8 percent glucose is rapid. Most sports drinks contain about 7 percent carbohydrate (about half the sugar of ordinary soft drinks, or about 5 teaspoons in each 355 millilitres). Less than 6 percent carbohydrate may not enhance performance, and more than 8 percent may cause abdominal cramps, nausea, and diarrhea. Although glucose can enhance endurance and performance in strenuous competitive events, for the moderate exerciser, it can be counterproductive if weight loss is the goal. Glucose is sugar, and like candy, it provides only empty kcalories—no vitamins or minerals. Most sports drinks provide between 50 and 100 kcalories per 250 millilitres.

Sodium and Other Electrolytes Sports drinks offer sodium and other electrolytes to help replace those lost during physical activity. Sodium in sports drinks also helps to increase the rate of fluid absorption from the GI tract and maintain plasma volume during activity and recovery. Most physically active people do not need to replace the minerals lost in sweat immediately; a meal eaten within hours of competition replaces these minerals soon enough. Most sports drinks are relatively low in sodium, however, so those who choose to use these beverages run little risk of excessive intake.

Good Taste Manufacturers reason that if a drink tastes good, people will drink more, thereby ensuring adequate hydration. For athletes who prefer the flavours of sports drinks over water, it may be worth paying for good taste to replace lost fluids.

For athletes who exercise for one hour or more or in high temperatures, sports drinks provide an advantage over water. For most physically active people, though, water is the best fluid to replenish lost fluids. The most important thing to do is drink—even if you don't feel thirsty.

Enhanced Water

Another beverage often marketed to athletes and active people is **enhanced water**, sometimes referred to as *vitamin water.* Enhanced waters are lightly flavoured waters with lower carbohydrate and electrolyte contents than traditional sports drinks. Marketers promote these beverages for the added vitamins, minerals, and in some cases, protein, they contain. In fact, most enhanced waters contain small amounts of only a few minerals, some of the B vitamins, and sometimes vitamin C or vitamin E. In the context of daily needs, the vitamins and minerals in these drinks do not add up to much. For example, it takes a litre of most of these beverages to provide only 10 percent of the RDA for iron or calcium. Quite simply, enhanced waters are not a substitute for eating nutrient-rich fruits and vegetables. Enhanced waters may not be harmful (except maybe to the wallet), but most people do not need them. Plain water can meet fluid needs. If the flavour of enhanced waters encourages greater fluid intake, then they may offer some advantage. Serious endurance athletes need the carbohydrate-electrolyte sports drinks discussed earlier.

Poor Beverage Choices: Caffeine and Alcohol

Athletes, like others, sometimes drink beverages that contain caffeine or alcohol. Each of these substances can influence physical performance.

Caffeine Caffeine is a stimulant, and athletes sometimes use it to enhance performance as Highlight 15 explains. Carbonated soft drinks, with or without caffeine, may not be a wise choice for athletes: bubbles make a person feel full quickly and so limit fluid intake. Some of the increasingly popular beverages, called *energy drinks*, contain amounts of caffeine equivalent to a cup or two of coffee. When used in excess or in combination with stimulants or other unregulated substances, energy drinks can hinder performance and are potentially

enhanced water: water that is fortified with ingredients such as vitamins, minerals, protein, oxygen, or herbs. Enhanced water is marketed as *vitamin water, sports water, oxygenated water,* and *protein water.*

dangerous.[61] Another reason energy drinks should not be used for fluid replacement during athletic events is that the carbohydrate concentrations are too high for optimal fluid absorption. The caffeine contents of selected energy drinks are listed in APPENDIX H.

Alcohol Some athletes mistakenly believe that they can replace fluids and load up on carbohydrates by drinking beer. ♦ A 355 millilitre beer provides 13 grams of carbohydrate—one-third the amount of carbohydrate in a glass of orange juice the same size. In addition to carbohydrate, beer also contains alcohol, of course. Energy from alcohol breakdown generates heat, but it does not fuel muscle work because alcohol is metabolized in the liver.

It is difficult to overstate alcohol's detrimental effects on physical activity. Alcohol's diuretic effect impairs the body's fluid balance, making dehydration likely; after physical activity, a person needs to replace fluids, not lose them by drinking beer. Alcohol also impairs the body's ability to regulate its temperature, increasing the likelihood of hypothermia or heat stroke.

Alcohol also alters perceptions; slows reaction time; reduces strength, power, and endurance; and hinders accuracy, balance, eye–hand coordination, and coordination in general—all opposing optimal athletic performance. In addition, it deprives people of their judgment, thereby compromising their safety in sports. Many sports-related fatalities and injuries involve alcohol or other drugs.

Clearly, alcohol impairs performance. For those who do drink, however, do not drink alcohol before exercising and drink plenty of water after exercising before drinking alcohol.

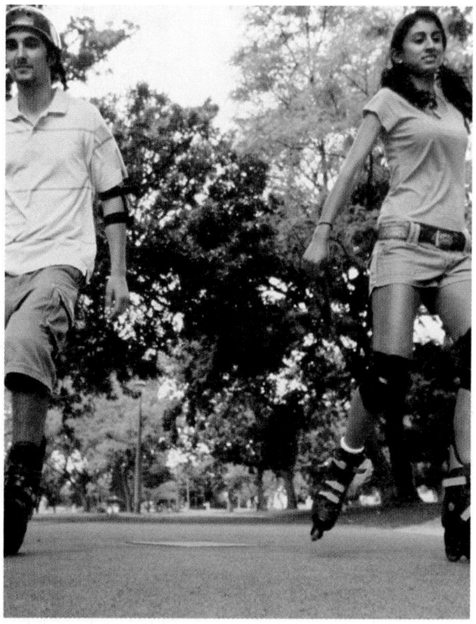
photos.com

Physical activity helps you look good, feel good, and have fun, and it brings many long-term health benefits as well.

IN SUMMARY **Active people need to drink plenty of water; endurance athletes need to drink both water and carbohydrate-containing beverages, especially during training and competition. During longer lasting events athletes need to pay special attention to replace sodium losses to prevent hyponatremia.**

♦ Beer facts:

- *Beer is not carbohydrate-rich.* Beer is *kcalorie-*rich, but only one-third of its kcalories are from carbohydrates. The other two-thirds are from alcohol.
- *Beer is mineral-poor.* Beer contains a few minerals, but to replace the minerals lost in sweat, athletes need good sources such as fruit juices.
- *Beer is vitamin-poor.* Beer contains traces of some B vitamins, but it cannot compete with food sources.
- *Beer causes fluid losses.* Beer is a fluid, but alcohol is a diuretic and causes the body to lose valuable fluid.

Diets for Physically Active People

No one diet best supports physical performance. Active people who choose foods within the framework of the diet-planning principles presented in Chapter 2 can design many excellent diets.

Choosing a Diet to Support Fitness

Above all, keep in mind that water is depleted more rapidly than any other nutrient. A diet to support fitness must provide water, energy, and all the other nutrients.

Water Even casual exercisers must attend conscientiously to their fluid needs. Physical activity blunts the thirst mechanism, especially in cold weather. During activity, thirst signals come too late, so don't wait to feel thirsty before drinking. To find out how much water is needed to replenish activity losses, weigh yourself before and after the activity—the difference is almost all water. One-half kilogram equals roughly 2 cups (500 millilitres) of fluid.

Nutrient Density A healthful diet is based on nutrient-dense foods—foods that supply adequate vitamins and minerals for the energy they provide. Active people need to eat both for nutrient adequacy and for energy. A diet that is high in carbohydrate (60 to 70 percent of total kcalories), moderate in fat (20 to 35 percent), and adequate in protein (10 to 20 percent) ensures full glycogen and other nutrient stores.

Carbohydrate On two occasions, the active person's regular high-carbohydrate, ♦ fibre-rich diet may require temporary adjustment. Both of these exceptions involve training for competition rather than for fitness in general. One special

♦ Carbohydrate recommendation for athletes in heavy training: 8 to 10 g/kg body weight

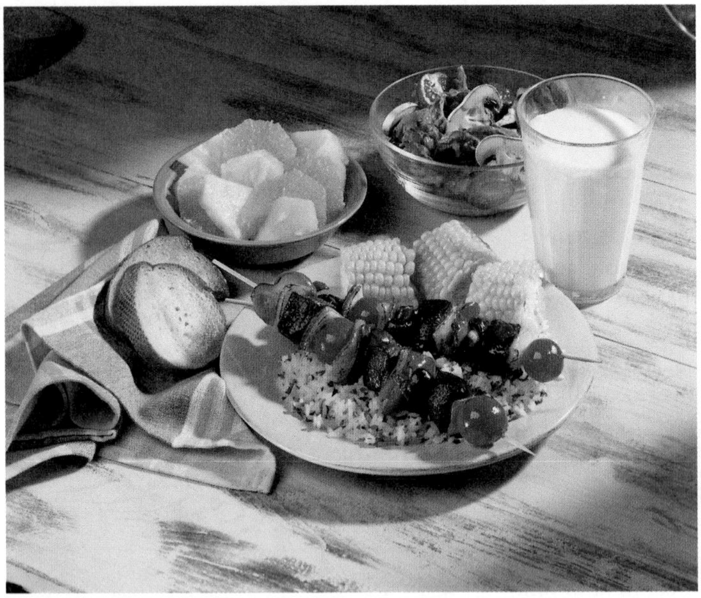

© Polara Studios, Inc.

A variety of foods is the best source of nutrients for athletes.

occasion is the pregame meal, when fibre-rich, bulky foods are best avoided. The pregame meal is discussed in a later section.

The other occasion is during intensive training, when energy needs may be so high ♦ as to outstrip the person's capacity to eat enough food to meet them. The athlete can add concentrated carbohydrate foods, such as dried fruits, sweet potatoes, and nectars, and even high-fat foods, such as avocados and nuts. Still, a nutrient-rich diet remains central for adequacy's sake. Though vital, energy alone is not enough to support performance.

Some athletes use commercial high-carbohydrate liquid supplements to obtain the carbohydrate and energy needed for heavy training and top performance. These supplements do not *replace* regular food; they are meant to be used in *addition* to it. Unlike the sports beverages discussed earlier, these high-carbohydrate supplements are too concentrated in carbohydrate to be used for fluid replacement.

♦ During training, meals for some Olympian athletes provide as much as 12 000 kcalories a day.

Protein In addition to carbohydrate and some fat (and the energy they provide), physically active people need protein. Meats and milk products are rich protein sources, but recommending that active people emphasize these foods is narrow advice. As mentioned repeatedly, active people need diets rich in carbohydrate, and of course, meats have none to offer. Legumes, whole grains, and vegetables provide some protein with abundant carbohydrate. Table 15-5 (p. 484) shows recommended protein intakes for active people.

A Performance Diet Example A person who engages in vigorous physical activity on a daily basis could easily require more than 3000 kcalories per day. To meet this need, the person can choose a variety of nutrient-dense foods. Figure 15-4

FIGURE 15-4 An Example of an Athlete's Meal Selections

This sample menu provides about 3000 kcalories, with almost 520 grams of carbohydrate (63 percent of total kcalories) and about 125 grams of protein (15 percent of total kcalories). In addition to meeting the carbohydrate and protein needs of an athlete, these meals also meet or exceed recommendations for all vitamins and minerals.

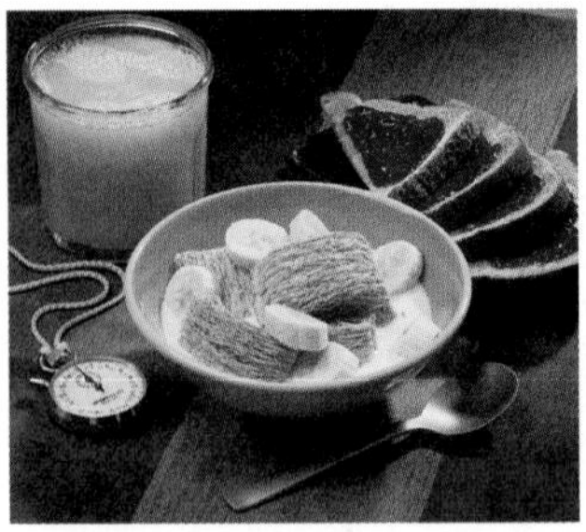

© Polara Studios, Inc

Breakfast
250 mL (1 c) shredded wheat with 1% milk and banana
2 slices whole-wheat toast with jelly
375 mL (1½ c) orange juice

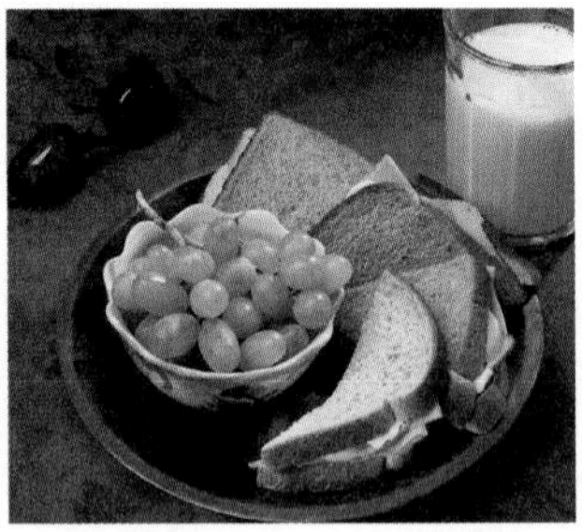

© Polara Studios, Inc

Lunch
2 turkey sandwiches
375 mL (1½ c) 1% milk
Large bunch of grapes

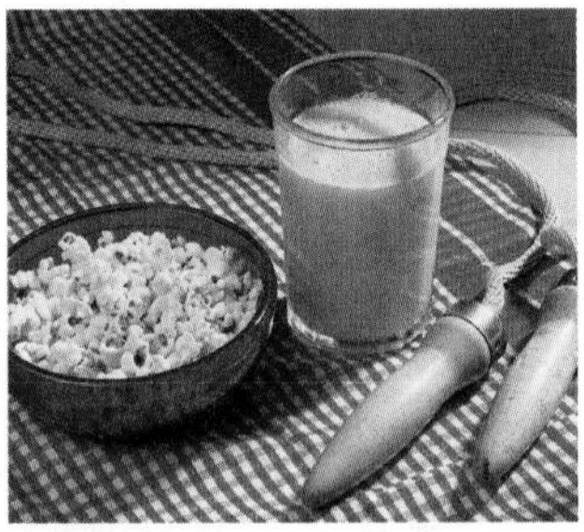

© Polara Studios, Inc

Snack
750 mL (3 c) plain popcorn
A smoothie made from:
375 mL (1½ c) apple juice
1½ frozen banana

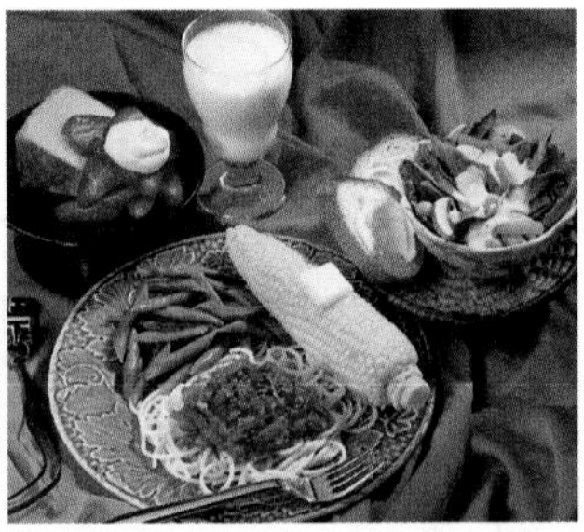

© Polara Studios, Inc

Dinner
Salad: 250 mL (1 c) spinach, carrots, and mushrooms with 125 mL (½ c) garbanzo beans, 15 mL (1 Tbsp) sunflower seeds, and 15 mL (1 Tbsp) ranch salad dressing
250 mL (1 c) spaghetti with meat sauce
250 mL (1 c) green beans
1 corn on the cob
2 slices Italian bread
20 mL (4 tsp) butter
1 piece angel food cake with fresh strawberries and whipping cream
250 mL (1 c) 1% milk

Total kcal: about 3000
63% kcal from carbohydrate
22% kcal from fat
15% kcal from protein
All vitamin and mineral intakes exceed the RDA for both men and women.

shows one example of meals that provide just over 3000 kcalories. These meals supply about 125 grams of protein, more than sufficient in meeting the recommended intake for an athlete weighing 72 kilograms (160 pounds). Obviously, the higher a person's energy intake, the more protein that person will receive, assuming the foods chosen are nutrient dense. This relationship between energy and protein intakes breaks down only when people meet their energy needs with high-fat, high-sugar confections. The meals shown in Figure 15-4 provide almost 520 grams of carbohydrate, or 63 percent of total kcalories. Athletes who train exhaustively for endurance events may want to aim for somewhat higher carbohydrate intakes. Beyond these specific concerns of total energy, protein, and carbohydrate, the diet most beneficial to athletic performance is remarkably similar to the diet recommended for most people.[62]

Meals before and after Competition

No single food improves speed, strength, or skill in competitive events, although some *kinds* of foods do support performance better than others as already explained. Still, a competitor may eat a particular food before or after an event for psychological reasons. One eats a steak the night before wrestling. Another eats a spoonful of honey within minutes of diving. As long as these practices remain harmless, they should be respected.

Pregame Meals Science indicates that the pregame meal or snack should include plenty of fluids and be light and easy to digest. It should provide between 300 and 800 kcalories, primarily from carbohydrate-rich foods that are familiar and well tolerated by the athlete. The meal should end three to four hours before competition to allow time for the stomach to empty before exertion.

Breads, potatoes, pasta, and fruit juices—that is, carbohydrate-rich foods low in fat and fibre—form the basis of the best pregame meal (see Figure 15-5 for some examples). Bulky, fibre-rich foods such as raw vegetables or high-bran cereals, although usually desirable, are best avoided just before competition. Fibre in the digestive tract attracts water and can cause stomach discomfort during performance. Liquid meals ♦ are easy to digest, and many such meals are commercially available. Alternatively, athletes can mix skim milk or juice, frozen fruits, and flavourings in a blender.

♦ High-carbohydrate, liquid pregame meal ideas:
- Apple juice, frozen banana, and cinnamon
- Papaya juice, frozen strawberries, and mint
- Skim milk, frozen banana, and vanilla

Postgame Meals As mentioned earlier, eating high-carbohydrate foods *after* physical activity enhances glycogen storage. Because people are usually not

FIGURE 15-5 Examples of High-Carbohydrate Pregame Meals

Pregame meals should be eaten three to four hours before the event and provide 300 to 800 kcalories, primarily from carbohydrate-rich foods. Each of these sample meals provides at least 65 percent of total kcalories from carbohydrate.

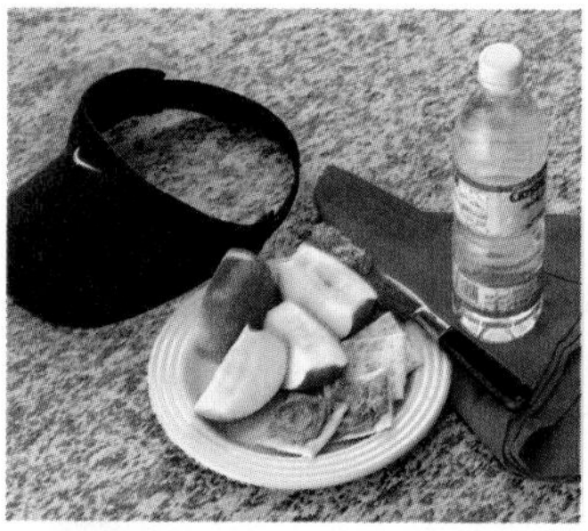
© Matt Farruggio

300-kcalorie meal
1 large apple
4 saltine crackers
22 mL (1 1/2 Tbsp) reduced-fat peanut butter

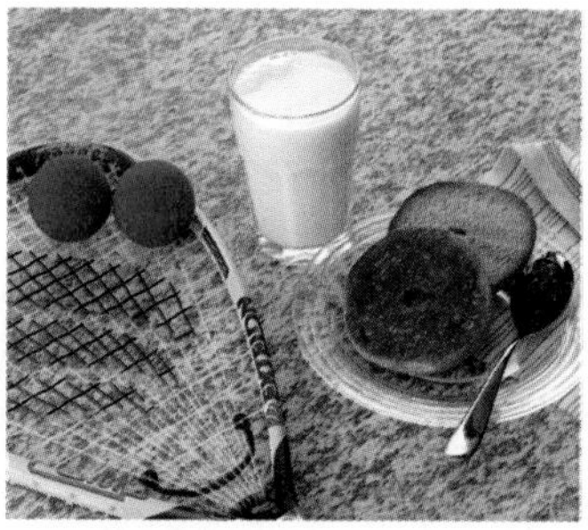
© Matt Farruggio

500-kcalorie meal
1 large whole-wheat bagel
30 mL (2 Tbsp) jelly
375 mL (1½ c) 1% milk

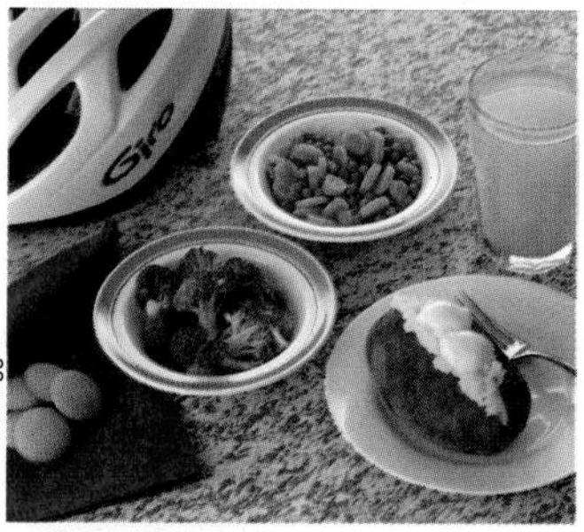
Giro
© Matt Farruggio

750-kcalorie meal
1 large baked potato
10 mL (2 tsp) margarine
250 mL (1 c) steamed broccoli
250 mL (1 c) mixed carrots and green peas
5 vanilla wafers
375 mL (1½ c) apple or pineapple juice

hungry immediately following physical activity, carbohydrate-containing beverages such as sports drinks or fruit juices may be preferred. If an active person does feel hungry after an event, then foods high in carbohydrate, moderate in protein, and low in fat and fibre are the ones to choose—similar to those recommended prior to competition.

IN SUMMARY **The person who wants to excel physically will apply accurate nutrition knowledge along with dedication to rigorous training. A diet that provides ample fluid and includes a variety of nutrient-dense foods in quantities to meet energy needs will enhance not only athletic performance, but overall health as well. Carbohydrate-rich foods that are light and easy to digest are recommended for both the pregame and the postgame meal. Training and genetics being equal, who will win a competition—the athlete who habitually consumes inadequate amounts of needed nutrients or the competitor who arrives at the event with a long history of full nutrient stores and well-met metabolic needs?**

Some athletes learn that nutrition can support physical performance and turn to pills and powders instead of foods. In case you need further convincing that a healthful diet surpasses such potions, the following highlight addresses this issue.

Nutrition Portfolio

The foods and beverages you eat and drink provide fuel and other nutrients to support your physical activity.

Go to Diet Analysis Plus and choose one of the days on which you tracked your diet and activity for an entire day. Select the Activities Spreadsheet report to help you answer the following.

- Describe your daily physical activities and how they compare with recommendations to engage in at least 150 minutes of moderate- to vigorous-intensity activity per week and strengthening activities at least twice per week.

Now click on the Intake vs. Goals report and consider the following:

- Estimate your daily fluid intake, making note of whether you drink fluids, especially water, before, during, and after physical activity.
- Evaluate the carbohydrate contents of your diet and consider whether it would meet the needs of a physically active person.

Diet Analysis PLUS **To complete this exercise, go to your Diet Analysis Plus at www.cengage.com/sso.**

Nutrition on the Net

CENGAGENOW™
For further study of topics covered in this chapter, log on to **www.cengage.com/sso.**

- Visit the Healthy Living, Physical Activity section of the Public Health Agency of Canada website: **www.phac-aspc.gc.ca/hp-ps/hl-mvs/pa-ap/index-eng.php**
- Learn about current research and trends in physical activity among Canadians at the Canadian Fitness and Lifestyle Research Institute: **www.cflri.ca**
- Find practical information on getting active at ParticipACTION: **www.participaction.com**
- Visit the Canadian Council of Sports Medicine: **www.ccsm.info**
- Find information at the American College of Sports Medicine: **www.acsm.org**
- Review resources offered on the Nutrition, Physical Activity, and Obesity division of the U.S. Centers for Disease Control and Prevention: **www.cdc.gov/nccdphp/dnpao**
- Find information on sports drinks and other nutrition and fitness topics at the Gatorade Sports Science Institute site: **www.gssiweb.com**

References

1. P. T. Katzmarzyk and coauthors, Sitting time and mortality from all causes, cardiovascular disease, and cancer, *Medicine & Science in Sports & Exercise* 41 (2009): 998–1005.
2. M. Hamer and E. Stamatakis, Physical activity and risk of cardiovascular disease events: Inflammatory and metabolic mechanisms, *Medicine & Science in Sports & Exercise* 41 (2009): 1206–1211; Centers for Disease Control and Prevention, www.cdc.gov/physicalactivity/everyone; site updated October 7, 2008, and accessed October 20, 2008; X. Yang and coauthors, The longitudinal effects of physical activity history on metabolic syndrome, *Medicine & Science in Sports & Exercise* 40 (2008): 1424–1431; L. B. Yates and coauthors, Exceptional longevity in men, *Archives of Internal Medicine* 168 (2008): 284–290; X. Sui and coauthors, Cardiorespiratory fitness and adiposity as mortality predictors in older adults, *Journal of the American Medical Association* 298 (2007): 2507–2516; T. S. Altena and coauthors, Lipoprotein subfraction changes after continuous or intermittent exercise training, *Medicine & Science in Sports & Exercise* 38 (2006): 367–372.; D. E. Warburton, C. W. Nicol, and S. S. Bredin, Health benefits of physical activity: The evidence, *Canadian Medical Association Journal* 174 (2006): 801–809; P.T. Katzmarzyk, N. Gledhill, and R. J. Shephard, The economic burden of physical inactivity in Canada, *Canadian Medical Association Journal* 163 (2000): 1435–1440; P. T. Katzmarzyk, T. S. Church, and S. N. Blair, Cardiorespiratory fitness attenuates the effects of the metabolic syndrome on all-cause and cardiovascular disease mortality in men, *Archives of Internal Medicine* 164 (2004): 1092–1097; J. A. Romijn and coauthors, Substrate metabolism during different exercise intensities in endurance-trained women, *Journal of Applied Physiology* 88 (2000): 1707–1714.
3. Canadian Fitness and Lifestyle Research Institute, Physical activity levels of Canadians, *2008 Physical Activity Monitor,* (2009): 1-2. http://72.10.49.94/node/82, accessed September 12, 2011; Human Resources and Skills Development Canada, Indicators of well-being in Canada: Physical activity (2005). www4.hrsdc.gc.ca/.3ndic.1t.4r@-eng .jsp?iid=8, accessed August 21, 2010.
4. V. A. Narkar and coauthors, AMPK and PPARδ agonists are exercise mimetics, *Cell* 134 (2008): 1–11.
5. P. Anand and coauthors, Cancer is a preventable disease that requires major lifestyle changes, *Pharmaceutical Research* 25 (2008): 2097–2116; N. Orsini and coauthors, Combined effects of obesity and physical activity in predicting mortality among men, *Journal of Internal Medicine* 264 (2008): 442–451; A. R. Weinstein and coauthors, The joint effects of physical activity and body mass index on coronary heart disease risk in women, *Archives of Internal Medicine* 168 (2008): 884–890; Yang and coauthors, 2008; R. D. Telford, Low physical activity and obesity: Causes of chronic disease or simply predictors? *Medicine & Science in Sports & Exercise* 39 (2007): 1233–1240.
6. M. J. Tremblay, New Canadian Physical Activity Guidelines, *Journal of Applied Physiology, Nutrition, and Metabolism* 36 (2011): 36–46; Canadian Society for Exercise Physiology, *Canadian Physical Activity Guidelines.* www.csep.ca/guidelines, accessed September 12, 2011.
7. S. J. Elder and S. B. Roberts, The effects of exercise on food intake and body fatness: A summary of published studies, *Nutrition* Reviews 65 (2007): 1–19; P. T. Williams, Maintaining vigorous activity attenuates 7-yr weight gain in 8340 runners, *Medicine & Science in Sports & Exercise* 39 (2007): 801–809; P. T. Williams and R. R. Pate, Cross-sectional relationships of exercise and age to adiposity in 60,617 male runners, *Medicine & Science in Sports & Exercise* 37 (2005): 1329–1337.
8. N. A. Lynch and coauthors, Older elite football players have reduced cardiac and osteoporosis risk factors, *Medicine & Science in Sports & Exercise* 39 (2007): 1124–1130; K. M. Shedd and coauthors, Quantifying leisure physical activity and its relation to bone density and strength, *Medicine & Science in Sports & Exercise* 39 (2007): 2189–2198; American College of Sports Medicine, Position stand: Physical activity and bone health, *Medicine & Science in Sports & Exercise* 36 (2004): 1985–1996.
9. M. Gleeson, Immune function in sport and exercise, *Journal of Applied Physiology* 103 (2007): 693–699; M. H Arai, A. J Duarte, and V. M. Natale, The effects of long-term training on the immune and endocrine systems of elderly men: The role of cytokines and anabolic hormones, *Immunity & Ageing* 3 (2006): 9.
10. World Cancer Research Fund/American Institute for Cancer Research, *Food, Nutrition, Physical Activity, and the Prevention of Cancer: A Global Perspective* (Washington, D.C.: AICR, 2007), pp. 244–321; B. Tehard and coauthors, Effect of physical activity on women at increased risk of breast cancer: Results from the E3N cohort study, *Cancer Epidemiology, Biomarkers, and Prevention* 15 (2006): 57–64.
11. P. T. Williams, Reduced diabetic, hypertensive, and cholesterol medication use with walking, *Medicine & Science in Sports & Exercise* 40 (2008): 433–443; S. Kodama and coauthors, Effect of aerobic exercise training on serum levels of high-density lipoprotein cholesterol, *Archives of Internal Medicine* 167 (2007): 999–1008; M. M. Lockard and coauthors, Exercise training-induced changes in coagulation factors in older adults, *Medicine & Science in Sports & Exercise* 39 (2007): 587–592; T. Rankinen and coauthors, Cardiorespiratory fitness, BMI, and risk of hypertension: The HYPGENE Study, *Medicine & Science in Sports & Exercise* 39 (2007): 1687–1692; J. W. Starnes and R. P. Taylor, Exercise-induced cardioprotection: Endogenous mechanisms, *Medicine & Science in Sports & Exercise* 39 (2007): 1537–1543; L. K. Stewart and coauthors, The influence of exercise training on inflammatory cytokines and C-reactive protein, *Medicine & Science in Sports & Exercise* 39 (2007): 1714–1719; M. B. Conroy and coauthors, Past physical activity, current physical activity, and risk of coronary heart disease, *Medicine & Science in Sports & Exercise* 37 (2005): 1251–1256.
12. M. Fogelhom, How physical activity can work? *International Journal of Pediatric Obesity* 3 (2008): 10–14; B. A. Irving and coauthors, Effect of exercise training intensity on abdominal visceral fat and body composition, *Medicine & Science in Sports & Exercise* 40 (2008): 1863–1872; K. Wijndaele and coauthors, Muscular strength, aerobic fitness, and metabolic syndrome risk in Flemish adults, *Medicine & Science in Sports & Exercise* 39 (2007): 233–240.
13. C. Y. Jeon and coauthors, Physical activity of moderate intensity and risk of type 2 diabetes: A systematic review, *Diabetes Care* 30 (2007): 744–752; S. A. Kavouras and coauthors, Physical activity, obesity status, and glycemic control: The ATTICA Study, *Medicine & Science in Sports & Exercise* 39 (2007): 606–611; R. J. Sigal and coauthors, Effects of aerobic training, resistance training, or both on glycemic control in type 2 diabetes, *Annals of Internal Medicine* 147 (2007): 357–369.
14. A. M. Kriska and coauthors, Physical activity and gallbladder disease determined by ultrasonography, *Medicine & Science in Sports & Exercise* 39 (2007): 1927–1932; K. L. Storti and coauthors, Physical activity and decreased risk of clinical gallstone disease among post-menopausal women, *Preventive Medicine* 41 (2005): 772–777.
15. D. B. Nelson and coauthors, Effect of physical activity on menopausal symptoms among urban women, *Medicine & Science in Sports & Exercise* 40 (2008): 50–58; J. A. Blumenthal and coauthors, Exercise and pharmacotherapy in the treatment of major depressive disorder, *Psychosomatic Medicine* 69 (2007): 587–596; D. I. Galper and coauthors, Inverse association between physical inactivity and mental health in men and women, *Medicine & Science in Sports & Exercise* 38 (2006): 173–178; J. B. Bartholomew, D. Morrison, and J. T. Ciccolo, Effects of acute exercise on mood and well-being in patients with major depressive disorder, *Medicine & Science in Sports & Exercise* 37 (2005): 2032–2037.
16. P. Kokkinos and coauthors, Exercise capacity and mortality in black and white men, *Circulation* 117 (2008): 614–622; Yates and coauthors, 2008; Sui and coauthors, 2007; T. M. Manini and coauthors, Daily activity energy expenditure and mortality among older adults, *Journal of the American Medical Association* 296 (2006): 171–179.
17. P. Aagaard and coauthors, Mechanical muscle function, morphology, and fiber type in lifelong trained elderly, *Medicine & Science in Sports & Exercise* 39 (2007): 1989–1996; M. E. Nelson and coauthors, Physical activity and public health in older adults: Recommendation from the American College of Sports Medicine and the American Heart Association, *Medicine & Science in Sports & Exercise* 39 (2007): 1435–1445; N. Takeshima and coauthors, Functional fitness gain varies in older adults

depending on exercise mode, *Medicine & Science in Sports & Exercise* 39 (2007): 2036–2043.

18. M. J. Tremblay, New Canadian Physical Activity Guidelines, *Journal of Applied Physiology, Nutrition, and Metabolism* 36 (2011): 36–46; D. E. R. Warburton, S. Charlesworth, A. Ivey, L. Nettlefold, and S. S. D. Bredin, A systematic review of the evidence for Canada's Physical Activity Guidelines for Adults, *International Journal of Behavioral Nutrition and Physical Activity* 7 (2010): 39; D. E. R. Warburton, C. W. Nicol, S. S. D. Bredin, Health benefits of physical activity: The evidence, *Canadian Medical Association Journal* 174 (2006): 801–809; Canadian Society for Exercise Physiology, *Canadian Physical Activity Guidelines*.
19. Canadian Society for Exercise Physiology, *Canadian Physical Activity Guidelines*; Public Health Agency of Canada, Tips to Get Active, www.phac-aspc.gc.ca/hp-ps/hl-mvs/pa-ap/04paap-eng.php.
20. Centers for Disease Control and Prevention, www.health.gov/paguidelines/guidelines/chapter2.aspx; site updated October 7, 2008, and accessed October 21, 2008; W. L. Haskell and coauthors, Physical activity and public health: Updated recommendation for adults from the American College of Sports Medicine and the American Heart Association, *Medicine & Science in Sports & Exercise* 39 (2007): 1423–1434; Warburton, Nicol, and Bredin, 2006.
21. M. S. Tremblay and coauthors, Physiological and health implications of a sedentary lifestyle, *Applied Physiology, Nutrition and Metabolism* 35 (2010): 725–740; D. E. R. Warburton, C. W. Nicol, S. S. D. Bredin, Prescribing exercise as preventive therapy, *Canadian Medical Association Journal* 174 (2006): 961–974; American College of Sports Medicine, *ACSM's Guidelines for Exercise Testing and Prescription,* 7th ed. (Philadelphia, Pa.: Lippincott, Williams, and Wilkins, 2006), pp. 19–35.
22. Rankinen and coauthors, 2007; American College of Sports Medicine, Position stand: Exercise and hypertension, *Medicine & Science in Sports & Exercise* 36 (2004): 533–553.
23. American College of Sports Medicine, 2004, pp. 1985–1996.
24. K. T. Borer, Physical activity in the prevention and amelioration of osteoporosis in women: Interaction of mechanical, hormonal and dietary factors, *Sports Medicine* 35 (2005): 779–830.
25. American College of Sports Medicine, Position stand: Progression models in resistance training for healthy adults, *Medicine & Science in Sports & Exercise* 41 (2009): 687–708; Haskell and coauthors, 2007; Nelson and coauthors, 2007.
26 S. Karikanta and coauthors, A multi-component exercise regimen to prevent functional decline and bone fragility in home-dwelling elderly women: Randomized, controlled trial, *Osteoporosis International* 18 (2007): 453–462; Nelson and coauthors, 2007; J. A. Katula and coauthors, Strength training in older adults: An empowering intervention, *Medicine & Science in Sports & Exercise* 38 (2006): 106–111.
27. American College of Sports Medicine, Position stand: Progression models in resistance training for healthy adults, *Medicine & Science in Sports & Exercise* 41 (2009): 687–708.
28. R. Beneke and D. Böning, The limits of human performance, *Essays in Biochemistry* 44 (2008): 11–25.
29. J. Bergstrom and coauthors, Diet, muscle glycogen and physical performance, *Acta Physiologica Scandanavica* 71 (1967): 140–150.
30. A. M. Bellinger and coauthors, Remodeling of ryanodine receptor complex causes "leaky" channels: A molecular mechanism for decreased exercise capacity, *Proceedings of the National Academy of Sciences* 105 (2008): 2198–2202; S. P. Cairns, Lactic acid and exercise performance: Culprit or friend? *Sports Medicine* 36 (2006): 279–291; J. P. Weir and coauthors, Is fatigue all in your head? A critical review of the central governor model, *British Journal of Sports Medicine* 40 (2006): 573–586; A. Philp, A. L. Macdonald, and P. W. Watt, Lactate: A signal coordinating cell and systemic function, *Journal of Experimental Biology* 208 (2005): 4561–4575.
31. A. Foskett and coauthors, Carbohydrate availability and muscle energy metabolism during intermittent running, *Medicine & Science in Sports & Exercise* 40 (2008): 96–103; S. G. Harger-Domitrovich and coauthors, Exogenous carbohydrate spares muscle glycogen in men and women during 10 h of exercise, *Medicine & Science in Sports & Exercise* 39 (2007): 2171–2179; J. J. Winnick and coauthors, Carbohydrate feedings during team sport exercise preserve physical and CNS function, *Medicine & Science in Sports & Exercise* 37 (2005): 306–315.
32. American College of Sports Medicine, Position stand: Exercise and fluid replacement, *Medicine & Science in Sports & Exercise* 39 (2007): 377–390.
33. American College of Sports Medicine, 2007, pp. 377–390.
34. B. C. Romano-Ely and coauthors, Effect of an isocaloric carbohydrate-protein antioxidant drink on cycling performance, *Medicine & Science in Sports & Exercise* 38 (2006): 1608–1616; M. Van Essen and M. J. Gibala, Failure of protein to improve time trial performance when added to a sports drink, *Medicine & Science in Sports & Exercise* 38 (2006): 1476–1483.
35. Van Essen and Gibala, 2006.
36. Position of the American Dietetic Association, Dietitians of Canada, and the American College of Sports Medicine: Nutrition and athletic performance, *Journal of the American Dietetic Association* 109 (2009): 509–527; G. A. Wallis and coauthors, Postexercise muscle glycogen synthesis with combined glucose and fructose ingestion, *Medicine & Science in Sports & Exercise* 40 (2008): 1789–1794.
37. E. J. Coleman, Carbohydrate and exercise, in *Sports Nutrition: A Practical Manual for Professionals,* 4th ed., ed. M. Dunford (Chicago: The American Dietetic Association, 2006), pp. 14–32.
38. S. L. Wee and coauthors, Ingestion of a high-glycemic index meal increases muscle glycogen storage at rest but augments its utilization during subsequent exercise, *Journal of Applied Physiology* 99 (2005): 707–714.
39. C. M. Cook and M. D. Haud, Low-carbohydrate diets and performance, *Current Sports Medicine Reports* 6 (2007): 225–229.
40. L. Havemann and coauthors, Fat adaptation followed by carbohydrate loading compromises high-intensity sprint performance, *Journal of Applied Physiology* 100 (2006): 194–202.
41. Position of the American Dietetic Association, Dietitians of Canada, and the American College of Sports Medicine, 2009.
42. K. D. Tipton and A. A. Ferrando, Improving muscle mass: Response of muscle metabolism to exercise, nutrition, and anabolic agents, *Essays in Biochemistry* 44 (2008): 85–98; T. G. Anthony and coauthors, Feeding meals containing soy or whey protein after exercise stimulates protein synthesis and translation initiation in the skeletal muscle of male rats, *Journal of Nutrition* 137 (2007): 357–362; N. R. Rodriguez, L. M. Vislocky, and P. Courtney Gaine, Dietary protein, endurance exercise, and human skeletal-muscle protein turnover, *Current Opinion in Clinical and Metabolic Care* 10 (2007): 40–45; R. R. Wolfe, Skeletal muscle protein metabolism and resistance exercise, *Journal of Nutrition* 136 (2006): 525S–528S.
43. S. M. Phillips, Dietary protein for athletes: From requirements to metabolic advantage, *Applied Physiology, Nutrition, and Metabolism* 31 (2006): 647–654.
44. Position of the American Dietetic Association, Dietitians of Canada, and the American College of Sports Medicine, 2009; Committee on Dietary Reference Intakes, *Dietary Reference Intakes for Energy, Carbohydrate, Fiber, Fat, Fatty Acids, Cholesterol, Protein, and Amino Acids* (Washington, D.C.: National Academies Press, 2005), pp. 660–661.
45. Position of the American Dietetic Association, Dietitians of Canada, and the American College of Sports Medicine, 2009.
46 Position of the American Dietetic Association, Dietitians of Canada, and the American College of Sports Medicine, 2009; American College of Sports Medicine, Position stand: The female athlete triad, *Medicine & Science in Sports & Exercise* 39 (2007): 1867–1882.
47. M. J. Jackson, Free radicals generated by contracting muscle; By-products of metabolism or key regulators of muscle function? *Free Radical Biology & Medicine* 44 (2008): 132–141; S. Sachdev and K. J. Davies, Production, detection, and adaptive responses to free radicals in exercise, *Free Radical Biology & Medicine* 44 (2008): 215–223; J. Finaud G. Lac, and E. Filaire, Oxidative stress: Relationship with exercise and training, *Sports Medicine* 36 (2006): 327–358; A. Mastaloudis and coauthors, Antioxidants did not prevent muscle damage in response to an ultramarathon run, *Medicine & Science in Sports & Exercise* 38 (2006): 72–80.
48. W. L. Knex, D. G. Jenkins, and J. S. Coombes, Oxidative stress in half and full ironman triathletes, *Medicine & Science in Sports & Exercise* 39 (2007): 283–288; S. L. Williams and coauthors, Antioxidant requirements of endurance athletes: Implications for health, *Nutrition Reviews* 64 (2006): 93–108.

49. M. C. Gomez-Cabrera, E. Domenech, and J. Vina, Moderate exercise is an antioxidant: Upregulation of antioxidant genes by training, *Free Radical Biology & Medicine* 44 (2008): 126–131; Jackson, 2008; Sachdev and Davies, 2008; J. Padilla and T. D. Mickleborough, Does antioxidant supplementation prevent favorable adaptations to exercise training? *Medicine & Science in Sports & Exercise* 39 (2007): 1887; L. L. Ji , M. C. Gomez-Cabrera, and J. Vina, Exercise and hormesis: Activation of cellular antioxidant signaling pathway, *Annals of the New York Academy of Sciences* 1067 (2006): 425–435.
50. S. S. Gropper and coauthors, Iron status of female collegiate athletes involved in different sports, *Biological Trace Element Research* 109 (2006): 1–14; S. L. Akabas and K. R. Dolins, Micronutrient requirements of physically active women: What can we learn from iron? *American Journal of Clinical Nutrition* 81 (2005): 1246S–1251S.
51. R. E. Rodenberg and S. Gustafson, Iron as an ergogenic aid: Ironclad evidence? *Current Sports Medicine Reports* 6 (2007): 258–264.
52. Position of the American Dietetic Association, Dietitians of Canada, and the American College of Sports Medicine, 2009; A. M. Venderley and W. W. Campbell, Vegetarian diets: Nutritional considerations for athletes, *Sports Medicine* 36 (2006): 293–305.
53. P. S. Hinton and L. M. Sinclair, Iron supplementation maintains ventilatory threshold and improves energetic efficiency in iron-deficient non-anemic athletes, *European Journal of Clinical Nutrition* 61 (2007): 30–39.
54. American College of Sports Medicine, 2007, pp. 377–390; D. J. Casa, P. M. Clarkson, and W. O. Roberts, American College of Sports Medicine Roundtable on Hydration and Physical Activity: Consensus Statements, *Current Sports Medicine Reports* 4 (2005): 115–127; Committee on Dietary Reference Intakes, *Dietary Reference Intakes for Water, Potassium, Sodium, Chloride, and Sulfate* (Washington, D.C.: National Academies Press, 2005), pp. 108–110; R. J. Maughan and S. M. Shirreffs, Development of individual hydration strategies for athletes, International Journal of Sport Nutrition and Exercise Metabolism 18 (2008): 457–472; B. Murray, Hydration and physical performance, Journal of the American College of Nutrition 26 (2007): 542S–548S.
55. C. K. Seto, D. Way, and N. O'Connor, Environmental illness in athletes, *Clinics in Sports Medicine* 24 (2005): 695–718.
56. Casa, Clarkson, and Roberts, 2005.
57. M. N. Sawka, L. M. Burke, E. R. Eichner, R. J. Maughan, S. J. Montain, and N. S. Stachenfeld, Exercise and fluid replacement, Medicine & Science in Sports & Exercise (2007). DOI: 10.1249/mss.0b013e31802ca597.
58. American College of Sports Medicine, 2007, pp. 377–390; Seto, Way, and O'Connor, 2005.
59. Committee on Dietary Reference Intakes, 2005.
60. American College of Sports Medicine, 2007, pp. 377–390.
61. Position of the American Dietetic Association, Dietitians of Canada, and the American College of Sports Medicine, 2009; S. L. Ballard, J. J. Wellborn-Kim, and K. A. Clauson, Effects of commercial energy drink consumption on athletic performance and body composition, *The Physician and Sportsmedicine* 38 (2010). DOI: 10.3810/psm.2010.04.1768; E. Duchan, N. D. Patel, and C. Feucht, Energy drinks: A review of use and safety for athletes, *The Physician and Sportsmedicine* 38 (2010). DOI: 10.3810/psm.2010.06.1796.
62. Position of the American Dietetic Association, Dietitians of Canada, and the American College of Sports Medicine, 2009.

HIGHLIGHT 15

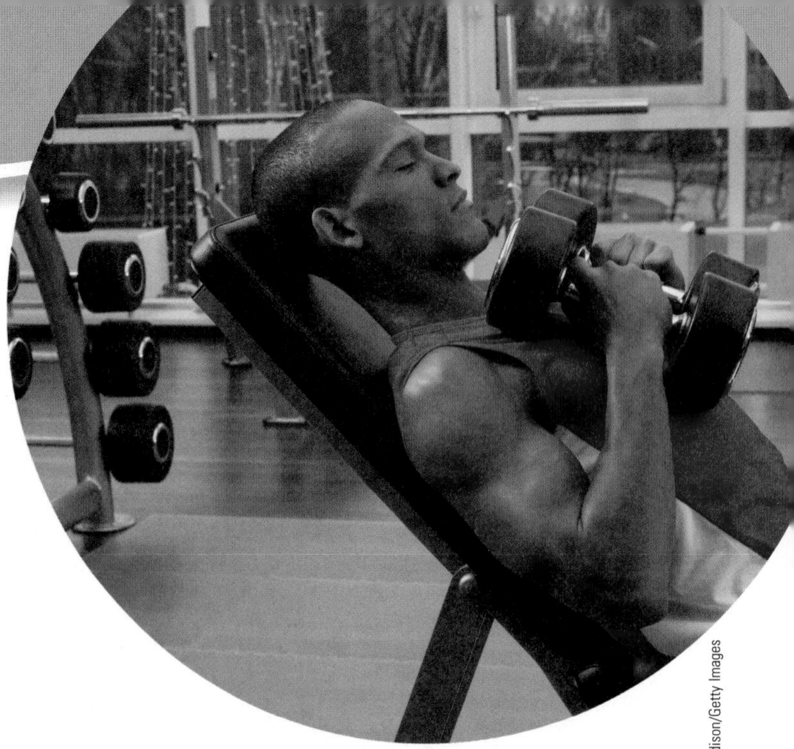

David Madison/Getty Images

Supplements as Ergogenic Aids

Athletes gravitate to promises that they can enhance their performance by taking pills, powders, or potions. Unfortunately, they often hear such promises from their coaches and peers, who advise them to use nutrient supplements, take drugs, or follow procedures that claim to deliver results with little effort.[1] When such performance-enhancing aids are harmless, they are only a waste of money; when they impair performance or harm health, they waste athletic potential and cost lives. This highlight looks at some promises of magic to enhance physical performance.

Ergogenic Aids

Many substances or treatments claim to be *ergogenic,* meaning work enhancing. The accompanying glossary defines several of the commonly used **ergogenic aids** discussed in this highlight. Table H15-1 presents additional substances promoted as ergogenic aids. For the large majority of these substances, research findings do not support those claims.[2] Athletes who hear that a product is ergogenic should ask who is making the claim and who will profit from the sale.

Athletes who supplement their diets with products promoted to improve athletic performance should be aware that some supplements are contaminated with illegal substances such as steroids that are not listed on the label.[3] In one study, researchers analysed the composition of more than 100 supplements (creatine, prohormones, "mental enhancers," and branched-chain amino acids).[4] Three of the supplements contained high levels of an anabolic steroid, several other products contained traces of hormones not listed on the label, and many contained other substances not declared on the label. Supplements contaminated with illegal substances pose health risks to those who use them as well as the risk of positive drug testing for athletes subject to such tests.

Sometimes it is difficult to distinguish valid claims from bogus ones. Fitness magazines and Internet websites are particularly troublesome because many of them present both valid and invalid nutrition information along with slick advertisements for nutrition products. Advertisements often feature colourful anatomical figures, graphs, and tables that appear scientific. Some ads even include references, citing or linking to such credible sources as the *American Journal of Clinical Nutrition* and the *Journal of the American Medical Association.* These ads create the illusion of endorsement and credibility to gain readers' trust. Keep in mind, however, that the ads are created not to teach, but to sell. A careful reading of the cited research might reveal that the ads have presented the research findings out of context. For example, an ad might use a research article to conclude that its human growth hormone supplement "increases lean body mass and bone mineral," when in fact,

GLOSSARY

Table H15-1 includes additional supplements commonly used to enhance performance.

anabolic steroids: drugs related to the male sex hormone, testosterone, that stimulate the development of lean body mass.

- **anabolic** = promoting growth
- **sterols** = compounds chemically related to cholesterol

androstenedione: *See DHEA.*

caffeine: a natural stimulant found in many common foods and beverages, including coffee, tea, and chocolate; may enhance endurance by stimulating fatty acid release. High doses cause headaches, trembling, rapid heart rate, and other undesirable side-effects.

carnitine: a nonessential nonprotein amino acid made in the body from lysine that helps transport fatty acids across the mitochondrial membrane. Carnitine supposedly "burns" fat and spares glycogen during endurance events, but in reality it does neither.

chromium picolinate (CROW-mee-um pick-oh-LYN-ate): a trace mineral supplement; falsely promoted as building muscle, enhancing energy, and burning fat. **Picolinate** is a derivative of the amino acid tryptophan that seems to enhance chromium absorption.

conjugated linoleic acid: a naturally occuring *trans* fatty acid with 18 carbons and 2 double bonds; sometimes taken as a supplement to improve body composition.

creatine (KREE-ah-tin): a nitrogen-containing compound that combines with phosphate to form the high-energy compound creatine phosphate (or phosphocreatine) in muscles. Claims that creatine enhances energy use and muscle strength need further confirmation.

DHEA (dehydroepiandrosterone) and **androstenedione:** hormones made in the adrenal glands that serve as precursors to the male hormone, testosterone; falsely promoted as burning fat, building muscle, and slowing aging. Side-effects include acne, aggressiveness, and liver enlargement.

ergogenic (ER-go-JEN-ick) **aids:** substances or techniques used in an attempt to enhance physical performance.

- **ergo** = work
- **genic** = gives rise to

hGH (human growth hormone): a hormone produced by the brain's pituitary gland that regulates normal growth and development; also called *somatotropin.* Some athletes misuse this hormone to increase their height and strength.

TABLE H15-1 Substances Promoted as Ergogenic Aids

Dietary Supplement	Claims	Research Findings	Risks
Arginine (an amino acid)	Increases muscle mass	Ineffective	Generally well tolerated; may be harmful to people with heart disease
Boron (trace mineral)	Increases muscle mass	Ineffective	No adverse effects reported with doses up to 10 mg/day; should be avoided by those with kidney disease or women with hormone-sensitive conditions
Coenzyme Q_{10} (carrier in the electron transport chain)	Enhances exercise performance	Ineffective	Mild indigestion
Gamma-oryzanol (plant sterol)	Increases muscle mass; mimics anabolic steroids without known side-effects	Ineffective	No adverse effects reported with short-term use; no long-term safety studies
Ginseng (plant)	Enhances exercise performance	Ineffective	No adverse effects reported with moderate doses; large doses may cause hypertension, nervousness, sleeplessness, acne, edema, headache, and diarrhea; those with diabetes should be aware of hypoglycemic effects; should be avoided by those at risk for estrogen-related cancers, those with blood clotting issues, and pregnant or lactating women
Glycerol (a 3-carbon molecule that is part of triglycerides and phospholipids)	Improves hydration during exercise; regulates body temperature during exercise; enhances exercise performance	Inconsistent findings for improving hydration and regulating body temperature; ineffective for enhancing exercise performance	May cause nausea, headaches, and blurred vision; should be avoided by those with edema, congestive heart failure, kidney disease, hypertension, and other conditions that may be aggravated by fluid retention
HMB (beta-hydroxy-beta-methylbutyrate) (a metabolite of the branched-chain amino acid leucine)	Increases muscle mass and strength	Inconsistent findings	No adverse effects with short-term use and doses up to 76 mg/kg of body weight
Pyruvate (a 3-carbon sugar)	Enhances exercise endurance	Ineffective	No long-term safety studies; digestive problems with short-term use (<6 weeks)
Ribose (a 5-carbon sugar)	Increases ATP production and enhances high-intensity exercise performance	Ineffective	Naturally generated in body
Royal jelly (produced by bees)	Enhances stamina and reduces fatigue	No studies on human beings to date	No adverse effects with doses up to 12 mg/day; should be avoided by those with a history of asthma or allergic reactions
Sodium bicarbonate (baking soda)	Reduces lactic acid and delays fatigue; enhances power and strength	May reduce lactic acid and muscle fatigue; more research is needed for definitive conclusions	Gastrointestinal distress including diarrhea, cramps, and bloating; should be avoided by those on sodium-restricted diets

SOURCES: Adapted from A. S. Fragakis and C. Thomson, *The Health Professional's Guide to Popular Dietary Supplements,* 3rd ed. (Chicago: American Dietetic Association, 2007); M. Dunford and M. Smith, Dietary supplements and ergogenic aids, in *Sports Nutrition: A Practice Manual for Professionals,* 4th ed., M. Dunford (Chicago: American Dietetic Association, 2006), pp. 116–141.

the researchers would conclude that "its general use now or in the immediate future is not justified." Scientific facts are often exaggerated and twisted to promote sales. Highlight 1 describes ways to recognize misinformation and quackery.

Dietary Supplements

A variety of supplements make claims based on misunderstood nutrition principles. The claims may sound good, but for the most part, they have little or no factual basis. Chapter 6 includes a discussion on protein powders and amino acid supplements (pp. 193–194).

Carnitine

Carnitine, a nonessential nutrient, is often promoted to bodybuilders as a "fat burner." Some endurance athletes believe carnitine will help them burn more fat, thereby sparing glycogen during long-distance events.

In the body, carnitine facilitates the transfer of fatty acids across the mitochondrial membrane. Supplement manufacturers suggest that with more carnitine available, fat oxidation will be enhanced, but this does not seem to be the case. Carnitine supplementation neither raises muscle carnitine concentrations nor enhances exercise performance.[5] Milk and meat products are good sources of carnitine, and supplements are not needed.

Chromium Picolinate

Chapter 10 introduces chromium as an essential trace mineral involved in carbohydrate and lipid metabolism. Advertisements in bodybuilding magazines claim that **chromium picolinate,** which is more easily absorbed than chromium alone, builds muscle, enhances energy, and burns fat. Such claims derive from one or two initial studies reporting that men who weight trained while taking chromium picolinate supplements increased lean body mass and reduced body fat. Most subsequent studies, however, show no effects of chromium picolinate supplementation on strength, lean body mass, or body fat.[6] Chromium-rich foods include whole grains, liver, and nuts. Athletes who have adequate energy intakes from a variety of foods are unlikely to be chromium deficient.

Complete Nutrition Supplements

Several drinks and chocolate bars appeal to athletes by claiming to provide "complete" nutrition. These products usually taste good and provide extra food energy, but they fall short of providing "complete" nutrition. They can be useful as a pregame meal or a between-meal snack, but they should not replace regular meals.

A nutritionally "complete" drink may help a nervous athlete who cannot tolerate solid food on the day of an event. A liquid meal two or three hours before competition can supply some of the fluid and carbohydrate needed in a pregame meal, but a shake of skim milk or juice (such as apple or papaya) and ice milk or frozen fruit (such as strawberries or bananas) can do the same thing less expensively.

Creatine

Interest in—and use of—**creatine** supplements to enhance performance during intense activity has grown dramatically in the last few years. Power athletes such as weight lifters use creatine supplements to enhance stores of the high-energy compound creatine phosphate (CP) in muscles. Theoretically, the more creatine phosphate in muscles, the higher the intensity at which an athlete can train. High-intensity training stimulates the muscles to adapt, which, in turn, improves performance.

The results of some studies suggest that creatine supplementation does enhance performance of short-term, repetitive, high-intensity activity such as weight lifting or sprinting.[7] Creatine may improve performance by increasing muscle strength and size, cell hydration, or glycogen loading capacity.[8] In contrast, creatine supplementation has not been shown to benefit endurance activity.[9]

The question of whether short-term use (up to a year) of creatine supplements (up to 5 grams per day) is safe continues to be studied, but so far, the supplements are viewed to be safe for healthy adults.[10] More research is needed, however, to confirm the safety of larger doses and long-term creatine use. Creatine supplementation may pose risks to athletes with kidney disease or other conditions.[11] One side-effect of creatine supplementation that no one disputes is weight gain. For some athletes, weight gain, especially muscle gain, is beneficial, but for others, it is not.

Some medical and fitness experts voice concern that, like many performance enhancement supplements before it, creatine is being taken in huge doses (up to 30 grams per day) before evidence of its value has been ascertained. Even people who eat red meat, which is a creatine-rich food, do not consume nearly the amount supplements provide. (Creatine content varies, but on average, pork, chicken, and beef provide 65 to 180 milligrams per 30 grams.) Despite the uncertainties, creatine supplements are not illegal in international competition. Many pediatricians strongly discourage the use of creatine supplements, as well as the use of any performance-enhancing substance in adolescents younger than 18 years old.[12]

Conjugated Linoleic Acid

Conjugated linoleic acid (CLA) derives from linoleic acid, which is an essential fatty acid. CLA is part of a group of naturally occurring polyunsaturated fatty acids found in beef, lamb, and dairy products. In animal studies, CLA has been shown to reduce body fat and increase lean body mass—findings that have sparked interest in CLA as a performance-enhancing aid.[13] The results of studies on the effects of supplemental CLA on body composition in human beings, however, have been less consistent.[14] A meta-analysis of carefully controlled studies of human beings in which CLA was given as a supplement to reduce body fat did find that CLA produced a modest loss of body fat compared to a placebo.[15] When researchers studied the combined effects of supplemental CLA and resistance training on body composition in men and women, they found small increases in lean body mass and reductions in body fat—but no improvements in strength.[16] The researchers noted that although the effects were statistically significant, they were nevertheless small and should be weighed against the relatively high cost of supplemental CLA.

Caffeine

Some research supports the use of **caffeine** to enhance endurance and, to some extent, to enhance short-term, high-intensity exercise performance.[17] Caffeine may stimulate fatty acid release during endurance activity, but in contrast to what was previously thought, caffeine does not slow muscle glycogen use. Light activity before a workout also stimulates fat release, but in addition, the activity warms the muscles and connective tissues, making them flexible and resistant to injury. Caffeine does not offer these added benefits.

Caffeine is a stimulant that elicits a number of physiological and psychological effects in the body. Caffeine enhances alertness and reduces fatigue.[18] The possible benefits of caffeine use must be weighed against its adverse effects—stomach upset, nervousness, irritability, headaches, and diarrhea. Caffeine-containing beverages should be used in moderation, if at all, and *in addition* to other fluids, not as a substitute for them. In 2004, the World Anti-Doping Agency (WADA), established by the International Olympic Committee, removed caffeine from its list of prohibited substances. Canadian Interuniversity Sport (CIS) works in cooperation with the Canadian Centre for Ethics in Sport to coordinate an anti-doping program for university athletes using the WADA prohibited substance list, which allows maximum urine caffeine concentrations of 12 micrograms per millilitre. Caffeine is a *restricted* substance by the U.S. National Collegiate Athletic Association, which allows urine concentrations of 15 milligrams per litre or less. This is equivalent to about 1250 mL (5 cups) of coffee consumed within a few hours before testing. Urine tests that detect more caffeine than this disqualify athletes from competition. (APPENDIX H provides a list of common caffeine-containing items and the doses they deliver.)

Hormonal Supplements

The dietary supplements discussed thus far may or may not help athletic performance, but in the doses commonly taken, they seem to cause little harm. The remaining discussion features supplements that are clearly harmful.

Anabolic Steroids

Among the most dangerous and illegal ergogenic practices is the taking of **anabolic steroids.** These drugs are derived from the male sex hormone testosterone, which promotes the development of male characteristics and lean body mass. The athletes who take steroids do so to stimulate muscle bulking.

To athletes struggling to excel, the promise of bigger, stronger muscles than training alone can produce is tempting. Athletes who lack superstar genetic material and who normally would not be able to break into the elite ranks can, with the help of steroids, suddenly compete with true champions. Especially in professional circles such as Major League Baseball and the National Football League in the United States, where monetary rewards for excellence are sky-high, steroid use is common despite its illegality and side-effects.

The World Anti-Doping Agency has released a set of international anti-doping rules known as the "Code." Around the world, sport organizations, including the Canadian Olympic Committee and International Olympic Committee, have adopted the code in an effort to make sport fair for all athletes. Banned substances such as anabolic steroids and growth factors appear on the prohibited list. The Canadian Centre for Ethics in Sport manages Canada's Anti-Doping program. Recently, the federal, provincial, and territorial governments developed and have committed to implementing the Canadian Policy Against Doping in Sport—2011, to ensure Canadian athletes participate in safe, ethical, and doping-free sports. These authorities cite the known toxic side-effects and maintain that taking these drugs is a form of cheating. Other athletes are put in the difficult position of either conceding an unfair advantage to competitors who use steroids or taking them and accepting the risk of harmful side-effects (see Table H15-2). Young athletes should not be forced to make such a choice.

The price for the potential competitive edge that steroids confer is high—sometimes it is life itself. Steroids are not simple pills that build bigger muscles. They are complex chemicals to which the body reacts in many ways, particularly when bodybuilders and other athletes take large amounts.[19] The safest, most effective way to build muscle has always been through hard training and a sound diet, and—despite popular misconceptions—it still is.

Some manufacturers peddle specific herbs as legal substitutes for steroid drugs. They falsely claim that these herbs contain hormones, enhance the body's hormonal activity, or both. In some cases, an herb may contain plant sterols, such as gamma-oryzanol, but these compounds are poorly absorbed. Even if absorption occurs, the body cannot convert herbal compounds to anabolic steroids. None of these products has any proven anabolic steroid activity, none enhances muscle strength, and some contain natural toxins. In short, "natural" does not mean "harmless."

TABLE H15-2 Anabolic Steroids: Side-Effects and Adverse Reactions

Mind
• Extreme aggression with hostility ("steroid rage"); mood swings; anxiety; dizziness; drowsiness; unpredictability; insomnia; psychotic depression; personality changes; suicidal thoughts
Face and Hair
• Swollen appearance; greasy skin; severe, scarring acne; mouth and tongue soreness; yellowing of whites of eyes (jaundice) • In females, male-pattern hair loss and increased growth of face and body hair
Voice
• In females, irreversible deepening of voice
Chest
• In males, breathing difficulty, breast development • In females, breast atrophy
Heart
• Heart disease; elevated or reduced heart rate; heart attack; stroke; hypertension; increased LDL; reduced HDL
Abdominal Organs
• Nausea; vomiting; bloody diarrhea; pain; edema; liver tumours (possibly cancerous); liver damage, disease, or rupture leading to fatal liver failure; kidney stones and damage; gallstones; frequent urination; possible rupture of aneurysm or hemorrhage
Blood
• Blood clots; high risk of blood poisoning; those who share needles risk contracting HIV (the AIDS virus) or other disease-causing organisms; septic shock (from injections)
Reproductive System
• In males, permanent shrinkage of testes; prostate enlargement with increased risk of cancer; sexual dysfunction; loss of fertility; excessive and painful erections • In females, loss of menstruation and fertility; permanent enlargement of external genitalia; fetal damage, if pregnant
Muscles, Bones, and Connective Tissues
• Increased susceptibility to injury with delayed recovery times; cramps; tremors; seizure-like movements; injury at injection site • In adolescents, failure to grow to normal height
Other
• Fatigue; increased risk of cancer

HIGHLIGHT 15

DHEA and Androstenedione

Some athletes use **DHEA** and **androstenedione** as alternatives to anabolic steroids. Androstenedione made headlines in the late 1990s when the media reported that baseball great Mark McGwire had been using it. DHEA (dehydroepiandrosterone) and androstenedione are hormones made in the adrenal glands that serve as precursors to the male hormone testosterone. Advertisements claim the hormones "burn fat," "build muscle," and "slow aging," but evidence to support such claims is lacking. In Canada, DHEA and androstenedione are controlled substances and only legally available by prescription. The Canadian Centre for Ethics in Sport is the body responsible for administering Canada's anti-doping program.

Short-term side-effects of DHEA and androstenedione may include oily skin, acne, body hair growth, liver enlargement, testicular shrinkage, and aggressive behaviour. Long-term effects, such as serious liver damage may take years to become evident. The potential for harm from DHEA and androstenedione supplements is great, and athletes, as well as others, should avoid them.

Canada's governing body for university sport (Canadian Interuniversity Sport), the U.S. National Collegiate Athletic Association, the Canadian Football League, the National Football League, and the International Olympic Committee have banned the use of androstenedione and DHEA in competition. In addition, many medical professional groups have spoken out against the use of these and other "hormone replacement" substances.

Human Growth Hormone

A wide range of athletes, including weight lifters, baseball players, cyclists, and track and field participants use **hGH (human growth hormone)** to build lean tissue and improve athletic performance. The athletes experiment with hGH, believing the injectable hormone will provide the benefits of anabolic steroids without the dangerous side-effects.

Taken in large quantities, hGH causes the disease acromegaly, in which the body becomes huge and the organs and bones overenlarge. Other effects include diabetes, thyroid disorder, heart disease, menstrual irregularities, diminished sexual desire, and shortened life span. The International Olympic Committee, the Canadian Football League, the National Football League, Major League Baseball, and most professional sports leagues ban hGH use, but its use is difficult to detect.[20] In 2011, the CFL began testing players year-round for hGH and other substances found on the WADA prohibited list. These organizations maintain that the use of hGH is a form of cheating that undermines the quest for physical excellence and that its use is coercive to other athletes.

The search for a single food, nutrient, drug, or technique that will safely and effectively enhance athletic performance will no doubt continue as long as people strive to achieve excellence in sports. When athletic performance does improve after use of an ergogenic aid, the improvement can often be attributed to the placebo effect, which is strongly at work in athletes. Even if a reliable source reports a performance boost from a newly tried product, give the effect time to fade away. Chances are excellent that it simply reflects the power of the mind over the body.

The overwhelming majority of performance-enhancing aids sold for athletes are frauds. Wishful thinking will not substitute for talent, hard training, adequate diet, and mental preparedness in competition. But don't discount the power of mind over body for a minute—it is formidable, and sports psychologists dedicate their work to harnessing it. You can use it by imagining yourself a winner and visualizing yourself excelling in your sport. You don't have to buy magic to obtain a winning edge; you already possess it—your physically fit mind and body.

Nutrition on the Net

CENGAGENOW™
For furthur study of topics covered in this Highlight, log on to **www.cengage.com/sso**.

- Learn more about the role of the Canadian Centre for Ethics in Sport in promoting a doping-free sport environment in Canada: **www.cces.ca**
- Find information on sports drinks and other nutrition and fitness topics at the Gatorade Sports Science Institute site: **www.gssiweb.com**

References

1. K. A. Erdman, T. S. Fung, and R. A. Reimer, Influence of performance level on dietary supplementation in elite Canadian athletes, *Medicine & Science in Sports & Exercise* 38 (2006): 349–356.
2. L. Di Luigi, Supplements and the endocrine system in athletes, *Clinics in Sports Medicine* 27 (2008): 131–151; R. Calfee and P. Fadale, Popular ergogenic drugs and supplements in young athletes, *Pediatrics* 117 (2006): e577–e589.
3. Position of the American Dietetic Association, Dietitians of Canada, and the American College of Sports Medicine: Nutrition and athletic performance, *Journal of the American Dietetic Association* 109 (2009): 509–527; Di Luigi, 2008.
4. N. Baume and coauthors, Research of stimulants and anabolic steroids in dietary supplements, *Scandinavian Journal of Medicine & Science in Sports* 16 (2006): 41–48.

5. L. L. Spriet, C. G. Perry, and J. L. Talanian, Legal pre-event nutritional supplements to assist energy metabolism, *Essays in Biochemistry* 44 (2008): 27–43; E. M. Broad, R. J. Maughan, and S. D. Galloway, Effects of four weeks L-carnitine L-tartrate ingestion on substrate utilization during prolonged exercise, *International Journal* of *Sport Nutrition and Exercise Metabolism* 15 (2005): 665–679.
6. Di Luigi, 2008; M. L. Diaz and coauthors, Chromium picolinate and conjugated linoleic acid do not synergistically influence diet- and exercise-induced changes in body composition and health indexes in overweight women, *Journal of Nutritional Biochemistry* 19 (2008): 61–68; H. C. Lukaski, W. A. Siders, and J. G. Penland, Chromium picolinate supplementation in women: Effects on body weight, composition, and iron status, *Nutrition* 23 (2007): 187–195.
7. Spriet, Perry, and Talanian, 2008; K. D. Tipton and A. A. Ferrando, Improving muscle mass: response of muscle metabolism to exercise, nutrition, and anabolic agents, *Essays in Biochemistry* 44 (2008): 85–98; P. J. Cribb, A. D. Williams, and A. Hayes, A creatine-protein-carbohydrate supplement enhances responses to resistance training, *Medicine & Science in Sports & Exercise* 39 (2007): 1960–1968; J. T. Brosnan and M. E. Brosnan, Creatine: Endogenous metabolite, dietary, and therapeutic supplement, *Annual Review of Nutrition* 27 (2007): 241–261; P. J. Cribb and coauthors, Effects of whey isolate, creatine, and resistance training on muscle hypertrophy, *Medicine & Science in Sports & Exercise* 39 (2007): 298–307; M. C. Peyrebrune and coauthors, Effect of creatine supplementation on training for competition in elite swimmers, *Medicine & Science in Sports & Exercise* 37 (2005): 2140–2147.
8. Brosnan and Brosnan, 2007.
9. Brosnan and Brosnan, 2007.
10. A. Shao and J. N. Hathcock, Risk assessment for creatine monohydrate, *Regulatory Toxicology and Pharmacology* 45 (2006): 242–251; M. Dunford and M. Smith, Dietary supplements and ergogenic aids, in *Sports Nutrition: A Practice Manual for Professionals*, 4th ed., ed. M. Dunford (Chicago: American Dietetic Association, 2006), pp. 116–141.
11. Position of the American Dietetic Association, Dietitians of Canada, and the American College of Sports Medicine, 2009.
12. American Academy of Pediatrics, Policy Statement, Committee on Sports Medicine and Fitness, Use of performance-enhancing substances, *Pediatrics* 115 (2005): 1103–1106.
13. B. A. Cori and coauthors, Conjugated linoleic acid reduces body fat accretion and lipogenic gene expression in neonatal pigs fed low- or high-fat formulas, *Journal of Nutrition* 138 (2008): 449–454; A. M. Bhattacharya and coauthors, The combination of dietary conjugated linoleic acid and treadmill exercise lowers gain in body fat mass and enhances lean body mass in high fat-fed male Balb/C mice, *Journal of Nutrition* 135 (2005): 1124–1130.
14. M. Plourde and coauthors, Conjugated linoleic acids: Why the discrepancy between animal and human studies? *Nutrition Reviews* 66 (2008): 415–421; S. E. Steck and coauthors, Conjugated linoleic acid supplementation for twelve weeks increases lean body mass in obese humans, *Journal of Nutrition* 137 (2007): 1188–1193; J. M. Gaullier and coauthors, Six months supplementation with conjugated linoleic acid (CLA) induces regional-specific fat mass decreases in overweight and obese, *British Journal of Nutrition* 97 (2007): 50–60; A. C. Watras and coauthors, The role of conjugated linoleic acid in reducing body fat and preventing holiday weight gain, *International Journal of Obesity* 31 (2007): 481–487; E. V. Lambert and coauthors, Conjugated linoleic acid versus high-oleic acid sunflower oil: Effects on energy metabolism, glucose tolerance, blood lipids, appetite, and body composition in regularly exercising individuals, *British Journal of Nutrition* 97 (2007): 1001–1111; T. M. Larsen and coauthors, Conjugated linoleic acid supplementation for 1 y does not prevent weight or body fat regain, *American Journal of Clinical Nutrition* 83 (2006): 606–612.
15. L. D. Whigham, A. C. Watras, and D. A. Schoeller, Efficacy of conjugated linoleic acid for reducing fat mass: A meta-analysis in humans, *American Journal of Clinical Nutrition* 85 (2007): 1203–1211.
16. C. Pinkoski and coauthors, The effects of conjugated linoleic acid supplementation during resistance training, *Medicine & Science in Sports & Exercise* 38 (2006): 339–348.
17. E. Hogervorst and coauthors, Caffeine improves physical and cognitive performance during exhaustive exercise, *Medicine & Science in Sports & Exercise* 40 (2008): 1841–1851; M. Glaister and coauthors, Caffeine supplementation and multiple sprint running performance, *Medicine & Science in Sports & Exercise* 40 (2008): 1835–1840; G. Jones, Caffeine and other sympathomimetic stimulants: Modes of action and effects on sports performance, *Essays in Biochemistry* 44 (2008): 109–123; K. T. Schneiker and coauthors, Effects of caffeine on prolonged intermittent-sprint ability in team-sport athletes, *Medicine & Science in Sports & Exercise* 38 (2006): 578–585; G. R. Stuart and coauthors, Multiple effects of caffeine on simulated high-intensity team-sport performance, *Medicine & Science in Sports & Exercise* 37 (2005): 1998–2005.
18. Jones, 2008; Stuart and coauthors, 2005.
19. Di Luigi, 2008; A. B. Parkinson and N. A. Evans, Anabolic androgenic steroids: A survey of 500 users, *Medicine & Science in Sports & Exercise* 38 (2006): 644–651.
20. H. Liu and coauthors, Systematic review: The effects of growth hormone on athletic performance, *Annals of Internal Medicine* 148 (2008): 747–758.

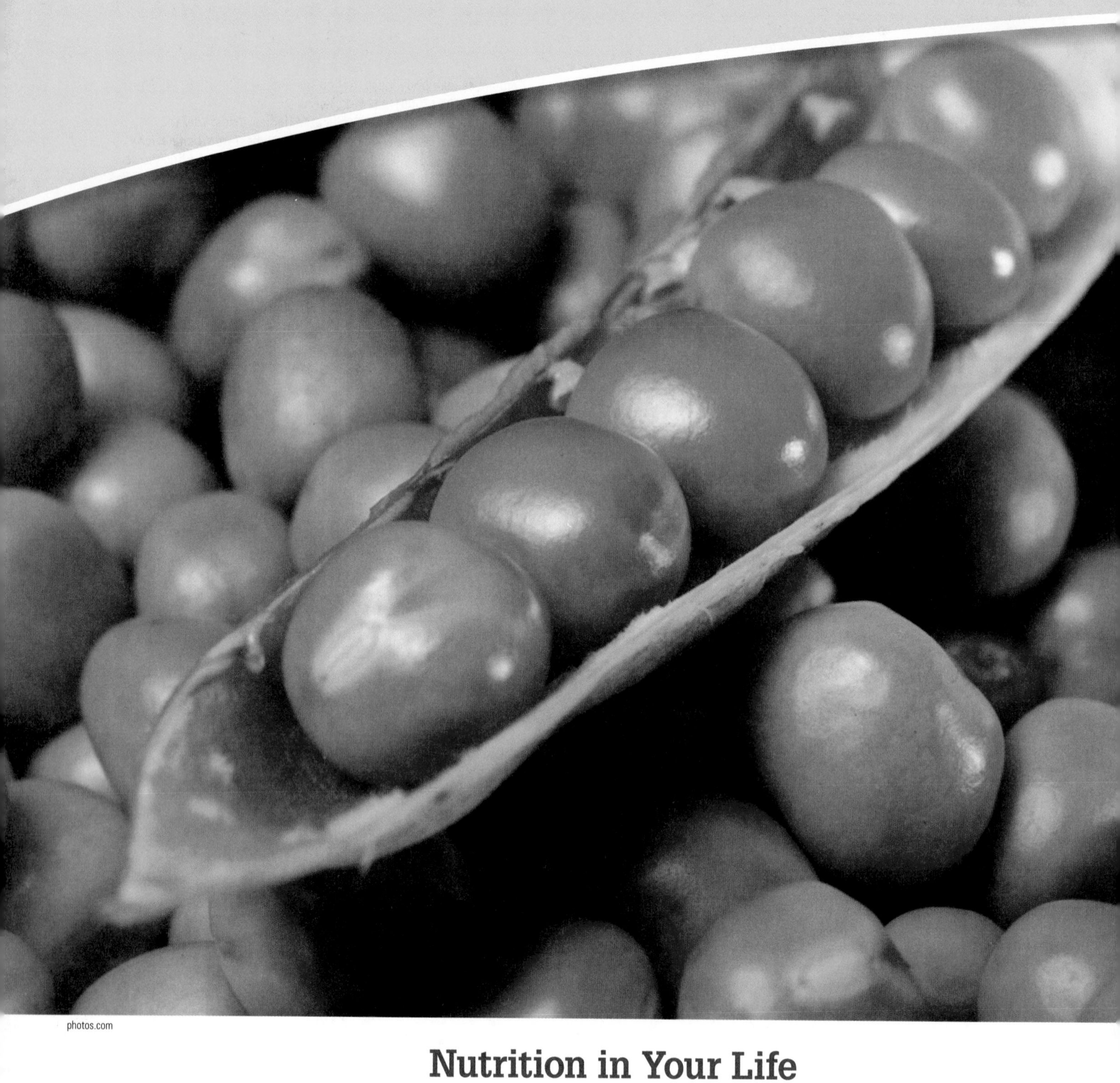

photos.com

Nutrition in Your Life

CENGAGENOW™

Throughout this chapter, the CengageNOW logo indicates an opportunity for online self-study, linking you to interactive tutorials, activities, and videos to increase your understanding of chapter concepts.
www.cengage.com/sso

Food choices have consequences. Sometimes they are immediate, as when you get heartburn after eating a pepperoni pizza. Other times they sneak up on you, as when you gain weight after repeatedly overindulging in double hot fudge sundaes. Quite often, they are temporary and easily resolved, as when hunger pangs strike after you skip lunch. During pregnancy, however, the consequences of a woman's food choices are dramatic. They affect not only her health, but also the growth and development of another human being—and not just for today, but for years to come. Making smart food choices is a huge responsibility, but fortunately, it's fairly simple.

CHAPTER 16

Life Cycle Nutrition: Pregnancy and Lactation

CHAPTER OUTLINE

All people—pregnant and lactating women, infants, children, adolescents, and adults—need the same nutrients, but the amounts they need vary depending on their stage of life. This chapter focuses on nutrition in preparation for, and support of, pregnancy and lactation. The next two chapters address the needs of infants, children, adolescents, and older adults.

Nutrition prior to Pregnancy

A section on nutrition prior to pregnancy must, by its nature, focus mainly on women. Both a man's and a woman's nutrition may affect **fertility** and possibly the genetic contributions they make to their children, but it is the woman's nutrition that has the most direct influence on the developing fetus. Her body provides the environment for the growth and development of a new human being. Prior to pregnancy, a woman has a unique opportunity to prepare herself physically, mentally, and emotionally for the many changes to come. In preparation for a healthy pregnancy, a woman can establish the following habits:[1]

- *Achieve and maintain a healthy body weight.* Both underweight and overweight are associated with infertility.[2] Overweight and obese men have low sperm counts and hormonal changes that reduce fertility.[3] Excess body fat in women disrupts menstrual regularity and ovarian hormone production.[4] Should a pregnancy occur, mothers, both underweight and overweight, and their newborns, face increased risks of complications.
- *Choose an adequate and balanced diet.* Malnutrition reduces fertility and impairs the early development of an infant should a woman become pregnant. In contrast, a healthy diet that emphasizes monounsaturated fats instead of *trans* fats, vegetable proteins instead of animal proteins, and low glycemic carbohydrates instead of simple sugars can favourably influence fertility.[5] Men with diets rich in antioxidant nutrients have higher sperm numbers and motility.[6]
- *Be physically active.* A woman who wants to be physically active *when* she is pregnant needs to become physically active *beforehand.*

fertility: the capacity of a woman to produce a normal ovum periodically and of a man to produce normal sperm; the ability to reproduce.

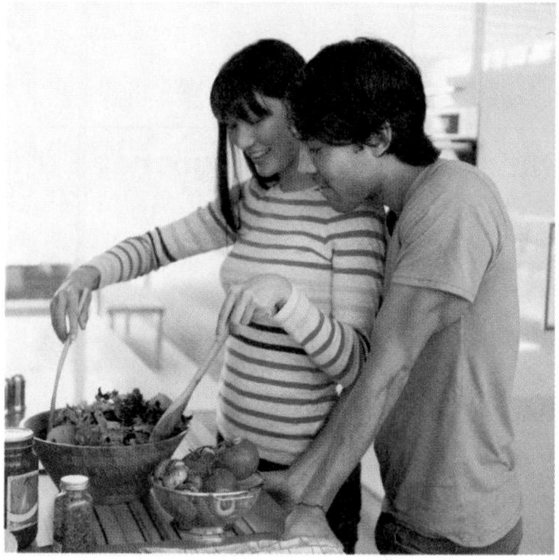
© Fancy/Alamy

Young adults can prepare for a healthy pregnancy by taking care of themselves today.

- *Receive regular medical care.* Regular health-care visits can help ensure a healthy start to pregnancy.
- *Manage chronic conditions.* Conditions such as diabetes, HIV/AIDS, phenylketonuria (PKU), and sexually transmitted infections can adversely affect a pregnancy and need close medical attention to help ensure a healthy outcome.
- *Avoid harmful influences.* Both maternal and paternal ingestion of or exposure to harmful substances (such as cigarettes, alcohol, drugs, or environmental contaminants) can cause miscarriage or abnormalities, alter genes or their expression, and interfere with fertility.[7]

Young adults who nourish and protect their bodies do so not only for their own sakes, but also for future generations.

Dietary Guidance for Canadians

According to *Eating Well with Canada's Food Guide:*[8]

- Pregnant and breastfeeding women need more calories. Include an extra two to three *Food Guide* Servings each day.
- All women who could become pregnant (e.g., three months before pregnancy) need a multivitamin containing folic acid every day.
- Pregnant women need to ensure that their multivitamin also contains iron.

Growth and Development during Pregnancy

A whole new life begins at **conception.** Organ systems develop rapidly, and nutrition plays many supportive roles. This section describes placental development and fetal growth, paying close attention to times of intense developmental activity.

Placental Development

In the early days of pregnancy, a spongy structure known as the **placenta** develops in the **uterus.** Two associated structures also form (see Figure 16-1). One is the **amniotic sac,** a fluid-filled balloonlike structure that houses the developing fetus. The other is the **umbilical cord,** a ropelike structure containing fetal blood vessels that extends through the fetus's "belly button" (the umbilicus) to the placenta. These three structures play crucial roles during pregnancy, and then are expelled from the uterus during childbirth.

The placenta develops as an interweaving of fetal and maternal blood vessels embedded in the uterine wall. The maternal blood transfers oxygen and nutrients to the fetus's blood and picks up fetal waste products. By exchanging oxygen, nutrients, and waste products, the placenta performs the respiratory, absorptive, and excretory functions that the fetus's lungs, digestive system, and kidneys will provide after birth.

The placenta is a versatile, metabolically active organ. Like all body tissues, the placenta uses energy and nutrients to support its work. It produces an array of hormones that maintain pregnancy and prepare the mother's breasts for lactation (making milk). A healthy placenta is essential for the developing fetus to attain its full potential.[9]

Fetal Growth and Development

Fetal development begins with the fertilization of an **ovum** by a **sperm.** Three stages follow: the zygote, the embryo, and the fetus (see Figure 16-2).

The Zygote The newly fertilized ovum is called a **zygote.** It begins as a single cell and rapidly divides to become a **blastocyst.** During that first week, the blastocyst floats down into the uterus where it will embed itself in the inner uterine

conception: the union of the male sperm and the female ovum; fertilization.

placenta (plah-SEN-tuh): the organ that develops inside the uterus early in pregnancy, through which the fetus receives nutrients and oxygen and returns carbon dioxide and other waste products to be excreted.

uterus (YOU-ter-us): the muscular organ within which the infant develops before birth.

amniotic (am-nee-OTT-ic) **sac:** the "bag of waters" in the uterus, in which the fetus floats.

umbilical (um-BILL-ih-cul) **cord:** the ropelike structure through which the fetus's veins and arteries reach the placenta; the route of nourishment and oxygen to the fetus and the route of waste disposal from the fetus. The scar in the middle of the abdomen that marks the former attachment of the umbilical cord is the *umbilicus* (um-BILL-ih-cus), commonly known as the "belly button."

ovum (OH-vum): the female reproductive cell, capable of developing into a new organism upon fertilization; commonly referred to as an egg.

sperm: the male reproductive cell, capable of fertilizing an ovum.

zygote (ZY-goat): the initial product of the union of ovum and sperm; a fertilized ovum.

blastocyst (BLASS-toe-sist): the developmental stage of the zygote when it is about five days old and ready for implantation.

FIGURE 16-1 The Placenta and Associated Structures

To understand how placental villi absorb nutrients without maternal and fetal blood interacting directly, think of how the intestinal villi work. The GI side of the intestinal villi is bathed in a nutrient-rich fluid (chyme). The intestinal villi absorb the nutrient molecules and release them into the body via capillaries. Similarly, the maternal side of the placental villi is bathed in nutrient-rich maternal blood. The placental villi absorb the nutrient molecules and release them to the fetus via fetal capillaries.

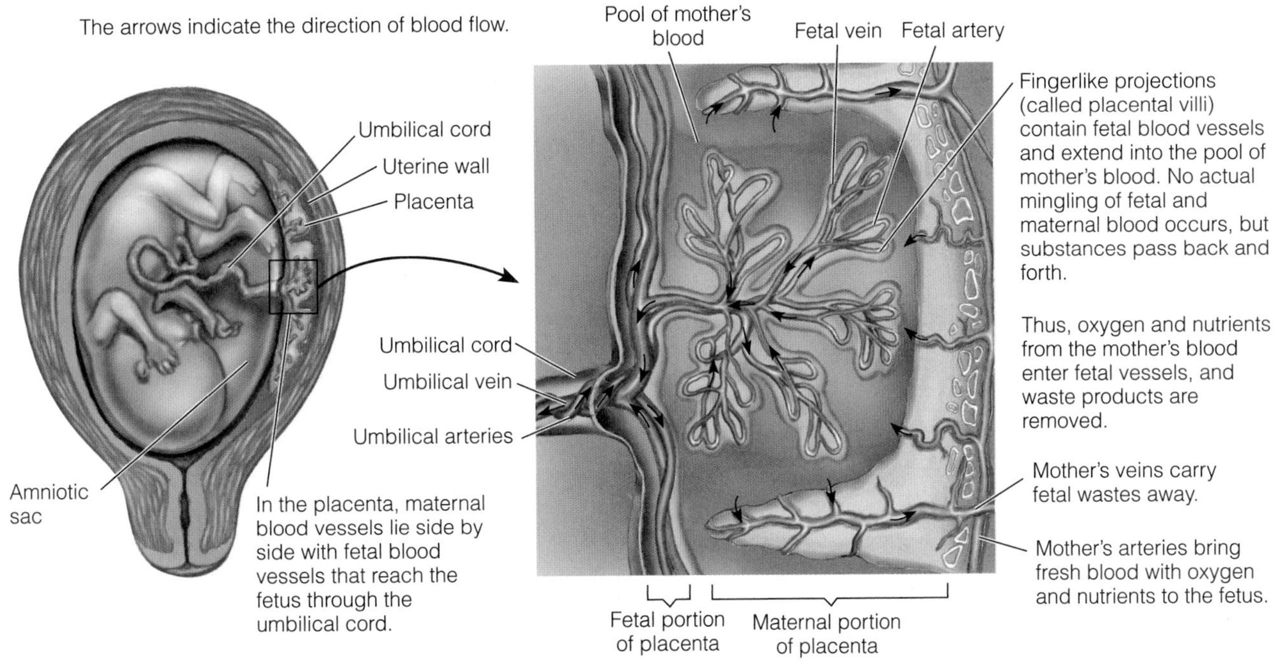
The arrows indicate the direction of blood flow.
Umbilical cord
Uterine wall
Placenta
Amniotic sac
In the placenta, maternal blood vessels lie side by side with fetal blood vessels that reach the fetus through the umbilical cord.
Pool of mother's blood
Fetal vein
Fetal artery
Fingerlike projections (called placental villi) contain fetal blood vessels and extend into the pool of mother's blood. No actual mingling of fetal and maternal blood occurs, but substances pass back and forth.
Thus, oxygen and nutrients from the mother's blood enter fetal vessels, and waste products are removed.
Umbilical cord
Umbilical vein
Umbilical arteries
Mother's veins carry fetal wastes away.
Mother's arteries bring fresh blood with oxygen and nutrients to the fetus.
Fetal portion of placenta
Maternal portion of placenta

FIGURE 16-2 Stages of Embryonic and Fetal Development

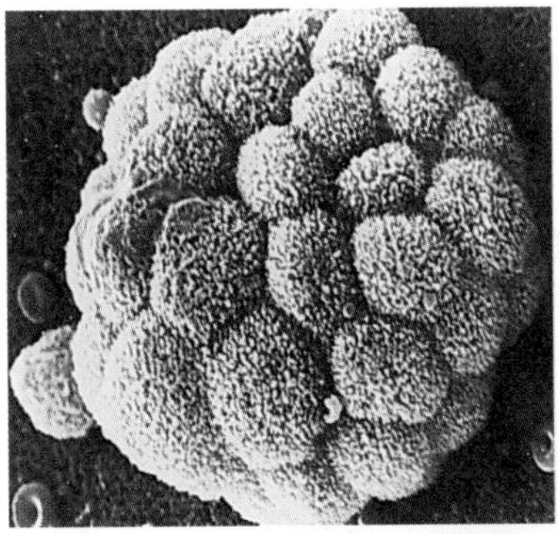

1 A newly fertilized ovum is called a **zygote** and is about the size of the period at the end of this sentence. Less than one week after fertilization, these cells have rapidly divided multiple times and are ready for implantation.

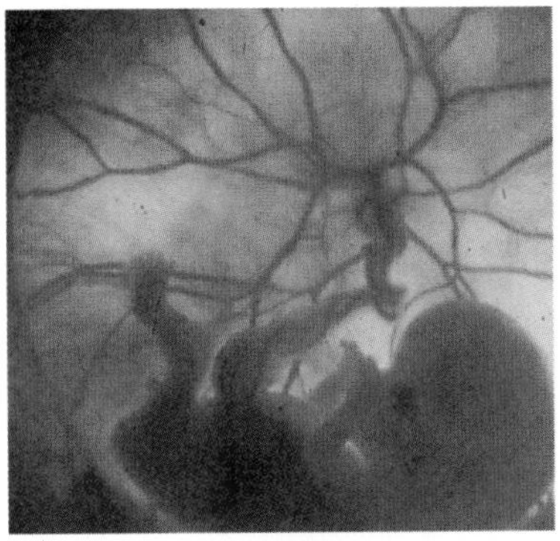

3 A **fetus** after 11 weeks of development is 4 centimetres long. Notice the umbilical cord and blood vessels connecting the fetus with the placenta.

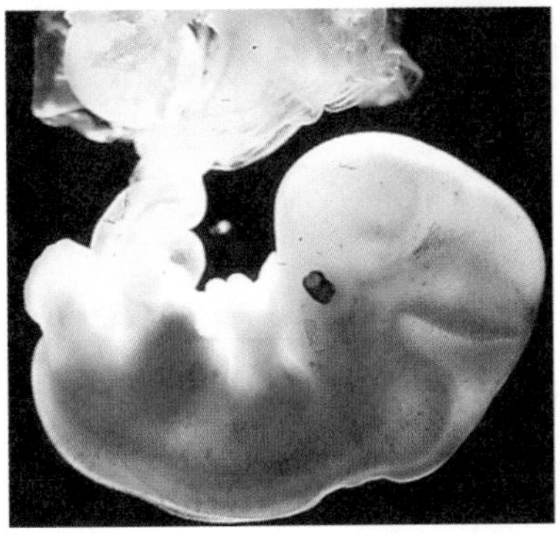

2 After implantation, the placenta develops and begins to provide nourishment to the developing embryo. An **embryo** 5 weeks after fertilization is about 1.25 centimetres long.

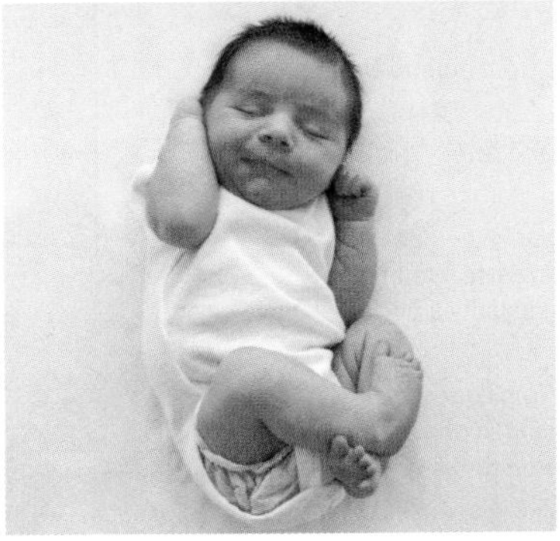

4 A **newborn infant** after nine months of development measures close to 50 centimetres in length. From 8 weeks to term, this infant grew 20 times longer and 50 times heavier.

FIGURE 16-3 The Concept of Critical Periods in Fetal Development

Critical periods occur early in fetal development. An adverse influence felt early in pregnancy can have a much more severe and prolonged impact than one felt later on.

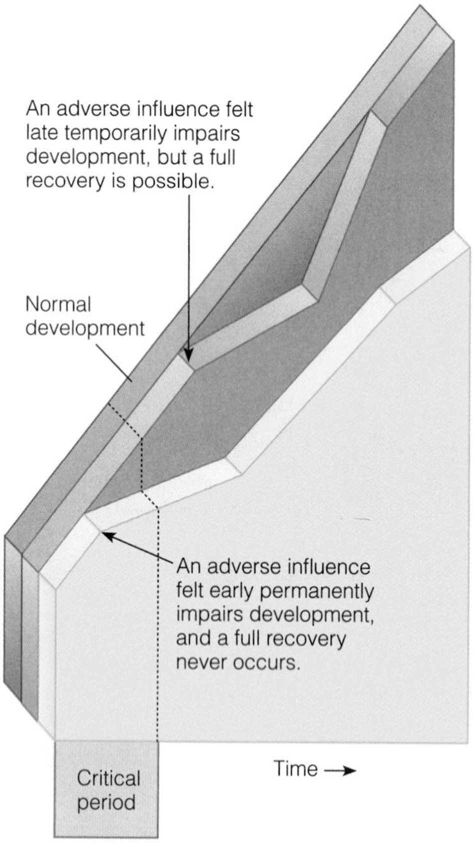
An adverse influence felt late temporarily impairs development, but a full recovery is possible.
Normal development
An adverse influence felt early permanently impairs development, and a full recovery never occurs.
Critical period
Time →

♦ The **neural tube** is the structure that eventually becomes the brain and spinal cord.

implantation (IM-plan-TAY-shun): the embedding of the blastocyst in the inner lining of the uterus.

embryo (EM-bree-oh): the developing infant from two to eight weeks after conception.

fetus (FEET-us): the developing infant from eight weeks after conception until term.

full term: between the thirty-eighth and forty-second week of pregnancy.

critical periods: finite periods during development in which certain events occur that will have irreversible effects on later developmental stages; usually a period of rapid cell division.

gestation (jes-TAY-shun): the period from conception to birth. For human beings, the average length of a healthy gestation is 40 weeks. Pregnancy is often divided into three-month periods, called *trimesters.*

wall—a process known as **implantation**. Cell division continues at an amazing rate as each set of cells divides into many other cells.

The Embryo At first, the number of cells in the **embryo** doubles approximately every 24 hours; later the rate slows, and only one doubling occurs during the final 10 weeks of pregnancy. At 8 weeks, the 3.2 cm embryo has a complete central nervous system, a beating heart, a digestive system, well-defined fingers and toes, and the beginnings of facial features.

The Fetus The **fetus** continues to grow during the next seven months. Each organ grows to maturity according to its own schedule, with greater intensity at some times than at others. As Figure 16-2 shows, fetal growth is phenomenal: weight increases from less than 30 grams (1 ounce) to about 3500 grams (7½ pounds). Most successful pregnancies are **full term**—lasting 38 to 42 weeks—and produce a healthy infant weighing between 3 and 3.5 kilograms (6½ and 8 pounds).

Critical Periods

Times of intense development and rapid cell division are called **critical periods**—critical in the sense that those cellular activities can occur only at those times. If cell division and number are limited during a critical period, full recovery is not possible (see Figure 16-3).

The development of each organ and tissue is most vulnerable to adverse influences (such as nutrient deficiencies or toxins) during its own critical period (see Figure 16-4). The critical period for neural tube ♦ development, for example, is from 17 to 30 days **gestation.** Consequently, neural tube development is most vulnerable to nutrient deficiencies, nutrient excesses, or toxins during this critical time—when most women do not even realize they are pregnant. Any abnormal development of the neural tube or its failure to close completely can cause a major defect in the central nervous system. Figure 16-5 shows photos of neural tube development in the early weeks of gestation.

FIGURE 16-4 Critical Periods of Development

During embryonic development (from two to eight weeks), many of the tissues are in their critical periods (purple area of the bars); events occur that will have irreversible effects on the development of those tissues. In the later stages of development (green area of the bars), the tissues continue to grow and change, but the events are less critical in that they are relatively minor or reversible.

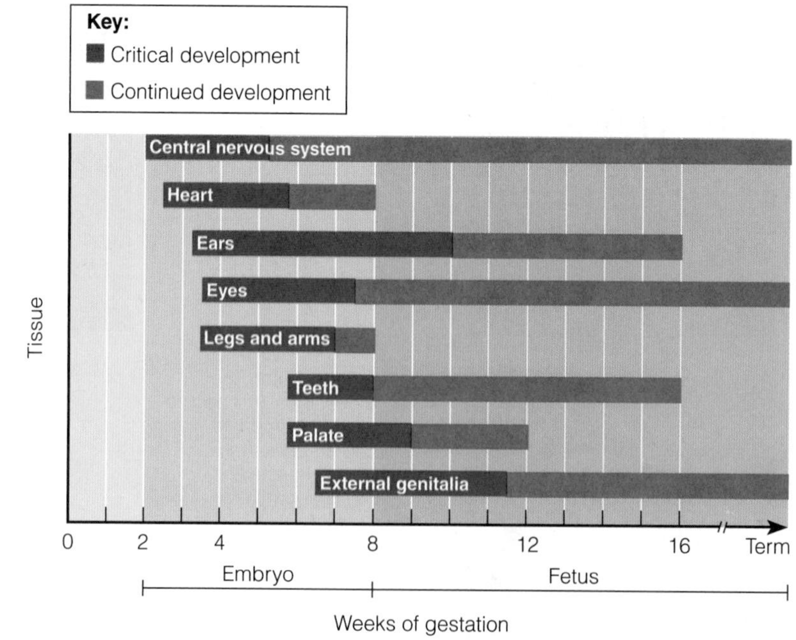
Key:
Critical development
Continued development
Central nervous system
Heart
Ears
Eyes
Legs and arms
Teeth
Palate
External genitalia
Tissue
0
2
4
8
12
16
Term
Embryo
Fetus
Weeks of gestation

SOURCE: Adapted from *Before We Are Born: Essentials of Embryology and Birth Defects* by K. L. Moore and T. V. N. Persaud (W. B. Saunders, 2003).

FIGURE 16-5 Neural Tube Development

The neural tube is the beginning structure of the brain and spinal cord. Any failure of the neural tube to close or to develop normally results in central nervous system disorders such as spina bifida and anencephaly. Successful development of the neural tube depends, in part, on the vitamin folate.

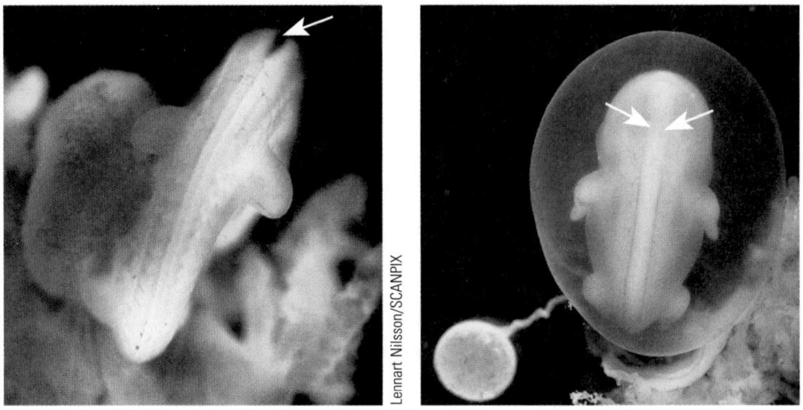

Lennart Nilsson/SCANPIX

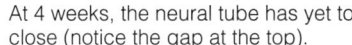

At 4 weeks, the neural tube has yet to close (notice the gap at the top).

Lennart Nilsson/SCANPIX

At 6 weeks, the neural tube (outlined by the delicate red vertebral arteries) has successfully closed.

Neural Tube Defects In Canada, the incidence of neural tube defects is between 1 and 4 cases per 1000 live births; ♦ worldwide, more than 300 000 infants are affected each year. Following mandatory fortification of wheat flour in 1998, the number of children born with neural tube defects has fallen by close to between two-fifths and one-half per 1000.[10] Many other pregnancies with neural tube defects end in abortions or stillbirths.

The two most common types of neural tube defects are anencephaly and spina bifida. In **anencephaly**, the upper end of the neural tube fails to close. Consequently, the brain is either missing or fails to develop. Pregnancies affected by anencephaly often end in miscarriage; infants born with anencephaly die shortly after birth.

Spina bifida is characterized by incomplete closure of the spinal cord and its bony encasement (see Figure 16-6 on p. 510). The meninges membranes covering the spinal cord often protrude as a sac, which may rupture and lead to meningitis, a life-threatening infection. Spina bifida is accompanied by varying degrees of paralysis, depending on the extent of the spinal cord damage. Mild cases may not even be noticed, but severe cases lead to death. Common problems include clubfoot, dislocated hip, kidney disorders, curvature of the spine, muscle weakness, mental handicaps, and motor and sensory losses.

The cause of neural tube defects is unknown, but researchers are examining several gene-gene, gene-nutrient, and gene-environment interactions.[11] A pregnancy affected by a neural tube defect can occur in any woman, but these factors make it more likely:[12]

- A personal or family history of a pregnancy affected by a neural tube defect
- Maternal diabetes
- Maternal use of certain antiseizure medications
- Mutations in folate-related enzymes
- Maternal obesity

Folate supplementation reduces the risk.

Folate Supplementation Chapter 10 describes how folate supplements taken one month before conception and continued throughout the first trimester can

♦ A **neural tube defect** is a malformation of the brain, spinal cord, or both during embryonic development. The two main types of neural tube defects are **spina bifida** (literally, "split spine") and **anencephaly** ("no brain").

anencephaly (AN-en-SEF-a-lee): an uncommon and always fatal type of neural tube defect; characterized by the absence of a brain.
- **an** = not (without)
- **encephalus** = brain

spina (SPY-nah) **bifida** (BIFF-ih-dah): one of the most common types of neural tube defects; characterized by the incomplete closure of the spinal cord and its bony encasement.
- **spina** = spine
- **bifida** = split

FIGURE 16-6 Spina Bifida–A Neural Tube Defect

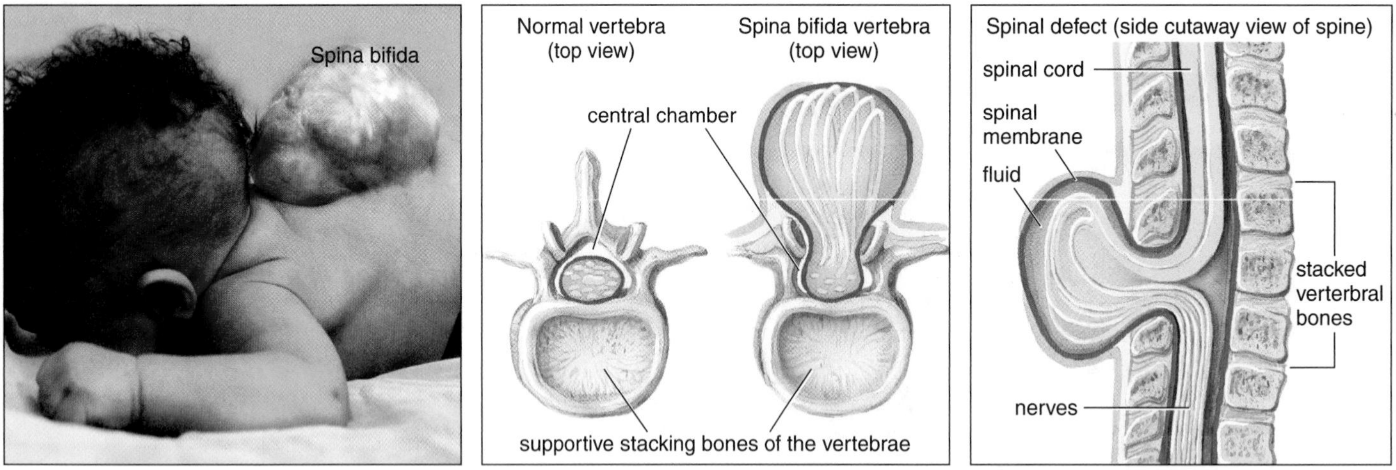
Spina bifida
Normal vertebra
(top view)
Spina bifida vertebra
(top view)
central chamber
supportive stacking bones of the vertebrae
Spinal defect (side cutaway view of spine)
spinal cord
spinal
membrane
fluid
stacked
verterbral
bones
nerves

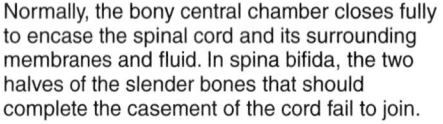

Normally, the bony central chamber closes fully to encase the spinal cord and its surrounding membranes and fluid. In spina bifida, the two halves of the slender bones that should complete the casement of the cord fail to join.

In the serious form shown here, membranes and fluid have bulged through the gap and nerves are exposed, invariably leading to some degree of paralysis and often to mental retardation.

help support a healthy pregnancy, prevent neural tube defects, and reduce the severity of those that do occur.[13] For this reason, all women of childbearing age ♦ who are capable of becoming pregnant should consume 400 micrograms (0.4 milligrams) of folate daily. A woman who has previously had an infant with a neural tube defect may be advised by her physician to take folate supplements in doses ten times larger—4 milligrams daily. Because high doses of folate can mask the symptoms of the pernicious anemia of a vitamin B_{12} deficiency, quantities of 1 milligram or more require a prescription. Most over-the-counter multivitamin-mineral supplements contain 400 micrograms of folate; prenatal supplements usually contain 800 micrograms.

♦ Folate RDA:
- For women: 400 μg (0.4 mg)/day
- During pregnancy: 600 μg (0.6 mg)/day

Dietary Guidance for Canadians

Folate, a B vitamin, is vital to the normal development of the fetus's spine, brain, and skull, especially during the first month of pregnancy. All women of childbearing age who are capable of becoming pregnant need a multivitamin containing 400 micrograms (0.4 milligrams) of folic acid in addition to their dietary folate intake every day of folate daily.[14]

Because half of the pregnancies each year are unplanned and because neural tube defects occur early in development before most women realize they are pregnant, bleached wheat flour—and thus other grain products made from it—are fortified with folate to help ensure an adequate intake. Although not yet the case in Canada, food labels in the United States on fortified products may claim that an "adequate intake of folate has been shown to reduce the risk of neural tube defects." Fortification has improved folate status in women of childbearing age and lowered the number of neural tube defects that occur each year, as shown in Figure 10-12 on p. 330.[15] Whether folate fortification should be increased further is still the subject of much debate.[16]

Chronic Diseases Much research suggests that adverse influences at critical times during fetal development set the stage for the infant to develop chronic diseases in adult life.[17] Poor maternal diet or health during pregnancy may alter the infant's bodily functions such as blood pressure, cholesterol metabolism, and immune functions that influence disease development.[18] For example, maternal malnutrition may alter blood vessel growth and program lipid metabolism and lean body mass development in such a way that the infant will develop risk factors for cardiovascular disease as an adult.[19]

Malnutrition during the critical period of pancreatic cell growth provides an example of how type 2 diabetes may develop in adulthood. The pancreatic cells responsible for producing insulin (the beta cells) normally increase more than 130-fold between 12 weeks gestation and 5 months after birth. Nutrition is a primary determinant of beta cell growth, and infants who have suffered prenatal malnutrition have significantly fewer beta cells than well-nourished infants. They are also more likely to be low-birthweight infants—and low birthweight and premature birth correlate with insulin resistance later in life.[20] One hypothesis suggests that diabetes may develop from the interaction of inadequate nutrition early in life with abundant nutrition later in life: the small mass of beta cells developed in times of undernutrition during fetal development may be insufficient in times of overnutrition during adulthood when the body needs more insulin.

Hypertension may develop from a similar scenario of inadequate growth during placental and gestational development followed by accelerated growth during early childhood: the small mass of kidney cells developed during malnutrition may be insufficient to handle the excessive demands of later life.[21] Low-birthweight infants who gain weight rapidly as young children are likely to develop hypertension and heart disease as adults.

Fetal Programming Recent genetic research may help to explain the phenomenon of substances such as nutrients influencing the development of obesity and diseases later on in adulthood—a process known as **fetal programming.** In the case of pregnancy, the mother's nutrition can change gene expression in the fetus.[22] Such epigenetic changes during pregnancy can affect the infant's development of obesity and related adult diseases.[23] Some research suggests that fetal programming may influence succeeding generations.[24]

IN SUMMARY **Maternal nutrition before and during pregnancy affects both the mother's health and the infant's growth. As the infant develops through its three stages—the zygote, embryo, and fetus—its organs and tissues grow, each on its own schedule. Times of intense development are critical periods that depend on nutrients to proceed smoothly. Without adequate folate, for example, the neural tube fails to develop completely during the first month of pregnancy, prompting recommendations that all women of childbearing age take folate daily.**

Because critical periods occur throughout pregnancy, a woman should continuously take good care of her health. That care should include achieving and maintaining a healthy body weight prior to pregnancy and gaining sufficient weight during pregnancy to support a healthy infant.

Maternal Weight

Birthweight is the most reliable indicator of an infant's health. As a later section of this chapter explains, compared with a normal-weight infant, an underweight infant is more likely to have physical and mental defects, become ill, and die. In general, higher birthweights present fewer risks for infants. Two characteristics of the mother's weight influence an infant's birthweight: her weight *prior* to conception and her weight gain *during* pregnancy.

Weight prior to Conception

A woman's weight ♦ prior to conception influences fetal growth. Even with the same weight gain during pregnancy, underweight women tend to have smaller babies than heavier women. Ideally, before a woman becomes pregnant, she will have established diet and activity habits to support an adequate, and not excessive, weight gain during pregnancy.[25]

Underweight An underweight woman has a high risk of having a low-birthweight infant, especially if she is malnourished or unable to gain sufficient weight during

♦ BMI is introduced in Chapter 8.
- Underweight = BMI <18.5
- Normal weight = BMI 18.5 to 24.9
- Overweight = BMI 25 to 29.9
- Obesity = BMI ≥ 30

fetal programming: the influence of substances during fetal growth on the development of diseases in later life.

pregnancy. In addition, the rates of **preterm** births and infant deaths are higher for underweight women. An underweight woman improves her chances of having a healthy infant by gaining sufficient weight prior to conception or by gaining extra pounds during pregnancy. To gain weight and ensure nutrient adequacy, an underweight woman can follow the dietary recommendations for pregnant women (described on pp. 503–507).

◆ The term *macrosomia* (mak-roh-SO-me-ah) describes high-birthweight infants (roughly 4000 g or 9 lb or more); macrosomia results from prepregnancy obesity, excessive weight gain during pregnancy, or uncontrolled diabetes.
- **macro** = large
- **oma** = body

Overweight and Obesity According to a recent national survey of mothers of a single child, an estimated one-third had a high prepregnancy body mass index (~20% overweight; ~14% obese) prior to becoming pregnant, which can create problems related to pregnancy and childbirth.[26] Obese women have an especially high risk of medical complications such as hypertension, gestational diabetes, and postpartum infections. Compared with other women, obese women are also more likely to have other complications of labour and delivery.[27] Complications in women after gastric bypass surgery and weight loss are lower than in obese women.[28]

Overweight women have the lowest rate of low-birthweight infants. In fact, infants of overweight women are more likely to be born **post term** and to weigh more than 4000 grams (9 pounds). ◆ Large newborns increase the likelihood of a difficult labour and delivery, birth trauma, and **cesarean section.**[29] Consequently, these infants have a greater risk of poor health and death than infants of normal weight.

Of greater concern than infant birthweight is the poor development of infants born to obese mothers.[30] Obesity may double the risk for neural tube defects. Folate's role has been examined, but a more likely explanation seems to be poor glycemic control.[31] Undiagnosed diabetes might also explain why obese women have a greater risk of giving birth to infants with heart defects and other abnormalities.[32]

Health-care providers have traditionally advised against weight-loss dieting during pregnancy. Limited research, however, suggests that obese women with gestational diabetes who follow a well-balanced, kcalorie-restricted diet and regular exercise program can gain little or no weight without adverse consequences.[33] Ideally, overweight women will achieve a healthy body weight before becoming pregnant, avoid excessive weight gain during pregnancy, and postpone weight loss until after childbirth.[34]

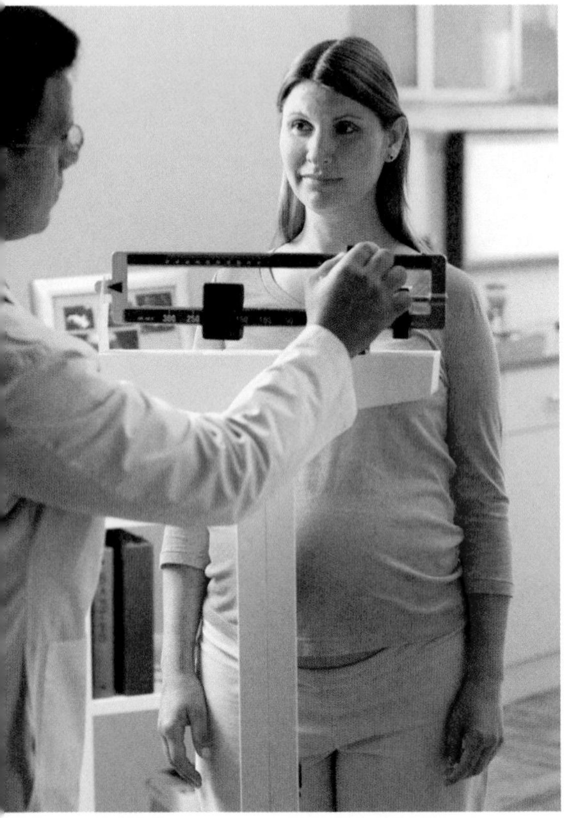

photos.com

Fetal growth and maternal health depend on a sufficient weight gain during pregnancy.

Weight Gain during Pregnancy

Fetal growth and maternal health depend on a sufficient weight gain during pregnancy. Maternal weight gain during pregnancy correlates closely with infant birthweight, which is a strong predictor of the health and subsequent development of the infant.

Dietary Guidance for Canadians

Pregnant women should ensure appropriate weight gain as specified by a health-care provider.

◆ Nutrient density = nutrient/kcal
Energy density = kcal/g

Recommended Weight Gains Table 16-1 presents recommended weight gains for various prepregnancy weights. The recommended gain for a woman who begins pregnancy at a healthy weight and is carrying a single fetus is 11.5–16.0 kilograms (25 to 35 pounds).[35] An underweight woman needs to gain 12.5–18.0 kilograms (28 to 40 pounds); and an overweight woman, 7.0–11.5 kilograms (15 to 25 pounds). About one-third of North American women gain weight within these recommended ranges; most gain more than recommended.[36] Appropriate weight gains help women limit weight retention after pregnancy and help their infants prevent obesity during childhood.[37] To limit excessive weight gains, pregnant women can select foods with a high nutrient density but a low energy density. ◆[38]

Weight-Gain Patterns For the normal-weight woman, weight gain ideally follows a pattern of 1.5 kilograms (3½ pounds) during the first trimester and 0.5 kilogram (1 pound) per week thereafter. Health-care professionals monitor weight gain using a prenatal weight-gain grid (see Figure 16-7).

preterm (premature): prior to the thirty-eighth week of pregnancy.

post term: after the forty-second week of pregnancy.

cesarean (si-ZAIR-ee-un) **section:** a surgically assisted birth involving removal of the fetus by an incision into the uterus, usually by way of the abdominal wall.

TABLE 16-1 Recommended Weight Gains Based on Prepregnancy Weight

	Recommended Weight Gain	
Prepregnancy Weight	*For single birth*	*For twin birth*
Underweight (BMI <18.5)	12.5 to 18.0 kg (28 to 40 lb)	Insufficient data to make recommendation
Healthy weight (BMI 18.5 to 24.9)	11.5 to 16.0 kg (25 to 35 lb)	17.0 to 25.0 kg (37 to 54 lb)
Overweight (BMI 25.0 to 29.9)	7.0 to 11.5 kg (15 to 25 lb)	14.0 to 23.0 kg (31 to 50 lb)
Obese (BMI ≥30)	5.0 to 9.0 kg (11 to 20 lb)	11.0 to 19.0 kg (25 to 42 lb)

SOURCE: Reprinted with permission from the Institute of Medicine, Weight Gain during Pregnancy: Reexamining the Guidelines, 2009 by the National Academy of Sciences, Courtesy of the National Academies Press, Washington, D.C.

FIGURE 16-7 Recommended Prenatal Weight Gain Based on Prepregnancy Weight

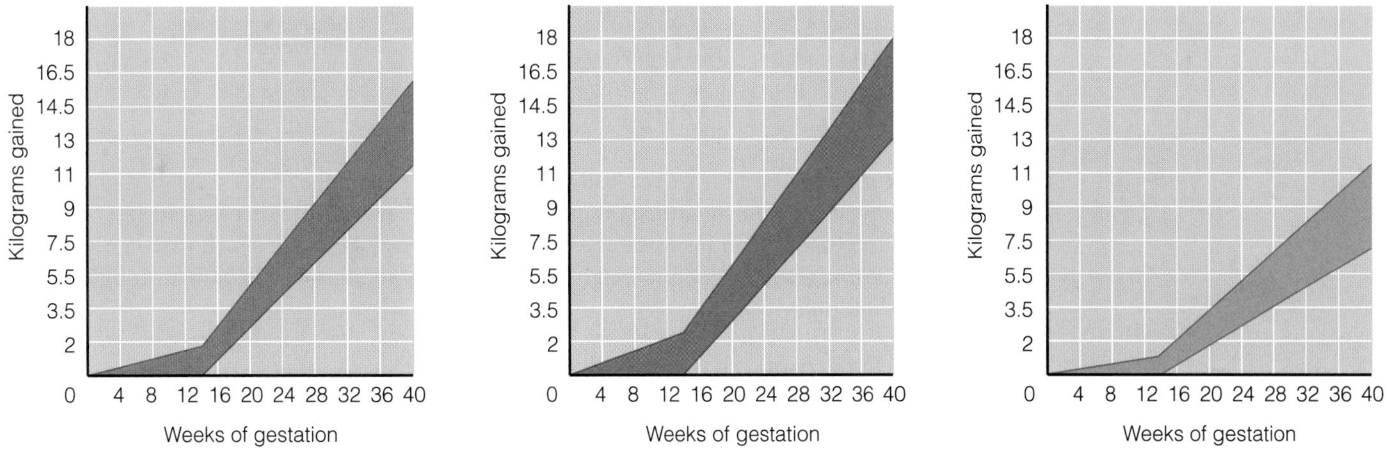
Kilograms gained
18
16.5
14.5
13
11
9
7.5
5.5
3.5
2
0
4 8 12 16 20 24 28 32 36 40
Weeks of gestation

Normal-weight women should gain about 1.5 kg/3.5 pounds in the first trimester and just under 0.5 kg/1 pound/week thereafter, achieving a total gain of 11.5–16.0 kg/25–35 pounds by term.

Underweight women should gain about 2.5 kg/5 pounds in the first trimester and just over 0.5 kg/1 pound/week thereafter, achieving a total gain of 12.5–18.0 kg/28–40 pounds by term.

Overweight women should gain about 1 kg/2 pounds in the first trimester and about 330 g/ ⅔ pound/week thereafter, achieving a total gain of 7.0–11.5 kg/15–25 pounds.

If a woman gains more than is recommended early in pregnancy, she should not restrict her energy intake later in order to lose weight. A large weight gain over a short time, however, indicates excessive fluid retention and may be the first sign of the serious medical complication preeclampsia, which is discussed later.

Components of Weight Gain Women often express concern about the weight gain that accompanies a healthy pregnancy. They may find comfort by remembering that most of the gain supports the growth and development of the placenta, uterus, blood, and breasts, the increase in blood supply and fluid volume, as well as a healthy 3.5 kilogram (7½-pound) infant. A small amount goes into maternal fat stores, and even that fat is there for a special purpose—to provide energy for labour and lactation. Figure 16-8 (p. 514) shows the components of a healthy 13.5 kilogram (30-pound) weight gain.

Weight Loss after Pregnancy The pregnant woman loses some weight at delivery. In the following weeks, she loses more as her blood volume returns to normal and she sheds accumulated fluids. The typical woman does not, however, return to her prepregnancy weight. In general, the more weight a woman gains beyond the needs of pregnancy, the more she retains—mostly as body fat.[39] Even with an average weight gain during pregnancy, most women tend to retain a couple of kilograms with each pregnancy. When those couple of kilograms become three

FIGURE 16-8 Components of Weight Gain during Pregnancy

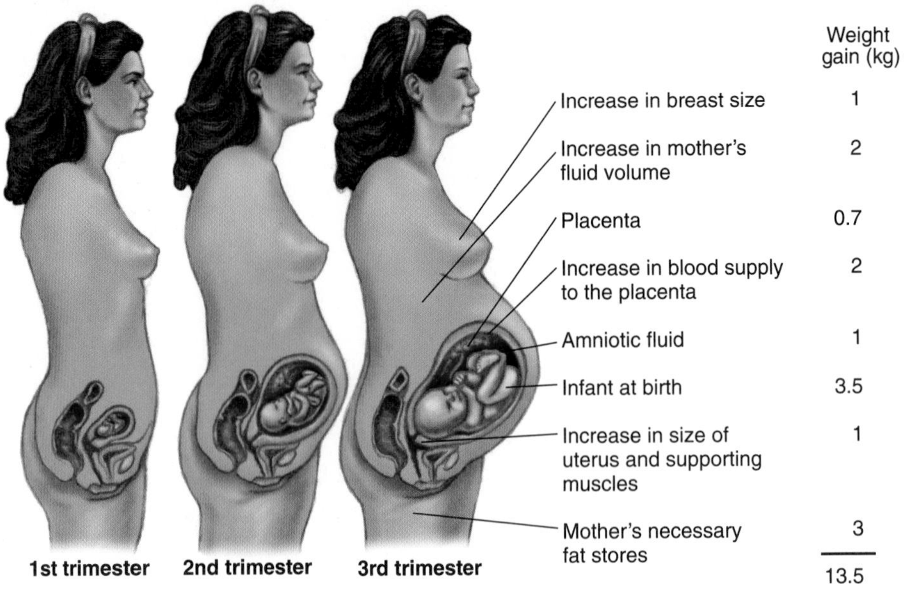
Weight gain (kg)
Increase in breast size 1
Increase in mother's fluid volume 2
Placenta 0.7
Increase in blood supply to the placenta 2
Amniotic fluid 1
Infant at birth 3.5
Increase in size of uterus and supporting muscles 1
Mother's necessary fat stores 3
13.5
1st trimester
2nd trimester
3rd trimester

or more and BMI increases by a unit or more, complications such as diabetes and hypertension in future pregnancies as well as chronic diseases in later life can increase—even for women who are not overweight.[40] Those who are successful in losing their pregnancy weight are more likely to limit weight gains through middle adulthood.[41]

Exercise during Pregnancy

An active, physically fit woman experiencing a normal pregnancy can continue to exercise throughout pregnancy, adjusting the duration and intensity of activity as the pregnancy progresses.[42] Inactive women and those experiencing pregnancy complications should discuss physical activity options with their health-care provider.

Staying active can improve fitness, prevent or manage gestational diabetes, facilitate labour, and reduce stress. Women who exercise during pregnancy report fewer discomforts throughout their pregnancies. Regular exercise develops the strength and endurance a woman needs to carry the extra weight through pregnancy and to labour through an intense delivery. It also maintains the habits that help a woman lose excess weight and get back into shape after the birth.

A pregnant woman should participate in "low-impact" activities and avoid sports in which she might fall or be hit by other people or objects. For example, playing singles tennis with one person on each side of the net is safer than a fast-moving game of racquetball in which the two competitors can collide. Swimming and water aerobics are particularly beneficial because they allow the body to remain cool and move freely with the water's support, thus reducing back pain.[43] Figure 16-9 provides some guidelines for exercise during pregnancy. Several of the guidelines are aimed at preventing excessively high internal body temperature and dehydration, both of which can harm fetal development. To this end, pregnant women should also stay out of saunas, steam rooms, and hot tubs or hot whirlpool baths.

Physical Activity Guidance for Canadians

- For uncomplicated pregnancies, women can participate in 30 minutes of aerobic activity sessions 3–4 times per week.[44]

FIGURE 16-9 Exercise Guidelines during Pregnancy

DO

Do begin to exercise gradually.

Do exercise regularly (most, if not all, days of the week).

Do warm up with 5 to 10 minutes of light activity.

Do 30 minutes of moderate physical activity.

Do cool down with 5 to 10 minutes of slow activity and gentle stretching.

Do drink water before, after, and during exercise.

Do eat enough to support the needs of pregnancy plus exercise.

Do rest adequately.

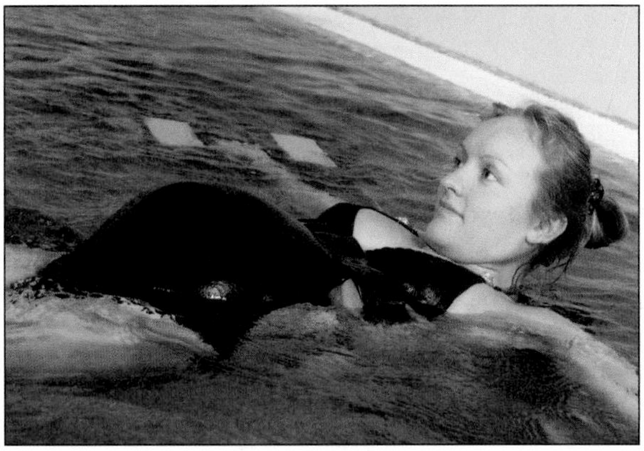

Sergey Chirkov/shutterstock

Pregnant women can enjoy the benefits of exercise.

DON'T

Don't exercise vigorously after long periods of inactivity.

Don't exercise in hot, humid weather.

Don't exercise when sick with fever.

Don't exercise while lying on your back after the 1st trimester of pregnancy or stand motionless for prolonged periods.

Don't exercise if you experience any pain, discomfort, or fatigue.

Don't participate in activities that may harm the abdomen or involve jerky, bouncy movements.

Don't scuba dive.

IN SUMMARY **A healthy pregnancy depends on a sufficient weight gain. Women who begin their pregnancies at a healthy weight need to gain about 13.5 kilograms (30 pounds), which covers the growth and development of the placenta, uterus, blood, breasts, and infant. By remaining active throughout pregnancy, a woman can develop the strength she needs to carry the extra weight and maintain habits that will help her lose it after the birth.**

Nutrition during Pregnancy

A woman's body changes dramatically during pregnancy. Her uterus and its supporting muscles increase in size and strength; her blood volume increases by half to carry the additional nutrients and other materials; her joints become more flexible in preparation for childbirth; her feet swell in response to high concentrations of the hormone estrogen, which promotes water retention and helps to ready the uterus for delivery; and her breasts enlarge in preparation for lactation. The hormones that mediate all these changes may influence her mood. She can best prepare to handle these changes given a nutritious diet, regular physical activity, plenty of rest, and caring companions. This section highlights the role of nutrition.

Energy and Nutrient Needs during Pregnancy

From conception to birth, all parts of the infant—bones, muscles, blood cells, skin, and all other tissues—are made from nutrients in the foods the mother eats. For most women, nutrient needs during pregnancy and lactation ♦ are higher than at any other time (see Figure 16-10 on page 516). To meet the high nutrient demands of pregnancy, a woman will need to make careful food choices, but her body will also help by maximizing absorption and minimizing losses.

♦ The Dietary Reference Intakes (DRI) table on the inside front cover provides separate listings for women during pregnancy and lactation, reflecting their heightened nutrient needs.

Energy The enhanced work of pregnancy raises the basal metabolic rate dramatically and demands extra energy.[45] Energy needs of pregnant women are greater than those of nonpregnant women—an additional 340 kcalories per day during the second trimester and an extra 450 kcalories per day during the third. ♦ A woman can easily get these added kcalories with nutrient-dense selections from the four food groups, although the *Food Guide* does recommend supplemental folate and iron during pregnancy. See Figure 16-11 (p. 517) for a sample menu for pregnant and lactating women.

♦ Energy requirement during pregnancy:
- 1st trimester: +0 kcal/day
- 2nd trimester: +340 kcal/day
- 3rd trimester: +450 kcal/day

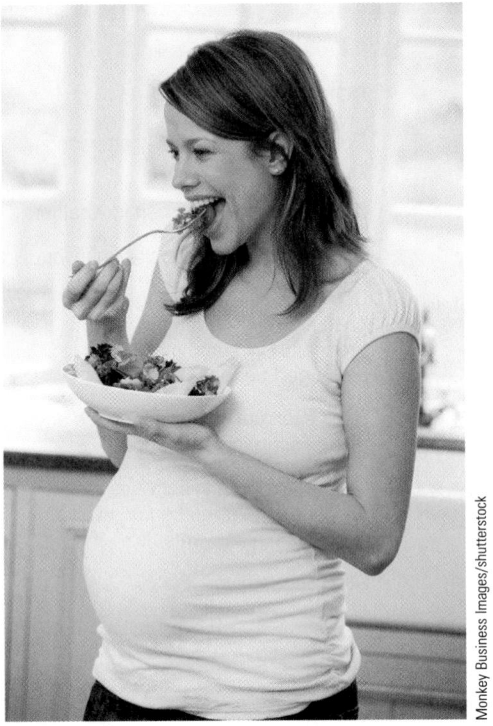
Monkey Business Images/shutterstock

A pregnant woman's food choices support both her health and her infant's growth and development.

For a 2000-kcalorie daily intake, these added kcalories represent about 15 to 20 percent more food energy than before pregnancy. The increase in nutrient needs is often greater than this, so nutrient-dense foods should be chosen to supply the extra kcalories: foods such as whole-grain breads and cereals, legumes, dark

FIGURE 16-10 Comparison of Nutrient Recommendations for Nonpregnant, Pregnant, and Lactating Women

For actual values, turn to the table on the inside front cover.

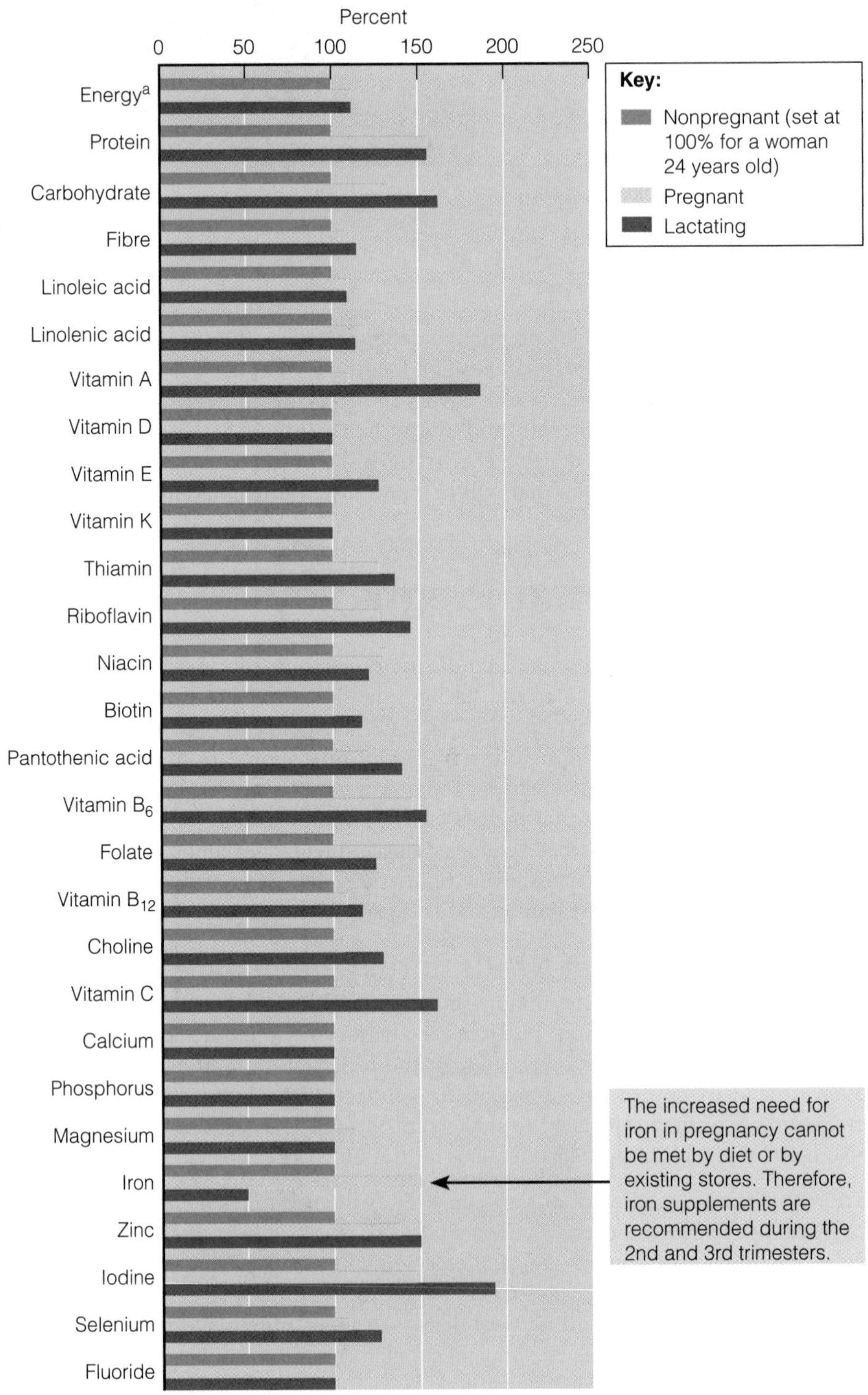
Percent
0
50
100
150
200
250
Energy[a]
Protein
Carbohydrate
Fibre
Linoleic acid
Linolenic acid
Vitamin A
Vitamin D
Vitamin E
Vitamin K
Thiamin
Riboflavin
Niacin
Biotin
Pantothenic acid
Vitamin B6
Folate
Vitamin B12
Choline
Vitamin C
Calcium
Phosphorus
Magnesium
Iron
Zinc
Iodine
Selenium
Fluoride
Key:
Nonpregnant (set at 100% for a woman 24 years old)
Pregnant
Lactating
The increased need for iron in pregnancy cannot be met by diet or by existing stores. Therefore, iron supplements are recommended during the 2nd and 3rd trimesters.

[a]Energy allowance during pregnancy is for second trimester; energy allowance during the third trimester is slightly higher; no additional allowance is provided during the first trimester. Energy allowance during lactation is for the first six months; energy allowance during the second six months is slightly higher.

green vegetables, citrus fruits, low-fat milk and milk products, and lean meats, fish, poultry, and eggs.

Carbohydrate Ample carbohydrate (ideally, 175 grams or more per day and certainly no less than 135 grams) is necessary to fuel the fetal brain. Sufficient carbohydrate also ensures that the protein needed for growth will not be broken down and used to make glucose.

Protein The protein RDA ♦ for pregnancy is an additional 25 grams per day higher than for nonpregnant women. Pregnant women can easily meet their protein needs by selecting meats, milk products, and protein-containing plant foods such as legumes, whole grains, nuts, and seeds. Because use of high-protein supplements during pregnancy may be harmful to the infant's development, it is discouraged.

♦ Protein RDA during pregnancy:
- +25 g/day

Essential Fatty Acids The high nutrient requirements of pregnancy leave little room in the diet for excess fat, but the essential long-chain polyunsaturated fatty acids are particularly important to the growth and development of the fetus.[46] The brain is largely made of lipid material, and it depends heavily on the long-chain omega-3 (e.g., eicosapentaenoic acid, EPA, and docosaheaxaenoic acid, DHA) and omega-6 (arachidonic acid, AA) fatty acids for its growth, function, and structure.[47] (See Table 5-2 on p. 149 for a list of good food sources of the omega fatty acids.)

Nutrients for Blood Production and Cell Growth New cells are laid down at a tremendous pace as the fetus grows and develops. At the same time, the mother's red blood cell mass expands. All nutrients are important in these processes, but for folate, vitamin B_{12}, iron, and zinc, the needs are especially great due to their key roles in the synthesis of DNA and new cells.

The requirement for folate increases dramatically during pregnancy. ♦ It is best to obtain sufficient folate from a combination of supplements, fortified foods, and a diet that includes fruits, juices, green vegetables, and whole grains.[48] The "How To" feature in Chapter 10 on p. 317 describes how folate from each of these sources contributes to a day's intake.

♦ Folate RDA during pregnancy:
- 600 µg/day

The pregnant woman also has a slightly greater need for the B vitamin that activates the folate enzyme—vitamin B_{12}. ♦ Generally, even modest amounts of meat, fish, eggs, or milk products together with body stores easily meet the need

♦ Vitamin B_{12} RDA during pregnancy:
- 2.6 µg/day

FIGURE 16-11 Daily Food Choices for Pregnancy (2nd and 3rd trimesters) and Lactation

Food Group	Amount
Fruits	500 mL (2 c)
Vegetables	750 mL (3 c)
Grains	240 g
Meats and legumes	200 g
Milk	750 mL (3 c)

SAMPLE MENU

Breakfast
1 whole-wheat English muffin
30 mL (2 Tbsp) peanut butter
250 mL (1 c) low-fat vanilla yogurt
125 mL (½ c) fresh strawberries
250 mL (1 c) orange juice

Midmorning snack
125 mL (½ c) cranberry juice
30 g pretzels

Lunch
Sandwich (tuna salad on whole-wheat bread)
½ carrot (sticks)
250 mL (1 c) 1% milk

Dinner
Chicken cacciatore
90 g chicken
125 mL (½ c) stewed tomatoes
250 mL (1 c) rice
125 mL (½ c) summer squash
125 mL (1½ c) salad (spinach, mushrooms, carrots)
15 mL (1 Tbsp) salad dressing
1 slice Italian bread
30 mL (2 tsp) soft margarine
250 mL (1 c) 1% milk

NOTE: This sample meal plan provides about 2500 kcalories (55% from carbohydrate, 20% from protein, and 25% from fat) and meets most of the vitamin and mineral needs of pregnant and lactating women.

for vitamin B_{12}. Vegans who exclude all foods of animal origin, however, need daily supplements of vitamin B_{12} or vitamin B_{12}–fortified foods to prevent the neurological complications of a deficiency.

♦ Iron RDA during pregnancy:
- 27 mg/day

Pregnant women need iron ♦ to support their enlarged blood volume and to provide for placental and fetal needs.[49] The developing fetus draws on maternal iron stores to create sufficient stores of its own to last through the first four to six months after birth. Even women with inadequate iron stores transfer significant amounts of iron to the fetus, suggesting that the iron needs of the fetus have priority over those of the mother. In addition, blood losses are inevitable at birth, especially during a cesarean section, and can further drain the mother's supply.*

During pregnancy, the body makes several adaptations to help meet the exceptionally high need for iron. Menstruation, the major route of iron loss in women, ceases, and iron absorption improves thanks to an increase in transferrin, the body's iron-absorbing and iron-carrying protein. Without sufficient intake, though, iron stores would quickly dwindle.

Few women enter pregnancy with adequate iron stores, so a daily iron supplement is recommended during the second and third trimesters for all pregnant women. For this reason, most prenatal supplements provide 30 to 60 milligrams of iron a day. To enhance iron absorption, the supplement should be taken between meals or at bedtime and with liquids other than milk, coffee, or tea, which inhibit iron absorption. Drinking orange juice does not enhance iron absorption from supplements as it does from foods; vitamin C enhances iron absorption by converting iron from ferric to ferrous, but supplemental iron is already in the ferrous form. Vitamin C is helpful, however, in preventing the premature rupture of amniotic membranes.[50]

♦ Zinc RDA during pregnancy:
- 12 mg/day (≤18 yr)
- 11 mg/day (19–50 yr)

Zinc ♦ is required for DNA and RNA synthesis and thus for protein synthesis and cell development. Typical zinc intakes for pregnant women are lower than recommendations, but fortunately, zinc absorption increases when zinc intakes are low.[51] Routine supplementation is not advised.[52] Women taking iron supplements (more than 30 milligrams per day), however, may need zinc supplementation because large doses of iron can interfere with the body's absorption and use of zinc.

Nutrients for Bone Development Vitamin D and the bone-building minerals calcium, phosphorus, magnesium, and fluoride are in great demand during pregnancy. Insufficient intakes may produce abnormal fetal bones and teeth.

♦ The RDA for vitamin D increases to 15 ug/600 IU per day during pregnancy.

Vitamin D ♦ plays a vital role in calcium absorption and utilization. Consequently, severe maternal vitamin D deficiency interferes with normal calcium metabolism, resulting in rickets in the infant and osteomalacia in the mother. Regular exposure to sunlight and consumption of vitamin D–fortified milk are usually sufficient to provide the recommended amount of vitamin D during pregnancy, although some researchers question whether current recommendations, even with prenatal supplements, are adequate.[53]

♦ The RDA for calcium does not increase during pregnancy.

Calcium absorption and retention increase dramatically in pregnancy, helping the mother to meet the calcium needs of pregnancy. ♦ During the last trimester, as the fetal bones begin to calcify, more than 300 milligrams a day are transferred to the fetus. Recommendations to ensure an adequate calcium intake during pregnancy help to conserve maternal bones while supplying fetal needs.[54]

♦ The *Food Guide* suggests consuming 500–1000 millilitres (2–4 cups) per day of skim or 1% milk or the equivalent in milk products.

Calcium intakes for pregnant women ♦ typically fall below recommendations. Because bones are still actively depositing minerals until about age 30, adequate calcium is especially important for young women. Pregnant women younger than age 25 who receive less than 600 milligrams of dietary calcium daily need to increase their intake of milk, cheese, yogurt, and other calcium-rich foods. Alternatively, and less preferably, they may need a daily supplement of 600 milligrams of calcium.

*On average, almost twice as much blood is lost during a cesarean delivery as during the average vaginal delivery of a single fetus.

Other Nutrients The nutrients mentioned here are those most intensely involved in blood production, cell growth, and bone growth. Of course, other nutrients are also needed during pregnancy to support the growth and health of both fetus and mother. Even with adequate nutrition, repeated pregnancies within a short time span can deplete nutrient reserves. When this happens, fetal growth may be compromised, and maternal health may decline. The optimal interval between pregnancies is 18 to 23 months.

Nutrient Supplements Pregnant women who make wise food choices can meet most of their nutrient needs, with the possible exception of folate and iron. Even so, physicians routinely recommend daily multivitamin-mineral supplements for pregnant women. Prenatal supplements typically contain greater amounts of folate, iron, and calcium than regular multivitamin-mineral supplements. These supplements are particularly beneficial for women who do not eat adequately and for those in high-risk groups: women carrying multiple fetuses, cigarette smokers, and alcohol and drug abusers. The use of prenatal supplements may help reduce the risks of preterm delivery, low infant birthweights, and birth defects. Supplement use *prior* to conception also seems to reduce the risk of preterm births. Figure 16-12 presents a label from a standard prenatal supplement.

FIGURE 16-12 **Example of a Prenatal Supplement**

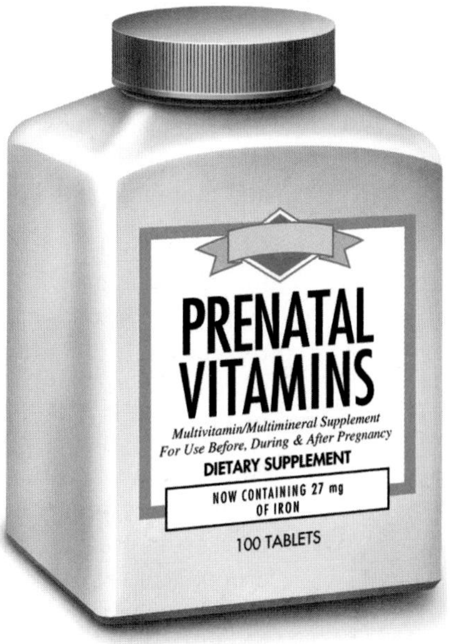
PRENATAL
VITAMINS
Multivitamin/Multimineral Supplement
For Use Before, During & After Pregnancy
DIETARY SUPPLEMENT
NOW CONTAINING 27 mg OF IRON
100 TABLETS

Supplement Facts
Serving Size 1 Tablet

Amount per Tablet	% Daily Value for Pregnant/ Lactating Women
Vitamin A 4000 IU	50%
Vitamin C 100 mg	167%
Vitamin D 400 IU	100%
Vitamin E 11 IU	37%
Thiamin 1.84 mg	108%
Riboflavin 1.7 mg	85%
Niacin 18 mg	90%
Vitamin B6 2.6 mg	104%
Folate 800 mcg	100%
Vitamin B12 4 mcg	50%
Calcium 200 mg	15%
Iron 27 mg	150%
Zinc 25 mg	167%

INGREDIENTS: calcium carbonate, microcrystalline cellulose, dicalcium phosphate, ascorbic acid, ferrous fumarate, zinc oxide, acacia, sucrose ester, niacinamide, modified cellulose gum, di-alpha tocopheryl acetate, hydroxypropyl methylcellulose, hydroxypropyl cellulose, artificial colours (FD&C blue no. 1 lake, FD&C red no. 40 lake, FD&C yellow no. 6 lake, titanium dioxide), polyethylene glycol, starch, pyridoxine hydrochloride, vitamin A acetate, riboflavin, thiamin mononitrate, folic acid, beta carotene, cholecalciferol, maltodextrin, gluten, cyanocobalamin, sodium bisulfite.

Vegetarian Diets during Pregnancy and Lactation

In general, a well-planned vegetarian diet can support a healthy pregnancy and successful lactation if it provides adequate energy and contains a wide variety of legumes, whole grains, nuts, seeds, fruits, and vegetables.[55] Many vegetarian women are well nourished, with nutrient intakes from diet alone exceeding the RDA for all vitamins and minerals except iron, which is low for most women. In contrast, vegan women who restrict themselves to an exclusively plant-based diet generally have low food energy intakes and are thin. For pregnant women, this can be a problem. Women with low prepregnancy weights and small weight gains during pregnancy jeopardize a healthy pregnancy.

Vegan diets may require supplementation with vitamin B_{12}, calcium, and vitamin D, or the addition of foods fortified with these nutrients. Infants of vegan parents may suffer spinal cord damage and develop severe psychomotor retardation due to a lack of vitamin B_{12} in the mother's diet during pregnancy. Breastfed infants of vegan mothers have been reported to develop vitamin B_{12} deficiency and severe movement disorders. Giving the infants vitamin B_{12} supplements corrects the blood and neurological symptoms of deficiency, as well as the structural abnormalities, but cognitive and language development delays may persist. A vegan mother needs a regular source of vitamin B_{12}–fortified foods or a supplement that provides 2.6 micrograms daily.

A pregnant woman who cannot meet her calcium needs through diet alone may need 600 milligrams of supplemental calcium daily, taken with meals. Pregnant women who do not receive sufficient dietary vitamin D or enough exposure to sunlight may need a supplement to achieve this level.

Common Nutrition-Related Concerns of Pregnancy

Nausea, constipation, heartburn, and food sensitivities are common nutrition-related concerns during pregnancy. A few simple strategies can help alleviate maternal discomforts (see Table 16-2 on page 520).

Nausea Not all women have queasy stomachs in the early months of pregnancy, but many do. The nausea of "morning sickness" may actually occur anytime and

TABLE 16-2 Strategies to Alleviate Maternal Discomforts

To Alleviate the Nausea of Pregnancy	To Prevent or Alleviate Constipation	To Prevent or Relieve Heartburn
• On waking, rise slowly. • Eat dry toast or crackers. • Chew gum or suck hard candies. • Eat small, frequent meals. • Avoid foods with offensive odours. • When nauseated, drink carbonated beverages instead of citrus juice, water, milk, coffee, or tea.	• Eat foods high in fibre (fruits, vegetables, and whole grains). • Exercise regularly. • Drink at least eight glasses of liquids a day. • Respond promptly to the urge to defecate. • Use laxatives only as prescribed by a physician; do not use mineral oil, because it interferes with absorption of fat-soluble vitamins.	• Relax and eat slowly. • Chew food thoroughly. • Eat small, frequent meals. • Drink liquids between meals. • Avoid spicy or greasy foods. • Sit up while eating; elevate the head while sleeping. • Wait 3 hours after eating before lying down. • Wait 2 hours after eating before exercising.

ranges from mild queasiness to debilitating nausea and vomiting. Severe and continued vomiting may require hospitalization if it results in acidosis, dehydration, or excessive weight loss. The hormonal changes of early pregnancy seem to be responsible for a woman's sensitivities to the appearance, texture, or smell of foods. Traditional strategies for quelling nausea are listed in Table 16-2, but many women benefit most from simply resting when nauseous and eating the foods they want when they feel like eating. They may also find comfort in a cleaner, quieter, and more temperate environment.

Constipation and Hemorrhoids As the hormones of pregnancy alter muscle tone and the growing fetus crowds intestinal organs, an expectant mother may experience constipation. She may also develop hemorrhoids (swollen veins of the rectum). Hemorrhoids can be painful, and straining during bowel movements may cause bleeding. She can gain relief by following the strategies listed in Table 16-2.

♦ Heartburn, medically known as **gastroesophageal reflux,** is discussed in Highlight 3.

Heartburn Heartburn ♦ is another common complaint during pregnancy. The hormones of pregnancy relax the digestive muscles, and the growing fetus puts increasing pressure on the mother's stomach. This combination causes gastroesophageal reflux, the painful sensation a person feels behind the breastbone when stomach acid splashes back up into the lower esophagus. Tips to help relieve heartburn are included in Table 16-2.

Food Cravings and Aversions Some women develop cravings for, or aversions to, particular foods and beverages during pregnancy. **Food cravings** and **food aversions** are fairly common, but they do not seem to reflect real physiological needs. In other words, a woman who craves pickles does not necessarily need salt. Similarly, cravings for ice cream are common in pregnancy but do not signify a calcium deficiency. Cravings and aversions that arise during pregnancy are most likely due to hormone-induced changes in sensitivity to taste and smell.

♦ **Pica** is the general term for eating nonfood items. The specific craving for nonfood items that come from the earth, such as clay or dirt, is known as **geophagia.**

Nonfood Cravings Some pregnant women develop cravings for nonfood items ♦ such as freezer frost, laundry starch, clay, soil, or ice—a practice known as pica. Pica is a cultural phenomenon that reflects a society's folklore; it is especially common among women of African descent. Pica is often associated with iron-deficiency anemia, but whether iron deficiency leads to pica or pica leads to iron deficiency is unclear. Eating clay or soil may interfere with iron absorption and displace iron-rich foods from the diet.

IN SUMMARY **Energy and nutrient needs are high during pregnancy. A balanced diet that includes an extra serving from each of the four food groups can usually meet these needs, with the possible exception of iron and folate (supplements are recommended). The nausea, constipation, and heartburn that sometimes accompany pregnancy can usually be alleviated with a few simple strategies. Food cravings do not typically reflect physiological needs.**

food cravings: strong desires to eat particular foods.

food aversions: strong desires to avoid particular foods.

High-Risk Pregnancies

Some pregnancies jeopardize the life and health of the mother and infant. Table 16-3 identifies several characteristics of a **high-risk pregnancy**. A woman with none of these risk factors is said to have a **low-risk pregnancy**. The more factors that apply, the higher the risk. All pregnant women, especially those in high-risk categories, need prenatal medical care, including dietary ♦ advice.

♦ Nutrition advice in prenatal care:
- Eat well-balanced meals.
- Gain enough weight to support fetal growth.
- Take prenatal supplements as prescribed.
- Stop drinking alcohol.

The Infant's Birthweight

A high-risk pregnancy is likely to produce an infant with **low birthweight** (LBW). Low-birthweight infants, defined as infants who weigh 2.5 kilograms (5½ pounds) or less, are classified according to their gestational age. Preterm infants are born before they are fully developed; they are often underweight and have trouble breathing because their lungs are immature. Preterm infants may be small, but if their size and weight are appropriate for their age, ♦ they can catch up in growth given adequate nutritional support. In contrast, small-for-gestational-age infants have suffered growth failure in the uterus and do not catch up as well. For the most part, survival improves with increased gestational age and birthweight.

♦ The weight of some preterm infants is **appropriate for gestational age (AGA);** others are **small for gestational age (SGA),** often reflecting malnutrition.

Low-birthweight infants are more likely to experience complications during delivery than normal-weight babies. They also have a statistically greater chance of having physical and mental birth defects, contracting diseases, and dying early in life. Of infants who die before their first birthdays, about two-thirds were low-birthweight newborns. Very-low-birthweight infants (1.5 kilograms/3½ pounds or less) struggle not only for their immediate physical health and survival, but for their future cognitive development and abilities as well.

A strong relationship is evident between socioeconomic disadvantage and low birthweight. Low socioeconomic status impairs fetal development by causing stress and by limiting access to medical care and to nutritious foods. Low socioeconomic status often accompanies teen pregnancies, smoking, and alcohol and drug abuse—all predictors of low birthweight.

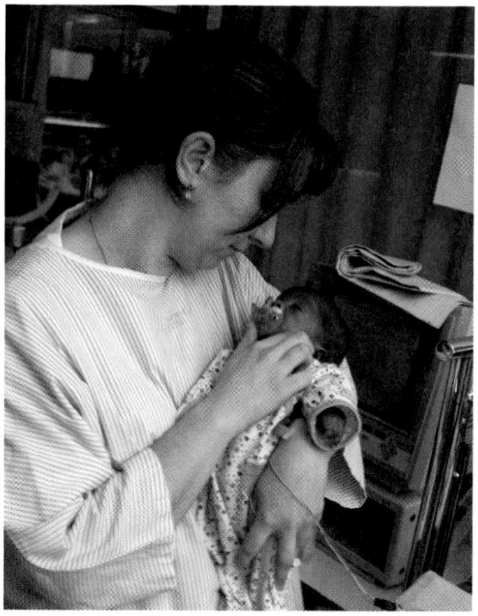
AJPhoto/Photo Researchers, Inc

Low-birthweight babies need special care and nourishment.

TABLE 16-3 High-Risk Pregnancy Factors

Factor	Condition that Raises Risk
Maternal weight	
• Prior to pregnancy	Prepregnancy BMI either <18.5 or ≥25
• During pregnancy	Insufficient or excessive pregnancy weight gain
Maternal nutrition	Nutrient deficiencies or toxicities; eating disorders
Socioeconomic status	Poverty, lack of family support, low level of education, limited food available
Lifestyle habits	Smoking, alcohol, or other drug use
Age	Teens, especially 15 years or younger; women 35 years or older
Previous pregnancies	
• Number	Many previous pregnancies (3 or more to mothers under age 20; 4 or more to mothers age 20 or older)
• Interval	Short or long intervals between pregnancies (<18 months or >59 months)
• Outcomes	Previous history of problems
• Multiple births	Twins or triplets
• Birthweight	Low- or high-birthweight infants
Maternal health	
• High blood pressure	Development of gestational hypertension
• Diabetes	Development of gestational diabetes
• Chronic diseases	Diabetes; heart, respiratory, and kidney disease; certain genetic disorders; special diets and medications

high-risk pregnancy: a pregnancy characterized by risk factors that make it likely the birth will be surrounded by problems such as premature delivery, difficult birth, retarded growth, birth defects, and early infant death.

low-risk pregnancy: a pregnancy characterized by factors that make it likely the birth will be normal and the infant healthy.

low birthweight (LBW): a birthweight of 2.5 kilograms (5½ pounds) or less; indicates probable poor health in the newborn and poor nutrition status in the mother during pregnancy, before pregnancy, or both. Optimal birthweight for a full-term baby is about 3100 to 3600 grams (6.8 to 7.9 pounds).

Malnutrition and Pregnancy Good nutrition clearly supports a healthy pregnancy. In contrast, malnutrition interferes with the ability to conceive, the likelihood of implantation, and the subsequent development of a fetus should conception and implantation occur.[56]

Malnutrition and Fertility The nutrition habits and lifestyle choices people make can influence the course of a pregnancy they are not even planning at the time. Severe malnutrition and food deprivation can reduce fertility because women may develop amenorrhea, ♦ and men may be unable to produce viable sperm. Furthermore, both men and women lose sexual interest during times of starvation. Starvation arises predictably during famines, wars, and droughts, but it can also occur amid peace and plenty. Many young women who diet excessively are starving and suffering from malnutrition (see Highlight 8).

♦ **Amenorrhea** is the temporary or permanent absence of menstrual periods. Amenorrhea is normal before puberty, after menopause, during pregnancy, and during lactation; otherwise it is abnormal.

Malnutrition and Early Pregnancy If a malnourished woman does become pregnant, she faces the challenge of supporting both the growth of a baby and her own health with inadequate nutrient stores. Malnutrition prior to and around conception prevents the placenta from developing fully. A poorly developed placenta cannot deliver optimum nourishment to the fetus, and the infant will be born small and possibly with physical and cognitive abnormalities. If this small infant is a female, she may develop poorly and have an elevated risk of developing a chronic condition that could impair her ability to give birth to a healthy infant. Thus a woman's malnutrition can adversely affect not only her children but her *grandchildren*.

Malnutrition and Fetal Development Without adequate nutrition during pregnancy, fetal growth and infant health are compromised. In general, consequences of malnutrition during pregnancy include fetal growth retardation, congenital malformations (birth defects), spontaneous abortion and stillbirth, preterm birth, and low infant birthweight. Malnutrition, coupled with low birthweight, is a factor in more than half of all deaths of children younger than four years of age worldwide.

Food Assistance Programs Women in high-risk pregnancies can find assistance from the Canada Prenatal Nutrition Program (CPNP)—a high-quality, cost-effective health-care and nutrition services program for women, infants, and children in Canada. It provides nutrition education and nutritious foods to infants, children, and pregnant and breastfeeding women who qualify and have a high risk of medical or nutritional problems. ♦ The program is both remedial and preventive: services include health-care referrals, nutrition education, prenatal vitamins, and food packages or vouchers for specific foods. These foods supply nutrients known to be lacking in the diets of the target population—most notably, protein, calcium, iron, vitamin A, and vitamin C. About 50 000 women receive CPNP benefits each year.

♦ Canada Prenatal Nutrition Program (CPNP)
- There are about 330 sites across Canada
- Serves about 2000 communities
- Serves close to 50 000 women each year

Maternal Health Medical disorders can threaten the life and health of both mother and fetus. If diagnosed and treated early, many diseases can be managed to ensure a healthy outcome—another strong argument for early prenatal care. Furthermore, the changes in pregnancy can reveal disease risks, making screening important and early intervention possible.[57]

Preexisting Diabetes The risks of diabetes depend on how well it is managed before and during pregnancy. Without proper management of maternal diabetes, women face high infertility rates, and those who do conceive may experience episodes of severe hypoglycemia or hyperglycemia, preterm labour, and pregnancy-related hypertension. Infants may be large, suffer physical and mental abnormalities, and experience other complications such as severe hypoglycemia or respiratory distress, both of which can be fatal. Signs of fetal health problems are apparent even when maternal glucose is above normal but still below the diagnosis of diabetes.[58] To minimize complications, a woman needs to achieve glucose control before conception and continued glucose control throughout pregnancy.[59]

Gestational Diabetes For every 25 women entering pregnancy, one will develop a condition known as **gestational diabetes** during pregnancy. Gestational diabetes usually develops during the second half of pregnancy, with subsequent return to normal after childbirth. Some women with gestational diabetes, however, develop diabetes (usually type 2) after pregnancy, especially if they are overweight.[60] For this reason, health-care professionals strongly advise against excessive weight gain during pregnancy.

The most common consequences of gestational diabetes are complications during labour and delivery and a high infant birthweight. Birth defects associated with gestational diabetes include heart damage, limb deformities, and neural tube defects. To ensure that the problems of gestational diabetes are dealt with promptly, physicians screen for the risk factors ♦ listed in the margin and test high-risk women for glucose intolerance immediately and average-risk women between 24 and 28 weeks gestation.[61]

Dietary recommendations should meet the needs of pregnancy and maternal blood glucose goals.[62] Diet and moderate exercise may control gestational diabetes, but if blood glucose fails to normalize, insulin or other drugs may be required. Importantly, treatment reduces birth complications, infant deaths, and maybe even postpartum depression.[63]

♦ Risk factors for gestational diabetes:
- Age 25 or older
- BMI ≥25 or excessive weight gain
- Complications in previous pregnancies, including gestational diabetes or high-birthweight infant
- Prediabetes or symptoms of diabetes
- Family history of diabetes
- Be of Aboriginal, Hispanic, South Asian, Asian, or African descent

Chronic Hypertension Hypertension complicates pregnancy and affects its outcome in different ways, depending on when the hypertension first develops and on how severe it becomes.[64] In addition to the threats hypertension always carries (such as heart attack and stroke), high blood pressure increases the risks of a low-birthweight infant or the separation of the placenta from the wall of the uterus before the birth, resulting in stillbirth. Ideally, before a woman with hypertension becomes pregnant, her blood pressure is under control.

Gestational Hypertension Some women develop **gestational hypertension**—high blood pressure during the second half of pregnancy.* For 50 percent of the women with gestational hypertension, the rise in blood pressure is mild and does not affect the pregnancy adversely. Blood pressure usually returns to normal during the first few weeks after childbirth. For the other 50 percent, gestational hypertension is an early sign of the most serious maternal complication of pregnancy—preeclampsia.

Preeclampsia **Preeclampsia** ♦ is a condition characterized not only by gestational hypertension but also by protein in the urine. The cause of preeclampsia remains unclear, but it usually occurs with first pregnancies ♦ and most often after 20 weeks gestation. Symptoms typically regress within two days of delivery. Both men and women who were born of pregnancies complicated by preeclampsia are more likely to have a child born of a pregnancy complicated by preeclampsia, suggesting a genetic predisposition. Black women have a much greater risk of preeclampsia than white women.

♦ Preeclampsia affects more than 10 000 pregnant women in Canada annually.[65]

♦ Signs and symptoms of preeclampsia:
- Hypertension
- Protein in the urine
- Upper abdominal pain
- Severe headaches
- Swelling of hands, feet, and face
- Vomiting
- Blurred vision
- Sudden weight gain 0.5 kilogram (1 lb) per day
- Fetal growth retardation

Preeclampsia affects almost all of the mother's organs—the circulatory system, liver, kidneys, and brain.[66] Blood flow through the vessels that supply oxygen and nutrients to the placenta diminishes. For this reason, preeclampsia often retards fetal growth. It also seems to increase the risk of epilepsy for the infant.[67] In some cases, the placenta separates from the uterus, resulting in preterm birth or stillbirth.

Preeclampsia can progress rapidly to **eclampsia**—a condition characterized by seizures and coma. Maternal death during pregnancy and childbirth is extremely rare in developed countries, but when it does occur, eclampsia is a common cause. The rate of death for black women with eclampsia is more than four times the rate for white women.

Preeclampsia demands prompt medical attention. Treatment focuses on controlling blood pressure and preventing seizures. If preeclampsia develops early and is severe, induced labour or cesarean section may be necessary, regardless of gestational age. The infant will be preterm, with all of the associated problems,

gestational diabetes: glucose intolerance with onset or first recognition during pregnancy.

gestational hypertension: high blood pressure that develops in the second half of pregnancy and resolves after childbirth, usually without affecting the outcome of the pregnancy.

preeclampsia (PRE-ee-KLAMP-see-ah): a condition characterized by hypertension and protein in the urine.

eclampsia (eh-KLAMP-see-ah): a severe stage of preeclampsia characterized by seizures.

*Blood pressure of 140/90 millimetres mercury or greater during the second half of pregnancy in a woman who has not previously exhibited hypertension indicates high blood pressure.

including poor lung development and special care needs. Several dietary factors have been studied, but none have proved beneficial in preventing preeclampsia.[68] Limited research suggests that exercise may protect against preeclampsia by stimulating placenta growth and vascularity and reducing oxidative stress.[69]

The Mother's Age

Maternal age also influences the course of a pregnancy. Compared with women of the physically ideal childbearing age of 20 to 25, both younger and older women face more complications of pregnancy.

Pregnancy in Adolescents Many adolescents become sexually active before age 19, and approximately 40 000 adolescent girls face pregnancies each year in Canada; slightly less than half of them give birth.[70] Nourishing a growing fetus adds to a teenage girl's nutrition burden, especially if her growth is still incomplete. Simply being young and physically immature increases the risks of pregnancy complications. Pregnant teens are less likely to receive early prenatal care and are more likely to smoke during pregnancy—two factors that predict low birthweight and infant death.[71]

Common complications among adolescent mothers include iron-deficiency anemia (which may reflect poor diet and inadequate prenatal care) and prolonged labour (which reflects the mother's physical immaturity). On a positive note, maternal death is lowest for mothers under age 20.

The rates of stillbirths, preterm births, and low-birthweight infants are high for teenagers—both for teen moms and for teen dads.[72] Many of these infants suffer physical problems, require intensive care, and die within the first year. Furthermore, their low economic status contributes significantly to the complications surrounding their pregnancies. At a time when prenatal care is most important, it is less accessible. And the pattern of teenage pregnancies continues from generation to generation, with almost 40 percent of the daughters born to teenage mothers becoming teenage mothers themselves. Clearly, teenage pregnancy is a major public health problem.

To support the needs of both mother and fetus, young teenagers (13 to 16 years old) are encouraged to strive for the highest weight gains recommended for pregnancy. For a teen who enters pregnancy at a healthy body weight, a weight gain of approximately 16 kilograms (35 pounds) is recommended; this amount minimizes the risk of delivering a low-birthweight infant. Pregnant and lactating teenagers can use the *Food Guide*, making sure to select a high enough kcalorie level to support adequate weight gain.

Without the appropriate economic, social, and physical support, a young mother will not be able to care for herself during her pregnancy and for her child after the birth. To improve her chances for a successful pregnancy and a healthy infant, she must seek prenatal care. CPNP provides health-care referrals and helps pregnant teenagers obtain adequate food for themselves and their infants. (CPNP is introduced on p. 522.)

Pregnancy in Older Women In the last several decades, many women have delayed childbearing while they pursue education and careers. As a result, the number of first births to women 35 and older has increased dramatically. Most of these women, even those older than age 50, have healthy pregnancies.

The few complications associated with later childbearing often reflect chronic conditions such as hypertension and diabetes, which can complicate an otherwise healthy pregnancy. These complications may result in a cesarean section, which is twice as common in women older than 35 as among younger women. For all these reasons, maternal death rates are higher in women older than 35 than in younger women.

The babies of older mothers face problems of their own including higher rates of preterm births and low birthweight. Their rates of birth defects are also high. Because 1 out of 50 pregnancies in older women produces an infant with genetic abnormalities, obstetricians routinely screen women older than 35. For a 40-year-old mother, the risk of having a child with **Down syndrome**, for example, is about

Down syndrome: a genetic abnormality that causes mental retardation, short stature, and flattened facial features.

1 in 100 compared with 1 in 300 for a 35-year-old and 1 in 10 000 for a 20-year-old. In addition, fetal death is twice as high for women 35 years and older than for younger women. Why this is so remains a bit of a mystery. One possibility is that the uterine blood vessels of older women may not fully adapt to the increased demands of pregnancy.

Practices Incompatible with Pregnancy

Besides malnutrition, a variety of lifestyle factors can have adverse effects on pregnancy, and some may be teratogenic. ♦ People who are planning to have children can make the choice to practice healthy behaviours.

♦ The word *teratogenic* describes a factor that causes abnormal fetal development and birth defects.

Alcohol Over 70 percent of women indicated that they would stop drinking if they became pregnant.[73] Alcohol consumption during pregnancy can cause irreversible mental and physical retardation of the fetus—fetal alcohol spectrum disorder (FASD). Of the leading causes of mental retardation, FASD is the only one that is totally *preventable*. To that end, Health Canada urges all pregnant women to refrain from drinking alcohol. Fetal alcohol spectrum disorder is the topic of Highlight 16, which includes mention of how alcohol consumption by men may also affect fertility and fetal development.

Medicinal Drugs Drugs other than alcohol can also cause complications during pregnancy, problems in labour, and serious birth defects. For these reasons, pregnant women should not take any medicines without consulting their physicians, who must weigh the benefits against the risks.

Herbal Supplements Similarly, pregnant women should seek a physician's advice before using herbal supplements. Women sometimes seek herbal preparations during their pregnancies to quell nausea, induce labour, aid digestion, promote water loss, support restful sleep, and fight depression. As Highlight 19 explains, some herbs may be safe, but many others are definitely harmful.

Illicit Drugs The recommendation to avoid drugs during pregnancy also includes illicit drugs, of course. Unfortunately, use of illicit drugs, such as cocaine and marijuana, is common among some pregnant women.

Drugs of abuse, such as cocaine, easily cross the placenta and impair fetal growth and development. Furthermore, they are responsible for preterm births, low-birthweight infants, perinatal deaths, ♦ and sudden infant deaths. If these newborns survive, central nervous system damage is evident: their cries, sleep, and behaviours early in life are abnormal, and their cognitive development later in life is impaired.[74] They may be hypersensitive or underaroused; those who test positive for drugs suffer the greatest effects of toxicity and withdrawal. Their growth throughout childhood continues at a slow rate.[75]

♦ The word *perinatal* refers to the time between the twenty-eighth week of gestation and one month after birth.

Smoking and Chewing Tobacco Unfortunately, an estimated 20–30 percent of pregnant women in Canada use tobacco.[76] Smoking cigarettes and chewing tobacco at any time exert harmful effects, and pregnancy dramatically magnifies the hazards of these practices. Smoking restricts the blood supply to the growing fetus and thus limits oxygen and nutrient delivery and waste removal. A mother who smokes is more likely to have a complicated birth and a low-birthweight infant. Indeed, of all preventable causes of low birthweight in Canada, smoking is at the top of the list. Although, most infants born to cigarette smokers are low birthweight, some are not, suggesting that the effect of smoking on birthweight also depends, in part, on genes involved in the metabolism of smoking toxins.

In addition to contributing to low birthweight, smoking interferes with lung growth and increases the risks of poor lung function, respiratory infections, and childhood asthma.[77] It can also cause death in an otherwise healthy fetus or newborn. A positive relationship exists between **sudden infant death syndrome** (SIDS) and both cigarette smoking during pregnancy and postnatal exposure to passive smoke. Smoking during pregnancy may reduce brain size and impair the intellectual and behavioural development of the child later in life.[78] The margin ♦ lists complications of smoking during pregnancy.

♦ Complications associated with smoking during pregnancy:
- Fetal growth retardation
- Low birthweight
- Complications at birth (prolonged final stage of labour)
- Mislocation of the placenta
- Premature separation of the placenta
- Vaginal bleeding
- Spontaneous abortion
- Fetal death
- Sudden infant death syndrome (SIDS)
- Middle ear diseases
- Cardiac and respiratory diseases

sudden infant death syndrome (SIDS): the unexpected and unexplained death of an apparently well infant; the most common cause of death of infants between the second week and the end of the first year of life; also called *crib death*.

Infants of mothers who chew tobacco also have low birthweights and high rates of fetal deaths. Any woman who smokes cigarettes or chews tobacco and is considering pregnancy or who is already pregnant needs to quit.

Environmental Contaminants Proving that environmental contaminants cause reproductive damage is difficult, but evidence is established for wildlife and seems likely for human beings. Infants and young children of pregnant women exposed to environmental contaminants such as lead show signs of delayed mental and psychomotor development. During pregnancy, lead readily moves across the placenta, inflicting severe damage on the developing fetal nervous system. In addition, infants exposed to even low levels of lead during gestation weigh less at birth and consequently struggle to survive. For these reasons, it is particularly important that pregnant women receive foods and beverages grown and prepared in environments free of contamination. A diet high in calcium will help to defend against lead contamination, and breastfeeding may help to counterbalance developmental damage incurred from contamination during pregnancy.[79]

Mercury is among the contaminants of concern. As Chapter 5 mentions, fatty fish are a good source of omega-3 fatty acids, but some fish contain large amounts of the pollutant mercury, which can impair fetal growth and harm the developing brain and nervous system.[80] Because the benefits of seafood consumption seem to outweigh the risks, pregnant (and lactating) women should do the following:[81]

- Avoid shark, swordfish, king mackerel, and tilefish (also called golden snapper or golden bass).
- Limit average weekly consumption to 350 grams (cooked or canned) of seafood *or* to 180 grams (cooked or canned) of white (albacore) tuna.

Supplements of fish oil are not recommended because they may contain concentrated toxins and because their effects on pregnancy remain unknown.

Foodborne Illness As Chapter 20 explains, foodborne illnesses arise when people eat foods that contain infectious microbes or microbes that produce toxins. At best, the vomiting and diarrhea associated with these illnesses can leave a pregnant woman exhausted and dehydrated; at worst, foodborne illnesses can cause meningitis, pneumonia, or even fetal death. Pregnant women are about 20 times more likely than other healthy adults to get the foodborne illness **listeriosis.** The margin ♦ presents tips to prevent listeriosis, and Chapter 20 includes precautions to minimize the risks of other common foodborne illnesses.

♦ Listeriosis can be prevented in the following ways:

- Use only pasteurized juices and dairy products; avoid Mexican soft cheeses, feta cheese, brie, Camembert, and blue-veined cheeses such as Roquefort.
- Thoroughly cook meat, poultry, eggs, and seafood.
- Thoroughly reheat hot dogs, luncheon meats, and deli meats, including cured meats such as salami.
- Wash all fruits and vegetables.
- Avoid refrigerated pâté, meat spreads, smoked seafood such as salmon or trout, and any fish labelled "nova," "lox," or "kippered," unless prepared in a cooked dish.

Dietary Guidance for Canadians

- Pregnant women should not eat or drink unpasteurized milk, milk products, or juices; raw or undercooked eggs, meat, or poultry; or raw sprouts.
- Pregnant women should eat only deli meats and frankfurters that have been reheated to steaming hot.

Vitamin-Mineral Megadoses The pregnant woman who is trying to eat well may mistakenly assume that more is better when it comes to multivitamin-mineral supplements. This is simply not true; many vitamins and minerals are toxic when taken in excess. Excessive preformed vitamin A is particularly infamous for its role in fetal malformations of the cranial nervous system. Intakes before the seventh week appear to be the most damaging. (Review Figure 16-4 on p. 508 to see how many tissues are in their critical periods prior to the seventh week.) For this reason, vitamin A supplements are not given during pregnancy unless there is specific evidence of deficiency, which is rare. A pregnant woman can obtain all the vitamin A and most of the other vitamins and minerals she needs by making wise food choices. She should take supplements only on the advice of a registered dietitian or physician.

listeriosis (lis-TEAR-ee-OH-sis): an infection caused by eating food contaminated with the bacterium *Listeria monocytogenes,* which can be killed by pasteurization and cooking but can survive at refrigerated temperatures; certain ready-to-eat foods, such as hot dogs and deli meats, may become contaminated after cooking or processing, but before packaging.

Caffeine Caffeine crosses the placenta, and the developing fetus has a limited ability to metabolize it. Research studies have not proved that caffeine (even in high doses) causes birth defects in human infants (as it does in animals), but limited evidence suggests that heavy use increases the risk of miscarriage and fetal death.[82] Depending on the quantities consumed and the mother's metabolism, caffeine may also interfere with fetal growth.[83] All things considered, it is most sensible to limit caffeine consumption to the equivalent of about 500 millilitres (two cups) of coffee a day. ♦ (The caffeine contents of selected beverages, foods, and drugs are listed in APPENDIX H.)

♦ The Public Health Agency of Canada recommends that "women of reproductive age consume no more than 300 mg of caffeine per day"

Weight-Loss Dieting Weight-loss dieting, even for short periods, can be hazardous during pregnancy. Low-carbohydrate diets or fasts that cause ketosis deprive the fetal brain of needed glucose and may impair cognitive development. Such diets are also likely to lack other nutrients vital to fetal growth. Regardless of prepregnancy weight, pregnant women need an adequate diet and sufficient weight gain to support healthy fetal development.

Sugar Substitutes Artificial sweeteners have been extensively investigated and found to be acceptable during pregnancy if used within Health Canada's guidelines.[84] Still, it is prudent for pregnant women to use sweeteners in moderation and within an otherwise nutritious and well-balanced diet. Women with the inherited disease phenylketonuria (PKU) should not use the artificial sweetener aspartame. Aspartame contains the amino acid phenylalanine, and people with PKU are unable to dispose of any excess phenylalanine. The accumulation of phenylalanine and its by-products is toxic to the developing nervous system, causing irreversible brain damage.

IN SUMMARY **High-risk pregnancies, especially for teenagers, threaten the life and health of both mother and infant. Proper nutrition and abstinence from smoking, alcohol, and other drugs improve the outcome. In addition, prenatal care includes monitoring pregnant women for gestational diabetes and preeclampsia.**

In general, the following guidelines will allow most women to enjoy a healthy pregnancy:[85]

- Strive for good nutrition and health prior to pregnancy and get prenatal care during pregnancy.
- Gain a healthy amount of weight.
- Eat a balanced diet, safely prepared, and engage in physical activity regularly.
- Take prenatal vitamin and mineral supplements as prescribed.
- Refrain from cigarettes, alcohol, and drugs (including herbal remedies, unless prescribed by a physician).

Childbirth marks the end of pregnancy and the beginning of a new set of parental responsibilities—including feeding the newborn.

Nutrition during Lactation

Before the end of her pregnancy, a woman needs to consider whether to feed her infant breast milk, ♦ infant formula, or both. These options are the only recommended foods for an infant during the first four to six months of life. The rate of breastfeeding initiation is just under 90 percent in Canada but it falls to about 25 percent at, six months.[86] This section focuses on how the mother's nutrition supports the making of breast milk, and the next chapter describes how the infant benefits from drinking breast milk.

♦ To learn about breastfeeding, a pregnant woman can read at least one of the many books available. At the end of this chapter, Nutrition on the Net provides a list of resources, including La Leche League International.

In many countries around the world, a woman breastfeeds her newborn without considering the alternatives or making a conscious decision. In other parts of the world, a woman feeds her newborn formula simply because she knows so little about breastfeeding. She may have misconceptions or feel uncomfortable about a process she has never seen or experienced. Breastfeeding offers many health benefits to both mother and infant, and every pregnant woman should seriously consider it (see Table 16-4).[87] Even so, women's choices are often influenced by factors other than health and science—factors such as culture, politics, religion, and marketing.[88] Mothers may have valid reasons for not breastfeeding, and formula-fed infants grow and develop into healthy children.

Lactation: A Physiological Process **Lactation** naturally follows pregnancy, as the mother's body continues to nourish the infant. The **mammary glands** secrete milk for this purpose. The mammary glands develop during puberty but remain fairly inactive until pregnancy. During pregnancy, hormones promote the growth and branching of a duct system in the breasts and the development of the milk-producing cells.

The hormones **prolactin** and **oxytocin** finely coordinate lactation. The infant's demand for milk stimulates the release of these hormones, which signal the mammary glands to supply milk. Prolactin is responsible for milk production. As long as the infant is nursing, prolactin concentrations remain high, and milk production continues.

The hormone oxytocin causes the mammary glands to eject milk into the ducts, a response known as the **let-down reflex.** The mother feels this reflex as a contraction of the breast, followed by the flow of milk and the release of pressure. By relaxing and eating well, the nursing mother promotes easy let-down of milk and greatly enhances her chances of successful lactation.

Breastfeeding: A Learned Behaviour Lactation is an automatic physiological process that virtually all mothers are capable of doing. Breastfeeding, on the other hand, is a learned behaviour that not all mothers decide to do. Of women who do breastfeed, those who receive early and repeated information

TABLE 16-4 Benefits of Breastfeeding

For Infants
• Provides the appropriate composition and balance of nutrients with high bioavailability • Provides hormones that promote physiological development • Improves cognitive development • Protects against a variety of infections • May protect against some chronic diseases—such as diabetes (both types), obesity, atherosclerosis, asthma, and hypertension—later in life • Protects against food allergies
For Mothers
• Contracts the uterus • Delays the return of regular ovulation, thus lengthening birth intervals (is not, however, a dependable method of contraception) • Conserves iron stores (by prolonging amenorrhea) • May protect against breast and ovarian cancer and reduce the risk of diabetes (type 2)
Other
• Cost savings from not needing medical treatment for childhood illnesses or time off work to care for them • Cost savings from not needing to purchase formula (even after adjusting for added foods in the diet of a lactating mother)[a] • Environmental savings to society from not needing to manufacture, package, and ship formula and dispose of the packaging • Convenience of not having to shop for and prepare formula

[a]A nursing mother produces close to 150 litres of milk during the first six months, saving roughly $450 in formula costs.

lactation: production and secretion of breast milk for the purpose of nourishing an infant.

mammary glands: glands of the female breast that secrete milk.

prolactin (pro-LAK-tin): a hormone secreted from the anterior pituitary gland that acts on the mammary glands to promote the production of milk. The release of prolactin is mediated by *prolactin-inhibiting hormone (PIH).*

- **pro** = promote
- **lacto** = milk

oxytocin (OCK-see-TOH-sin): a hormone that stimulates the mammary glands to eject milk during lactation and the uterus to contract during and after childbirth.

let-down reflex: the reflex that forces milk to the front of the breast when the infant begins to nurse.

TABLE 16-5 Ten Steps to Successful Breastfeeding

To promote breastfeeding, every maternity facility should:

- Develop a written breastfeeding policy that is routinely communicated to all health-care staff
- Train all health-care staff in the skills necessary to implement the breastfeeding policy
- Inform all pregnant women about the benefits and management of breastfeeding
- Help mothers initiate breastfeeding within ½ hour of birth
- Show mothers how to breastfeed and how to maintain lactation, even if they need to be separated from their infants
- Give newborn infants no food or drink other than breast milk, unless medically indicated
- Practise rooming-in, allowing mothers and infants to remain together 24 hours a day
- Encourage breastfeeding on demand
- Give no artificial nipples or pacifiers to breastfeeding infants[a]
- Foster the establishment of breastfeeding support groups and refer mothers to them at discharge from the facility

[a]Compared with nonusers, infants who use pacifiers breastfeed less frequently and stop breastfeeding at a younger age.
SOURCE: From the Baby-Friendly Hospital Initiative, "Ten Steps to Successful Breastfeeding", p.11. United Nations Children's Fund, 2009. http://www.unicef.org/nutrition/files/BFHI_2009_s1.pdf Reprinted by permission of the World Health Organization.

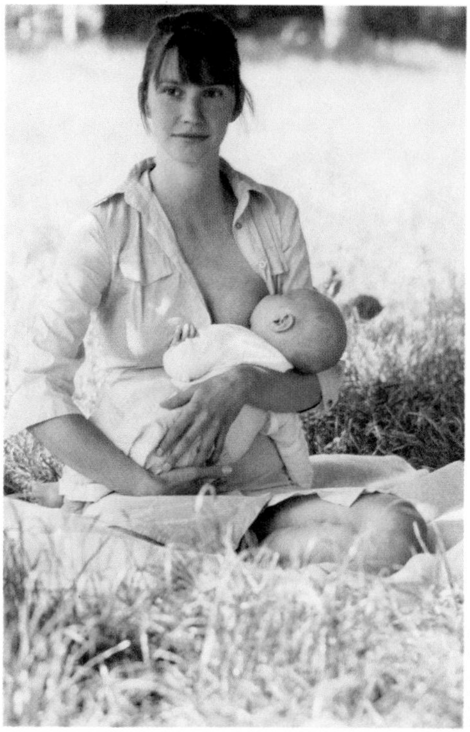

A woman who decides to breastfeed offers her infant a full array of nutrients and protective factors to support optimal health and development.

and support breastfeed their infants longer than others. Health-care professionals ♦ play an important role in providing encouragement and accurate information on breastfeeding.[89] Women who have been successful breastfeeding can offer advice and dispel misperceptions about lifestyle issues. Table 16-5 lists ten steps maternity facilities and health-care professionals can take to promote successful breastfeeding among new mothers.[90]

The mother's partner also plays an important role in encouraging breastfeeding.[91] When partners support the decision, mothers are more likely to start and continue breastfeeding. Clearly, educating those closest to the mother could change attitudes and promote breastfeeding.

Most healthy women who want to breastfeed can do so with a little preparation. Physical obstacles to breastfeeding are rare, although most nursing mothers quit before the recommended six months because of perceived difficulties. Obese mothers seem to have a particularly difficult time because of both biological and sociocultural factors.[92] Successful breastfeeding requires adequate nutrition and rest. This, plus the support of all who care, will help to enhance the well-being of mother and infant.

♦ Some hospitals employ **certified lactation consultants** who specialize in helping new mothers establish a healthy breastfeeding relationship with their newborn. These consultants are often registered nurses and dietitians with specialized training in breast and infant anatomy and physiology.

Maternal Energy and Nutrient Needs during Lactation

Ideally, the mother who chooses to breastfeed her infant will continue to eat nutrient-dense foods throughout lactation. An adequate diet is needed to support the stamina, patience, and self-confidence that nursing an infant demands.

Energy Intake and Exercise A nursing mother produces about 750 millilitres of milk per day, with considerable variation from woman to woman and in the same woman from time to time, depending primarily on the infant's demand for milk. To produce an adequate supply of milk, a woman needs extra energy—almost 500 kcalories a day above her regular need during the first six months of lactation. To meet this energy need, ♦ she can eat an extra 330 kcalories of food each day and let the fat reserves she accumulated during pregnancy provide the rest. Most women need at least 1800 kcalories a day to receive all the nutrients required for successful lactation. Severe energy restriction may hinder milk production.

♦ Energy requirement during lactation:
- 1st 6 mo: +330 kcal/day
- 2nd 6 mo: +400 kcal/day

After the birth of the infant, many women actively try to lose the extra weight and body fat they accumulated during pregnancy. How much weight a woman retains after pregnancy depends on her gestational weight gain and the duration and intensity of breastfeeding. Many women who follow recommendations for gestational weight gain and breastfeeding can readily return to prepregnancy weight by six months.[93] Neither the quality nor the quantity of breast milk is adversely affected by moderate weight loss, and infants grow normally.

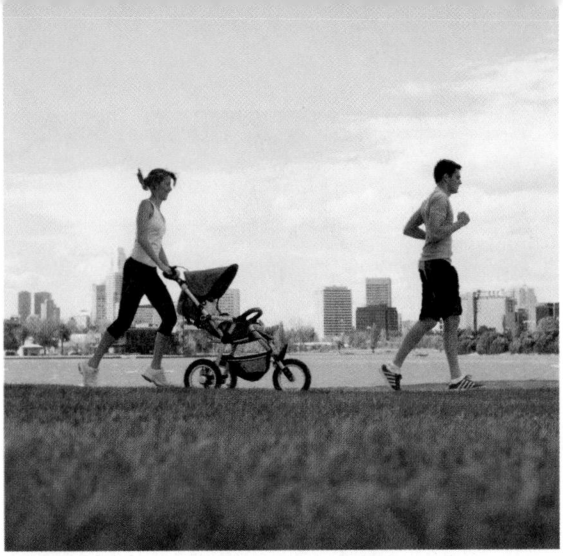
© eyetrigger Pty Ltd/Corbis

A jog through the park provides an opportunity for physical activity and fresh air.

Women often exercise to lose weight and improve fitness, and this is compatible with breastfeeding and infant growth. Because intense physical activity can raise the lactate concentration of breast milk and influence the milk's taste, some infants may prefer milk produced prior to exercise. In these cases, mothers can either breastfeed before exercise or express their milk before exercise for use afterward.

Dietary Guidance for Canadians

- Moderate weight reduction is safe for breastfeeding women and does not compromise weight gain of the nursing infant.
- Regular exercise does not adversely affect the mother's ability to successfully breastfeed.

Energy Nutrients Recommendations for protein and fatty acids intakes remain about the same during lactation as during pregnancy, but they increase for carbohydrates and fibres. Nursing mothers need additional carbohydrate to replace the glucose used to make the lactose in breast milk. The fibre recommendation is 1 gram higher simply because it is based on kcalorie intake, which increases during lactation. While Health Canada also recommends that women continue to eat fish during lactation (150 grams of cooked fish per week as recommended in *Canada's Food Guide*), they also mention that women pay special attention to the types of fish they consume during this time. For example, it is recommended that they choose the types of fish generally known to have low levels of contaminants, such as salmon, trout, and canned light tuna.[94]

Vitamins and Minerals A question often raised is whether a mother's milk may lack a nutrient if she fails to get enough in her diet. The answer differs from one nutrient to the next, but in general, nutritional inadequacies reduce the *quantity*, not the *quality*, of breast milk. Women can produce milk with adequate protein, carbohydrate, fat, and most minerals, even when their own supplies are limited. For these nutrients and for the vitamin folate as well, milk quality is maintained at the expense of maternal stores. This is most evident in the case of calcium: dietary calcium has no effect on the calcium concentration of breast milk, but maternal bones lose some density during lactation if calcium intakes are inadequate.[95] Bone density increases again when lactation ends; breastfeeding has no long-term harmful effects on bones. The nutrients in breast milk that are most likely to decline in response to prolonged inadequate intakes are the vitamins—especially vitamins B_6, B_{12}, A, and D. Review Figure 16-10 (p. 516) to compare a lactating woman's nutrient needs with those of pregnant and nonpregnant women.

Water Despite misconceptions, a mother who drinks more fluid does not produce more breast milk. To protect herself from dehydration, however, a lactating woman needs to drink plenty of fluids. ♦ A sensible guideline is to drink a glass of milk, juice, or water at each meal and each time the infant nurses.

♦ AI for *total* water (including drinking water, other beverages, and foods) during lactation: 3.8 L/day. Because foods provide about 20 percent of total water intake, beverages—including drinking water—should provide 3.1 L/day (≈13 cups).

Nutrient Supplements Most lactating women can obtain all the nutrients they need from a well-balanced diet without taking multivitamin-mineral supplements, although *Canada's Food Guide* does recommend a multivitamin containing folic acid every day while breastfeeding. Nevertheless, some may need iron supplements, not to enhance the iron in their breast milk, but to refill their depleted iron stores. The mother's iron stores dwindle during pregnancy as she supplies the developing fetus with enough iron to last through the first four to six months of the infant's life. In addition, childbirth may have incurred blood losses. Thus a woman may need iron supplements during lactation even though, until menstruation resumes, her iron requirement is about half that of other nonpregnant women her age.

Food Assistance Programs In general, women most likely to participate in the food assistance program CPNP—those who are poor and have little education—are less likely to breastfeed. Because CPNP recognizes the many benefits of breastfeeding, efforts are made to overcome this dilemma.[96] In addition to nutrition education and encouragement, breastfeeding mothers receive the following:

- More foods and larger quantities
- Breast pumps and other support materials

Together, these efforts help to provide nutrition support and encourage CPNP mothers to breastfeed.

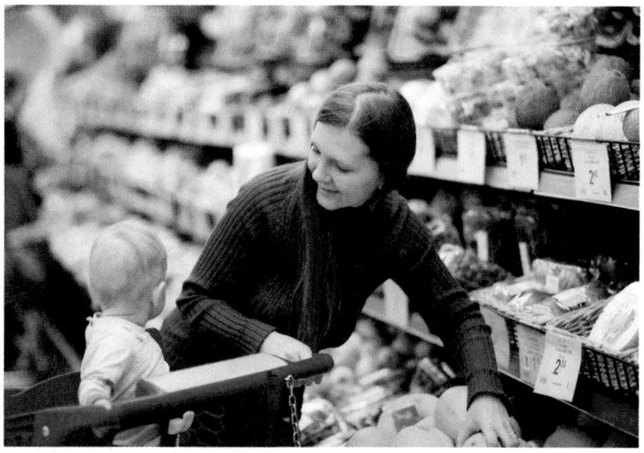
BlueOrange Studio/shutterstock

Nutritious foods support successful lactation.

Particular Foods Foods with strong or spicy flavours (such as garlic) may alter the flavour of breast milk. A sudden change in the taste of the milk may annoy some infants. Familiar flavours may enhance enjoyment.

Current evidence does not support a major role for maternal dietary restrictions during lactation to prevent or delay the onset of food allergy in infants.[97] Infants who develop symptoms of food allergy, however, may be more comfortable if the mother's diet excludes the most common offenders—cow's milk, eggs, fish, peanuts, and tree nuts. Generally, infants with a strong family history of food allergies benefit from breastfeeding.[98]

A nursing mother can usually eat whatever nutritious foods she chooses. If she suspects a particular food is causing the infant discomfort, her physician may recommend a dietary challenge: eliminate the food from the diet to see if the infant's reactions subside; then return the food to the diet and again monitor the infant's reactions. If a food must be eliminated for an extended time, appropriate substitutions must be made to ensure nutrient adequacy.

Maternal Health

If a woman has an ordinary cold, she can continue nursing without worry. If susceptible, the infant will catch it from her anyway. (Thanks to the immunological protection of breast milk, the baby may be less susceptible than a formula-fed baby would be.) With appropriate treatment, a woman who has an infectious disease such as tuberculosis or hepatitis can breastfeed; transmission is rare. Women with HIV (human immunodeficiency virus) infections, however, should consider other options.

HIV Infection and AIDS Mothers with HIV infections can transmit the virus (which causes AIDS) to their infants through breast milk, especially during the early months of breastfeeding. In developed countries such as Canada, where safe alternatives are available, HIV-positive women should *not* breastfeed their infants.[99] In developing countries, where the feeding of inappropriate or contaminated formulas causes 1.5 million infant deaths each year, breastfeeding can be critical to infant survival. Thus the decision of whether HIV-infected women in developing countries should breastfeed must consider the potential risks and benefits. The World Health Organization (WHO) recommends exclusive breastfeeding for infants of HIV-infected women for the first six months of life unless formula feeding is acceptable, feasible, affordable, sustainable, and safe before that time.[100] Alternatively, HIV-exposed infants may be protected by receiving antiretroviral treatment while being breastfed.[101]

Diabetes Women with diabetes (type 1) may need careful monitoring and counseling to ensure successful lactation. These women need to adjust their energy intakes and insulin doses to meet the heightened needs of lactation. Maintaining good glucose control helps to initiate lactation and support milk production.

Postpartum Amenorrhea Women who breastfeed experience prolonged **postpartum amenorrhea.** Absent menstrual periods, however, do not protect a woman from pregnancy. To prevent pregnancy, a couple must use some form of contraception. Breastfeeding women who use oral contraceptives should use progestin-only agents for at least the first six months.[102] Estrogen-containing oral contraceptives reduce the volume and the protein content of breast milk.

Breast Health Some women fear that breastfeeding will cause their breasts to sag. The breasts do swell and become heavy and large immediately after the birth,

postpartum amenorrhea (ay-MEN-oh-REE-ah): the normal temporary absence of menstrual periods immediately following childbirth.

but even when they produce enough milk to nourish a thriving infant, they eventually shrink back to their prepregnant size. Given proper support, diet, and exercise, breasts often return to their former shape and size when lactation ends. Breasts change their shape as the body ages, but breastfeeding does not accelerate this process.

Whether the physical and hormonal events of pregnancy and lactation protect women from later breast cancer is an area of active research.[103] Some research suggests no association between breastfeeding and breast cancer, whereas other research suggests a protective effect. Protection against breast cancer is most apparent for premenopausal women who were young when they breastfed and who breastfed for a long time.

Practices Incompatible with Lactation

Some substances impair milk production or enter breast milk and interfere with infant development. This section discusses practices that a breastfeeding mother should avoid.

Alcohol Alcohol easily enters breast milk, and its concentration peaks within an hour of ingestion. Infants drink less breast milk when their mothers have consumed even small amounts of alcohol (equivalent to a can of beer). Three possible reasons, acting separately or together, may explain why. For one, the alcohol may have altered the flavour of the breast milk and thereby the infants' acceptance of it. For another, because infants metabolize alcohol inefficiently, even low doses may be potent enough to suppress their feeding and cause sleepiness. Third, the alcohol may have interfered with lactation by inhibiting the hormone oxytocin.

In the past, alcohol has been recommended to mothers to facilitate lactation despite a lack of scientific evidence that it does so. The research summarized here suggests that alcohol actually hinders breastfeeding. An occasional alcoholic beverage may be within safe limits, but breastfeeding should be delayed for at least two hours afterward.

Medicinal Drugs Most medicines are compatible with breastfeeding, but some are contraindicated, either because they suppress lactation or because they are secreted into breast milk and can harm the infant. As a precaution, a nursing mother should consult with her physician prior to taking any drug, including herbal supplements.

Illicit Drugs Illicit drugs, of course, are harmful to the physical and emotional health of both the mother and the nursing infant. Breast milk can deliver such high doses of illicit drugs as to cause irritability, tremors, hallucinations, and even death in infants. Women on methadone maintenance can safely breastfeed their infants.[104]

Smoking Because cigarette smoking reduces milk volume, smokers may produce too little milk to meet their infants' energy needs. The milk they do produce contains nicotine, which alters its smell and flavour. Furthermore, infants of breastfeeding mothers who smoke sleep less than infants of those who do not smoke.[105] Infant exposure to passive smoke negates the protective effect breastfeeding offers against SIDS and increases the risks dramatically.

Environmental Contaminants Chapter 20 discusses environmental contaminants in the food supply. Some of these environmental contaminants, such as DDT, PCBs, and dioxin, can find their way into breast milk. Inuit mothers living in Arctic Quebec who eat seal and beluga whale blubber have high concentrations of DDT and PCBs in their breast milk, but the impact on infant development is unclear. Preliminary studies indicate that the children of these Inuit mothers are developing normally. Researchers speculate that the abundant omega-3 fatty acids of the Inuit diet may protect against damage to the central nervous system. Breast milk tainted with dioxin interferes with tooth development during early infancy, producing soft, mottled teeth that are vulnerable to dental caries. To limit mercury intake, lactating women should heed the fish restrictions mentioned earlier for pregnant women (see p. 514).

Caffeine Caffeine enters breast milk and may make an infant irritable and wakeful. As during pregnancy, caffeine consumption should be moderate (but less than 300 mg/day)—the equivalent of up to 500 millilitres (two cups) of coffee a day. Larger doses of caffeine may interfere with the bioavailability of iron from breast milk and impair the infant's iron status.

IN SUMMARY **The lactating woman needs extra fluid and enough energy and nutrients to produce about 750 millilitres of milk a day. Breastfeeding is contraindicated for those with HIV/AIDS. Alcohol, other drugs, smoking, and contaminants may reduce milk production or enter breast milk and impair infant development.**

This chapter has focused on the nutrition needs of the mother during pregnancy and lactation. The next chapter explores the dietary needs of infants, children, and adolescents.

Nutrition Portfolio

The choices a woman makes in preparation for, and in support of, pregnancy and lactation can influence both her health and her infant's development—today and for decades to come.

Go to Diet Analysis Plus and choose one of the days on which you tracked your diet and activity for an entire day. Select the Intake vs. Goals report to help you answer the following questions:

- For women of childbearing age, determine whether you consume at least 400 micrograms of dietary folate equivalents daily.
- For women who are pregnant, evaluate whether you are meeting your nutrition needs and gaining the amount of weight recommended.
- For women who are about to give birth, carefully consider all the advantages of breastfeeding your infant and obtain the needed advice to support you.

Diet Analysis PLUS **To complete this exercise, go to your Diet Analysis Plus at www.cengage.com/sso.**

Nutrition on the Net

CENGAGENOW™
For further study of topics covered in this chapter, log on to **www.cengage.com/sso.**

- Learn more about having a healthy baby and about birth defects from the March of Dimes and the U.S. National Center on Birth Defects and Developmental Disabilities: **www.marchofdimes.com** and **www.cdc.gov/ncbddd**
- Learn more about neural tube defects from the Spina Bifida Association of America: **www.spinabifidaassociation.org**
- Search for "birth defect," "pregnancy," "teenage pregnancy," "maternal health," and "breastfeeding" on Health Canada's website: **www.hc-sc.gc.ca**
- Search for "pregnancy" on the Dietitians of Canada's website: **www.dietitians.ca**
- Learn more about the Canadian Prenatal Nutrition Program on the Public Health Agency of Canada's website: **www.phac-aspc.gc.ca/hp-ps/dca-dea/prog-ini/cpnp-pcnp/index-eng.php**
- Visit the Canadian Paediatric Society's website: **www.cps.ca**
- Learn more about gestational diabetes from the Canadian Diabetes Association: **www.diabetes.ca**
- Learn more about breastfeeding from La Leche League Canada: **www.lllc.ca**
- Obtain prenatal nutrition guidelines from Health Canada: **www.hc-sc.gc.ca**
- Visit the U.S. Women's Health Information Center: **www.womenshealth.gov**

References

1. Health Canada, Food and Nutrition, Prenatal nutrition. www.hc-sc.gc.ca/fn-an/nutrition/prenatal/index-eng.php, accessed September 15, 2011; A Report of the CDC/ATSDR Preconception Care Work Group and the Select Panel on Preconception Care prepared by K. Johnson and coauthors, Recommendations to improve preconception health and health care: United States, *Morbidity and Mortality Weekly Report* 55 (2006): 1–23.
2. Health Canada, Food and Nutrition, Prenatal nutrition guidelines for health professionals: Gestational weight gain. www.hc-sc.gc.ca/fn-an/nutrition/prenatal/ewba-mbsa-eng.php#t2, accessed September 15, 2011; M. Jokela, M. Elovainio, and M. Kivimäki, Lower fertility associated with obesity and underweight: The U.S. National Longitudinal Survey of Youth, *American Journal of Clinical Nutrition* 88 (2008): 886–893; M. J. Davies, Evidence for effects of weight on reproduction in women, *Reproductive Biomedicine Online* 12 (2006): 552–561.
3. M. Sallmén and coauthors, Reduced fertility among overweight and obese men, *Epidemiology* 17 (2006): 520–523; H. I. Kort and coauthors, Impact of body mass index values on sperm quantity and quality, *Journal of Andrology* 27 (2006): 450–452.
4. R. Pasquali and A. Gambineri, Metabolic effects of obesity on reproduction, *Reproductive Biomedicine Online* 12 (2006): 542–551.
5. B. Eskenazi and coauthors, Antioxidant intake is associated with semen quality in healthy men, *Human Reproduction* 20 (2005): 1006–1012.
6. J. Mendiola and coauthors, A low intake of antioxidant nutrients is associated with poor semen quality in patients attending fertility clinics, *Fertility and Sterility,* http://doi:10.1016/j.fertnstert.2008.10.075; J. E. Chavarro and coauthors, Diet and lifestyle in the prevention of ovulatory disorder infertility, *Obstetrics and Gynecology* 110 (2007): 1050–1058.
7. S. Cordier, Evidence for a role of paternal exposures in developmental toxicity, *Basic and Clinical Pharmacology and Toxicology* 102 (2008): 176–181; S. Sépaniak, T. Forges, and P. Monnier-Barbarino, Cigarette smoking and fertility in women and men, *Gynécologie, Obstétrique and Fertilité* 34 (2006): 945–949.
8. Health Canada, *Eating Well with Canada's Food Guide.* www.hc-sc.gc.ca/fn-an/food-guide-aliment/index-eng.php and www.hc-sc.gc.ca/fn-an/pubs/nutrition/folate-eng.php, accessed September 12, 2011.
9. J. C. Cross and L. Mickelson, Nutritional influences on implantation and placental development, *Nutrition Reviews* 64 (2006): S12–S18.
10. P. De Wals and coauthors, Spina bifida before and after folic acid fortification in Canada, *Birth Defects Research Part A: Clinical and Molecular Teratology* 82:9 (2008): 622–626. http://onlinelibrary.wiley.com/doi/10.1002/bdra.20485/pdf, accessed September 12, 2011.
11. R. Padmanabhan, Etiology, pathogenesis and prevention of neural tube defects, *Congenital Anomalies* 46 (2006): 55–67.
12. U.S. Preventive Services Task Force, Folic acid for the prevention of neural tube defects: U.S. Preventive Services Task Force recommendation statement, *Annals of Internal Medicine* 150 (2009): 626–631; Canadian Paediatric Society, Periconceptional use of folic acid for the reduction of the risk of neural tube defects. www.cps.ca/english/statements/DT/dt95-01.htm#Neural tube defects, accessed September 12, 2011.
13. K. A. Bol, J. S. Collins, and R. S. Kirby, Survival of infants with neural tube defects in the presence of folic acid fortification, *Pediatrics* 117 (2006): 803–813; T. Tamura and M. F. Picciano, Folate and human reproduction, *American Journal of Clinical Nutrition* 83 (2006): 993–1016; L. B. Bailey and R. J. Berry, Folic acid supplementation and the occurrence of congenital heart defects, orofacial clefts, multiple births, and miscarriage, *American Journal of Clinical Nutrition* 81 (2005): 1213S–1217S; Canadian Paediatric Society, Periconceptional use of folic acid for the reduction of the risk of neural tube defects.
14. Health Canada, Food and Nutrition, Prenatal nutrition guidelines for health professionals: Folate contributes to a healthy pregnancy. www.hc-sc.gc.ca/fn-an/pubs/nutrition/folate-eng.php, accessed September 12, 2011.
15. Public Health Agency of Canada, Folic acid and the Prevention of neural tube defects—Information update from PHAC-2008. www.phac-aspc.gc.ca/fa-af/fa-af08-eng.php, accessed September 15, 2011; J. G. Ray, C. Meier, M. J. Vermeulen, S. Boss, P. R. Wyatt, and D. E. C. Cole, Association of neural tube defects and folic acid fortification in Canada, *New England Journal of Medicine* 350:9350 (2002): 2047–2048; P. Mersereau and coauthors, Spina bifida and anencephaly before and after folic acid mandate: United States, 1995–1996 and 1999–2000, *Morbidity and Mortality Weekly Report* 53 (2004): 362–365; J. Erickson, Folic acid and prevention of spina bifida and anencephaly, *Morbidity and Mortality Weekly Report* 51 (2002): 1–3.
16. C. K. Colapinto, D. L. O'Connor, and M. S. Tremblay, Folate status of adults in the Canadian Health Measures Survey, *Canadian Medical Association Journal* (early release December 13, 2010); Y. A. Shakur, D. Garrigeut, P. Corey, and D. L. O'Connor, Folic acid fortification above mandated levels results in a low prevalence of folate inadequacy among Canadians, *American Journal of Clinical Nutrition* 92 (2010): 818–825; R. L. Brent and G. P. Oakley, The folate debate, *Pediatrics* 117 (2006): 1418–1419; J. I. Rader and B. O. Schneeman, Prevalence of neural tube defects, folate status, and folate fortification of enriched cereal-grain products in the United States, *Pediatrics* 117 (2006): 1394–1399.
17. P. D. Gluckman and coauthors, Effect of in utero and early-life conditions on adult health and disease, *New England Journal of Medicine* 359 (2008): 61–73.
18. W. Palinski and coauthors, Developmental programming: Maternal hypercholesterolemia and immunity influence susceptibility to atherosclerosis, *Nutrition Reviews* 65 (2007): S182–S187.
19. F. Lussana and coauthors, Prenatal exposure to the Dutch famine is associated with a preference for fatty foods and a more atherogenic lipid profile, *American Journal of Clinical Nutrition* 88 (2008): 1648–1652; R. C. Painter and coauthors, Early onset of coronary artery disease after prenatal exposure to the Dutch famine, *American Journal of Clinical Nutrition* 84 (2006): 322–327; O. A. Kensara and coauthors, Fetal programming of body composition: Relation between birth weight and body composition measured with dual-energy X-ray absorptiometry and anthropometric methods in older Englishmen, *American Journal of Clinical Nutrition* 82 (2005): 980–987.
20. J. Rotteveel and coauthors, Infant and childhood growth patterns, insulin sensitivity, and blood pressure in prematurely born young adults, *Pediatrics* 122 (2008): 313–321.
21. L. Adair and D. Dahly, Developmental determinants of blood pressure in adults, *Annual Review of Nutrition* 25 (2005): 407–434.
22. J. C. Mathers, Early nutrition: Impact on epigenetics, *Forum of Nutrition* 60 (2007): 42–48.
23. B. Delage and R. H. Dashwood, Dietary manipulation of histone structure and function, *Annual Review of Nutrition* 28 (2008): 347–366; W. Kiess and coauthors, Adipocytes and adipose tissues, *Best Practice and Research. Clinical Endocrinology and Metabolism* 22 (2008): 135–153; W. S. Cutfield and coauthors, Could epigenetics play a role in the developmental origins of health and disease? *Pediatric Research* 61 (2007): 68R–75R; C. Junien and P. Nathanielsz, Report on the IASO Stock Conference 2006: Early and lifelong environmental epigenomic programming of metabolic syndrome, obesity and type II diabetes, *Obesity Review* 8 (2007): 487–502; D. A. Lawlor and coauthors, Epidemiologic evidence for the fetal overnutrition hypothesis: Findings from the Mater-University Study of Pregnancy and its Outcomes, *American Journal of Epidemiology* 165 (2007): 418–424; R. A. Waterland and K. B. Michels, Epigenetic epidemiology of the developmental origins hypothesis, *Annual Review of Nutrition* 27 (2007): 363–388.
24. G. K. Swamy, T. Østbye, and R. Skjærven, Association of preterm birth with long-term survival, reproduction, and next-generation preterm birth, *Journal of the American Medical Association* 299 (2008): 1429–1436.
25. Health Canada, Food and Nutrition, Prenatal Nutrition; Position of the American Dietetic Association and American Society for Nutrition: Obesity, reproduction, and pregnancy outcomes, *Journal of the American Dietetic Association* 109 (2009): 918–927; P. Brawarsky and coauthors, Pre-pregnancy and pregnancy-related factors and the risk of excessive or inadequate gestational weight gain, *International Journal of Gynaecology and Obestetrics* 91 (2005): 125–131.
26. Public Health Agency of Canada, What mothers say: The Canadian Maternity Experience Survey (2009). www.phac-aspc.gc.ca/rhs-ssg/pdf/survey-eng.pdf, accessed September 21, 2011; T. Henriksen, Nutrition

and pregnancy outcome, *Nutrition Reviews* 64 (2006): S19–S23; J. C. King, Maternal obesity, metabolism, and pregnancy outcomes, *Annual Review of Nutrition* 26 (2006): 271–291; D. B. Sarwer and coauthors, Pregnancy and obesity: A review and agenda for future research, *Journal of Women's Health* 15 (2006): 720–733.

27. S. Y. Chu and coauthors, Association between obesity during pregnancy and increased use of health care, *New England Journal of Medicine* 358 (2008): 1444–1453.
28. M. A. Maggard and coauthors, Pregnancy and fertility following bariatric surgery: A systematic review, *Journal of the American Medical Association* 300 (2008): 2286–2296.
29. E. A. Nohr and coauthors, Combined associations of prepregnancy body mass index and gestational weight gain with the outcome of pregnancy, *American Journal of Clinical Nutrition* 87 (2008): 1750–1759.
30. K. J. Stothard and coauthors, Maternal overweight and obesity and the risk of congenital anomalies: A systematic review and meta-analysis, *Journal of the American Medical Association* 301 (2009): 636–650.
31. King, 2006.
32. D. K. Waller and coauthors, Prepregnancy obesity as a risk factor for structural birth defects, *Archives of Pediatric and Adolescent Medicine* 161 (2007): 745–750.
33. R. Artal and coauthors, A lifestyle intervention of weight-gain restriction: Diet and exercise in obese women with gestational diabetes mellitus, *Applied Physiology, Nutrition, and Metabolism* 32 (2007): 596–601.
34. J. H. Cohen and H. Kim, Sociodemographic and health characteristics associated with attempting weight loss during pregnancy, *Preventing Chronic Disease* 6 (2009): A07.
35. Institute of Medicine, *Weight Gain during Pregnancy: Reexamining the Guidelines* (Washington, D.C.: National Academies Press, 2009).
36. C. M. Olson, Achieving a healthy weight gain during pregnancy, *Annual Review of Nutrition* 28 (2008): 411–423.
37. B. H. Wrotniak and coauthors, Gestational weight gain and risk of overweight in the offspring at age 7 y in a multicenter, multiethnic cohort study, *American Journal of Clinical Nutrition* 87 (2008): 1818–1824.
38. Health Canada, Food and Nutrition, Prenatal nutrition guidelines for health professionals: Gestational weight gain; A. L. Deierlein, A. M. Siega-Riz, and A. Herring, Dietary energy density but not glycemic load is associated with gestational weight gain, *American Journal of Clinical Nutrition* 88 (2008): 693–699.
39. J. L. Baker and coauthors, Breastfeeding reduces postpartum weight retention, *American Journal of Clinical Nutrition* 88 (2008): 1543–1551; N. F. Butte and coauthors, Composition of gestational weight gain impacts maternal fat retention and infant birth weight, *American Journal of Obstetrics and Gynecology* 189 (2003): 1423–1432.
40. D. A. Krummel, Postpartum weight control: A vicious cycle, *Journal of the American Dietetic Association* 107 (2007): 37–40; E. Villamor and S. Cnattingius, Interpregnancy weight change and risk of adverse pregnancy outcomes: A population-based study, *Lancet* 368 (2006): 1164–1170.
41. A. R. Amorium and coauthors, Does excess pregnancy weight gain constitute a major risk for increasing long-term BMI? *Obesity* 15 (2007): 1278–1286.
42. Health Canada, Food and Nutrition, Prenatal nutrition guidelines for health professionals: Gestational weight gain; Position of the American Dietetic Association: Nutrition and lifestyle for a healthy pregnancy outcome, *Journal of the American Dietetic Association* 108 (2008): 553–561; U.S. Department of Health and Human Services, *2008 Physical Activity Guidelines for Americans*, www.health.gov/paguidelines/guidelines/chapter7.aspx, accessed June 26, 2009.
43. A. B. Granath, M. S. Hellgren, and R. K. Gunnarsson, Water aerobics reduces sick leave due to low back pain during pregnancy, *Journal of Obstetrics, Gynecology, and Neonatal Nursing* 35 (2006): 465–471; S. A. Smith and Y. Michel, A pilot study on the effects of aquatic exercises on discomforts of pregnancy, *Journal of Obstetrics, Gynecology, and Neonatal Nursing* 35 (2006): 315–323.
44. Health Canada, Food and Nutrition, Draft prenatal nutrition guidelines for health professionals: Maternal weight and weight gain in pregnancy. www.hc-sc.gc.ca/fn-an/consult/_matern-weight-poids2009/draft-ebauche-eng.php, accessed September 12, 2011.
45. E. Forsum and M. Löf, Energy metabolism during human pregnancy, *Annual Review of Nutrition* 27 (2007): 277–292; M. Löf and coauthors, Changes in basal metabolic rate during pregnancy in relation to changes in body weight and composition, cardiac output, insulin-like growth factor I, and thyroid hormones and in relation to fetal growth, *American Journal of Clinical Nutrition* 81 (2005): 678–685.
46. S. M. Innis and R. W. Freisen, Essential n-3 fatty acids in pregnant women and early visual acuity maturation in term infants, *American Journal of Clinical Nutrition* 87 (2008): 548–557; M. von Eijsden and coauthors, Maternal n-3, n-6, and *trans* fatty acid profile early in pregnancy and term birth weight: A prospective cohort study, *American Journal of Clinical Nutrition* 87 (2008): 887–895.
47. R. Uauy and A. D. Dangour, Nutrition in brain development and aging: Role of essential fatty acids, *Nutrition Reviews* 64 (2006): S24–S33; Health Canada, Food and Nutrition, Prenatal nutrition guidelines for health professionals: Fish and Omega 3 fatty acids. www.hc-sc.gc.ca/fn-an/pubs/nutrition/omega3-eng.php, accessed September 15, 2011.
48. Health Canada, Food and Nutrition, *Eating Well with Canada's Food Guide* (2007). www.hc-sc.gc.ca/fn-an/food-guide-aliment/index-eng.php, accessed September 15, 2011; Health Canada, Food and Nutrition: Prenatal nutrition guidelines for health professionals: Folate contributes to a healthy pregnancy. www.hc-sc.gc.ca/fn-an/pubs/nutrition/folate-eng.php, accessed September 15, 2011; Committee on Dietary Reference Intakes, *Dietary Reference Intakes for Thiamin, Riboflavin, Niacin, Vitamin B_6, Folate, Vitamin B_{12}, Pantothenic Acid, Biotin, and Choline* (Washington, D.C.: National Academies Press, 1998), pp. 196–305.
49. T. O. Scholl, Iron status during pregnancy: Setting the stage for mother and infant, *American Journal of Clinical Nutrition* 81 (2005): 1218S–1222S.
50. E. Casanueva and coauthors, Vitamin C supplementation to prevent premature rupture of the chorioamniotic membranes: A randomized trial, *American Journal of Clinical Nutrition* 81 (2005): 859–863.
51. C. M. Donangelo and coauthors, Zinc a.bsorption and kinetics during pregnancy and lactation in Brazilian women, *American Journal of Clinical Nutrition* 82 (2005): 118–124.
52. D. Shah and H. P. S. Sachdev, Zinc deficiency in pregnancy and fetal outcome, *Nutrition Reviews* 64 (2006): 15–30.
53. C. S. Kovacs, Vitamin D in pregnancy and lactation: Maternal, fetal, and neonatal outcomes from human and animal studies, *American Journal of Clinical Nutrition* 88 (2008): 520S–528S; L. M. Bodnar and coauthors, High prevalence of vitamin D insufficiency in black and white pregnant women residing in the northern United States and their neonates, *Journal of Nutrition* 137 (2007): 447–452.
54. K. O. O'Brien and coauthors, Bone calcium turnover during pregnancy and lactation in women with low calcium diets is associated with calcium intake and circulating insulin-like growth factor 1 concentrations, *American Journal of Clinical Nutrition* 83 (2006): 317–323.
55. Position of the American Dietetic Association: Vegetarian diets, *Journal of the American Dietetic Association* 109 (2009): 1266–1282.
56. L. H. Allen, Multiple micronutrients in pregnancy and lactation: An overview, *American Journal of Clinical Nutrition* 81 (2005): 1206S–1212S.
57. R. J. Kaaja and I. A. Greer, Manifestations of chronic disease during pregnancy, *Journal of the American Medical Association* 294 (2005): 2751–2757.
58. The HAPO Study Cooperative Research Group, Hyperglycemia and adverse pregnancy outcomes, *New England Journal of Medicine* 358 (2008): 1991–2002.
59. Canadian Diabetes Association, Canadian Diabetes Association 2008 Clinical Practice Guidelines (2008). www.diabetes.ca/for-professionals/resources/2008-cpg/, accessed September 15, 2011; J. L. Kitzmiller and coauthors, Managing preexisting diabetes for pregnancy: Summary of evidence and consensus recommendations for care, *Diabetes Care* 31 (2008): 1060–1079; C. Mulholland and coauthors, Comparison of guidelines available in the United States for diagnosis and management of diabetes before, during, and after pregnancy, *Journal of Women's Health* 16 (2007): 790–801.
60. Y. Yogev and G. H. Visser, Obesity, gestational diabetes and pregnancy outcome, *Seminars in Fetal and Neonatal Medicine,* available online October 2008.
61. Canadian Diabetes Association, 2008; American Diabetes Association, Diagnosis and classification of diabetes mellitus, *Diabetes Care* 31 (2008): S55–S60.

62. Position of the American Diabetes Association: Nutrition recommendations and interventions for diabetes, *Diabetes Care* 31 (2008): S61–S78.
63. C. A. Crowther and coauthors, Effect of treatment of gestational diabetes mellitus on pregnancy outcomes, *New England Journal of Medicine* 352 (2005): 2477–2486; O. Langer and coauthors, Overweight and obese in gestational diabetes: The impact on pregnancy outcomes, *American Journal of Obstetrics and Gynecology* 192 (2005): 1768–1776.
64. P. E. Marik, Hypertensive disorders of pregnancy, *Postgraduate Medicine* 121 (2009): 69–76.
65. Mount Sinai Hospital. Mount Sinai researcher discovers how genetic link causes preeclampsia in pregnant women (Feb. 12, 2009). www.mountsinai.on.ca/about_us/news/2009/mount-sinai-researcher-discovers-how-genetic-link-causes-preeclampsia-in-pregnant-women, accessed September 12, 2011.
66. B. E. Vikse and coauthors, Preeclampsia and the risk of end-stage renal disease, *New England Journal of Medicine* 359 (2008): 800–809.
67. C. S. Wu and coauthors, Preeclampsia and risk for epilepsy in offspring, *Pediatrics* 122 (2008): 1072–1078.
68. P. R. Trumbo and K. C. Ellwood, Supplemental calcium and risk reduction of hypertension, pregnancy-induced hypertension, and preeclampsia: An evidence-based review by the U.S. Food and Drug Administration, *Nutrition Reviews* 65 (2007): 78–87; L. Poston and coauthors, Vitamin C and vitamin E in pregnant women at risk for preeclampsia (VIP trial): Randomized placebo-controlled trial, *Lancet* 367 (2006): 1145–1154.
69. C. B. Rudra and coauthors, A prospective analysis of recreational physical activity and preeclampsia risk, *Medicine & Science in Sports & Exercise* 40 (2008): 1581–1588.
70. Statistics Canada, Teenage pregnancy. www.statcan.gc.ca/kits-trousses/preg-gross/preg-gross-eng.htm, accessed September 15, 2011.
71. Quickstats—Birthrates among females aged 15–19 years, by state: United States, 2004, *Morbidity and Mortality Weekly Report* 55 (2007): 1383.
72. X. Chen and coauthors, Paternal age and adverse birth outcomes: Teenager or 40+, who is at risk? *Human Reproduction* 23 (2008): 1290–1296.
73. Public Health Agency of Canada, Alcohol use during pregnancy and awareness of Fetal Alcohol Spectrum Disorder—Results of a national survey. www.phac-aspc.gc.ca/publicat/fas-saf-natsurv-2006/index-eng.php, accessed September 15, 2011.
74. M. J. Rivkin and coauthors, Volumetric MRI study of brain in children with intrauterine exposure to cocaine, alcohol, tobacco, and marijuana, *Pediatrics* 121 (2008): 741–750; H. S. Bada and coauthors, Impact of prenatal cocaine exposure on child behavior problems through school age, *Pediatrics* 119 (2007): e348; B. A. Lewis and coauthors, Prenatal cocaine and tobacco effects on children's language trajectories, *Pediatrics* 120 (2007): e78.
75. G. A. Richardson, L. Goldschmidt, and C. Larkby, Effects of prenatal cocaine exposure on growth: A longitudinal analysis, *Pediatrics* 120 (2007): e1017.
76. Health Canada, Health concerns—Pregnancy. www.hc-sc.gc.ca/hc-ps/tobac-tabac/body-corps/preg-gros-eng.php, accessed September 15, 2011.
77. H. Moshhammer and coauthors, Parental smoking and lung function in children: An international study, *American Journal of Respiratory and Critical Care Medicine* 173 (2006): 1255–1263.
78. Rivkin and coauthors, 2008.
79. N. Ribas-Fitó and coauthors, Breastfeeding, exposure to organochlorine compounds, and neurodevelopment in infants, *Pediatrics* 111 (2003): e580–e585.
80. T. I. Halldorsson and coauthors, Is high consumption of fatty fish during pregnancy a risk factor for fetal growth retardation? A study of 44,824 Danish pregnant women, *American Journal of Epidemiology* 166 (2007): 687–696.
81. Health Canada, Food and Nutrition, Prenatal nutrition guidelines for health professionals: Fish and omega 3 fatty acids; E. Oken and coauthors, Maternal fish intake during pregnancy, blood mercury levels, and child cognition at age 3 years in a U.S. cohort, *American Journal of Epidemiology* 167 (2008): 1171–1181; J. R. Hibbeln and coauthors, Maternal seafood consumption in pregnancy and neurodevelopmental outcomes in childhood (ALSPAC study): An observational cohort study, *Lancet* 369 (2007): 578–585; D. Mozaffarian and E. B. Rimm, Fish intake, contaminants, and human health: Evaluating the risks and the benefits, *Journal of the American Medical Association* 296 (2006): 1885–1899; Institute of Medicine report brief, *Seafood Choices: Balancing Benefits and Risks*, October 2006.
82. Health Canada, Healthy living: Caffeine. www.hc-sc.gc.ca/hl-vs/iyh-vsv/food-aliment/caffeine-eng.php#he; accessed September 15, 2011; X. Weng, R. Odouli, and D. Li, Maternal caffeine consumption during pregnancy and the risk of miscarriage: A prospective cohort study, *American Journal of Obstetrics and Gynecology* 198 (2008): 279.e1–279.e8; M. L. Browne, Maternal exposure to caffeine and risk of congenital anomalies: A systematic review, *Epidemiology* 17 (2006): 324–331; A. Matijasevich and coauthors, Maternal caffeine consumption and fetal death: A case-control study in Uruguay, *Paediatric and Perinatal Epidemiology* 20 (2006): 100–109; B. H. Bech and coauthors, Coffee and fetal death: A cohort study with prospective data, *American Journal of Epidemiology* 162 (2005): 983–990.
83. CARE Study Group, Maternal caffeine intake during pregnancy and risk of fetal growth restriction: A large prospective observational study, *British Medical Journal* 337 (2008): a2332.
84. Health Canada, Healthy living: The safety of sugar substitutes. www.hc-sc.gc.ca/hl-vs/iyh-vsv/food-aliment/sugar_sub_sucre-eng.php, accessed September 15, 2011; Position of the American Dietetic Association: Use of nutritive and nonnutritive sweeteners, *Journal of the American Dietetic Association* 104 (2004): 255–275.
85. Health Canada, Healthy living: Healthy pregnancy. www.hc-sc.gc.ca/hl-vs/preg-gros/index-eng.php, accessed September 15, 2011; Position of the American Dietetic Association, 2008.
86. Statistics Canada. Breastfeeding, 2009. www.statcan.gc.ca/pub/82-625-x/2010002/article/11269-eng.htm, accessed September 15, 2011; Public Health Agency of Canada, What mothers say: The Canadian Experiences Survey.
87. Health Canada, Food and Nutrition, Breastfeeding; American Academy of Pediatrics, Breastfeeding and the use of human milk, *Pediatrics* 115 (2005): 496–506; Position of the American Dietetic Association: Promoting and supporting breastfeeding, *Journal of the American Dietetic Association* 105 (2005): 810–818.
88. D. Thulier, Breastfeeding in America: A history of influencing factors, *Journal of Human Lactation* 25 (2009): 85–94.
89. K. A. Bonuck and coauthors, Randomized, controlled trial of a prenatal and postnatal lactation consultant intervention on duration and intensity of breastfeeding up to 12 months, *Pediatrics* 116 (2005): 1413–1426; J. Labarere and coauthors, Efficacy of breastfeeding support provided by trained clinicians during an early, routine, preventive visit: A prospective, randomized, open trial of 226 mother-infant pairs, *Pediatrics* 115 (2005): e139.
90. S. Merten, J. Dratva, and U. Ackermann-Liebrich, Do baby-friendly hospitals influence breastfeeding duration on a national level? *Pediatrics* 116 (2005): e702; A. Merewood and coauthors, Breastfeeding rates in U.S. baby-friendly hospitals: Results of a national survey, *Pediatrics* 116 (2005): 628–634.
91. A. Pisacane and coauthors, A controlled trial of the father's role in breastfeeding promotion, *Pediatrics* 116 (2005): e494.
92. K. M. Rasmussen, Association of maternal obesity before conception with poor lactation performance, *Annual Review of Nutrition* 27 (2007): 103–121; C. A. Lovelady, Is maternal obesity a cause of poor lactation performance? *Nutrition Reviews* 63 (2005): 352–355.
93. Baker and coauthors, 2008.
94. Health Canada, Prenatal nutrition: Fish and omega-3 fatty acids.
95. O'Brien and coauthors, 2006.
96. Public Health Agency of Canada, Canadian Prenatal Nutrition Program. www.phac-aspc.gc.ca/hp-ps/dca-dea/prog-ini/cpnp-pcnp/index-eng.php, accessed September 21, 2011.
97. F. R. Greer, S. H. Sicherer, A. Wesley Burks, and the Committee on Nutrition and Section on Allergy and Immunology, Effects of early nutritional interventions on the development of atopic disease in infants and children: The role of maternal dietary restriction, breastfeeding, timing of introduction of complementary foods, and hydrolyzed formulas, *Pediatrics* 121 (2008): 183–191.
98. Greer, Sicherer, Wesley Burks, and the Committee on Nutrition and Section on Allergy and Immunology, 2008.

99. P. L. Havens, L. M. Mofenson, and the Committee on Pediatric AIDS, Evaluation and management of the infant exposed to HIV-1 in the United States, *Pediatrics* 123 (2009): 175–187.
100. World Health Organization, *HIV and Infant Feeding,* www.who.int/child_adolescent_health/topics/prevention_care/child/nutrition/hivif/en/, accessed June 1, 2009; M. W. Kline, Early exclusive breast-feeding: Still the cornerstone of child survival, *American Journal of Clinical Nutrition* 89 (2009): 1281–1282.
101. G. E. Gray and H. Saloojee, Breast-feeding, antiretroviral prophylaxis, and HIV, *New England Journal of Medicine* 359 (2008): 189–191; N. I. Kumwenda and coauthors, Extended antiretroviral prophylaxis to reduce breast-milk HIV-1 transmission, *New England Journal of Medicine* 359 (2008): 119–129; W. T. Shearer, Breastfeeding and HIV infection, *Pediatrics* 121 (2008): 1046–1047.
102. R. Lesnewski and L. Prine, Initiating hormonal contraception, *American Family Physician* 74 (2006): 105–112.
103. S. Cnattingius and coauthors, Pregnancy characteristics and maternal risk of breast cancer, *Journal of the American Medical Association* 294 (2005): 2474–2480.
104. L. M. Jansson and coauthors, Methadone maintenance and breastfeeding in the neonatal period, *Pediatrics* 121 (2008): 106–114.
105. J. A. Mennella, L. M. Yourshaw, and L. K. Morgan, Breastfeeding and smoking: Short-term effects on infant feeding and sleep, *Pediatrics* 120 (2007): 497–502.

HIGHLIGHT 16

Fetal Alcohol Syndrome

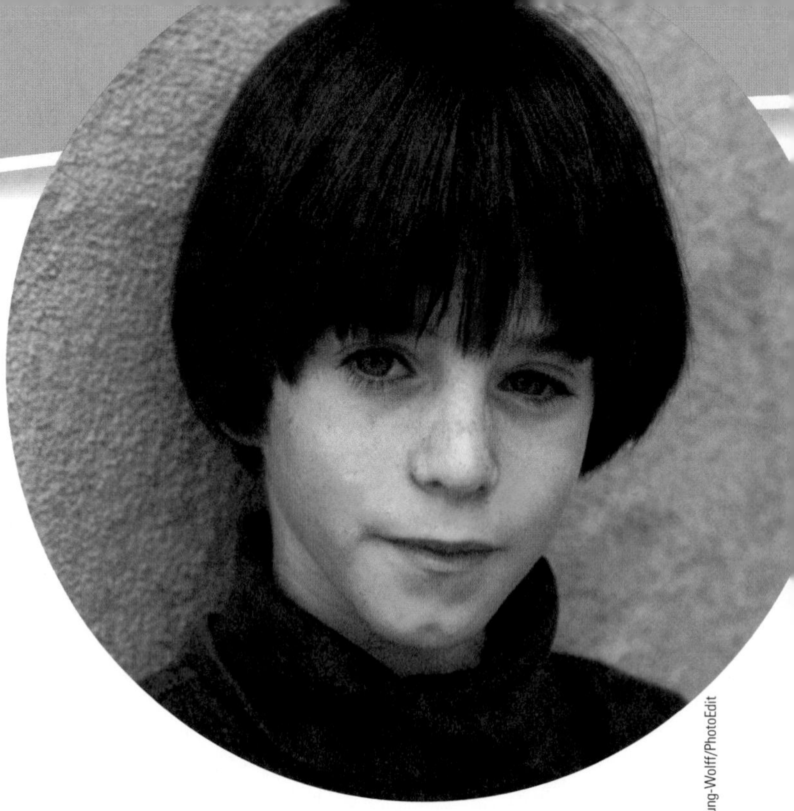
© David Young-Wolff/PhotoEdit

As Chapter 16 mentions, drinking alcohol during pregnancy endangers the fetus. Alcohol crosses the placenta freely and deprives the developing fetus of both nutrients and oxygen. The damaging effects of alcohol on the developing fetus cover a range of abnormalities referred to as **fetal alcohol spectrum disorder** (see the accompanying glossary).[1] Those at the most severe end of the spectrum are described as having **fetal alcohol syndrome (FAS),** a cluster of physical, mental, and neurobehavioural symptoms that includes:

- Prenatal and postnatal growth retardation
- Impairment of the brain and central nervous system, with consequent mental retardation, poor motor skills and coordination, and hyperactivity
- Abnormalities of the face and skull (see Figure H16-1)
- Increased frequency of major birth defects: cleft palate, heart defects, and defects in ears, eyes, genitals, and urinary system

Those with more severe physical abnormalities have more cognitive limitations.[2] Tragically, the damage evident at birth persists: children with FASD never fully recover.

Each year, as many as 9 of every 1000 babies are affected by FASD because their mothers drank too much alcohol during pregnancy.[3] The cluster of mental problems associated with **prenatal alcohol exposure** is known as **alcohol-related neurodevelopmental disorder (ARND),** and the physical malformations are referred to as **alcohol-related birth defects (ARBD).** Some children with ARBD and ARND have no outward signs; others may be short or have only minor facial abnormalities. They often go undiagnosed even when they develop learning difficulties in the early school years. Mood disorders and problem behaviours, such as aggression, are common. They typically need support and guidance to function and participate in daily activities.[4]

Health Canada and the Canadian Public Health Agency of Canada state that pregnant women should abstain from alcohol. Abstinence from alcohol is the best policy for pregnant women both because alcohol consumption during pregnancy has such severe consequences and because FASD can only be prevented—it cannot be treated. Further, because the most severe damage occurs around the time of conception—*before a woman may even realize that she is pregnant*—the warning to abstain includes women who may become pregnant.

Drinking during Pregnancy

One out of 12 pregnant women drinks alcohol at some time during her pregnancy; 1 out of 30 U.S. women uses alcohol frequently and admits to binge drinking.[5] When a woman drinks during pregnancy, she causes damage in two ways: directly, by intoxication, and indirectly, by malnutrition. Prior to the complete formation of the placenta (approximately 12 weeks), alcohol diffuses directly into the tissues of the developing embryo, causing incredible damage. (Review Figure 16-4 on p. 508 and note that the critical periods for most tissues occur during embryonic development.) Alcohol interferes with the orderly development of tissues during their critical periods, reducing the number of cells and damaging those that are produced. The damage of alcohol toxicity during brain development is apparent in its reduced size and impaired function.

When alcohol crosses the placenta, fetal blood alcohol rises until it reaches equilibrium with maternal blood alcohol. The

GLOSSARY

alcohol-related birth defects (ARBD): malformations in the skeletal and organ systems (heart, kidneys, eyes, ears) associated with prenatal alcohol exposure.

alcohol-related neurodevelopmental disorder (ARND): abnormalities in the central nervous system and cognitive development associated with prenatal alcohol exposure.

fetal alcohol spectrum disorder (FASD): a range of physical, behavioural, and cognitive abnormalities caused by prenatal alcohol exposure.

fetal alcohol syndrome (FAS): a cluster of physical, behavioural, and cognitive abnormalities associated with prenatal alcohol exposure, including facial malformations, growth retardation, and central nervous disorders.

prenatal alcohol exposure: subjecting a fetus to a pattern of excessive alcohol intake characterized by substantial regular use or heavy episodic drinking.

Note: See Highlight 7 for other alcohol-related terms and information.

mother may not even appear drunk, but the fetus may be poisoned. The fetus's body is small, its detoxification system is immature, and alcohol remains in fetal blood long after it has disappeared from maternal blood.

A pregnant woman harms her unborn child not only by consuming alcohol but also by not consuming food. This combination enhances the likelihood of malnutrition and a poorly developed infant. It is important to realize, however, that malnutrition is not the cause of FASD. It is true that mothers of FASD children often have unbalanced diets and nutrient deficiencies. It is also true that nutrient deficiencies may exacerbate the clinical signs seen in these children, but it is the *alcohol* that causes the damage.[6] An adequate diet alone will not prevent FASD if alcohol abuse continues.

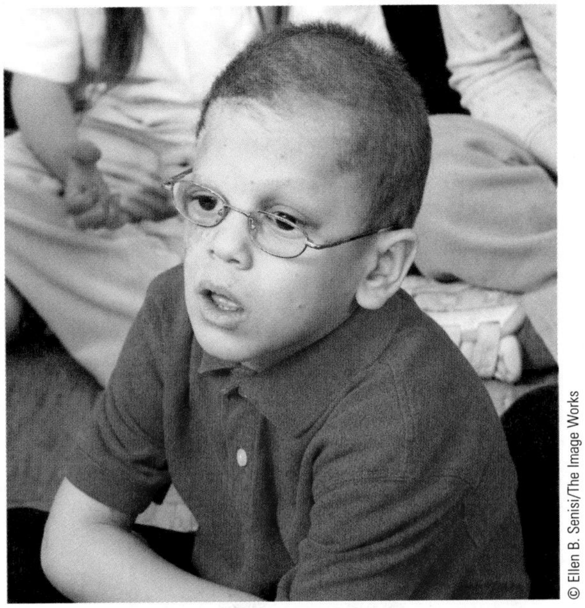
© Ellen B. Senisi/The Image Works

Characteristic facial features may diminish with time, but children with FAS typically continue to be short and underweight for their age.

How Much Is Too Much?

A pregnant woman need not have an alcohol-abuse problem to give birth to a baby with FASD. She need only drink in excess of her liver's capacity to detoxify alcohol. Even one drink a day threatens neurological development and behaviours. Four drinks a day dramatically increase the risk of having an infant with physical malformations.

FIGURE H16-1 Typical Facial Characteristics of FAS

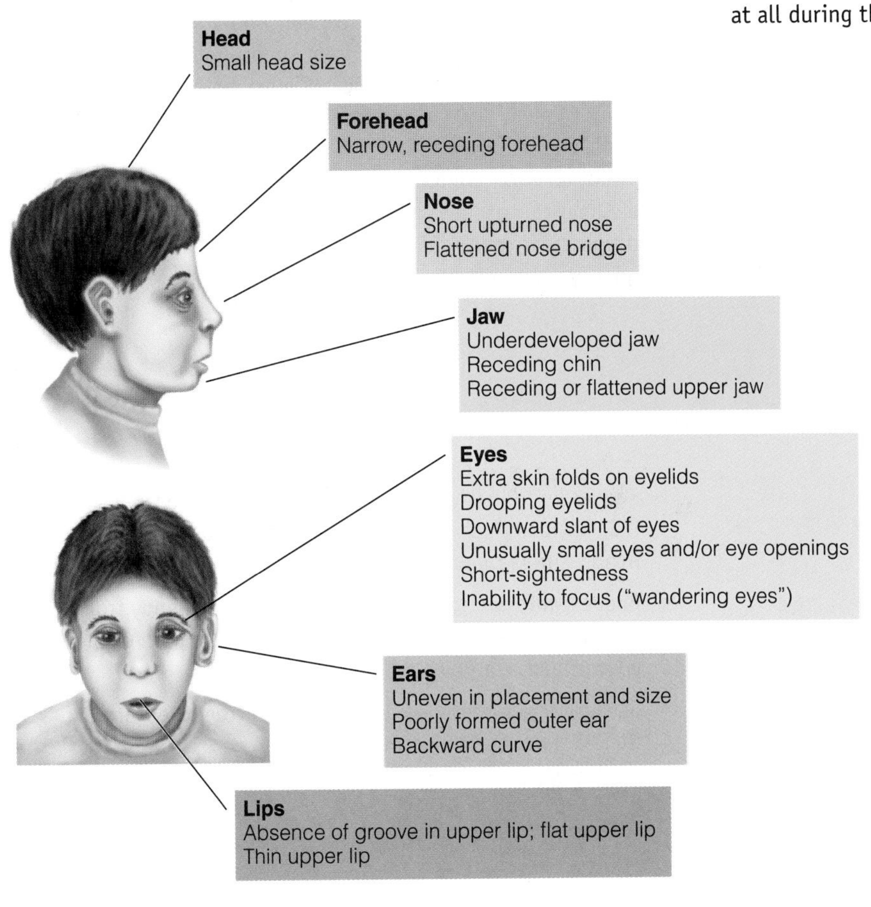
Head
Small head size
Forehead
Narrow, receding forehead
Nose
Short upturned nose
Flattened nose bridge
Jaw
Underdeveloped jaw
Receding chin
Receding or flattened upper jaw
Eyes
Extra skin folds on eyelids
Drooping eyelids
Downward slant of eyes
Unusually small eyes and/or eye openings
Short-sightedness
Inability to focus ("wandering eyes")
Ears
Uneven in placement and size
Poorly formed outer ear
Backward curve
Lips
Absence of groove in upper lip; flat upper lip
Thin upper lip

In addition to total alcohol intake, drinking patterns play an important role. Most FASD studies report their findings in terms of average intake per day, but people usually drink more heavily on some days than on others. For example, a woman who drinks an *average* of 30 millilitres of alcohol (2 drinks) a day may not drink at all during the week, but then have 10 drinks on Saturday night, exposing the fetus to extremely toxic quantities of alcohol. Whether various drinking patterns incur damage depends on the frequency of consumption, the quantity consumed, and the stage of fetal development at the time of each drinking episode.

An occasional drink may be innocuous, but researchers are unable to say how much alcohol is safe to consume during pregnancy. For this reason, health-care professionals urge women to stop drinking alcohol as soon as they realize they are pregnant, or better, as soon as they *plan* to become pregnant. Why take any risk? The only sure way to protect an infant from alcohol damage is for the mother to abstain.[7]

When Is the Damage Done?

The first month or two of pregnancy is a critical period of fetal development (refer back to Figures 16-3 and 16-4). Because pregnancy usually cannot be confirmed before five to six weeks, a woman may not even realize she is pregnant during that critical time. Therefore, it is advisable for women who are trying to conceive, or who suspect they

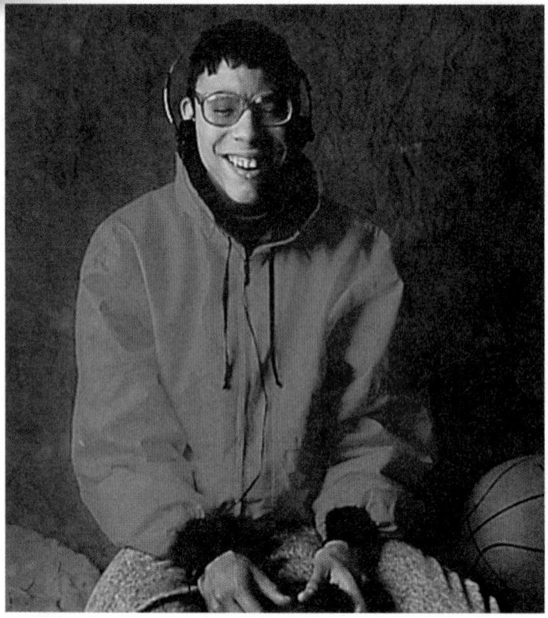

Children born with FASD must live with the long-term consequences of prenatal brain damage.

© 1995 George Steinmetz

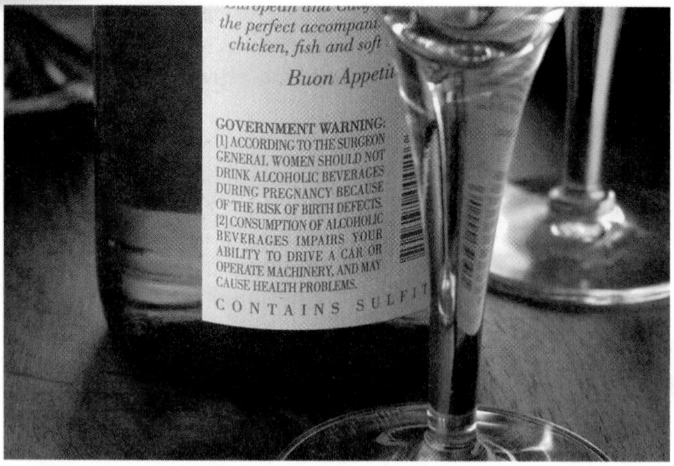
the perfect accompani
chicken, fish and soft
Buon Appetit
GOVERNMENT WARNING:
(1) ACCORDING TO THE SURGEON GENERAL WOMEN SHOULD NOT DRINK ALCOHOLIC BEVERAGES DURING PREGNANCY BECAUSE OF THE RISK OF BIRTH DEFECTS.
(2) CONSUMPTION OF ALCOHOLIC BEVERAGES IMPAIRS YOUR ABILITY TO DRIVE A CAR OR OPERATE MACHINERY, AND MAY CAUSE HEALTH PROBLEMS.
CONTAINS SULFIT

All containers of beer, wine, and liquor warn women not to drink alcoholic beverages during pregnancy because of the risk of birth defects.

© Matt Farruggio

might be pregnant, to abstain or curtail their alcohol intakes to ensure a healthy start.

The type of abnormality observed in an FASD infant depends on the developmental events occurring at the times of alcohol exposure. During the first trimester, developing organs such as the brain, heart, and kidneys may be malformed. During the second trimester, the risk of spontaneous abortion increases. During the third trimester, body and brain growth may be retarded.

Male alcohol ingestion may also affect fertility and fetal development. Animal studies have found smaller litter sizes, lower birthweights, reduced survival rates, and impaired learning ability in the offspring of males consuming alcohol prior to conception. An association between paternal alcohol intake one month prior to conception and low infant birthweight is also apparent in human beings. (Paternal alcohol intake was defined as an average of two or more drinks daily or at least five drinks on one occasion.) This relationship was independent of either parent's smoking and of the mother's use of alcohol, caffeine, or other drugs.

In view of the damage caused by FASD, prevention efforts focus on educating women not to drink during pregnancy. Everyone should know of the potential dangers. Women who drink alcohol and who are sexually active may benefit from counseling and effective contraception to prevent pregnancy. Almost half of all pregnancies are unintended, with many conceived during a binge-drinking episode.

Public service announcements and alcohol beverage warning labels help to raise awareness. Everyone should hear the message loud and clear: don't drink alcohol prior to conception or during pregnancy.

Nutrition on the Net

CENGAGENOW™
For further study of topics covered in this Highlight, log on to **www.cengage.com/sso**.

- Learn more about Fetal Alcohol Spectrum Disorder (FASD) from the Public Health Agency of Canada: **www.phac-aspc.gc.ca/hp-ps/dca-dea/prog-ini/fasd-etcaf/index-eng.php**
- Request information on fetal alcohol syndrome from the U.S. National Clearinghouse for Alcohol and Drug Information: **ncadi.samhsa.gov**
- Request information on drinking during pregnancy from the U.S. National Institute on Alcohol Abuse and Alcoholism: **www.niaaa.nih.gov**
- Gather facts on fetal alcohol syndrome from the March of Dimes: **www.marchofdimes.com**

References

1. Public Health Agency of Canada, Fetal alcohol spectrum disorder (FASD). www.phac-aspc.gc.ca/hp-ps/dca-dea/prog-ini/fasd-etcaf/index-eng.php, accessed September 15, 2011; H. E. Hoyme and coauthors, A practical clinical approach to diagnosis of fetal alcohol spectrum disorders: Clarification of the 1996 Institute of Medicine Criteria, *Pediatrics* 115 (2005): 39–47.
2. N. Ervalahti and coauthors, Relationship between dysmorphic features and general cognitive function in children with fetal alcohol spectrum disorders, *American Journal of Medical Genetics* 143A (2007): 2916–2923.
3. G. Koren, I. Nulman, A. E. Chudley, and C. Looke, Fetal alcohol spectrum disorder, *Canadian Medical Association Journal* 169 (2003): 1181–1185; Fetal Alcohol Spectrum Disorders, *Department of Health and Human Services,* www.cdc.gov/ncbddd, created September 9, 2005; Guidelines for identifying and referring persons with fetal alcohol syndrome, *Morbidity and Mortality Weekly Report* 54 (2005): 1–10.
4. T. Jirikowic, D. Kartin, and H. C. Olsen, Children with fetal alcohol spectrum disorders: A descriptive profile of adaptive function, *Canadian Journal of Occupational Therapy* 75 (2008): 238–248.
5. Public Health Agency of Canada, What mothers say: The Canadian Maternity Experience Survey (2009). www.phac-aspc.gc.ca/rhs-ssg/pdf/survey-eng.pdf, accessed September 21, 2011; Alcohol use and pregnancy, *Department of Health and Human Services,* www.cdc.gov/ncbddd, created September 15, 2005.
6. R. C. Carter and coauthors, Fetal alcohol exposure, iron-deficiency anemia, and infant growth, *Pediatrics* 120 (2007): 559–567.
7. R. A. S. Mukherjee and coauthors, Low level alcohol consumption and the fetus, *British Medical Journal* 330 (2005): 375–376.

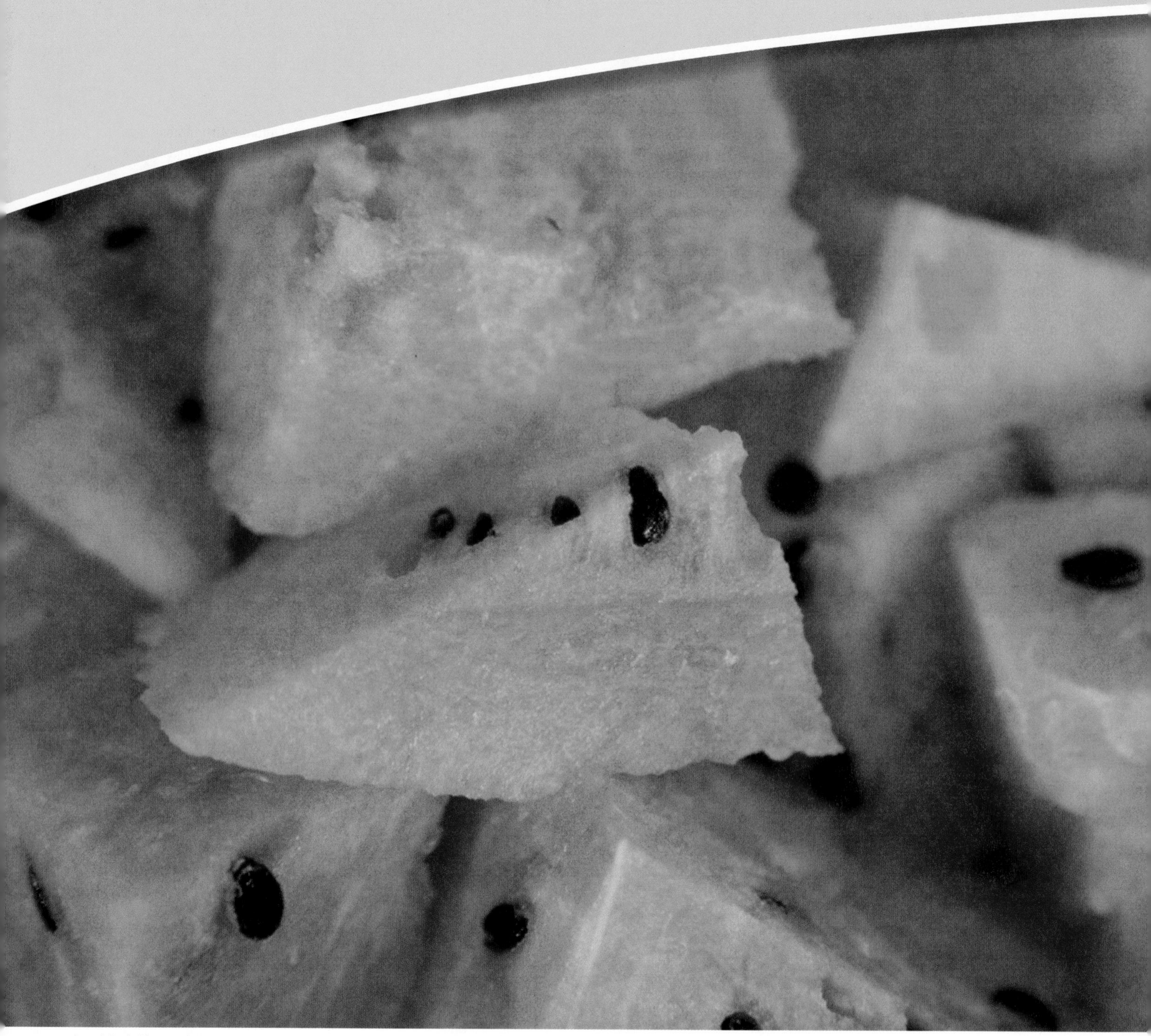

Anna Jurkovska/shutterstock

CENGAGENOW™

Throughout this chapter, the CengageNOW logo indicates an opportunity for online self-study, linking you to interactive tutorials, activities, and videos to increase your understanding of chapter concepts.
www.cengage.com/sso

Nutrition in Your Life

Much of this book has focused on you—your food choices and how they might affect your health. This chapter shifts the focus from you the recipient to you the caregiver. One day (if not already), children will depend on you to feed them well and teach them wisely. The responsibility of nourishing children can seem overwhelming at times, but the job is fairly simple. Offer children a variety of nutritious foods to support their growth, and teach them how to make healthy food and activity choices. Presenting foods in a relaxed and supportive environment nourishes both physical and emotional well-being.

CHAPTER

17

Life Cycle Nutrition: Infancy, Childhood, and Adolescence

CHAPTER OUTLINE

The first year of life (infancy) is a time of phenomenal growth and development. After the first year, a child continues to grow and change, but more slowly. Still, the cumulative effects over the next decade are remarkable. Then, as the child enters the teen years, the pace toward adulthood accelerates dramatically. This chapter examines the special nutrient needs of infants, children, and adolescents.

Nutrition during Infancy

Initially, the infant drinks only breast milk or formula but later begins to eat some foods, as appropriate. Common sense in the selection of infant foods along with a nurturing, relaxed environment support an infant's health and well-being.

Energy and Nutrient Needs

An infant grows fast during the first year, as Figure 17-1 shows. Growth directly reflects nutrient intake and is an important parameter in assessing the nutrition status of infants and children. Health-care professionals measure the heights and weights of infants and children at intervals and compare the measurements with standard growth curves for gender and age and with previous measures of each child (see the "How To" on p. 544).

Energy Intake and Activity A healthy infant's birthweight doubles by about 5 months of age and triples by 1 year, typically reaching 9 to 11 kilograms (20 to 25 pounds). The infant's length changes more slowly than weight, increasing about 25 centimetres (10 inches) from birth to 1 year. By the end of the first year, infant growth slows considerably; during the second year, an infant typically gains less than 4.5 kilograms (10 pounds) and grows about 12.5 centimetres (5 inches) in length.

Not only do infants grow rapidly, but their energy requirement is remarkably high—about twice that of an adult (i.e., a much higher metabolic rate), based on body weight. A newborn baby requires about 450 kcalories per day, whereas most adults require about 2000 kcalories per day. In terms of body weight, the

FIGURE 17-1 Weight Gain of Infants in Their First Five Years of Life

In the first year, an infant's birthweight may triple, but over the following several years, the rate of weight gain gradually diminishes.

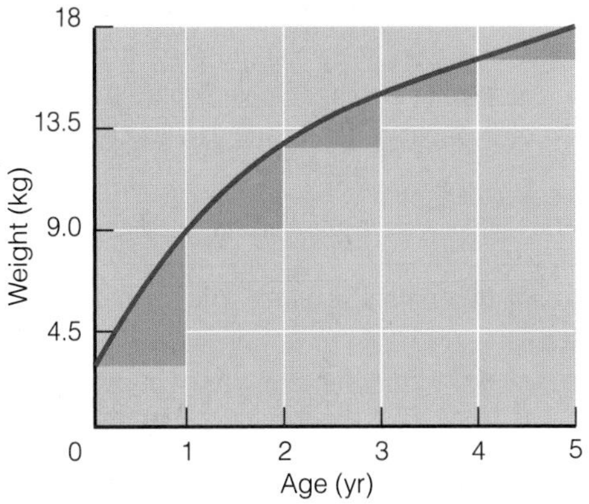
18
13.5
9.0
4.5
Weight (kg)
0
1
2
3
4
5
Age (yr)

HOW TO Plot Measures on a Growth Chart

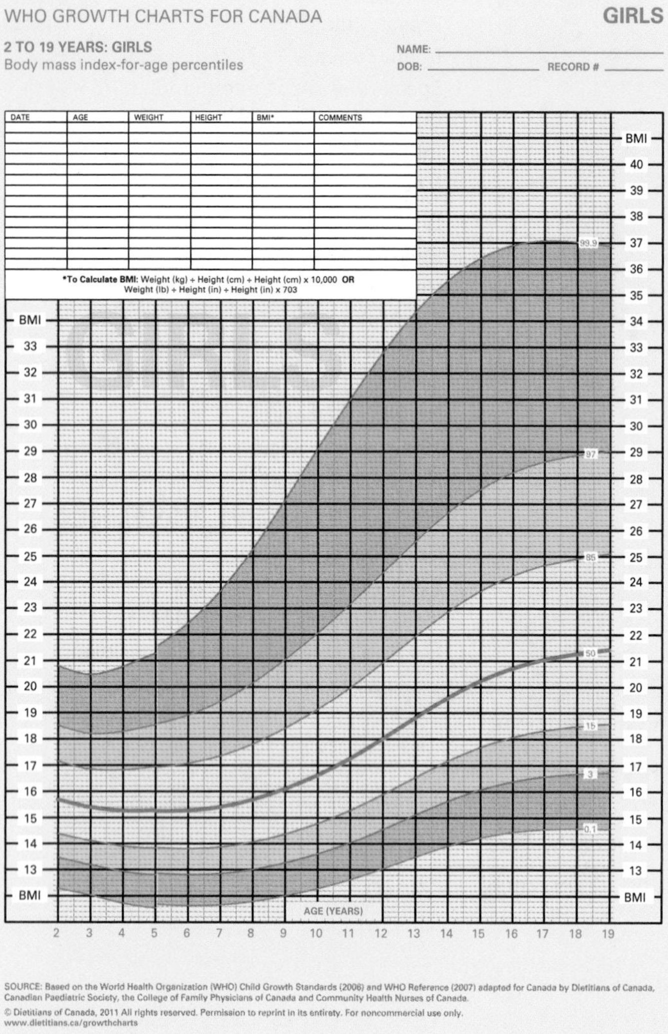
WHO GROWTH CHARTS FOR CANADA
GIRLS
2 TO 19 YEARS: GIRLS
Body mass index-for-age percentiles
NAME:
DOB:
RECORD #
DATE
AGE
WEIGHT
HEIGHT
BMI*
COMMENTS
*To Calculate BMI: Weight (kg) ÷ Height (cm) ÷ Height (cm) x 10,000 OR Weight (lb) ÷ Height (in) ÷ Height (in) x 703
BMI
AGE (YEARS)
SOURCE: Based on the World Health Organization (WHO) Child Growth Standards (2006) and WHO Reference (2007) adapted for Canada by Dietitians of Canada, Canadian Paediatric Society, the College of Family Physicians of Canada and Community Health Nurses of Canada.
© Dietitians of Canada, 2011 All rights reserved. Permission to reprint in its entirety. For noncommercial use only.
www.dietitians.ca/growthcharts

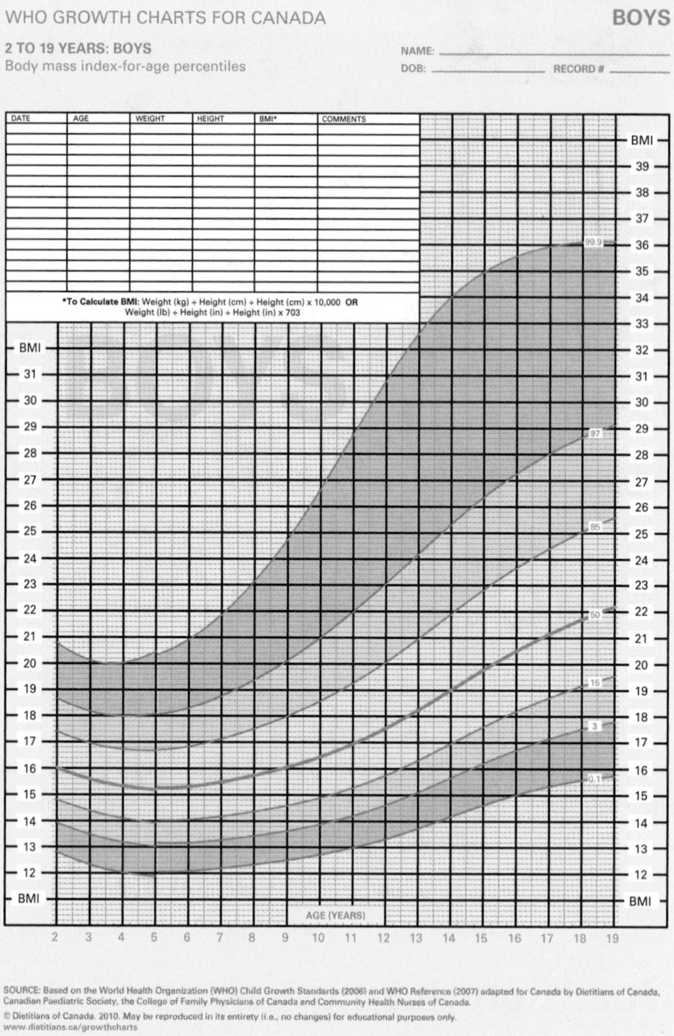
WHO GROWTH CHARTS FOR CANADA
BOYS
2 TO 19 YEARS: BOYS
Body mass index-for-age percentiles
NAME:
DOB:
RECORD #
DATE
AGE
WEIGHT
HEIGHT
BMI*
COMMENTS
*To Calculate BMI: Weight (kg) ÷ Height (cm) ÷ Height (cm) x 10,000 OR Weight (lb) ÷ Height (in) ÷ Height (in) x 703
BMI
AGE (YEARS)
SOURCE: Based on the World Health Organization (WHO) Child Growth Standards (2006) and WHO Reference (2007) adapted for Canada by Dietitians of Canada, Canadian Paediatric Society, the College of Family Physicians of Canada and Community Health Nurses of Canada.
© Dietitians of Canada, 2010. May be reproduced in its entirety (i.e., no changes) for educational purposes only.
www.dietitians.ca/growthcharts

You can assess the growth of infants and children by plotting their measurements on a percentile graph. Percentile graphs divide the measures of a population into 100 equal divisions so that half of the population falls at or above the 50th percentile and half falls below. Using percentiles allows for comparisons among people of the same age and gender.

To plot measures on a growth chart, follow these steps:

- Select the appropriate chart based on age and gender. For this example, use the accompanying chart, which gives percentiles for weight for girls and boys from birth to 19 years based on age and BMI.
- Calculate the child's/adolescent's BMI using the formula at the top of the chart then locate it on vertical axis. Next locate the child's/adolescent's age along the horizontal axis at the bottom of the chart then follow the line to the right hand side of the graph to find the percentile the child/adolescent falls into. If, for example, the child/adolescent falls above the 85th percentile she/he may be regarded as overweight or obese, and parents should then check with their health care provider to confirm this finding and seek appropriate advice.

CENGAGENOW™
For additional practice log on to **www.cengage.com/sso**.

TRY IT Determine the percentile for a 12-month-old girl who weighs 9.5 kilograms (21 pounds).

difference is remarkable. Infants require about 100 kcalories per kilogram of body weight per day, whereas most adults need fewer than 40 (see Table 17-1). If an infant's energy needs were applied to an adult, a 77 kilogram (170-pound) adult would require more than 7000 kcalories a day. After 6 months, the infant's energy needs decline as the growth rate slows, but some of the energy saved by slower growth is spent in increased activity.

TABLE 17-1 Infant and Adult Heart Rate, Respiration Rate, and Energy Needs Compared

	Infants	Adults
Heart rate (beats/minute)	120 to 140	70 to 80
Respiration rate (breaths/minute)	20 to 40	15 to 20
Energy needs (kcal/body weight)	100/kg (45/lb)	<40/kg (<18/lb)

Energy Nutrients Recommendations for the energy nutrients—carbohydrate, fat, and protein—during the first six months of life are based on the average intakes of healthy, full-term infants fed breast milk.[1] During the second six months of life, recommendations reflect typical intakes from solid foods as well as breast milk.

As Chapter 4 discusses, carbohydrates provide energy to all the cells of the body, especially those in the brain, which depend primarily on glucose to fuel activities. Relative to the size of the body, ♦ the size of an infant's brain is greater than that of an adult's. Thus, an infant's brain uses *relatively* more glucose—about 60 percent of the day's total energy intake.[2]

♦ An infant's brain weight is about 12% of its body weight, whereas an adult's brain weight is about 2%.

Fat provides most of the energy in breast milk and standard infant formula. Its high energy density supports the rapid growth of early infancy.

No single nutrient is more essential to growth than protein. All of the body's cells and most of its fluids contain protein; it is the basic building material of the body's tissues. Chapter 6 details the problems inadequate protein can cause. Excess dietary protein can cause problems, too, especially in a small infant. Too much protein stresses the liver and kidneys, which have to metabolize and excrete the excess nitrogen. Signs of protein overload include acidosis, dehydration, diarrhea, elevated blood ammonia, elevated blood urea, and fever. Such problems are not common, but they have been observed in infants fed inappropriate foods, such as skim milk or concentrated formula.

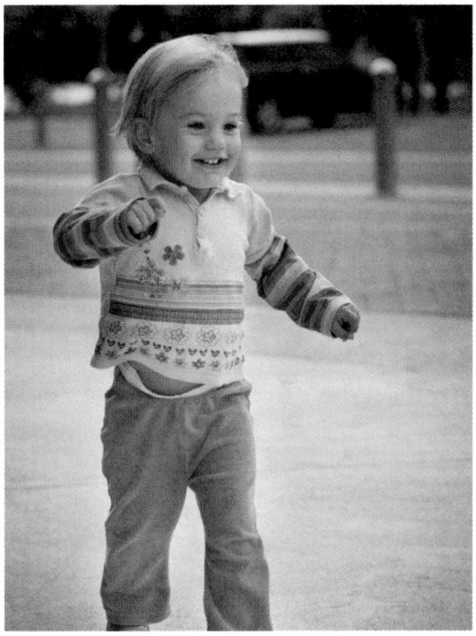

Jandrie Lombard/shutterstock

After 6 months, energy saved by slower growth is spent in increased activity.

Vitamins and Minerals An infant's needs for most nutrients, in proportion to body weight, are more than double those of an adult. Figure 17-2 (p. 246) illustrates this by comparing a 5-month-old infant's needs per unit of body weight with those of an adult man. Some of the differences are extraordinary. Infant recommendations are based on the average amount of nutrients consumed by thriving infants breastfed by well-nourished mothers.

Water One of the most essential nutrients for infants, as for everyone, is water. The younger the infant, the greater the percentage of body weight is water. During early infancy, breast milk or infant formula normally provides enough water to replace fluid losses in a healthy infant. If the environmental temperature is extremely high, however, infants need supplemental water.[3] Because much of the fluid in an infant's body is located *outside* the cells—between the cells and in the blood vessels—rapid fluid losses and the resulting dehydration can be life-threatening. Conditions that cause rapid fluid loss, such as diarrhea or vomiting, require treatment with an electrolyte solution designed for infants.

Breast Milk

In Canada and the United States the two dietary practices that have the most significant effect on an infant's nutrition are the milk the infant receives and the age at which solid foods are introduced. A later section discusses the introduction of solid foods, but as to the milk, both the Canadian Paediatric Society (CPS) and American Academy of Pediatrics (AAP) strongly recommend breastfeeding for healthy full-term infants, except where specific contraindications exist. The Dietitians of Canada and the American Dietetic Association (ADA) also advocates breastfeeding for the nutritional health it confers on the infant as well as for the many other benefits it provides both infant and mother (review Table 16-4 on p. 528).[4]

Breast milk excels as a source of nutrients for infants. Its unique nutrient composition and protective factors promote optimal infant health and development throughout the first year of life. Health Canada, the Canadian Paediatric Society (CPS), and the Dietitians of Canada recommend exclusive breastfeeding for 6 months, and breastfeeding with complementary foods for at least 12 months,

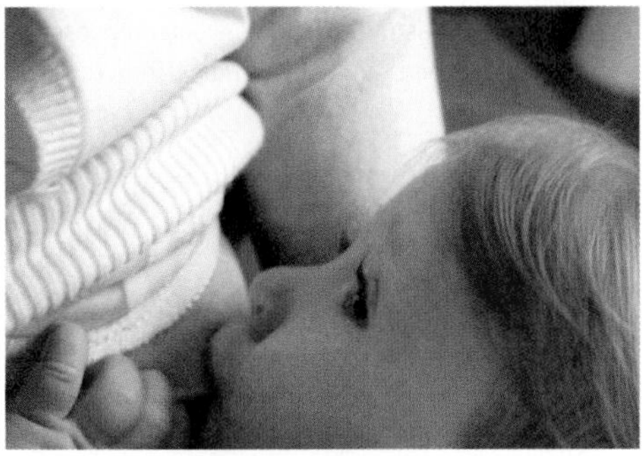

© Christina Kennedy/Alamy

Women are encouraged to breastfeed whenever possible because breast milk offers infants many nutrient and health advantages.

FIGURE 17-2 Recommended Intakes of an Infant and an Adult Compared on the Basis of Body Weight

Because infants are small, they need smaller total amounts of the nutrients than adults do, but when comparisons are based on body weight, infants need more than twice as much of many nutrients. Infants use large amounts of energy and nutrients, in proportion to their body size, to keep all their metabolic processes going.

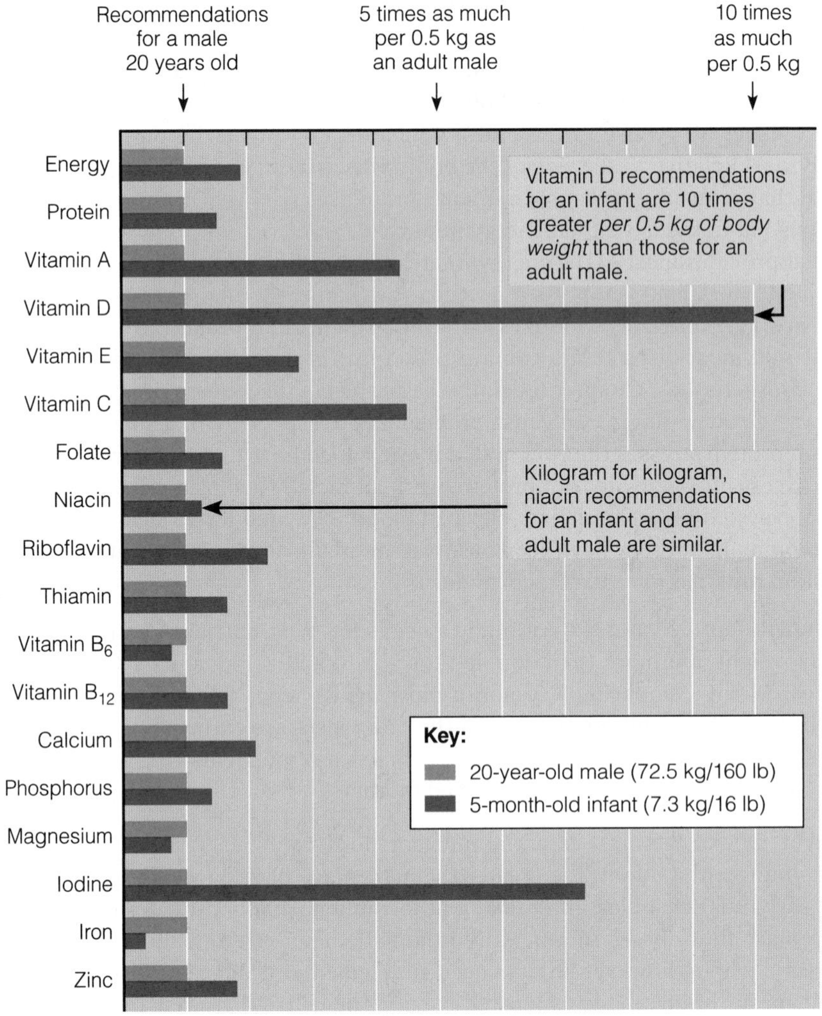
Recommendations for a male 20 years old
5 times as much per 0.5 kg as an adult male
10 times as much per 0.5 kg
Energy
Protein
Vitamin A
Vitamin D
Vitamin E
Vitamin C
Folate
Niacin
Riboflavin
Thiamin
Vitamin B6
Vitamin B12
Calcium
Phosphorus
Magnesium
Iodine
Iron
Zinc
Vitamin D recommendations for an infant are 10 times greater per 0.5 kg of body weight than those for an adult male.
Kilogram for kilogram, niacin recommendations for an infant and an adult male are similar.
Key:
20-year-old male (72.5 kg/160 lb)
5-month-old infant (7.3 kg/16 lb)

SOURCE: Used with permission of the American Academy of Pediatrics, *Pediatric Nutrition Handbook*, 6th ed. American Academy of Pediatrics © 2009.

but Health Canada also recommends that exclusively breastfed infants receive a vitamin D supplement of 10 ug (400 IU)/day for the first year of life.[5] Experts add, though, that iron-fortified formula, which imitates the nutrient composition of breast milk, is an acceptable alternative. After all, the primary goal is to provide the infant nourishment in a relaxed and loving environment. ♦

♦ Chapter 16 discusses breastfeeding, breastfeeding support, reasons why some women choose not to breastfeed, and contraindications to breastfeeding.

Frequency and Duration of Breastfeeding Breast milk is more easily and completely digested than formula, so breastfed infants usually need to eat more frequently than formula-fed infants do. During the first few weeks, approximately 8 to 12 feedings a day, on demand, as soon as the infant shows early signs of hunger such as increased alertness, activity, or suckling motions, promote optimal milk production and infant growth.[6] Crying is a late indicator of hunger. An infant who nurses every two to three hours and sleeps contentedly between feedings is adequately nourished. As the infant gets older, stomach capacity enlarges and the mother's milk production increases, allowing for longer intervals between feedings.

Even though the infant obtains about half the milk from the breast during the first two or three minutes of sucking, breastfeeding is encouraged for about 10 to

15 minutes on each breast. The infant's sucking, as well as the complete removal of milk from the breast, stimulates lactation.

Energy Nutrients The energy-nutrient composition of breast milk differs dramatically from that recommended for adult diets (see Figure 17-3). Yet for infants, breast milk is nature's most nearly perfect food, providing the clear lesson that people at different stages of life have different nutrient needs.

The main carbohydrate in breast milk (and infant formula) is the disaccharide lactose. In addition to being easily digested, lactose enhances calcium absorption. The carbohydrate component of breast milk also contains abundant oligosaccharides, which are present only in trace amounts in cow's milk and infant formula made from cow's milk.[7] Human milk oligosaccharides help protect the infant from infection by preventing the binding of pathogens to the infant's intestinal cells.[8]

The amount of protein in breast milk is less than in cow's milk, but this quantity is actually beneficial because it places less stress on the infant's immature kidneys to excrete the major end product of protein metabolism, urea. Much of the protein in breast milk is **alpha-lactalbumin**, which is efficiently digested and absorbed.

As for the lipids, breast milk contains a generous proportion of the essential fatty acids linoleic acid and linolenic acid, as well as their longer-chain derivatives arachidonic acid and DHA (docosahexaenoic acid). In the past, infant formula provided only linoleic acid and linolenic acid, but now arachidonic acid and DHA are also added. Infants can make arachidonic acid and DHA from linoleic acid and linolenic acid, respectively, but some infants may need more than they can make.

As Chapters 5 and 16 mention, DHA is the most abundant fatty acid in the brain and is also present in the retina of the eye. DHA accumulation in the brain is greatest during fetal development and early infancy.[9] Research has focused on the mental and visual development of breastfed infants and infants fed standard formula with and without DHA added.[10] One group of researchers found that infants fed formula fortified with DHA had sharper vision at 1 year of age than those who were fed standard formula.[11] Most studies, however, show no beneficial effect of DHA supplementation of formula for term infants.[12] Adding DHA to standard infant formulas has no adverse effects, however, and most standard formulas are currently fortified with both DHA and arachidonic acid.

Vitamins With the exception of vitamin D, the vitamins in breast milk are ample to support infant growth. The vitamin D in breast milk is low, and vitamin D deficiency impairs bone mineralization. Vitamin D deficiency is most likely in infants who are not exposed to sunlight daily, have darkly pigmented skin, and receive breast milk without vitamin D supplementation.[13] Reports of infants in the United States developing the vitamin D–deficiency disease rickets and recommendations by the AAP to keep infants under 6 months of age out of direct sunlight prompted revisions in vitamin D guidelines. Health Canada currently recommends a vitamin D supplement for all infants who are breastfed exclusively, and for any infants who do not receive at least 1 litre (1000 millilitres, roughly 32 ounces) of vitamin D–fortified formula daily.[14]

Minerals The calcium content of breast milk is ideal for infant bone growth, and the calcium is well absorbed. Breast milk contains relatively small amounts of iron, but the iron has a high bioavailability. Zinc also has a high bioavailability, thanks to the presence of a zinc-binding protein. Breast milk is low in sodium, another benefit for immature kidneys. Fluoride promotes the development of strong teeth, but breast milk is not a good source.

Supplements Pediatricians may routinely prescribe liquid supplements containing vitamin D, iron, and fluoride. Table 17-2 (p. 548) offers a schedule of supplements that are recommended during infancy. In addition, the Canadian Paediatric Society recommends giving a single dose of vitamin K to infants at birth to protect them from developing hemorrhagic disease of the newborn (HDNB). (See Chapter 12 for a description of vitamin K's role in blood clotting.)

Immunological Protection In addition to its nutritional benefits, breast milk offers immunological protection. Not only is breast milk sterile, but it actively

FIGURE 17-3 Percentages of Energy-Yielding Nutrients in Breast Milk and in Recommended Adult Diets

The proportions of energy-yielding nutrients in human breast milk differ from those recommended for adults.[a]

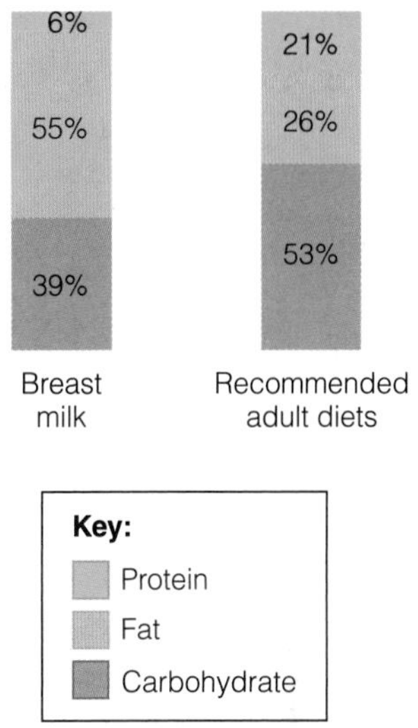

6%
55%
39%
21%
26%
53%
Breast milk
Recommended adult diets
Key:
Protein
Fat
Carbohydrate

[a]The values listed for adults represent approximate midpoints of the acceptable ranges for protein (10 to 35 percent), fat (20 to 35 percent), and carbohydrate (45 to 65 percent).

alpha-lactalbumin (lact-AL-byoo-min): a major protein in human breast milk, as opposed to *casein* (CAY-seen), a major protein in cow's milk.

TABLE 17-2 Supplements for Full-Term Infants

	Vitamin D[a]	Iron[b]	Fluoride[c]
Breastfed infants			
Birth to 6 months of age	✓		
6 months to 1 year	✓	✓	✓
Formula-fed infants			
Birth to 6 months of age			
6 months to 1 year		✓	✓

[a]Vitamin D supplements are recommended for all infants who are exclusively breastfed and for any infants who do not receive at least 1 litre (1000 millilitres or 32 ounces) of vitamin D–fortified formula per day.
[b]All infants 6 months of age need additional iron, preferably in the form of iron-fortified infant cereal and/or infant meats. Formula-fed infants need iron-fortified infant formula.
[c]At 6 months of age, breastfed infants and formula-fed infants who receive ready-to-use formulas (these are prepared with water low in fluoride) or formula mixed with water that contains little or no fluoride (less than 0.3 ppm) need supplements.
SOURCE: Adapted from Committee on Nutrition, American Academy of Pediatrics, *Pediatric Nutrition Handbook,* 6th ed., ed. R. E. Kleinman (Elk Grove Village, Ill.: American Academy of Pediatrics, 2009).

fights disease and protects infants from illnesses.[15] Such protection is most valuable during the first year, when the infant's immune system is not fully prepared to mount a response against infections.

During the first two or three days after delivery, the breasts produce **colostrum**, a premilk substance containing mostly serum with antibodies and white blood cells. Colostrum (like breast milk) helps protect the newborn from infections against which the mother has developed immunity. The maternal antibodies in the breast milk inactivate disease-causing bacteria within the infant's digestive tract before they can start infections.[16] This explains, in part, why breastfed infants have fewer intestinal infections than formula-fed infants.

In addition to antibodies, colostrum and breast milk provide other powerful agents ♦ that help to fight against bacterial infection. Among them are the oligosaccharides, described earlier, that prevent pathogens from binding to intestinal cells. Also present are **bifidus factors**, which favour the growth of the "friendly" bacterium *Lactobacillus bifidus* in the infant's digestive tract, so that other, harmful bacteria cannot become established. An iron-binding protein in breast milk, **lactoferrin**, keeps bacteria from getting the iron they need to grow, helps absorb iron into the infant's intestinal cells, and kills some bacteria directly.[17] The protein **lactadherin** in breast milk binds to, and inhibits replication of, the virus that causes most infant diarrhea.[18] Breastfeeding also protects against other common illnesses of infancy such as middle ear infection and respiratory illness.[19] In addition, a growth factor that is present in breast milk stimulates the development and maintenance of the infant's digestive tract and its protective factors. Several breast milk enzymes such as lipase also help protect the infant against infection. Clearly, breast milk is a very special substance.

♦ Protective factors in breast milk:
- Antibodies
- Oligosaccharides
- Bifidus factors
- Lactoferrin
- Lactadherin
- Growth factor
- Lipase enzyme

Allergy and Disease Protection In addition to protection against infection, breast milk may offer protection against the development of allergies.[20] Compared with formula-fed infants, breastfed infants have a lower incidence of allergic reactions, such as recurrent wheezing and skin rashes.[21] This protection is especially noticeable among infants with a family history of allergies.[22] Similarly, breast milk may offer protection against the development of cardiovascular disease. Compared with formula-fed infants, breastfed infants have lower blood pressure and lower blood cholesterol as adults.[23]

Other Potential Benefits Breastfeeding may offer some protection against excessive weight gain later, although findings are inconsistent.[24] One extensive review suggests that initial breastfeeding protects against obesity in later life.[25] Another study confirms this finding and adds that the longer the duration of breastfeeding, the lower the risk of overweight in childhood.[26] Still another review reports a protective effect, a protective effect only in certain groups, or no effect.[27] Researchers note that many other factors—socioeconomic status, other infant and child feeding practices, and especially the mother's weight—strongly predict a child's body weight.

colostrum (ko-LAHS-trum): a milklike secretion from the breast, present during the first few days after delivery before milk appears; rich in protective factors.

bifidus (BIFF-id-us, by-FEED-us) **factors:** factors in colostrum and breast milk that favour the growth of the "friendly" bacterium *Lactobacillus* (lack-toh-ba-SILL-us) *bifidus* in the infant's intestinal tract, so that other, less desirable intestinal inhabitants will not flourish.

lactoferrin (lack-toh-FERR-in): a protein in breast milk that binds iron and keeps it from supporting the growth of the infant's intestinal bacteria.

lactadherin (lack-tad-HAIR-in): a protein in breast milk that attacks diarrhea-causing viruses.

Many studies suggest a beneficial effect of breastfeeding on intelligence, but when subjected to strict standards of methodology (e.g., large sample size and appropriate intelligence testing), the evidence is less convincing.[28] Nevertheless, the possibility that breastfeeding may positively affect later intelligence is intriguing. It may be that some specific component of breast milk, such as DHA, stimulates brain development or that certain factors associated with the feeding process itself promote intellect.[29] Most likely, a combination of factors is involved. More large, well-controlled studies are needed to confirm the effects, if any, of breastfeeding on later intelligence.

Breast Milk Banks Similar to blood banks that collect blood from individuals to give to others in need, **breast milk banks** (about one dozen in North America, with one operating in Canada and another in the developmental stage) receive milk from lactating women who have an abundant supply to give to infants whose own mothers' milk is unavailable or insufficient. The women who donate breast milk are carefully screened to exclude those who smoke cigarettes, use illicit drugs, take medications (including high doses of dietary supplements), drink more than two alcoholic beverages a day, or have communicable diseases. The breast milk from several donors is pooled to ensure an even distribution of all components, pasteurized to destroy bacteria, checked for contamination, and frozen before being shipped overnight to hospitals, where it is dispensed by physician prescription. In the absence of a mother's own breast milk, donor milk may be the life-saving solution for fragile infants, most notably those with very low birthweight or unusual medical conditions.[30]

Infant Formula

A woman who breastfeeds for a year can **wean** her infant to cow's milk, bypassing the need for infant formula. However, a woman who decides to feed her infant formula from birth, to wean to formula after less than a year of breastfeeding, or to substitute formula for breastfeeding on occasion must select an appropriate infant formula and learn to prepare it. Cow's milk is inappropriate.

breast milk bank: a service that collects, screens, processes, and distributes donated human milk.

wean: to gradually replace breast milk with infant formula or other foods appropriate to an infant's diet.

Infant Formula Composition Formula manufacturers attempt to copy the nutrient composition of breast milk as closely as possible. Figure 17-4 illustrates the energy-nutrient balance of both. The CPS recommends that all formula-fed infants receive iron-fortified infant formulas.[31] The increasing use of iron-fortified formulas during the past few decades is a major reason for the decline in iron-deficiency anemia among infants in North America.

FIGURE 17-4 Percentages of Energy-Yielding Nutrients in Breast Milk, Infant Formula, and Cow's Milk

The average proportions of energy-yielding nutrients in human breast milk and formula differ slightly. In contrast, cow's milk provides too much protein and too little carbohydrate.

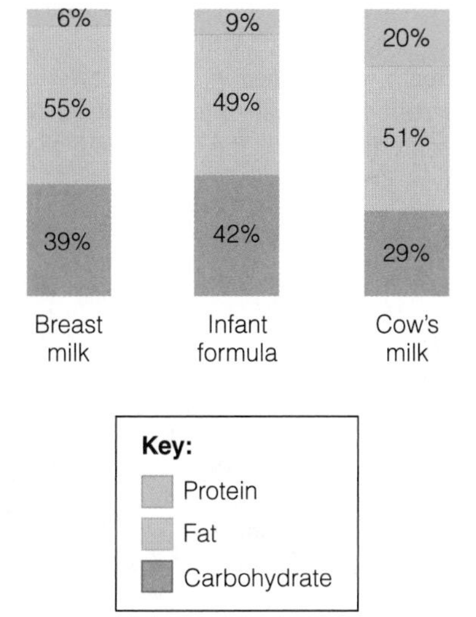
6%
55%
39%
Breast milk
9%
49%
42%
Infant formula
20%
51%
29%
Cow's milk
Key:
Protein
Fat
Carbohydrate

Risks of Formula Feeding Infant formulas contain no protective antibodies for infants, but in general, vaccinations, purified water, and clean environments in developed countries help protect infants from infections. Formulas can be prepared safely by following the rules of proper food handling and by using water that is free of contamination. Of particular concern is lead-contaminated water, a major source of lead poisoning in infants. Because the first water drawn from the tap each day is highest in lead, a person living in a house with old, lead-soldered plumbing should let the water run a few minutes before drinking or using it to prepare formula or food.

In developing countries, formula may be unavailable, prepared with contaminated water, or overdiluted in an attempt to save money. Contaminated formulas often cause infections, leading to diarrhea, dehydration, and malabsorption. Without sterilization and refrigeration, formula is an ideal breeding ground for bacteria. Whenever such risks are present, breastfeeding can be a life-saving option: breast milk is sterile, and its antibodies enhance an infant's resistance to infections . To this end, Health Canada guidelines recommend using boiled water to make infant formula from either powdered or concentrated formula, whereas guidelines in other countries may not be as strict.[32]

Infant Formula Standards National and international standards have been set for the nutrient contents of infant formulas. In the United States, the standard developed by the AAP reflects "human milk taken from well-nourished mothers

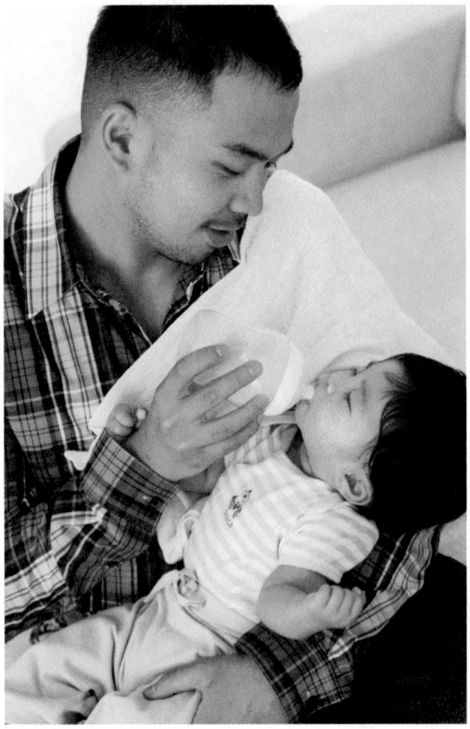
Ruth Jenkinson/Getty Images

The infant thrives on infant formula offered with affection.

during the first or second month of lactation, when the infant's growth rate is high." Health Canada mandates the safety and nutritional quality of infant formulas. Formulas meeting these standards have similar nutrient compositions. Small differences among formulas are sometimes confusing, but they are usually unimportant.

Special Formulas Standard formulas are inappropriate for some infants. Special formulas have been designed to meet the dietary needs of infants with specific conditions such as prematurity or inherited diseases. Most infants allergic to milk protein can drink formulas based on soy protein.[33] Soy formulas also use cornstarch and sucrose instead of lactose and so are recommended for infants with lactose intolerance as well. They are also useful as an alternative to milk-based formulas for vegan families. Despite these limited uses, soy formulas account for one-fourth of the infant formulas sold today. Although soy formulas support the normal growth and development of infants, for infants who don't need them, they offer no advantage over milk formulas.

Some infants who are allergic to cow's milk protein may also be allergic to soy protein.[34] For these infants, special formulas based on hydrolyzed protein are available.

Inappropriate Formulas Caregivers must use only products designed for infants; soy *beverages*, for example, are nutritionally incomplete and inappropriate for infants. Goat's milk is also inappropriate for infants in part because of its low folate content. An infant receiving goat's milk is likely to develop "goat's milk anemia," an anemia characteristic of folate deficiency.

Nursing Bottle Tooth Decay An infant cannot be allowed to sleep with a bottle because of the potential damage to developing teeth. Salivary flow, which normally cleanses the mouth, diminishes as the infant falls asleep. Prolonged sucking on a bottle of formula, milk, or juice bathes the upper teeth in a carbohydrate-rich fluid that nourishes decay-producing bacteria. (The tongue covers and protects most of the lower teeth, but they, too, may be affected.) The result is extensive and rapid tooth decay (see Figure 17-5). To prevent **nursing bottle tooth decay**, no infant should be put to bed with a bottle of nourishing fluid.

nursing bottle tooth decay: extensive tooth decay due to prolonged tooth contact with formula, milk, fruit juice, or other carbohydrate-rich liquid offered to an infant in a bottle.

FIGURE 17-5 Nursing Bottle Tooth Decay

This child was frequently put to bed sucking on a bottle filled with apple juice, so the teeth were bathed in carbohydrate for long periods of time—a perfect medium for bacterial growth. The upper teeth show signs of decay.

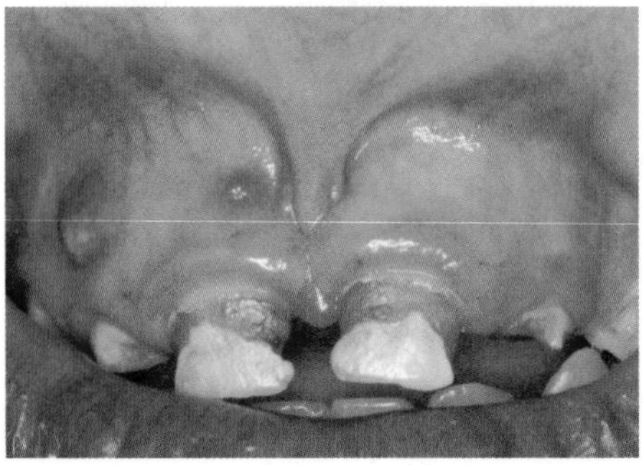
© E. H. Gill/Custom Medical Stock Photo

Special Needs of Preterm Infants

An estimated one out of sixteen pregnancies (~6 percent) in Canada results in a preterm birth.[35] The terms *preterm* and *premature* imply incomplete fetal development, or immaturity, of many body systems. As might be expected, preterm birth is a leading cause of infant deaths. Preterm infants face physical independence from their mothers before some of their organs and body tissues are ready. The rate of weight gain in the fetus is greater during the last trimester of gestation than at any other time. Therefore, a preterm infant is most often a low-birthweight infant as well. A premature birth deprives the infant of the nutritional support of the placenta during a time of maximal growth.

The last trimester of gestation is also a time of building nutrient stores. Being born with limited nutrient stores intensifies the already precarious situation for the infant. The physical and metabolic immaturity of preterm infants further compromises their nutrition status. Nutrient absorption, especially of fat and calcium, from an immature GI tract is limited. Consequently, preterm, low-birthweight infants are candidates for nutrient imbalances. Deficiencies of the fat-soluble vitamins, calcium, iron, and zinc are common.

Preterm breast milk is well suited to meet a preterm infant's needs. During early lactation, preterm breast milk contains higher concentrations of protein and is lower in volume than term breast milk. The low milk volume is advantageous because preterm infants consume small quantities of milk per feeding, and the higher protein concentration allows for better growth. In many instances, supplements of nutrients specifically designed for preterm infants are added to the mother's expressed breast milk and fed to the infant from a bottle. When fortified with a preterm supplement, preterm breast milk supports growth at a rate that approximates the growth rate that would have occurred within the uterus.[36]

Introducing Cow's Milk The age at which whole cow's milk should be introduced to the infant's diet has long been a source of controversy. The CPS advises that whole cow's milk is not appropriate during the first year.[37] Children 1 to 2 years of age should not be given 2%, 1%, or skim milk routinely; they need whole milk. Between the ages of 2 and 5 years, a gradual transition from whole milk to the lower-fat milks can take place, but care should be taken to avoid excessive restriction of dietary fat.

Dietary Guidance for Canadians
Children 2 to 8 years should consume 500 millilitres (2 cups) per day of milk and milk alternatives, such as 1% or 2% milk or fortified soy beverage.

In some infants, particularly those younger than 6 months of age, whole cow's milk may cause intestinal bleeding, which can lead to iron deficiency. Cow's milk is also a poor source of iron. Consequently, it both causes iron loss and fails to replace iron. Furthermore, the bioavailability of iron from infant cereal and other foods is reduced when cow's milk replaces breast milk or iron-fortified formula during the first year. Compared with breast milk or iron-fortified formula, cow's milk is higher in calcium and lower in vitamin C, characteristics that reduce iron absorption. Furthermore, the higher protein concentration of cow's milk can stress the infant's kidneys. In short, cow's milk is a poor choice during the first year of life; infants need breast milk or iron-fortified infant formula.

Introducing Solid Foods The high nutrient needs of infancy are met first by breast milk or formula only and then by the limited addition of selected foods over time. Infants gradually develop the ability to chew, swallow, and digest the wide variety of foods available to adults. The caregiver's selection of appropriate foods at the appropriate stages of development is prerequisite to the infant's optimal growth and health.

When to Begin In addition to breast milk or formula, an infant can begin eating solid foods at 6 months.[38] The CPS supports exclusive breastfeeding for 6 months. The main purpose of introducing solid foods is to provide needed nutrients that are no longer supplied adequately by breast milk or formula alone. The foods ♦ chosen must be those that the infant is developmentally capable of handling both physically and metabolically. The exact timing depends on the individual infant's needs and developmental readiness (see Table 17-3 on page 552), ♦ which vary from infant to infant because of differences in growth rates, activities, and environmental conditions. In addition to the infant's nutrient needs and physical readiness to handle different forms of foods, the introduction of solid foods should consider the need to detect and control allergic reactions.

♦ The German word *beikost* (BYE-cost) describes any nonmilk foods given to an infant.

♦ Digestive secretions gradually increase throughout the first year of life, making the digestion of solid foods more efficient.

Food Allergies To prevent allergy and to facilitate its prompt identification should it occur, experts recommend introducing single-ingredient foods, one at a time, in small portions, and waiting three to five days before introducing the next new food.[39] For example, rice cereal is usually the first cereal introduced because it is the least allergenic. When it is clear that rice cereal is not causing an allergy, another grain, perhaps barley or oat, is introduced. Wheat cereal is offered last because it is the most common offender. If a cereal causes an allergic reaction such as a skin rash, digestive upset, or respiratory discomfort, it should be discontinued before introducing the next food. A later section in this chapter offers more information about food allergies.

Choice of Infant Foods Infant foods should be selected to provide variety, balance, and moderation. Commercial baby foods offer a wide variety of palatable, nutritious foods in a safe and convenient form. Homemade infant foods can be as nutritious as commercially prepared ones, as long as the cook minimizes nutrient losses during preparation. Ingredients for homemade foods should be fresh, whole foods without added salt, sugar, or seasonings. Pureed food can be frozen in ice cube trays, providing convenient-size blocks of food that can be thawed,

TABLE 17-3 Infant Development and Recommended Foods

Because each stage of development builds on the previous stage, the foods from an earlier stage continue to be included in all later stages.

Age (mo)	Feeding Skill	Appropriate Foods Added to the Diet
0–4	Turns head toward any object that brushes cheek. Initially swallows using back of tongue; gradually begins to swallow using front of tongue as well. Strong reflex (extrusion) to push food out during first 2 to 3 months.	Feed breast milk or infant formula.
4–6	Extrusion reflex diminishes, and the ability to swallow nonliquid foods develops. Indicates desire for food by opening mouth and leaning forward. Indicates satiety or disinterest by turning away and leaning back. Sits erect with support at 6 months. Begins chewing action. Brings hand to mouth. Grasps objects with palm of hand.	Begin iron-fortified cereal mixed with breast milk, formula, or water. Begin pureed meats, legumes, vegetables, and fruits.
6–8	Able to self-feed finger foods. Develops pincer (finger to thumb) grasp. Begins to drink from cup.	Begin textured vegetables and fruits. Begin unsweetened, diluted fruit juices from cup.
8–10	Begins to hold own bottle. Reaches for and grabs food and spoon. Sits unsupported.	Begin breads and cereals from table. Begin yogurt. Begin pieces of soft, cooked vegetables and fruit from table. Gradually begin finely cut meats, fish, casseroles, cheese, eggs, and mashed legumes.
10–12	Begins to master spoon, but still spills some.	Add variety. Gradually increase portion sizes.[a]

[a]Portion sizes for infants and young children are smaller than those for an adult. For example, a grain serving might be ½ slice of bread instead of 1 slice, or 60 mL (¼ cup) rice instead of 125 mL (½ cup).

SOURCE: Adapted in part from Committee on Nutrition, American Academy of Pediatrics, *Pediatric Nutrition Handbook,* 6th ed., ed. R. E. Kleinman (Elk Grove Village, Ill.: American Academy of Pediatrics, 2009), pp. 113–142.

warmed, and fed to the infant. To guard against foodborne illnesses, hands and equipment must be kept clean.

Because recommendations to restrict fat do not apply to children younger than age 2, labels on foods for children younger than 2 (such as infant meats and cereals) cannot carry information about fat. Fat information is omitted from infant food labels to prevent parents from restricting fat in infants' diets. Fearing that their infant will become overweight, parents may unintentionally malnourish the infant by limiting fat. In fact, infants and young children, because of their rapid growth, need more fat than older children and adults.

Foods to Provide Iron Rapid growth demands iron. At about 4 to 6 months of age, the infant begins to need more iron than body stores plus breast milk or iron-fortified formula can provide. In addition to breast milk or iron-fortified formula, infants can receive iron from iron-fortified cereals and, once they readily accept solid foods, from meat or meat alternates such as legumes. Iron-fortified cereals contribute a significant amount of iron to an infant's diet, but the iron's bioavailability is poor.[40] Caregivers can enhance iron absorption from iron-fortified cereals by serving vitamin C–rich foods with meals.

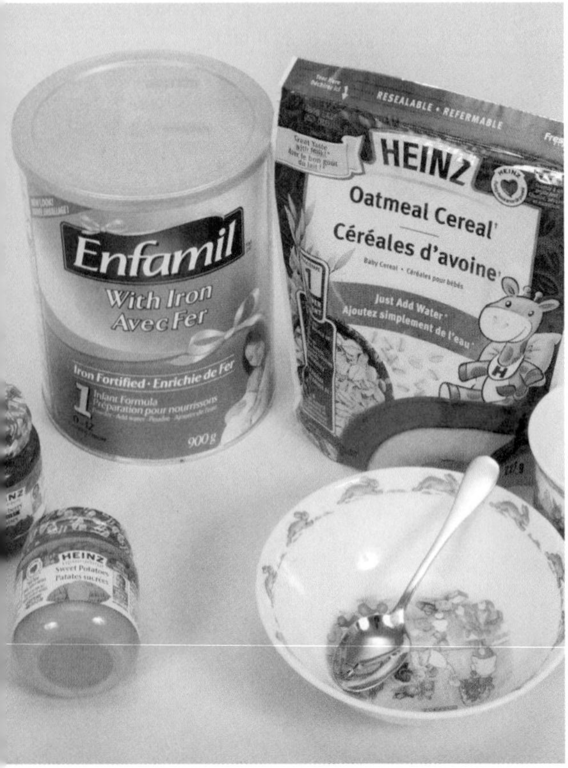
Enfamil
With Iron
Avec Fer
HEINZ
Oatmeal Cereal
Céréales d'avoine
Just Add Water
RESEALABLE • REFERMABLE
Dick Hemingway

Foods such as iron-fortified cereals and formulas, mashed legumes, and strained meats provide iron.

Foods to Provide Vitamin C The best sources of vitamin C are fruits and vegetables (see pp. 395–396 in Chapter 12). It has been suggested that infants who are introduced to fruits before vegetables may develop a preference for sweets and find the vegetables less palatable, but there is no evidence to support offering these foods in a particular order.[41]

Fruit juice is a good source of vitamin C, but drinking too much juice can lead to diarrhea in infants and young children.[42] CPS recommendations limit juice consumption for infants to between 60 and 125 mL (2 and 4 ounces) per day.[43] Too much fruit juice contributes excessive kcalories and displaces other nutrient-rich foods. Fruit juices should be diluted and served in a cup, not a bottle, once the infant is 6 months of age or older.

Foods to Omit Concentrated sweets, including baby food "desserts," have no place in an infant's diet. They convey no nutrients to support growth, and the extra food energy can promote obesity. Products containing sugar alcohols such as sorbitol should also be limited, as they may cause diarrhea. Canned vegetables are also inappropriate for infants, as they often contain too much sodium. Honey and corn syrup should never be fed to infants because of the risk of **botulism**.* Infants and young children are vulnerable to foodborne illnesses, and the *Dietary Guidance for Canadians* address this risk.

Dietary Guidance for Canadians

Infants and young children should not eat or drink unpasteurized milk, milk products, or juices; raw or undercooked eggs, meat, poultry, fish, or shellfish; or raw sprouts.

Infants and even young children cannot safely chew and swallow any of the foods listed in the margin; ♦ they can easily choke on these foods, a risk not worth taking. Nonfood items may present even greater choking hazards to infants and young children. Parents and caregivers must pay careful attention to eliminate choking hazards in children's environments.

♦ To prevent choking, do not give infants or young children:

- Cherries
- Gum
- Hard or gel-type candies
- Hot dog slices
- Marshmallows
- Nuts
- Peanut butter
- Popcorn
- Raw carrots
- Raw celery
- Whole beans
- Whole grapes

Keep these nonfood items out of their reach:

- Balloons
- Coins
- Pen tops
- Small balls and marbles

Vegetarian Diets during Infancy The newborn infant is a lacto-vegetarian. As long as the infant has access to sufficient quantities of either iron-fortified infant formula or breast milk (plus a vitamin D supplement) from a mother who eats an adequate diet, the infant will thrive during the early months. "Health-food beverages," such as rice milk, are inappropriate choices because they lack the protein, vitamins, and minerals infants and toddlers need; in fact, their use can lead to severe nutritional deficiencies.

Infants beyond about 6 months of age present a greater challenge in terms of meeting nutrient needs by way of vegetarian and, especially, vegan diets. Continued breastfeeding or formula feeding is recommended, but supplementary feedings are necessary to ensure adequate energy and iron intakes. Infants and young children in vegetarian families should be given iron-fortified infant cereals well into the second year. Mashed or pureed legumes, tofu, and cooked eggs can be added to their diets in place of meat.

The risks of malnutrition in infants increase with weaning and reliance on table foods. Infants who receive a well-balanced vegetarian diet that includes milk products and a variety of other foods can easily meet their nutritional requirements for growth. This is not always true for vegan infants; the growth of vegan infants slows significantly around the time of transition from breast milk to solid foods. Protein-energy malnutrition and deficiencies of vitamin D, vitamin B_{12}, iron, and calcium have been reported in infants fed vegan diets. Vegan diets that are high in fibre, other complex carbohydrates, and water will fill infants' stomachs before meeting their energy needs. This problem can be partially alleviated by providing more energy-dense foods, such as nut butters, legumes, dried fruit spreads, and mashed avocado. Using soy formulas (or milk) fortified with calcium, vitamin B_{12}, and vitamin D and including vitamin C–containing foods at meals to enhance iron absorption will help prevent some nutrient deficiencies in vegan diets. Parents or caregivers who choose to feed their infants vegan diets should consult with their pediatrician and a registered dietitian frequently to ensure a nutritionally adequate diet that will support growth.

botulism (BOT-chew-lism): an often fatal foodborne illness caused by the ingestion of foods containing a toxin produced by bacteria that grow without oxygen. (See Chapter 20 for details.)

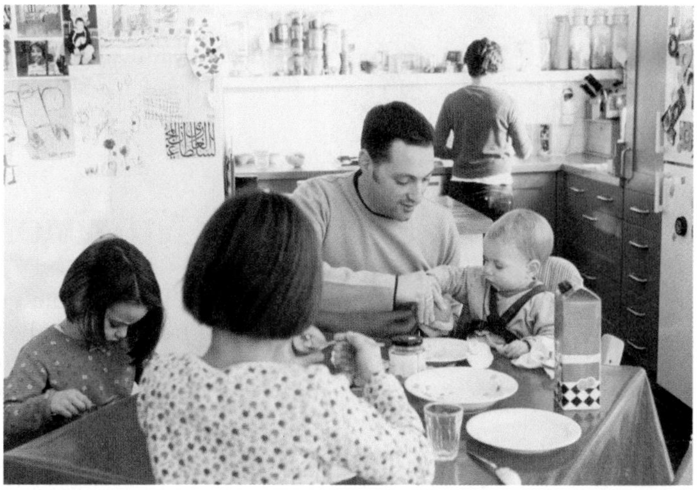
Ruth Jenkinson/Getty Images

Ideally, a 1-year-old eats many of the same foods as the rest of the family.

Foods at 1 Year At 1 year of age, whole cow's milk can become a primary source of most of the nutrients an infant needs; 500–750 millilitres (2 to 3 cups) a day meets those needs sufficiently. Ingesting more milk than this can displace

*In infants, but not in older individuals, ingestion of *Clostridium botulinum* spores can cause illness when the spores germinate in the intestine and produce a toxin, which is absorbed. Symptoms include poor feeding, constipation, loss of tension in the arteries and muscles, weakness, and respiratory compromise. Infant botulism has been implicated in 5 percent of cases of sudden infant death syndrome (SIDS).

FIGURE 17-6 Sample Meal Plan for a 1 Year Old

SAMPLE MENU

Breakfast	1 scrambled egg 1 slice whole-wheat toast 125 mL (½ c) whole milk
Morning snack	125 mL (½ c) yogurt 60 mL (¼ c) fruit[a]
Lunch	½ grilled cheese sandwich: 1 slice whole-wheat bread with 1 slice cheese 125 mL (½ c) vegetables[b] (steamed carrots) 60 mL (¼ c) 100% fruit juice
Afternoon snack	125 mL (½ c) fruit[a] 125 mL (½ c) toasted oat cereal
Dinner	30 g chopped meat or 60 mL (¼ c) well-cooked mashed legumes 125 mL (½ c) rice or pasta 125 mL (½ c) vegetables[b] (chopped broccoli) 125 mL (½ c) whole milk

NOTE: This sample menu provides about 1000 kcalories.
[a]Include citrus fruits, melons, and berries.
[b]Include dark green, leafy, and deep yellow vegetables.

iron-rich foods, which can lead to **milk anemia.** If powdered milk is used, it should contain fat.

Other foods—meats, iron-fortified cereals, enriched or whole-grain breads, fruits, and vegetables—should be supplied in variety and in amounts sufficient to round out total energy needs. Ideally, a 1-year-old will sit at the table, eat many of the same foods everyone else eats, and drink liquids from a cup, not a bottle. Figure 17-6 shows a meal plan that meets a 1-year-old's requirements.

milk anemia: iron-deficiency anemia that develops when an excessive milk intake displaces iron-rich foods from the diet.

Mealtimes with Toddlers

The nurturing of a young child involves more than nutrition. Those who care for young children are responsible for providing not only nutritious foods, milk, and water, but also a safe, loving, secure environment in which the children may grow and develop. In light of toddlers' developmental and nutrient needs and their often contrary and willful behaviour, a few feeding guidelines may be helpful:

- *Discourage unacceptable behaviour, such as standing at the table or throwing food.* Be consistent and firm, not punitive. For example, instead of saying "You make me mad when you don't sit down," say "The fruit salad tastes good, please sit down and eat some with me." The child will soon learn to sit and eat.
- *Let toddlers explore and enjoy food, even if this means eating with fingers for a while.* Learning to use a spoon will come in time. Children who are allowed to touch, mash, and smell their food while exploring it are more likely to accept it.
- *Don't force food on children.* Rejecting new foods is normal and acceptance is more likely as children become familiar with new foods through repeated opportunities to taste them. Instead of saying "You cannot go outside to play until you taste your carrots," say "You can try the carrots again another time."
- *Provide nutritious foods, and let children choose which ones, and how much, they will eat.* Gradually, they will acquire a taste for different foods.
- *Limit sweets.* Infants and young children have little room for empty-kcalorie foods in their daily energy allowance. Do not use sweets as a reward for eating meals.
- *Don't turn the dining table into a battleground.* Make mealtimes enjoyable. Teach healthy food choices and eating habits in a pleasant environment. Mealtimes are not the time to fight, argue, or scold.

IN SUMMARY **The primary food for infants during the first 12 months is either breast milk or iron-fortified formula. In addition to nutrients, breast milk also offers immunological protection. At about 4 to 6 months of age, infants should gradually begin eating solid foods. By 1 year, they are drinking from a cup and eating many of the same foods as the rest of the family.**

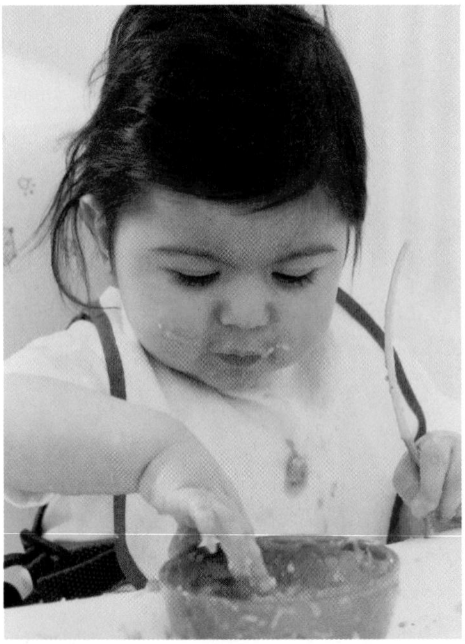
Ruth Jenkinson/Getty Images

Let toddlers explore and enjoy their food.

Nutrition during Childhood

Each year from age 1 to adolescence, a child typically grows taller by 5 to 7 centimetres (2 to 3 inches) and heavier by 2 to 3 kilograms (5 to 6 pounds). Growth charts provide valuable clues to a child's health. Weight gains out of proportion to height gains may reflect overeating and inactivity, whereas measures significantly below the standard suggest malnutrition.

Increases in height and weight are only two of the many changes growing children experience (see Figure 17-7). At age 1, children can stand alone and are beginning to toddle; by 2, they can walk and are learning to run; and by 3, they can jump and climb with confidence. Bones and muscles increase in mass and density to make these accomplishments possible. Thereafter, lengthening of the long bones and increases in musculature proceed unevenly and more slowly until adolescence.

FIGURE 17-7 Body Shape of 1-Year-Old and 2-Year-Old Compared

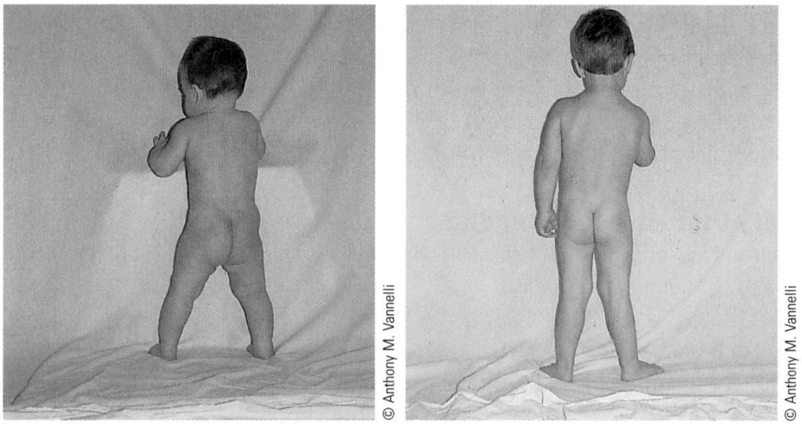
© Anthony M. Vannelli
© Anthony M. Vannelli

The body shape of a 1-year-old (left) changes dramatically by age 2 (right). The 2-year-old has lost much of the baby fat; the muscles (especially in the back, buttocks, and legs) have firmed and strengthened; and the leg bones have lengthened.

Energy and Nutrient Needs

Children's appetites begin to diminish around 1 year, consistent with the slowing growth. Thereafter, children spontaneously vary their food intakes to coincide with their growth patterns; they demand more food during periods of rapid growth than during slow growth. Sometimes they seem insatiable, and other times they seem to live on air and water.

Children's energy intakes also vary widely from meal to meal. Even so, their total daily intakes remain remarkably constant.[44] If children eat less at one meal, they typically eat more at the next, and vice versa. Overweight children do not always adjust their energy intakes appropriately, however, and may eat in response to external cues, disregarding hunger and satiety signals.[45]

Energy Intake and Activity Individual children's energy needs vary widely, depending on their growth and physical activity. A 1-year-old child needs about 800 kcalories a day; an active 6-year-old child needs twice as many kcalories a day. By age 10, an active child needs about 2000 kcalories a day. Total energy needs increase slightly with age, but energy needs per kilogram of body weight actually decline gradually.

Physically active children of any age need more energy because they expend more, and inactive children can become obese even when they eat less food than the average. Unfortunately, our nation's children are less active than they were a couple decades ago and our schools would serve them well by offering more activities to promote physical fitness on a regular basis.[46] Children who learn to enjoy physical play and exercise, both at home and at school, are best prepared to maintain active lifestyles as adults.

Physical Activity Guidance for Canadians

Although Physical Activity Guidelines for pre-schoolers are pending, children (5–11 years old) and youth (12–17 years old) should accumulate at least 60 minutes of moderate-to vigorous-intensity physical activity daily. Note: There are also *Canadian Sedentary Behaviour Guidelines* for children (5–11) youth (12–17) that recommend limiting recreational screen time to less than 2 hours per day.[47]

Some children, notably those adhering to a vegan diet, may have difficulty meeting their energy needs. Grains, vegetables, and fruits provide plenty of fibre, adding bulk, but may provide too little energy to support growth. Soy products, other legumes, and nut or seed butters offer more concentrated sources of energy to support optimal growth and development.[48]

♦ Fibre recommendations for children:

Age (yr)	AI (g)
1–3	19
4–8	25
9–13	
Boys	31
Girls	26
14–18	
Boys	38
Girls	26

♦ There are special regulations for labelling foods manufactured for children under 2 years of age. For example, the expression of nutrients in terms of %DV for the upper part of the Nutrition Facts Table is not allowed. Thus, only the amount of total fat is given per serving, but the %DV for fat is not listed.[51]

Carbohydrate and Fibre Carbohydrate recommendations are based on glucose use by the brain. After 1 year of age, brain glucose use remains fairly constant and is within the adult range. Carbohydrate recommendations for children after 1 year are therefore the same as for adults (see inside front cover).[49]

Fibre recommendations ♦ derive from adult intakes shown to reduce the risk of coronary heart disease and are based on energy intakes. Consequently, fibre recommendations for younger children with low energy intakes are less than those for older ones with high energy intakes.[50]

Dietary Guidance for Canadians

Children and adolescents should consume whole-grain products often, and at least half of the grains should be whole grains.

Fat and Fatty Acids No RDA for total fat has been established, but the DRI Committee recommends a fat intake of 30 to 40 percent of energy for children 1 to 3 years of age ♦ and 25 to 35 percent for children 4 to 18 years of age.[52] As long as children's energy intakes are adequate, however, fat intakes below 30 percent of total energy do not impair growth.[53] Children who eat low-fat diets, however, tend to have low intakes of some vitamins and minerals. Recommended intakes of the essential fatty acids are based on average intakes (see inside front cover).

Dietary Guidance for Canadians

Keep total fat intake between 30 to 35 percent of kcalories for children 2 to 3 years of age and between 25 and 35 percent of kcalories for children and adolescents 4 to 18 years of age, with most fats coming from sources of polyunsaturated and monounsaturated fatty acids, such as fish, nuts, and vegetable oils.

Protein Like energy needs, total protein needs increase slightly with age, but when the child's body weight is considered, the protein requirement actually declines slightly (see inside front cover). Protein recommendations must consider the requirements for maintaining nitrogen balance, the quality of protein consumed, and the added needs of growth.

Vitamins and Minerals The vitamin and mineral needs of children increase with age (see inside front cover). A balanced diet of nutritious foods can meet children's needs for these nutrients, with the notable exception of iron, and possibly vitamin D. Iron-deficiency anemia is a major problem worldwide, and is prevalent among both Canadian and American children, especially toddlers 1 to 3 years of age.[54] During the second year of life, toddlers progress from a diet of iron-rich infant foods such as breast milk, iron-fortified formula, and iron-fortified infant cereal to a diet of adult foods and iron-poor cow's milk. In addition, their appetites often fluctuate—some become finicky about the foods they eat, and others prefer milk and juice to solid foods. These situations can interfere with children eating iron-rich foods at a critical time for brain growth and development.

To prevent iron deficiency, children's foods must deliver 7 to 10 milligrams of iron per day. To achieve this goal, snacks and meals should include iron-rich foods, and milk intake should be reasonable so that it will not displace lean meats, fish, poultry, eggs, legumes, and whole-grain or enriched products. (Chapter 14 describes iron-rich foods and ways to maximize iron absorption.)

As for vitamin D, the Canadian Paediatric Society recently updated guidelines for children. Children who do not obtain 10 micrograms of vitamin D per day by drinking vitamin D–fortified milk (2.5 micrograms per 250 mL/1 cup serving) and eating fortified foods such as dry cereals (1 microgram per 125 mL/½ cup serving) should receive a vitamin D supplement of 10 micrograms (400 IU on labels) per day.[55]

Supplements With the exception of specific recommendations for fluoride, iron, and vitamin D during infancy and childhood, the CPS and other professional groups agree that well-nourished children do not need vitamin and mineral supplements. Despite this, many children and adolescents take supplements.[56] Ironically, children with poor nutrient intakes typically do not receive supplements,

TABLE 17-4 Recommended Number of *Food Guide* Servings for Children 2–3 Years of Age

Food Group	Number of *Food Guide* Servings	Examples of One Child-Size Serving
Vegetables and Fruit	4 • Eat at least one dark green and one orange vegetable each day • Choose vegetables and fruit prepared with little or no added fat • Have vegetables and fruit more often than juice	125 mL (1/2 cup) fresh, frozen, or canned vegetables 125 mL (1/2 cup) cooked or 250 mL (1 cup) raw leaf vegetables 1 fruit or 125 mL (1/2 cup) fresh, frozen, or canned fruit 125 mL (1/2 cup) 100% juice
Grain Products	3 • Make at least half of your grain products whole grain each day • Choose grain products that are lower in fat, sugar, or salt	1 slice bread 1/2 bagel, 1/2 pita, or tortilla 125 mL (1/2 cup) cooked rice, bulgur, or quinoa 185 mL (3/4 cup) hot cereal or 30 g cold cereal 125 mL (1/2 cup) cooked pasta or couscous
Milk and Alternatives	2 • Drink skim, 1%, or 2% milk each day • Select lower-fat milk alternatives	250 mL (1 cup) milk or powdered milk (reconstituted) 125 mL (1/2 cup) canned milk (evaporated) 250 mL (1 cup) fortified soy beverage 185 mL (3/4 cup) yogurt
Meat and Alternatives	1 • Have meat alternatives such as beans, lentils, and tofu often • Eat at least two *Food Guide* Servings of fish each week • Select lean meat and alternatives prepared with little or no added fat	125 mL (1/2 cup) or 75 g cooked fish, shellfish, poultry, lean meat 185 mL (3/4 cup) legumes; 185 mL (3/4 cup) tofu 2 eggs 30 mL (2 Tbsp) peanut or nut butter; 60 mL (1/4 cup) shelled nuts and seeds

SOURCE: *Eating Well with Canada's™ Food Guide* (2007), Health Canada. Reproduced with the permission of the Minister of Public Works and Government Services Canada, 2010.

and those who do take supplements typically receive extra nutrients they do not need.[57] Furthermore, researchers are still studying the safety of supplement use by children. The Federal Trade Commission has warned parents about giving supplements advertised to prevent or cure childhood illnesses such as colds, ear infections, and asthma. Dietary supplements on the market today include many herbal products that have not been tested for safety and effectiveness in children.

Planning Children's Meals Table 17-4 lists recommended amounts from each food group for children 2–3 years of age. Estimated daily kcalorie needs for active and sedentary children of various ages are shown in Table 17-5. To provide all the needed nutrients, children's meals should include a variety of foods from each food group—in amounts suited to their appetites and needs.

Parents and caregivers of infants and toddlers need to offer a much greater variety of nutrient-dense vegetables and fruits at meals and snacks to help ensure adequate nutrition. Among other nutrition concerns for Canadian children are that they may not be meeting their needs for potassium and fibre, and that 75 percent of them have intakes of sodium that exceed the Tolerable Upper Intake Level (UL).[58]

Hunger and Malnutrition in Children

Most children in Canada have access to regular meals, but hunger and malnutrition do appear in certain circumstances. Children in very low-income families, for example, are more likely to be hungry and malnourished. More than 1 million Canadian children are living in poverty.[59] Chapter 21 examines the causes and consequences of hunger in Canada and around the world.

Hunger and Behaviour Even when hunger is temporary, as when a child misses one meal, behaviour and academic performance are affected. Children who eat nutritious breakfasts improve their school performance and are tardy or absent significantly less often than their peers who do not.[60] A nutritious breakfast is a central feature of a diet that meets the needs of children and supports their

TABLE 17-5 Estimated Daily kCalorie Needs for Children

Children	Sedentary[a]	Active[b]
2 to 3 yr	1000	1400
Females		
4 to 8 yr	1200	1800
9 to 13 yr	1600	2200
Males		
4 to 8 yr	1400	2000
9 to 13 yr	1800	2600

[a]*Sedentary* describes a lifestyle that includes only the activities typical of day-to-day life.
[b]*Active* describes a lifestyle that includes at least 60 minutes per day of moderate physical activity (equivalent to walking more than 5 kilometres/3 miles per day at 5 to 6 km/h or 3 to 4 mph) in addition to the activities of day-to-day life.

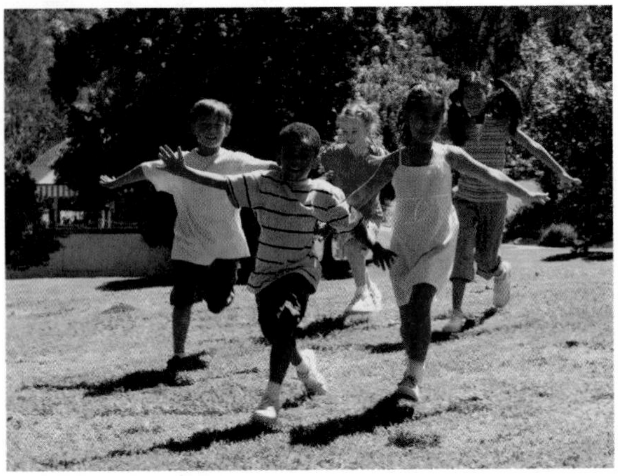
© Ocean/Corbis

Healthy, well-nourished children are alert in the classroom and energetic at play.

healthy growth and development.[61] Children who skip breakfast typically do not make up the deficits at later meals—they simply have lower intakes of energy, vitamins, and minerals than those who eat breakfast. Without breakfast, children perform poorly in tasks requiring concentration, their attention spans are shorter, and they even score lower on intelligence tests than their well-fed peers. Malnourished children are particularly vulnerable. Common sense dictates that it is unreasonable to expect anyone to learn and perform without fuel. For the child who hasn't had breakfast, the morning's lessons may be lost altogether. Even if a child has eaten breakfast, discomfort from hunger may become distracting by late morning. Teachers aware of the late-morning slump in their classrooms wisely request that midmorning snacks be provided; snacks improve classroom performance all the way to lunchtime.

Iron Deficiency and Behaviour Iron deficiency has well-known and widespread effects on children's behaviour and intellectual performance.[62] In addition to carrying oxygen in the blood, iron transports oxygen within cells, which use it for energy metabolism. Iron is also used to make neurotransmitters—most notably, those that regulate the ability to pay attention, which is crucial to learning. Consequently, iron deficiency not only causes an energy crisis, but also directly impairs attention span and learning ability.

Iron deficiency is often diagnosed by a quick, easy, inexpensive hemoglobin or hematocrit test that detects a deficit of iron in the *blood*. A child's *brain*, however, is sensitive to low iron concentrations long before the blood effects appear. Iron deficiency lowers the "motivation to persist in intellectually challenging tasks" and impairs overall intellectual performance. Anemic children perform poorly on tests and are disruptive in the classroom; iron supplementation improves learning and memory. When combined with other nutrient deficiencies, iron-deficiency anemia has synergistic effects that are especially detrimental to learning. Furthermore, children who had iron-deficiency anemia *as infants* continue to perform poorly as they grow older, even if their iron status improves.[63] The long-term damaging effects on mental development make prevention and treatment of iron deficiency during infancy and early childhood a high priority.

Other Nutrient Deficiencies and Behaviour A child with any of several nutrient deficiencies may be irritable, aggressive, and disagreeable, or sad and withdrawn. Such a child may be labelled "hyperactive," "depressed," or "unlikable," when in fact these traits may be due to simple, even marginal, malnutrition. Parents and medical practitioners often overlook the possibility that malnutrition may account for abnormalities of appearance and behaviour. Any departure from normal healthy appearance and behaviour is a sign of possible poor nutrition (see Table 17-6). In any such case, inspection of the child's diet by a registered dietitian or other qualified health-care professional is in order. Any suspicion of dietary inadequacies, no matter what other causes may be implicated, should prompt steps to correct those inadequacies immediately.

The Malnutrition-Lead Connection

Children who are malnourished are vulnerable to lead poisoning. They absorb more lead if their stomachs are empty; if they have low intakes of calcium, zinc, vitamin C, or vitamin D; and, of greatest concern because it is so common, if they have an iron deficiency. Iron deficiency weakens the body's defences against lead absorption, and lead poisoning can cause iron deficiency. Common to both iron deficiency and lead poisoning are a low socioeconomic background and a lack of immunizations against infectious diseases. Another common factor is pica—a craving for nonfood items. Many children with lead poisoning eat dirt or chips of old paint, two common sources of lead.

The anemia brought on by lead poisoning may be mistaken for a simple iron deficiency and therefore may be incorrectly treated. Like iron deficiency, mild lead toxicity has nonspecific symptoms, including diarrhea, irritability, and fatigue. Adding iron to the diet does not reverse the symptoms; exposure to lead must stop and treatment for lead poisoning must begin. With further exposure, the

TABLE 17-6 Physical Signs of Malnutrition in Children

	Well-Nourished	Malnourished	Possible Nutrient Deficiencies
Hair	Shiny, firm in the scalp	Dull, brittle, dry, loose; falls out	PEM
Eyes	Bright, clear pink membranes; adjust easily to light	Pale membranes; spots; redness; adjust slowly to darkness	Vitamin A, the B vitamins, zinc, and iron
Teeth and gums	No pain or caries, gums firm, teeth bright	Missing, discoloured, decayed teeth; gums bleed easily and are swollen and spongy	Minerals and vitamin C
Face	Clear complexion without dryness or scaliness	Off-colour, scaly, flaky, cracked skin	PEM, vitamin A, and iron
Glands	No lumps	Swollen at front of neck, cheeks	PEM and iodine
Tongue	Red, bumpy, rough	Sore, smooth, purplish, swollen	B vitamins
Skin	Smooth, firm, good colour	Dry, rough, spotty; "sandpaper" feel or sores; lack of fat under skin	PEM, essential fatty acids, vitamin A, B vitamins, and vitamin C
Nails	Firm, pink	Spoon-shaped, brittle, ridged	Iron
Internal systems	Regular heart rhythm, heart rate, and blood pressure; no impairment of digestive function, reflexes, or mental status	Abnormal heart rate, heart rhythm, or blood pressure; enlarged liver, spleen; abnormal digestion; burning, tingling of hands, feet; loss of balance, coordination; mental confusion, irritability, fatigue	PEM and minerals
Muscles and bones	Muscle tone; posture, long bone development appropriate for age	"Wasted" appearance of muscles; swollen bumps on skull or ends of bones; small bumps on ribs; bowed legs or knock-knees	PEM, minerals, and vitamin D

symptoms become more pronounced, and children develop learning disabilities and behavioural problems. Still more severe lead toxicity can cause irreversible nerve damage, paralysis, mental retardation, and death.

Recent research suggests that childhood lead exposure disrupts normal brain development—a finding that may partially explain the impaired cognitive and behavioural abilities of lead-exposed children. For six years, researchers measured blood lead levels at intervals in young children who lived in lead-contaminated houses.[64] Years later, brain images revealed that the higher the blood lead concentrations during childhood, the smaller the brain size as a young adult. The brains of boys were more affected than the brains of girls.

Lead may also leach into a home's water supply from old lead pipes. Recently, the water flowing into older homes in London, Ontario, was found to contain elevated levels of lead, and since this is a matter of concern to everyone, especially pregnant women and children, the chief drinking water inspector for Ontario ordered three dozen municipalities from across the province "to conduct immediate drinking water tests for lead in older homes." The results of testing during 2008–2009 revealed that, of the 70000 samples tested, 98 percent met the provincial standard of less than 10 mg/L. In addition, the most recent Canadian Health Measures Survey (CHMS) revealed that "Less than 1% of Canadians aged 6 to 79 had concentrations of lead at or above the intervention level of 10 micrograms per decilitre of blood."[65] Lead toxicity in young children comes from their own behaviours and activities—putting their hands in their mouths, playing in dirt and dust, and chewing on nonfood items.[66] Unfortunately, the body readily absorbs lead during times of rapid growth and hoards it possessively thereafter. Lead is not easily excreted and accumulates mainly in the bones, but also in the brain, teeth, and kidneys. Tragically, a child's neuromuscular system is also maturing during these first few years of life. No wonder children with elevated lead levels experience impairment of balance, motor development, and the relaying of nerve messages to and from the brain. Deficits in intellectual development are only partially reversed when lead levels decline.[67]

Federal laws mandating reductions in leaded gasoline, lead-based solder, and other products over the past four decades have helped to

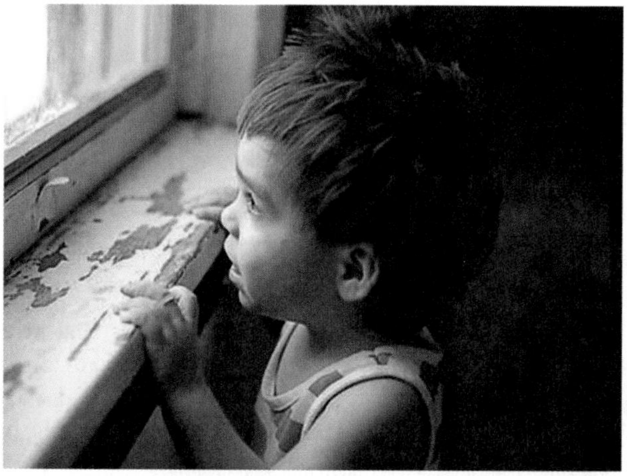

Old, lead-based paint threatens the health of an exploring child.

reduce the amounts of lead in food and in the environment. The accompanying "How To" presents strategies for defending children against lead toxicity.

Hyperactivity and "Hyper" Behaviour

All children are naturally active, and many of them become overly active on occasion—for example, in anticipation of a birthday party. Such behaviour is markedly different from true **hyperactivity.**

Hyperactivity Hyperactive children have trouble sleeping, cannot sit still for more than a few minutes at a time, act impulsively, and have difficulty paying attention. These behaviours interfere with social development and academic progress. The cause of hyperactivity remains unknown, but it affects about 5 to 10 percent of young school-age children.[68] To resolve the problems surrounding hyperactivity, physicians often recommend specific behavioural strategies, special educational programs, and psychological counselling. In many cases, they prescribe medication.[69]

Researchers have debated whether hyperactivity is due to a brain deficit or to a delay in brain development. Recent research supports the view that some areas in the brains of children with hyperactivity develop more slowly than those of other children.[70] Such findings remain controversial, but further support comes from the fact that hyperactivity symptoms tend to improve as children get older.

Parents of hyperactive children often blame sugar as the cause. They mistakenly believe that simply eliminating candy and other sweet treats will solve the problem. This dietary change will not solve the problem, however, and studies have consistently found no convincing evidence that sugar causes hyperactivity or worsens behaviour. Such speculation has been based on personal stories. No scientific evidence supports a relationship between sugar and hyperactivity or other misbehaviours.

Food additives have also been blamed for hyperactivity and other behaviour problems in children, but scientific evidence to substantiate the connection has been elusive—until recently. A well-controlled study of close to 300 children suggests that food additives such as artificial colours or sodium benzoate preservative (or both) exacerbate hyperactive symptoms such as inattention and impulsivity.[71] Additional studies are needed to confirm the findings and to determine which additives studied might be responsible for negative behaviours.

Misbehaving Even a child who is not truly hyperactive can be difficult to manage at times. Michael may act unruly out of a desire for attention, Jessica may be cranky because of a lack of sleep, Christopher may react violently after watching too much television, and Sheila may be unable to sit still in class due to a lack of exercise. All of these children may benefit from more consistent care—regular hours of sleep, regular mealtimes, and regular outdoor activity.

Food Allergy and Intolerance

Food allergy is frequently blamed for physical and behavioural abnormalities in children, but just 6 to 8 percent of children younger than 4 years of age are diagnosed with true food allergies.[72] Food allergies diminish with age, until in adulthood they affect less than 4 percent of the population.[73] The prevalence of food allergy, especially peanut allergy, is on the rise, however.[74] Reasons for an increase in peanut allergy are not yet clear, but possible contributing factors include genetics, food preparation methods (roasting peanuts at very high temperatures makes them more allergenic), and exposure to medicinal skin creams containing peanut oil.[75]

A true food allergy occurs when fractions of a food protein or other large molecule are absorbed into the blood and elicit an immunologic response. (Recall that proteins are normally dismantled in the digestive tract to amino acids that are absorbed without such a reaction.) The body's immune system reacts to these large food molecules as it does to other antigens—by producing antibodies, histamines, or other defensive agents.

Detecting Food Allergy Allergies may have one or two components. They always involve antibodies, but they may or may not involve symptoms. ♦ This

♦ A person who produces antibodies *without* having any symptoms has an **asymptomatic allergy;** a person who produces antibodies *and* has symptoms has a **symptomatic allergy.**

hyperactivity: inattentive and impulsive behaviour that is more frequent and severe than is typical of others a similar age; professionally called *attention-deficit/hyperactivity disorder (ADHD).*

food allergy: an adverse reaction to food that involves an immune response; also called *food-hypersensitivity reaction.*

HOW TO Protect against Lead Toxicity

Researchers simultaneously made three major discoveries about lead toxicity: lead poisoning has *subtle* effects, the effects are *permanent,* and they occur at *low levels of exposure.* The amount of lead recognized to cause harm is only 10 micrograms per 100 millilitres of blood. Some research shows that blood lead concentrations *below* this amount may adversely affect children's physical and mental development.[a] Consequently, consumers should take ultraconservative measures to protect themselves, and especially their infants and young children, from lead poisoning. The American Academy of Pediatrics and the Centers for Disease Control recommend screening in communities with a substantial number of houses built before 1950 and in those with a substantial number of children with elevated lead levels. In addition to screening children most likely to be exposed, pediatricians should alert all parents to the possible dangers of lead exposure and explain prevention strategies.

Preventive strategies include:

- In contaminated environments, keep small children from putting dirty or old painted objects in their mouths, and make sure children wash their hands before eating. Similarly, keep small children from eating any nonfood items. Lead poisoning has been reported in young children who have eaten crayons or pool cue chalk.
- Wet-mop floors and damp-sponge walls regularly. Children's blood lead levels decline when the homes they live in are cleaned regularly.
- Be aware that other countries do not have the same regulations protecting consumers against lead. Children have been poisoned by eating crayons made in China and drinking fruit juice canned in Mexico.
- Do not use lead-contaminated water to make infant formula.
- Once you have opened canned food, store it in a lead-free container to prevent lead migration into the food.
- Do not store acidic foods or beverages (such as vinegar or orange juice) in ceramic dishware or alcoholic beverages in pewter or crystal decanters.
- Many manufacturers are now making lead-safe products. Old, handmade, or imported ceramic cups and bowls may contain lead and should not be used to heat coffee or tea or acidic foods such as tomato soup.
- Feed children nutritious meals regularly.
- Before using your newspaper to wrap food, mulch garden plants, or add to your compost, confirm with the publisher that the paper uses no lead in its ink.

The Environmental Protection Agency (EPA) also publishes a booklet, *Lead and Your Drinking Water,* in which the following cautions appear:

- Have the water in your home tested by a competent laboratory.
- Use only cold water for drinking, cooking, and making formula (cold water absorbs less lead).
- When water has been standing in pipes for more than two hours, flush the cold-water pipes by running water through them for 30 seconds before using it for drinking, cooking, or mixing formulas.
- If lead contamination of your water supply seems probable, obtain additional information and advice from the EPA and your local public health agency.

By taking these steps, parents can protect themselves and their children from this preventable danger.[b]

CENGAGENOW™
For additional practice log on to **www.cengage.com/sso.**

TRY IT Visit the website for the U.S. Environmental Protection Agency (www.epa.gov/lead) and identify the most common sources of lead poisoning.

[a]Centers for Disease Control and Prevention, Interpreting and managing blood lead levels <10μg/dL in children and reducing childhood exposures to lead: Recommendations of CDC's Advisory Committee on Childhood Lead Poisoning Prevention, *Morbidity and Mortality Weekly Report* 56/RR-8 (2007): 1–16; Policy of Committee on Environmental Health, American Academy of Pediatrics: Lead exposure in children: Prevention, detection, and management, *Pediatrics* 116 (2005): 1036–1046.

[b]If you have concerns about lead in your drinking water contact your local Health Unit and visit Health Canada's Lead and Human Health website: www.hc-sc.gc.ca/hl-vs/iyh-vsv/environ/lead-plomb-eng.php, or call the U.S. National Lead Information Center hotline at (800) 424-LEAD (424-5323) for general information.

means that allergies can be diagnosed only by testing for antibodies. Even symptoms exactly like those of an allergy may not be caused by an allergy. Once a food allergy has been diagnosed, the required treatment is strict elimination of the offending food. Children with allergies, like all children, need all their nutrients, so it is important to include other foods that offer the same nutrients as the omitted foods.[76]

Allergic reactions to food may be immediate or delayed. In either case, the antigen interacts immediately with the immune system, but the timing of symptoms varies from minutes to 24 hours after consumption of the antigen. Identifying the food that causes an immediate allergic reaction is fairly easy because the symptoms appear shortly after the food is eaten. Identifying the food that causes a delayed reaction is more difficult because the symptoms may not appear until much later. By this time, many other foods may have been eaten, complicating the picture.

Anaphylactic Shock The life-threatening food allergy reaction of **anaphylactic shock** is most often caused by peanuts, tree nuts, milk, eggs, wheat, soybeans,

anaphylactic (ana-fill-LAC-tic) **shock:** a life-threatening, whole-body allergic reaction to an offending substance.

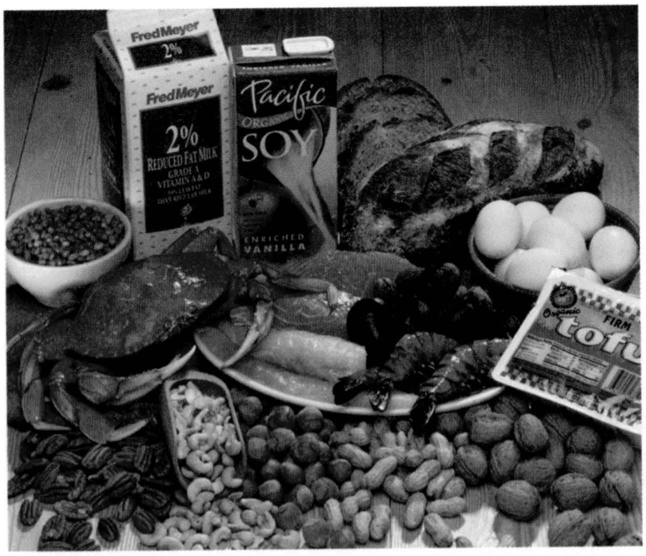
Fred Meyer
2%
REDUCED FAT MILK
Pacific
SOY
ENRICHED
VANILLA
tofu
© Polara Studios, Inc.

These normally wholesome foods may cause life-threatening symptoms in people with allergies.

fish, or shellfish. Among these foods, eggs, milk, soy, and peanuts most often cause problems in children.[77] Children are more likely to outgrow allergies to eggs, milk, and soy than allergies to peanuts. Peanuts cause more life-threatening reactions than do all other food allergies combined. Research is currently under way to help people with peanut allergies tolerate small doses, thus saving lives and minimizing reactions.[78] One possible solution depends on finding a natural, hypoallergenic peanut among the 14 000 varieties of peanuts. Families of children with a life-threatening food allergy and the school personnel who supervise those children must guard them against any exposure to the allergen. The child must learn to identify which foods pose a problem and then learn and use refusal skills for all foods that may contain the allergen.

Parents of children with allergies can pack safe foods for lunches and snacks and ask school officials to strictly enforce a "no swapping" policy in the lunchroom. The child must be able to recognize the symptoms of impending anaphylactic shock, ♦ such as a tingling of the tongue, throat, or skin, or difficulty breathing. Any person with food allergies severe enough to cause anaphylactic shock should wear a medical alert bracelet or necklace. Finally, the responsible child and the school staff should be prepared with injections of epinephrine, ♦ which prevents anaphylaxis after exposure to the allergen. Many preventable deaths occur each year when people with food allergies accidentally ingest the allergen but have no epinephrine available.

♦ Symptoms of impending anaphylactic shock:
- Tingling sensation in mouth
- Swelling of the tongue and throat
- Irritated, reddened eyes
- Difficulty breathing, asthma
- Hives, swelling, rashes
- Vomiting, abdominal cramps, diarrhea
- Drop in blood pressure
- Loss of consciousness
- Death

♦ **Epinephrine** is a hormone of the adrenal gland that modulates the stress response; formerly called *adrenaline*. When administered by injection, epinephrine counteracts anaphylactic shock by opening the airways and maintaining heartbeat and blood pressure.

Food Labelling Food labels must list the presence of common allergens in plain language, using the names of the nine most common/priority allergy-causing foods.[79] For example, a food containing "textured vegetable protein" must say "soy" on its label. Similarly, "casein" must be identified as "milk," and so forth. Food producers must also prevent cross-contamination during production and clearly label foods in which it is likely to occur. For example, equipment used for making peanut butter must be scrupulously clean before being used to pulverize cashew nuts for cashew butter to protect unsuspecting cashew butter consumers from peanut allergens.

Technology may soon offer new solutions. New drugs are being developed that may interfere with the immune response that causes allergic reactions.[80] Also, through genetic engineering, scientists may one day create allergen-free peanuts, soybeans, and other foods to make them safer.

Food Intolerances Not all **adverse reactions** to foods are food allergies, although even physicians may describe them as such. Signs of adverse reactions to foods include stomachaches, headaches, rapid pulse rate, nausea, wheezing, hives, bronchial irritation, coughs, and other such discomforts. Among the causes may be reactions to chemicals in foods, such as the flavour enhancer monosodium glutamate (MSG), the natural laxative in prunes, or the mineral sulphur; digestive diseases, obstructions, or injuries; enzyme deficiencies, such as lactose intolerance; and even psychological aversions. These reactions involve symptoms but no antibody production. Therefore, they are **food intolerances**, not allergies.

Pesticides on produce may also cause adverse reactions. Pesticides that were applied in the fields may linger on the foods. Health risks from pesticide exposure may be low for healthy adults, but children are vulnerable. Therefore, government agencies have set a **tolerance level** for each pesticide by first identifying foods that children commonly eat in large amounts and then considering the effects of pesticide exposure during each developmental stage. Chapter 20 revisits the issues surrounding the use of pesticides on food crops.

adverse reactions: unusual responses to food (including intolerances and allergies).

food intolerances: adverse reactions to foods that do not involve the immune system.

tolerance level: the maximum amount of residue permitted in a food when a pesticide is used according to the label directions.

Hunger, lead poisoning, hyperactivity, and allergic reactions can all adversely affect a child's nutrition status and health. Fortunately, each of these problems has solutions. They may not be easy solutions, but at least we have a reasonably good understanding of the problems and ways to correct them. Such is not the case with the most pervasive health problem for children in North America—obesity.

Childhood Obesity The number of overweight children has increased dramatically over the past three decades (see Figure 17-8). Like their parents, children in Canada are becoming fatter. An estimated 18 percent of Canadian children and adolescents 2 to 17 years of age are overweight and 7 percent are obese.[81] Based on data from the BMI-for-age growth charts, children and adolescents are categorized as *overweight* above the 85th percentile and as *obese* at the 95th percentile and above.[82] There are exceptions to the use of the 85th and 95th percentile cutoff points. For older adolescents, a BMI at the 95th percentile is higher than a BMI of 30, the adult obesity cutoff point. Therefore, obesity is defined as a BMI at the 95th percentile or a BMI of 30 or greater, whichever is lower. For children younger than 2 years of age, BMI values are not available. For this age group, weight-for-height values above the 95th percentile are classified as overweight. Figure 17-9 (p. 564) presents the BMI for children and adolescents, indicating cutoff points for obesity and overweight.

The Expert Committee of the American Medical Association recommends a third cutoff point (99th percentile) to define severe obesity in childhood.[83] Unfortunately, severe obesity in children is becoming more prevalent. Many of these children have multiple risk factors for cardiovascular disease and a high risk of severe obesity in adulthood.[84] The special risks and treatment needs of severely obese children need to be recognized.

The problem of obesity in children is especially troubling because overweight children have the potential of becoming obese adults with all the social, economic, and medical ramifications that often accompany obesity. They have additional problems, too, arising from differences in their growth, physical health, and psychological development. In trying to explain the rise in childhood obesity, researchers point to both genetic and environmental factors.

FIGURE 17-8 Trends in Childhood Obesity

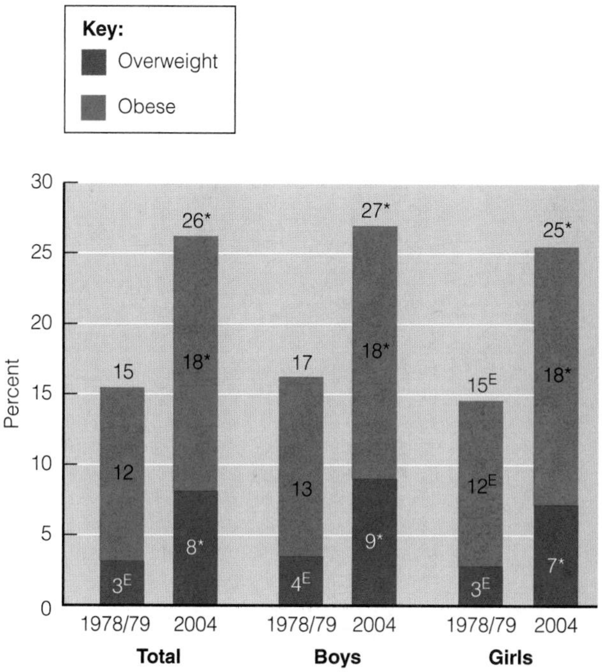
Key:
Overweight
Obese
Percent
30
25
20
15
10
5
0
15
12
3E
26*
18*
8*
17
13
4E
27*
18*
9*
15E
12E
3E
25*
18*
7*
1978/79
2004
1978/79
2004
1978/79
2004
Total
Boys
Girls

SOURCE: M Tjepkema, M Shields. Measured Obesity: Overweight Canadian Children and Adolescents. Canadian Community Health Survey: Obesity among Children and Adults. Statistics Canada - Cat. No. 82-620-MWE (2004).

*Significantly different from 1978/79 ($p < 0.05$)

E Data are highly variable, interpret with caution

Genetic and Environmental Factors Parental obesity predicts an early increase in a young child's BMI, and it more than doubles the chances that a young child will become an obese adult. Children with neither parent obese have a less than 10 percent chance of becoming obese in adulthood, whereas overweight teens with at least one obese parent have a greater than 80 percent chance of being obese adults. The chances of an obese child becoming an obese adult grow greater as the child grows older.[85] The link between parental and child obesity reflects both genetic and environmental factors (as described in Chapter 9).

Diet and physical inactivity must also play a role in explaining why children are heavier today than they were 40 or so years ago. As the prevalence of childhood obesity throughout North America has more than doubled for young children and more than tripled for children 6 to 11 years of age and adolescents, the society our children live in has changed considerably.[86] In many families today, both parents work outside the home and work longer hours; more emphasis is placed on convenience foods and foods eaten away from home; meal choices at school are more diverse and often less nutritious; sedentary activities such as watching television and playing video or computer games occupy much of children's free time; and opportunities for physical activity and outdoor play both during and after school have declined.[87] All of these factors—and many others—influence children's eating and activity patterns.

Children learn food behaviours from their families, and research confirms the significant roles parents play in teaching their children about healthy food choices, providing nutrient-dense foods, and serving as role models.[88] When parents eat fruits and vegetables frequently, their children do, too.[89] The more fruits and vegetables children eat, the more vitamins, minerals, and fibres, and the less saturated fat in their diets.[90]

Research shows that one in four toddlers (19 to 24 months of age) exceeds estimated energy requirements as a result of eating such foods as candy, pizza, chicken nuggets, soft drinks, sweet tea, and salty snacks such as cheese puffs and

FIGURE 17-9 Body Mass Index-for-Age Percentiles: Boys and Girls, Age 2 to 19

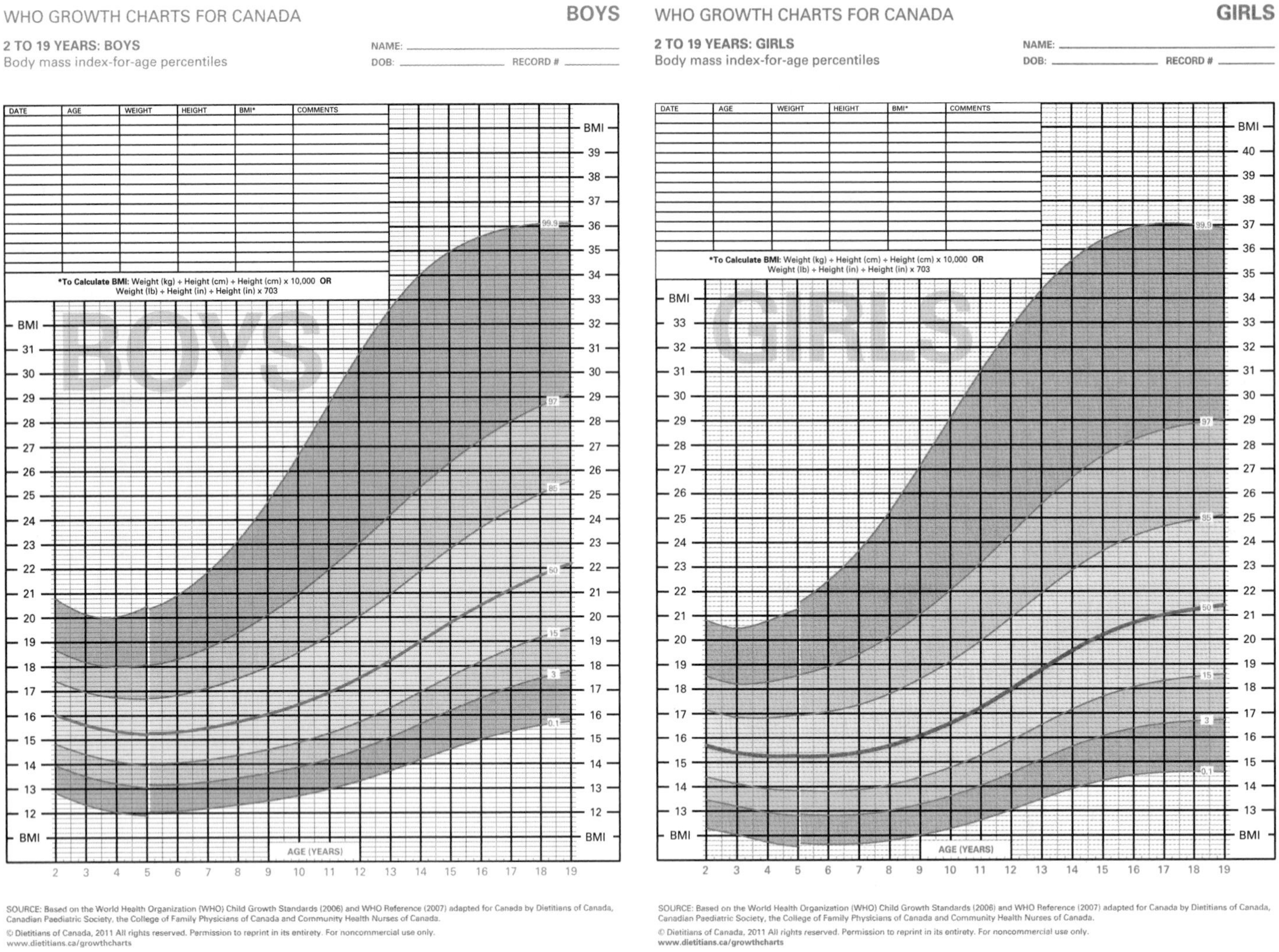
WHO GROWTH CHARTS FOR CANADA
BOYS
2 TO 19 YEARS: BOYS
Body mass index-for-age percentiles
NAME:
DOB:
RECORD #
DATE
AGE
WEIGHT
HEIGHT
BMI*
COMMENTS
*To Calculate BMI: Weight (kg) ÷ Height (cm) ÷ Height (cm) x 10,000 OR Weight (lb) ÷ Height (in) ÷ Height (in) x 703
BMI
AGE (YEARS)
WHO GROWTH CHARTS FOR CANADA
GIRLS
2 TO 19 YEARS: GIRLS
Body mass index-for-age percentiles

SOURCE: © Dietitians of Canada, 2011 All rights reserved. Permission to reprint in its entirety. For noncommercial use only.

chips.[91] Not surprisingly, when researchers ask, "Are today's children eating more kcalories than those of 40 years ago?" the answer is, "Yes."

As Highlight 4 discusses, as the prevalence of obesity among both children and adults has surged over the past four decades, so has the consumption of added sugars and, especially, high-fructose corn syrup—the easily consumed, energy-dense liquid sugar added to soft drinks.[92] Each 355 millilitre (12-ounce) can of soft drink provides the equivalent of about 50 millilitres (10 teaspoons) of sugar and 150 kcalories. More than half of U.S. school-age children consume at least one soft drink each day at school; adolescent males consume the most—four or more cans daily.[93] Research shows that soft drink consumption is associated with increased energy intake and body weight.[94] According to one estimate, the risk of obesity increases by 60 percent with each sugared soft drink consumed daily.

No doubt, the tremendous increase in soft drink consumption plays a role, but much of the obesity epidemic can be explained by lack of physical activity. Children have become more sedentary, and sedentary children are more often overweight.[95] Television watching and playing video games ♦ may contribute most to physical inactivity. Longer television time is linked with overweight in children.[96] A child who spends more than an hour or two each day in front of a television, computer monitor, or other media can become overweight even while eating fewer kcalories than a more active child. Too much screen time and not enough activity time also contributes to a child's psychological distress.[97]

♦ TV fosters obesity because it:
- Requires no energy beyond basal metabolism
- Replaces vigorous activities
- Encourages snacking
- Promotes a sedentary lifestyle

Playing video games influences children's activity patterns similarly.

Children who have television sets in their bedrooms spend more time watching TV, are less physically active, and are more likely to be overweight than children who do not have televisions in their rooms.[98] Watching television influences food intake as well as physical activity.[99] Children who watch a great deal of television are most likely to be overweight and least likely to eat family meals or fruits and vegetables.[100] They often snack on the nutrient-poor, energy-dense foods that are advertised.[101] The average child in North America sees an estimated 40 000 TV commercials a year—many peddling foods high in sugar, saturated fat, and salt such as sugar-coated breakfast cereals, chocolate bars, chips, fast foods, and carbonated beverages.[102] More than half of all food advertisements are aimed specifically at children and market their products as fun and exciting.[103] Not surprisingly, the more time children spend watching television, the more they request these advertised foods and beverages—and they get their requests about half of the time.[104] The most popular foods and beverages are marketed to children and adolescents on the Internet as well, using "advergaming" (advertised product as part of a game), cartoon characters or "spokes-characters," and designated children's areas.[105]

The physically inactive time spent watching television is second only to time spent sleeping. Children also spend more time playing video games. These activities use no more energy than resting, displace participation in more vigorous activities, and foster snacking on high-fat foods.[106] Simply reducing the amount of time spent watching television (and playing video games) can improve a child's BMI. The Canadian Paediatric Society (CPS) and the Canadian Sedentary Behaviour Guidelines for "recreational screen time" for children (5–11 years old) and youth (12–17 years old) released in 2011 by the Canadian Society for Exercise Physiology recommend limiting television and video time to two hours per day as a strategy to help prevent childhood obesity.[107]

Growth Overweight children develop a characteristic set of physical traits. They typically begin puberty earlier and so grow taller than their peers at first, but then they stop growing at a shorter height. They develop greater bone and muscle mass in response to the demand of having to carry more weight—both fat and lean weight. Consequently, they appear "stocky" even when they lose their excess fat.

Physical Health Like overweight adults, overweight children display a blood lipid profile indicating that atherosclerosis is beginning to develop—high levels of total cholesterol, triglycerides, and LDL cholesterol. Overweight children also tend to have high blood pressure; in fact, obesity is a leading cause of pediatric hypertension.[108] Their risks for developing type 2 diabetes and respiratory diseases (such as asthma) are also exceptionally high.[109] These relationships between childhood obesity and chronic diseases are discussed fully in Highlight 17.

Psychological Development In addition to the physical consequences, childhood obesity brings a host of emotional and social problems.[110] Because people frequently judge others on appearance more than on character, overweight children are often victims of prejudice. Many suffer discrimination by adults and rejection by their peers. They may have poor self-images, a sense of failure, and a passive approach to life. Television shows, which are a major influence in children's lives, often portray the fat person as the bumbling misfit.[111] Overweight children may come to accept this negative stereotype in themselves and in others, which can lead to additional emotional and social problems. Researchers investigating children's reactions to various body types find that both normal-weight and underweight children respond unfavourably to overweight bodies.

Prevention and Treatment of Obesity Medical science has worked wonders in preventing or curing many of even the most serious childhood diseases, but obesity remains a challenge.[112] Once excess fat has been stored, it is difficult to lose. In light of all this, parents are encouraged to make major efforts to prevent childhood obesity, starting at birth, or to begin treatment early—before adolescence.[113] The Expert Committee of the American Medical Association recommends specific eating and physical activity behaviours to prevent obesity, for all children (see Table 17-7 on page 566).

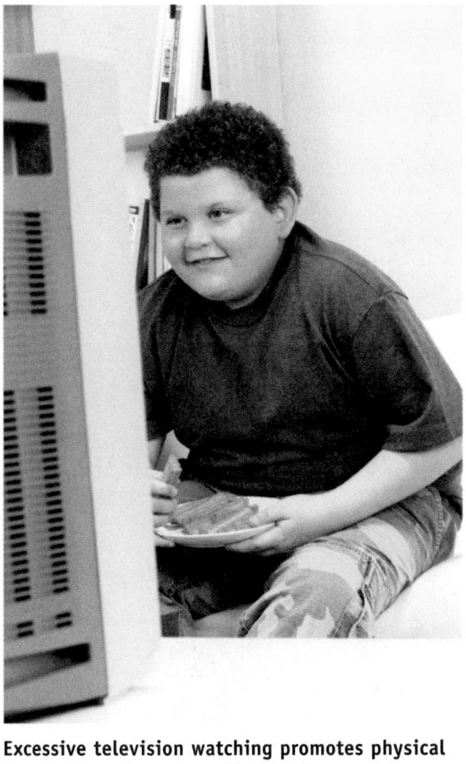

Excessive television watching promotes physical inactivity and poor snacking habits.

TABLE 17-7 Recommended Eating and Physical Activity Behaviours to Prevent Obesity

The Expert Committee of the American Medical Association recommends the following healthy habits for children 2 to 18 years of age to help prevent childhood obesity:

- Limit consumption of sugar-sweetened beverages, such as soft drinks and fruit flavoured punches.
- Eat the recommended amounts of fruits and vegetables every day (500 to 1125 mL/2 to 4.5 cups per day based on age).
- Learn to eat age-appropriate portions of foods.
- Eat foods low in energy density such as those high in fibre and/or water and modest in fat.
- Eat a nutritious breakfast every day.
- Eat a diet rich in calcium.
- Eat a diet balanced in recommended proportions for carbohydrate, fat, and protein.
- Eat a diet high in fibre.
- Eat together as a family as often as possible.
- Limit the frequency of restaurant meals.
- Limit television watching or other screen time to no more than 2 hours per day and do not have televisions or computers in bedrooms.
- Engage in at least 60 minutes of moderate to vigorous physical activity every day.

SOURCES: D. C. W. Lau and co-authors, 2006 Canadian clinical practice guidelines on the management and prevention of obesity in adults and children. http://www.cmaj.ca/content/176/8/S1.full; Canadian Paediatric Society, Healthy active living for children and youth. http://www.cps.ca/english/statements/HAL/HAL02-01.htm; Canadian Society for Exercise Physiology (CSEP), 2011 Canadian Physical Activity and Sedentary Behaviour Guidelines. http://www.csep.ca/english/view.asp?x=804; S. E. Barlow, Expert Committee recommendations regarding the prevention, assessment, and treatment of child and adolescent overweight and obesity: Summary report, *Pediatrics* 120 (2007): S164–S192.

Treatment of obesity must consider the many aspects of the problem and possible solutions. The main goal of obesity treatment is to improve long-term physical health through permanent healthy lifestyle habits.[114] The most successful approach integrates diet, physical activity, psychological support, and behavioural changes.[115] As a first step, the Expert Committee recommends that overweight and obese children and their families adopt the same healthy eating and activity behaviours presented in Table 17-7 for obesity prevention. The goal for overweight and obese children is to improve BMI. If the child's BMI does not improve after several months, the Expert Committee recommends increasing the intensity of the treatment. The level of intensity depends on treatment response, age, degree of obesity, health risks, and the family's readiness to change. Advanced treatment involves close follow-up monitoring by a health-care provider and greater support and structure for the child.[116]

Diet The initial goal for overweight children is to reduce the rate of weight gain; that is, to maintain weight as the child grows taller. Continued growth will then accomplish the desired change in BMI. Weight loss is usually not recommended because diet restriction can interfere with growth and development. Intervention for some overweight children with accompanying medical conditions may warrant weight loss, but this treatment requires an individualized approach based on the degree of overweight and severity of the medical conditions.[117] Dietary strategies begin with those listed in Table 17-7 and progress to more structured family meal plans when necessary. For example, the child or the parent may be instructed to keep detailed records of dietary intake and physical activity.

Dietary Guidance for Canadians

Help overweight children reduce the rate of body weight gain while allowing growth and development. Consult a health-care provider and the Canadian Clinical Practice Guidelines on the Prevention and Management of Obesity in Adults and Children[118] before placing a child on a weight-reduction diet.

Physical Activity The many benefits of physical activity are well known but often are not enough to motivate overweight people, especially children. Yet regular vigorous activity can improve a child's weight, body composition, and physical fitness.[119] Ideally, parents will limit sedentary activities and encourage at least one hour of daily physical activity to promote strong skeletal, muscular, and cardiovascular development and instill in their children the desire to be physically active

FIGURE 17-10 ***Canadian Physical Activity Guidelines***

Canadian Physical Activity Guidelines

FOR CHILDREN - 5–11 YEARS

Guidelines

For health benefits, children aged 5-11 years should accumulate at least 60 minutes of moderate- to vigorous-intensity physical activity daily. This should include:

Vigorous-intensity activities at least 3 days per week.

Activities that strengthen muscle and bone at least 3 days per week.

More daily physical activity provides greater health benefits.

Let's Talk Intensity!

Moderate-intensity physical activities will cause children to sweat a little and to breathe harder. Activities like:

- Bike riding
- Playground activities

Vigorous-intensity physical activities will cause children to sweat and be 'out of breath'. Activities like:

- Running
- Swimming

Being active for at least **60 minutes** daily can help children:

- Improve their health
- Do better in school
- Improve their fitness
- Grow stronger
- Have fun playing with friends
- Feel happier
- Maintain a healthy body weight
- Improve their self-confidence
- Learn new skills

Parents and caregivers can help to plan their child's daily activity. Kids can:

☑ Play tag – or freeze-tag!
☑ Go to the playground after school.
☑ Walk, bike, rollerblade or skateboard to school.
☑ Play an active game at recess.
☑ Go sledding in the park on the weekend.
☑ Go "puddle hopping" on a rainy day.

60 minutes a day. You can help your child get there!

PARTICIPACTION

CSEP | SCPE
THE GOLD STANDARD IN EXERCISE SCIENCE AND PERSONAL TRAINING
www.csep.ca/guidelines

Canadian Physical Activity Guidelines

FOR YOUTH - 12–17 YEARS

Guidelines

For health benefits, youth aged 12-17 years should accumulate at least 60 minutes of moderate- to vigorous-intensity physical activity daily. This should include:

Vigorous-intensity activities at least 3 days per week.

Activities that strengthen muscle and bone at least 3 days per week.

More daily physical activity provides greater health benefits.

Let's Talk Intensity!

Moderate-intensity physical activities will cause teens to sweat a little and to breathe harder. Activities like:

- Skating
- Bike riding

Vigorous-intensity physical activities will cause teens to sweat and be 'out of breath'. Activities like:

- Running
- Rollerblading

Being active for at least **60 minutes** daily can help teens:

- Improve their health
- Do better in school
- Improve their fitness
- Grow stronger
- Have fun playing with friends
- Feel happier
- Maintain a healthy body weight
- Improve their self-confidence
- Learn new skills

Parents and caregivers can help to plan their teen's daily activity. Teens can:

☑ Walk, bike, rollerblade or skateboard to school.
☑ Go to a gym on the weekend.
☑ Do a fitness class after school.
☑ Get the neighbours together for a game of pick-up basketball, or hockey after dinner.
☑ Play a sport such as basketball, hockey, soccer, martial arts, swimming, tennis, golf, skiing, snowboarding…

Now is the time. 60 minutes a day can make a difference.

PARTICIPACTION

CSEP | SCPE
THE GOLD STANDARD IN EXERCISE SCIENCE AND PERSONAL TRAINING
www.csep.ca/guidelines

SOURCE: Canadian Physical Activity Guidelines, © 2011. Used with permission from the Canadian Society for Exercise Physiology, www.csep.ca/guidelines.

throughout life. Opportunities to be physically active can include team, individual, and recreational activities (see Figure 17-10). Most importantly, parents need to set a good example, especially since parents as well as children are spending many hours a week engaged in screen-viewing activities.[120] Physical activity is a natural and lifelong behaviour of healthy living. It can be as simple as riding a bike, playing tag, jumping rope, or doing chores. The AAP supports the efforts of schools to include more physical activity in the curriculum and encourages parents to support their children's participation.[121]

Psychological Support Weight-loss programs that involve parents and other caregivers in treatment report greater success than those without parental involvement. Because obesity in parents and their children tends to be positively correlated, both benefit when parents participate in a weight-loss program. Parental attitudes about food greatly influence children's eating behaviour, so it is important that the influence be positive. Otherwise, eating problems may become exacerbated.

Behavioural Changes In contrast to traditional weight-loss programs that focus on *what* to eat, behavioural programs focus on *how* to eat. These techniques involve changing learned habits that lead a child to eat excessively.

Drugs The use of weight-loss drugs to treat obesity in children merits special concern because the long-term effects of these drugs on growth and development have not been studied.[122] The drugs may be used in addition to structured lifestyle changes for carefully selected children or adolescents who are at high risk for severe obesity in adulthood. One anti-obesity drug that is available for use in adults is Xenical (Orlistat); it has also recently been tested in adolescents.

♦ Surgery may be an option for adolescents who meet the following criteria:

- Have reached physical maturity
- BMI ≥50 or BMI ≥40 with significant weight-related health problems
- Have experienced failure in a formal, six-month weight-loss program
- Are capable of adhering to the long-term lifestyle changes required after surgery

Surgery The use of surgery to treat severe obesity in adults (see Chapter 9) has created interest in its use for adolescents. Limited research shows that after surgery extremely obese adolescents lose significant weight and experience improvements in type 2 diabetes and cardiovascular risk factors.[123] The selection criteria for surgery to treat obesity in adolescents ♦ are based on recommendations of a panel of pediatricians and surgeons.[124]

Obesity is prevalent in our society. Because treatment of obesity is frequently unsuccessful, it is most important to prevent its onset. Above all, be sensible in teaching children how to maintain appropriate body weight. Children can easily get the impression that their worth is tied to their body weight. Parents and the media are most influential in shaping self-concept, weight concerns, and dieting practices.[125] Some parents fail to realize that society's ideal of slimness can be perilously close to starvation and that a child encouraged to "diet" cannot obtain the energy and nutrients required for normal growth and development. Even healthy children without diagnosable eating disorders have been observed to limit their growth through "dieting." Weight loss in truly overweight children can be managed without compromising growth, but it should be overseen by a health-care professional.

Mealtimes at Home

Traditionally, parents served as **gatekeepers**, determining what foods and activities were available in their children's lives. Then the children made their own selections. Gatekeepers who wanted to promote nutritious choices and healthful habits provided access to nutrient-dense, delicious foods and opportunities for active play at home.

In today's consumer-oriented society, children have greater influence over family decisions concerning food—the fast-food restaurant the family chooses when eating out, the type of food the family eats at home, and the specific brands the family purchases at the grocery store. Parental guidance in food choices is still necessary, but teaching children consumer skills to help them make informed choices is equally important.

Honouring Children's Preferences Researchers attempting to explain children's food preferences encounter contradictions. Children say they like colourful foods, yet they most often reject green and yellow vegetables in favour of brown peanut butter and white potatoes, apple wedges, and bread. They seem to like raw vegetables better than cooked ones, so it is wise to offer vegetables that are raw or slightly undercooked, served separately, and easy to eat. Foods should be warm, not hot, because a child's mouth is much more sensitive than an adult's. The flavour should be mild because a child has more taste buds, and smooth foods such as mashed potatoes or split-pea soup should contain no lumps (a child wonders, with some disgust, what the lumps might be).

Make mealtimes fun for children. Young children like to eat at little tables and to be served small portions of food. They like sandwiches cut in different geometric shapes and common foods called silly names. They also like to eat with other children, and they tend to eat more when in the company of their friends. Children are also more likely to give up their prejudices against foods when they see their peers eating them.

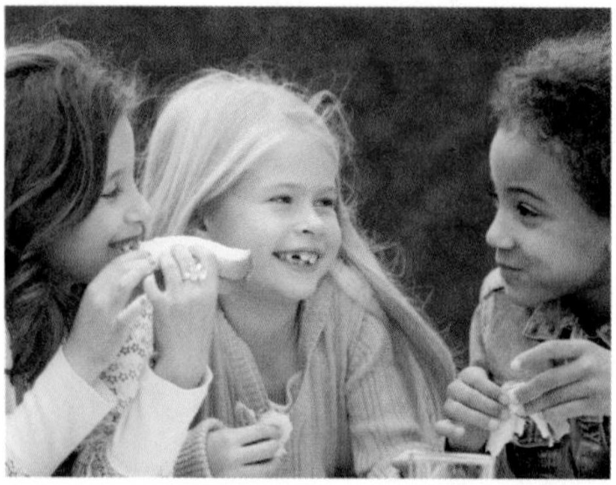
JGI/Getty Images

Eating is more fun for children when friends are there.

Learning through Participation Allowing children to help plan and prepare the family's meals provides enjoyable learning experiences and encourages children to eat the foods they have prepared. Vegetables are pretty, especially when fresh, and provide opportunities for children to learn about colour, seeds, growing vegetables, and shapes and textures—all of which are fascinating to young children. Measuring, stirring, washing, and arranging foods are skills that even a young child can practise with enjoyment and pride (see Table 17-8).

Avoiding Power Struggles Problems over food often arise during the second or third year, when children begin asserting their independence. Many of these problems stem from the conflict between children's developmental stages and capabilities and parents who, in attempting to do what they think is best for their

gatekeepers: with respect to nutrition, key people who control other people's access to foods and thereby exert profound impacts on their nutrition. Examples are the spouse who buys and cooks the food, the parent who feeds the children, and the caregiver in a day care centre.

children, try to control every aspect of eating. Such conflicts can disrupt children's abilities to regulate their own food intakes or to determine their own likes and dislikes. For example, many people share the misconception that children must be persuaded or coerced to try new foods. In fact, the opposite is true. When children are forced to try new foods, even by way of rewards, they are less likely to try those foods again than are children who are left to decide for themselves. Similarly, when children are restricted from eating their favourite foods, they are more likely to want those foods.[126] Wise parents provide healthful foods and allow their child to determine *how much* and even *whether* to eat.

When introducing new foods, offer them one at a time and only in small amounts such as one bite at first. The more often a food is presented to a young child, the more likely the child will accept that food.[127] Offer the new food at the beginning of the meal, when the child is hungry, and allow the child to make the decision to accept or reject it. Never make an issue of food acceptance.

Choking Prevention Parents must always be alert to the dangers of choking. A choking child is silent, so an adult should be present whenever a child is eating. Make sure the child sits when eating; choking is more likely when a child is running or falling. (See the margin list on p. 553 for foods and nonfood items most likely to cause choking.)

Playing First Children may be more relaxed and attentive during meals if outdoor play or other fun activities are scheduled before, rather than immediately after, mealtimes. Otherwise children "hurry up and eat" so that they can go play.

Snacking Parents may find that when their children snack, they aren't hungry at mealtimes. Instead of teaching children *not* to snack, parents are wise to teach them *how* to snack. Provide snacks that are as nutritious as the foods served at mealtime. Snacks can even be mealtime foods served individually over time, instead of all at once on one plate. When providing snacks to children, think of the four food groups and offer such snacks as pieces of cheese, tangerine slices, and egg salad on whole-wheat crackers (see Table 17-9, p. 570). Snacks that are easy to prepare should be readily available to children, especially if they arrive home from school before their parents.

To ensure that children have healthy appetites and plenty of room for nutritious foods when they are hungry, parents and teachers must limit access to candy, soft drinks, and other concentrated sweets. Limiting access includes limiting the amount of pocket money children have to buy such foods themselves. If these foods are permitted in large quantities, the only possible outcomes are nutrient deficiencies, obesity, or both. The preference for sweets is innate; most children do not naturally select nutritious foods on the basis of taste. When children are allowed to create meals freely from a variety of foods, they typically select foods that provide a lot of sugar. When their parents are watching, or even when they only think their parents are watching, children improve their selections.

Sweets need not be banned altogether. Children who are exceptionally active can enjoy high-kcalorie foods such as ice cream or pudding from the milk group or pancakes from the bread group. Sedentary children need to become more active so they can also enjoy some of these foods without unhealthy weight gain.

Preventing Dental Caries Children frequently snack on sticky, sugary foods that stay on the teeth and provide an ideal environment for the growth of bacteria that cause dental caries. Teach children to brush and floss after meals, to brush or rinse after eating snacks, to avoid sticky foods, and to select crisp or fibrous foods frequently.

Serving as Role Models In an effort to practise these many tips, parents may overlook perhaps the single most important influence on their children's food habits—themselves.[128] Parents who don't eat carrots shouldn't be surprised when their children refuse to eat carrots. Likewise, parents who comment negatively on the smell of Brussels sprouts may not be able to persuade children to try them. Children learn much through imitation. It is not surprising that children prefer

TABLE 17-8 Food Skills of Preschool Children[a]

Age 2 years, when large muscles develop:

- Uses a spoon
- Helps feed self
- Lifts and drinks from a cup
- Helps scrub fruits and vegetables, tear lettuce or greens, snap green beans, or dip foods
- Wipes table
- Places items in recycle bin or trash

Age 3 years, when medium hand muscles develop:

- Spears food with a fork
- Feeds self independently
- Adds ingredients to pancake batters, cookie recipes, salads, or other mixed dishes
- Helps wrap, pour, mix, shake, stir, or spread foods
- Helps crack nuts with supervision

Age 4 years, when small finger muscles develop:

- Uses all utensils and napkin
- Helps roll, juice, or mash foods
- Helps measure dry ingredients
- Cracks egg shells
- Helps make sandwiches and toss salads
- Peels foods such as hard-boiled eggs and bananas

Age 5 years, when fine coordination of fingers and hands develops:

- Measures liquids
- Helps grind, grate, and cut (soft foods with dull knife)
- Uses hand mixer with supervision

[a]These ages are approximate. Healthy, normal children develop at their own pace.

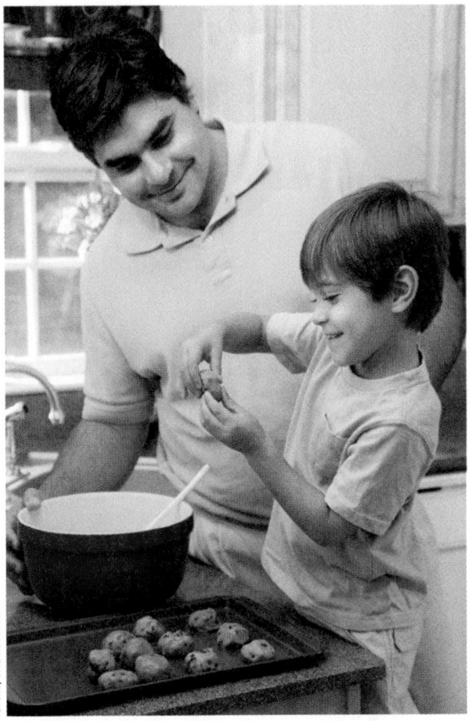

iofoto/shutterstock

Children enjoy eating the foods they help to prepare.

TABLE 17-9 Healthful Snack Ideas—Think Food Groups, Alone and in Combination

Selecting two or more foods from different food groups adds variety and nutrient balance to snacks. The combinations are endless, so be creative. Whenever possible, choose whole grains, 1% or 2% or milk products, and lean meats.
Grain Products
Grain products are filling snacks, especially when combined with other foods: • Cereal with fruit and milk • Crackers and cheese • Whole-grain toast with peanut butter • Popcorn with grated cheese • Oatmeal raisin cookies with milk
Vegetables and Fruit
Cut-up, fresh, raw vegetables make great snacks alone or in combination with foods from other food groups: • Celery with peanut butter • Broccoli, cauliflower, and carrot sticks with a flavoured cottage cheese dip Fruits are delicious snacks and can be eaten alone—fresh, dried, or juiced—or combined with other foods: • Apples and cheese • Bananas and peanut butter • Peaches with yogurt • Raisins mixed with sunflower seeds or nuts
Meat and Alternatives
Meats and legumes add protein to snacks: • Refried beans with nachos and cheese • Tuna on crackers • Luncheon meat on whole-grain bread
Milk and Alternatives
Milk can be used as a beverage with any snack, and many other milk products, such as yogurt and cheese, can be eaten alone or with other foods as listed above.

the foods other family members enjoy and dislike foods that are never offered to them.[129] Parents, older siblings, and other caregivers set an irresistible example by sitting with younger children, eating the same foods, and having pleasant conversations during mealtimes.

While serving and enjoying food, caregivers can promote both physical and emotional growth at every stage of a child's life. They can help their children develop both a positive self-concept and a positive attitude toward food. With good beginnings, children will grow without the conflicts and confusions about food that can lead to nutrition and health problems.

Nutrition at School

While parents are doing what they can to establish good eating habits in their children at home, others are preparing and serving foods to their children at daycare centres and schools. ♦ In addition, children begin to learn about food and nutrition in the classroom. Meeting the nutrition ♦ and education needs of children is critical to supporting their healthy growth and development.[130]

♦ For Breakfast for Learning Canada child nutrition programs, see www.breakfastforlearning.ca

♦ Breakfast for Learning's "Breakfast Program" provide foods from at least 3 of the 4 Food Groups described in the *Food Guide*, while a "Snack" must provide foods from at least 2 of the 4 Food Groups.[131]

Competing Influences at School Serving healthful lunches is only half the battle; students need to eat them, too. Short lunch periods and long waiting lines prevent some students from eating a school lunch and leave others with too little time to complete their meals.[132] Nutrition efforts at schools are also undermined when students can buy foods such as pizza or snack foods and carbonated beverages from snack bars, school stores, and vending machines.[133] In one study, students who selected competitive foods in addition to, or instead of, school meals consumed more energy and fat and less calcium and vitamin A than those who selected only the school lunch.[134]

Increasingly, school-based nutrition issues are being addressed by legislation. Some provinces restrict the sale of less nutritious "junk foods." In Ontario, for example, a new School Food and Beverage Policy came into effect September 1, 2011. According to the Ontario Ministry of Education website, "The nutrition standards embody the principles of healthy eating outlined in *Canada's Food Guide*."[135]

IN SUMMARY **Children's appetites and nutrient needs reflect their stage of growth. Those who are chronically hungry and malnourished suffer growth retardation; when hunger is temporary and nutrient deficiencies are mild, the problems are usually more subtle—such as poor academic performance. Iron deficiency is widespread and has many physical and behavioural consequences. "Hyper" behaviour is not caused by poor nutrition; misbehaviour may be due to lack of sleep, too little physical activity, or too much television, among other factors. Childhood obesity has become a major health problem. Adults at home and at school need to provide children with nutrient-dense foods and teach them how to make healthful diet and activity choices.**

Nutrition during Adolescence

Teenagers make many more choices for themselves than they did as children. They are not fed, they eat; they are not sent out to play, they choose to go. At the same time, social pressures thrust choices at them, such as whether to drink alcoholic beverages and whether to develop their bodies to meet extreme ideals of slimness or athletic prowess. Their interest in nutrition—both valid information and misinformation—derives from personal, immediate experiences. They are concerned with how diet can improve their lives now—they engage in fad dieting in order to fit into a new bathing suit, avoid greasy foods in an effort to clear acne, or eat a pile of spaghetti to prepare for a big sporting event. In presenting information on the nutrition and health of adolescents, this section includes many topics of interest to teens.

Growth and Development

With the onset of **adolescence**, the steady growth of childhood speeds up abruptly and dramatically, and the growth patterns of females and males become distinct. Hormones direct the intensity of the adolescent growth spurt, profoundly affecting every organ of the body, including the brain. After two to three years of intense growth and a few more at a slower pace, physically mature adults emerge.

In general, the adolescent growth spurt begins at age 10 or 11 for females and at 12 or 13 for males. It lasts about two and a half years. Before **puberty**, male and female body compositions differ only slightly, but during the adolescent spurt, differences between the genders become apparent in the skeletal system, lean body mass, and fat stores. In females, fat assumes a larger percentage of total body weight, and in males, the lean body mass—principally muscle and bone—increases much more than in females (review Figure 8-6 on p. 254). On average, males grow 20 centimetres (8 inches) taller, and females, 15 centimetres (6 inches) taller. Males gain approximately 20 kilograms (45 pounds), and females, about 16 kilograms (35 pounds).

Energy and Nutrient Needs

Energy and nutrient needs are greater during adolescence than at any other time of life, except pregnancy and lactation. In general, nutrient needs rise throughout childhood, peak in adolescence, and then level off or even diminish as the teen becomes an adult.

Energy Intake and Activity

The energy needs of adolescents vary greatly, depending on their current rate of growth, gender, body composition, and physical

adolescence: the period from the beginning of puberty until maturity.

puberty: the period in life in which a person becomes physically capable of reproduction.

activity.[136] Boys' energy needs may be especially high; they typically grow faster than girls and, as mentioned, develop a greater proportion of lean body mass. An exceptionally active boy of 15 may need 3500 kcalories or more a day just to maintain his weight. Girls start growing earlier than boys and attain shorter heights and lower weights, so their energy needs peak sooner and decline earlier than those of their male peers. A sedentary girl of 15 whose growth is nearly at a standstill may need fewer than 1800 kcalories a day if she is to avoid excessive weight gain. Thus adolescent girls need to pay special attention to being physically active and selecting foods of high nutrient density so as to meet their nutrient needs without exceeding their energy needs.

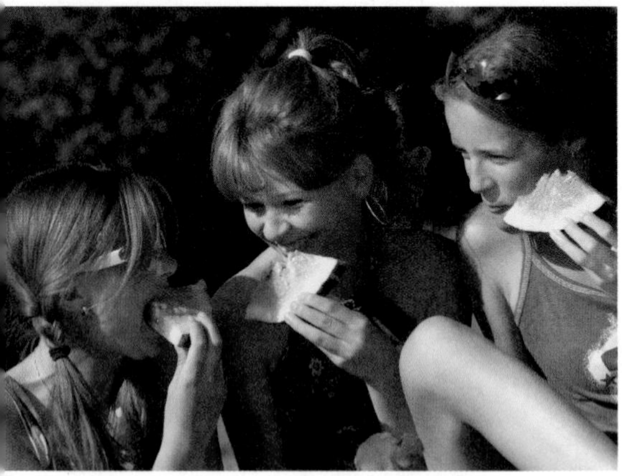
Mediaimages/Photodisc

Nutritious snacks contribute valuable nutrients and energy to an active teen's diet.

Physical Activity Guidance for Canadians

Adolescents should engage in at least 60 minutes of physical activity on most, preferably all, days of the week.

The insidious problem of obesity becomes ever more apparent in adolescence and often continues into adulthood. The problem is most evident in females of African descent and in Hispanic children of both genders. Without intervention, overweight adolescents face numerous physical and socioeconomic consequences for years to come. The consequences of obesity are so dramatic and our society's attitude toward obese people is so negative that even teens of normal or below-normal weight may perceive a need to lose weight. When taken to extremes, restrictive diets bring dramatic physical consequences of their own, as Highlight 8 explains.

Vitamins The RDA (or AI) for most vitamins increases during the adolescent years (see the table on the inside front cover). Several of the vitamin recommendations for adolescents are similar to those for adults, including the recommendations for vitamin D. Vitamin D is essential for bone growth and development. Although in the United States, as many as half of adolescents are vitamin D deficient,[137] this is not the case in Canada. Recent studies of vitamin D status in Canadian adolescents show that only about 5 percent of adolescents have vitamin D levels below 27.5 nmol/L, indicating deficiency.[138] Evidence that adequate vitamin D may help prevent diseases such as diabetes and cancer has led to revised recommendations.[139] The 2010 DRI report now recommends tripling the previous amount, from 5 micrograms per day to 15 micrograms per day. Adolescents who do not receive 15 micrograms of vitamin D from minimal sun exposure, vitamin D–fortified milk (2.5 micrograms per 250 millilitres) and vitamin D–or other fortified foods each day may be at risk for getting too little vitamin D.[140] Although drinking one litre of vitamin D–fortified milk will provide the recommended amount, the majority of adolescents in Canada drink much less than this.

Iron The need for iron increases during adolescence for both females and males, but for different reasons. Iron needs increase for females as they start to lose blood through menstruation and for males as their lean body mass develops. Hence, the RDA increases at age 14 for both males and females. For females, the RDA remains high into late adulthood. For males, the RDA returns to preadolescent values in early adulthood.

In addition, iron needs increase when the adolescent growth spurt begins, whether that occurs before or after age 14. Therefore, boys in a growth spurt need an additional 2.9 milligrams of iron per day above the RDA for their age; girls need an additional 1.1 milligrams per day.[141]

Furthermore, iron recommendations for girls before age 14 do not reflect the iron losses of menstruation. The average age of menarche (first menstruation) in North America is 12.5 years. Therefore, for girls younger than the age of 14 who have started to menstruate, an additional 2.5 milligrams of iron per day is recommended.[142] Thus the RDA for iron depends not only on age and gender but also on whether the individual is in a growth spurt or has begun to menstruate, as listed in the margin. ♦

♦ Iron RDA for males:
- 9–13 yr: 8 mg/day
- 9–13 yr in growth spurt: 10.9 mg/day
- 14–18 yr: 11 mg/day
- 14–18 yr in growth spurt: 13.9 mg/day

Iron RDA for females:
- 9–13 yr: 8 mg/day
- 9–13 yr in menarche: 10.5 mg/day
- 9–13 yr in menarche and growth spurt: 11.6 mg/day
- 14–18 yr: 15 mg/day
- 14–18 yr in growth spurt: 16.1 mg/day

Iron intakes often fail to keep pace with increasing needs, especially for females, who typically consume fewer iron-rich foods such as meat and fewer total kcalories than males. Not surprisingly, iron deficiency is most prevalent among adolescent girls. Iron-deficient children and teens score lower on standardized tests than those who are not iron deficient.

Calcium Adolescence is a crucial time for bone development, and the requirement for calcium reaches its peak during these years.[143] Unfortunately, low calcium intakes among adolescents (14–19 years) is a concern since only about 17 percent of females and 50 percent of males exceeded the recommended level of 1300 mg/day.[144] ♦ Low calcium intakes during times of active growth, especially if paired with physical inactivity, can compromise the development of peak bone mass, which is considered the best protection against adolescent fractures and adult osteoporosis. Increasing milk products in the diet to meet calcium recommendations greatly increases bone density.[145] Once again, however, teenage girls are most vulnerable, for their milk—and therefore their calcium—intakes begin to decline at the time when their calcium needs are greatest. Furthermore, women have much greater bone losses than men in later life. In addition to dietary calcium, bones grow stronger with physical activity. However, because most high schools do not require students to attend physical education classes, many adolescents are not as physically active as healthy bones demand.

♦ Calcium RDA for males and females:
- 9–13 yr: 1300 mg/day

Dietary Guidance for Canadians

Children 9 years of age and older should consume 750 to 1000 millilitres (3–4 cups) per day of skim or 1% milk or equivalent milk products.

Food Choices and Health Habits

Teenagers like the freedom to come and go as they choose. They eat what they want if it is convenient and if they have the time. With a multitude of after school, social, and job activities, they almost inevitably fall into irregular eating habits. At any given time on any given day, a teenager may be skipping a meal, eating a snack, preparing a meal, or consuming food prepared by a parent or restaurant. Adolescents who frequently eat meals with their families, however, eat more fruits, vegetables, grains, and calcium-rich foods, and drink fewer soft drinks, than those who seldom eat with their families.[146] Some research shows that the more often teenagers eat dinner with their families, the less likely they are to smoke, drink, or use drugs; other research supports these findings only in teenage girls.[147] Many adolescents also begin to skip breakfast on a regular basis, missing out on important nutrients that are not made up at later meals during the day. Compared with those who skip breakfast, teenagers who do eat breakfast have higher intakes of vitamin A, vitamin C, and riboflavin, as well as calcium, iron, and zinc, while some subgroups of adolescents had inadequate intakes of magnesium and phosphorous.[148] Teenagers who eat breakfast are therefore more likely to meet their nutrient recommendations.

Breakfast skipping may also lead to weight gain in adolescents. Research shows a dose-response, inverse relationship between breakfast eating and BMI.[149] As adolescents make the transition to adulthood, not only do they skip breakfast more often, they also eat fast food more often. Both skipping breakfast and eating fast foods lead to weight gain.[150]

Ideally, in light of adolescents' busy schedules and desire for freedom, parents continue to play the role of gatekeepers, controlling the type and availability of food in the teenager's environment. Teenagers should find plenty of nutritious, easy-to-grab foods in the refrigerator (meats for sandwiches; low-fat cheeses; fresh, raw vegetables and fruits; fruit juices; and milk) and more in the cabinets (whole-grain breads and crackers, peanut butter, nuts, popcorn, and cereal). In many households today, with adults working outside the home, teenagers perform some of the gatekeepers' roles, such as shopping for groceries or choosing fast or prepared foods.

Snacks Snacks typically provide at least one-fourth of the average teenager's daily food energy intake. Often, favourite snacks are too high in added sugars, saturated fat, and sodium and too low in fibre.[151] A survey of more than 4000 U.S. adolescents, however, found that those who ate snacks more often had higher intakes of fruit compared with those who ate snacks less often.[152] Table 17-9 on p. 570 shows how to combine foods from different food groups to create healthy snacks.

Beverages Most frequently, adolescents drink soft drinks instead of fruit juice or milk with lunch, supper, and snacks. About the only time they select fruit juices is at breakfast. When teens drink milk, they are more likely to consume it with a meal (especially breakfast) than as a snack. Because of their greater food intakes, boys are more likely than girls to drink enough milk to meet their calcium needs.

Soft drinks, when chosen as the primary beverage, may affect bone density, partly because they displace milk from the diet.[153] Over the past three decades, teens (especially girls) have been drinking more soft drinks and less milk. Adolescents who drink soft drinks regularly have a higher energy intake and a lower calcium intake than those who do not; they are also more likely to be overweight.[154]

Soft drinks containing caffeine ♦ present a different problem if caffeine intake becomes excessive. ♦ Caffeine seems to be relatively harmless when used in moderate doses (the equivalent of fewer than three 355 millilitre/12-ounce cola beverages a day). In greater amounts, however, it can cause the symptoms associated with anxiety, such as sweating, tenseness, and inability to concentrate.

♦ For perspective, caffeine-containing soft drinks typically deliver between 30 and 55 mg of caffeine per 355 mL (12-ounce) can. A pharmacologically active dose of caffeine is defined as 200 mg. APPENDIX H lists the caffeine contents of selected foods, beverages, and drugs.

♦ Maximum Caffeine Recommendations for Children and Adolescents:[155] Children 4–6 yrs: 45 mg/day Children 7–9 yrs: 62.5 mg/day Children 10–12 yrs: 85 mg/day Adolescents: 2.5 mg/kg body weight/day

Eating Away from Home Adolescents eat about one-third of their meals away from home, and their nutritional welfare is enhanced or hindered by the choices they make. A lunch consisting of a hamburger, a chocolate shake, and french fries supplies substantial quantities of many nutrients at a kcalorie cost of about 800, an energy intake some adolescents can afford. When they eat this sort of lunch, teens can adjust their breakfast and dinner choices to include fruits and vegetables for vitamin A, vitamin C, folate, and fibre and lean meats and legumes for iron and zinc. (See APPENDIX H for the nutrient contents of fast foods.) Fortunately, many fast-food restaurants are offering more nutritious choices than the standard hamburger meal.

Peer Influence Physical maturity and growing independence present adolescents with new choices. The consequences of those choices will influence their health and nutrition status both today and throughout life. Many of the food and health choices adolescents make reflect the opinions and actions of their peers. When others perceive milk as "babyish," a teen may choose soft drinks instead; when others skip lunch and hang out in the parking lot, a teen may join in for the camaraderie, regardless of hunger. Some teenagers begin using drugs, alcohol, and tobacco; others wisely refrain. Adults can set up the environment so that nutritious foods are available and can stand by with reliable information and advice about health and nutrition, but the rest is up to the adolescents. Ultimately, they make the choices. (Highlight 8 examines the influence of social pressures on the development of eating disorders.)

Drug Abuse The nutrition problems associated with drugs vary in degree, but drug abusers in general face multiple nutrition problems. ♦ During withdrawal from drugs, an important part of treatment is to identify and correct nutrient deficiencies.

♦ Nutrition problems of drug abusers:
- They buy drugs with money that could be spent on food.
- They lose interest in food during "highs."
- They use drugs that suppress appetite.
- Their lifestyle fails to promote good eating habits.
- If they use intravenous (IV) drugs, they may contract AIDS, hepatitis, or other infectious diseases, which increase their nutrient needs. Hepatitis also causes taste changes and loss of appetite.
- Medicines used to treat drug abuse may alter nutrition status.

Alcohol Abuse Sooner or later all teenagers face the decision of whether to drink alcohol. Depending on the province, the law forbids the sale of alcohol to people younger than 18 or 19, but most adolescents who want it can get it. By the end of high school, 77 percent of students have tried alcohol, and about half have been drunk at least once.[156] Highlight 7 describes how alcohol affects nutrition status. To sum it up, alcohol provides energy but no nutrients, and it can displace nutritious foods from the diet. Alcohol alters nutrient absorption and metabolism, so imbalances develop. People who cannot keep their alcohol use moderate must abstain to maintain their health. Highlight 7 lists resources for people with alcohol-related problems.

Smoking According to Physicians for a Smoke-Free Canada, smoking has declined from about 50 percent of girls and boys 15–19 years old in 1975 to about 15 percent in 2009.[157] Cigarette smoking is a pervasive health problem causing thousands of people to suffer from cancer and diseases of the cardiovascular, digestive, and respiratory systems. These effects are beyond the scope of nutrition, but smoking cigarettes does influence hunger, body weight, and nutrient status.

Smoking a cigarette eases feelings of hunger. When smokers receive a hunger signal, they can quiet it with cigarettes instead of food. Such behaviour ignores body signals and postpones energy and nutrient intake. Indeed, smokers tend to weigh less than nonsmokers and to gain weight when they stop smoking. People contemplating giving up cigarettes should know that the average weight gain is about 4.5 kilograms (10 pounds) in the first year. Smokers wanting to quit should prepare for the possibility of weight gain and adjust their diet and activity habits so as to maintain weight during and after quitting. Smoking cessation programs need to include strategies for weight management.

Nutrient intakes of smokers and nonsmokers differ. Smokers tend to have lower intakes of dietary fibre, vitamin A, beta-carotene, folate, and vitamin C. In fact, due in part to increased oxidative stress, the recommendation for vitamin C for smokers is higher by 35 mg/day. The association between smoking and low intakes of fruits and vegetables rich in these nutrients may be noteworthy, considering their protective effect against lung cancer (see Highlight 12).

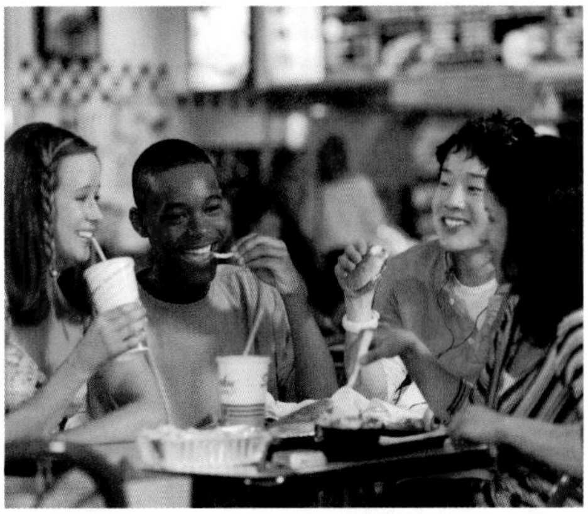

© White Packert/Getty Images

Because their lunches rarely include fruits, vegetables, or milk, many teens fail to get all the vitamins and minerals they need each day.

Smokeless Tobacco Like cigarettes, smokeless tobacco use is linked to many health problems, from minor mouth sores to tumours in the nasal cavities, cheeks, gums, and throat. The risk of mouth and throat cancers is even greater than for smoking tobacco. Other drawbacks to tobacco chewing and snuff dipping include bad breath, stained teeth, and blunted senses of smell and taste. Tobacco chewing also damages the gums, tooth surfaces, and jawbones, making tooth loss later in life likely.

The nutrition and lifestyle choices people make as children and adolescents have long-term, as well as immediate, effects on their health. Highlight 17 describes how sound choices and good habits during childhood and adolescence can help prevent chronic diseases later in life.

Nutrition Portfolio

Encouraging children to eat nutritious foods today helps them learn how to make healthy food choices tomorrow.

- If there are children in your life, think about the food they eat and consider whether they receive enough food for healthy growth, but not so much as to lead to obesity.
- Describe the advantages of physical activity to children's health and well-being.
- Plan a day's menu for a child 4 to 8 years of age, making sure to include foods that provide enough calcium and iron.
- Now, go to Diet Analysis Plus and create a profile for a child 4 to 8 years of age. Enter the day's menu you suggested in the previous exercise and see if you met the basic requirements for that child.

Diet Analysis PLUS **To complete this exercise, go to your Diet Analysis Plus at www.cengage.com/sso.**

Nutrition on the Net

CENGAGENOW™
For further study of topics covered in this chapter, log on to **www.cengage.com/sso.**

- Learn more about breast milk banks from the Human-Milk Banking Association of North America: **www.hmbana.org**
- See breastfeeding recommendations from the Canadian Paediatric Society and Dietitians of Canada: **www.cps.ca/english/statements/n/breastfeedingmar05.htm** and **www.dietitians.ca/Your-Health/Nutrition-A-Z/Breastfeeding.aspx?categoryID=7**
- Learn how to care for infants, children, and adolescents from the American Academy of Pediatrics and the Canadian Paediatric Society: **www.aap.org** and **www.cps.ca**
- Download growth charts and learn more about them: **www.cdc.gov/growthcharts**
- See recommendations on vitamin D supplement for breastfed babies at Health Canada, Food and Nutrition: **www.hc-sc.gc.ca/fn-an/nutrition/infant-nourisson/vita_d_supp-eng.php**
- Get tips on feeding babies from the Canadian Paediatric Society: **www.caringforkids.cps.ca/pregnancybabies/Feeding.htm**
- See results from the 2007–2009 Canadian Health Measures Survey on the fitness of Canadian children and youth from Statistics Canada: **www.statcan.gc.ca/pub/82-003-x/2010001/article/11065-eng.htm**
- Visit the U.S. National Center for Education in Maternal and Child Health and the U.S. National Institute of Child Health and Human Development: **www.ncemch.org** and **www.nichd.nih.gov**
- Learn about child nutrition programs: **www.fns.usda.gov/fns**
- Learn how UNICEF works to protect children: **www.unicef.org**
- Learn how to reduce lead exposure in your home from the U.S. Department of Housing and Urban Development Office of Lead Hazard Control: **www.hud.gov/lead**
- Learn more about food allergies from the American Academy of Allergy, Asthma, and Immunology; the Food Allergy and Anaphylaxis Network; and the International Food Information Council: **www.aaaai.org**, **www.foodallergy.org**, and **www.foodinsight.org**
- Learn more about hyperactivity from Children and Adults with Attention Deficit/Hyperactivity Disorder: **www.chadd.org**
- Visit the Milk Matters section of the U.S. National Institute of Child Health and Human Development: **www.nichd.nih.gov/milk**
- Learn more about caffeine recommendations for Canadians from Health Canada: **www.hc-sc.gc.ca/hl-vs/iyh-vsv/food-aliment/caffeine-eng.php**
- To learn about healthy foods and to find recipes and ideas for physical activities, visit: **www.kidnetic.com**
- Promote good television habits with tips from the Canadian Paediatric Society: **www.caringforkids.cps.ca/growinglearning/GoodTelevision.htm**
- Get help quitting smoking at Health Canada, Quit 4 Life: **www.quit4life.com**
- Visit the Tobacco Information and Prevention Source (TIPS) of the U.S. Centers for Disease Control and Prevention: **www.cdc.gov/tobacco**

References

1. Committee on Dietary Reference Intakes, *Dietary Reference Intakes for Energy, Carbohydrate, Fiber, Fat, Fatty Acids, Cholesterol, Protein, and Amino Acids* (Washington, D.C.: National Academies Press, 2005).
2. Committee on Dietary Reference Intakes, 2005, pp. 280–281.
3. Formula feeding of term infants, in *Pediatric Nutrition Handbook,* 6th ed., ed. R. E. Kleinman (Elk Grove Village, Ill.: American Academy of Pediatrics, 2009), pp. 61–78.
4. Dietitians of Canada, Breastfeeding. www.dietitians.ca/Your-Health/Nutrition-A-Z/Breastfeeding.aspx?categoryID=7, accessed September 15, 2011; Position of the American Dietetic Association: Promoting and supporting breastfeeding, *Journal of the American Dietetic Association* 105 (2005): 810–818.
5. Health Canada, Food and Nutrition, Vitamin D supplementation for breastfed infants–2004 Health Canada recommendation. www.hc-sc.gc.ca/fn-an/nutrition/infant-nourisson/vita_d_supp-eng.php, accessed September 15, 2011; Canadian Paediatric Society, Exclusive breastfeeding should continue to six months (2009). www.cps.ca/english/statements/n/breastfeedingmar05.htm, accessed September 15, 2011; Dietitians of Canada, Breastfeeding; Breastfeeding, in *Pediatric Nutrition Handbook,* 6th ed., ed. R. E. Kleinman (Elk Grove Village, Ill.: American Academy of Pediatrics, 2009), pp. 29–59; Position of the American Academy of Pediatrics: Breastfeeding and the use of human milk, *Pediatrics* 115 (2005): 496–506; M. Boland, Exclusive breastfeeding should continue to six months, *Paediatrics and Child Health* 10 (2005): 148–149; Position of the American Dietetic Association: Promoting and supporting breastfeeding, 2005.
6. Canadian Paediatric Society, 2009.
7. L. Bode, Recent advances on structure, metabolism, and function of human milk oligosaccharides, *Journal of Nutrition* 136 (2006): 2127–2130.
8. S. M. Donovan, Human milk oligosaccharides: The plot thickens, *British Journal of Nutrition* 101 (2009): 1267–1269.
9. S. M. Innis, Dietary (n-3) fatty acids and brain development, *Journal of Nutrition* 137 (2007): 855–859.
10. K. Simmer, S. K. Patole, and S. C. Rao, Longchain polyunsaturated fatty acid supplementation in infants born at term, *Cochrane Database of Systematic Reviews,* January 23, 2008, CD000376; Innis, 2007; M. S. Fewtrell, Long-chain polyunsaturated fatty acids in early life: Effects on multiple health outcomes, in *Primary Prevention by Nutrition Intervention in Infancy and Childhood,* eds. A. Lucas and H. A. Sampson, *Nestle Nutrition Workshop Series Pediatric Program* 57 (2006): 203–221; W. C. Heird and A. Lapillonne, The role of essential fatty acids in development, *Annual Review of Nutrition* 25 (2005): 549–571; J. C. McCann and B. N. Ames, Is docosahexaenoic acid, an n-3 long-chain polyunsaturated fatty acid, required for development of normal brain function? An overview of evidence from cognitive and behavioral tests in humans and animals, *American Journal of Clinical Nutrition* 82 (2005): 281–295.

11. E. E. Birch and coauthors, Visual maturation of term infants fed long-chain polyunsaturated fatty acid-supplemented or control formula for 12 mo, *American Journal of Clinical Nutrition* 81 (2005): 871–879.
12. Simmer, Patole, and Rao, 2008.
13. Fat-soluble vitamins, in *Pediatric Nutrition Handbook,* 6th ed., ed. R. E. Kleinman (Elk Grove Village, Ill.: American Academy of Pediatrics, 2009), pp. 461–474.
14. Health Canada, Food and Nutrition, Vitamin D supplementation for breastfed infants–2004 Health Canada recommendation.
15. Breastfeeding, in *Pediatric Nutrition Handbook,* 2009; American Academy of Pediatrics, 2005; Position of the American Dietetic Association: Promoting and supporting breastfeeding, 2005.
16. K. Sadeharju and coauthors, Maternal antibodies in breast milk protect the child from enterovirus infections, *Pediatrics* 119 (2007): 941–946.
17. L. A. Hanson, Session 1: Feeding and infant development breast-feeding and immune function, *Proceedings of the Nutrition Society* 66 (2007): 384–396.
18. D. S. Newburg, G. M. Ruiz-Palacios, and A. L. Morrow, Human milk glycans protect infants against enteric pathogens, *Annual Review of Nutrition* 25 (2005): 37–58.
19. Breastfeeding, in *Pediatric Nutrition Handbook,* 2009; Hanson, 2007; C. J. Chantry, C. R. Howard, and P. Auinger, Full breastfeeding duration and associated decrease in respiratory tract infection in U.S. children, *Pediatrics* 117 (2006): 425–432; American Academy of Pediatrics, 2005; Position of the American Dietetic Association: Promoting and supporting breastfeeding, 2005.
20. F. R. Greer, S. H. Sicherer, A. W. Burks, and the Committee on Nutrition and Section on Allergy and Immunology, Effects of early nutritional interventions on the development of atopic disease in infants and children: The role of maternal dietary restriction, breastfeeding, timing of introduction of complementary foods, and hydrolyzed formulas, *Pediatrics* 121 (2008): 183–191.
21. Greer, Sicherer, Burks, and the Committee on Nutrition and Section on Allergy and Immunology, 2008; R. S. Zeiger and N. J. Friedman, The relationship of breastfeeding to the development of atopic disorders, *Nestle Nutrition Workshop Series: Pediatric Program* 57 (2006): 93–108.
22. Greer, Sicherer, Burks, and the Committee on Nutrition and Section on Allergy and Immunology, 2008; A. C. Krakowski and coauthors, Management of atopic dermatitis in the pediatric population, *Pediatrics* 122 (2008): 812–824.
23. C. G. Owen and coauthors, Does initial breastfeeding lead to lower blood cholesterol in adult life? A quantitative review of the evidence, *American Journal of Clinical Nutrition* 88 (2008): 305–314; L. Schack-Nielsen and K. F. Michaelsen, Advances in our understanding of the biology of human milk and its effects on the offspring, *Journal of Nutrition* 137 (2007): 503S–510S; R. A. Singhal, Early nutrition and long-term cardiovascular health, *Nutrition Reviews* 64 (2006): S44–S49; M. Martin, D. Gunnell, and G. D. Smith, Breastfeeding in infancy and blood pressure in later life: Systematic review and meta-analysis, *American Journal of Epidemiology* 161 (2005): 15–26.
24. A. S. Ryan, Breastfeeding and the risk of childhood obesity, *Collegium Antropologicum* 31 (2007): 19–28; S. Scholtens and coauthors, Breastfeeding, weight gain in infancy, and overweight at seven years of age: The prevention and incidence of asthma and mite allergy birth cohort study, *American Journal of Epidemiology* 165 (2007): 919–926; A. M. Toschke and coauthors, Infant feeding method and obesity: Body mass index and dual-energy X-ray absorptiometry measurements at 9–10 y of age from the Avon Longitudinal Study of Parents and Children (ALSPAC), *American Journal of Clinical Nutrition* 85 (2007): 1578–1585; R. Novotny and coauthors, Breastfeeding is associated with lower body mass index among children of the Commonwealth of the Northern Mariana Islands, *Journal of the American Dietetic Association* 107 (2007): 1743–1746; K. B. Michels and coauthors, A longitudinal study of infant feeding and obesity throughout life course, *International Journal of Obesity* advance online publication, April 24, 2007.
25. C. G. Owen and coauthors, Effect of infant feeding on the risk of obesity across the life course: A quantitative review of published evidence, *Pediatrics* 115 (2005): 1367–1377.
26. T. Harder and coauthors, Duration of breastfeeding and risk of overweight: A meta-analysis, *Journal of Epidemiology* 162 (2005): 397–403.
27. Ryan, 2007.
28. Schack-Nielsen and Michaelsen, 2007; G. Der, G. D. Batty, and I. J. Deary, Effect of breast feeding on intelligence in children; prospective study, sibling pairs analysis, and meta-analysis, *British Medical Journal* 333 (2006): 929–930; M. C. Daniels and L. S. Adair, Breastfeeding influences cognitive development in Filipino children, *Journal of Nutrition* 135 (2005): 2589–2595.
29. Schack-Nielsen and Michaelsen, 2007.
30. K. Woo and D. Spatz, Human milk donation: What do you know about it? *American Journal of Maternal and Child Nursing* 32 (2007): 150–155.
31. Canadian Paediatric Society, Breastfeeding. www.caringforkids.cps.ca/pregnancybabies/Breastfeeding.htm, accessed September 15, 2011.
32. Health Canada, Food and Nutrition, Recommendations for the preparation and handling of powdered infant formula (PIF). www.hc-sc.gc.ca/fn-an/nutrition/infant-nourisson/pif-ppn-recommandations-eng.php, accessed September 15, 2011.
33. Formula feeding of term infants, in *Pediatric Nutrition Handbook,* 2009; L. Seppo and coauthors, A follow-up study of nutrient intake, nutritional status, and growth in infants with cow milk allergy fed either a soy formula or an extensively hydrolyzed whey formula, *American Journal of Clinical Nutrition* 82 (2005): 140–145.
34. Formula feeding of term infants, in *Pediatric Nutrition Handbook,* 2009; Seppo and coauthors, 2005.
35. Canadian Paediatric Society, Safe discharge of late preterm infant, *Paediatrics and Child Health* 15:10 (2010):655–660. www.cps.ca/english/statements/FN/fn10-01.htm#Definition, accessed September 15, 2011.
36. D. L. O'Connor and coauthors, Growth and nutrient intakes of human milk-fed preterm infants provided with extra energy and nutrients after hospital discharge, *Pediatrics* 121 (2008): 766–776.
37. Canadian Paediatric Society, Breastfeeding. Complementary feeding, in Pediatric Nutrition Handbook, 2009; A. Fiocchi, A. Assa'ad, and S. Bahna, Food allergy and the introduction of solid foods to infants: A consensus document, Annals of Allergy, Asthma and Immunology 97 (2006): 10–21.
38. Canadian Paediatric Society, Feeding your baby (2010). www.caringforkids.cps.ca/pregnancybabies/Feeding.htm, accessed September 15, 2011.
39. Canadian Paediatric Society, Feeding your baby, 2010; Complementary feeding, in *Pediatric Nutrition Handbook*, 2009; A. Fiocchi, A. Assa'ad, and S. Bahna, Food allergy and the introduction of solid foods to infants: A consensus document, *Annals of Allergy, Asthma and Immunology* 97 (2006): 10–21.
40. Iron, in *Pediatric Nutrition Handbook,* 6th ed., ed. R. E. Kleinman (Elk Grove Village, Ill.: American Academy of Pediatrics, 2009), pp. 403–422.
41. Canadian Paediatric Society, Feeding your baby, 2010; Complementary feeding, in *Pediatric Nutrition Handbook,* 2009.
42. Feeding the child, in *Pediatric Nutrition Handbook,* 6th ed., ed. R. E. Kleinman (Elk Grove Village, Ill.: American Academy of Pediatrics, 2009), pp. 145–174.
43. Canadian Paediatric Society, Position statment: Weaning from the breast. www.cps.ca/english/statements/CP/cp04-01.htm, accessed September 15, 2011; Canadian Paediatric Society, Feeding your baby, 2010.
44. M. K. Fox and coauthors, Relationship between portion size and energy intake among infants and toddlers: Evidence of self-regulation, *Journal of the American Dietetic Association* 106 (2006): S77–S83.
45. Position of the American Dietetic Association: Nutrition guidance for healthy children ages 2 to 11 years, *Journal of the American Dietetic Association* 108 (2008): 1038–1047; Position of the American Dietetic Association: Individual-, family-, school-, and community-based interventions for pediatric overweight, *Journal of the American Dietetic Association* 106 (2006): 925–945.
46. M. S. Tremblay and coauthors, Fitness of Canadian children and youth: Results from the 2007–2009 Canadian Health Measures Survey, Statistics Canada. www.statcan.gc.ca/pub/82-003-x/2010001/article/11065-eng.htm, accessed September 15, 2011.
47. Canadian Society for Exercise Physiology, Canadian Sedentary Behaviour Guidelines for children and youth. www.csep.ca/CMFiles/Guidelines/SBGuidelinesChildandYouth_E.pdf, accessed September 15, 2011.
48. Nutritional aspects of vegetarian diets, in *Pediatric Nutrition Handbook,* 6th ed., ed. R. E. Kleinman (Elk Grove Village, Ill.: American Academy of Pediatrics, 2009), pp. 201–224.
49. Committee on Dietary Reference Intakes, 2005, Chapter 6.
50. Committee on Dietary Reference Intakes, 2005, Chapter 7.

51. Department of Justice, Food and Drug Regulations, Foods for children under two years of age. http://lois-laws.justice.gc.ca/eng/regulations/C.R.C.%2C_c._870/page-29.html, accessed September 15, 2011.
52. Committee on Dietary Reference Intakes, 2005, Chapter 11.
53. Committee on Dietary Reference Intakes, 2005, Chapter 8.
54. J. M. Brotanek and coauthors, Iron deficiency in early childhood in the United States: Risk factors and racial/ethnic disparities, *Pediatrics* 120 (2007): 568–575; K. C. White, Anemia is a poor predictor of iron deficiency among toddlers in the United States: For heme the bell tolls, *Pediatrics* 115 (2005): 315–320.
55. Wagner and Greer, and the Section on Breastfeeding and Committee on Nutrition, 2008.
56. Feeding the child, in *Pediatric Nutrition Handbook*, 2009.
57. U. Shaikh, R. S. Byrd, and P. Auinger, Vitamin and mineral supplement use by children and adolescents in the 1999–2004 National Health and Nutrition Examination survey: Relationship with nutrition, food security, physical activity, and health care access, *Archives of Pediatrics and Adolescent Medicine* 163 (2009): 150–157; R. Briefel and coauthors, Feeding Infants and Toddlers Study: Do vitamin and mineral supplements contribute to nutrient adequacy or excess among U.S. infants and toddlers? *Journal of the American Dietetic Association* 106 (2006): S52–S65.
58. Health Canada, Food and Nutrition, Do Canadian children meet their nutrient requirements through food intake alone? (2009). www.hc-sc.gc.ca/fn-an/surveill/nutrition/commun/art-nutr-child-enf-eng.php, accessed September 15, 2011.
59. Canadian Children's Rights Council, Child poverty in Canada. www.canadiancrc.com/child_poverty_in_canada.aspx, accessed September 15, 2011.
60. K. Widenhorn-Muller and coauthors, Influence of having breakfast on cognitive performance and mood in 13- to 20-year-old high school students: Results of a crossover trial, *Pediatrics* 122 (2008): 279–284.
61. W. O. Song and coauthors, Ready-to-eat breakfast cereal consumption enhances milk and calcium intake in the U.S. population, *Journal of the American Dietetic Association* 106 (2006): 1783–1789; S. G. Affenito and coauthors, Breakfast consumption by African-American and white adolescent girls correlates positively with calcium and fiber intake and negatively with body mass index, *Journal of the American Dietetic Association* 105 (2005): 938–945; G. C. Rampersaud and coauthors, Breakfast habits, nutritional status, body weight, and academic performance in children and adolescents, *Journal of the American Dietetic Association* 105 (2005): 743–760.
62. J. C. McCann and B. N. Ames, An overview of evidence for a causal relation between iron deficiency during development and deficits in cognitive or behavioral function, *American Journal of Clinical Nutrition* 85 (2007): 931–945.
63. B. Lozhoff and coauthors, Long-lasting neural and behavioral effects of iron deficiency in infancy, *Nutrition Reviews* 64 (2006): S34–S43.
64. K. M. Cecil and coauthors, Decreased brain volume in adults with childhood lead exposure, *PLoS Medicine* 27 (2008): e112.
65. Ontario Ministry of the Environment, Chief Drinking Water Inspector issues municipalities orders to do lead testing, news release (May 27, 2007). www.ene.gov.on.ca/en/news/2007/052502.php; Chief Drinking Water Inspector (Ontario): Annual Report 2008–2009. www.offlaio.ca/distributer/dw_el_prd_039637.pdf; Statistics Canada, Canadian Health Measures Survey: Lead, bisphenol A and mercury. www.statcan.gc.ca/daily-quotidien/100816/dq100816a-eng.htm#il, accessed September 21, 2011.
66. Centers for Disease control and Prevention, Interpreting and managing blood lead levels 10μg/dL in children and reducing childhood exposures to lead: Recommendations of DCD's Advisory Committee on Childhood Lead Poisoning Prevention, *Morbidity and Mortality Weekly Report* 56/RR-8 (2007): 1–16; Position of the Committee on Environmental Health, American Academy of Pediatrics: Lead exposure in children: Prevention, detection, and management, *Pediatrics* 116 (2005): 1036–1046.
67. Committee on Environmental Health, American Academy of Pediatrics, 2005.
68. P. N. Pastor and C. A. Reuben, Diagnosed attention deficit hyperactivity disorder and learning disability: United States, 2004–2006, *Vital and Health Statistics, Series 10, Data from the National Health Survey* 237 (2008): 1–14; E. Romano and coauthors, Development and prediction of hyperactive symptoms from 2 to 7 years in a population-based sample, *Pediatrics* 117 (2006): 2101–2109.
69. M. L. Wolraich and coauthors, Attention-deficit/hyperactivity disorder among adolescents: A review of the diagnosis, treatment, and clinical implications, *Pediatrics* 115 (2005): 1734–1746.
70. K. Rubia, Neuro-anatomic evidence for the maturational delay hypothesis of ADHD, *Proceedings of the National Academy of Sciences* 104 (2007): 19663–19664.
71. D. McCann and coauthors, Food additives and hyperactive behaviour in 3-year-old and 8/9-year-old children in the community: A randomized, double-blinded, placebo-controlled trial, *Lancet* 370 (2007): 1560–1567.
72. National Institutes of Health, National Institute of Allergy and Infectious Diseases, *Food Allergy: Report of the NIH Expert Panel on Food Allergy Research,* March 13–14, 2006, www.naid.nih.gov.
73. National Institutes of Health, National Institute of Allergy and Infectious Diseases, 2006.
74. U.S. Food and Drug Administration, Food allergies; Reducing the risks, January 23, 2009, www.fda.gov/consumer/updates/foodallergies012209.html.
75. A. Boulay and coauthors, A EuroPrevall review of factors affecting incidence of peanut allergy: Priorities for research and policy, *Allergy* 63 (2008): 797–809; L. A. Lee and A. W. Burks, Food allergies: Prevalence, molecular characterization, and treatment/prevention strategies, *Annual Review of Nutrition* 26 (2006): 539–565.
76. M. Boguniewicz, N. Moore, and K. Paranto, Allergic diseases, quality of life, and the role of the dietitian, *Nutrition Today* 43 (2008): 6–10.
77. S. Ramesh, Food allergy overview in children, *Clinical Reviews in Allergy & Immunology* 34 (2008): 217–230.
78. Lee and Burks, 2006.
79. Canadian Food Inspection Agency, Questions and answers regarding the labelling of food allergens and the use of precautionary statements—Priority food allergens. www.inspection.gc.ca/english/fssa/labeti/allerg/allergee.shtml, accessed September 15, 2011; Lee and Burks, 2006.
80. National Institutes of Health, National Institute of Allergy and Infectious Diseases, 2006.
81. M. Tjepkema and M. Shields, Measured obesity: Overweight Canadian children and adolescents. Canadian Community Health Survey: Obesity among Children and Adults. Statistics Canada, Cat. No. 82-620-MWE (2004).
82. S. E. Barlow and the Expert Committee, Expert Committee recommendations regarding the prevention, assessment, and treatment of child and adolescent overweight and obesity: Summary report, *Pediatrics* 120 (2007): S164–S192.
83. Barlow and the Expert Committee, 2007.
84. D. S. Freedman and coauthors, Cardiovascular risk factors and excess adiposity among overweight children and adolescents: The Bogalusa Heart Study, *Journal of Pediatrics* 150 (2007): 12–17.
85. A.S. Singh and coauthors, Tracking of childhood overweight into adulthood: A systematic review of the literature. Obesity Review 9:5 (2008): 474–488; N. F. Krebs and coauthors, Assessment of child and adolescent overweight and obesity, *Pediatrics* 120 (2007): S193–S228.
86. Barlow and the Expert Committee, 2007.
87. M. He, L. Piché, C. Beynon, and S. B. Harris, Screen-related sedentary behaviors: Children's and parents' attitudes, social influence and intention, Journal of Nutrition Education and Behavior 42 (2010): 17–25; M. He, S. B. Harris, L. A. Piché, and C. Beynon, Understanding screen-related sedentary behavior and its contributing factors among school-aged children: A social-ecological exploration, American Journal of Health Promotion 23:5 (2009): 299–308; B. A. Spear and coauthors, Recommendations for treatment of child and adolescent overweight and obesity, *Pediatrics* 120 (2007): S254–S287; S. L. Martin, S. M. Lee, and R. Lowry, National prevalence and correlates of walking and bicycling to school, *American Journal of Preventive Medicine* 33 (2007): 98–105; American Academy of Pediatrics, Council on Sports Medicine and Fitness and Council on School Health, Active healthy living: Prevention of childhood obesity through increased physical activity, *Pediatrics* 117 (2006): 1834–1842; J. P. Koplan, C. T. Liverman, and V. I. Kraak, eds., *Preventing Childhood Obesity: Health in the Balance* (Washington, D.C.: National Academies Press, 2005), pp. 79–123.
88. K. J. Campbell and coauthors, Associations between the home food environment and obesity-promoting eating behaviors in adolescence, *Obesity* 15 (2007): 719–730; Barlow and the Expert Commit-tee, 2007.

89. K. S. Geller and D. A. Dzewaltowski, Longitudinal and cross-sectional influences on youth fruit and vegetable consumption, *Nutrition Reviews* 67 (2009): 65–76; J. Brug and coauthors, Taste preferences,liking and other factors related to fruit and vegetable intakes among schoolchildren: Results from observational studies, *British Journal of Nutrition* 99 (2008): S7–S14; C. A. Forestell and J. A. Mennella, Early determinants of fruit and vegetable acceptance, *Pediatrics* 120 (2007): 1247–1254; C. Arcan and coauthors, Parental eating behaviours, home food environment and adolescent intakes of fruits, vegetables and dairy foods: Longitudinal finding form Project EAT, *Public Health Nutrition* 11 (2007): 1257–1265; M. Wind and coauthors, Correlates of fruit and vegetable consumption among 11-year-old Belgina-Flemish and Dutch schoolchildren, *Journal of Nutrition Education and Behavior* 38 (2006): 211–221.
90. K. E. Leahy, L. L. Birch, and B. Rolls, Reducing the energy density of multiple meals decreases the energy intake of preschool-age children, *American Journal of Clinical Nutrition* 88 (2008): 1459–1468.
91. S. A. Lederman and coauthors, Summary of the presentations at the Conference on Preventing Childhood Obesity, December 8, 2003, *Pediatrics* 114 (2004): 1146–1173.
92. S. N. Bleich and coauthors, Increasing consumption of sugar-sweetened beverages among U.S. adults: 1988–1994 to 1999–2004, *American Journal of Clinical Nutrition* 89 (2009): 372–381; Spear and coauthors, 2007; L. Dubois and coauthors, Regular sugar-sweetened beverage consumption between meals increases risk of overweight among preschool-aged children, *Journal of the American Dietetic Association* 107 (2007): 924–934; V. S. Malik, M. B. Schultz, and F. B. Hu, Intake of sugar-sweetened beverages and weight gain: A systematic review, *American Journal of Clinical Nutrition* 84 (2006): 274–288.
93. S. Harrington, The role of sugar-sweetened beverage consumption in adolescent obesity: A review of the literature, *Journal of School Nursing* 24 (2008): 3–12; Committee on School Health, American Academy of Pediatrics, Soft drinks in schools, *Pediatrics* 113 (2004): 152–154.
94. L. R. Vartanian, M. B. Schwartz, and K. D. Brownell, Effects of soft drink consumption on nutrition and health: A systematic review and meta-analysis, *American Journal of Public Health* 97 (2007): 667–675.
95. American Academy of Pediatrics, Council on Sports Medicine and Fitness and Council on School Health, Active healthy living: Prevention of childhood obesity through increased physical activity, *Pediatrics* 117 (2006): 1834–1842.
96. He and coauthors, 2009; V. J. Rideout, U. G. Foehr, and D. F. Roberts, GENERATION M2–Media in the lives of 8- to 18-year-olds, *Kaiser Family Foundation Study* (Jan. 2010). S. Gable, Y. Chang, and J. L. Krull, Television watching and frequency of family meals are predictive of overweight onset and persistence in a national sample of school-aged children, *Journal of the American Dietetic Association* 107 (2007): 53–61; Spear and coauthors, 2007.
97. M. Hamer, E. Stamsatakis, and G. Mishra, Psychological distress, television viewing, and physical activity in children aged 4 to 12 years, *Pediatrics* 123 (2009): 1263–1268.
98. He and coauthors, 2009; D. J. Barr-Anderson and coauthors, Characteristics associated with older adolescents who have a television in their bedrooms, *Pediatrics* 121 (2008): 718–724; A. M. Adachi-Mejia and coauthors, Children with a TV in their bedroom at higher risk for being overweight, *International Journal of Obesity* 31 (2007): 644–651.
99. He and coauthors, 2009; D. M. Jackson and coauthors, Increased television viewing is associated with elevated body fatness but not with lower total energy expenditure in children, *American Journal of Clinical Nutrition* 89 (2009): 1031–1036.
100. L. Dubois and coauthors, Social factors and television use during meals and snacks is associated with higher BMI among pre-school children, *Public Health Nutrition* 11 (2008): 1267–1279; Gable, Chang, and Krull, 2007.
101. J. L. Wiecha and coauthors, When children eat what they watch: Impact of television viewing on dietary intake in youth, *Archives of Pediatrics & Adolescent Medicine* 160 (2006): 436–442; S. C. Folta and coauthors, Food advertising targeted at school-age children: A content analysis, *Journal of Nutrition Education and Behavior* 38 (2006): 244–248.
102. A. Batada and coauthors, Nine out of 10 food advertisements shown during Saturday morning children's television programming are for foods high in fat, sodium, or added sugars, or low in nutrients, *Journal of the American Dietetic Association* 108 (2008): 673–678; L. M. Powell and coauthors, Nutritional content of television food advertisements seen by children and adolescents in the United States, *Pediatrics* 120 (2007): 576–583; Wiecha and coauthors, 2006.
103. S. M. Connor, Food-related advertising on preschool television: Building brand recognition in young viewers, *Pediatrics* 118 (2006): 1478–1485; Folta and coauthors, 2006.
104. L. J. Chamberlain, Y. Wang, and T. N. Robinson, Does children's screen time predict requests for advertised products? Cross-sectional and prospective analyses, *Archives of Pediatrics & Adolescent Medicine* 160 (2006): 363–368; Y. Aktas-Arnas, the effects of television food advertisement on children's food purchasing requests, *Pediatrics International* 48 (2006): 138–145; M. O'Dougherty, M. Story, and J. Stang, Observations of parent-child co-shoppers in supermarkets: Children's involvement in food selections, parental yielding, and refusal strategies, *Journal of Nutrition Education and Behavior* 38 (2006): 183–188.
105. K. Weber, M. Story, and L. Harnack, Internet food marketing strategies aimed at children and adolescents: A content analysis of food and beverage brand web sites, *Journal of the American Dietetic Association* 106 (2006): 1463–1466.
106. Spear and coauthors, 2007.
107. Canadian Paediatric Society, How to promote good television habits (2010). www.caringforkids.cps.ca/growinglearning/GoodTelevision.htm, accessed September 15, 2011; Canadian Society for Exercise Physiology, *Canadian Sedentary Behaviour Guidelines* (Feb. 2011). www.csep.ca/english/view.asp?x=804, accessed September 15, 2011.
108. M. Salvadori and coauthors, Elevated blood pressure in relation to overweight and obesity among children in a rural Canadian community, *Pediatrics* 122 (2008): e821–e827; R. Jago and coauthors, Prevalence of abnormal lipid and blood pressure values among an ethnically diverse population of eighth-grade adolescents and screening implications, *Pediatrics* 117 (2006): 2065–2073.
109. S. Cook and coauthors, Metabolic Syndrome rates in United States adolescents, from the National Health and Nutrition Examination Survey, 1999–2002, *Journal of Pediatrics* 152 (2008): 165–170; K. L. Jones, Role of obesity in complicating and confusing the diagnosis and treatment of diabetes in children, *Pediatrics* 121 (2008): 361–368; C. L. Carroll and coauthors, Childhood overweight increases hospital admission rates for asthma, *Pediatrics* 120 (2007): 734–740; M. L. Cruz and coauthors, Pediatric obesity and insulin resistance: Chronic disease risk and implications for treatment and prevention beyond body weight modification, *Annual Review of Nutrition* 25 (2005):v 435–468.
110. D. S. Ludwig, Childhood obesity: The shape of things to come, *New England Journal of Medicine* 357 (2007): 2325–2326; A. J. Daley and coauthors, Exercise therapy as a treatment for psychopathologic conditions in obese and morbidly obese adolescents: A randomized, controlled trial, *Pediatrics* 118 (2006): 2126–2134; J. Franklin and coauthors, Obesity and risk of low self-esteem: A statewide survey of Australian children, *Pediatrics* 118 (2006): 2481–2487.
111. S. M. Himes and J. K. Thompson, Fat stigmatization in television shows and movies: A content analysis, *Obesity* 15 (2007): 712–718.
112. Barlow and the Expert Committee, 2007.
113. M. M. Davis and coauthors, Recommendations for prevention of childhood obesity, *Pediatrics* 120 (2007): S229–S253; Position of the American Dietetic Association: Individual-, family-, school-, and community-based interventions for pediatric overweight, 2006.
114. Barlow and the Expert Committee, 2007.
115. Spear and coauthors, 2007.
116. Barlow and the Expert Committee, 2007.
117. Barlow and the Expert Committee, 2007.
118. D. C. W. Lau and coauthors, 2006 Canadian clinical practice guidelines on the management and prevention of obesity in adults and children, *Canadian Medical Association Journal* 176 (8 suppl) (2007): S1-13. www.cmaj.ca/cgi/content/full/176/8/S1/DC1, accessed September 15, 2011.
119. American Academy of Pediatrics, 2006.
120. M. Shields and M. S. Tremblay, Screen time among Canadian adults: A profile, Statistics Canada, Health Reports 19:2 (2008). www.statcan.gc.ca/pub/82-003-x/2008002/article/10600/5202425-eng.htm, accessed September 15, 2011; R. C. Colley and coauthors, Physical activity of Canadian children and youth: Accelerometer results from the 2007 to 2009 Canadian Health Measures Survey, Statistics

Canada, Health Reports 22:1 (2011). www.statcan.gc.ca/pub/82-003-x/2011001/article/11397-eng.htm, accessed September 15, 2011.
121. American Academy of Pediatrics, 2006.
122. Spear and coauthors, 2007.
123. T. H. Inge and coauthors, Reversal of type 2 diabetes mellitus and improvements in cardiovascular risk factors after surgical weight loss in adolescents, *Pediatrics* 123 (2009): 214–222.
124. Spear and coauthors, 2007.
125. Position of the American Dietetic Association, 2008; Position of the American Dietetic Association: Individual-, family-, school-, and community-based interventions for pediatric overweight, 2006.
126. E. Jansen and coauthors, From the Garden of Eden to the land of plenty: Restriction of fruit and sweets intake leads to increased fruit and sweets consumption in children, *Appetite* 51 (2008): 570–575; E. Jansen, S. Mulkens, and A. Jansen, Do not eat the red food: Prohibition of snacks leads to their relatively higher consumption in children, *Appetite* 49 (2007): 572–577.
127. Position of the American Dietetic Association, 2008.
128. Position of the American Dietetic Association, 2008; J. Wardle, S. Carnell, and L. Cooke, Parental control over feeding and children's fruit and vegetable intake: How are they related? *Journal of the American Dietetic Association* 105 (2005): 227–232; A. T. Galloway and coauthors, Parental pressure, dietary patterns, and weight status among girls who are "picky eaters," *Journal of the American Dietetic Association* 105 (2005): 541–548.
129. L. Cooke, The importance of exposure for healthy eating in childhood: A review, *Journal of Human Nutrition and Dietetics* 20 (2007): 294–301.
130. Position of the American Dietetic Association: Benchmarks for nutrition programs in child care settings, *Journal of the American Dietetic Association* 105 (2005): 979–986; Position of the American Dietetic Association, Society of Nutrition Education, and American School Food Service Association—Nutrition services: An essential component of comprehensive school health programs, *Journal of the American Dietetic Association* 103 (2003): 505–514.
131. Breakfast for Learning, Menu planner. www.breakfastforlearning.ca/images/pdfs/Services_and_Information/menuplanner.pdf, accessed September 15, 2011.
132. Position of the American Dietetic Association: Local support for nutrition integrity in schools, 2006.
133. Centers for Disease Control and Prevention, Competitive foods and beverages available for purchase in secondary schools—selected sites, United States, 2006, *Morbidity and Mortality Weekly Report* 57 (2008): 935–938; Position of the American Dietetic Association: Local support for nutrition integrity in schools, 2006; C. Probart and coauthors, Competitive foods available in Pennsylvania public high schools, *Journal of the American Dietetic Association* 105 (2005): 1243–1249.
134. S. B. Templeton and coauthors, Competitive foods increase the intake of energy and decrease the intake of certain nutrients by adolescents consuming school lunch, *Journal of the American Dietetic Association* 105 (2005): 215–220.
135. Ontario Ministry of Education, Policy/Program Memorandum No. 150 (October 4, 2010). www.edu.gov.on.ca/extra/eng/ppm/150.html, accessed September 15, 2011.
136. Committee on Dietary Reference Intakes, 2005, Chapter 5.
137. S. Saintonge, H. Bang, and L. M. Gerber, Implications of a new definition of vitamin D deficiency in a multiracial US adolescent population: The National Health and Nutrition Examination Survey III, *Pediatrics* 123 (2009): 797–803; Wagner, Greer, and the Section on Breastfeeding and Committee on Nutrition, 2008.
138. K. Langlois, L. Greene-Finestone, J. Little, N. Hidiroglou, and S. Whiting, Vitamin D status of Canadians as measured in the 2007 to 2009 Canadian Health Measures Survey. Statistics Canada, *Health Reports* (March 2010), Cat No. 82-003-X.
139. C. D. Davis, Vitamin D and cancer: Current dilemmas and future research needs, *American Journal of Clinical Nutrition* 88 (2008): 565S–569S; Wagner, Greer, and the Section on Breastfeeding and Committee on Nutrition, 2008.
140. Institute of Medicine, Dietary Reference Intakes for calcium and vitamin D (Nov 2010). www.iom.edu/Reports/2010/Dietary-Reference-Intakes-for-Calcium-and-Vitamin-D.aspx, accessed September 15, 2011.
141. Committee on Dietary Reference Intakes, *Dietary Reference Intakes for Vitamin A, Vitamin K, Arsenic, Boron, Chromium, Copper, Iodine, Iron, Manganese, Molybdenum, Nickel, Silicon, Vanadium, and Zinc* (Washington, D.C.: National Academies Press, 2001), pp. 290–393.
142. Committee on Dietary Reference Intakes, 2001.
143. F. R. Greer, N. F. Krebs, and the Committee on Nutrition, American Academy of Pediatrics, Optimizing bone health and calcium intakes of infants, children, and adolescents, *Pediatrics* 117 (2006): 578–585.
144. Health Canada and Statistics Canada, Canadian Community Health Survey Cycle 2.2, Nutrition (2004) vol 1. www.hc-sc.gc.ca/fn-an/surveill/nutrition/commun/cchs_focus-volet_escc-eng.php, accessed September 15, 2011.
145. L. Esterie and coauthors, Milk, rather than other foods, is associated with vertebral bone mass and circulating IGF-1 in female adolescents, *Osteoporosis International* 2008 20 (2009): 567–575; M. M. Murphy and coauthors, Drinking flavored or plain milk is positively associated with nutrient intake and is not associated with adverse effects on weight status in U.S. children and adolescents, *Journal of the American Dietetic Association* 108 (2008): 631–639; M. L. Savaiano and coauthors, Perceived milk intolerance is related to bone mineral content in 10- to 13-year-old female adolescents, *Pediatrics* 120 (2007): e669–e677.
146. N. I. Larson and coauthors, Family meals during adolescence are associated with higher diet quality and healthful meal patterns during young adulthood, *Journal of the American Dietetic Association* 107 (2007): 1502–1510.
147. M. E. Eisenberg and coauthors, Family meals and substance use: Is there a long-term association? *Journal of Adolescent Health* 43 (2008): 151–156; National Center on Addiction and Substance Abuse (CASA) at Columbia University, *The Importance of Family Dinners*, September, 2003.
148. Health Canada and Statistics Canada, Canadian Community Health Survey Cycle 2.2, Nutrition, 2004; Rampersaud and coauthors, 2005.
149. M. T. Timlin and coauthors, Breakfast eating and weight change in a 5-year prospective analysis of adolescents: Project EAT (Eating Among Teens), *Pediatrics* 121 (2008): e638–e645.
150. C. M. McDonald and coauthors, Overweight is more prevalent than stunting and is associated with socioeconomic status, maternal obesity, and a snacking dietary pattern in school children from Bogota, Colombia, *Journal of Nutrition* 139 (2009): 370–376; H. M. Niemeier and coauthors, Fast food consumption and breakfast skipping: Predictors of weight gain from adolescence to adulthood in a nationally representative sample, *Journal of Adolescent Health* 39 (2006): 842–849.
151. American Heart Association, S. S. Gidding, and coauthors, Dietary recommendations for children and adolescents: A guide for practitioners, *Pediatrics* 117 (2006): 544–559
152. R. S. Sebastian, L. E. Cleveland, and J. D. Goldman, Effect of snacking frequency on adolescents' dietary intakes and meeting national recommendations, *Journal of Adolescent Health* 42 (2008): 503–511.
153 L. Libuda and coauthors, Association between long-term consumption of soft drinks and variables of bone modeling and remodeling in a sample of healthy German children and adolescents, *American Journal of Clinical Nutrition* 88 (2008): 1670–1677; Greer, Krebs, and the Committee on Nutrition, 2006; H. Vatanparast and coauthors, Positive effects of vegetable and fruit consumption and calcium intake on bone mineral accrual in boys during growth from childhood to adolescence: The University of Saskatchewan Pediatric Bone Mineral Accrual Study, *American Journal of Clinical Nutrition* 82 (2005): 700–706.
154. Vartanian, Schwartz, and Brownell, 2007; Malik, Schulze, and Hu, 2006.
155. Health Canada, Health Canada reminds Canadians to manage caffeine consumption (March 19, 2010). www.hc-sc.gc.ca/ahc-asc/media/advisories-avis/_2010/2010_40-eng.php, accessed September 30, 2011.
156. J. W. Kulig and the Committee on Substance Abuse, Tobacco, alcohol, and other drugs: The role of the pediatrician in prevention, identification, and management of substance abuse, *Pediatrics* 115 (2005): 816–821.
157. Physicians for a Smoke-Free Canada, Smoking prevalence: Girls and boys, aged 15–19 (Feb. 2011). www.smoke-free.ca/factsheets/pdf/prevalence.pdf, accessed September 15, 2011.

HIGHLIGHT 17

Childhood Obesity and the Early Development of Chronic Diseases

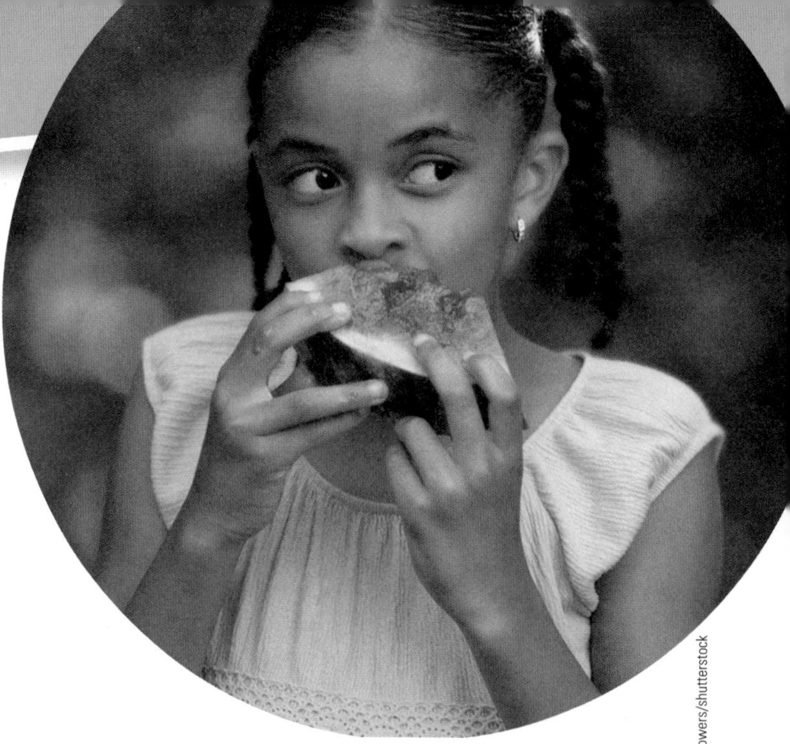

Glenda M. Powers/shutterstock

When people think about the health problems of children and adolescents, they typically think of ear infections, colds, and acne—not heart disease, diabetes, or hypertension. Today, however, unprecedented numbers of North American children are being diagnosed with obesity and the serious "adult diseases," such as type 2 diabetes, that accompany overweight.[1] When type 2 diabetes develops before the age of 20, the incidence of diabetic kidney disease and death in middle age increases dramatically, largely because of the long duration of the disease.[2] For children born in North America in the year 2000, the risk of developing type 2 diabetes sometime in their lives is estimated to be 30 percent for boys and 40 percent for girls.[3] North American children are not alone—rapidly rising rates of obesity threaten the health of an alarming number of children around the globe.[4] Without immediate intervention, millions of children are destined to develop type 2 diabetes and hypertension in childhood followed by **cardiovascular disease (CVD)** in early adulthood.[5] (See the accompanying glossary for this and related terms.)

This highlight focuses on efforts to prevent childhood obesity and the development of heart disease and type 2 diabetes, but the benefits extend to other obesity-related diseases as well. The years of childhood (ages 2 to 18) are emphasized here, because the earlier in life health-promoting habits become established, the better they will stick. Chapter 19 fills in the rest of the story of nutrition's role in reducing chronic disease risk.

Invariably, questions arise as to what extent genetics is involved in disease development. For heart disease and type 2 diabetes, genetics does not appear to play a *determining* role; that is, a person is not simply destined at birth to develop these diseases. Instead, genetics appears to play a *permissive* role—the potential is inherited and will develop if given a push by poor health choices such as excessive weight gain, poor diet, sedentary lifestyle, and cigarette smoking.

Many experts agree that preventing or treating obesity in childhood will reduce the rate of chronic diseases in adulthood. Without intervention, most overweight children become overweight adolescents who become overweight adults, and being overweight exacerbates every chronic disease that adults face.[6] Fatty liver, a condition that correlates directly with BMI, was not even recognized in pediatric research until recently. Today, fatty liver disease affects about one in three obese children.[7]

Early Development of Type 2 Diabetes

In recent years, type 2 diabetes, a chronic disease closely linked with obesity, has been on the rise among children and adolescents as the prevalence of obesity in North American youth has increased.[8] Obesity is the most important risk factor for type 2 diabetes—most of the children diagnosed with it are obese.[9] Most are diagnosed during puberty, but as younger children become more obese and less active, the trend is shifting to younger ages. Type 2

GLOSSARY

atherosclerosis (ATH-er-oh-scler-OH-sis): a type of artery disease characterized by plaques (accumulations of lipid-containing material) on the inner walls of the arteries (see Chapter 19).

- **athero** = porridge or soft
- **scleros** = hard
- **osis** = condition

cardiovascular disease (CVD): a general term for all diseases of the heart and blood vessels. Atherosclerosis is the main cause of CVD. When the arteries that carry blood to the heart muscle become blocked, the heart suffers damage known as **coronary heart disease (CHD).**

- **cardio** = heart
- **vascular** = blood vessels

fatty streaks: accumulations of cholesterol and other lipids along the walls of the arteries.

plaque (PLACK): an accumulation of fatty deposits, smooth muscle cells, and fibrous connective tissue that develops in the artery walls in atherosclerosis. Plaque associated with atherosclerosis is known as **atheromatous** (ATH-er-OH-ma-tus) **plaque.**

diabetes is most likely to occur in those who are obese and sedentary and have a family history of diabetes.

In type 2 diabetes, the cells become insulin-resistant—that is, the cells become less sensitive to insulin, reducing the amount of glucose entering the cells from the blood. The combination of obesity and insulin resistance produces a cluster of symptoms, including high blood cholesterol and high blood pressure, which, in turn, promotes the development of atherosclerosis and the early development of CVD.[10] Other common problems evident by early adulthood include kidney disease, blindness, and miscarriages. The complications of diabetes, especially when encountered at a young age, can shorten life expectancy.

Prevention and treatment of type 2 diabetes depend on weight management, which can be particularly difficult in a youngster's world of food advertising, video games, and pocket money for chocolate bars. The activity and dietary suggestions to help defend against heart disease later in this highlight apply to type 2 diabetes as well.

Early Development of Heart Disease

Most people consider heart disease to be an adult disease because its incidence rises with advancing age, and symptoms rarely appear before age 30. The disease process actually begins much earlier.

Atherosclerosis

Most cardiovascular disease involves **atherosclerosis.** Atherosclerosis develops when regions of an artery's walls become progressively thickened with **plaque**—an accumulation of fatty deposits, smooth muscle cells, and fibrous connective tissue. If it progresses, atherosclerosis may eventually block the flow of blood to the heart and cause a heart attack or cut off blood flow to the brain and cause a stroke. Infants are born with healthy, smooth, clear arteries, but within the first decade of life, **fatty streaks** may begin to appear (see Figure H17-1). During adolescence, these fatty streaks may begin to accumulate fibrous connective tissue. By early adulthood, the fibrous plaques may begin to calcify and become raised lesions, especially in boys and young men. As the lesions grow more numerous and enlarge, the heart disease rate begins to rise, most dramatically at about age 45 in men and 55 in women. From this point on, arterial damage and blockage progress rapidly, and heart attacks and strokes threaten life. In short, the consequences of atherosclerosis, which become apparent only in adulthood, have their beginnings in the first decades of life.[11]

Atherosclerosis is not inevitable; people can grow old with relatively clear arteries. Early lesions may either progress or regress, depending on several factors, many of which reflect lifestyle behaviours. Smoking, for example, is strongly associated with the prevalence of fatty streaks and raised lesions, even in young adults.

Blood Cholesterol

As blood cholesterol rises, atherosclerosis worsens. Cholesterol values at birth are similar in all populations; differences emerge in early childhood. Standard values for cholesterol in children and adolescents (ages 2 to 18 years) are listed in Table H17-1. Cholesterol concentrations change with age in children and adolescents, however, and are especially variable during puberty.[12] Thus, using a single cut point for all pediatric age groups has limitations.

In general, blood cholesterol tends to rise as dietary saturated fat intakes increase. Blood cholesterol also correlates with childhood obesity, especially abdominal obesity.[13] LDL cholesterol rises with obesity, and HDL declines. These relationships are apparent throughout childhood, and their magnitude increases with age.

Children who are both overweight and have high blood cholesterol are likely to have parents who develop heart disease early. For this reason, selective screening is recommended for children

FIGURE H17-1 The Formation of Plaques in Atherosclerosis

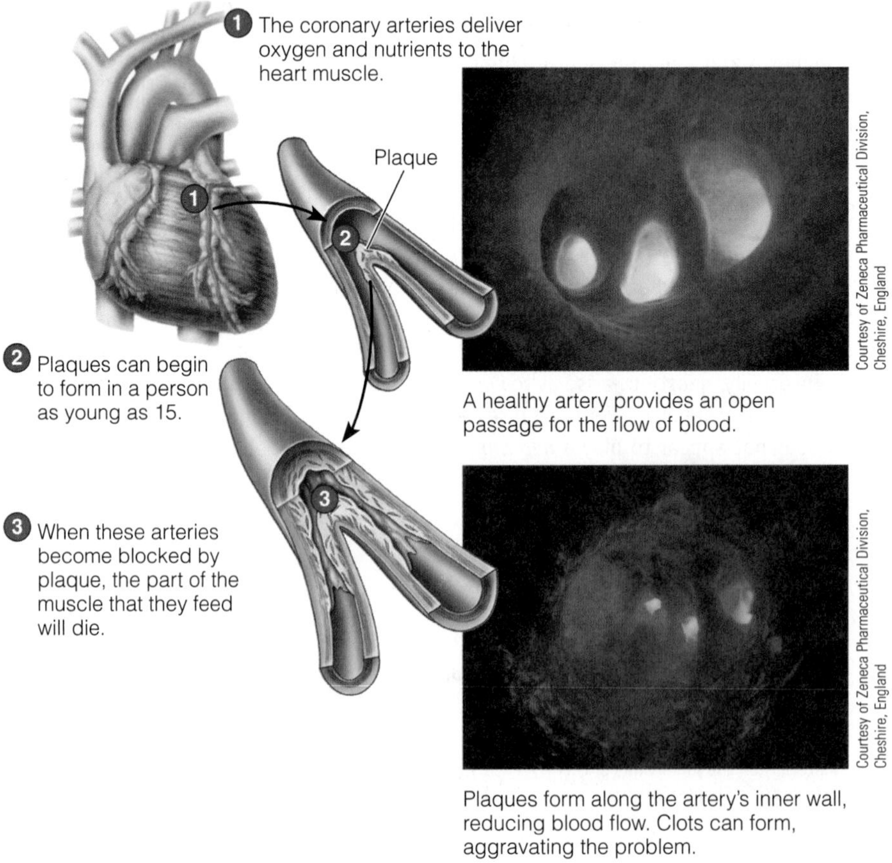
1 The coronary arteries deliver oxygen and nutrients to the heart muscle.
Plaque
1
2
2 Plaques can begin to form in a person as young as 15.
3
3 When these arteries become blocked by plaque, the part of the muscle that they feed will die.
Courtesy of Zeneca Pharmaceutical Division, Cheshire, England
A healthy artery provides an open passage for the flow of blood.
Courtesy of Zeneca Pharmaceutical Division, Cheshire, England
Plaques form along the artery's inner wall, reducing blood flow. Clots can form, aggravating the problem.

TABLE H17-1 Cholesterol Values for Children and Adolescents

Disease Risk	Total Cholesterol (mmol/L)	LDL Cholesterol (mmol/L)
Acceptable	<4.4	<2.8
Borderline	4.4–5.1	2.8–3.3
High	≥5.2	≥3.4

NOTE: Adult values appear in Chapter 19.

and adolescents who are overweight or obese; those whose parents (or grandparents) have premature (≤55 years of age for men and ≤65 years of age for women) heart disease; those whose parents have elevated blood cholesterol; those who have other risk factors for heart disease such as hypertension, cigarette smoking, or diabetes; and those whose family history is unavailable.[14] Because blood cholesterol in children is a good predictor of adult values, some experts recommend universal screening for all children, and particularly for those who are overweight, smoke, are sedentary, or consume diets high in saturated fat.

Early—but not advanced—atherosclerotic lesions are reversible, making screening and education a high priority. Both those with family histories of heart disease and those with multiple risk factors need intervention. Children with the highest risks of developing heart disease are sedentary and obese, with high blood pressure and high blood cholesterol. In contrast, children with the lowest risks of heart disease are physically active and of normal weight, with low blood pressure and favourable lipid profiles. Routine pediatric care should identify these known risk factors and provide intervention when needed.

Blood Pressure

Pediatricians routinely monitor blood pressure in children and adolescents. High blood pressure may signal an underlying disease or the early onset of hypertension. Hypertension accelerates the development of atheroscerlosis.[15] Diagnosing hypertension in children and adolescents requires consideration of age, gender, and height and cannot be assessed using simple tables applied to adults.[16]

Like atherosclerosis and high blood cholesterol, hypertension may develop in the first decades of life, especially among obese children, and worsen with time. Children can control their hypertension by participating in regular aerobic activity and by losing weight or maintaining their weight as they grow taller. Restricting dietary sodium also causes an immediate drop in most children's and adolescents' blood pressure.[17]

Physical Activity

Research has also confirmed an association between blood lipids and physical activity in children, similar to that seen in adults. Physically active children have a better lipid profile and lower blood pressure than physically inactive children, and these positive findings often persist into adulthood. The *Canadian Physical Activity Guidelines, 2011,* recommendations for children and adolescents are listed in Chapter 17 on pp. 555 and 567.

Just as blood cholesterol and obesity track over the years, so does a child's level of physical activity. Those who are inactive now are likely to still be inactive years later. Similarly, those who are physically active now tend to remain so. Compared with inactive teens, those who are physically active weigh less, smoke less, eat a diet lower in saturated fats, and have better blood lipid profiles. Both obesity and blood cholesterol correlate with the inactive pastime of watching television. The message is clear: physical activity offers numerous health benefits, and children who are active today are most likely to be active for years to come.

Dietary Recommendations for Children

Regardless of family history, experts in North America agree that all children older than age 2 should eat a variety of foods and maintain desirable weight (see Table H17-2). Children (4 to 18 years of age) should receive at least 25 percent and no more than 35 percent of total energy from fat, less than 10 percent from saturated fat, and less than 300 milligrams of cholesterol per day.[18] Recommendations

TABLE H17-2 Dietary Guidelines and Strategies for Children[a]

- Balance dietary kcalories with physical activity to maintain normal growth.
- Every day, engage in 60 minutes of moderate to vigorous play or physical activity.
- Eat vegetables and fruits daily. Use fresh, frozen, and canned vegetables and fruits and serve at every meal; limit those with added fats, salt, and sugar.
- Limit juice intake (125 to 175 mL per day for children 1 to 6 years of age, 250 to 355 mL for children 7 to 18 years of age).
- Use vegetable oils (canola, soybean, olive, safflower, or other unsaturated oils) and soft margarines low in saturated fat and *trans*-fatty acids instead of butter or most other animal fats in the diet.
- Choose whole-grain breads and cereals rather than refined products; read labels and make sure that "whole grain" is the first ingredient.
- Reduce the intake of sugar-sweetened beverages and foods.
- Consume 1% and skim milk and milk products daily.
- Include two servings of fish per week, especially fatty fish such as broiled or baked salmon.
- Choose legumes and tofu in place of meat for some meals.
- Choose only lean cuts of meat and reduced-fat meat products; remove the skin from poultry.
- Use less salt, including salt from processed foods. Breads, breakfast cereals, and soups may be high in salt and/or sugar so read food labels and choose high-fibre, low-salt, low-sugar alternatives.
- Limit the intake of high-kcalorie add-ons such as gravy, Alfredo sauce, cream sauce, cheese sauce, and hollandaise sauce.
- Serve age-appropriate portion sizes on appropriately sized plates and bowls.

[a] These guidelines are for children 3 years of age and older.

SOURCES: Adapted from Health Camada, *Eating Well with Canada's Food Guide* (2007). www.hc-sc.gc.ca/fn-an/food-guide-aliment/index-eng.php, accessed September 15, 2011; American Heart Association, Samuel S. Gidding, and coauthors, Dietary recommendations for children and adolescents: A guide for practitioners, *Pediatrics* 117 (2006): 544–559.

Smoking

limiting fat and cholesterol are not intended for infants or children younger than 2 years old. Infants and toddlers need a higher percentage of fat to support their rapid growth. For children between 1 year of age and 2 years of age who are overweight or obese, or have a family history of heart disease, obesity, or abnormal blood lipids, however, the use of 2% milk is recommended.[19]

Moderation, Not Deprivation

Healthy children older than age 2 can begin the transition to eating according to recommendations by eating fewer foods high in saturated fat and selecting more fruits and vegetables. Healthy meals can occasionally include moderate amounts of a child's favourite foods, even if they are high in saturated fat such as french fries and ice cream. A steady diet from some "children's menus" in restaurants such as chicken nuggets, hot dogs, and french fries easily exceeds a prudent intake of saturated fat, *trans* fat, and kcalories, however, and invites both nutrient shortages and weight gains.[20] Fortunately, most restaurants chains are changing children's menus to include steamed vegetables, fruit cups, and broiled or grilled chicken—additions welcomed by busy parents who often dine out or purchase take-out foods.

Other fatty foods, such as nuts, vegetable oils, and some varieties of fish such as tuna or salmon, contribute essential fatty acids. Low-fat or 1% milk and milk products also deserve special attention in a child's diet for the needed calcium and other nutrients they supply.[21]

Parents and caregivers play a key role in helping children establish healthy eating habits. Balanced meals need to provide lean meat, poultry, fish, and legumes; fruits and vegetables; whole grains; and 1% milk products. Such meals can provide enough energy and nutrients to support growth and maintain blood cholesterol within a healthy range.

Pediatricians warn parents to avoid extremes. Although intentions may be good, excessive food restriction may create nutrient deficiencies and impair growth. Furthermore, parental control over eating may instigate battles and foster attitudes about foods that can lead to inappropriate eating behaviours.

Diet First, Drugs Later

Experts agree that children with high blood cholesterol should first be treated with diet. If high blood cholesterol persists despite dietary intervention in children 8 years of age and older, then drugs may be necessary to lower blood cholesterol. Drugs can effectively lower blood cholesterol without interfering with adolescent growth or development.[22]

Even though the focus of this text is nutrition, another risk factor for heart disease that starts in childhood and carries over into adulthood must also be addressed—cigarette smoking. It is somewhat encouraging to note that, according to Physicians for a Smoke-Free Canada, smoking amongst teenagers has declined from about 50 percent of girls and boys 15–19 years old in 1975 to about 15 percent in 2009.[23] Approximately 80 percent of all adult smokers began smoking before the age of 18.

Of those teenagers who continue smoking, half will eventually die of smoking-related causes. Efforts to teach children about the dangers of smoking need to be aggressive. Children are not likely to consider the long-term health consequences of tobacco use. They are more likely to be struck by the immediate health consequences, such as shortness of breath when playing sports, or social consequences, such as having bad breath. Whatever the context, the message to all children and teens should be clear: don't start smoking. If you've already started, quit.

In conclusion, *adult* heart disease is a major *pediatric* problem. Without intervention, some 60 million North American children are destined to suffer its consequences within the next 30 years. Optimal prevention efforts focus on children, especially on those who are overweight.[24] Just as young children receive vaccinations against infectious diseases, they need screening for, and education about, chronic diseases. Many health education programs have been implemented in schools around the country. These programs are most effective when they include education in the classroom, heart-healthy meals in the lunch room, fitness activities on the playground, and parental involvement at home.

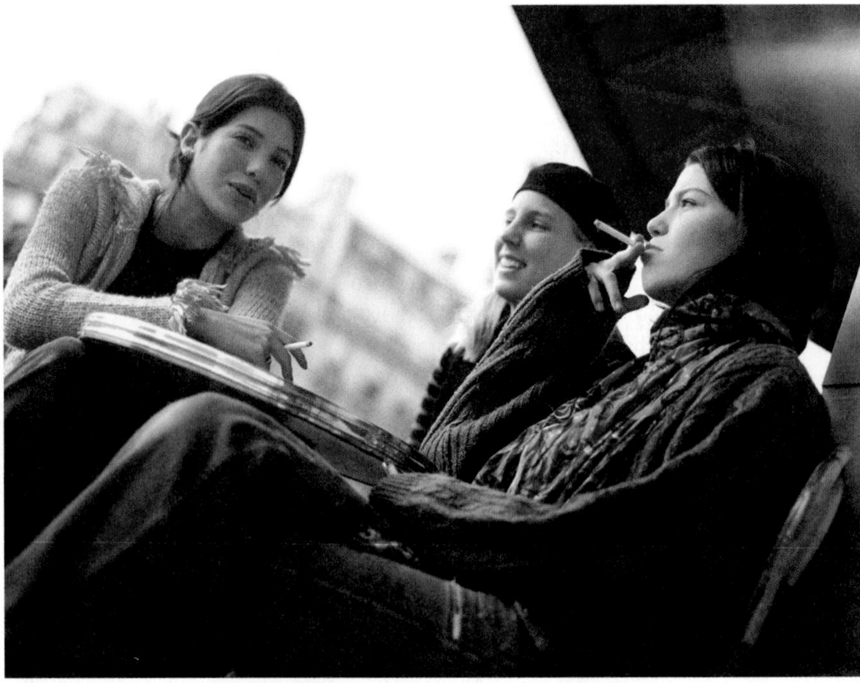

Cigarette smoking is the number-one preventable cause of deaths.

Nutrition on the Net

CENGAGENOW™
For further study of topics covered in this Highlight, log on to **www.cengage.com/sso**.

- Get weight-loss tips for children and adolescents: **www.shapedown.com**
- Visit the Nemours Foundation: **www.kidshealth.org**
- Find information on diabetes in children at the Canadian Diabetes Association: **www.diabetes.ca/diabetes-and-you/youth/diagnosis/**

References

1. D. S. Freedman and coauthors, Risk factors and adult body mass index among overweight children: The Bogalusa Heart Study, *Pediatrics* 123 (2009): 750–757; S. Cook and coauthors, Metabolic syndrome rates in United States adolescents, from the National Health and Nutrition Examination survey, 1999–2002, *Journal of Pediatrics* 152 (2008): 165–170; M. Gardner, D. W. Gardner, and J. R. Sowers, The cardiometabolic syndrome in the adolescent, *Pediatric Endocrinology Reviews* Suppl. 4 (2008): 964–968; K. L. Jones, Role of obesity in complicating and confusing the diagnosis and treatment of diabetes in children, *Pediatrics* 121 (2008): 361–368; C. L. Ogden, M. D. Carroll, and K. M. Flegal, High body mass index for age among U.S. children and adolescents, 2003–2006, *Journal of the American Medical Association* 299 (2008): 2401–2405; D. S. Ludwig, Childhood obesity: The shape of things to come, *New England Journal of Medicine* 357 (2007): 2325–2327; J. P. Kaplan, C. T. Liverman, and V. I. Kraak, eds., *Preventing Childhood Obesity: Health in the Balance* (Washington, D.C.: National Academies Press, 2005), pp. 1–20; M. L. Cruz and coauthors, Pediatric obesity and insulin resistance: Chronic disease risk and implications for treatment and prevention beyond body weight modification, *Annual Review of Nutrition* 25 (2005): 435–468.
2. M. E. Pavkov and coauthors, Effect of youth-onset type 2 diabetes mellitus on incidence of end-stage renal disease and mortality in young and middle-aged Pima Indians, *Journal of the American Medical Association* 296 (2006): 421–426.
3. Kaplan, Liverman, and Kraak, 2005.
4. W. Maziak, K. D. Ward, and M. B. Stockton, Childhood obesity: Are we missing the big picture? *Obesity Reviews* 9 (2008): 35–42; Y. Wang and T. Lobstein, Worldwide trends in childhood overweight and obesity, *International Journal of Pediatric Obesity* 1 (2006): 11–25; Cruz and coauthors, 2005.
5. Freedman and coauthors, 2009; H. Zhu and coauthors, Relationships of cardiovascular phenotypes with healthy weight, at risk of overweight, and overweight in U.S. youths, *Pediatrics* 121 (2008): 115–122; D. S. Freedman and coauthors, Cardiovascular risk factors and excess adiposity among overweight children and adolescents: The Bogalusa Heart Study, *Journal of Pediatrics* 150 (2007): 12–17.
6. S. E. Barlow, and the Expert Committee, Expert Committee recommendations regarding the prevention, assessment, and treatment of child and adolescent overweight and obesity: Summary report, *Pediatrics* 120 (2007): S164–S192; Ludwig, 2007.
7. Ludwig, 2007.
8. Jones, 2008; T. S. Hannon, G. Rao, and S. A. Arslanian, Childhood obesity and type 2 diabetes mellitus, *Pediatrics* 116 (2005): 473–480; Cruz and coauthors, 2005.
9. Jones, 2008; Hannon, Rao, and Arslanian, 2005; Cruz and coauthors, 2005.
10. Cook and coauthors, 2008; G. S. Boyd and coauthors, Effect of obesity and high blood pressure on plasma lipid levels in children and adolescents, *Pediatrics* 116 (2005): 473–480.
11. Zhu and coauthors, 2008; Freedman and coauthors, 2007; D. R. Thompson and coauthors, Childhood overweight and cardiovascular disease risk factors: The National Heart, Lung, and Blood Institute Growth and Health Study, *Journal of Pediatrics* 150 (2007): 18–25; J. Botton and coauthors, Cardiovascular risk factor levels and their relationships with overweight and fat distribution in children: The Fleurbaix Laventie Ville Sante II Study, *Metabolism* 56 (2007): 614–622; J. C. Eisenmann and coauthors, Fatness, fitness, and cardiovascular disease risk factors in children and adolescents, *Medicine & Science in Sports & Exercise* 39 (2007): 1251–1256.
12. S. R. Daniels, F. R. Greer, and the Committee on Nutrition, Lipid screening and cardiovascular health in childhood, *Pediatrics* 122 (2008): 198–208.
13. Freedman and coauthors, 2009; Cook and coauthors, 2008; Botton and coauthors, 2007; Thompson and coauthors, 2007.
14. Daniels, Greer, and the Committee on Nutrition, 2008.
15. National High Blood Pressure Education Program Working Group on High Blood Pressure in Children and Adolescents, The fourth report on the diagnosis, evaluation, and treatment of high blood pressure in children and adolescents, *Pediatrics* 114 (2004): 555S–576S.
16. National High Blood Pressure Education Program Working Group on High Blood Pressure in Children and Adolescents, 2004.
17. F. J. He and G. A. MacGregor, Importance of salt in determining blood pressure in children: Meta-analysis of controlled trials, *Hypertension* 48 (2006): 861–869.
18. Committee on Dietary Reference Intakes, *Dietary Reference Intakes for Energy, Carbohydrate, Fiber, Fat, Fatty Acids, Cholesterol, Protein, and Amino Acids* (Washington, D.C.: National Academies Press, 2005), pp. 769–879.
19. Daniels, Greer, and the Committee on Nutrition, 2008.
20. L. Johnson and coauthors, Energy-dense, low-fiber, high-fat dietary pattern is associated with increased fatness in childhood, *American Journal of Clinical Nutrition* 87 (2008): 846–854; J. Hurley and B. Liebman, Kids' cuisine: "What would you like with your fries?" *Nutrition Action Healthletter* 31 (2004): 12–15.
21. F. R. Greer, N. F. Krebs, and the Committee on Nutrition, American Academy of Pediatrics, Optimizing bone health and calcium intakes of infants, children, and adolescents, *Pediatrics* 117 (2006): 578–585.
22. Daniels, Greer, and the Committee on Nutrition, 2008.
23. Physicians for a Smoke-Free Canada, Smoking in Canada (Feb. 2011). www.smoke-free.ca/factsheets/pdf/prevalence.pdf, accessed September 15, 2011; Centers for Disease Control and Prevention, Youth tobacco surveillance: United States, 2001–2002, *Morbidity and Mortality Weekly Report* 55 (2006): entire supplement.
24. Daniels, Greer, and the Committee on Nutrition, 2008; Barlow and the Expert Committee, 2007.

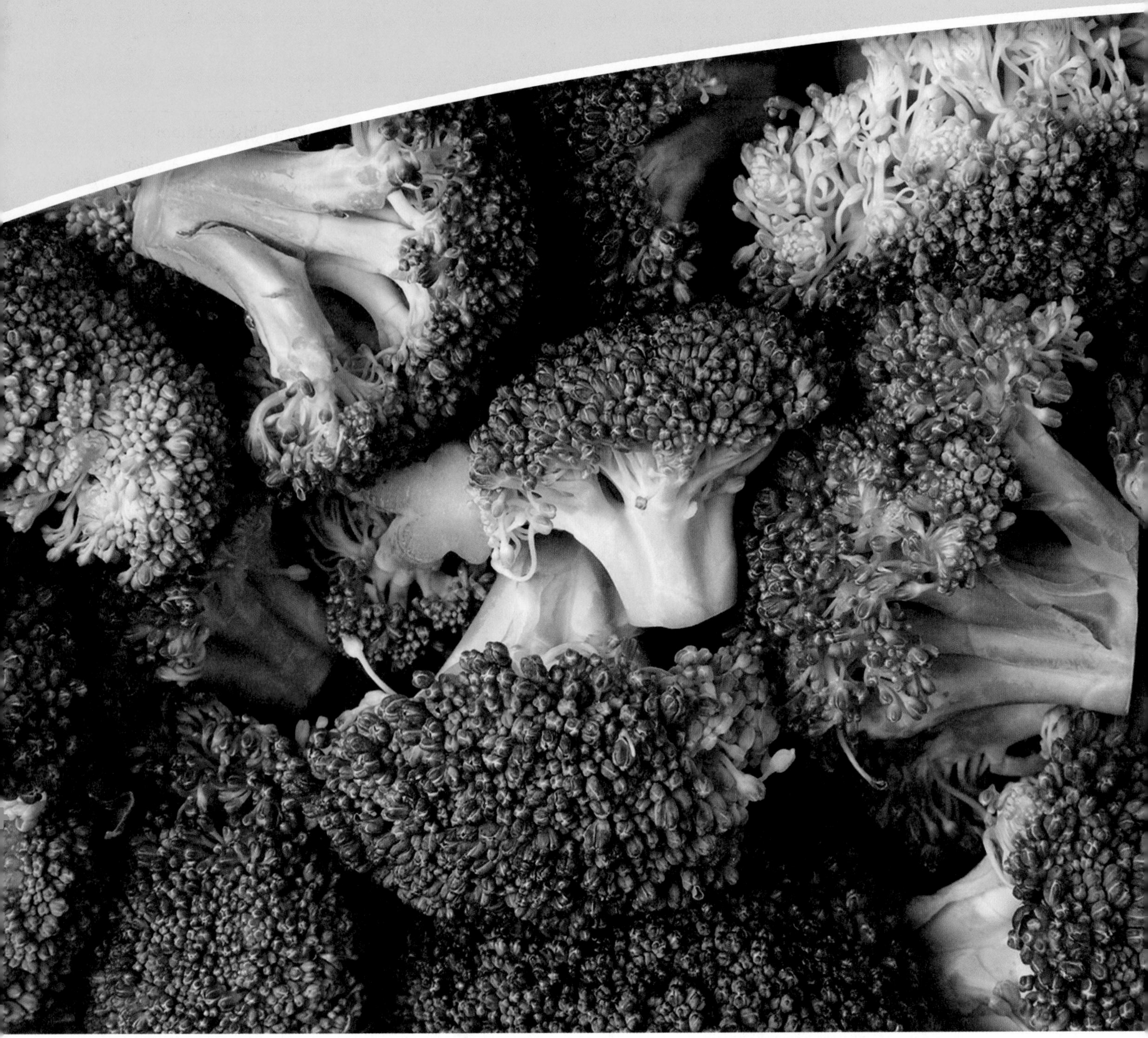

Kongsak/shutterstock

Nutrition in Your Life

CENGAGENOW™

Throughout this chapter, the CengageNOW logo indicates an opportunity for online self-study, linking you to interactive tutorials, activities, and videos to increase your understanding of chapter concepts.
www.cengage.com/sso

Take a moment to envision yourself at age 60, 75, or even 90. Are you physically fit and healthy? Can you see yourself walking on the beach with friends or tossing a ball with children? Are you able to climb stairs and carry your own groceries? Importantly, are you enjoying life? If you're lucky, you will enjoy old age in good health. Making nutritious foods and physical activities a priority in your life can help bring rewards of continued health and enjoyment throughout life.

CHAPTER 18

Life Cycle Nutrition: Adulthood and the Later Years

CHAPTER OUTLINE

Wise food choices, made throughout adulthood, can support a person's ability to meet physical, emotional, and mental challenges and to enjoy freedom from disease.[1] Two goals motivate adults to pay attention to their diets: promoting health and slowing aging. Much of this text has focused on nutrition to support health, and Chapter 19 features prevention of chronic diseases such as cancer and heart disease. This chapter focuses on aging and the nutrition needs of older adults. As you will see, the same diet and behaviours that reduce disease risks also slow aging.

The Canadian population is growing older. The majority is now middle-aged, and the percentage of seniors making up the population is increasing, as Figure 18-1 (p. 588) shows. In 1921, only 1 out of 20 people was 65 or older. In 2001, 1 out of 8 had reached age 65. Projections for 2031 are 1 out of 5. Also note that the vast majority of our seniors (5 out of 6) live in our four most populated provinces: Ontario, Quebec, British Columbia, and Alberta.[2]

Our society uses the arbitrary age of 65 years ♦ to define the transition point between middle age and old age, but growing "old" happens day by day, with changes occurring gradually over time. Since 1950 the population of those older than 65 has almost tripled. Remarkably, the fastest-growing age group has been people older than 85 years; since 1950 their numbers have increased sevenfold. The number of people in Canada age 100 or older increased nearly 50 percent (from ~3000 to ~4500) between 1996 and 2006. Similar trends are occurring in populations worldwide.

♦ Commonly used age groups:
- young old (65–74 years)
- old old (75–84 years)
- oldest old (≥85 years)

Life expectancy in the Canada is 83 years for women, 79 years for men. All of these record highs are much higher than the average life expectancy of 47 years for men and 50 years for women in 1900.[3] Women who live to 70 can expect to survive an additional 20 years, on average; men, an additional 16 years. Advances in medical science—antibiotics and other treatments—are largely responsible for almost doubling the life expectancy in the 20th century. Improved nutrition and an abundant food supply have also

life expectancy: the average number of years lived by people in a given society.

FIGURE 18-1 The Aging of the Canadian Population

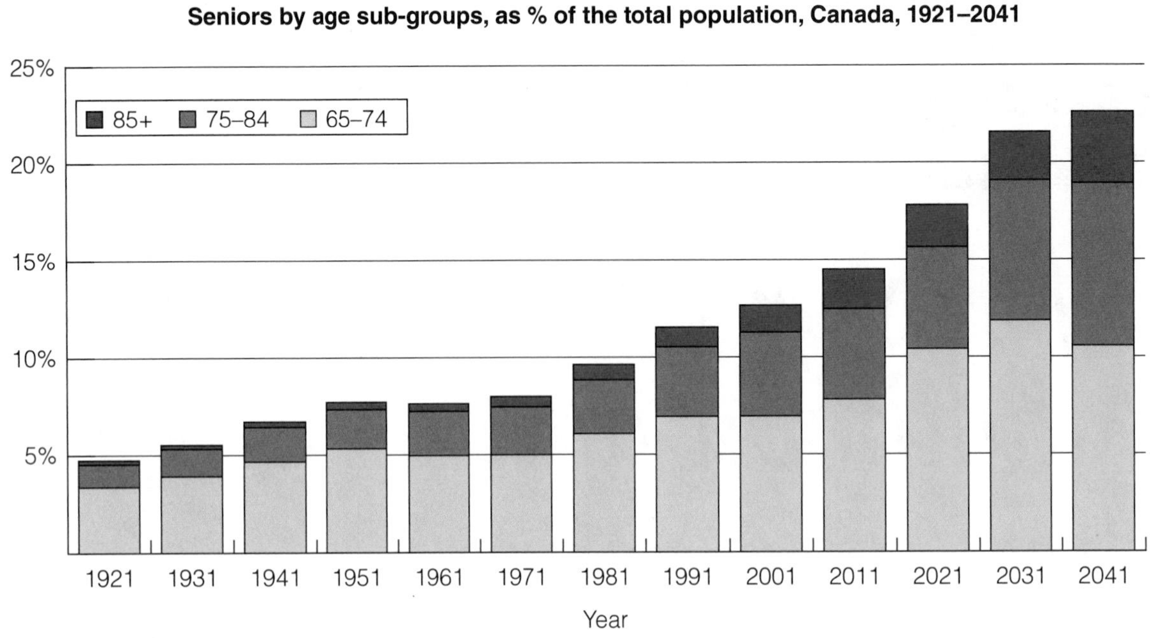
Seniors by age sub-groups, as % of the total population, Canada, 1921–2041
25%
20%
15%
10%
5%
85+
75–84
65–74
1921
1931
1941
1951
1961
1971
1981
1991
2001
2011
2021
2031
2041
Year

contributed to lengthening life expectancy. Ironically, an abundant food supply has also jeopardized the chances of lengthening life expectancy as obesity rates increase.[4]

The **life span** has not lengthened as dramatically; human **longevity** appears to have an upper limit. The maximum potential human life span is currently about 130 years. The verifiably oldest person died in 1997 at age 122. With recent advances in medical technology and genetic knowledge, researchers may one day be able to extend the life span even further by slowing, or perhaps preventing, aging and its accompanying diseases.[5]

Nutrition and Longevity

Research in the field of aging is active—and difficult. Researchers are challenged by the diversity of older adults. When older adults experience health problems, it is hard to know whether to attribute these problems to genetics, aging, or environmental factors such as nutrition. The idea that nutrition can influence the aging process is particularly appealing because people can control and change their eating habits. The questions being asked include:

- To what extent is aging inevitable, and can it be slowed through changes in lifestyle and environment?
- What role does nutrition play in the aging process, and what role can it play in slowing aging?

With respect to the first question, it seems that aging is an inevitable, natural process, programmed into the genes at conception. People can, however, slow the process within genetic limits by adopting healthy lifestyle habits such as eating nutritious foods and engaging in physical activities. In fact, an estimated 70 to 80 percent of the average person's life expectancy may depend on individual health-related behaviours; genes determine the remaining 20 to 30 percent.

With respect to the second question, good nutrition helps to maintain a healthy body and can therefore ease the aging process in many significant ways. Clearly, nutrition can improve the **quality of life** in the later years.

life span: the maximum number of years of life attainable by a member of a species.

longevity: long duration of life.

quality of life: a person's perceived physical and mental well-being.

Observation of Older Adults

The strategies adults use to meet the two goals mentioned at the start of this chapter—promoting health and slowing aging—are actually very much the same. What to eat, how physically active to be, and other lifestyle choices greatly influence both physical health and the aging process.

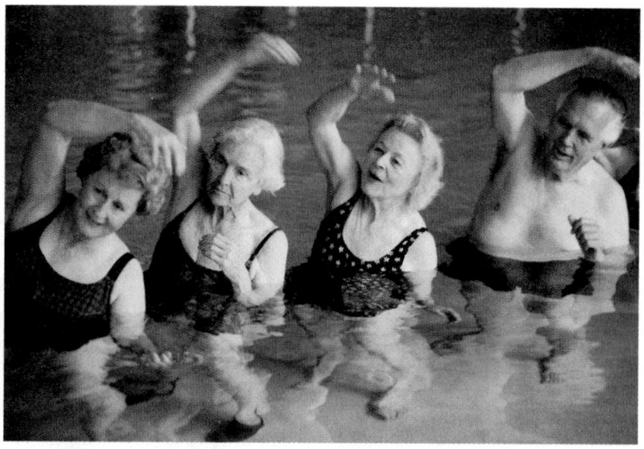

Purestock/Getty Images

Growing old can be enjoyable for people who take care of their health and live each day fully.

Healthy Habits A person's **physiological age** reflects his or her health status and may or may not reflect the person's **chronological age.** Quite simply, some people seem younger, ♦ and others older, than their years. Six lifestyle behaviours seem to have the greatest influence on people's health and therefore on their physiological age:[6]

- Eating well-balanced meals rich in fruits and vegetables regularly
- Engaging in physical activity regularly
- Not smoking
- Not using alcohol, or using it in moderation
- Maintaining a healthy body weight
- Sleeping regularly and adequately

♦ Older adults who lead active lives contrary to stereotypes of diminished abilities are sometimes referred to as the *young old.*

Over the years, the effects of these lifestyle choices accumulate—that is, people who follow most of these practices live longer and have fewer disabilities as they age. They are in better health, even when older in chronological age, than people who do not adopt these behaviors.[7] Even though people cannot change their birth dates, they may be able to add years to, and enhance the quality of, their lives.[8] Physical activity seems to be most influential in preventing or slowing the many changes that define a stereotypical "old" person. After all, many of the physical limitations that accompany aging occur because people become inactive, not because they become older.

Physical Activity The many remarkable benefits of regular physical activity outlined in Chapter 15 are not limited to the young. Compared with those who are inactive, older adults who are active weigh less; have greater flexibility, more endurance, better balance, and better health; and live longer.[9] They reap additional benefits from various activities as well: aerobic activities improve cardiorespiratory endurance, blood pressure, and blood lipid concentrations; moderate endurance activities improve the quality of sleep; and strength training improves posture and mobility. ♦ In fact, regular physical activity is the most powerful predictor of a person's mobility in the later years. Physical activity also increases blood flow to the brain, thereby preserving mental ability, alleviating depression, supporting independence, and improving quality of life.[11]

♦ Canadian Health Measures Survey (2007–2009) data for those 60–69 years old:[10]

- females were significantly more flexible than males
- Percentage able to complete 25 partial curl-ups in 1 minute: females 4%, males 12%
- males had significantly greater hand grip strength than females

Muscle mass and muscle strength tend to decline with aging, making older people vulnerable to falls and immobility. Falls are a major cause of fear, injury, disability, and even death among older adults.[12] Many lose their independence as a result of falls. Regular physical activity tones, firms, and strengthens muscles, helping to improve balance, restore confidence, reduce the risk of falling, and lessen the risk of injury should a fall occur.

Even without a fall, older adults may become so weak that they can no longer perform life's daily tasks, such as climbing stairs, carrying packages, and opening jars. Resistance training helps older adults to maintain independence by improving muscle strength to perform these tasks. Even in frail, elderly people older than 85 years of age, strength training not only improves balance, muscle strength, and mobility, but it also increases energy expenditure and energy intake, thereby enhancing nutrient intakes. This finding highlights another reason to be physically active: a person expending energy can afford to eat more food and thus receives more nutrients. People who are committed to an ongoing fitness program can benefit from higher energy and nutrient intakes and still maintain their body weights.

Ideally, physical activity should be part of each day's schedule and should be intense enough to prevent muscle atrophy and to speed the heartbeat and

physiological age: a person's age as estimated from her or his body's health and probable life expectancy.

chronological age: a person's age in years from his or her date of birth.

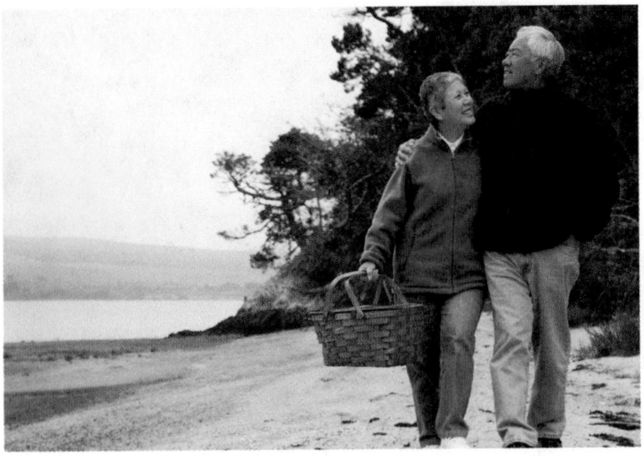

© Kris Timken/Blend Images/Corbis

Regular physical activity promotes a healthy, independent lifestyle.

respiration rate. Although aging reduces both speed and endurance to some degree, older adults can still train and achieve exceptional performances. Healthy older adults who have not been active can ease into a suitable routine, becoming as physically active as their abilities allow. They can start by walking short distances until they are walking at least 10 minutes continuously and then gradually increase their distance to add up to at least 150 minutes per a week. Figure 18-2 provides exercise goals and guidelines for seniors.[13] People with medical conditions should check with a physician before beginning an exercise routine, as should sedentary men older than 40 and sedentary women older than 50 who want to participate in a vigorous program.

Physical Activity Guidance for Canadians

Older adults should participate in regular physical activity to reduce the functional declines associated with aging and to achieve the other benefits of physical activity identified for all adults.

Manipulation of Diet

In their efforts to understand longevity, researchers have not only observed people, but they have also manipulated influencing factors, such as diet, in animals. This research has given rise to some interesting and suggestive findings.

Energy Restriction in Animals Animals live longer and have fewer age-related diseases when their energy intakes are restricted. These life-prolonging benefits become evident when the diet provides enough food to prevent malnutrition and an energy intake of about 70 percent of normal; benefits decline as the age of starting the energy restriction is delayed.[14] Exactly how energy restriction prolongs life remains unexplained, although gene activity appears to play a key role. The genetic activity of old mice differs from that of young mice, with some genes becoming more active with age and others less active. With an energy-restricted diet, many of the genetic activities of older mice revert to those of younger mice. These "slow-aging" genetic changes are apparent in as little as one month on an energy-restricted, but still nutritionally adequate, diet.

The consequences of energy restriction in animals include a delay in the onset, or prevention, of chronic diseases such as cancer and atherosclerosis and age-related conditions such as neuron degeneration; prolonged growth and development; and improved blood glucose, insulin sensitivity, and blood lipids.[15] In addition, energy metabolism slows and body temperature drops—indications of a reduced rate of oxygen consumption. Oxygen consumption is lower in mice prone to obesity, and they benefit more from energy-restricted diets than other mice.[16] As Highlight 12 explains, the use of oxygen during energy metabolism produces free radicals, which have been implicated in the aging process. Restricting energy intake in animals, not only produces fewer free radicals, but also increases antioxidant activity and enhances DNA repair. Reducing oxidative stress may at least partially explain how restricting energy intake lengthens life expectancy.

Interestingly, longevity appears to depend on restricting energy intake and not on the amount of body fat. Genetically obese rats live longer when given a restricted diet even though their body fat is similar to that of other rats allowed to eat freely.

♦ kCalorie-restricted research has been conducted on various species, including mice, rats, rhesus monkeys, cynomolgus monkeys, spiders, and fish.

Energy Restriction in Human Beings Research on a variety of animals ♦ confirms the relationship between energy restriction and longevity. Applying the results of animal studies to human beings is problematic, however, and conducting studies on human beings raises numerous questions—beginning with how to define energy restriction. Does it mean eating less or just weighing less? Is it less than you want or less than the average? Does eating less have to result in weight loss?

FIGURE 18-2 ***Canadian Physical Activity Guidelines* for Older Adults—65 Years and Older**

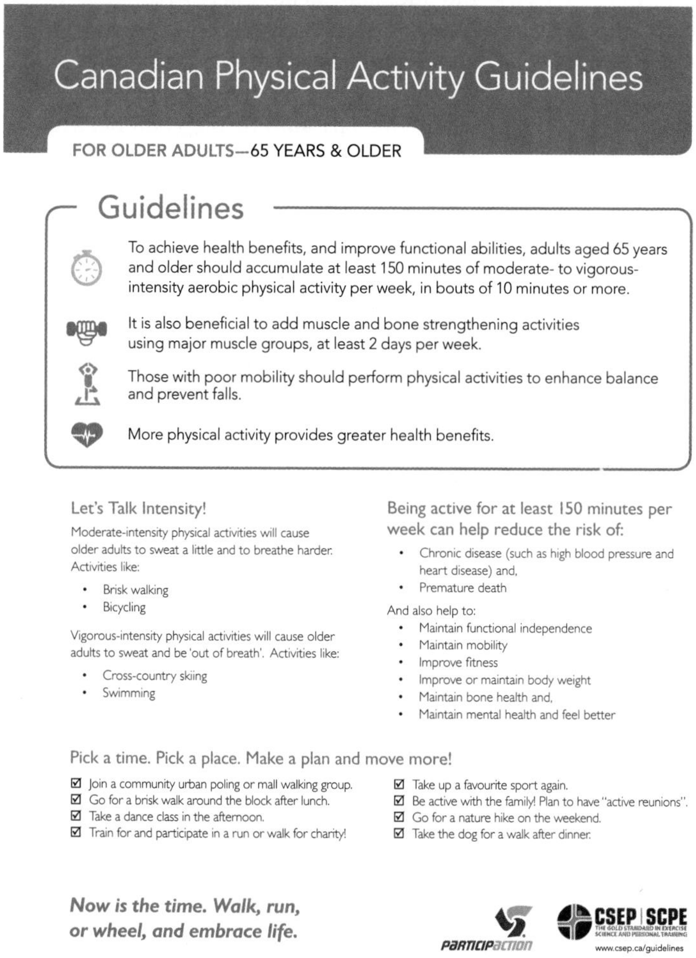
Canadian Physical Activity Guidelines
FOR OLDER ADULTS—65 YEARS & OLDER
Guidelines
To achieve health benefits, and improve functional abilities, adults aged 65 years and older should accumulate at least 150 minutes of moderate- to vigorous-intensity aerobic physical activity per week, in bouts of 10 minutes or more.
It is also beneficial to add muscle and bone strengthening activities using major muscle groups, at least 2 days per week.
Those with poor mobility should perform physical activities to enhance balance and prevent falls.
More physical activity provides greater health benefits.
Let's Talk Intensity!
Moderate-intensity physical activities will cause older adults to sweat a little and to breathe harder. Activities like:
• Brisk walking
• Bicycling
Vigorous-intensity physical activities will cause older adults to sweat and be 'out of breath'. Activities like:
• Cross-country skiing
• Swimming
Being active for at least 150 minutes per week can help reduce the risk of:
• Chronic disease (such as high blood pressure and heart disease) and,
• Premature death
And also help to:
• Maintain functional independence
• Maintain mobility
• Improve fitness
• Improve or maintain body weight
• Maintain bone health and,
• Maintain mental health and feel better
Pick a time. Pick a place. Make a plan and move more!
☑ Join a community urban poling or mall walking group.
☑ Go for a brisk walk around the block after lunch.
☑ Take a dance class in the afternoon.
☑ Train for and participate in a run or walk for charity!
☑ Take up a favourite sport again.
☑ Be active with the family! Plan to have "active reunions".
☑ Go for a nature hike on the weekend.
☑ Take the dog for a walk after dinner.
Now is the time. Walk, run, or wheel, and embrace life.
PARTICIPACTION
CSEP | SCPE
THE GOLD STANDARD IN EXERCISE SCIENCE AND PERSONAL TRAINING
www.csep.ca/guidelines

SOURCE: Canadian Physical Activity Guidelines, © 2011. Used with permission from the Canadian Society for Exercise Physiology, www.csep.ca/guidelines.

Does it matter whether weight loss results from more exercise or from less food? Or whether weight loss is intentional or unintentional? Answers await research.

Extreme starvation to extend life, like any extreme, is rarely, if ever, worth the price. Hunger is persistent when energy is restricted by 30 percent. Furthermore, using animal data to extrapolate to humans, researchers estimate that it would take 30 years of such energy-restricted dieting to increase life expectancy by less than 3 years.[17]

Moderation, on the other hand, may be valuable. Many of the physiological responses to energy restriction seen in animals also occur in people whose intakes are *moderately* restricted. When people cut back on their usual energy intake by 10 to 20 percent, ♦ body weight, body fat, and blood pressure drop, and blood lipids and insulin response improve—favourable changes for preventing chronic diseases.[18] Some research suggests that fasting on alternative days may provide similar benefits.[19]

♦ For perspective, a person with a usual energy intake of 2000 kcalories might cut back to 1600 to 1800 kcalories.

The reduction in oxidative damage that occurs with energy restriction in animals also occurs in people whose diets include antioxidant nutrients and phytochemicals. Diets, such as the Mediterranean diet, which include an abundance of fruits, vegetables, olive oil, and red wine—with their array of phytochemicals that have antioxidant activity—support good health and long life. Clearly, nutritional adequacy is essential to living a long and healthy life.

IN SUMMARY Life expectancy in Canada increased dramatically in the 20th century. Factors that enhance longevity include limited or no alcohol use, regular balanced meals, weight control, abstinence from smoking, regular physical activity, and adequate sleep. Energy restriction in animals seems to lengthen their lives. Whether such dietary intervention in human beings is beneficial remains unknown. At the very least, nutrition—especially when combined with regular physical activity—can influence aging and longevity in human beings by supporting good health and preventing disease.

The Aging Process

As people get older, each person becomes less and less like anyone else. The older people are, the more time has elapsed for such factors as nutrition, genetics, physical activity, and everyday **stress** to influence physical and psychological aging.

Stress contributes to a variety of age-related diseases.[20] Both physical **stressors** (such as alcohol abuse, other drug abuse, smoking, pain, and illness) and psychological stressors (such as exams, divorce, moving, and the death of a loved one) elicit the body's **stress response.** The body responds to such stressors with an elaborate series of physiological steps, as the nervous and hormonal systems bring about defensive readiness in every body part. These effects favour physical action—the classic fight-or-flight response. Prolonged or severe stress can drain the body of its reserves and leave it weakened, aged, and vulnerable to illness, especially if physical action is not taken. As people age, they lose their ability to adapt to both external and internal disturbances. When disease strikes, the reduced ability to adapt makes the aging individual more vulnerable to death than a younger person. Measures to preserve health forestall disease, disability, and death.[21]

Because the stress response is mediated by hormones, it differs between men and women. The fight-or-flight response may be more typical of men than of women. Women's reactions to stress more typically follow a pattern of "tend-and-befriend." Women *tend* by nurturing and protecting themselves and their children. These actions promote safety and reduce stress. Women *befriend* by creating and maintaining a social group that can help in the process.

Highlight 12 describes the oxidative stresses and cellular damage that occur when free radicals exceed the body's ability to defend itself. Increased free-radical activity and decreased antioxidant protection are common features of aging—and foods rich in antioxidants seem to help slow the aging process and improve cognition.[22] Such findings seem to suggest that the fountain of youth may actually be a cornucopia of fruits and vegetables rich in antioxidants. (Return to Highlight 12 for more details on the antioxidant action of fruits and vegetables in defending against oxidative stress.)

Physiological Changes

As aging progresses, inevitable changes in each of the body's organs contribute to the body's declining function. These physiological changes influence nutrition status, just as growth and development do in the earlier stages of the life cycle.

Body Weight Twenty-four percent of older adults (74 plus) Canada are now considered obese. Chapter 8 presents the many health problems that accompany obesity and the BMI guidelines for a healthy body weight (18.5–24.9). These guidelines apply to all adults, regardless of age, but they may be too restrictive for older adults. The importance of body weight in defending against chronic diseases differs for older adults. Being moderately *overweight* may not be harmful. For adults older than 65, health risks do not become apparent until BMI reaches at least 27—and the relationship tends to diminish with age until it disappears by age 75. Older adults who are *obese*, however, face serious medical complications and can significantly improve their quality of life with weight loss.[23]

stress: any threat to a person's well-being; a demand placed on the body to adapt.

stressors: environmental elements, physical or psychological, that cause stress.

stress response: the body's response to stress, mediated by both nerves and hormones.

For some older adults, a low body weight may be more detrimental than a high one. Low body weight often reflects malnutrition and the trauma associated with a fall. Many older adults experience unintentional weight loss, in large part because of an inadequate food intake.[24] Without adequate nutrient reserves, an underweight person may be unprepared to fight against diseases. For underweight people, even a slight weight loss (5 percent) increases the likelihood of disease and premature death, making every meal a life-saving event. Snacking between meals can help older adults obtain needed nutrients and energy.[25]

Body Composition In general, older people tend to lose bone and muscle and gain body fat. Many of these changes occur because some hormones that regulate appetite and metabolism become less active with age, whereas others become more active.*

Loss of muscle, known as **sarcopenia**, can be significant in the later years, and its consequences can be quite dramatic (see Figure 18-3). As muscles diminish and weaken, people lose the ability to move and maintain balance—making falls likely. The limitations that accompany the loss of muscle mass and strength play a key role in the diminishing health that often accompanies aging.[26] Optimal nutrition with sufficient protein and regular physical activity can help maintain muscle mass and strength and minimize the changes in body composition associated with aging.[27]

FIGURE 18-3 Sarcopenia

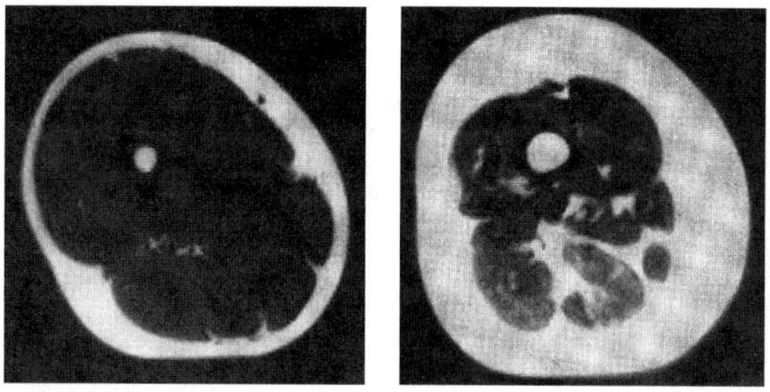
Courtesy of Dr. William Evans (both)

These cross sections of two women's thighs may appear to be about the same size from the outside, but the 20-year-old woman's thigh (left) is dense with muscle tissue. The 64-year-old woman's thigh (right) has lost muscle and gained fat, changes that may be largely preventable with strength-building physical activities.

Risk factors for sarcopenia include weight loss, little physical activity, and cigarette smoking.[28] Obesity and the inflammation that accompanies it may also contribute to sarcopenia.[29]

Immunity and Inflammation As people age, the immune system loses function. As they become ill, the immune system becomes overstimulated. The combination of an inefficient and overactive response in aging—known as "inflammaging"—results in a chronic inflammation that accompanies frailty, illness, and death.[30]

Most diseases common in older adults—such as atherosclerosis, Alzheimer's disease, obesity, and rheumatoid arthritis—are different in obvious ways, but they all reflect an underlying inflammatory process.[31] Because of this association with diseases, inflammation is often perceived as a harmful process, yet it is critical in supporting health as the immune system destroys invading organisms and repairs damaged tissues.[32] Thus inflammation presents a challenge to identify factors that will both protect the beneficial effects and limit the harmful consequences.

In addition to aging and diseases, the immune system is compromised by nutrient deficiencies. Thus the combination of age, illness, and malnutrition makes older people particularly vulnerable to infectious diseases. Adding insult to injury, antibiotics often are not effective against infections in people with compromised immune systems. Consequently, infectious diseases are a major cause of death in older adults. Older adults may improve their immune system responses with regular physical activity.[33]

GI Tract In the GI tract, the intestinal wall loses strength and elasticity with age, and GI hormone secretions change. All of these actions slow motility. Constipation is much more common in the elderly than in the young. Changes in GI hormone secretions also diminish appetite, leading to decreased energy intake and unintentional weight loss.

*Causes of diminished appetite in older adults include increased cholecystokinin, leptin, and cytokines and decreased ghrelin and testosterone. Additional examples of hormones that change with age include growth hormone and androgens, which decline with advancing age, thus contributing to the decrease in lean body mass, and prolactin, which increases with age, helping to maintain body fat. Insulin sensitivity also diminishes as people grow older, most likely because of increases in body fat and decreases in physical activity.

sarcopenia (SAR-koh-PEE-nee-ah): loss of skeletal muscle mass, strength, and quality.
- **sarco** = flesh
- **penia** = loss or lack

♦ Consequences of atrophic gastritis:
- Inflamed stomach
- Increased bacterial growth
- Reduced hydrochloric acid
- Reduced intrinsic factor
- Increased risk of nutrient deficiencies, notably of vitamin B_{12}

Atrophic gastritis, a condition that affects almost one-third of those older than 60, is characterized ♦ by an inflamed stomach, bacterial overgrowth (in some cases), and a lack of hydrochloric acid and intrinsic factor. All of these can impair the digestion and absorption of nutrients, most notably, vitamin B_{12}, but also biotin, folate, calcium, iron, and zinc.

Difficulty swallowing, medically known as **dysphagia**, occurs in all age groups, but especially in the elderly. Being unable to swallow a mouthful of food can be scary, painful, and dangerous. Even swallowing liquids can be a problem for some people. Consequently, the person may eat less food and drink fewer beverages, resulting in weight loss, malnutrition, and dehydration. Dietary intervention for dysphagia is highly individualized based on the person's abilities and tolerances. The diet typically provides moist, soft-textured, tender-cooked, or pureed foods and thickened liquids.

Tooth Loss Regular dental care over a lifetime protects against tooth loss and gum disease, which are common in old age. These conditions make chewing difficult or painful. Dentures, even when they fit properly, are less effective than natural teeth, and inefficient chewing can cause choking. Inefficient chewing can also interfere with protein digestibility.[34]

♦ The medical term for lack of teeth is **edentulous** (ee-DENT-you-lus).
- **e** = without
- **dens** = teeth

People with tooth loss, ♦ gum disease, and ill-fitting dentures tend to limit their food selections to soft foods. If foods such as corn on the cob, apples, and hard rolls are replaced by creamed corn, applesauce, and rice, then nutrition status may not be greatly affected. However, when food groups are eliminated and variety is limited, poor nutrition follows. People without teeth typically eat fewer fruits and vegetables and have less variety in their diets. Consequently, they have low intakes of fibre and vitamins, which exacerbates their dental and overall health problems. To determine whether a visit to the dentist is needed, an older adult can check the conditions listed in the margin. ♦ Also, note that some Meals on Wheels programs offer "soft diet" choices to home-bound seniors who require them for dental or other reasons.

♦ Conditions requiring dental care:
Dry mouth
Eating difficulty
No dental care within two years
Tooth or mouth pain
Altered food selections
Lesions, sores, or lumps in mouth

Sensory Losses and Other Physical Problems Sensory losses and other physical problems can also interfere with an older person's ability to obtain adequate nourishment. Failing eyesight, for example, can make driving to the grocery store impossible and shopping for food a frustrating experience. It may become so difficult to read food labels and count money that the person doesn't buy needed foods. Carrying bags of groceries may be an unmanageable task. Similarly, a person with limited mobility may find cooking and cleaning up too hard to do. Not too surprisingly, the prevalence of undernutrition is high among those who are homebound.

Sensory losses can also interfere with a person's ability or willingness to eat. Taste and smell sensitivities tend to diminish with age and may make eating less enjoyable. If a person eats less, then weight loss and nutrient deficiencies may follow. Loss of vision and hearing may contribute to social isolation, and eating alone may lead to poor intake.

Other Changes

In addition to the physiological changes that accompany aging, adults change in many other ways that influence their nutrition status.[35] Psychological, economic, and social factors play big roles in a person's ability and willingness to eat.

Psychological Changes Although not an inevitable component of aging, depression is common among older adults. Depressed people, even those without disabilities, lose their ability to perform simple physical tasks. They frequently lose their appetite and the motivation to cook or even to eat. An overwhelming sense of grief and sadness at the death of a spouse, friend, or family member may leave a person, especially an elderly person, feeling powerless to overcome depression. When a person is suffering the heartache and loneliness of bereavement, cooking meals may not seem worthwhile. The support and companionship

dysphagia (dis-FAY-jah): a common term used to describe problems with swallowing.

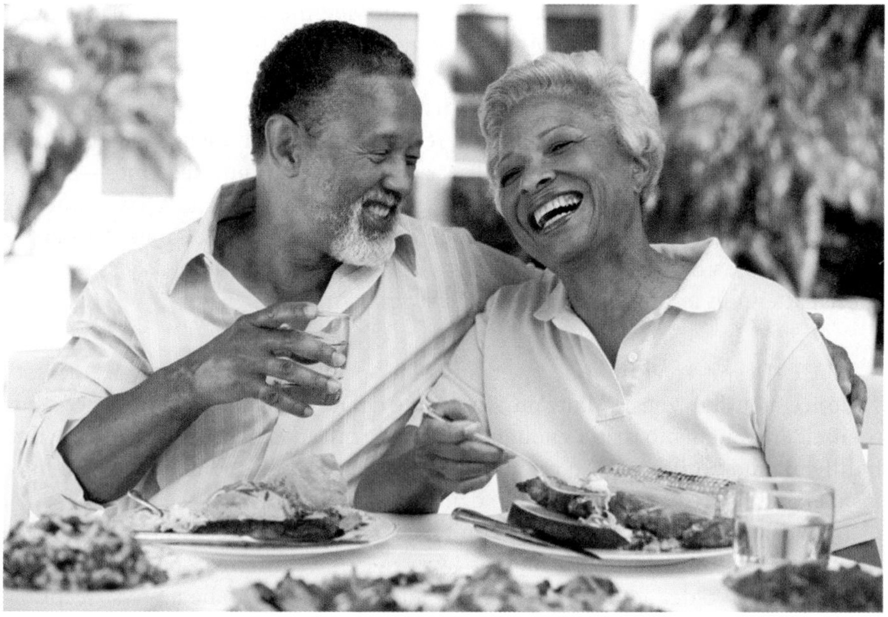
Monkey Business Images/shutterstock

Shared meals can brighten the day and enhance the appetite.

of family and friends, especially at mealtimes, can help overcome depression and enhance appetite.

Economic Changes Overall, older adults today have higher incomes than their cohorts of previous generations. Still, 10 percent of the people older than age 65 live in poverty. Factors such as living arrangements and income make significant differences in the food choices, eating habits, and nutrition status of older adults, especially those older than age 80. People of low socioeconomic means are likely to have inadequate food and nutrient intakes.

Social Changes Malnutrition among older adults is most common in hospitals and nursing homes.[36] In the community, malnutrition is most likely to occur among those living alone, especially men; those with the least education; those living in subsidized housing (an indicator of low income); and those who have recently experienced a change in lifestyle. Adults who live alone do not necessarily make poor food choices, but they often consume too little food. Loneliness is directly related to nutritional inadequacies, especially of energy intake.

IN SUMMARY **Many changes that accompany aging can impair nutrition status. Among physiological changes, hormone activity alters body composition, immune system changes raise the risk of infections, atrophic gastritis interferes with digestion and absorption, and tooth loss limits food choices. Psychological changes such as depression, economic changes such as loss of income, and social changes such as loneliness contribute to poor food intake.**

Energy and Nutrient Needs of Older Adults

Knowledge about the nutrient needs and nutrition status of older adults has grown considerably in recent years. The Dietary Reference Intakes (DRI) cluster people older than 50 into two age categories—one group of 51 to 70 years and one of 71 and older.

Setting standards for older people is difficult because individual differences become more pronounced as people grow older.[37] People start out with different genetic predispositions and ways of handling nutrients, and the effects of these

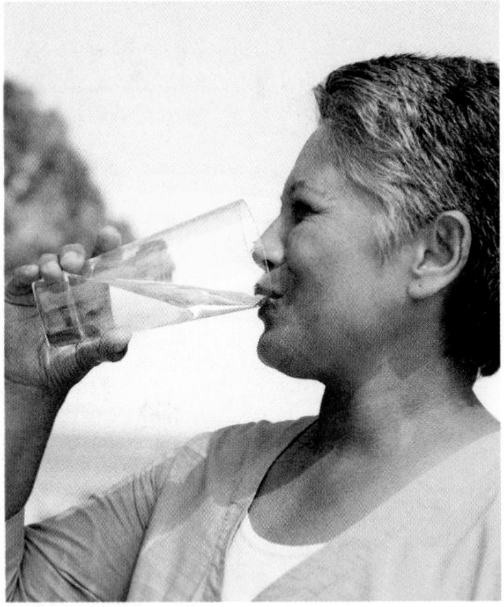
© Masterfile Corporation

To ensure adequate hydration, keep a glass of water next to you at home, drink from water fountains whenever you walk by, and put a bottle of water in your car.

differences become magnified with years of unique dietary habits. For example, one person may tend to omit fruits and vegetables from his diet, and by the time he is old, he may have a set of nutrition problems associated with a lack of fibre and antioxidants. Another person may have omitted milk and milk products all her life—her nutrition problems may be related to a lack of calcium. Also, as people age, they suffer different chronic diseases and take various medicines—both of which will affect nutrient needs. For all of these reasons, researchers have difficulty even defining "healthy aging," a prerequisite to developing recommendations to meet the "needs of practically all healthy persons." The following discussion gives special attention to the nutrients of greatest concern.

Water

Despite real fluid needs, many older people do not seem to feel thirsty or notice mouth dryness. Many nursing home employees say it is hard to persuade their elderly clients to drink enough water and fruit juices. Older adults may find it difficult and bothersome to get a drink or to get to a bathroom. Those who have lost bladder control may be afraid to drink too much water.

Dehydration is a risk for older adults.[38] Total body water decreases as people age, so even mild stresses such as fever or hot weather can precipitate rapid dehydration in older adults. Dehydrated older adults seem to be more susceptible to urinary tract infections, pneumonia, **pressure ulcers**, and confusion and disorientation. To prevent dehydration, older adults need to drink *at least* six glasses of water or other beverages every day. ♦ Emphasizing foods with high-water content, such as melons and soups, can also be helpful.

♦ Total Water (fluid) recommendation for adults 51+ yr:
- Men: 3700 mL (15 cups)/day
- Women: 2700 mL (11 cups)/day

A person we know uses this trick to ensure getting enough water: he keeps six 250 millilitre cups in the cupboard. Through the day he uses each to drink one cup of fluid, including juices and other beverages, collecting the used cups in the dish drain. (For clear soups and other hot beverages, he simply moves one of his cups for each 250 millilitres consumed from his bowl or mug.) In the afternoon, he checks the cupboard and drinks from any remaining cups. For him, drinking enough fluid has become a habit, and seldom are any cups left in the cupboard after supper.

Energy and Energy Nutrients

On average, energy needs decline an estimated 5 percent per decade. One reason is that people usually reduce their physical activity as they age, although they need not do so. Another reason is that basal metabolic rate declines 1 to 2 percent per decade in part because lean body mass and thyroid hormones diminish.[39]

The lower energy expenditure of older adults means that they need to eat less food to maintain their weights. Accordingly, the estimated energy requirements for adults decrease steadily after age 19. The accompanying "How To" explains how to estimate energy requirements for older adults.

Older adults need fewer kcalories as they age, but their nutrient needs remain high. For this reason, it is most important that they select mostly nutrient-dense foods from the *Food Guide* and obtain the number of *Food Guide* Servings depicted for their age group in Figure 18-4.[40]. There is little leeway for added sugars, solid fats, or alcohol. Such nutrient-poor selections can easily lead to weight gain and malnutrition.

Protein

Because energy needs decrease, protein must be obtained from low-kcalorie sources of high-quality protein, such as lean meats, poultry, fish, and eggs; skim and 1% milk products; and legumes. Protein is especially important for the elderly to support a healthy immune system, prevent muscle wasting, and optimize bone mass.[41] Maintaining muscles helps to support protein metabolism and immune function.

Underweight or malnourished older adults need protein- and energy-dense snacks such as hard-boiled eggs, tuna salad, peanut butter on whole-grain toast, and hearty soups. Drinking liquid nutritional formulas between meals can also boost energy and nutrient intakes. Importantly, the diet should provide enjoyment as well as nutrients.[42]

pressure ulcers: damage to the skin and underlying tissues as a result of compression and poor circulation; commonly seen in people who are bedridden or chairbound.

HOW TO Estimate Energy Requirements for Older Adults

The "How To" on p. 250 described how to estimate the energy requirements for adults using an equation that accounts for age, physical activity, weight, and height. Alternatively, energy requirements for older adults can be "guesstimated" by using the values listed in the tables in APPENDIX F for adults 30 years of age and subtracting 7 kcalories for women and 10 kcalories for men per day for each year older than 30.

For example, Table F-4 lists 2556 kcalories per day for a 30-year-old woman who is 165 centimetres (5 feet 5 inches) tall, weighs 68 kilograms (150 pounds), and has a low activity level. To estimate the energy requirements of a similar 50-year-old woman, subtract 7 kcalories per day for each year over 30:

$$50 - 30 = 20 \text{ yr}$$
$$20 \text{ yr} \times 7 \text{ kcal/day} = 140 \text{ kcal/day}$$
$$2556 \text{ kcal/day (at age 30)} - 140 \text{ kcal/day} = 2416 \text{ kcal/day (at age 50)}$$

Similarly, using Table F-5 to estimate the energy requirements of a sedentary 65-year-old man who is 180 centimetres (5 feet 11 inches) tall and weighs 113 kilograms (250 pounds), subtract 10 kcalories per day for each year over 30:

$$65 - 30 = 35 \text{ yr}$$
$$35 \text{ yr} \times 10 \text{ kcal/day} = 350 \text{ kcal/day}$$
$$3088 \text{ kcal/day (at age 30)} - 350 \text{ kcal/day} = 2738 \text{ kcal/day (at age 65)}$$

Adults between the ages of 19 and 30 can also use the values listed in the tables in APPENDIX F by adding 7 kcalories for women and 10 kcalories for men per day for each year below 30.

CENGAGENOW™
For additional practice log on to **www.cengage.com/sso**.

TRY IT Use APPENDIX F to calculate your energy requirements.

FIGURE 18-4 Recommended *Food Guide* Servings

Recommended Number of Food Guide Servings per Day

	Children			Teens		Adults			
Age in Years	2–3	4–8	9–13	14–18		19–50		51+	
Sex	Girls and Boys			Females	Males	Females	Males	Females	Males
Vegetables and Fruit	4	5	6	7	8	7–8	8–10	7	7
Grain Products	3	4	6	6	7	6–7	8	6	7
Milk and Alternatives	2	2	3–4	3–4	3–4	2	2	3	3
Meat and Alternatives	1	1	1–2	2	3	2	3	2	3

The chart above shows how many Food Guide Servings you need from each of the four food groups every day.

Having the amount and type of food recommended and following the tips in *Canada's Food Guide* will help:

- Meet your needs for vitamins, minerals, and other nutrients.
- Reduce your risk of obesity, type 2 diabetes, heart disease, certain types of cancer, and osteoporosis.
- Contribute to your overall health and vitality.

♦ **CCHS, Cycle 2.2, Nutrition (2004),[44] fibre intakes (grams/day):**

Age	Females	Males
51–70	16.6	19.0
>70	15.2	17.9

Carbohydrate and Fibre As always, abundant carbohydrate is needed to protect protein from being used as an energy source. Carbohydrate-rich foods such as legumes, vegetables, whole grains, and fruits are also rich in fibre and essential vitamins and minerals. Average fibre intakes among older adults (see margin) are lower than current recommendations (14 grams per 1000 kcalories).[43] ♦ Eating high-fibre foods and drinking water can alleviate constipation—a condition common among older adults, especially nursing home residents. Physical inactivity and medications also contribute to the high incidence of constipation.

Fat As is true for people of all ages, fat intake needs to be moderate in the diets of most older adults—enough to enhance flavours and provide valuable nutrients, but not so much as to raise the risks of atherosclerosis and other degenerative diseases. This recommendation should not be taken too far; limiting fat too severely may lead to nutrient deficiencies and weight loss—two problems that carry greater health risks in the elderly than overweight.

Vitamins and Minerals

Most people can achieve adequate vitamin and mineral intakes simply by including foods from all food groups in their diets, but older adults often omit fruits and vegetables. Similarly, few older adults consume the recommended amounts of milk or milk products.

♦ **Atrophic gastritis** is a chronic inflammation of the stomach characterized by inadequate hydrochloric acid and intrinsic factor—two key players in vitamin B_{12} absorption.

Vitamin B_{12} An estimated 10 to 30 percent of adults older than 50 have atrophic gastritis. ♦ As Chapter 10 explains, people with atrophic gastritis are particularly vulnerable to vitamin B_{12} deficiency. The bacterial overgrowth that accompanies this condition uses up the vitamin, and without hydrochloric acid and intrinsic factor, digestion and absorption of vitamin B_{12} are inefficient. Given the poor cognition, anemia, and devastating neurological effects associated with a vitamin B_{12} deficiency, an adequate intake is imperative.[45] The RDA for older adults is the same as for younger adults, but with the added suggestion to obtain most of a day's intake from vitamin B_{12}–fortified foods and supplements.[46] The bioavailability of vitamin B_{12} from these sources is better than from foods.

Dietary Guidance for Canadians

People older than age 50 should consume vitamin B_{12} from fortified foods or supplements.

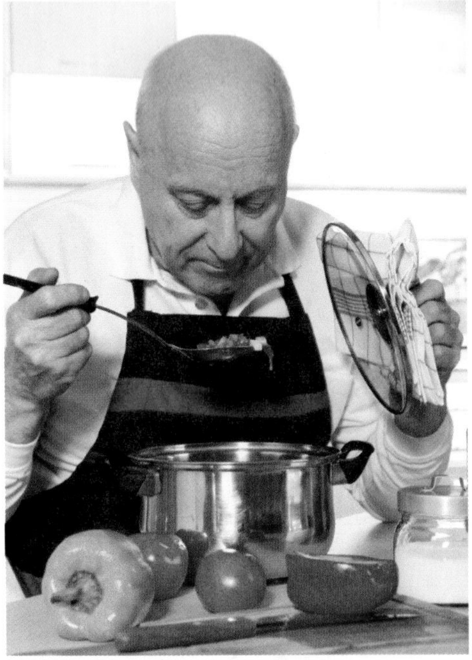

Larisa Lofitskaya/shutterstock

Taking time to nourish your body well is a gift you give yourself.

Vitamin D Vitamin D deficiency is a problem among older adults. Vitamin D–fortified milk is the most reliable source of vitamin D, but many older adults drink little or no milk. Further compromising the vitamin D status of many older people, especially those in nursing homes, is their limited exposure to sunlight. Finally, aging reduces the skin's capacity to make vitamin D and the kidneys' ability to convert it to its active form. Not only are older adults not getting enough vitamin D, but they may actually need more to improve both muscle and bone strength. To prevent bone loss and to maintain vitamin D status, especially in those who engage in minimal outdoor activity, adults 51 to 70 years old need 15 micrograms daily, and those older than 70 need 20 micrograms.[47]

Dietary Guidance for Canadians

Older adults should consume extra vitamin D from vitamin D–fortified foods and/or supplements.

Folate As is true of vitamin B_{12}, folate intakes of older adults typically fall short of recommendations. The elderly are also more likely to have medical conditions or to take medications that can compromise folate status (see Highlight 18).

♦ **CCHS, Cycle 2.2, Nutrition (2004),[49] calcium intakes (mg/day):**

Age	Females	Males
51–70	740	832
>70	690	762

Calcium Chapter and Highlight 13 emphasize the importance of abundant dietary calcium throughout life, especially for women after menopause, to protect against osteoporosis. The DRI Committee recommends 1200 milligrams of calcium daily, but the calcium intakes of older people in Canada are well below recommendations.[48] ♦ Some older adults avoid milk and milk products because they dislike these foods or associate them with stomach discomfort. Simple solutions include using calcium-fortified juices, adding powdered milk to recipes, and taking supplements. Chapter 13 offers many other strategies for including nonmilk sources of calcium for those who do not drink milk.

Iron The iron needs of men remain unchanged throughout adulthood. For women, iron needs decrease substantially when blood loss through menstruation ceases. Consequently, iron-deficiency anemia is less common in older adults than in younger people. In fact, elevated iron stores are more likely than deficiency in older people, especially those who take iron supplements, eat red meat regularly, and include vitamin C–rich fruits in their daily diet.

Nevertheless, iron deficiency may develop in older adults, especially when their food energy intakes are low. Aside from diet, two other factors may lead to iron deficiency in older people: chronic blood loss from diseases and medicines and poor iron absorption due to reduced stomach acid secretion and antacid use. Iron deficiency impairs immunity and leaves older adults vulnerable to infectious diseases. Anyone concerned with older people's nutrition should keep these possibilities in mind.

Zinc Zinc intake is commonly low in older people. Zinc deficiency can depress the appetite and blunt the sense of taste, thereby reducing food intake and worsening zinc status. Many medications that older adults commonly use can impair zinc absorption or enhance its excretion and thus lead to deficiency.

Nutrient Supplements

People judge for themselves how to manage their nutrition, and many older adults turn to dietary supplements. When recommended by a physician or registered dietitian, vitamin D and calcium supplements for osteoporosis or vitamin B_{12} for pernicious anemia may be beneficial. Many health-care professionals recommend a daily multivitamin-mineral supplement that provides 100 percent or less of the Daily Value for the listed nutrients. They reason that such a supplement is more likely to be beneficial than to cause harm. Although supplement use does help many older adults meet their calcium, vitamin C, and magnesium needs, many still do not meet the DRI recommendations even with supplementation.[50]

People with small energy allowances would do well to become more active so they can afford to eat more food. Food is the best source of nutrients for everybody. Supplements are just that—supplements to foods, not substitutes for them. For anyone who is motivated to obtain the best possible health, it is never too late to learn to eat well, drink water, exercise regularly, and adopt other lifestyle habits such as quitting smoking and moderating alcohol use.

IN SUMMARY The accompanying table provides a summary of the nutrient concerns of aging. Although some nutrients need special attention in the diet (e.g., a vitamin D supplement as identified in the *Food Guide*), supplements are not routinely recommended to otherwise healthy individuals. The ever-growing number of older people creates an urgent need to learn more about how their nutrient requirements differ from those of others and how such knowledge can enhance their health.

Nutrient	Effect of Aging	Comments
Water	Lack of thirst and decreased total body water make dehydration likely.	Mild dehydration is a common cause of confusion. Difficulty obtaining water or getting to the bathroom may compound the problem.
Energy	Need decreases as muscle mass decreases (sarcopenia).	Physical activity moderates the decline.
Fibre	Likelihood of constipation increases with low intakes and changes in the GI tract.	Inadequate water intakes and lack of physical activity, along with some medications, compound the problem.
Protein	Needs may stay the same or increase slightly.	Low-fat, high-fibre legumes and grains meet both protein and other nutrient needs.
Vitamin B_{12}	Atrophic gastritis is common.	Deficiency causes neurological damage; supplements may be needed.
Vitamin D	Increased likelihood of inadequate intake; skin synthesis declines.	Daily sunlight exposure in moderation (between mid-March and mid-October in most of Canada) or supplements may be beneficial.
Calcium	Intakes may be low; osteoporosis is common.	Stomach discomfort commonly limits milk intake; calcium substitutes or supplements may be needed.
Iron	In women, status improves after menopause; deficiencies are linked to chronic blood losses and low stomach acid output.	Adequate stomach acid is required for absorption; antacid or other medicine use may aggravate iron deficiency; vitamin C and meat increase absorption.

Nutrition-Related Concerns of Older Adults

Nutrition may play a greater role than has been realized in preventing many changes once thought to be inevitable consequences of growing older. The following discussions of vision, arthritis, and the aging brain show that nutrition may provide at least some protection against some of the conditions associated with aging.

Vision

One key aspect of healthy aging is maintaining good vision.[51] Age-related eye diseases that impair vision, such as cataract and macular degeneration, correlate with poor survival that cannot be explained by other risk factors.[52] Following a healthy diet as described by *Canada's Food Guide* is one way to protect against these age-related vision problems. Foods containing phytochemicals that act as antioxidants or anti-inflammatory agents may be especially beneficial.[53]

Cataracts

Cataracts are age-related clouding of the lenses of the eyes that impairs vision. If not surgically removed, they ultimately lead to blindness. Cataracts may develop as a result of ultraviolet light exposure, oxidative stress, injury, viral infections, toxic substances, and genetic disorders. Most cataracts, however, are vaguely called *senile cataracts*—meaning "caused by aging." In Canada, more than one million adults 65 and older have a cataract.

Oxidative stress appears to play a significant role in the development of cataracts, and the antioxidant nutrients may help minimize the damage. Studies have reported an inverse relationship between cataracts and dietary intakes of vitamin C, vitamin E, and carotenoids; taking supplements or eating fruits and vegetables rich in these antioxidant nutrients seems to slow the progression or reduce the risk of developing cataracts.[54]

One other diet-related factor may play a role in the development of cataracts—obesity. Obesity appears to be associated with cataracts, but its role has not been identified. Risk factors that typically accompany overweight, such as inactivity, diabetes, or hypertension, do not explain the association.

Macular Degeneration

The leading cause of visual loss among older people is age-related **macular degeneration**, a deterioration of the macular region of the retina.[55] As with cataracts, risk factors for age-related macular degeneration include oxidative stress from sunlight, and preventive factors may include supplements of the omega-3 fatty acid DHA and the carotenoids lutein and zeaxanthin.[56]

Arthritis

According to Health Canada, about 4 million people in Canada have some form of **arthritis**.[57] As the population ages, it is expected that the prevalence will increase to 7 million by 2031.

Osteoarthritis

The most common type of arthritis that disables older people is **osteoarthritis**, a painful deterioration of the cartilage in the joints. During movement, the ends of bones are normally protected from wear by cartilage and by small sacs of fluid that act as a lubricant. With age, the cartilage sometimes disintegrates, and the joints become malformed and painful to move.

One known connection between osteoarthritis ♦ and nutrition is overweight. Weight loss may relieve some of the pain for overweight persons with osteoarthritis, partly because the joints affected are often weight-bearing joints that are stressed and irritated by having to carry excess pounds. Interestingly, though, weight loss often relieves much of the pain of arthritis in the hands as well, even though they are not weight-bearing joints. Jogging and other weight-bearing exercises do not worsen arthritis. In fact, both aerobic activity and strength training offer improvements in physical performance and pain relief, especially when accompanied by even modest weight loss.[58]

♦ Risk factors for osteoarthritis:
- Age
- Smoking
- High BMI at age 40
- Lack of hormone therapy (in women)

cataracts (KAT-ah-rakts): clouding of the eye lenses that impairs vision and can lead to blindness.

macular (MACK-you-lar) **degeneration:** deterioration of the macular area of the eye that can lead to loss of central vision and eventual blindness. The **macula** is a small, oval, yellowish region in the centre of the retina that provides the sharp, straight-ahead vision so critical to reading and driving.

arthritis: inflammation of a joint, usually accompanied by pain, swelling, and structural changes.

osteoarthritis: a painful, degenerative disease of the joints that occurs when the cartilage in a joint deteriorates; joint structure is damaged, with loss of function; also called *degenerative arthritis*.

Rheumatoid Arthritis Another type of arthritis known as **rheumatoid arthritis** has possible links to diet through the immune system. In rheumatoid arthritis, the immune system mistakenly attacks the bone coverings as if they were made of foreign tissue. In some individuals, certain foods, notably a Mediterranean-type diet of fish, vegetables, and olive oil, may moderate the inflammatory response and provide some relief.[59]

The omega-3 fatty acids commonly found in fatty fish reduce joint tenderness and improve mobility in some people with rheumatoid arthritis. The same diet recommended for heart health—one low in saturated fat from meats and milk products and high in omega-3 fats from fish—helps prevent or reduce the inflammation in the joints that makes arthritis so painful.

Another possible link between nutrition and rheumatoid arthritis involves the oxidative damage to the membranes within joints that causes inflammation and swelling. The antioxidant vitamins C and E and the carotenoids defend against oxidation, and increased intakes of these nutrients may help prevent or relieve the pain of rheumatoid arthritis.[60]

Gout Another form of arthritis, which most commonly affects men, is **gout**, a condition characterized by deposits of uric acid crystals in the joints. Uric acid derives from the breakdown of **purines**, primarily from those made by the body but also from those found in foods.[61] Foods such as meat and seafood that are rich in purines increase uric acid levels and the risk of gout, whereas milk products seem to lower uric acid levels and the risk of gout.[62]

Treatment Treatment for arthritis—dietary or otherwise—may help relieve discomfort and improve mobility, but it does not cure the condition. Traditional medical intervention for arthritis includes medication and surgery. Alternative therapies to treat arthritis abound, but none have proved safe and effective in scientific studies. Popular supplements—glucosamine, chondroitin, or a combination—may relieve pain and improve mobility as well as over-the-counter pain relievers, but mixed reports from studies emphasize the need for additional research.[63] Drugs and supplements used to relieve arthritis can impose nutrition risks; many affect appetite and alter the body's use of nutrients, as Highlight 18 explains.

The Aging Brain

The brain, like all of the body's organs, responds to both genetic and environmental factors ♦ that can enhance or diminish its amazing capacities. One of the challenges researchers face when studying the human brain is to distinguish among normal age-related physiological changes, changes caused by diseases, and changes that result from cumulative, environmental factors such as diet.

♦ Factors that protect brain function:
- Physical activities
- Intellectual challenges
- Social interactions
- Balanced diet rich in antioxidants

The brain normally changes in some characteristic ways as it ages. For one thing, its blood supply decreases. For another, the number of **neurons**, the brain cells that specialize in transmitting information, diminishes as people age. When the number of nerve cells in one part of the cerebral cortex diminishes, hearing and speech are affected. Losses of neurons in other parts of the cortex can impair memory and cognitive function. When the number of neurons in the cerebellum diminishes, balance and posture are affected. Losses of neurons in other parts of the brain affect still other functions. Some of the cognitive loss and forgetfulness generally attributed to aging may be due in part to environmental, and therefore controllable, factors—including nutrient deficiencies.

Nutrient Deficiencies and Brain Function Nutrients influence the development and activities of the brain. The ability of neurons to synthesize specific neurotransmitters depends in part on the availability of precursor nutrients that are obtained from the diet. The neurotransmitter serotonin, for example, derives from the amino acid tryptophan. To function properly, the enzymes involved in neurotransmitter synthesis require vitamins and minerals. Thus nutrient deficiencies may contribute to the loss of memory and cognition that some older adults experience. Such losses may be preventable or at least diminished or delayed through

rheumatoid (ROO-ma-toyd) **arthritis:** a disease of the immune system involving painful inflammation of the joints and related structures.

gout (GOWT): a common form of arthritis characterized by deposits of uric acid crystals in the joints.

purines: compounds of nitrogen-containing bases such as adenine, guanine, and caffeine. Purines that originate from the body are *endogenous* and those that derive from foods are *exogenous*.

neurons: nerve cells; the structural and functional units of the nervous system. Neurons initiate and conduct nerve impulse transmissions.

TABLE 18-1 Summary of Nutrient-Brain Relationships

Brain Function	Adequate Intake of
Short-term memory	Vitamin B_{12}, vitamin C, vitamin E
Performance in problem-solving tests	Riboflavin, folate, vitamin B_{12}, vitamin C
Mental health	Thiamin, niacin, zinc, folate
Cognition	Folate, vitamin B_6, vitamin B_{12}, iron, vitamin E , long-chain omega-3 fatty acids, and foods rich in antioxidants
Vision	Essential fatty acids, vitamin A
Neurotransmitter synthesis	Tyrosine, tryptophan, choline

TABLE 18-2 Common Signs of Dementia

- Agitated behaviour
- Becoming lost in familiar surroundings or circumstances
- Confusion
- Delusions
- Loss of interest in daily activities
- Loss of memory
- Loss of problem-solving skills
- Unclear thinking

diet and exercise. Table 18-1 summarizes some of the better-known connections between brain function and nutrients.

In some instances, the degree of cognitive loss is extensive. Such **senile dementia** may be attributable to a specific disorder such as a brain tumour or Alzheimer's disease. Table 18-2 lists common signs of dementia.

Alzheimer's Disease Much attention has focused on the *abnormal* deterioration of the brain called **Alzheimer's disease**, which affects about 1.5 percent of Canadians. Diagnosis of Alzheimer's disease depends on its characteristic symptoms: the victim gradually loses memory and reasoning, the ability to communicate, physical capabilities, and eventually life itself. Nerve cells in the brain die, and communication between the cells breaks down.

Researchers are closing in on the exact cause of Alzheimer's disease.* Clearly, genetic factors are involved.[64] Free radicals and oxidative stress also seem to be involved.[65] Nerve cells in the brains of people with Alzheimer's disease show evidence of free-radical attack—damage to DNA, cell membranes, and proteins.[66] They also show evidence of the minerals that trigger free-radical attacks—iron, copper, zinc, and aluminum. Increasing evidence also suggests that overweight and obesity in middle age are associated with dementia in general, and with Alzheimer's disease in particular.[67]

In Alzheimer's disease, the brain develops **senile plaques** and **neurofibrillary tangles.** Senile plaques are clumps of a protein fragment called beta-amyloid, whereas neurofibrillary tangles are snarls of the fibres that extend from the nerve cells. Both seem to occur in response to oxidative stress.[68] Researchers question whether these characteristics are the cause or the result of Alzheimer's disease.[69] In fact, scientists are unsure whether these plaques and tangles are causing the damage, serving as markers, or even protecting by sequestering the proteins that begin the dementia process.[70] In any case, treatment research focuses on lowering beta-amyloid levels.[71]

Late in the course of the disease there is a decline in the activity of the enzyme that assists in the production of the neurotransmitter acetylcholine from choline and acetyl CoA. Acetylcholine is essential to memory, but supplements of choline (or of lecithin, which contains choline) have no effect on memory or on the progression of the disease. Drugs, such as donepezil, that inhibit the breakdown of acetylcholine, on the other hand, have proved beneficial.[72]

Research suggests that cardiovascular disease risk factors such as high blood pressure, diabetes, and elevated levels of homocysteine may be related to the development of Alzheimer's disease.[73] Numerous studies have revealed that diets designed to support a healthy heart, including the omega-3 fatty acids of oily fish, may benefit brain health as well.[74] Similarly, physical activity supports heart health and slows the cognitive decline of Alzheimer's disease.[75]

Treatment for Alzheimer's disease involves providing care to clients and support to their families. Drugs are used to improve or at least to slow the loss of short-term memory and cognition, but they do not cure the disease. Other drugs may be used to control depression, anxiety, and behaviour problems.

Maintaining appropriate body weight may be the most important nutrition concern for the person with Alzheimer's disease. Depression and forgetfulness can lead to changes in eating behaviours and poor food intake. Furthermore, changes in the body's weight-regulation system may contribute to weight loss. Perhaps the best that a caregiver can do nutritionally for a person with Alzheimer's disease is to supervise food planning and mealtimes. Providing well-liked and well-balanced meals and snacks in a cheerful atmosphere encourages food consumption. To minimize confusion, offer a few ready-to-eat foods, in bite-size pieces, with seasonings and sauces. To avoid mealtime disruptions, control distractions such as music, television, children, and the telephone.

*A report on the genetic and other aspects of Alzheimer's is available from Alzheimer's Disease Education and Referral Center, P.O. Box 8250, Silver Springs, MD 20907-8250.

senile dementia: the loss of brain function beyond the normal loss of physical adeptness and memory that occurs with aging.

Alzheimer's (AHLZ-high-merz) **disease:** a degenerative disease of the brain involving memory loss and major structural changes in neuron networks; also known as *senile dementia of the Alzheimer's type (SDAT), primary degenerative dementia of senile onset,* or *chronic brain syndrome.*

senile plaques: clumps of the protein fragment beta-amyloid on the nerve cells, commonly found in the brains of people with Alzheimer's dementia.

neurofibrillary tangles: snarls of the threadlike strands that extend from the nerve cells, commonly found in the brains of people with Alzheimer's dementia.

IN SUMMARY Senile dementia and other losses of brain function afflict millions of older adults, and others face loss of vision due to cataracts or macular degeneration or cope with the pain of arthritis. As the number of people older than age 65 continues to grow, the need for solutions to these problems becomes urgent. Some problems may be inevitable, but others are preventable and good nutrition may play a key role.

Food Choices and Eating Habits of Older Adults

Older people are an incredibly diverse group, and for the most part, they are independent, socially sophisticated, mentally lucid, fully participating members of society who report themselves to be happy and healthy. In fact, the quality of life among the elderly has improved, and their chronic disabilities have declined dramatically in recent years. By practising stress-management skills, maintaining physical fitness, participating in activities of interest, and cultivating spiritual health, as well as obtaining adequate nourishment, people can support a high quality of life into old age (see Table 18-3 for some strategies).

Older people spend more money per person on foods to eat at home than other age groups and less money on foods away from home. Manufacturers would be wise to cater to the preferences of older adults by providing good-tasting, nutritious foods in easy-to-open, single-serving packages with labels that are easy to read. Such services enable older adults to maintain their independence and to feel a sense of control and involvement in their own lives. Another way older adults can take care of themselves is by remaining or becoming physically active. As mentioned earlier, physical activity helps preserve one's ability to perform daily tasks and so promotes independence.

Familiarity, taste, and health beliefs are most influential on older people's food choices. Eating foods that are familiar, especially ethnic foods that recall family meals and pleasant times, can be comforting. People 65 and older are less likely to diet to lose weight than younger people are, but they are more likely to diet in pursuit of medical goals such as controlling blood glucose and cholesterol.

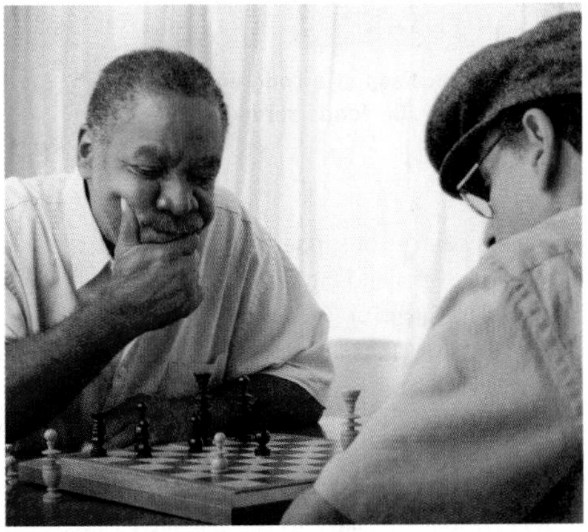

Both foods and mental challenges nourish the brain.

TABLE 18-3 Strategies for Growing Old Healthfully

- Choose nutrient-dense foods.
- Be physically active. Walk, run, dance, swim, bike, or row for aerobic activity. Lift weights, do calisthenics, or pursue some other activity to tone, firm, and strengthen muscles. Practise balancing on one foot or doing simple movements with your eyes closed. Modify activities to suit changing abilities and preferences.
- Maintain appropriate body weight.
- Reduce stress—cultivate self-esteem, maintain a positive attitude, manage time wisely, know your limits, practise assertiveness, release tension, and take action.
- For women, discuss with a physician the risks and benefits of estrogen replacement therapy.
- For people who smoke, discuss with a physician strategies and programs to help you quit.
- Expect to enjoy sex, and learn new ways of enhancing it.
- Use alcohol only moderately, if at all; use drugs only as prescribed.
- Take care to prevent accidents.
- Expect good vision and hearing throughout life; obtain glasses and hearing aids if necessary.
- Take care of your teeth; obtain dentures if necessary.
- Be alert to confusion as a disease symptom, and seek diagnosis.
- Take medications as prescribed; see a physician before self-prescribing medicines or herbal remedies and a registered dietitian before self-prescribing supplements.
- Control depression through activities and friendships; seek professional help if necessary.
- Drink six to eight glasses of water every day.
- Practise mental skills. Keep on solving math problems and crossword puzzles, playing cards or other games, reading, writing, imagining, and creating.
- Make financial plans early to ensure security.
- Accept change. Work at recovering from losses; make new friends.
- Cultivate spiritual health. Cherish personal values. Make life meaningful.
- Go outside for sunshine and fresh air as often as possible.
- Be socially active—play bridge, join an exercise or dance group, take a class, teach a class, eat with friends, volunteer time to help others.
- Stay interested in life—pursue a hobby, spend time with grandchildren, take a trip, read, grow a garden, or go to the movies.
- Enjoy life.

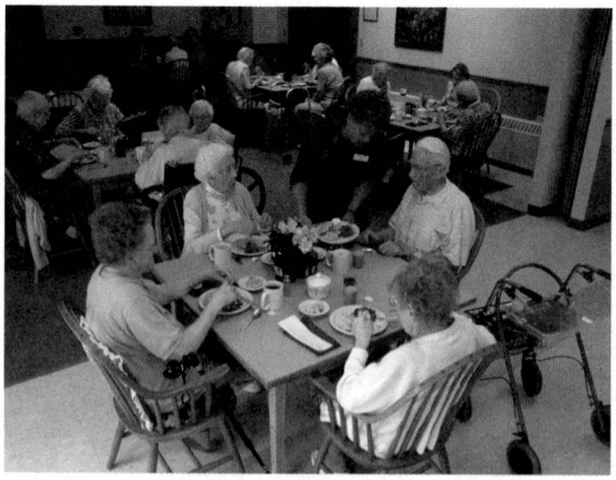
© Jeff Greenberg/Alamy

Social interactions at a congregate meal site can be as nourishing as the foods served.

Nutrition Screening of Older Adults In Canada, a tool called "Seniors in the Community: Risk Evaluation for Eating and Nutrition (SCREEN)" was developed to assess "weight change, food intake, and risk factors for impaired food intake"[76] ♦. In fact, an abbreviated version of SCREEN II© was recently used by Statistics Canada in the 2008-2009 Canadian Community Health Survey—Healthy Aging in those 45 years and over; approximately one-third were classified as at "nutritional risk."[77] Also, in the United States, the Nutrition Screening Initiative is part of a national effort to identify and treat nutrition problems in older persons; it uses a screening checklist. To *determine* the risk of malnutrition in older clients, health-care professionals can keep in mind the characteristics and questions listed in Table 18-4.

Programs That Help Federal programs can provide help for older people. ♦ Canada Pension provides income to retired people over age 62 who paid into the system during their working years, and the Old Age Security pension scheme was set up to guarantee a fixed minimum income for Canadian residents over 65 years old. For the homebound, **Meals on Wheels** volunteers deliver meals to the door, a benefit even though the recipients miss out on the social atmosphere of the congregate meals. Nutritionists are wise not to focus solely on nutrient and food intakes of the elderly because enjoyment and social interactions may be as important as food itself.

♦ Federal sources of support for older adults:
- Canada Pension Plan (CPP)
- Old Age Security (OAS)
- Guaranteed Income Supplement (GSI)
- Allowance for the Survivor Program (ASP)

♦ For the latest developments in terms of research, SCREEN tool applications (i.e., SCREEN™ I & SCREEN™ II), and copyright licence for your site or community, see Dr Keller's SCREEN website at www.drheatherkeller.com/SCREEN.htm.

Meals for Singles

Many older adults live alone, and singles of all ages face challenges in purchasing, storing, and preparing food. Large packages of meat and vegetables are often intended for families of four or more, and even a head of lettuce can spoil before one person can use it all. Many singles live in small dwellings and have little storage space for foods. A limited income presents additional obstacles. This section offers suggestions that can help to solve some of the problems singles face, beginning with a special note about the dangers of foodborne illness.

Foodborne Illness The risk of older adults getting a foodborne illness is greater than for other adults. The consequences of an upset stomach, diarrhea, fever, vomiting, abdominal cramps, and dehydration are oftentimes more severe, sometimes leading to paralysis, meningitis, or even death. For these reasons, older adults need to carefully follow the food-safety suggestions presented in Chapter 20.

TABLE 18-4 Risk Factors for Malnutrition in Older Adults

	These questions help *determine* the risk of malnutrition in older adults:
Disease	• Do you have an illness or condition that changes the types or amounts of foods you eat?
Eating poorly	• Do you eat fewer than two meals a day? Do you eat fruits, vegetables, and milk products daily?
Tooth loss or mouth pain	• Is it difficult or painful to eat?
Economic hardship	• Do you have enough money to buy the food you need?
Reduced social contact	• Do you eat alone most of the time?
Multiple medications	• Do you take three or more different prescribed or over-the-counter medications daily?
Involuntary weight loss or gain	• Have you lost or gained 5 kilograms (10 pounds) or more in the last 6 months?
Needs assistance	• Are you physically able to shop, cook, and feed yourself?
Elderly person	• Are you older than 80?

NOTE: A complete description of DETERMINE and its scoring system are available online from the American Academy of Family Physicians: www.aafp.org/afp/980301ap/edits.html

Courtesy Abbott Nutrition

Meals on Wheels: a nutrition program that delivers food for the elderly to their homes.

Dietary Guidance for Canadians

- Older adults should not eat or drink unpasteurized milk, milk products, or juices; raw or undercooked eggs, meat, poultry, fish, or shellfish; or raw sprouts.
- Older adults should only eat deli meats and frankfurters that have been reheated to steaming hot.

Spend Wisely People who have the means to shop and cook for themselves can cut their food bills simply by being wise shoppers. Large supermarkets are usually less expensive than convenience stores. A grocery list helps reduce impulse buying, and specials and coupons can save money when the items featured are those that the shopper needs and uses.

Buying the right amount so as not to waste any food is a challenge for people eating alone. They can buy fresh milk in the size best suited for personal needs. Cup-size cartons ♦ of milk are available and can be stored unopened on a shelf for as long as three months without refrigeration.

♦ Boxes of milk that can be stored at room temperature have been exposed to temperatures above those of pasteurization just long enough to sterilize the milk—a process called **ultrahigh temperature (UHT).**

Many foods that offer a variety of nutrients for practically pennies have a long shelf life; staples such as rice, pastas, dry powdered milk, and dried legumes can be purchased in bulk and stored for months at room temperature. Other foods that are usually a good buy include whole pieces of cheese rather than sliced or shredded cheese, fresh produce in season, variety meats such as chicken livers, and cereals that require cooking instead of ready-to-serve cereals.

A person who has ample freezer space can buy large packages of meat, such as pork chops, ground beef, or chicken, when they are on sale. Then the meat can be immediately wrapped into individual servings for the freezer. All the individual servings can be put in a bag marked appropriately with the contents and the date.

Frozen vegetables are more economical in large bags than in small boxes. After the amount needed is taken out, the bag can be closed tightly with a twist tie or rubber band. If the package is returned quickly to the freezer each time, the vegetables will stay fresh for a long time.

Finally, breads and cereals usually must be purchased in larger quantities. Again the amount needed for a few days can be taken out and the rest stored in the freezer.

Grocers will break open a package of wrapped meat and rewrap the portion needed. Similarly, eggs can be purchased by the half-dozen. Eggs do keep for long periods, though, if stored properly in the refrigerator.

Fresh fruits and vegetables can be purchased individually. A person can buy fresh fruit at various stages of ripeness: a ripe one to eat right away, a semiripe one to eat soon after, and a green one to ripen on the windowsill. If vegetables are packaged in large quantities, the grocer can break open the package so that a smaller amount can be purchased. Small cans of fruits and vegetables, even though they are more expensive per unit, are a reasonable alternative, considering that it is expensive to buy a regular-size can and let the unused portion spoil.

Be Creative Creative chefs think of various ways to use foods when only large amounts are available. For example, a head of cauliflower can be divided into thirds. Then one-third is cooked and eaten hot. Another third is put into a vinegar and oil marinade for use in a salad. And the last third can be used in a casserole or stew.

A variety of vegetables and meats can be enjoyed stir-fried; inexpensive vegetables such as cabbage, celery, and onion are delicious when crisp cooked in a little oil with herbs or lemon added. Interesting frozen vegetable mixtures are available in larger grocery stores. Cooked, leftover vegetables can be dropped in at the last minute. A bonus of a stir-fried meal is that there is only one pan to wash. Similarly, a microwave oven allows a chef to use fewer pots and pans. Meals and leftovers can also be frozen or refrigerated in microwavable containers to reheat as needed.

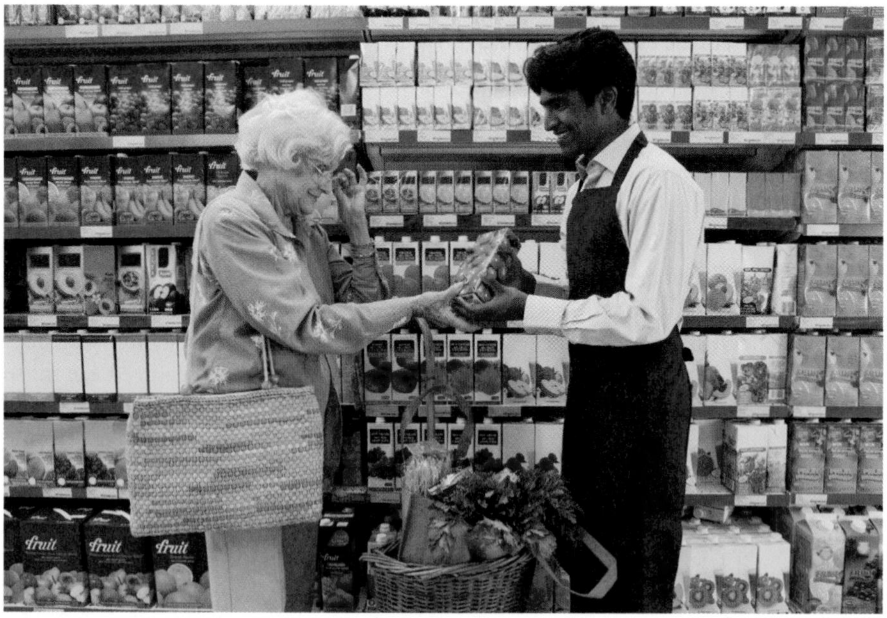
photos.com

Buy only what you will use.

Many frozen dinners offer nutritious options. Adding a fresh salad, a whole-wheat roll, and a glass of milk can make a nutritionally balanced meal.

Also, single people shouldn't hesitate to invite someone to share meals with them whenever there is enough food. It's likely that the person will return the invitation, and both parties will get to enjoy companionship and a meal prepared by others.

IN SUMMARY **Older people may benefit from being screened for "nutritional risk" and some would also benefit from programs such as Meals on Wheels. With creativity and careful shopping, those living alone can prepare nutritious, inexpensive meals. Physical activity, mental challenges, stress management, and social activities can also help people grow old comfortably.**

Nutrition Portfolio

By eating a balanced diet, maintaining a healthy body weight, and engaging in a variety of physical, social, and mental activities, you can enjoy good health in later life.

Visit older adults in your community and . . .

- Consider whether they have the financial means, physical ability, and social support they need to eat adequately.
- Note whether they have experienced an unintentional loss of weight recently.
- Discuss how they occupy their time physically, socially, and mentally.
- Offer to analyze the diet of an older adult who you care about using Diet Analysis Plus. Have the person write down one, two, or even three days of their food and beverage intake, and then enter it into the program and print out a three-day average report of the results. It will be fun and educational to go over it together. Remind the person that you are not a doctor and that this is a learning tool for an introductory nutrition course.

Diet Analysis PLUS **To complete this exercise, go to your Diet Analysis Plus at www.cengage.com/sso.**

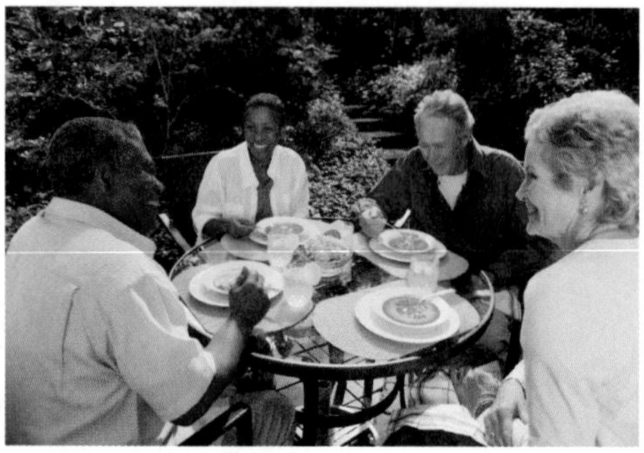
Fancy Photography/Veer

Invite guests to share a meal.

Nutrition on the Net

CENGAGENOW™
For further study of topics covered in this chapter, log on to **www.cengage.com/sso.**

- Search for "aging," "arthritis," and "Alzheimer's" on the Public Health Agency of Canada's website: **www.phac-aspc.gc.ca**
- Visit the Canadian Institutes of Health Research's Institute of Aging: **www.cihr-irsc.gc.ca**
- Visit the Arthritis Society of Canada's website: **www.arthritis.ca**
- Visit the U.S. National Institute on Aging: **www.nia.nih.gov**
- Visit the American Association of Retired Persons: **www.aarp.org**
- Get nutrition tips for growing older in good health from Dietitians of Canada: **www.dietitians.ca**
- Learn more about cataracts and macular degeneration from the U.S. National Eye Institute, the Macular Degeneration Partnership, and the American Society of Cataract and Refractive Surgery: **www.nei.nih.gov**, **www.amd.org**, and **www.ascrs.org**
- Learn more about arthritis from the Arthritis Foundation and the National Institute of Arthritis and Musculoskeletal and Skin Diseases: **www.arthritis.org** and **www.niams.nih.gov**
- Learn more about Alzheimer's disease from the Alzheimer's Society of Canada: **www.alzheimer.ca**
- Find out about the Government of Canada's services for seniors: **www.seniors.gc.ca**
- Learn more about cognitive impairment from the U.S. National Institute of Neurological Disorders and Stroke: **www.ninds.nih.gov**
- Visit the U.S. National Council on Aging: **www.ncoa.org**

References

1. D. E. King, A. G. Mainous, and M. E. Geesey, Turning back the clock: Adopting a healthy lifestyle in middle age, *American Journal of Medicine* 120 (2007): 598–603.
2. Division of Aging and Seniors, Health Canada, Canada's aging population (2002). http://dsp-psd.pwgsc.gc.ca/Collection/H39-608-2002E.pdf, accessed September 18, 2011.
3. S. Norris and T. Williams, Healthy aging: Adding life to years and years to life, Government of Canada (October 21, 2000). http://dsp-psd.pwgsc.gc.ca/Collection-R/LoPBdP/BP/prb0023-e.htm, accessed September 18, 2011; Statistics Canada. Life expectancy at birth, by sex, by province. http://www40.statcan.ca/l01/cst01/health26-eng.htm
4. R. S. Blacklow, Actuarially speaking: An overview of life expectancy. What can we expect? *American Journal of Clinical Nutrition* 86 (2007): 1560S–1562S.
5. Living well to 100: Nutrition, genetics, inflammation, supplement to *American Journal of Clinical Nutrition* 83 (2006): 401S–490S.
6. N. M. Peel, R. J. McClure, and H. P. Bartlett, Behavioral determinants of healthy aging, *American Journal of Preventive Medicine* 28 (2005): 298–304.
7. K. Khaw and coauthors, Combined impact of health behaviours and mortality in men and women: The EPIC-Norfolk Prospective Population Study, *PLoS Medicine* 5 (2008): e12.
8. L. B. Yates and coauthors, Exceptional longevity in men—Modifiable factors associated with survival and function to age 90 years, *Archives of Internal Medicine* 168 (2008): 284–290.
9. P. Kokkinos and coauthors, Exercise capacity and mortality in black and white men, *Circulation* 117 (2008): 614–622.
10. Statistics Canada, Canadian Health Measures Survey 2007–2009. www.statcan.gc.ca/daily-quotidien/100113/dq100113a-eng.htm, accessed September 18, 2011.
11. R. C. Cassilhas and coauthors, The impact of resistance exercise on the cognitive function of the elderly, *Medicine & Science in Sports & Exercise* 39 (2007): 1401–1407.
12. J. A. Stevens, G. Ryan, and M. Kresnow, Fatalities and injuries from falls among older adults: United States, 1993–2003 and 2001–2005, *Morbidity and Mortality Weekly Report* 55 (2006): 1221–1224.
13. Canadian Society for Exercise Physiology, Guidelines (2011). www.csep.ca/english/view.asp?x=804, accessed September 18, 2011; M. E. Nelson and coauthors, Physical activity and public health in older adults: Recommendation from the American College of Sports Medicine and the American Heart Association, *Medicine & Science in Sports & Exercise* 39 (2007): 1435–1445.
14. J. R. Speakman and C. Hambly, Starving for life: What animal studies can and cannot tell us about the use of caloric restriction to prolong human lifespan, *Journal of Nutrition* 137 (2007): 1078–1086.
15. C. W. Levenson and N. J. Rich, Eat less, live longer? New insights into the role of caloric restriction in the brain, *Nutrition Reviews* 65 (2007): 412–415; S. R. Spindler and J. M. Dhahbi, Conserved and tissue-specific genic and physiologic responses to caloric restriction and altered IGFI signaling in mitotic and postmitotic tissues, *Annual Review of Nutrition* 27 (2007): 193–217.
16. R. S. Sohal and coauthors, Life span extension in mice by food restriction depends on an energy imbalance, *Journal of Nutrition* 139 (2009): 533–539.
17. Speakman and Hambly, 2007.
18. L. Fontana and S. Klein, Aging, adiposity, and calorie restriction, *Journal of the American Medical Association* 297 (2007): 986–994; G. Wolf, Calorie restriction increases life span: A molecular mechanism, *Nutrition Reviews* 64 (2006): 89–92.
19. K. A. Varaday and M. K. Hellerstein, Do calorie restriction or alternate-day fasting regimens modulate adipose tissue physiology in a way that reduces chronic disease risk? *Nutrition Reviews* 66 (2008): 333–342; L. K. Heilbronn and coauthors, Alternate-day fasting in nonobese subjects: Effects on body weight, body composition, and energy metabolism, *American Journal of Clinical Nutrition* 81 (2005): 69–73; M. P. Mattson, Energy intake, meal frequency, and health: A neurobiological perspective, *Annual Review of Nutrition* 25 (2005): 237–260.
20. S. Cohen, D. Janicki-Deverts, and G. E. Miller, Psychological stress and disease, *Journal of the American Medical Association* 298 (2007): 1685–1687.
21. R. S. Rivlin, Keeping the young-elderly healthy: Is it too late to improve our health through nutrition? *American Journal of Clinical Nutrition* 86 (2007): 1572S–1576S.
22. L. M. Willis, B. Shukitt-Hale, and J. A. Joseph, Recent advances in berry supplementation and age-related cognitive decline, *Current Opinion in Clinical Nutrition and Metabolic Care* 12 (2009): 91–94; E. Head, Combining an antioxidant-fortified diet with behavioral enrichment leads to cognitive improvement and reduced brain pathology in aging canines: Strategies for healthy aging, *Annals of the New York Academy of Sciences* 1114 (2007): 398–406; D. P. Jones, Extracellular redox state: Refining the definition of oxidative stress in aging, *Rejuvenation Research* 9 (2006): 169–181; F. Sierra, Is (your cellular response to) stress killing you? *Journals of Gerontology. Series A, Biological Sciences*

and Medical Sciences 61 (2006): 557–561; B. P. Yu and H. Y. Chung, Adaptive mechanisms to oxidative stress during aging, *Mechanisms of Ageing and Development* 127 (2006): 436–443.
23. Public Health Agency of Canada, Healthy eating and healthy aging (2009). www.phac-aspc.gc.ca/seniors-aines/publications/pro/healthy-sante/haging_newvision/vison-rpt/eating-alimentation-eng.php, accessed September 18, 2011; D. T. Villareal and coauthors, Obesity in older adults: Technical review and position statement of the American Society for Nutrition and NAASO, The Obesity Society, *American Journal of Clinical Nutrition* 82 (2005): 923–934.
24. S. M. H. Alibhai, C. Greenwood, and H. Payette, An approach to the management of unintentional weight loss in elderly people, *Canadian Medical Association Journal* 172 (2005): 773–780.
25. C. A. Zizza, F. A. Tayie, and M. Lino, Benefits of snacking in older Americans, *Journal of the American Dietetic Association* 107 (2007): 800–806.
26. M. Cesari and coauthors, Frailty syndrome and skeletal muscle: Results from the Invecchiare in Chianti Study, *American Journal of Clinical Nutrition* 83 (2006): 1142–1148.
27. D. K. Houston and coauthors, Dietary protein intake is associated with lean mass change in older, community-dwelling adults: The Health, Aging, and Body Composition (Health ABC) Study, *American Journal of Clinical Nutrition* 87 (2008): 150–155; D. Paddon-Jones and coauthors, Role of dietary protein in the sarcopenia of aging, *American Journal of Clinical Nutrition* 87 (2008): 1562S–1566S; H. B. Iglay and coauthors, Resistance training and dietary protein: Effects on glucose tolerance and contents of skeletal muscle insulin signaling proteins in older persons, *American Journal of Clinical Nutrition* 85 (2007): 1005–1013; K. S. Nair, Aging muscle, *American Journal of Clinical Nutrition* 81 (2005): 953–963.
28. A. B. Newman and coauthors, Weight change and the conservation of lean mass in old age: The Health, Aging and Body Composition Study, *American Journal of Clinical Nutrition* 82 (2005): 872–878; P. Szulc and coauthors, Hormonal and lifestyle determinants of appendicular skeletal muscle mass in men: The MINOS Study, *American Journal of Clinical Nutrition* 80 (2004): 496–503.
29. M. Cesari and coauthors, Sarcopenia, obesity, and inflammation—Results from the Trial of Angiotensin Converting Enzyme Inhibition and Novel Cardiovascular Risk Factors Study, *American Journal of Clinical Nutrition* 82 (2005): 428–434.
30. C. Franceschi, Inflammaging as a major characteristic of old people: Can it be prevented or cured? *Nutrition Reviews* 65 (2007): S173–S176.
31. P. Libby, Inflammatory mechanisms: The molecular basis of inflammation and disease, *Nutrition Reviews* 65 (2007): S140–S146.
32. J. Gauldie, Inflammation and the aging process: Devil or angel, *Nutrition Reviews* 65 (2007): S167–S169.
33. R. Roubenoff, Physical activity, inflammation, and muscle loss, *Nutrition Reviews* 65 (2007): S208–S212.
34. D. Rémond and coauthors, Postprandial whole-body protein metabolism after a meat meal is influenced by chewing efficiency in elderly subjects, *American Journal of Clinical Nutrition* 85 (2007): 1286–1292.
35. Position paper of the American Dietetic Association: Nutrition across the spectrum of aging, *Journal of the American Dietetic Association* 105 (2005): 616–633.
36. H. Keller, A Canadian response to malnutrition in hospitals. Canadian Medical Association (Dec 13, 2010) eLetters. canadianmedicaljournal.ca/cgi/eletters/182/17/1843; M. A. Bocock and H. H. Keller, Hospital diagnosis of malnutrition: A call for action. *Canadian Journal of Dietetic Practice and Research* 70:1 (2009): 37–41; N. Kagansky and coauthors, Poor nutritional habits are predictors of poor outcome in very old hospitalized patients, *American Journal of Clinical Nutrition* 82 (2005): 784–791.
37. R. Chernoff, Micronutrient requirements in older women, *American Journal of Clinical Nutrition* 81 (2005): 1240S–1245S.
38. M. Ferry, Strategies for ensuring good hydration in the elderly, *Nutrition Reviews* 63 (2005): S22–S29.
39. N. Meunier and coauthors, Basal metabolic rate and thyroid hormones of late-middle-aged and older human subjects: The ZENITH Study, *European Journal of Clinical Nutrition* 59 (2005): S53–S57.
40. Health Canada, Food and Nutrition, *Eating Well with Canada's Food Guide* (2007). www.hc-sc.gc.ca/fn-an/food-guide-aliment/index-eng.php, accessed September 18, 2011.
41. R. P. Heaney and D. K. Layman, Amount and type of protein influences bone health, *American Journal of Clinical Nutrition* 87 (2008): 1567S–1570S; A. E. Thalacker-Mercer and coauthors, Inadequate protein intake affects skeletal muscle transcript profiles in older humans, *American Journal of Clinical Nutrition* 85 (2007): 1344–1352; R. R. Wolfe, The underappreciated role of muscle in health and disease, *American Journal of Clinical Nutrition* 84 (2006): 475–482.
42. Public Health Agency of Canada, 2009; Dietitians of Canada, Upcoming events, Moving beyond dietary requirements: Optimal eating (and exercise) to age successfully (Feb. 24, 2011). www.dietitians.ca/Events/Workshops/General-Workshops/Moving-Beyond-Dietary-Requirements—Optimal-Ea-(2).aspx; Position of the American Dietetic Association: Liberalization of the diet prescription improves quality of life for older adults in long-term care, *Journal of the American Dietetic Association* 105 (2005): 1955–1965.
43. Committee on Dietary Reference Intakes, *Dietary Reference Intakes for Energy, Carbohydrate, Fiber, Fat, Fatty Acids, Cholesterol, Protein, and Amino Acids* (Washington, D.C.: National Academies Press, 2002).
44. Health Canada, Canadian Community Health Survey Cycle 2.2 Nutrition—Nutrient Intakes from Food Volume 1 (2004). www.hc-sc.gc.ca/fn-an/surveill/nutrition/commun/cchs_focus-volet_escc-eng.php#p1, accessed September 18, 2011.
45. R. Clarke and coauthors, Low vitamin B-12 status and risk of cognitive decline in older adults, *American Journal of Clinical Nutrition* 86 (2007): 1384–1391.
46. Committee on Dietary Reference Intakes, *Dietary Reference Intakes for Thiamin, Riboflavin, Niacin, Vitamin B_6, Folate, Vitamin B_{12}, Pantothenic Acid, Biotin, and Choline* (Washington, D.C.: National Academies Press, 2000), p. 338.
47. Institute of Medicine, Dietary Reference Intakes for Calcium and Vitamin D (Nov. 2010). www.iom.edu/Reports/2010/Dietary-Reference-Intakes-for-Calcium-and-Vitamin-D.aspx, accessed September 18, 2011.
48. Health Canada, Canadian Community Health Survey 2.2 (2004), Focus (Vol 1); Institute of Medicine, Dietary Reference Intakes for Calcium and Vitamin D (Nov 2010).
49. Health Canada, Canadian Community Health Survey Cycle 2.2 Nutrition—Nutrient Intakes from Food Volume 1 (2004).
50. A. N. Burnett-Hartman and coauthors, Supplement use contributes to meeting recommended dietary intakes for calcium, magnesium, and vitamin C in four ethnicities of middle-aged and older Americans: The Multi-Ethnic Study of Atherosclerosis, *Journal of the American Dietetic Association* 109 (2009): 422–429.
51. T. Ostbye and coauthors, Ten dimensions of health and their relationships with overall self-reported health and survival in a predominately religiously active elderly population: The Cache County Memory Study, *Journal of the American Geriatrics Society* 54 (2006): 199–209.
52. M. D. Knudtson, B. E. Klein, and R. Klein, Age-related disease, visual impairment, and survival: The Beaver Dam Eye Study, *Archives of Ophthalmology* 124 (2006): 243–249.
53. M. Rhone and A. Basu, Phytochemicals and age-related eye diseases, *Nutrition Reviews* 66 (2008): 465–472.
54. W. G. Christen and coauthors, Dietary carotenoids, vitamins C and E, and risk of cataract in women. A Prospective Study, *Archives of Ophthalmology* 126 (2008): 102–109; A. G. Tan and coauthors, Antioxidant nutrient intake and the long-term incidence of age-related cataract: The Blue Mountains Eye Study, *American Journal of Clinical Nutrition* 87 (2008): 1899–1905; W. G. Christen and coauthors, Fruit and vegetable intake and the risk of cataract in women, *American Journal of Clinical Nutrition* 81 (2005): 1417–1422.
55. R. D. Jager, W. F. Mieler, and J. W. Miller, Age-related macular degeneration, *New England Journal of Medicine* 358 (2008): 2606–2617.
56. C. Augood and coauthors, Oily fish consumption, dietary docosahexaenoic acid and eicosapentaenoic acid intakes, and associations with neovascular age-related macular degeneration, *American Journal of Clinical Nutrition* 88 (2008): 398–406; E. J. Johnson and coauthors, The influence of supplemental lutein and docosahexaenoic acid on serum, lipoproteins, and macular pigmentation, *American Journal of Clinical*

Nutrition 87 (2008): 1521–1529; E. D. O'Connell and coauthors, Diet and risk factors for age-related maculopathy, *American Journal of Clinical Nutrition* 87 (2008): 712–722; H. Coleman and E. Chew, Nutritional supplementation in age-related macular degeneration, *Current Opinion in Ophthalmology* 18 (2007): 220–223; P. R. Trumbo and K. C. Ellwood, Lutein and zeaxanthin intakes and risk of age-related macular degeneration and cataracts: An evaluation using the Food and Drug Administration's evidence-based review system for health claims, *American Journal of Clinical Nutrition* 84 (2006): 971–974; S. S. Ahmed, M. N. Lott, and D. M. Marcus, The macular xanthophylls, *Survey of Ophthalmology* 50 (2005): 183–193; R. van Leeuwen and coauthors, Dietary intake of antioxidants and risk of age-related macular degeneration, *Journal of the American Medical Association* 294 (2005): 3101–3107.

57. Health Canada, Message from Leona Aglukkaq, Minister of Health--Arthritis awareness month. www.hc-sc.gc.ca/ahc-asc/minist/messages/_2010/2010_09_09-eng.php, accessed September 18, 2011.
58. L. Devos-Comby, T. Cronan, and S. C. Roesch, Do exercise and self-management interventions benefit patients with osteoarthritis of the knee? A metaanalytic review, *Journal of Rheumatology* 33 (2006): 744–756.
59. G. McKellar and coauthors, A pilot study of a Mediterranean-type diet intervention in female patients with rheumatoid arthritis living in areas of social deprivation in Glasgow, *Annals of the Rheumatic Disease* 66 (2007): 1239–1243.
60. D. J. Pattison and coauthors, Dietary β-cryptoxanthin and inflammatory polyarthritis: Results from a population-based prospective study, *American Journal of Clinical Nutrition* 82 (2005): 451–455.
61. N. Schlesinger, Dietary factors and hyperuricaemia, *Current Pharmaceutical Design* 11 (2005): 4133–4138.
62. H. K. Choi, S. Liu, and G. Curhan, Intake of purine-rich foods, protein, and dairy products and relationship to serum levels of uric acid: The Third National Health and Nutrition Examination Survey, *Arthritis and Rheumatism* 52 (2005): 283–289.
63. D. O. Clegg and coauthors, Glucosamine, chondroitin sulfate, and the two in combination for painful knee osteoarthritis, *New England Journal of Medicine* 354 (2006): 795–808.
64. T. D. Bird, Genetic factors in Alzheimer's disease, *New England Journal of Medicine* 352 (2005): 862–864; P. M. Kidd, Neurodegeneration from mitochondrial insufficiency: Nutrients, stem cells, growth factors, and prospects for brain rebuilding using integrative management, *Alternative Medicine Review* 10 (2005): 268–293.
65. P. I. Moreira and coauthors, Oxidative stress: The old enemy in Alzheimer's disease pathophysiology, *Current Alzheimer Research* 2 (2005): 403–408.
66. P. I. Moreira and coauthors, Alzheimer disease and the role of free radicals in the pathogenesis of the disease, *CNS and Neurological Disorders Drug Targets* 7 (2008): 3–10; A. Nunomura and coauthors, Involvement of oxidative stress in Alzheimer disease, *Journal of Neuropathology and Experimental Neurology* 65 (2006): 631–641.
67. J. A. Luchsinger and D. R. Gustafon, Adiposity and Alzheimer's disease, *Current Opinion in Clinical Nutrition and Metabolic Care* 12 (2009): 15–21; D. B. Miller and J. P. O'Callaghan, Do early-life insults contribute to the late-life development of Parkinson's and Alzeimer disease? *Metabolism* 57 (2008): S44–S49; R. A. Whitmer, The epidemiology of adiposity and dementia, *Current Alzheimer Research* 4 (2007): 117–122.
68. R. J. Castellani and coauthors, Antioxidant protection and neurodegenerative disease: The role of amyloid-beta and tau, *American Journal of Alzheimer's Disease and Other Dementias* 21 (2006): 126–130; P. Zafrilla and coauthors, Oxidative stress in Alzheimer patients in different stages of the disease, *Current Medicinal Chemistry* 13 (2006): 1075–1083.
69. R. A. Armstrong, Plaques and tangles and the pathogenesis of Alzheimer's disease, *Folia Neuropathologica* 44 (2006): 1–11; G. L. Wenk, Neuropathologic changes in Alzheimer's disease: Potential targets for treatment, *Journal of Clinical Psychiatry* 67 (2006): 3–7.
70. A. Nunomura and coauthors, Neuropathology in Alzheimer's disease: Awaking from a hundred-year-old dream, *Science of Aging Knowledge Environment* (2006): pe10; R. E. Tanzi, Tangles and neurodegenerative disease: A surprising twist, *New England Journal of Medicine* 353 (2005): 1853–1855.
71. D. J. Selkoe, Developing preventive therapies for chronic diseases: Lessons learned from Alzheimer's disease, *Nutrition Reviews* 65 (2007): S239–S243.
72. B. Benjamin and A. Burns, Donepezil for Alzheimer's disease, *Expert Review of Neurotherapeutics* 7 (2007): 1243–1249.
73. G. Ravaglia and coauthors, Homocysteine and folate as risk factors for dementia and Alzheimer disease, *American Journal of Clinical Nutrition* 82 (2005): 636–643; K. L. Tucker and coauthors, High homocysteine and low B vitamins predict cognitive decline in aging men: The Veterans Affairs Normative Aging Study, *American Journal of Clinical Nutrition* 82 (2005): 627–635.
74. DHA/EPA Omega-3 Institute, Requirements and Importance of DHA plus EPA omega-3 for heart, brain and visual functions. www.dhaomega3.org, accessed September 18, 2011; L. J. Whalley and coauthors, n-3 Fatty acid erythrocyte membrane content, APOE ε4, and cognitive variation: An observational follow-up study in late adulthood, *American Journal of Clinical Nutrition* 87 (2008): 449–454; M. A. Beydoun and coauthors, Plasma n-3 fatty acids and the risk of cognitive decline in older adults: The Atherosclerosis Risk in Communities Study, *American Journal of Clinical Nutrition* 85 (2007): 1103–1111; W. E. Connor and S. L. Connor, The importance of fish and docosahexaenoic acid in Alzheimer disease, *American Journal of Clinical Nutrition* 85 (2007): 929–930; C. Dullemeijer and coauthors, n-3 Fatty acid proportions in plasma and cognitive performance in older adults, *American Journal of Clinical Nutrition* 86 (2007): 1479–1485; B.M.V. Gelder and coauthors, Fish consumption, n-3 fatty acids, and subsequent 5-y cognitive decline in elderly men: The Zutphen Elderly Study, *American Journal of Clinical Nutrition* 85 (2007): 1142–1147; E. Nurk and coauthors, Cognitive performance among the elderly and dietary fish intake: The Hordaland Health Study, *American Journal of Clinical Nutrition* 86 (2007): 1470–1478; E. J. Schaefer and coauthors, Plasma phosphatidylcholin docosahexaenoic acid content and risk of dementia and Alzheimer disease, *Archives of Neurology* 63 (2006): 1545–1550; R. Uauy and A. D. Dangour, Nutrition in brain development and aging: Role of essential fatty acids, *Nutrition Reviews* 64 (2006): S24–S33; F. Calon and coauthors, Docosahexaenoic acid protects from dendritic pathology in an Alzheimer's disease mouse model, *Neuron* 43 (2004): 633–645; T. den Heijer and coauthors, Alcohol intake in relation to brain magnetic resonance imaging findings in older persons without dementia, *American Journal of Clinical Nutrition* 80 (2004): 992–997.
75. E. B. Larson, Physical activity for older adults at risk for Alzheimer disease, *Journal of the American Medical Association* 300 (2008): 1077–1079; N. T. Lautenschlager and coauthors, Effect of physical activity on cognitive function in older adults at risk for Alzheimer disease, *Journal of the American Medical Association* 300 (2008): 1027–1037.
76. H. H. Keller, M. R. Hedley, and S. Wong-Brownlee, The development of Seniors in the Community: Risk Evaluation for Eating and Nutrition (SCREEN), Canadian Journal of Dietetic Practice and Research 61 (2000): 62–72; H. Keller, Nutrition risk screening, Dr. Heather Keller, RD, PhD, FDC. www.drheatherkeller.com/risk.htm, accessed September 18, 2011.
77. Statistics Canada, Canadian Community Health Survey—Healthy Aging 2008-2009 Table 105-1200.

Nutrient–Drug Interactions

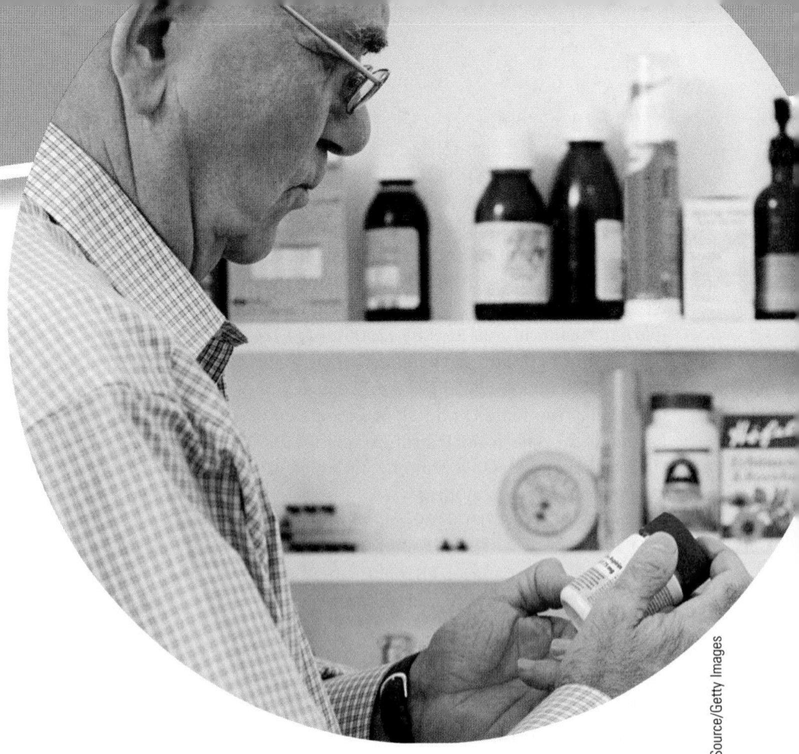

Image Source/Getty Images

According to a 2008 study by the Canadian Institute for Health Information, over 60 percent of seniors living in the community in six provinces take five or more prescription drugs (regarded as polypharmacy).[1] Most often, they take these drugs and other supplements for heart disease, but also to treat arthritis, respiratory problems, and gastrointestinal disorders. Furthermore, physiologic changes associated with aging may alter drug metabolism and excretion, which may, in turn, diminish drug effectiveness or create potential toxicities.[2] For all these reasons, physicians and other health-care providers need to "start low and go slow" when prescribing for older adults.[3]

To avoid harmful drug interactions, consumers need to inform all of their physicians, pharmacists, dietitians, and other health-care providers of all the medicines being taken. These medicines enable people of all ages to enjoy better health, but they also bring side effects and risks.

This highlight focuses on some of the nutrition-related consequences of medical drugs, both prescription drugs and nonprescription (over-the-counter) drugs. Highlight 7 describes the relationships between nutrition and the drug alcohol, and Highlight 19 presents information on herbal supplements and other alternative therapies.

The Actions of Drugs

Most people think of drugs either as medicines that help them recover from illnesses or as illegal substances that lead to bodily harm and addiction. Actually, both uses of the term *drug* are correct because any substance that modifies one or more of the body's functions is, technically, a drug. Even prescription drugs and Natural Health Products (NHPs) alone or in combination with other medications or even foods can have both desirable and undesirable consequences within the body.

Consider aspirin. One action of aspirin is to limit the production of certain prostaglandins. Some prostaglandins help to produce fevers, some sensitize pain receptors, some cause contractions of the uterus, some stimulate digestive tract motility, some control nerve impulses, some regulate blood pressure, some promote blood clotting, and some cause inflammation. By interfering with prostaglandin actions, aspirin reduces fever and inflammation, relieves pain, and slows blood clotting, among other things.

A person cannot use aspirin to produce one of its effects without producing all of its other effects. Someone who is prone to strokes and heart attacks might take aspirin to prevent blood clotting, but it will also dull that person's sense of pain. Another person who takes aspirin only for pain will also experience slow blood clotting. The anticlotting effect might be dangerous if it causes abnormal bleeding. A single two-tablet dose of aspirin doubles the bleeding time of wounds, an effect that lasts from four to seven hours. For this reason, physicians instruct clients to refrain from taking aspirin before surgery.

The Interactions between Drugs and Nutrients

Hundreds of drugs and nutrients interact, and these interactions can lead to nutrient imbalances or interfere with drug effectiveness. Adverse nutrient–drug interactions are most likely if drugs are taken over long periods, if several drugs are taken, or if nutrition status is poor or deteriorating. Understandably, then, elderly people with chronic diseases are most vulnerable.

Nutrients and medications may interact in many ways:

- Drugs can alter food intake and the absorption, metabolism, and excretion of nutrients.
- Foods and nutrients can alter the absorption, metabolism, and excretion of drugs.
- Combinations can be toxic.

The following paragraphs describe these interactions, and Table H18-1 summarizes this information and provides specific examples.

Drugs Alter Food Intake

Some medications can make eating difficult or unpleasant. They may suppress appetite, alter taste sensations, induce nausea or vomiting, cause mouth dryness, or create inflammation or lesions in the mouth, stomach, or intestinal lining. Side effects, such as abdominal discomfort, constipation, and diarrhea may worsen when food is eaten. Medications that cause drowsiness may make a person too tired to eat. All of these complications limit food intake and can lead to weight loss and malnutrition if not resolved.

TABLE H18-1 Examples of Diet–Drug Interactions

Drugs May Alter Food Intake by
• Altering the appetite (Amphetamines suppress appetite; corticosteroids increase appetite.) • Interfering with taste or smell (Amphetamines change taste perceptions.) • Inducing nausea or vomiting (Digitalis may do both.) • Interfering with oral function (Some antidepressants may cause dry mouth.) • Causing sores or inflammation in the mouth (Methotrexate may cause painful mouth ulcers.)
Drugs May Alter Nutrient Absorption by
• Changing the acidity of the digestive tract (Antacids may interfere with iron and folate absorption.) • Damaging mucosal cells (Cancer chemotherapy may damage mucosal cells.) • Binding to nutrients (Bile acid binders bind to fat-soluble vitamins.)
Foods and Nutrients May Alter Drug Absorption by
• Stimulating secretion of gastric acid (The antifungal agent ketoconazole is absorbed better with meals due to increased acid secretion.) • Altering rate of gastric emptying (Intestinal absorption of drugs may be delayed when they are taken with food.) • Binding to drugs (Calcium binds to tetracycline, reducing drug, and calcium absorption.) • Competing for absorption sites in the intestines (Dietary amino acids interfere with levodopa absorption.)
Drugs and Nutrients May Interact and Alter Metabolism by
• Acting as structural analogues (Warfarin and vitamin K are structural analogues.) • Using similar enzyme systems (Phenobarbital induces liver enzymes that increase metabolism of folate, vitamin D, and vitamin K.) • Competing for transport on plasma proteins (Fatty acids and drugs may compete for the same sites on the plasma protein albumin.)
Drugs May Alter Nutrient Excretion by
• Altering reabsorption in the kidneys (Some diuretics increase the excretion of sodium and potassium.) • Causing diarrhea or vomiting (Diarrhea and vomiting may cause electrolyte losses.)
Foods May Alter Medication Excretion by
• Inducing activities of liver enzymes that metabolize drugs to allow their excretion (Components of charcoal-broiled meats increase metabolism of warfarin, theophylline, and acetominophen.)
Toxicity May Occur from Diet and Drug Interactions by
• Increasing side effects of the drug (Caffeine in beverages can increase adverse effects of stimulants.) • Increasing drug action to excessive levels (Grapefruit components may block metabolism of drugs and enhance drugs' actions and side effects.)

Some medications stimulate appetite and cause weight gain. Unintentional weight gain may result from the use of some antipsychotics, antidepressants, and corticosteroids (e.g., prednisone). People using these drugs do not feel satiated and sometimes gain 20 to 30 kilograms (40 to 60 pounds) in just a few months. Patients with diseases that cause wasting, such as cancer or AIDS, may be prescribed appetite enhancers, such as megestrol acetate.

Medications prescribed for obesity intentionally suppress the appetite and promote weight loss. Examples include sibutramine, amphetamines, and amphetamine-like compounds such as phentermine. When amphetamines are prescribed for other purposes, such as narcolepsy or attention-deficit/hyperactivity disorder, appetite suppression and weight loss may be unwanted side effects.

Drugs Alter Nutrient Absorption

Nutrient malabsorption is most likely to occur with medications that damage the intestinal mucosa. Antineoplastic and antiretroviral drugs are especially detrimental; nonsteroidal anti-inflammatory drugs (NSAIDS) and some antibiotics can have similar, though milder, effects.

Some medications bind nutrients in the GI tract, preventing their absorption. For example, bile acid binders, used to reduce cholesterol levels, also bind to the fat-soluble vitamins A, D, E, and K. Some antibiotics, notably tetracycline and ciprofloxacin, bind to the calcium in foods and supplements, which reduces the absorption of both the drug and the calcium. Other minerals, such as iron, magnesium, and zinc, may also bind to antibiotics. For this reason, pharmacists advise consumers to use dairy products and all mineral supplements at least two hours apart from these medications.

Medications that reduce stomach acidity may interfere with the absorption of vitamin B_{12}, folate, and iron. Examples include antacids, which neutralize stomach acid by acting as weak bases, and antiulcer drugs (such as proton pump inhibitors and H_2 blockers), which interfere with acid secretion.

Several drugs impede absorption by interfering with the intestinal metabolism or transport of nutrients into mucosal cells. For example, the antibiotics trimethoprim and pyrimethamine compete with folate for absorption into intestinal cells.

Diets Alter Drug Absorption

Most drugs are absorbed in the upper small intestine. Major influences on drug absorption include the stomach emptying rate, level of acidity, and direct interactions with dietary components. The drug's formulation also influences its absorption, and pharmacists often provide instructions advising whether food should be eaten or avoided when using a medication.

Drugs reach the small intestine more quickly when the stomach is empty. Therefore, taking a medication with meals may delay its absorption, although the total amount absorbed may not be lower. As an example, aspirin works faster when taken on an empty stomach, but taking it with food is often encouraged to reduce stomach irritation.

Both nutrients and nonnutrients may bind to drugs and inhibit their absorption. For example, high-fibre diets may decrease the absorption of some tricyclic antidepressants. Phytates in foods can bind to digoxin, a drug prescribed for heart disease. As mentioned earlier, calcium and other minerals may bind to some antibiotics, reducing absorption of both the minerals and the drug.

HIGHLIGHT 18

Drugs Alter Nutrient Metabolism

Drugs and nutrients share many of the same enzyme systems in the small intestine and the liver. Consequently, some drugs may enhance or inhibit the activities of enzymes that are needed for nutrient metabolism. For example, the anticonvulsants phenobarbital and phenytoin increase levels of the liver enzymes that metabolize folate, vitamin D, and vitamin K; therefore, persons using these drugs may require supplements of these vitamins.

The drug methotrexate, used to treat cancer and inflammatory conditions, acts by interfering with folate metabolism and thus depriving rapidly dividing cancer cells of the folate they need to multiply. Methotrexate resembles folate in structure (see Figure H18-1) and competes with folate for the enzyme that converts folate to its active form.* The adverse effects of using methotrexate therefore include symptoms of folate deficiency. These adverse effects can be reduced by using a pre-activated form of folate (called leucovorin), which is often prescribed along with methotrexate to ensure that the body's rapidly dividing cells (such as cells of the digestive tract, skin cells, and red blood cells) receive adequate folate.

Isoniazid (INH), an antituberculosis drug, can induce a vitamin B_6 deficiency. Because isoniazid is similar in structure to vitamin B_6, it interferes with the vitamin's conversion to its active form. Because the drug must be taken for at least six months to treat infection, vitamin B_6 supplements are routinely given to prevent deficiency.[4]

FIGURE H18-1 Folate and Methotrexate

By competing for the enzyme that activates folate, methotrexate prevents cancer cells from obtaining the folate they need to multiply. This interference with folate metabolism creates a secondary deficiency of folate that deprives normal cells of the folate they need as well. Notice the similarities in their chemical structures.

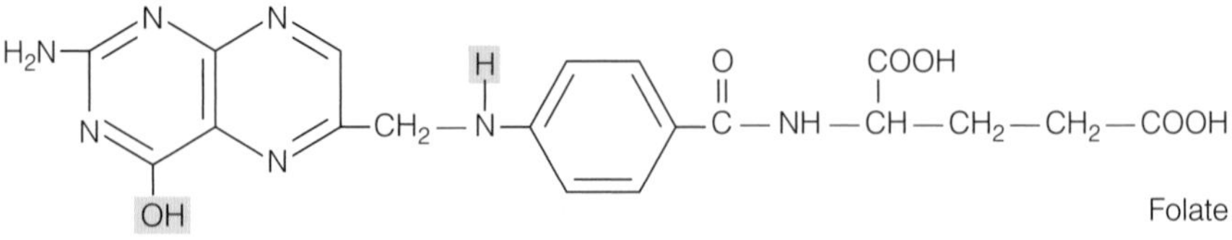

Folate

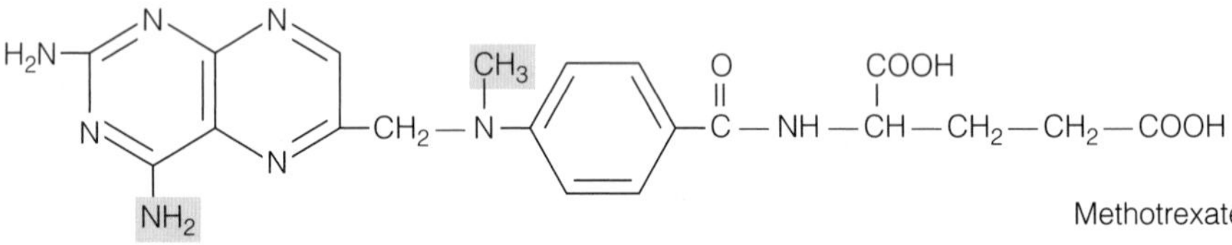

Methotrexate

Diet Alters Drug Metabolism

Some foods affect the activities of enzymes that metabolize drugs or may counteract the drugs' effects in other ways. For example, compounds in grapefruit and grapefruit juice interfere with enzymes that metabolize a number of drugs.[5] As a result of reduced enzyme action, blood concentrations of the drugs increase, leading to stronger physiological effects. The effect of the grapefruit juice lasts for a substantial period after the juice is consumed. Table H18-2 provides examples of drugs that interact with grapefruit juice, as well as some that are not affected.

TABLE H18-2 Grapefruit Juice–Drug Interactions—Selected Examples

Drug Category	Drugs Affected by Grapefruit Juice	Drugs Unaffected by Grapefruit Juice
Cardiovascular drugs	Felodipine Nicardipine Nifedipine Verapamil	Amlodipine Diltiazem Propafenone Quinidine
Cholesterol-lowering drugs	Atorvastatin Lovastatin Simvastatin	Pravastatin
Central nervous system drugs	Buspirone Carbamazepine Diazepam Triazolam	Clomipramine Haloperidol
Anti-infective drugs	Saquinavir	Clarithromycin Itraconazole
Estrogens	Ethinylestradiol	17-β-estradiol
Anticoagulants	—	Acenocoumarol Warfarin
Immunosuppressants	Cyclosporine Tacrolimus	Prednisone
Antiasthmatic drugs	—	Theophylline

SOURCE: D. G. Bailey, M. O. Arnold, and J. D. Spence, Inhibitors in the diet: Grapefruit juice–drug interactions, in R. H. Levy and coeditors, Metabolic Drug Interactions (Philadelphia, Pa.: Lippincott Williams & Wilkins, 2000), pp. 661–669.

A number of dietary factors affect the activity of the anticoagulant drug warfarin. The most important interaction is with vitamin K, which is structurally similar to warfarin. Warfarin acts by blocking the enzyme that activates vitamin K, thereby preventing the synthesis of blood-clotting factors. The amount of warfarin prescribed is dependent, in part, on how much vitamin K is in the diet. If vitamin K consumption from foods or supplements increases substantially, it can weaken the effect of the drug. Individuals using warfarin are advised to consume similar amounts of vitamin K daily to keep warfarin activity stable. The dietary sources highest in vitamin K are green leafy vegetables. Because large quantities of cranberry juice also interfere with warfarin therapy, patients should avoid their concurrent use.[6]

*Other folate antagonists include aminopterin, sulfasalazine, pyrimethamine, trimethoprim, triamterene, carbamazepine, phenytoin, phenobarbital, and primidone.

Some interactions between foods and drugs can cause toxicity or exacerbate a drug's side effects. The combination of tyramine, a compound in some foods, and monoamine oxidase (MAO) inhibitors, which include some medications that treat depression and Parkinson's disease, can be fatal. MAO inhibitors block an enzyme that normally inactivates tyramine, as well as the hormones epinephrine and norepinephrine. When people who take MAO inhibitors consume excessive tyramine, the increase in tyramine can cause a sudden release of accumulated norepinephrine. This surge in norepinephrine results in severe headaches, rapid heartbeat, and a dangerous increase in blood pressure. For this reason, people taking MAO inhibitors are advised to restrict their intakes of foods with substantial amounts of tyramine (see Table H18-3).

TABLE H18-3 Examples of Foods with a High Tyramine Content[a]

• Aged cheeses	• Feta cheese
• Aged meats	• Lima beans
• Alcoholic beverages (beer, wine)	• Mushrooms
• Anchovies	• Pickled fish or meat
• Caviar	• Prepared soy foods (miso, tempeh, tofu)
• Fava beans	• Smoked fish or meat
• Fermented foods (sauerkraut, sausages)	• Soy sauce
	• Yeast extract (Marmite)

[a]The tyramine content of foods depends on storage conditions and processing; thus the amounts in similar products can vary substantially.

Drugs Alter Nutrient Excretion

Drugs that enhance urinary excretion may interfere with nutrient reabsorption in the kidneys, resulting in greater urinary losses. For example, some diuretics accelerate the excretion of calcium, potassium, and magnesium. Risk of mineral depletion is highest if multiple drugs with the same effect are used, if kidney function is impaired, or if medications are used for a long time. Note that some diuretics may cause mineral retention instead.[7]

Diets Alter Drug Excretion

Inadequate excretion of medications can cause toxicity, whereas excessive losses may reduce the amount available for therapeutic effect. Some food components can alter drug reabsorption by the kidneys. For example, the amount of the medication lithium that is reabsorbed by the kidneys correlates with the amount of sodium reabsorbed. Consequently, both dehydration and sodium depletion, which increase sodium reabsorption, may result in lithium retention. Similarly, a person with a high sodium intake will excrete more sodium in the urine, and therefore more lithium. Individuals using lithium are advised to maintain a consistent sodium intake from day to day in order to maintain a stable blood level of lithium.[8]

Urine acidity can also affect drug excretion due to the effects of pH on a compound's chemical structure. The medication quinidine, used to treat arrhythmias, is excreted more readily in acidic urine. Foods or drugs that cause urine to become more alkaline (e.g., sodium bicarbonate) may reduce quinidine excretion and raise its blood levels.

The Inactive Ingredients in Drugs

Besides the active ingredients, medicines may contain other substances such as sugar, sorbitol, lactose, and sodium. For most people who use medicines on occasion and in small amounts, such ingredients pose no problem. When medicines are taken regularly or in large doses, however, people on special diets may need to be aware of these additional ingredients and their effects.

Sugar, Sorbitol, and Lactose

Many liquid preparations contain sugar or sorbitol to make them taste better. For people who must regulate their intakes of carbohydrates, such as people with diabetes, the amount of sugar in these medicines may need to be considered. Large doses of liquids containing sorbitol may cause diarrhea. The lactose added as filler to some medications may cause problems for people who are lactose intolerant.

Sodium

Antibiotics and antacids often contain sodium. People who take Alka Seltzer, for example, may not realize that a single two-tablet dose may exceed their recommended sodium intake for a whole day. In addition, antacids neutralize stomach acid, and many nutrients depend on acid for their digestion. Taking any antacid regularly will reduce the absorption of many nutrients.

Nutrient interactions and risks are not unique to prescription drugs. People who buy over-the-counter drugs or NHPs also need to protect themselves. The increasing availability of over-the-counter drugs and NHPs allows people to treat themselves for many ailments from arthritis to yeast infections. Consumers need to ask their physicians or other health-care providers about potential interactions and check with their pharmacists for instructions on taking drugs with foods. If problems arise, they should seek professional care without delay.

References

1. Canadian Institute of Health Information, Nearly two thirds of seniors using five or more types of prescription drugs (2008). www.cihi.ca/CIHI-ext-portal/internet/en/Document/types+of+care/pharmaceutical/RELEASE_18MAR2010, accessed September 18, 2011.
2. A. Bhutto and J. E. Morley, The clinical significance of gastrointenstinal changes with aging, *Current Opinion in Clinical and Nutritional Metabolism* 11 (2008): 651–660; J. Tam-McDevitt, Polypharmacy, aging, and cancer, *Oncology* 22 (2008): 1052–1055; E. Perucca, Age-related changes in pharmacokinetics: Predictability and assessment methods, *International Review of Neurobiology* 81 (2007): 183–199.
3. E. S. ElDesoky, Pharmacokinetic-pharmacodynamic crisis in the elderly, *American Journal of Therapeutics* 14 (2007): 488–498.
4. I. F. Btaiche and M. D. Kraft, Nutrients that may optimize drug effects, in J. I. Boullata and V. T. Armenti, eds., *Handbook of Drug-Nutrient Interactions* (Totowa, N.J.: Humana Press, 2004), pp. 195–216.
5. D. G. Bailey, J. Malcolm, O. Arnold, and J. D. Spence, Grapefruit juice-drug interactions, *British Journal of Clinical Pharmacology* 46:2 (1998): 101–110; W. W. McCloskey, K. Zaiken, and R. R. Couris, Clinically significant grapefruit juice: Drug interactions, *Nutrition Today* 43 (2008): 19–26; M. F. Paine and coauthors, Further characterization of a furanocoumarin-free grapefruit juice on drug disposition: Studies with cyclosporine, *American Journal of Clinical Nutrition* 87 (2008): 863–871; R. Bressler, Grapefruit juice and drug interactions. Exploring mechanisms of this interaction and potential toxicity for certain drugs, *Geriatrics* 61 (2006): 12–18.
6. J. L. Aston, A. E. Lodolce, and N. L. Shapiro, Interaction between warfarin and cranberry juice, *Pharmacotherapy* 26 (2006): 1314–1319.
7. S. A. Shapses, Y. R. Schlussel, and M. Cifuentes, Drug-nutrient interactions that impact mineral status, in J. I. Boullata and V. T. Armenti, eds., *Handbook of Drug-Nutrient Interactions* (Totowa, N.J.: Humana Press, 2004), pp. 301–328; B. J. McCabe, E. H. Frankel, and J. J. Wolfe, Monitoring nutritional status in drug regimens, in B. J. McCabe, E. H. Frankel, and J. J. Wolfe, eds., *Handbook of Food-Drug Interactions* (Boca Raton, Fla.: CRC Press, 2003), pp. 73–108.
8. McCabe, Frankel, and Wolfe, 2003.

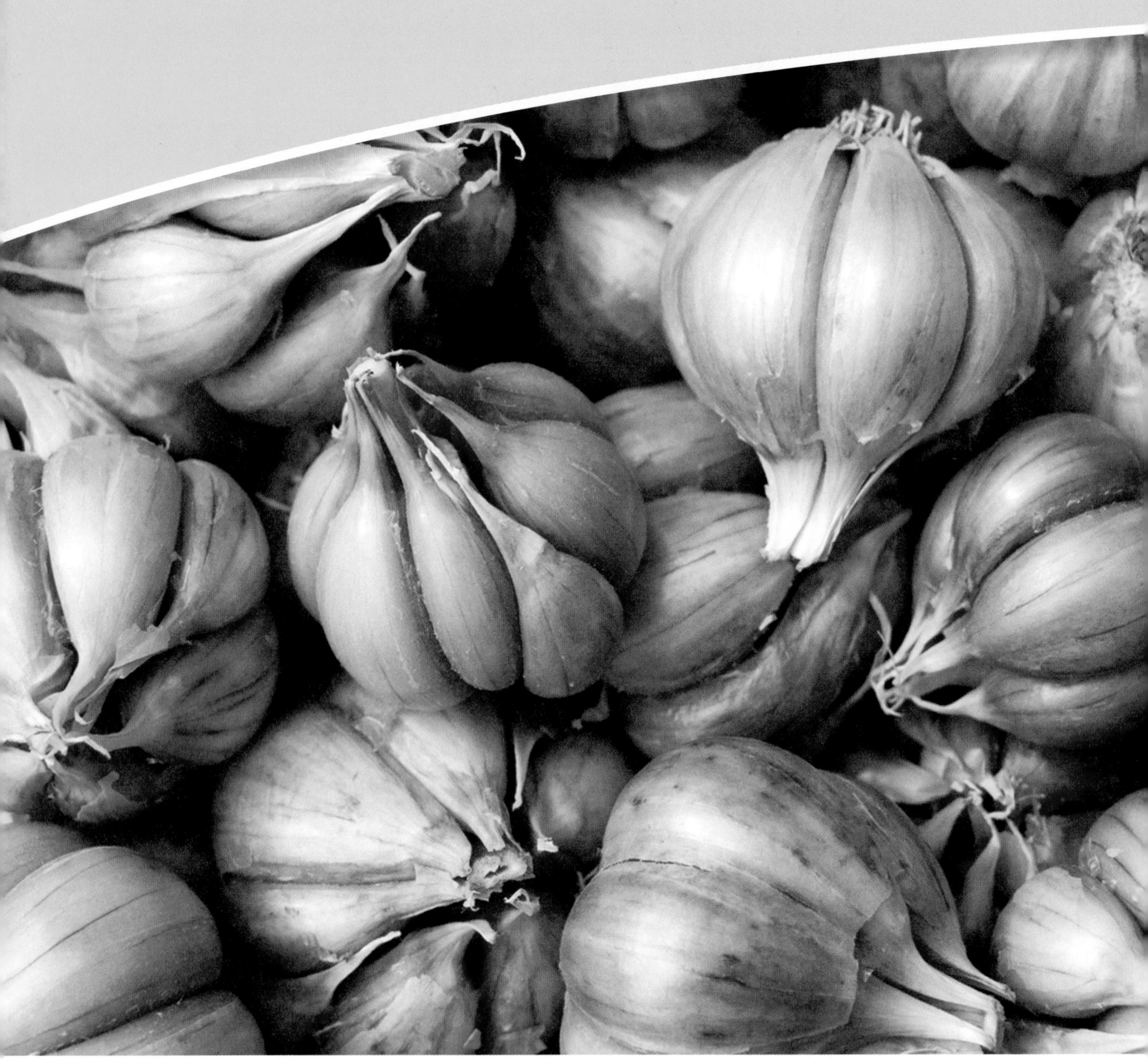

romvo/shutterstock

Nutrition in Your Life

CENGAGENOW™

Throughout this chapter, the CengageNOW logo indicates an opportunity for online self-study, linking you to interactive tutorials, activities, and videos to increase your understanding of chapter concepts.
www.cengage.com/sso

No doubt, you're familiar with the following recommendations for the primary prevention of chronic diseases: Eat more veggies. Eat more fibre. Eat more fish. Put down the saltshaker. Limit the fat. Be active. Don't smoke. And don't drink too much alcohol. What's the deal? If you follow this advice, will it really make a difference in how well or how long you live? In a word, yes. You can bet your life on it. If you could grow old in good health without having a heart attack or stroke, or getting diabetes, hypertension, or cancer, wouldn't you be willing to do just about anything—including improving your diet and activity habits? Of course, you would. And you can start today.

CHAPTER

19

Diet and Health

CHAPTER OUTLINE

Infectious diseases such as smallpox once claimed the lives of many children and limited the average life expectancy of adults. Thanks to medical science's ability to identify disease-causing microorganisms and develop preventive strategies, most people now live well into their later years, and the average life expectancy far exceeds that of our ancestors. In developed nations, purification of water and safe handling of foods help prevent the spread of infection. Antibiotics and immunizations provide additional protection for individuals.

Despite these advances, some infectious diseases still endanger many lives today. Disease strains such as tuberculosis and some foodborne infections, for example, have become resistant to antibiotics.[1] Nutrition cannot directly prevent or cure infectious diseases, but good nutrition can strengthen, and malnutrition can weaken, the body's defences against them.

The bulk of this chapter focuses on the chronic diseases that pose the greatest threat to the lives of most people in developed countries, but it begins with a description of the immune system and its inflammatory response. As you will see, inflammation underlies the development of many chronic diseases. Chronic diseases develop over a lifetime as a result of metabolic abnormalities induced by such factors as genetics, age, gender, and lifestyle. As you have learned, diet is among the many lifestyle factors ♦ that influence the development of chronic diseases.[2]

♦ Lifestyle factors that contribute to the development of chronic diseases:
- Diet
- Physical inactivity
- Overweight
- Tobacco use
- Alcohol and drug abuse

Nutrition and Infectious Diseases

It is difficult to know exactly where infectious diseases fall among the leading causes of death. Compared with chronic diseases, infectious diseases pose a much greater challenge for public health officials who track disease prevalence. One physician might classify an ear infection as an infectious disease, whereas another calls it a disease of the ear. Trends change quickly as well. A disease, such as AIDS, that did not even exist until the early 1980s may suddenly appear and become one of the leading causes of death. A preventive strategy, such as food irradiation, may just as quickly eliminate hundreds of thousands of cases of foodborne infections each year. Public health strategies help the entire country defend against the

infectious diseases: diseases caused by bacteria, viruses, parasites, or other microorganisms that can be transmitted from one person to another through air, water, or food; by contact; or through vector organisms such as mosquitoes.

spread of infection, and each individual's immune system provides a personal line of defence. A strong immune system depends on adequate nutrition. Poor nutrition weakens the immune system, which increases susceptibility to infections.

The Immune System

The **immune system** defends the body so diligently and silently that people do not even notice the thousands of enemy attacks mounted against them every day (the accompanying glossary defines immune system terms). If the immune system fails, though, the body suddenly becomes vulnerable to every wayward disease-causing agent that comes its way. Infectious disease invariably follows.

The body's first lines of defence—the skin, mucous membranes, and GI tract—normally deter foreign substances. If these barriers fail, then the organs ♦ and cells of the immune system race into action. Foreign substances that gain entry into the body and elicit such a response are called **antigens.** Examples include bacteria, viruses, toxins, and food proteins that cause allergies.

♦ Organs of the immune system:
- Spleen
- Lymph nodes
- Thymus

Of the 100 trillion cells that make up the human body, one in every hundred is a white blood cell. Two types of white blood cells, ♦ the phagocytes and lymphocytes, defend the body against infectious diseases.

♦ Cells of the immune system:
- Phagocytes
  - Neutrophils
  - Macrophages
- Lymphocytes
  - B-cells
  - T-cells

Phagocytes

Phagocytes, the scavengers of the immune system, are the first to arrive at the scene if an invader, such as a microorganism, gains entry. Upon recognizing the foreign invader, the phagocyte engulfs and digests it, if possible, in a process called **phagocytosis.** ♦ Phagocytes also secrete special proteins called **cytokines** that activate the metabolic and immune responses to infection.

♦ Two types of immune system cells ingest and destroy foreign antigens by phagocytosis: **neutrophils** and **macrophages.**

Lymphocytes: B-cells

There are two distinct types of **lymphocytes:** B-cells and T-cells. **B-cells** respond to infection by rapidly dividing and producing large proteins known as **antibodies.** Antibodies travel in the bloodstream to the site of the infection. There they stick to the surfaces of antigens and kill or otherwise inactivate them, making it easy for the phagocytes to ingest.

The antibodies are members of a class of proteins known as **immunoglobulins**—literally, large globular proteins that produce immunity. Antibodies react selectively to a specific foreign organism, and the B-cells retain a memory of how to make them. Consequently, the immune system can respond with greater speed the next time it encounters the same foreign organism. By doing so, B-cells play a major role in resistance to infection.

Lymphocytes: T-cells

The **T-cells** travel directly to the invasion site to battle the invaders. T-cells recognize the antigens displayed on the surfaces of phagocyte cells and multiply in response. Then they release powerful chemicals to destroy all the foreign particles that have this antigen on their surfaces. As the T-cells begin to win the battle against infection, they release signals to slow down the immune response.

Unlike the phagocytes, which are capable of inactivating many different types of invaders, T-cells are highly specific. Each T-cell can attack only one type of antigen. This specificity is remarkable, for nature creates millions of antigens. After destroying a particular antigen, some T-cells retain the necessary information to

GLOSSARY OF IMMUNE SYSTEM TERMS

antibodies: large proteins of the blood and body fluids, produced by the immune system in response to the invasion of the body by foreign molecules (usually proteins called *antigens*). Antibodies combine with and inactivate the foreign invaders, thus protecting the body.

antigens: substances that elicit the formation of antibodies or an inflammation reaction from the immune system.

B-cells: lymphocytes that produce antibodies. *B* stands for *bone marrow,* where the B-cells develop and mature.

cytokines (SIGH-toe-kines): special proteins that direct immune and inflammatory responses.

immune system: the body's natural defence against foreign materials that have penetrated the skin or mucous membranes.

immunoglobulins (IM-you-noh-GLOB-you-linz): proteins capable of acting as antibodies.

lymphocytes (LIM-foh-sites): white blood cells that participate in acquired immunity; B-cells and T-cells.

phagocytes (FAG-oh-sites): white blood cells (neutrophils and macrophages) that have the ability to ingest and destroy foreign substances.
- **phagein** = to eat

phagocytosis (FAG-oh-sigh-TOH-sis): the process by which phagocytes engulf and destroy foreign materials.

T-cells: lymphocytes that attack antigens. *T* stands for the *thymus gland,* where the T-cells mature.

serve as memory cells so that the immune system can rapidly produce the same type of T-cells again if the identical infection recurs.

T-cells actively defend the body against fungi, viruses, parasites, and a few types of bacteria; they can also destroy cancer cells. In organ transplant patients, T-cells participate in the rejection of newly transplanted tissues, which is why physicians prescribe immunosuppressive drugs following such surgery.

Nutrition and Immunity Of all the body's systems, the immune system responds most sensitively to subtle changes in nutrition status. Malnutrition compromises immunity.[3] Impaired immunity opens the way for infectious diseases, which typically raise nutrient needs and lower food intake. Consequently, nutrition status suffers further.[4] Thus disease and malnutrition create a **synergistic** downward spiral that must be broken for recovery to occur (see Figure 19-1).

Impaired immunity is a hallmark of protein-energy malnutrition (PEM). Table 19-1 presents the effects of PEM on the body's defences. As Chapter 6 explains, without sufficient protein to make antibodies, the immune system loses its ability to fight infections. Deficiencies of vitamins and minerals also diminish the immune response, as may excesses.[5] Likewise, interactions between nutrients may enhance or impair immunity. Quite simply, optimal immunity depends on optimal nutrition—enough, but not too much, of each of the nutrients. ♦ People with weakened immune systems, such as the elderly, may benefit from a nutritious diet and supplements of selected nutrients.

HIV and AIDS Perhaps the most infamous infectious disease today is **AIDS (acquired immune deficiency syndrome).** AIDS develops from infection by **HIV (human immunodeficiency virus)**, which is transmitted by direct contact with contaminated body fluids, including semen, vaginal secretions, and blood (but not saliva), or by passage of the infection from a mother to her infant during pregnancy, birth, or breastfeeding. HIV attacks the immune system and disables the body's defences against other diseases. Then these diseases, which would produce only mild, if any, illness in people with healthy immune systems, destroy health and life.

Table 19-2 (p. 620) shows the impact of AIDS worldwide and in North America. For many years, the devastating effects of HIV infection seemed unstoppable. However, in the mid-to-late 1990s, the death rate in the United States from AIDS began to decline, and the progression from HIV to AIDS slowed dramatically.[6] Even though remarkable progress has been made in understanding and treating HIV infection, the disease still has no cure. Without a cure, the best course is prevention. Unlike the chronic diseases featured in the remainder of this chapter, AIDS prevention does not in any way depend on good nutrition. Although good nutrition cannot prevent or cure AIDS, an adequate diet may improve responses to drugs, shorten hospital stays, promote independence, and improve the quality of life. In addition, because common food bacteria can easily overwhelm a compromised immune system, attention to food safety is critical. (Chapter 20 provides food-safety strategies.)

TABLE 19-1 Effects of Protein-Energy Malnutrition (PEM) on the Body's Defence Systems

Body's Defence System	Effects of PEM
Skin	Thinned, with less connective tissue to serve as a barrier to protect underlying tissues; delayed skin sensitivity reaction to antigens
Digestive tract and other body linings	Antibody secretions and immune cell number reduced
Lymph tissues[a]	Immune system organs reduced in size; cells of immune defence depleted
General response	Invader kill time prolonged; circulating immune cells reduced; antibody response impaired

[a]Lymph tissues include the thymus, lymph nodes, and spleen.

FIGURE 19-1 Nutrition and Immunity

Regardless of where a person enters the spiral, malnutrition, illness, and weakened immunity interact to compromise recovery and worsen malnutrition.

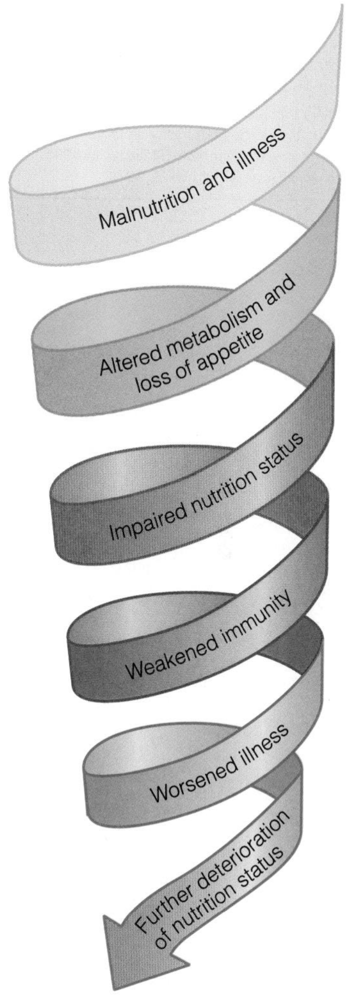
Malnutrition and illness
Altered metabolism and loss of appetite
Impaired nutrition status
Weakened immunity
Worsened illness
Further deterioration of nutrition status

♦ Nutrients known to affect immunity:
- Fatty acids
- Folate
- Iron
- Protein
- Selenium
- Vitamin A
- Vitamin B_6
- Vitamin C
- Vitamin E
- Zinc

synergistic (SIN-er-JIS-tick): multiple factors operating together in such a way that their combined effects are greater than the sum of their individual effects.

AIDS (acquired immune deficiency syndrome): the late stage of HIV infection, in which severe complications develop.

HIV (human immunodeficiency virus): the virus that causes AIDS. The infection progresses to become an immune system disorder that leaves its victims defenseless against numerous infections.

TABLE 19-2 The HIV and AIDS Epidemic at a Glance, 2007

Stage of Epidemic	World	North America
Individuals living with HIV infection or AIDS	33 200 000	1 300 000
Individuals newly infected with HIV	2 500 000	46 000
AIDS deaths	2 100 000	21 000

SOURCE: Joint United Nations Programme on HIV/AIDS and World Health Organization, *AIDS epidemic update: December 2007*, http://data.unaids.org/pub/EPISlides/2007/2007_epiupdate_en.pdf, accessed March 23, 2009.

Inflammation and Chronic Diseases The immune system's response to infection or injury results in inflammation. The blood supply to the area increases and the blood vessels become permeable, which allows the white blood cells to rush to the site. As phagocytes engulf the offending microbes, they release oxidative products, such as hydrogen peroxide, that kill the microbes. In this acute phase, inflammation fights off the infection or injury, removes damaged tissue, heals wounds, and promotes recovery from external stressors.[7] In this way, acute inflammation is beneficial.

When the inflammatory process persists, however, chronic inflammation is harmful. Cells of chronically inflamed tissues produce cytokines, oxidative products, blood clotting factors, and other bioactive chemicals that sustain the inflammatory response.[8] Such sustained inflammation threatens health and worsens the development of each of the chronic diseases discussed in the remainder of this chapter.

IN SUMMARY **Public health measures such as purification of water and safe handling of food help prevent the spread of infection in developed nations, and immunizations and antibiotics protect individuals. Nevertheless, some infectious diseases still endanger people today. Nutrition cannot prevent or cure infectious diseases, but adequate intakes of all the nutrients can help support the immune system as the body defends against disease-causing agents. If the immune system is impaired because of malnutrition or diseases such as AIDS, a person becomes vulnerable to infectious disease. Inflammation underlies many chronic diseases.**

Nutrition and Chronic Diseases

Figure 19-2 shows the four leading causes of death in Canada.[9] Three of these causes have some relationship with diet. Taken together, these three conditions account for almost 135 000 (57 percent) of deaths each year. Worldwide, statistics are similar, with developing nations sharing many of the same chronic diseases as developed nations.[10]

This chapter explains how the major chronic diseases develop and summarizes their major links with nutrition. Earlier chapters that describe the connections between individual nutrients and diseases did not focus on the mistaken impression of "one disease–one nutrient" relationships. Indeed, valid links do exist between saturated fat and heart disease, calcium and osteoporosis, and antioxidant nutrients and cancer, but focusing only on these links oversimplifies the story. In reality, each nutrient may have connections with several diseases

FIGURE 19-2 The Four Leading Causes of Death in Canada for 2007

Many deaths have multiple causes, but diet influences the development of several chronic diseases—notably, heart disease, some types of cancer, stroke, and diabetes.

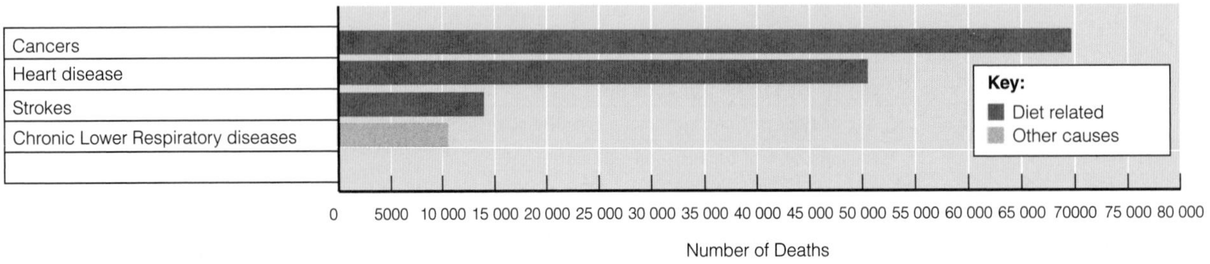
Cancers
Heart disease
Strokes
Chronic Lower Respiratory diseases
Key:
Diet related
Other causes
0
5000
10 000
15 000
20 000
25 000
30 000
35 000
40 000
45 000
50 000
55 000
60 000
65 000
70000
75 000
80 000
Number of Deaths

SOURCE: Statistics Canada, Leading Causes of Death 2007, Catalogue no. 84-215-X, http://www.statcan.gc.ca/pub/84-215-x/2010001/table-tableau/tbl001-eng.htm

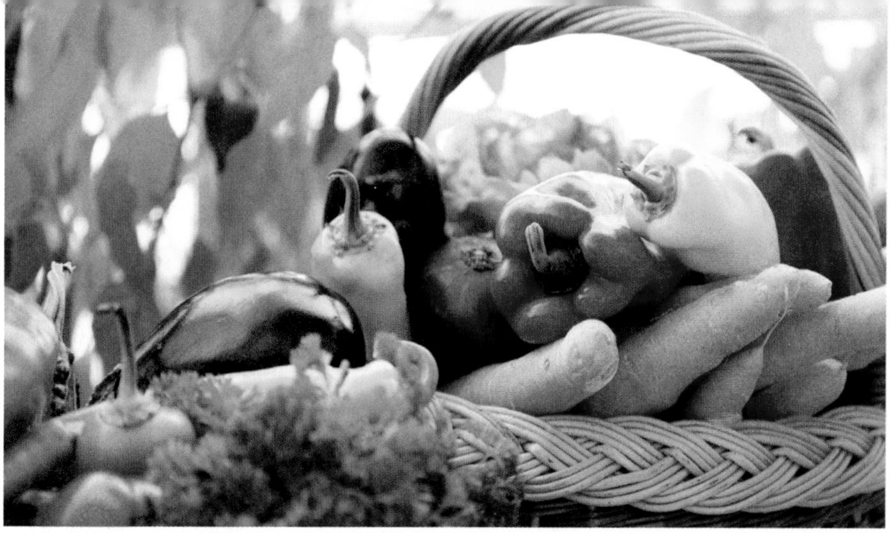

© Jasmina/iStockphoto

Vegetables rich in fibre, phytochemicals, and the antioxidant nutrients (beta-carotene, vitamin C, and vitamin E) help to protect against chronic diseases.

because its role in the body is not specific to a disease but to a body function. Furthermore, each of the chronic diseases develops in response to multiple risk factors, including many nondietary factors such as genetics, physical inactivity, and smoking. This chapter presents an integrated and balanced approach to primary prevention of disease, paying careful attention to all of the factors involved. Table 19-3 presents some of the relationships between risk factors and chronic diseases. Figure 19-3 shows how many of the diseases themselves are risk factors for other chronic diseases. For example, a person with diabetes is likely to develop atherosclerosis and hypertension.

Notice how many of the diseases listed in Table 19-3 have a genetic component. A family history of a certain disease is a powerful indicator of a person's tendency to contract that disease. Still, lifestyle factors are often pivotal in determining whether that tendency will be expressed.[11] Genetics and lifestyle often work synergistically; for instance, cigarette smoking is especially likely to bring on heart disease in people who are genetically predisposed to develop it. Not smoking would benefit everyone's health, of course, regardless of genetic predis-

FIGURE 19-3 Interrelationships among Chronic Diseases

Notice that many chronic diseases are themselves risk factors for other chronic diseases and that all of them are linked to obesity. The risk factors highlighted in blue define the metabolic syndrome.

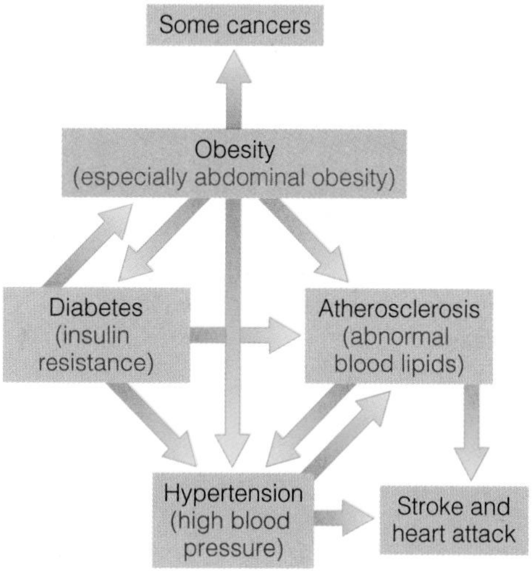
Some cancers
Obesity (especially abdominal obesity)
Diabetes (insulin resistance)
Atherosclerosis (abnormal blood lipids)
Hypertension (high blood pressure)
Stroke and heart attack

TABLE 19-3 Risk Factors and Chronic Diseases

	Cancers	Hypertension	Diabetes (type 2)	Atherosclerosis	Obesity	Stroke
Dietary Risk Factors						
Diets high in added sugars (e.g., beverages)				✓*	✓	
Diets high in salty or pickled foods	✓	✓				
Diets high in saturated and/or *trans* fat	✓	✓	✓	✓	✓	✓
Diets low in fruits, vegetables, and other foods rich in fibre and phytochemicals	✓		✓	✓	✓	✓
Diets low in vitamins and/or minerals	✓	✓		✓		
Excessive alcohol intake	✓	✓		✓	✓	✓
Other Risk Factors						
Age	✓	✓	✓	✓		✓
Environmental contaminants	✓					
Genetics	✓	✓	✓	✓	✓	✓
Sedentary lifestyle	✓	✓	✓	✓	✓	✓
Smoking and tobacco use	✓	✓		✓		✓
Stress		✓		✓		✓

* Emerging evidence.

position, but some recommendations to prevent chronic diseases best meet an individual's needs when family history is considered. For example, women with a family history of breast cancer might reduce their risks if they abstain from alcohol, whereas those with a family history of heart disease might benefit from one or two glasses of wine a week.

IN SUMMARY **Cancer, heart disease, and strokes are the three leading causes of death in the Canada and diabetes also ranks among the top 10. All of these chronic diseases have significant links with nutrition. Other lifestyle risk factors and genetics are also important.**

Cardiovascular Disease

The major causes of death around the world today are diseases of the heart and blood vessels, collectively known as **cardiovascular disease (CVD)**. (The accompanying glossary defines this and other heart disease terms.) In Canada cardiovascular disease claims the lives of over 50 000 people each year.[12]

Coronary heart disease (CHD) is the most common form of cardiovascular disease and is usually caused by **atherosclerosis** in the **coronary arteries** that supply blood to the heart muscle. Atherosclerosis is the accumulation of lipids and other materials in the arteries.

How Atherosclerosis Develops

As Highlight 17 points out, no one is free of the fatty streaks that may one day become the **plaques** ♦ of atherosclerosis. For most adults, the question is not whether you have plaques, but how advanced they are and what you can do to slow or reverse their progression.

♦ Plaques associated with atherosclerosis are known as **atheromatous** (ATH-er-OH-ma-tus) **plaques.**

Atherosclerosis or "hardening of the arteries" usually begins with the accumulation of soft fatty streaks along the inner arterial walls, especially at branch points (review Figure H17-1 on p. 582). These fatty streaks gradually enlarge and harden as they fill with cholesterol, other lipids, and calcium, and they become encased in fibrous connective tissue, forming plaques. Plaques stiffen the arteries and narrow the passages through them. Most people have well-developed plaques by the age of 30. As Chapter 5 points out, a diet high in saturated fat is a major contributor to the development of plaques and the progression of atherosclerosis.[13] But atherosclerosis is much more than the simple accumulation of lipids

GLOSSARY OF HEART DISEASE TERMS

aneurysm (AN-you-rizm): an abnormal enlargement or bulging of a blood vessel (usually an artery) caused by damage to or weakness in the blood vessel wall.

angina (an-JYE-nah or AN-ji-nah): a painful feeling of tightness or pressure in and around the heart, often radiating to the back, neck, jaw, and arms; caused by a lack of oxygen to an area of heart muscle.

atherosclerosis: a type of artery disease characterized by plaques along the inner walls of the arteries.

cardiovascular disease (CVD): a general term for all diseases of the heart and blood vessels.

CHD risk equivalents: disorders that raise the risk of heart attacks, strokes, and other complications associated with cardiovascular disease to the same degree as existing CHD. These disorders include symptomatic carotid artery disease, peripheral arterial disease, abdominal aortic aneurysm, and diabetes mellitus.

coronary arteries: blood vessels that supply blood to the heart.

coronary heart disease (CHD): the damage that occurs when the blood vessels carrying blood to the heart (the **coronary arteries**) become narrow and occluded.

embolism (EM-boh-lizm): the obstruction of a blood vessel by an *embolus* (EM-boh-luss), or travelling clot, causing sudden tissue death.
- **embol** = to insert, plug

heart attack: sudden tissue death caused by blockages of vessels that feed the heart muscle; also called *myocardial* (my-oh-KAR-dee-al) *infarction* (in-FARK-shun) or *cardiac arrest*.
- **myo** = muscle
- **cardial** = heart
- **infarct** = tissue death

hypertension: higher-than-normal blood pressure. Hypertension that develops without an identifiable cause is known as *essential* or *primary hypertension;* hypertension that is caused by a specific disorder such as kidney disease is known as *secondary hypertension*.

plaques (PLACK): an accumulation of fatty deposits, smooth muscle cells, calcium, and fibrous connective tissue that develops in the artery walls in atherosclerosis. Plaque associated with atherosclerosis is known as *atheromatous* (ATH-er-OH-mat-tus) *plaque*.

prehypertension: slightly higher than normal blood pressure, but not as high as hypertension (see Table 19-5).

stroke: an event in which the blood flow to a part of the brain is cut off; also called *cerebrovascular accident (CVA)*.
- **cerebro** = brain
- **vascular** = blood vessels

thrombosis (throm-BOH-sis): the formation of a *thrombus* (THROM-bus), or a blood clot, that may obstruct a blood vessel, causing gradual tissue death.
- **thrombo** = clot

transient ischemic (is-KEY-mik) **attack (TIA):** a temporary reduction in blood flow to the brain, which causes temporary symptoms that vary depending on the part of the brain affected. Common symptoms include light-headedness, visual disturbances, paralysis, staggering, numbness, and inability to swallow.

within the artery wall—it is a complex inflammatory response to tissue damage. Indeed, extensive evidence confirms that inflammation is centrally involved in all stages of atherosclerosis.[14]

Inflammation The cells lining the blood vessels may incur damage from high LDL cholesterol, hypertension, toxins from cigarette smoking, elevated homocysteine, or some viral and bacterial infections.[15] Such damage increases the permeability of the blood vessel walls and elicits an inflammatory response. The immune system sends in macrophages, ♦ and the smooth muscle cells of the artery wall try to repair the damage. Particles of LDL cholesterol become trapped in the blood vessel walls. Free radicals produced during inflammatory responses oxidize the LDL cholesterol, and the macrophages engulf it. The macrophages swell with large quantities of oxidized LDL cholesterol and eventually become the cells of plaque. Arterial damage and the inflammatory response also favour the formation of blood clots and allow minerals to harden plaque and form the fibrous connective tissue that encapsulates it.

The inflammatory response of atherosclerosis weakens the walls of the arteries and may cause an **aneurysm**—the abnormal bulging of a blood vessel wall. Aneurysms can rupture and lead to massive bleeding and death, particularly when a large blood vessel such as the aorta is affected. The central role of the inflammatory response in atherosclerosis has led researchers to look for signs or markers of inflammation in the blood vessel walls. One of the most promising of these markers is a protein known as **C-reactive protein (CRP)**. Recent studies have revealed that high levels of CRP, non-HDL cholesterol (non-HDL-C), and other bio-markers of cardiovascular disease may prove to more accurately predict future heart attack and mortality than high LDL cholesterol, which has a strong relationship with atherosclerosis, as a later section explains.[16]

Emerging evidence points to another important inflammatory marker, **lipoprotein-associated phospholipase A(2)** or **Lp-PLA(2)**. Lp-PLA(2) appears to be a highly specific marker of plaque inflammation and the formation of plaques that are most susceptible to rupture.[17] ♦ In addition to traditional risk assessment, Lp-PLA(2) is recommended as a diagnostic test for vascular inflammation to better identify people at high or very high risk of cardiovascular disease.[18]

Plaques Once a plaque has formed, a sudden spasm or surge in blood pressure in an artery can tear away part of its fibrous coat/cap, causing it to rupture. Some types of plaque are more unstable than others and are therefore more vulnerable to rupture.[19] Such plaques have a thin fibrous cap, a large lipid core, and an abundance of macrophages—characteristics that undermine plaque stability.[20] Researchers now know that the *composition* of plaques—rather than the *size* of plaques—is a key predictor of plaque rupture and subsequent clot formation.[21] When plaques rupture, the immune system responds to the damage as it would to other tissue injuries.

Blood Clots **Platelets** are tiny disc-shaped bodies that cover an injured or damaged area. Together with other factors, platelets form blood clots. Abnormal blood clotting can trigger life-threatening events. For example, a blood clot may gradually grow large enough to restrict or close off a blood vessel (**thrombosis**). ♦ A clot may also break free from an artery wall and travel through the circulatory system until it lodges in a small artery and suddenly shuts off blood flow to the tissues (**embolism**).

The action of platelets is under the control of certain eicosanoids, known as prostaglandins and thromboxanes, which are made from the 20-carbon omega-6 and omega-3 fatty acids (introduced in Chapter 5). Each eicosanoid plays a specific role in helping to regulate ♦ many of the body's activities. Sometimes their actions oppose each other.[22] For example, one eicosanoid prevents clot formation, and another promotes it. Similarly, one dilates the blood vessels, and another constricts them. When omega-3 fatty acids are abundant in the diet, ♦ they make more of the kinds of eicosanoids that favour heart health.[23]

♦ **Macrophages** are large, phagocytic cells of the immune system.
- **macro** = large
- **phagein** = to eat

♦ A plaque that is susceptible to rupture because it has only a thin fibrous barrier between its lipid-rich core and the artery lining is called **vulnerable plaque.**

♦ A **coronary thrombosis** blocks blood flow through an artery that feeds the heart muscle. A **cerebral thrombosis** blocks blood flow through an artery that feeds the brain.

♦ Eicosanoids help to regulate:
- Blood pressure
- Blood clot formation
- Blood vessel contractions
- Immune response
- Nerve impulse transmissions

♦ Major sources of omega-3 fatty acids:
- Vegetable oils (canola, soybean, flaxseed)
- Walnuts, flaxseeds
- Fatty fish (mackerel, salmon, sardines)

C-reactive protein (CRP): a protein released during the acute phase of infection or inflammation that enhances immunity by promoting phagocytosis and activating platelets. Its presence may be used to assess a person's risk of an impending heart attack or stroke.

lipoprotein-associated phospholipase A(2) or **Lp-PLA(2):** a lipoprotein-bound enzyme that generates potent proinflammatory and proatherogenic products such as oxidized free fatty acids and lysophosphatidylcholine. Lp-PLA(2) is a specific marker of plaque inflammation.

platelets: tiny, disc-shaped bodies in the blood, important in blood clot formation.

Blood Pressure and Atherosclerosis The heart must create enough pressure to push blood around the body through the circulatory system. When arteries are narrowed by plaques, clots, or both, blood flow is restricted, and the heart must then work harder to generate more pressure to deliver blood to the tissues. This higher blood pressure further damages the artery walls, and plaques and clots are especially likely to form at damage points. Thus the development of atherosclerosis is a self-accelerating process. (A later section describes additional consequences of high blood pressure.)

The Result: Heart Attacks and Strokes When atherosclerosis in the coronary arteries becomes severe enough to restrict blood flow and deprive the heart muscle of oxygen, CHD develops. The person with CHD often experiences pain and pressure in the area around the heart (**angina**). A **heart attack** occurs when blood flow to the heart is cut off and that area of the heart muscle dies. Restricted blood flow to the brain causes a **transient ischemic attack (TIA)** or **stroke**. Right behind cancer, coronary heart disease and strokes are the leading causes of death for adults in Canada.

♦ Some risk factors, such as diet and physical activity, are *modifiable,* meaning that they can be changed; others, such as genetics, age, and gender, are not modifiable.

Risk Factors for Coronary Heart Disease

Although atherosclerosis can develop in any blood vessel, the coronary arteries are most often affected, leading to CHD. Table 19-4 lists the major risk factors ♦ for CHD. The criteria for defining blood lipids, blood pressure, and obesity in relation to CHD risk are shown in Table 19-5; Table H17-1 on p. 583 presents cholesterol standards for children and adolescents.

By middle age, most adults have at least one risk factor for CHD, and many have more than one.[24] Public health officials in both Canada and the United States recommend screening to identify risk factors in individuals and offer preventive advice for the population.[25] Regular screening and early detection have proven successful: for the last couple decades, both blood cholesterol levels and deaths from cardiovascular disease among Canadian adults have shown a continuous and substantial downward trend.[26] These trends also reflect behaviour changes in individuals. As adults grow older, many of them stop smoking, limit alcohol consumption, and become mindful that their food choices can improve their cardiovascular health.

TABLE 19-4 Risk Factors for CHD

Major Risk Factors for CHD (not modifiable)
• Increasing age
• Male gender
• Family history of premature heart disease
Major Risk Factors for CHD (modifiable)
• High blood LDL cholesterol
• Low blood HDL cholesterol
• High blood pressure (hypertension)
• Diabetes
• Obesity (especially abdominal obesity)
• Physical inactivity
• Cigarette smoking
• An "atherogenic" diet (high in saturated fats and low in vegetables, fruits, and whole grains)

NOTE: Risk factors highlighted in yellow have relationships with diet.
SOURCE: National Heart, Lung, and Blood Institute, National Institutes of Health, U.S. Department of Health and Human Services. Expert Panel on Detection, Evaluation, and Treatment of High Blood Cholesterol in Adults (Adult Treatment Panel III), Third Report of the National Cholesterol Education Program (NCEP), NIH publication no. 02-5215 (Bethesda, Md.: National Heart, Lung, and Blood Institute, 2002), pp. II-15–II-20.

Age, Gender, and Family History A review of Table 19-4 shows that three of the major risk factors for CHD cannot be modified by diet or otherwise: age, gender, and family history. As men and women grow older, the risk of CHD rises. The increasing risk of CHD with advancing age reflects the steady progression of atherosclerosis.[27] On average, older people have more atherosclerosis than younger people do.

In men, aging becomes a significant risk factor at age 45 and older. CHD occurs about 10 to 15 years later in women than in men. Women younger than 45 tend to have lower LDL cholesterol than men of the same age, but women's blood cholesterol typically begins to rise between ages 45 and 55. Thus aging becomes a significant risk factor for women who are 55 and older. The gender difference has been attributed to a protective effect of estrogen in women, but CHD rates do not suddenly accelerate at menopause as naturally occurring estrogen levels taper off.[28] Rather, as in men, heart disease rates increase linearly with age. And, as

TABLE 19-5 Adult Standards for Blood Lipids, Body Mass Index (BMI), and Blood Pressure

	Total Blood Cholesterol (mmol/L)	LDL Cholesterol (mmol/L)	HDL Cholesterol (mmol/L)	Total Cholesterol to HDL Cholesterol Ratio	Triglycerides, Fasting (mmol/L)	Body Mass Index (BMI)[a]	Blood Pressure Systolic/Diastolic (mmHg)
Low risk	≤4.1	<5.0	>1.2	<6.0	<1.7	<25	<120/90

[a]Body mass index (BMI) was defined in Chapter 9; BMI standards are found on the inside back cover.

SOURCE: Data from Genest J. and co-authors. 2009 Canadian Cardiovascular Society/Canadian guidelines for the diagnosis and treatment of dyslipidemia and prevention of cardiovascular disease in the adult—2009 recommendations. Canadian Journal of Cardiology 25 (10): 567–579.

in men, all of the major risk factors raise the risk of CHD in women. Ultimately, CHD kills as many women as men.

Nonetheless, at every age, men have a greater risk of CHD than women do. The reasons for this gender difference are not completely understood, but they can be partly explained by the earlier onset of risk factors such as elevated LDL cholesterol and blood pressure in men. Levels of the amino acid homocysteine, which may damage artery walls and increase oxidative stress, rise with age and are generally higher in men. Researchers have not determined whether the damage is caused by homocysteine itself or by a factor associated with it.[29]

A history of early CHD in immediate family members is an independent risk factor even when other risk factors are considered. The more family members affected and the earlier the age of onset, the greater the risk.[30]

High LDL and Low HDL Cholesterol In population studies, the relationship between total blood cholesterol and atherosclerosis is strong ♦ —and most of the total cholesterol is made up of LDL cholesterol. The higher the LDL cholesterol, the greater the risk of CHD. In contrast, the lower the LDL cholesterol and blood pressure, the slower the progression of atherosclerosis.[32]

♦ More than 40 percent of Canadian adults have high plasma Total Cholesterol levels.[31]

The LDL are clearly the most atherogenic lipoproteins. As Chapter 5 explains, HDL also carry cholesterol, but raised HDL represents cholesterol returning from the cells to the liver where it will be used to make bile acids and excreted in the GI tract. Thus high HDL indicates a *reduced* risk of atherosclerosis and heart attack. High LDL and low HDL correlate *directly* with heart disease, ♦ whereas low LDL and high HDL correlate *inversely* with risk.

♦ Cholesterol is carried in several lipoproteins, chief among them LDL and HDL (see Chapter 5 for details). Remember them this way:
- **LDL** = **L**ow-density lipoproteins = **L**ess healthy
- **HDL** = **H**igh-density lipoproteins = **H**ealthy

Any LDL cholesterol that remains in the blood after the body's cells take up the amount they need becomes vulnerable to oxidation. High blood levels of LDL cholesterol, especially oxidized LDL, trigger a series of events that promote plaque development and contribute to plaque instability.[33] Oxidized LDL cholesterol stimulates production of atherogenic signalling molecules. These signalling molecules attract immune cells and allow them to adhere to, and penetrate, the innermost layer of the arterial wall. Within the arterial wall, these immune cells undergo transformation and replication into macrophages that form the lipid-rich foam cells characteristic of fatty streaks. Macrophages within the arterial wall perpetuate chronic inflammation by releasing inflammatory cytokines that contribute to plaque rupture.[34] When plaques rupture, a heart attack or stroke may occur. In the early stages of atherosclerosis, the goal of treatment is to slow plaque development. In the later stages, the goal of treatment is to stabilize plaques.

Research shows that atherosclerosis is reversible by removing the trapped macrophages from the arterial wall.[35] Key antioxidants such as resveratrol (found in red grapes and wine made from red grapes) break the adhesion, releasing the macrophages from the arterial wall and promoting healing.

High Blood Pressure (Hypertension) Atherosclerosis is frequently accompanied by chronic high blood pressure (**hypertension**). The higher blood pressure is above normal, the greater the risk of heart disease. However, even values only slightly higher than desirable—classified as **prehypertension** in Table 19-5—increase the risk of heart attack and stroke.[36] This relationship between hypertension and heart disease risk holds true for men and women, young and old. High blood pressure injures the artery walls and accelerates plaque formation, thus initiating or worsening the progression of atherosclerosis. Then the plaques and reduced blood flow raise blood pressure further, and hypertension and atherosclerosis become mutually aggravating conditions.

Diabetes Diabetes—a major independent risk factor for all forms of cardiovascular disease—substantially increases the risk of death from CHD.[37] In diabetes, blood vessels often become blocked and circulation diminishes. Atherosclerosis progresses rapidly. For many people with diabetes, the risk of heart attack is similar to that of people with established CHD.[38] In fact, physicians describe diabetes and other disorders that have risks similar to CHD as **CHD risk equivalents.** Treatment to lower LDL cholesterol in diabetes follows the same recommendations as in CHD.

Obesity and Physical Inactivity Obesity, especially abdominal obesity, and physical inactivity significantly increase the risk for CHD, contributing to high LDL cholesterol, low HDL cholesterol, hypertension, and diabetes.[39] Conversely, weight loss and physical activity protect against CHD by lowering LDL, raising HDL, improving insulin sensitivity, and lowering blood pressure.[40] Regular physical activity also increases energy expenditure and builds lean body mass, thereby improving body composition and physical fitness.

Cigarette Smoking Cigarette smoking is a powerful risk factor for CHD and other forms of cardiovascular disease. The risk increases the more a person smokes and is the same for men and women. Smoking damages the heart directly by increasing blood pressure and the heart's workload. It deprives the heart of oxygen and damages platelets, making blood clot formation likely. Toxins in cigarette smoke damage blood vessels, setting the stage for atherosclerosis. When people quit smoking, their risk of CHD begins to decline within a few months.[41]

Atherogenic Diet Diet also influences the risk of CHD. An "atherogenic diet"—high in saturated fats, *trans* fats, and cholesterol and low in vegetables, fruits, and whole grains—elevates LDL cholesterol. Conversely, diets rich in fruits, vegetables, and whole grains seem to lower the risk of CHD even more than might be expected based on risk factors such as LDL cholesterol alone.[42] Dietary strategies to reduce the risk of CHD are discussed in a later section.

Other Risk Factors The major risk factors for CHD listed in Table 19-4 (p. 624) and discussed in the previous sections have solid associations with the development of CHD. Nevertheless, other factors also seem to influence a person's risk of CHD. These factors, known as **emerging risk factors,** may be helpful in assessing an individual's risk of CHD. For example, some people with CHD, especially those with diabetes and those who are overweight, have elevated triglycerides. Whether elevated triglycerides represent an independent risk factor for CHD remains controversial.[43] Part of the controversy arises from the role that elevated triglyceride levels play in lipoprotein metabolism. When triglycerides are moderately high, remnants of very-low-density lipoproteins (VLDL) increase in the blood. These small, triglyceride-rich lipoproteins are highly atherogenic.[44]

A second part of the controversy has to do with the way triglycerides are currently measured. National guidelines recommend drawing blood for lipid profiles after a 12-hour fast to provide consistent risk assessment. Recent research, however, suggests that *nonfasting* triglyceride levels more strongly predict CHD risk than fasting levels.[45] The latest report by the U.S. National Cholesterol Education Program Expert Panel considers elevated blood triglycerides a marker for other risk factors (high LDL, low HDL, overweight, and diabetes), but does not designate them as a major risk factor.

Metabolic Syndrome As Table 19-4 shows, most of the modifiable risk factors for CHD are directly related to diet. Several of these diet-related risk factors—low HDL, high blood pressure, insulin resistance, ♦ and abdominal obesity—along with high blood triglycerides comprise a cluster of health risks known as **metabolic syndrome.** As Figure 19-3 (p. 621) shows, the risks that define metabolic syndrome ♦ underlie several chronic diseases and increase the risks of CHD and type 2 diabetes.[46] Metabolic syndrome, like the chronic diseases associated with it, also includes markers of inflammation and thrombosis.[47] Overeating and physical inactivity play a major role in the development of metabolic syndrome. A new definition of the metabolic syndrome has recently been proposed to include greater emphasis on central obesity.[48] Regardless of slight differences in defining *metabolic syndrome,* experts agree that the prevalence of metabolic syndrome among Canadian adults is high, and that treatment to reduce these risk factors for heart disease and diabetes should begin early and focus on changes in lifestyle.

♦ **Insulin resistance** is the condition in which a normal amount of insulin is ineffective in lowering blood glucose. Thus insulin resistance results in an elevated fasting glucose. Insulin resistance develops as a metabolic consequence of obesity that precedes type 2 diabetes.

♦ Metabolic syndrome includes any three of the following:

- Abdominal obesity: waist circumference >102 cm (for men) or >89 cm (for women)
- Triglycerides: ≥1.7 mmol/L
- HDL: <1.03 mmol/L (in men) or <1.3 mmol/L (in women)
- Blood pressure: ≥130/85 mmHg
- Fasting glucose: ≥6.1 mmol/L

emerging risk factors: recently identified factors that enhance the ability to predict disease risk in an individual.

metabolic syndrome: a combination of risk factors—insulin resistance, hypertension, abnormal blood lipids, and abdominal obesity—that greatly increase a person's risk of developing coronary heart disease; also called *Syndrome X, insulin resistance syndrome,* or *dysmetabolic syndrome.*

Recommendations for Reducing Coronary Heart Disease Risk

Recommendations to reduce CHD risk include both screening and intervention. The "How To" on p. 628 provides a tool to assess a person's 10-year heart disease risk. Notice that total cholesterol and HDL cholesterol are included in the assessment, but LDL cholesterol is not. LDL cholesterol is routinely estimated from measures of total cholesterol and HDL cholesterol and thus would not add information to this assessment.[49] Once a person's risks have been identified, treatment focuses on lowering LDL cholesterol. Lowering LDL cholesterol significantly reduces the incidence of CHD.[50] Treatment plans may include major lifestyle changes in diet, physical activity, and smoking cessation; medications; or combinations. The LDL cholesterol goals and treatment plans are specific to individuals, so they are best prescribed by a qualified health-care provider.

Cholesterol Screening To determine an individual's risk of CHD, health-care professionals review the person's health history and measure several blood lipids including total cholesterol, LDL cholesterol, HDL cholesterol, and triglycerides. Ideally, at least two measurements are taken at least one week apart and then compared to standards (shown earlier in Table 19-5 on p. 624). Single measurements may fail to identify those at risk or may misclassify them because blood cholesterol and other lipid concentrations vary significantly from day to day.

Lifestyle Changes Recommendations to reduce the risk of CHD focus first on lifestyle changes. To that end, people are encouraged to increase physical activity, lose weight (if necessary), implement dietary changes, and reduce exposure to tobacco smoke either by quitting smoking or by avoiding secondhand smoke.[51] Altering one's lifestyle is challenging, and instruction and counselling, including assessing the client's or patient's "stage of change," are critical for success. Health-care professionals can explain the reasons for change, set obtainable goals, and offer practical suggestions. If lifestyle changes fail to lower LDL or blood pressure to acceptable levels, then medications are prescribed. Table 19-6 summarizes strategies to reduce the risk of heart disease.[52] The "How To" on p. 629 offers suggestions for implementing a heart-healthy diet, most of which are aligned with the *Food Guide*.

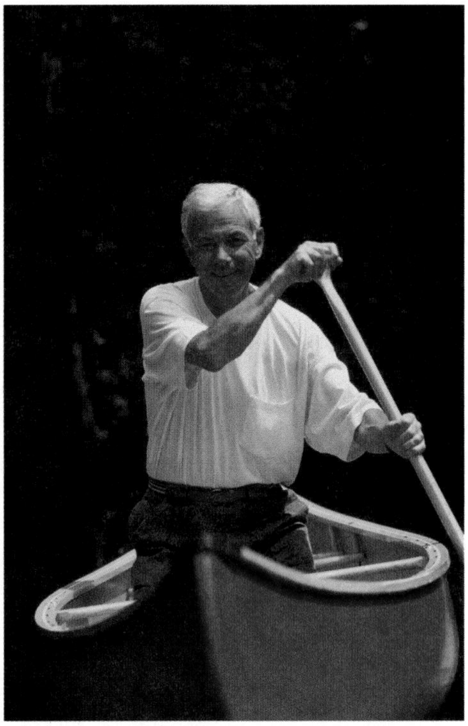

photos.com

Regular aerobic exercise can help to defend against heart disease by strengthening the heart muscle, promoting weight loss, and improving blood lipid and blood glucose levels.

IN SUMMARY **Atherosclerosis is characterized by plaque build-up in artery walls. Rupture of plaques or abnormal blood clotting can cause heart attacks and strokes. Dietary recommendations to lower the risks of cardiovascular disease are summarized in Table 19-6. Quitting smoking and engaging in regular physical activity also improve heart health.**

TABLE 19-6 Primary and Secondary Prevention Strategies to Reduce Risk of CHD

Dietary Strategies

- **Energy:** Balance energy intake and physical activity to prevent weight gain and to achieve or maintain a healthy body weight.
- **Saturated fat, *trans* fat, and cholesterol:** Choose lean meats, vegetables, and 1% milk products; minimize intake of hydrogenated fats. Limit saturated fats to less than 7 percent of total kcalories, *trans* fat to less than 1 percent of total kcalories, and cholesterol to less than 300 milligrams a day.
- **Soluble fibres:** Choose a diet rich in vegetables, fruits, whole grains, and other foods such as oat products high in soluble fibres and look for this type of Health Claim on foods.
- **Potassium and sodium:** Choose a diet high in potassium-rich fruits and vegetables, 1% milk products, nuts, and whole grains. Choose and prepare foods with little or no salt (limit sodium intake to 2300 mg/day) and look for this type of Health Claim on foods.
- **Added sugars:** Minimize intake of beverages and foods with added sugars (e.g., keep added sugars to less than 100 kcal/day for females and 150 kcals/day for men).
- **Fish and omega-3 fatty acids:** Consume fatty fish rich in omega-3 fatty acids (salmon, tuna, sardines) at least twice a week (see Table H5-1).
- **Plant sterols and stanols:** Consume food products that contain added plant sterols or stanols and look for this type of Health Claim on foods.
- **Soy:** Consume soy foods more often to replace animal and dairy products that contain saturated fat and cholesterol.
- **Alcohol:** If alcohol is consumed, limit it to one drink daily for women and two drinks daily for men.

Lifestyle Choices

- **Physical activity:** Participate in at least 30 minutes of moderate- to vigorous-intensity endurance activity on most days of the week. The eventual goal should be an expenditure of at least 2000 kcalories weekly.
- **Smoking cessation:** Minimize exposure to any form of tobacco or tobacco smoke.

SOURCES: AHA Scientific Statement: Diet and lifestyle recommendations revision 2006, *Circulation* 114 (2006): 82–96; F. M. Sacks and coauthors for the American Heart Association Nutrition Committee, Soy protein, isoflavones, and cardiovascular health, *Circulation* 113 (2006): 1034–1044; Expert Panel on Detection, Evaluation, and Treatment of High Blood Cholesterol in Adults (Adult Treatment Panel III) *Third Report of the National Cholesterol Education Program (NCEP)*, NIH publication No. 02-5215 (Bethesda, Md.: National Heart, Lung, and Blood Institute, 2002), pp. V1–V28; J. Genest, R. McPherson, J. Frohlich, et al. 2009 Canadian Cardiovascular Society/Canadian guidelines for the diagnosis and treatment of dyslipidemia and prevention of cardiovascular disease in the adult—2009 recommendations. *Canadian Journal of Cardiology* 25:10 (2009): 567–579.

HOW TO

HOW TO ASSESS YOUR RISK OF HEART DISEASE

Do you know your heart disease risk score? This assessment estimates your ten-year risk for heart disease using charts from the Framingham Heart Study.* Be aware that a high score does not mean that you will develop heart disease, but it should warn you of the possibility and prompt you to consult a physician about your health. You will need to know your blood cholesterol (ideally, the average of at least two recent measurements) and blood pressure (ideally, the average of several recent measurements). With this information in hand, find yourself in the charts below and add the points for each risk factor.

Age (years)	Points	
	Men	Women
30—34	0	0
35—39	2	2
40—44	5	4
45—49	7	5
50—54	8	7
55—59	10	8
60—64	11	9
65—69	13	10
70—74	14	11
75+	16	12

HDL Cholesterol Level (mmol/L)	Points	
HDL-C (mmol/L)	Men	Women
>1.6	—2	—2
1.3—1.6	—1	—1
1.2—1.3	0	0
0.9—1.2	1	1
<0.9	2	2

Systolic Blood Pressure (mm Hg)	Points			
	Untreated		Treated	
	Men	*Women*	*Men*	*Women*
<120	—2	—3	0	—1
120—129	0	0	2	2
130—139	1	1	3	3
140—149	2	2	4	5
150—159	2	4	4	6
>160	3	5	5	7

Total Cholesterol (mmol/L)	Points	
Total-C (mmol/L)	Men	Women
<4.1	0	0
4.1—5.2	1	1
5.2—6.2	2	3
6.2—7.2	3	4
>7.2	4	5

Scoring Your 10-Year Heart Disease Risk

From the four panels above add up the total points for your gender: _____. Now find your 10-year risk score in the panel below.

- <10 = Low Risk
- 10 – 20 = Moderate Risk
- >20 = High Risk

Cardiovascular Disease Risk		
Total Points	Men (Risk, %)	Women (Risk, %)
—3 or less	<1	<1
—2	1.1	<1
—1	1.4	1.0
0	1.6	1.2
1	1.9	1.5
2	2.3	1.7
3	2.8	2.0
4	3.3	2.4
5	3.9	2.8
6	4.7	3.3
7	5.6	3.9
8	6.7	4.5
9	7.9	5.3
10	9.4	6.3
11	11.2	7.3
12	13.3	8.6
13	15.6	10.0
14	18.4	11.7
15	21.6	13.7
16	25.3	15.9
17	29.4	18.5
18	>30	21.5
19	>30	24.8
20	>30	27.5
21+	>30	>30

*An electronic version of this assessment is available on the Canadfan Journal of Cardiology website at http:/Awnv.ccs.ca/download/consensus_conference/consensus_conference_ archives/2009_Dyslipidemia-Guidelines.pdf. Another risk inventory is available from the Heart and Stroke Foundation of Canada at http://vnv2.heartandstroke.ca/Page.asp?PagelD=1 969 &CategorylD=1 &Src=heart.

TRY IT

SOURCE: Reprinted from *Canadian Journal of Cardiology* 25 (10), Canadian guidelines for the diagnosis and treatment of dyslipidemia and prevention of cardiovascular disease in the adult–2009 recommendations, pp. 567–579, 2009, with permission from Elsevier.

HOW TO

Implement a Heart-Healthy Diet

Following a heart-healthy diet can require major changes in dietary choices. It helps to make a few changes at a time and to focus on positive choices (what to eat) first, rather than negative ones (what not to eat).

Breads, Cereals, and Pasta

- Choose whole-grain breads and cereals that list "whole grain wheat" as the first ingredient on labels.
- Choose foods whose labels *do not* list any *trans* fat in the Nutrition Facts panel or "hydrogenated oil" in the ingredients list.
- Avoid products that contain tropical oils (coconut, palm, and palm kernel oil), which are high in saturated fat.
- Choose oat products that provide at least 0.75 g of beta-glucan oat fibre.

Vegetables and Fruits

- Consume fruits and vegetables frequently. Keep the refrigerator stocked with a variety of colourful fruits and vegetables (baby carrots, grapes, blueberries, melon).
- Incorporate at least one or two servings of fruits and vegetables into each meal.
- Choose canned products carefully. Canned vegetables (especially tomato-based products) may be high in sodium. Fruits that are canned in juice are higher in nutrient density than those canned in syrup.
- Restrict high-sodium foods such as pickles, olives, sauerkraut, and kimchee.
- Avoid french fries from fast-food restaurants, which may be loaded with *trans* fats.
- Choose foods that are low or lower in salt.

Lunch and Dinner Entrées

- Limit meat, fish, and poultry servings to 150 g/day.
- Select lean cuts of beef, such as sirloin tip, round steak, and arm roast, and lean cuts of pork, such as centre-cut ham, loin chops, and tenderloin. Trim visible fat before cooking.
- Select extra-lean ground meat and drain well after cooking. Use lean ground turkey, without skin added, in place of ground beef.
- Limit cholesterol-rich organ meats (liver, brain, sweetbreads).
- Limit egg yolks to no more than two per week; replace whole eggs in recipes with egg whites or commercial egg substitutes.
- Include more vegetarian entrées or legume dishes to reduce meat intake and boost vegetable, soluble fibre, and soy protein intakes.
- Restrict these high-sodium foods:
  - Cured or smoked meats such as beef jerky, bologna, corned or chipped beef, frankfurters, ham, luncheon meats, salt pork, and sausage
  - Salty or smoked fish, such as anchovies, caviar, salted or dried cod, herring, sardines, and smoked salmon
  - Packaged, canned, or frozen soups, sauces, and entrées

Milk Products

- To obtain two to three servings of milk products daily, include a portion of skim or 1% milk, yogurt, or cottage cheese in each meal.
- Use yogurt or fat-free sour cream to make dips or salad dressings. Substitute evaporated skim milk for heavy cream.
- Restrict foods high in saturated fat or sodium, such as cheese, processed cheeses, ice cream, and other milk-based desserts.

Fats and Oils

- Add nuts (not salted) and avocados to meals to increase monounsaturated fat intakes and make meals more appetizing.
- Include vegetable oils in salad dressings and recipes, such as canola, corn, olive, peanut, flaxseed, safflower, sesame, soybean, and sunflower oils.
- Use margarines with added plant sterols or stanols regularly.
- Select soft margarines in tubs or liquid form; avoid stick margarines and solid vegetable shortenings.
- Avoid products that contain tropical oils (coconut, palm, and palm kernel oil), which are high in saturated fat.

Spices and Seasonings

- Use salt only at the end of cooking, and you will need to add much less. Use salt substitutes at the table.
- Spices and herbs improve the flavour of foods without adding sodium. Try using more garlic, ginger, basil, curry or chili powder, cumin, pepper, lemon, mint, oregano, rosemary, and thyme.
- Check the sodium content on labels. Flavourings and sauces that are usually high in sodium include bouillon cubes, soy sauce, steak and barbecue sauces, relishes, mustard, and catsup.

Snacks and Desserts

- Select low-sodium and low–saturated fat choices such as unsalted pretzels, nuts, popcorn, chips, and crackers.
- Choose canned or dried fruits and some raw vegetables to boost fruit and vegetable intake.
- Enjoy angel food cake, which is made without egg yolks and added fat.
- Select low-fat frozen desserts such as sherbet, sorbet, fruit bars, and some low-fat ice creams.

CENGAGENOW™
For additional practice log on to **www.cengage.com/sso.**

TRY IT Plan heart-healthy meals for a day and analyze them using your personal profile. Discuss whether these meals meet the strategies listed in Table 19-6 (p. 627) and how to improve any shortcomings.

Hypertension

Anyone concerned about atherosclerosis and the risk it presents must also be concerned about hypertension. Together, the two are a life-threatening combination. The higher the blood pressure is above normal, ♦ the greater the risk. For each 20 point increase in systolic blood pressure and 10 point increase in diastolic blood pressure, the risk of death from CVD doubles.[53] Low blood pressure, on the other hand, is generally a sign of long life expectancy and low heart disease risk.[54]

♦ Optimal resting blood pressure for adults is 120 over 80 mmHg (120/80). Blood pressure is measured in millimetres of mercury (mmHg). Blood pressure is measured both when the heart muscle contracts (*systolic* blood pressure) and when it relaxes (*diastolic* blood pressure).

Hypertension affects over 4.5 million adults in Canada; however, a similar number of adults had blood pressure readings in the prehypertension range.[55] It contributes to more than 50 000 heart attacks and almost 15 000 strokes each year. People cannot feel the physical effects of high blood pressure, but it can impair life's quality and end life prematurely.

How Hypertension Develops

The underlying causes of most cases of hypertension are not fully understood, but much is known about the physiological factors that affect blood pressure. Blood pressure arises from contractions in the heart muscle that pump blood away from the heart (**cardiac output**) and the resistance blood encounters in the arterioles (**peripheral resistance**). When either cardiac output or peripheral resistance increases, blood pressure rises. ♦ Cardiac output is raised when heart rate or blood volume increases; peripheral resistance is affected mostly by the diameters of the arterioles. Blood pressure is therefore influenced by the nervous system, which regulates heart muscle contractions and the arterioles' diameters, and hormonal signals, which may cause fluid retention or blood vessel constriction. The kidneys also play a role in regulating blood pressure by controlling the secretion of the hormones involved in vasoconstriction and retention of sodium and water (review Figure 11-4 on p. 360).[56]

♦ The equation describing this relationship is blood pressure = cardiac output × peripheral resistance.

Risk Factors for Hypertension

Several major risk factors predicting the development of hypertension have been identified, including:

- *Aging.* Hypertension risk increases with age. Individuals who have normal blood pressure at age 55 still have a 90 percent risk of developing high blood pressure during their lifetimes.[57]
- *Genetics.* Hypertension risk is similar among family members. It is also more prevalent and severe in certain ethnic groups: for African Americans in the United States, the prevalence of high blood pressure is among the highest in the world.[58] Compared with others, African Americans typically develop high blood pressure earlier in life, and their average blood pressure is much higher.
- *Obesity.* Most people with hypertension—an estimated 60 percent—are obese.[59] Obesity raises blood pressure in part by altering kidney function and promoting fluid retention.[60]
- *Salt sensitivity.* Approximately 50 percent of those with hypertension have blood pressure that is sensitive to salt.[61] These people can improve their blood pressure by reducing salt in their diets.[62]
- *Alcohol.* Alcohol consumption, especially if consumed regularly in amounts greater than two drinks per day, ♦ is strongly associated with hypertension. Alcohol is also associated with strokes independently of hypertension, and its use may interfere with drug therapy.

♦ One *drink* delivers 15 mL of pure ethanol:
- 150 mL wine
- 300 mL wine cooler
- 360 mL beer
- 50 mL distilled liquor (80 proof whiskey, scotch, rum, or vodka)

cardiac output: the volume of blood pumped out by the heart each minute.

peripheral resistance: the resistance to pumped blood by the small arterial branches (arterioles) that carry blood to tissues.

Treatment of Hypertension

The single most effective step people can take against hypertension is to find out whether they have it. At checkup time, a health-care professional can provide an accurate resting blood pressure reading. Under normal conditions, blood pressure fluctuates continuously in response to a variety of factors including stress and such actions as talking or shifting position. Some people react emotionally to the procedure, which raises the blood pressure

TABLE 19-7 Lifestyle Modifications to Reduce Blood Pressure

Modification	Recommendation	Expected Reduction in Systolic Blood Pressure
Weight reduction	Maintain healthy body weight (BMI below 25).	5–20 mmHg/10 kg lost
DASH eating plan	Adopt a diet rich in fruits, vegetables, and 1% milk products with reduced saturated fat intake.	8–14 mmHg
Sodium restriction	Reduce dietary sodium intake to less than 2400 milligrams sodium (less than 6 grams salt) per day.[a]	2–8 mmHg
Physical activity	Perform aerobic physical activity for at least 30 minutes per day, most days of the week.	4–9 mmHg
Moderate alcohol consumption	Men: Limit to two drinks per day. Women and lighter-weight men: Limit to one drink per day.	2–4 mmHg

[a]According to the DRI recommendations, sodium intake should be limited to 2300 milligrams daily.

SOURCE: Adapted from *Reference Card from the Seventh Report of the Joint National Committee on Prevention, Detection, Evaluation, and Treatment of High Blood Pressure (JNC 7),* NIH publication No. 03-5231 (Bethesda, Md.: National Institutes of Health, National Heart, Lung, and Blood Institute, and National High Blood Pressure Education Program, May 2003).

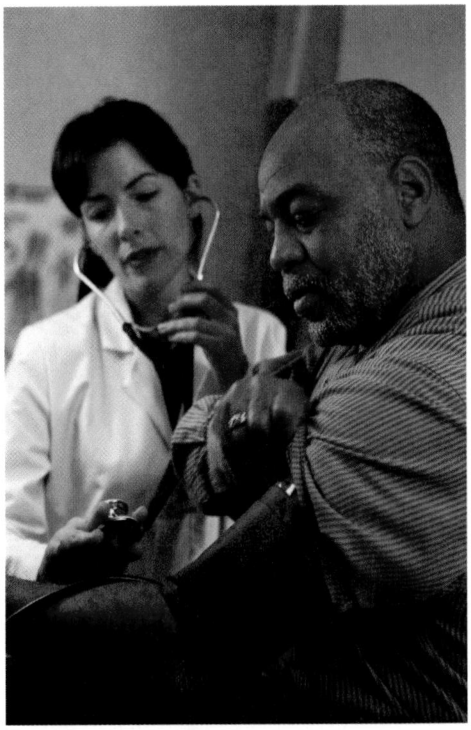

Charles Thatcher/Getty Images

To guard against hypertension, have your blood pressure checked regularly.

reading. For these reasons, if the resting blood pressure is above normal, the reading should be repeated before confirming the diagnosis of hypertension (see Table 19-5 on p. 624 for blood pressure standards). Thereafter, the blood pressure should be checked regularly. Both lifestyle modifications and drug therapies are used to treat hypertension. Table 19-7 describes the lifestyle changes that reduce blood pressure and the expected reduction in systolic blood pressure for each change.

Weight Control Efforts to reduce high blood pressure focus on weight control. Weight loss alone is one of the most effective nondrug treatments for hypertension. Those who are using drugs to control their blood pressure can often reduce or discontinue the drugs when they lose weight. Even a modest weight loss of 5 kilograms (10 pounds) can lower blood pressure significantly.

Physical Activity The higher the blood pressure and the less active a person is to begin with, the greater the effect physical activity has in reducing blood pressure. Physical activity helps with weight control, of course, but moderate aerobic activity, such as 30 to 60 minutes of brisk walking most days, also helps to lower blood pressure directly.[63] Those who engage in regular aerobic activity may not need medication for mild hypertension.[64]

The DASH Diet The results of the Dietary Approaches to Stop Hypertension (DASH) trial show that a diet rich in fruits, vegetables, nuts, and 1% milk products and low in total fat and saturated fat can significantly lower blood pressure. In addition to lowering blood pressure, the DASH diet lowers total cholesterol and LDL cholesterol.[65] Compared to the typical North American diet, the DASH eating plan provides more fibre, potassium, magnesium, and calcium and less red meat, sweets, and sugar-containing beverages. Table 19-8 shows the DASH eating plan.[66]

Salt/Sodium Intake For many years, controversy surrounded recommendations to restrict sodium and/or salt, but strong evidence supports the important role this strategy plays in preventing and reducing hypertension. Lowering sodium intake reduces blood pressure regardless of gender or race, presence or absence of hypertension, or whether people follow the DASH diet or a typical North American diet. The combination of the DASH diet with a limited intake of sodium, however,

TABLE 19-8 The DASH Eating Plan

Food Group	DASH
Grains	180–240 g
Vegetables	500–625 mL (2–2½ c)
Fruits	500–625 mL (2–2½ c)
Milk (skim/1%)	500–750 mL (2–3 c)
Lean meats, poultry, fish	180 g or less
Nuts, seeds, legumes	120–150 g per week

NOTE: This diet plan is based on 2000 kcal/day. The DASH recommended that fats and sugars be used sparingly and with discretion.

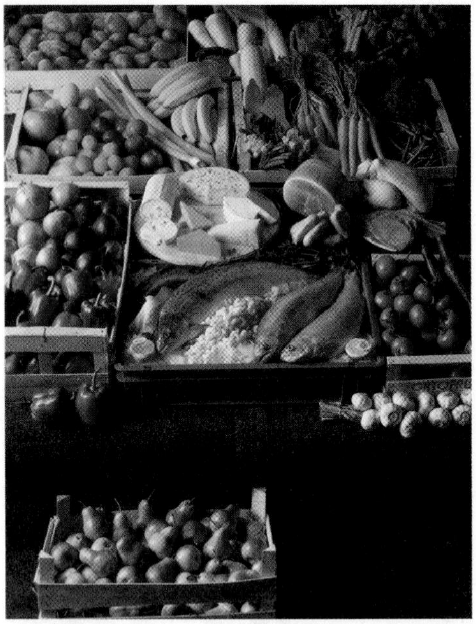

© Masterfile Corporation/foodanddrinkphotos

The richest sources of potassium are fresh foods of all kinds.

improves blood pressure better than either strategy alone.[67] Furthermore, the lower the sodium intake, the greater the drop in blood pressure. (See the "How To" in Chapter 11 on p. 367 for suggestions about limiting sodium intake. Readers interested in finding out more about how to reduce sodium intake can go to www.sodium101.ca; they may be surprised to find that "Yes, there's an App for that!" and that it is FREE.) Research shows salt reduction provides additional protection against heart disease, beyond lowering blood pressure.[68]

Dietary Guidance for Canadians

Individuals with hypertension, black people, and middle-aged and older adults should aim to consume no more than 1500 mg of sodium per day and to meet the potassium recommendation (4700 mg/day) with food.

Drug Therapy When diet and physical activity fail to reduce blood pressure, diuretics and antihypertensive drugs may be prescribed. Diuretics lower blood pressure by increasing fluid loss and lowering blood volume.

Some diuretics can lead to a potassium deficiency. People taking these diuretics need to include rich food sources of potassium or supplements daily and watch for signs of potassium imbalances such as weakness (particularly of the legs), unexplained numbness or tingling sensation, cramps, irregular heartbeats, and excessive thirst and urination. Blood potassium should be monitored regularly. Although some diuretics can lead to a potassium deficiency, others spare potassium. A combination of these two types of diuretics may be prescribed to prevent potassium deficiency.

Most people with hypertension use two or more medications to meet their blood pressure goals. Using a combination of drugs with different modes of action can reduce the doses needed and minimize side effects. In addition to diuretics, other medications ♦ commonly prescribed include ACE inhibitors, beta-blockers, and calcium channel blockers; these drugs are also used to treat various heart conditions.

♦ Hypertension medications:
- ACE inhibitors interfere with the conversion of angiotensin I to angiotensin II, a peptide that constricts blood vessels and releases hormones that increase blood pressure (review Figure 11-4 on p. 360). (*ACE* stands for *angiotensin-converting enzyme*.)
- Beta-blockers cause the heart to beat more slowly and with less force and the blood vessels to open up, which improves blood flow.
- Calcium channel blockers relax blood vessels and decrease the heart's pumping strength.

IN SUMMARY **The most effective dietary strategy for preventing hypertension is weight control. Also beneficial are diets rich in fruits, vegetables, nuts, and 1% milk products and low in fat, saturated fat, and sodium.**

Diabetes Mellitus

The incidence of diabetes among children and adults has risen dramatically in the last decade. Figure 19-4 shows statistics regarding the mortality rate per 100 000 in 16 peer countries where Canada ranks 14th out of 16. Also, note that while the statistics for Canada are currently similar to those of the United States, our rate is about triple those of the United Kingdom—at close to 20/100 000. More than 3 million people in Canada have been diagnosed with diabetes.[69] Of those with diabetes, about 10 percent have type 1 diabetes; about 90 percent have type 2 diabetes. Gestational diabetes affects 2–4 percent of all pregnancies, but many Canadians also have **prediabetes**—their blood glucose is elevated but not to such an extent as to be classified as diabetes (an estimated 9 million Canadians are living with diabetes or prediabetes).[70] ♦ People with prediabetes have a high risk of developing diabetes. The glossary on p. 634 defines diabetes terms.

♦ Fasting plasma glucose
- Normal: 4.0–6.0 mmol/L
- Prediabetes: 6.1–6.9 mmol/L
- Diabetes: ≥7.0 mmol/L

Diabetes ranks sixth among the leading causes of death (review Figure 19-2 on p. 620). In addition, diabetes underlies, or contributes to, several other major diseases, including heart disease, stroke, hypertension, blindness, and kidney failure. Heart disease is the leading cause of diabetes-related deaths. In fact, people with diabetes are two to three times as likely to develop cardiovascular problems as those without diabetes.

How Diabetes Develops **Diabetes mellitus** is the formal name of a group of metabolic disorders characterized by high blood glucose concentrations and disordered insulin metabolism. People with diabetes may have insufficient insulin, ineffective insulin, or a combination of the two. The result is **hyperglycemia**, a marked elevation in blood glucose that can ultimately cause damage to blood vessels, nerves, and tissues.

Table 19-9 shows the distinguishing features of type 1 diabetes and type 2 diabetes. As the following pages explain, the development of type 1 and type 2 diabetes differs, but some of their complications are similar.

To appreciate the problems presented by an absolute or relative lack of insulin, consider insulin's normal action. After a meal, insulin signals the body's cells to receive the energy nutrients from the blood—amino acids, glucose, and fatty acids. Insulin helps to maintain blood glucose within normal limits and stimulates protein synthesis, glycogen synthesis in liver and muscle, and fat synthesis. Without insulin, glucose regulation falters, and metabolism of the energy-yielding nutrients changes.

Type 1 Diabetes In **type 1 diabetes**, the less common type of diabetes (about 10 percent of all diagnosed cases), the pancreas loses its ability to synthesize the hormone insulin. Type 1 diabetes is an **autoimmune disorder**.[71] In most cases, the individual inherits a defect in which immune cells mistakenly attack and destroy the insulin-producing beta cells of the pancreas. The rate of beta cell destruction in type 1 diabetes varies. In some people (mainly infants and children), destruction is rapid; in others (mainly adults), it is slow. Type 1 diabetes commonly occurs in childhood and adolescence, but it can occur at any age, even late in life.[72]

Without insulin, the body's energy metabolism changes, with such severe consequences as to threaten survival. The cells must have insulin to take up the needed fuels from the blood. People with type 1 diabetes must receive insulin either by injection or external pumps; insulin cannot be taken orally because it is a protein, and the enzymes of the GI tract would digest it.

Type 2 Diabetes **Type 2 diabetes** is the most prevalent form of diabetes, accounting for about 90 percent of cases.[73] The primary defect in type 2 diabetes is insulin resistance, a reduced sensitivity to insulin. Consequently, muscle and adipose cells cannot remove glucose from the blood, and liver cells continue to make glucose. To compensate, the pancreas secretes larger amounts of insulin, and plasma insulin concentrations can rise to abnormally high levels (hyperinsulinemia). Over time, the pancreas becomes less able to compensate for the cells' reduced sensitivity to insulin, and hyperglycemia worsens. The high demand for insulin can eventually

FIGURE 19-4 Mortality Due to Diabetes, 2006, by Country

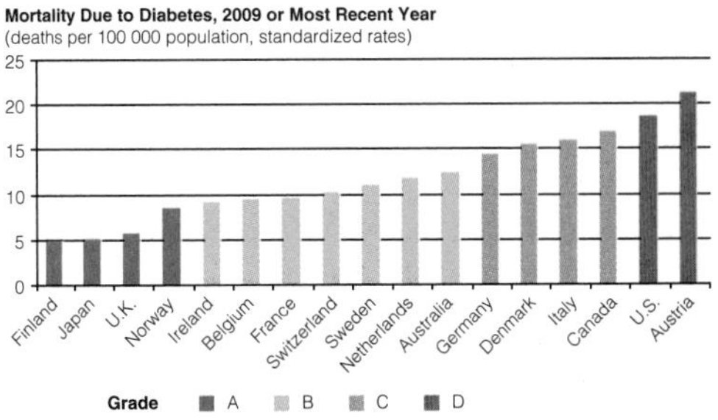
Mortality Due to Diabetes, 2009 or Most Recent Year
(deaths per 100 000 population, standardized rates)
25
20
15
10
5
0
Finland
Japan
U.K.
Norway
Ireland
Belgium
France
Switzerland
Sweden
Netherlands
Australia
Germany
Denmark
Italy
Canada
U.S.
Austria
Grade
A
B
C
D

SOURCE: Reprinted by permission of the Conference Board of Canada. Source of data: OECD.

TABLE 19-9 Features of Type 1 and Type 2 Diabetes

	Type 1	Type 2
Prevalence in diabetic population	~10 percent of cases	~90 percent of cases
Age of onset	<30 years	>40 years[a]
Associated conditions	Autoimmune diseases, viral infections, inherited factors	Obesity, aging, inherited factors
Major defect	Destruction of pancreatic beta cells; insulin deficiency	Insulin resistance; insulin deficiency (relative to needs)
Insulin secretion	Little or none	Varies; may be normal, increased, or decreased
Requirement for insulin therapy	Always	Sometimes
Older names	Juvenile-onset diabetes Insulin-dependent diabetes mellitus (IDDM)	Adult-onset diabetes Noninsulin-dependent diabetes mellitus (NIDDM)

[a]Incidence of type 2 diabetes is increasing in children and adolescence; in more than 90 percent of these cases, it is associated with overweight or obesity and a family history of type 2 diabetes.

hyperglycemia: elevated blood glucose concentrations.

autoimmune disorder: a condition in which the body develops antibodies to its own proteins and then proceeds to destroy cells containing these proteins. In type 1 diabetes, the body develops antibodies to its insulin and destroys the pancreatic cells that produce the insulin, creating an insulin deficiency.

exhaust the beta cells of the pancreas and lead to impaired insulin secretion and reduced plasma insulin concentrations. Type 2 diabetes is therefore associated both with insulin resistance and with relative insulin deficiency; that is, the amount of insulin is insufficient to compensate for its diminished effect in cells.

Although the actual causes of type 2 diabetes are unknown, the risk is substantially increased by obesity (especially abdominal obesity), poor dietary habits, smoking, excessive alcohol consumption, aging, and physical inactivity. When people take action to control their lifestyle choices, prevention of type 2 diabetes is not only possible, but likely. ♦ Even older adults can lower their diabetes risk by changing their lifestyles.[74]

♦ Lifestyle factors that lower diabetes risk:
- Healthy body weight
- Diet that follows *Canada's Food Guide*
- Never smoking
- Limited alcohol intake
- Physical activity

Most people with type 2 diabetes are obese, and obesity itself can directly cause some degree of insulin resistance.[75] As discussed in Highlight 17, obesity has led to a dramatic rise in the incidence of type 2 diabetes among children and adolescents during the past two decades.[76] Inherited factors also strongly influence risk, and type 2 diabetes is more common in certain ethnic populations, including those of Aboriginal, Hispanic, African, Asian, or South Asian descent.

Inflammation contributes to insulin resistance, and its many links with obesity, metabolic syndrome, and CVD make inflammation central to the development of diabetes as well.[77] Chronic inflammation correlates with increases in blood glucose and decreases in insulin effectiveness.

Complications of Diabetes

In both types of diabetes, glucose fails to gain entry into the cells and consequently accumulates in the blood. These two problems lead to both acute and chronic complications. Figure 19-5 summarizes the metabolic changes and acute complications that can arise in uncontrolled diabetes. Notice that when some glucose enters the cells, as in type 2 diabetes, many of the symptoms of type 1 do not occur.

Over the long term, the person with diabetes suffers not only from the acute complications shown in Figure 19-5, but also from its chronic effects. Chronically elevated blood glucose alters glucose metabolism in virtually every cell of the body. Some cells begin to convert excess glucose to sugar alcohols, for example, causing toxicity and cell distention—distended cells in the lenses of the eyes, for example, cause blurry vision. Some cells produce glycoproteins by attaching excess glucose to an amino acid in a protein; the altered proteins cannot function normally, which leads to a host of other problems. The structures of the blood vessels and nerves become damaged, leading to loss of circulation and nerve function. Infections occur due to poor circulation coupled with glucose-rich blood and urine. People with diabetes must pay special attention to hygiene and keep alert for early signs of infection. Early, aggressive treatment to control blood glucose significantly reduces the risk of long-term diabetes-related complications.

Diseases of the Large Blood Vessels As mentioned, atherosclerosis tends to develop early, progress rapidly, and be more severe in people with diabetes. The interrelationships among insulin resistance, obesity, hypertension, and atherosclerosis help explain why about 75 percent of people with diabetes die as a consequence of cardiovascular diseases, especially heart attacks. Intensive diabetes treatment that keeps blood glucose levels tightly controlled can reduce the risk of cardiovascular disease among those with type 1 diabetes.[78]

GLOSSARY OF DIABETES TERMS

diabetes (DYE-uh-BEET-eez) **mellitus** (MELL-ih-tus or mell-EYE-tus): a group of metabolic diseases characterized by hyperglycemia resulting from defects in insulin secretion, insulin action, or both.
- **mellitus** = honey-sweet (sugar in urine)

prediabetes: condition in which blood glucose levels are higher than normal but not high enough to be diagnosed as diabetes; considered a major risk factor for future diabetes and cardiovascular diseases; formerly called *impaired glucose tolerance*.

type 1 diabetes: the type of diabetes that accounts for 10 percent of diabetes cases and usually results from autoimmune destruction of pancreatic beta cells. In this type of diabetes, the pancreas produces little or no insulin.

type 2 diabetes: the type of diabetes that accounts for 90 percent of diabetes cases and usually results from insulin resistance coupled with insufficient insulin secretion. Obesity is present in 80 to 90 percent of cases.

FIGURE 19-5 Metabolic Consequences of Untreated Diabetes

The metabolic consequences of type 1 diabetes differ from those of type 2. In type 1, no insulin is available to allow any glucose to enter the cells. When glucose cannot enter the cells, a cascade of metabolic changes quickly follows. In type 2 diabetes, some glucose enters the cells. Because the cells are not "starved" for glucose, the body does not shift into the metabolism of fasting (losing weight and producing ketones).

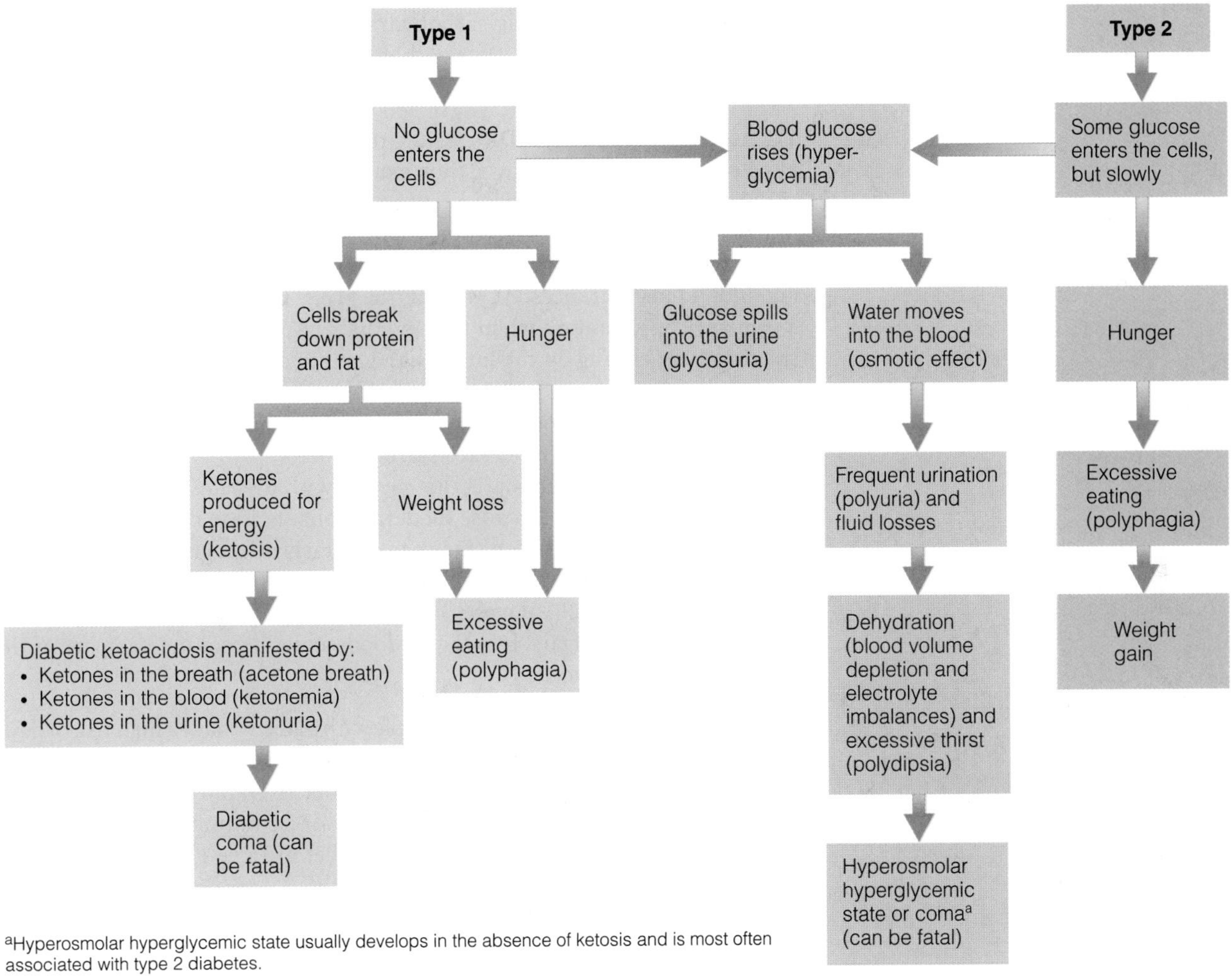
Type 1
Type 2
No glucose enters the cells
Blood glucose rises (hyperglycemia)
Some glucose enters the cells, but slowly
Cells break down protein and fat
Hunger
Glucose spills into the urine (glycosuria)
Water moves into the blood (osmotic effect)
Hunger
Ketones produced for energy (ketosis)
Weight loss
Frequent urination (polyuria) and fluid losses
Excessive eating (polyphagia)
Diabetic ketoacidosis manifested by:
• Ketones in the breath (acetone breath)
• Ketones in the blood (ketonemia)
• Ketones in the urine (ketonuria)
Excessive eating (polyphagia)
Dehydration (blood volume depletion and electrolyte imbalances) and excessive thirst (polydipsia)
Weight gain
Diabetic coma (can be fatal)
Hyperosmolar hyperglycemic state or coma[a] (can be fatal)

[a]Hyperosmolar hyperglycemic state usually develops in the absence of ketosis and is most often associated with type 2 diabetes.

Diseases of the Small Blood Vessels For people with diabetes, disorders of the small blood vessels (capillaries) ♦ may also develop and lead to loss of kidney function and retinal degeneration with accompanying loss of vision. About 85 percent of people with diabetes have impaired kidney function, loss of vision, or both. Consequently, diabetes is a leading cause of both kidney failure and blindness.[79]

♦ Disorders of the small blood vessels are called **microangiopathies.**
- **micro** = small
- **angeion** = vessel
- **pathos** = disease

Diseases of the Nerves Nerve tissues may also deteriorate with diabetes, expressed at first as a painful prickling sensation, often in the arms and legs. Later, the person loses sensation in the hands and feet. Injuries to these areas may go unnoticed, and infections can progress rapidly. With loss of both circulation and nerve function, undetected injury and infection may lead to death of tissue (gangrene), ♦ necessitating amputation of the limbs (most often the legs or feet). People with diabetes are advised to take conscientious care of their feet and visit a podiatrist regularly.

♦ The death of tissue, usually due to deficient blood supply, is **gangrene** (GANG-green).

Recommendations for Diabetes

Diet is an important component of diabetes treatment. To maintain near-normal blood glucose levels, the diet is designed to deliver the same amount of carbohydrate each day, spaced evenly throughout the day. Several approaches can be used to plan such diets, but many people with diabetes learn to count carbohydrates using the exchange system that is presented in APPENDIX G.

Total Carbohydrate Intake Providing a consistent carbohydrate intake spaced throughout the day helps to maintain appropriate blood glucose levels and maximize the effectiveness of drug therapy. Eating too much carbohydrate at one time can raise blood glucose too high, stressing the already-compromised insulin-producing cells. Eating too little carbohydrate can lead to abnormally low blood glucose (hypoglycemia). The *amount* of carbohydrate affects blood glucose levels and so can the *source* of the carbohydrate—for example, foods with a lower glycemic index (see below).[80] Low-carbohydrate diets (less than 45 percent of total energy from carbohydrate per day) are not recommended.[81]

Carbohydrate Sources Different carbohydrate-containing foods have varying effects on blood glucose levels; for example, consuming a portion of white rice may cause blood glucose to rise higher and quicker than would a similar portion of barley. As Chapter 4 describes, this *glycemic effect* of foods is influenced by a food's fibre content, the preparation method, the other foods included in a meal, and individual tolerances. At present, the glycemic effect of individual foods is not a primary consideration when treating diabetes; however, they may be part of the treatment depending on the interest and ability of individual patients.[82] However, as for others, people with diabetes should derive at least half of their grain intake from high-fibre, whole-grain products that have more moderate effects on blood glucose than do highly processed starchy foods.

A common misconception is that people with diabetes need to avoid sugar and sugar-containing foods. Because moderate consumption of sugar (up to 10 percent of total calories) has not been shown to adversely affect glycemic control, however, sugar recommendations for people with diabetes are similar to those for the general population, which suggests choosing foods and beverages with little added sugars. Of course, sugars and sugary foods must be counted as part of the daily carbohydrate allowance.

Dietary Fat As mentioned earlier, people with diabetes have a high risk of developing cardiovascular diseases, and their guidelines for dietary fat are similar to those for others with high risks. Saturated fat intake should be limited to less than 7 percent of kcalories, *trans* fat and cholesterol intake should be minimized.[83] Dietary strategies for cardiovascular disease were presented earlier in Table 19-6 (p. 627).

Protein Protein intakes in North America generally range from 15 to 20 percent of total kcalories. Protein intakes in this range need not be modified for individuals with diabetes and normal kidney function.[84] Higher protein intakes are discouraged because they may be detrimental to kidney function.

Alcohol Adults with diabetes can drink alcohol in moderation. Guidelines are similar to those for the general population, which advise a daily limit of one drink for women and two drinks for men.[85]

Recommendations for Type 1 Diabetes Normally, the body secretes a constant baseline amount of insulin at all times and secretes more as blood glucose rises following meals. People with type 1 diabetes, however, produce little or no insulin. They must learn to adjust the amount and schedule of their insulin doses to accommodate meals, physical activity, and health status. To maintain blood glucose within a fairly normal range requires a lifelong commitment to a carefully coordinated program of diet, physical activity, and insulin.

Nutrition therapy for type 1 diabetes focuses on maintaining optimal nutrition status, controlling blood glucose, achieving a desirable blood lipid profile, controlling blood pressure, and preventing and treating the complications of diabetes. In addition to meeting basic nutrient requirements, the diet must provide a fairly consistent carbohydrate intake from day to day and at each meal and snack to help minimize fluctuations in blood glucose. Further alterations in diet may be necessary for the person with chronic complications such as cardiovascular or kidney disease.

Participation in all levels of physical activity is possible for people with type 1 diabetes who have good blood glucose control and no complications, but they should check with their physician first. One potential problem is hypoglycemia, which can occur during, immediately after, or many hours after physical activity.[86] To avoid hypoglycemia, the person must monitor blood glucose before and after activity to identify when adjustments in insulin or food intake are needed. Carbohydrate-rich foods should be readily available during and after activity.

Recommendations for Type 2 Diabetes In overweight people with type 2 diabetes, even moderate weight loss (5 to 10 kilograms) can help improve insulin resistance, blood lipids, and blood pressure. Together with diet, a regular routine of moderate physical activity not only supports weight loss, but also improves blood glucose control, blood lipid profiles, and blood pressure. Thus the benefits of regular, long-term physical activity (e.g., 150 minutes of moderate- to vigorous-intensity exercise per week) for the treatment and prevention of type 2 diabetes are substantial.[87]

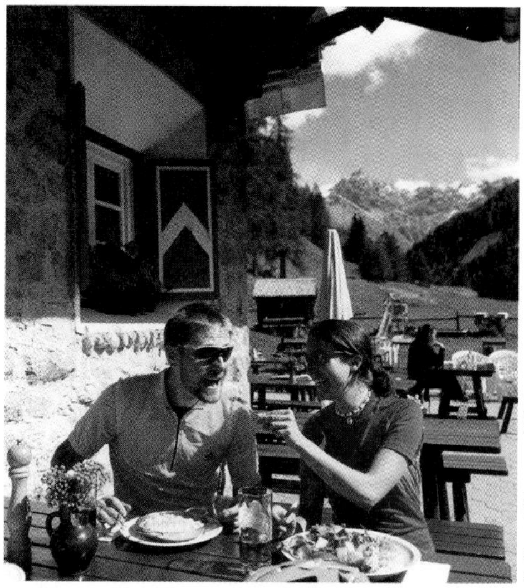

For a person with type 1 diabetes, good health depends on coordinating the timing of meals, activities, and insulin.

IN SUMMARY **Diabetes is characterized by high blood glucose and either insufficient insulin, ineffective insulin, or a combination of the two. People with type 1 diabetes coordinate diet, insulin, and physical activity to help control their blood glucose. Those with type 2 diabetes benefit most from a diet and physical activity program that controls glucose fluctuations and promotes weight loss.**

Cancer

Cancer, the growth of **malignant** tissue, ranks just above cardiovascular disease as a cause of death in Canada. (See the accompanying glossary of cancer terms.) As with cardiovascular disease, the prognosis for cancer today is far brighter than in the past. Identification of risk factors, new detection techniques, and innovative therapies offer hope and encouragement.

Cancer is not a single disorder. There are many **cancers**, that is, many different kinds of malignant growths. They have different characteristics, occur in different locations in the body, take different courses, and require different treatments.

How Cancer Develops The development of cancer, called **carcinogenesis**, often proceeds slowly and continues for several decades. A cancer arises from mutations in the genes that control cell division in a single cell. These mutations may promote cellular growth, interfere with growth restraint, or prevent cellular death.[88] The affected cell thereby loses its built-in capacity for halting cell division, and it produces daughter cells with the same genetic defects. As the abnormal mass of cells, called a **tumour**, ♦ grows, a network of blood vessels develops to supply the tumour with the nutrients it needs to support its growth. The tumour can disrupt the functioning of the normal tissue around it, and some tumour cells

♦ An abnormal mass of cells that is noncancerous is called a **benign** tumour.

GLOSSARY OF CANCER TERMS

antipromoters: factors that oppose the development of cancer.

cancers: malignant growths or tumours that result from abnormal and uncontrolled cell division.

carcinogenesis (CAR-sin-oh-JEN-eh-sis): the process of cancer development.

carcinogens (CAR-sin-oh-jenz or car-SIN-oh-jenz): substances that can cause cancer (the adjective is *carcinogenic*).
- **carcin** = cancer
- **gen** = gives rise to

initiators: factors that cause mutations that give rise to cancer, such as radiation and carcinogens.

malignant (ma-LIG-nant): describes a cancerous cell or tumour, which can injure healthy tissue and spread cancer to other regions of the body.

metastasize (me-TAS-tah-size): the spread of cancer from one part of the body to another.

promoters: factors that favour the development of cancers once they have begun.

tumour: an abnormal tissue mass with no physiological function; also called a *neoplasm* (NEE-oh-plazm).

Cancers are classified by the tissues or cells from which they develop:
- *adenomas* (ADD-eh-NOH-mahz): cancers that arise from glandular tissues.
- *carcinomas* (KAR-see-NOH-mahz): cancers that arise from epithelial tissues.
- *gliomas* (gly-OH-mahz): cancers that arise from glial cells of the central nervous system.
- *leukemias* (loo-KEE-mee-ahz): cancers that arise from white blood cell precursors.
- *lymphomas* (lim-FOH-mahz): cancers that arise from lymph tissue.
- *melanomas* (MEL-ah-NOH-mahz): cancers that arise from pigmented skin cells.
- *sarcomas* (sar-KOH-mahz): cancers that arise from connective tissues, such as muscle or bone.

FIGURE 19-6 Cancer Development

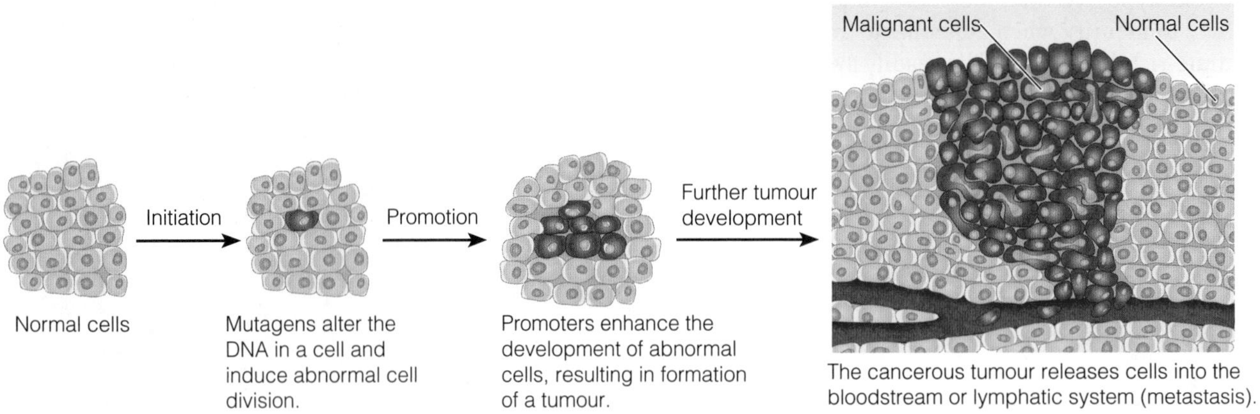
Malignant cells
Normal cells
Initiation
Promotion
Further tumour development
Normal cells
Mutagens alter the DNA in a cell and induce abnormal cell division.
Promoters enhance the development of abnormal cells, resulting in formation of a tumour.
The cancerous tumour releases cells into the bloodstream or lymphatic system (metastasis).

may **metastasize** to other regions of the body.[89] Figure 19-6 illustrates cancer development. In leukemia (cancer affecting the white blood cells), the cells do not form a tumour, but rather accumulate in blood and other tissues.

The reasons cancers develop are numerous and varied. Vulnerability to cancer is sometimes inherited, as when a person is born with a genetic defect that alters DNA structure, function, or repair. Certain metabolic processes may initiate carcinogenesis, as when phagocytes of the immune system produce oxidants that cause DNA damage or when chronic inflammation enhances the rate of cell division and the risk of a damaging mutation. More often, cancers are caused by interactions between a person's genes and the environment. Exposure to cancer-causing substances, or **carcinogens**, may either induce genetic mutations that lead to cancer or promote proliferation of cancerous cells.

Environmental Factors Among environmental factors, exposure to radiation and sun, water and air pollution, and smoking are known to cause cancer. Lack of physical activity may also play a role in the development of some cancers.[90] Men and women whose lifestyles include regular, vigorous physical activity have the lowest risk of colon cancer.[91] Physical activity may also protect against breast cancer by reducing body weight and by other mechanisms not related to body weight.[92]

Obesity itself is clearly a risk factor for certain cancers (such as colon, breast in postmenopausal women, endometrial, pancreas, kidney, and esophageal) and possibly for other types (such as gallbladder) as well.[93] Because different cancers have various causes, obesity's influence on cancer development depends on the site as well as other factors such as hormonal interactions. In the case of breast cancer in postmenopausal women, for example, the hormone estrogen is implicated. Obese postmenopausal women have much higher levels of estrogen than lean women do because fat tissue produces estrogen. Researchers believe that the extended exposure to estrogen in obese women is linked to the increased risk of breast cancer after menopause.[94] The relationships between excessive body weight and certain cancers provide yet another reason to adopt a lifestyle that embraces physical activity and good nutrition.

As Table 19-10 shows, specific dietary constituents are associated with probable increased or decreased risk of certain cancers. Some dietary factors may initiate cancer development **(initiators)**, others may promote cancer development once it has started **(promoters)**, and still others may protect against the development of cancer **(antipromoters)**.

Dietary Factors—Cancer Initiators We do not know to what extent diet contributes to cancer development, although some experts estimate that diet may be linked to as many as one-third of all cases.[95] Consequently, many people think that certain foods are carcinogenic, especially those that contain additives or

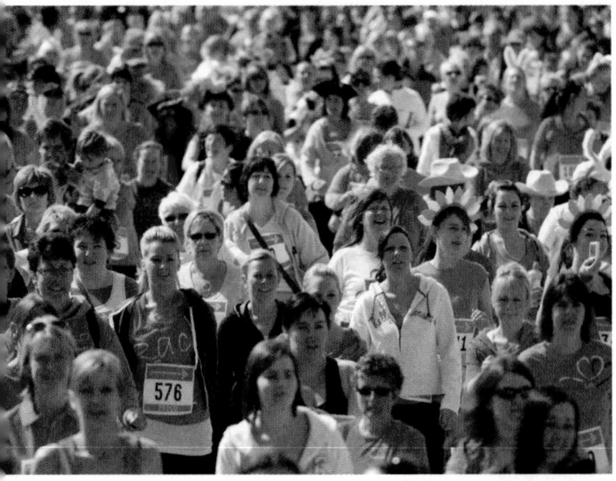
576

People with cancer take comfort from the support of others and from the knowledge that medical science is waging an unrelenting battle in their defence.

TABLE 19-10 Factors Associated with Cancers at Specific Sites

	Convincing or Probable Increased Risk	Convincing or Probable Decreased Risk
Breast Cancer (Premenopausal)	Alcohol	Breastfeeding, body fatness
Breast Cancer (Postmenopausal)	Alcohol, body/abdominal fatness	Breastfeeding, physical activity
Colorectal Cancer	Red and processed meat, body/abdominal fatness, alcohol	Foods containing dietary fibre, physical activity, garlic, diets high in calcium
Mouth and Throat Cancer	Alcohol	Fruits, nonstarchy vegetables
Esophagus Cancer	Body fatness, maté*, alcohol	Fruits, nonstarchy vegetables
Liver Cancer	Mould aflatoxin, alcohol	
Lung Cancer	Beta-carotene supplements (in smokers), arsenic in drinking water	Fruits
Pancreatic Cancer	Body/abdominal fatness	Foods containing folate
Prostate Cancer	Diets high in calcium	Foods combining lycopene, foods containing selenium
Stomach Cancer	Salt, salted and salty foods	Fruits, nonstarchy vegetables, foods in the allium family (e.g., onion and garlic)

*Herbal beverage in parts of South America that is drunk while it is very hot through a metal straw.

SOURCE: This material has been adapted from the 2009 WCRF/AICR Report Food, Nutrition, Physical Activity and the Prevention of Cancer: A Global Perspective. http://www.dietandcancerreport.org/ (accessed June 07, 2010). Please visit HYPERLINK "http://www.wcrf.org" www.wcrf.org and HYPERLINK "http://www.aicr.org" www.aicr.org.

pesticides. As Chapter 20 explains, our food supply is one of the safest in the world. Additives that have been approved for use in foods are not carcinogens. Some pesticides are carcinogenic at high doses, but not at the concentrations allowed on fruits and vegetables. The benefits of eating fruits and vegetables are far greater than any potential risk.

Cancers of the head and neck correlate strongly with the combination of alcohol and tobacco use and with low intakes of fruits and vegetables. Alcohol intake alone is associated with cancers of the mouth, throat, and breast, and alcoholism often damages the liver and precedes the development of liver cancer.[96] These findings illustrate clearly why any potential benefit of moderate alcohol consumption on cardiovascular disease must be weighed against the potential dangers.

Cooking meats at high temperatures (frying, broiling) causes amino acids and creatine in the meats to react together and form carcinogens.* Grilling meat, ♦ fish, or other foods over a direct flame causes fat and added oils to splash on the fire and then vaporize, creating other carcinogens that rise and stick to the food.** Eating grilled food introduces these carcinogens to the digestive system, where they may damage the stomach and intestinal lining. Once these compounds are absorbed into the blood, however, they are detoxified by the liver.

♦ To minimize carcinogen formation during cooking:
- Roast or bake meats in the oven.
- When grilling, line the grill with foil, or wrap the food in foil.
- Take care not to burn foods.
- Marinate meats beforehand.

Evidence from population studies spanning the globe for more than 30 years strongly suggests that diets high in red meat and processed meat (meat preserved by smoking, curing, or salting, or by the addition of preservatives) are a cause of colon cancer.[97] Based on such evidence, replacing most servings of red meat with poultry, fish, or legumes and choosing only occasional servings of grilled, fried, highly browned, or smoked foods is in the best interest of health.

Another reason to moderate consumption of fried foods such as french fries and potato chips is the presence of acrylamide, a potential carcinogen. Acrylamide is produced when certain starches such as potatoes are fried or baked at high temperatures. Chapter 20 discusses acrylamide in foods.

Dietary Factors—Cancer Promoters Unlike carcinogens, which initiate cancers, some dietary components promote cancers. That is, once the initiating step has taken place, these components may accelerate tumour development.

Although studies of animals suggest that high-fat diets may promote cancer, studies of human beings have not proved that the effects of fat are independent of

*These carcinogens are heterocyclic amines.
**These carcinogens are polycyclic aromatic hydrocarbons.

the effects of energy intake and physical activity.[98] Recent studies have weakened the overall evidence associating fats and oils with cancer risk.[99]

The type of fat in the diet, however, may influence cancer promotion or prevention. Studies of colon cancer implicate animal fats but not vegetable fats, and a number of studies suggest that omega-3 fatty acids from fish may protect against some cancers.[100] Thus the same dietary fat advice applies to cancer protection as to heart health: reduce saturated fat intake and increase omega-3 fatty acids.

Dietary Factors—Antipromoters Some foods may contain antipromoters—dietary compounds that defend against cancer. Table 19-10 (p. 639) includes these protective dietary factors. Research on dietary patterns of populations has led to recommendations aimed at reducing cancer risks.

Recommendations for Reducing Cancer Risks

Almost without exception, epidemiological studies find a link between eating plenty of fruits and vegetables and a low incidence of cancers. Fruits and vegetables contain both nutrients and phytochemicals with antioxidant activity, and these substances may prevent or reduce the oxidative reactions in cells that cause DNA damage. Phytochemicals may also help to inhibit carcinogen production in the body, enhance immune functions that protect against cancer development, and promote enzyme reactions that inactivate carcinogens.[101] For example, the **cruciferous vegetables**—cabbage, cauliflower, broccoli, and Brussels sprouts—contain a variety of phytochemicals that defend against cancers of the esophagus and endometrium.[102]

In addition, fruits and vegetables, as well as legumes and whole grains, are rich in fibre. As Chapter 4 explains, fibre may protect against cancer by binding, diluting, and rapidly removing potential carcinogens from the GI tract. High-fibre and whole-grain foods also help a person to maintain a healthy body weight—another preventive measure against cancer. Physical activity also helps maintain a healthy body weight and reduce the risk of some cancers. Table 19-11 summarizes dietary and lifestyle recommendations for reducing cancer risk.

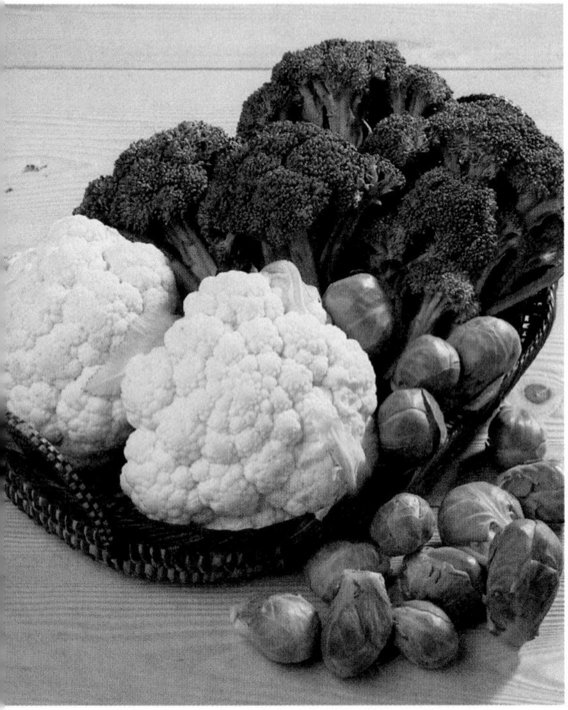

Cruciferous vegetables, such as cauliflower, broccoli, and Brussels sprouts, contain nutrients and phytochemicals that may inhibit cancer development.

IN SUMMARY **Some dietary factors, such as alcohol and heavily smoked foods, may initiate cancer development; others, such as animal fats, may promote cancer once it has gotten started; and still others, such as fibre, omega-3 fatty acids from fish, antioxidant nutrients, and phytochemicals, may serve as antipromoters that protect against the development of cancer. By eating many fruits, vegetables, legumes, and whole grains and reducing saturated fat intake, people obtain the best possible nutrition at the lowest possible risk. Minimizing weight gain through regular physical activity and a healthy diet is also beneficial.**

Recommendations for Chronic Diseases

This chapter's discussion of chronic diseases began with the major cardiovascular diseases, described diabetes, and then went on to cancer—three different conditions with distinct sets of causes. Yet dietary excesses, particularly excess food energy and saturated fat intakes, increase the likelihood of all three diseases.[103] Similarly, all are responsive to diet, and in most cases, the beneficial foods are similar.

Not all diet recommendations apply equally to all of the diseases or to all people with a particular disease, but fortunately for the consumer, dietary recommendations ♦ do not contradict one another. In fact, they support one another. Most people can gain some disease-prevention benefits by making dietary changes. To that end, the recommendations presented earlier for reducing the risks of heart disease (Table 19-6 on p. 627), hypertension (Table 19-8 on p. 631), and cancer (Table 19-11) describe the kinds of foods people should include or limit. Table 19-12 compares current recommendations for the prevention of chronic diseases.

♦ A summary of the *Diet, Nutrition, and Prevention of Chronic Diseases* report from the World Health Organization (WHO) is presented in APPENDIX I.

Critics have noted several shortcomings with the USDA MyPyramid, which was recently replaced by MyPlate (see Nutrition on the Net); MyPlate has also been critically assessed by nutrition experts. An alternative pyramid was created

cruciferous vegetables: vegetables of the cabbage family, including cauliflower, broccoli, and Brussels sprouts.

TABLE 19-11 Recommendations for Reducing Cancer Risk

Body fatness: Be as lean as possible within the normal range of body weight.

- Ensure that body weight throughout childhood and adolescence projects toward the lower end of the normal adult BMI range by age 21.
- Maintain body weight within the normal range from age 21.
- Avoid weight gains and increases in waist circumference throughout adulthood.

Physical activity: Be physically active as part of everyday life.

- Be moderately physically active, equivalent to brisk walking, for at least 30 minutes every day.
- As fitness improves, aim for at least 60 minutes of moderate, or at least 30 minutes of vigorous, physical activity every day.
- Limit sedentary habits such as watching television.

Foods and drinks that promote weight gain: Limit consumption of energy-dense foods and avoid sugary drinks.

- Consume energy-dense foods (>225 kcal/100 grams food), sparingly.
- Avoid drinks with added sugar and limit fruit juices.
- Consume "fast foods" sparingly, if at all.

Plant foods: Eat mostly foods of plant origin.

- Eat at least five servings of a variety of nonstarchy vegetables and fruits every day.
- Eat relatively unprocessed grains and/or legumes with every meal.
- Limit refined starchy foods.

Animal foods: Limit intake of red meat and avoid processed meat.

- Eat no more than 540 grams of red meat a week, very little if any of which is processed.

Alcoholic drinks: Limit alcoholic drinks.

- If alcoholic drinks are consumed, limit consumption to no more than two drinks a day for men and one drink a day for women.

Preservation, processing, preparation: Limit consumption of salt and avoid mouldy grains or legumes.

- Avoid salt-preserved, salted, or salty foods.
- Limit consumption of processed foods with added salt to ensure an intake of less than 6 grams of salt (2.4 grams of sodium) a day.
- Do not eat mouldy grains or legumes.

Dietary supplements: Aim to meet nutritional needs through diet.

- Dietary supplements are not recommended for cancer prevention.

SOURCE: World Cancer Research Fund/American Institute for Cancer Research, Food, Nutrition, Physical Activity and the Prevention of Cancer: A Global Perspective (Washington, D.C.: AICR, 2007).

by the nutrition faculty from the Harvard School of Public Health. The internationally renowned Healthy Eating Pyramid (Figure 19-7 on page 642) is based on their critical review of links between diet and health.[104]

Several recommendations are aimed at weight control. Obesity is common in Canada, and it is linked with most of the chronic diseases that threaten life (review Figure 19-3 on p. 621). The problems of overweight multiply when medical conditions develop. For example, overweight people readily develop diabetes, which is often accompanied by high blood pressure and high blood cholesterol. Such a combination of problems may require only one treatment: adopting a healthful diet and regular exercise program.

Dietary Guidance for Canadians

To reduce the risk of chronic disease in adulthood, engage in at least 30 minutes of moderate-to vigorous-intensity physical activity, above usual activity, at work or at home on most days of the week. For most people, greater health benefits can be obtained by engaging in physical activity of more vigorous intensity or longer duration.

TABLE 19-12 Recommendations for the Prevention and Treatment of Chronic Diseases Compared

Dietary Guidelines	Heart Disease	Hypertension	Diabetes	Cancer
Maintain a healthy body weight	✓	✓	✓	✓
Engage in regular physical activity	✓	✓	✓	✓
Keep total fat 20–35 percent	✓			
Limit saturated and *trans* fats	✓			
Select fibre-rich fruits, vegetables, and whole grains	✓	✓	✓	✓
Use little sugar	✓		✓	
Use little salt	✓	✓		✓
Drink alcohol in moderation	✓	✓	✓	✓

FIGURE 19-7 **The Healthy Eating Pyramid**

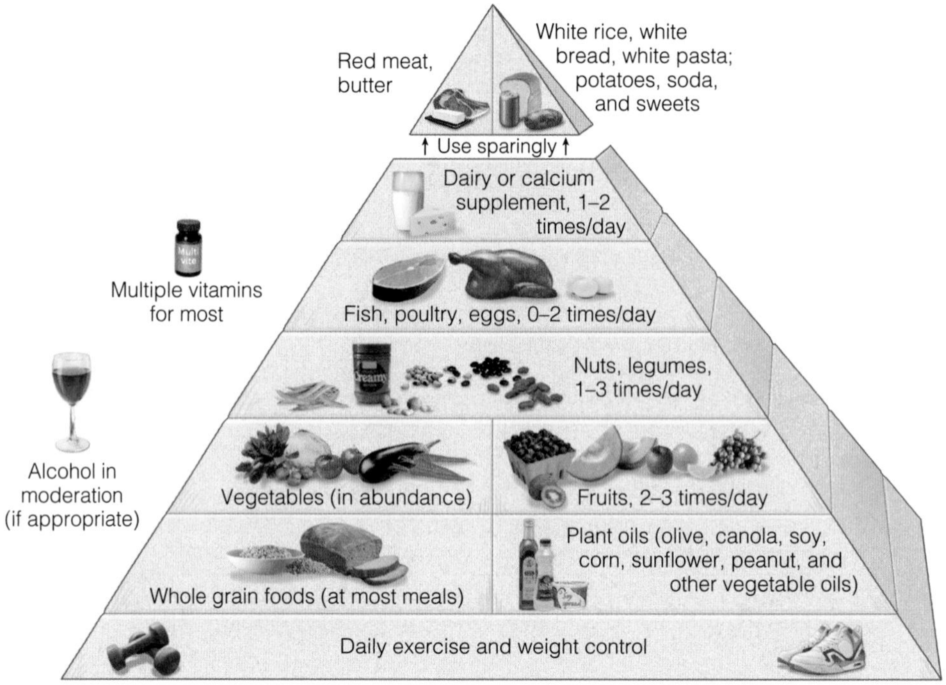
Red meat, butter
White rice, white bread, white pasta; potatoes, soda, and sweets
Use sparingly
Dairy or calcium supplement, 1–2 times/day
Multiple vitamins for most
Fish, poultry, eggs, 0–2 times/day
Nuts, legumes, 1–3 times/day
Alcohol in moderation (if appropriate)
Vegetables (in abundance)
Fruits, 2–3 times/day
Plant oils (olive, canola, soy, corn, sunflower, peanut, and other vegetable oils)
Whole grain foods (at most meals)
Daily exercise and weight control

SOURCE: Copyright © 2008 Harvard University. For more information about The Healthy Eating Pyramid, please see The Nutrition Source, Department of Nutrition, Harvard School of Public Health, http://www.thenutritionsource.org, and Eat, Drink, and Be Healthy, by Walter C. Willett, M.D. and Patrick J. Skerrett (2005), Free Press/Simon & Schuster Inc.

♦ Recommendations that urge all people to make dietary changes believed to forestall or prevent diseases are taking a *preventive* or *population approach.* Alternatively, recommendations that urge dietary changes only for people who are known to need them are taking a *medical* or *individual approach.*

Recommendations for the Population The recommendations to prevent chronic diseases address the general population ♦ in the hope that all people at all levels of risk may benefit. Such a strategy is similar to national efforts to vaccinate to prevent measles, fluoridate water to prevent dental caries, and fortify grains with folate to prevent neural tube defects.

Recommendations for Individuals People's hereditary susceptibility to diseases and their responsiveness to dietary measures vary. Unlike nutrient-deficiency diseases, which develop when nutrients are lacking and disappear when the nutrients are provided, chronic diseases are neither caused nor prevented by diet alone. Many people have followed dietary advice and developed heart disease or cancer anyway; others have ignored all advice and lived long and healthy lives. For many people, though, diet does influence the time of onset and course of some chronic diseases, and many health-care professionals urge dietary measures as part of a disease-prevention strategy.

To determine whether dietary recommendations are important to you personally, look at your family history to see which diseases are common to your relatives. In addition, examine your personal history, taking note of your blood pressure, blood lipid profile, and lifestyle habits such as smoking and physical activity.

Recommendations for Each Individual Even when recommendations are made "for individuals," they apply to large groups of people—those with hypertension or those with diabetes, for example. But that's expected to change in the next decade or so as research on the human genome provides the knowledge needed to create *specific* recommendations for *each* individual (as Highlight 6 explains).[105]

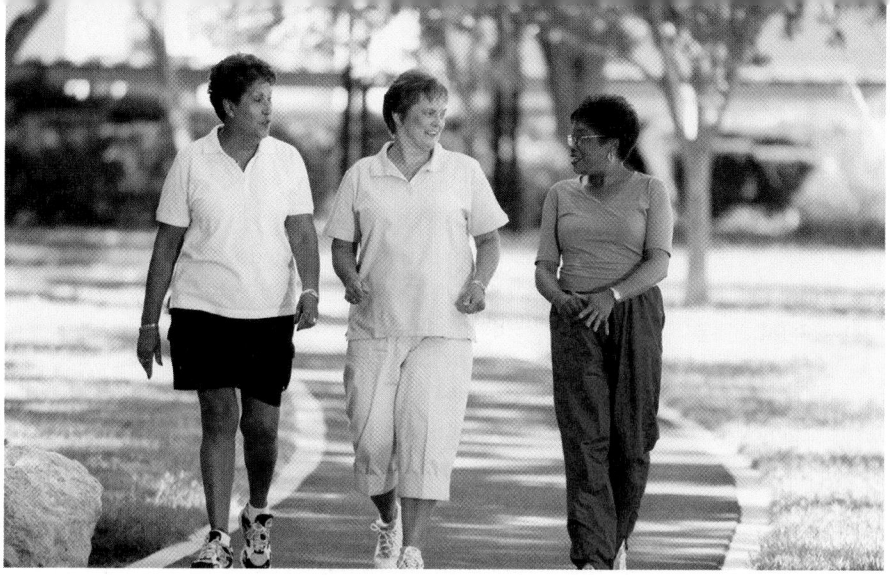

Physical activity and a moderate weight loss of even 5 to 10 kilograms (10 to 20 pounds) can help improve blood glucose, blood lipids, and blood pressure.

IN SUMMARY **Clearly, optimal nutrition plays a key role in keeping people healthy and reducing the risk of chronic diseases. To have the greatest impact possible, dietary recommendations are aimed at the entire population, not just at the individuals who might benefit most. Recommendations focus on weight control and urge people to limit saturated and *trans* fat; increase fibre-rich fruits, vegetables, and whole grains; and balance food intake with physical activity. A person can do no better than to incorporate those suggestions into his or her daily life.**

Nutrition Portfolio

Identifying your risk factors is the first step in taking action to defend yourself against heart attack, stroke, hypertension, diabetes, and cancer.

- Review your personal and family history of heart disease, hypertension, diabetes, and cancer.

Go to Diet Analysis Plus and choose one of the days on which you tracked your diet and activity for an entire day. Select the Energy Balance report to help you answer the following questions:

- In this report, did you expend more energy (kcalories) than you consumed or vice versa? Consider whether you are sedentary or overweight and how you might become more physically active and achieve a healthy body weight. If you smoke cigarettes, develop a reasonable plan for quitting.
- Learn whether you have high blood cholesterol or high blood pressure.

Go to Diet Analysis Plus and choose the Intake vs. Goals report to help you answer the following questions:

- In this report many dietary factors related to heart disease are assessed: sodium intake, fat intake, cholesterol intake, vitamin and mineral intake, and more. Please comment on how your Intake vs. Goals report relates to your risk factors. Is your diet helping to protect you or could it be putting you at higher risk?

Finally, go to Diet Analysis Plus and choose the Fat Breakdown report.

- We know from Chapter 5 that some types of fats appear to be protective against heart disease (monounsaturated and polyunsaturated) and some appear to put us more at risk (saturated fats and cholesterol). How was your intake for each type of fat?

Diet Analysis PLUS **To complete this exercise, go to your Diet Analysis Plus at www.cengage.com/sso.**

Nutrition on the Net

CENGAGENOW™
For further study of topics covered in this chapter, log on to **www.cengage.com/sso.**

- Find AIDS information and learn about HIV infections at the Public Health Agency of Canada: **www.phac-aspc.gc.ca/aids-sida/publication/index-eng.php**
- Review resources offered by the Centre for Chronic Diseases Prevention and Control of the Public Health Agency of Canada: **www.phac-aspc.gc.ca/ccdpc-cpcmc/index_e.html**
- Find information on health in Canada and health statistics at Statistics Canada: **www.statcan.gc.ca**
- Visit the Canadian Cancer Society: **www.cancer.ca**
- Search for "chronic diseases," "disease prevention," "men's health," "women's health," "heart disease," "stroke," "high blood pressure," "cancer," and "diabetes" at Health Canada's website: **www.hc-sc.gc.ca**
- Learn about women's health from the Canadian Women's Health Network: **www.cwhn.ca**
- Review the National Strategy to Reduce Tobacco Use in Canada: **www.hc-sc.gc.ca/hc-ps/pubs/tobac-tabac/ns-sn/preface-eng.php**
- Visit the Heart & Stroke Foundation of Canada: **www.heartandstroke.ca**
- Find information on the DASH diet: **www.dashdiet.org**
- Read about the Canadian Guidelines for Cardiovascular Disease for Canada: **www.ccs.ca/download/consensus_conference/consensus_conference_archives/2009_Dyslipidemia-Guidelines.pdf**
- Learn about diabetes prevention from the Canadian Diabetes Association: **www.diabetes.ca**
- Learn more about the USDA MyPlate: **www.choosemyplate.gov**

References

1. Centers for Disease Control and Prevention, Plan to combat extensively drug-resistant tuberculosis: Recommendations of the Federal Tuberculosis Task Force, *Morbidity and Mortality Weekly Report* 58 (2009): 1–43.
2. A. Flood and coauthors, Dietary patterns as identified by factor analysis and colorectal cancer among middle-aged Americans, *American Journal of Clinical Nutrition* 88 (2008): 176–184; P. L. Lutsey, L. M. Steffen, and J. Stevens, Dietary intake and the development of the metabolic syndrome: The Atherosclerosis Risk in Communities Study, *Circulation* 117 (2008): 754–761; World Cancer Research Fund/American Institute for Cancer Research, *Summary: Food, Nutrition, Physical Activity, and the Prevention of Cancer: A Global Perspective* (Washington, D.C.: AICR, 2007); P. B. Mellen and coauthors, Whole-grain intake and carotid artery atherosclerosis in a multiethnic cohort: The Insulin Resistance Atherosclerosis Study, *American Journal of Clinical Nutrition* 85 (2007): 1495–1502; Position of the American Dietetic Association: The roles of registered dietitians and dietetic technicians, registered in health promotion and disease prevention, *Journal of the American Dietetic Association* 106 (2006): 1875–1884; Committee on Dietary Reference Intakes, *Dietary Reference Intakes for Energy, Carbohydrate, Fiber, Fat, Fatty Acids, Cholesterol, Protein, and Amino Acids* (Washington, D.C.: National Academies Press, 2005), Chapter 11; B. E. Millen and coauthors, Unique dietary patterns and chronic disease risk profiles of adult men: The Framingham Nutrition Studies, *Journal of the American Dietetic Association* 105 (2005): 1723–1734.
3. E. S. Wintergerst, S. Maggini, and D. H. Hornig, Contribution of selected vitamins and trace elements to immune function, *Annals of Nutrition & Metabolism,* 51 (2007): 301–323; B. W. Ritz and E. M. Gardner, Malnutrition and energy restriction differentially affect viral immunity, *Journal of Nutrition* 136 (2006): 1141–1144.
4. Wintergerst, Maggini, and Hornig, 2007.
5. A. L. Webb and E. Villamor, Update: Effects of antioxidant and non-antioxidant vitamin supplementation on immune function, *Nutrition Reviews* 65 (2007): 181–217; Position of the American Dietetic Association and Dietitians of Canada: Nutrition intervention in the care of persons with human immunodeficiency virus infection, *Journal of the American Dietetic Association* 104 (2004): 1425–1441.
6. Centers for Disease Control and Prevention, Twenty-five years of HIV/AIDS: United States, 1981–2006, *Morbidity and Mortality Weekly Report* 55 (2006): 586–603.
7. B. Bistrian, Systemic response to inflammation, *Nutrition Reviews* 65 (2007): S170–S172.
8. P. Libby, Inflammatory mechanisms: The molecular basis of inflammation and disease, *Nutrition Reviews* 65 (2007): S140–S146.
9. Statistics Canada, Leading causes of death 2007, Catalogue no. 84-215-X. www.statcan.gc.ca/pub/84-215-x/2010001/table-tableau/tbl001-eng.htm, accessed September 20, 2011.
10. World Health Organization, Chronic diseases and health promotion, www.who.int/chp/en, accessed March 3, 2009.
11. A. Trichopoulou and coauthors, Genetic predisposition, nongenetic risk factors, and coronary infarct, *Archives of Internal Medicine* 168 (2008): 891–96.
12. Statistics Canada, Mortality, summary list of causes, 2005, Catalogue no. 84F0209X. www.statcan.gc.ca/pub/84f0209x/84f0209x2005000-eng.pdf, accessed September 20, 2011.
13. E. Warensjo and coauthors, Markers of dietary fat quality and fatty acid desaturation as predictors of total and cardiovascular mortality: A population-based prospective study, *American Journal of Clinical Nutrition* 88 (2008): 203–209; R. De Caterina and coauthors, Nutritional mechanisms that influence cardiovascular disease, *American Journal of Clinical Nutrition* 83 (2006): 421S–426S; J. Xu, and coauthors, Dietary fat intake and risk of coronary heart disease: The Strong Heart Study, *American Journal of Clinical Nutrition* 84 (2006): 894–902.
14. Libby, 2007; G. Davi and C. Patrono, Platelet activation and atherothrombosis, *New England Journal of Medicine* 357 (2007): 2482–2494; P. Libby, Inflammation and cardiovascular disease mechanisms, *American Journal of Clinical Nutrition* 83 (2006): 456S–460S; M. S. Elkind, Inflammation, atherosclerosis, and stroke, *Neurologist* 12 (2006): 140–148.
15. Libby, 2006.
16. S. Devaraj, U. Singh, and I. Jialal, The evolving role of C-reactive protein in atherothrombosis, *Clinical Chemistry* 55 (2009): 229–238; P. M. Ridker, Inflammatory biomarkers and risks of myocardial infarction, stroke, diabetes, and total mortality: Implications for longevity, *Nutrition Reviews* 65 (2007): S253–S259; M. S. Sabatine and coauthors, Prognostic significance of the Centers for Disease Control/American Heart Association high-sensitivity C-reactive protein cut points for cardiovascular and other outcomes in patients with stable coronary artery disease, *Circulation* 115 (2007): 1528–1536; N. R. Cook, J. E. Buring, and P. M. Ridker, The effect of including C-reactive protein in cardiovascular risk prediction models for women, *Annals of Internal Medicine* 145 (2006): 21–29; Y. Cui and coauthors, Non-high-density lipoprotein cholesterol level as a predictor of cardiovascular disease mortality,

Archives of Internal Medicine 161 (2001): 1413–1419; J. Lui and coauthors, Non-high-density lipoprotein and very-low-density lipoprotein cholesterol and their risk predictive values in coronary heart disease, *American Journal of Cardiology* 98:10 (2006):1363–1368.

17. J. Y. Kim and coauthors, Lipoprotein-associated phospholipase A_2 activity is associated with coronary artery disease and markers of oxidative stress: A case-control study, *American Journal of Clinical Nutrition* 88 (2008): 630–637; H. S. Weintraub, Identifying the vulnerable patient with rupture-prone plaque, *American Journal of Cardiology* (12A) 101 (2008): 3F–10F.
18. M. H. Davidson and coauthors, Consensus panel recommendation for incorporating lipoprotein-associated phospholipase A2 testing into cardiovascular disease risk assessment guidelines, *American Journal of Cardiology* (12A) 101 (2008): 51F–57F.
19. W. Insull, The pathology of atherosclerosis: Plaque development and plaque responses to medical treatment, *American Journal of Medicine* 122 (2009): S3–S14; V. E. Friedewald and coauthors, The Editor's Roundtable: The vulnerable plaque, *American Journal of Cardiology* 102 (2008): 1644–1653.
20. Friedewald and coauthors, 2008.
21. Friedewald and coauthors, 2008.
22. W. S. Harris and coauthors, Omega-6 fatty acids and risk for cardiovascular disease, A Science Advisory from the American Heart Association Nutrition Subcommittee of the Council on Nutrition, Physical Activity, and Metabolism; Council on Cardiovascular Nursing; and Council on Epidemiology and Prevention, *Circulation* 119 (2009): 902–907; P. C. Calder, n-3 Polyunsaturated fatty acids, inflammation, and inflammatory diseases, *American Journal of Clinical Nutrition* 83 (2006): 1505S–1519S; B. Holub, Clinical nutrition: 4. Omega-3 Fatty acids and cardiovascular care (Review), *Canadian Medical Association Journal* 166 (2002): 609-615; Dietitians of Canada, Position of the American Dietetic Association and Dietitians of Canada (2007): Dietary fatty acids. www.dietitians.ca/Downloadable-Content/Public/dietaryfats-position-paper.aspx, accessed September 20, 2011.
23. D. S. Kelley and coauthors, Docosahexaenoic acid supplementation improves fasting and postprandial lipid profiles in hypertriglyceridemic men, *American Journal of Clinical Nutrition* 86 (2007): 324–333; R. G. Metcalf and coauthors, Effects of fish-oil supplementation on myocardial fatty acids in humans, *American Journal of Clinical Nutrition* 85 (2007): 222–228; C. Chrysohoou and coauthors, Long-term fish consumption is associated with protection against arrhythmia in healthy persons in a Mediterranean region: The ATTICA Study, *American Journal of Clinical Nutrition* 85 (2007): 1385–1391; J. L. Breslow, n-3 Fatty acids and cardiovascular disease, *American Journal of Clinical Nutrition* 83 (2006): 1477S–1482S; C. Wang and coauthors, n-3 Fatty acids from fish or fish-oil supplements, but not α-linolenic acid, benefit cardiovascular disease outcomes in primary- and secondary-prevention studies: A systematic review, *American Journal of Clinical Nutrition* 84 (2006): 5–17; B. Holub, 2002; Dietitians of Canada, 2007.
24. N. T. Nguyen and coauthors, Association of hypertension, diabetes, dyslipidemia, and metabolic syndrome with obesity: Findings from the National Health and Nutrition Examination Survey, 1999 to 2004, *Journal of the American College of Surgeons* 207 (2008): 928–934; S. C. Smith, Multiple risk factors for cardiovascular disease and diabetes mellitus, *American Journal of Medicine* 120 (2007): S3–S11.
25. J. Genest, R. McPherson, J. Frohlich, et al. 2009 Canadian Cardiovascular Society/Canadian guidelines for the diagnosis and treatment of dyslipidemia and prevention of cardiovascular disease in the adult—2009 recommendations, *Canadian Journal of Cardiology* 25:10 (2009): 567–579.
26. J. V. Tu, C. A. Jackevicius, D. S. Lee, and L. R. Donovan for the Canadian Cardiovascular Outcomes Research Team, National trends and cardiovascular care and outcomes, *Healthcare Quarterly* 13(2010): 22–25.
27. Expert Panel on Detection, Evaluation, and Treatment of High Blood Cholesterol in Adults (Adult Treatment Panel III), *Third Report of the National Cholesterol Education Program (NCEP),* NIH publication No. 02-5215 (Bethesda, Md.: National Heart, Lung, and Blood Institute, 2002), p. II–18.
28. Expert Panel on Detection, Evaluation, and Treatment of High Blood Cholesterol in Adults (Adult Treatment Panel III), 2002, p. VIII-2.
29. L. L. Humphrey and coauthors, Homocysteine level and coronary heart disease incidence: A systematic review and meta-analysis, *Mayo Clinic Proceedings* 83 (2008): 3-16; M. A. Albert, Inflammatory biomarkers, race/ethnicity and cardiovascular disease, *Nutrition Reviews* 65 (2007): S234–S238; K. S. McCully, Homocysteine, vitamins, and vascular disease prevention, *American Journal of Clinical Nutrition* 86 (2007): 1563S–1568S; D. S. Wald and coauthors, Folic acid, homocysteine, and cardiovascular disease: Judging causality in the face of inconclusive trial evidence, *BMJ* 333 (2006): 1114–1117; A. M. Gori and coauthors, A proinflammatory state is associated with hyperhomocysteinemia in the elderly, *American Journal of Clinical Nutrition* 82 (2005): 335–341.
30. Expert Panel on Detection, Evaluation, and Treatment of High Blood Cholesterol in Adults (Adult Treatment Panel III), 2002, p. II-19.
31. Statistics Canada, Canadian Health Measures Survey 2007–2009. www.statcan.gc.ca/daily-quotidien/100323/dq100323a-eng.htm, accessed September 20, 2011.
32. A. K. Chhatriwalla and coauthors, Low levels of low-density lipoprotein cholesterol and blood pressure and progression of coronary atherosclerosis, *Journal of the American College of Cardiology* 53 (2009): 1110–1115.
33. De Caterina and coauthors, 2006; Expert Panel on Detection, Evaluation, and Treatment of High Blood Cholesterol in Adults (Adult Treatment Panel III), pp. II-2–II-3.
34. M. H. Beers and coeditors, *The Merck Manual of Diagnosis and Therapy* (Whitehouse Station, N.J: Merck Research Laboratories, 2006), pp. 570–772; De Caterina and coauthors, 2006.
35. L. K. Curtiss, Reversing atherosclerosis? *New England Journal of Medicine* 360 (2009): 1144–1146; Y. M. Prak, M. Febbraio, and R. L. Silverstein, CD36 modulates migration of mouse and human macrophages in response to oxidized LDL and may contribute to macrophage trapping in the arterial intima, *Journal of Clinical Investigation* 119 (2009): 136–145.
36. Joint National Committee, *Prevention, Detection, Evaluation, and Treatment of High Blood Pressure, Seventh Report,* NIH publication No. 03-5233 (Bethesda, Md.: National Heart, Lung, and Blood Institute, 2003), pp. 1–3; Hypertension Canada, 2011 Canadian Hypertension Education Program (CHEP) Recommendations. www.hypertension.ca/chep-recommendations, accessed September 20, 2011.
37. Genest and coauthors, 2009; Canadian Diabetes Association Clinical Practice Guidelines Expert Committee, Canadian Diabetes Association 2008 clinical practice guidelines for the prevention and management of diabetes in Canada. *Canadian Journal of Diabetes* 32 (Supp 1)(2008): S1–S201. O. H. Franco and coauthors, Associations of diabetes mellitus with total life expectancy and life expectancy with and without cardiovascular disease, *Archives of Internal Medicine* 167 (2007): 1145–1151; De Caterina and coauthors, 2006.
38. Genest and coauthors, 2009; Canadian Diabetes Association Clinical Practice Guidelines Expert Committee, 2008; Expert Panel on Detection, Evaluation, and Treatment of High Blood Cholesterol in Adults (Adult Treatment Panel III), pp. II-16, 11-50–11-53.
39. N. Orsini and coauthors, Combined effects of obesity and physical activity in predicting mortality among men, *Journal of Internal Medicine* 264 (2008): 442–451; A. R. Weinstein and coauthors, The joint effects of physical activity and body mass index on coronary heart disease risk in women, *Archives of Internal Medicine* 168 (2008): 884–890; T. S. Altena and coauthors, Lipoprotein subfraction changes after continuous or intermittent exercise training, *Medicine & Science in Sports & Exercise* 38 (2006): 367–372; C. E. Finley and coauthors, Cardiorespiratory fitness, macronutrient intake, and the metabolic syndrome: The Aerobics Center Longitudinal Study, *Journal of the American Dietetic Association* 106 (2006): 673–679; T. Weinbrenner and coauthors, Circulating oxidized LDL is associated with increased waist circumference independent of body mass index in men and women, *American Journal of Clinical Nutrition* 83 (2006): 30–35.
40. R. Silvestre and coauthors, Effects of exercise at different times on postprandial lipemia and endothelial function, *Medicine & Science in Sports & Exercise* 40 (2008): 264–274; P. T. Williams, Reduced diabetic, hypertensive, and cholesterol medication use with walking, *Medicine & Science in Sports & Exercise* 40 (2008): 433–443; T. A. Lakka and

D. E. Laaksonen, Physical activity in prevention and treatment of metabolic syndrome, *Applied Physiology, Nutrition, and Metabolism* 32 (2007): 76–88.

41. S. A. Kenfield, Smoking and smoking cessation in relation to mortality in women, *JAMA* 299 (2008): 2037–2047; Expert Panel on Detection, Evaluation, and Treatment of High Blood Cholesterol in Adults (Adult Treatment Panel III), p. II-16.
42. A. Mente and coauthors, A systematic review of the evidence supporting a causal link between dietary factors and coronary heart disease, *Archives of Internal Medicine* 169 (2009): 659-669.
43. J. D. Brunzell, Hypertriglyceridemia, *New England Journal of Medicine* 357 (2007): 1009–1017.
44. P. E. McBride, Triglycerides and risk for coronary heart disease, *JAMA* 298 (2007): 336–338.
45. S. Bansal and coauthors, Fasting compared with nonfasting triglycerides and risk of cardiovascular events in women, *JAMA* 298 (2007): 309–316; B. G. Nordestgaard and coauthors, Nonfasting triglycerides and risk of myocardial infarction, ischemic heart disease, and death in men and women, *JAMA* 298 (2007): 299–308.
46. D. M. Minich and J. S. Bland, Dietary management of the metabolic syndrome beyond macronutrients, *Nutrition Reviews* 66 (2008): 429–444; C. Day, Metabolic syndrome, or what you will: Definitions and epidemiology, *Diabetes and Vascular Disease Research* 4 (2007): 32–38; D. J. Magliano, J. E. Shaw, and P. Z. Zimmet, How to best define the metabolic syndrome, *Annals of Medicine* 38 (2006): 34–41.
47. Minich and Bland, 2008; P. Meerarani and coauthors, Metabolic syndrome and diabetic atherothrombosis: Implications in vascular complications, *Current Molecular Medicine* 6 (2006): 501–514; American Heart Association/National Heart, Lung, and Blood Institute Scientific Statement, Diagnosis and management of metabolic syndrome, *Circulation* 112 (2005): 2735–2752; Genest and coauthors, 2009.
48. E. S. Ford, Prevalence of the metabolic syndrome defined by the International Diabetes Federation among adults in the U.S., *Diabetes Care* 28 (2005): 2745–2749; Expert Panel on Detection, Evaluation, and Treatment of High Blood Cholesterol in Adults (Adult Treatment Panel III), pp. II-26–II-28.
49. Genest and coauthors, 2009; Expert Panel on Detection, Evaluation, and Treatment of High Blood Cholesterol in Adults (Adult Treatment Panel III), p. III-6.
50. E. Ingelsson and coauthors, Clinical utility of different lipid measures for prediction of coronary heart disease in men and women, *JAMA* 298 (2007): 776–785; Expert Panel on Detection, Evaluation, and Treatment of High Blood Cholesterol in Adults (Adult Treatment Panel III), pp. II-1–II-4; Genest and coauthors, 2009.
51. S. S. Gidding and coauthors, Implementing American Heart Association pediatric and adult nutrition guidelines: A Scientific Statement from the American Heart Association Nutrition Committee of the Council on Nutrition, Physical Activity and Metabolism, Council on Cardiovascular Disease in the Young, Council on Arteriosclerosis, Thrombosis and Vascular Biology, Council on Cardiovascular Nursing, Council on Epidemiology and Prevention, and Council for High Blood Pressure Research, *Circulation* 119 (2009): 1161–1175; Genest and coauthors, 2009.
52. AHA Scientific Statement: Diet and lifestyle recommendations revision 2006, *Circulation* 114 (2006): 82–96; Expert Panel on Detection, Evaluation, and Treatment of High Blood Cholesterol in Adults (Adult Treatment Panel III), pp. V-1–V-28; Genest and coauthors, 2009.
53. C. Rosendorff and coauthors, Treatment of hypertension in the prevention and management of ischemic heart disease: A Scientific Statement from the American Heart Association Council for High Blood Pressure Research and the Councils on Clinical Cardiology and Epidemiology and Prevention, *Circulation* 115 (2007): 2761–2788.
54. Chhatriwalla and coauthors, 2009.
55. Statistics Canada, Canadian Health Measures Survey: Blood pressure in adults 2007–2009, *The Daily*. www.statcan.gc.ca/daily-quotidien/100217/dq100217b-eng.htm, accessed September 20, 2011.
56. B. Rodriquez-Iturbe and N. D. Vaziri, Salt-sensitive hypertension: Update on novel findings, *Nephrology Dialysis Transplantation* 22 (2007): 992–995; K. M. O'Shaughnessy and F. E. Karet, Salt handling and hypertension, *Annual Review of Nutrition* 26 (2006): 343–365.
57. Beers and coeditors, 2006.
58. American Heart Association, *Know the Facts, Get the Stats*. www.americanheart.org, accessed March 18, 2009.
59. T. A. Kotchen and J. M. Kotchen, Nutrition, diet, and hypertension, in M. E. Shils and coeditors, *Modern Nutrition in Health and Disease*, 10th ed. (Philadelphia: Lippincott Williams & Wilkins, 2006), pp. 1095–1107.
60. J. Redon and coauthors, Mechanisms of hypertension in the cardiometabolic syndrome, *Journal of Hypertension* 27 (2009): 441–451; F. W. Visser and coauthors, Rise in extracellular fluid volume during high sodium depends on BMI in healthy men, *Obesity (Silver Spring)*, March 2009, e-pub ahead of print.
61. Rodriquez-Iturbe and Vaziri, 2007.
62. Kotchen and Kotchen, 2006.
63. N. L. Chase and coauthors, The association of cardiorespiratory fitness and physical activity with incidence of hypertension in men, *American Journal of Hypertension* February 5, 2009, advance online publication; T. Rankinen and coauthors, Cardiorespiratory fitness, BMI, and risk of hypertension: The HYPGENE Study, *Medicine & Science in Sports & Exercise* 39 (2007): 1687–1692.
64. P. T. Williams, Reduced diabetic, hypertensive, and cholesterol medication use with walking, *Medicine & Science in Sports & Exercise* 40 (2008): 433–443.
65. J. F. Swain and coauthors, Characteristics of the diet patterns tested in the optimal macronutrient intake trial to prevent heart disease (OmniHeart): Options for a heart-healthy diet, *Journal of the American Dietetic Association* 108 (2008): 257–265; National Institutes of Health, National Heart, Lung, and Blood Institute, *Your Guide to Lowering Your Blood Pressure with DASH* (NIH Publication No. 06-4082, 2006).
66. National Institutes of Health, National Heart, Lung, and Blood Institute, *Your Guide to Lowering Your Blood Pressure with DASH* (NIH Publication No. 06-4082, 2006).
67. F. Dumier, Dietary sodium intake and arterial blood pressure, *Journal of Renal Nutrition* 19 (2009): 57–60; National Institutes of Health, National Heart, Lung, and Blood Institute, 2006.
68. K. M. Dickinson, J. B. Keogh, and P. M. Clifton, Effects of a low-salt diet on flow-mediated dilation in humans, *American Journal of Clinical Nutrition* 89 (2009); 485–490.
69. Canadian Diabetes Association, Diabetes—Facts (Dec. 2009). www.diabetes.ca/files/Diabetes_Fact_Sheet.pdf, accessed September 20, 2011.
70. Canadian Diabetes Association, The prevalence and cost of diabetes (2011). www.diabetes.ca/diabetes-and-you/what/prevalence/, accessed September 20, 2011.
71. E. Lefebvre and coauthors, Dietary proteins as environmental modifiers of type 1 diabetes mellitus, *Annual Review of Nutrition* 26 (2006): 175–202; Canadian Diabetes Association, Canadian Diabetes Association 2008 clinical practice guidelines for the prevention and management of diabetes in Canada. *Canadian Journal of Diabetes* 32 (Suppl 1, 2008): S1–S201.
72. Canadian Diabetes Association, 2011.
73. Canadian Diabetes Association, 2011.
74. D. Mozaffarian and coauthors, Lifestyle risk factors and new-onset diabetes mellitus in older adults: The Cardiovascular Health Study, *Archives of Internal Medicine* 169 (2009): 798–807; Canadian Diabetes Association, 2008.
75. Canadian Diabetes Association, 2008.
76. K. L. Jones, Role of obesity in complicating and confusing the diagnosis and treatment of diabetes in children, *Pediatrics* 121 (2008): 361–368; J. A. Morrison and coauthors, Pre-teen insulin resistance predicts weight gain, impaired fasting glucose, and type 2 diabetes at age 18-19 y: A 10-y prospective study of black and white girls, *American Journal of Clinical Nutrition* 88 (2008): 778–788; Canadian Diabetes Association, 2008.
77. A. Pradhan, Obesity, metabolic syndrome, and type 2 diabetes: Inflammatory basis of glucose metabolic disorders, *Nutrition Reviews* 65 (2007): S152–S156.
78. Canadian Diabetes Association, 2008; The Juvenile Diabetes Research Foundation Continuous Glucose Monitoring Study Group, Continuous glucose monitoring and intensive treatment of type 1 diabetes, *New England Journal of Medicine* 359 (2008): 1464–1476; R. R. Holman, 10-year follow-up of intensive glucose control in type 2 diabetes, *New*

England Journal of Medicine 15 (2008): 1577–1589; The Diabetes Control and Complications Trial/Epidemiology of Diabetes Interventions and Complications (DCCT/EDIC) Study Research Group, Intensive diabetes treatment and cardiovascular disease in patients with type 1 diabetes, *New England Journal of Medicine* 353 (2005): 2643–2653.
79. A. Whaley-Connell and coauthors, Diabetes mellitus and CKD awareness: The Kidney Early Evaluation Program (KEEP) and National Health and Nutrition Examination Survey (NHANES), *American Journal of Kidney Diseases* 53 (2009): S11–S21; Centers for Disease Control, *National Diabetes Fact Sheet, 2007.*
80. Canadian Diabetes Association, 2008.
81. Canadian Diabetes Association, 2008.
82. Canadian Diabetes Association, 2008.
83. Canadian Diabetes Association, 2008.
84. Canadian Diabetes Association, 2008.
85. Canadian Diabetes Association, 2008.
86. Canadian Diabetes Association, 2008.
87. C. Hayes and A. Kriska, Role of physical activity in diabetes management and prevention, *Journal of the American Dietetic Association* 108 (2008): S19–S23; Canadian Diabetes Association, 2008; Canadian Society for Exercise Physiology (CSEP). *Canadian Physical Activity Guidelines* (2011). www.csep.ca/english/view.asp?x=587, accessed September 1, 2011.
88. C. M. Croce, Oncogenes and cancer, *New England Journal of Medicine* 358 (2008): 502–511.
89. A. C. Chiang and J. Massague, Molecular basis of metastasis, *New England Journal of Medicine* 359 (2008): 2814–2823.
90. World Cancer Research Fund/American Institute for Cancer Research, *Policy and Action for Cancer Prevention. Food, Nutrition, and Physical Activity: A Global Perspective* (Washington, D.C.: AICR, 2009), pp. 12–28; L. Dossus and R. Kaaks, Nutrition, metabolic factors and cancer risk, *Best Practice & Research: Clinical Endocrinology & Metabolism* 22 (2008): 551–571; Orsini and coauthors, 2008; K. C. Westerlind and N. I. Williams, Effect of energy deficiency on estrogen metabolism in premenopausal women, *Medicine & Science in Sports & Medicine* 39 (2007): 1090–1097.
91. S. Y. Pan and M. DesMeules, Energy intake, physical activity, energy balance, and cancer: Epidemiologic evidence, *Methods in Molecular Biology* 472 (2009): 191–215; J. B. Peel and coauthors, Cardiorespiratory fitness and digestive cancer mortality: Findings from the Aerobics Center Longitudinal Study, *Cancer Epidemiology Biomarkers Prevention,* March 17, 2009, advance online publication; K. Y. Wolin and coauthors, Physical activity and colon cancer prevention: A meta-analysis, *British Journal of Cancer* 100 (2009): 611–616.
92. J. B. Peel and coauthors, A prospective study of cardiorespiratory fitness and breast cancer mortality, *Medicine & Science in Sports & Exercise* 41 (2009): 742–748; Westerlind and Williams, 2007; World Cancer Research Fund/American Institute for Cancer Research, 2007.
93. S. Larsson and A. Wolk, Obesity and colon and rectal cancer risk: A meta-analysis of prospective studies, *American Journal of Clinical Nutrition* 86 (2007): 556–565; C. Liu and R. M. Russell, Nutrition and gastric cancer risk: An update, *Nutrition Reviews* 66 (2008): 237–249; World Cancer Research Fund/American Institute for Cancer Research, 2007, pp. 211–242.
94. N. H. Rod and coauthors, Low-risk factor profile, estrogen levels, and breast cancer risk among postmenopausal women, *International Journal of Cancer* 124 (2009): 1935–1940; World Cancer Research Fund/American Institute for Cancer Research, 2007, pp. 30–46.
95. World Cancer Research Fund/American Institute for Cancer Research, 2007, pp. xiv–xxiv.
96. World Cancer Research Fund/American Institute for Cancer Research, 2007, pp. 277–280; P. Boffetta and M. Hashibe, Alcohol and cancer, *Lancet Oncology* 7 (2006): 149–156.
97. R. Sinha and coauthors, Meat intake and mortality: A prospective study of over half a million people, *Archives of Internal Medicine* 169 (2009): 562–571; J. Hu and coauthors, Meat and fish consumption and cancer in Canada, *Nutrition and Cancer* 60 (2008): 313–324; R. L. Santarelli, F. Pierre, and D. E. Corpet, Processed meat and colorectal cancer: A review of epidemiologic and experimental evidence, *Nutrition and Cancer* 60 (2008): 131–144; World Cancer Research Fund/American Institute for Cancer Research, 2007, pp. 280–288; A. J. Cross and coauthors, A prospective study of red and processed meat intake in relation cancer risk, *PLoS Medicine* 4 (2007): e325.
98. W. C. Willett and E. Giovannucci, Epidemiology of diet and cancer risk, in M. E. Shils and coeditors, *Modern Nutrition in Health and Disease* (Philadelphia: Lippincott Williams & Wilkins, 2006), pp. 1267–1279.
99. World Cancer Research Fund/American Institute for Cancer Research, 2007, pp. 135–140; S. A. A. Beresford and coauthors, Low-fat dietary pattern and risk of colorectal cancer: The Women's Health Initiative Randomized Controlled Dietary Modification Trial, *JAMA* 295 (2006): 634–654; R. L. Prentice and coauthors, Low-fat dietary pattern and risk of invasive breast cancer: The Women's Health Initiative Randomized Controlled Dietary Modification Trial, *JAMA* 295 (2006): 629–642.
100. World Cancer Research Fund/American Institute for Cancer Research, 2007, pp. 280–288; R. S. Chapkin, D. N. McMurray, and J. R. Lupton, Colon cancer, fatty acids and anti-inflammatory compounds, *Current Opinion in Gastroenterology* 23 (2007): 48–54; J. Shannon and coauthors, Erythrocyte fatty acids and breast cancer risk: A case-control study in Shanghai, China, *American Journal of Clinical Nutrition* 85 (2007): 1090–1097; E. Theodoratou and coauthors, Dietary fatty acids and colorectal cancer: A case-control study, *American Journal of Epidemiology* 166 (2007): 181–195.
101. World Cancer Research Fund/American Institute for Cancer Research, 2007, pp. 75–115, 182.
102. World Cancer Research Fund/American Institute for Cancer Research 2007, pp. 75–115.
103. A. Galimanis and coauthors, Lifestyle and stroke risk: A review, *Current Opinion in Neurology* 22 (2009): 60–68; Gidding and coauthors, 2009; American Diabetes Association, 2008, pp. S61–S78; Lutsey, Steffen, and Stevens, 2008; World Cancer Research Fund/American Institute for Cancer Research, 2007, pp. 373–390.
104. W. C. Willett and P. J. Skerrett, *Eat, Drink, and Be Healthy* (New York, N.Y.: Free Press, 2005).
105. L. R. Ferguson and M. Philpott, Nutrition and mutagenesis, *Annual Review of Nutrition* 28 (2008): 313–329; S. H. Zeisel, Nutrigenomics and metabolomics will change clinical nutrition and public health practice: Insights from studies on dietary requirements for choline, *American Journal of Clinical Nutrition* 86 (2007): 542–548.

HIGHLIGHT 19

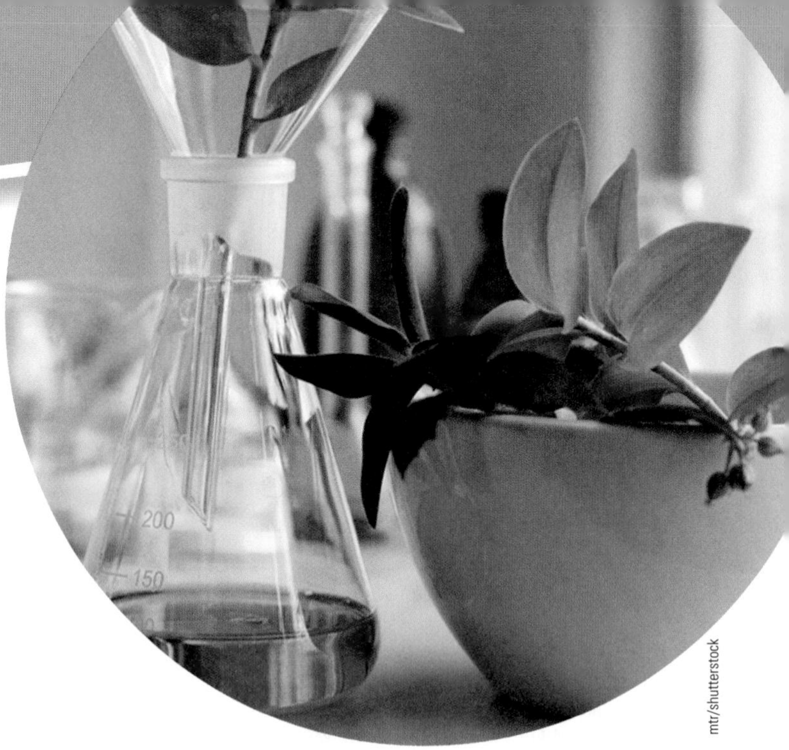
200
150

mt/shutterstock

Complementary and Alternative Medicine

If you suffered from migraine headaches or severe joint pain, where would you turn for relief? Would you visit a physician? Or are you more likely to go to an herbalist or an acupuncturist? Most physicians diagnose and treat medical conditions in ways that are accepted by the established medical community; herbalists and acupuncturists, among others, offer alternatives to standard medical practice. Instead of taking two aspirin, for example, you might be advised to chew two fresh leaves of the herb feverfew or to swallow a tincture of white willow bark. Or you might receive a massage and several acupuncture needles.

Complementary and alternative medicine (CAM) has become increasingly popular in recent decades (see the accompanying glossary for this and related terms).[1] People use these therapies for a variety of reasons. Some want to take more responsibility for both maintaining their own health and finding cures for their own diseases, especially when traditional medical therapies prove ineffective. Others have become distrustful of, and feel overwhelmed by, the high-tech diagnostic tests and costly treatments that **conventional medicine** offers. This highlight explores alternative therapies in search of their possible benefits and with an awareness of their potential harms.

Defining Complementary and Alternative Medicine

By definition, **complementary** and alternative **medicine** is not conventional medicine because for some treatments there is insufficient evidence that they are safe and effective. It includes a variety of approaches, philosophies, and treatments, some of which are defined in the accompanying glossary of alternative therapies on p. 649. When these therapies are used instead of conventional medicine, they are called *alternative;* when used together with conventional medicine, they are called *complementary.* **Integrative medicine** combines conventional medicine and CAM treatments for which there is some high-quality scientific evidence of safety and effectiveness.[2]

A growing number of health-care professionals are learning about alternative therapies; all Canadian medical schools now offer courses in alternative medicine. More than ever before, health-care professionals are incorporating some of the beneficial alternative therapies into their practices; thus the gap between conventional medicine and CAM is narrowing.

For some alternative therapies, preliminary and limited scientific evidence suggests some effectiveness; but for most, well-designed scientific studies have yet to determine safety and effectiveness. If proved safe and effective, an alternative therapy may be adopted by conventional medicine. Cancer radiation therapy, for example, was once considered an unconventional therapy, but it proved its clinical value and became part of accepted medical practice. In some cases, a therapy that is accepted by conventional medicine for a specific ailment is used for a different purpose in an alternative therapy. For example, chelation therapy, the preferred medical treatment for lead poisoning, is a common alternative therapy for cardiovascular disease.

GLOSSARY

complementary and alternative medicine (CAM): diverse medical and health-care systems, practices, and products that are not currently considered part of conventional medicine; also called *adjunctive, unconventional,* or *unorthodox therapies.*

complementary medicine: an approach that uses alternative therapies as an adjunct to, and not simply a replacement for, conventional medicine.

conventional medicine: diagnosis and treatment of diseases as practised by medical doctors (M.D.) and doctors of osteopathy (D.O.) and allied health professionals such as physical therapists and registered nurses; also called *allopathy; Western, mainstream, orthodox,* or *regular medicine;* and *biomedicine.*

integrative medicine: care that combines conventional and complementary therapies for which there is some high-quality scientific evidence of safety and effectiveness. Integrative medicine emphasizes the importance of the relationship between the practitioner and the patient and focuses on wellness, healing, and the whole person.

Sound Research, Loud Controversy

Much information on alternative therapies comes from folklore, tradition, and testimonial accounts. Relatively few clinical trials have been conducted. Consequently, scientific evidence proving the safety and effectiveness of many alternative therapies is lacking. Some say that alternative therapies simply do not work; others suggest that these therapies have not been given a fair trial. In an effort to "explore complementary and alternative healing practices through vigorous science," the U.S. National Center for Complementary and Alternative Medicine supports clinical trials of these therapies. Articles reporting the results of these clinical trials are available in a subset of PubMed *(CAM on PubMed)* created specifically for scientifically based, peer-reviewed journals on complementary and alternative therapies.

Sound research would answer two important questions. First, does the treatment offer better results than either doing nothing or giving a placebo? Second, do the benefits clearly outweigh the risks? Each of these points is worthy of elaboration.

Placebo Effect

Stories abound that credit alternative therapies with miraculous cures. Without scientific research to determine effectiveness, however, one is left to wonder whether it is the therapies or the placebo effect that produces the cure. Recall from Chapter 1 that giving a placebo often brings about a healing effect in people who believe they are receiving the treatment. Traditional medicine tends to neglect this powerful remedy, whereas many alternative therapies embrace it.

Risks versus Benefits

Ideally, a therapy provides benefits with little or no risk. Figure H19-1 (p. 650) presents several examples of herbal remedies that appear to be generally safe and possibly effective in treating various conditions.[3] Such findings, if replicated, hold promise that these alternative therapies may one day be integrated into conventional medicine.

Some alternative therapies are innocuous, providing little or no benefit for little or no risk. Sipping a cup of warm tea with a pleasant aroma, for example, won't cure heart disease, but it may improve one's mood and help relieve tension. Given no physical hazard and little financial risk, such therapies are acceptable.

In contrast, other products and procedures are downright dangerous, posing great risks while providing no benefits. One example is the folk practice of geophagia (eating earth or clay), which can cause GI impaction and impair iron absorption. Another is the taking of laetrile to treat cancer, which can cause cyanide poisoning. Clearly, such therapies are too harmful to be used.

Perhaps most controversial are alternative therapies that may provide benefits, but also carry significant, unknown, or debatable

GLOSSARY OF ALTERNATIVE THERAPIES

acupuncture (AK-you-PUNK-cher): a technique that involves piercing the skin with long thin needles at specific anatomical points to relieve pain or illness. Acupuncture sometimes uses heat, pressure, friction, suction, or electromagnetic energy to stimulate the points.

aroma therapy: a technique that uses oil extracts from plants and flowers (usually applied by massage or baths) to enhance physical, psychological, and spiritual health.

ayurveda (AH-your-VAY-dah): a traditional Hindu system of improving health by using herbs, diet, meditation, massage, and yoga to stimulate the body, mind, and spirit to prevent and treat disease.

bioelectromagnetic medical applications: the use of electrical energy, magnetic energy, or both to stimulate bone repair, wound healing, and tissue regeneration.

biofeedback: the use of special devices to convey information about heart rate, blood pressure, skin temperature, muscle relaxation, and the like to enable a person to learn how to consciously control these medically important functions.

biofield therapeutics: a manual healing method that directs a healing force from an outside source (commonly God or another supernatural being) through the practitioner and into the client's body; commonly known as "laying on of hands."

cartilage therapy: the use of cleaned and powdered connective tissue, such as collagen, to improve health.

chelation (kee-LAY-shun) **therapy:** the use of ethylene diamine tetraacetic acid (EDTA) to bind with metallic ions, thus healing the body by removing toxic metals.

chiropractic (KYE-roh-PRAK-tik): a manual healing method of manipulating the spine to restore health.

faith healing: healing by invoking divine intervention without the use of medical, surgical, or other traditional therapy.

herbal (ERB-al) **medicine:** the use of plants to treat disease or improve health; also known as *botanical medicine* or *phytotherapy.*

homeopathy (hoh-me-OP-ah-thee): a practice based on the theory that "like cures like," that is, that substances that cause symptoms in healthy people can cure those symptoms when given in very dilute amounts.

- **homeo** = like
- **pathos** = suffering

hydrotherapy: the use of water (in whirlpools, as douches, or packed as ice, for example) to promote relaxation and healing.

hypnotherapy: a technique that uses hypnosis and the power of suggestion to improve health behaviours, relieve pain, and heal.

imagery: a technique that guides clients to achieve a desired physical, emotional, or spiritual state by visualizing themselves in that state.

iridology: the study of changes in the iris of the eye and their relationships to disease.

macrobiotic diet: a philosophical approach of eating mostly plant-based foods such as whole grains, legumes, and vegetables, with small amounts of fish, fruits, nuts, and seeds.

- **macro** = large, great
- **biotic** = life

massage therapy: a healing method in which the therapist manually kneads muscles to reduce tension, increase blood circulation, improve joint mobility, and promote healing of injuries.

meditation: a self-directed technique of relaxing the body and calming the mind.

naturopathic (nay-chur-oh-PATH-ick) **medicine:** a system that taps the natural healing forces within the body by integrating several practices, including traditional medicine, herbal medicine, clinical nutrition, homeopathy, acupuncture, East Asian medicine, hydrotherapy, and manipulative therapy.

orthomolecular medicine: the use of large doses of vitamins to treat chronic disease.

ozone therapy: the use of ozone gas to enhance the body's immune system.

qi gong (chée GUNG): a Chinese system that combines movement, meditation, and breathing techniques to enhance the flow of qi (vital energy) in the body.

FIGURE H19-1 Examples of Herbal Remedies

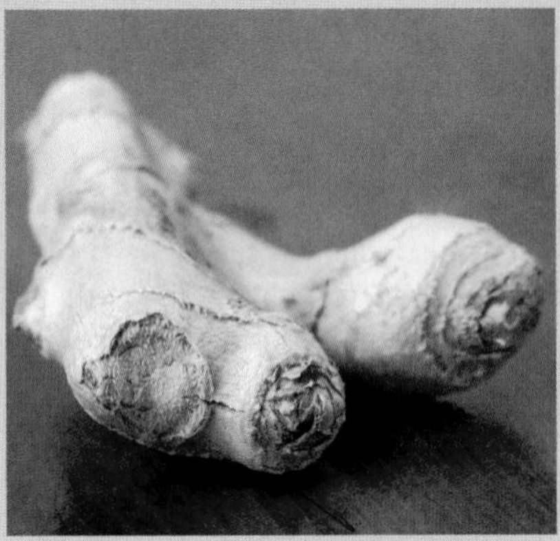
IngridHS/shutterstock

Ginger may relieve nausea and vomiting due to motion sickness or pregnancy.

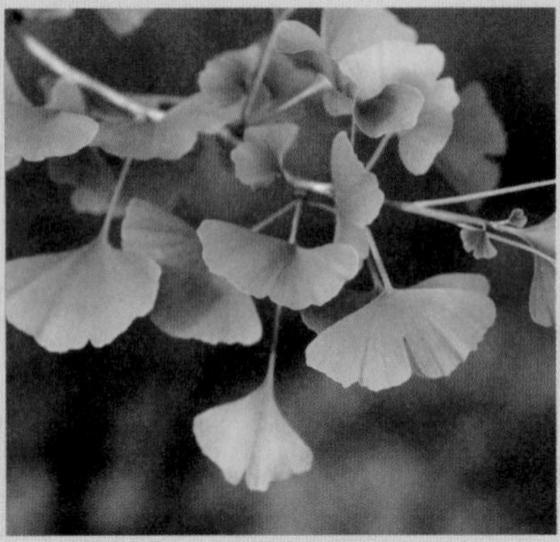
Michael Pettigrew/shutterstock

Ginkgo may slow the loss of cognitive function associated with age.

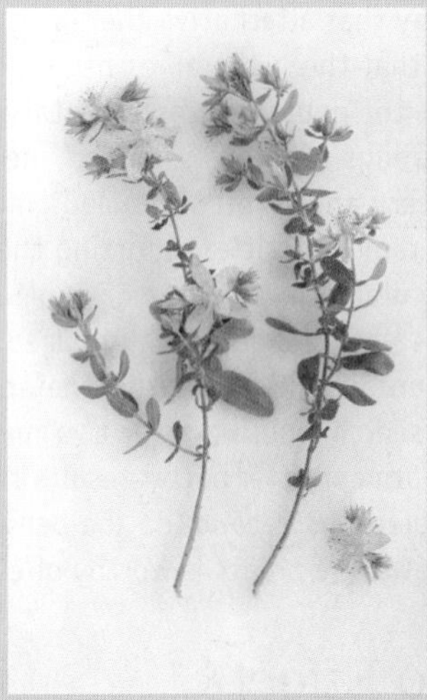
Michael Rosenfeld/Getty Images

St. John's wort may be effective in treating mild depression.

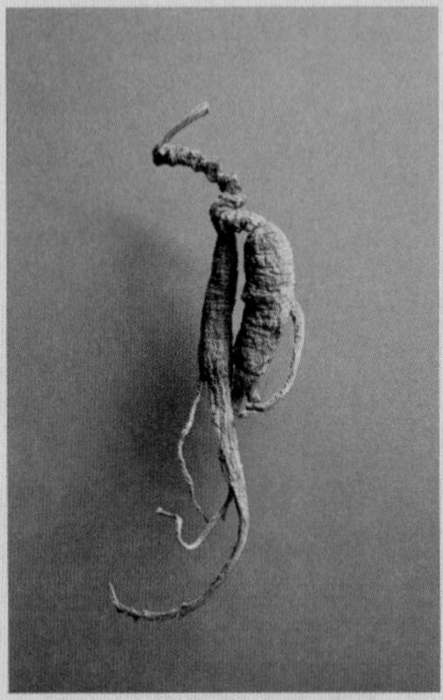
Ross M Horowitz/Getty Images

American ginseng may improve glucose control in people with type 2 diabetes.

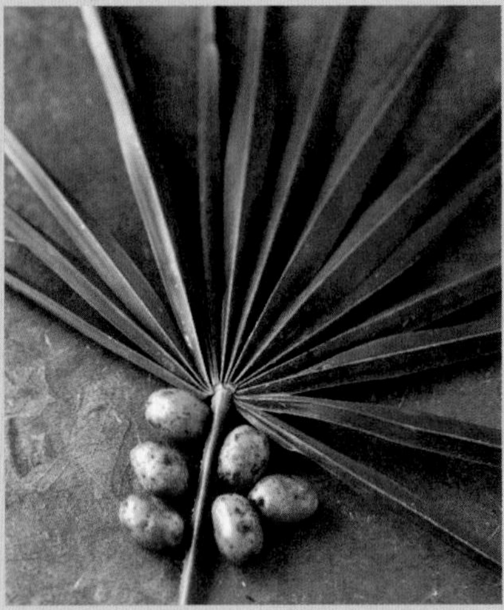
© James Worrell/Time/Getty Images

Saw palmetto may improve the symptoms associated with an enlarged prostate.

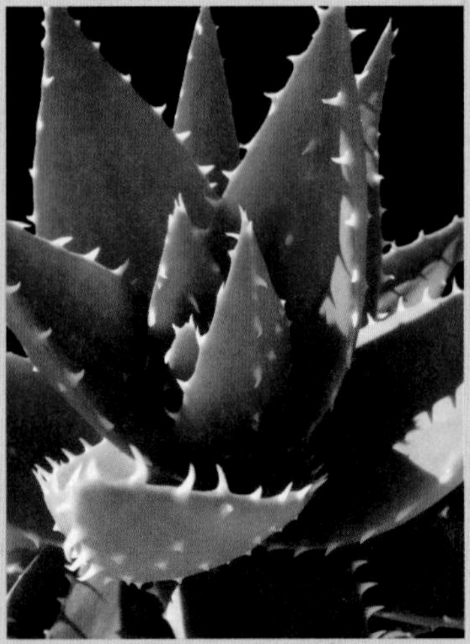
Colour/shutterstock

The gel of an aloe vera plant soothes a minor burn.

risks. Smoking marijuana is an example of such an alternative therapy.[4] The compounds in marijuana seem to provide relief from symptoms such as nausea, vomiting, and pain that commonly accompany cancer, AIDS, and other diseases, but marijuana use also poses risks that some people consider acceptable whereas others deem intolerable. Figure H19-2 summarizes the relationships between risks and benefits.

Nutrition-Related Alternative Therapies

Most alternative therapies fall outside the field of nutrition, but nutrition itself can be an alternative therapy. Furthermore, many alternative therapies prescribe specific dietary regimens even though most practitioners are not registered dietitians (see Highlight 1). Nutrition-related alternative therapies include the use of foods, vitamin and mineral supplements, and herbs to prevent and treat illnesses.

FIGURE H19-2 Risk-Benefit Relationships

RISK: No (or little) → Much; BENEFIT: No (or little) → Much

Ideal situation Benefits with little or no risk (Accept)	**Cautionary situation** Possible benefits with great or unknown risks (Consider carefully)
Neutral situation Little or no benefit with little or no risk (Accept or reject as preferred)	**Dangerous situation** No benefits with great risks (Reject)

Foods

The many dietary recommendations presented throughout this text are based on scientific evidence and do *not* fall into the alternative therapies category; strategies that are still experimental, however, do. For example, alternative therapists may recommend macrobiotic diets to help prevent chronic diseases, whereas most registered dietitians would advise people to eat a balanced diet that includes 1000–1250 millilitres (4 to 5 cups) of fresh vegetables and fruits daily. Similarly, enough scientific evidence is available to recommend including soy foods in the diet to protect against heart disease—but not to determine whether the phytoestrogens of soy are safe or beneficial in managing the symptoms of menopause.

Highlight 14 explores the potential health benefits of soy and many other functional foods and concludes that no one food is magical. As part of a balanced diet, these foods can support good health and protect against disease. Importantly, the benefits derive from a variety of *foods.* More research is needed to determine the safety and effectiveness of taking supplements of the phytochemicals found in these foods.

Natural Health Products

According to Health Canada, natural health products (NHPs) include homeopathic preparations; substances used in traditional medicines (e.g., herbal remedies); vitamins; minerals or trace elements; amino acids; essential fatty acids; or other botanical, animal-, or microorganism-derived (e.g., probiotics) substances. These products are generally sold in medicinal or "dosage" form to diagnose, treat, or prevent disease; restore or correct function; or maintain or promote health. As a product group, NHPs include nutraceuticals.

NPN Labelling

All licensed NHPs must bare the following information[5]:

- product name
- product licence number: ♦
- a Natural Product Number (NPN) (i.e., NPN followed by an 8-digit code)
- a Homeopathic Medicine Number (DIN-HM) (i.e., DIN-HM followed by an 8-digit code)
- an Exemption Number (EN) (i.e., EN followed by a 6-digit code)
- quantity in the bottle/package
- list of both medicinal and non-medicinal ingredients
- recommended use
- cautionary statements, warnings, contra-indications, possible adverse reactions associated with the product
- any special storage conditions

Vitamin and Mineral Supplements Are Regulated as Natural Health Products Like foods, vitamin and mineral supplements may fall into either the conventional or the alternative realm of medicine. For example, conventional advice recommends consuming 400 micrograms of folate to prevent neural tube defects, but not the taking of 1000 milligrams of vitamin C to prevent the common cold. Highlight 10 examines the appropriate use of supplements and potential dangers of excessive intakes.

As research on nutrition and chronic diseases has revealed many of the roles played by the vitamins and minerals in supporting health, conventional medicine has warmed up to the

♦ See Health Canada's website (www.hc-sc-gc.ca) for access to the databases of licensed Natural Health Products & Exempted Products.

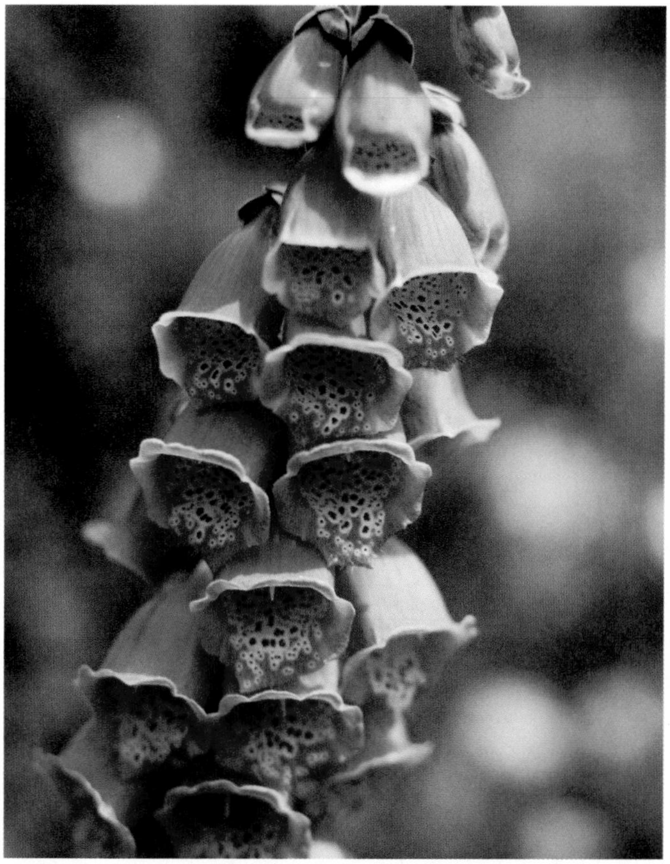

Rowland Roques O'Neil/Photo Researchers, Inc

Digoxin, the most commonly prescribed heart medication, derives from the leaves of the foxglove plant *(Digitalis purpurea).*

possibility that vitamin and mineral supplements might be an appropriate preventive therapy.[6] Some vitamin and mineral supplements appear to be in transition from alternative medicine to conventional medicine; that is, they have begun to prove their safety and effectiveness. Table H19-1 includes several nutrition-related therapies among those recognized to slow the progression of cancer and treat related symptoms. Herbal remedies, however, still remain clearly in the realm of complementary and alternative medicine.

Herbal Remedies Are Regulated as Natural Health Products From earliest times, people have used myriad herbs and other plants to cure aches and ills with varying degrees of success (review Figure H19-1). In fact, today's pharmaceutical industry originated from the use of plant-derived products for human health.[7] Upon scientific study, dozens of these folk remedies reveal their secrets. For example, myrrh, a plant resin used as a painkiller in ancient times, does indeed have an analgesic effect. The herb valerian, which has long been used as a tranquilizer, contains oils that have a sedative effect. Senna leaves, brewed as a laxative tea, produce compounds that act as a potent cathartic drug. Green tea, brewed from the dried leaves of *Camellia sinensis,* contains phytochemicals that induce cancer cells to self-destruct. Naturally occurring salicylates provide the same protective effects as low doses of aspirin. Salicylates are found in spices such as curry, paprika, and thyme; fruits; vegetables; teas; and candies flavoured with wintergreen (methylsalicylate).

Beneficial compounds from wild species contribute to about half of our modern medicines. By analyzing these compounds, pharmaceutical labs can synthesize pure forms of the drugs. Unlike herbs and wild species, which vary from batch to batch, synthesized medicines deliver exact dosages. By synthesizing drugs, we are also able to conserve endangered species. Consider that it took all of the bark from one 12-metre-tall, 100-year-old Pacific yew tree to produce one 300 milligram dose of the anticancer drug paclitaxel (Taxol), until scientists learned how to synthesize it. Many yet undiscovered cures may be forever lost as wild species are destroyed, long before their secrets are revealed to medicine.

TABLE H19-1 Advice and Precautions on Alternative Therapies for Cancer and Related Conditions

Therapy	Precautions
Accept/Consider Recommending—Evidence supports effectiveness and safety.	
Vitamin E (for prostate cancer)	Not appropriate for people with a low platelet count; those taking anticoagulant medications; or those undergoing radiation, chemotherapy, or surgery
Acupuncture (for nausea and vomiting)	Not appropriate for people with a low platelet count or those taking anticoagulant medications
Massage (for anxiety, nausea, and lymph drainage)	Not appropriate directly over tumours, stents, or prosthetic devices and in areas damaged by surgery or radiation; or in people with bleeding abnormalities
Accept—Evidence supports safety, but inconclusive on effectiveness.	
Low-fat diet (for breast and prostate cancer)	Not appropriate for people with poor nutrition status
Macrobiotic diet[a]	Not appropriate for people with poor nutrition status or those who have breast or endometrial cancer
Vitamin E (for some cancers)	Not appropriate for people with a low platelet count; those taking anticoagulant medications; or those undergoing radiation, chemotherapy, or surgery
Soy (for prostate cancer)	Not appropriate for people with a low platelet count or those taking anticoagulant medications or undergoing surgery
Mind-body therapies	Not appropriate for people who do not have reasonable expectations
Acupuncture (for chronic pain)	Not appropriate for people with a low platelet count or those taking anticoagulant medications
Massage (for pain)	Not appropriate directly over tumours, stents, or prosthetic devices and in areas damaged by surgery or radiation; or in people with bleeding abnormalities
Discourage—Evidence indicates either ineffectiveness or serious risk.	
Vitamin A supplements	May increase the incidence of cancer in high-risk populations (both retinols and carotenoid precursors)
Vitamin C supplements	May have anticoagulant effects
Soy (for breast or endometrial cancer)	May stimulate tumour growth and inhibit platelet aggregation

NOTE: Alternative therapies may be appropriate as an adjunct to, not a replacement of, conventional treatment; physicians need to monitor progress and revise recommendations as needed.
[a]When carefully planned, macrobiotic diets can provide adequate nutrition, little fat, and abundant phytoestrogens from soy. Restrictive macrobiotic diets, however, can cause malnutrition.
SOURCE: Adapted from W. A. Weiger and coauthors, Advising patients who seek complementary and alternative medical therapies for cancer, Annals of Internal Medicine 137 (2002): 889–903.

TABLE H19-2 Selected Herbs, Their Common Use, and Risks

Common and Scientific Names	Claims	Research Findings	Risks[a]
Aloe (gel) *Aloe vera*	Promote wound healing	May help heal minor burns and abrasions; may cause infections in severe wounds	Generally considered safe
Black cohosh (stems and roots) *Actaea racemosa, Cimifuga racemosa*	Ease menopause symptoms	Conflicting evidence	May cause headaches, stomach discomfort, liver damage
Chamomile (flowers) *Matricaria recutita, Chamomilla recutita*	Relieve indigestion	Little evidence available	Generally considered safe
Chaparral (leaves and twigs) *Larrea tridentata*	Slow aging, "cleanse" blood, heal wounds, cure cancer, treat acne	No evidence available	Acute, toxic hepatitis; liver damage
Cinnamon (bark) *Cinnamomum zeylanicum, Cinnamomum cassia*	Relieve indigestion, lower blood glucose and blood lipids	May lower blood glucose in type 2 diabetes	May have a blood-thinning effect; not safe for pregnant women or those taking diabetes medication
Comfrey (leafy plant) *Symphytum officinale, Symphytum asperum, Symphytum x uplandicum*	Soothe nerves	No evidence available	Liver damage
Echinacea (roots) *Enchinacea angustifolia, Enchinacea pallida, Enchinacea purpurea*	Alleviate symptoms of colds, flus, and infections; promote wound healing; boost immunity	Ineffective in preventing colds or other infections	Generally considered safe; may cause headache, dizziness, nausea
Ephedra (stems) *Ephedra sinica*	Promote weight loss	Little evidence available. While the U.S. FDA has banned the sale of ephedra-containing products, low-dose licensed Natural Health Products are available in Canada where it is used in herbal medicine as a decongestant. However, be sure to read the numerous Cautions/Warnings/Contraindications/Known Adverse Reactions that appear on product labels	Rapid heart rate, tremors, seizures, insomnia, headaches, hypertension
Feverfew (leaves) *Tanacetum parthenium*	Prevent migraine headaches	May prevent migraine headaches	Generally considered safe; may cause mouth irritation, swelling, ulcers, and GI distress
Garlic (bulbs) *Allium sativum*	Lower blood lipids and blood pressure	May lower blood cholesterol slightly; conflicting evidence on blood pressure	Generally considered safe; may cause garlic breath, body odour, gas, and GI distress; inhibits blood clotting
Ginger (roots) *Zingiber officinale*	Prevent motion sickness, nausea	May relieve pregnancy-induced nausea; conflicting evidence on nausea caused by motion, chemotherapy, or surgery	Generally considered safe
Ginkgo (tree leaves) *Ginkgo biloba*	Improve memory, relieve vertigo	Little evidence available	Generally considered safe; may cause headache, GI distress, dizziness; may inhibit blood clotting
Ginseng (roots) *Panax ginseng* (Asian), *Panax quinquefolius* (American)	Boost immunity, increase endurance	Little evidence available	Generally considered safe; may cause insomnia, headaches, and high blood pressure
Goldenseal (roots) *Hydrastis canadensis*	Relieve indigestion, treat urinary infections	Little evidence available	Generally considered safe; not safe for people with hypertension or heart disease
Kava (roots) *Piper methysticum*	Relieves anxiety, promotes relaxation	Little evidence available	Liver failure
Saw palmetto (ripe fruits) *Serenoa repens*	Relieve symptoms of enlarged prostate; diuretic; enhance sexual vigour	Little evidence available	Generally considered safe; may cause nausea, vomiting, diarrhea
St. John's wort (leaves and tops) *Hypericum perforatum*	Relieve depression and anxiety	May relieve mild depression	Generally considered safe; may cause fatigue, increased sensitivity to sunlight, and GI distress
Turmeric (roots) *Curcuma longa*	Reduces inflammation; relieves heartburn; prevents or treats cancer	No evidence available	Generally considered safe; may cause indigestion; not safe for people with gallbladder disease
Valerian (roots) *Valeriana officinalis*	Calm nerves, improve sleep	Little evidence available	Long-term use associated with liver damage
Yohimbe (tree bark) *Pausinystalia yohimbe*	Enhance "male performance"	No evidence available	Kidney failure, seizures

[a]Allergies are always a possible risk; see Table H18-3 (p. 612) and the appropriate Natural Health Product Directorate Monographs for drug interactions. Pregnant women should not use herbal supplements.

HIGHLIGHT 19

Herbal Precautions

Plants are "natural," but that does not mean all plants are beneficial or even safe. Nothing could be more natural—and deadly—than the poisonous herb hemlock. Several herbal remedies have toxic effects. The popular Chinese herbal potion jin bu huan, which is used as a pain and insomnia remedy, has been linked with several cases of acute hepatitis. Germanium, a nonessential mineral commonly found in many herbal products, has been associated with chronic kidney failure. Paraguay tea produces symptoms of agitation, confusion, flushed skin, and fever. Kombucha tea, commonly used in the hopes of preventing cancer, relieving arthritis, curing insomnia, and stimulating hair regrowth, can cause severe metabolic acidosis. Table H19-2 lists selected herbs, their common uses, and risks.[8]

Although some people use herbs to treat or prevent disease, and while herbal preparations are considered Natural Health Products in Canada (where they must be approved prior to sale), in the United States herbs are not regulated as drugs where they are considered dietary supplements. Thus, consumers who purchase licensed Canadian Natural Health Products do not share many of the concerns (as outlined below) as those who buy similar herbal products in the United States. Indeed, prior to purchasing a Natural Health Product in Canada, consumers can search online to find out whether a particular herbal preparation has been licensed for sale by Health Canada by going to their online NHP database (see Nutrition on the Net). Consumers can also receive notices about any herbal or other therapeutic products that may have been recalled by Health Canada.

The U.S. Food and Drug Administration (FDA) does not evaluate dietary supplements for safety or effectiveness, nor does it monitor their contents. Under the Dietary Supplement Health and Education Act, rather than the herb manufacturers having to prove the safety of their products, the FDA has the burden of proving that a product is not safe. Consequently, consumers who purchase herbal products from U.S. retailers or via the Internet may lack information about or find discrepancies regarding:

- *True identification of herbs.* Most mint teas are safe, for instance, but some varieties contain the highly toxic pennyroyal oil. Mistakenly used to soothe a colicky baby, mint tea laden with pennyroyal has been blamed for the liver and neurological injuries of at least two infants, one of whom died.
- *Purity of herbal preparations.* A young child diagnosed with lead poisoning had taken an herbal vitamin that contained large quantities of lead and mercury for four years. Twelve cases of lead poisoning among adults using Ayurvedic remedies were reported to the Centers for Disease Control and Prevention in recent years.[9] One-fifth of Ayurvedic medicines purchased via the Internet for analyses contained detectable levels of lead, mercury, or arsenic.[10] Another herbal supplement, sold worldwide, is implicated in ten cases of severe liver toxicity.[11] The suspected cause of the toxicity is unintended contamination or overdose of an ingredient that can lead to liver toxicity.
- *Appropriate uses and contraindications of herbs.* Herbal remedies alone may be appropriate for minor ailments—a cup of chamomile tea to ease gastric discomfort or the gel of an aloe vera plant to soothe a sunburn, for example—but not for major health problems such as cancer or AIDS.
- *Effectiveness of herbs.* Herbal remedies may claim to work wonders without having to prove effectiveness. Research studies often report conflicting findings, with some suggesting a benefit and others indicating no effectiveness.[12]
- *Variability of herbs.* Not all species are created equal. The various species of coneflower provide an example. *Echinacea purpurea,* for example, may help in the early treatment of colds, but *Echinacea augustifolia* may not.[13] Similarly, not all parts of a plant provide the same compounds. Leaves, roots, and oils contain different compounds and extracts, and the temperatures used during manufacturing may affect their potency. Consumers are not always aware of such differences, and manufacturers do not always make such distinctions when preparing and labelling supplements.
- *Accuracy of labels.* Supplements may contain none of an herb or mixed species, and labels are often inaccurate. More often than not, supplements do not contain the species or the quantities of active ingredients stated on their labels.[14] In several cases, supplements did not even contain herbs, but drugs that can interact with prescription medicines and lower blood pressure to dangerous levels.[15] Such discrepancies in the contents of supplements can be dangerous to the consumer, interfere with scientific research, and make it difficult to interpret the findings. Consumers may want to shop for supplements bearing a logo from either U.S. Pharmacopeia or Consumer Lab indicating that the contents have been analyzed and found to contain the ingredients and quantities listed on the label.
- *Safe dosages of herbs.* Herbs may contain active ingredients—compounds that affect the body. Each of these active ingredients has a different potency, time of onset, duration of activity, and consequent effects, making the plant itself too unpredictable to be useful. Foxglove leaves, for example, contain dozens of compounds that have an effect on the heart; digoxin, a drug derived from foxglove, offers a standard dosage that allows for a more predictable cardiac response. Even when herbs are manufactured into capsules or liquids, their concentrations of active ingredients differ dramatically from batch to batch and from the quantities stated on the labels.[16]
- *Interactions of herbs with medicines and other herbs.* Like drugs, herbs may interfere with, or potentiate, the effects of other herbs and drugs (see Table H19-3).[17] A person taking both cardiac medication and the herb foxglove may be headed for disaster from the combined effect on the heart. Similarly, taking St. John's wort with medicines used to treat heart disease, depression, seizures, and certain cancers might

TABLE H19-3 Herb and Drug Interactions

Herb	Drug	Interaction
American ginseng	Estrogens, corticosteroids	Enhances hormonal response
American ginseng	Breast cancer therapeutic agent	Synergistically inhibits cancer cell growth
American ginseng, karela	Blood glucose regulators	Affect blood glucose levels
Echinacea (possible immunostimulant)	Cyclosporine and corticosteroids (immunosuppressants)	May reduce drug effectiveness
Evening primrose oil, borage	Anticonvulsants	Lower seizure threshold
Feverfew	Aspirin, ibuprofen, and other nonsteroidal anti-inflammatory drugs	Negates the effect of the herb in treating migraine headaches
Feverfew, garlic, ginkgo, ginger, and Asian ginseng	Warfarin, coumarin (anticlotting drugs, "blood thinners")	Prolong bleeding time; increase likelihood of hemorrhage
Garlic	Protease inhibitor (HIV drug)	May reduce drug effectiveness
Kava, valerian	Anesthetics	May enhance drug action
Kelp (iodine source)	Synthroid or other thyroid hormone replacers	Interferes with drug action
Kyushin, licorice, plantain, uzara root, hawthorn, Asian ginseng	Digoxin (cardiac antiarrhythmic drug derived from the herb foxglove)	Interfere with drug action and monitoring
St. John's wort, saw palmetto, black tea	Iron	Tannins in herbs inhibit iron absorption
St. John's wort	Protease inhibitors (HIV drugs), warfarin (anticlotting drug), digoxin (cardiac antiarrhythmic drug), oral contraceptives, tamoxifen (breast cancer drug)	May enhance or reduce drug effectiveness
Valerian	Barbiturates	Causes excessive sedation

diminish or exaggerate the intended effects.[18] Because *Ginkgo biloba* impairs blood clotting, it can cause bleeding problems for people taking aspirin or other blood-thinning medicines regularly.[19]

- *Adverse reactions and toxicity levels of herbs.* Herbs may produce undesirable reactions. The herbal root kava, commonly used to treat anxiety and insomnia, can cause liver abnormalities and may have such a sedating effect as to impair driving. Chinese herbal treatments containing *Aristolochia fangchi* are notorious for causing kidney damage and cancers.[20] Table H19-2 (p. 653) includes risks associated with commonly used herbs.

Because herbal medicines are sold as dietary supplements in the United States, their labels cannot claim to cure a disease, but they can make various other claims. Not surprisingly, when a label claims that an herbal product may strengthen immunity, improve memory, support eyesight, or maintain heart health, consumers believe that taking the product will provide those benefits. Beware. Manufacturers need not prove effectiveness; they need only state on the product label that this claim "Has not been evaluated by the FDA." Consumers who decide to use herbs need to become informed of the possible risks. To ensure the safety and standardization of herbal remedies on the U.S. market, the U.S. Congress needs to establish new regulations.[21]

Internet Precautions

As Highlight 1 points out, just because something appears on the Internet, "it ain't necessarily so." Keep in mind that the thousands of websites touting the benefits of herbal medicines and other dietary supplements are marketing their products. Most product advertisements claim to prevent or treat specific diseases, but few include the U.S. FDA disclaimer statement. Many of the websites promote products by quoting researchers or physicians. Such quotations lend an air of authority to advertisements, but be aware that these sources may not even exist—and if they do, their comments may have been taken out of context. When asked, they may not agree at all with the claims attributed to them by the manufacturer.

Other deceits and dangers lurk in cyberspace as well. Potentially toxic substances, illegal and unavailable in many countries, are now easy to obtain via the Internet. Electronic access to products such as absinthe and oil of wormwood could be deadly. When the FDA discovers websites selling unapproved drugs, such as laetrile, it can order the business to shut down. But consumers need to remain vigilant because other similar businesses pop up quickly.

The Consumer's Perspective

Some health-care professionals may dismiss alternative therapies as ineffective and perhaps even dangerous, but many consumers think otherwise. In a U.S. survey of more than 20 000 people, almost 40 percent of adults had used at least one alternative therapy for a variety of medical complaints ranging from back pain and anxiety to heart disease and cancer, while in a similar Canadian survey over 70 percent indicated they regularly took Natural Health Products such as vitamins and herbal products.[22] Interestingly, those who seek alternative therapies seem to do so not so much because they are dissatisfied with conventional medicine as because they find these alternatives more in line with their beliefs about health and life.

Most often, people use alternative therapies in addition to, rather than in place of, conventional therapies. Few consult an alternative therapist without also seeing a physician. In fact, most people seek alternative therapies for nonserious medical conditions or for health promotion. They simply want to feel better and access is easy. Sometimes their symptoms are chronic and subjective, such as pain and fatigue, and difficult to treat. In these cases, the chances of finding relief are often as good with a placebo, standard medical intervention, or even nonintervention.

Consumers spend billions of dollars on alternative health services and related products such as herbs, crystals, and aromas.[23] As Highlight 1 points out, selecting a reliable practitioner depends on finding out about training, qualifications, and licences. (To review how a person can identify health fraud and quackery, turn to pp. 32–33. For a list of credible sources of nutrition information, see p. 32.)

In addition, consumers should inform their physicians, dietitians, and other health-care providers about the use of any alternative therapies so that a comprehensive treatment plan can be developed and potential problems can be averted. When considering herbal products, remember to include supplements, teas, and garden plants. Sometimes herbal products may need to be discontinued during pregnancy and lactation and especially before surgery when interactions with anesthesia or normal blood clotting can be life-threatening.[24]

Alternative therapies come in a variety of shapes and sizes. Both their benefits and their risks may be small, none, or great. Wise consumers and health-care professionals accept the beneficial, or even neutral, practices with an open mind and reject those practices known to cause harm. Making healthful choices requires understanding all the choices.

Nutrition on the Net

CENGAGENOW™
For further study of topics covered in this Highlight, log on to **www.cengage.com/sso**.

- Visit Health Canada's Natural Health Products Directorate: **www.hc-sc.gc.ca/dhp-mps/prodnatur/index-eng.php**
- Check online to see if a NHP has been licensed by Health Canada: **www.hc-sc.gc.ca/dhp-mps/prodnatur/applications/licen-prod/lnhpd-bdpsnh-eng.php**
- Sign up to receive notices of recalls on NHPs: **www.hc-sc.gc.ca/dhp-mps/medeff/subscribe-abonnement/index-eng.php**
- Visit the Canadian Alternative Medicine website: **CAMline.ca**
- Learn about complementary and alternative medicine from the U.S. National Institutes of Health's National Center for Complementary and Alternative Medicine: **http://nccam.nih.gov**
- Search CAM on PubMed for a literature search of the complementary and alternative subset of PubMed: **http://nccam.nih.gov/research/camonpubmed**
- Find out more about herbs from the American Botanical Council: **http://abc.herbalgram.org**
- Report adverse effects associated with herbal remedies to the FDA MedWatch: **www.fda.gov/Safety/MedWatch**
- Obtain information on herbal medications from HerbMed or from the Integrative Medicine Service at Memorial Sloan-Kettering Cancer Center: **www.herbmed.org** or **www.mskcc.org/aboutherbs**
- Get dietary supplement information from the U.S. National Institutes of Health's Office of Dietary Supplements: **http://dietary-supplements.info.nih.gov**
- Review the backgrounds and practices of many popular practitioners of alternative treatments: **www.quackwatch.com**

References

1. Complementary and Alternative Medicine, www.CAMline.ca, accessed September 20, 2011; P. M. Barnes, B. Bloom, and R. L. Nahin, Complementary and alternative medicine use among adults and children: United States, 2007, *National Health Statistics Reports*, December 10, 2008; K. J. Kemper, S. Vohra, R. Walls, and the Task Force on Complementary and Alternative Medicine, the Provisional Section on Complementary, Holistic, and Integrative Medicine, *Pediatrics* 122 (2008): 1374–1386.
2. National Institutes of Health, National Center for Complementary and Alternative Medicine, The use of complementary and alternative medicine in the United States. http://nccam.nih.gov/news/camstats/2007/camsurvey_fs1.htm, accessed December 2008.

3. Health Canada, Drugs and health products: Natural Health Products. www.hc-sc.gc.ca/dhp-mps/prodnatur/index-eng.php, accessed September 20, 2011; Complementary and Alternative Medicine. CAMline.ca; C. Andreescu, B. H. Mulsant, and J. E. Emanuel, Complementary and alternative medicine in the treatment of bipolar disorder: A review of the evidence, *Journal of Affective Disorders* 110 (2008): 1–2; S. T. DeKosky and C. D. Furberg, Turning over a new leaf: Ginkgo biloba in prevention of dementia? *Neurology* 70 (2008): 1730–1731; S. Kasper and coauthors, Efficacy of St. John's wort extract WS 5570 in acute treatment of mild depression: A reanalysis of data from controlled clinical trials, *European Archives of Psychiatry and Clinical Neuroscience* 258 (2008): 59–63; T. Hoffman, Ginger: An ancient remedy and modern miracle drug, *Hawaii Medical Journal* 66 (2007): 326–327; B. White, Ginger: An overview, *American Family Physician* 75 (2007): 1689–1691; A. L. Avins, and S. Bent, Saw palmetto and lower urinary tract symptoms: What is the latest evidence? *Current Urology Reports* 7 (2006): 260–265; R. S. DiPaola and R. A. Morton, Proven and unproven therapy for benign prostatic hyperplasia, *New England Journal of Medicine* 354 (2006): 632–634; M. D. Kostka-Rokosz and coauthors, Selected herbal therapies, *Nutrition Today* 40 (2005): 17–28; S. Lawvere and M. C. Mahoney, St. John's wort, *American Family Physician* 72 (2005): 2249–2254.
4. L. O. Gostin, Medical marijuana, American federalism, and the Supreme Court, *JAMA* 294 (2005): 842–844.
5. Health Canada, Drugs and health products: About Natural Health Product regulation in Canada. www.hc-sc.gc.ca/dhp-mps/prodnatur/about-apropos/index-eng.php, accessed September 20, 2011.
6. National Institutes of Health State-of-the-Science Panel, National Institutes of Health State-of-the-Science Conference Statement: Multivitamin/mineral supplements and chronic disease prevention, *Annals of Internal Medicine* 145 (2006): 364–371; H. Huang and coauthors, The efficacy and safety of multivitamin and mineral supplement use to prevent cancer and chronic disease in adults: A systematic review for a National Institutes of Health State-of-the-Science Conference, *Annals of Internal Medicine* 145 (2006): 372–385; R. D. Jackson and coauthors, Calcium plus vitamin D supplementation and the risk of fractures, *New England Journal of Medicine* 354 (2006): 669–683.
7. D. M. Ribnicky and coauthors, Evaluation of botanicals for human health, *American Journal of Clinical Nutrition* 87 (2008): 472S–475S.
8. National Institutes of Health, National Center for Complementary and Alternative Medicine, Herbs at a glance. http://nccam.nih.gov/health/herbsataglance.htm, accessed February 18, 2009; Kostka-Rokosz and coauthors, 2005.
9. Centers for Disease Control and Prevention, Lead poisoning associated with ayurvedic medications—five states, 2000–2003, *Morbidity and Mortality Weekly Report* 53 (2004): 582–584.
10. R. B. Saper and coauthors, Lead, mercury, and arsenic in U.S.- and Indian-manufactured Ayurvedic medicines sold via the Internet, *JAMA* 300 (2008): 915–923.
11. A. M. Schoepfer and coauthors, Herbal does not mean innocuous: Ten cases of severe hepatotoxicity associated with dietary supplements from Herbalife® products, *Journal of Hepatology* 47 (2007): 521–526.
12. S. T. DeKosky and coauthors, *Ginkgo biloba* for prevention of dementia: A randomized controlled trial, *JAMA* 300 (2008): 2253–2262; DeKosky and Furberg, 2008; W. Weber and coauthors, *Hypericum perforatum* (St John's Wort) for attention-deficit/hyperactivity disorder in children and adolescents: A randomized controlled trial, *JAMA* 299 (2008): 2633–2641; Kasper and coauthors, 2008; White, 2007.
13. D. F. Birt and coauthors, *Echinacea* in infection, *American Journal of Clinical Nutrition* 87 (2008): 488S–492S; K. Linde and coauthors, Echinacea for preventing and treating the common cold, *Cochrane Database of Systematic Reviews* 25 (2006): CD000530; B. A. M. Messina, Herbal supplements: Facts and myths—talking to your patients about herbal supplements, *Journal of PeriAnesthesia Nursing* 21 (2006): 268–278.
14. Ribnicky and coauthors, 2008; M. Meadows, Cracking down on health fraud, *FDA Consumer,* November–December, 2006, pp. 17–23.
15. Meadows, 2006.
16. Ribnicky and coauthors, 2008.
17. National Institutes of Health, National Center for Complementary and Alternative Medicine, Herbs at a glance: A quick guide to herbal supplements, NIH Publication No. 09-6248.
18. National Institutes of Health, National Center for Complementary and Alternative Medicine, Herbs at a glance, St. John's wort. http://nccam.nih.gov/health/stjohnswort/ataglance.htm, accessed March 2008; S. F. Zhou and X. Lai, An update on clinical drug interactions with the herbal antidepressant St. John's wort, *Current Drug Metabolism* 9 (2008): 394–409; Messina, 2006.
19. National Institutes of Health, National Center for Complementary and Alternative Medicine, Herbs at a glance: Ginkgo. http://nccam.nih.gov/health/ginkgo/ataglance.htm, accessed November 2008; Messina, 2006.
20. F. D. Debelle, J. L. Vanherweghem, and J. L. Nortier, Aristolochic acid nephropathy: A worldwide problem, *Kidney International* 74 (2008): 158–169.
21. K. A. Clauson, M. L. Santamarina, and J. C. Rutledge, Clinically relevant safety issues associated with St. John's wort product labels, *BMC Complementary and Alternative Medicine* 8 (2008): 42.
22. Barnes, Bloom, and Nahin, 2008; Health Canada, Drugs and health products: Natural Health Products..
23. M. A. Alsawaf and A. Jatoi, Shopping for nutrition-based complementary and alternative medicine on the Internet: How much money might cancer patients be spending online? *Journal of Cancer Education* 22 (2007): 174–176.
24. Messina, 2006.

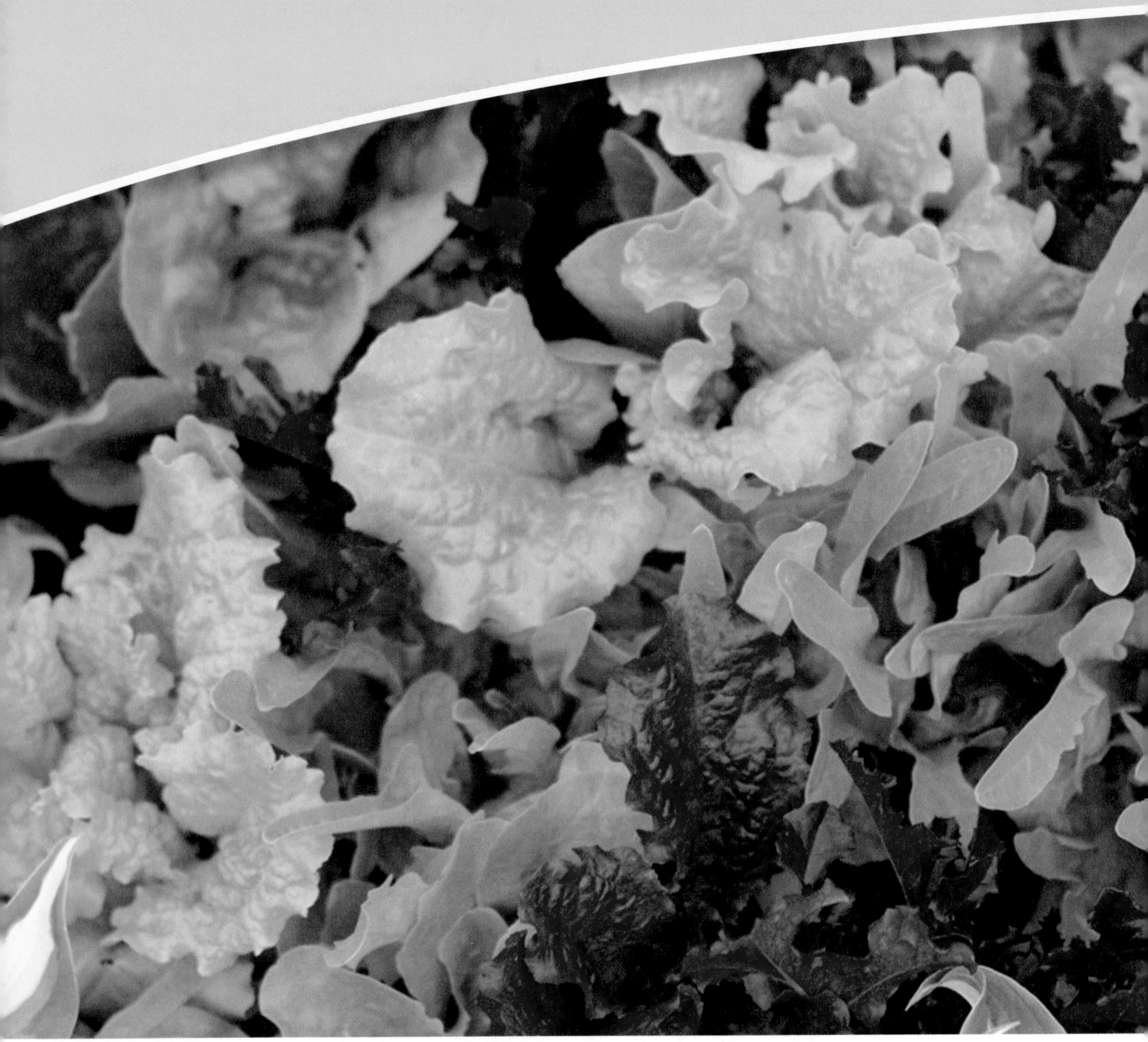

fotique/shutterstock

Nutrition in Your Life

CENGAGENOW™

Throughout this chapter, the CengageNOW logo indicates an opportunity for online self-study, linking you to interactive tutorials, activities, and videos to increase your understanding of chapter concepts.
www.cengage.com/sso

Do you know what causes food poisoning and how to protect yourself against it? Were you alarmed to learn that french fries contain acrylamide or that fish contain mercury? Are you concerned about the pesticides that might linger on fruits and vegetables—or the hormones and antibiotics that remain in beef and chicken? Do you wonder whether foods contain enough nutrients—or too many additives? Making informed choices and practicing a few food-safety tips will allow you to enjoy a variety of foods while limiting your risks of experiencing food-related illnesses.

CHAPTER 20

Consumer Concerns about Foods and Water

CHAPTER OUTLINE

Take a moment to consider the task of supplying food to over 37 million people in Canada (and millions more in all corners of the world). To feed this nation, farmers grow and harvest crops; dairy producers supply milk products; ranchers raise livestock; shippers deliver foods to manufacturers by land, sea, and air; manufacturers prepare, process, preserve, and package products for refrigerated food cases and grocery-store shelves; and grocers store the food and supply it to consumers. After much time, much labour, and extensive transport, an abundant supply of a large variety of safe foods finally reaches consumers at reasonable market prices.

Consumers in Canada and the United States enjoy food supplies ranking among the safest (both ranked 4th out of 17 in the world in 2010), most pleasing, and most abundant in the world. With this benefit, though, comes the consumer's responsibility to distinguish between paths leading to food **safety** and those that pose a **hazard**. The agencies that regulate the safety of the Canadian food supply at the federal level are shown in the Glossary on p. 660. These agencies monitor all aspects of food safety, including the use of pesticides, which are primarily regulated by Agriculture and Agri-Food Canada. Provincial departments of health, agriculture, and the environment and municipal health departments also share responsibilities for the safety of the food and water supply.

Government agencies focus on the potential hazard of foods, which differs from the **toxicity** of a substance—a distinction worth understanding. Anything can be toxic. Toxicity simply means that a substance *can* cause harm *if* enough is consumed. We consume many substances that are toxic, without **risk**, because the amounts are so small. The term *hazard,* on the other hand, is more relevant to our daily lives because it refers to the harm that is *likely* under real-life conditions. Consumers rely on these monitoring agencies to set safety standards and can learn to protect themselves from food hazards by taking a few preventive measures.

safety: the condition of being free from harm or danger.

hazard: a source of danger; used to refer to circumstances in which harm is possible under normal conditions of use.

toxicity: the ability of a substance to harm living organisms. All substances are toxic if high enough concentrations are used.

risk: a measure of the probability and severity of harm.

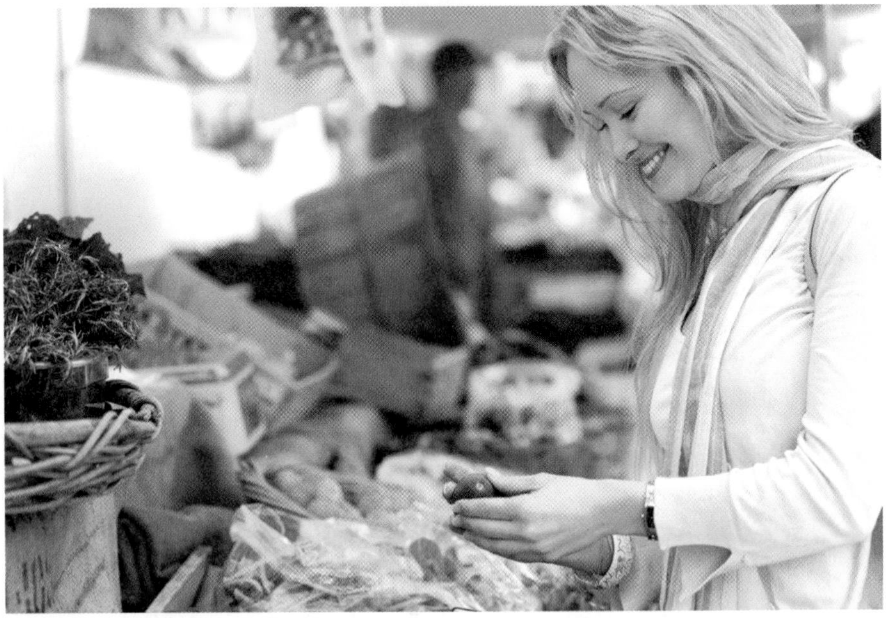
Yuri Arcurs/Veer

With the benefits of a safe and abundant food supply comes the responsibility to select, prepare, and store foods safely.

Microbial foodborne illness, commonly called *food poisoning*, is a priority for the agencies listed in the Glossary below because episodes of food poisoning far outnumber any other kind of food contamination. Canada has had a Foodborne Illness Outbreak Response Protocol (FIORP) in place since the summer of 2004, updated in June 2010 in light of the tragic events that took place during the summer 2008 Listeriosis outbreak,[1] a protocol undoubtedly affected by the events of 9/11 and SARS. The Federal, Provincial, and Territorial Committee on Food Safety and Policy views it as a "key procedural document in national emergency preparedness." Many agencies are taking ongoing action to protect the food supply, and Canada and the U.S. Food and Drug Administration (FDA) have developed broad strategies for countering bioterrorism.[2] Undoubtably, the recent outbreak of *Escherichia coli* [0104:H4] infection in Germany that is linked to organic sprouts in Germany where over 4000 individuals have reportedly been infected (with almost 50 deaths in Germany alone) will further impact food-safety policies globally.

This chapter focuses on actions of individuals to promote food safety. It addresses the following food-safety concerns:

- Foodborne illnesses
- Nutritional adequacy of foods
- Environmental contaminants
- Naturally occurring toxicants
- Pesticides

GLOSSARY OF FOOD REGULATORY AGENCIES

Agriculture and Agri-Food Canada (AAFC): "provides information, research and technology, and policies and programs to achieve an environmentally sustainable agriculture, agri-food and agri-based products sector, a competitive agriculture, agri-food and agri-based products sector that proactively manages risk, and an innovative agriculture, agri-food and agri-based products sector." **www.agr.gc.ca**

Canadian Food Inspection Agency: This federal agency works with other agencies from the farm gate to the consumer's plate to protect public health, and the safety of Canada's food supply is central to everything they do. **www.inspection.gc.ca**

Environment Bureau of Agriculture and Agri-Food Canada: "is an integration of three existing components—Prairie Farm Rehabilitation Administration (PFRA), National Land and Water Information Service (NLWIS) and Agri-Environmental Policy Bureau (AEPB) to address Agriculture and Agri-Food Canada (AAFC)'s agri-environmental issues." **www.agr.gc.ca/policy/environment/**

Environment Canada: "is a science-based department (that provides) the science and technology information needed so that Canadians can make informed decisions about the environment. In addition, Environment Canada's science and technology work helps us to protect and conserve our air, water, wildlife and spaces." **www.ec.gc.ca**

FAO (Food and Agriculture Organization): an international agency (part of the United Nations) that has adopted standards to regulate pesticide use among other responsibilities.

Health Canada: "is the Federal department responsible for helping Canadians maintain and improve their health, while respecting individual choices and circumstances." **www.hc-sc.gc.ca**

WHO (World Health Organization): an international agency concerned with promoting health and eradicating disease.

- Food additives
- Water safety

The chapter begins with one of our government's highest priorities—the serious and prevalent threat of foodborne illnesses. The highlight that follows looks at genetically engineered foods.

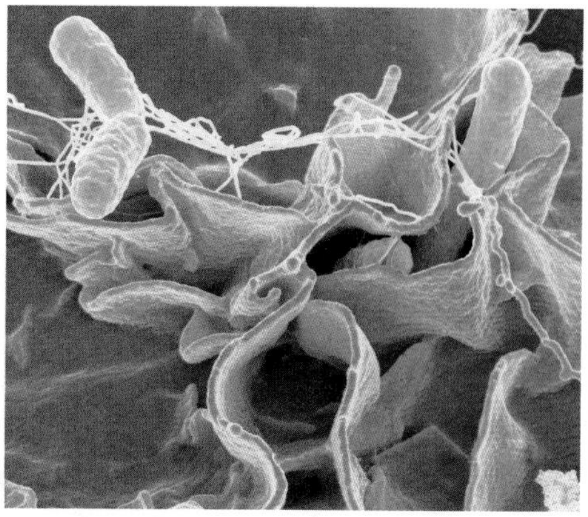

Science Source/Photo Researchers, Inc.

An infection with *Salmonella* bacteria typically causes diarrhea, fever, and abdominal cramps for 12 to 72 hours.

Foodborne Illnesses

The Canadian Food Inspection Agency lists **foodborne illness** as the leading food-safety concern because **outbreaks** of food poisoning far outnumber episodes of any other kind of food contamination. Public Health experts estimate that between 11 and 13 million people experience foodborne illness each year in Canada.[3] For some people, the symptoms ♦ can be so severe as to cause death. Most vulnerable are pregnant women; very young, very old, sick, or malnourished people; and those with a weakened immune system (as in AIDS). By taking the proper precautions, people can minimize their chances of contracting foodborne illnesses.

♦ Get medical help for these symptoms:
- Bloody diarrhea
- Diarrhea lasting more than 3 days
- Difficulty breathing
- Difficulty swallowing
- Double vision
- Fever lasting more than 24 hours
- Headache, muscle stiffness, and fever
- Numbness, muscle weakness, and tingling sensations in the skin
- Rapid heart rate, fainting, and dizziness

foodborne illness: illness transmitted to human beings through food and water, caused by either an infectious agent (foodborne infection) or a poisonous substance (food intoxication); commonly known as *food poisoning.*

outbreaks: two or more cases of a similar illness resulting from the ingestion of a common food.

Foodborne Infections and Food Intoxications

Foodborne illness can be caused by either an infection or an intoxication. Table 20-1 (pp. 662–663) summarizes the most common and most severe foodborne illnesses, along with their food sources, general symptoms, and prevention methods.

Foodborne Infections Foodborne infections are caused by eating foods contaminated by infectious microbes. Among foodborne infections, *Salmonella* is a major cause of illness and *Listeria* infection may be fatal in more than 20 percent of high-risk individuals.[4] These **pathogens** enter the GI tract in contaminated foods such as hot dogs, deli meats, undercooked poultry, and unpasteurized milk. Symptoms generally include abdominal cramps, fever, vomiting, and diarrhea.

Food Intoxications Food intoxications are caused by eating foods containing natural toxins or, more likely, microbes that produce toxins. The most common food toxin is produced by *Staphylococcus aureus;* it affects more than one million people each year. Other foods such as shellfish may be contaminated by toxic algal blooms (e.g., Red Tides) that occur off the shores of various countries, including Canada. These toxins can build up in the tissues of clams and oysters and if eaten can result in symptoms from stomachache to paralysis, and may even result in death. Less common, but more infamous, is *Clostridium botulinum,* an organism that produces a deadly toxin in anaerobic conditions such as improperly canned (especially home-canned) foods and homemade garlic or herb-flavoured oils stored at room temperature. Because the toxin paralyzes muscles, a person with botulism has difficulty seeing, speaking, swallowing, and breathing. Because death can occur within 24 hours of onset, botulism demands immediate medical attention. Even then, survivors may suffer the effects for months or years.

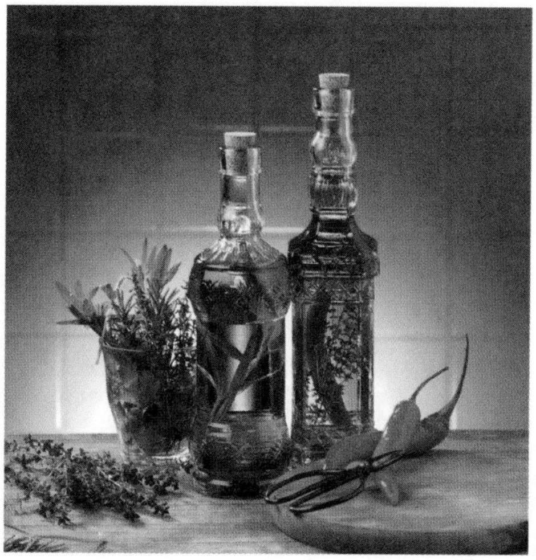

Polara Studios, Inc.

To prevent food intoxication from homemade flavoured oils, wash and dry the herbs before adding them to the oil and keep the oil refrigerated.

Food Safety in the Marketplace

Transmission of foodborne illness has changed as our food supply and lifestyles have changed.[5] In the past, foodborne illness was caused by one person's error in a small setting, such as improperly refrigerated egg salad at a family picnic, and affected only a few victims. Today, we eat more foods that have been prepared and packaged by others. Consequently, when a food manufacturer or restaurant chef makes an error, foodborne illness can become epidemic. Foodborne illnesses may also be caused by errors in a commercial setting, such as nonpasteurization or improper **pasteurization** of milk products or juices.

The listeriosis outbreak in Canada in 2008 resulted in 23 deaths and made 35 others seriously ill. In the 2006 *E. coli* outbreak due to contaminated fresh spinach, nearly 200 people became sick, including one confirmed case in Canada; 2 elderly women and a 2-year-old boy died before consumers got the U.S. FDA message to not eat fresh spinach. In 2009, *Salmonella* was found in peanut butter that

pathogens (PATH-oh-jenz): a microorganism capable of producing disease.

pasteurization: heat processing of food that inactivates some, but not all, microorganisms in the food; not a sterilization process. Bacteria that cause spoilage are still present.

TABLE 20-1 Foodborne Illnesses

Disease and Organism that Causes It	Most Frequent Food Sources	Onset and General Symptoms	Prevention Methods[a]
Foodborne Infections			
Campylobacteriosis (KAM-pee-loh-BAK-ter-ee-OH-sis) *Campylobacter* bacterium	Raw and undercooked poultry, unpasturized milk, contaminated water	Onset: 2 to 5 days. Diarrhea, vomiting, abdominal cramps, fever; sometimes bloody stools; lasts 2 to 10 days	Cook foods thoroughly; use pasteurized milk; use sanitary food-handling methods
Cryptosporidiosis (KRIP-toe-spo-rid-ee-OH-sis) *Crytosporidium parvum* parasite	Contaminated swimming or drinking water, even from treated sources; highly chlorine-resistant; contaminated raw produce and unpasteurized juices and ciders	Onset: 2 to 10 days. Diarrhea, stomach cramps, upset stomach, slight fever; symptoms may come and go for weeks or months	Wash all raw vegetables and fruits before peeling; use pasteurized milk and juice; do not swallow drops of water while using pools, hot tubs, ponds, lakes, rivers, or streams for recreation
Cyclosporiasis (sigh-clo-spore-EYE-uh-sis) *Cyclospora cayetanensis* parasite	Contaminated water, contaminated fresh produce	Onset: 1 to 14 days. Diarrhea, loss of appetite, weight loss, stomach cramps, nausea, vomiting, fatigue; symptoms may come and go for weeks or months	Use treated, boiled, or bottled water; cook foods thoroughly; peel fruits
***E. coli* infection** *Escherichia coli*[b] bacterium	Undercooked ground beef, unpasteurized milk and juices, raw fruits and vegetables, contaminated water, and person-to-person contact	Onset: 1 to 8 days. Severe bloody diarrhea, abdominal cramps, vomiting; lasts 5 to 10 days	Cook ground beef thoroughly; use pasteurized milk; use sanitary food-handling methods; use treated, boiled, or bottled water
Gastroenteritis[c] Norwalk virus	Person-to-person contact; raw foods, salads, sandwiches	Onset: 1 to 2 days. Vomiting; lasts 1 to 2 days	Use sanitary food-handling methods
Giardiasis (JYE-are-DYE-ah-sis) *Giardia intestinalis* parasite	Contaminated water; uncooked foods	Onset: 7 to 14 days. Diarrhea (but occasionally constipation), abdominal pain, gas	Use sanitary food-handling methods; avoid raw fruits and vegetables where parasites are endemic; dispose of sewage properly
Hepatitis (HEP-ah-TIE-tis) Hepatitis A virus	Undercooked or raw shellfish	Onset: 15 to 50 days (28 days average). Diarrhea, dark urine, fever, headache, nausea, abdominal pain, jaundice (yellowed skin and eyes from build-up of wastes); lasts 2 to 12 weeks	Cook foods thoroughly
Listeriosis (lis-TER-ee-OH-sis) *Listeria monocytogenes* bacterium	Unpasteurized milk; fresh soft cheeses; luncheon meats, hot dogs	Onset: 1 to 21 days. Fever, muscle aches; nausea, vomiting, blood poisoning, complications in pregnancy, and meningitis (stiff neck, severe headache, and fever)	Use sanitary food-handling methods; cook foods thoroughly; use pasteurized milk
Perfringens (per-FRINGE-enz) **food poisoning** *Clostridium perfringens* bacterium	Meats and meat products stored at between 50°C (120°F) and 55°C (130°F)	Onset: 8 to 16 hours. Abdominal pain, diarrhea, nausea; lasts 1 to 2 days	Use sanitary food-handling methods; use pasteurized milk; cook foods thoroughly; regrigerate foods promptly and properly
Salmonellosis (sal-moh-neh-LOH-sis) *Salmonella* bacteria (>2300 types)	Raw or undercooked eggs, meats, poultry, raw milk and other dairy products, shrimp, frog legs, yeast, coconut, pasta, and chocolate	Onset: 1 to 3 days. Fever, vomiting, abdominal cramps, diarrhea; lasts 4 to 7 days; can be fatal	Use sanitary food-handling methods; use pasteurized milk; cook foods thoroughly; refrigerate foods promptly and properly
Shigellosis (shi-gel-LOH-sis) *Shigella* bacteria (>30 types)	Person-to-person contact, raw foods, salads, sandwiches, and contaminated water	Onset: 1 to 2 days. Bloody diarrhea, cramps, fever; lasts 4 to 7 days	Use sanitary food-handling methods; cook foods thoroughly; use proper refrigeration
Vibrio (VIB-ree-oh) **infection** *Vibrio vulnificus*[d] bacterium	Raw or undercooked seafood, contaminated water	Onset: 1 to 7 days. Diarrhea, abdominal cramps, nausea, vomiting; lasts 2 to 5 days; can be fatal	Use sanitary food-handling methods; cook foods thoroughly
Yersiniosis (yer-SIN-ee-OH-sis) *Yersinia enterocolitica* bacterium	Raw and undercooked pork, unpasteurized milk	Onset: 1 to 2 days. Diarrhea, vomiting, fever, abdominal pain; lasts 1 to 3 weeks	Cook foods thoroughly; use pasteurized milk; use treated, boiled, or bottled water
Food Intoxications			
Botulism (BOT-chew-lizm) Botulinum toxin produced by *Clostridium botulinum* bacterium, which grows without oxygen, in low-acid foods, and at temperatures between 40°F and 120°F; the **botulinum** (BOT-chew-line-um) **toxin** responsible for botulism is called **botulin** (BOT-chew-lin)	Anaerobic environment of low acidity (canned corn, peppers, green beans, soups, beets, asparagus, mushrooms, ripe olives, spinach, tuna, chicken, chicken liver, liver pâté, luncheon meats, ham, sausage, stuffed eggplant, lobster, and smoked and salted fish)	Onset: 4 to 36 hours. Nervous system symptoms, including double vision, inability to swallow, speech difficulty, and progressive paralysis of the respiratory system; often fatal; leaves prolonged symptoms in survivors	Use proper canning methods for low-acid foods; refrigerate homemade garlic and herb oils; avoid commercially prepared foods with leaky seals or with bent, bulging, or broken cans Do not give infants honey because it may contain spores of *Clostridium botulinum,* which is a common source of infection for infants

TABLE 20-1 Foodborne Illnesses *(continued)*

Disease and Organism that Causes It	Most Frequent Food Sources	Onset and General Symptoms	Prevention Methods[a]
Food Intoxications			
Staphylococcal (STAF-il-oh-KOK-al) **food poisoning** Staphylococcal toxin (produced by *Staphylococcus aureus* bacterium)	Toxin produced in improperly refrigerated meats; egg, tuna, potato, and macaroni salads; cream-filled pastries	Onset: 1 to 6 hours. Diarrhea, nausea, vomiting, abdominal cramps, fever; lasts 1 to 2 days	Use sanitary food-handling methods; cook food thoroughly; refrigerate foods promptly and properly; use proper home-canning methods

NOTE: Travellers' diarrhea is most commonly caused by *E. coli, Campylobacter jejuni, Shigella,* and *Salmonella.*
[a]The "How To" on pp. 666–667 provides more details on the proper handling, cooking, and refrigeration of foods.
[b]The most serious strain is *E. coli* 0104:H4 Entero-hemorrhagic E. Coli [EHEC 0104:H4] outbreak resulted from Europe in spring of 2011).
[c]Gastroenteritis refers to an inflammation of the stomach and intestines but is the most common name used for illnesses caused by Norwalk viruses.
[d]Most cases of *Vibrio vulnificus* infection occur in persons with underlying illness, particularly those with liver disorders, diabetes, cancer, and AIDS, and those who require long-term steroid use. The fatality rate is 50 percent for this population.
SOURCE: From SIZER/WHITNEY/PICHE. Nutrition, 2E. © 2012 Nelson Education Ltd. Reproduced by permission. www.cengage.com/permissions

had been used in more than 2100 products (the CFIA issued a Health Hazard Alert about nine such products) made by more than 200 companies. In 2011, there was an outbreak of *E. coli* [0104:H4] infection in Germany that was linked to organic sprouts grown there where over 4000 individuals in Europe have reportedly been infected (with almost 50 deaths in Germany, 1 in Sweden, and 1 in the United States). In cases like this, where there is an outbreak of a newly identified disease in a limited geographic location, the Canadian Public Health Agency would issue a Travel Health Notice for that part of the world (see Nutrition on the Net). These incidents and others focus the national spotlight on two important safety issues: disease-causing organisms are commonly found in foods, and safe food-handling practices can minimize harm from most of these foodborne pathogens.

Industry Controls—Government Inspections and HACCP Under the mandatory Food Safety Enhancement Program (FSEP), all federally registered meat and poultry establishments and storages are being encouraged to implement and maintain a **Hazard Analysis Critical Control Point (HACCP)** plan to help prevent foodborne illnesses at their source.[6] Each slaughterhouse, producer, packer, distributor, and transporter of susceptible foods must identify "critical control points" in its procedures where the risk of food contamination is high and then devise and implement ways of minimizing contamination.

This example raises another issue regarding the safety of imported foods. To this end, in 2008, the CFIA announced its "CFIA Renewal Plan 2008–2013" and listed as the first of the agency's priorities was to "Enhance regulatory compliance, with a focus on safety of domestic and imported food."[7] The CFIA is working with other countries to adopt the safe food-handling practices used in Canada, especially since more than 70 percent of products sold in Canada are imported and most domestic products contain ingredients that have been imported from more than 190 countries (Figure 20-1).

FIGURE 20-1 Percent of Food Imported, 2007 (From Top 10 Countries)

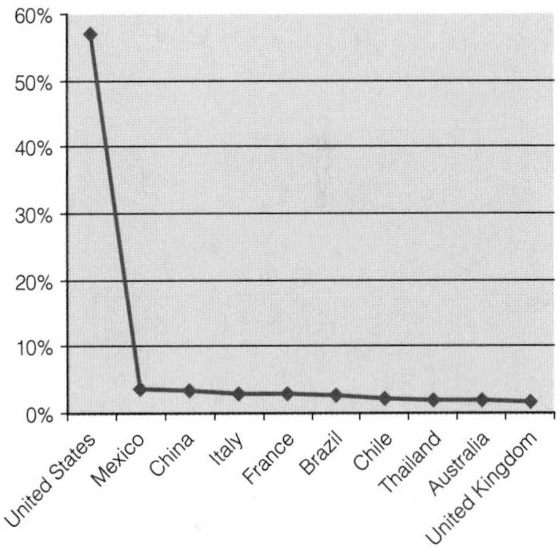
60%
50%
40%
30%
20%
10%
0%
United States
Mexico
China
Italy
France
Brazil
Chile
Thailand
Australia
United Kingdom

SOURCE: Adapted from Statistics Canada, Human Activity and the Environment: Annual Statistics, 16-201-XIE2009000, June 2009; http://www.statcan.gc.ca/bsolc/olc-cel/olc-cel?lang=eng&catno=16-201-X

Consumer Awareness Canned and packaged foods sold in grocery stores are easily controlled, but rare accidents do happen. Batch numbering makes it possible to recall contaminated foods through public announcements via Internet, newspapers, television, and radio. In the grocery store, consumers can buy items before the "Best Before" date and inspect the safety seals and wrappers of packages. A broken seal, bulging can lid, or mangled package fails to protect the consumer against microbes, insects, spoilage, or even vandalism.

State and local health regulations provide guidelines on the cleanliness of facilities and the safe preparation of foods for restaurants, cafeterias, and fast-food establishments. Even so, consumers can also take these actions to help prevent foodborne illnesses when dining out:

- Wash hands with hot, soapy water before meals.
- Expect clean tabletops, dinnerware, utensils, and food preparation areas.
- Expect cooked foods to be served piping hot and salads to be fresh and cold.
- Refrigerate take-home items within two hours.

Hazard Analysis Critical Control Points (HACCP): a systematic plan to identify and correct potential microbial hazards in the manufacturing, distribution, and commercial use of food products; commonly referred to as "HASS-ip."

FIGURE 20-2 **Food Safety from Farms to Consumers**

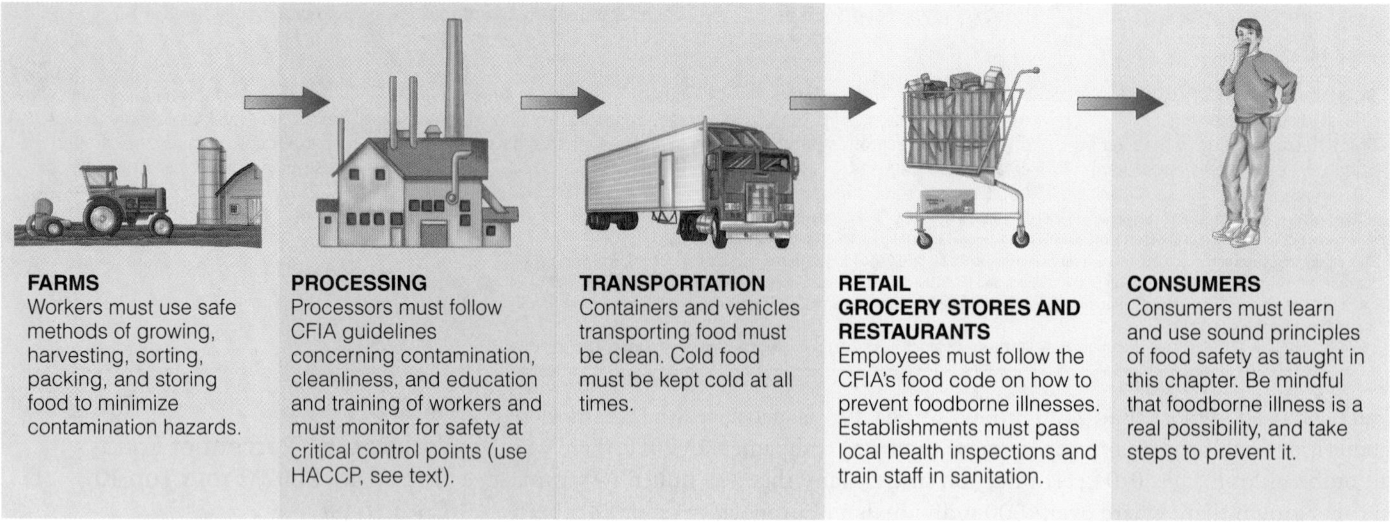
FARMS
Workers must use safe methods of growing, harvesting, sorting, packing, and storing food to minimize contamination hazards.
PROCESSING
Processors must follow CFIA guidelines concerning contamination, cleanliness, and education and training of workers and must monitor for safety at critical control points (use HACCP, see text).
TRANSPORTATION
Containers and vehicles transporting food must be clean. Cold food must be kept cold at all times.
RETAIL
GROCERY STORES AND RESTAURANTS
Employees must follow the CFIA's food code on how to prevent foodborne illnesses. Establishments must pass local health inspections and train staff in sanitation.
CONSUMERS
Consumers must learn and use sound principles of food safety as taught in this chapter. Be mindful that foodborne illness is a real possibility, and take steps to prevent it.

Improper handling of foods can occur anywhere along the line from commercial manufacturers to large supermarkets to small restaurants to private homes. Maintaining a safe food supply requires everyone's efforts (see Figure 20-2).

Food Safety in the Kitchen Whether microbes multiply and cause illness depends, in part, on a few key food-handling behaviours in the kitchen—whether the kitchen is in your home, a school cafeteria, a gourmet restaurant, or a canning manufacturer. Figure 20-3 summarizes the four simple things that can help most to prevent foodborne illness , an initiative supported by Health Canada:

- *Keep a clean, safe kitchen.* Wash countertops, cutting boards, hands, sponges, and utensils in hot, soapy water before and after each step of food preparation. Hand sanitizers are as effective as hand washing in reducing bacterial contamination on hands.[8]
- *Avoid cross-contamination.* Keep raw eggs, meat, poultry, and seafood separate from other foods. Wash all utensils and surfaces (such as cutting boards or platters) that have been in contact with these foods with hot, soapy water before using them again. Bacteria inevitably left on the surfaces from the raw meat can recontaminate the cooked meat or other foods—a problem known as **cross-contamination.** Washing raw eggs, meat, and poultry is not recommended because the extra handling increases the risk of cross-contamination.
- *Keep hot foods hot.* Cook foods long enough to reach internal temperatures that will kill microbes, and maintain adequate temperatures to prevent bacterial growth until the foods are served.
- *Keep cold foods cold.* Go directly home upon leaving the grocery store and immediately place foods in the refrigerator or freezer. After a meal, refrigerate any leftovers immediately.

Unfortunately, consumers commonly fail to follow these simple food-handling recommendations. See the "How To" on pp. 666–667 for additional food-safety tips.

Safe Handling of Meats and Poultry Figure 20-4 presents label instructions for the safe handling of foods (e.g., raw meat and poultry). Meats and poultry contain bacteria and provide a moist, nutrient-rich environment that favours microbial growth. Ground meat is especially susceptible because it receives more handling than other kinds of meat and has more surface exposed to bacterial contamination. Consumers cannot detect the harmful bacteria in or on meat. For safety's sake, cook meat thoroughly, using a thermometer to test the internal temperature (see Figure 20-5).

FIGURE 20-3 **Fight Bac!**

Four ways to keep food safe. The Fight Bac! website is at www.fightbac.org.

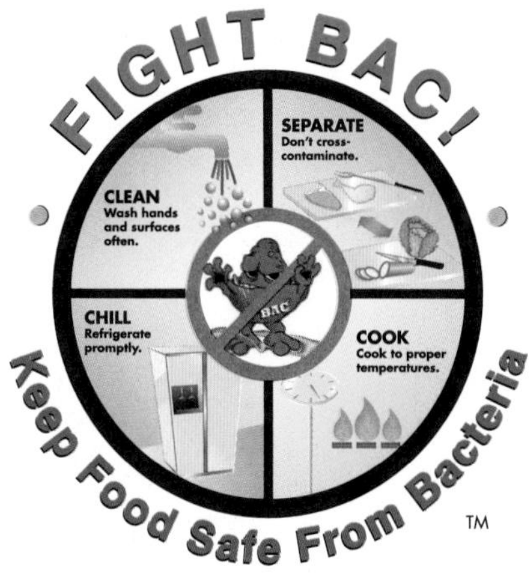
FIGHT BAC!
SEPARATE
Don't cross-contaminate.
CLEAN
Wash hands and surfaces often.
CHILL
Refrigerate promptly.
COOK
Cook to proper temperatures.
BAC
Keep Food Safe From Bacteria
TM

SOURCE: Reprinted by permission of the Partnership for Food Safety Education.

cross-contamination: the contamination of food by bacteria that occurs when the food comes into contact with surfaces previously touched by raw meat, poultry, or seafood.

FIGURE 20-4 Meat and Poultry Safety

Inspection is mandatory; grading is voluntary. Neither guarantees that the product will not cause foodborne illnesses, but consumers can help to prevent foodborne illnesses by following the safe handling instructions. The CFIA recommends that safe handling instructions appear on all packages of raw/ground meat and poultry.

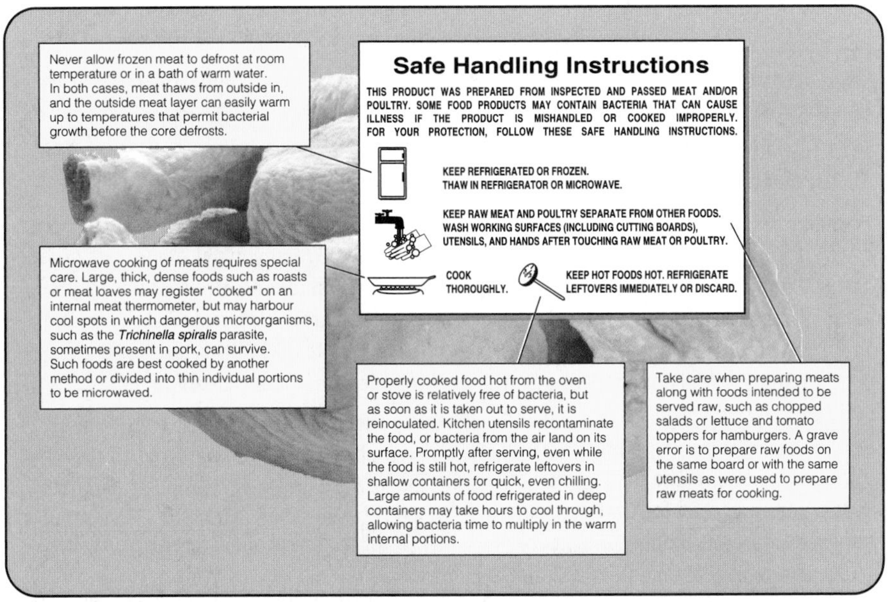
Never allow frozen meat to defrost at room temperature or in a bath of warm water. In both cases, meat thaws from outside in, and the outside meat layer can easily warm up to temperatures that permit bacterial growth before the core defrosts.
Safe Handling Instructions
THIS PRODUCT WAS PREPARED FROM INSPECTED AND PASSED MEAT AND/OR POULTRY. SOME FOOD PRODUCTS MAY CONTAIN BACTERIA THAT CAN CAUSE ILLNESS IF THE PRODUCT IS MISHANDLED OR COOKED IMPROPERLY. FOR YOUR PROTECTION, FOLLOW THESE SAFE HANDLING INSTRUCTIONS.
KEEP REFRIGERATED OR FROZEN. THAW IN REFRIGERATOR OR MICROWAVE.
KEEP RAW MEAT AND POULTRY SEPARATE FROM OTHER FOODS. WASH WORKING SURFACES (INCLUDING CUTTING BOARDS), UTENSILS, AND HANDS AFTER TOUCHING RAW MEAT OR POULTRY.
COOK THOROUGHLY.
KEEP HOT FOODS HOT. REFRIGERATE LEFTOVERS IMMEDIATELY OR DISCARD.
Microwave cooking of meats requires special care. Large, thick, dense foods such as roasts or meat loaves may register "cooked" on an internal meat thermometer, but may harbour cool spots in which dangerous microorganisms, such as the *Trichinella spiralis* parasite, sometimes present in pork, can survive. Such foods are best cooked by another method or divided into thin individual portions to be microwaved.
Properly cooked food hot from the oven or stove is relatively free of bacteria, but as soon as it is taken out to serve, it is reinoculated. Kitchen utensils recontaminate the food, or bacteria from the air land on its surface. Promptly after serving, even while the food is still hot, refrigerate leftovers in shallow containers for quick, even chilling. Large amounts of food refrigerated in deep containers may take hours to cool through, allowing bacteria time to multiply in the warm internal portions.
Take care when preparing meats along with foods intended to be served raw, such as chopped salads or lettuce and tomato toppers for hamburgers. A grave error is to prepare raw foods on the same board or with the same utensils as were used to prepare raw meats for cooking.

SOURCE: Safe Handling Instructions: From SIZER/WHITNEY/PICHE. Nutrition, 2E. © 2012 Nelson Education Ltd. Reproduced by permission. www.cengage.com/permissions

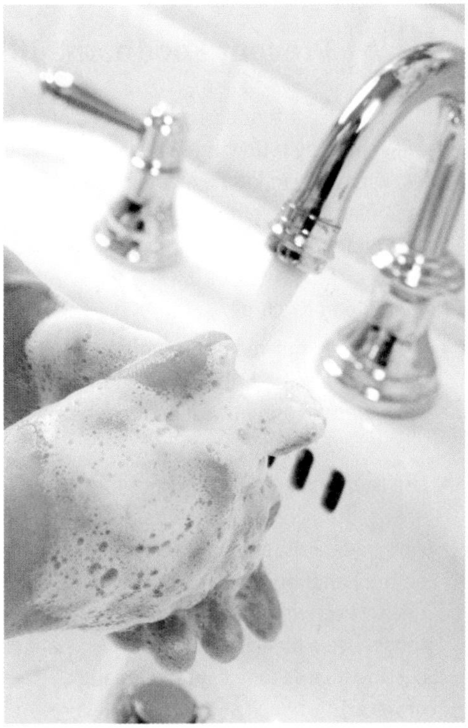

© Michael Krinke/iStockphoto

Wash your hands with warm water and soap for at least 20 seconds before preparing or eating food to reduce the chance of microbial contamination.

FIGURE 20-5 Food Safety Temperatures and Household Thermometers

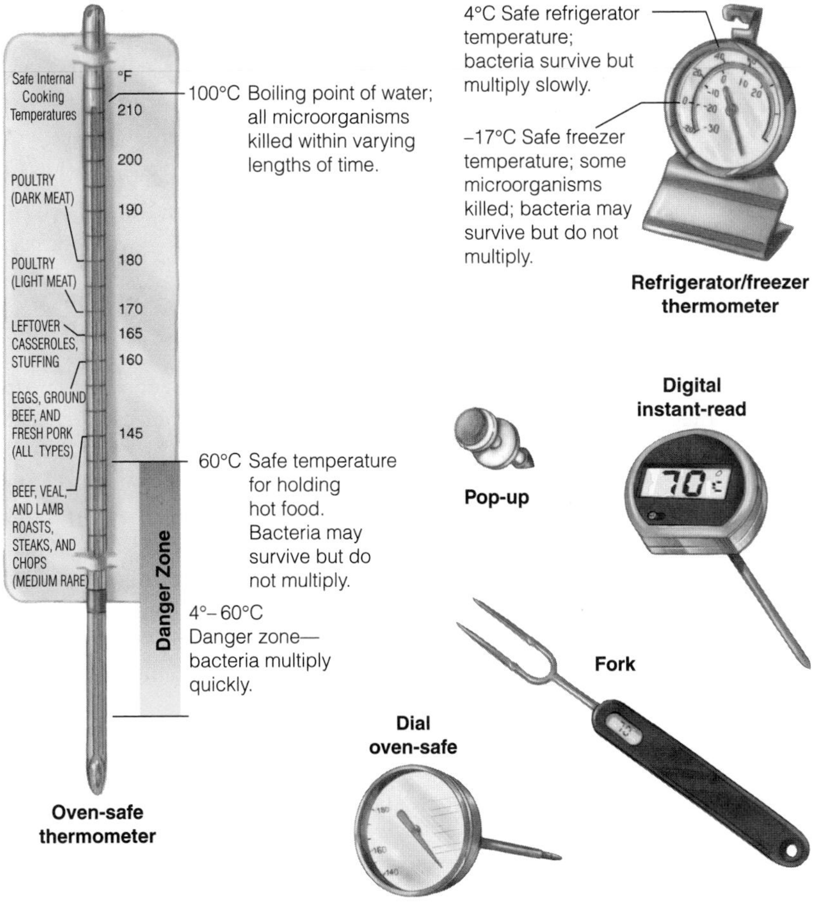
Safe Internal Cooking Temperatures
°F
210
200
190
180
170
165
160
145
POULTRY (DARK MEAT)
POULTRY (LIGHT MEAT)
LEFTOVER CASSEROLES, STUFFING
EGGS, GROUND BEEF, AND FRESH PORK (ALL TYPES)
BEEF, VEAL, AND LAMB ROASTS, STEAKS, AND CHOPS (MEDIUM RARE)
Danger Zone
100°C Boiling point of water; all microorganisms killed within varying lengths of time.
60°C Safe temperature for holding hot food. Bacteria may survive but do not multiply.
4°–60°C Danger zone—bacteria multiply quickly.
Oven-safe thermometer
4°C Safe refrigerator temperature; bacteria survive but multiply slowly.
−17°C Safe freezer temperature; some microorganisms killed; bacteria may survive but do not multiply.
Refrigerator/freezer thermometer
Digital instant-read
70°C
Pop-up
Fork
Dial oven-safe

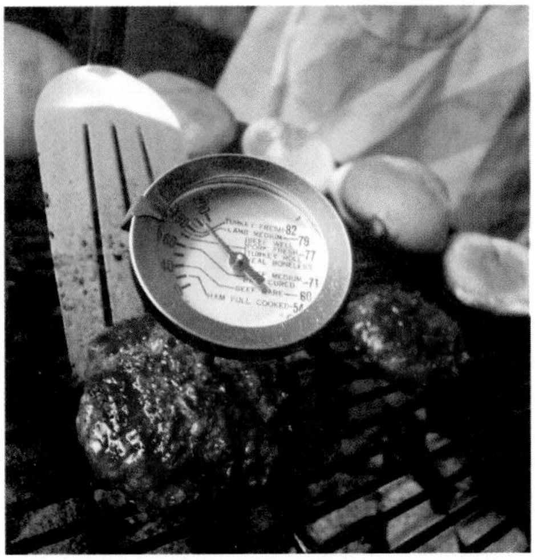

Eric O'Connell/Getty Images

Cook hamburgers to 70°C; colour alone cannot determine doneness. Some burgers will turn brown before reaching 70°C, whereas others may retain some pink colour, even when cooked to 80°C.

HOW TO Prevent Foodborne Illnesses

Most foodborne illnesses can be prevented by following four simple rules: keep a clean kitchen, avoid cross-contamination, keep hot foods hot, and keep cold foods cold.

Keep a Clean Kitchen

- Wash fruits and vegetables in a clean sink with a scrub brush and warm water; store washed and unwashed produce separately.
- Use hot, soapy water to wash hands, utensils, dishes, nonporous cutting boards, and countertops before handling food and between tasks when working with different foods. Use a bleach solution on cutting boards (one capful per gallon of water).
- Cover cuts with clean bandages before food preparation; dirty bandages carry harmful microorganisms.
- Mix foods with utensils, not hands; keep hands and utensils away from mouth, nose, and hair.
- Anyone may be a carrier of bacteria and should avoid coughing or sneezing over food. A person with a skin infection or infectious disease should not prepare food.
- Wash or replace sponges and towels regularly.
- Clean up food spills and crumb-filled crevices.

Avoid Cross-Contamination

- Wash all surfaces that have been in contact with raw meats, poultry, eggs, fish, and shellfish before reusing.
- Serve cooked foods on a clean plate with a clean utensil. Separate raw foods from those that have been cooked.
- Don't use marinade that was in contact with raw meat for basting or sauces.

Keep Hot Foods Hot

- When cooking meats or poultry, use a thermometer to test the internal temperature. Insert the thermometer between the thigh and the body of a turkey or into the thickest part of other meats, making sure the tip of the thermometer is not in contact with bone or the pan. Cook to the temperature indicated for that particular meat (see Figure 20-5 on p. 665); cook hamburgers to at least medium well done. If you have food safety questions, call CFIA: 1-800-442-2342 between 8:00 am and 4:00 pm (EST) Monday to Friday.
- Cook stuffing separately, or stuff poultry just prior to cooking.
- Do not cook large cuts of meat or turkey in a microwave oven; it leaves some parts undercooked while overcooking others.
- Cook eggs before eating them (soft-boiled for at least 3½ minutes; scrambled until set, not runny; fried for at least 3 minutes on one side and 1 minute on the other).
- Cook seafood thoroughly. If you have safety questions about seafood, call CFIA: 1-800-442-2342.
- When serving foods, maintain temperatures at 60°C (140°F) or higher.
- Heat leftovers thoroughly to at least 75°C (165°F).

Keep Cold Foods Cold

- When running errands, stop at the grocery store last. When you get home, refrigerate the perishable groceries (such as meats and dairy products) immediately. Do not leave perishables in the car any longer than it takes for ice cream to melt.
- Put packages of raw meat, fish, or poultry on a plate before refrigerating to prevent juices from dripping on food stored below.
- Buy only foods that are solidly frozen in store freezers.
- Keep cold foods at 5°C (40°F) or less; keep frozen foods at –18°C (0°F) or less (keep a thermometer in the refrigerator).
- Marinate meats in the refrigerator, not on the counter.
- Look for "Keep Refrigerated" or "Refrigerate After Opening" on food labels.
- Refrigerate leftovers promptly; use shallow containers to cool foods faster; use leftovers within three to four days.
- Thaw meats or poultry in the refrigerator, not at room temperature. If you must

(continued)

Mad Cow Disease Reports on mad cow disease from dozens of countries, including Canada and the United States, have sparked consumer concerns.[9] Mad cow disease is a slowly progressive, fatal condition that affects the central nervous system of cattle.* A similar disease develops in people who have eaten contaminated beef from infected cows (milk products appear to be safe).** Approximately 150 cases have been reported worldwide, primarily in the United Kingdom. The CFIA has taken numerous steps to prevent the transmission of mad cow disease in cattle, and if these measures are followed, then risks from Canadian cattle are low. Because the infectious agents occur in the intestines, central nervous system, and other organs, but not in muscle meat, concerned consumers may want to select whole cuts of meat instead of ground beef or sausage. A few reports of hunters developing fatal neurological disorders have raised concerns about a similar disease in wild game. Hunters and consumers who regularly eat elk, deer, or antelope should check the advisories of their state department of agriculture.

*Mad cow disease is technically known as bovine spongiform encephalopathy (BSE).
**The human form of BSE is called variant Creutzfeldt–Jakob Disease (vCJD).

HOW TO Prevent Foodborne Illnesses *(continued)*

hasten thawing, use cool water (changed every 30 minutes) or a microwave oven.
- Freeze meat, fish, or poultry immediately if not planning to use within a few days.

In General

- Do not reuse disposable containers; use nondisposable containers or recycle instead.
- Do not taste food that is suspect. "If in doubt, throw it out."
- Throw out foods with danger-signalling odours. Be aware, though, that most food-poisoning bacteria are odourless, colourless, and tasteless.
- Do not buy or use items that have broken seals or mangled packaging; such containers cannot protect against microbes, insects, spoilage, or even vandalism. Check safety seals, buttons, and expiration dates.
- Follow label instructions for storing and preparing packaged and frozen foods; throw out foods that have been thawed or refrozen.
- Discard foods that are discoloured, mouldy, or decayed or that have been contaminated by insects or rodents.

For Specific Food Items

- *Canned goods.* Carefully discard food from cans that leak or bulge so that other people and animals will not accidentally ingest it; before canning, seek professional advice from the CFIA by calling toll-free 1-800-442-2342.
- *Milk and cheeses.* Use only pasteurized milk and milk products. Aged cheeses, such as cheddar and Swiss, do well for an hour or two without refrigeration, but they should be refrigerated or stored in an ice chest for longer periods.
- *Eggs.* Use clean eggs with intact shells. Do not eat eggs, even pasteurized eggs, raw; raw eggs are commonly found in Caesar salad dressing, eggnog, cookie dough, hollandaise sauce, and key lime pie. Cook eggs until whites are firmly set and yolks begin to thicken.
- *Honey.* Honey may contain dormant bacterial spores, which can awaken in the human body to produce botulism. In adults, this poses little hazard, but infants younger than 1 year of age should never be fed honey. Honey can accumulate enough toxin to kill an infant; it has been implicated in several cases of sudden infant death. (Honey can also be contaminated with environmental pollutants picked up by the bees.)
- *Mayonnaise.* Commercial mayonnaise may actually help a food to resist spoilage because of the acid content. Still, keep it refrigerated after opening.
- *Mixed salads.* Mixed salads of chopped ingredients spoil easily because they have extensive surface area for bacteria to invade, and they have been in contact with cutting boards, hands, and kitchen utensils that easily transmit bacteria to food (regardless of their mayonnaise content). Chill them well before, during, and after serving.
- *Picnic foods.* Choose foods that last without refrigeration, such as fresh fruits and vegetables, breads and crackers, and canned spreads and cheeses that can be opened and used immediately. Pack foods cold, layer ice between foods, and keep foods out of water.
- *Seafood.* Buy only fresh seafood that has been properly refrigerated or iced. Cooked seafood should be stored separately from raw seafood to avoid cross-contamination.

TRY IT After cutting the fat from a pork loin, you rinse the wooden cutting board under warm water before using it to chop vegetables. Discuss whether this precaution is adequate to protect against cross-contamination.

H1N1 Virus Originally called "swine flu," H1N1 is a very contagious and life-threatening viral infection. Because the virus is contagious, scientists are concerned that it could spread rapidly from person to person, creating a pandemic. Like other flu viruses, H1N1 is spread mainly through the coughs and sneezes of people who are sick with the virus. Table 20-2 lists ways to protect against H1N1 infection. Importantly, H1N1 virus is *not* transmitted by eating pork.

Safe Handling of Seafood Most seafood available in Canada is safe, but eating it undercooked or raw can cause severe illnesses—hepatitis, worms, parasites, viral intestinal disorders, and other diseases.* Rumour has it that freezing fish will make it safe to eat raw, but this is only partly true. Commercial freezing kills mature parasitic worms, but only cooking can kill all worm eggs and other microorganisms that can cause illness. For safety's sake, all seafood should be

TABLE 20-2 Prevention of H1N1 Infection

- Cover your nose and mouth with a tissue when you cough or sneeze. Throw the tissue in the trash after you use it.
- Wash your hands often with soap and warm water for 20 seconds, especially after you cough or sneeze. Alternatively, clean hands with alcohol-based wipes or gel sanitizers.
- Minimize spreading germs by not touching your eyes, nose, or mouth.
- Avoid close contact with sick people.
- If you are sick, limit contact with other people as much as possible.
- If you are sick, seek medical care.

*Diseases caused by toxins from the sea include ciguatera poisoning, scombroid poisoning, and paralytic and neurotoxic shellfish poisoning.

TABLE 20-3 Safe Refrigerator Storage Times (≤5°C)

One to Two Days
Raw ground meats, breakfast or other raw sausages, raw fish or poultry; gravies
Three to Five Days
Raw steaks, roasts, or chops; cooked meats, poultry, vegetables, and mixed dishes; lunchmeats (packages opened); mayonnaise salads (chicken, egg, pasta, tuna)
One Week
Hard-cooked eggs, bacon or hot dogs (opened packages); smoked sausages or seafood
Two to Four Weeks
Raw eggs (in shells); lunchmeats, bacon, or hot dogs (packages unopened); dry sausages (pepperoni, hard salami); most aged and processed cheeses (Swiss, brick)
Two Months
Mayonnaise (opened jar); most dry cheeses (Parmesan, Romano)

cooked until it is opaque. Even **sushi** can be safe to eat when chefs combine cooked seafood and other ingredients into these delicacies.

Eating raw oysters can be dangerous for anyone, but people with liver disease and weakened immune systems are most vulnerable.[10] At least 10 species of bacteria found in raw oysters can cause serious illness and even death.* Raw oysters may also carry the hepatitis A virus, which can cause liver disease. Some hot sauces can kill many of these bacteria, but not the virus; alcohol inactivates some bacteria, but not enough to guarantee protection (or to recommend drinking alcohol).[11] Pasteurization of raw oysters—holding them at a specified temperature for a specified time—holds promise for killing bacteria without cooking the oyster or altering its texture or flavour.

As population density increases along the shores of seafood-harvesting waters, pollution inevitably invades the sea life there. Preventing seafood-borne illness is in large part a task of controlling water pollution. To help ensure a safe seafood market, the CFIA requires processors to adopt food-safety practices based on the HACCP system mentioned earlier.

Chemical pollution and microbial contamination lurk not only in the water, but also in the boats and warehouses where seafood is cleaned, prepared, and refrigerated. Because seafood is one of the most perishable foods, time and temperature are critical to its freshness, flavour, and safety. To keep seafood as fresh as possible, people in the industry must "keep it cold, keep it clean, and keep it moving." Wise consumers eat it cooked.

Other Precautions and Procedures Fresh food generally smells fresh. Not all types of food poisoning are detectable by odour, but some bacterial wastes produce "off" odours. If an abnormal odour exists, the food is spoiled. Throw it out or, if it was recently purchased, return it to the grocery store. Do not taste it. Table 20-3 lists safe refrigerator storage times for selected foods.

Local health departments, Health Canada, and the CFIA can provide additional information about food safety (e.g., see Health Canada's Safe Food Handing Interactive Guide—see Nutrition on the Net). If precautions fail and a mild foodborne illness develops, drink clear liquids to replace fluids lost through vomiting and diarrhea. If serious foodborne illness is suspected, first call a physician. Then wrap the remainder of the suspected food and label the container so that the food cannot be mistakenly eaten, place it in the refrigerator, and hold it for possible inspection by health authorities.

Dietary Guidance for Canadians

To avoid microbial foodborne illness:

- Clean hands, food contact surfaces, and fruits and vegetables.
- Separate raw, cooked, and ready-to-eat foods while shopping, preparing, or storing foods.
- Cook foods to a safe temperature to kill microorganisms.
- Chill (refrigerate) perishable foods promptly and defrost foods properly.
- Meat and poultry should *not* be washed or rinsed.
- Avoid raw (unpasteurized) milk or any products made from unpasteurized milk, raw or partially cooked eggs or foods containing raw eggs, raw or undercooked meat and poultry, unpasteurized juices, and raw sprouts.

Consumers can find out about food recalls and allergy alerts by visiting Canadian Food Inspection Agency's website (see Nutrition on the Net).

Food Safety While Travelling

People who travel to other countries have a 50–50 chance of contracting a foodborne illness, commonly described as **travellers' diarrhea**. Like many other foodborne illnesses, travellers' diarrhea is a

sushi: vinegar-flavoured rice and seafood, typically wrapped in seaweed and stuffed with colourful vegetables. Some sushi is stuffed with raw fish; other varieties contain cooked seafood.

travellers' diarrhea: nausea, vomiting, and diarrhea caused by consuming food or water contaminated by any of several organisms, most commonly, *E. coli*, *Shigella*, *Campylobacter jejuni*, and *Salmonella*.

*Raw oysters can carry the bacterium *Vibrio vulnificus*; see Table 20-1 (pp. 662–663) for details.

sometimes serious, always annoying bacterial infection of the digestive tract. The risk is high because, for one thing, some countries' cleanliness standards for food and water are lower than those in Canada and the United States. For another, every region's microbes are different, and although people are immune to the microbes in their own neighbourhoods, they have had no chance to develop immunity to the pathogens in places they are visiting for the first time. In addition to the food-safety tips outlined in the "How To" on pp. 666–667, precautions while travelling include:

- Wash hands frequently with soap and hot water, especially before handling food or eating. Use antiseptic gel or hand wipes regularly.
- Eat only well-cooked and hot or canned foods. Eat raw fruits or vegetables only if washed in purified water and peeled with clean hands.
- Use purified, bottled water for drinking, making ice cubes, and brushing teeth. Alternatively, use disinfecting tablets or boil water.
- Refuse dairy products that have not been pasteurized and refrigerated properly.
- Travel with antidiarrheal medication in case efforts to avoid illness fail.

To sum up these recommendations, "Boil it, cook it, peel it, or forget it."

Advances in Food Safety

Advances in technology have dramatically improved the quality and safety of foods available on the market. From pasteurization in the early 1900s ♦ to irradiation in the early 2000s, these advances offer numerous benefits, but they also raise consumer concerns.

♦ During the last century, pasteurization of milk helped to control typhoid fever, tuberculosis, scarlet fever, diphtheria, and other infectious diseases.

Irradiation

The use of low-dose **irradiation** protects consumers from foodborne illnesses by[12]:

- Controlling mould in grains
- Sterilizing spices and teas for storage at room temperature
- Controlling insects and extending shelf life in fresh fruits and vegetables (inhibits the growth of sprouts on potatoes and onions and delays ripening in some fruits such as strawberries and mangoes)
- Destroying harmful bacteria in fresh and frozen beef, poultry, lamb, and pork

Some foods, however, are not candidates for irradiation. For example, when irradiated, high-fat meats develop off-odours, egg whites turn milky, grapefruits become mushy, and milk products change flavour. (Incidentally, the milk in those boxes kept at room temperature on grocery-store shelves is not irradiated; it is sterilized with an **ultrahigh temperature treatment.**)

The use of food irradiation has been extensively evaluated over the past 50 years; approved for use in more than 40 countries; and supported by numerous health agencies, including the **FAO, WHO**, and the Canadian Medical Association. Irradiation does not make foods radioactive, nor does it noticeably change the taste, texture, or appearance of approved foods. ♦ Vitamin loss is minimal and comparable to amounts lost in other food-processing methods such as canning. Because irradiation kills bacteria without the use of heat, it is sometimes called "cold pasteurization."

♦ Foods approved for irradiation[13]:
- Whole and ground spices, dehydrated seasonings
- Vegetables (potatoes, onions)
- Wheat, flour, whole-wheat flour

Note: It was recently proposed that ground beef, poultry, and mangoes also be irradiated.

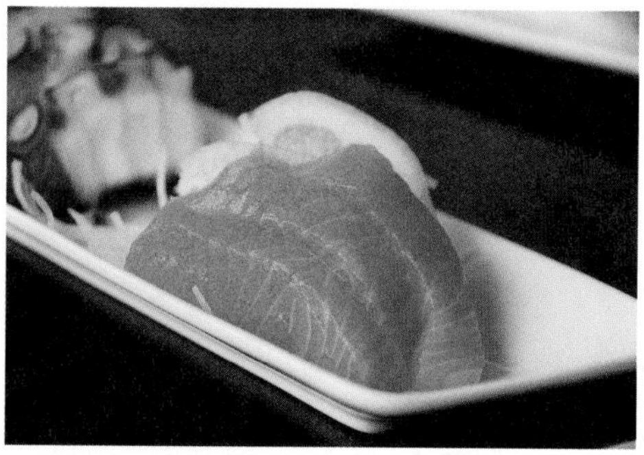
sbarabu/shutterstock

Eating raw seafood is a risky proposition.

Consumer Concerns about Irradiation

Many consumers associate the term *radiation* with cancer, birth defects, and mutations, and consequently have strong negative emotions about using irradiation on foods. Some may mistakenly fear that irradiated food has been contaminated by radioactive particles, such as occurs in the aftermath of a nuclear accident. Some balk at the idea of irradiating, and thus sterilizing, contaminated foods and prefer instead the elimination of unsanitary slaughtering and food preparation conditions. Food producers, on the other hand, are eager to use irradiation, but they hesitate to do so until consumers are ready to accept it and willing to pay for it. Once consumers understand the benefits of irradiation, about half are willing to use irradiated foods, but only one-quarter are willing to pay more.[14]

Regulation of Irradiation

Health Canada establishes regulations governing the specific uses of irradiation and allowed doses. Each prepackaged food that

irradiation: sterilizing a food by exposure to energy waves, similar to ultraviolet light and microwaves; sometimes called *ionizing radiation.*

ultrahigh temperature (UHT) treatment: sterilizing a food by brief exposure to temperatures above those normally used.

♦ This international symbol, called the **radura,** identifies retail foods that have been irradiated. The phrases "Treated by irradiation" or "Treated with radiation" must accompany the symbol. The irradiation label is not required on commercially prepared foods that contain irradiated ingredients, such as spices.

has been wholly treated with irradiation must display the international radiation symbol. ♦ Labels of food that contain irradiated foods that make up more than 10 percent of the product must indicate in the Ingredients List that the particular component has been irradiated.

IN SUMMARY **Millions of people suffer mild to life-threatening symptoms caused by foodborne illnesses (review Table 20-1). As the "How To" on pp. 666–667 describes, most of these illnesses can be prevented by storing and cooking foods at their proper temperatures and by preparing them in sanitary conditions. Irradiation of certain foods protects consumers from foodborne illnesses, but it also raises some concerns.**

Nutritional Adequacy of Foods and Diets

In years past, when most foods were whole and farm fresh, the task of meeting nutrient needs primarily involved balancing servings from the various food groups. Today, however, foods have changed. Many "new" foods are available to appeal to consumers' demands for convenience and flavour, but not necessarily to deliver a balanced assortment of needed nutrients.

Obtaining Nutrient Information To help consumers find their way among these foods and combine them into healthful diets, Health Canada has developed extensive nutrition labelling regulations, as Chapter 2 describes. In addition, Health Canada's nutrition recommendations help consumers "eat to stay healthy," and the *Food Guide* helps them to put those recommendations into practice (see Chapter 2).

Minimizing Nutrient Losses In addition to selecting nutritious foods and preparing them safely, consumers can improve their nutritional health by learning to store and cook foods in ways that minimize nutrient losses. Water-soluble vitamins are the most vulnerable of the nutrients, but both vitamins and minerals can be lost when they dissolve in water that is then discarded.

Fruits and vegetables contain enzymes that both synthesize and degrade vitamins. After a fruit or vegetable has been picked, vitamin synthesis stops, but degradation continues. To slow the degradation of vitamins, most fruits and vegetables should be kept refrigerated until used. (Degradative enzymes are most active at warmer temperatures.)

Some vitamins are easily destroyed by oxygen. To minimize the destruction of vitamins, store fruits and vegetables that have been cut and juice that has been opened in airtight containers and refrigerate them.

Water-soluble vitamins readily dissolve in water. To prevent losses during washing, wash fruits and vegetables before cutting. To minimize losses during cooking, steam or microwave vegetables. Alternatively, use the cooking water when preparing meals such as casseroles and soups.

Finally, keep in mind that most vitamin losses are not catastrophic and that a law of diminishing returns operates. Do not fret over small losses or waste time that may be valuable in improving your health in other ways. Be assured that if you start with plenty of fruits and vegetables and are reasonably careful in their safe storage and preparation, you will receive a sufficient supply of all the nutrients they provide.

IN SUMMARY **In the marketplace, food labels, Health Canada's nutrition recommendations, and the *Food Guide* all help consumers learn about nutrition and how to plan healthy diets. At home, consumers can minimize nutrient losses from fruits and vegetables by safely refrigerating them, washing them before cutting them, storing them in airtight containers, and cooking them for short times in minimal water.**

Environmental Contaminants

Concern about environmental contamination of foods is growing as the world becomes more populated and more industrialized. Industrial processes pollute the air, water, and soil. Plants absorb the **contaminants**, and people consume the plants (grains, vegetables, legumes, and fruits) or the meat and milk products from livestock that have eaten the plants. Similarly, polluted water contaminates the fish and other seafood that people eat. Environmental contaminants present in air, water, and foods find their way into our bodies and have the potential to cause numerous health problems but together Health Canada and Environment Canada set maximum allowable levels in our food and environment.[15]

Harmfulness of Environmental Contaminants

The potential harmfulness of a contaminant depends in part on its **persistence**—the extent to which it lingers in the environment or in the body. Some contaminants in the environment are short-lived because microorganisms or agents such as sunlight or oxygen can break them down. Some contaminants in the body may linger for only a short time because the body rapidly excretes them or metabolizes them to harmless compounds. These contaminants present little cause for concern. Some contaminants, however, resist breakdown and can accumulate. Each level of the **food chain**, then, has a greater concentration than the one below (**bioaccumulation**). Figure 20-6 shows how bioaccumulation leads to high concentrations of toxins in people at the top of the food chain.

contaminants: substances that make a food impure and unsuitable for ingestion.

persistence: stubborn or enduring continuance; with respect to food contaminants, the quality of persisting, rather than breaking down, in the bodies of animals and human beings.

food chain: the sequence in which living things depend on other living things for food.

bioaccumulation: the accumulation of contaminants in the flesh of animals high on the food chain.

FIGURE 20-6 Bioaccumulation of Toxins in the Food Chain

This example features fish as the food for human consumption, but bioaccumulation of toxins occurs on land as well when cows, pigs, and chickens eat or drink contaminated foods or water.

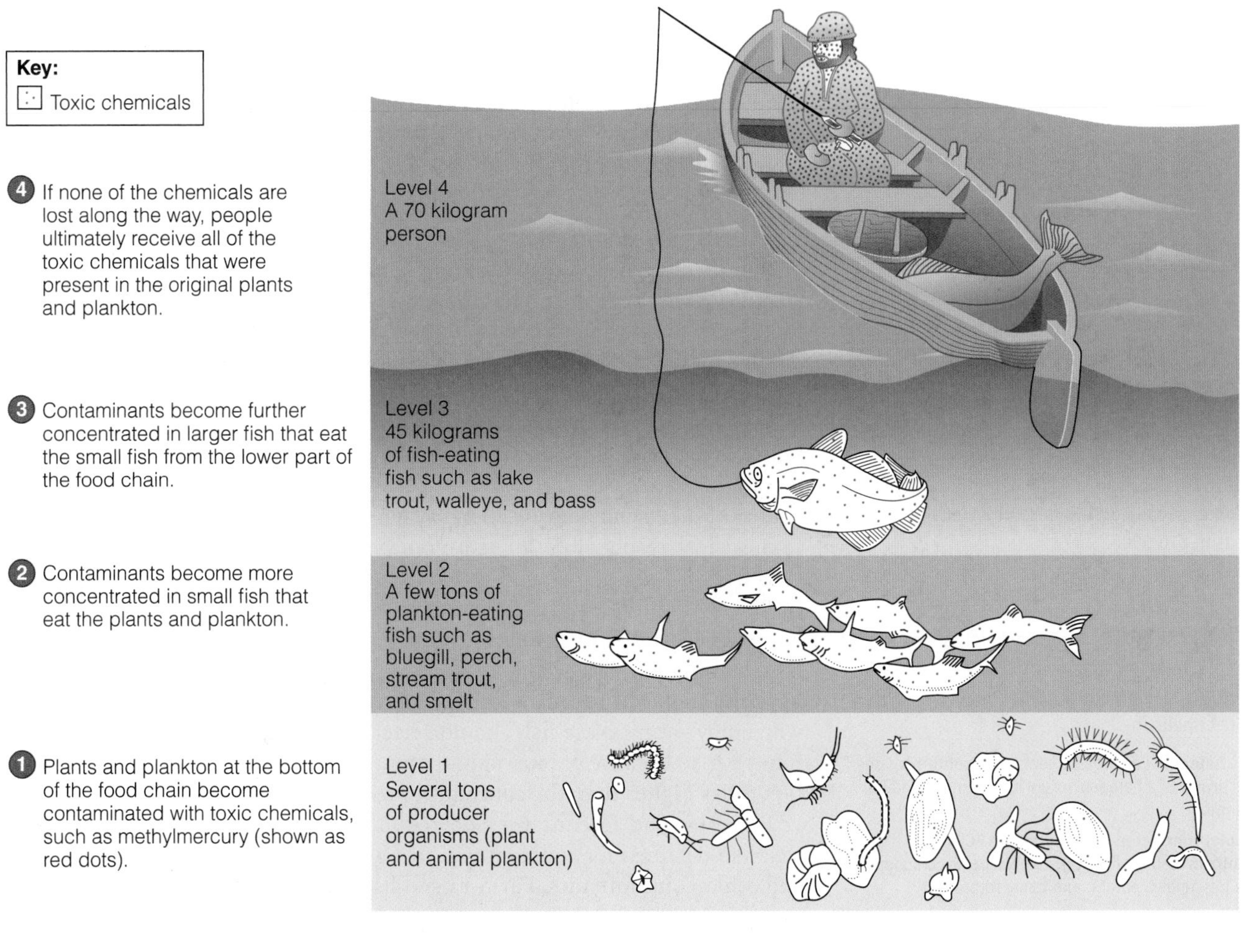
Key:
Toxic chemicals
4 If none of the chemicals are lost along the way, people ultimately receive all of the toxic chemicals that were present in the original plants and plankton.
3 Contaminants become further concentrated in larger fish that eat the small fish from the lower part of the food chain.
2 Contaminants become more concentrated in small fish that eat the plants and plankton.
1 Plants and plankton at the bottom of the food chain become contaminated with toxic chemicals, such as methylmercury (shown as red dots).
Level 4
A 70 kilogram person
Level 3
45 kilograms of fish-eating fish such as lake trout, walleye, and bass
Level 2
A few tons of plankton-eating fish such as bluegill, perch, stream trout, and smelt
Level 1
Several tons of producer organisms (plant and animal plankton)

Contaminants enter the environment in various ways. Accidental spills are rare but can have devastating effects. More commonly, small amounts are released over long periods. The following paragraphs describe how three contaminants found their way into the food supply in the past. The first example involves a heavy metal; ♦ the others involve **organic halogens.**

♦ **A heavy metal** is any of a number of mineral ions such as mercury or lead, so called because they are of relatively high atomic weight. Many heavy metals are poisonous.

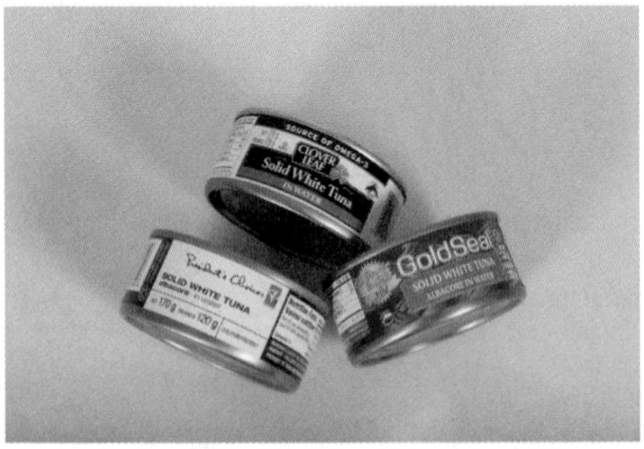
Solid White Tuna
GoldSeal
SOLID WHITE TUNA

Dick Hemingway

Because albacore ("white") tuna has more mercury than canned light tuna, consumers should limit their intake to no more than 150 grams of albacore tuna per week.

Methylmercury A classic example of acute contamination occurred in 1953 when a number of people in Minamata, Japan, became ill with a disease no one had seen before. By 1960, 121 cases had been reported, including 23 in infants. Mortality was high; 46 died, and the survivors suffered blindness, deafness, lack of coordination, and intellectual deterioration. The cause was ultimately revealed to be methylmercury contamination of fish from the bay where these people lived. The infants who contracted the disease had not eaten any fish, but their mothers had, and even though the mothers exhibited no symptoms during their pregnancies, the poison affected their unborn babies. Manufacturing plants in the region were discharging mercury-containing waste into the waters of the bay, the mercury was turning into methylmercury, and the fish in the bay were accumulating this poison in their bodies. Some of the affected families had been eating fish from the bay every day.

PBB and PCB In 1973, half a ton of **PBB (polybrominated biphenyls)**, toxic organic compounds, were accidentally mixed into some livestock feed that was distributed throughout the state of Michigan. The PBB found its way into millions of animals and then into the people who ate the meat. The seriousness of the accident came to light when dairy farmers reported that their cows were going dry, aborting their calves, and developing abnormal growths on their hooves. Although more than 30 000 cattle, sheep, and swine and more than a million chickens were destroyed, an estimated 97 percent of Michigan's residents had been exposed to PBB. Some of the exposed farm residents suffered nervous system aberrations and liver disorders.

A similar accident occurred in 1979 when **PCB (polychlorinated biphenyls)** contaminated rice oil in Taiwan. Women who had eaten the tainted rice oil gave birth to children with developmental problems. Decades later, young men who were exposed to PCB during gestation had reduced fertility. The interactive effects of PCB and mercury—two environmental contaminants found in fish—are especially damaging to brain functions such as balance and coordination.[16]

Guidelines for Consumers

How much of a threat do environmental contaminants pose to the food supply? For the most part, the hazards appear to be small. Health Canada regulates the presence of contaminants in foods and requires foods with unsafe amounts to be removed from the market. Similarly, health agencies may issue advisories informing consumers about the potential dangers of eating contaminated foods.

Most recently, mercury poisoning has aroused concerns—even at levels one-tenth of those in the Minamata catastrophe. Virtually all fish have at least trace amounts of mercury (on average, 0.12 parts per million). ♦ Fish is the main source of dietary mercury.[17] Mercury, PCB, chlordane, dioxins, and DDT are the toxins most responsible for fish contamination, but mercury leads the list by threefold.

♦ For perspective, 1 ppm (part per million) is equivalent to about 1 minute in 2 years or 1 cent in $10 000.

Review Figure 20-6 (p. 671) and notice how toxins such as mercury become more concentrated in animals and in people high in the food chain. Because of bioaccumulation, large game fish at the top of the aquatic food chain ♦ generally have the highest concentrations of mercury (10 times the average). Consumers who enjoy eating these fish should select the smaller, younger ones (within legal limits). Also because of bioaccumulation, the concentrations in fish may be a million times higher than the concentrations in the water itself.

♦ Fish relatively high in mercury:
- Tilefish, swordfish, king mackerel, shark

Fish relatively low in mercury:
- Cod, haddock, pollock, salmon, sole, tilapia
- Most shellfish

organic halogens: an organic compound containing one or more atoms of a halogen—fluorine, chlorine, iodine, or bromine.

PBB (polybrominated biphenyls) and **PCB (polychlorinated biphenyls):** toxic organic compounds used in pesticides, paints, and flame retardants.

Fisheries and Oceans Canada regulates commercial fishing to help ensure that fish destined for consumption in Canada meet safety standards for mercury and other contaminants. Farm-raised fish usually have lower concentrations of mercury than fish caught in the wild. Consequently, most consumers in Canada are not in danger of receiving harmful levels of mercury from fish.

The potential harm from contaminants must be balanced against the potential benefits from nutrients.[18] Pregnant and lactating women and young children are most vulnerable because mercury toxicity damages the developing brain. Yet they are also likely to benefit from consuming seafood rich in omega-3 fatty acids. To receive the benefits and minimize the risks, pregnant and lactating women and young children can safely consume up to 150 grams of seafood per month.[19] In addition, they should limit their intake of albacore tuna and avoid eating large predatory fish altogether. ♦ Average blood levels of mercury in young children and women of child-bearing age are currently below levels of concern.

♦ Pregnant and lactating women and young children should limit their intake of the following:
- Tilefish (also called golden snapper or golden bass), swordfish, king mackerel, shark to 150 g monthly

And limit weekly consumption of the following:
- 300 g (4 *Food Guide* Servings) (cooked or canned) commercial fish and shellfish (such as shrimp, salmon, pollock, and catfish), canned albacore "white" tuna

What about the noncommercial fish a person catches from a local lake, river, or ocean? After all, it's almost impossible to tell whether water is contaminated without sophisticated equipment. Together the federal and provincial/territorial governments monitor the waters and issue advisories to inform the public if chemical contaminants have been found in the local fish. To find out whether a fish advisory has been posted in your region, call the provincial/territorial environmental health department.

All things considered, fish continue to support a healthy diet, providing valuable protein, omega-3 fatty acids, and minerals. For most adults, the benefits of protecting against heart disease outweigh the risks of consuming seafood regularly. Ideally, consumers would select fish ♦ with high levels of omega-3 fatty acids and low levels of mercury.[20] In addition, they should select a variety of seafood to reduce the risk of exposure to contaminants from a single source.

♦ Fish relatively high in omega-3 fatty acids and low in mercury:
- Salmon, herring, sardines, shad, lake trout, mackerel, whitefish, flounder/sole, pollock

IN SUMMARY **Environmental contamination of foods is a concern, but so far, the hazards appear relatively small. In all cases, two principles apply. First, remain alert to the possibility of contamination of foods, and keep an ear open for public health announcements and advice. Second, eat a variety of foods. Varying food choices is an effective defensive strategy against the accumulation of toxins in the body. Each food eaten dilutes contaminants that may be present in other components of the diet.**

Natural Toxicants in Foods

Consumers concerned about food contamination may think that they can eliminate all poisons from their diets by eating only "natural" foods. On the contrary, nature has provided plants with an abundant array of toxicants. A few examples will show how even "natural" foods may contain potentially harmful substances. They also show that although the *potential* for harm exists, *actual* harm rarely occurs.

Poisonous mushrooms are a familiar example of plants that can be harmful when eaten. Few people know, though, that other commonly eaten foods contain substances that can cause illnesses. Cabbage, turnips, mustard greens, kale, Brussels sprouts, cauliflower, broccoli, kohlrabi, and radishes contain small quantities of goitrogens—compounds that can enlarge the thyroid gland. Eating exceptionally large amounts of goitrogen-containing vegetables can aggravate a preexisting thyroid problem, but it usually does not initiate one.

Lima beans and fruit seeds such as apricot pits contain cyanogens—inactive compounds that produce the deadly poison cyanide upon activation by a specific plant enzyme. For this reason, many countries restrict commercially grown lima beans to those varieties with the lowest cyanogen contents. As for fruit seeds, they are seldom deliberately eaten. An occasional swallowed seed or two presents no danger, but a couple of dozen seeds can be fatal to a small child. Perhaps the most infamous cyanogen in seeds is laetrile—a compound erroneously represented as a cancer cure. True, laetrile kills cancer, but only at doses that kill the person, too. The combination of cyanide poisoning and lack of medical attention is life-threatening.

♦ Average solanine content: 8 mg/100 g potato
Toxic solanine dose: 20 to 25 mg/100 g potato

The humble potato contains many natural poisons including **solanine**, a powerful narcotic-like substance. ♦ Most of a potato's solanine is found in the sprouts and in the green layer that develops just beneath the skin. Solanine poisoning is extremely rare, however, because the small amounts of solanine normally found in potatoes are harmless—even when the potato skin is eaten. Solanine can be toxic, however, and presents a hazard when consumed in large quantities. Cooking does not destroy solanine, but it can be removed by peeling the potato. Symptoms of solanine poisoning include gastrointestinal disturbances and neurological disorders.

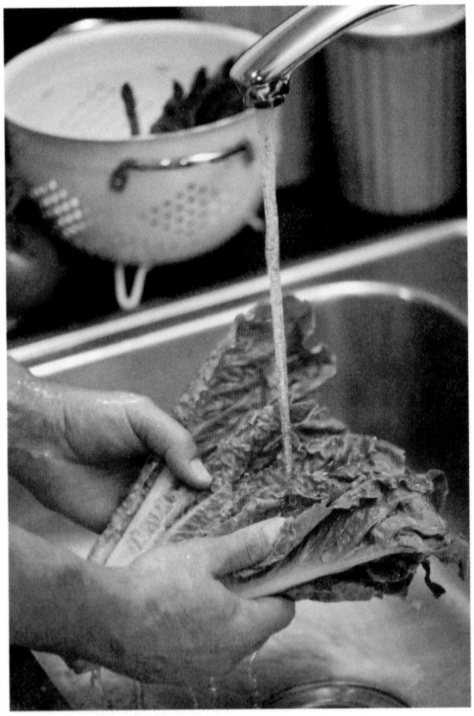
Tom Grill/Getty Images

Washing fresh fruits and vegetables removes most, if not all, of the pesticide residues that might have been present.

IN SUMMARY **Natural toxicants include the goitrogens in cabbage, cyanogens in lima beans, and solanine in potatoes. These examples of naturally occurring toxicants illustrate two familiar principles. First, any substance can be toxic when consumed in excess. Second, poisons are poisons, whether made by people or by nature. Remember: it is not the source of a chemical that makes it hazardous, but its chemical structure and the quantity consumed.**

Pesticides

The use of **pesticides** in agriculture is controversial. They help to ensure the survival of crops, but they leave **residues** in the environment and on some of the foods we eat.

Hazards and Regulation of Pesticides

Ideally, a pesticide destroys the pest and quickly degenerates to nontoxic products without accumulating in the food chain. Then, by the time consumers eat the food, no harmful residues remain. Unfortunately, no such perfect pesticide exists. As new pesticides are developed, government agencies assess their risks and benefits and vigilantly monitor their use.

Hazards of Pesticides Pesticides applied in the field may linger on the foods. Health risks from pesticide exposure are probably small for healthy adults, but children, the elderly, and people with weakened immune systems may be vulnerable to some types of pesticide poisoning. To protect infants and children, government agencies set a **tolerance level** for each pesticide by first identifying foods that children commonly eat in large amounts and then considering the effects of pesticide exposure during each developmental stage.

Regulation of Pesticides Consumers depend on Health Canada to set regulations for pesticide levels in foods and the CFIA to monitor and enforce these regulations (interested readers can stay up-to-date and even subscribe to Real Simple Syndicated [RSS] feeds regarding pesticide use in Canada through Health Canada's website [see Nutrition on the Net]). These agencies evaluate the risks and benefits of a pesticide's use by asking such questions as: How dangerous is it? How much residue is left on the crop? How much harm does the pesticide do to the environment? How necessary is it? What are the alternatives to its use?

If the pesticide is approved, Health Canada establishes a tolerance level for its presence in foods, well below the level at which it could cause any conceivable harm. Tolerance regulations also state the specific crops to which each pesticide can be applied. If a pesticide is misused, growers risk fines, lawsuits, and destruction of their crops.

Once tolerances are set, the CFIA enforces them by monitoring domestic and imported foods and livestock feeds for the presence of pesticides. Indeed, as part of CFIA's "National Chemical Residue Monitoring Program for Fresh Fruit and Vegetables," approximately 10 000 samples of domestic and imported fruits and vegetables are analyzed each year for over 260 agricultural chemical residues (e.g., pesticides and toxic metals) to verify they are safe to eat (i.e., do not exceed Canadian maximum residue limits, MRL).[21] Over the past several decades of

solanine (SOH-lah-neen): a poisonous narcotic-like substance present in potato peels and sprouts.

pesticides: chemicals used to control insects, weeds, fungi, and other pests on plants, vegetables, fruits, and animals. Used broadly, the term includes herbicides (to kill weeds), insecticides (to kill insects), and fungicides (to kill fungi).

residues: whatever remains. In the case of pesticides, those amounts that remain on or in foods when people buy and use them.

tolerance level: the maximum amount of a residue permitted in a food when a pesticide is used according to label directions.

testing, the CFIA has seldom found residues (less than 1 percent during 2006/2007 testing[22]) above tolerance levels, so it appears that pesticides are generally used according to regulations. Minimal pesticide use means lower costs for growers. In addition to costs, many farmers are also concerned about the environment, the quality of their farmland, and a safe food supply. Where violations are found, they are usually due to unusual weather conditions, use of unapproved pesticides, or misuse—for example, application of a particular pesticide to a crop for which it has not been approved.

Pesticides from Other Countries Federal inspectors sample imported foods and refuse entry if they are found to contain illegal pesticide residues. Canada, the United States, and Mexico work together to establish a pesticide policy for all of North America.

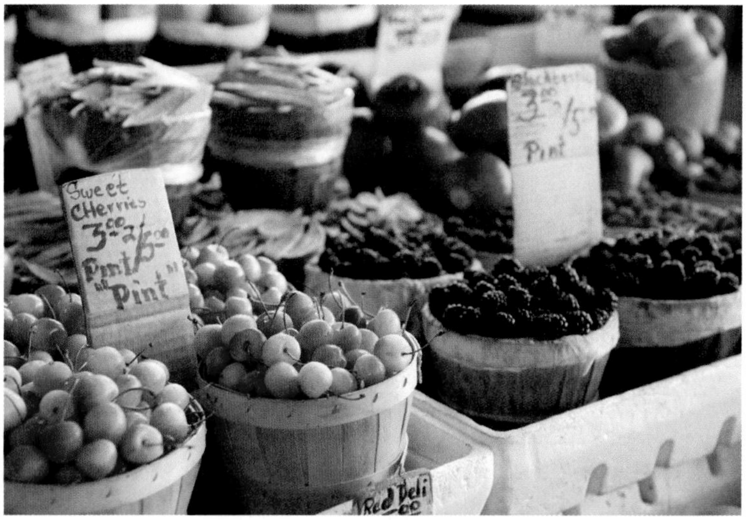
Sweet
Cherries
Pint
Red Deli

Dallas Events Inc/shutterstock

As many as 400 varieties of fruits and vegetables are imported from other countries.

Monitoring Pesticides

The CFIA collects and analyzes samples of both domestic and imported foods. If the agency finds samples in violation of regulations, it can seize the products or order them destroyed.

Food in the Fields In addition to its ongoing surveillance, the CFIA conducts selective surveys to determine the presence of particular pesticides in specific crops.

Food on the Plate Health Canada's Pest Management Regulatory Agency (PMRA) is responsible for regulating the nature and amount of pesticide residues in domestic and imported food. Their scientists conduct *dietary risk assessments* "to quantify the level of food residue exposures to consumers of all ages."[23]

All in all, these findings confirm the safety of Canada's food supply and ensure that the levels of any residues in our food are unlikely to cause health concerns.

Consumer Concerns

Despite these reassuring reports, consumers still worry that food monitoring may not be adequate. For one thing, manufacturers develop new pesticides all the time. For another, other countries use pesticides that are illegal for use here.

The CFIA does not sample *all* food shipments or test for *all* pesticides in each sample. The CFIA is a *monitoring* agency, and as such, it cannot, nor can it be expected to, guarantee 100 percent safety in the food supply. Instead, it checks enough samples to adequately assess average food safety, and acts promptly when problems or suspicions arise.

Minimizing Risks Whether consumers ingest pesticide residues depends on a number of factors. How much of a given food does the consumer eat? What pesticide was used on it? How much was used? How long ago was the food last sprayed? Did environmental conditions promote pest growth or pesticide breakdown? How well was the produce washed? Was it peeled or cooked? With so many factors, consumers cannot know for sure whether pesticide residues remain on foods, but they can minimize their risks by following the guidelines offered in Table 20-4 (p. 676). The food supply is protected well enough that consumers who take these precautions can feel secure that the foods they eat are safe.

Alternatives to Pesticides The use of pesticides has helped to generate higher crop yields that feed the world and protect against diseases transmitted by insects. Still, many consumers are leery. To feed a nation while using fewer pesticides requires creative farming methods. Highlight 20 describes how scientists can genetically alter plants to enhance their production of natural pesticides, and Chapter 21 presents alternative, or sustainable, agriculture methods. These methods include such practices as rotating crops, releasing organisms into fields

TABLE 20-4 Minimize Pest Residues

When Shopping for Foods

- Select fruits and vegetables that do not have holes.
- Select a variety of foods to minimize exposure to any one pesticide.
- Consider buying certified organic foods when shopping for produce most likely to be contaminated (see Table 20-5).

When Preparing Foods

- Trim the fat from meat, and remove the skin from poultry and fish; discard fats and oils in broths and pan drippings (pesticide residues concentrate in the animal's fat).
- Wash fresh produce in warm running water, use a scrub brush, and rinse thoroughly.
- Use a knife to peel an orange and grapefruit; do not bite into the peel.
- Discard the outer leaves of leafy vegetables such as cabbage and lettuce.
- Peel waxed fruits and vegetables; waxes don't wash off and can seal in pesticide residues.
- Peel vegetables such as carrots and fruits such as apples when possible (peeling removes dirt, bacteria, and pesticides that remain in or on the peel, but also removes fibres, vitamins, and minerals).

to destroy pests, and planting nonfood crops nearby to kill pests or attract them away from the food crops. For example, releasing sterile male fruit flies into orchards helps to curb the population growth of these pests; some flowers, such as marigolds, release natural insecticides and are often planted near crops such as tomatoes. Such alternative farming methods are more labour-intensive and may produce smaller yields than conventional methods, at least initially. Over time, though, by eliminating expensive pesticides, fertilizers, and fuels, these alternatives may actually cut costs more than they cut yields.

Organically Grown Crops Scientists and shoppers have strong opinions about groceries these days. Sales of all kinds of certified **organic** foods are skyrocketing, making **organic** foods one of the fastest growing segments of the Canadian food industry.[24] Figure 20-7 shows examples of food labels for products using organic ingredients.

Canadian organic food sales now exceed 1 billion dollars.[25] Consumers purchase organic foods primarily to avoid pesticides. Other reasons for buying organic include benefitting the environment, protecting animals, improving worker safety, and obtaining safer and more nutritious foods.[26] That organic products are safer (e.g., conventionally grown foods have higher pesticide residues than organically grown foods) or healthier for consumers than those grown using other methods, however, may not be the case. Using unprocessed animal manure as an organic fertilizer, for example, may transmit bacteria, such as *E. coli*, to human beings. For this reason, animal manure must be aged or composted before being used as fertilizer. Some research indicates that bacterial contamination from manure more likely reflects the type of crop than the type of farm.[27] Both organic and conventional methods may have advantages and disadvantages, and consumers must remain informed.

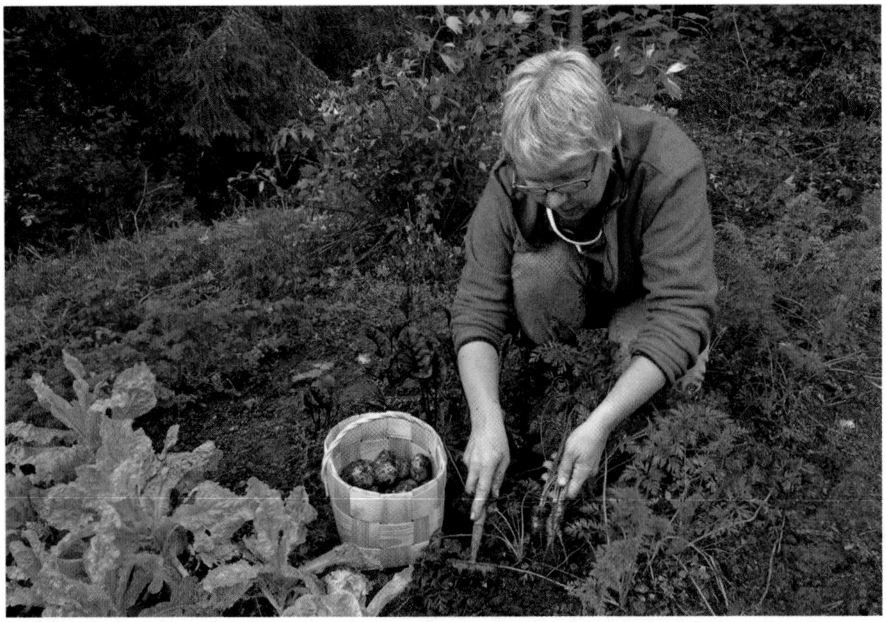

© superclic/Alamy

People can grow organic crops when their gardens or farms are relatively small.

organic: in agriculture, crops grown and processed according to Canada's Organic Product Regulations defining the use of fertilizers, herbicides, insecticides, fungicides, preservatives, and other chemical ingredients.

FIGURE 20-7 Food Labels for Organic Products

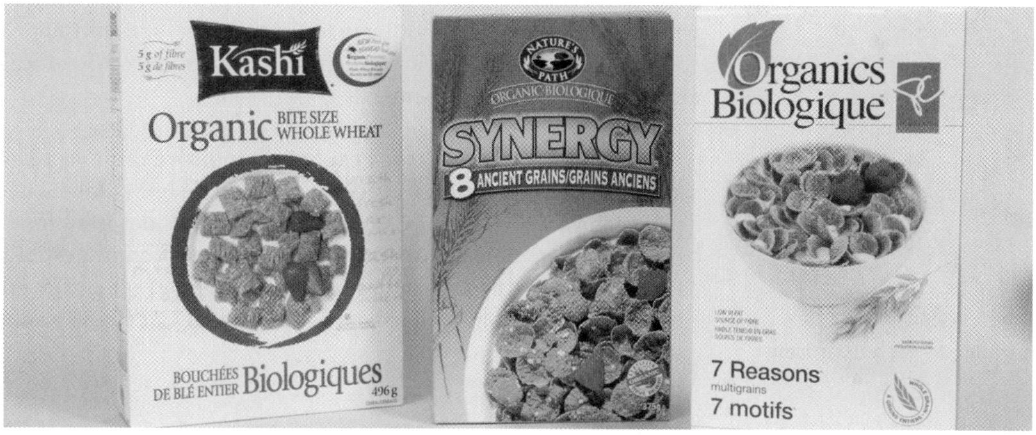
Kashi
Organic BITE SIZE WHOLE WHEAT
BOUCHÉES DE BLÉ ENTIER Biologiques
496 g
NATURE'S PATH
ORGANIC/BIOLOGIQUE
SYNERGY
8 ANCIENT GRAINS/GRAINS ANCIENS
Organics Biologique
7 Reasons
multigrains
7 motifs

Dick Hemingway

Whether buying conventionally grown or organically grown produce, consumers benefit most from eating the recommended number of servings of fruits and vegetables daily.

A shopper picks up two fragrant, orange-yellow mangoes, one from a bin marked "organic" and another from a regular bin; both bear stickers identifying them as the "Hayden" variety. Both may be sweet and succulent. Both may have been kept in storage or shipped from faraway destinations. In fact, both may have been harvested from the same grove, separated by only a thin strip of land. The only obvious differences are the organic label and the cost: the organic mango costs more. The not-so-obvious differences are the methods used to produce them. A farmer wishing to grow and market organic foods must receive certification by the CFIA. To be sold or labelled as organic, or to bear the Canada Organic seal, a food must be produced according to the principles outlined in Table 20-5. Organic foods must be free of ingredients produced by way of specified technologies, such as irradiation and genetic engineering. In contrast, foods bearing "natural" or "free-range" or other wholesome-sounding labels are not required to meet these standards.

Standards for Organic Foods The Canadian General Standards Board worked with the Canadian Organic Advisory Board to develop national standards for organic agriculture, which are included on their website (see Nutrition on the Net). The Organic Agriculture Centre of Canada also provide current information on the latest proposed documents on standards regarding Canadian Organic Production Systems, for example, the Canadian Organic Standards (see Nutrition on the Net). Canada, like the United States and various European countries, has a "Canada organic" seal/symbol ♦. According to information from the Canada Organic Office of the Canadian Food Inspection Agency, there are just under 4000 organic farms in Canada[28] and numerous certified "Canada Organic" products have appeared on store shelves since the Organic Product Regulations were released. These products can only bear the "Canada Organic" logo if they have been approved by a CFIA-accredited certification body.

As mentioned earlier, infants and children may be particularly vulnerable to the effects of pesticides. To determine whether organic foods might reduce their exposure to pesticides, children were given a five-day diet composed entirely of organic foods.[29] Before, during, and after the organic diet period, researchers tested the children's urine for chemicals known to arise from the ingestion of common pesticides. The results were dramatic and immediate: the concentrations of chemicals fell and remained low during the organic diet and increased again when the conventional diet resumed.

♦ Organic foods that have met Canada's Organic Product Regulations may use this logo on their labels.

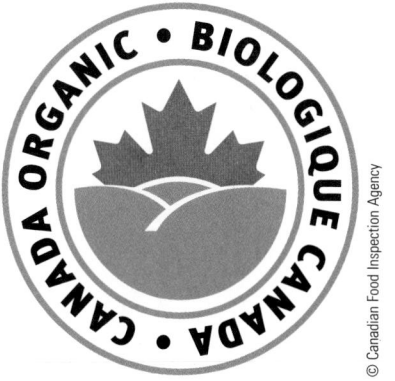

CANADA ORGANIC • BIOLOGIQUE CANADA •

© Canadian Food Inspection Agency

TABLE 20-5 General Principles of Organic Production

1. Protect the environment, minimize soil degradation and erosion, decrease pollution, optimize biological productivity and promote a sound state of health.
2. Maintain long-term soil fertility by optimizing conditions for biological activity within the soil.
3. Maintain biological diversity within the system.
4. Recycle materials and resources to the greatest extent possible within the enterprise.
5. Provide attentive care that promotes the health and meets the behavioural needs of livestock.
6. Prepare organic products, emphasizing careful processing, and handling methods in order to maintain the organic integrity and vital qualities of the products at all stages of production.
7. Rely on renewable resources in locally organized agricultural systems.

SOURCE: Adapted from Organic Production Systems General Principles and Management Standards ICS 67.040, Canadian General Standards Board, CAN/CGSB-32.310-2006, http://www.pwgsc.gc.ca/cgsb/on_the_net/organic/032_0310_2006-e.pdf.

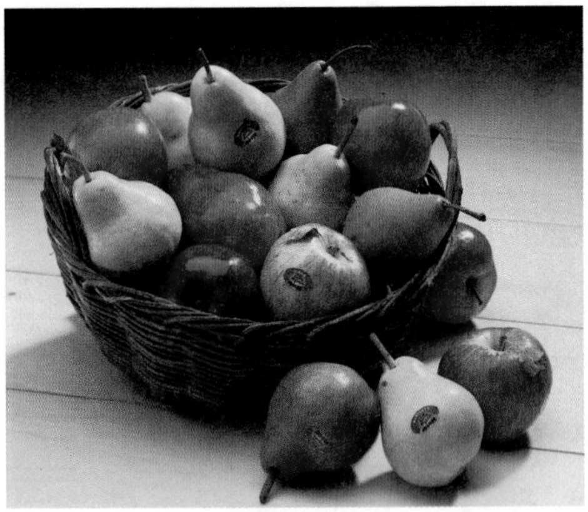
Polara Studios, Inc.

Many consumers are willing to pay a little more for organic produce.

Are organic foods nutritionally superior to conventional foods? For the most part, any nutrient differences reported have been within the range that normally occurs in crops. When results have been significant, it is difficult to determine whether they were due to differences in soil type, soil nutrients, or environmental conditions.[30] Limited research suggests foods produced organically have increased amounts of some phytochemicals.[31]

IN SUMMARY **Pesticides can safely improve crop yields when used according to regulations, but they can also be hazardous when used inappropriately. The CFIA tests both domestic and imported foods for pesticide residues. Consumers can minimize their ingestion of pesticide residues on foods by following the suggestions in Table 20-4 on p. 676. Alternative farming methods may allow farmers to grow crops with few or no pesticides.**

Food Additives

Additives confer many benefits on foods. Some reduce the risk of foodborne illness (e.g., nitrites used in curing meat prevent poisoning from the botulinum toxin). Others enhance nutrient quality (as in vitamin D–fortified milk). Most additives are **preservatives** that help prevent spoilage during the time it takes to deliver foods long distances to grocery stores and then to kitchens. Some additives simply make foods look and taste good.

Intentional additives are put into foods on purpose, whereas indirect additives may get in unintentionally before or during processing. This discussion begins with the regulations that govern additives, then presents intentional additives class by class, and finally goes on to say a word about indirect additives.

Regulations Governing Additives

What are additives, why are they there, and are they dangerous in any way? Food additives are regulated in Canada under the Food and Drugs Act and Regulations and those allowed and their maximum levels are listed in Division 16 of these regulations.[32] The approach and regulations are similar to those of the United States. The policy on the use of food additives in Canada is consistent with the FAO/WHO Joint Expert Committee on Food Additives.

The safety of food additives is a concern for individuals with allergies or hypersensitivities.

The requirement that all ingredients and food additives be included on labels of prepackaged foods helps these individuals select foods that they can tolerate. Health Canada publishes warnings with product recalls; foods or beverages are recalled when nuts or other common allergens are found in them but are not listed as ingredients. Food recalls, health hazard alerts, safety alerts, and allergy alerts can be accessed from the CFIA's website (see Nutrition on the Net).

Manufacturers use food additives to give foods desirable characteristics: colour, flavour, texture, stability, enhanced nutrient composition, or resistance to spoilage. Some classes of additives along with their purpose and examples are listed in Table 20-6 (p. 680), and some are also discussed in the following sections. Food manufacturers must follow Health Canada's Good Manufacturing Practice Regulations and only add the minimum amount of additive needed to achieve the desired effect.[33]

The U.S. FDA's concern with additives hinges primarily on their safety. To receive permission to use a new additive in food products, a manufacturer must satisfy the FDA that the additive is:

- Effective (it does what it is supposed to do)
- Detectable and measurable in the final food product
- Safe (when fed in large doses to animals under strictly controlled conditions, it causes no cancer, birth defects, or other injury)

additives: substances not normally consumed as foods but added to food either intentionally or by accident.

preservatives: antimicrobial agents, antioxidants, and other additives that retard spoilage or maintain desired qualities, such as softness in baked goods.

On approving an additive's use, the FDA writes a regulation stating in what amounts and in what foods the additive may be used. No additive receives permanent approval, and all must undergo periodic review.

The GRAS List Many familiar substances are exempted from complying with the FDA's approval procedure because they are **generally recognized as safe (GRAS)**, based either on their extensive, long-term use in foods or on current scientific evidence. Several hundred substances are on the GRAS list, including such items as salt, sugar, caffeine, and many spices. Whenever substantial scientific evidence or public outcry has questioned the safety of any substance on the GRAS list, it has been re-evaluated. If a legitimate question has been raised about a substance, it has been removed or reclassified. Meanwhile, the entire GRAS list is subjected to ongoing review.

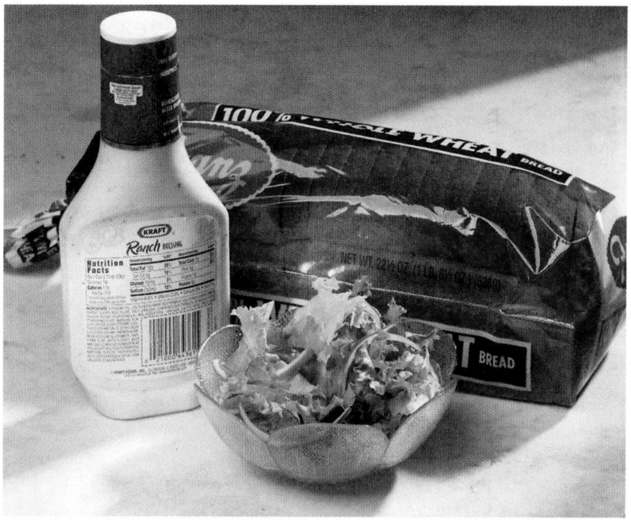
KRAFT
Ranch
Nutrition Facts
100%
WHEAT
BREAD

Polara Studios, Inc

Without additives, bread would quickly get mouldy, and salad dressing would go rancid.

The Delaney Clause One risk that the U.S. law on additives refuses to tolerate at any level is the risk of cancer. To remain on the GRAS list, an additive must not have been found to be a carcinogen in any test on animals or human beings. The **Delaney Clause** (the part of the law that states this criterion) is uncompromising in addressing carcinogens in foods and drugs; in fact, it has been under fire for many years for being too strict and inflexible.

The Delaney Clause is best understood as a product of a different historical era. It was adopted decades ago at a time when scientists knew less about the relationships between carcinogens and cancer development. At that time, most substances were detectable in foods only in relatively large amounts, such as parts per thousand. Today, scientific understanding of cancer has progressed, and technology has advanced so that carcinogens in foods can be detected even when they are present only in parts per billion or even per trillion. ♦ Earlier, "zero risk" may have seemed attainable, but today we know it is not: all substances, no matter how pure, can be shown to be contaminated at some level with one carcinogen or another. For these reasons, the FDA prefers to deem additives (and pesticides and other contaminants) safe if lifetime use presents no more than a one-in-a-million risk of cancer to human beings. Thus, instead of the "zero-risk" policy of the Delaney Clause, the FDA uses a "negligible-risk" standard, sometimes referred to as the *de minimis* rule. ♦

♦ For perspective, one part per trillion is equivalent to about 1 inch in 16 million miles; or 1 second in 32 000 years.

♦ The *de minimis* rule defines risk as a cancer rate of less than one cancer per million people exposed to a contaminant over a 70-year lifetime.

Margin of Safety Whatever risk level is permitted, actual risks must be determined by experiments. To determine risks posed by an additive, researchers feed test animals the additive at several concentrations throughout their lives. The additive is then permitted in foods in amounts 100 times *below* the lowest level that is found to cause any harmful effect, that is, at a 1/100 **margin of safety.** In many foods, *naturally* occurring substances occur with narrower margins of safety. Even nutrients pose risks at dose levels above those recommended and normally consumed: for young adults, the recommendation for vitamin D is only 1/10 of the Upper Level. People consume common table salt daily in amounts only three to five times less than those that pose a hazard.

Risks versus Benefits Of course, additives would not be added to foods if they only presented risks. In general, additives are used in foods when they offer benefits that outweigh the risks, or make the risks worth taking. No amount of risk may be worth taking in the case of colour additives that only enhance appearance but do not improve health or safety. In contrast, Health Canada allows the use of nitrites on meat products, for example, because nitrites inhibit the formation of the deadly botulinum toxin. The choice involves a compromise between the risks of using additives and the risks of doing without them.

It is the manufacturers' responsibility to use only the amounts of additives that are necessary to achieve the needed effect, and no more. The FDA also requires that additives *not* be used:

generally recognized as safe (GRAS): food additives that have long been in use and are believed to be safe. First established by the U.S. FDA in 1958, the GRAS list is subject to revision as new facts become known.

Delaney Clause: a clause in the U.S. Food Additive Amendment to the Food, Drug, and Cosmetic Act that states that no substance that is known to cause cancer in animals or human beings at any dose level shall be added to foods.

margin of safety: when speaking of food additives, a zone between the concentration normally used and that at which a hazard exists. For common table salt, for example, the margin of safety is 1/5 (five times the amount normally used would be hazardous).

TABLE 20-6 Intentional Food Additives

Food Additive	Purpose	Common Examples
Antimicrobial agents	Prevent microorganisms from growing	Salt, sugar, nitrites, and nitrates (such as sodium nitrate)
Antioxidants	Delay or prevent rancidity of fats and other damage to foods caused by oxygen	Vitamin C (erythorbic acid, sodium ascorbate), vitamin E (tocopherol), sulphites, BHA, and BHT
Colours	Enhance appearance	Artificial: indigotine, erythrosine, tartrazine Natural: annatto (yellow), caramel (yellowish brown), carotenoids (yellowish orange), dehydrated beets (reddish brown), grape skins (red, green)
Flavours	Enhance taste	Salt, sugar, spices, artificial sweeteners, MSG
Emulsifiers and gums	Thicken, stabilize, or otherwise improve the consistency	Emulsifiers: lecithin, alginates, mono- and diglycerides Gums: agar, alginates, carrageenan, guar, locust bean, psyllium, pectin, xanthan gum, gum arabic, cellulose derivatives
Nutrients (vitamins and minerals)	Improve the nutritive value	Thiamin, niacin, riboflavin, folate, iron (in grain products); iodine (in salt); vitamins A and D (in milk); vitamin C and calcium (in fruit drinks); vitamin B_{12} (in vegetarian foods)

- To disguise faulty or inferior products
- To deceive the consumer
- When they significantly destroy nutrients
- When their effects can be achieved by economical, sound manufacturing processes

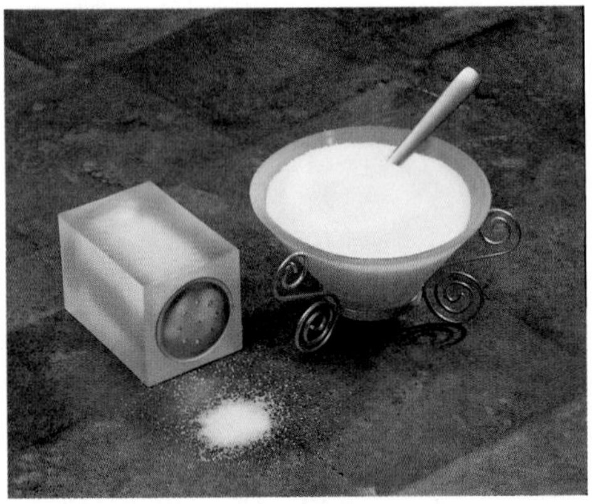

Polara Studios, Inc.

Both salt and sugar act as preservatives by withdrawing water from food; microbes cannot grow without water.

Intentional Food Additives

Intentional food additives are added to foods to give them some desirable characteristic: resistance to spoilage, colour, flavour, texture, stability, or nutritional value. Table 20-6 presents an overview of additives, and the next sections describe additives people most often ask about.

Foods can go bad in two ways. One way is relatively harmless: by losing their flavour and attractiveness. (Additives to prevent this kind of spoilage include antioxidants, discussed later.) The other way is by becoming contaminated with microbes that cause foodborne illnesses, a hazard that justifies the use of antimicrobial agents.

Antimicrobial Agents

The most widely used antimicrobial agents are ordinary salt and sugar. Salt has been used throughout history to preserve meat and fish (note, however, the links between salt intake and hypertension and cancer from Chapter 19); sugar serves the same purpose in canned and frozen fruits and in jams and jellies. Both exert their protective effect primarily by capturing water and making it unavailable to microbes.

Other antimicrobial agents, the **nitrites,** are added to foods for three main purposes: to preserve colour, especially the pink colour of hot dogs and other cured meats; to enhance flavour by inhibiting rancidity, especially in cured meats and poultry; and to protect against bacterial growth. In amounts smaller than those needed to confer colour, nitrites prevent the growth of the bacteria that produce the deadly botulinum toxin.

Nitrites clearly serve a useful purpose, but their use has been controversial. During the curing process and in the human body, nitrites can be converted to **nitrosamines.** Because some nitrosamines are known to cause cancer, Health Canada regulates and the CFIA monitors the use of nitrites in foods and beverages.

Detectable amounts of nitrosamine-related compounds are found in malt beverages (beer) and cured meats (primarily bacon). Exposure to nitrosamine-related compounds from beer and bacon are relatively small, however, compared with nitrosamine exposure from tobacco, new car interiors, and cosmetics.

In their efforts to further combat the potentially life-threatening foodborne illness, listeriosis, the U.S. FDA recently approved a mixture of viruses as a food additive for ready-to-eat meat and poultry products.[34] ♦ These viruses, known

♦ Ready-to-eat products include sausages, turkey, soups, stews, hot dogs, bologna, and ham.

intentional food additives: additives intentionally added to foods, such as nutrients, colours, and preservatives.

nitrites (NYE-trites): salts added to food to prevent botulism. One example is sodium nitrite, which is used to preserve meats.

nitrosamines (nye-TROHS-uh-meens): derivatives of nitrites that may be formed in the stomach when nitrites combine with amines. Nitrosamines are carcinogenic in animals.

as **bacteriophages**, destroy the bacterium *Listeria monocytogenes*, thus protecting consumers from listeriosis. These additives are included in the ingredients list on food labels as a "bacteriophage preparation."

Antioxidants Another way food can go bad is by exposure to oxygen (oxidation). Often, these changes involve no hazard to health, but they damage the food's appearance, flavour, and nutritional quality. Oxidation is easy to detect when sliced apples or potatoes turn brown or when oil goes rancid. Antioxidants prevent these reactions. Among the antioxidants approved for use in foods are vitamin C (ascorbate) and vitamin E (tocopherol).

Another group of antioxidants, the **sulphites**, ♦ cost less than the vitamins. Sulphites prevent oxidation in many processed foods, alcoholic beverages (especially wine), and drugs. Sulphites were used to keep the raw vegetables and fruits in salad bars looking fresh, but this practice was banned after a few people experienced dangerous food sensitivity reactions to the sulphites. Health Canada requires foods to list on their labels any sulphites that are present in quantities greater than 10 ppm.[35] For most people, sulphites pose no hazard in the amounts used in products, but there is one more consideration—sulphites destroy the B vitamin thiamin.

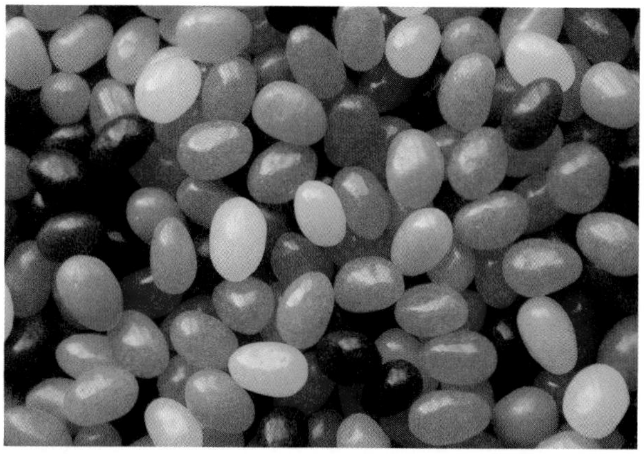
Dee Golden/shutterstock

Colour additives not only make foods attractive, but they identify flavours as well. Everyone agrees that yellow jellybeans should taste lemony and black ones should taste like licorice.

♦ Sulphites appear on food labels as:
- Sulphur dioxide
- Sodium suphite
- Sodium bisulphite
- Potassium bisulphite
- Sodium metabisulphite
- Potassium metabisulphite

Two other antioxidants in wide use are **BHA** and **BHT**, which prevent rancidity in baked goods and snack foods.* Several tests have shown that animals fed large amounts of BHT develop *less* cancer when exposed to carcinogens and live *longer* than controls. Apparently, BHT protects against cancer through its antioxidant effect, which is similar to that of the antioxidant nutrients. A caution: at intakes higher than those that protect against cancer, BHT has *produced* cancer. Vitamins E and C remain the most important dietary antioxidants to strengthen defences against cancer. (See Highlight 12 for a full discussion.)

Colours Only about two dozen natural and ten artificial colours are on Health Canada's list of additives approved for use in foods—a highly select group that has survived considerable testing.[36] Colours derived from the natural pigments of plants must also meet standards of purity and safety. Examples of natural pigments commonly used by the food industry are the caramel that tints cola beverages and baked goods and the carotenoids that colour margarine, cheeses, and pastas. Carotenoids are also added to the feed for farm-raised salmon, which deepens the pink flesh colour.

Artificial Flavours and Flavour Enhancers Natural flavours, artificial flavours, and flavour enhancers are the largest single group of food additives. Many foods taste wonderful because manufacturers have added the natural flavours of spices, herbs, essential oils, fruits, and fruit juices. Some spices, notably those used in Mediterranean cooking, provide antioxidant protection as well as flavours. Often, natural flavours are used in combination with artificial flavours.

One of the best-known flavour enhancers is **monosodium glutamate**, or **MSG**—a sodium salt of the amino acid glutamic acid. MSG is used widely in a number of foods, especially Asian foods, canned vegetables, soups, and processed meats. Besides enhancing the well-known sweet, salty, bitter, and sour tastes, MSG itself may possess a pleasant flavour, a basic taste (termed *umami*) independent of the well-known sweet, salty, bitter, and sour tastes. Adverse reactions to MSG—known as the **MSG symptom complex**—may occur in people with asthma and in sensitive individuals who consume large amounts of MSG, especially on an empty stomach. Otherwise, MSG is considered safe for adults.[37] Food labels require ingredient lists to itemize all additives, including MSG.

Sugar Alternatives The sugar alternatives, introduced in Chapter 4, are among the most widely used artificial flavour additives. Table 4-2 (pp. 113–114) provides a summary of the sugar alternatives. This section presents safety issues surrounding a few of the most controversial ones.

bacteriophages (bak-TIR-ee-oh-fayjz): viruses that infect bacteria.
- **bacterio** = bacteria
- **phage** = eat

sulphites: salts containing sulphur that are added to foods to prevent spoilage.

BHA and **BHT:** preservatives commonly used to slow the development of off-flavours, odours, and colour changes caused by oxidation.

monosodium glutamate (MSG): a sodium salt of the amino acid glutamic acid commonly used as a flavour enhancer. The FDA classifies MSG as a "generally recognized as safe" ingredient.

MSG symptom complex: an acute, temporary intolerance reaction that may occur after the ingestion of the additive MSG (monosodium glutamate). Symptoms include burning sensations, chest and facial flushing and pain, and throbbing headaches.

*BHA is butylated hydroxyanisole; BHT is butylated hydroxytoluene.

Questions about saccharin's safety surfaced in 1977, when experiments suggested that large doses of **saccharin** (equivalent to hundreds of cans of diet soda daily for a lifetime) increased the risk of bladder cancer in rats. As a result, Health Canada delisted saccharin as a food additive (but can still be used as a table-top sweetener) and the U.S. FDA proposed banning it. Public outcry in favour of saccharin was so loud in the United States, however, that the U.S. Congress imposed a moratorium on the ban while additional safety studies were conducted. Products containing saccharin were required to carry a warning label until 2001, when studies concluded that saccharin did not cause cancer in humans. Common sense dictates that consuming large amounts of any substance is probably not wise, but at current, moderate intake levels, saccharin appears to be safe for most people. In December 2009, Health Canada announced that it intended to reinstate saccharin as a food additive in a restricted number of foods and beverages.[38]

Aspartame—a simple chemical compound made of two amino acids (phenylalanine and aspartic acid) and a methyl group (CH_3)—must bear a warning label for people with the inherited disease phenylketonuria (PKU): "contains phenylalanine". People with PKU are unable to dispose of any excess phenylalanine. The accumulation of phenylalanine and its by-products is toxic to the developing nervous system, causing irreversible brain damage. The little extra phenylalanine from aspartame poses only a small risk, even in heavy aspartame users, but people with PKU need to get all their required phenylalanine from protein- and nutrient-rich foods instead of from an artificial sweetener.

During metabolism in the body, the methyl group of aspartame momentarily becomes methyl alcohol (methanol)—a potentially toxic compound. This breakdown also occurs in aspartame-sweetened beverages when they are stored at warm temperatures over time. The amount of methanol produced may be safe to consume, but a person may not want to, considering that the beverage has lost its sweetness. In the body, enzymes convert methanol to formaldehyde, another toxic compound. Finally, formaldehyde is broken down to carbon dioxide. Before aspartame could be approved, the quantities of these products generated during metabolism had to be determined, and they were found to fall below the threshold at which they would cause harm. In fact, millilitre for millilitre, tomato juice yields six times as much methanol as a diet soda.

In 2005, an Italian study found that aspartame caused cancer in female rats and fuelled controversies surrounding aspartame's safety.[39] Statements from the U.S. FDA and others, however, indicate that such a conclusion is not supported by the data and Health Canada concluded that it would not change the way aspartame is used in Canada.[40] The only valid scientific concern is that for people with epilepsy, excessive intake of aspartame may decrease their threshold for seizures; this does not appear to be a problem when intakes are within recommended amounts.

The amount of artificial sweetener considered safe is called the **Acceptable Daily Intake (ADI)** and represents the amount of consumption that, if maintained every day throughout a person's life, would still be considered safe by a wide margin. It usually reflects an amount 100 times less than the level at which no observed effects occur in animal research studies. The ADI for aspartame, for example, is 40 milligrams per kilogram of body weight. For a 68 kilogram (150-pound) adult, the ADI is equivalent to 97 packets of Equal or 20 cans of soft drinks sweetened only with aspartame every day for a lifetime. Most people who use aspartame consume less than 5 milligrams per kilogram of body weight per day. Table 4-2 (pp. 113–114) includes the ADI for approved sweeteners.

Texture and Stability Some additives help to maintain a desirable consistency in foods. Emulsifiers keep mayonnaise stable, control crystallization in syrups, keep spices dispersed in salad dressings, and allow powdered coffee creamer to dissolve easily. Gums are added to thicken foods and help form gels. Yeast may be added to provide leavening, and bicarbonates and acids may be used to control acidity.

Nutrient Additives As mentioned earlier, manufacturers sometimes add nutrients to fortify or maintain the nutritional quality of foods. Included among nutrient additives are the five nutrients added to bleached wheat flour (thiamin,

saccharin (SAK-ah-ren)**:** an artificial sweetener that has been approved for use in the United States. In Canada, approval for use in foods and beverages is pending; currently available only in pharmacies and only as a tabletop sweetener, not as an additive.

aspartame (ah-SPAR-tame or ASS-par-tame)**:** an artificial sweetener composed of two amino acids (phenylalanine and aspartic acid); approved for use in both the United States and Canada.

Acceptable Daily Intake (ADI): the estimated amount of a sweetener that individuals can safely consume each day over the course of a lifetime without adverse effect.

riboflavin, niacin, folate, and iron), the iodine added to salt, the vitamins A and D added to milk, and other nutrients added to other foods such as orange juice. A nutrient-poor food with nutrients added may appear to be nutrient-rich, but it is rich only in those nutrients chosen for addition. Appropriate uses of nutrient additives are to:

- Correct dietary deficiencies known to result in diseases
- Restore nutrients to levels found in the food before storage, handling, and processing
- Balance the vitamin, mineral, and protein contents of a food in proportion to the energy content
- Correct nutritional inferiority in a food that replaces a more nutritious traditional food

As mentioned earlier, nutrients are sometimes also added for other purposes. For example, vitamins C and E are used for their antioxidant properties, and beta-carotene and other carotenoids are sometimes used for colour.

Indirect Food Additives

Indirect or **incidental additives** find their way into foods during harvesting, production, processing, storage, or packaging. Incidental additives may include tiny bits of plastic, glass, paper, tin, and other substances from packages as well as chemicals from processing, such as the solvent used to decaffeinate coffee. The following paragraphs discuss six different types of indirect additives that sometimes make headline news.

Acrylamide Raw potatoes don't have it, but french fries do—acrylamide, a compound that forms when carbohydrate-rich foods containing sugars and the amino acid asparagine ♦ are cooked at high temperatures.[41] Apparently, acrylamide has been in foods ever since we started baking, frying, and roasting, but only recently has its presence been analyzed. At high doses, acrylamide causes cancer in animals and nerve damage in people. As such, scientists classify it as both a carcinogen and a genotoxicant, ♦ but quantities commonly found in foods appear to be well below the amounts that cause such damage. Health Canada is investigating how acrylamide is formed in foods, how its formation can be limited, and whether its presence is harmful. To this end, Health Canada implemented an "Acrylamide Monitoring Program" in August 2009 (see http://www.hc-sc.gc.ca/fn-an/securit/chem-chim/food-aliment/acrylamide/sampling-plan-echantillonnage-eng.php).

♦ Common foods containing acrylamide:
- French fries
- Potato chips
- Breakfast cereals
- Cookies

♦ A **carcinogen** is a substance that causes cancer, and a **genotoxicant** is a substance that mutates or damages genetic material.

Food Packaging You may have heard about the recent BPA (Bisphenol A) controversy (e.g., potential negative effects during neurological development and reproductive problems in animal studies). BPA is a chemical used in the production of polycarbonate plastic and exopy resins. It is used in the production of items such as infant feeding bottles (Health Canada banned the import and sale of polycarbonate baby bottles containing BPA in October 2008), beverage bottles, and the protective linings of food containers. While Health Canada's Food Directorate recently concluded that "the current dietary exposure to BPA through food packaging uses is not expected to pose a health risk to the general population, including newborns and infants," the Canadian government has recommended that "the general principle of ALARA (as low as reasonably achievable) be applied to continue efforts on limiting BPA exposure from food packaging applications to infants and newborns."[42] (Furthermore, Health Canada hosted an international meeting to review the toxicological and health aspects of BPA in late fall 2010.)

Some microwave products are sold in "active packaging" that helps to cook the food; for example, pizzas are often heated on a metalized film laminated to paperboard. This film absorbs the microwave energy in the oven and reaches temperatures as high as 260°C (500°F). At such temperatures, packaging components migrate into the food. For this reason, manufacturers must perform specific tests to determine whether materials are migrating into foods. If they are, their safety must be confirmed by strict procedures similar to those governing intentional additives.

indirect or **incidental additives:** substances that can get into food as a result of contact during growing, processing, packaging, storing, cooking, or some other stage before the foods are consumed; sometimes called *accidental additives.*

♦ Quick test for using glass or ceramic containers in a microwave oven: Microwave the empty container for 1 minute.

- If it's hot, it's unsafe for the microwave.
- If it's warm, it's safe for short-term heating in the microwave.
- If it's cool, it's safe for long-term cooking in the microwave.

Most microwave products are sold in "passive packaging" that is transparent to microwaves and simply holds the food as it cooks. These containers don't get much hotter than the foods, but materials still migrate at high temperatures. Consumers should not reuse these containers in the microwave oven. Instead they should use only glass or ceramic containers labelled as microwave safe; ♦ tiny air bubbles in some glass may expand when microwaved, causing the glass to break, and glazes on some ceramics may leach when microwaved, contaminating the food. Thus use only plastic wraps labelled as microwave-safe. Avoid using disposable styrofoam or plastic containers such as those used for carryout or margarine.

Dioxins Coffee filters, milk cartons, paper plates, and frozen food packages, if made from bleached paper, can contaminate foods with small quantities of **dioxins**—compounds formed during chlorine treatment of wood pulp during paper manufacture. Dioxin contamination of foods from such products appears only in trace quantities—in the parts-per-trillion range (recall, for perspective, that one part per trillion is equal to 1 second in 32 000 years). Such levels appear to present no health risks to people, but scientists recognize that dioxins are extremely toxic and are likely to cause cancer in humans.[43] Accordingly, the paper industry has reduced its use of chlorine to cut dioxin exposure. In the meantime, the U.S. FDA has concluded that drinking milk from bleached-paper cartons presents no health hazard. Contrary to e-mail warnings, plastics do not yield dioxins when broken down and dioxins are not released from plastic wrap when microwaved.[44] Human exposure to dioxins comes primarily from foods such as beef, milk products, pork, fish, and shellfish.[45]

Decaffeinated Coffee Many consumers have tried to eliminate caffeine from their diets by selecting decaffeinated coffee. To remove caffeine from coffee beans, manufacturers often use methylene chloride in a process that leaves traces of the chemical in the final product. A person drinking decaffeinated coffee containing 100 times as much methylene chloride every day for a lifetime has a one-in-a-million chance of developing cancer from it. People are exposed to much more methylene chloride from other sources such as hair sprays and paint-stripping solutions. Still, some consumers prefer either to return to caffeine or to select coffee decaffeinated in another way, perhaps by steam. Unfortunately, manufacturers are not required to state on their labels the type of decaffeination process used in their products. Many labels provide consumer-information telephone numbers for those who have such questions.

Hormones Hormones are a unique type of incidental additive in that their use is intentional, but their presence in the final food product is not. For instance, **growth hormone—bovine somatotropin (bST)**—is used in the United States to promote lean tissue growth and milk production. Canada and the European Union ban the use of bST for milk cows on the grounds that bST stimulates the release of another bovine hormone, insulin-like growth factor I (IGF-I), and some questions have been raised about its effects on human health. IGF-I is produced naturally in people, with levels declining as they age. After a thorough review of the literature, the U.S. FDA concluded that IGF-I levels in milk from bST-treated cows are within the normal range of variation seen in milk from untreated cows and therefore that IGF-I from this source presents no additional risk. Because all cows make bST, the U.S. FDA prohibits milk processors from stating "hormone free" on milk labels. The World Health Organization's expert committee on food additives concurs.

Antibiotics Like hormones, antibiotics are also intentionally given to livestock, and residues may remain in the meats and milks. Consequently, people consuming these foods receive tiny doses of antibiotics regularly, and those with sensitivity to antibiotics may suffer allergic reactions. To minimize drug residues in foods, the CFIA requires a specified time between the time of medication and the time of slaughter to allow for drug metabolism and excretion.

Of greater concern to the public's health is the development of antibiotic resistance, which occurs when antibiotics are overused. Physicians and veterinarians use antibiotics to treat infections in people and animals. Not surprisingly,

dioxins (dye-OCK-sins): a class of chemical pollutants created as by-products of chemical manufacturing, incineration, chlorine bleaching of paper pulp, and other industrial processes. Dioxins persist in the environment and accumulate in the food chain.

bovine growth hormone (BGH): a hormone produced naturally in the pituitary gland of a cow that promotes growth and milk production; now produced for agricultural use by bacteria.

- **bovine** = of cattle

meat from these animals contains resistant bacteria. Such indiscriminate use of antibiotics can be catastrophic to the treatment of disease in human beings. Antibiotics are less effective in treating people who are infected with resistant bacteria. The CFIA continues to monitor the use of antibiotics in the food industry with the goal of ensuring that antibiotics remain effective in treating human disease. The results of such monitoring also become part of the Canadian Integrated Program for Antimicrobial Resistance Surveillance (CIPARS) reports published by the Public Health Agency of Canada, which inform us about the "trends in antimicrobial use and antimicrobial resistance in selected bacterial organisms from human, animal and food sources across Canada."[46]

IN SUMMARY **On the whole, the benefits of food additives seem to justify the risks associated with their use. The CFIA regulates the use of the following intentional additives: antimicrobial agents (such as nitrites) to prevent microbial spoilage; antioxidants (such as vitamins C and E, sulphites, and BHA and BHT) to prevent oxidative changes; colours (such as tartrazine) and flavour enhancers (such as MSG) to appeal to senses; and nutrients (such as iodine in salt) to enrich or fortify foods. Incidental additives sometimes get into foods during processing, but rarely present a hazard.**

Consumer Concerns about Water

Foods are not alone in transmitting diseases; water is guilty, too.[47] In fact, *Cryptosporidium* and *Cyclospora,* commonly found in fresh fruits and vegetables, and *Vibrio vulnificus,* found in raw oysters, are commonly transmitted through contaminated water. In addition to microorganisms, water may contain many of the same impurities that foods do: environmental contaminants, pesticides, and additives such as chlorine used to kill pathogenic microorganisms and fluoride used to protect against dental caries. A glass of "water" is more than just H_2O. This discussion examines the sources of drinking water, ♦ harmful contaminants, and ways to ensure water safety.

♦ Water that is suitable for drinking is called **potable** (POT-ah-bul). Only 1 percent of all the earth's water is potable.

Sources of Drinking Water

Drinking water comes from two sources—surface water (~88 percent) and groundwater (~12 percent).

Most major cities obtain their drinking water from surface water—the water in lakes, rivers, and reservoirs. Surface water is readily contaminated because it is directly exposed to acid rain, runoff from highways and urban areas, pesticide runoff from agricultural areas, and industrial wastes that are dumped directly into it. Surface water contamination is reversible, however, because fresh rain constantly replaces the water. It is also cleansed to some degree by aeration, sunlight, and plants and microorganisms that live in it.

Groundwater is the water in underground aquifers—rock formations that are saturated with and yield usable water. People who live in rural areas rely mostly on groundwater pumped up from private wells. Groundwater is contaminated more slowly than surface water, but also more permanently. Contaminants deposited on the ground migrate slowly through the soil before reaching groundwater. Once there, the contaminants break down less rapidly than in surface water due to the lack of aeration, sunlight, and aerobic microorganisms. The slow replacement of groundwater also helps contaminants remain for a long time. Groundwater is especially susceptible to contamination from hazardous waste sites, dumps and landfills, underground tanks storing gasoline and other chemicals, and improperly discarded household chemicals and solvents.

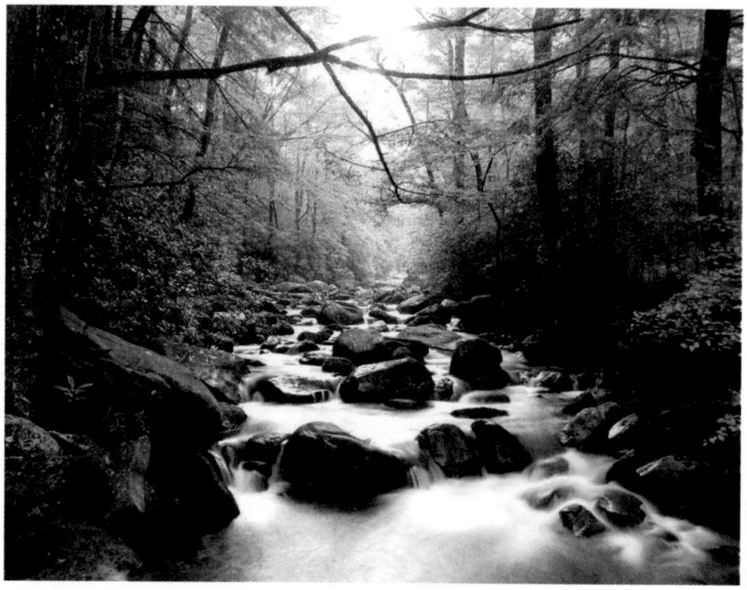

Ishbukar Yalilfatar/shutterstock

Clean rivers represent irreplaceable water resources.

Water Systems and Regulations Public water systems treat water to remove contaminants that have been detected above acceptable levels. During treatment, a disinfectant (usually, chlorine) is added to kill bacteria. The addition of chlorine to public water is an important public health measure that appears to offer great benefits and small risks. On the one hand, chlorinated water has eliminated such waterborne diseases as typhoid fever, which once ravaged communities, killing thousands of people. On the other hand, it has been associated with an increase in bladder cancer and dioxin contamination of the environment.[48] Safe drinking water is the shared responsibility of the federal, provincial/territorial, and municipal governments ♦.

♦ Freshwater supply and demand in Canada: According to Statistics Canada "In 2005, Canadians withdrew about 42 cubic kilometres of water from the environment, roughly 1.2% of the total average water yield. More than 90% of this volume went to support economic activity, while about 9% was used directly by the residential sector."[49]

Even safe water may have characteristics that some consumers find unpleasant. Most of these problems reflect the mineral content of the water. For example, manganese and copper give water a metallic taste, and sulphur produces a "rotten egg" odour. Iron leaves a rusty brown stain on plumbing fixtures and laundry. Calcium and magnesium (commonly found in "hard water") build up in coffeemakers and hot water heaters. Similarly, soap is not easily rinsed away in hard water, leaving bathtubs and laundry looking dingy. For these and other reasons, some consumers have adopted alternatives to the public water system.

Home Water Treatments To ease concerns about the quality of drinking water, some people purchase home water-treatment systems. Manufacturers offer a variety of units for removing contaminants from drinking water. None of them removes all contaminants, and each has its own advantages and disadvantages. Choosing the right treatment unit depends on the kinds of contaminants in the water. For example, activated carbon filters are particularly effective in removing chlorine, heavy metals such as mercury, and organic contaminants from sediment. Reverse osmosis forces pressurized water through a membrane, flushing out minerals such as sodium and some microorganisms such as *Giardia*. Ozonation uses ozone gas to disinfect water. And distillation systems, which boil water and condense the steam to water, leave behind minerals such as lead and kill microorganisms in the process. Therefore, before purchasing a home water-treatment unit, a consumer must first determine the quality of the water. In some cases, a state or county health department will test water samples or can refer the consumer to a certified laboratory. Consumers need to be aware that unscrupulous vendors may use scare tactics during home inspections to prompt sales.

Bottled Water Despite the higher cost, many people turn to bottled water as an alternative to tap water. Canadians consume an average of about 65 litres per person each year.[50] Health Canada regulates bottled drinking water and has established quality and safety standards.[51] In addition, all bottled waters are considered foods and must be processed, packaged, and labelled in accordance with these regulations, which are enforced by the CFIA. Water quality varies among brands because of variations in the source water used and company practices.

As Chapter 15 discusses, some bottled waters are marketed as "enhanced water"—water that has been enhanced with sweeteners, juices, colouring, flavours, vitamins, minerals, protein, and extra oxygen. Consumers perceive these bottled waters as healthful and sales have skyrocketed.

Labels on bottled water must identify the water's source. Approximately 75 percent of bottled waters derive from protected groundwater (from springs or wells) that has been disinfected with ozone rather than chlorine. Ozone kills microorganisms, then disintegrates spontaneously into water and oxygen, leaving behind no toxic by-products. Other bottled waters derive from municipal tap water that has been treated by carbon filtration to remove chlorine and inorganic compounds. Bottled waters may also be treated by reverse osmosis or ion exchange to remove inorganic compounds. Alternatively, the water may be distilled or deionized to remove dissolved solids. Most bottled waters do not contain fluoride; consequently, they do not provide the tooth protection of fluoridated water from community public water systems. Furthermore, while about 45 percent of Canadians receive fluoridated water, and some municipalities across the country have or are considering removing it. The recent CHMS (2007–2009) reveals that one third of Canadians have no dental insurance and that over 50 percent of children and youth have or have had a cavity—facts to keep in mind when considering the controversy over fluoridated water supplies.

Bottled water is considered a food and should be handled like other foods and be refrigerated after opening.

Protection of drinking water is the subject of ongoing concern and controversy. It may soon become a source of conflict between the world's nations as the population continues to grow and the renewable water supply remains constant. Estimates are that within the next 50 years, half of the world's people will not have enough clean water to meet their needs. To avert this potential calamity, we must take active steps to conserve water, clean polluted water, desalinate seawater, and curb population growth.[52]

IN SUMMARY **Like foods, water may contain infectious microorganisms, environmental contaminants, pesticide residues, and additives. The EPA monitors the safety of the public water system, but many consumers choose home water-treatment systems or bottled water instead of tap water.**

As this chapter said at the start, supplying food safely to hundreds of millions of people is an incredible challenge—one that is met, for the most part, with incredible efficiency. The following chapter describes a contrasting situation—that of the food supply not reaching the people.

Nutrition Portfolio

Practising food safety allows you to eat a variety of foods, with little risk of food-related illnesses.

- Review your food-handling practices and describe how effectively you wash your hands, utensils, and kitchen surfaces when preparing foods.
- Describe the steps you take to separate raw and cooked foods while storing and preparing them.
- Describe how you can ensure that you cook foods to a safe temperature and refrigerate perishable foods promptly.

Go to Diet Analysis Plus and choose one of the days on which you tracked your diet and activity for an entire day. Select the Intake Spreadsheet report to help you answer the following questions:

- Imagine for a moment that you got a foodborne illness on this particular day. Which food would you most suspect to have contained the illness-causing organism or toxin? Why would you suspect that food more than the other foods you ate that day?

Diet Analysis PLUS **To complete this exercise, go to your Diet Analysis Plus at www.cengage.com/sso.**

Nutrition on the Net

CENGAGENOW™
For further study of topics covered in this chapter, log on to **www.cengage.com/sso.**

- Check out Health Canada's interactive guide for safe food handling: **www.hc-sc.gc.ca/fn-an/securit/kitchen-cuisine/interact/index-eng.php**
- Find out about health hazards alerts, food recalls, and allergy alerts (including Twitter and RSS feeds) at Canadian Food Inspection Agency's website: **www.inspection.gc.ca/english/corpaffr/recarapp/recaltoce.shtml**
- Get food-safety tips from the U.S. Gateway to Government Food Safety Information site or from the Fight BAC!

campaign of the Partnership for Food Safety Education: **www.foodsafety.gov** or **www.fightbac.org**

- Learn about food safety from Health Canada: **www.hc-sc.gc.ca/fn-an/securit/index-eng.php**
- Find commonsense health tips for travellers at the U.S. Centers for Disease Control and Prevention: **wwwnc.cdc.gov/travel**
- Learn more about food irradiation from Health Canada: **www.hc-sc.gc.ca/fn-an/securit/irridation/index-eng.php**
- Report adverse reactions to Health Canada, MedEffect Canada, Adverse reaction reporting: **www.hc-sc.gc.ca/dhp-mps/medeff/report-declaration/index-eng.php**
- Get advisories and recalls about food from Health Canada by subscribing to RSS feeds: **www.hc-sc.gc.ca/ahc-asc/media/sub-abonn/index-eng.php#rss**
- Review tips from Health Canada about pesticides and subscribe to RSS feeds about pesticides and pest management: **www.hc-sc.gc.ca/cps-spc/pest/index-eng.php**
- Visit the Canadian Food Inspection Agency (CFIA): **www.inspection.gc.ca**
- Learn more about food safety in the marketplace from the Food Safety and Inspection Service: **www.fsis.usda.gov**
- Learn more about the organic foods logo and regulations: **www.inspection.gc.ca/english/fssa/orgbio/orgbioe.shtml**
- Find current information on the proposed documents on standards regarding Canadian organic production: **www.organicagcentre.ca/Standards/std_canadian.asp**
- Find information on foodborne illnesses and safe food handling from the American Dietetic Association: **www.homefoodsafety.org**
- Learn more about safe drinking water from the U.S. Environmental Protection Agency: **www.epa.gov/safewater**

References

1. Public Health Agency of Canada, Foodborne illness outbreak response protocol (FIORP 2010) (June 11, 2010). www.phac-aspc.gc.ca/zoono/fiorp-pritioa/fiorp-pritioa-eng.php, accessed September 21, 2011.
2. Federal Drug Administration, Consumer Magazine (January–February 2004). www.fda.gov/ForConsumers/default.htm), accessed September 21, 2011.
3. Canadian Food Inspection Agency, Causes of foodborne illness (2010). www.inspection.gc.ca/english/fssa/concen/causee.shtml, accessed September 21, 2011.
4. Canadian Food Inspection Agency, Causes of foodborne illness (2010).
5. Position of the American Dietetic Association: Food and water safety, *Journal of the American Dietetic Association* 109 (2009): 1449–1460.
6. Canadian Food Inspection Agency, Implementation of Mandatory Food Safety Enhancement Program (FSEP), Meat Inspection Regulations (Nov. 2005). www.inspection.gc.ca/english/fssa/polstrat/haccp/manue/app8e.shtml.
7. Canadian Food Inspection Agency, CFIA renewal plan 2008–2013. www.inspection.gc.ca/english/hrrh/renpla/renplane.shtml, accessed September 30, 2011; Canadian Food Inspection Agency, Imported food sector regulatory proposal: Questions and answers (October 2010). www.inspection.gc.ca/english/fssa/imp/lic/queste.shtml, accessed September 30, 2011.
8. D. W. Schaffner and K. M. Schaffner, Management of risk of microbial cross-contamination from uncooked frozen hamburgers by alcohol-based hand sanitizer, *Journal of Food Protection* 70 (2007): 109–113.
9. Canadian Food Inspection Agency, Bovine Spongyform Encephalopathy (BSE) in North America (September 2009). www.inspection.gc.ca/english/anima/disemala/bseesb/bseesbe.shtml, accessed September 21, 2011; U.S. Food and Drug Administration, Consumer asked questions about BSE in products regulated by FDA's Center for Food Safety and Applied Nutrition (CFSAN), www.cfsan.fda.gov/~comm/bsefaq.html, updated September 14, 2005, accessed December 6, 2006; U.S. Department of Agriculture, Bovine spongiform encephalopathy (BSE) Q & A's, www.aphis.usda.gov/lpa/issues/bse/bse_q&a.html, updated January 21, 2004, accessed December 6, 2006.
10. S. M. Haq and H. H. Dayal, Chronic liver disease and consumption of raw oysters: A potentially lethal combination: A review of *Vibrio vulnificus* septicemia, *American Journal of Gastroenterology* 100 (2005): 1195–1199.
11. C. Liu, R. Chen, and Y. C. Su, Bactericidal effects of wine on *Vibrio parahaemolyticus* in oysters, *Journal of Food Protection* 69 (2006): 1823–1828.
12. Canadian Food Inspection Agency, Food safety tips: Food irradiation (November 2010). www.inspection.gc.ca/english/fssa/concen/tipcon/irrade.shtml, accessed September 21, 2011; Position of the American Dietetic Association: Food irradiation, *Journal of the American Dietetic Association* 100 (2000): 246–253.
13. Canadian Food Inspection Agency, Food safety tips: Food irradiation, 2010.
14. P. Frenzen and coauthors, Consumer acceptance of irradiated meat and poultry products, www.cdc.gov/foodnet/pub/publications.
15. Health Canada, Food and Nutrition, Environmental contaminants. www.hc-sc.gc.ca/fn-an/securit/chem-chim/environ/index-eng.php, accessed September 21, 2011.
16. C. S. Roegge and S. L. Schantz, Motor function following developmental exposure to PCBS and/or MEHG, *Neurotoxicology and Teratology* 28 (2006): 260–277.
17. Health Canada, Food and Nutrition, Human health risk assessment of mercury in fish and health benefits of fish consumption. www.hc-sc.gc.ca/fn-an/pubs/mercur/merc_fish_poisson-eng.php, accessed September 21, 2011.
18. A. Tsuchiya and coauthors, Fish intake guidelines: Incorporating n-3 fatty acid intake and contaminant exposure in the Korean and Japanese communities, *American Journal of Clinical Nutrition* 87 (2008): 1867–1875; A. L. Yaktine, M. C. Nesheim, and C. A. James, Nutrient and contaminant tradeoffs: Exchanging meat, poultry, or seafood for dietary protein, *Nutrition Reviews* 66 (2008): 113–122.
19. Health Canada, Food and Nutrition, Mercury in fish—Consumption advice: Making informed choices about fish. www.hc-sc.gc.ca/fn-an/securit/chem-chim/environ/mercur/cons-adv-etud-eng.php, accessed September 21, 2011; Institute of Medicine, *Seafood Choices: Balancing Benefits and Risks*, October 2006.
20. C. W. Levenson and D. M. Axelrad, Too much of a good thing? Update on fish consumption and mercury exposure, *Nutrition Reviews* 64 (2006): 139–145.
21. Canadian Food Inspection Agency, National chemical residue monitoring program for fresh fruit and vegetables. www.inspection.gc.ca/english/fssa/frefra/safsal/cheme.shtml, accessed September 21, 2011.
22. Health Canada, Pesticides and food. www.hc-sc.gc.ca/cps-spc/pubs/pest/_fact-fiche/pesticide-food-alim/index-eng.php, accessed September 21, 2011.
23. Health Canada, Consumer Safety, Science policy note: Assessing exposure from pesticides in food—A user's suide. www.hc-sc.gc.ca/cps-spc/pubs/pest/_pol-guide/spn2003-03/index-eng.php, accessed September 21, 2011.

24. Canadian Food Inspection Agency, Organic products. www.inspection.gc.ca/english/fssa/orgbio/orgbioe.shtml, accessed September 21, 2011.
25. Organic Agriculture Centre of Canada. Canadian organic food sales grow past $1 billion (June 2007). www.organicagcentre.ca/MarketInfo/mkt_press_release_may07.asp, accessed September 21, 2011.
26. C. K. Winter and S. F. Davis, Organic foods, *Journal of Food Science* 71 (2006): R117–R124.
27. A. Mukherjee and coauthors, Longitudinal microbiological survey of fresh produce grown by farmers in the upper Midwest, *Journal of Food Protection* 69 (2006): 1928–1936.
28. Canadian Food Inspection Agency, Organic products.
29. C. Lu and coauthors, Organic diets significantly lower children's dietary exposure to organophosphorus pesticides, *Environmental Health Perspectives* 114 (2006): 260–263.
30. D. M. Barrett and coauthors, Qualitative and nutritional differences in processing tomatoes grown under commercial organic and conventional production systems, *Journal of Food Science* 72 (2007): C441–C451.
31. A. E. Mitchell and coauthors, Ten-year comparison of the influence of organic and conventional crop management practices on the content of flavonoids in tomatoes, *Journal of Agricultural and Food Chemistry* 55 (2007): 6154–6159.
32. Department of Justice, Food and Drug Regulations (C.R.C., c870): Division 16, Food additives. http://lois-laws.justice.gc.ca/eng/regulations/C.R.C.%2C_c._870/page-145.html, accessed September 21, 2011.
33. Health Canada, Health Products and Food Branch Inspectorate, Good Manufacturing Practices (GMP) Guidelines—2009 Edition Version 2 (GUI-0001) March 2011. www.hc-sc.gc.ca/dhp-mps/alt_formats/pdf/compli-conform/gmp-bpf/docs/gui-0001-eng.pdf, accessed September 30, 2011.
34. L. Bren, Bacteria-eating virus approved as food additive, *FDA Consumer,* January/February 2007, pp. 20–22.
35. Health Canada, Food and Nutrition, Health Canada continues to urge food manufacturers to label priority food allergens, gluten sources and added sulphites in the interim period of the Food Allergen Labelling Regulatory Amendments coming into force (2011). www.hc-sc.gc.ca/fn-an/label-etiquet/allergen/guide_ligne_direct_indust-eng.php, accessed September 21, 2011.
36. Canadian Food Inspection Agency, Food colours: Permitted synthetic colours in Canada and corresponding United States and European names. www.inspection.gc.ca/english/fssa/labeti/decisions/coloure.shtml, accessed September 21, 2011.
37. K. Beyreuther and coauthors, Consensus meeting: Monosodium glutamate: An update, *European Journal of Clinical Nutrition* 61 (2007): 304–313.
38. Health Canada, Summary of input received on Health Canada's consultation to reinstate saccharin as a food additive. www.hc-sc.gc.ca/fn-an/securit/addit/sweeten-edulcor/saccharin-summary-eng.php, accessed September 21, 2011.
39. M. Soffritti and coauthors, Aspartame induces lymphomas and leukaemias in rats, *European Journal of Oncology* 10 (2005): 107–116.
40. U.S. Food and Drug Administration, FDA statement on European aspartame study, posted May 8, 2006, www.fda.gov; M. R. Weihrauch and V. Diehl, Artificial sweeteners: Do they bear a carcinogenic risk? *Annals of Oncology* 15 (2004): 1460–1465; Health Canada, Food and Nutrition, Health Canada comments on the recent study relating to the safety of Aspartame (May 2006). www.hc-sc.gc.ca/fn-an/securit/addit/sweeten-edulcor/aspartame_statement-eng.php, accessed September 21, 2011.
41. M. DiNovi, The 2006 exposure assessment for acrylamide, July 2006, www.cfsan.fda.gov/~dms/acryexpo.html.
42. Health Canada, Food and Nutrition, Bisphenol A. www.hc-sc.gc.ca/fn-an/securit/packag-emball/bpa/index-eng.php, accessed September 21, 2011.
43. National Academy of Sciences, EPA assessment of dioxin understates uncertainty about health risks and may overstate human cancer risk, 2006, http://national-academies.org.
44. D. Schardt, Microwave myths: Fact vs. fiction, *Nutrition Action Healthletter,* April 2005, pp. 10–12.
45. National Academy of Sciences, *Health Risks from Dioxin and Related Compounds: Evaluation of the EPA Reassessment,* July 2006.
46. Public Health Agency of Canada, Canadian Integrated Program for Antimicrobial Resistance Surveillance (CIPARS). www.phac-aspc.gc.ca/cipars-picra/index-eng.php, accessed September 21, 2011.
47. B. G. Blackburn and coauthors, Surveillance for waterborne disease and outbreaks associated with drinking water and water not intended for drinking: United States, 2003–2004, *Morbidity and Mortality Weekly Report* 55 (2006): 31–58.
48. C. M. Villanueva and coauthors, Bladder cancer and exposure to water disinfection byproducts through ingestion, bathing, showering, and swimming in pools, *American Journal of Epidemiology* 165 (2007): 148–156.
49. Statistics Canada, Study: Freshwater supply and demand in Canada, *The Daily* (2010). www.statcan.gc.ca/daily-quotidien/100913/dq100913b-eng.htm, accessed September 21, 2011.
50. Agriculture and Agri-Food Canada, The Canadian bottled water industry. www4.agr.gc.ca/AAFC-AAC/display-afficher.do?id=1171644581795&lang=eng, accessed September 30, 2011.
51. Health Canada, Food and Nutrition, Bottled water. www.hc-sc.gc.ca/fn-an/securit/facts-faits/bottle_water-eau_embouteillee-eng.php, accessed September 30, 2011.
52. D. D. Marino, Water and food safety in the developing world: Global implications for health and nutrition of infants and young children, *Journal of the American Dietetic Association* 107 (2007): 1930–1934.

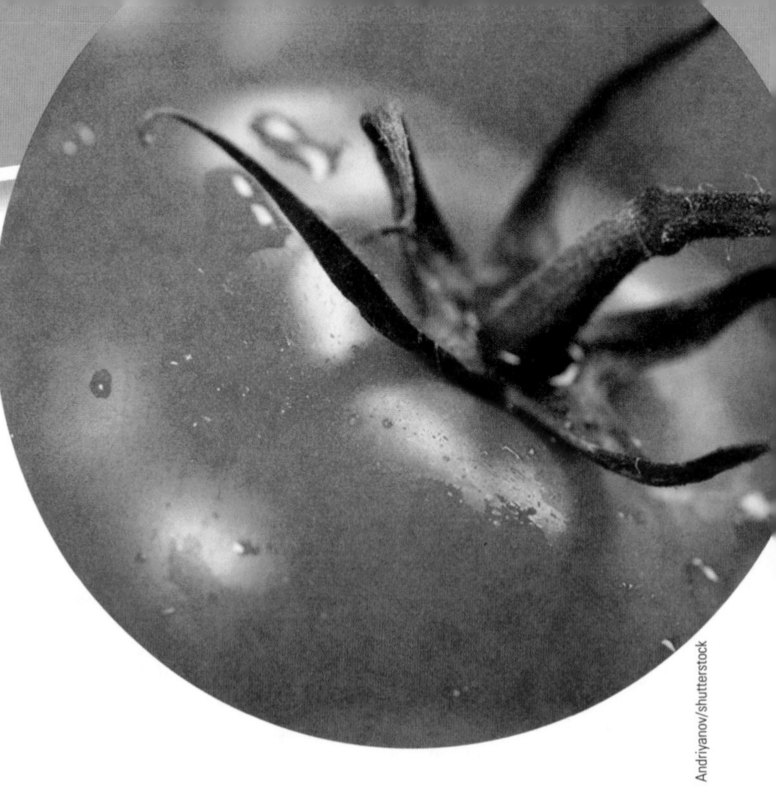

Ilya Andriyanov/shutterstock

Food Biotechnology

Advances in food **biotechnology** promise just about everything from the frivolous (a tear-free onion) to the profound (a hunger-free world). Already biotechnology has produced leaner meats, longer shelf lives, better nutrient composition, and greater crop yields grown with fewer pesticides. Overall, biotechnology offers numerous opportunities to overcome food shortages, improve the environment, and eliminate disease. But it also raises concerns about possible risks to the environment and human health. Critics assert that biotechnology will exacerbate world hunger, destroy the environment, and endanger health. This highlight presents some of the many issues surrounding genetically engineered foods, and the accompanying glossary defines the terms used.

The Promises of Genetic Engineering

For centuries, farmers have been selectively breeding plants and animals to shape the characteristics of their crops and livestock. They have created prettier flowers, hardier vegetables, and leaner animals. Consider the success of selectively breeding corn. Early farmers in Mexico began with a wild, native plant called teosinte (tay-oh-SEEN-tay) that bears only five or six kernels on each small spike. Many years of patient selective breeding have produced large ears filled with hundreds of plump kernels aligned in perfect formation, row after row.

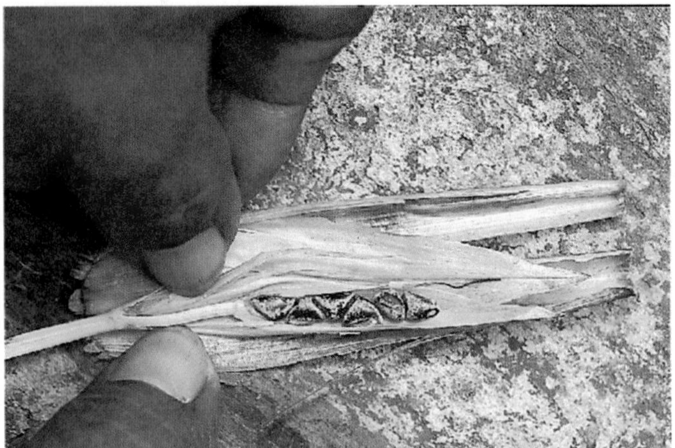

Courtesy of © Smithsonian Tropical Research Institute/Antonio Mortaner, photographer

This wild predecessor of corn, with its sparse five or six kernels, bears little resemblance to today's large, full, sweet ears.

Such genetic improvements, together with the use of irrigation, fertilizers, and pesticides, were responsible for more than half of the increases in U.S. crop yields in the 20th century. Farmers still use selective breeding, but now, in the 21st century, advances in **genetic engineering** have brought rapid and dramatic changes to agriculture and food production.

Although selective breeding works, it is slow and imprecise because it involves mixing thousands of genes from two plants and hoping for the best. With genetic engineering, scientists can improve crops (or livestock) by introducing a copy of the specific gene needed to produce the desired trait. Figure H20-1 illustrates the difference. Once introduced, the selected gene acts like any other gene—it provides instructions for making a protein. The protein then determines a characteristic in the genetically modified plant or animal. In short, the process is now faster and more refined. Farmers no longer need to wait patiently for breeding to yield improved crops and animals, nor must they even respect natural lines of reproduction among species. Laboratory scientists can copy genes from one organism and insert them into almost any other organism—plant, animal, or microbe. Their work is changing not only the way farmers plant, fertilize, and harvest their crops, but also the ways the food industry processes food and consumers receive nutrients, phytochemicals, and drugs.

GLOSSARY

biotechnology: the use of biological systems or organisms to create or modify products. Examples include the use of bacteria to make yogurt, yeast to make beer, and cross-breeding to enhance crop production.

clone: a genetic copy of an animal, similar to identical twins but born at different times.

genetic engineering: the use of biotechnology to modify the genetic material of living cells so that they will produce new substances or perform new functions. Foods produced via this technology are called *genetically modified (GM)* or *genetically engineered (GE) foods.*

plant-pesticides: pesticides made by the plants themselves.

rennin: an enzyme that coagulates milk; found in the gastric juice of cows, but not human beings.

FIGURE H20-1 Selective Breeding and Genetic Engineering Compared

Traditional Selective Breeding

Traditional selective breeding combines many genes from two varieties of the same species to produce one with the desired characteristics.

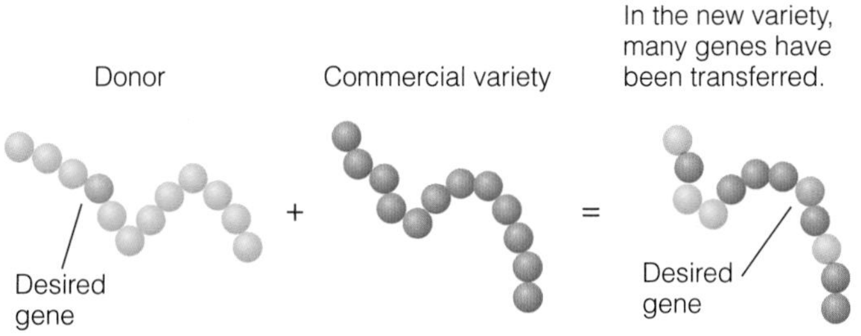
Donor
Commercial variety
In the new variety, many genes have been transferred.
Desired gene
Desired gene

Genetic Engineering

Through genetic engineering, a single gene is (or several are) transferred from the same or different species to produce one with the desired characteristics.

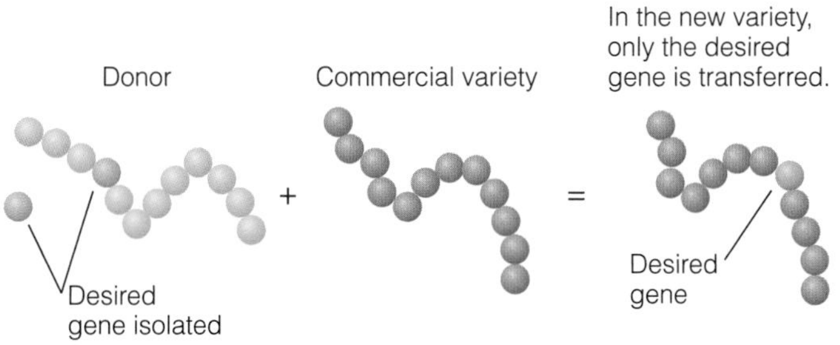
Donor
Commercial variety
In the new variety, only the desired gene is transferred.
Desired gene isolated
Desired gene

SOURCE: © 1995 Monsanto Company

Extended Shelf Life

Among the first products of genetic engineering to hit the market were tomatoes that stay firm and ripe longer than regular tomatoes that are typically harvested green and ripened in the stores. These genetically modified tomatoes promise less waste and higher profits. Normally, tomatoes produce a protein that softens them after they have been picked. Scientists can now introduce into a tomato plant a gene that is a mirror image of the one that codes for the "softening" enzyme. This gene fastens itself to the RNA of the native gene and blocks synthesis of the softening protein. Without this protein, the genetically altered tomato softens more slowly than a regular tomato, allowing growers to harvest it at its most flavourful and nutritious vine-ripe stage.

Improved Nutrient Composition

Genetic engineering can also improve the nutrient composition of foods. Instead of manufacturers adding nutrients to foods during processing, plants can be genetically altered to do their own fortification work—a strategy called *biofortification.*[1] Biofortification of staple crops with key vitamins and minerals can effectively combat the nutrient deficiency diseases that claim so many lives

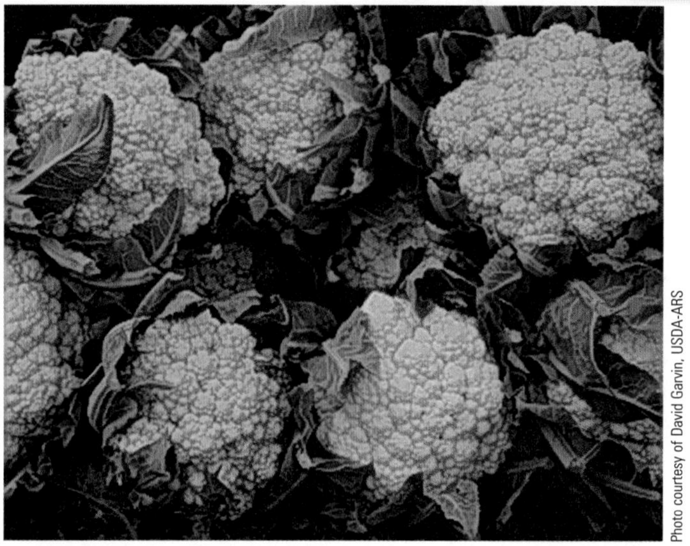
Photo courtesy of David Garvin, USDA-ARS

Genetically modified cauliflower is orange, reflecting a change in a single gene that increases its production of beta-carotene hundredfold.

worldwide. Genetically modifying wheat can improve its protein, zinc, and iron content.[2] Soybeans may be implanted with a gene that upgrades soy protein to a quality approaching that of milk. Corn may be modified to contain lysine and tryptophan, its two limiting amino acids. Soybean and canola plants can be genetically modified to alter the composition of their oils, making them richer in the heart-healthy monounsaturated fatty acids. "Golden rice," which has received genes from a daffodil and a bacterium that enable it to make beta-carotene, offers some promise in helping to correct vitamin A deficiency worldwide. (Chapter 12 describes how vitamin A deficiency contributes to the deaths of two million children and the blindness of a half million each year.) Of course, increasing nutrients in crops may have unintended consequences as well. For example, when broccoli is manipulated to increase its selenium content, production of the cancer-fighting phytochemical sulphoraphane declines.[3]

As you might predict, enhancing the chemical composition of plants is not limited to the essential nutrients. Genetically modified crops can also produce more of the phytochemicals that help maintain health and reduce the risks of chronic diseases (see Highlight 14). They can also be coaxed to produce less phytate, which allows more zinc to be absorbed. The possibilities seem endless.

Efficient Food Processing

Genetic engineering also helps to process foods more efficiently, which saves money. For example, the protein **rennin,** which is used to coagulate milk in the production of cheese, has traditionally been harvested from the stomachs of calves, a costly process. Now scientists can insert a copy of the rennin gene into bacteria and then use bacterial cultures to mass-produce rennin—saving time, money, space, and animals.

Genetic engineering can also help to bypass costly food-processing steps. At present, people who are lactose intolerant can buy milk that has been treated with the lactase enzyme. Wouldn't it be more convenient, and less expensive, if scientists could induce cows to make lactose-free milk directly? They're working on it. They have already successfully inserted into mice the genetic material needed to make lactase in their mammary glands, thereby producing low-lactose milk. Decaffeinated coffee beans are another real possibility.

Genetic research today has progressed well beyond tweaking a gene here and there to produce a desired trait. Scientists can now **clone** animals. By cloning animals, scientists have the ability to produce both needed food and pharmaceutical products. While the U.S. FDA has declared that food from cloned livestock is safe to eat, none are presently on the market in either Canada or the United States. Cloned animals are used primarily for breeding; their offspring are used primarily for food. The percentage of consumers who have a favourable impression of eating food from cloned animals or their offspring is small, but increasing. The industry does not track cloned offspring entering the market. Because U.S. FDA does not distinguish between foods from cloned animals or their offspring and foods from conventional animals, food labels are not required to provide this information.[4]

Efficient Drug Delivery

Using cloned animals and other organisms in the development of pharmaceuticals is whimsically called "biopharming." For example, a cow cloned with the genetic equipment to make a vaccine in its milk could provide both nourishment and immunization to a whole village of people now left unprotected because they lack food and medical help. Similarly, researchers have figured out how to induce hens to produce eggs with a drug to treat multiple sclerosis. Bananas and potatoes have been designed to make hepatitis vaccines, and tobacco leaves to make AIDS drugs. Researchers can also harvest vaccines by genetically altering hydroponically grown tomato plants to secrete a protein through their root systems into the water. Using foods to deliver drugs is only a small part of the promise and potential biotechnology offers the field of medicine.[5]

Genetically Assisted Agriculture

Genetic engineering has helped farmers to increase yields, extend growing seasons, and grow crops that resist herbicides. About half of the soybean crops in the United States have been genetically engineered to withstand a potent herbicide. As a result, farmers can spray whole fields with this herbicide and kill the weeds without harming the soybeans.

Similarly, farmers can grow crops that produce their own pesticides—substances known as **plant-pesticides.** Corn, broccoli, and potatoes have received a gene from a bacterium that produces a protein that is toxic to leaf-chewing caterpillars (but not to humans). Yellow squash has been given two viral genes that confer resistance to the most common viral diseases. Potatoes can now produce a beetle-killing toxin in their leaves. These crops and many others like them are currently being grown or tested in fields around the United States. Growing crops that make their own pesticides allows farmers to save time, increase yields, and use fewer, or less harmful, pesticides. Genetically modified crops have decreased the environmental impact associated with pesticide use over the past decade by more than 15 percent.[6]

Other Possibilities

Many other biotechnology possibilities are envisioned for the near future. Shrimp may be empowered to fight diseases with genetic ammunition borrowed from sea urchins. Plants may be given special molecules to help them grow in polluted soil. With these and other advances, farmers may reliably produce bumper crops of food every year on far fewer acres of land, with less loss of water and topsoil, and far less use of toxic pesticides and herbicides. Supporters of biotechnology predict that these efforts will enhance food production and help meet the challenge of feeding an ever-increasing world population. They contend that genetically modified crops have the potential to eliminate hunger and starvation. Others suggest that the problems of world hunger are more complex than biotechnology alone can resolve and that the potential risks of genetic engineering may outweigh the potential benefits.

The projects mentioned in this highlight are already in progress. Close on their heels are many more ingenious ideas. What if salt tolerance could be transplanted from a coastal marsh plant into crop plants? Could crops then be irrigated with seawater, thus conserving dwindling freshwater supplies? Or could crops be genetically designed to use less water? Would the world food supply increase if rice farmers could grow plants that were immune to disease? What if consumers could dictate which traits scientists insert into food plants? Would they choose to add phytochemicals to fight cancer or reduce the risk of heart disease? These and other possibilities seem unlimited, and though they may sound incredible, many such products have already been developed and are awaiting approval from the FDA, EPA, and USDA.

The Potential Problems and Concerns

Although many scientists hail biotechnology with confidence, others have reservations.[7] Most consumers know little about biotechnology or the extent to which their foods contain genetically modified foods.[8] Some consumers have concerns about what they call "Frankenfoods." Those who oppose biotechnology fear for the safety of a world where genetic tampering produces effects that are not yet fully understood. They suspect that the food industry may be driven by potential profits, without ethical considerations or laws to harness its effects. They point out that even the scientists who developed the techniques cannot predict the ultimate outcomes of their discoveries. These consumers don't want to eat a scientific experiment or interfere with natural systems. Genetic decisions, they say, are best left to the powers of nature.

If science and the marketplace are allowed to drive biotechnology without restraint, critics fear that these problems may result in:

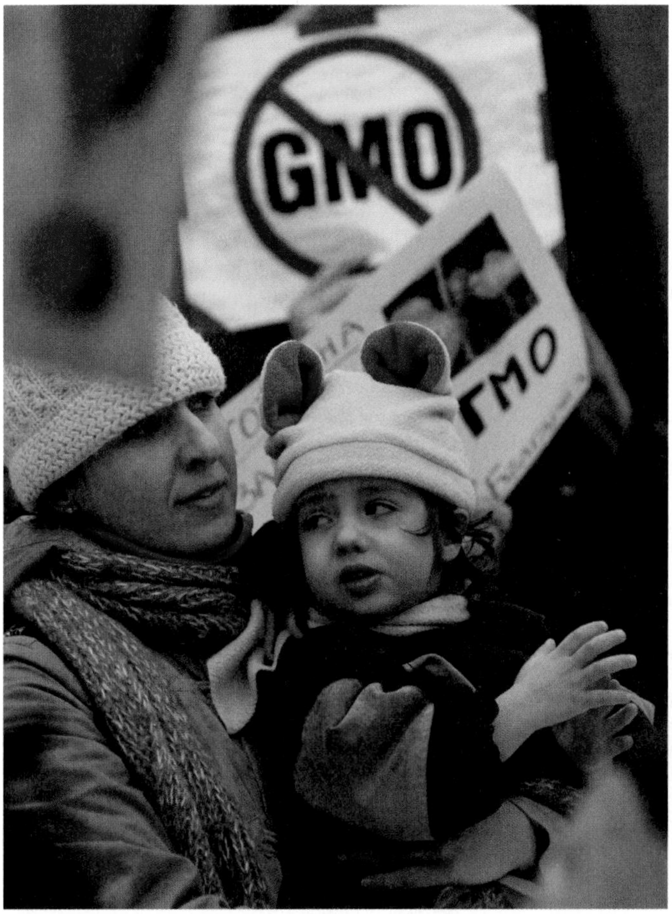
GMO
ГМО

AP Photo/Petar Petrov/CP Images

Some consumers believe that food biotechnology will cause more harm than good.

- *Disruption of natural ecosystems.* New, genetically unique organisms that have no natural place in the food chain or evolutionary biological systems could escape into the environment and reproduce.
- *Introduction of diseases.* Newly created viruses may mutate to cause deadly diseases that may attack plants, animals, or human beings. Genetically modified bacteria may develop resistance to antibiotics, making the drugs useless in fighting infections.
- *Introduction of allergens and toxins.* Genetically modified crops may contain new substances that have consequences, such as causing allergies.[9]
- *Creation of biological weapons.* Fatal bacterial and viral diseases may be developed for use as weapons.
- *Ethical dilemmas.* Critics pose the question, "How many human genes does an organism have to contain before it is considered human? For instance, how many human genes would a green pepper have to contain before one would have qualms about eating it?"

Proponents of biotechnology respond that evidence to date does not justify these concerns. Opponents counter that the lack of evidence showing harm does not provide evidence showing safety. These opposing views illustrate the tension between the forward thrust of science and the hesitation of consumers. Both positions highlight the need for more research on the safety and effectiveness of genetically modified food. In addition to evaluating the potential risks and benefits, genetically modified crops need to be closely monitored by the international community.[10] Table H20-1 summarizes the issues.

From another perspective, some argue that the concerns expressed by those protesting genetically engineered foods reflect prejudices acquired in an elitist world of fertile land and abundant food. Those living in poverty-stricken areas of the world do not have the luxury of determining how to grow crops and process foods. They cannot afford the delays created when protesters destroy test crops and disrupt scientific meetings. They need solutions now. People are starving, and genetic engineering holds great promise for providing them with food.

The work of Nobel Prize winner Dr. Norman Borlaug and his team over the past four decades attests to the benefits of using technology to defend against hunger. By developing grains that resist pests and diseases, they have been able to increase yields and provide real solutions to global hunger problems. When Mexico used Borlaug's special breed of dwarf wheat, yields increased threefold compared with traditional varieties. India increased wheat production tenfold and became self-sufficient in its grain production. Pakistan increased its wheat production fivefold, and sub-Saharan Africa more than tripled crop yields by changing farming practices. The combination of improved conventional systems and biotechnology produces more food to meet the nutritional needs of more people.

At a minimum, critics of biotechnology have made a strong case for rigorous safety testing and labelling of new products. They contend, for example, that when a new gene has been introduced into a food, tests should ensure that other, unwanted genes have not accompanied it. If a disease-producing microorganism has donated genetic material, scientists must prove that no dangerous characteristic from the microorganism has also entered the food. If the inserted genetic material comes from a source to which some people develop allergies, such as nuts, then the new product should be labelled to alert them. Furthermore, if the newly altered genetic material creates proteins that have never before been encountered by the human body, their effects should be studied to ensure that people can eat them safely.

Canadian Regulations

Health Canada and the Canadian Food Inspection Agency (CFIA) have responsibilities for regulating products derived through biotechnology. Health Canada is responsible for assessing the human health and safety of products derived from biotechnology including foods, drugs, cosmetics, medical devices, and pest control products. CFIA is responsible for regulating products derived through biotechnology, including plants, animal feeds and animal feed ingredients, fertilizers, and veterinary biologics. For genetically modified crop plants, CFIA assesses the potential risk of adverse environmental effects and authorizes and oversees import permits, confined trials, unconfined release, and variety registration.

TABLE H20-1 Food Biotechnology: Point, Counterpoint

Arguments in Opposition to Genetic Engineering	Arguments in Support of Genetic Engineering
1. **Ethical and moral issues.** It's immoral to "play God" by mixing genes from organisms unable to do so naturally. Religious and vegetarian groups object to genes from prohibited species occurring in their allowable foods.	1. **Ethical and moral issues.** Scientists throughout history have been persecuted and even put to death by fearful people who accuse them of playing God. Yet, today many of the world's citizens enjoy a long and healthy life of comfort and convenience due to once-feared scientific advances put to practical use.
2. **Imperfect technology.** The technology is young and imperfect—genes rarely function in just one way, their placement is imprecise ("shotgun"), and all of their potential effects are impossible to predict. Toxins are as likely to be produced as the desired trait. More than 95 percent of DNA is called "junk" because scientists have not yet determined its function.	2. **Advanced technology.** Recombinant DNA technology is precise and reliable. Many of the most exciting recent advances in medicine, agriculture, and technology were made possible by the application of this technology.
3. **Environmental concerns.** Environmental side effects are unknown. The power of a genetically modified organism to change the world's environments is unknown until such changes actually occur—then the "genie is out of the bottle." Once out, insects, birds, and the wind distribute genetically altered seed and pollen to points unknown.	3. **Environmental protection.** Genetic engineering may be the only hope of saving rain forest and other habitats from destruction. Through genetic engineering, farmers can make use of previously unproductive lands such as salt-rich soils and arid areas.
4. **"Genetic pollution."** Other kinds of pollution can often be cleaned up with money, time, and effort. Once genes are spliced into living things, those genes forever bear the imprint of human tampering.	4. **Genetic improvements.** Genetic side effects are more likely to benefit the environment than to harm it.
5. **Crop vulnerability.** Pests and diseases can quickly adapt to overtake genetically identical plants or animals around the world. Diversity is key to defence.	5. **Improved crop resistance.** Pests and diseases can be specifically fought on a case-by-case basis. Biotechnology is the key to defence.
6. **Loss of gene pool.** Loss of genetic diversity threatens to deplete valuable gene banks from which scientists can develop new agricultural crops.	6. **Gene pool preserved.** Thanks to advances in genetics, laboratories around the world are able to stockpile the genetic material of millions of species that, without such advances, would have been lost forever.
7. **Profit motive.** Genetic engineering will profit industry more than the world's poor and hungry.	7. **Everyone profits.** Industries benefit from genetic engineering, and a thriving food industry benefits the nation and its people, as witnessed by countries lacking such industries. Genetic engineering promises to provide adequate nutritious food for millions who lack such food today. Developed nations gain cheaper, more attractive, more delicious foods with greater variety and availability year round.
8. **Unproven safety for people.** Human safety testing of genetically altered products is generally lacking. The population is an unwitting experimental group in a nationwide laboratory study for the benefit of industry.	8. **Safe for people.** Human safety testing of genetically altered products is unneeded because the products are essentially the same as the original foodstuffs.
9. **Increased allergens.** Allergens can unwittingly be transferred into foods.	9. **Control of allergens.** A few allergens can be transferred into foods, but these are known. Also, foods likely to contain them are clearly labelled to warn consumers.
10. **Decreased nutrients.** A fresh-looking tomato or other produce held for several weeks may have lost substantial nutrients.	10. **Increased nutrients.** Genetic modifications can easily enhance the nutrients in foods.
11. **No product tracking.** Without labelling, the food industry cannot track problems to the source.	11. **Excellent product tracking.** The identity and location of genetically altered foodstuffs are known, and they can be tracked should problems arise.
12. **Overuse of herbicides.** Farmers, knowing that their crops resist herbicide effects, will use them liberally.	12. **Conservative use of herbicides.** Farmers will not waste expensive herbicides in second or third applications when the prescribed amount gets the job done the first time.
13. **Increased consumption of pesticides.** When a pesticide is produced by the flesh of produce, consumers cannot wash it off the skin of the produce with running water as they can with ordinary sprays.	13. **Reduced pesticides on foods.** Pesticides produced by produce in tiny amounts known to be safe for consumption are more predictable than applications by agricultural workers who make mistakes. Because other genetic manipulations will eliminate the need for postharvest spraying, fewer pesticides will reach the dinner table.
14. **Lack of oversight.** Government oversight is run by industry people for the benefit of industry—no one is watching out for the consumer.	14. **Sufficient regulation and rapid response.** Government agencies are efficient in identifying and correcting problems as they occur in the industry.

The Canadian General Standards Board approved standards for voluntary labelling and advertising of foods that are and are not products of genetic engineering. These standards were published in April 2004 and can be accessed via the Canadian General Standards Board website.

Note: It is mandatory to label all foods that have significant nutritional or compositional changes due to this technology or where health or safety risk exists, such as the presence of an allergen. Today, more than 50 genetically modified (GM) foods (e.g., canola, corn, potatoes, tomatoes, and soybeans) have been approved for sale in Canada.[11] Any substances introduced into a food (such as a hormone or protein) by way of bioengineering must meet the same safety standards applied to all additives. A tomato plant with a gene that, for example, produces a pesticide cannot be marketed until tests prove it safe for consumption. Such testing assures consumers that all bioengineered foods on the market today are as safe as their traditional counterparts.

Foods produced through biotechnology that are substantially different from others must be labelled to identify that difference. For example, if the nutrient composition of the new product differs from its traditional counterpart, as in the soybean and canola oils mentioned earlier, then labelling is required. Similarly, if an allergy-causing protein has been introduced to a nonallergenic food, then labelling must warn consumers.

Most consumers want all genetically altered products clearly labelled. Consumer advocacy groups claim that by not requiring such labelling, forces millions of consumers to be guinea pigs, unwittingly testing genetically engineered foods. Additionally, they say, people who have religious objections to consuming foods to which genes of prohibited organisms have been added have no way of identifying those foods. For example, someone keeping a kosher kitchen may unknowingly use a food containing genes from a pig. Currently, labelling is voluntary. Manufacturers may state that a product has been "genetically engineered." Those who do would be wise to explain its purpose and benefit. When consumers recognize a personal health benefit, most tend to accept genetically engineered foods.

Speaking in defence of the U.S. FDA's position are the FDA itself, recognized as that nation's leading expert and advocate for food safety, and the American Dietetic Association, which represents current scientific thinking in nutrition.[12] Many other scientific organizations agree, contending that biotechnology can deliver an improved food supply if we give it a fair chance to do so.

Will these new technologies provide foods to meet the needs of the future? Some would say yes. Biotechnology holds a world of promise, and with proper safeguards and controls, it may yield products that meet the needs of consumers almost perfectly.

Nutrition on the Net

CENGAGENOW™

For further study of topics covered in this Highlight, log on to **www.cengage.com/sso**.

- Search for "biotechnology" on Health Canada's website: **www.hc-sc.gc.ca**
- Get a "pro" biotechnology perspective from the Council for Biotechnology Information: **www.whybiotech.com**
- For another "for" view, search for "biotechnology" at the International Food Information Council: **www.foodinsight.org**
- Get a "con" biotechnology perspective from the Genetic Engineering section of Greenpeace Canada: **www.greenpeace.org/canada/**
- Another "against" view is available from the Union of Concerned Scientists: **www.ucsusa.org**

References

1. R. M. Welch, Biotechnology, biofortification, and global health, *Food and Nutrition Bulletin* 26 (2005): 419–421.
2. C. Uauy and coauthors, A NAC gene regulating senescence improves grain protein, zinc, and iron content in wheat, *Science* 314 (2006): 1298–1301.
3. J. W. Finley, Selenium accumulation in plant foods, *Nutrition Reviews* 63 (2005): 196–202.
4. U.S. Food and Drug Administration, Animal cloning and food safety, posted January 15, 2008, www.fda.gov/consumer/updates/cloning011508.html.
5. P. B. Fontanarosa and C. D. DeAngelis, Medical applications of biotechnology, *JAMA* 293 (2005): 866–867.
6. G. Brookes and P. Barfoot, Global impact of biotech crops: Socio-economic and environmental effects in the first ten years of commercial use, *Journal of Agrobiotechnology Management and Economics* 9 (2006): 139–151.
7. P. G. Lemaux, Genetically engineered plants and foods: A scientist's analysis of the issues (part I), *Annual Review of Plant Biology* 59 (2008): 771–812.
8. Pew initiative on food and biotechnology, 2007, www.pewagbiotech.org.
9. H. V. Davies, GM organisms and the EU regulatory environment: Allergenicity as a risk component, *Proceedings of the Nutrition Society* 64 (2005): 481–486; R. Mazza and coauthors, Assessing the transfer of genetically modified DNA from feed to animal tissues, *Transgenic Research* 14 (2005): 775–784.
10. O. V. Singh and coauthors, Genetically modified crops: Success, safety assessment, and public concern, *Applied Microbiology and Technology* 71 (2006): 598–607.
11. Health Canada, Genetically modified foods: Approved products. www.hc-sc.gc.ca/fn-an/gmf-agm/appro/index-eng.php, accessed September 21, 2011.
12. Position of the American Dietetic Association: Agricultural and food biotechnology, *Journal of the American Dietetic Association* 106 (2006): 285–293.

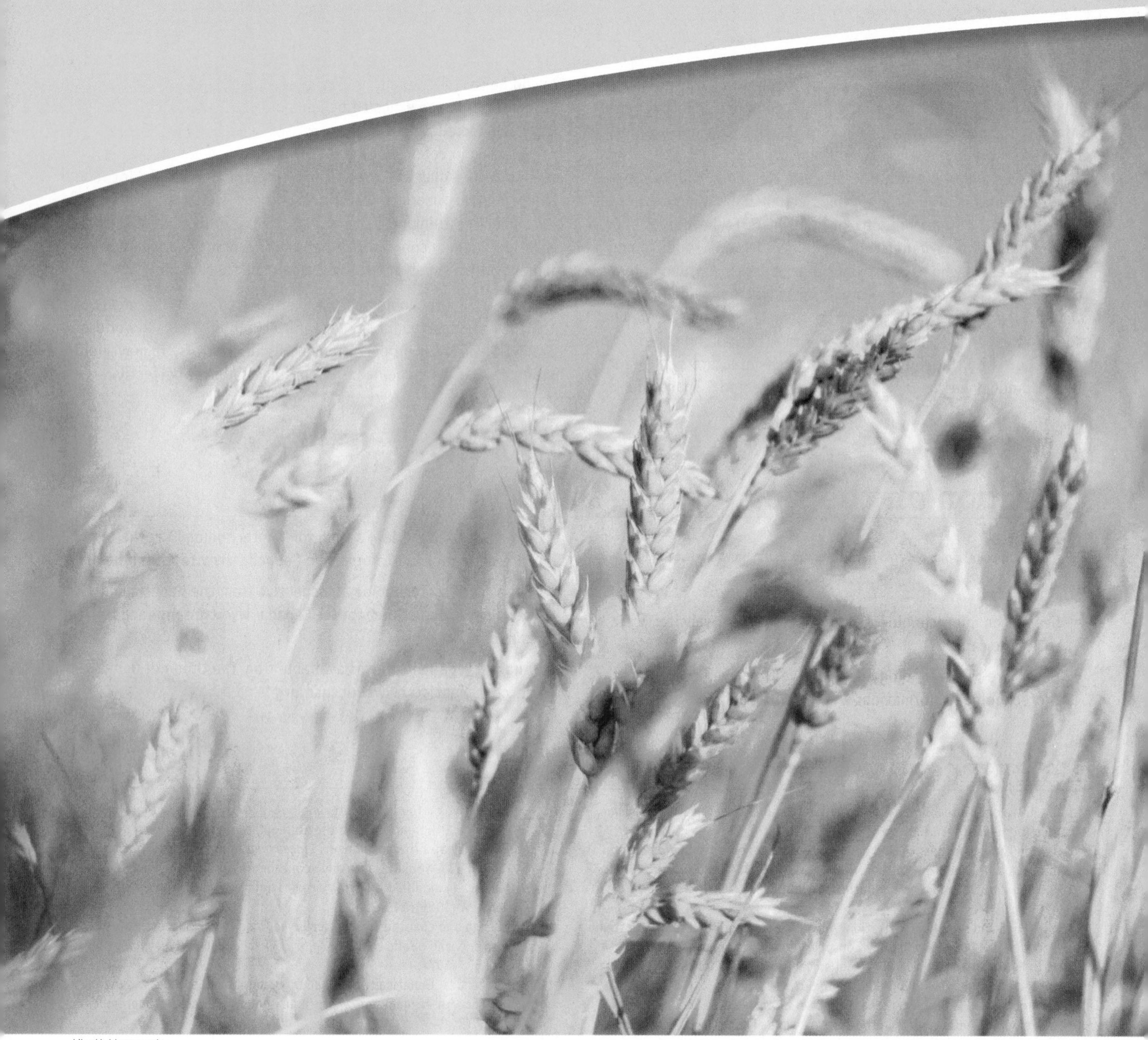

biletskiy/shutterstock

Nutrition in Your Life

Imagine living with hunger from the moment you wake up until the time you thankfully fall asleep—and all through your dreams as well. Meal after meal, day after day, you have little or no food to eat. You know you need food, but you have no money. Would you beg on the street corner or go "dumpster diving" at the nearest fast-food restaurant? And then where would you find your next meal? How will you ever get enough to eat as long as you live in poverty? Resolving the hunger problem—whether in your community or on the other side of the world—depends on alleviating poverty and using resources wisely.

CENGAGENOW™

Throughout this chapter, the CengageNOW logo indicates an opportunity for online self-study, linking you to interactive tutorials, activities, and videos to increase your understanding of chapter concepts.
www.cengage.com/sso

CHAPTER

21

Hunger and the Global Environment

CHAPTER OUTLINE

Worldwide, one person in every seven ♦ experiences persistent hunger—not the healthy appetite triggered by anticipation of a hearty meal, but the painful sensation caused by a lack of food.[1] In this chapter, **hunger** takes on the greater meaning—hunger that develops from prolonged, recurrent, and involuntary lack of food and results in discomfort, illness, weakness, or pain that exceeds the usual uneasy sensation. Such hunger deprives a person of the physical and mental energy needed to enjoy a full life and often leads to severe malnutrition and death. Tens of thousands of people die of hunger-related causes each day—one child every five seconds.

♦ 963 million of the world's 6.7 billion people (14%)

The enormity of the world hunger problem is reflected not only by huge numbers, but also by major challenges. As people populate and pollute the Earth, resources become depleted, making food less available. Hunger and poverty, population growth, and environmental degradation are linked together; thus they tend to worsen one another. Because their causes overlap, so do their solutions; any initiative a person takes to help solve one problem will help solve many others. Eliminating hunger requires a balance among the distribution of food, the numbers of people, and the care of the environment.

Resolving the hunger problem may seem at first beyond the influence of the ordinary person. Can one person's choice to limit family size or to recycle a bottle or to volunteer at a food recovery program make a difference? ♦ In truth, such choices produce several benefits. For one, a person's action may influence many other people over time. For another, a repeated action becomes a habit, with compounded benefits. For still another, making choices with an awareness of the consequences gives a person a sense of personal control, hope, and effectiveness. The daily actions of many concerned people can help solve the problems of hunger in their own neighbourhoods or on the other side of the world.

♦ "Never doubt that a small group of thoughtful, committed people can change the world. Indeed, it is the only thing that ever has." —Margaret Mead

hunger: consequence of food insecurity that, because of prolonged, involuntary lack of food, results in discomfort, illness, weakness, or pain that goes beyond the usual uneasy sensation.

Hunger in Canada

Ideally, all people at all times would have access to enough food to support an active, healthy life. In other words, they would experience **food security.** ♦ Hunger is a concern in Canada. Poverty among women with young children is one important factor related to hunger. ♦ According to Statistics Canada, in 2006 just over 11 percent of children under 18 years lived in low-income families.[2] The percentage is even greater for children in single-parent households. Given the agricultural bounty and enormous wealth in this country, do these numbers surprise you? The limited or uncertain availability of nutritionally adequate and safe foods is known as **food insecurity** ♦ and is a major social problem in our nation today. Inadequate diets lead to poor health in adults and impaired physical, psychological, and cognitive development in children.

About 18 percent of the Canadian population lives in a general state of poverty. Furthermore, Figure 21-1 shows that about 7.5 percent of Canadians live in "food insecure" households.

Based on the National Nutritious Food Basket, Health Canada provides the framework for "stakeholders at the local, provincial and federal level to develop their own food costing protocols and monitor the cost of a nutritious diet in their jurisdiction."[3] Since each jurisdiction may use slightly different protocols, check with your local health unit for the cost of a nutritious food basket in your area. In Ontario, for example the average cost of a nutritious food basket for a week in 2010 for a family of four (mother, father, female child, and teenage boy) was just under $170.00.

♦ **Food security** categories:
- **High food security:** no indications of food-access problems or limitations
- **Marginal food security:** one or two indications of food-access problems but with little or no change in food intake

♦ An estimated one out of seven children lives in poverty.

♦ **Food insecurity** categories:
- **Low food security:** reduced quality of life with little or no indication of reduced food intake; formerly known as *food insecurity without hunger*
- **Very low food security:** multiple indications of disrupted eating patterns and reduced food intake; formerly known as *food insecurity with hunger*

FIGURE 21-1 Household Food Insecurity in Canada, 2007–2008

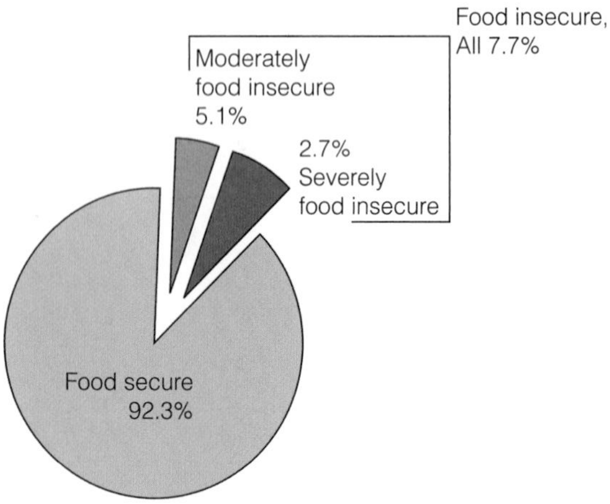
Food insecure, All 7.7%
Moderately food insecure 5.1%
2.7% Severely food insecure
Food secure 92.3%

SOURCE: Household Food Insecurity in Canada, 2007–2008: Key Statistics and Graphic. Health Canada, 2011. Reproduced with the permission of the Minister of Health, 2011.

Other Aspects of Hunger in Canada

At its most extreme, people experience hunger because they have absolutely no food. More often, they have too little food (**food insufficiency**) and try to stretch their limited resources by eating small meals or skipping meals—often for days at a time. Sometimes hungry people obtain enough food to satisfy their hunger, perhaps by seeking food assistance or finding food through socially unacceptable ways—begging from strangers, stealing from markets, or scavenging through garbage cans, for example. Sometimes obtaining food raises concerns for food safety—for example, when rot, slime, mould, or insects have damaged foods or when people eat others' leftovers or meat from roadkill.

Hunger has many causes, but in developed countries, the primary cause is **food poverty.** People are hungry not because there is no food nearby to purchase, but because they lack money. For a sample of the many programs in Canada that promote food security, see Table 21-1; to keep abreast of food insecurity in Canada, see Statistics Canada's website (see Nutrition on the Net). In 2005, two reports on household food insecurity in Canada were published.[4] Dietitians of Canada (DC) also wrote a position statement entitled "Individual and Household Food Insecurity in Canada: Position of Dietitians of Canada."[5] The full report is available at the DC website (www.dietitians.ca), although a summary has also been published. According to these reports, the households most at risk include one-parent families with one or more young children, those receiving social assistance, and Aboriginal people living off reserves. DC also holds that access to adequate amounts of safe, nutritious, and culturally appropriate food at all times is a fundamental human right. More recently (April 2007), DC also released their position statement on community food security (CFS), where they advocate that "CFS involves long-term planning with a wide range of stakeholders working toward a healthy, just, and sustainable food system."[6] Eradicating hunger is in everyone's interest because the hunger of individual families affects the nation as a whole. Even those who fall into the low-income bracket ♦ may not have food security. Physical and mental illnesses and disabilities, unemployment, low-paying jobs, unexpected or ongoing medical expenses, and high living expenses threaten financial stability. When money

♦ Almost 10% of Canadians fall into the low-income bracket.

food security: access to enough food to sustain a healthy and active life.

food insecurity: limited or uncertain access to foods of sufficient quality or quantity to sustain a healthy and active life.

food insufficiency: an inadequate amount of food due to a lack of resources.

food poverty: hunger resulting from inadequate access to available food for various reasons, including inadequate resources, political obstacles, social disruptions, poor weather conditions, and lack of transportation.

is tight, people are forced to choose between food and life's other necessities—utilities, housing, and medical care. Food costs are more variable and flexible; people can purchase fewer groceries to lower the monthly food bill, but they usually can't pay only a portion of the bills for electricity, rent, or medication. Other problems further contribute to food poverty, such as abuse of alcohol and other drugs; lack of awareness of available food assistance programs; and the reluctance of people, particularly the elderly, to accept what they perceive as "welfare" or "charity." Lack of resources remains the major cause of food poverty in developed countries, and solving this problem would do a lot to relieve hunger.

Ideally, all people would always have enough nutritious food to support an active, healthy life; in other words, they would experience food security. Yet, according to Food Banks Canada's national survey of emergency food programs, HungerCount, the number of food bank users in Canada more than doubled from 378 000 in March 1989 to almost 870 000 in March 2010 (highest number on record) and to just over 850 000 in 2011. These numbers are released on World Food Day (October 16) each year; watch for them in the coming year.

Ironically, hunger and obesity exist side by side—sometimes within the same household or even the same person.[7] That hunger reflects an inadequate food intake and obesity implies an excessive intake seems paradoxical, but research studies have confirmed the relationship.[8] The highest rates of obesity occur among those living in the greatest poverty—the same people who live with food insecurity.[9] Unfortunately, many healthful food choices, such as fruits and vegetables, are not readily available in low-income or rural neighbourhoods.[10] Furthermore, fruits and vegetables tend to cost more than the energy-dense foods that foster weight gain but offer few, if any, nutrients. Foods such as doughnuts, pizzas, and hamburgers provide the most energy and satiety for the least cost. Quite simply, poor-quality diets deliver more kcalories, but fewer nutrients, for less money; high-quality diets deliver fewer kcalories, but more nutrients, for more money.[11] People who are unsure about their next meal may overeat when food or money are available. Interestingly, food insecure people who do not participate in food assistance programs have a greater risk of obesity than those who do participate—illustrating that providing food actually helps to prevent obesity.[12] Figure 21-2 shows how poverty and food insecurity can lead to both malnutrition and obesity.[13]

FIGURE 21-2 The Poverty-Obesity Paradox

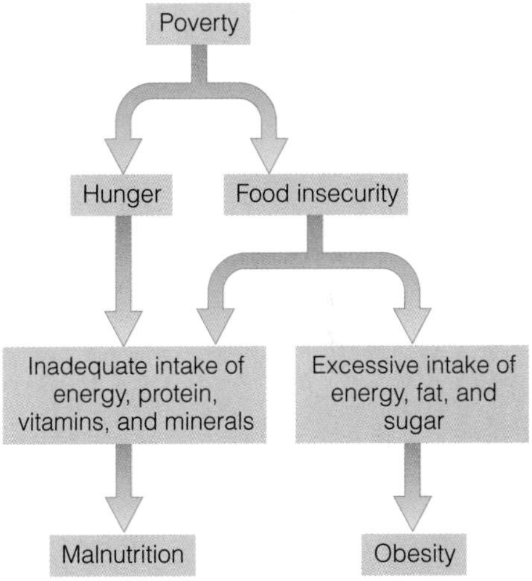
Poverty
Hunger
Food insecurity
Inadequate intake of energy, protein, vitamins, and minerals
Excessive intake of energy, fat, and sugar
Malnutrition
Obesity

Canadian Programs Promoting Food Security

According to Food Banks Canada's 2010 national survey of emergency food programs, HungerCount, due in part to the recent economic downturn, there was an increase of over 75 000 users in 2009; 38 percent of those helped by a **food bank** during 2010 were children and 38 percent were individuals who were single while over 50 percent were receiving social assistance (see Figure 21-3 on page 700).[14] The Canadian Living Foundation's "Breakfast for Learning" program is "Canada's only national, non-profit organization dedicated to supporting child nutrition,"[15] Help from industry is also available—for example, according to Food & Consumer Products of Canada, "The manufacturing sector of the food, beverage and consumer product industry ... [donated] more than 5 million bags of groceries to food banks in Canada."[16]

Food Recovery Programs Food recovery programs ♦, such as Second Harvest, collect and distribute good food that would otherwise go to waste; those donating the food often qualify for tax deductions for their donations. Although these efforts provide emergency relief to hungry people, they leave unsolved the greater problems of low wages and poverty among people who lack higher education or training.

Food Assistance Programs For a sample of the many programs in Canada that promote food security, see Table 21-1 (p. 700); to keep abreast of food insecurity in Canada, see Statistics Canada's website (see Nutrition on the Net).

♦ Four common methods of food recovery:
- *Field gleaning:* Collecting crops from fields that either have already been harvested or are not profitable to harvest.
- *Perishable food rescue or salvage:* Collecting perishable produce from wholesalers and markets.
- *Prepared food rescue:* Collecting prepared foods from commercial kitchens.
- *Nonperishable food collection:* Collecting processed foods from wholesalers and markets.

food bank: a facility that collects and distributes food donations to authorized organizations feeding the hungry.

TABLE 21-1 Examples of Canadian Programs that Promote Food Security

- Food Skills Programs: e.g., A Seat at the Table-Resource guide for local governments to promote food secure communities
- Community Kitchens
- Community Gardens
- FoodShare: www.foodshare.net
- Hunger Relief Advisory Committee of London
- Meals on Wheels: www.mealcall.org/canada/
- School Feeding Programs: e.g., www.breakfastforlearning.ca
- Wheels to Meals: www.wheelstomeals.org

SOURCE: From SIZER/WHITNEY/PICHE. Nutrition, 2E. © 2012 Nelson Education Ltd. Reproduced by permission. www.cengage.com/permissions

FIGURE 21-3 Household Composition of Food Bank Clients: March 2010 (percent)

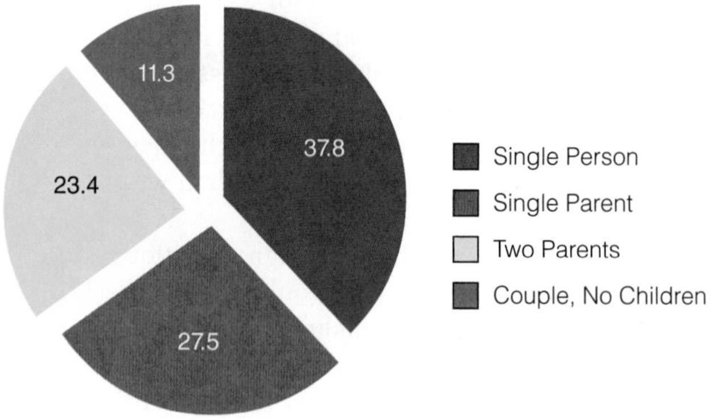
11.3
37.8
23.4
27.5
Single Person
Single Parent
Two Parents
Couple, No Children

SOURCE: Food Banks Canada (2010). HungerCount 2010. Toronto: Food Banks Canada.

Community Efforts **Food recovery** programs depend on volunteers. Concerned citizens work through local agencies and churches to feed the hungry. Community-based **food pantries** provide groceries, and **soup kitchens** and **emergency shelters** serve prepared meals. Meals often deliver adequate nourishment, but most homeless people receive fewer than one and a half meals a day, so many are still inadequately nourished. A combination of various strategies helps to build food security in a community.[17]

IN SUMMARY **Food insecurity is widespread in Canada, especially among those living in poverty. Government and other assistance programs help to relieve poverty and hunger. Food recovery programs and other community efforts are equally important.**

World Hunger

As distressing as hunger is in Canada, the prevalence is greater and the consequences more severe in developing countries. Although hunger in developing countries has diverse causes, once again, the primary cause is poverty, ♦ and the poverty is far more extreme than in Canada. Most people cannot grasp the severity of poverty in the developing world. One-sixth of the world's 6.7 billion people have no land and no possessions *at all*. They are the "poorest poor." They survive on less than $1 a day each, and they lack safe housing, clean water, and health care. They cannot read or write. The average North American housecat receives twice as much protein every day as one of these people, and the cost of keeping that cat is greater than such a person's annual income.

♦ The international poverty line for an individual is $1.08 a day or about $394 a year.

The "poorest poor" are usually female. Many societies around the world undervalue females, providing girls with poorer diets and fewer opportunities than boys. Malnourished girls become malnourished mothers who give birth to low-birthweight infants—and the cycle of hunger, malnutrition, and poverty continues.

Not only does poverty cause hunger, but tragically, hunger worsens poverty by robbing a person of the good health and the physical and mental energy needed to be active and productive. Hungry people simply cannot work hard enough to get themselves out of poverty. Economists calculate that cutting world hunger and malnutrition in half by 2015 would generate a value of more than $120 billion in longer, healthier, and more productive lives.

Food Shortages

World hunger brings to mind victims of **famine**, a severe food shortage in an area that causes widespread starvation and death. In recent

food recovery: collecting wholesome food for distribution to low-income people who are hungry.

food pantries: programs that provide groceries to be prepared and eaten at home.

soup kitchens: programs that provide prepared meals to be eaten on site.

emergency shelters: facilities that are used to provide temporary housing.

famine: widespread and extreme scarcity of food in an area that causes starvation and death in a large portion of the population.

HOW TO Plan Healthy, Thrifty Meals

Chapter 2 introduces *Canada's Food Guide* and principles for planning a healthy diet. Meeting that goal on a limited budget adds to the challenge. To save money and spend wisely, plan and shop for healthy meals with the following tips in mind:

Planning

- Make a grocery list before going to the store to avoid expensive "impulse" items.
- Do not shop when hungry.
- Use leftovers.
- Centre meals on rice, noodles, and other grains.
- Use small quantities of meat, poultry, fish, or eggs.
- Use legumes instead of meat, poultry, fish, or eggs several times a week.
- Use cooked cereals such as oatmeal instead of ready-to-eat breakfast cereals.
- Cook large quantities when time and money allow.
- Check for sales and clip coupons for products you need; plan meals to take advantage of sale items.

Shopping

- Buy day-old bread and other products from the bakery outlet.
- Select whole foods instead of convenience foods (potatoes instead of instant mashed potatoes, for example).
- Try store brands.
- Buy fresh produce that is in season; buy canned or frozen items at other times.
- Buy only the amount of fresh foods that you will eat before it spoils. Buy large bags of frozen items or dry goods; when cooking, take out the amount needed and store the remainder.
- Buy powdered skim milk; mix and refrigerate quantities needed for a day or two. Buy fresh milk in 2 or 4 litres.
- Buy less expensive cuts of meat. Chuck and bottom round roast are usually inexpensive; cover during cooking and cook long enough to make meat tender. Buy whole chickens instead of pieces.
- Compare the unit price (cost per ounce, for example) of similar foods so that you can select the least expensive brand or size.
- Buy nonfood items such as toilet paper and laundry detergent at discount stores instead of grocery stores.

For daily menus and recipes for healthy, thrifty meals, visit the Heart & Stroke Foundation's HealthCheck Program **(www.healthcheck.org, where you will also find My Heart&Stroke HealthCheck Recipe Helper app for your mobile phone).**

TRY IT For readers interested in better understanding their personal eating pattern (e.g., the nutrient content of their meals relative to current recomendations) and physical activity choices, sign up to use the Dietitians of Canada's 'eaTracker' program at **www.eatracker.ca.** Also, if you wish to speak to a Registered Dietitian about nutrition and healthy eating, some provinces have a toll-free number you can call (e.g., EatRight Ontario: 1-877-510-5102) and website with valuable information on healthy menu planning, healthy recipes, and videos on proper food handing (e.g., www.eatrightontario.ca).

years, the natural causes of famine—drought, flood, and pests—have become less important than the political causes created by people. Figure 21-4 (p. 702) shows the hunger hotspots in the world.

Political Turbulence A sudden increase in food prices, a drop in workers' incomes, or a change in government policy can quickly leave millions hungry. An estimated 30 million people died during the Chinese famine of 1959 through 1961, the worst famine of the 20th century. The main cause was government policies associated with the Great Leap Forward, a government initiative that was intended to transform China's economy. However, the poorly planned communal farm system and the widespread waste of resources devastated the Chinese agricultural system.

Armed Conflicts In the past decade, armed conflict and political unrest were the dominant cause of famine worldwide. In times of war, farmers become warriors, their agricultural fields become battlegrounds, the citizens go hungry, and the warring factions often block famine relief. The world continues to struggle to find a middle ground between respecting the sovereignty of nations and insisting that all nations allow humanitarian assistance to reach the people. When supplementary food programs reach the people in war-torn countries, the children benefit.

Natural Disasters Natural disasters and other poor weather conditions create food shortages. In 2007, a cyclone and flooding in Bangladesh dramatically

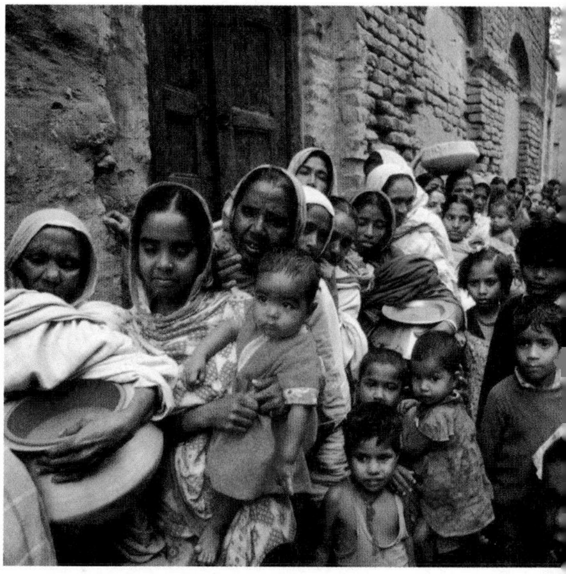

Tim Graham/Getty Images

Feeding the hungry—in Calcutta, India.

FIGURE 21-4 Hunger Hotspots

Hunger is prevalent in the developing world, with some countries reporting hunger and malnutrition in more than half of their population.

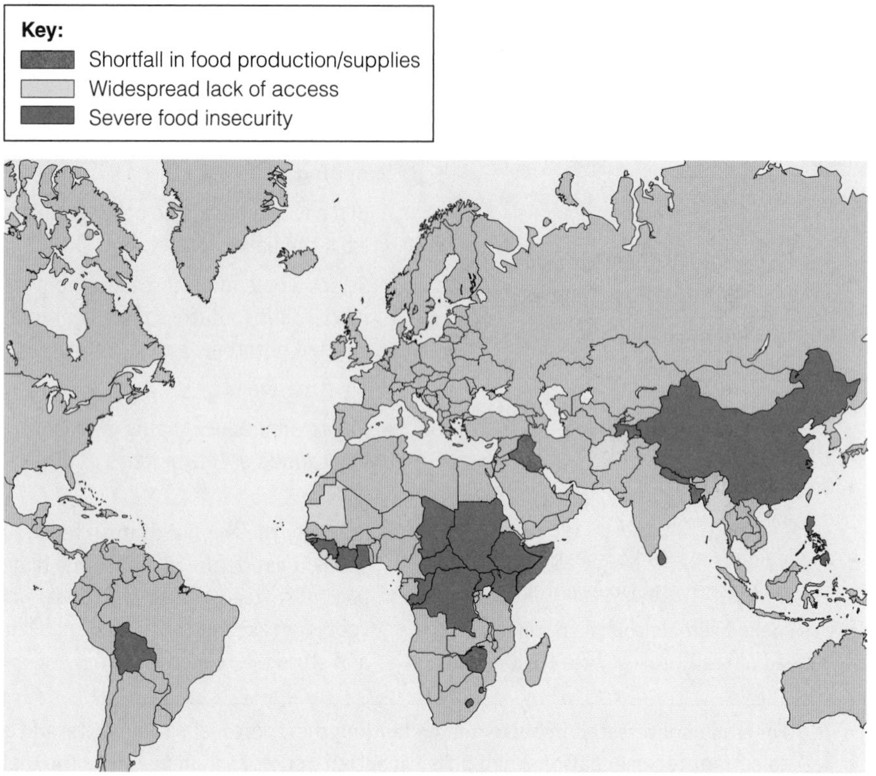
Key:
Shortfall in food production/supplies
Widespread lack of access
Severe food insecurity

SOURCE: *The State of Food Insecurity in the World* published by the Food and Agriculture Organization of the United Nations © 2010 FAO.

reduced food supplies. During such natural disasters, emergency food relief from countries around the world provides a safety net for countries in need. International food relief programs also provide ongoing food assistance to countries, such as Ethiopia, that are chronically short of food because of ongoing drought and poverty.

♦ To help prevent blindness and reduce measles mortality, health-care workers distribute vitamin A supplements to millions of children worldwide.

Malnutrition

Although we usually associate world hunger with famine, the numbers affected by famine are relatively small compared with those suffering from persistent hunger and malnutrition. The nutrients most likely to be lacking are iron, iodine, and vitamin A. The prevalence and consequences of these deficiencies stagger the mind.[18] More than 30 percent of the world's population have iron-deficiency anemia, a leading cause of maternal deaths, premature births, low birthweights, infections, and premature deaths. Iodine deficiency affects one out of seven, resulting in stillbirths and irreversible mental retardation (cretinism) in 37 million newborns every year. Almost 80 million children (younger than age five) suffer from symptoms of vitamin A deficiency—blindness, growth retardation, and poor resistance to common childhood infections such as measles. ♦ The deficiency symptoms of these nutrients and those of the other vitamins and minerals are presented in Chapters 10 through 14; Chapter 6 describes protein-energy malnutrition; and Chapters 16 through 18 examine the effects of malnutrition during various stages of the life cycle. The consequences of nutrient deficiencies are felt not only by individuals, but by entire nations. When people suffer from mental retardation, growth failure, blindness, infections, and other consequences of malnutrition, the economy of their country declines as productivity decreases and health-care costs increase. The dramatic signs of malnutrition are most evident at each end of the life span in a nation's high infant mortality rate and short life expectancy.

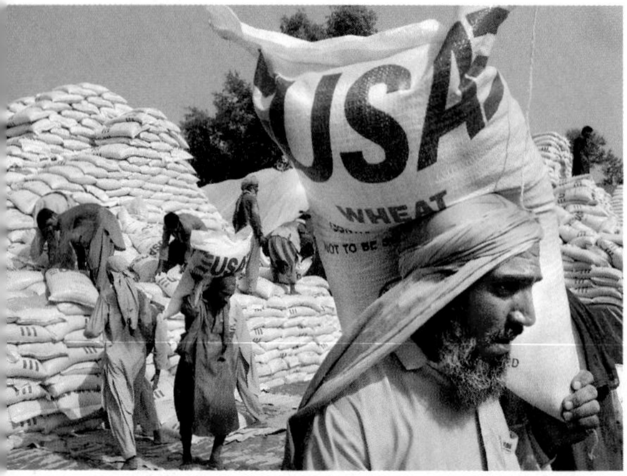
USA
WHEAT

International efforts help to relieve hunger and poverty in Afghanistan and around the world.

In addition to specific nutrient deficiencies, one child in six worldwide is born underweight, and one in four children is underweight by the age of five. ♦ These underweight children are malnourished and readily develop the diseases of poverty: parasitic and infectious diseases that cause diarrhea (dysentery and cholera), acute respiratory illnesses (pneumonia and whooping cough), measles, and malaria. The synergistic combination of infectious disease and malnutrition dramatically increases the likelihood of early death.[19] Compared with adequately nourished children, the risk of death is 2.5 times greater for children with mild malnutrition, 4.6 times greater for children with moderate malnutrition, and 8.4 times greater for children with severe malnutrition. Each year, 5.6 million children die as a result of hunger and malnutrition. Most of them do not starve to death—they die from the diarrhea and dehydration that accompany infections. Health-care workers around the world save millions of lives ♦ each year by effectively reversing dehydration and correcting the diarrhea with **oral rehydration therapy (ORT).** ORT is a simple, inexpensive, and effective treatment that consists of giving a sugar and salt solution orally.

♦ More than half of the world's underweight children live in just three countries:
- Bangladesh
- India
- Pakistan

♦ To prevent death from diarrheal disease, provide:
- Adequate sanitation
- Safe water
- Oral rehydration therapy

Diminishing Food Supply The demand for food is great and continues to increase. But crop **yields** have levelled off. Environmental degradation and dwindling water supplies may limit further growth in the world's food production in many agricultural areas. No part of the world is safely insulated against future food shortages. Developed countries may be the last to feel the effects, but they will ultimately go as the world goes. Presently, Canada ranks seventh globally in terms of arable land and our rank in the world in terms of the production of cereals, meat, and fish/aquaculture is 8th, 10th, and 19th, respectively.[20]

IN SUMMARY **Natural causes such as drought, flood, and pests and political causes such as armed conflicts and government policies all contribute to the extreme hunger and poverty seen in the developing countries. To meet future demands for food, technology must improve food production, and nations must control overpopulation.**

Poverty and Overpopulation

The world's population is rising at an alarming rate, as Figure 21-5 (p. 704) shows. Skyrocketing numbers threaten the Earth's capacity ♦ to provide safe water and adequate food for its inhabitants. Contaminated water and food shortages are responsible for much of the world's disease and death.[21]

♦ The maximum number of people the Earth can support over time is its **human carrying capacity.**

The sheer magnitude of the world's annual population increase of more than 70 million people is difficult to comprehend. Every half-second, the world's population increases by another person. Every six months, the world adds the equivalent of another California.

As the world's population continues to grow, much of the increase is occurring in developing countries where hunger and malnutrition are already widespread. More people sharing the little food available can only worsen the problem. Stabilizing the population may be the only way the world's food production will be able to keep up with demands. Without population stabilization, the world can neither support the lives of people nor halt environmental degradation. Before the population problem can be resolved, it may be necessary to remedy the poverty problem. In countries around the world, economic growth has been accompanied by slowed population growth.

Population growth is a central factor contributing to poverty and hunger. The reverse is also true: poverty and hunger contribute to population growth.

Population Growth Leads to Hunger and Poverty The first of these cause-and-effect relationships is easy to understand. As a population grows larger, more mouths must be fed, and the worse poverty and hunger become.

oral rehydration therapy (ORT): the administration of a simple solution of sugar, salt, and water, taken by mouth, to treat dehydration caused by diarrhea. A simple ORT recipe:
- ½ L boiling water
- 20 mL sugar
- 2.5 mL salt

yields: production per acre.

FIGURE 21-5 World Population Totals and Projections

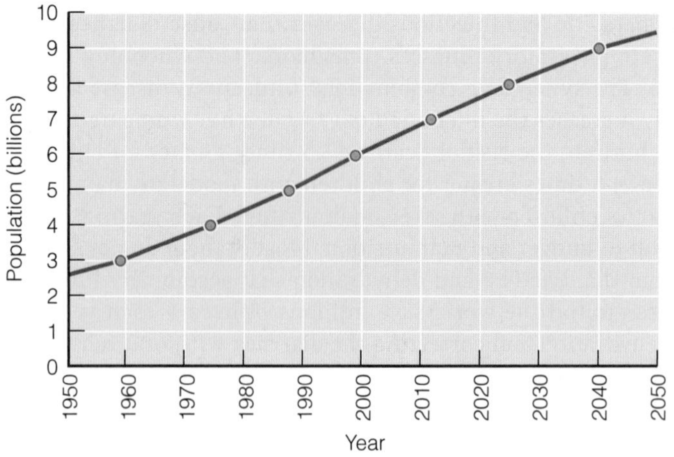
10
9
8
7
6
5
4
3
2
1
0
Population (billions)
1950
1960
1970
1980
1990
2000
2010
2020
2030
2040
2050
Year

SOURCE: U.S. Census Bureau, International Data Base, updated December 2008.

Population growth also contributes to hunger indirectly by using agricultural land for growing cities and industry. Remaining lands are insufficient to produce enough food for the people. The world's poorest people live in the world's most damaged and inhospitable environments.

Hunger and Poverty Lead to Population Growth How does poverty lead to overpopulation? Poverty and its consequences—inadequate food and shelter—leave women vulnerable to physical abuse, forced marriages, and prostitution. Furthermore, they lack access to reproductive health care and family planning counseling. Also, in some regions of the world, families depend on children to farm the land, haul water, and care for adults in their old age. Children are an economic asset for these families. Poverty claims many young children, who are among the most likely to die from malnutrition and disease. If a family faces ongoing poverty, the parents often choose to have many children to ensure that some will survive to adulthood. People are willing to risk having fewer children only if they are sure that their children will live and that the family can develop other economic assets (skills, businesses, land).

Breaking the Cycle Relieving poverty and hunger may be a necessary first step in curbing population growth. When people attain better access to health care, education, and family planning, the death rate falls. At first, births outnumber deaths, but as the standard of living continues to improve, families become willing to risk having fewer children. Then the birthrate falls. Thus improvements in living standards help stabilize the population.

The link between improved economic status and slowed population growth has been demonstrated in several countries. Central to achieving this success is sustainable development that includes not only economic growth, but a sharing of resources among all groups. Where this has happened, population growth has slowed the most: in parts of Sri Lanka, Taiwan, Malaysia, and Costa Rica, for example. Where economic growth has occurred but only the rich have grown richer, population growth has remained high. Examples include Brazil, the Philippines, and Thailand, where large families continue to be a major economic asset for the poor.

As a society gains economic footing, education also becomes a higher priority. A society that educates its children, both males and females, experiences a drop in birthrates. Education, particularly for girls and women, brings improvements in family life, including improved nutrition, better sanitation, effective birth control, and elevated status. With improved conditions, more infants live to adulthood, making smaller families feasible.

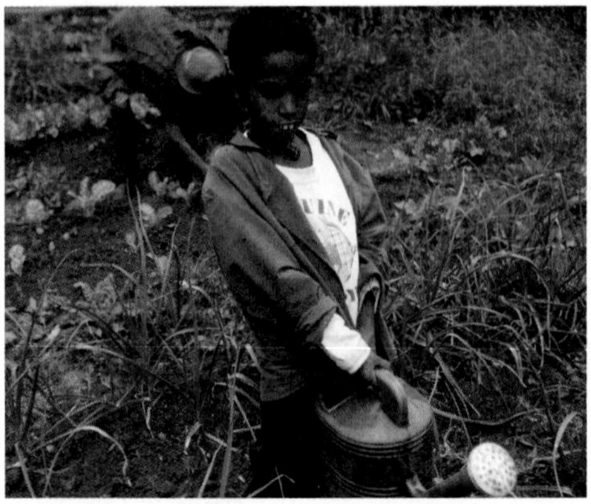

Families in developing countries depend on their children to help provide for daily needs.

IN SUMMARY **More people means more mouths to feed, which worsens the problems of poverty and hunger. Poverty and hunger, in turn, encourage parents to have more children. Breaking this cycle requires improving the economic status of the people and providing them with health care, education, and family planning.**

The Global Environment

The world currently produces enough food to feed all of its people, ♦ and the problem of hunger today remains a problem of unequal distribution of land to grow crops or income to purchase foods. If present trends continue, however, the time is fast approaching when there will be an absolute deficit of food. This conclusion seems inescapable. The world's increasing population threatens the world's capacity to produce adequate food. Until the nations of the world resolve the population problem, they can neither support the lives of people already born nor remedy global trends toward environmental deterioration. And to resolve the population problem, a necessary first step is to remedy the poverty problems, for reasons already discussed. Of the 70 million people being added to the population each year, 95 percent are born in the most poverty-stricken areas of the world.

♦ World agriculture produces enough food to provide each person with 3747 kcal/day. Food consumption in North America averages 2720 kcal/day.

In recent years, even as crop yields set new record highs, more people needed more food and reserves dwindled. Food prices skyrocketed as the costs of energy and fertilizer increased dramatically. Hunger worsened as the world experienced its worst food crisis in a generation. Efforts to identify some of the causes of, and possible solutions for, hunger have focused on the environment.

Hunger and Environment Connections

Hunger interacts with the environment in two major ways:

- Producing enough food to feed billions of people around the world damages the environment.
- A damaged environment cannot adequately support the production of enough food to feed billions of people around the world.

Without concerted efforts to improve food production in ways that will protect the environment, the vicious cycle of hunger and environmental degradation will continue, and poverty and population growth will escalate.

Planting Crops Producing food costs the Earth dearly. To grow food, we clear land—prairie, wetland, and forest—losing native ecosystems and wildlife. Then we plough the fields and plant crops. The soil loses nutrients as each crop is harvested, so fertilizer is applied. Some fertilizer runs off, polluting the waterways and stimulating algae growth. Some soil erodes into the waterways and interferes with the growth of aquatic plants and animals. By the time the water reaches the seas, it is unsuitable for most marine life. Agriculture is the largest single source of **nonpoint water pollution.** Pollution from "point sources," such as sewage plants or factories, is relatively easy to control, but runoff from fields and pastures enters waterways from so many broad regions that it is nearly impossible to control.

To protect crops against weeds and pests, farmers apply herbicides and pesticides. These chemicals also pollute the water and, wherever the wind carries them, the air. Most herbicides and pesticides injure more than weeds and pests; they also injure native plants, native insects, and animals that eat those plants and insects. Ironically, widespread use of pesticides and herbicides causes pests and weeds to evolve, becoming more resistant. Consequently, farmers must use more pesticides and herbicides. These chemicals pose hazards for farm workers who handle them, and the residues can create health problems for consumers as well (as Chapter 20 discusses).

nonpoint water pollution: water pollution caused by runoff from all over an area rather than from discrete "point" sources. An example is the pollution caused by runoff from agricultural fields.

FIGURE 21-6 Kilograms of Grain Needed to Produce One Kilogram of Bread and One Kilogram of Animal Weight Gain

To gain one kilogram, animals raised for food have to eat many more kilograms of grain than it takes to make a kilogram of bread.

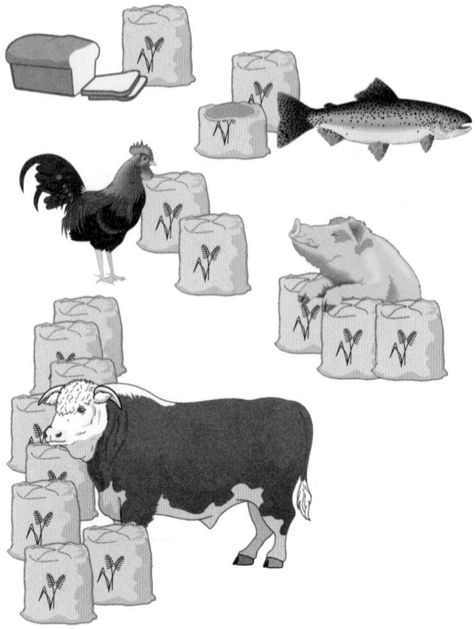

SOURCE: Idea and data from T. R. Reid, Feeding the planet, *National Geographic,* October 1998, pp. 58–74

♦ Excessive fishing, or **overfishing,** means catching fish at a faster rate than they can reproduce.

♦ The practice of fish farming is called **aquaculture.**

♦ Litres of water to produce 1 serving of:

- Lettuce: 23
- Milk: 185
- Steak: 9900

fossil fuels: coal, oil, and natural gas.

Finally, when fields are irrigated, the water evaporates, but the salts do not. Consequently, salts accumulate on the soil surface. As the surface soil becomes increasingly salty, plant growth suffers. Irrigation can also deplete the water supply over time as it drains water from surface waters or from underground; then, the water evaporates or runs off. Excessive irrigation can dry up rivers and lakes and lower the water table of a whole region. A vicious cycle develops. The drier the region becomes, the more farmers irrigate, and the more they irrigate, the drier the region becomes.

Raising Livestock Raising livestock also takes a toll. Like plant crops, herds of livestock occupy land that once maintained itself in a natural state. The land suffers the losses of native plants and animals, soil erosion, water depletion, and desert formation. Alternatively, animals in large concentrated areas such as cattle feedlots create environmental problems when huge masses of animal wastes are produced. To prevent contamination of local soils and water supplies, the U.S. Environmental Protection Agency suggests several strategies for managing livestock, poultry, and horse waste. In addition to manure, cows produce large quantities of methane—a potent gas that may contribute to climate change.

In addition to the waste problems, animals must be fed; grain is grown for them on other land. That land may require fertilizers, herbicides, pesticides, and irrigation, too. In North America, more cropland is used to produce grains for livestock than to produce grains for people. Figure 21-6 compares the grain required to produce various foods.

Fishing Fishing also incurs environmental costs. On the sea, we harvest fish with little thought of the dwindling supplies or the environmental damage incurred. Excessive fishing ♦ diminishes the availability of seafood for people to eat, upsets the balance of marine life, and reduces water quality.[22] Some fishing methods, such as nets and filament line, kill nonfood species and deplete large populations of aquatic animals, such as dolphins. Some fishing methods damage the ocean floor. Environmental habitats can also be destroyed by irresponsible fish farms. ♦ Table H21-1 (p. 714) in the highlight that follows this chapter presents lists of seafood sorted from an environmental perspective.

Fishing is also energy-intensive, requiring fuel for boats, refrigeration, processing, packing, and transport. Water pollution incurs health risks when people eat contaminated fish. Bioaccumulation of toxins in fish is a serious problem in some areas; in others it rules out fish consumption altogether.

Energy Overuse The entire food industry, whether based on growing crops, raising livestock, or fishing, requires energy, which primarily entails burning **fossil fuels.** Massive fossil fuel use threatens the environment by causing air and water pollution, changing climate patterns, depleting the ozone layer, and more. In the United States, for example, the food industry consumes about 20 percent of all the energy the nation uses. Most of this energy is used to run farm machinery and to produce fertilizers and pesticides. Energy is also used to process, package, transport, refrigerate, store, and prepare foods.

Water Misuse Food production uses an enormous amount of water. It takes an estimated 5.7 million litres ♦ of water to produce the food for one U.S. consumer for one year.[23] According to the U.S. Environmental Protection Agency, current farming practices are also responsible for an estimated 70 percent of the pollution in U.S. rivers and streams. Growing crops adds sediment, nutrients, and pesticides to the water. Irrigating crops depletes groundwater supplies, causing the land to become desert, which ironically can lead to flooding.

Biodiversity By the year 2050, some 40 000 plant species may become extinct. Traditional agricultural practices and the increasing uniformity of global food habits have failed to conserve species diversity. Wheat, rice, and maize provide more than half of the food energy around the world; only two dozen other crops provide the remainder. As people everywhere eat the same limited array of foods, local regions' native, genetically diverse plants no longer seem worth preserving. Yet, in the future, as the climate and environment change, those may be the very plants that people will need for food sources. A wild species of corn that grows in a dry climate, for example, might contain the genetic information necessary to help make domestic corn resistant to drought. (Highlight 20 offers several examples of how biotechnology is being used to improve food crops.)

In short, food production has taken a tremendous toll on the environment. And environmental problems are reducing the world's ability to feed its people and keep them healthy.[24] For the most part, our food production systems are not **sustainable.**

Sustainable Solutions

Can advances in agriculture compensate for the increases in population growth and the losses caused by environmental degradation? Historically, agricultural yields improved with advances in irrigation systems, fertilizers, and genetic strains. Today, however, the contributions these measures can make are reaching their limits, in part because they have also created environmental problems.

Irrigation can no longer increase crop yields because almost all the land that can benefit from irrigation is already receiving it. In fact, rising concentrations of salt in the soil—a by-product of irrigation—are *lowering* yields on many of the world's irrigated croplands.

Nor can fertilizer use significantly enhance agricultural production. Much of the fertilizing that can be done is being done—and with great effect; fertilizers support some 40 percent of the world's total crop yields. Using more fertilizer, however, will not increase yields further and adds to the pollution of nearby waterways.

As for the development of high-yielding strains of crops, recent advances have been dramatic, but even they may be inadequate to change the overall trends. Furthermore, the raw materials necessary for developing new crops have become less available as genetic variation for many plant species is lost. Of the 5000 food plants grown throughout the world a few centuries ago, only 150 are cultivated in commercial agriculture today. Most of the world's population relies on only five cereals, three legumes, and three root crops to meet their energy needs. Even among these, valuable strains are vanishing.

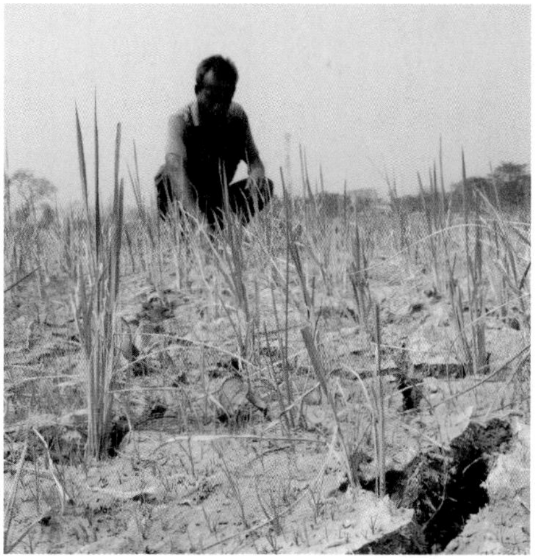
© epa/Corbis

Without water, croplands become deserts.

Sustainable Agriculture

For each environmental problem, agricultural solutions are being considered. Many farmers are implementing **sustainable agriculture** practices that can be adapted to meet the particular needs of a local area. The crop yields from farms that employ these practices often compare favourably with those from farms using less sustainable methods. Table 21-2 (p. 708) contrasts low-input, sustainable agriculture methods with high-input, unsustainable methods. Many sustainable practices are not really new, incidentally; they would be familiar to our great-grandparents. Farmers today are rediscovering the benefits of traditional techniques as they adapt and experiment with them in search of sustainable methods. According to Agriculture and Agri-Food Canada's Sustainable Development Strategy 2007–2009, "in environmental terms, sustainable agriculture and agri-food production is built on the sustainable use of natural resources, such as land, air, water, and genetic resources; the protection of soil, water, and air quality; and the conservation of the rich biodiversity found on agricultural lands and in the wide array of agricultural crops and animals."[25]

Sustainable Development

The keys to solving the world's hunger, poverty, and environmental problems are in the hands of both the poor and the rich nations but require different efforts from them. The poor nations need to provide contraceptive technology and family planning information to their citizens, develop better programs to assist the poor, and slow and reverse the destruction of environmental resources. The rich nations need to stem their wasteful and

sustainable: able to continue indefinitely; using resources at such a rate that the Earth can keep on replacing them and producing pollutants at a rate with which the environment and human cleanup efforts can keep pace, so that no net accumulation of pollution occurs.

sustainable agriculture: ability to produce food indefinitely, with little or no harm to the environment.

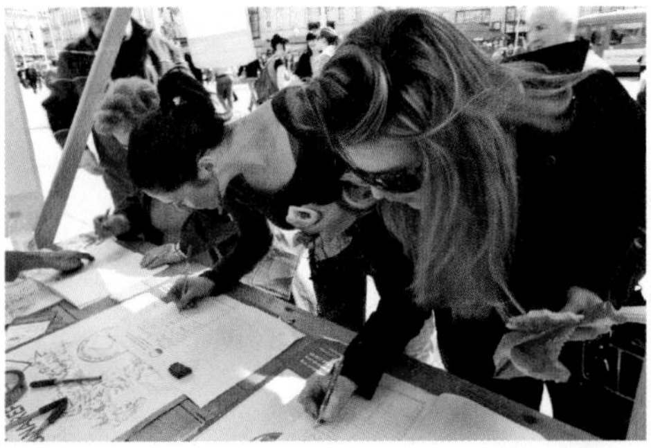
© NIKOLA SOLIC/Reuters/Corbis

Each person's choice to get involved and be heard can help lead to needed change.

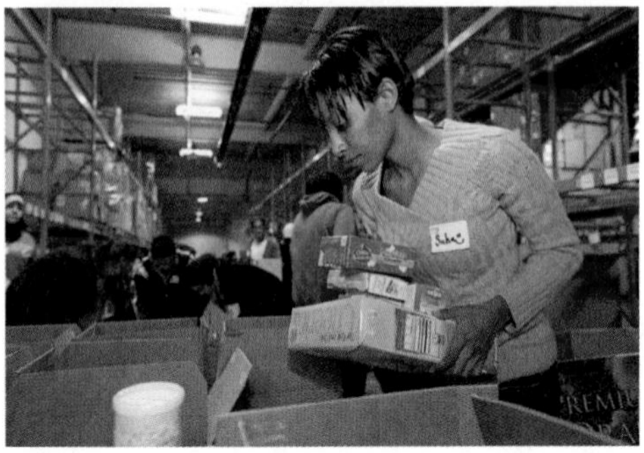
Jim West/GetStock

The fight against hunger depends on the helping hands of caring volunteers.

polluting uses of resources and energy, which are contributing to global environmental degradation. They also must become willing to ease the debt burden that many poor nations face. Relieving poverty will help relieve environmental degradation and hunger.

To rephrase a well-known adage: If you give a man a fish, he will eat for a day. If you teach him to fish and enable him to buy and maintain his own gear and bait, he will eat for a lifetime and help to feed others. Unlike food giveaways and money doles, which are only stop-gap measures, social programs that permanently improve the lives of the poor can permanently solve the hunger problem.

Sustainable Actions Every segment of our society can join in the fight against hunger, poverty, and environmental degradation. The federal government, the states, local communities, big business and small companies, educators, and all individuals have many opportunities to resolve these problems.

Dietitians have a special role to play, and their efforts can make an impressive difference. Their professional organization, the Dietitians of Canada (DC), urges members to conserve resources and minimize waste in both their professional and their personal lives.[26] In addition, the ADA urges its members to educate themselves and others on hunger, its consequences, and programs to fight it; to conduct research on the effectiveness and benefits of programs; and to serve as advocates to help end hunger in Canada.[27] Globally, DC supports programs that combat malnutrition, provide food security, promote self-sufficiency, respect local cultures, protect the environment, and sustain the economy.[28]

TABLE 21-2 Agricultural Methods Compared

Environmental Issues	Unsustainable Methods	Sustainable Methods
Soil	Growing the same crop repeatedly on the same land takes nutrients out of the soil, making fertilizer use necessary; favours soil erosion; and invites weeds and pests to become established, making pesticide use necessary. Plowing the same way everywhere, allows water runoff and erosion.	Rotating crops increases nitrogen in the soil so there is less need to use fertilizers. Using appropriate plowing methods reduces soil erosion problems caused by weeds and pests. Using cover crops, crop rotation, no-till planting, contour planting, ridge till, mulch, terraces, and grass strips conserves both soil and water.
Fertilizer	Using fertilizers pollutes ground and surface water and increases costs as fossil fuels become scarce.	Reducing the use of fertilizers and using livestock manure more effectively lowers costs. Planting cover crops, such as legumes, after harvest restores nutrients and reduces erosion. Composting all plant residues not harvested into the soil improves its nutrient content and water-holding capacity.
Livestock	Feeding livestock in feedlots concentrates manure that pollutes water and releases methane, a global warming gas. Injecting animals with antibiotics prevents diseases.	Feeding livestock or buffalo on the open range allows their manure to fertilize the ground and releases no methane. Collecting feedlot animals' manure enables it to be used as fertilizer or treated before it is released. Maintaining animals' health can prevent disease.
Herbicide/ pesticide	Spraying herbicides and pesticides over large areas wipes out weeds, pests, and other plants and insects.	Using crop rotations, cover crops, and mechanical cultivation can control weeds. Using resistant crops and rotating crops foils pests that lay their eggs in the soil where last year's crop was grown. Using biological controls such as predators can destroy pests.
Water	Irrigating on a large scale depletes water supplies and concentrates salts in the soil.	Irrigating only during dry spells and applying only spot irrigation conserves water.
Energy	Using only fossil fuels depletes resources.	Using renewable energy technologies such as hydroelectric, biomass, photovoltaics, wind power, solar thermal, geothermal, biogas, and methanol conserves resources. Using machinery scaled to the job at hand, and operating it at efficient speeds conserves energy. Combining operations such as harrowing, planting, and fertilizing in the same operation conserves energy.

Individuals can assist the global community in solving its poverty and hunger problems by joining and working for hunger-relief organizations (see Table 21-3). They can also support organizations that lobby for the needed changes in economic policies toward developing countries.

Most importantly, all individuals can try to make lifestyle choices ♦ that consider the environmental consequences. Many small decisions each day have major consequences for the environment. Highlight 21 describes how consumers can conserve resources and minimize waste when making food-related choices.

The personal rewards of making environmentally friendly food choices are many, from saving money to the satisfaction of knowing that you are treading lightly on the Earth. But do they really help? They do, if enough people join in. Because we number more than six billion, individual actions can add up to exert an immense impact.

Individuals: What Can You Do? There are many things you can do to help our environment and reduce our ecological footprint globally, such as eating meat-free meals more often and using less pesticides. You might consider, from a nutrition standpoint, visiting the David Suzuki Foundation website and checking out the "Food and climate change" webpage (see Nutrition on the Net). All individuals can become involved in these large trends. Many small decisions each day add up to large impacts on the environment.

♦ "Be part of the solution, not part of the problem" another adage says. In other words, don't waste time or energy moaning and groaning about how bad things

♦ A popular adage urges us to "Think globally, act locally."

TABLE 21-3 Hunger-Relief Organizations

Organization	Mission Statement
Action without Borders www.idealist.org	International organization seeking to connect people, organizations, and resources to help build a world where all people can live free and dignified lives.
Bread for the World www.bread.org	Nonpartisan, Christian citizens' movement seeking to influence reform in policies, programs, and conditions that allow hunger and poverty to persist globally.
Catholic Relief Services www.crs.org	Humanitarian service agency assisting the impoverished and disadvantaged through community-based, sustainable development initiatives.
Community Food Security Coalition www.foodsecurity.org	North American coalition of diverse people and organizations working from the local to the international levels to build community food security.
Congressional Hunger Center www.hungercenter.org	Bipartisan organization training and inspiring leaders with the intent to end hunger, and advocating public policies to create a food-secure world.
Feeding America www.feedingamerica.org	U.S. charity organization providing food assistance through a nationwide network of member food banks and facilitating education to end hunger nationally.
Food and Agriculture Organization (FAO) of the United Nations www.fao.org	International organization leading efforts to defeat hunger by helping to develop and modernize countries' agriculture, forestry, and fishery practices.
Oxfam Canada www.oxfam.ca	International relief and development organization aiming to create lasting solutions to poverty, hunger, and injustice.
Pan American Health Organization www.paho.org	International public health agency aiming to strengthen national and local health systems with the purpose of improving the quality of, and lengthening, the lives of peoples in the Americas.
Society of St. Andrew www.endhunger.org	Ecumenical Christian ministry salvaging and redirecting large amounts of fresh produce to hunger agencies for distribution to the poor.
The Hunger Project www.thp.org	International relief organization emphasizing sustainable solutions such as rural development and self-reliance to facilitate food security.
United Nations Children's Fund (UNICEF) www.unicef.org	International organization advocating for the protection of children's rights, to help meet their basic needs and to expand their opportunities to reach their full potentials.
World Food Program www.wfp.org	Food aid branch of the United Nations aiming to prepare for, protect during, and provide assistance after, emergencies, as well as reducing hunger and undernutrition.
World Health Organization (WHO) www.who.int	United Nations agency acting as the authority on international public health by influencing policy, setting research agendas, establishing standards, and providing technical support to monitor and assess health trends.
World Hunger Year (WHY) www.whyhunger.org	U.S. organization supporting and funding community-based organizations intent on empowering individuals and building self-reliance to provide long-term solutions to hunger and poverty.

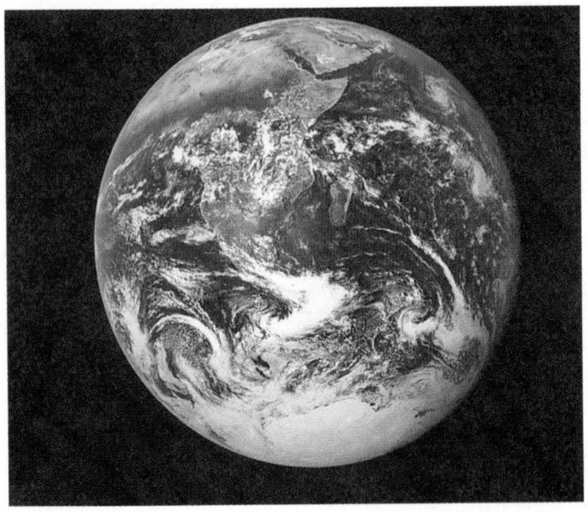
NASA

"We do not inherit the earth from our ancestors, we borrow it from our children." Ascribed to Chief Seattle, a 19th-century Native American leader.

are: do something to improve them. They are our problems: human beings created them, and human beings must solve them, especially in light of the recent estimate in a global report that 30 percent of food is wasted.[29]

IN SUMMARY **Environmental degradation reduces our ability to produce enough food to feed the world's people. The rapid increase in the world's population exacerbates the situation. The global environment, which supports all life, is deteriorating, largely because of our irresponsible use of resources and energy. Governments, businesses, and all individuals have many opportunities to make environmentally conscious choices, which may help solve the hunger problem, improve the quality of life, and generate jobs. Personal choices, made by many people, can have a great impact.**

Nutrition on the Net

CENGAGENOW™
For further study of topics covered in this chapter, log on to **www.cengage.com/sso.**

- For updates on hunger statistics, see Statistics Canada: **www.statcan.ca**
- Explore the problems of hunger, malnutrition, and food insecurity at the Feeding Minds, Fighting Hunger site: **www.feedingminds.org**
- Learn about constructive, community-based solutions to the problems of poverty and hunger within and between the public and private sectors from the National Hunger Clearinghouse: **www.whyhunger.org**
- Visit the USDA Supplemental Nutrition Assistance Program: **www.fns.usda.gov/snap**
- Download recipes, sample menus, and numerous tips for planning, shopping for, and cooking healthy meals that are kind to your waistline: **www.dietitians.ca/Your-Health/Plan-Shop-Cook/Cook-Healthy.aspx**
- Review the Best Practices Manual for Food Recovery and Gleaning at the USDA Food and Nutrition Service site: **www.fns.usda.gov/fdd/gleaning/gleanintro.htm**
- Find information on feeding the hungry from the Emergency Food and Shelter National Board Program: **www.efsp.unitedway.org**
- Donate free food at The Hunger Site: **www.thehungersite.com**
- Learn more about soil conservation and sustainable agriculture: **www4.agr.gc.ca/AAFC-AAC/display-afficher.do?id=1175526032952&lang=eng**
- Find information on food production and distribution from the Institute for Food and Development Policy: **www.foodfirst.org**
- Visit the David Suzuki Foundation website to help reduce your carbon footprint regarding food and climate change: **www.davidsuzuki.org/what-you-can-do/eat-for-a-healthy-planet/food-and-climate-change/**
- See Table 21-3 (on p. 709) for additional websites.

References

1. *State of Food Insecurity in the World, 2008,* Food Security Statistics, available from Food and Agriculture Organization, www.fao.org.
2. Statistics Canada, Census-related topics: Income in Canada 2006, www12.statcan.ca/census-recensement/2006/consultation/qz-135/topic-themeeng.cfm; Canadian Social Research Links, Poverty Measures – Canadian Resources, www.canadiansocialresearch.net/poverty.htm, accessed October 2, 2011.
3. Health Canada, Food and Nutrition, National nutritious food basket. www.hc-sc.gc.ca/fn-an/surveill/basket-panier/index-eng.php, accessed September 21, 2011.
4. Statistics Canada, Study: Food insecurity in Canadian households, *The Daily* (May 5, 2005). www.statcan.ca/Daily/English/050503/d050503b.htm, accessed September 21, 2011.
5. Dietitians of Canada, Individual and household food insecurity in Canada: Position of Dietitians of Canada (2005). See especially Tables 2 and 3 of this resource for numerous Canadian food security initiatives that involve dietitians. www.dietitians.ca/Downloadable-Content/Public/householdfoodsec-position-paper.aspx, accessed September 21, 2011.
6. Dietitians of Canada, Community Food Security Position of Dietitians of Canada (2007). www.dietitians.ca/Downloadable-Content/Public/cfs-position-paper.aspx, accessed September 21, 2011.
7. E. T. Kennedy, The global face of nutrition: What can governments and industry do? *Journal of Nutrition* 135 (2005): 913–915.
8. S. A. Tanumihardjo and coauthors, Poverty, obesity, and malnutrition: An international perspective recognizing the paradox, *Journal of the American Dietetic Association* 107 (2007): 1966–1972; P. H. Casey and coauthors, The association of child and household food insecurity with childhood overweight status, *Pediatrics* 118 (2006): e1406; L. M. Scheier, What is the hunger-obesity paradox? *Journal of the American Dietetic Association* 105 (2005): 883–886.
9. L. M. Dinour, D. Bergen, and M. Yeh, The food insecurity-obesity paradox: A review of the literature and the role food stamps may play, *Journal of the American Dietetic Association* 107 (2007): 1952–1961;

P. E. Wilde and J. N. Peterman, Individual weight change is associated with household food security status, *Journal of Nutrition* 136 (2006): 1395–1400.
10. A. D. Liese and coauthors, Food store types, availability, and cost of foods in a rural environment, *Journal of the American Dietetic Association* 107 (2007): 1916–1923; J. P. Stimpson and coauthors, Neighborhood deprivation is associated with lower levels of serum carotenoids among adults participating in the Third National Health and Nutrition Examination Survey, *Journal of the American Dietetic Association* 107 (2007): 1895–1902; S. N. Zenk and coauthors, Fruit and vegetable intake in African Americans—Income and store characteristics, *American Journal of Preventive Medicine* 29 (2005): 1–9.
11. M. S. Townsend and coauthors, Less-energy-dense diets of low-income women in California are associated with higher energy-adjusted diet costs, *American Journal of Clinical Nutrition* 89 (2009): 1220–1226.
12. S. J. Jones and E. A. Frongillo, The modifying effects of Food Stamp program participation on the relation between food insecurity and weight change in women, *Journal of Nutrition* 136 (2006): 1091–1094; S. J. Jones and coauthors, Lower risk of overweight in school-aged food insecure girls who participate in food assistance, *Archives of Pediatrics and Adolescent Medicine* 157 (2003): 780–784.
13. Tanumihardjo and coauthors, 2007.
14. Food Banks Canada, HungerCount 2010 (2010). www.foodbankscanada.ca/documents/HungerCount2010_web.pdf, accessed September 21, 2011.
15. Canadian Living Foundation, Breakfast for Learning. www.breakfastforlearning.ca, accessed September 21, 2011.
16. Food & Consumer Products of Canada, About us. www.fcpc.ca/about/index.html, accessed September 21, 2011.
17. C. McCullum and coauthors, Evidence-based strategies to build community food security, *Journal of the American Dietetic Association* 105 (2005): 278–283.
18. I. Darnton-Hill and coauthors, Micronutrient deficiencies and gender: Social and economic costs, *American Journal of Clinical Nutrition* 81 (2005): 1198S–1205S.
19. R. L. Guerrant and coauthors, Malnutrition as an enteric infectious disease with long-term effects on child development, *Nutrition Reviews* 66 (2008): 487–505.
20. Statistics Canada, Human activity and the environment: Annual statistics (2009) – Section 1: Food in Canada. www.statcan.gc.ca/pub/16-201-x/2009000/part-partie1-eng.htm, accessed September 21, 2011.
21. D. D. Marino, Water and food safety in the developing world: Global implications for health and nutrition of infants and young children, *Journal of the American Dietetic Association* 107 (2007): 1930–1934.
22. B. Worm and coauthors, Impacts of biodiversity loss on ocean ecosystem services, *Science* 314 (2006): 787–790.
23. Don Hinrichsen, Water pressure, www.nwf.org/nationalwildlife/article.cfm, accessed March 2009.
24. B. M. Kuehn, Desertification called global health threat, *Journal of the American Medical Association* 295 (2006): 2463–2465.
25. Agriculture and Agri-food Canada, Sustainable Development Strategy 2007–2009: Making Progress Together. www4.agr.gc.ca/resources/prod/doc/policy/environment/pdfs/sds/sds4_e.pdf, accessed September 21, 2011.
26. Dietitians of Canada, Individual and household food insecurity in Canada: Position of the Dietitians of Canada (2005). www.dietitians.ca/Downloadable-Content/Public/householdfoodsec-position-paper.aspx, accessed September 21, 2011.
27. Dietitians of Canada, 2005.
28. Dietitians of Canada, 2005.
29. Foresight. The Future of Food and Farming (2011) Executive Summary. The Government Office for Science, London. www.bis.gov.uk/assets/bispartners/foresight/docs/food-and-farming/11-547-future-of-food-and-farming-summary, accessed September 21, 2011.

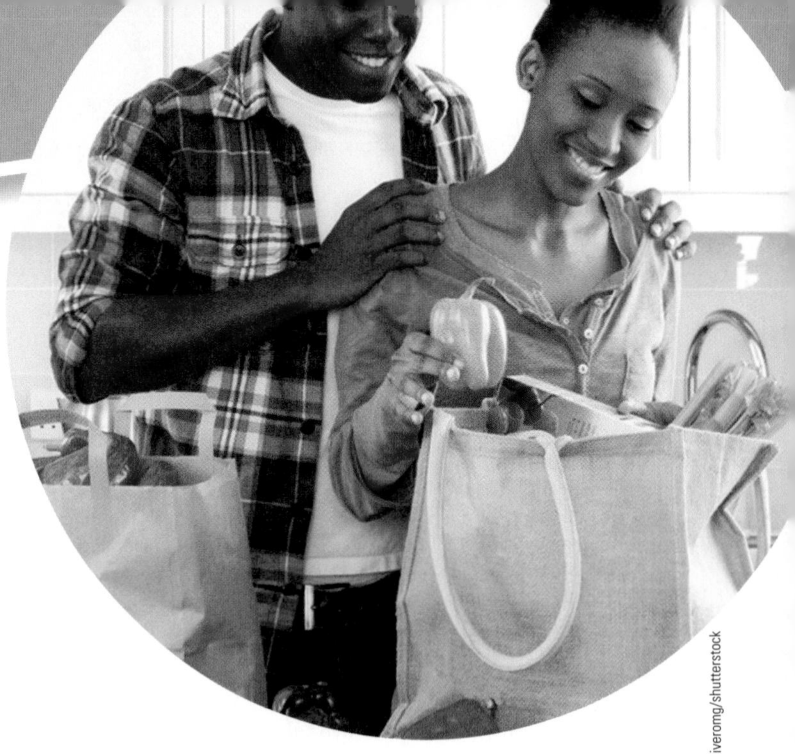

oliveromg/shutterstock

Environmentally Friendly Food Choices

Chapter 21 concludes its examination of Canada and the United States and world hunger by focusing on the environment. It explains how producing enough food to feed billions of people around the world damages the environment—and how a damaged environment cannot adequately feed billions of people around the world. Efforts to resolve hunger and protect the environment demand improvements in our ways of producing, processing, packaging, transporting, storing, and preparing foods.[1]

The United Nations describes a nation's impact on the environment as its "ecological footprint"—a measure of the resources used to support a nation's consumption of food, materials, and energy. This measure takes into account the two most challenging aspects of sustainability—per capita resource consumption and population growth. As Figure H21-1 shows, the people of North America are the world's greatest consumers on a per capita basis. Some have estimated that it would take four more planet Earths to accommodate every person in the world using resources at the level currently used in North America. This highlight explores ways that consumers can conserve resources when making food-related choices. Such conscientious food choices can reduce pollution production and resource use.[2]

Choice: Animal or Vegetable?

Some foods require more water, more fertilizer, more pesticides, and more energy for their production than others. One way to reduce these costs of food production is for consumers to eat low on the food chain. For the most part, that means eating more foods derived from plants and fewer foods derived from animals.[3]

Relatively little energy is needed to produce grains: it takes about one-third kcalorie of fuel to produce each kcalorie of grain. Fruits and vegetables are intermediate, and most animal-derived foods require from 10 to 90 kcalories of fuel per kcalorie of edible food. In general, meat-based foods require much more energy, as well as more land and water, than do plant-based foods. An exception is livestock raised on the open range; these animals require about as much energy as most plant foods.[4] Because we raise so much more grain-fed, than range-fed, livestock, however, the average energy requirement for meat production is high. Figure H21-2 shows how much less fuel vegetarian diets require than meat-based diets and shows that vegan diets require the least fuel of all.

To support our meat intake, we maintain several billion livestock, about four times our own weight in animals. Livestock consume 10 times as much grain each day as we do. We could use much of that grain to make grain products for ourselves and for others around the

FIGURE H21-1 Ecological Footprints

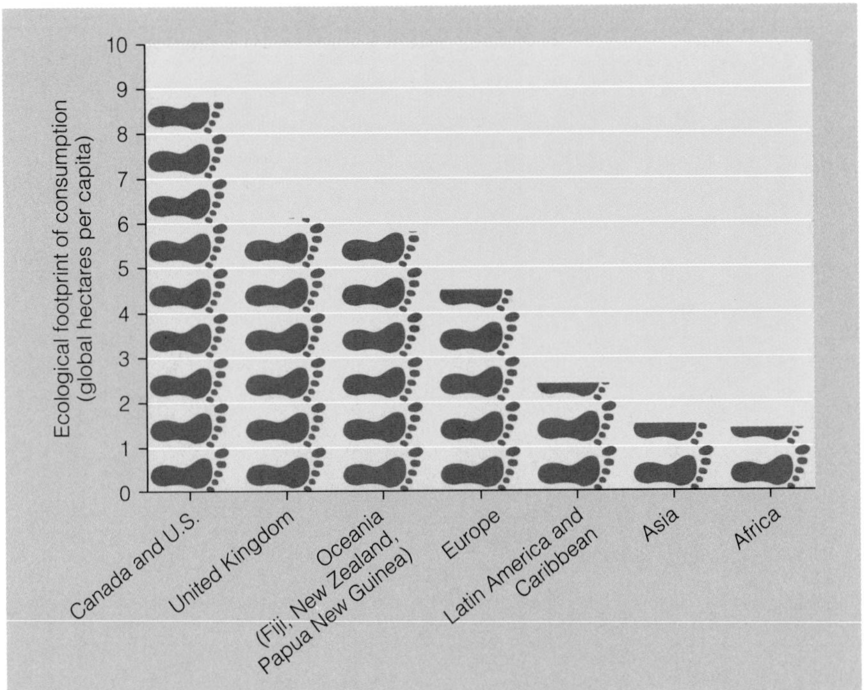
Ecological footprint of consumption (global hectares per capita)
0
1
2
3
4
5
6
7
8
9
10
Canada and U.S.
United Kingdom
Oceania (Fiji, New Zealand, Papua New Guinea)
Europe
Latin America and Caribbean
Asia
Africa

SOURCE: Data from Global Footprint Network, *Ecological Footprint Atlas,* 2008. From SIZER, WHITNEY, PICHE; *Nutrition: Concepts and Controversies,* Nelson Education Ltd., © 2012. Reprinted with permission. www.cengage.com/permissions.

FIGURE H21-2 Amounts of Fuel Required to Feed People Eating at Different Points on the Food Chain

Three people who eat differently are compared here. Each has the same energy intake: 3300 kcalories a day. The fossil fuel amounts necessary to produce these different diets are calculated based on North American conditions.

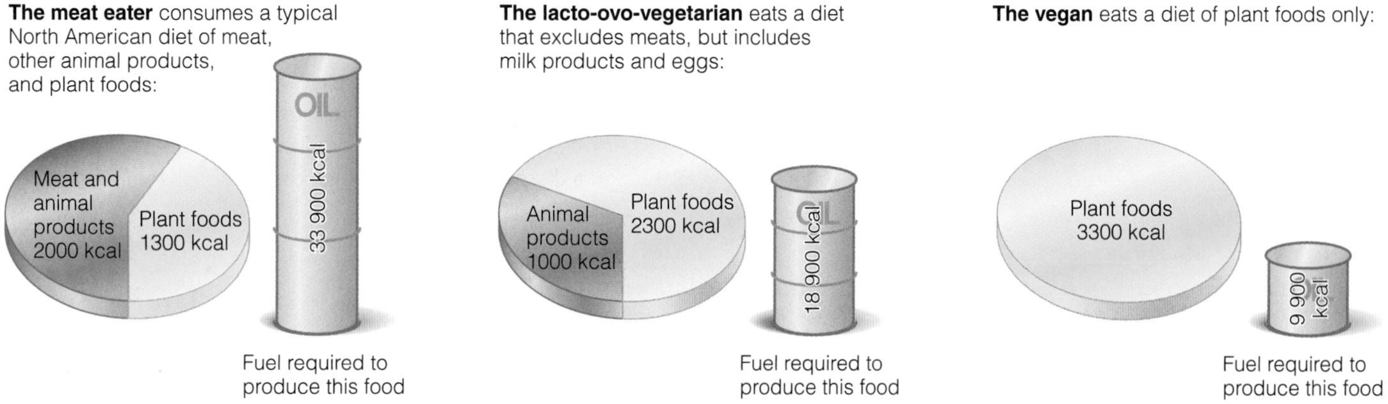
The meat eater consumes a typical North American diet of meat, other animal products, and plant foods:
Meat and animal products 2000 kcal
Plant foods 1300 kcal
OIL
33 900 kcal
Fuel required to produce this food
The lacto-ovo-vegetarian eats a diet that excludes meats, but includes milk products and eggs:
Animal products 1000 kcal
Plant foods 2300 kcal
OIL
18 900 kcal
Fuel required to produce this food
The vegan eats a diet of plant foods only:
Plant foods 3300 kcal
9 900 kcal
Fuel required to produce this food

SOURCE: Adapted from D. Pimentel, *Food, Energy and the Future of Society* (Boulder, Colo.: Associated University Press, 1980), Figure 5, p. 27.

world. Making this shift could free up enough grain to feed 400 million people while using less fuel, water, and land.

Part of the solution to the livestock problem may be to cease feeding grain to animals and return to grazing them on the open range, which can be a sustainable practice. Ranchers have to manage the grazing carefully to hold the cattle's numbers to what the land can support without environmental degradation. To accomplish this, the economic benefits of traditional livestock and feed-growing operations would have to end. If producers were to pay the true costs of the environmental damage incurred by irrigation water, fertilizers, pesticides, and fuels, the price of meats might double or triple. According to classic economic theory, people would then buy less meat (reducing demand), and producers would respond by producing less meat (reducing supply). Meat production would then fall to a sustainable level.

Some consumers are trying to help solve some of these problems by choosing smaller portions of meat or selecting range-fed beef or buffalo only. Livestock on the range eat grass, which people cannot eat. "Rangeburger" buffalo also offers nutrient advantages over grain-fed beef because it is lower in fat and because the fat has more polyunsaturated fatty acids, including the omega-3 type.

Some consumers are opting for vegetarian, and even vegan, diets—at least occasionally. Vegetarian diets have less of an environmental impact than meat-based diets. Shifting to a fish diet may be a practical alternative if seafood is selected with an awareness of the environmental consequences. Table H21-1 (p. 714) presents seafood options grouped according to their impact on the environment.

Choice: Global or Local?

Plant-centred diets have an environmental advantage over meat-based diets, but some would argue that they don't go far enough. A more ecologically responsible diet is also based on locally grown products. The average meal travels 1200 kilometres before it is eaten—when the crops are grown and the final destination are both in Canada. That "our foods now travel more than we do" has several costly ramifications:

- *Energetically costly.* Foods must be refrigerated and transported thousands of miles to provide a full array of all produce all year round.
- *Socially unjust.* Farmers in impoverished countries, where the people are malnourished, are paid meagre wages to grow food for wealthy nations.
- *Economically unwise.* It supports agribusinesses that buy land and labour cheaply in foreign countries instead of supporting local farmers raising crops in our communities.
- *Biologically risky.* Highly perishable foods are shipped from countries with unsafe drinking water and sanitation practices.

For all these reasons, consumers may want to improve the global environment by buying locally. The "How To" on p. 715 lists some of the ways consumers can "tread lightly on the Earth" through their daily food choices.

Buying locally offers other benefits as well. Families buying homegrown produce tend to eat a greater quantity and selection of fruits and vegetables.[5]

Adopting a local diet presents a bit of a challenge at first, especially when local fruits and vegetables are "out of season." But a nutritionally balanced diet of delicious foods is quite possible with a little creative planning.

Defining Local

Consumers shopping for "locally grown" produce are often trying to find fresh foods that will both help support small farms and protect the environment. Grocers tapping into this "local" marketing concept have seen significant increases in sales. But what exactly does "local" mean? How far is "locally grown" from the farm to the market? Given that *local* is not defined by Health Canada, consumers and grocers do not always share the same understanding of the term. Some would say *local* means reasonably nearby—say, within 10 to 20 kilometres, or up to 150 kilometres (or 100 miles). Others say it means within a day's drive, or within the province or a geographic region, thus, beyond what would be considered a 100-mile-diet. Without agreement, consumers are left to identify which goods meet their limited definition and grocers are free to market their goods with a broad definition.

Consumers who think of "local" as "fresh from a small farm" may be surprised to learn that is not always the case. Local may be a corporate-managed 1000-acre tomato farm or a family-run 3-acre blueberry farm. Because large retail stores need large volumes, they tend to deal with a few large producers. Shipments typically go through a distribution centre, which can delay deliveries for several

TABLE H21-1 Environmental Impact of Commonly Eaten Seafood Choices

Seafood	Abundant, Well-Managed, and Fished or Farmed Using Methods that Are Environmentally Friendly	Fished or Farmed Using Methods that Raise Some Environmental Concerns	Overfished and/or Fished or Farmed Using Methods that Harm Other Marine Life or the Environment
Catfish	U.S. farmed	—	—
Clams	Worldwide farmed, U.S. Pacific and Atlantic wild-caught	U.S. Atlantic wild-caught	—
Cod	U.S. Pacific longline, jig, and trap-caught	U.S. Pacific trawl-caught	U.S. Atlantic wild-caught
Crab, blue	—	U.S. trap-caught	—
Crab, Dungeness	U.S. and Canada trap-caught	—	—
Crab, Jonah	—	U.S. Atlantic wild-caught	—
Crab, king	—	U.S. trap-caught	Imported trap-caught
Crab, kona	Australia wild-caught	Hawaii wild-caught	—
Crab, snow	—	Alaska and Canada wild-caught	—
Crab, stone	U.S. Atlantic and Gulf of Mexico trap-caught	—	—
Flatfish, flounder	—	—	Atlantic wild-caught
Flatfish, halibut	U.S. and Canadian Pacific wild-caught	U.S. Pacific hook-and-line or bottom trawl, wild-caught	U.S. Atlantic wild-caught, U.S. Pacific set gillnet
Flatfish, plaice	—	U.S. Pacific wild-caught	U.S. Atlantic wild-caught
Pollock	Alaska wild-caught	—	—
Salmon	Alaska wild-caught	Washington wild-caught	Worldwide farmed
Scallops, bay	Worldwide farmed	—	—
Scallops, sea	—	Atlantic U.S. and Canada wild-caught	—
Shrimp	Oregon wild-caught	U.S. and Canada wild-caught, U.S. Gulf of Mexico and South Atlantic wild-caught, U.S. farmed	Imported farmed and wild-caught
Tilapia	U.S. farmed	Central and South America farmed	China and Taiwan farmed
Tuna, albacore	British Columbia U.S. troll/pole, Hawaii troll/pole or handline	Hawaii longline	Worldwide except Hawaii longline
Tuna, bigeye[a]	—	Hawaii pole/troll or handline, worldwide troll/poll, U.S. Atlantic longline	Worldwide except U.S. Atlantic longline
Tuna, bluefin	—	—	Worldwide wild-caught
Tuna, canned[a]	—	Worldwide wild-caught	—
Tuna, skipjack	Worldwide troll/pole, Hawaii troll/pole or handline	Hawaii longline	Imported longline
Tuna, yellowfin[a]	U.S. Atlantic troll/pole	Hawaii troll/pole or handline, worldwide troll/pole, U.S. Atlantic longline	Worldwide except U.S. Atlantic longline

[a]Canned tuna is predominantly sold as either "chunk white" (albacore) or "chunk light" (yellowfin and skipjack tuna).

SOURCE: Adapted from the Seafood Guide of the Monterey Bay Aquarium Foundation, www.montereybayaquarium.org, accessed March 2009.

hours or even days. In contrast, small producers tend to sell to farmers' markets and small stores. Deliveries often arrive within hours of harvest. A growing number of consumers do, however, appreciate knowing how their food is grown and handled and urban consumers often relish a trip to the local farmers' market or to the "country" to pick up locally grown foods (see Nutrition on the Net and a recent national bestseller about locavores by Sarah Elton [2011] *Locavore: From Farmers' Fields to Rooftop Gardens–How Canadians Are Changing the Way We Eat*. Toronto: Harper-Perenial).

Eco-Friendly Miles

Consumers who support the concept of purchasing local foods may believe that the fewer miles a food travels, the better for the environment—but this is not always the case. The type of transportation also contributes to environmental costs. In general, transporting by ship is cleaner than by airplane; by train is cleaner than by truck. It may be obvious that the eco-friendly choice for a person living in Toronto is a Niagra wine, but what about a person

HOW TO Make Environmentally Friendly Food-Related Choices

Food production taxes environmental resources and causes pollution. Consumers can make environmentally friendly choices at every step from food shopping to cooking and use of kitchen appliances to serving, cleanup, and waste disposal.

Food Shopping

Transportation

- Whenever possible, walk or ride a bicycle; use car pools and mass transit.
- Shop only once a week, share trips, or take turns shopping for each other.
- When buying a car, choose an energy-efficient one.

Food Choices

- Choose foods low on the food chain; that is, eat more plants and fewer animals that eat plants.
- Eat small portions of meat; select range-fed beef and poultry.
- Shop at farmers' markets and roadside stands for local foods; they require less transportation, packaging, and refrigeration.
- Limit use of imported canned beef products such as stews, chili, and corned beef that frequently come from cleared rain forest land.
- Choose seafood that has been farmed or fished in environmentally responsible ways (see Table H21-1).
- Choose chickens from local farms.

Food Packages

- Whenever possible, select foods with no packages; next best are minimal, reusable, or recyclable ones.
- Buy juices and soft drinks in large glass or recyclable plastic bottles (not small individual cans or cartons); grains, legumes, and nuts in bulk (not separate little packages); and eggs in pressed fibre cartons (not foam, unless it is recycled locally).
- Carry reusable string or cloth shopping bags; alternatively, reuse plastic bags.

Gardening

- Grow some of your own food, even if it is only herbs planted in pots on your kitchen windowsill.
- Compost all vegetable scraps, fruit peelings, and leftover plant foods.

Cooking Food

- Cook foods quickly in a stir-fry, pressure cooker, or microwave oven.
- When using the oven, bake a lot of food at one time and keep the door closed tightly.
- Use nondisposable utensils, dishes, and pans.
- Use pumps instead of spray products.

Kitchen Appliances

- Use fewer small electrical appliances; open cans, mix batters, sharpen knives, and chop vegetables by hand.
- When buying a large appliance, choose an energy-efficient one.
- Consider solar power to meet home electrical needs.
- Set the water heater at 54°C ≤ 134°F, no hotter; put it on a timer; wrap it and the hot-water pipes in insulation; install water-saving faucets.
- Set the refrigerator at 4°C to 6°C (37°F to 40°F) and the freezer to -18°C (0°F).
- Keep all appliances clean and in good repair.

Food Serving, Dish Washing, and Waste Disposal

- Use "real" plates, cups, and glasses instead of disposable ones.
- Use cloth towels and napkins, reusable storage containers with lids, reusable pans, and dishcloths instead of paper towels, plastic wrap, plastic storage bags, aluminum foil, and sponges.
- Run the dishwasher only when it is full.
- Recycle all paper, glass, plastic, and aluminum.

These suggested lifestyle changes can easily be extended from food to other areas.

TRY IT Find out if you are living a sustainable life from a food standpoint by visiting "Eat for a healthy planet" on the David Suzuki Foundation website: www.davidsuzuki.org/what-you-can-do/eat-for-a-healthy-planet/.

living in Winnipeg? Is it "greener" to buy wine trucked across the country from Ontario or British Columbia or shipped across the ocean from France?

Other Food-Related Choices

Eating more foods derived from plants and produced locally are two major trends that can influence the food industry. Consumers can also make dozens of other smaller decisions every day to help conserve resources and protect the environment.

Chapter 21 and this highlight have presented many problems and have suggested that, although many of the problems are global in scope, the solutions depend on the actions of individual people at the local level. On learning of this, concerned people may take a perfectionist attitude, believing that they "should" be doing more than they realistically can, and so feel defeated. Keep in mind that striving for perfection even while falling short is progress. A positive attitude can bring about improvement, and sometimes improvement is enough. Celebrate the changes that are possible today by making them a permanent part of your life; do the same with changes that become possible tomorrow and every day thereafter. The results may surprise you.

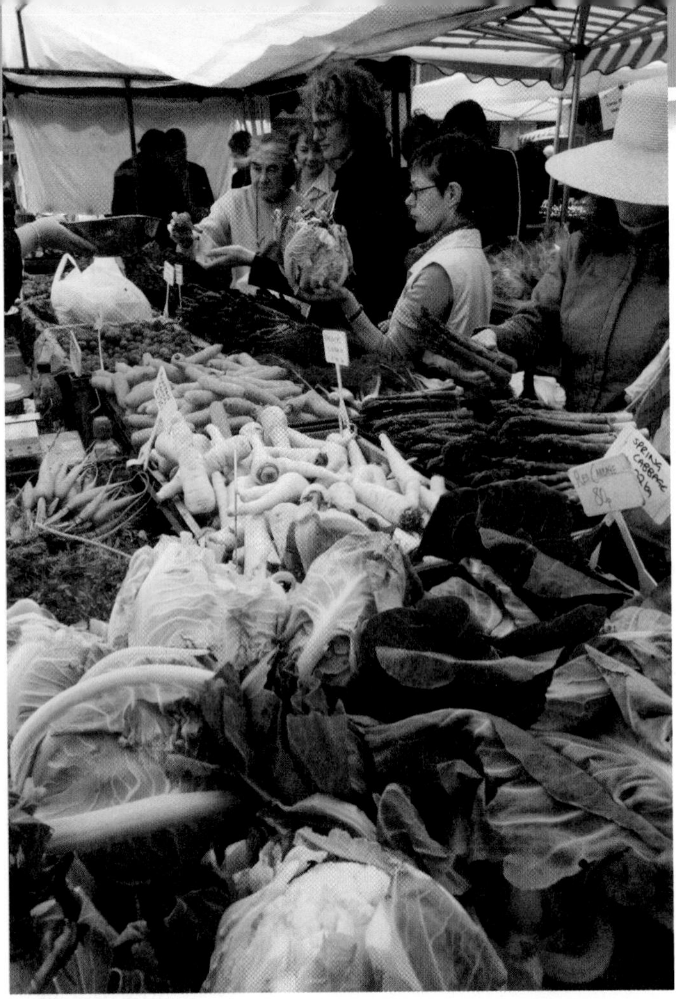

Locally grown foods offer benefits to both the local economy and the global environment.

Nutrition on the Net

CENGAGENOW™
For further study of topics covered in this Highlight, log on to **www.cengage.com/sso**.

- Check out the list of interactive and static local food maps in Ontario: **http://brescia.uwo.ca/about/our_people/our_faculty/food_nutrition/local_food_maps_ontario.html**
- Look for a farmers' market near you: **www.farmersmarkets-canada.ca**
- Visit Agriculture Agri-Food Canada's website for information about Canada's Organic Food Industry: **www4.agr.gc.ca/AAFC-AAC/display-afficher.do?id=1276292934938&lang=eng**
- Visit the Sustainable Development Strategies for Canada on the Agriculture Agri-Food website: **www4.agr.gc.ca/AAFC-AAC/display-afficher.do?id=1175526032952&lang=eng**

References

1. D. Pimentel and coauthors, Reducing energy inputs in the U.S. food system, *Human Ecology* 36 (2008): 459–461.
2. A. Carlsson-Kanyama and A. D. González, Potential contributions of food consumption patterns to climate change, *American Journal of Clinical Nutrition* 89 (2009): 1704S–1709S.
3. David Suzuki Foundation, What You Can Do: Eat for a healthy planet. www.davidsuzuki.org/what-you-can-do/eat-for-a-healthy-planet/, accessed September 21, 2011; H. J. Marlow and coauthors, Diet and the environment: Does what you eat matter? *American Journal of Clinical Nutrition* 89 (2009): 1699S–1703S.
4. J. Robinson, Grass fed basics: Key differences between conventional and pasture animal production, 2002–2003, www.eatwild.com/basics.html.
5. M. S. Nanney and coauthors, Frequency of eating homegrown produce is associated with higher intake among parents and their preschool-aged children in rural Missouri, *Journal of the American Dietetic Association* 107 (2007): 577–584.

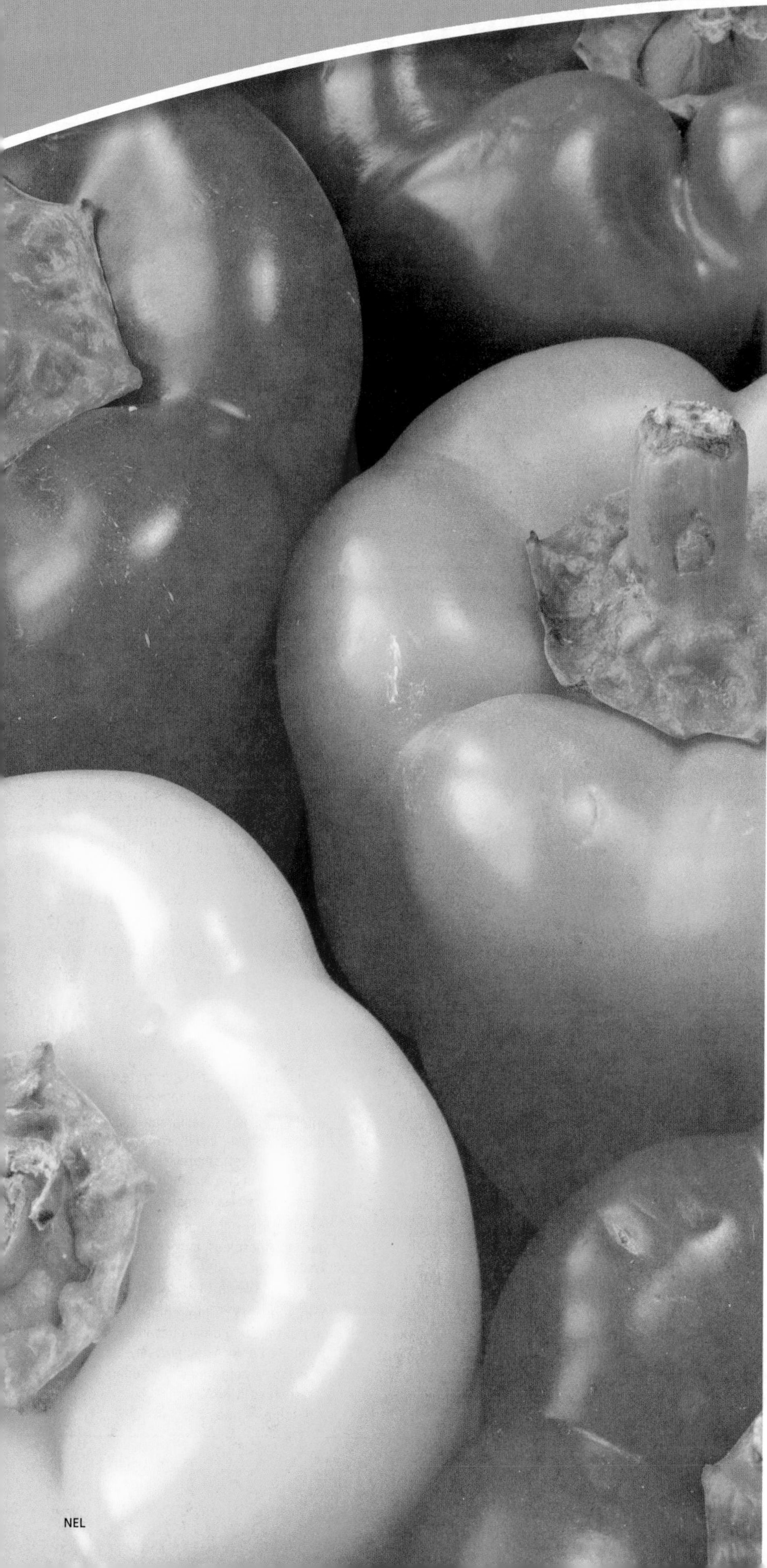

Malgorzata Kistryn/shutterstock

Appendixes

APPENDIX A

CONTENTS

Cells, Hormones, and Nerves

This appendix is offered as an optional chapter for readers who want to enhance their understanding of how the body coordinates its activities. It presents a brief summary of the structure and function of the body's basic working unit (the cell) and of the body's two major regulatory systems (the hormonal system and the nervous system).

Cells

The body's organs are made up of millions of cells and of materials produced by them. Each **cell** is specialized to perform its organ's functions, but all cells have common structures (see the accompanying glossary and Figure A-1). Every cell is contained within a **cell membrane**. The cell membrane assists in moving materials into and out of the cell, and some of its special proteins act as "pumps" (described in Chapter 6). Some features of cell membranes, such as microvilli (Chapter 3), permit cells to interact with other cells and with their environments in highly specific ways.

Inside the membrane lies the **cytoplasm**, which is filled with **cytosol**, a jelly-like fluid. The cytoplasm contains much more than just cytosol, though. It is a highly organized system of fibres, tubes, membranes, particles, and subcellular **organelles** as complex as a city. These parts intercommunicate, manufacture and exchange materials, package and prepare materials for export, and maintain and repair themselves.

Within each cell is another membrane-enclosed body, the **nucleus**. Inside the nucleus are the **chromosomes**, which contain the genetic material, DNA. The DNA encodes all the instructions for carrying out the cell's activities. The role of DNA in coding for cell proteins is summarized in Figure 6-7 on p. 177. Chapter 6

GLOSSARY OF CELL STRUCTURES

cell: the basic structural unit of all living things.

cell membrane: the thin layer of tissue that surrounds the cell and encloses its contents; made primarily of lipid and protein.

chromosomes: a set of structures within the nucleus of every cell that contains the cell's genetic material, DNA, associated with other materials (primarily proteins).

cytoplasm (SIGH-toh-plazm): the cell contents, except for the nucleus.
- **cyto** = cell
- **plasm** = a form

cytosol: the fluid of cytoplasm; contains water, ions, nutrients, and enzymes.

endoplasmic reticulum (en-doh-PLAZ-mic reh-TIC-you-lum): a complex network of intracellular membranes. The *rough endoplasmic reticulum* is dotted with ribosomes, where protein synthesis takes place. The *smooth endoplasmic reticulum* bears no ribosomes.
- **endo** = inside
- **plasm** = the cytoplasm

Golgi (GOAL-gee) **apparatus:** a set of membranes within the cell where secretory materials are packaged for export.

lysosomes (LYE-so-zomes): cellular organelles; membrane-enclosed sacs of degradative enzymes.
- **lysis** = dissolution

mitochondria (my-toh-KON-dree-uh); singular *mitochondrion:* the cellular organelles responsible for producing ATP aerobically; made of membranes (lipid and protein) with enzymes mounted on them.
- **mitos** = thread (referring to their slender shape)
- **chondros** = cartilage (referring to their external appearance)

nucleus: a major membrane-enclosed body within every cell, which contains the cell's genetic material, DNA, embedded in chromosomes.
- **nucleus** = a kernel

organelles: subcellular structures such as ribosomes, mitochondria, and lysosomes.
- **organelle** = little organ

ribosomes (RYE-boh-zomes): protein-making organelles in cells; composed of RNA and protein.
- **ribo** = containing the sugar ribose (in RNA)
- **some** = body

FIGURE A-1 The Structure of a Typical Cell

The cell shown might be one in a gland (such as the pancreas) that produces secretory products (enzymes) for export (to the intestine). The rough endoplasmic reticulum with its ribosomes produces the enzymes; the smooth reticulum conducts them to the Golgi region; the Golgi membranes merge with the cell membrane, where the enzymes can be released into the extracellular fluid.

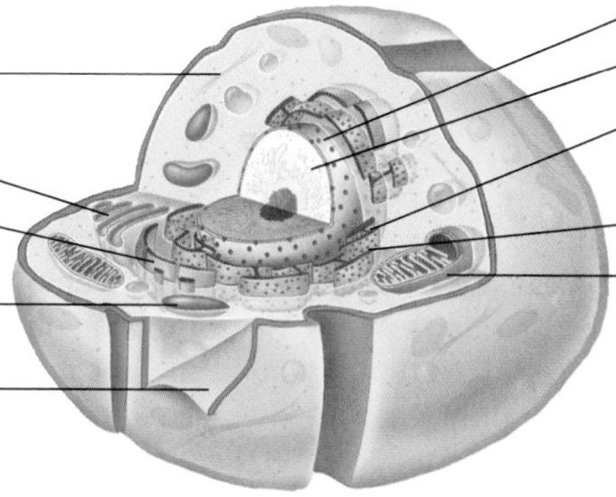
Nucleus
Chromosomes
Rough endoplasmic reticulum
Ribosomes
Mitochondrion
Cytoplasm
Golgi apparatus
Smooth endoplasmic reticulum
Lysosome
Cell membrane

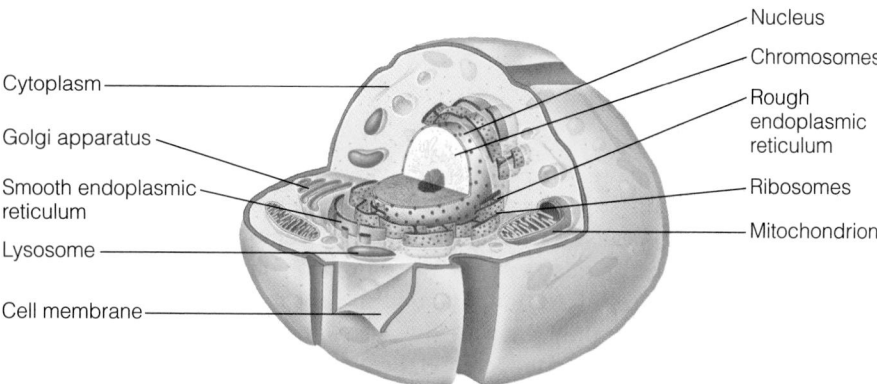

also describes the variety of proteins produced by cells and the ways they perform the body's work.

Among the organelles within a cell are ribosomes, mitochondria, and lysosomes. Figure 6-7 briefly refers to the **ribosomes**; they assemble amino acids into proteins, following directions conveyed to them by RNA.

The **mitochondria** are made of intricately folded membranes that bear thousands of highly organized sets of enzymes on their inner and outer surfaces. Mitochondria are crucial to energy metabolism (described in Chapter 7) and muscles conditioned to work aerobically are packed with them. Their presence is implied whenever the TCA cycle and electron transport chain are mentioned because the mitochondria house the needed enzymes.*

The **lysosomes** are membranes that enclose degradative enzymes. When a cell needs to self-destruct or to digest materials in its surroundings, its lysosomes free their enzymes. Lysosomes are active when tissue repair or remodelling is taking place—for example, in cleaning up infections, healing wounds, shaping embryonic organs, and remodelling bones.

Besides these and other cellular organelles, the cell's cytoplasm contains a highly organized system of membranes, the **endoplasmic reticulum.** The ribosomes may either float free in the cytoplasm or be mounted on these membranes. A membranous surface dotted with ribosomes looks speckled under the microscope and is called "rough" endoplasmic reticulum; such a surface without ribosomes is called "smooth." Some intracellular membranes are organized into tubules that collect cellular materials, merge with the cell membrane, and discharge their contents to the outside of the cell; these membrane systems are named the **Golgi apparatus**, after the scientist who first described them. The rough and smooth endoplasmic reticula and the Golgi apparatus are continuous with one another, so secretions produced deep in the interior of the cell can be efficiently transported to the outside and released. These and other cell structures enable cells to perform the multitudes of functions for which they are specialized.

*For the reactions of glycolysis, the TCA cycle, and the electron transport chain, see Chapter 7 and APPENDIX C. The reactions of glycolysis take place in the cytoplasm; the conversion of pyruvate to acetyl CoA takes place in the mitochondria, as do the TCA cycle and electron transport chain reactions. The mitochondria then release carbon dioxide, water, and ATP as their end products.

◆ The study of hormones and their effects is *endocrinology*.

The actions of cells are coordinated by both hormones and nerves, as the next sections show. Among the types of cellular organelles are receptors for the hormones delivering instructions that originate elsewhere in the body. Some hormones penetrate the cell and its nucleus and attach to receptors on chromosomes, where they activate certain genes to initiate, stop, speed up, or slow down synthesis of certain proteins as needed. Other hormones attach to receptors on the cell surface and transmit their messages from there. The hormones ◆ are described in the next section; the nerves, in the one following.

Hormones

A chemical compound—a **hormone**—originates in a gland and travels in the bloodstream. The hormone flows everywhere in the body, but only its target organs respond to it because only they possess the receptors to receive it.

The hormones, the glands they originate in, their target organs, and their effects are described in this section. Many of the hormones you might be interested in are included, but only a few are discussed in detail. Figure A-2 identifies the glands that produce the hormones, and the accompanying glossary defines the hormones discussed in this section.

◆ The *pituitary gland* in the brain has two parts—the *anterior* (front) and the *posterior* (hind).

hormone: a chemical messenger. Hormones are secreted by a variety of endocrine glands in response to altered conditions in the body. Each hormone travels to one or more specific target tissues or organs, where it elicits a specific response to maintain homeostasis.

Hormones of the Pituitary Gland and Hypothalamus

The anterior pituitary gland ◆ produces the following hormones, each of which acts on one or more target organs and elicits a characteristic response:

- **Adrenocorticotropin (ACTH)** acts on the adrenal cortex, promoting the production and release of its hormones.
- **Thyroid-stimulating hormone (TSH)** acts on the thyroid gland, promoting the production and release of thyroid hormones.

GLOSSARY OF HORMONES

adrenocorticotropin (ad-REE-noh-KORE-tee-koh-TROP-in) or **ACTH:** a hormone, so named because it stimulates *(trope)* the adrenal cortex. The adrenal gland, like the pituitary, has two parts, in this case an outer portion *(cortex)* and an inner core *(medulla)*. The release of ACTH is mediated by *corticotropin-releasing hormone (CRH)*.

aldosterone: a hormone from the adrenal gland involved in blood pressure regulation.
- **aldo** = aldehyde

angiotensin: a hormone involved in blood pressure regulation that is activated by **renin** (REN-in), an enzyme from the kidneys.
- **angio** = blood vessels
- **tensin** = pressure
- **ren** = kidneys

antidiuretic hormone (ADH): the hormone that prevents water loss in urine (also called **vasopressin**).
- **anti** = against
- **di** = through
- **ure** = urine
- **vaso** = blood vessels
- **pressin** = pressure

calcitonin (KAL-see-TOH-nin): a hormone secreted by the thyroid gland that regulates (tones) calcium metabolism.

erythropoietin (eh-RITH-ro-POY-eh-tin): a hormone that stimulates red blood cell production.
- **erythro** = red (blood cell)
- **poiesis** = creating (like poetry)

estrogens: hormones responsible for the menstrual cycle and other female characteristics.
- **oestrus** = the egg-making cycle
- **gen** = gives rise to

follicle-stimulating hormone (FSH): a hormone that stimulates maturation of the ovarian follicles in females and the production of sperm in males. (The ovarian follicles are part of the female reproductive system where the eggs are produced.) The release of FSH is mediated by *follicle-stimulating hormone releasing hormone (FSH–RH)*.

glucocorticoids: hormones from the adrenal cortex that affect the body's management of glucose.
- **gluco** = glucose
- **corticoid** = from the cortex

growth hormone (GH): a hormone secreted by the pituitary that regulates the cell division and protein synthesis needed for normal growth (also called **somatotropin**). The release of GH is mediated by *GH-releasing hormone (GHRH)* and *GH-inhibiting hormone (GHIH)*.

luteinizing (LOO-tee-in-EYE-zing) **hormone (LH):** a hormone that stimulates ovulation and the development of the corpus luteum (the small tissue that develops from a ruptured ovarian follicle and secretes hormones); so called because the follicle turns yellow as it matures. In men, LH stimulates testosterone secretion. The release of LH is mediated by *luteinizing hormone–releasing hormone (LH–RH)*.
- **lutein** = a yellow pigment

oxytocin (OCK-see-TOH-sin): a hormone that stimulates the mammary glands to eject milk during lactation and the uterus to contract during and after childbirth.
- **oxy** = quick
- **tocin** = childbirth

progesterone: the hormone of gestation (pregnancy).
- **pro** = promoting
- **gest** = gestation (pregnancy)
- **sterone** = a steroid hormone

prolactin (proh-LAK-tin): a hormone so named because it promotes *(pro)* the production of milk *(lacto)*. The release of prolactin is mediated by *prolactin-inhibiting hormone (PIH)*.

relaxin: the hormone of late pregnancy.

somatostatin (GHIH): a hormone that inhibits the release of growth hormone; the opposite of *somatotropin (GH)*.
- **somato** = body
- **stat** = keep the same
- **tropin** = make more

testosterone: a steroid hormone from the testicles, or testes. The steroids, as explained in Chapter 5, are chemically related to, and some are derived from, the lipid cholesterol.
- **sterone** = a steroid hormone

thyroid-stimulating hormone (TSH): a hormone secreted by the pituitary that stimulates the thyroid gland to secrete its hormones—thyroxine and triiodothyronine. The release of TSH is mediated by *TSH-releasing hormone (TRH)*.

FIGURE A-2 The Endocrine System

These organs and glands release hormones that regulate body processes. An *endocrine gland* secretes its product directly into *(endo)* the blood; for example, the pancreas cells that produce insulin. An *exocrine gland* secretes its product(s) out *(exo)* to an epithelial surface either directly or through a duct; the sweat glands of the skin and the enzyme-producing glands of the pancreas are both examples. The pancreas is therefore both an endocrine and an exocrine gland.

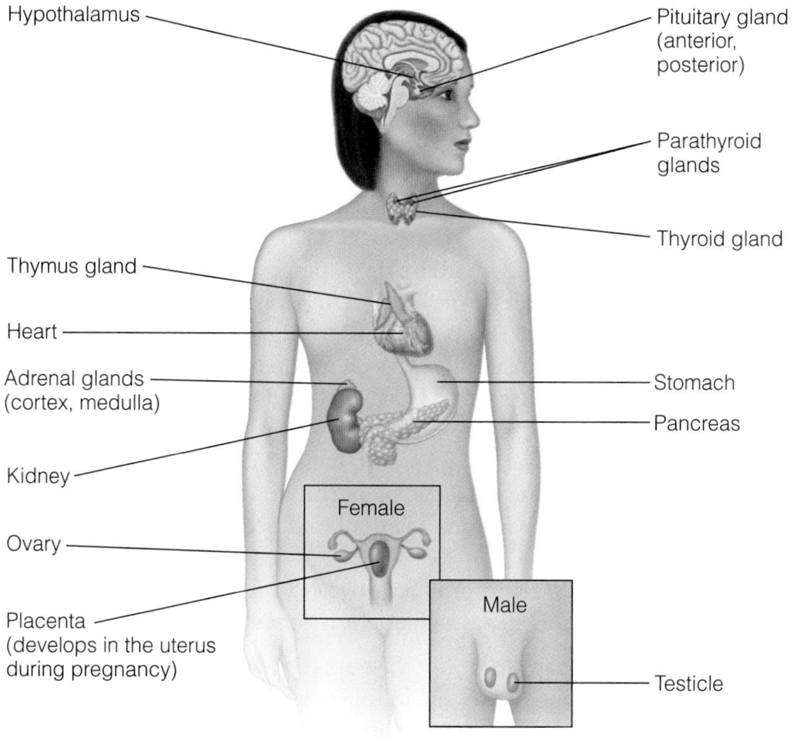
Hypothalamus
Pituitary gland (anterior, posterior)
Parathyroid glands
Thyroid gland
Thymus gland
Heart
Adrenal glands (cortex, medulla)
Stomach
Pancreas
Kidney
Female
Ovary
Placenta (develops in the uterus during pregnancy)
Male
Testicle

- **Growth hormone (GH)** or **somatotropin** acts on all tissues, promoting growth, fat breakdown, and the formation of antibodies.
- **Follicle-stimulating hormone (FSH)** acts on the ovaries in the female, promoting their maturation, and on the testicles in the male, promoting sperm formation.
- **Luteinizing hormone (LH)** also acts on the ovaries, stimulating their maturation, the production and release of progesterone and estrogens, and ovulation; and on the testicles, promoting the production and release of testosterone.
- **Prolactin,** secreted in the female during pregnancy and lactation, acts on the mammary glands to stimulate their growth and the production of milk.

Each of these hormones has one or more signals that turn it on and another (or others) that turns it off. ♦ Among the controlling signals are several hormones from the hypothalamus:

- **Corticotropin-releasing hormone (CRH)**, which promotes release of ACTH, is turned on by stress and turned off by ACTH when enough has been released.
- **TSH-releasing hormone (TRH)**, which promotes release of TSH, is turned on by large meals or low body temperature.
- **GH-releasing hormone (GHRH)**, which stimulates the release of growth hormone, is turned on by insulin.

♦ Hormones that are turned off by their own effects are said to be regulated by *negative feedback* (see Figure 3-13 on p. 80).

- **GH-inhibiting hormone** (**GHIH** or **somatostatin**), which inhibits the release of GH and interferes with the release of TSH, is turned on by hypoglycemia and/or physical activity and is rapidly destroyed by body tissues so that it does not accumulate.
- **FSH/LH–releasing hormone** (**FSH/LH–RH**) is turned on in the female by nerve messages or low estrogen and in the male by low testosterone.
- **Prolactin-inhibiting hormone** (**PIH**) is turned on by high prolactin levels and off by estrogen, testosterone, and suckling (by way of nerve messages).

Let's examine some of these controls. PIH, for example, responds to high prolactin levels (remember, prolactin promotes milk production). High prolactin levels ensure that milk is made and—by calling forth PIH—ensure that prolactin levels don't get too high. But when the infant is suckling—and creating a demand for milk—PIH is not allowed to work (suckling turns off PIH). The consequence: prolactin remains high, and milk production continues. Demand from the infant thus directly adjusts the supply of milk. The need is met through the interaction of the nerves and hormones.

As another example, consider CRH. Stress, perceived in the brain and relayed to the hypothalamus, switches on CRH. On arriving at the pituitary, CRH switches on ACTH. Then ACTH acts on its target organ, the adrenal cortex, which responds by producing and releasing stress hormones. The stress hormones trigger a cascade of events involving every body cell and many other hormones.

The numerous steps required to set the stress response in motion make it possible for the body to fine-tune the response; control can be exerted at each step. These two examples illustrate what the body can do in response to two different stimuli—producing milk in response to an infant's need and gearing up for action in an emergency.

The posterior pituitary gland produces two hormones, each of which acts on one or more target cells and elicits a characteristic response:

- **Antidiuretic hormone** (**ADH**), or **vasopressin**, acts on the arteries, promoting their contraction, and on the kidneys, preventing water excretion. ADH is turned on whenever the blood volume is low, the blood pressure is low, or the salt concentration of the blood is high (see Chapter 11). It is turned off by the return of these conditions to normal.
- **Oxytocin** acts during late pregnancy on the uterus, inducing contractions, and during lactation on the mammary glands, causing milk ejection. Oxytocin is produced in response to reduced progesterone levels, suckling, or the stretching of the cervix.

Hormones that Regulate Energy Metabolism

Hormones produced by a number of different glands have effects on energy metabolism:

- Insulin from the pancreas beta cells is turned on by many stimuli, including high blood glucose. It acts on cells to increase glucose and amino acid uptake into them and to promote the secretion of GHRH.
- Glucagon from the pancreas alpha cells responds to low blood glucose and acts on the liver to promote the breakdown of glycogen to glucose, the conversion of amino acids to glucose, and the release of glucose into the blood.
- Thyroxine from the thyroid gland responds to TSH and acts on many cells to increase their metabolic rate, growth, and heat production.
- Norepinephrine and epinephrine ♦ from the adrenal medulla respond to stimulation by sympathetic nerves and produce reactions in many cells that facilitate the body's readiness for fight or flight: increased heart activity, blood vessel constriction, breakdown of glycogen and glucose, raised blood glucose levels, and fat breakdown. Norepinephrine and epinephrine also influence the secretion of the many hormones from the hypothalamus that exert control on the body's other systems.

♦ Norepinephrine and epinephrine were formerly called *noradrenalin* and *adrenalin*, respectively.

- Growth hormone (GH) from the anterior pituitary (already mentioned).
- **Glucocorticoids** from the adrenal cortex become active during times of stress and carbohydrate metabolism.

Every body part is affected by these hormones. Each different hormone has unique effects; and hormones that oppose each other are produced in carefully regulated amounts, so each can respond to the exact degree that is appropriate to the condition.

Hormones that Adjust Other Body Balances

Hormones are involved in moving calcium into and out of the body's storage deposits in the bones:

- **Calcitonin** from the thyroid gland acts on the bones, which respond by storing calcium from the bloodstream whenever blood calcium rises above the normal range. It also acts on the kidneys to increase excretion of both calcium and phosphorus in the urine. Calcitonin plays a major role in infants and young children, but is less active in adults.
- Parathyroid hormone (parathormone or PTH) from the parathyroid gland responds to the opposite condition—lowered blood calcium—and acts primarily on two targets: the bones, which release stored calcium into the blood; and the kidneys, which slow the excretion of calcium and activate vitamin D.
- Vitamin D from the skin or diet and activated in the liver and kidneys acts with parathyroid hormone and is essential for the absorption of calcium in the intestine, release of calcium from bone into the blood, and retention of calcium in the blood by the kidneys.

Figure 13-1 on p. 411 diagrams the ways vitamin D and the hormones calcitonin and parathyroid hormone regulate calcium homeostasis.

Another hormone has effects on blood-making activity:

- **Erythropoietin** from the kidneys is responsive to oxygen depletion of the blood and to anemia. It acts on the bone marrow to stimulate the making of red blood cells.

Another hormone is special for pregnancy:

- **Relaxin** from the ovaries is secreted in response to the raised progesterone and estrogen levels of late pregnancy. This hormone acts on the cervix and pelvic ligaments to allow them to stretch so that they can accommodate the birth process without strain.

Other agents help regulate blood pressure:

- **Renin** (an enzyme), from the kidneys, in cooperation with **angiotensin** in the blood responds to a reduced blood supply experienced by the kidneys and acts in several ways to increase blood pressure. Renin and angiotensin also stimulate the adrenal cortex to secrete the hormone aldosterone.
- **Aldosterone**, a hormone from the adrenal cortex, targets the kidneys, which respond by reabsorbing sodium. The effect is to retain more water in the bloodstream—thus, again, raising the blood pressure. Figure 11-4 (on p. 360) in Chapter 11 provides more details.

The Gastrointestinal Hormones

Several hormones are produced in the stomach and intestines in response to the presence of food or the components of food:

- Gastrin from the stomach and duodenum stimulates the production and release of gastric acid and other digestive juices and the movement of the GI contents through the system.
- Cholecystokinin from the duodenum signals the gallbladder and pancreas to release their contents into the intestine to aid in digestion.

- Secretin from the duodenum calls forth acid-neutralizing bicarbonate from the pancreas into the intestine and slows the action of the stomach and its secretion of acid and digestive juices.
- Gastric-inhibitory peptide from the duodenum and jejunum inhibits the secretion of gastric acid and slows the process of digestion.

These hormones are defined and discussed in Chapter 3.

The Sex Hormones There are three major sex hormones:

- **Testosterone** from the testicles is released in response to LH (described earlier) and acts on all the tissues that are involved in male sexuality, promoting their development and maintenance.
- **Estrogens** from the ovaries are released in response to both FSH and LH and act similarly in females.
- **Progesterone** from the ovaries' corpus luteum and from the placenta acts on the uterus and mammary glands, preparing them for pregnancy and lactation.

This brief description of the hormones and their functions should suffice to provide an awareness of the enormous impact these compounds have on body processes. The other overall regulating agency is the nervous system.

Nerves

The nervous system has a central control system that can evaluate information about conditions within and outside the body, and a vast system of wiring that receives information and sends instructions. The control unit is the brain and spinal cord, called the **central nervous system;** and the vast complex of wiring between the centre and the parts is the **peripheral nervous system.** The smooth functioning that results from the systems' adjustments to changing conditions is homeostasis.

The nervous system has two general functions: it controls voluntary muscles in response to sensory stimuli from them, and it controls involuntary, internal muscles and glands in response to nerve-borne and chemical signals about their status. In fact, the nervous system is best understood as two systems that use the same or similar pathways to receive and transmit their messages. The **somatic nervous system** controls the voluntary muscles; the **autonomic nervous system** controls the internal organs.

When scientists were first studying the autonomic nervous system, they noticed that when something hurt one organ of the body, some of the other organs reacted as if in sympathy for the afflicted one. They therefore named the nerve network they were studying the sympathetic nervous system. The term is still used today to refer to that branch of the autonomic nervous system that responds to pain and stress. The other branch is called the parasympathetic nervous system. (Think of the sympathetic branch as the responder when homeostasis needs restoring and the parasympathetic branch as the commander of function during normal times.) Both systems transmit their messages through the brain and spinal cord. Nerves of the two branches travel side by side along the same pathways to transmit their messages, but they oppose each other's actions (see Figure A-3).

GLOSSARY OF NERVOUS SYSTEM

autonomic nervous system: the division of the nervous system that controls the body's automatic responses. Its two branches are the *sympathetic* branch, which helps the body respond to stressors from the outside environment, and the *parasympathetic* branch, which regulates normal body activities between stressful times.
- **autonomous** = self-governing

central nervous system: the central part of the nervous system; the brain and spinal cord.

peripheral (puh-RIFF-er-ul) **nervous system:** the peripheral (outermost) part of the nervous system; the vast complex of wiring that extends from the central nervous system to the body's outermost areas. It contains both somatic and autonomic components.

somatic (so-MAT-ick) **nervous system:** the division of the nervous system that controls the voluntary muscles, as distinguished from the autonomic nervous system, which controls involuntary functions.
- **soma** = body

FIGURE A-3 **The Organization of the Nervous System**

The brain and spinal cord evaluate information about conditions within and outside the body, and the peripheral nerves receive information and send instructions.

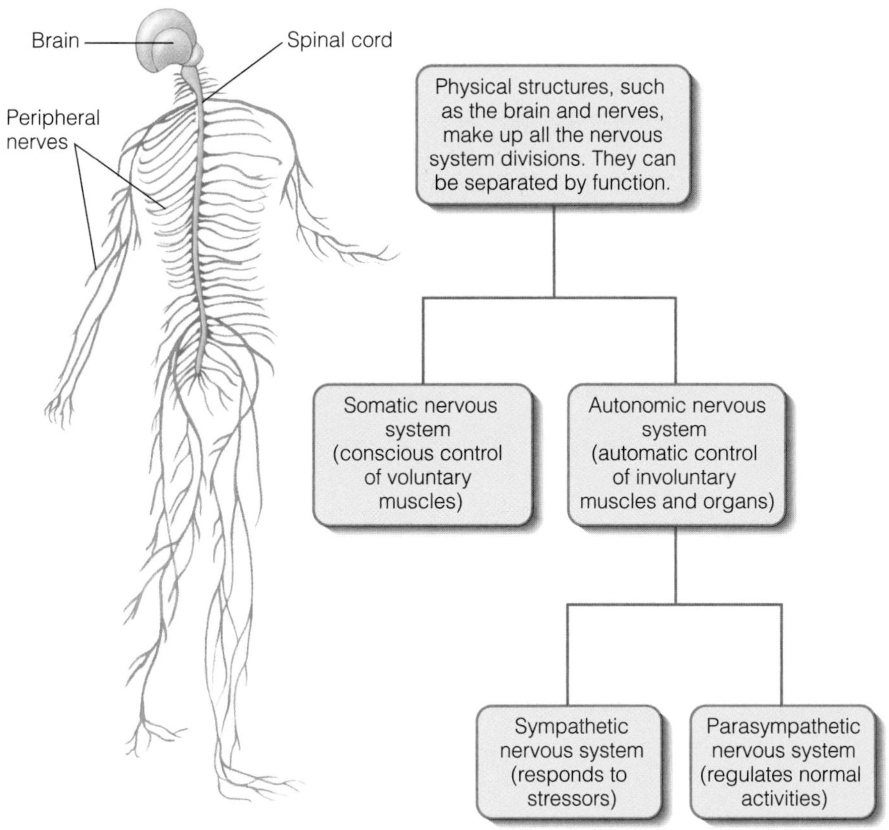
Brain
Spinal cord
Peripheral nerves
Physical structures, such as the brain and nerves, make up all the nervous system divisions. They can be separated by function.
Somatic nervous system (conscious control of voluntary muscles)
Autonomic nervous system (automatic control of involuntary muscles and organs)
Sympathetic nervous system (responds to stressors)
Parasympathetic nervous system (regulates normal activities)

An example will show how the sympathetic and parasympathetic nervous systems work to maintain homeostasis. When you go outside in cold weather, your skin's temperature receptors send "cold" messages to the spinal cord and brain. Your conscious mind may intervene at this point to tell you to zip your jacket, but let's say you have no jacket. Your sympathetic nervous system reacts to the external stressor, the cold. It signals your skin-surface capillaries to shut down so that your blood will circulate deeper in your tissues, where it will conserve heat. Your sympathetic nervous system also signals involuntary contractions of the small muscles just under the skin surface. The product of these muscle contractions is heat, and the visible result is goose bumps. If these measures do not raise your body temperature enough, then the sympathetic nerves signal your large muscle groups to shiver; the contractions of these large muscles produce still more heat. All of this activity helps to maintain your homeostasis (with respect to temperature) under conditions of external extremes (cold) that would throw it off balance. The cold was a stressor; the body's response was resistance.

Now let's say you come in and sit by a fire and drink hot cocoa. You are warm and no longer need all that sympathetic activity. At this point, your parasympathetic nerves take over; they signal your skin-surface capillaries to dilate again, your goose bumps to subside, and your muscles to relax. Your body is back to normal. This is recovery.

Putting It Together

The hormonal and nervous systems coordinate body functions by transmitting and receiving messages. The point-to-point messages of the nervous system travel through a central switchboard (the spinal cord and brain), whereas the messages of the hormonal system are broadcast over the airways (the bloodstream), and any organ with the appropriate receptors can pick them up. Nerve impulses travel faster than hormonal messages do—although both are remarkably swift. Whereas your brain's command to wiggle your toes reaches the toes within a fraction of a second and stops as quickly, a gland's message to alter a body condition may take several seconds or minutes to get started and may fade away equally slowly.

Together, the two systems possess every characteristic a superb communication network needs: varied speeds of transmission, along with private communication lines or public broadcasting systems, depending on the needs of the moment. The hormonal system, together with the nervous system, integrates the whole body's functioning so that all parts act smoothly together.

Basic Chemistry Concepts

APPENDIX B

CONTENTS

This appendix is intended to provide the background in basic chemistry you need to understand the nutrition concepts presented in this book. Chemistry is the branch of natural science that is concerned with the description and classification of **matter**, the changes that matter undergoes, and the **energy** associated with these changes. The accompanying glossary defines matter, energy, and other related terms.

GLOSSARY

atoms: the smallest components of an element that have all of the properties of the element.

compound: a substance composed of two or more different atoms—for example, water (H_2O).

element: a substance composed of atoms that are alike—for example, iron (Fe).

energy: the capacity to do work.

matter: anything that takes up space and has mass.

molecule: two or more atoms of the same or different elements joined by chemical bonds. Examples are molecules of the element oxygen, composed of two oxygen atoms (O_2), and molecules of the compound water, composed of two hydrogen atoms and one oxygen atom (H_2O).

Matter: The Properties of Atoms

Every substance has physical and chemical properties that distinguish it from all other substances and thus give it a unique identity. The physical properties include such characteristics as colour, taste, texture, and odour, as well as the temperatures at which a substance changes its state (from a solid to a liquid or from a liquid to a gas) and the weight of a unit volume (its density). The chemical properties of a substance have to do with how it reacts with other substances or responds to a change in its environment so that new substances with different sets of properties are produced.

A physical change does not change a substance's chemical composition. The three physical states—ice, water, and steam—all consist of two hydrogen atoms and one oxygen atom bound together. In contrast, a chemical change occurs when an electric current passes through water. The water disappears, and two different substances are formed: hydrogen gas, which is flammable, and oxygen gas, which supports life.

Substances: Elements and Compounds

The smallest part of a substance that can exist separately without losing its physical and chemical properties is a **molecule.** If a molecule is composed of **atoms** that are alike, the substance is an **element** (e.g., O_2). If a molecule is composed of two or more different kinds of atoms, the substance is a **compound** (e.g., H_2O).

Just over 100 elements are known, and these are listed in Table B-1 (pp. B-2–B-3). A familiar example is hydrogen, whose molecules are composed only of hydrogen atoms linked together in pairs (H_2). On the other hand, more than a million compounds are known. An example is the sugar glucose. Each of its molecules is composed of 6 carbon, 6 oxygen, and 12 hydrogen atoms linked together in a specific arrangement (as described in Chapter 4).

The Nature of Atoms

Atoms themselves are made of smaller particles. Within the atomic nucleus are protons (positively charged particles), and surrounding the nucleus are electrons (negatively charged particles). The number of protons (+) in the nucleus of an atom determines the number of electrons (−) around it. The positive charge on a proton is equal to the negative charge on an electron, so the charges cancel each other out and leave the atom neutral to its surroundings.

The nucleus may also include neutrons, subatomic particles that have no charge. Protons and neutrons are of equal mass, and together they give an atom its weight. Electrons bond atoms together to make molecules, and they are involved in chemical reactions.

Each type of atom has a characteristic number of protons in its nucleus. The hydrogen atom is the simplest of all. It possesses a single proton, with a single electron associated with it:

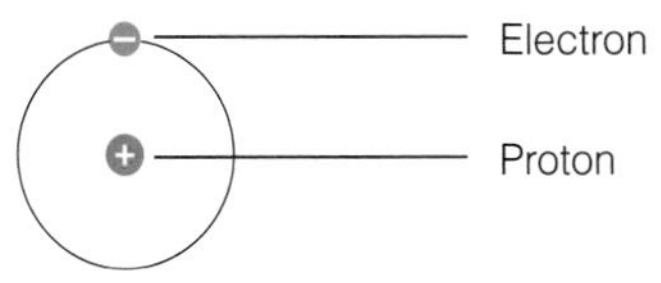
Electron
Proton

Hydrogen atom (H), atomic number 1.

Just as hydrogen always has one proton, helium always has two, lithium three, and so on. The atomic number of each element is the number of protons in the nucleus of that atom, and

TABLE B-1 Chemical Symbols for the Elements

Number of Protons (Atomic Number)	Element	Number of Electrons in Outer Shell	Number of Protons (Atomic Number)	Element	Number of Electrons in Outer Shell
1	Hydrogen (H)	1	50	Tin (Sn)	4
2	Helium (He)	2	51	Antimony (Sb)	5
3	Lithium (Li)	1	52	Tellurium (Te)	6
4	Beryllium (Be)	2	53	Iodine (I)	7
5	Boron (B)	3	54	Xenon (Xe)	8
6	Carbon (C)	4	55	Cesium (Cs)	1
7	Nitrogen (N)	5	56	Barium (Ba)	2
8	Oxygen (O)	6	57	Lanthanum (La)	2
9	Fluorine (F)	7	58	Cerium (Ce)	2
10	Neon (Ne)	8	59	Praseodymium (Pr)	2
11	Sodium (Na)	1	60	Neodymium (Nd)	2
12	Magnesium (Mg)	2	61	Promethium (Pm)	2
13	Aluminum (Al)	3	62	Samarium (Sm)	2
14	Silicon (Si)	4	63	Europium (Eu)	2
15	Phosphorus (P)	5	64	Gadolinium (Gd)	2
16	Sulphur (S)	6	65	Terbium (Tb)	2
17	Chlorine (Cl)	7	66	Dysprosium (Dy)	2
18	Argon (Ar)	8	67	Holmium (Ho)	2
19	Potassium (K)	1	68	Erbium (Er)	2
20	Calcium (Ca)	2	69	Thulium (Tm)	2
21	Scandium (Sc)	2	70	Ytterbium (Yb)	2
22	Titanium (Ti)	2	71	Lutetium (Lu)	2
23	Vanadium (V)	2	72	Hafnium (Hf)	2
24	Chromium (Cr)	1	73	Tantalum (Ta)	2
25	Manganese (Mn)	2	74	Tungsten (W)	2
26	Iron (Fe)	2	75	Rhenium (Re)	2
27	Cobalt (Co)	2	76	Osmium (Os)	2
28	Nickel (Ni)	2	77	Iridium (Ir)	2
29	Copper (Cu)	1	78	Platinum (Pt)	1
30	Zinc (Zn)	2	79	Gold (Au)	1
31	Gallium (Ga)	3	80	Mercury (Hg)	2
32	Germanium (Ge)	4	81	Thallium (Tl)	3
33	Arsenic (As)	5	82	Lead (Pb)	4
34	Selenium (Se)	6	83	Bismuth (Bi)	5
35	Bromine (Br)	7	84	Polonium (Po)	6
36	Krypton (Kr)	8	85	Astatine (At)	7
37	Rubidium (Rb)	1	86	Radon (Rn)	8
38	Strontium (Sr)	2	87	Francium (Fr)	1
39	Yttrium (Y)	2	88	Radium (Ra)	2
40	Zirconium (Zr)	2	89	Actinium (Ac)	2
41	Niobium (Nb)	1	90	Thorium (Th)	2
42	Molybdenum (Mo)	1	91	Protactinium (Pa)	2
43	Technetium (Tc)	1	92	Uranium (U)	2
44	Ruthenium (Ru)	1	93	Neptunium (Np)	2
45	Rhodium (Rh)	1	94	Plutonium (Pu)	2
46	Palladium (Pd)	—	95	Americium (Am)	2
47	Silver (Ag)	1	96	Curium (Cm)	2
48	Cadmium (Cd)	2	97	Berkelium (Bk)	2
49	Indium (In)	3	98	Californium (Cf)	2

(continued)

TABLE B-1 Chemical Symbols for the Elements (*continued*)

Number of Protons (Atomic Number)	Element	Number of Electrons in Outer Shell	Number of Protons (Atomic Number)	Element	Number of Electrons in Outer Shell
99	Einsteinium (Es)	2	105	Dubnium (Db)	2
100	Fermium (Fm)	2	106	Seaborgium (Sg)	2
101	Mendelevium (Md)	2	107	Bohrium (Bh)	2
102	Nobelium (No)	2	108	Hassium (Hs)	2
103	Lawrencium (Lr)	2	109	Meitnerium (Mt)	2
104	Rutherfordium (Rf)	2	110	Darmstadtium (Ds)	2

Key
Elements found in energy-yielding nutrients, vitamins, and water
Major minerals
Trace minerals

this never changes in a chemical reaction; it gives the atom its identity. The atomic numbers for the known elements are listed in Table B-1.

Besides hydrogen, the atoms most common in living things are carbon (C), nitrogen (N), and oxygen (O), whose atomic numbers are 6, 7, and 8, respectively. Their structures are more complicated than that of hydrogen, but each of them possesses the same number of electrons as there are protons in the nucleus. These electrons are found in orbits, or shells (shown below).

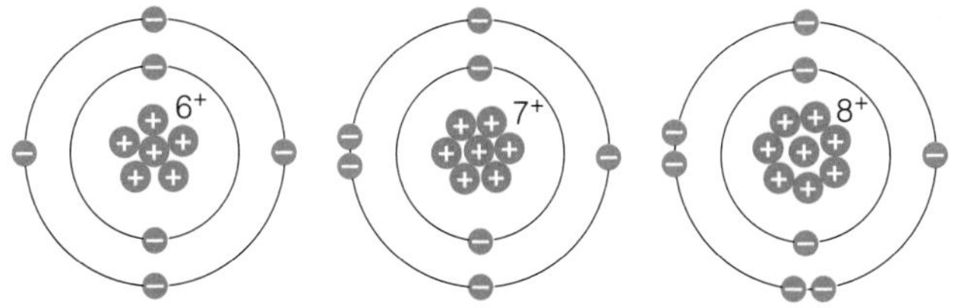
6+
7+
8+
Carbon atom (C), atomic number 6
Nitrogen atom (N), atomic number 7
Oxygen atom (O), atomic number 8

In these and all diagrams of atoms that follow, only the protons and electrons are shown. The neutrons, which contribute only to atomic weight, not to charge, are omitted.

The most important structural feature of an atom for determining its chemical behaviour is the number of electrons in its outermost shell. The first, or innermost, shell is full when it is occupied by two electrons; so an atom with two or more electrons has a filled first shell. When the first shell is full, electrons begin to fill the second shell.

The second shell is completely full when it has eight electrons. A substance that has a full outer shell tends not to enter into chemical reactions. Atomic number 10, neon, is a chemically inert substance because its outer shell is complete. Fluorine, atomic number 9, has a great tendency to draw an electron from other substances to complete its outer shell, and thus it is highly reactive. Carbon has a half-full outer shell, which helps explain its great versatility; it can combine with other elements in a variety of ways to form a large number of compounds.

Atoms seek to reach a state of maximum stability or of lowest energy in the same way that a ball will roll down a hill until it reaches the lowest place. An atom achieves a state of maximum stability:

- By gaining or losing electrons to either fill or empty its outer shell.
- By sharing its electrons with other atoms and thereby completing its outer shell.

The number of electrons determines how the atom will chemically react with other atoms. The atomic number, not the weight, is what gives an atom its chemical nature.

Chemical Bonding

Atoms often complete their outer shells by sharing electrons with other atoms. In order to complete its outer shell, a carbon atom requires four electrons. A hydrogen atom requires one. Thus, when a carbon atom shares electrons with four hydrogen atoms, each completes its outer shell (as shown below). Electron sharing binds the atoms together and satisfies the conditions of maximum stability for the molecule. The outer shell of each atom is complete because hydrogen effectively has the required 2 electrons in its first (outer) shell, and carbon has 8 electrons in its second (outer) shell; and the molecule is electrically neutral, with a total of 10 protons and 10 electrons.

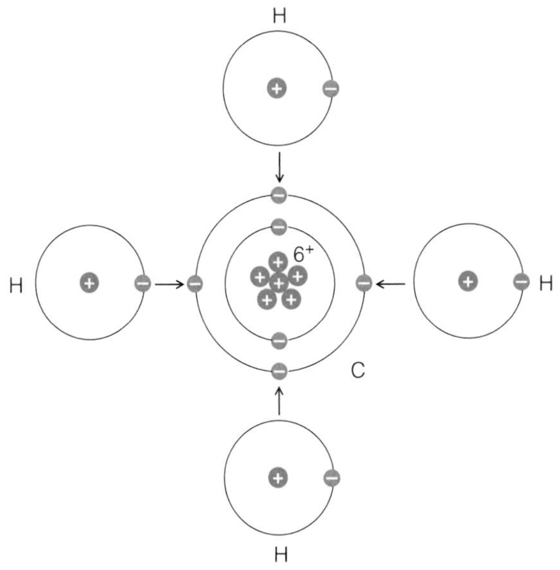
H
H
6+
H
C
H

When a carbon atom shares electrons with four hydrogen atoms, a methane molecule is made.

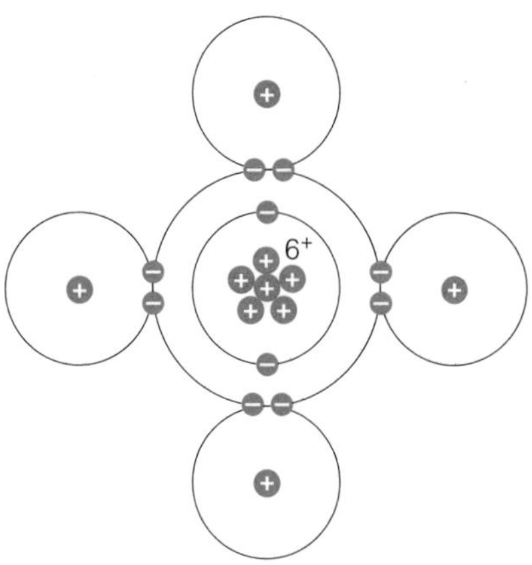
6+

The chemical formula for methane is CH_4. Note that by sharing electrons, every atom achieves a filled outer shell.

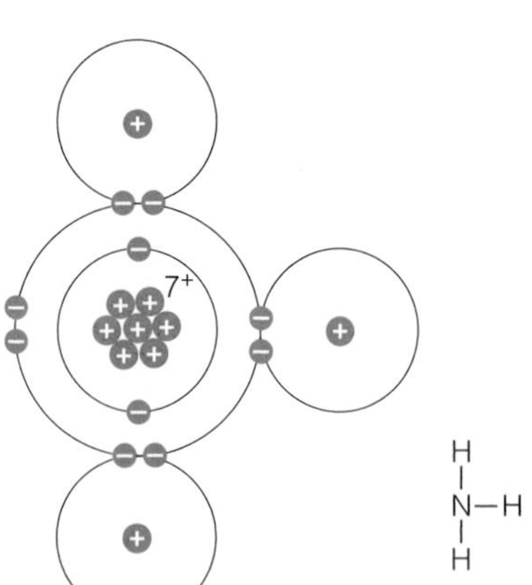
7+
H
N—H
H

Ammonia (NH_3)

The chemical formula for ammonia is NH_3. Count the electrons in each atom's outer shell to confirm that it is filled.

Bonds that involve the sharing of electrons, like the bonds between carbon and the four hydrogens, are the most stable kind of association that atoms can form with one another. These bonds are called covalent bonds, and the resulting combination of atoms is called a molecule. A single pair of shared electrons forms a single bond. A simplified way to represent a single bond is with a single line. Thus the structure of methane (CH_4) could be represented like this:

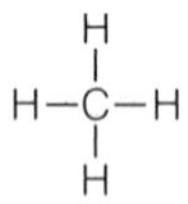
H
H—C—H
H

Methane (CH_4)

Similarly, one nitrogen atom and three hydrogen atoms can share electrons to form one molecule of ammonia (NH_3):

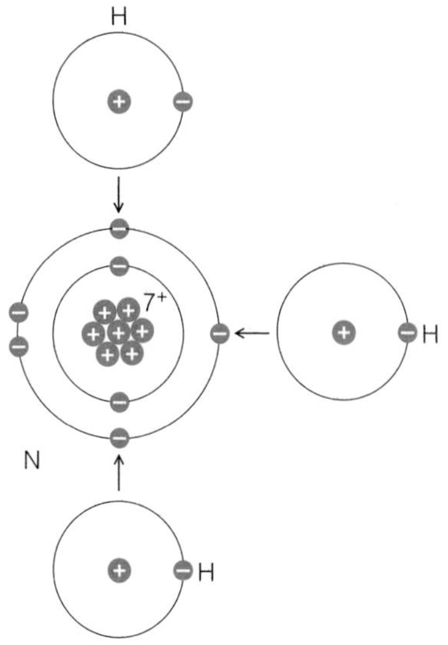
H
7+
H
N
H

When a nitrogen atom shares electrons with three hydrogen atoms, an ammonia molecule is made.

One oxygen atom may be bonded to two hydrogen atoms to form one molecule of water (H_2O):

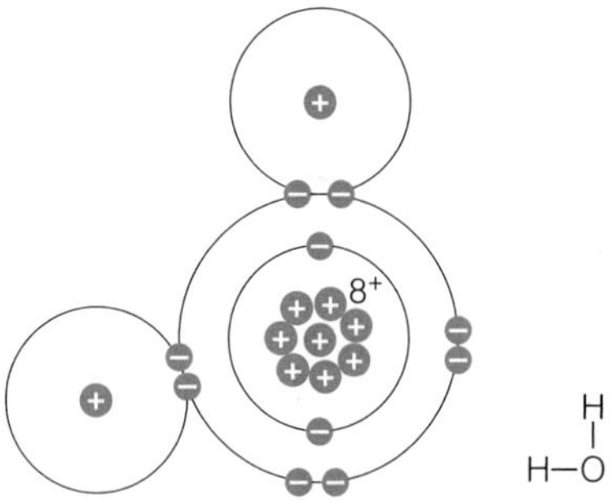
8+
H
H—O

Water molecule (H_2O)

When two oxygen atoms form a molecule of oxygen, they must share two pairs of electrons. This double bond may be represented as two single lines:

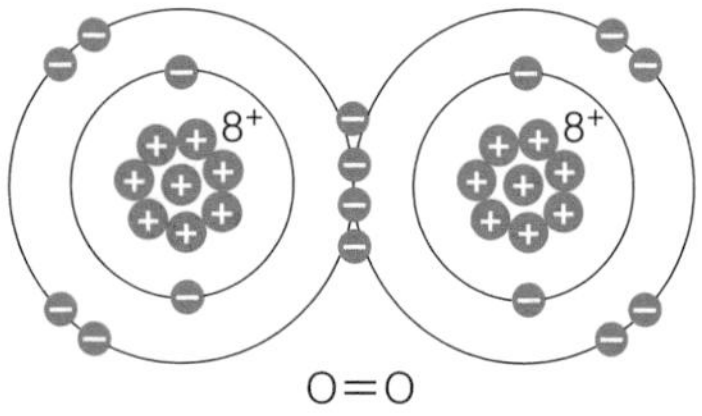
8+
8+
O=O

Oxygen molecule (O_2)

Small atoms form the tightest, most stable bonds. H, O, N, and C are the smallest atoms capable of forming one, two, three, and four electron-pair bonds, respectively. This is the basis for the statement in Chapter 4 that in drawings of compounds containing these atoms, hydrogen must always have one, oxygen two, nitrogen three, and carbon four bonds radiating to other atoms:

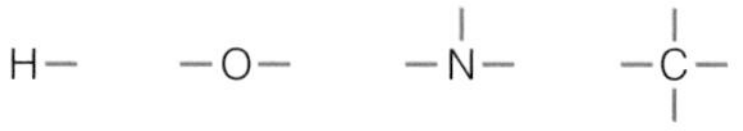
H—
—O—
—N—
—C—

TABLE B-2 Elemental Composition of the Human Body

Element	Chemical Symbol	By Weight (%)
Oxygen	O	65.0
Carbon	C	18.0
Hydrogen	H	10.0
Nitrogen	N	3.0
Calcium	Ca	1.5
Phosphorus	P	1.0
Potassium	K	0.4
Sulphur	S	0.3
Sodium	Na	0.2
Chloride	Cl	0.1
Magnesium	Mg	0.1
Total		99.6[a]

[a]The remaining 0.4 percent by weight is contributed by the trace elements: chromium (Cr), copper (Cu), zinc (Zn), selenium (Se), molybdenum (Mo), fluorine (F), iodine (I), manganese (Mn), and iron (Fe). Cells may also contain variable traces of some of the following: boron (B), cobalt (Co), lithium (Li), strontium (Sr), aluminum (Al), silicon (Si), lead (Pb), vanadium (V), arsenic (As), bromine (Br), and others.

The stability of the associations between these small atoms and the versatility with which they can combine make them very common in living things. Interestingly, all cells, whether they come from animals, plants, or bacteria, contain the same elements in very nearly the same proportions. The elements commonly found in living things are shown in Table B-2.

Formation of Ions

An atom such as sodium (Na, atomic number 11) cannot easily fill its outer shell by sharing. Sodium possesses a filled first shell of two electrons and a filled second shell of eight; there is only one electron in its outermost shell:

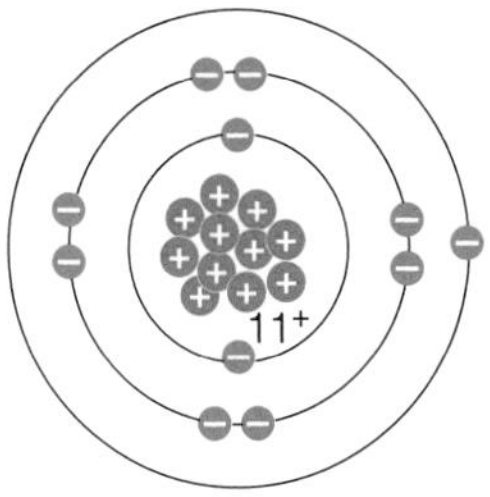
11+

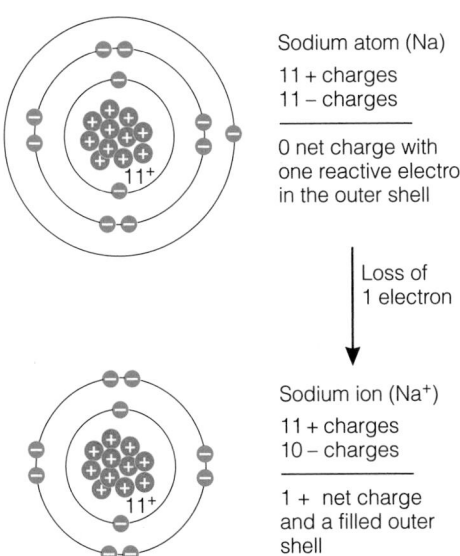

Sodium atom (Na)

11 + charges
11 – charges

0 net charge with one reactive electron in the outer shell

Loss of 1 electron

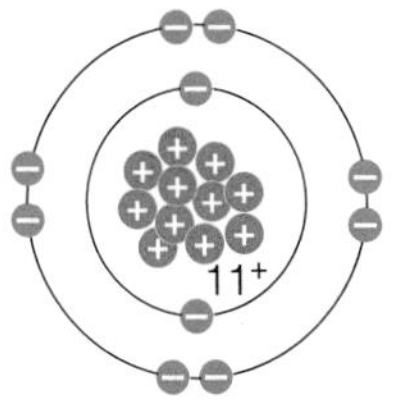
11+

Sodium ion (Na^+)

11 + charges
10 – charges

1 + net charge and a filled outer shell

If sodium loses this electron, it satisfies one condition for stability: a filled outer shell (now its second shell counts as the outer shell). However, it is not electrically neutral. It has 11 protons (positive) and only 10 electrons (negative). It therefore has a net positive charge. An atom or molecule that has lost or gained one or more electrons and so is electrically charged is called an ion.

An atom such as chlorine (Cl, atomic number 17), with seven electrons in its outermost shell, can share electrons to fill its outer shell, or it can gain one electron to complete its outer shell and thus give it a negative charge:

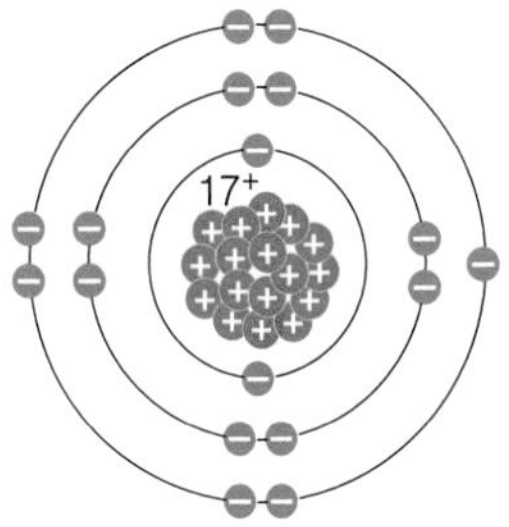
17+

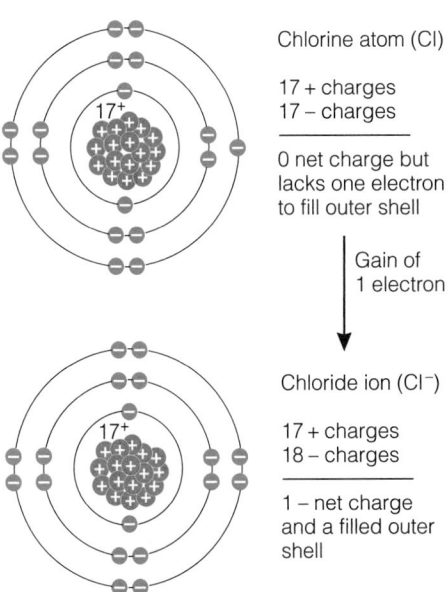

Chlorine atom (Cl)

17 + charges
17 – charges

0 net charge but lacks one electron to fill outer shell

Gain of 1 electron

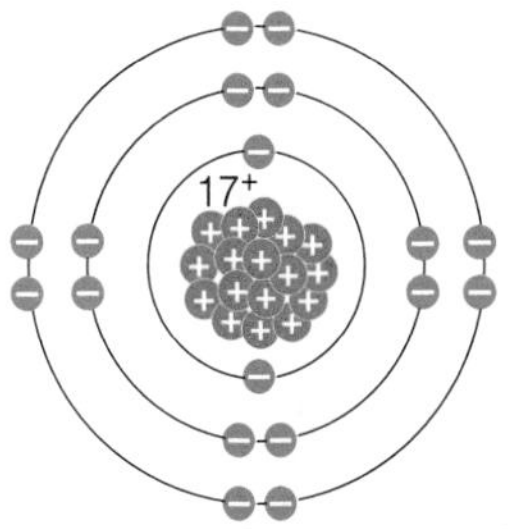
17+

Chloride ion (Cl^-)

17 + charges
18 – charges

1 – net charge and a filled outer shell

A positively charged ion such as sodium ion (Na^+) is called a cation; a negatively charged ion such as a chloride ion (Cl^-) is called an anion. Cations and anions attract one another to form salts:

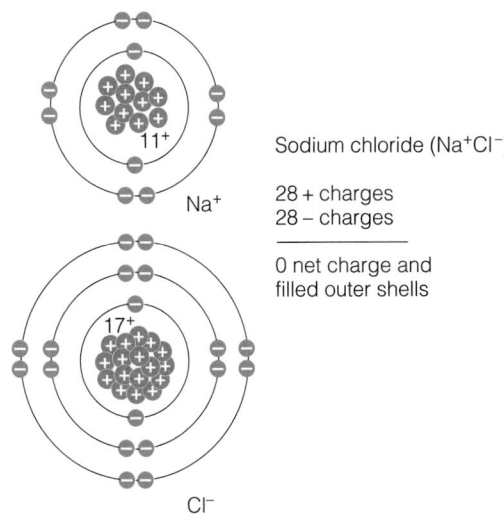

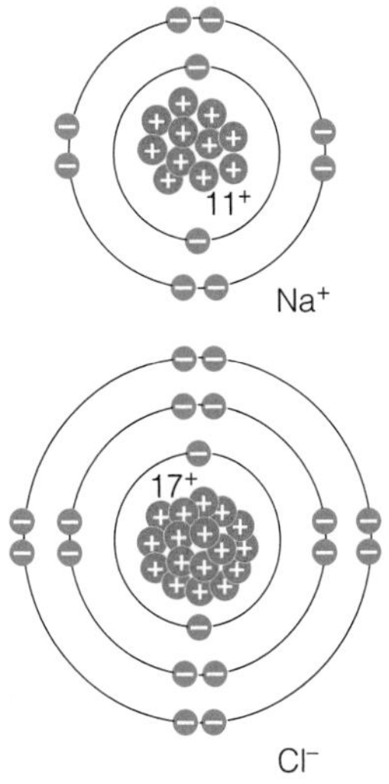
11+
Na+
17+
Cl−

Sodium chloride (Na^+Cl^-)

28 + charges
28 – charges

0 net charge and filled outer shells

With all its electrons, sodium is a shiny, highly reactive metal; chlorine is the poisonous greenish yellow gas that was used in World War I. But after sodium and chlorine have transferred electrons, they form the stable white salt familiar to you as table salt, or sodium chloride (Na^+Cl^-). The dramatic difference illustrates how profoundly the electron arrangement can influence the nature of a substance. The wide distribution of salt in nature attests to the stability of the union between the ions. Each meets the other's needs (a good marriage).

When dry, salt exists as crystals; its ions are stacked very regularly into a lattice, with positive and negative ions alternating in a three-dimensional checkerboard structure. In water, however, the salt quickly dissolves, and its ions separate from one another, forming an electrolyte solution in which they move about freely. Covalently bonded molecules rarely dissociate like this in a water solution. The most common exception is when they behave like acids and release H^+ ions, as discussed in the next section.

An ion can also be a group of atoms bound together in such a way that the group has a net charge and enters into reactions as a single unit. Many such groups are active in the fluids of the body. The bicarbonate ion is composed of five atoms—one H, one C, and three Os—and has a net charge of −1 (HCO_3^-). Another important ion of this type is a phosphate ion with one H, one P, and four O, and a net charge of −2 (HPO_4^{2-}).

Whereas many elements have only one configuration in the outer shell and thus only one way to bond with other elements, some elements have the possibility of varied configurations. Iron is such an element. Under some conditions iron loses two electrons, and under other circumstances it loses three. If iron loses two electrons, it then has a net charge of +2, and we call it ferrous iron (Fe^{++}). If it donates three electrons to another atom, it becomes the +3 ion, or ferric iron (Fe^{+++}).

Ferrous iron (Fe^{++})	Ferric iron (Fe^{+++})
(had 2 outer-shell electrons but has lost them)	(had 3 outer-shell electrons but has lost them)
26 + charges	26 + charges
24 − charges	23 − charges
2 + net charge	3 + net charge

Remember that a positive charge on an ion means that negative charges—electrons—have been lost and not that positive charges have been added to the nucleus.

Water, Acids, and Bases

Water The water molecule is electrically neutral, having equal numbers of protons and electrons. When a hydrogen atom shares its electron with oxygen, however, that electron will spend most of its time closer to the positively charged oxygen nucleus. This leaves the positive proton (nucleus of the hydrogen atom) exposed on the outer part of the water molecule. We know, too, that the two hydrogens both bond toward the same side of the oxygen. These two facts explain why water molecules are polar: they have regions of more positive and more negative charge.

Polar molecules like water are drawn to one another by the attractive forces between the positive polar areas of one and the negative poles of another. These attractive forces, sometimes known as polar bonds or hydrogen bonds, occur among many molecules and also within the different parts of single large molecules. Although very weak in comparison with covalent bonds, polar bonds may occur in such abundance that they become exceedingly important in determining the structure of such large molecules as proteins and DNA.

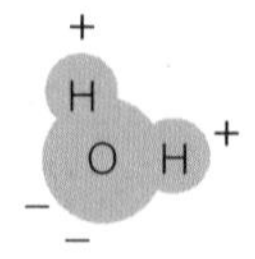
+
H
O H
+
−
−

This diagram of the polar water molecule shows displacement of electrons toward the O nucleus; thus the negative region is near the O and the positive regions are near the H atoms.

Water molecules have a slight tendency to ionize, separating into positive (H^+) and negative (OH^-) ions. In pure water, a small but constant number of these ions is present, and the number of positive ions exactly equals the number of negative ions.

Acid An acid is a substance that releases H^+ ions (protons) in a water solution. Hydrochloric acid (HCl^-) is such a substance because it dissociates in a water solution into H^+ and Cl^- ions. Acetic acid is also an acid because it dissociates in water to acetate ions and free H^+:

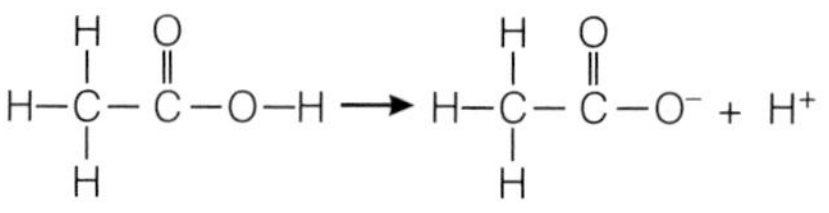

Acetic acid dissociates into an acetate ion and a hydrogen ion.

The more H^+ ions released, the stronger the acid.

pH Chemists define degrees of acidity by means of the pH scale, which runs from 0 to 14. The pH expresses the concentration of H^+ ions: a pH of 1 is extremely acidic, 7 is neutral, and 13 is very basic. There is a tenfold difference in the concentration of H^+ ions between points on this scale. A solution with pH 3, for example, has 10 times as many H^+ ions as a solution with pH 4. At pH 7, the concentrations of free H^+ and OH^- are exactly the same—1/10 000 000 moles per litre (1027 moles per litre).* At pH 4, the concentration of free

*A mole is a certain number (about 6×10^{23}) of molecules. The pH of a solution is defined as the negative logarithm of the hydrogen ion concentration of the solution. Thus, if the concentration is 10^{-2} (moles per litre), the pH is 2; if 10^{-8}, the pH is 8; and so on.

H^+ ions is 1/10 000 (1024) moles per litre. This is a higher concentration of H^+ ions, and the solution is therefore acidic. Figure 3-7 on p. 72 presents the pH scale.

Bases A base is a substance that can combine with H^+ ions, thus reducing the acidity of a solution. The compound ammonia is such a substance. The ammonia molecule has two electrons that are not shared with any other atom; a hydrogen ion (H^+) is just a naked proton with no shell of electrons at all. The proton readily combines with the ammonia molecule to form an ammonium ion; thus a free proton is withdrawn from the solution and no longer contributes to its acidity. Many compounds containing nitrogen are important bases in living systems. Acids and bases neutralize each other to produce substances that are neither acid nor base.

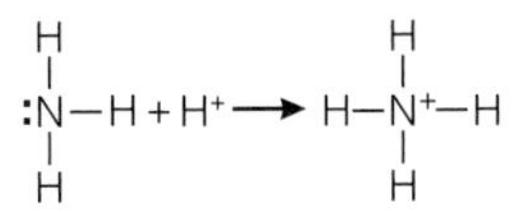

Ammonia captures a hydrogen ion from water. The two dots here represent the two electrons not shared with another atom. These dots are ordinarily not shown in chemical structure drawings. Compare this drawing with the earlier diagram of an ammonia molecule (p. B-4).

Chemical Reactions

A chemical reaction, or chemical change, results in the breakdown of substances and the formation of new ones. Almost all such reactions involve a change in the bonding of atoms. Old bonds are broken, and new ones are formed. The nuclei of atoms are never involved in chemical reactions—only their outer-shell electrons take part. At the end of a chemical reaction, the number of atoms of each type is always the same as at the beginning. For example, two hydrogen molecules ($2H_2$) can react with one oxygen molecule (O_2) to form two water molecules ($2H_2O$). In this reaction two substances (hydrogen and oxygen) disappear, and a new one (water) is formed, but at the end of the reaction there are still four H atoms and two O atoms, just as there were at the beginning. Because the atoms are now linked in a different way, their characteristics or properties have changed.

In many instances chemical reactions involve not the relinking of molecules but the exchanging of electrons or protons among them. In such reactions the molecule that gains one or more electrons (or loses one or more hydrogen ions) is said to be reduced; the molecule that loses electrons (or gains protons) is oxidized. A hydrogen ion is equivalent to a proton. Oxidation and reduction reactions take place simultaneously because an electron or proton that is lost by one molecule is accepted by another. The addition of an atom of oxygen is also oxidation because oxygen (with six electrons in the outer shell) accepts two electrons in becoming bonded. Oxidation, then, is loss of electrons, gain of protons, or addition of oxygen (with six electrons); reduction is the opposite—gain of electrons, loss of protons, or loss of oxygen. The addition of hydrogen atoms to oxygen to form water can thus be described as the reduction of oxygen *or* the oxidation of hydrogen.

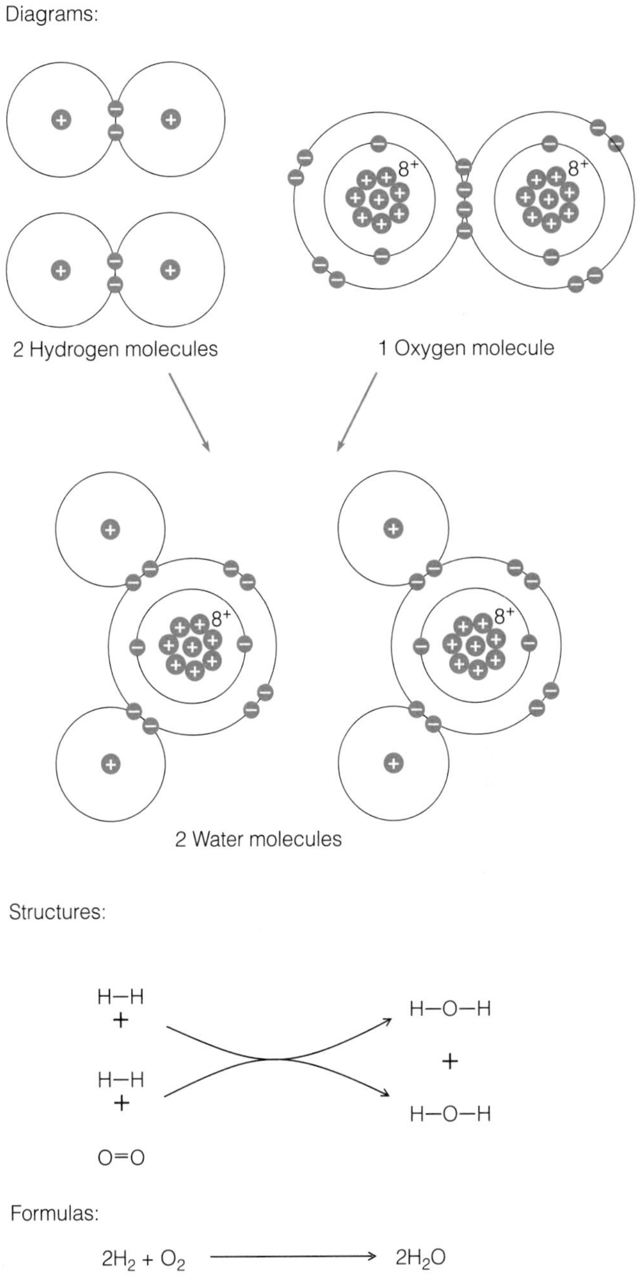
Diagrams:
8+
2 Hydrogen molecules
1 Oxygen molecule
2 Water molecules
Structures:
H—H
+
H—H
+
O=O
H—O—H
+
H—O—H
Formulas:
2H2 + O2
2H2O

Hydrogen and oxygen react to form water.

If a reaction results in a net increase in the energy of a compound, it is called an endergonic, or "uphill," reaction (energy, *erg,* is added into, *endo,* the compound). An example is the chief result of photosynthesis, the making of sugar in a plant from carbon dioxide and water using the energy of sunlight. Conversely, the oxidation of sugar to carbon dioxide and water is an exergonic, or "downhill," reaction because the end products have less energy than the starting products. Oftentimes, but not always, reduction reactions are endergonic, resulting in an increase in the energy of the products. Oxidation reactions often, but not always, are exergonic.

Chemical reactions tend to occur spontaneously if the end products are in a lower energy state and therefore are more stable than the reacting compounds. These reactions often give off energy in the form of heat as they occur. The generation of heat by wood burning in a fireplace and the maintenance of human body warmth both depend on energy-yielding chemical reactions. These downhill reactions occur easily, although they may require some activation energy to get them started, just as a ball requires a push to start rolling.

Uphill reactions, in which the products contain more energy than the reacting compounds started with, do not occur until an energy source is provided. An example of such an energy source is the sunlight used in photosynthesis, where carbon dioxide and water (low-energy compounds) are combined to form the sugar glucose (a higher-energy compound). Another example is the use of the energy in glucose to combine two low-energy compounds in the body into the high-energy compound ATP (see Chapter 7). The energy in ATP may be used to power many other energy-requiring, uphill reactions. Clearly, any of many different molecules can be used as a temporary storage place for energy.

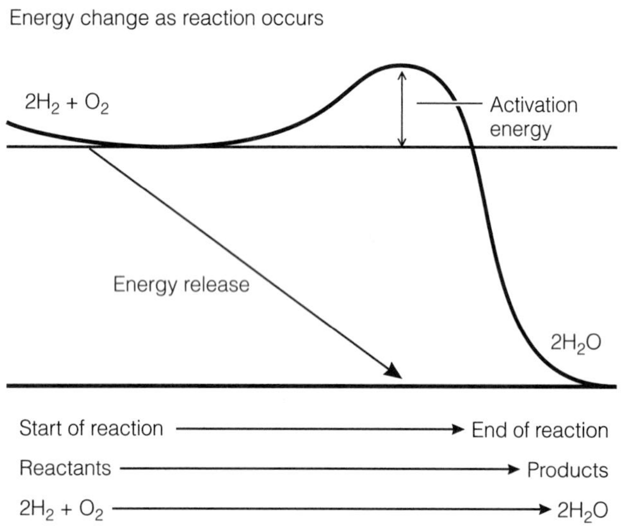
Energy change as reaction occurs
$2H_2 + O_2$
Activation energy
Energy release
$2H_2O$
Start of reaction → End of reaction
Reactants → Products
$2H_2 + O_2$ → $2H_2O$

Formation of Free Radicals

Normally, when a chemical reaction takes place, bonds break and re-form with some redistribution of atoms and rearrangement of bonds to form new, stable compounds. Normally, bonds don't split in such a way as to leave a molecule with an odd, unpaired electron. When they do, free radicals are formed. Free radicals are highly unstable and quickly react with other compounds, forming more free radicals in a chain reaction. A cascade may ensue in which many highly reactive radicals are generated, resulting finally in the disruption of a living structure such as a cell membrane.

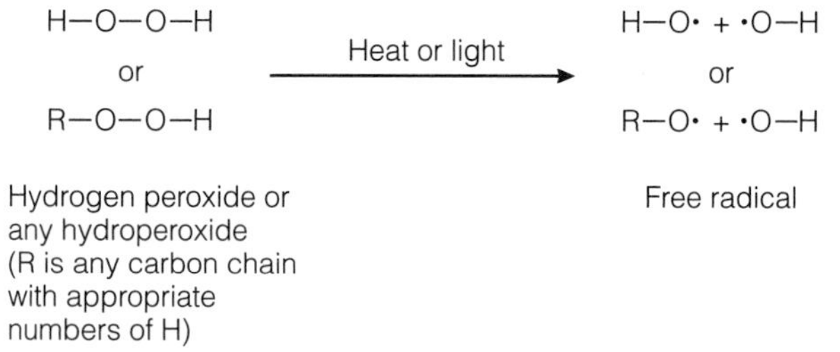
H—O—O—H
or
R—O—O—H
Heat or light
H—O• + •O—H
or
R—O• + •O—H
Hydrogen peroxide or any hydroperoxide (R is any carbon chain with appropriate numbers of H)
Free radical

Free radicals are formed. The dots represent single electrons that are available for sharing (the atom needs another electron to fill its outer shell).

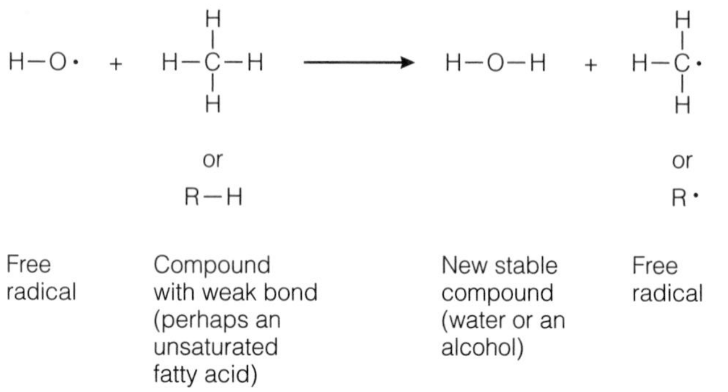
H—O• + H—C—H (with H above and below C) or R—H → H—O—H + H—C• (with H above and below C) or R•
Free radical
Compound with weak bond (perhaps an unsaturated fatty acid)
New stable compound (water or an alcohol)
Free radical

Free radicals destroy biological compounds. The free radical attacks a weak bond in a biological compound, disrupting it and forming a new stable molecule and another free radical. This free radical can attack another biological compound, and so on.

Oxidation of some compounds can be induced by air at room temperature in the presence of light. Such reactions are thought to take place through the formation of compounds called peroxides:

Peroxides:

H—O—O—H	Hydrogen peroxide
R—O—O—H	Hydroperoxides (R is any carbon chain with appropriate numbers of H)
R—O—O—R	Peroxide

Some peroxides readily disintegrate into free radicals, initiating chain reactions like those just described.

Free radicals are of special interest in nutrition because the antioxidant properties of vitamins C and E as well as beta-carotene and the mineral selenium are thought to protect against the destructive effects of these free radicals (see Highlight 12). For example, vitamin E on the surface of the lungs reacts with, and is destroyed by, free radicals, thus preventing the radicals from reaching underlying cells and oxidizing the lipids in their membranes.

Biochemical Structures and Pathways

APPENDIX C

CONTENTS

The diagrams of nutrients presented here are meant to enhance your understanding of the most important organic molecules in the human diet. Following the diagrams of nutrients are sections on the major metabolic pathways mentioned in Chapter 7—glycolysis, fatty acid oxidation, amino acid degradation, the TCA cycle, and the electron transport chain—and a description of how alcohol interferes with these pathways. Discussions of the urea cycle and the formation of ketone bodies complete the appendix.

Carbohydrates

Monosaccharides

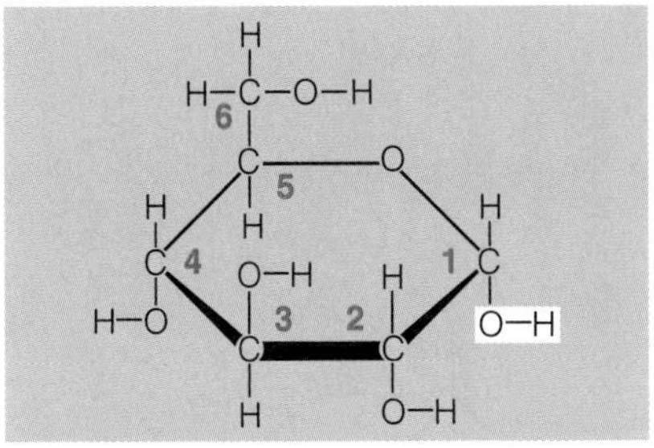

Glucose (alpha form). The ring would be at right angles to the plane of the paper. The bonds directed upward are above the plane; those directed downward are below the plane. This molecule is considered an alpha form because the OH on carbon 1 points downward.

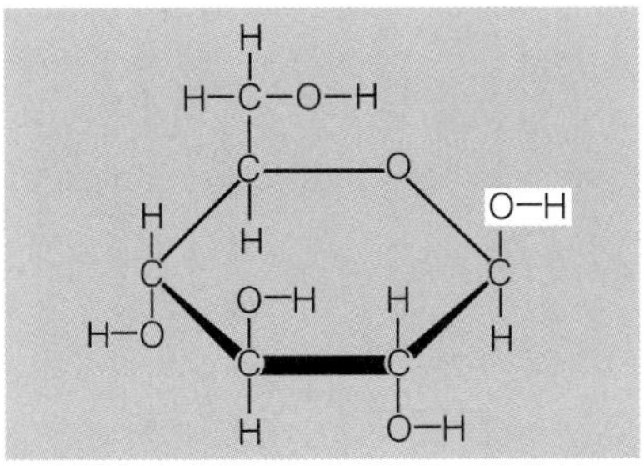

Glucose (beta form). The OH on carbon 1 points upward.
Fructose, galactose: see Chapter 4.

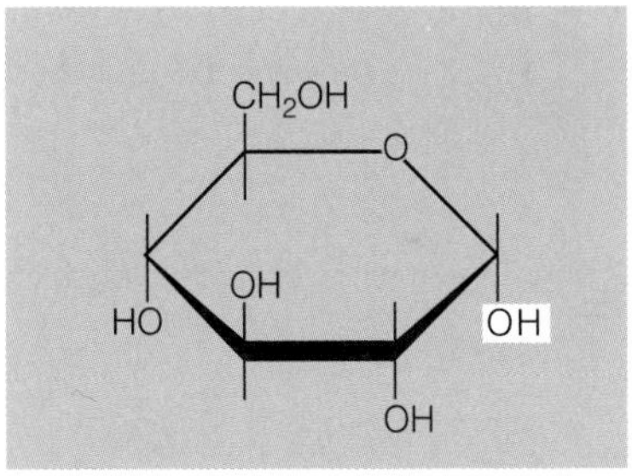

Glucose (alpha form) shorthand notation. This notation, in which the carbons in the ring and single hydrogens have been eliminated, will be used throughout this appendix.

Disaccharides

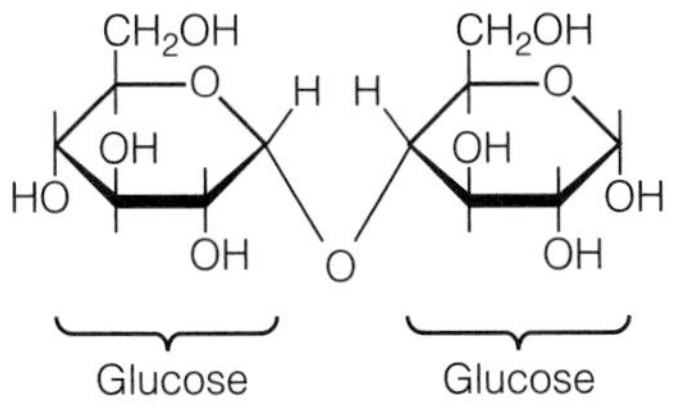
Glucose
Glucose

Maltose.

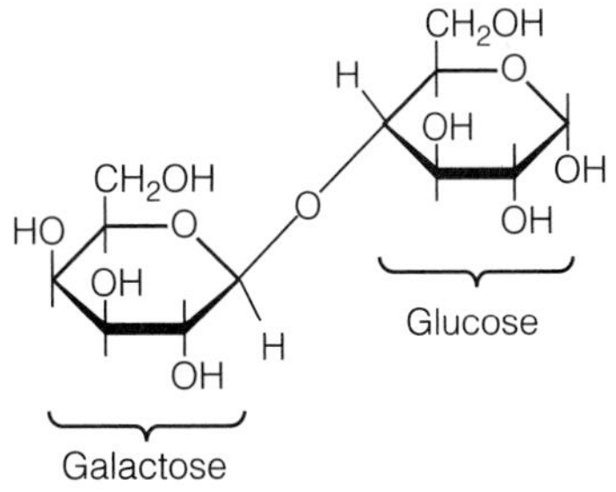
Galactose
Glucose

Lactose (alpha form).

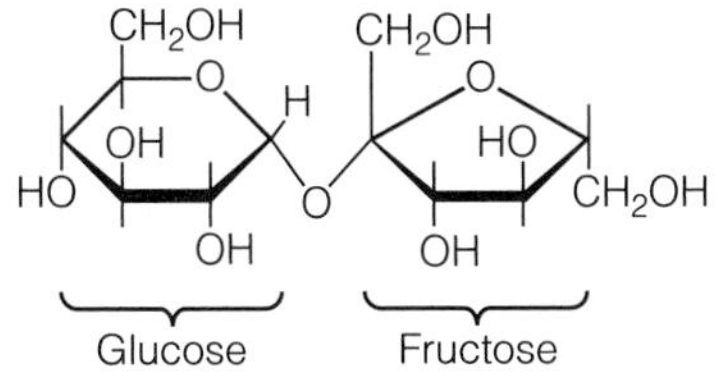
Glucose
Fructose

Sucrose.

Polysaccharides As described in Chapter 4, starch, glycogen, and cellulose are all long chains of glucose molecules covalently linked together.

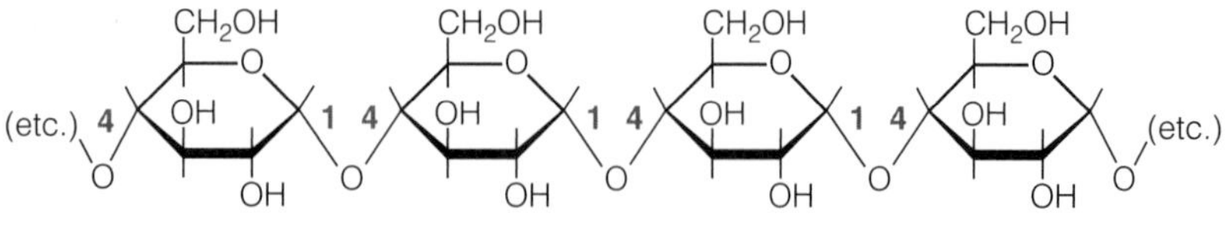

Amylose (unbranched starch)

Starch. Two kinds of covalent linkages occur between glucose molecules in starch, giving rise to two kinds of chains. Amylose is composed of straight chains, with carbon 1 of one glucose linked to carbon 4 of the next (α-1,4 linkage). Amylopectin is made up of straight chains like amylose but has occasional branches arising where the carbon 6 of a glucose is also linked to the carbon 1 of another glucose (α-1,6 linkage).

Glycogen. The structure of glycogen is like amylopectin but with many more branches.

Cellulose. Like starch and glycogen, cellulose is also made of chains of glucose units, but there is an important difference: in cellulose, the OH on carbon 1 is in the beta position (see p. C-1). When carbon 1 of one glucose is linked to carbon 4 of the next, it forms a β-1,4 linkage, which cannot be broken by digestive enzymes in the human GI tract.

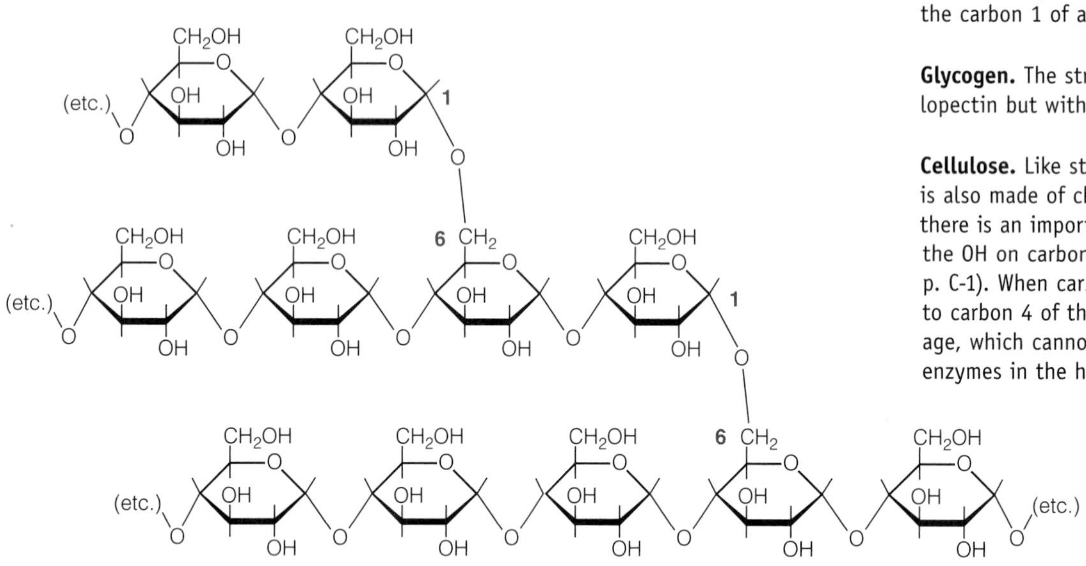

Amylopectin (branched starch)

Fibres, such as hemicelluloses, consist of long chains of various monosaccharides.

Monosaccharides common in the backbone chain of hemicelluloses:

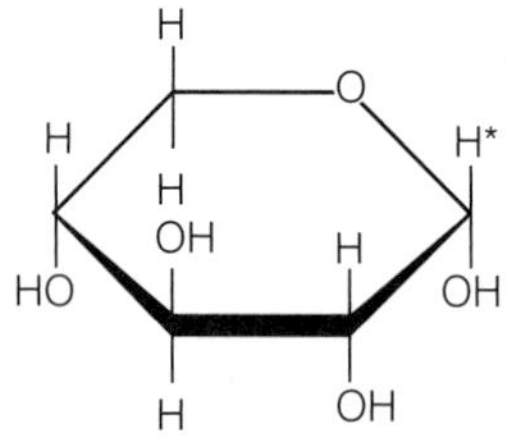

Xylose

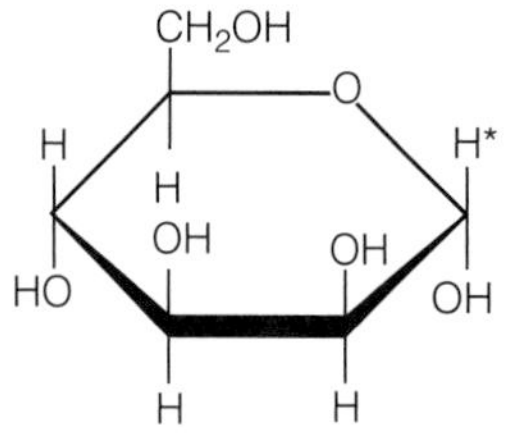

Mannose

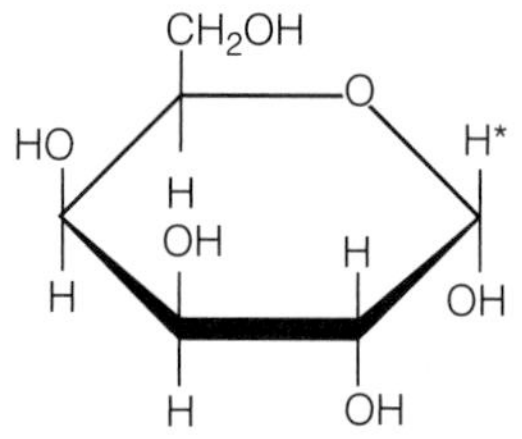

Galactose

Monosaccharides common in the side chains of hemicelluloses:

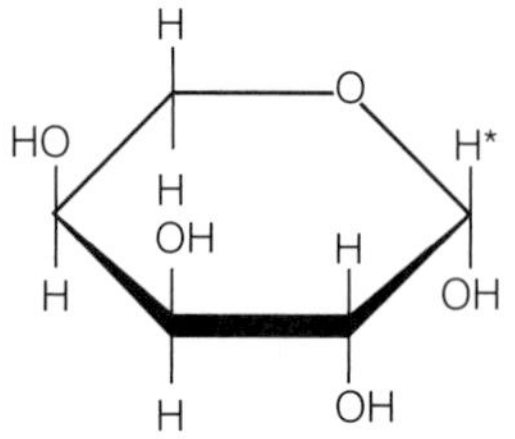

Arabinose

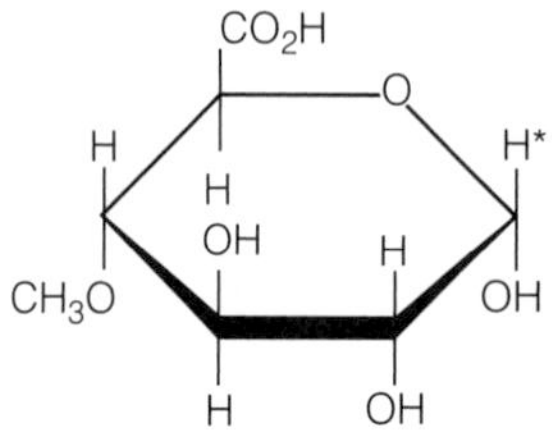

Glucuronic acid

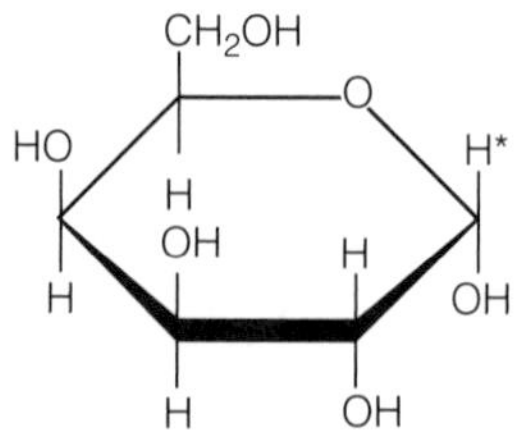

Galactose

Hemicelluloses. The most common hemicelluloses are composed of a backbone chain of xylose, mannose, and galactose, with branching side chains of arabinose, glucuronic acid, and galactose.

*These structures are shown in the alpha form with the H on the carbon pointing upward and the OH pointing downward, but they may also appear in the beta form with the H pointing downward and the OH upward.

Lipids

TABLE C-1 Saturated Fatty Acids Found in Natural Fats

Saturated Fatty Acids	Chemical Formulas	Number of Carbons	Major Food Sources
Butyric	C_3H_7COOH	4	Butterfat
Caproic	$C_5H_{11}COOH$	6	Butterfat
Caprylic	$C_7H_{15}COOH$	8	Coconut oil
Capric	$C_9H_{19}COOH$	10	Palm oil
Lauric	$C_{11}H_{23}COOH$	12	Coconut oil, palm oil
Myristic[a]	$C_{13}H_{27}COOH$	14	Coconut oil, palm oil
Palmitic[a]	$C_{15}H_{31}COOH$	16	Palm oil
Stearic[a]	$C_{17}H_{35}COOH$	18	Most animal fats
Arachidic	$C_{19}H_{39}COOH$	20	Peanut oil
Behenic	$C_{21}H_{43}COOH$	22	Seeds
Lignoceric	$C_{23}H_{47}COOH$	24	Peanut oil

[a]Most common saturated fatty acids.

TABLE C-2 Unsaturated Fatty Acids Found in Natural Fats

Unsaturated Fatty Acids	Chemical Formulas	Number of Carbons	Number of Double Bonds	Standard Notation[a]	Omega Notation[b]	Major Food Sources
Palmitoleic	$C_{15}H_{29}COOH$	16	1	16:1;9	16:1ω7	Seafood, beef
Oleic	$C_{17}H_{33}COOH$	18	1	18:1;9	18:1ω9	Olive oil, canola oil
Linoleic	$C_{17}H_{31}COOH$	18	2	18:2;9,12	18:2ω6	Sunflower oil, safflower oil
Linolenic	$C_{17}H_{29}COOH$	18	3	18:3;9,12,15	18:3ω3	Soybean oil, canola oil
Arachidonic	$C_{19}H_{31}COOH$	20	4	20:4;5,8,11,14	20:4ω6	Eggs, most animal fats
Eicosapentaenoic	$C_{19}H_{29}COOH$	20	5	20:5;5,8,11,14,17	20:5ω3	Seafood
Docosahexaenoic	$C_{21}H_{31}COOH$	22	6	22:6;4,7,10,13,16,19	22:6ω3	Seafood

NOTES: A fatty acid has two ends; designated the methyl (CH_3) end and the carboxyl, or acid (COOH), end.

[a]Standard chemistry notation begins counting carbons at the acid end. The number of carbons the fatty acid contains comes first, followed by a colon and another number that indicates the number of double bonds; next comes a semicolon followed by a number or numbers indicating the positions of the double bonds. Thus the notation for linoleic acid, an 18-carbon fatty acid with two double bonds between carbons 9 and 10 and between carbons 12 and 13, is 18:2;9,12.

[b]Because fatty acid chains are lengthened by adding carbons at the acid end of the chain, chemists use the omega system of notation to ease the task of identifying them. The omega system begins counting carbons at the methyl end. The number of carbons the fatty acid contains comes first, followed by a colon and the number of double bonds; next come the omega symbol (ω) and a number indicating the position of the double bond nearest the methyl end. Thus linoleic acid with its first double bond at the sixth carbon from the methyl end would be noted 18:2ω6 in the omega system.

Protein: Amino Acids

The common amino acids may be classified into the seven groups listed below. Amino acids marked with an asterisk (*) are indispensable/essential.

1. Amino acids with aliphatic side chains, which consist of hydrogen and carbon atoms (hydrocarbons):

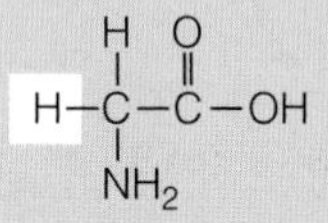

Glycine (Gly)

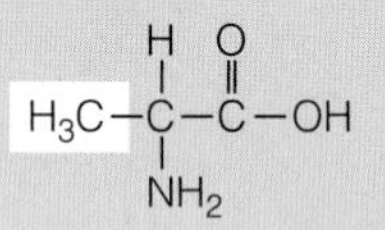

Alanine (Ala)

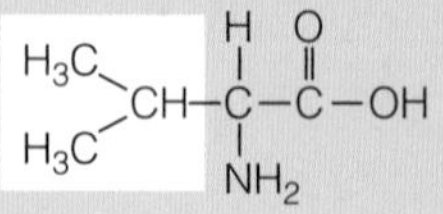

Valine* (Val)

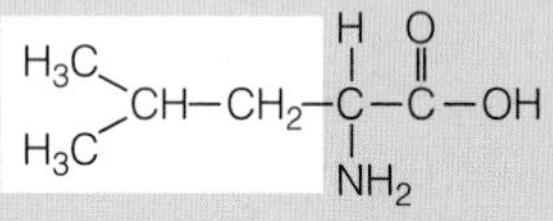

Leucine* (Leu)

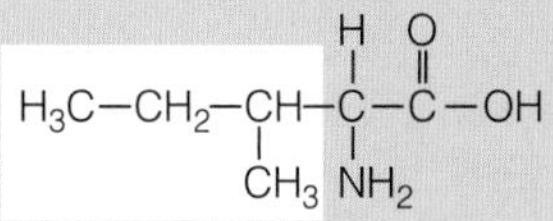

Isoleucine* (Ile)

2. Amino acids with hydroxyl (OH) side chains:

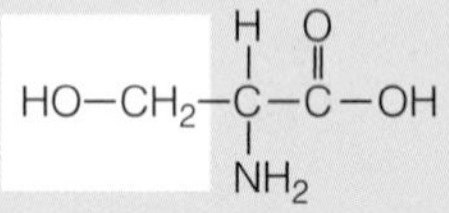

Serine (Ser)

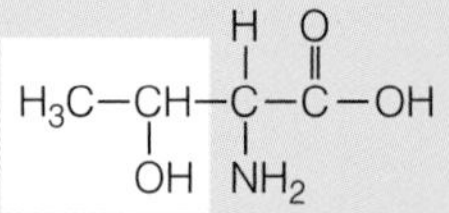

Threonine* (Thr)

3. Amino acids with side chains containing acidic groups or their amides, which contain the group NH_2:

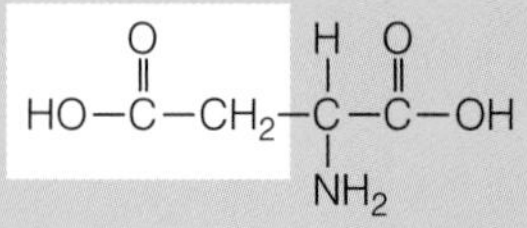

Aspartic acid (Asp)

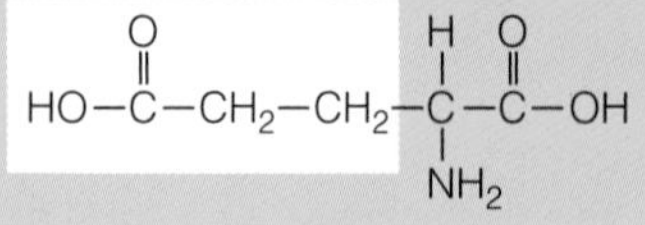

Glutamic acid (Glu)

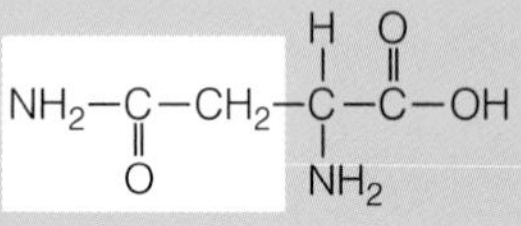

Asparagine (Asn)

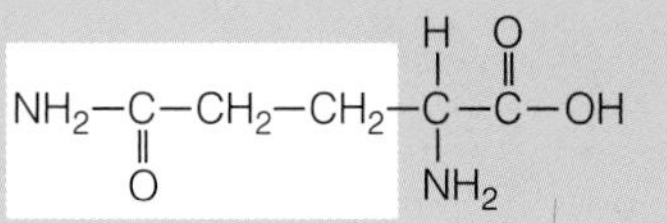

Glutamine (Gln)

4. Amino acids with basic side chains:

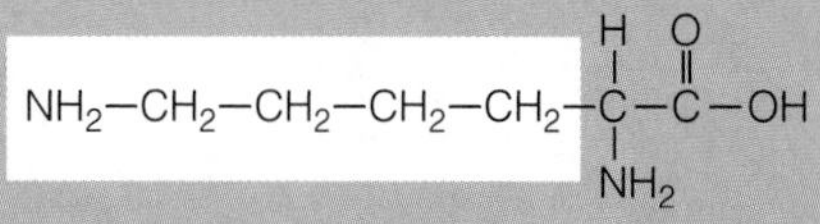

Lysine* (Lys)

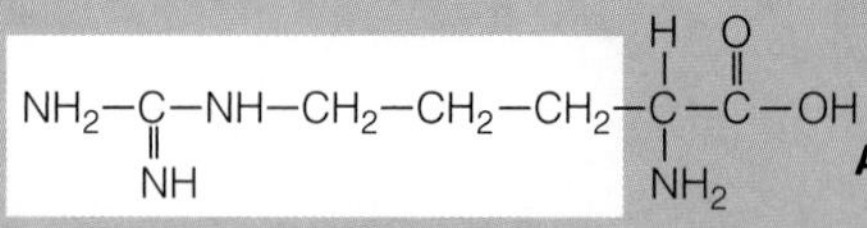

Arginine (Arg)

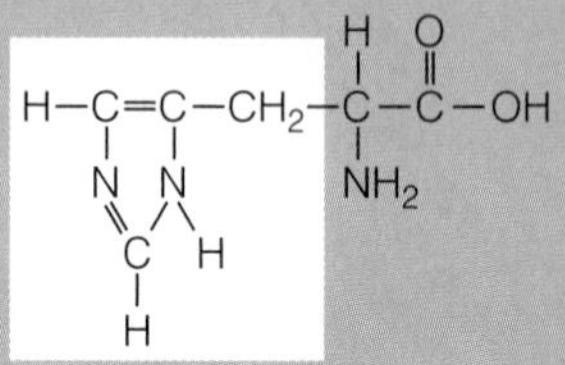

Histidine* (His)

5. Amino acids with aromatic side chains, which are characterized by the presence of at least one ring structure:

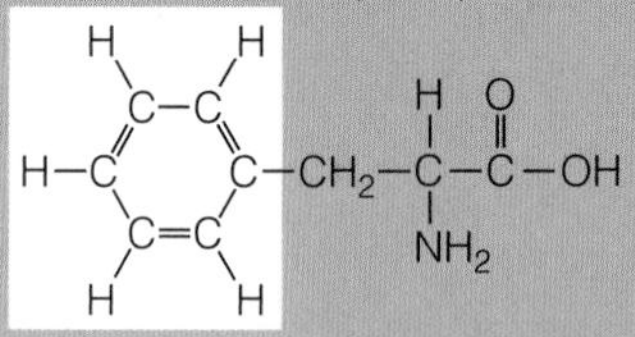

Phenylalanine* (Phe)

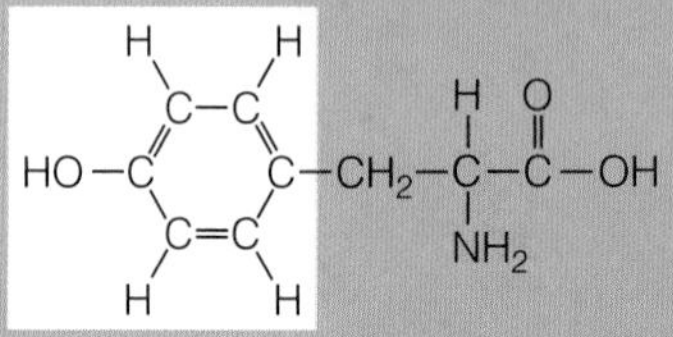

Tyrosine (Tyr)

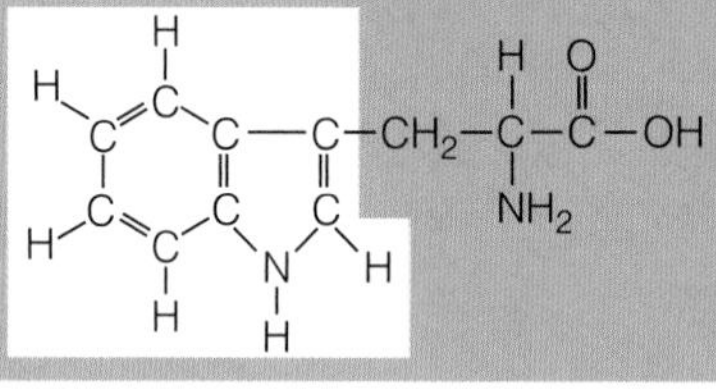

Tryptophan* (Trp)

6. Amino acids with side chains containing sulphur atoms:

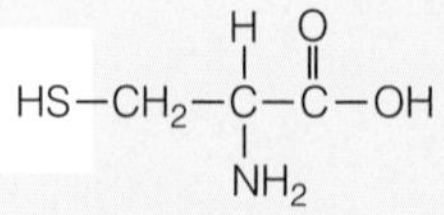

Cysteine (Cys)

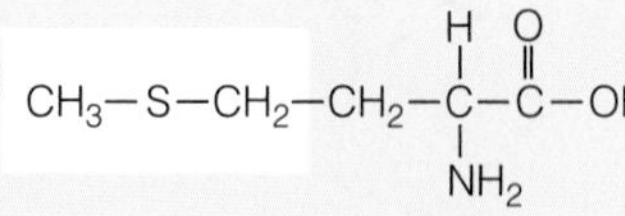

Methionine* (Met)

7. Imino acid:

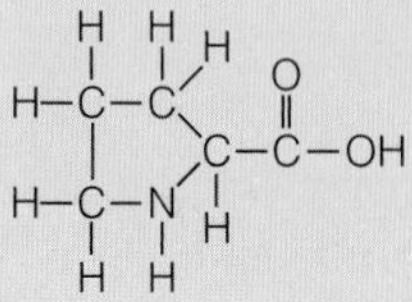

Proline (Pro)

Proline has the same chemical structure as the other amino acids, but its amino group has given up a hydrogen to form a ring.

Vitamins and Coenzymes

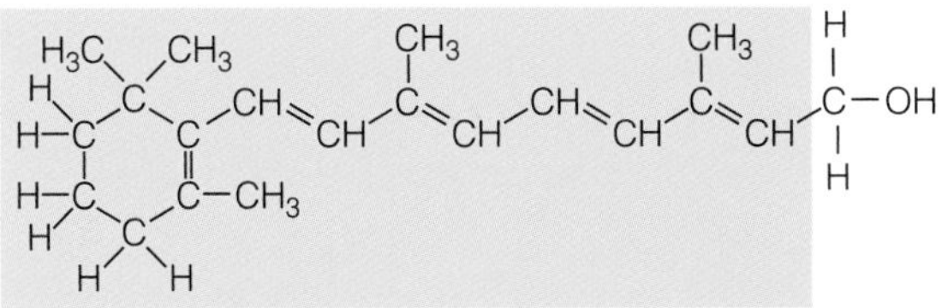

Vitamin A: retinol. This molecule is the alcohol form of vitamin A.

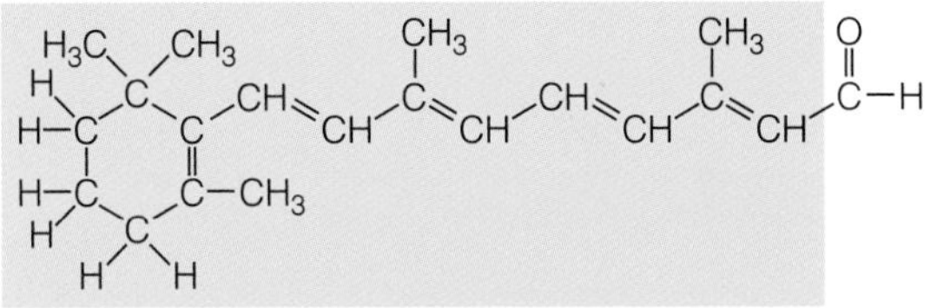

Vitamin A: retinal. This molecule is the aldehyde form of vitamin A.

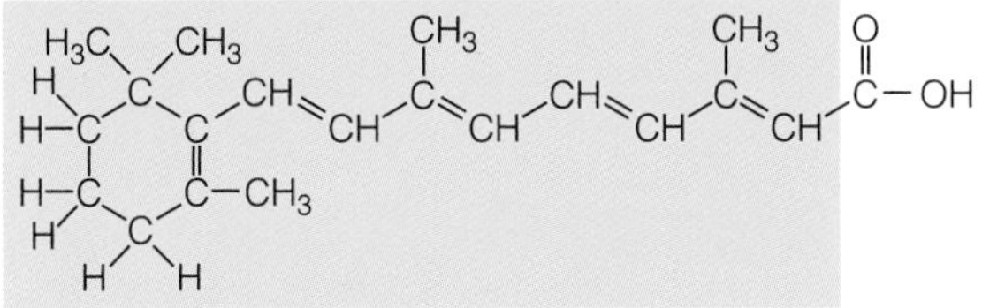

Vitamin A: retinoic acid. This molecule is the acid form of vitamin A.

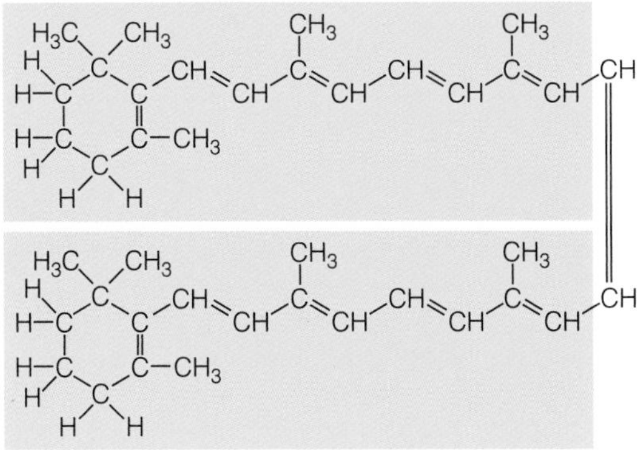

Vitamin A precursor: beta-carotene. This molecule is the carotenoid with the most vitamin A activity.

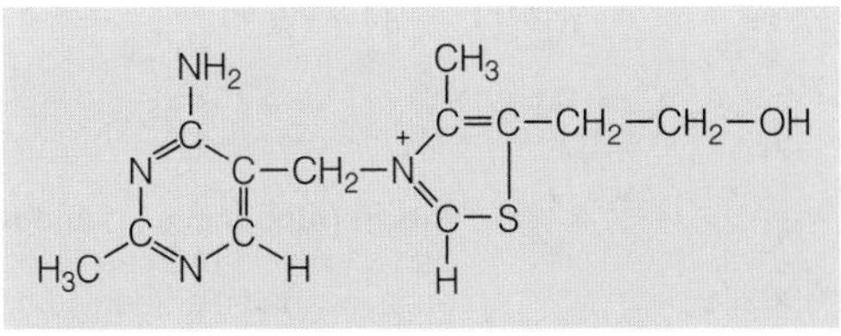

Thiamin. This molecule is part of the coenzyme thiamin pyrophosphate (TPP).

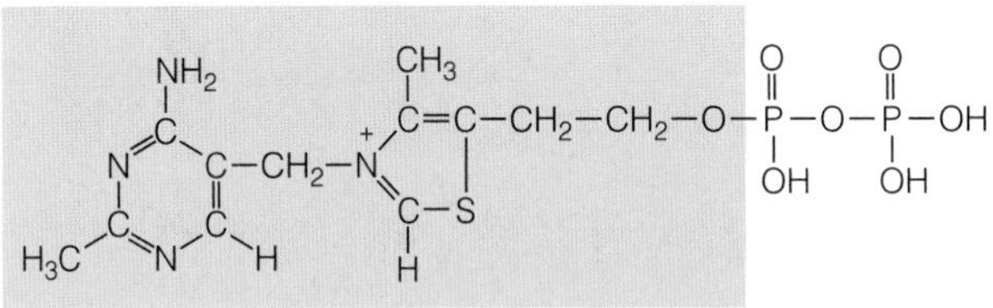

Thiamin pyrophosphate (TPP). TPP is a coenzyme that includes the thiamin molecule as part of its structure.

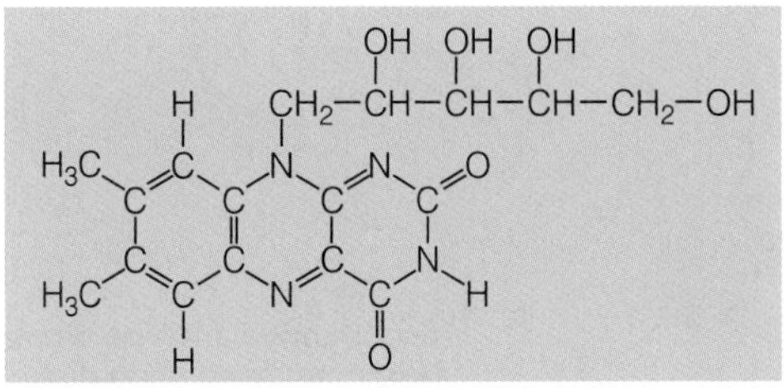

Riboflavin. This molecule is a part of two coenzymes—flavin mononucleotide (FMN) and flavin adenine dinucleotide (FAD).

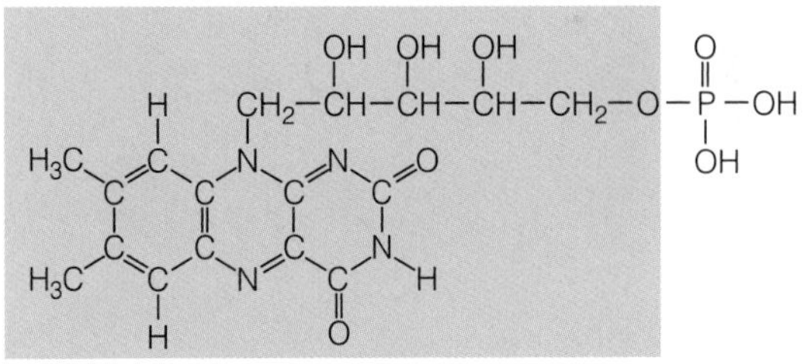

Flavin mononucleotide (FMN). FMN is a coenzyme that includes the riboflavin molecule as part of its structure.

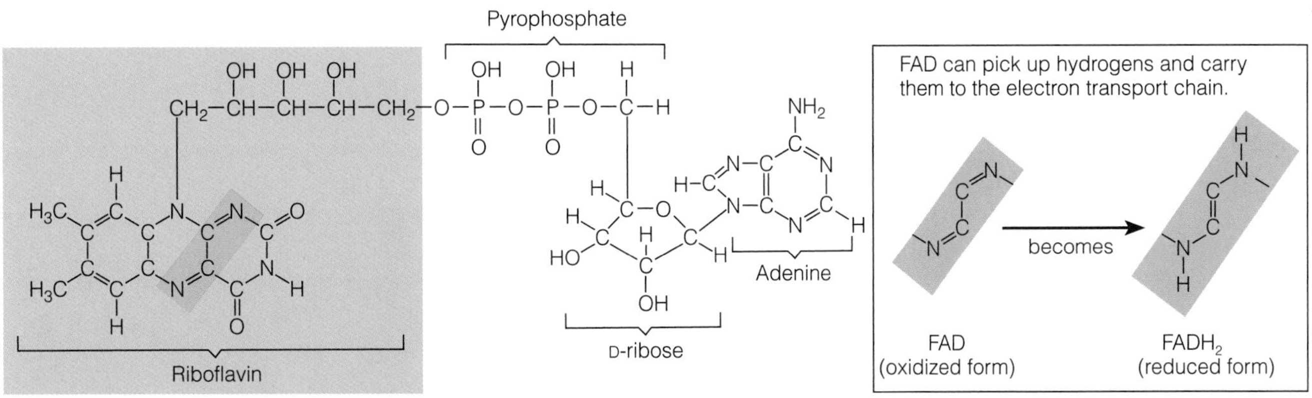
Pyrophosphate
Riboflavin
D-ribose
Adenine
FAD can pick up hydrogens and carry them to the electron transport chain.
becomes
FAD
(oxidized form)
FADH2
(reduced form)

Flavin adenine dinucleotide (FAD). FAD is a coenzyme that includes the riboflavin molecule as part of its structure.

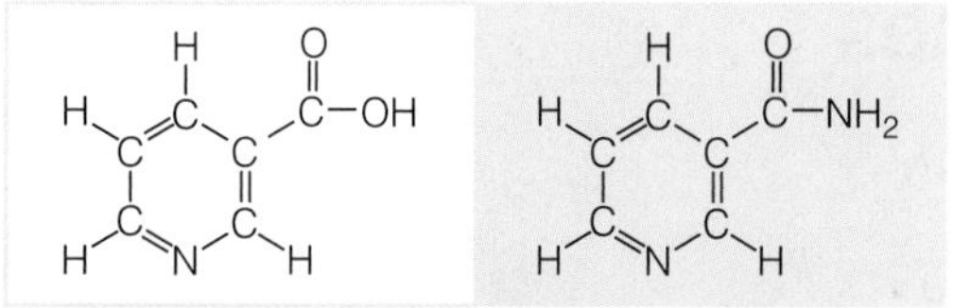

Nicotinic acid Nicotinamide

Niacin (nicotinic acid and nicotinamide). These molecules are a part of two coenzymes—nicotinamide adenine dinucleotide (NAD^+) and nicotinamide adenine dinucleotide phosphate ($NADP^+$).

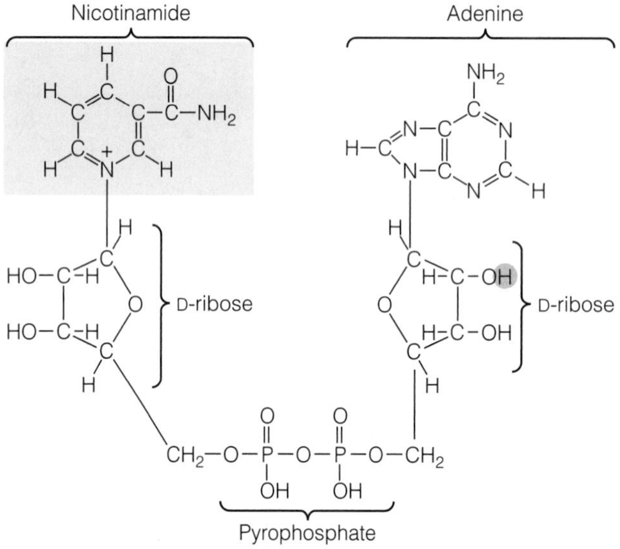
Nicotinamide
Adenine
D-ribose
D-ribose
Pyrophosphate

Nicotinamide adenine dinucleotide (NAD^+) and nicotinamide adenine dinucleotide phosphate ($NADP^+$). NADP has the same structure as NAD but with a phosphate group attached to the O instead of the H.

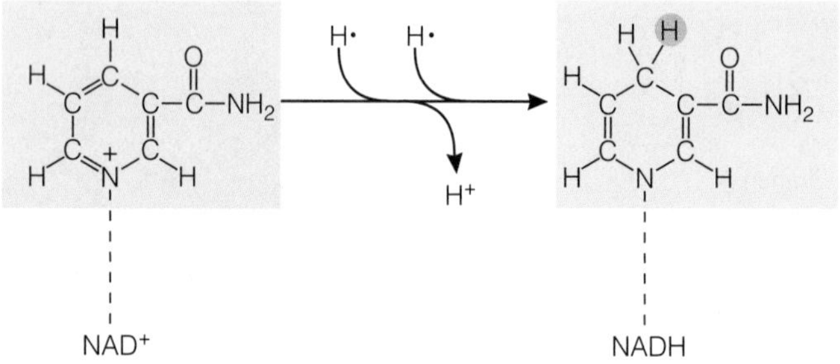
NAD+
NADH

Reduced NAD^+ (NADH). When NAD^+ is reduced by the addition of H^+ and two electrons, it becomes the coenzyme NADH. (The dots on the H entering this reaction represent electrons—see APPENDIX B.)

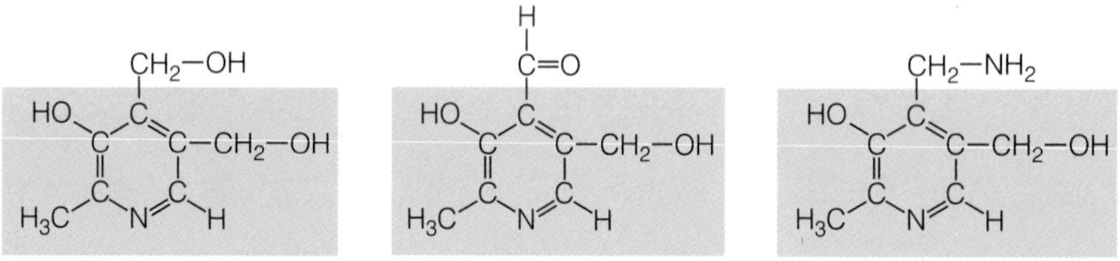

Pyridoxine Pyridoxal Pyridoxamine

Vitamin B_6 (a general name for three compounds—pyridoxine, pyridoxal, and pyridoxamine). These molecules are a part of two coenzymes—pyridoxal phosphate and pyridoxamine phosphate.

APPENDIX C

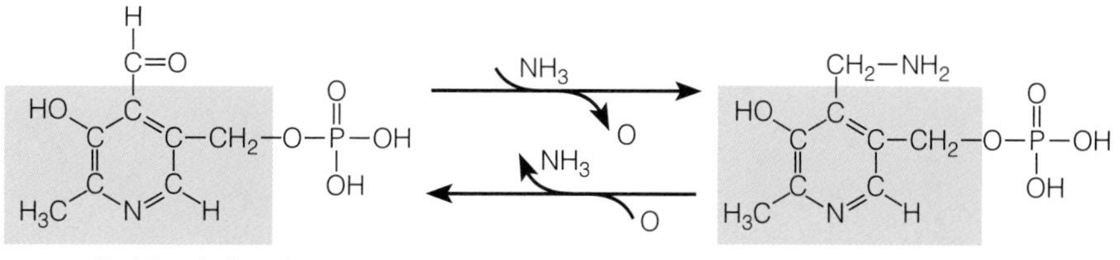
Pyridoxal phosphate
Pyridoxamine phosphate

Pyridoxal phosphate (PLP) and pyridoxamine phosphate. These coenzymes include vitamin B_6 as part of their structures.

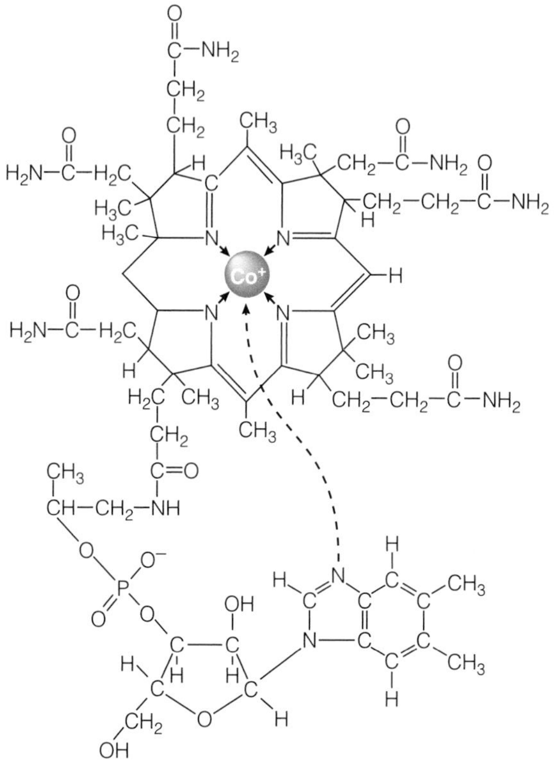

Vitamin B_{12} (cyanocobalamin). The arrows in this diagram indicate that the spare electron pairs on the nitrogens attract them to the cobalt.

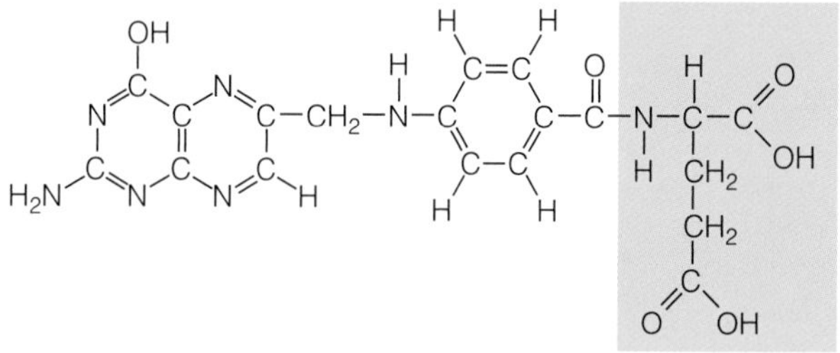

Folate (folacin or folic acid). This molecule consists of a double ring combined with a single ring and at least one glutamate (a nonessential amino acid marked in the box). Folate's biologically active form is tetrahydrofolate.

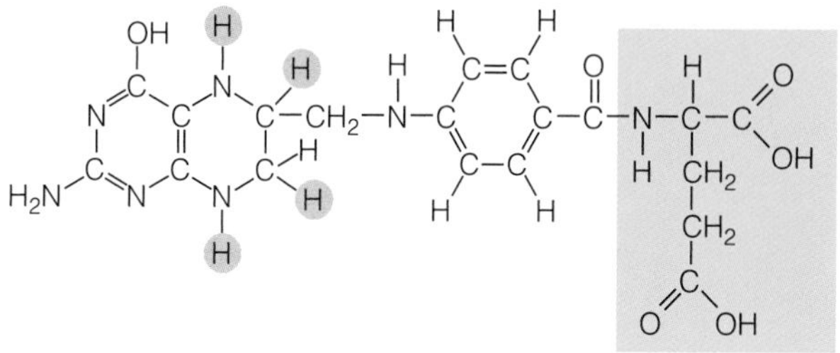

Tetrahydrofolate. This active coenzyme form of folate has four added hydrogens. An intermediate form, dihydrofolate, has two added hydrogens.

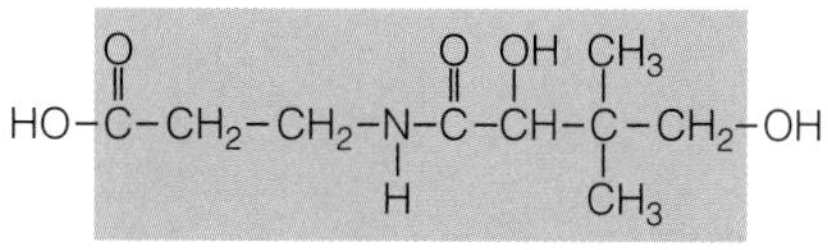

Pantothenic acid. This molecule is part of coenzyme A (CoA).

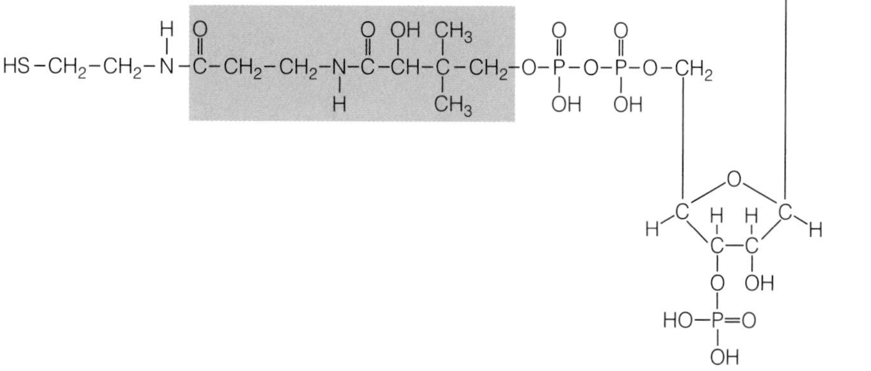

Coenzyme A (CoA). Coenzyme A is a coenzyme that includes pantothenic acid as part of its structure.

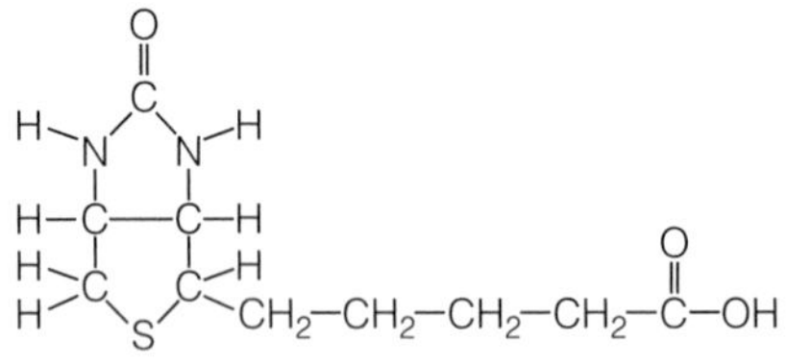

Biotin.

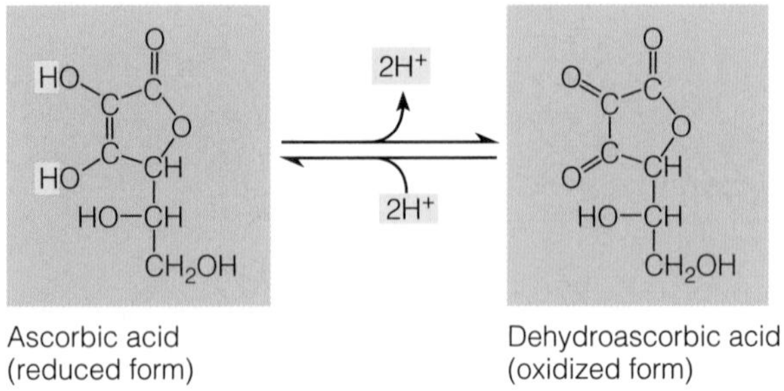
2H+
2H+
Ascorbic acid
(reduced form)
Dehydroascorbic acid
(oxidized form)

Vitamin C. Two hydrogen atoms with their electrons are lost when ascorbic acid is oxidized and gained when it is reduced again.

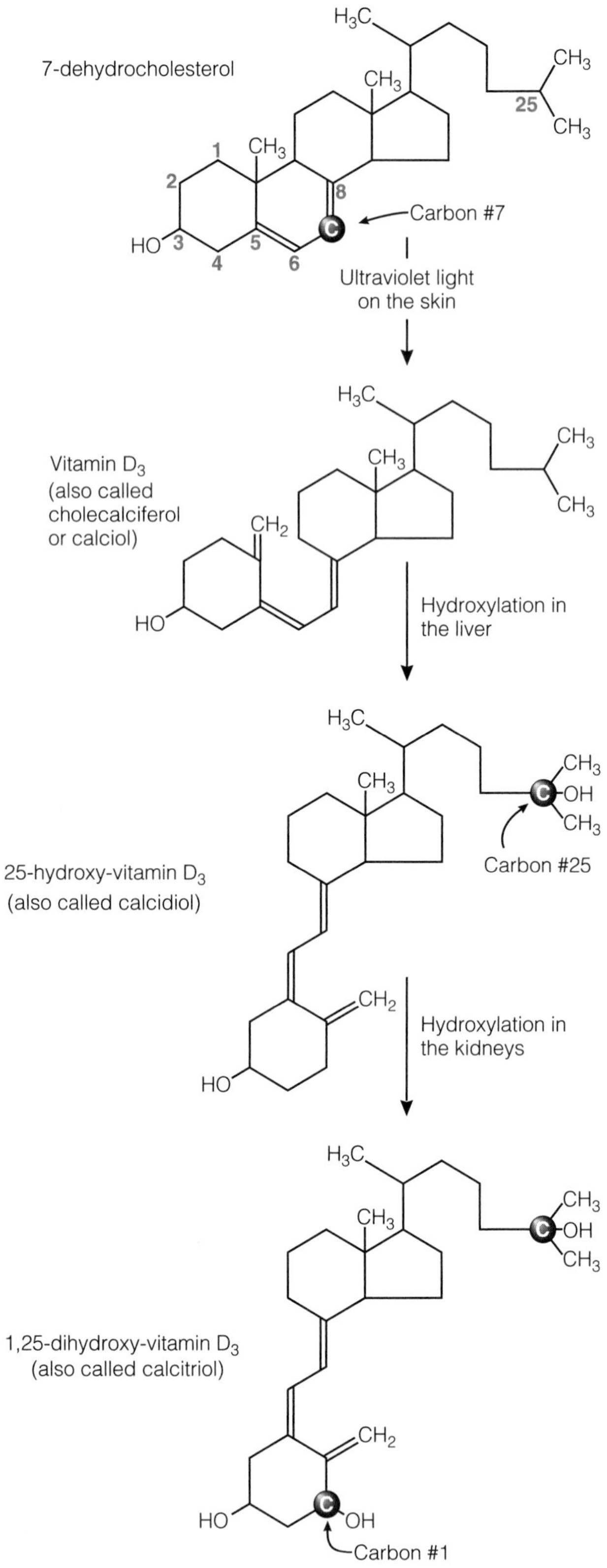
7-dehydrocholesterol
Carbon #7
Ultraviolet light
on the skin
Vitamin D3
(also called
cholecalciferol
or calciol)
Hydroxylation in
the liver
25-hydroxy-vitamin D3
(also called calcidiol)
Carbon #25
Hydroxylation in
the kidneys
1,25-dihydroxy-vitamin D3
(also called calcitriol)
Carbon #1

Vitamin D. The synthesis of active vitamin D begins with 7-dehydrocholesterol. (The carbon atoms at which changes occur are numbered.)

APPENDIX C

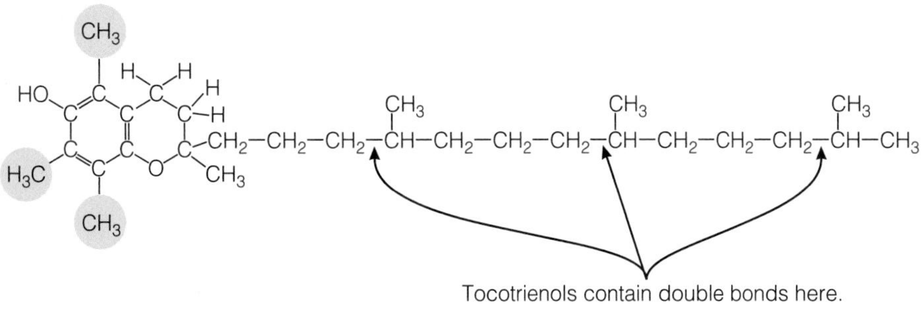
Tocotrienols contain double bonds here.

Vitamin E (alpha-tocopherol). The number and position of the methyl groups (CH_3) bonded to the ring structure differentiate among the tocopherols.

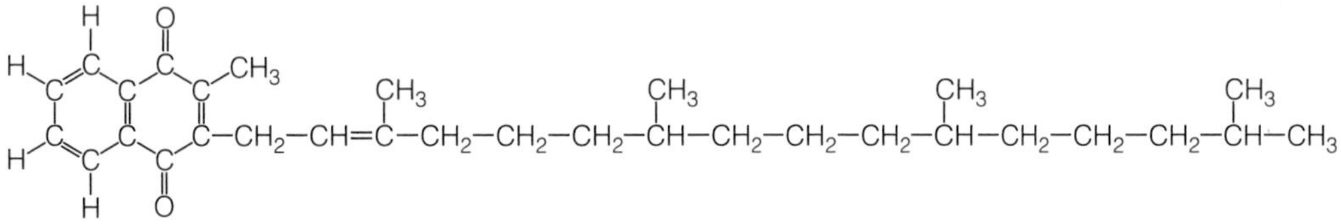

Vitamin K. Naturally occurring compounds with vitamin K activity include phylloquinones (from plants) and menaquinones (from bacteria).

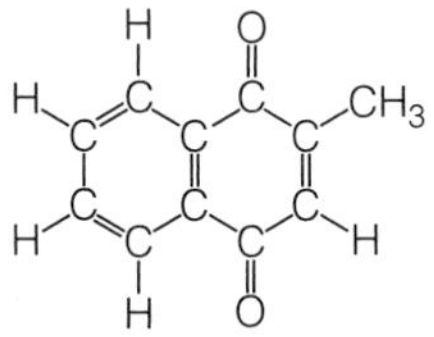

Menadione. This synthetic compound has the same activity as natural vitamin K.

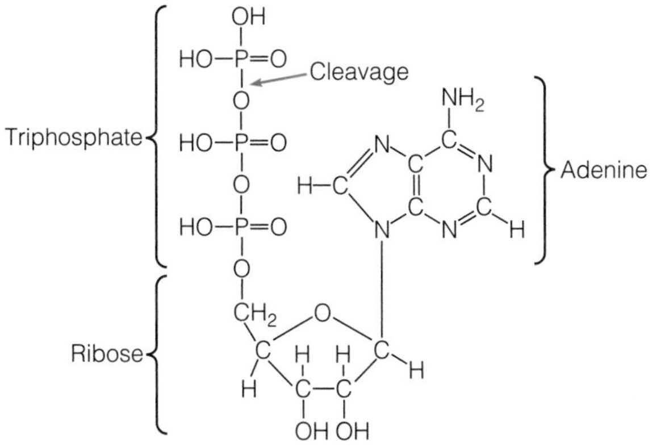
Triphosphate
Cleavage
Adenine
Ribose

Adenosine triphosphate (ATP), the energy carrier. The cleavage point marks the bond that is broken when ATP splits to become ADP + P.

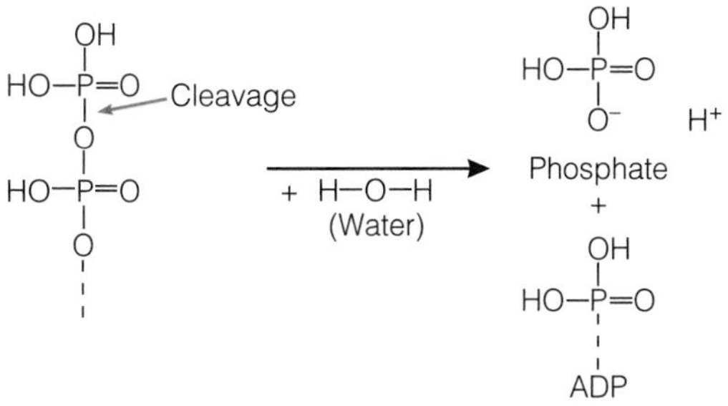
Cleavage
+ H—O—H
(Water)
Phosphate
ADP

Adenosine diphosphate (ADP).

Glycolysis

Figure C-1 depicts glycolysis. The following text describes key steps as numbered on the figure.

FIGURE C-1 **Glycolysis**

Notice that galactose and fructose enter at different places but continue on the same pathway.

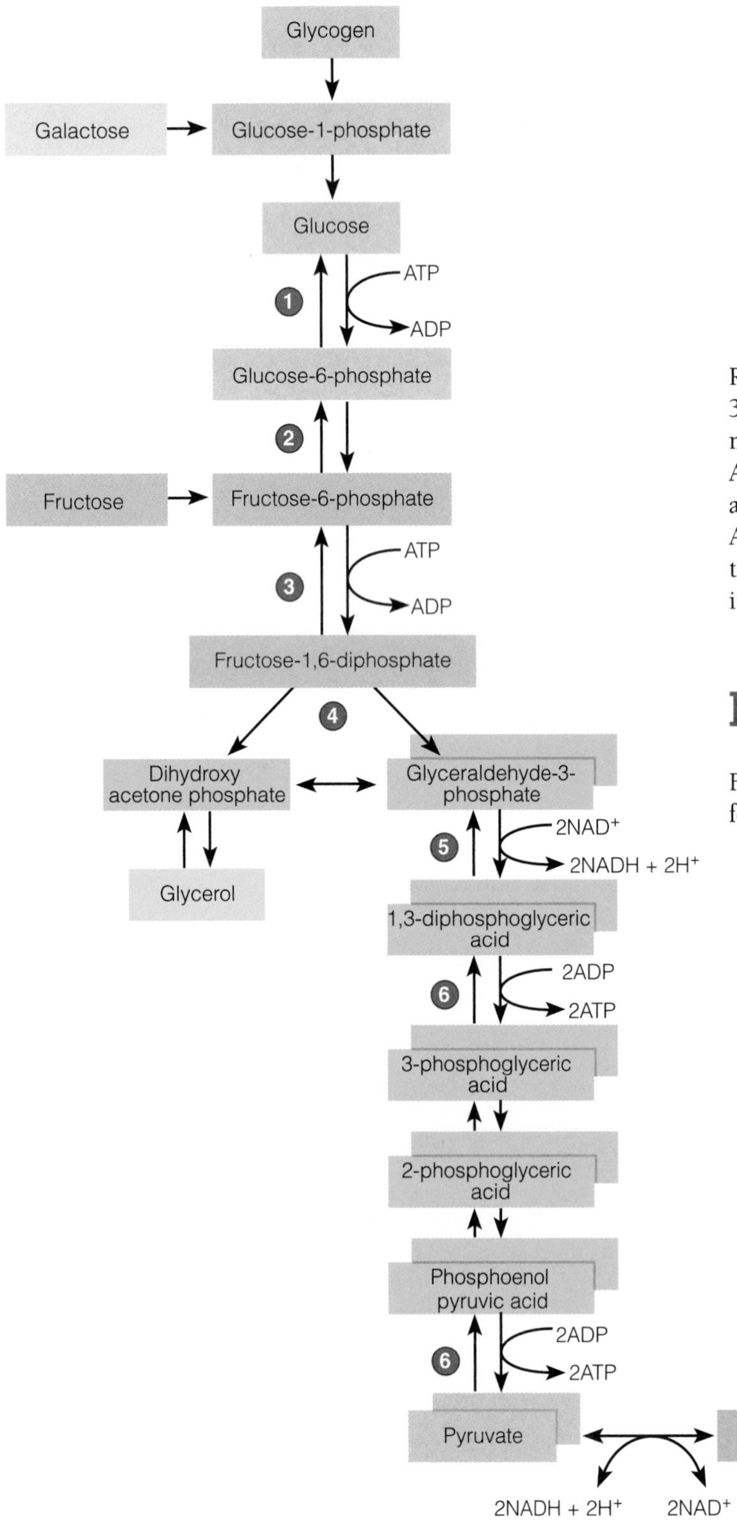
Glycogen
Galactose
Glucose-1-phosphate
Glucose
ATP
1
ADP
Glucose-6-phosphate
2
Fructose
Fructose-6-phosphate
ATP
3
ADP
Fructose-1,6-diphosphate
4
Dihydroxy acetone phosphate
Glyceraldehyde-3-phosphate
Glycerol
2NAD⁺
5
2NADH + 2H⁺
1,3-diphosphoglyceric acid
2ADP
6
2ATP
3-phosphoglyceric acid
2-phosphoglyceric acid
Phosphoenol pyruvic acid
2ADP
6
2ATP
Pyruvate
Lactate
2NADH + 2H⁺
2NAD⁺

1. A phosphate is attached to glucose at the carbon that chemists call number 6 (review the first diagram of glucose on p. C-1 to see how chemists number the carbons in a glucose molecule). The product is called, logically enough, glucose-6-phosphate. One ATP molecule is used to accomplish this.
2. Glucose-6-phosphate is rearranged by an enzyme.
3. A phosphate is added in another reaction that uses another molecule of ATP. The product this time is fructose-1,6-diphosphate. At this point the 6-carbon sugar has a phosphate group on its first and sixth carbons and is ready to break apart.
4. When fructose-1,6-diphosphate breaks in half, the two 3-carbon compounds are not identical. Each has a phosphate group attached, but only glyceraldehyde-3-phosphate converts directly to pyruvate. The other compound, however, converts easily to glyceraldehyde-3-phosphate.
5. In the next step, enough energy is released to convert NAD^+ to $NADH + H^+$.
6. In two of the following steps ATP is regenerated.

Remember that in effect two molecules of glyceraldehyde-3-phosphate are produced from glucose; therefore, four ATP molecules are generated from each glucose molecule. Two ATP were needed to get the sequence started, so the net gain at this point is two ATP and two molecules of $NADH + H^+$. As you will see later, each $NADH + H^+$ moves to the electron transport chain to unload its hydrogens onto oxygen, producing more ATP.

Fatty Acid Oxidation

Figure C-2 presents fatty acid oxidation. The sequence is as follows.

1. The fatty acid is activated by combining with coenzyme A (CoA). In this reaction, ATP loses two phosphorus atoms (PP, or pyrophosphate) and becomes AMP (adenosine monophosphate)—the equivalent of a loss of two ATP.
2. In the next reaction, two H with their electrons are removed and transferred to FAD, forming $FADH_2$.
3. In a later reaction, two H are removed and go to NAD^+ (forming $NADH + H^+$).
4. The fatty acid is cleaved at the "beta" carbon, the second carbon from the carboxyl (COOH) end. This break results in a fatty acid that is two carbons shorter than the previous one and a 2-carbon molecule of acetyl CoA.

FIGURE C-2 Fatty Acid Oxidation

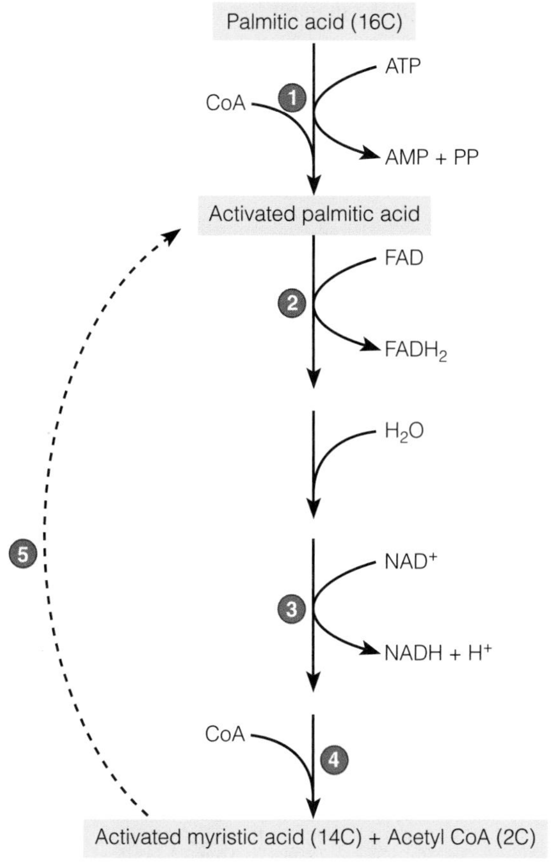
Palmitic acid (16C)
ATP
CoA
1
AMP + PP
Activated palmitic acid
FAD
2
$FADH_2$
H_2O
NAD+
3
NADH + H+
5
CoA
4
Activated myristic acid (14C) + Acetyl CoA (2C)

At the same time, another CoA is attached to the fatty acid, thus activating it for its turn through the series of reactions.

5. The sequence is repeated with each cycle producing an acetyl CoA and a shorter fatty acid until only a 2-carbon fatty acid remains—acetyl CoA.

In the example shown in Figure C-2, palmitic acid (a 16-carbon fatty acid) will go through this series of reactions seven times, using the equivalent of two ATP for the initial activation and generating seven $FADH_2$, seven NADH + H^+, and eight acetyl CoA. As you will see later, each of the seven $FADH_2$ will enter the electron transport chain to unload its hydrogens onto oxygen, yielding two ATP (for a total of 14). Similarly, each NADH + H^+ will enter the electron transport chain to unload its hydrogens onto oxygen, yielding three ATP (for a total of 21). Thus the oxidation of a 16-carbon fatty acid uses 2 ATP and generates 35 ATP. When the eight acetyl CoA enter the TCA cycle, even more ATP will be generated, as a later section describes.

Amino Acid Degradation

The first step in amino acid degradation is the removal of the nitrogen-containing amino group through either deamination (Figure 6-11 on p. 183) or transamination (Figure 6-12 on p. 184) reactions. Then the remaining carbon skeletons may enter the metabolic pathways at different places, as shown in Figure C-3 (p. C-12).

The TCA Cycle

The tricarboxylic acid, or TCA, cycle is the set of reactions that break down acetyl CoA to carbon dioxide and hydrogens. To link glycolysis to the TCA cycle, pyruvate enters the mitochondrion, loses a carbon group, and bonds with a molecule of CoA to become acetyl CoA. The TCA cycle uses any substance that can be converted to acetyl CoA directly or indirectly through pyruvate.

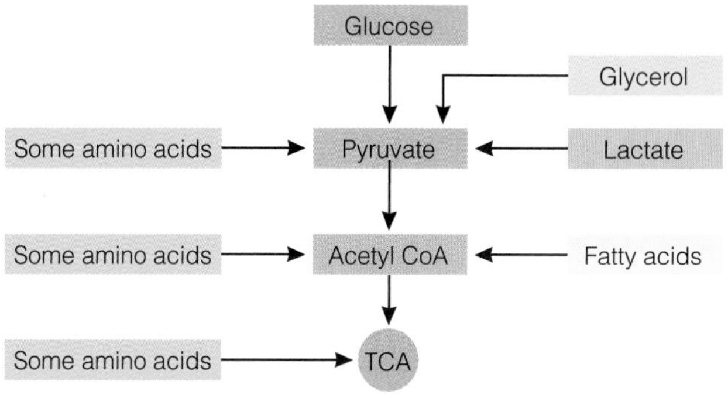
Glucose
Glycerol
Some amino acids
Pyruvate
Lactate
Some amino acids
Acetyl CoA
Fatty acids
Some amino acids
TCA

Any substance that can be converted to acetyl CoA directly, or indirectly through pyruvate, may enter the TCA cycle.

The step from pyruvate to acetyl CoA is complex. We have included only those substances that will help you understand the transfer of energy from the nutrients. Pyruvate loses a carbon to carbon dioxide and is attached to a molecule of CoA. In the process, NAD^+ picks up two hydrogens with their associated electrons, becoming NADH + H^+.

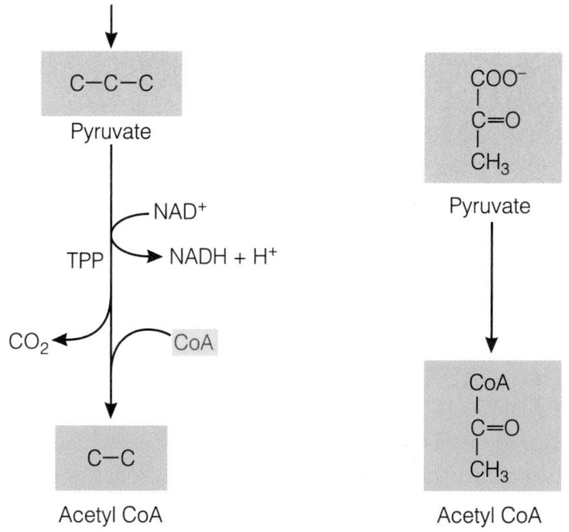
C–C–C
Pyruvate
NAD^+
TPP
NADH + H^+
CO_2
CoA
C–C
Acetyl CoA
COO^-
C=O
CH_3
Pyruvate
CoA
C=O
CH_3
Acetyl CoA

The step from pyruvate to acetyl CoA. (TPP and NAD are coenzymes containing the B vitamins thiamin and niacin, respectively.)

FIGURE C-3 Amino Acids Enter the Metabolic Pathways

After losing their amino groups, carbon skeletons can be converted to one of seven molecules that can enter the TCA cycle (presented in Figure C-4).

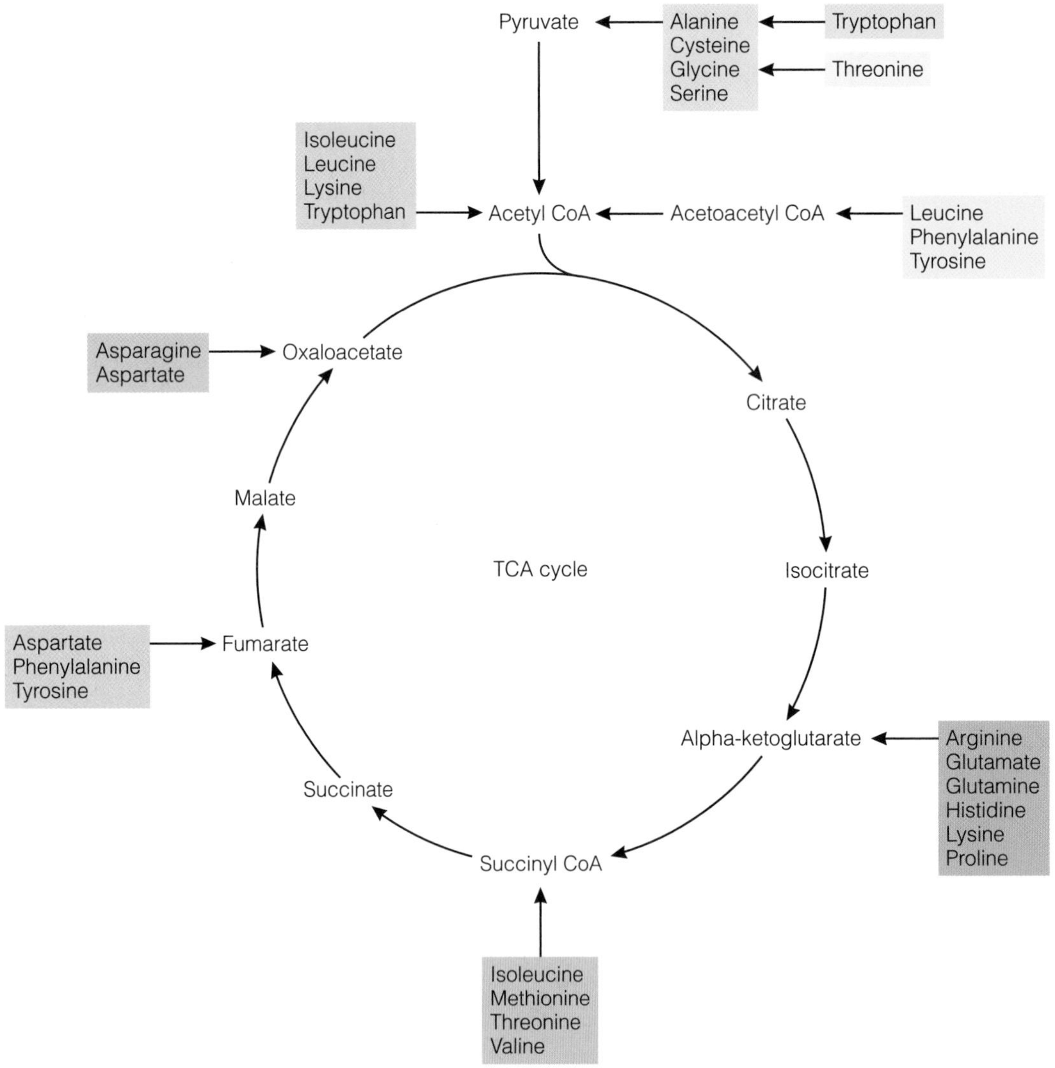
Pyruvate
Alanine
Cysteine
Glycine
Serine
Tryptophan
Threonine
Isoleucine
Leucine
Lysine
Tryptophan
Acetyl CoA
Acetoacetyl CoA
Leucine
Phenylalanine
Tyrosine
Asparagine
Aspartate
Oxaloacetate
Citrate
Malate
TCA cycle
Isocitrate
Aspartate
Phenylalanine
Tyrosine
Fumarate
Alpha-ketoglutarate
Arginine
Glutamate
Glutamine
Histidine
Lysine
Proline
Succinate
Succinyl CoA
Isoleucine
Methionine
Threonine
Valine

Let's follow the steps of the TCA cycle (see the corresponding numbers in Figure C-4).

1. The 2-carbon acetyl CoA combines with a 4-carbon compound, oxaloacetate. The CoA comes off, and the product is a 6-carbon compound, citrate.
2. The atoms of citrate are rearranged to form isocitrate.
3. Now two H (with their two electrons) are removed from the isocitrate. One H becomes attached to the NAD^+ with the two electrons; the other H is released as H^+. Thus NAD^+ becomes NADH + H^+. (Remember this NADH + H^+, but let's follow the carbons first.) Carbon dioxide is released during this reaction (which diffuses away into the blood and is exhaled). What is left is the 5-carbon compound alpha-ketoglutarate.
4. Now two compounds interact with alpha-ketoglutarate — a molecule of CoA and a molecule of NAD^+. In this complex reaction, another carbon dioxide molecule is released; two hydrogens are removed and go to NAD^+ (forming NADH + H^+); and the remaining 4-carbon compound is attached to the CoA, forming succinyl CoA. (Remember this NADH + H^+ also. You will see later what happens to it.)
5. Now two molecules react with succinyl CoA—a molecule called GDP and one of phosphate (P). The CoA comes off, the GDP and P combine to form the high-energy compound GTP (similar to ATP), and succinate remains. (Remember this GTP.)
6. In the next reaction, two H with their electrons are removed from succinate and are transferred to a molecule of FAD (a coenzyme like NAD^+) to form $FADH_2$. The product that remains is fumarate. (Remember this $FADH_2$.)
7. Next a molecule of water is added to fumarate, forming malate.

FIGURE C-4 The TCA Cycle

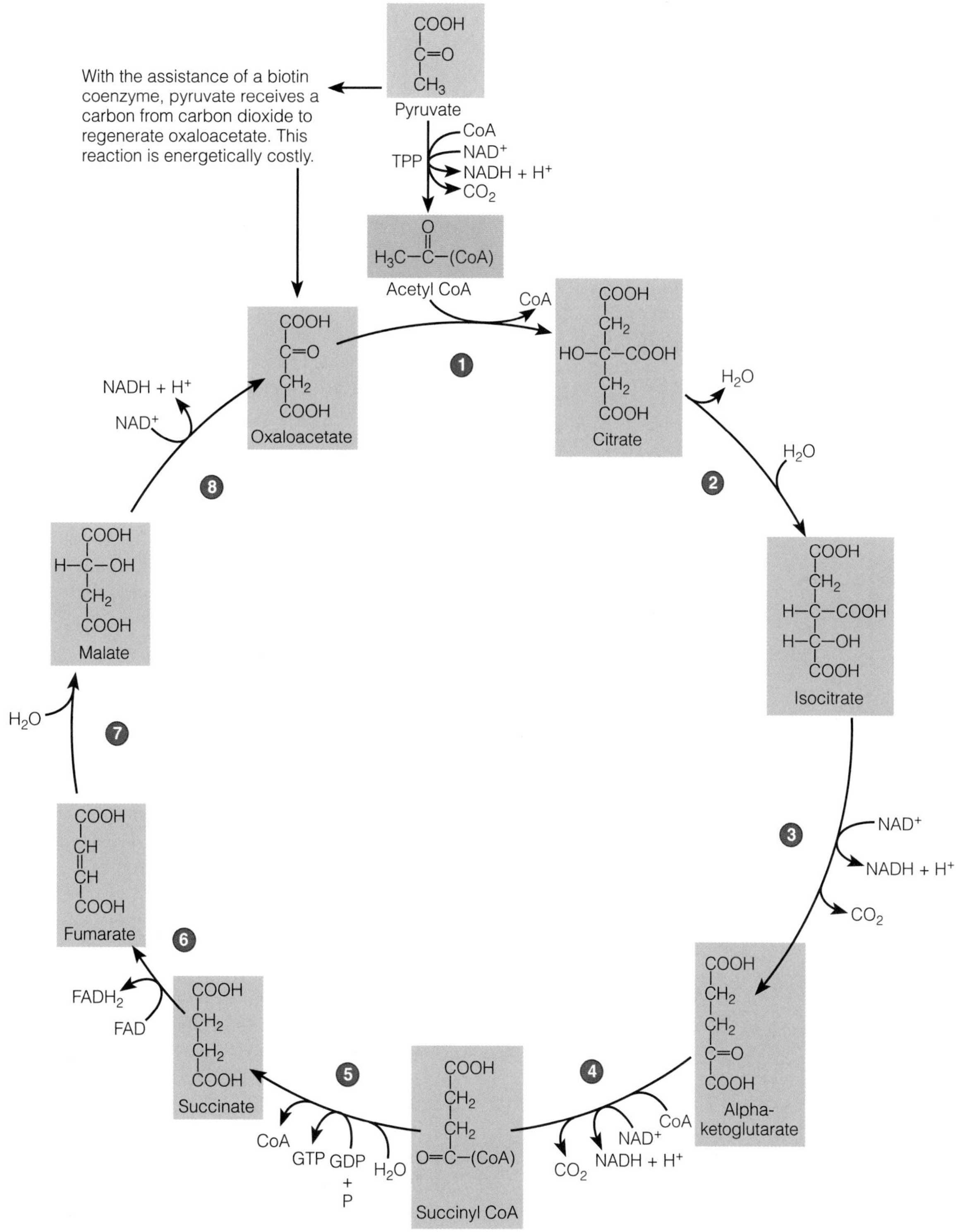

With the assistance of a biotin coenzyme, pyruvate receives a carbon from carbon dioxide to regenerate oxaloacetate. This reaction is energetically costly.
Pyruvate
TPP
CoA
NAD+
NADH + H+
CO2
Acetyl CoA
CoA
Citrate
H2O
H2O
Isocitrate
NAD+
NADH + H+
CO2
Alpha-ketoglutarate
CoA
NAD+
NADH + H+
CO2
Succinyl CoA
H2O
GDP + P
GTP
CoA
Succinate
FAD
FADH2
Fumarate
H2O
Malate
NAD+
NADH + H+
Oxaloacetate

8. A molecule of NAD^+ reacts with the malate; two H with their associated electrons are removed from the malate and form $NADH + H^+$. The product that remains is the 4-carbon compound oxaloacetate. (Remember this $NADH + H^+$.)

We are back where we started. The oxaloacetate formed in this process can combine with another molecule of acetyl CoA (step 1), and the cycle can begin again, as shown in Figure C-4.

So far, we have seen two carbons brought in with acetyl CoA and two carbons ending up in carbon dioxide. But where are the energy and the ATP we promised?

A review of the eight steps of the TCA cycle shows that the compounds $NADH + H^+$ (three molecules), $FADH_2$, and

GTP capture energy originally found in acetyl CoA. To see how this energy ends up in ATP, we must follow the electrons further—into the electron transport chain.

The Electron Transport Chain

The six reactions described here are those of the electron transport chain, which is shown in Figure C-5. Since oxygen is required for these reactions, and ADP and P are combined to form ATP in several of them (ADP is phosphorylated), these reactions are also called oxidative phosphorylation.

An important concept to remember at this point is that an electron is not a fixed amount of energy. The electrons that bond the H to NAD^+ in NADH have a relatively large amount

FIGURE C-5 The Electron Transport Chain

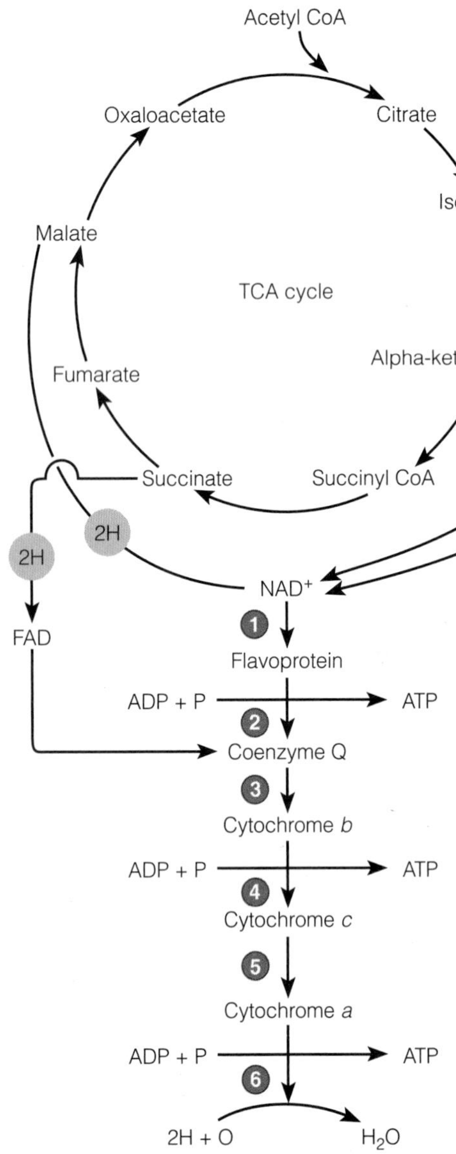
Acetyl CoA
Citrate
Oxaloacetate
Isocitrate
Malate
TCA cycle
Alpha-ketoglutarate
Fumarate
Succinate
Succinyl CoA
2H
2H
2H
2H
NAD+
FAD
Flavoprotein
ADP + P
ATP
Coenzyme Q
Cytochrome b
ADP + P
ATP
Cytochrome c
Cytochrome a
ADP + P
ATP
2H + O
H2O

of energy. In the series of reactions that follow, they release this energy in small amounts, until at the end they are attached (with H) to oxygen (O) to make water (H_2O). In some of the steps, the energy they release is captured in high-energy bonds in ATP-coupled reactions.

1. In the first step of the electron transport chain, NADH reacts with a molecule called a flavoprotein, losing its electrons (and their H). The products are NAD^+ and reduced flavoprotein. A little energy is released as heat in this reaction.
2. The flavoprotein passes on the electrons to a molecule called coenzyme Q. Again they release some energy as heat, but the phosphorylation of ADP to form ATP allows for the, storing much of the energy. This is a coupled reaction: ADP + P → ATP.
3. Coenzyme Q passes the electrons to cytochrome *b*. Again the electrons release energy.
4. Cytochrome *b* passes the electrons to cytochrome *c* in a coupled reaction in which ATP is formed: ADP + P → ATP.
5. Cytochrome *c* passes the electrons to cytochrome *a*.
6. Cytochrome *a* passes them (with their H) to an atom of oxygen (O), forming water (H_2O). This is a coupled reaction in which ATP is formed: ADP + P → ATP.

As Figure C-5 shows, each time NADH is oxidized (loses its electrons) by this means, the energy it releases is captured into three ATP molecules. When the electrons are passed on to water at the end, they are much lower in energy than they were originally. This completes the story of the electrons from NADH.

As for $FADH_2$, its electrons enter the electron transport chain at coenzyme Q. From coenzyme Q to water, ATP is generated in only two steps. Therefore, $FADH_2$ coming out of the TCA cycle yields just two ATP molecules.

One energy-receiving compound of the TCA cycle (GTP) does not enter the electron transport chain but gives its energy directly to ADP in a simple phosphorylation reaction. This reaction yields one ATP.

It is now possible to draw up a balance sheet of glucose metabolism (see Table C-3). Glycolysis has yielded 4 NADH + H^+ and 4 ATP molecules and has spent 2 ATP. The 2 acetyl CoA going through the TCA cycle have yielded 6 NADH + H^+, 2 $FADH_2$, and 2 GTP molecules. After the NADH + H^+ and $FADH_2$ have gone through the electron transport chain, there are 28 ATP. Added to these are the 4 ATP from glycolysis and the 2 ATP from GTP, making the total 34 ATP generated from one molecule of glucose. After the expense of 2 ATP is subtracted, there is a net gain of 32 ATP.*

*The total may sometimes be 30 ATP. The NADH + H^+ generated in the cytoplasm during glycolysis pass their electrons on to shuttle molecules, which move them into the mitochondria. One shuttle, malate, contributes its electrons to the electron transport chain before the first site of ATP synthesis, yielding 5 ATP. Another, glycerol phosphate, adds its electrons into the chain beyond that first site, yielding 3 ATP. Thus sometimes 5, and sometimes 3, ATP result from the NADH + H^+ that arise from glycolysis. The amount depends on the cell.

TABLE C-3 Balance Sheet for Glucose Metabolism

		ATP
Glycolysis:	4 ATP − 2 ATP	2
1 glucose to 2 pyruvate	2 NADH + H^+	3–5[a]
2 pyruvate to 2 acetyl CoA	2 NADH + H^+	5
TCA cycle and electron transport chain:		
2 isocitrate	2 NADH + H^+	5
2 alpha-ketoglutarate	2 NADH + H^+	5
2 succinyl CoA	2 GTP	2
2 succinate	2 $FADH_2$	3
2 malate	2 NADH + H^+	5
Total ATP collected from one molecule of glucose:		30–32

[a]Each NADH + H^+ from glycolysis can yield 1.5 or 2.5 ATP. See the accompanying text.

A similar balance sheet from the complete breakdown of one 16-carbon fatty acid would show a net gain of 129 ATP. As mentioned earlier, 35 ATP were generated from the 7 $FADH_2$ and 7 NADH + H^+ produced during fatty acid oxidation. The 8 acetyl CoA produced will each generate 12 ATP as they go through the TCA cycle and the electron transport chain, for a total of 96 more ATP. After subtracting the 2 ATP needed to activate the fatty acid initially, the net yield from one 16-carbon fatty acid: 35 + 96 − 2 = 129 ATP.

These calculations help explain why fat yields more energy (measured as kcalories) per gram than carbohydrate or protein. The more molecular bond energy conserved (e.g., during the capture of energy when carbon-carbon bonds are broken) and available hydrogen atoms a fuel contains, the more ATP will be generated during oxidation. The 16-carbon fatty acid molecule, with its 32 hydrogen atoms, generates 129 ATP, whereas glucose, with its 12 hydrogen atoms, yields only 32 ATP.

The TCA cycle and the electron transport chain are the body's major means of capturing the energy from nutrients in ATP molecules. Other means, such as anaerobic glycolysis, contribute energy quickly, but the aerobic processes are the most efficient. Biologists and chemists understand much more about these processes than has been presented here.

Alcohol's Interference with Energy Metabolism

Highlight 7 provides an overview of how alcohol interferes with energy metabolism. With an understanding of the TCA cycle, a few more details may be appreciated. During alcohol metabolism, the enzyme alcohol dehydrogenase oxidizes alcohol to acetaldehyde while it simultaneously reduces a molecule of NAD^+ to NADH + H^+. The related enzyme acetaldehyde dehydrogenase reduces another NAD^+ to NADH + H^+ while it oxidizes acetaldehyde to acetyl CoA, the compound that enters the TCA cycle to generate energy. Thus, whenever alcohol is being metabolized in the body, NAD^+ diminishes, and NADH + H^+ accumulates. Chemists say that the body's "redox state" is altered, because NAD^+ can oxidize, and NADH + H^+ can reduce, many other body compounds. During alcohol metabolism, NAD^+ becomes unavailable for the multitude of reactions for which it is required.

As the previous sections just explained, for glucose to be completely metabolized, the TCA cycle must be operating, and NAD^+ must be present. If these conditions are not met (and when alcohol is present, they may not be), the pathway will be blocked, and traffic will back up—or an alternate route will be taken. Think about this as you follow the pathway shown in Figure C-6.

In each step of alcohol metabolism in which NAD^+ is converted to NADH + H^+, hydrogen ions accumulate, resulting in a dangerous shift of the acid–base balance toward acid (Chapter 12 explains acid–base balance). The accumulation of NADH + H^+ slows TCA cycle activity, so pyruvate and acetyl

FIGURE C-6 Ethanol Enters the Metabolic Pathways

This is a simplified version of the glucose-to-energy pathway showing the entry of ethanol. The coenzyme NAD (which is the active form of the B vitamin niacin) is the only one shown here; however, many others are involved.

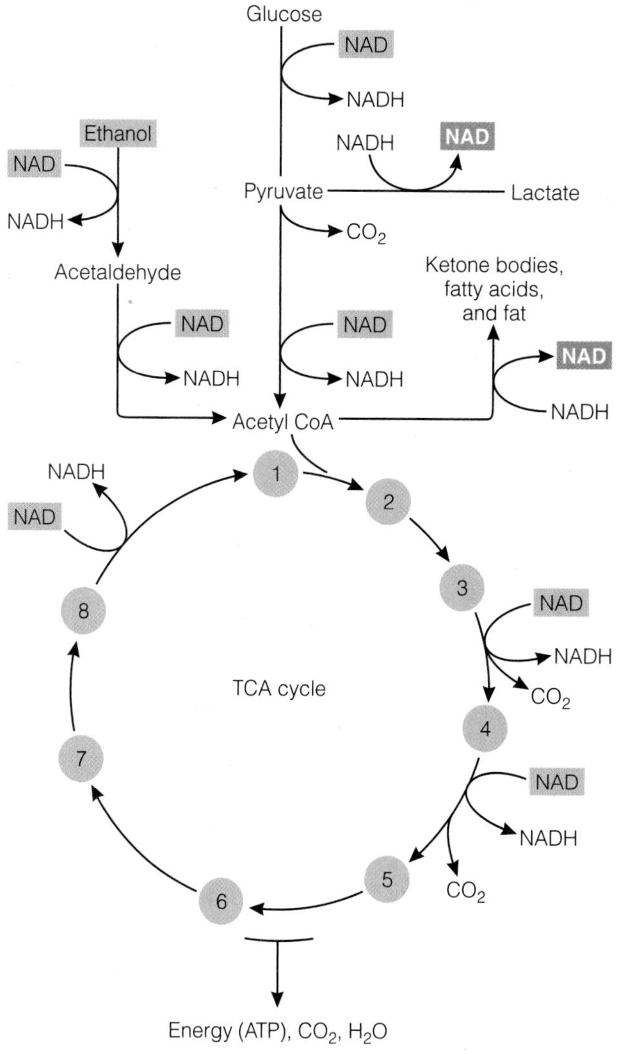
Glucose
NAD
NADH
Ethanol
NAD
NADH
NADH
NAD
Pyruvate
Lactate
CO_2
Acetaldehyde
Ketone bodies, fatty acids, and fat
NAD
NADH
NAD
NADH
NAD
NADH
Acetyl CoA
NADH
NAD
1
2
3
8
NAD
NADH
CO_2
TCA cycle
4
7
NAD
NADH
5
CO_2
6
Energy (ATP), CO_2, H_2O

CoA build up. This condition favours the conversion of pyruvate to lactate, which serves as a temporary storage place for hydrogens from NADH + H^+. The conversion of pyruvate to lactate restores some NAD^+, but a lactate buildup has serious consequences of its own. It adds to the body's acid burden and interferes with the excretion of uric acid, causing gout-like symptoms. Molecules of acetyl CoA become building blocks for fatty acids or ketone bodies. The making of ketone bodies consumes acetyl CoA and generates NAD^+; but some ketone bodies are acids, so they push the acid–base balance further toward acid.

Thus alcohol cascades through the metabolic pathways, wreaking havoc along the way. These consequences have physical effects, which Highlight 7 describes.

The Urea Cycle

Chapter 6 sums up the process by which waste nitrogen is eliminated from the body by stating that ammonia molecules combine with carbon dioxide to produce urea. This is true, but it is not the whole story. Urea is produced in a multistep process within the cells of the liver.

Ammonia, freed from an amino acid or other compound during metabolism anywhere in the body, arrives at the liver by way of the bloodstream and is taken into a liver cell. There, it is first combined with carbon dioxide and a phosphate group from ATP to form carbamoyl phosphate:

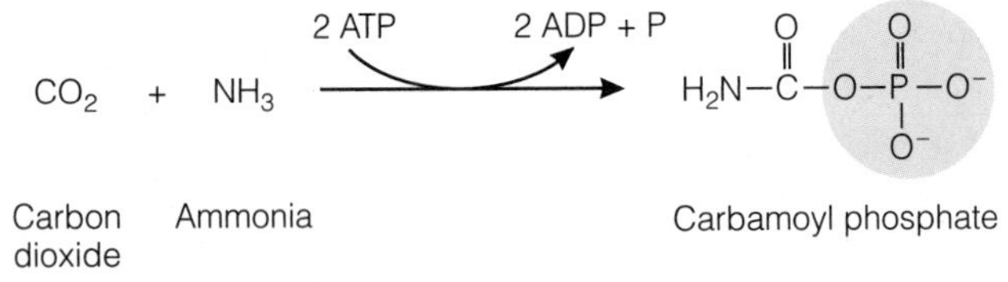
2 ATP
2 ADP + P
CO2 + NH3
Carbon dioxide
Ammonia
Carbamoyl phosphate

Figure C-7 shows the cycle of four reactions that follow.

1. Carbamoyl phosphate combines with the amino acid ornithine, losing its phosphate group. The compound formed is citrulline.
2. Citrulline combines with the amino acid aspartic acid, to form argininosuccinate. The reaction requires energy from ATP. (ATP was shown earlier losing one phosphorus atom in a phosphate group, P, to become ADP. In this reaction, it loses two phosphorus atoms joined together, PP, and becomes adenosine monophosphate, AMP.)
3. Argininosuccinate is split, forming another acid, fumarate, and the amino acid arginine.
4. Arginine loses its terminal carbon with two attached amino groups and picks up an oxygen from water. The

FIGURE C-7 The Urea Cycle

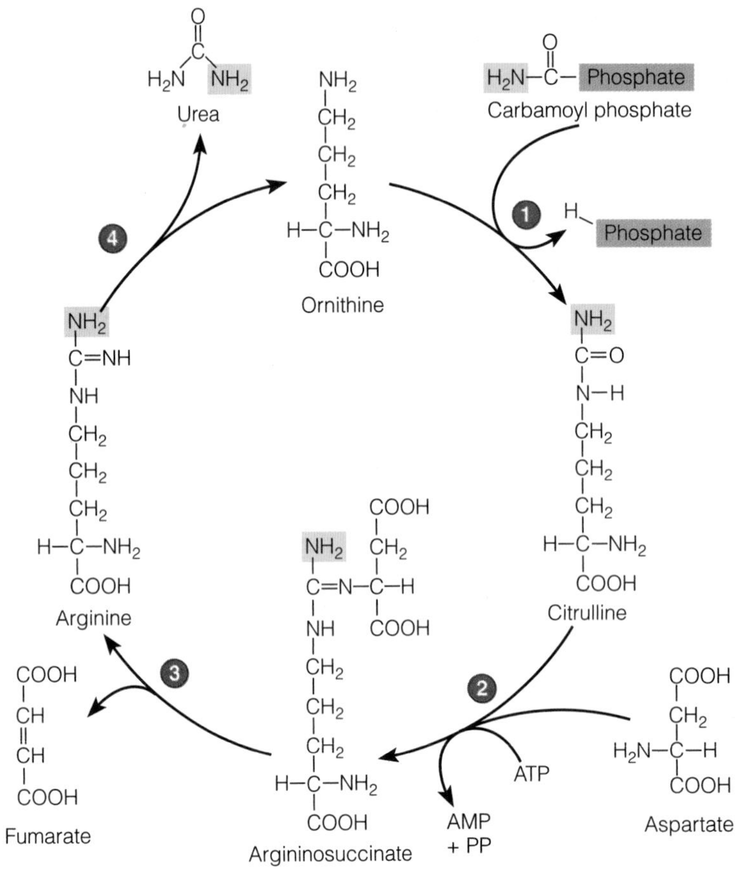
Urea
Ornithine
Carbamoyl phosphate
Phosphate
Citrulline
ATP
AMP + PP
Aspartate
Argininosuccinate
Fumarate
Arginine

APPENDIX C

end product is urea, which the kidneys excrete in the urine. The compound that remains is ornithine, identical to the ornithine with which this series of reactions began, and ready to react with another molecule of carbamoyl phosphate and turn the cycle again.

Formation of Ketone Bodies

Normally, fatty acid oxidation proceeds all the way to carbon dioxide and water. However, in ketosis (discussed in Chapter 7), an intermediate is formed from the condensation of two molecules of acetyl CoA: acetoacetyl CoA. Figure C-8 shows the formation of ketone bodies from that intermediate.

1. Acetoacetyl CoA condenses with acetyl CoA to form a 6-carbon intermediate, beta-hydroxy-beta-methylglutaryl CoA.
2. This intermediate is cleaved to acetyl CoA and acetoacetate.
3. Acetoactate can be metabolized either to beta-hydroxybutyrate (step 3a) or to acetone (3b).

Acetoacetate, beta-hydroxybutyrate, and acetone are the ketone bodies of ketosis. Two are real ketones (they have a C=O group between two carbons); the other is an alcohol that has been produced during ketone formation—hence the term *ketone bodies*, rather than ketones, to describe the three of them. There are many other ketones in nature; these three are characteristic of ketosis in the body.

FIGURE C-8 The Formation of Ketone Bodies

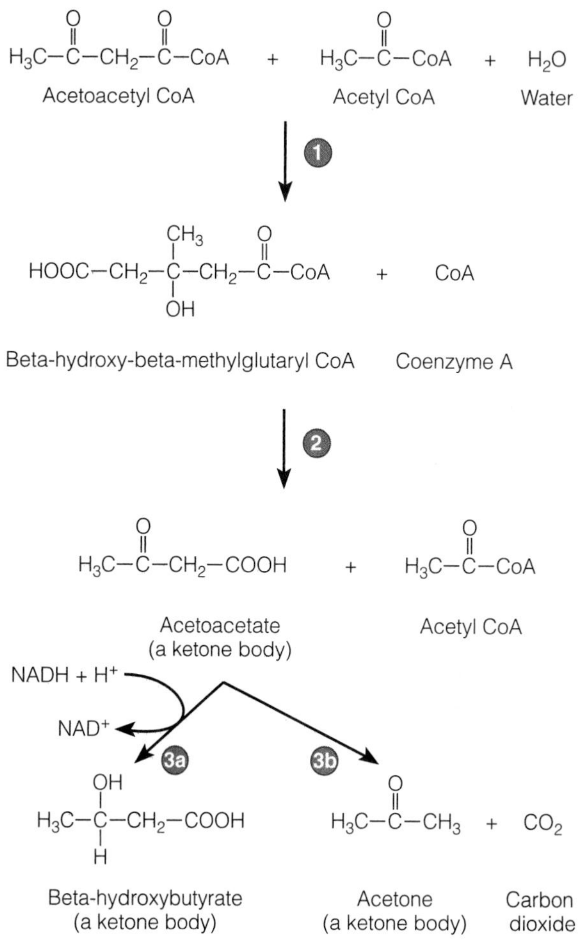

H3C–C–CH2–C–CoA + H3C–C–CoA + H2O
Acetoacetyl CoA
Acetyl CoA
Water
1
HOOC–CH2–C–CH2–C–CoA + CoA
Beta-hydroxy-beta-methylglutaryl CoA
Coenzyme A
2
H3C–C–CH2–COOH + H3C–C–CoA
Acetoacetate (a ketone body)
Acetyl CoA
NADH + H+
NAD+
3a
3b
H3C–C–CH2–COOH
H3C–C–CH3 + CO2
Beta-hydroxybutyrate (a ketone body)
Acetone (a ketone body)
Carbon dioxide

APPENDIX D

Measures of Protein Quality

CONTENTS

In a world where food is scarce and many people's diets contain marginal or inadequate amounts of protein, it is important to know which foods contain the highest-quality protein. Chapter 6 describes protein quality, and this appendix presents different measures researchers use to assess the quality of a food protein. The accompanying glossary defines related terms.

Amino Acid Scoring

Amino acid scoring evaluates a protein's quality by determining its amino acid composition and comparing it with that of a reference protein. The advantages of amino acid scoring are that it is simple and inexpensive, it easily identifies the limiting amino acid, and it can be used to score mixtures of different proportions of two or more proteins mathematically without having to make up a mixture and test it. Its chief weaknesses are that it fails to estimate the digestibility of a protein, which may strongly affect the protein's quality; it relies on a chemical procedure in which certain amino acids may be destroyed, making the pattern that is analyzed inaccurate; and it is blind to other features of the protein (such as the presence of substances that may inhibit the digestion or utilization of the protein) that would only be revealed by a test in living animals.

Table D-1 shows the reference pattern for the nine indispensible/essential amino acids. To interpret the table, read, "For every 3210 units of indispensable/essential amino acids, 145 must be histidine, 340 must be isoleucine, 540 must be leucine," and so on. To compare a test protein with the reference protein, the experimenter first obtains a chemical analysis of the test protein's amino acids. Then, taking 3210 units of the amino acids, the experimenter compares the amount of each amino acid to the amount found in 3210 units of essential amino acids in egg protein. For example, suppose the test protein contained (per 3210 units) 360 units of isoleucine; 500 units of leucine; 350 of lysine; and for each of the other amino acids, more units than egg protein contains. The two amino acids that are low are leucine (500 as compared with 540 in egg) and lysine (350 versus 440 in egg). The ratio, amino acid in the test protein

TABLE D-1 A Reference Pattern for Amino Acid Scoring of Proteins

Indispensable/Essential Amino Acids	Reference Protein—Whole Egg (mg amino acid/g nitrogen)
Histidine	145
Isoleucine	340
Leucine	540
Lysine	440
Methionine + cystine[a]	355
Phenylalanine + tyrosine[b]	580
Threonine	294
Tryptophan	106
Valine	410
Total	3210

[a]Methionine is essential and is also used to make cystine. Thus the methionine requirement is lower if cystine is supplied.
[b]Phenylalanine is essential and is also used to make tyrosine if not enough of the latter is available. Thus the phenylalanine requirement is lower if tyrosine is also supplied.

GLOSSARY

amino acid scoring: a measure of protein quality assessed by comparing a protein's amino acid pattern with that of a reference protein; sometimes called *chemical scoring.*

biological value (BV): a measure of protein quality assessed by measuring the amount of protein nitrogen that is retained from a given amount of protein nitrogen absorbed.

net protein utilization (NPU): a measure of protein quality assessed by measuring the amount of protein nitrogen that is retained from a given amount of protein nitrogen eaten.

PDCAAS (protein digestibility–corrected amino acid score): a measure of protein quality assessed by comparing the amino acid score of a food protein with the amino acid requirements of preschool-age children and then correcting for the true digestibility of the protein; recommended by the FAO/WHO and used to establish protein quality of foods for Daily Value percentages on food labels.

protein efficiency ratio (PER): a measure of protein quality assessed by determining how well a given protein supports weight gain in growing rats; used to establish the protein quality for infant formulas and baby foods.

divided by amino acid in egg, is 500/540 (or about 0.93) for leucine and 350/440 (or about 0.80) for lysine. Lysine is the limiting amino acid (the one that falls shortest compared with egg). If the protein's limiting amino acid is 80 percent of the amount found in the reference protein, it receives a score of 80.

PDCAAS

The **protein digestibility–corrected amino acid score,** or **PDCAAS,** compares the amino acid composition of a protein with human amino acid requirements and corrects for digestibility. First the protein's amino acid composition is determined, and then it is compared against the amino acid requirements of preschool-aged children. This comparison reveals the most limiting amino acid—the one that falls shortest compared with the reference. If a food protein's limiting amino acid is 70 percent of the amount found in the reference protein, it receives a score of 70. The amino acid score is multiplied by the food's protein digestibility percentage to determine the PDCAAS. The accompanying "How To" provides an example of how to calculate the PDCAAS, and Table D-2 lists the PDCAAS values of selected foods.

TABLE D-2 PDCAAS Values of Selected Foods

Casein (milk protein)	1.00
Egg white	1.00
Soybean (isolate)	0.99
Beef	0.92
Pea flour	0.69
Kidney beans (canned)	0.68
Chickpeas (canned)	0.66
Pinto beans (canned)	0.66
Rolled oats	0.57
Lentils (canned)	0.52
Peanut meal	0.52
Whole wheat	0.40

NOTE: 1.0 is the maximum PDCAAS a food protein can receive.

HOW TO Measure Protein Quality Using PDCAAS

To calculate the PDCAAS (protein digestibility–corrected amino acid score), researchers first determine the amino acid profile of the test protein (in this example, pinto beans). The second column of the table below presents the indispensable/essential amino acid profile for pinto beans. The third column presents the amino acid reference pattern.

To determine how well the food protein meets human needs, researchers calculate the ratio by dividing the second column by the third column (e.g., 30 ÷ 18 = 1.67 for histidine). The amino acid with the lowest ratio is the most limiting amino acid—in this case, methionine. Its ratio is the amino acid score for the protein—in this case, 0.84.

The amino acid score alone, however, does not account for digestibility. Protein digestibility, as determined by rat studies, yields a value of 79 percent for pinto beans. Together, the amino acid score and the digestibility value determine the PDCAAS:

$$\text{PDCAAS} = \text{protein digestibility} \times \text{amino acid score}$$

$$\text{PDCAAS for pinto beans} = 0.79 \times 0.84 = 0.66$$

Thus the PDCAAS for pinto beans is 0.66. Table D-2 lists the PDCAAS values of selected foods.

The PDCAAS is used to determine the percent Daily Value on food labels. To calculate the percent Daily Value for protein for canned pinto beans, multiply the number of grams of protein in a standard serving (in the case of pinto beans, 7 grams per 125 mL/½ cup) by the PDCAAS:

$$7 \text{ g} \times 0.66 = 4.62$$

This value is then divided by the recommended standard for protein (for children over age four and adults, 50 grams):

$$4.62 \div 50 = 0.09 \text{ (or 9\%)}$$

The food label for this can of pinto beans would declare that one serving provides 7 grams protein, and if the label included a percent Daily Value for protein (which is optional), the value would be 9 percent.

Indispensable/Essential Amino Acids	Amino Acid Profile of Pinto Beans (mg/g protein)	Amino Acid Reference Pattern (mg/g protein)	Amino Acid Score
Histidine	30.0	18	1.67
Isoleucine	42.5	25	1.70
Leucine	80.4	55	1.46
Lysine	69.0	51	1.35
Methionine (+ cystine)	21.1	25	0.84
Phenylalanine (+ tyrosine)	90.5	47	1.93
Threonine	43.7	27	1.62
Tryptophan	8.8	7	1.26
Valine	50.1	32	1.57

Biological Value

The **biological value (BV)** of a protein measures its efficiency in supporting the body's needs. In a test of biological value, two nitrogen balance studies are done. In the first, no protein is fed, and nitrogen (N) excretions in the urine and feces are measured. It is assumed that under these conditions, N lost in the urine is the amount the body always necessarily loses by filtration into the urine each day, regardless of what protein is fed (endogenous N). The N lost in the feces (called metabolic N) is the amount the body invariably loses into the intestine each day, whether or not food protein is fed. (To help you remember the terms: endogenous N is "urinary N on a zero-protein diet"; metabolic N is "fecal N on a zero-protein diet.")

In the second study, an amount of protein slightly below the requirement is fed. Intake and losses are measured; then the BV is derived using this formula:

$$\text{BV} = \frac{\text{N retained}}{\text{N absorbed}} \times 100$$

The denominator of this equation expresses the amount of nitrogen *absorbed:* food N minus fecal N (excluding the metabolic N the body would lose in the feces anyway, even without food). The numerator expresses the amount of N *retained* from the N absorbed: absorbed N (as in the denominator) minus the N excreted in the urine (excluding the endogenous N the body would lose in the urine anyway, even without food). The more nitrogen retained, the higher the protein quality. (Recall that when an essential amino acid is missing, protein synthesis stops, and the remaining amino acids are deaminated and the nitrogen excreted.)

Egg protein has a BV of 100, indicating that 100 percent of the nitrogen absorbed is retained. Supplied in adequate quantity, a protein with a BV of 70 or greater can support human growth as long as energy intake is adequate. Table D-3 presents the BV for selected foods.

TABLE D-3 Biological Values (BV) of Selected Foods

Egg	100
Milk	93
Beef	75
Fish	75
Corn	72

NOTE: 100 is the maximum BV a food protein can receive.

This method has the advantages of being based on experiments with human beings (it can be done with animals, too, of course) and of measuring actual nitrogen retention. But it is also cumbersome, expensive, and often impractical, and it is based on several assumptions that may not be valid. For example, the physiology, normal environment, or typical food intake of the subjects used for testing may not be similar to those for whom the test protein may ultimately be used. For another example, the retention of protein in the body does not necessarily mean that it is being well utilized. Considerable exchange of protein among tissues (protein turnover) occurs, but is hidden from view when only N intake and output are measured. The test of biological value wouldn't detect if one tissue were shorted.

Net Protein Utilization

Like BV, **net protein utilization (NPU)** measures how efficiently a protein is used by the body and involves two balance studies. The difference is that NPU measures retention of food nitrogen rather than food nitrogen absorbed (as in BV). The formula for NPU is:

$$\text{NPU} = \frac{\text{N retained}}{\text{N intake}} \times 100$$

The numerator is the same as for BV, but the denominator represents food N intake only—not N absorbed.

This method offers advantages similar to those of BV determinations and is used more frequently, with animals as the test subjects. A drawback is that if a low NPU is obtained, the test results offer no help in distinguishing between two possible causes: a poor amino acid composition of the test protein or poor digestibility. There is also a limit to the extent to which animal test results can be assumed to be applicable to human beings.

Protein Efficiency Ratio

The **protein efficiency ratio (PER)** measures the weight gain of a growing animal and compares it to the animal's protein intake. Until recently, the PER was generally accepted in Canada and the United States as the official method for assessing protein quality, and it is still used to evaluate proteins for infants.

Young rats are fed a measured amount of protein and weighed periodically as they grow. The PER is expressed as:

$$\text{PER} = \frac{\text{weight gain (g)}}{\text{protein intake (g)}}$$

This method has the virtues of economy and simplicity, but it also has many drawbacks. The experiments are time-consuming; the amino acid needs of rats are not the same as those of human beings; and the amino acid needs for growth are not the same as for the maintenance of adult animals (growing animals need more lysine, for example). Table D-4 presents PER values for selected foods.

TABLE D-4 Protein Efficiency Ratio (PER) Values of Selected Proteins

Casein (milk)	2.8
Soy	2.4
Gluten (wheat)	0.4

APPENDIX E

CONTENTS

Nutrition Assessment

Nutrition assessment evaluates a person's health from a nutrition perspective. Many factors influence or reflect nutrition status. Consequently, the assessor, usually a registered dietitian assisted by other qualified health-care professionals, gathers information from many sources, including:

- Historical information.
- Anthropometric measurements.
- Physical examinations.
- Biochemical analyses (laboratory tests).

Each of these methods involves collecting data in a variety of ways and interpreting each finding in relation to the others to create a total picture.

The accurate gathering of this information and its careful interpretation are the basis for a meaningful evaluation. The more information gathered about a person, the more accurate the assessment will be. Gathering information is a time-consuming process, however, and time is often a rare commodity in the health-care setting. Nutrition care is only one part of total care. It may not be practical or essential to collect detailed information on each person.

A strategic compromise is to screen clients by collecting preliminary data. Data such as height-weight and hematocrit are easy to obtain and can alert health-care workers to potential problems. **Nutrition screening** identifies clients who will require additional nutrition assessment. This appendix provides a sample of the procedures, standards, and charts commonly used in nutrition assessment.

Historical Information

Clues about present nutrition status become evident with a careful review of a person's historical data (see Table E-1). Even when the data are subjective, they reveal important facts about a person. A thorough history identifies risk factors associated with poor nutrition status (see Table E-2) and provides a sense of the

TABLE E-1 Historical Data Used in Nutrition Assessments

Type of History	What It Identifies
Health history	Current and previous health problems and family health history that affect nutrient needs, nutrition status, or the need for intervention to prevent or alleviate health problems
Socio-economic history	Personal, cultural, financial, and environmental influences on food intake, nutrient needs, and diet therapy options
Drug history	Medications (prescription and over-the-counter), illicit drugs, dietary supplements, and alternative therapies that affect nutrition status
Diet history	Nutrient intake excesses or deficiencies and reasons for imbalances

nutrition screening: the use of preliminary nutrition assessment techniques to identify people who are malnourished or are at risk for malnutrition.

TABLE E-2 Risk Factors for Poor Nutrition Status

Health History

- Acquired immune deficiency syndrome (AIDS)
- Alcoholism
- Anorexia (lack of appetite)
- Anorexia nervosa
- Bulimia nervosa
- Burns
- Cancer
- Chewing or swallowing difficulties (including poorly fitted dentures, dental caries, missing teeth, and mouth ulcers)
- Chronic obstructive pulmonary disease
- Circulatory problems
- Constipation
- Crohn's disease
- Cystic fibrosis
- Decubitus ulcers (pressure sores)
- Dementia
- Depleted blood proteins
- Depression
- Diabetes mellitus
- Diarrhea, prolonged or severe
- Drug addiction
- Dysphagia
- Failure to thrive
- Feeding disabilities
- Fever
- GI tract disorders or surgery
- Heart disease
- HIV infection
- Hormonal imbalance
- Hyperlipidemia
- Hypertension
- Infections
- Kidney disease
- Liver disease
- Lung disease
- Malabsorption
- Mental illness
- Mental retardation
- Multiple pregnancies
- Nausea
- Neurologic disorders
- Organ failure
- Overweight
- Pancreatic insufficiency
- Paralysis
- Physical disability
- Pneumonia
- Pregnancy
- Radiation therapy
- Recent major illness
- Recent major surgery
- Recent weight loss or gain
- Tobacco use
- Trauma
- Ulcerative colitis
- Ulcers
- Underweight
- Vomiting, prolonged or severe

Socio-economic History

- Access to groceries
- Activities
- Age
- Education
- Ethnic identity
- Income
- Kitchen facilities
- Number of people in household
- Occupation
- Religious affiliation

Drug History

- Amphetamines
- Analgesics
- Antacids
- Antibiotics
- Anticonvulsant agents
- Antidepressant agents
- Antidiabetic agents
- Antidiarrheals
- Antifungal agents
- Antihyperlipemics
- Antihypertensives
- Antineoplastics
- Antiulcer agents
- Antiviral agents
- Catabolic steroids
- Diuretics
- Hormonal agents
- Immunosuppressive agents
- Laxatives
- Oral contraceptives
- Vitamin and other dietary supplements

Diet History

- Deficient or excessive food intakes
- Frequently eating out
- Intravenous fluids (other than total parenteral nutrition) for 7 or more days
- Monotonous diet (lacking variety)
- No intake for 7 or more days
- Poor appetite
- Restricted or fad diets
- Unbalanced diet (omitting any food group)
- Recent weight gains or losses

whole person. As you can see, many aspects of a person's life influence nutrition status and provide clues to possible problems.

An adept history taker uses the interview both to gather facts and to establish a rapport with the client. This section briefly reviews the major areas of nutrition concern in a person's history: health, socio-economic factors, drugs, and diet.

Health History

The assessor can obtain a **health history** from records completed by the attending physician, nurse, or other health-care professional. In addition, conversations with the client can uncover valuable information previously overlooked because no one thought to ask or because the client was not thinking clearly when asked.

An accurate, complete health history can reveal conditions that increase a client's risk for malnutrition (review Table E-2). Diseases and their therapies can

health history: an account of a client's current and past health status and disease risks.

have either immediate or long-term effects on nutrition status by interfering with ingestion, digestion, absorption, metabolism, or excretion of nutrients.

Socio-economic History A **socio-economic history** reveals factors that profoundly affect nutrition status. The ethnic background and educational level of both the client and the other members of the household influence food availability and food choices. An understanding of the community environment is also important in assessing nutrition status. For example, the interviewer should be familiar with the food habits of the major ethnic groups within the locale, regional food preferences, and nutrition resources and programs available in the community. Local health departments and social agencies often can provide such information.

Level of income also influences the diet. In general, the quality of the diet declines as income falls. At some point, the ability to purchase the foods required to meet nutrient needs is lost; an inadequate income puts an adequate diet out of reach. Agencies use poverty indexes to identify people at risk for poor nutrition and to qualify people for government food assistance programs.

Low income affects not only the power to purchase foods but also the ability to shop for, store, and cook them. A skilled assessor will note whether a person has transportation to a grocery store that sells a sufficient variety of low-cost foods, and whether the person has access to a refrigerator and stove.

Drug History The many interactions of foods and drugs require that health-care professionals take a **drug history** and pay special attention to any client who takes drugs routinely. If a person is taking any drug, the assessor records the name of the drug; the dose, frequency, and duration of intake; the reason for taking the drug; and signs of any adverse effects.

The interactions of drugs and nutrients may take many forms:

- Drugs can alter food intake and the absorption, metabolism, and excretion of nutrients.
- Foods and nutrients can alter the absorption, metabolism, and excretion of drugs.

Highlight 18 discusses nutrient-drug interactions in more detail, and Table H18-1 (p. 611) summarizes the mechanisms by which these interactions occur and provides specific examples.

Diet History A **diet history** provides a record of a person's eating habits and food intake and can help identify possible nutrient imbalances. Food choices are an important part of lifestyle and often reflect a person's philosophy. The assessor who asks nonjudgmental questions about eating habits and food intake encourages trust and enhances the likelihood of obtaining accurate information.

Assessors evaluate food intake using various tools such as the 24-hour recall, the usual intake record, the food record, and the food frequency questionnaire. Food models or photos and measuring devices can help clients identify the types of foods and quantities consumed. The assessor also needs to know how the foods are prepared and when they are eaten. In addition to asking about foods, assessors will ask about beverage consumption, including beverages containing alcohol or caffeine.

Besides identifying possible nutrient imbalances, diet histories provide valuable clues about how a person will accept diet changes should they be necessary. Information about what and how a person eats provides the background for realistic and attainable nutrition goals.

24-Hour Recall The **24-hour recall** provides data for one day only and is commonly used in nutrition surveys to obtain estimates of the typical food intakes for a population. The assessor asks the client to recount everything eaten or drunk in the past 24 hours or for the previous day.

An advantage of the 24-hour recall is that it is easy to obtain. It is also more likely to provide accurate data, at least about the past 24 hours, than estimates

socio-economic history: a record of a person's social and economic background, including such factors as education, income, and ethnic identity.

drug history: a record of all the drugs, over-the-counter and prescribed, that a person takes routinely.

diet history: a record of eating behaviours and the foods a person eats.

24-hour recall: a record of foods eaten by a person for one 24-hour period.

of average intakes over long periods. It does not, however, provide enough information to allow accurate generalizations about an individual's usual food intake. The previous day's intake may not be typical, for example, or the person may be unable to report portion sizes accurately or may conceal or forget information about foods eaten. This limitation is partially overcome when 24-hour recalls are collected on several nonconsecutive days.

Usual Intake To obtain data about a person's usual intake, an inquiry might begin with "What is the first thing you usually eat or drink during the day?" Similar questions follow until a typical daily intake pattern emerges. This method can be useful, especially in verifying food intake when the past 24 hours have been atypical. It also helps the assessor verify food habits. For example, one person may always eat an afternoon snack; another may never eat breakfast. A person whose intake varies widely from day to day, however, may find it difficult to answer such general questions, and in that case, another food intake tool should be used to estimate nutrient intake.

Food Record Another tool for history taking is the **food record**, in which the person records food eaten, including the quantity and method of preparation. Figure 9-9 (p. 294) provides an example. A food record can help both the assessor and the client to determine factors associated with eating that may affect dietary balance and adequacy.

Food records work especially well with cooperative people but require considerable time and effort on their part. A prime advantage is that the record keeper assumes an active role and may for the first time become aware of personal food habits and assume responsibility for them. It also provides the assessor with an accurate picture of the person's lifestyle and factors that affect food intake. For these reasons, a food record can be particularly useful in outpatient counselling for such nutrition problems as overweight, underweight, or food allergy. The major disadvantages stem from poor compliance in recording the data and conscious or unconscious changes in eating habits that may occur while the person is keeping the record.

Food Frequency Questionnaire An assessor uses a **food frequency questionnaire** to compare a client's food intake with *Eating Well with Canada's Food Guide.* Clients may be asked how many servings of each of the following they eat in a typical day: vegetables and fruits, grain products, milk and alternatives, and meat and alternatives, as well as oils and sweets. This information helps pinpoint food groups, and therefore nutrients, that may be excessive or deficient in the diet. That a person ate no vegetables yesterday may not seem particularly significant, but never eating vegetables is a warning of possible nutrient deficiencies. When used with the usual intake or 24-hour recall approach, the food frequency questionnaire enables the assessor to double-check the accuracy of the information obtained.

Analysis of Food Intake Data After collecting food intake data, the assessor estimates nutrient intakes, either informally by using food guides or formally by using food composition tables. The assessor compares these intakes with standards, usually nutrient recommendations or dietary guidelines, to determine how closely the person's diet meets the standards. Are the types and amounts of proteins, carbohydrates (including fibre), and fats (including cholesterol) appropriate? Are all food groups included in appropriate amounts? Is caffeine or alcohol consumption excessive? Are intakes of any vitamins or minerals (including sodium and iron) excessive or deficient? An informal evaluation is possible only if the assessor has enough prior experience with formal calculations to "see" nutrient amounts in reported food intakes without calculations. Even then, such an informal analysis is best followed by a spot check for key nutrients by actual calculation.

Formal calculations can be performed either manually (by looking up each food in a table of food composition, recording its nutrients, and adding them up)

food record: an extensive, accurate log of all foods eaten over a period of several days or weeks. A food record that includes associated information such as when, where, and with whom each food is eaten is sometimes called a *food diary.*

food frequency questionnaire: a checklist of foods on which a person can record the frequency with which he or she eats each food.

or by using a computer diet analysis program. The assessor then compares the intakes with standards such as the RDA or AI.

Limitations of Food Intake Analysis Diet histories can be superbly informative, but the skillful assessor also keeps their limitations in mind. For example, a computer diet analysis tends to imply greater accuracy than is possible to obtain from data as uncertain as the starting information. Nutrient contents of foods listed in tables of food composition or stored in computer databases are averages and, for some nutrients, incomplete. In addition, the available data on nutrient contents of foods do not reflect the amounts of nutrients a person actually absorbs. Iron is a case in point: its availability from a given meal may vary depending on the person's iron status; the relative amounts of heme iron, nonheme iron, vitamin C, meat, fish, and poultry eaten at the meal; and the presence of inhibitors of iron absorption such as tea, coffee, and nuts. (Chapter 14 describes the many factors that influence iron absorption from a meal.)

Furthermore, reported portion sizes may not be correct. The person who reports eating "a serving" of greens may not distinguish between 125 millilitres (¼ cup) and 500 millilitres (2 cups); only trained individuals can accurately report serving sizes. Children tend to remember the serving sizes of foods they like as being larger than serving sizes of foods they dislike.

An estimate of nutrient intakes from a diet history, combined with other sources of information, allows the assessor to confirm or eliminate the possibility of suspected food intake problems. The assessor must constantly remember that nutrient intakes in adequate amounts do not guarantee adequate nutrient status for an individual. Likewise, insufficient intakes do not always indicate deficiencies, but instead alert the assessor to possible problems. Each person digests, absorbs, metabolizes, and excretes nutrients in a unique way; individual needs vary. In-takes of nutrients identified by diet histories are only pieces of a puzzle that must be put together with other indicators of nutrition status in order to extract meaning.

Anthropometric Measurements

Anthropometrics are physical measurements that reflect body composition and development (see Table E-3). They serve three main purposes: first, to evaluate the progress of growth in pregnant women, infants, children, and adolescents; second, to detect undernutrition and overnutrition in all age groups; and third, to measure changes in body composition over time.

Health-care professionals compare anthropometric measurements taken on an individual with population standards specific for gender and age or with previous measures of the individual. Measurements taken periodically and compared with previous measurements reveal changes in an individual's status.

TABLE E-3 Anthropometric Measurements Used in Nutrition Assessments

Type of Measurement	What It Reflects
Abdominal girth measurement	Abdominal fluid retention and abdominal organ size
Height-weight	Overnutrition and undernutrition; growth in children
Head circumference	Brain growth and development in infants and children under age 2
Skinfold	Subcutaneous and total body fat
Waist circumference	Body fat distribution

anthropometrics: measurements of the physical characteristics of the body, such as height and weight.
- **anthropos** = human
- **metric** = measuring

Mastering the techniques for taking anthropometric measurements requires proper instruction and practice to ensure reliability. Once the correct techniques are learned, taking measurements is easy and requires minimal equipment.

Height and weight are well-recognized anthropometrics; other anthropometrics include skinfold measurements and various measures of lean tissue. Other measures are useful in specific situations. For example, a head circumference measurement may help to assess brain development in an infant, and an abdominal girth measurement supplies information about abdominal fluid retention in individuals with liver disease.

Measures of Growth and Development

Height and weight are among the most common and useful anthropometric measurements. Length measurements for infants and children up to age 3 and height measurements for children over 3 are particularly valuable in assessing growth and therefore nutrition status. For adults, height measurements alone are not critical, but help to estimate healthy weight and to interpret other assessment data. Once adult height has been reached, changes in body weight provide useful information in assessing overnutrition and undernutrition.

Height For infants and children younger than 3, health-care professionals may use special equipment to measure length. The assessor lays the barefoot infant on a measuring board that has a fixed headboard and movable footboard attached at right angles to the surface (see Figure E-1). Often two people are needed to obtain an accurate measurement: one to hold the infant's head against the headboard, and the other to keep the legs straight and do the measuring. This method provides the most accurate measure possible, but many health-care professionals use a less exacting method. They may simply hold the infant straight with its head against the headboard or other vertical support, mark the blanket with a chalk or pen at the infant's heel, and then measure the distance from the headboard to the mark. Even more informally and less accurately, they may lay the infant on a flat surface and extend a nonstretchable measuring tape along the side of the infant from the top of the head to the heel of the foot.

FIGURE E-1 Length Measurement of an Infant

An infant is measured lying down on a measuring board with a fixed headboard and a movable footboard. Note that two people are needed to measure the infant's length.

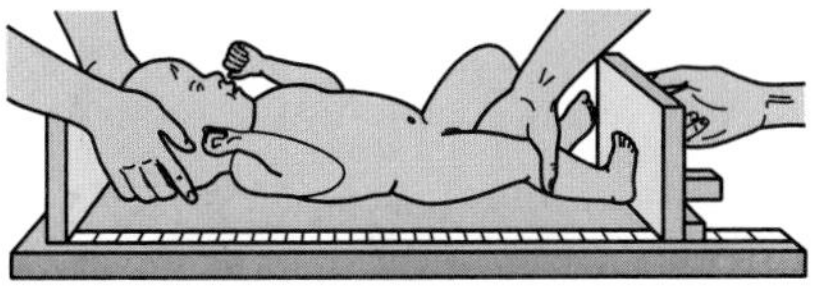

The procedure for measuring a child who can stand erect and cooperate is the same as for an adult. The best way to measure standing height is with the person's back against a flat wall to which a nonstretchable measuring tape or stick has been fixed (see Figure E-2). The person stands erect, without shoes, with heels together. The person's line of sight should be horizontal, with the heels, buttocks, shoulders, and head touching the wall. The assessor places a ruler, book, or other inflexible object on top of the head at a right angle to the wall; carefully checks the height measurement; and records it immediately in either inches or centimetres so that the correct measurement will not be forgotten.

FIGURE E-2 Height Measurement of an Older Child or Adult

Height is measured most accurately when the person stands against a flat wall to which a measuring tape has been affixed.

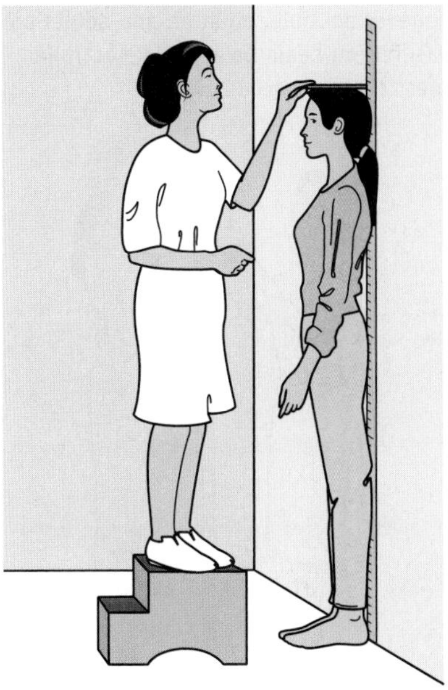

The measuring rod of a scale is commonly used, but is less accurate because it bends easily. The assessor follows the same general procedure, asking the person to face away from the scale and to take extra care to stand erect.

Unfortunately, many health-care professionals merely ask clients how tall they are rather than measuring their height. Self-reported height is often inaccurate and should be used only as a last resort when measurement is impractical (in the case of an uncooperative client, an emergency admission, or the like).

Weight Valid weight measurements require scales that have been carefully maintained, calibrated, and checked for accuracy at regular intervals. Beam balance and electronic scales are the most accurate types of scales. To measure infants' weight, assessors use special scales that allow infants to lie or sit (see Figure E-3 on p. E-6). Weighing infants naked, without diapers, is standard procedure. Children who can stand are weighed in the same way as adults (see Figure E-4 on p. E-6). To make repeated measures useful, standardized conditions are necessary. Each weighing should take place at the same time of day (preferably before breakfast), in the same amount of clothing (without shoes), after the person has voided, and on

FIGURE E-3 Weight Measurement of an Infant

Infants sit or lie down on scales that are designed to hold them while they are being weighed.

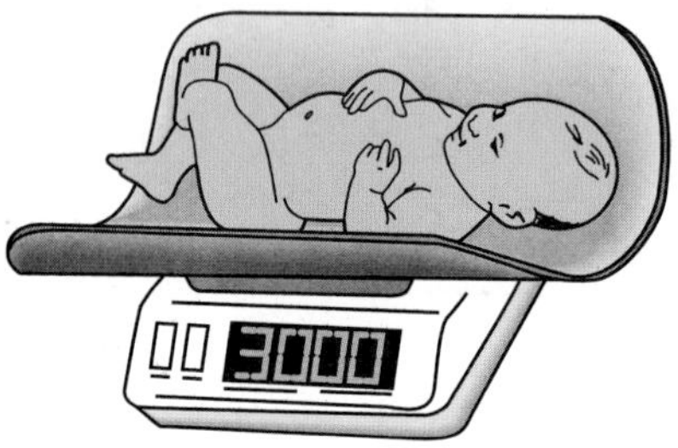

♦ Chapter 17 presents BMI charts for children and adolescents.

♦ The *body mass index (BMI)* is an index of a person's weight in relation to height, determined by dividing the weight in kilograms by the square of the height in metres:

$$\text{BMI} = \frac{\text{Weight (kg)}}{\text{Height (m)}^2}$$

FIGURE E-4 Weight Measurement of an Older Child or Adult

Whenever possible, children and adults are measured on beam balance or electronic scales to ensure accuracy.

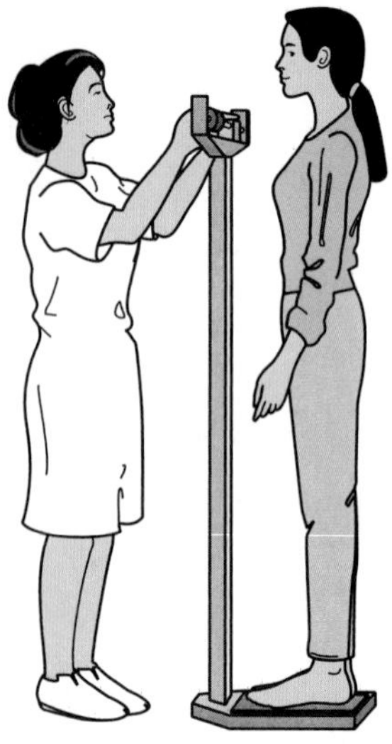

the same scale. Special scales and hospital beds with built-in scales are available for weighing people who are bedridden. Bathroom scales are inaccurate and inappropriate in a professional setting. As with all measurements, the assessor records the observed weight immediately in grams or kilograms.

Head Circumference Assessors may also measure head circumference to confirm that infant growth is proceeding normally or to help detect protein-energy malnutrition (PEM) and evaluate the extent of its impact on brain size. To measure head circumference, the assessor places a nonstretchable tape so that it encircles the largest part of the infant's or child's head: just above the eyebrow ridges, just above the point where the ears attach, and around the occipital prominence at the back of the head. To ensure accurate recording, the assessor immediately notes the measure in centimetres.

Analysis of Measures in Infants and Children Growth retardation is a sign of poor nutrition status. Obesity is also a sign that dietary intervention may be needed.

Health-care professionals generally evaluate physical development by monitoring the growth rate of a child and comparing this rate with standard charts. Standard charts compare weight to age, height to age, and weight to height; ideally, height and weight are in roughly the same percentile. Although individual growth patterns may vary, a child's growth curve will generally stay at about the same percentile throughout childhood. In children whose growth has been retarded, nutrition rehabilitation will ideally induce height and weight to increase to higher percentiles. In overweight children, the goal is for weight to remain stable as height increases, until weight becomes appropriate for height.

To evaluate growth in infants, an assessor uses charts such as those in Figures E-5 and E-6 (p. E-8). ♦ Growth charts of height-for-age, weight-for-age, and BMI for children and adolescents are found in Figures E-7 (p. E-9) and E-8 (p. E-10). To plot a weight measurement on a percentile chart, the assessor follows these steps:

- Select the appropriate chart based on age and gender.
- Locate the child's age along the horizontal axis on the bottom of the chart.
- Locate the child's weight in kilograms along the vertical axis.
- Mark the chart where the age and weight lines intersect, and read off the percentile.

To assess length, height, or head circumference, the assessor follows the same procedure, using the appropriate chart. (When length is measured, use the chart for birth to 24 months; when height is measured, use the chart for 2 to 19 years.) Head circumference percentile should be similar to the child's height and weight percentiles. With height, weight, and head circumference measures plotted on growth percentile charts, a skilled clinician can begin to interpret the data.

Percentile charts divide the measures of a population into 100 equal divisions. Thus half of the population falls above the 50th percentile, and half falls below. The use of percentile measures allows for comparisons among people of the same age and gender. For example, a 6-month-old female infant whose weight is at the 75 percentile weighs more than 75 percent of the female infants her age.

Head circumference is generally measured in children under 2 years of age. Because the brain grows rapidly before birth and during early infancy, extreme and chronic malnutrition during these times can impair brain development, curtailing the number of brain cells and the size of head circumference. Nonnutritional factors, such as certain disorders and genetic variation, can also influence head circumference.

Analysis of Measures in Adults For adults, health-care professionals typically compare weights with weight-for-height standards. One such standard is the body mass index (BMI), ♦ described in Chapter 8, which is useful for estimating the risk to health associated with overnutrition and undernutrition. The back cover shows BMI for various heights and weights.

FIGURE E-5A Length- and Weight-for-Age Percentiles, Boys Birth–24 Months

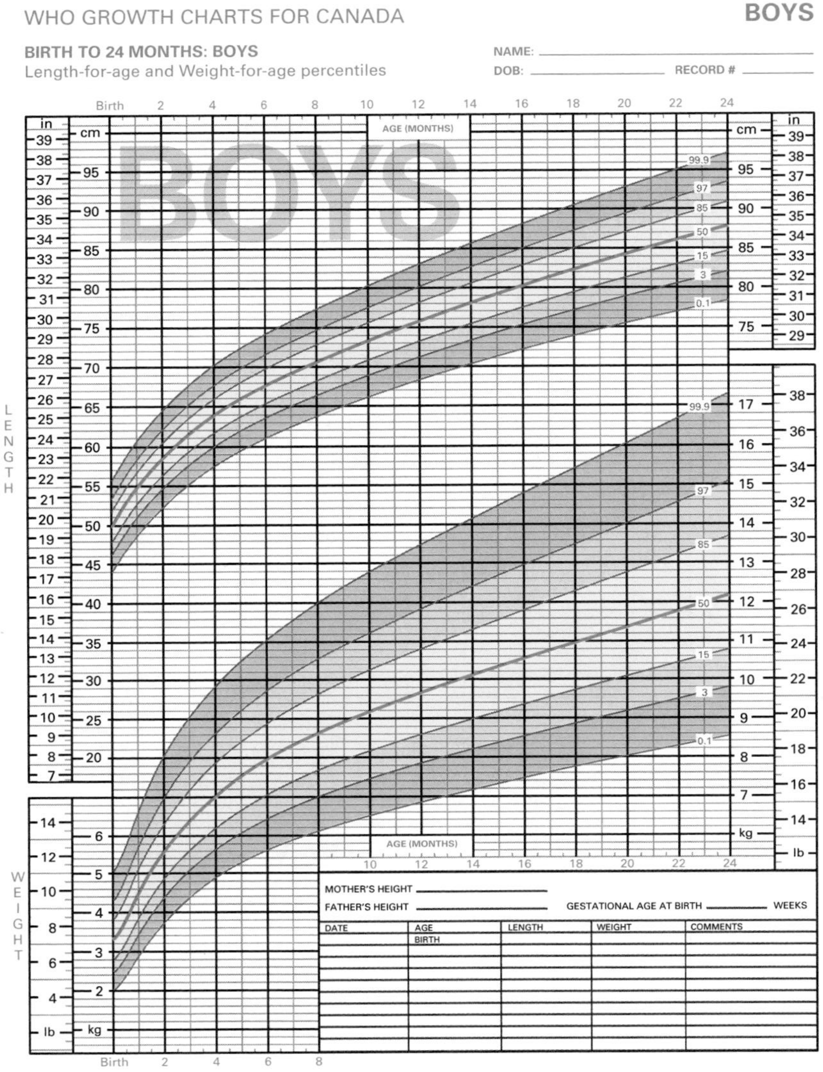
WHO GROWTH CHARTS FOR CANADA
BOYS
BIRTH TO 24 MONTHS: BOYS
Length-for-age and Weight-for-age percentiles
NAME:
DOB:
RECORD #
AGE (MONTHS)
LENGTH
WEIGHT
BOYS
MOTHER'S HEIGHT
FATHER'S HEIGHT
GESTATIONAL AGE AT BIRTH
WEEKS
DATE
AGE
BIRTH
LENGTH
WEIGHT
COMMENTS

FIGURE E-5B Length- and Weight-for-Age Percentiles, Girls Birth–24 Months

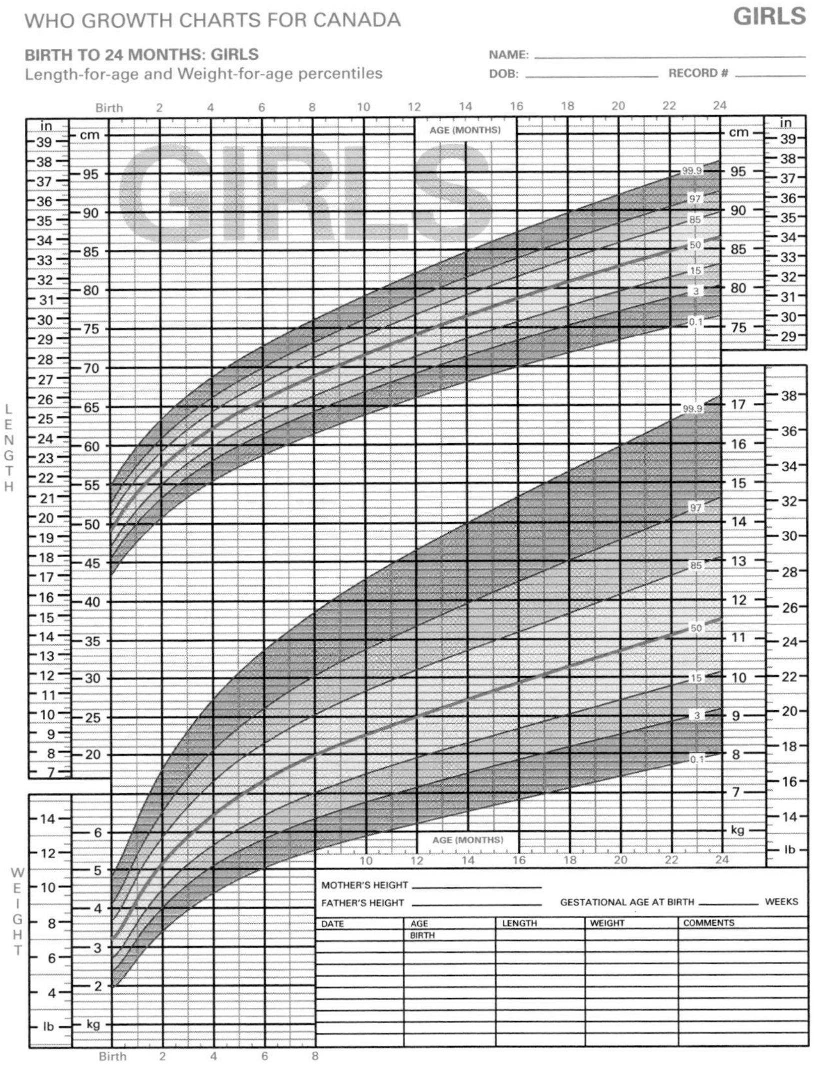
WHO GROWTH CHARTS FOR CANADA
GIRLS
BIRTH TO 24 MONTHS: GIRLS
Length-for-age and Weight-for-age percentiles
NAME:
DOB:
RECORD #
AGE (MONTHS)
LENGTH
WEIGHT
GIRLS
MOTHER'S HEIGHT
FATHER'S HEIGHT
GESTATIONAL AGE AT BIRTH
WEEKS
DATE
AGE
BIRTH
LENGTH
WEIGHT
COMMENTS

FIGURE E-6A **Head Circumference and Weight-for-Length Percentiles, Boys Birth–24 Months**

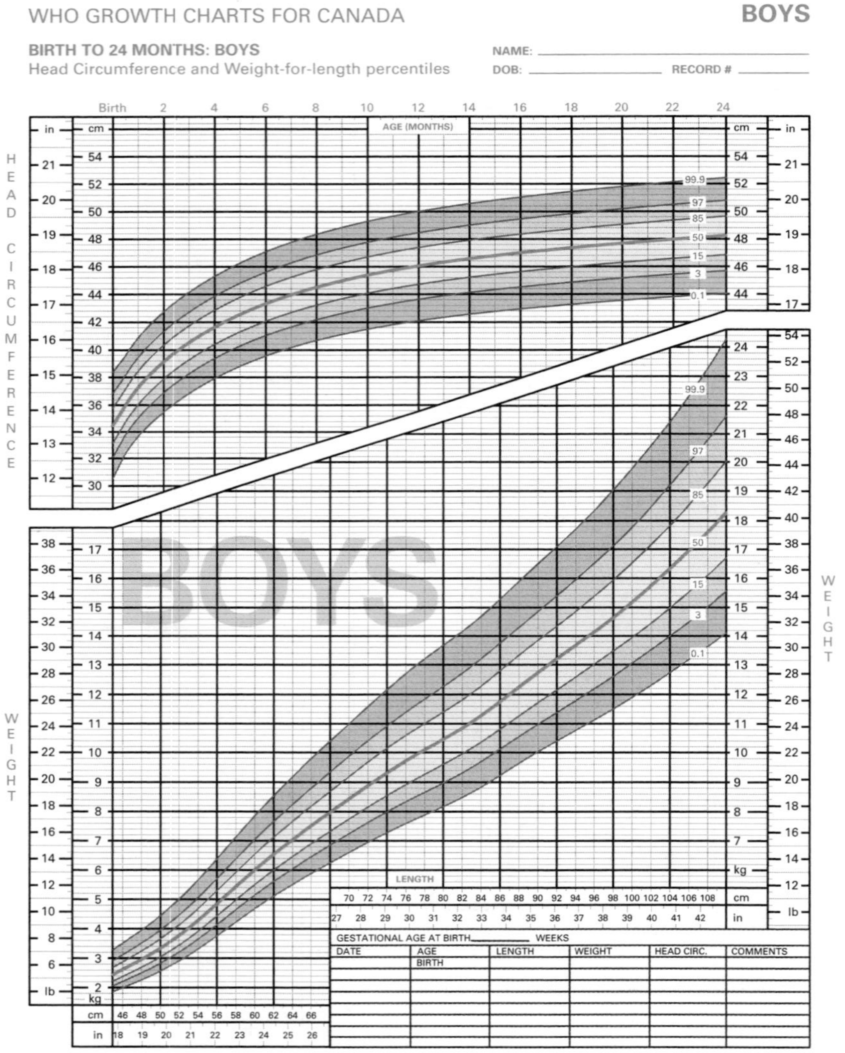
WHO GROWTH CHARTS FOR CANADA
BOYS
BIRTH TO 24 MONTHS: BOYS
Head Circumference and Weight-for-length percentiles
NAME:
DOB:
RECORD #
AGE (MONTHS)
HEAD CIRCUMFERENCE
WEIGHT
LENGTH
GESTATIONAL AGE AT BIRTH ____ WEEKS
DATE
AGE
BIRTH
LENGTH
WEIGHT
HEAD CIRC.
COMMENTS

FIGURE E-6B **Head Circumference and Weight-for-Length Percentiles, Girls Birth–24 Months**

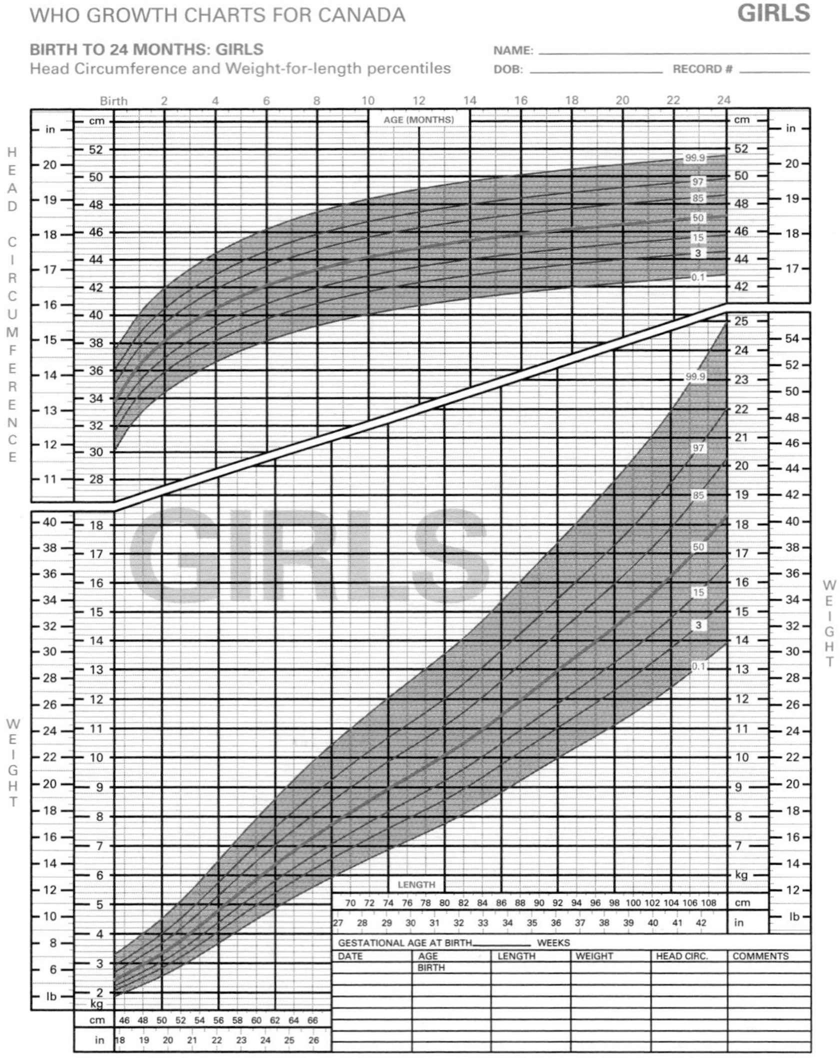
WHO GROWTH CHARTS FOR CANADA
GIRLS
BIRTH TO 24 MONTHS: GIRLS
Head Circumference and Weight-for-length percentiles
NAME:
DOB:
RECORD #
AGE (MONTHS)
HEAD CIRCUMFERENCE
WEIGHT
LENGTH
GESTATIONAL AGE AT BIRTH ____ WEEKS
DATE
AGE
BIRTH
LENGTH
WEIGHT
HEAD CIRC.
COMMENTS

FIGURE E-7A Height- and Weight-for-Age Percentiles, Boys 2–19 Years

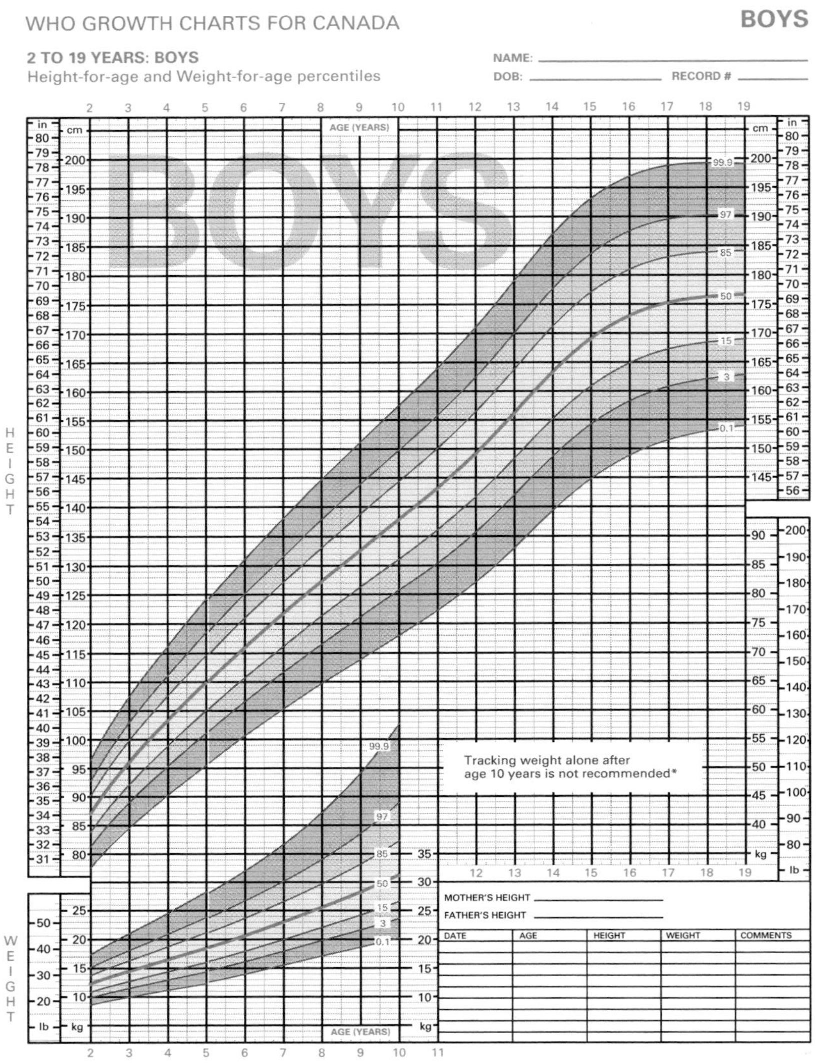
WHO GROWTH CHARTS FOR CANADA
BOYS
2 TO 19 YEARS: BOYS
Height-for-age and Weight-for-age percentiles
NAME:
DOB:
RECORD #
AGE (YEARS)
HEIGHT
WEIGHT
Tracking weight alone after age 10 years is not recommended*
MOTHER'S HEIGHT
FATHER'S HEIGHT
DATE
AGE
HEIGHT
WEIGHT
COMMENTS

FIGURE E-7B Height- and Weight-for-Age Percentiles, Girls 2–19 Years

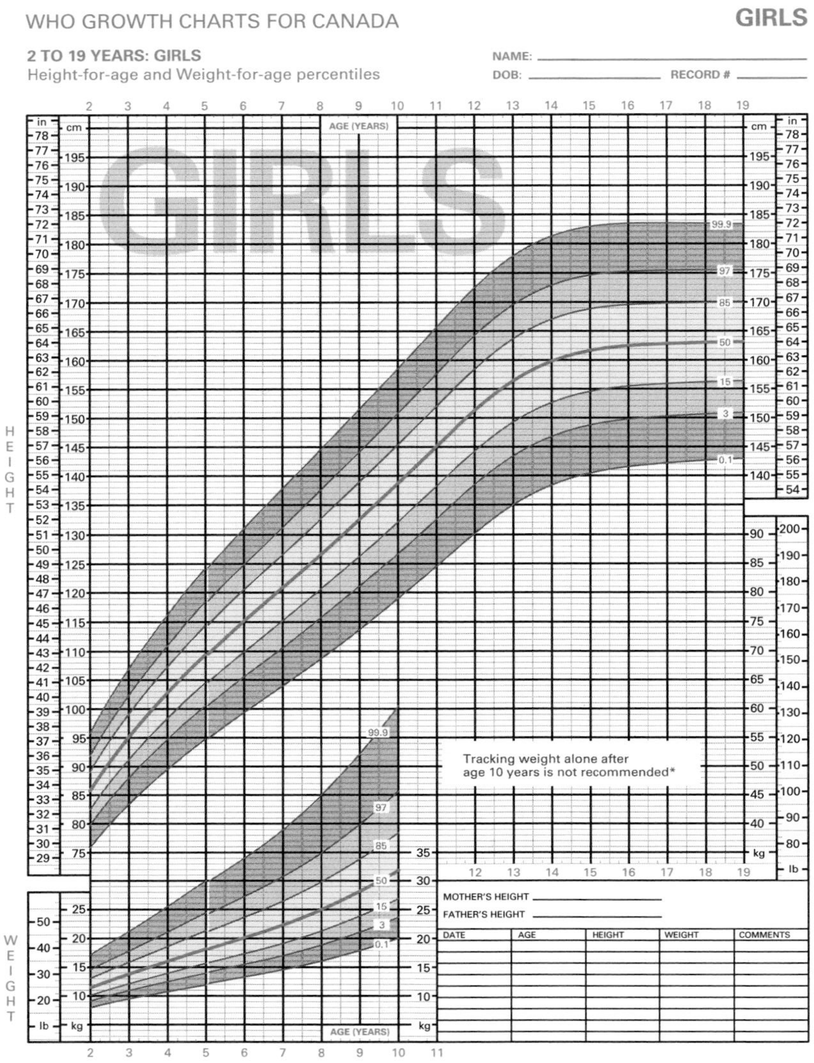
WHO GROWTH CHARTS FOR CANADA
GIRLS
2 TO 19 YEARS: GIRLS
Height-for-age and Weight-for-age percentiles
NAME:
DOB:
RECORD #
AGE (YEARS)
HEIGHT
WEIGHT
Tracking weight alone after age 10 years is not recommended*
MOTHER'S HEIGHT
FATHER'S HEIGHT
DATE
AGE
HEIGHT
WEIGHT
COMMENTS

FIGURE E-8A Body Mass Index-for-Age Percentiles, Boys 2–19 Years

WHO GROWTH CHARTS FOR CANADA

BOYS

2 TO 19 YEARS: BOYS
Body mass index-for-age percentiles

NAME: ______
DOB: ______ RECORD # ______

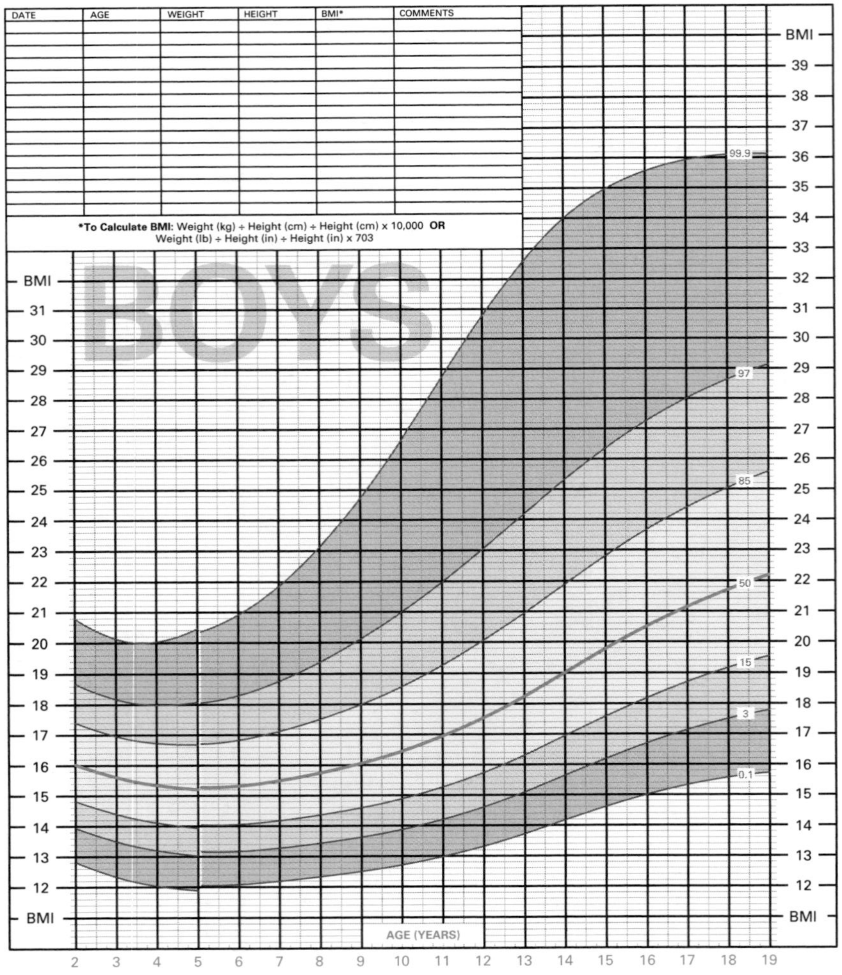
DATE
AGE
WEIGHT
HEIGHT
BMI*
COMMENTS
*To Calculate BMI: Weight (kg) ÷ Height (cm) ÷ Height (cm) x 10,000 OR
Weight (lb) ÷ Height (in) ÷ Height (in) x 703
BOYS
BMI
99.9
97
85
50
15
3
0.1
AGE (YEARS)

FIGURE E-8B Body Mass Index-for-Age Percentiles, Girls 2–19 Years

WHO GROWTH CHARTS FOR CANADA

GIRLS

2 TO 19 YEARS: GIRLS
Body mass index-for-age percentiles

NAME: ______
DOB: ______ RECORD # ______

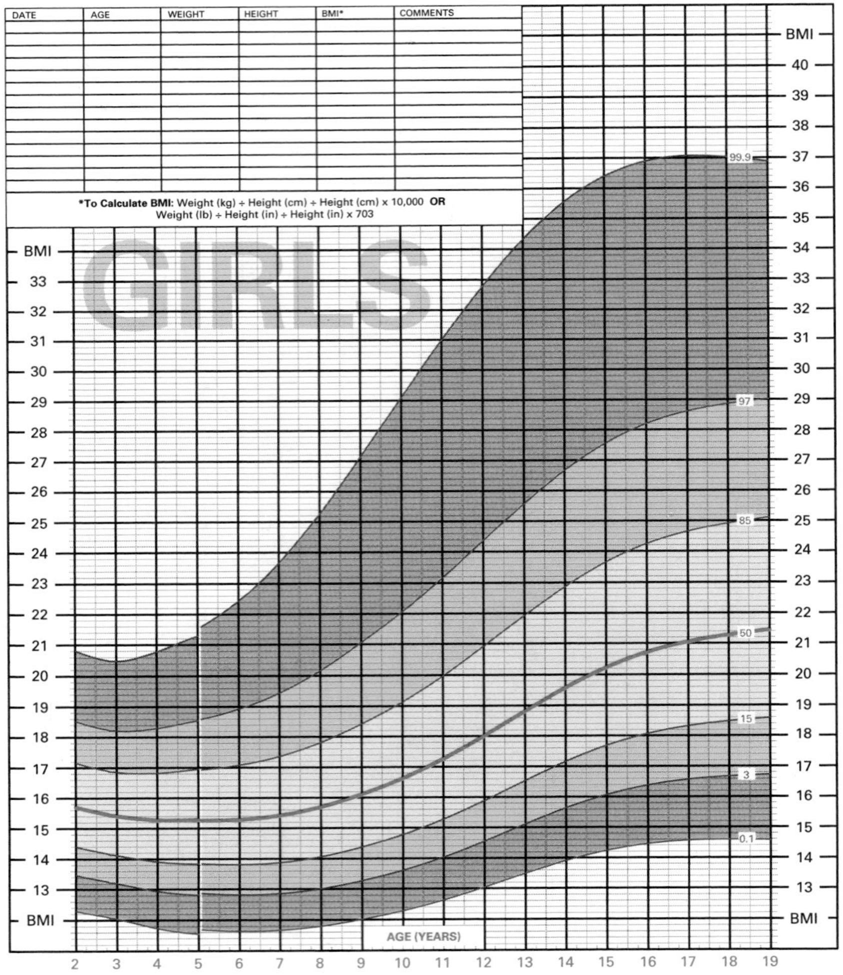
DATE
AGE
WEIGHT
HEIGHT
BMI*
COMMENTS
*To Calculate BMI: Weight (kg) ÷ Height (cm) ÷ Height (cm) x 10,000 OR
Weight (lb) ÷ Height (in) ÷ Height (in) x 703
GIRLS
BMI
99.9
97
85
50
15
3
0.1
AGE (YEARS)

Measures of Body Fat and Lean Tissue Significant weight changes in both children and adults can reflect overnutrition and undernutrition with respect to energy and protein. To estimate the degree to which fat stores or lean tissues are affected by overnutrition or malnutrition, several anthropometric measurements are useful (review Table E-3 on p. E-4).

Skinfold Measures Skinfold measures provide a good estimate of total body fat and a fair assessment of the fat's location. Approximately half the fat in the body lies directly beneath the skin, and the thickness of this subcutaneous fat reflects total body fat. In some parts of the body, such as the back and the back of the arm over the triceps muscle, this fat is loosely attached; ♦ a person can pull it up between the thumb and forefinger to obtain a measure of skinfold thickness. To measure skinfold, a skilled assessor follows a standard procedure using reliable calipers (illustrated in Figure E-9) and then compares the measurement with standards. Triceps skinfold measures greater than 15 millimetres in men or 25 millimetres in women suggest excessive body fat.

♦ Common sites for skinfold measures:
- Triceps
- Biceps
- Subscapular (below shoulder blade)
- Suprailiac (above hip bone)
- Abdomen
- Upper thigh

Skinfold measurements correlate directly with the risk of heart disease. They assess central obesity and its associated risks better than do weight measures alone. If a person gains body fat, the skinfold increases proportionately; if the person loses fat, it decreases. Measurements taken from central-body sites (around the abdomen) better reflect changes in fatness than those taken from upper sites (arm and back). A major limitation of the skinfold test is that fat may be thicker under the skin in one area than in another. A pinch at the side of the waistline may not yield the same measurement as a pinch on the back of the arm. This limitation can be overcome by taking skinfold measurements at several (often three) differ-

FIGURE E-9 How to Measure the Triceps Skinfold

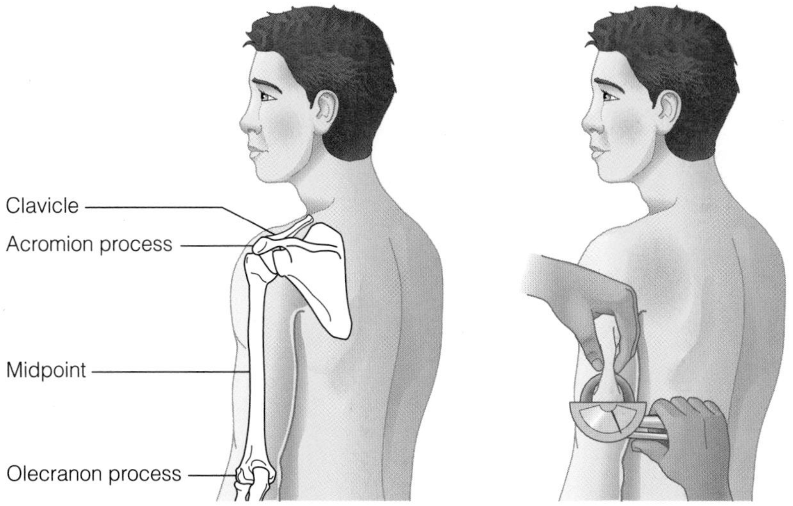
Clavicle
Acromion process
Midpoint
Olecranon process

A. Find the midpoint of the arm:
1. Ask the subject to bend his or her arm at the elbow and lay the hand across the stomach. (If he or she is right-handed, measure the left arm, and vice versa.)
2. Feel the shoulder to locate the acromion process. It helps to slide your fingers along the clavicle to find the acromion process. The olecranon process is the tip of the elbow.
3. Place a measuring tape from the acromion process to the tip of the elbow. Divide this measurement by 2, and mark the midpoint of the arm with a pen.

B. Measure the skinfold:
1. Ask the subject to let his or her arm hang loosely to the side.
2. Grasp a fold of skin and subcutaneous fat between the thumb and forefinger slightly above the midpoint mark. Gently pull the skin away from the underlying muscle. (This step takes a lot of practice. If you want to be sure you don't have muscle as well as fat, ask the subject to contract and relax the muscle. You should be able to feel if you are pinching muscle.)
3. Place the calipers over the skinfold at the midpoint mark, and read the measurement to the nearest 1.0 millimetre in two to three seconds. (If using plastic calipers, align pressure lines, and read the measurement to the nearest 1.0 millimetre in two to three seconds.)
4. Repeat steps 2 and 3 twice more. Add the three readings, and then divide by 3 to find the average.

ent places on the body (including upper-, central-, and lower-body sites) and comparing each measurement with standards for that site. Multiple measures are not always practical in clinical settings, however, and most often, the triceps skinfold measurement alone is used because it is easily accessible. Skinfold measures are not useful in assessing changes in body fat over time.

Waist Circumference Chapter 8 describes how fat distribution correlates with health risks and mentioned that the waist circumference is a valuable indicator of fat distribution. To measure waist circumference, the assessor places a non-stretchable tape around the person's body, crossing just above the upper hip bones and making sure that the tape remains on a level horizontal plane on all sides (see Figure E-10). The tape is tightened slightly, but without compressing the skin.

Waist-to-Hip Ratio Alternatively, some clinicians measure both the waist and the hips. The waist-to-hip ratio ♦ also assesses abdominal obesity, but provides no more information than using the waist circumference alone. In general, women with a waist-to-hip ratio of 0.80 or greater and men with a waist-to-hip ratio of 1.0 or greater have a high risk of health problems.

♦ To calculate the waist-to-hip ratio, divide the waistline measurement by the hip measurement. For example, a woman with a 71 centimetre waist and 97 centimetre hips would have a ratio of 71 ÷ 97 = 0.73.

Dual Energy X-ray Absorptiometry DEXA (dual energy X-ray absorptionmetry) provides a very accurate measure of body compartments: fat, lean tissue, and bone density. Using two different energies of X-rays, body scan measures of how different body tissues attenuate the X-rays provide an accurate determination of body composition. A full body scan takes between 10–20 minutes and the dose of radiation is less than a chest X-ray. Although DEXA is a very accurate clinical tool, the equipment is expensive and not portable, limiting its use to clinical settings.

FIGURE E-10 How to Measure Waist Circumference

Place the measuring tape around the waist just above the bony crest of the hip. The tape runs parallel to the floor and is snug (but does not compress the skin). The measurement is taken at the end of normal expiration.

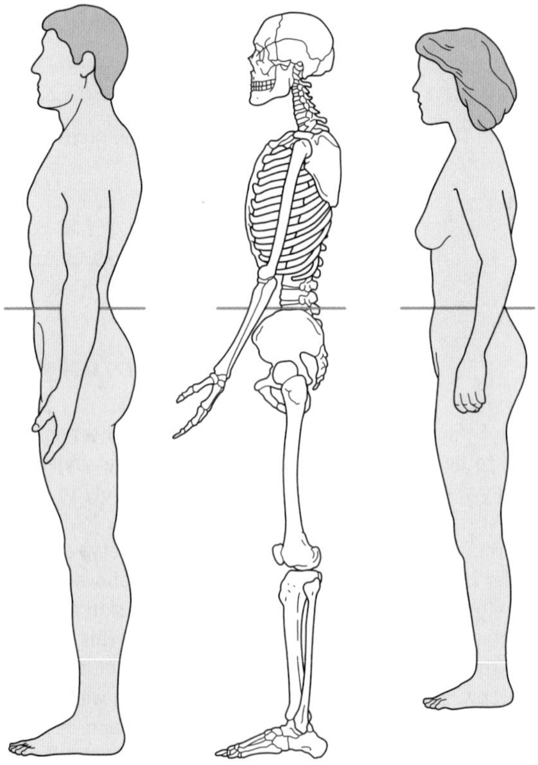

SOURCE: National Institutes of Health Obesity Education Initiative, *Clinical Guidelines on the Identification, Evaluation, and Treatment of Overweight and Obesity in Adults* (Washington, D.C.: U.S. Department of Health and Human Services, 1998), p. 59.

TABLE E-4 Methods of Estimating Body Fat and Its Distribution

Method	Cost	Ease of Use	Accuracy	Measures Fat Distribution
Height and weight	Low	Easy	High	No
Skinfolds	Low	Easy	Low	Yes
Circumferences	Low	Easy	Moderate	Yes
Ultrasound	Moderate	Moderate	Moderate	Yes
Hydrodensitometry	Low	Moderate	High	No
Heavy water tritiated	Moderate	Moderate	High	No
Deuterium oxide, or heavy oxygen	High	Moderate	High	No
Potassium isotope (^{40}K)	Very high	Difficult	High	No
Total body electrical conductivity (TOBEC)	High	Moderate	High	No
Bioelectric impedance (BIA)	Moderate	Easy	High	No
Dual-energy X-ray absorptiometry (DEXA)	High	Easy	High	No
Computed tomography (CT)	Very high	Difficult	High	Yes
Magnetic resonance imaging (MRI)	Very high	Difficult	High	Yes

SOURCE: Adapted with permisssion from G. A. Bray, a handout presented at the North American Association for the Study of Obesity and Emory University School of Medicine Conference on Obesity. Update: Pathophysiology, Clinical Consequences, and Therapeutic Options, Atlanta, Georgia, August 31–September 2, 1992.

Hydrodensitometry To estimate body density using hydrodensitometry, the person is weighed twice—first on land and then again when submerged under water. Underwater weighing usually generates a good estimate of body fat and is useful in research, although the technique has drawbacks: it requires bulky, expensive, and nonportable equipment. Furthermore, submerging some people (especially those who are very young, very old, ill, or fearful) under water is not always practical.

Bioelectric Impedance To measure body fat using the bioelectric impedance technique, a very-low-intensity electrical current is briefly sent through the body by way of electrodes placed on the wrist and ankle. As is true of other anthropometric techniques, bioelectrical impedance requires standardized procedures and calibrated instruments to provide reliable results. Recent food intake and hydration status, for example, influence results. Bioelectrical impedance is most accurate for people within a normal fat range; it tends to overestimate fat in lean people and underestimate fat in obese people.

Clinicians use many other methods to estimate body fat and its distribution. Each has its advantages and disadvantages as Table E-4 summarizes.

Physical Examinations

An assessor can use a physical examination to search for signs of nutrient deficiency or toxicity. Like the other assessment methods, such an examination requires knowledge and skill. Many physical signs are nonspecific; they can reflect any of several nutrient deficiencies as well as conditions not related to nutrition (see Table E-5 on p. E-14). For example, cracked lips may be caused by sunburn, windburn, dehydration, or any of several B vitamin deficiencies, to name just a few possible causes. For this reason, physical findings are most valuable in revealing problems for other assessment techniques to confirm or for confirming other assessment measures.

With this limitation understood, physical symptoms can be most informative and communicate much information about nutrition health. Many tissues and organs can reflect signs of malnutrition. The signs appear most rapidly in parts of the body where cell replacement occurs at a high rate, such as in the hair, skin, and digestive tract (including the mouth and tongue). The summary tables in Chapters 10 through 14 list additional physical signs of vitamin and mineral malnutrition.

TABLE E-5 Physical Findings Used in Nutrition Assessments

Body System	Healthy Findings	Malnutrition Findings	What the Findings Reflect
Hair	Shiny, firm in the scalp	Dull, brittle, dry, loose; falls out	PEM
Eyes	Bright, clear pink membranes; adjust easily to light	Pale membranes; spots; redness; adjust slowly to darkness	Vitamin A, B vitamin, zinc, and iron status
Teeth and gums	No pain or caries, gums firm, teeth bright	Missing, discoloured, decayed teeth; gums bleed easily and are swollen and spongy	Mineral and vitamin C status
Glands	No lumps	Swollen at front of neck	PEM and iodine status
Tongue	Red, bumpy, rough	Sore, smooth, purplish, swollen	B vitamin status
Skin	Smooth, firm, good colour	Off-colour, scaly, flaky, cracked, dry, rough, spotty; "sandpaper" feel or sores; lack of fat under skin	PEM, essential fatty acid, vitamin A, B vitamin, and vitamin C status
Nails	Firm, pink	Spoon-shaped, brittle, ridged, pale	Iron status
Internal systems	Regular heart rhythm, heart rate, and blood pressure; no impairment of digestive function, reflexes, or mental status	Abnormal heart rate, heart rhythm, or blood pressure; enlarged liver, spleen; abnormal digestion; burning, tingling of hands, feet; loss of balance, coordination; mental confusion, irritability, fatigue	PEM and mineral status
Muscles and bones	Muscle tone; posture, long bone development appropriate for age	"Wasted" appearance of muscles; swollen bumps on skull or ends of bones; small bumps on ribs; bowed legs or knock-knees	PEM, mineral, and vitamin D status

Biochemical Analyses

All of the approaches to nutrition assessment discussed so far are external approaches. Biochemical analyses or laboratory tests help to determine what is happening to the body internally. Common tests are based on analysis of blood and urine samples, which contain nutrients, enzymes, and metabolites that reflect nutrition status. Other tests, such as blood glucose, help pinpoint disease-related problems with nutrition implications. Tests that define fluid and electrolyte balance, acid–base balance, and organ function also have nutrition implications. Table E-6 lists biochemical tests most useful for assessing vitamin and mineral status.

The interpretation of biochemical data requires skill. Long metabolic sequences lead to the production of the end-products and metabolites seen in blood and urine. No single test can reveal nutrition status because many factors influence test results. The low blood concentration of a nutrient may reflect a primary deficiency of that nutrient, but it may also be secondary to the deficiency of one or several other nutrients or to a disease. Taken together with other assessment data, however, laboratory test results help to create a picture that becomes clear with careful interpretation. They are especially useful in helping to detect subclinical malnutrition by uncovering early signs of malnutrition before the clinical signs of a classic deficiency disease appear.

Laboratory tests used to assess vitamin and mineral status (review Table E-6) are particularly useful when combined with diet histories and physical findings. Vitamin and mineral levels present in the blood and urine sometimes reflect recent rather than long-term intakes. This makes detecting subclinical deficiencies ♦ difficult. Furthermore, many nutrients interact; therefore, the amounts of other nutrients in the body can affect a lab value for a particular nutrient. It is also important to remember that nonnutrient conditions such as diseases influence biochemical measures.

♦ A *subclinical deficiency* is a nutrient deficiency in the early stages before the outward signs have appeared.

It is beyond the scope of this text to describe all lab tests and their relations to nutrition status. Instead, the emphasis is on lab tests used to detect protein-energy malnutrition (PEM) and nutritional anemias.

TABLE E-6 Biochemical Tests Useful for Assessing Vitamin and Mineral Status

Nutrient	Assessment Tests
Vitamins	
Vitamin A	Serum retinol, retinol-binding protein
Thiamin[a]	Erythrocyte (red blood cell) transketolase activity, erythrocyte thiamin pyrophosphate
Riboflavin[a]	Erythrocyte glutathione reductase activity
Vitamin B_6[a]	Urinary xanthurenic acid excretion after tryptophan load test, erythrocyte transaminase activity, plasma pyridoxal 5′-phosphate (PLP)
Niacin	Plasma or urinary metabolites NMN (N-methyl nicotinamide) or 2-pyridone, or preferably both expressed as a ratio
Folate[b]	Serum folate, erythrocyte folate (reflects liver stores)
Vitamin B_{12}[b]	Serum vitamin B_{12}, serum and urinary methylmalonic acid, Schilling test
Biotin	Urinary biotin, urinary 3-hydroxyisovaleric acid
Vitamin C	Plasma vitamin C[c], leukocyte vitamin C
Vitamin D	Serum vitamin D
Vitamin E	Serum α-tocopherol, erythrocyte hemolysis
Vitamin K	Serum vitamin K, plasma prothrombin; blood-clotting time (prothrombin time) is not an adequate indicator
Minerals	
Phosphorus	Serum phosphate
Sodium	Serum sodium
Chloride	Serum chloride
Potassium	Serum potassium
Magnesium	Serum magnesium, urinary magnesium
Iron	Hemoglobin, hematocrit, serum ferritin, total iron-binding capacity (TIBC), erythrocyte protoporphyrin, serum iron, transferrin saturation
Iodine	Serum thyroxine or thyroid-stimulating hormone (TSH), urinary iodine
Zinc	Plasma zinc, hair zinc
Copper	Erythrocyte superoxide dismutase, serum copper, serum ceruloplasmin
Selenium	Erythrocyte selenium, glutathione peroxidase activity

[a]Urinary measurements for these vitamins are common, but may be of limited use. Urinary measurements reflect recent dietary intakes and may not provide reliable information concerning the severity of a deficiency.
[b]Folate assessments should always be conducted in conjunction with vitamin B_{12} assessments (and vice versa) to help distinguish the cause of common deficiency symptoms.
[c]Vitamin C shifts between the plasma and the white blood cells known as leukocytes; thus a plasma determination may not accurately reflect the body's pool. A measurement of leukocyte vitamin C can provide information about the body's stores of vitamin C. A combination of both tests may be more reliable than either one alone.
SOURCE: Adapted from H. E. Sauberlich, *Laboratory Tests for the Assessment of Nutritional Status* (Boca Raton, Fla.: CRC Press, 1999).

TABLE E-7 Normal Values for Serum Proteins

Indicator	Normal
Albumin (g/dL)	3.5–5.4
Transferrin (mg/dL)	200–400
Transthyretin (mg/dL)	23–43
Retinol-binding protein (mg/dL)	3–7
IGF-1 (μg/L)	300

NOTE: Levels less than normal suggest compromised protein status.

Protein-Energy Malnutrition

No single biochemical analysis can adequately evaluate protein-energy malnutrition (PEM). Numerous procedures have been used over the years. This discussion focuses on the measures commonly used today—transthyretin, retinol-binding protein, serum transferrin, ♦ and IGF-1 (insulin-like growth factor 1). Table E-7 provides standards for these indicators. Although serum albumin is easily and routinely measured, it lacks the sensitivity to assess PEM because of its long turnover rate.*

Transthyretin and Retinol-Binding Protein Transthyretin ♦ and retinol-binding protein occur as a complex in the plasma. They have a rapid turnover and thus respond quickly to dietary protein inadequacy and therapy.** Conditions other than malnutrition that lower transthyretin include metabolic stress,

*The half-life of albumin is 18 days, an indication of a slow degradation rate.
**The half-lives of transthyretin and retinol-binding protein are 2 days and 12 hours, respectively.

♦ The *serum* is the watery portion of the blood that remains after removal of the cells and clot-forming material; *plasma* is the fluid that remains when unclotted blood is centrifuged. In most cases, serum and plasma concentrations are similar, but plasma samples are more likely to clog mechanical blood analyzers, so serum samples are preferred.

♦ Transthyretin is also known as *prealbumin* or *thyroxine-binding prealbumin.*

hemodialysis, and hypothyroidism; those that raise transthyretin include kidney disease and corticosteroid use. Conditions other than protein malnutrition that lower retinol-binding protein include vitamin A deficiency, metabolic stress, hyperthyroidism, liver disease, and cystic fibrosis; kidney disease raises retinol-binding protein levels.

Serum Transferrin Serum transferrin transports iron; consequently, its concentrations reflect both protein and iron status. Using transferrin as an indicator of protein status is complicated when an iron deficiency is present. Transferrin rises as iron deficiency grows worse and falls as iron status improves. Markedly reduced transferrin levels indicate severe PEM; in mild-to-moderate PEM, transferrin levels may vary, limiting their usefulness. Conditions other than protein malnutrition that lower transferrin include liver disease, kidney disease, and metabolic stress; those that raise transferrin include pregnancy, iron deficiency, hepatitis, blood loss, and oral contraceptive use. Although transferrin breaks down in the body more quickly than albumin, it is still relatively slow to respond to changes in protein intake and is not a sensitive indicator of the response to therapy.*

Insulin-like Growth Factor 1 IGF-1 (insulin-like growth factor 1) declines in PEM. IGF-1 has a relatively short half-life and responds specifically to dietary protein rather than energy.** For these reasons, it is a sensitive indicator of protein status and response to therapy. Conditions that decrease IGF-1 include anorexia nervosa, inflammatory bowel disease, celiac disease, HIV infection, and fasting.

Nutritional Anemias

Anemia, a symptom of a wide variety of nutrition- and nonnutrition-related disorders, is characterized by a reduced number of red blood cells. Iron, folate, and vitamin B_{12} deficiencies caused by inadequate intake, poor absorption, or abnormal metabolism of these nutrients are the most common nutritional anemias. Some nonnutrition-related causes of anemia include massive blood loss, infections, hereditary blood disorders such as sickle-cell anemia and chronic liver or kidney disease.

Assessment of Iron-Deficiency Anemia

Iron deficiency, a common mineral deficiency, develops in stages. ♦ Chapter 14 describes iron deficiency in detail. This section describes tests used to uncover iron deficiency as it progresses. Table E-8 shows which laboratory tests detect various nutrition-related anemias, and Table E-9 provides values used for assessing iron status. Although other tests are more specific in detecting early deficiencies, hemoglobin and hematocrit are the commonly available tests.

♦ Stages of iron deficiency:
1. Iron stores diminish.
2. Transport iron decreases.
3. Hemoglobin production falls.

Hemoglobin Iron forms an integral part of the hemoglobin molecule that transports oxygen to the cells. In iron deficiency, the body cannot synthesize hemoglobin. Low hemoglobin values signal depleted iron stores. Table E-9 provides hemoglobin values used in nutrition assessment. Hemoglobin's usefulness in evaluating iron status is limited, however, because hemoglobin concentrations drop fairly late in the development of iron deficiency, and other nutrient deficiencies and medical conditions can also alter hemoglobin concentrations.

Hematocrit Hematocrit is commonly used to diagnose iron deficiency, even though it is an inconclusive measure of iron status. To measure the hematocrit, a clinician spins a volume of blood in a centrifuge to separate the red blood cells from the plasma. The hematocrit is the percentage of red blood cells in the total blood volume. Table E-9 includes values used to assess hematocrit status. Low values indicate incomplete hemoglobin formation, which is manifested by microcytic (abnormally small-celled), hypochromic (abnormally lacking in colour) red blood cells.

*The half-life of transferrin is 8 days.
**The half-life of IGF-1 is 12 to 15 hours.

TABLE E-8 Laboratory Tests Useful in Evaluating Nutrition-Related Anemias

Test or Test Result	What It Reflects
For Anemia (general)	
Hemoglobin (Hg)	Total amount of hemoglobin in the red blood cells (RBC)
Hematocrit (Hct)	Percentage of RBC in the total blood volume
Red blood cell (RBC) count	Number of RBC
Mean corpuscular volume (MCV)	RBC size; helps to determine if anemia is microcytic (iron deficiency) or macrocytic (folate or vitamin B_{12} deficiency)
Mean corpuscular hemoglobin concentration (MCHC)	Hemoglobin concentration within the average RBC; helps to determine if anemia is hypochromic (iron deficiency) or normochromic (folate or vitamin B_{12} deficiency)
Bone marrow aspiration	The manufacture of blood cells in different developmental states
For Iron-Deficiency Anemia	
↓ Serum ferritin	Early deficiency state with depleted iron stores
↓ Transferrin saturation	Progressing deficiency state with diminished transport iron
↑ Erythrocyte protoporphyrin	Later deficiency state with limited hemoglobin production
For Folate-Deficiency Anemia	
↓ Serum folate	Progressing deficiency state
↓ RBC folate	Later deficiency state
For Vitamin B_{12}–Deficiency Anemia	
↓ Serum vitamin B_{12}	Progressing deficiency state
Schilling test	Absorption of vitamin B_{12}

TABLE E-9 Common Criteria Used for Assessing Iron Status

Test	Age (yr)	Gender	Deficiency Value
Hemoglobin (g/dL)	0.5–10	M–F	<11
	11–15	M	<12
		F	<11.5
	>15	M	<13
		F	<12
	Pregnancy		<11
Hematocrit (%)	0.5–4	M–F	<32
	5–10	M–F	<33
	11–15	M	<35
		F	<34
	>15	M	<40
		F	<36
Serum ferritin (µg/L)	0.5–15	M–F	<10
	>15	M–F	<12
Total iron-binding capacity (µg/dL)	>15	M–F	>400
Serum iron (µg/dL)	>15	M–F	<60
Transferrin saturation (%)	0.5–4	M–F	<12
	5–10	M–F	<14
	>10	M–F	<16
Erythrocyte protoporphyrin (µg/dL RBC)	0.5–4	M–F	>80
	>4	M–F	>70

Low hemoglobin and hematocrit values alert the assessor to the possibility of iron deficiency. However, many nutrients and other conditions can affect hemoglobin and hematocrit. The other tests of iron status help pinpoint true iron deficiency.

Serum Ferritin In the first stage of iron deficiency, iron stores diminish. Measures of serum ferritin provide an estimate of iron stores. Such information is most valuable to iron assessment. Table E-9 (p. E-17) shows serum ferritin cutoff values that indicate iron store depletion in children and adults. Serum ferritin is not reliable for diagnosing iron deficiency in infants, since normal serum ferritin values are often present in conjunction with iron-responsive anemia.

A decrease in transport iron characterizes the second stage of iron deficiency. This is revealed by an increase in the iron-binding capacity of the protein transferrin and a decrease in serum iron. These changes are reflected by the transferrin saturation, which is calculated from the ratio of the other two values as described in the following paragraphs.

Total Iron-Binding Capacity Iron travels through the blood bound to the protein transferrin. Total iron-binding capacity (TIBC) is a measure of the total amount of iron that transferrin can carry. Lab technicians measure iron-binding capacity directly. Table E-9 includes the cutoff for TIBC.

Serum Iron Lab technicians can also measure serum iron directly. Elevated values indicate iron overload; reduced values indicate iron deficiency. Table E-9 shows the deficient value for serum iron.

Transferrin Saturation The percentage of transferrin that is saturated with iron is an indirect measure that is derived from the serum iron and total iron-binding capacity measures as follows:

$$\text{Percentage of Transferrin} = \frac{\text{serum iron}}{\text{total iron-binding capacity}} \times 100$$

Table E-9 shows deficient transferrin saturation values for various age groups.

The third stage of iron deficiency occurs when the supply of transport iron diminishes to the point that it limits hemoglobin production. It is characterized by increases in erythrocyte protoporphyrin, a decrease in mean corpuscular volume, and decreased hemoglobin and hematocrit.

Erythrocyte Protoporphyrin The iron-containing portion of the hemoglobin molecule is heme. Heme is a combination of iron and protoporphyrin. Protoporphyrin accumulates in the blood when iron supplies are inadequate for the formation of heme. Lab technicians can measure erythrocyte protoporphyrin directly in a blood sample. The cutoffs for abnormal values of erythrocyte protoporphyrin are shown in Table E-9.

Mean Corpuscular Volume A direct or calculated measure of the mean corpuscular volume (MCV) determines the average size of a red blood cell. Such a measure helps to classify the type of nutrient anemia. In iron deficiency, the red blood cells are smaller than average.

Assessment of Folate and Vitamin B_{12} Anemias

Folate deficiency and vitamin B_{12} deficiency present a similar clinical picture—an anemia characterized by abnormally large red blood cell precursors (megaloblasts) in the bone marrow and abnormally large, mature red blood cells (macrocytic cells) in the blood. Distinguishing between these two deficiencies is particularly important because their treatments differ. Giving folate to a person with vitamin B_{12} deficiency improves many of the lab test results indicative of vitamin B_{12} deficiency, but this is a dangerous error because vitamin B_{12} deficiency causes nerve damage that folate cannot correct. Thus inappropriate folate administration masks vitamin B_{12}–deficiency anemia, and nerve damage worsens. For this

TABLE E-10 Criteria for Assessing Folate and Vitamin B_{12}

	Deficient	Borderline	Acceptable
Serum folate (ng/mL)[a]	<3.0	3.0–5.9	>6.0
Erythrocyte folate (ng/mL)[a]	<140	140–159	>160
Serum vitamin B_{12} (pg/mL)	<150	150–200	≥201
Serum methylmalonic acid (nmol/L)	<376	—	—

NOTE: A nanogram (ng) is one-billionth of a gram; a picogram (pg) is one-trillionth of a gram.
[a]To convert folate values (ng/mL) to international standard units (nmol/L), multiply by 2.266.

reason, it is critical to determine whether the anemia results from a folate deficiency or from a vitamin B_{12} deficiency. The following biochemical assessment techniques help to make this distinction.

Mean Corpuscular Volume As previously mentioned, the mean corpuscular volume (MCV) is a measure of red blood cell size. In folate and vitamin B_{12} deficiencies, the red blood cells are larger than average (macrocytic). Additional tests must be performed to differentiate folate from vitamin B_{12} deficiency.

Folate Levels Serum folate levels fluctuate with changes in folate intake and metabolism. Thus serum folate concentrations reflect current status, but provide little information about folate stores. As folate deficiency progresses and low serum levels persist, folate stores decline, resulting in folate depletion. Folate depletion is characterized by a fall in the folate concentrations of red blood cells (erythrocytes). As erythrocyte folate levels diminish, folate-deficiency anemia develops. Because low erythrocyte folate concentrations also occur with vitamin B_{12} deficiency, serum vitamin B_{12} concentrations must also be measured. Table E-10 shows standards for folate assessment.

Vitamin B_{12} Levels Serum and urinary methylmalonic acid are elevated in vitamin B_{12} deficiency, but not in folate deficiency. Thus this measure is useful in distinguishing between the two. Vitamin B_{12} deficiency usually arises from malabsorption. To determine whether malabsorption is the cause, a small oral dose of vitamin B_{12} is given, and urinary excretion is measured. This procedure measures vitamin B_{12} absorption and is called a Schilling test.

Early stages of vitamin B_{12} deficiency can be detected by a low percentage saturation of its transport protein, a measure similar to iron's transferrin saturation. As the deficiency progresses, serum vitamin B_{12} concentrations fall. Table E-10 shows standards for vitamin B_{12} assessment.

Cautions about Nutrition Assessment

To give all the details of nutrition assessment procedures would entail writing another textbook. Nevertheless, any student of nutrition should know the basics of a proper nutrition assessment procedure for two reasons.

First, competent medical care includes attention to nutrition. Physicians should either employ a person skilled in nutrition assessment techniques or refer all clients to such a person to ensure the sound nutrition health of their clients. Health-care facilities should make nutrition assessment a routine part of the initial workup on every client so that poor nutrition will not hinder the response to medical treatment and the recovery from illness.

Second, because nutrition is such a popular subject today, fraudulent practices are even more abundant than they have been in the past (and they have always been rampant). The knowledgeable consumer needs to know what procedures to expect in a nutrition assessment and what kinds of information they yield. This appendix has presented the basics of nutrition assessment for these reasons.

This caution is added: the tests outlined here yield information that becomes meaningful only when integrated into a whole picture by a skilled, experienced, and educated interpreter. Potential sources of error are many, from the taking of the initial data to their reporting and analysis. Each assessment method and measure is useful only as a part of the whole to confirm or eliminate the possibility of suspected nutrition problems. For example, the assessor must constantly remember that a sufficient intake of a nutrient does not guarantee adequate nutrient status for an individual. Conversely, the apparent inadequate intake of a nutrient does not, by itself, establish that a deficiency exists.

Similarly, many uncertainties, such as the calibration of the equipment, the skills of the measurer, and the perspective of the interpreter, limit the accuracy and value of anthropometric measures. This is also true of the results of the physical examination. Physical signs suggestive of malnutrition are nonspecific: they can reflect nutrient deficiencies or may be totally unrelated to nutrition. Assessors must interpret physical findings in light of other assessment findings. Finally, the usefulness of biochemical tests is also limited; the assessor must use caution in interpreting results. Vitamin and mineral blood concentrations may reflect disease processes, abnormal hormone levels, or other aberrations rather than dietary intake. Even if concentrations do reflect dietary intake, they may reflect what the person has been eating recently and not give a true picture of the person's nutrient status. Such complications sometimes make it difficult to detect a subclinical deficiency. Furthermore, many nutrients interact. The assessor has to keep in mind that an abnormal lab value for one nutrient may reflect abnormal status of other nutrients. The final diagnosis is therefore appropriately tentative, and its confirmation comes only after careful remedial steps successfully alleviate the observed problems.

Physical Activity and Energy Requirements

APPENDIX F

CONTENTS

Chapter 8 describes how to calculate estimated energy requirements (EER) for adults by using an equation that accounts for gender, age, weight, height, and physical activity level. Table F-1 (p. F-2) presents additional equations to determine the EER for infants, children, adolescents, and pregnant and lactating women.

This appendix helps you determine the correct physical activity (PA) factor to use in the equations, either by calculating the physical activity level or by estimating it. For those who prefer to bypass these steps, the appendix presents tables that provide a shortcut to estimating total energy expenditure.*

Calculating Physical Activity Level

To calculate your physical activity level, record all of your activities for a typical 24-hour day, noting the type of activity, the level of intensity, and the duration. Then, using a copy of Table F-2 (pp. F-2–F-3), find your activity in the first column (or an activity that is reasonably similar) and multiply the number of minutes spent on that activity by the factor in the third column. Put your answer in the last column and total the accumulated values for the day. Now add the subtotal of the last column to 1.1 (to account for basal energy and the thermic effect of food) as shown. This score indicates your physical activity level. Using Table F-3 (p. F-3), find the PA factor for your age and gender that correlates with your physical activity level and use it in the energy equations presented in Table F-1.

Estimating Physical Activity Level

As an alternative to recording your activities for a day, you can use the third column of Table F-3 to decide if your daily activity is sedentary, low active, active, or very active. Find the PA factor for your age and gender that correlates with your typical physical activity level and use it in the energy equations presented in Table F-1.

Using a Shortcut to Estimate Total Energy Expenditure

The DRI Committee has developed estimates of total energy expenditure based on the equations for adults presented in Table F-1. These estimates are presented in Table F-4 (pp. F-4–F-5) for women and Table F-5 (pp. F-5–F-6) for men. You can use these tables to estimate your energy requirement—that is, the number of kcalories needed to maintain your current body weight. On the table appropriate for your gender, find your height in metres (or inches) in the left-hand column. Then follow

*This appendix, including the tables, is adapted from Committee on Dietary Reference Intakes, *Dietary Reference Intakes for Energy, Carbohydrate, Fiber, Fat, Fatty Acids, Cholesterol, Protein, and Amino Acids* (Washington, D.C.: National Academies Press, 2005).

the row across to find your weight in kilograms (or pounds). (If you can't find your exact height and weight, choose a value between the two closest ones.) Look down the column to find the number of kcalories that corresponds to your activity level.

Importantly, the values given in the tables are for 30-year-old people. Women 19 to 29 should add 7 kcalories per day for each year younger than age 30; older women should subtract 7 kcalories per day for each year older than age 30. Similarly, men 19 to 29 should add 10 kcalories per day for each year younger than age 30; older men should subtract 10 kcalories per day for each year older than age 30.

TABLE F-1 Equations to Determine Estimated Energy Requirement (EER)

Infants	
0–3 months	EER = (89 × weight − 100) + 175
4–6 months	EER = (89 × weight − 100) + 56
7–12 months	EER = (89 × weight − 100) + 22
13–15 months	EER = (89 × weight − 100) + 20
Children and Adolescents	
Boys	
3–8 years	EER = 88.5 − (61.9 × age) + PA × [(26.7 × weight) + (903 × height)] + 20
9–18 years	EER = 88.5 − (61.9 × age) + PA × [(26.7 × weight) + (903 × height)] + 25
Girls	
3–8 years	EER = 135.3 − (30.8 × age) + PA × [(10.0 × weight) + (934 × height)] + 20
9–18 years	EER = 135.3 − (30.8 × age) + PA × [(10.0 × weight) + (934 × height)] + 25
Adults	
Men	EER = 662 − (9.53 × age) + PA × [(15.91 × weight) + (539.6 × height)]
Women	EER = 354 − (6.91 × age) + PA × [(9.36 × weight) + (726 × height)]
Pregnancy	
1st trimester	EER = nonpregnant EER + 0
2nd trimester	EER = nonpregnant EER + 340
3rd trimester	EER = nonpregnant EER + 452
Lactation	
0–6 months postpartum	EER = nonpregnant EER + 500 − 170
7–12 months postpartum	EER = nonpregnant EER + 400 − 0

NOTE: Select the appropriate equation for gender and age and insert weight in kilograms, height in metres, and age in years. See the text and Table F-3 to determine PA.

TABLE F-2 Physical Activities and Their Scores

If your activity was equivalent to this . . .	Then list the number of minutes here and . . .	Multiply by this factor . . .	Add this column to get your physical activity level score:
Activities of Daily Living			
Gardening (no lifting)		0.0032	
Household tasks (moderate effort)		0.0024	
Lifting items continuously		0.0029	
Loading/unloading car		0.0019	
Lying quietly		0.0000	
Mopping		0.0024	
Mowing lawn (power mower)		0.0033	
Raking lawn		0.0029	
Riding in a vehicle		0.0000	
Sitting (idle)		0.0000	
Sitting (doing light activity)		0.0005	
Taking out trash		0.0019	
Vacuuming		0.0024	
Walking the dog		0.0019	
Walking from house to car or bus		0.0014	
Watering plants		0.0014	

(continued)

TABLE F-2 Physical Activities and Their Scores (*continued*)

If your activity was equivalent to this . . .	Then list the number of minutes here and . . .	Multiply by this factor . . .	Add this column to get your physical activity level score:
Additional Activities			
Billiards		0.0013	
Calisthenics (no weight)		0.0029	
Canoeing (leisurely)		0.0014	
Chopping wood		0.0037	
Climbing hills (carrying 5 kg load)		0.0061	
Climbing hills (no load)		0.0056	
Cycling (leisurely)		0.0024	
Cycling (moderately)		0.0045	
Dancing (aerobic or ballet)		0.0048	
Dancing (ballroom, leisurely)		0.0018	
Dancing (fast ballroom or square)		0.0043	
Golf (with cart)		0.0014	
Golf (without cart)		0.0032	
Horseback riding (walking)		0.0012	
Horseback riding (trotting)		0.0053	
Jogging (10 km/h)		0.0088	
Music (playing accordion)		0.0008	
Music (playing cello)		0.0012	
Music (playing flute)		0.0010	
Music (playing piano)		0.0012	
Music (playing violin)		0.0014	
Rope skipping		0.0105	
Skating (ice)		0.0043	
Skating (roller)		0.0052	
Skiing (water or downhill)		0.0055	
Squash		0.0106	
Surfing		0.0048	
Swimming (slow)		0.0033	
Swimming (fast)		0.0057	
Tennis (doubles)		0.0038	
Tennis (singles)		0.0057	
Volleyball (noncompetitive)		0.0018	
Walking (3 km/h)		0.0014	
Walking (5 km/h)		0.0022	
Walking (6 km/h)		0.0033	
Walking (8 km/h)		0.0067	
Subtotal			
Factor for basal energy and the thermic effect of food			**1.1**
Your physical activity level score			

TABLE F-3 Physical Activity Equivalents and Their PA Factors

Physical Activity Level	Description	Physical Activity Equivalents	Men, 19+ yr PA Factor	Women, 19+ yr PA Factor	Boys, 3–18 yr PA Factor	Girls, 3–18 yr PA Factor
1.0 to 1.39	Sedentary	Only those physical activities required for typical daily living	1.0	1.0	1.0	1.0
1.4 to 1.59	Low active	Daily living + 30–60 min moderate activity[a]	1.11	1.12	1.13	1.16
1.6 to 1.89	Active	Daily living + ≥60 min moderate activity	1.25	1.27	1.26	1.31
1.9 and above	Very active	Daily living + ≥60 min moderate activity *and* ≥60 min vigorous activity *or* ≥120 min moderate activity	1.48	1.45	1.42	1.56

[a]Moderate activity is equivalent to walking at a pace of 5 to 7 kilometres per hour.

TABLE F-4 Total Energy Expenditure (TEE in kCalories per Day) for Women 30 Years of Age[a] at Various Levels of Activity and Various Heights and Weights

Heights m (in)	Physical Activity Level	Weights[b] kg (lb)					
1.45 (57)		38.9 (86)	45.2 (100)	52.6 (116)	63.1 (139)	73.6 (162)	84.1 (185)
					kCalories		
	Sedentary	1564	1623	1698	1813	1927	2042
	Low active	1734	1800	1912	2043	2174	2304
	Active	1946	2021	2112	2257	2403	2548
	Very active	2201	2287	2387	2553	2719	2886
1.50 (59)		41.6 (92)	48.4 (107)	56.3 (124)	67.5 (149)	78.8 (174)	90.0 (198)
					kCalories		
	Sedentary	1625	1689	1771	1894	2017	2139
	Low active	1803	1874	1996	2136	2276	2415
	Active	2025	2105	2205	2360	2516	2672
	Very active	2291	2382	2493	2671	2849	3027
1.55 (61)		44.4 (98)	51.7 (114)	60.1 (132)	72.1 (159)	84.1 (185)	96.1 (212)
					kCalories		
	Sedentary	1688	1756	1846	1977	2108	2239
	Low active	1873	1949	2081	2230	2380	2529
	Active	2104	2190	2299	2466	2632	2798
	Very active	2382	2480	2601	2791	2981	3171
1.60 (63)		47.4 (104)	55.0 (121)	64.0 (141)	76.8 (169)	89.6 (197)	102.4 (226)
					kCalories		
	Sedentary	1752	1824	1922	2061	2201	2340
	Low active	1944	2025	2168	2327	2486	2645
	Active	2185	2276	2396	2573	2750	2927
	Very active	2474	2578	2712	2914	3116	3318
1.65 (65)		50.4 (111)	58.5 (129)	68.1 (150)	81.7 (180)	95.3 (210)	108.9 (240)
					kCalories		
	Sedentary	1816	1893	1999	2148	2296	2444
	Low active	2016	2102	2556	2425	2594	2763
	Active	2267	2364	2494	2682	2871	3059
	Very active	2567	2678	2824	3039	3254	3469
1.70 (67)		53.5 (118)	62.1 (137)	72.3 (159)	86.7 (191)	101.2 (223)	115.6 (255)
					kCalories		
	Sedentary	1881	1963	2078	2235	2393	2550
	Low active	2090	2180	2345	2525	2705	2884
	Active	2350	2453	2594	2794	2994	3194
	Very active	2662	2780	2938	3166	3395	3623
1.75 (69)		56.7 (125)	65.8 (145)	76.6 (169)	91.9 (202)	107.2 (236)	122.5 (270)
					kCalories		
	Sedentary	1948	2034	2158	2325	2492	2659
	Low active	2164	2260	2437	2627	2817	3007
	Active	2434	2543	2695	2907	3119	3331
	Very active	2758	2883	3054	3296	3538	3780
1.80 (71)		59.9 (132)	69.7 (154)	81.0 (178)	97.2 (214)	113.4 (250)	129.6 (285)
					kCalories		
	Sedentary	2015	2106	2239	2416	2593	2769
	Low active	2239	2341	2529	2731	2932	3133
	Active	2519	2634	2799	3023	3247	3472
	Very active	2855	2987	3172	3428	3684	3940

(*continued*)

[a]For each year younger than 30, add 7 kcalories/day to TEE. For each year older than 30, subtract 7 kcalories/day from TEE.
[b]These columns represent a BMI of 18.5, 22.5, 25, 30, 35, and 40, respectively.

TABLE F-4 Total Energy Expenditure (TEE in kCalories per Day) for Women 30 Years of Age[a] at Various Levels of Activity and Various Heights and Weights (*continued*)

Heights m (in)	Physical Activity Level	Weights[b] kg (lb)					
1.85 (73)		63.3 (139)	73.6 (162)	85.6 (189)	102.7 (226)	119.8 (264)	136.9 (302)
		kCalories					
	Sedentary	2083	2179	2322	2509	2695	2882
	Low active	2315	2422	2624	2836	3049	3262
	Active	2605	2727	2904	3141	3378	3615
	Very active	2954	3093	3292	3562	3833	4103
1.90 (75)		66.8 (147)	77.6 (171)	90.3 (199)	108.3 (239)	126.4 (278)	144.4 (318)
		kCalories					
	Sedentary	2151	2253	2406	2603	2800	2996
	Low active	2392	2505	2720	2944	3168	3393
	Active	2693	2821	3011	3261	3511	3760
	Very active	3053	3200	3414	3699	3984	4270
1.95 (77)		70.3 (155)	81.8 (180)	95.1 (209)	114.1 (251)	133.1 (293)	152.1 (335)
		kCalories					
	Sedentary	2221	2328	2492	2699	2906	3113
	Low active	2470	2589	2817	3053	3290	3526
	Active	2781	2917	3119	3383	3646	3909
	Very active	3154	3309	3538	3838	4139	4439

[a]For each year younger than 30, add 7 kcalories/day to TEE. For each year older than 30, subtract 7 kcalories/day from TEE.
[b]These columns represent a BMI of 18.5, 22.5, 25, 30, 35, and 40, respectively.

TABLE F-5 Total Energy Expenditure (TEE in kCalories per Day) for Men 30 Years of Age[a] at Various Levels of Activity and Various Heights and Weights

Heights m (in)	Physical Activity Level	Weights[b] kg (lb)					
1.45 (57)		38.9 (86)	47.3 (100)	52.6 (116)	63.1 (139)	73.6 (163)	84.1 (185)
		kCalories					
	Sedentary	1777	1911	2048	2198	2347	2496
	Low active	1931	2080	2225	2393	2560	2727
	Active	2127	2295	2447	2636	2826	3015
	Very active	2450	2648	2845	3075	3305	3535
1.50 (59)		41.6 (92)	50.6 (107)	56.3 (124)	67.5 (149)	78.8 (174)	90.0 (198)
		kCalories					
	Sedentary	1848	1991	2126	2286	2445	2605
	Low active	2009	2168	2312	2491	2670	2849
	Active	2215	2394	2545	2748	2951	3154
	Very active	2554	2766	2965	3211	3457	3703
1.55 (61)		44.4 (98)	54.1 (114)	60.1 (132)	72.1 (159)	84.1 (185)	96.1 (212)
		kCalories					
	Sedentary	1919	2072	2205	2376	2546	2717
	Low active	2089	2259	2401	2592	2783	2974
	Active	2305	2496	2646	2862	3079	3296
	Very active	2660	2887	3087	3349	3612	3875

(*continued*)

[a]For each year younger than 30, add 10 kcalories/day to TEE. For each year older than 30, subtract 10 kcalories/day from TEE.
[b]These columns represent a BMI of 18.5, 22.5, 25, 30, 35, and 40, respectively.

TABLE F-5 Total Energy Expenditure (TEE in kCalories per Day) for Men 30 Years of Age[a] at Various Levels of Activity and Various Heights and Weights (*continued*)

Heights m (in)	Physical Activity Level	Weights[b] kg (lb)					
1.60 (63)		47.4 (104)	57.6 (121)	64.0 (141)	76.8 (169)	89.6 (197)	102.4 (226)
		kCalories					
	Sedentary	1993	2156	2286	2468	2650	2831
	Low active	2171	2351	2492	2695	2899	3102
	Active	2397	2601	2749	2980	3210	3441
	Very active	2769	3010	3211	3491	3771	4051
1.65 (65)		50.4 (111)	61.3 (129)	68.1 (150)	81.7 (180)	95.3 (210)	108.9 (240)
		kCalories					
	Sedentary	2068	2241	2369	2562	2756	2949
	Low active	2254	2446	2585	2801	3017	3234
	Active	2490	2707	2854	3099	3345	3590
	Very active	2880	3136	3339	3637	3934	4232
1.70 (67)		53.5 (118)	65.0 (137)	72.3 (159)	86.7 (191)	101.2 (223)	115.6 (255)
		kCalories					
	Sedentary	2144	2328	2454	2659	2864	3069
	Low active	2338	2542	2679	2909	3139	3369
	Active	2586	2816	2961	3222	3483	3743
	Very active	2992	3265	3469	3785	4101	4417
1.75 (69)		56.7 (125)	68.9 (145)	76.6 (169)	91.9 (202)	107.2 (236)	122.5 (270)
		kCalories					
	Sedentary	2222	2416	2540	2757	2975	3192
	Low active	2425	2641	2776	3020	3263	3507
	Active	2683	2927	3071	3347	3623	3900
	Very active	3108	3396	3602	3937	4272	4607
1.80 (71)		59.9 (132)	72.9 (154)	81.0 (178)	97.2 (214)	113.4 (250)	129.6 (285)
		kCalories					
	Sedentary	2301	2507	2628	2858	3088	3318
	Low active	2513	2741	2875	3132	3390	3648
	Active	2782	3040	3183	3475	3767	4060
	Very active	3225	3530	3738	4092	4447	4801
1.85 (73)		63.3 (139)	77.0 (162)	85.6 (189)	102.7 (226)	119.8 (264)	136.9 (302)
		kCalories					
	Sedentary	2382	2599	2718	2961	3204	3447
	Low active	2602	2844	2976	3248	3520	3792
	Active	2883	3155	3297	3606	3915	4223
	Very active	3344	3667	3877	4251	4625	4999
1.90 (75)		66.8 (147)	81.2 (171)	90.3 (199)	108.3 (239)	126.4 (278)	144.4 (318)
		kCalories					
	Sedentary	2464	2693	2810	3066	3322	3579
	Low active	2693	2948	3078	3365	3652	3939
	Active	2986	3273	3414	3739	4065	4390
	Very active	3466	3806	4018	4413	4807	5202
1.95 (77)		70.3 (155)	85.6 (180)	95.1 (209)	114.1 (251)	133.1 (293)	152.1 (335)
		kCalories					
	Sedentary	2547	2789	2903	3173	3443	3713
	Low active	2786	3055	3183	3485	3788	4090
	Active	3090	3393	3533	3875	4218	4561
	Very active	3590	3948	4162	4578	4993	5409

[a]For each year younger than 30, add 10 kcalories/day to TEE. For each year older than 30, subtract 10 kcalories/day from TEE.
[b]These columns represent a BMI of 18.5, 22.5, 25, 30, 35, and 40, respectively.

Beyond the Basics: Meal Planning for Healthy Eating, Diabetes Prevention and Management

Beyond the Basics: Meal Planning for Healthy Eating, Diabetes Prevention and Management is a system of meal planning used in Canada.[1] Similar to the U.S. exchange system, *Beyond the Basics* sorts foods into groups and defines portion sizes to help people manage their blood glucose and maintain a healthy weight. Because foods that contain carbohydrate raise blood glucose, the food groups are organized into two sections—those that contain carbohydrate (presented in Table G-1 on pages G-2–G-3) and those that contain little or no carbohydrate (shown in Table G-2 on pages G-3–G-5). One portion from any of the food groups listed in Table G-1 provides about 15 grams of available carbohydrate (total carbohydrate minus fibre) and counts as one carbohydrate choice. Within each group, foods are identified as those to "choose more often" (generally higher in vitamins, minerals, and fibre) and those to "choose less often" (generally higher in sugar, saturated fat, or *trans* fat). Note that there are now resources available for multicultural populations—for example, people of South Asian descent—at www.diabetes.ca/for-professionals/resources/nutrition/tools/.

[1]The tables for the Canadian meal planning system are adapted from *Beyond the Basics: Meal Planning for Healthy Eating, Diabetes Prevention and Management,* copyright 2008, with permission of the Canadian Diabetes Association. Additional information is available from www.diabetes.ca.

KEY

● Choose more often
▲ Choose less often

APPENDIX G

TABLE G-1 Food Groups that Contain Carbohydrate

1 serving = 15 g carbohydrate or 1 carbohydrate choice

Food	Measure
Grains and starches: 15 g carbohydrate, 3 g protein, 0 g fat, 286 kJ (68 kcal)	
▲ Bagel, large (11 cm, 4.5″)	¼
▲ Bagel, small (8 cm, 3″)	½
▲ Bannock, fried	4 cm x 6 cm (1.5″ × 2.5″)
● Bannock, whole grain baked	4 cm x 6 cm (1.5″ × 2.5″)
● Barley, pearled, cooked	125 mL (½ c)
▲ Bread, white	1 slice (30 g)
● Bread, whole grain	1 slice (30 g)
● Bulghur, cooked	125 mL (½ c)
▲ Bun, hamburger or hotdog	½
▲ Cereal, flaked unsweetened	125 mL (½ c)
● Cream of Wheat, cooked	175 mL (¾ c)
● Red River, cooked	125 mL (½ c)
● Chapati (15 cm, 6″)	1 (44 g)
● Corn	125 mL (½ c)
● Couscous, cooked	125 mL (½ c)
▲ Crackers, soda type	7
▲ Croutons	175 mL (¾ c)
● English muffin, whole grain	½ (28 g)
▲ French fries	10 (50 g)
● Millet, cooked	75 mL (⅓ c)
▲ Naan bread (15 cm, 6″)	¼
▲ Pancake (10 cm, 4″)	1
● Pasta, cooked	125 mL (½ c)
▲ Pita bread, white (15 cm, 6″)	½
● Pita bread, whole wheat (15 cm, 6″)	½
▲ Pizza crust (30 cm, 12″)	1/12 (90 g)
● Plantain, cooked, mashed	75 mL (⅓ c)
● Potatoes, boiled or baked	½ medium (84 g)
● Rice, white or brown, cooked	75 mL (⅓ c)
● Roti (15 cm, 6″)	1 (44 g)
● Soup, thick, chunky type	250 mL (1 c)
● Sweet potato, mashed	75 mL (⅓ c)
▲ Taco shells (13 cm, 5″)	2 (17 g)
● Tortilla, wheat flour (25 cm, 10″)	½
▲ Waffle (medium)	1 (39 g)
Fruits: 15 g carbohydrate, 1–2 g protein, 0 g fat, 269 kJ (64 kcal)	
● Apple	1 medium (138 g)
● Applesauce, unsweetened	125 mL (½ c)
● Banana	1 small or ½ large
● Blackberries	500 mL (2 c)
● Cherries	15 (102 g)
● Fruit, canned in juice	125 mL (½ c)
▲ Fruit, dried	60 mL (¼ c)
● Grapefruit	1 small
● Grapes	15 or ½ c (80 g)

(continued)

TABLE G-1 Food Groups that Contain Carbohydrate (*continued*)

Food	Measure
Fruits: 15 g carbohydrate, 1–2 g protein, 0 g fat, 269 kJ (64 kcal)	
● Kiwi	2 medium (150 g)
▲ Juice	125 mL (½ c)
● Mango	½ medium
● Melon	250 mL (1 c)
● Orange	1 medium
● Other berries	250 mL (1 c)
● Pear	1 medium
● Pineapple	175 mL (¾ c)
● Plum	2 medium
● Raspberries	500 mL (2 c)
● Strawberries	500 mL (2 c)
Milk and alternatives: 15 g carbohydrate, 7 g protein, variable fat, 386–651 kJ (92–155 kcal)	
● Evaporated milk, canned	125 mL (½ c)
● Milk, fluid	250 mL (1 c)
● Milk powder, skim	60 mL (4 Tbsp)
● Soy beverage, flavoured	125 mL (½ c)
● Soy beverage, plain	250 mL (1 c)
● Soy yogurt, flavoured	75 mL (⅓ c)
● Yogurt, nonfat, plain	175 mL (¾ c)
● Yogurt, skim, artificially sweetened	250 mL (1 c)
Other choices (sweet foods and snacks): 15 g carbohydrate, variable protein and fat	
▲ Brownies, unfrosted	5 cm × 5 cm (2″ × 2″)
▲ Cake, unfrosted	5 cm × 5 cm (2″ × 2″)
▲ Cookies, arrowroot or gingersnap	3
▲ Jam, jelly, marmalade	15 mL (1 Tbsp)
● Milk pudding, skim, no sugar added	125 mL (½ c)
▲ Muffin, plain	½ small (30 g)
▲ Oatmeal granola bar	1 (28 g)
● Popcorn, low fat, air popped	750 mL (3 c)
▲ Pretzels, low fat, large	7
▲ Pretzels, low fat, sticks	30
▲ Sugar, white	15 mL (1 Tbsp, 3 tsp, or 3 packets)
▲ Syrup, honey, molasses	1 Tbsp (15 mL)

KEY

● Choose more often
▲ Choose less often

TABLE G-2 Food Groups that Contain Little or No Carbohydrate

Food	Measure
Vegetables: To encourage consumption, most vegetables are considered "free"	
▲ Artichokes, Jerusalem[a]	
● Asparagus	
● Beans, yellow or green	
● Bean sprouts	
● Beets	
● Broccoli	

(*continued*)

[a]These vegetables contain enough carbohydrate to be counted as one carbohydrate choice (15 g of available carbohydrate) when the portion size eaten is 250 mL (1 cup) or more.

KEY

● Choose more often
▲ Choose less often

KEY

● Choose more often
▲ Choose less often

TABLE G-2 Food Groups that Contain Little or No Carbohydrate (*continued*)

Food	Measure
Vegetables: To encourage consumption, most vegetables are considered "free"	
● Cabbage	
● Carrots	
● Cauliflower	
● Celery	
● Cucumber	
● Eggplant	
● Kale	
● Leeks	
● Mushrooms	
● Okra	
● Onions	
● Parsnips[a]	
● Peas[a]	
● Peppers	
● Rutabagas	
● Salad vegetables	
● Squash, Hubbard, pumpkin, spaghetti	
● Squash, acorn[a], butternut[a]	
● Tomatoes, fresh	
● Tomatoes, canned, regular	
▲ Tomatoes, canned, stewed[a]	
● Turnips	
Meat and alternatives: 0 g carbohydrate, 7 g protein, 3–5 g fat, 307 kJ (73 kcal)	
● Cheese, skim (<7% milk fat)	2.5 cm × 2.5 cm × 2.5 cm (1″ × 1″ × 1″)
● Cheese, light (<20% milk fat)	2.5 cm × 2.5 cm × 2.5 cm (1″ × 1″ × 1″)
▲ Cheese, regular (≥21% milk fat)	2.5 cm × 2.5 cm × 2.5 cm (1″ × 1″ × 1″)
● Cottage cheese (1–2% milk fat)	60 mL (¼ c)
● Egg	1 medium-large
● Fish, canned in oil or water	60 mL (¼ c)
● Fish, fresh or frozen, cooked	30 g (1 oz)
● Hummus	90 g (⅓ c)
● Legumes, cooked	125 mL (½ c)
● Meat, game, cooked	30 g (1 slice)
● Meat, ground, lean or extra lean, cooked	30 g (2 Tbsp)
● Meat, lean, cooked	30 g (1 slice)
● Meat, organ or tripe, cooked	30 g (1 slice)
● Meat, prepared, low fat	30 g (1–3 slices)
▲ Meat, prepared, regular fat	30 g (1–3 slices)
▲ Meat, regular, cooked	30 g (1–3 slices)
● Peameal/back bacon, cooked	30 g (1–2 slices)
● Poultry, ground, lean, cooked	30 g (2 Tbsp)
● Poultry, skinless, cooked	30 g (1 slice)
▲ Poultry/wings, skin on, cooked	45 g (2)
● Shellfish, cooked	30 g (3 medium)
● Tofu (soybean)	½ block (100 g)
● Vegetarian meat alternatives	30 g (1 oz)

(continued)

TABLE G-2 **Food Groups that Contain Little or No Carbohydrate (*continued*)**

Food	Measure
Fats: 0 g carbohydrate, 0 g protein, 5 g fat, 189 kJ (45 kcal)	
▲ Avocado	34 g (1/6)
▲ Bacon	30 g (1 slice)
▲ Butter	5 mL (1 tsp)
▲ Cheese, spreadable	15 mL (1 Tbsp)
▲ Margarine, non-hydrogenated, regular	5 mL (1 tsp)
▲ Mayonnaise, light	15 mL (1 Tbsp)
▲ Nuts	15 mL (1 Tbsp)
▲ Oil, canola or olive	5 mL (1 tsp)
▲ Salad dressing, regular	5 mL (1 tsp)
▲ Seeds	15 g (1 Tbsp)
▲ Tahini	8 mL (1/2 Tbsp)
Extras: <5 g carbohydrate, 84 kJ (20 kcal)	
Broth	
Coffee	
Herbs and spices	
Ketchup	
Mustard	
Relish	
Sugar-free gelatin	
Sugar-free soft drinks	
Tea	

KEY

● Choose more often
▲ Choose less often

APPENDIX H

Health Canada Santé Canada

Your health and safety… our priority. *Votre santé et votre sécurité… notre priorité.*

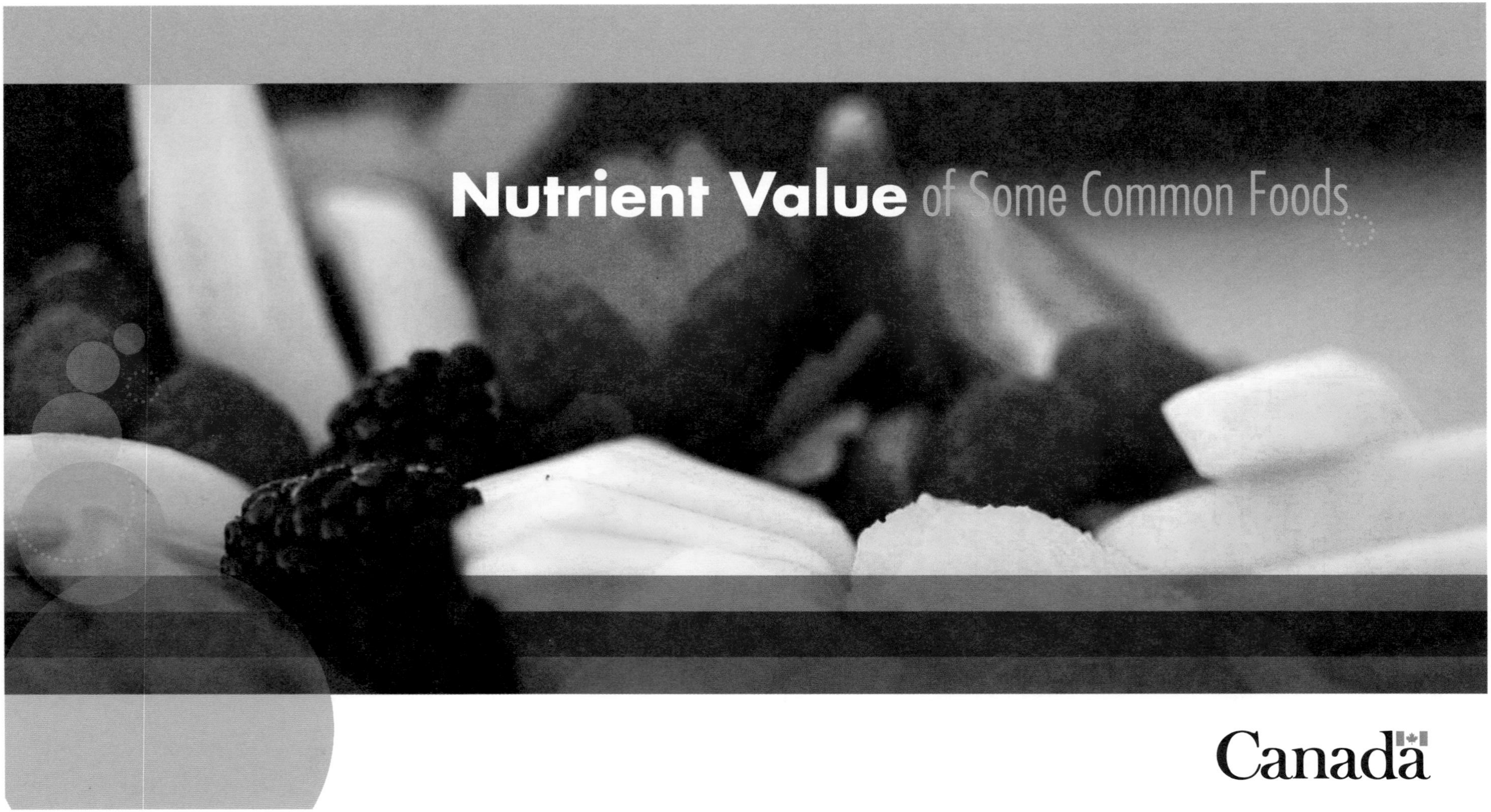
Nutrient Value of Some Common Foods

Canada

Nutrient Value of Some Common Foods

Nutrient Value of Some Common Foods

Health Canada is the federal department responsible for helping Canadians maintain and improve their health.
We assess the safety of drugs and many consumer products, help improve the safety of food, and provide information to Canadians to help them make healthy decisions. We provide health services to First Nations people and to Inuit communities. We work with the provinces to ensure our health care system serves the needs of Canadians.

Published by authority of the Minister of Health.

Nutrient Value of Some Common Foods
is available on Internet at the following address:
www.healthcanada.gc.ca/cnf

Également disponible en français sous le titre :
Valeur nutritive de quelques aliments usuels

This publication can be made available by request on
diskette, large print, audio-cassette and braille.

For further information or to obtain additional copies, please contact:
Publications
Health Canada
Ottawa, Ontario K1A 0K9
Tel.: (613) 954-5995 or 1-866-225-0709
Fax: (613) 941-5366
E-Mail: publications@hc-sc.gc.ca

HC Pub.: 4771
Cat.: H164-49/2008E-PDF
ISBN: 978-0-662-48082-2

APPENDIX H

Nutrient Value of Some Common Foods

Introduction

As Canadians recognize the crucial role of nutrition in the maintenance of good health, they increasingly seek information regarding the nutrient density of foods on the Canadian market.

Health Canada publishes two databases which list nutrient values in Canadian foods. The first is a large, comprehensive, computerized database called the Canadian Nutrient File (CNF). The 2007b version reports up to 143 nutrients in 5516 foods. The CNF can be accessed on the Internet at www.healthcanada.gc.ca/cnf. While this format and detail are useful to health professionals and food industry personnel, a second abbreviated, printed version is a more practical reference for many Canadians.

For this reason we have produced this booklet entitled *Nutrient Value of Some Common Foods.* This publication lists the nutrients most relevant in terms of public health and contribution to the food supply of 1100 of the most commonly consumed foods in Canada. Nutrient values taken from the CNF are calculated in terms of reasonable average household measures of the ready-to-eat form of the food. These amounts are not always identical to the serving sizes displayed on Canada's Food Guide, which are determined for the purpose of providing healthy patterns of eating for a wide range of ages and gender.

Nutrient Value of Some Common Foods

Contents

Facts About the Foods

This edition of the *Nutrient Value of Some Common Foods* is an update to the 1999 version. During this interval, changes have taken place in the food supply, in our understanding of nutrition with regards to health and disease prevention, and to nutrition recommendations.

In this updated version of the *Nutrient Value of Some Common Foods*, the emphasis has been placed on mixed dishes rather than individual ingredients. Detailed ingredient information is available on the CNF website.

Common recipes have been used to calculate nutrient profiles of mixed dishes. As there are multiple variations possible for recipes and ingredients, values given may not precisely match the profile of food you consume. For example, a lasagna prepared with veal and white sauce would differ somewhat from one prepared with the more common ground beef and tomato sauce. Please use these recipes as a general reference not a specific match to what you are eating.

Users may find some foods have been re-categorized, to better allow comparison between similar foods. For this reason, foods found in some categories will not match those displayed in Canada's Food Guide.

Foods commonly consumed by Canadians have been chosen and listed alphabetically under 17 general food headings. This classification allows the user to easily locate a particular food and to compare its nutrient values to similar foods. The index should be used to locate foods whose classification may not be apparent.

Products such as infant formulas, baby foods and frozen dinners are not included. Nutrient values for these products are well documented by the manufacturers, and can be found on the labels.

Nutrient values are given for the weight of the edible portion as described. This is the portion remaining after inedible or refuse parts are discarded, and cooking losses are calculated. This is especially important to note in the meat groupings, where descriptive measure and nutrients are for the cooked product unless raw is specifically stated in the food name.

Because of the condensed version of this booklet, composites have been used in several categories. These composites are an averaging of the most common cuts or brands. The resulting nutrient profiles give approximate values that can be used if a more precise match cannot be found.

Facts About the Nutrients

The approach to choosing nutrients for inclusion in the booklet has changed. The set of 19 nutrients now varies for different food groupings. Nutrients relevant to one specific food group may not be as important to another. For example, cholesterol is present in meats but is not present in fruits and vegetables. When nutrients do not contribute significantly, emphasis is now directed towards components more specific to the group. This allows the addition of more detailed information on the types of fats in the fats and oils group, reporting of beta-carotene and lycopene in the fruit and vegetable groups, and inclusion of values for alcohol and caffeine in the beverage group.

Although trans fatty acids are of public interest, these values cannot be included in this publication. Most food values in the CNF and therefore in this booklet, are generic. For example, chocolate cookies are a representative average of the most popular selling brands in Canada and do not correspond to a specific brand name. The fatty acid content of individual brands can vary widely, and many companies are in the process of re-formulating due to consumer demand. For these reasons, the most reliable way to determine trans fat content of your pre-packaged food is to check the mandatory Nutrition Facts table found on the package.

Trace indicates a measurable quantity in the food, but too small to be included. Zeros indicate a true zero content of the nutrient. N/A indicates a lack of data or "missing value" for a nutrient. Do not assume that missing values are zeros.

The values presented are mean values for a nationwide representative sample. Some of them have a wide range of deviation based on a variation in contributing samples due to such factors as soil type, season, geography, genetics and diet.

DHA and EPA (docosahexanoic acid and eicosapentanoic acid) are long chain omega-3 fatty acids that are known to have positive effects on health. The major dietary source of these fatty acids is fatty fish.

Vitamin E is the common name for the family of antioxidants called tocopherols. Nutrition recommendations are based solely on alpha-tocopherol as this naturally occurring form is the most biologically active. Vitamin E in this booklet refers to alpha-tocopherols only.

Nutrients and Other Components

Nutrient	Unit of measure
Energy	kcal
Energy	kJ
Protein	g
Carbohydrate	g
Total Fat	g
Total Dietary Fibre	g
Saturated Fat	g
Cholesterol	mg
Calcium	mg
Iron	mg
Sodium	mg
Potassium	mg
Magnesium	mg
Phosphorus	mg
Vitamin A	mcg RAE
Vitamin C	mg
Vitamin B12	mcg

Nutrient	Unit of measure
Folate	mcg DFE
Total Sugar	g
Thiamin	mg
Niacin	NE
Lycopene	mcg
Beta-carotene	mcg
Vitamin D	mcg
Caffeine	mg
DHA	g
EPA	g
Trans Fat	g
Monounsaturated Fat	g
Polyunsaturated Fat	g
Vitamin E	mg
Alcohol	g
Riboflavin	mg

Abbreviations and Symbols

cm	centimetre
DFE	dietary folate equivalent
DHA	docosahexaenoic fatty acid (22:6n-3)
diam	diameter
EPA	eicosapentaenoic fatty acid (20:5n-3)
g	gram
kcal	kilocalories
kJ	kilojoules
mcg	microgram
M.F.	milk fat
mg	milligram
mL	millilitre
N/A	no suitable value available
NE	niacin equivalent
RAE	retinol activity equivalent
tr	trace
TM	trademark (Brand name)
%	percent

Breads, Cereals and Other Grain Products

Food Name	Measure	Weight	Energy	Energy	Protein	Carbohydrate	Total Sugar	Total Dietary Fibre	Total Fat	Saturated Fat	Cholesterol	Calcium	Iron	Sodium	Potassium	Magnesium	Phosphorus	Thiamin	Riboflavin	Niacin	Folate
		g	kcal	kJ	g	g	g	g	g	g	mg	mg	mg	mg	mg	mg	mg	mg	mg	NE	DFE
Breads, Cereals and Other Grain Products																					
Flours and Brans																					
Chickpea flour	125mL	49	188	786	11	28	5	5.2	3	0.3	0	22	2.4	31	411	81	155	0.2	0.05	2.9	212
Cornmeal, dry	125mL	73	267	1116	6	57	1	5.4	1	0.2	0	4	0.8	2	118	29	61	0.1	0.04	1.9	35
Oat bran, dry	125mL	50	122	511	9	33	1	5.2	3	0.7	0	29	2.7	2	281	117	365	0.6	0.11	3.2	26
Oat flour	125mL	53	200	838	7	35	1	5.3	4	0.7	0	27	2.2	2	199	78	226	0.3	0.08	1.8	15
Potato flour	125mL	85	302	1262	6	70	3	0.1	tr	0.1	0	55	1.2	46	846	55	142	0.2	0.04	4.6	21
Rice flour	125mL	83	305	1278	5	67	tr	2.0	1	0.3	0	8	0.3	0	63	29	82	0.1	0.02	3.2	3
Rye flour, light	125mL	54	198	827	5	43	1	7.9	1	0.1	0	11	1.0	1	126	38	105	0.2	0.05	1.3	12
Soy flour	125mL	53	174	729	25	20	11	9.2	1	0.1	0	127	4.9	11	1259	153	356	0.4	0.13	7.4	161
Wheat bran	15mL	4	8	33	1	2	tr	1.6	tr	tr	0	3	0.4	tr	43	22	37	tr	0.02	0.7	3
Wheat flour, all purpose	125mL	66	240	1005	7	50	tr	2.0	1	0.1	0	10	3.1	1	71	15	71	0.5	0.33	5.3	192
Wheat flour, bread	125mL	72	261	1093	9	52	tr	1.7	1	0.2	0	11	3.2	1	72	18	70	0.6	0.37	7.1	208
Wheat flour, cake	125mL	72	262	1096	6	56	tr	1.2	1	0.1	0	10	5.3	1	76	12	62	0.6	0.31	6.3	204
Wheat flour, whole grain	125mL	63	215	899	9	46	tr	7.7	1	0.2	0	22	2.5	3	257	87	219	0.3	0.14	6.3	28
Wheat germ, toasted	15mL	7	27	114	2	4	1	1.1	1	0.1	0	3	0.7	tr	68	23	82	0.1	0.06	0.9	25
Breads and Buns																					
Bagel, plain (10cm diam)	1	71	195	817	7	38	4	1.6	1	0.2	0	53	2.5	379	72	21	68	0.4	0.22	4.7	117
Bannock	1 medium	37	84	353	2	19	N/A	0.5	tr	0	1	84	0.7	N/A	N/A	N/A	60	0.1	0.06	1.4	N/A
Bread, French or Vienna	1 slice	35	96	401	3	18	tr	1.1	1	0.2	0	26	0.9	213	40	9	37	0.2	0.12	2.3	80
Bread, Italian	1 slice	35	95	397	3	18	tr	0.9	1	0.3	0	27	1.0	204	39	9	36	0.2	0.10	2.1	106
Bread, mixed-grain	1 slice	35	88	366	4	16	4	2.2	1	0.3	0	32	1.2	170	71	19	62	0.1	0.12	2.3	58
Bread, naan	1/2	63	192	803	7	36	2	1.4	2	0.8	3	78	2.3	208	115	16	89	0.3	0.33	5.6	115
Bread, oatmeal	1 slice	35	94	394	3	17	3	1.4	2	0.2	0	23	0.9	210	50	13	44	0.1	0.08	1.8	30
Bread, pita, white (17cm diam)	1	60	165	690	5	33	1	1.3	1	0.1	0	52	1.6	322	72	16	58	0.4	0.20	3.8	99

Food Name	Measure	Weight	Energy	Energy	Protein	Carbohydrate	Total Sugar	Total Dietary Fibre	Total Fat	Saturated Fat	Cholesterol	Calcium	Iron	Sodium	Potassium	Magnesium	Phosphorus	Thiamin	Riboflavin	Niacin	Folate
		g	kcal	kJ	g	g	g	g	g	g	mg	mg	mg	mg	mg	mg	mg	mg	mg	NE	DFE
Breads, Cereals and Other Grain Products																					
Bread, pita, whole wheat (17cm diam)	1	64	170	712	6	35	1	4.7	2	0.3	0	10	2.0	340	109	44	115	0.2	0.05	3.4	22
Bread, pumpernickel	1 slice	35	88	366	3	17	tr	2.3	1	0.2	0	24	1.0	235	73	19	62	0.1	0.11	1.6	47
Bread, raisin	1 slice	35	96	401	3	18	2	1.5	2	0.4	0	23	1.0	137	79	9	38	0.1	0.14	1.7	55
Bread, rye	1 slice	35	91	379	3	17	1	2.0	1	0.2	0	26	1.0	231	58	14	44	0.2	0.12	1.9	53
Bread, white, Calorie-reduced	1 slice	35	72	303	3	16	2	3.4	1	0.2	0	33	1.1	159	27	8	42	0.1	0.10	1.9	48
Bread, white, commercial	1 slice	35	93	389	3	18	2	0.8	1	0.3	0	53	1.3	238	35	8	35	0.2	0.12	2.1	60
Bread, white, homemade with 2% milk	1 slice	35	100	417	3	17		0.7	2	0.4	1	20	1.0	126	51	7	40	0.1	0.13	1.8	44
Bread, whole wheat, commercial	1 slice	35	86	360	3	16	7	2.4	1	0.3	0	25	1.2	184	88	30	80	0.1	0.07	2.2	18
Bread, whole wheat, homemade with 2% milk	1 slice	35	97	407	3	18	1	2.1	2	0.3	0	12	1.1	121	110	28	65	0.1	0.08	2.1	27
English muffin, white, toasted	1	52	133	554	4	26	2	1.5	1	0.1	0	98	1.4	262	74	11	75	0.2	0.14	2.8	65
English muffin, whole wheat, toasted	1	52	126	528	5	25	1	2.6	1	0.2	0	100	1.6	216	105	22	65	0.2	0.15	2.8	41
Fry bread	1	37	122	511	2	18	1	1.0	5	1.7	3	21	1.5	122	28	7	46	0.2	0.08	2.2	73
Roll, crusty (kaiser)	1	57	167	698	6	30	1	1.3	2	0.3	0	54	1.9	310	62	15	57	0.3	0.19	3.5	86
Roll, dinner, white	1	28	85	356	2	14	2	0.9	2	0.5	tr	34	0.9	148	38	7	33	0.1	0.09	1.6	41
Roll, dinner, whole wheat	1	28	75	315	2	14	2	2.1	1	0.2	0	30	0.7	136	77	24	64	0.1	0.04	1.7	9
Roll, hamburger or hotdog, white	1	43	120	502	4	21	3	0.9	2	0.5	0	59	1.4	206	40	9	27	0.2	0.14	2.5	73
Roll, hamburger or hotdog, whole wheat	1	43	113	473	4	19	3	1.6	3	0.6	0	41	1.7	197	69	19	52	0.2	0.13	2.8	74
Other Bread Products																					
Bread stick, plain (19cm X 2cm)	1	10	41	172	1	7	tr	0.3	1	0.1	0	2	0.4	66	12	3	12	0.1	0.06	0.8	25
Bread stuffing, dry mix, prepared	125mL	106	188	786	3	23	2	3.1	9	1.8	0	34	1.2	574	78	13	44	0.1	0.11	2.3	56
Croutons, plain	60mL	8	31	129	1	6	N/A	0.4	1	0.1	0	6	0.3	53	9	2	9	tr	0.02	0.6	16
Dumpling	1 dumpling	35	69	289	1	8	tr	0.3	4	1.0	1	23	0.4	138	23	3	22	0.1	0.06	0.8	19
Matzo, plain	1	28	112	468	3	24	tr	0.9	tr	0.1	0	4	0.9	1	32	7	25	0.1	0.08	1.7	5
Taco shell, baked (13cm diam)	1 shell	13	61	254	1	8	tr	1.0	3	0.4	0	21	0.3	48	23	14	32	tr	0.01	0.3	28
Tortilla, corn (15cm diam)	1	19	41	173	1	8	tr	1.2	1	0.1	0	15	0.2	9	35	14	60	tr	0.01	0.4	1
Tortilla, wheat (20cm diam)	1	49	159	666	4	27	N/A	1.6	3	0.9	0	19	1.6	234	64	13	61	0.3	0.14	2.6	98
Pancakes, Waffles and French Toast																					
French toast, frozen, ready to heat, heated	1 slice	59	126	526	4	19	N/A	0.6	4	0.9	48	63	1.3	292	79	10	82	0.2	0.22	2.5	42

Food Name	Measure	Weight	Energy	Energy	Protein	Carbohydrate	Total Sugar	Total Dietary Fibre	Total Fat	Saturated Fat	Cholesterol	Calcium	Iron	Sodium	Potassium	Magnesium	Phosphorus	Thiamin	Riboflavin	Niacin	Folate
		g	kcal	kJ	g	g	g	g	g	g	mg	mg	mg	mg	mg	mg	mg	mg	mg	NE	DFE
Breads, Cereals and Other Grain Products																					
French toast, homemade	1 slice	65	149	623	5	16	N/A	0.7	7	1.8	75	65	1.1	311	87	11	76	0.1	0.21	2.1	37
Pancake, buckwheat, prepared from mix (13cm diam)	1	40	73	305	3	10	2	1.1	3	0.6	20	89	0.7	191	80	27	143	0.1	0.09	1.2	9
Pancake, homemade with butter and syrup (13cm diam)	1	50	112	468	3	20	2	0.8	3	1.0	11	85	0.5	211	78	9	118	0.1	0.11	1.1	23
Pancake, plain, from complete mix (13cm diam)	1	40	64	266	1	11	N/A	0.4	2	0.2	3	36	0.4	180	50	6	96	0.1	0.06	0.8	15
Pancake, plain, frozen, ready-to-heat (13cm diam), heated	1	41	94	393	2	18	4	0.7	1	0.3	4	25	1.4	209	30	6	153	0.2	0.19	2.1	27
Pancake, plain, homemade (13cm diam)	1	38	86	361	2	11	N/A	0.5	4	0.8	22	83	0.7	167	50	6	60	0.1	0.11	1.1	21
Potato pancake, homemade (8cm diam)	1	37	112	467	2	13	1	1.0	6	0.6	23	12	0.7	191	277	16	46	0.1	0.06	1.4	15
Waffle, homemade	1	37	103	432	3	14	2	0.5	4	0.7	33	44	0.9	146	58	7	53	0.1	0.15	1.7	37
Waffle, plain, frozen, ready-to-heat, heated	1	33	87	364	2	13	2	0.8	3	0.5	8	77	1.5	260	42	7	139	0.1	0.16	1.9	22
Rice, Pasta and Other Grains																					
Barley, pearled, cooked	125mL	83	102	426	2	23	tr	2.0	tr	0.1	0	9	1.1	2	77	18	45	0.1	0.05	2.2	13
Bulgur, cooked	125mL	96	80	334	3	18	tr	2.7	tr	tr	0	10	0.9	5	65	31	38	0.1	0.03	1.7	17
Couscous, cooked	125mL	83	93	388	3	19	tr	0.7	tr	tr	0	7	0.3	4	48	7	18	0.1	0.02	1.5	12
Quinoa, cooked	125mL	73	70	293	2	13	N/A	1.3	1	0.1	0	11	1.7	4	138	39	77	tr	0.07	1.0	9
Macaroni, cooked	250mL	148	209	873	7	42	1	1.8	1	0.1	0	10	2.1	1	46	27	80	0.3	0.14	4.0	184
Noodles, Chinese, chow mein	60mL	11	60	252	1	7	tr	0.4	4	0.5	0	2	0.5	50	14	6	18	0.1	0.05	0.9	16
Noodles, egg, cooked	250mL	169	225	940	8	42	1	1.9	2	0.5	56	20	2.7	12	47	32	117	0.3	0.14	4.3	176
Pasta, fresh-refrigerated, cooked	250mL	169	220	920	9	40	N/A	3.7	3	0.7	69	17	2.0	140	36	24	88	0.3	0.29	4.0	101
Pasta, fresh-refrigerated, spinach, cooked	250mL	169	223	933	9	41	1	2.2	3	0.6	56	32	1.8	20	63	41	96	0.4	0.21	4.4	159
Ramen noodles, chicken flavour, dry	1 package	85	371	1554	9	54	1	2.0	13	6.0	N/A	23	3.3	1760	147	19	100	0.5	0.21	3.8	150
Rice noodles, cooked	250mL	186	203	848	2	46	N/A	1.9	tr	tr	0	7	0.3	35	7	6	37	tr	0.01	0.5	6
Rice, brown, long-grain, cooked	125mL	103	115	479	3	24	tr	1.5	1	0.2	0	10	0.4	5	44	44	86	0.1	0.03	2.1	4
Rice, white, long-grain, cooked	125mL	83	109	454	2	24	tr	0.4	tr	0.1	0	8	0.2	1	29	10	36	tr	0.01	0.8	3
Rice, white, long-grain, instant, prepared	125mL	87	85	357	2	19	0	0.5	tr	tr	0	7	0.2	3	3	4	12	tr	0.04	0.9	7
Rice, white, long-grain, parboiled, cooked	125mL	92	105	441	2	23	tr	0.4	tr	0.1	0	18	0.2	3	34	11	39	tr	0.02	1.7	4
Rice, wild, cooked	125mL	87	88	366	3	18	1	1.6	tr	tr	0	3	0.5	3	88	28	71	tr	0.08	1.8	23

Food Name	Measure	Weight	Energy	Energy	Protein	Carbohydrate	Total Sugar	Total Dietary Fibre	Total Fat	Saturated Fat	Cholesterol	Calcium	Iron	Sodium	Potassium	Magnesium	Phosphorus	Thiamin	Riboflavin	Niacin	Folate
		g	kcal	kJ	g	g	g	g	g	g	mg	mg	mg	mg	mg	mg	mg	mg	mg	NE	DFE
Breads, Cereals and Other Grain Products																					
Soba noodles, cooked	250mL	120	119	499	6	26	N/A	N/A	tr	tr	0	5	0.6	72	42	11	30	0.1	0.03	2.1	8
Spaghetti, cooked	250mL	148	209	873	7	42	1	2.5	1	0.1	0	10	2.1	1	46	27	80	0.3	0.14	4.0	184
Spaghetti, whole wheat, cooked	250mL	148	183	768	8	39	1	4.8	1	0.1	0	22	1.6	4	65	44	132	0.2	0.07	2.7	7
Breakfast Cereals																					
Hot Cereal, cooked																					
Cream of wheat, regular	175mL	186	46	195	2	9	tr	0.7	tr	0	0	2	1.6	tr	15	2	17	tr	0.01	0.4	N/A
Oat bran, cooked	175mL	179	73	306	3	12	tr	3.4	1	0.3	0	17	1.3	1	120	N/A	127	0.2	0.06	0.9	9
Oatmeal, instant, apple-cinnamon	1 packet	186	141	592	3	29	12	2.8	2	0.3	0	21	5.0	256	108	36	88	0.8	0.03	1.4	50
Oatmeal, instant, regular	1 packet	186	112	468	4	20	1	2.7	2	0.4	0	21	4.0	241	112	45	132	0.6	0.04	1.5	N/A
Oatmeal, large flakes/quick	175mL	173	99	412	4	17	tr	2.6	2	0.3	0	13	1.0	1	98	N/A	111	0.2	0.04	0.9	8
Red River, Robin Hood™	175mL	180	115	482	4	24	N/A	4.0	1	0.1	tr	15	1.3	27	N/A	18	63	0.1	0.02	1.4	19
Ready-to-eat																					
All Bran Buds with psyllium, Kellogg's™	75mL	27	70	292	2	22	7	11.3	1	N/A	0	17	3.5	181	242	74	242	0.5	0.09	2.5	38
All Bran, Kellogg's™	125mL	35	92	384	4	27	6	11.8	1	N/A	0	30	4.7	305	408	130	350	0.7	0.07	6.0	50
Almond Raisin Muslix, Kellogg's™	175mL	44	173	722	4	34	13	3.0	3	N/A	0	24	5.9	140	191	30	86	0.9	0.07	2.1	N/A
Alpha-Bits, Post™	250mL	34	139	580	2	30	14	1.1	1	0.2	0	3	4.5	126	21	24	74	0.7	0	2.0	41
Bran Flakes, Post™	250mL	53	185	776	5	41	9	7.4	1	0.2	0	24	7.0	302	253	121	276	1.1	0.08	3.5	64
Cap'n Crunch, Quaker™	175mL	27	108	452	1	23	10	0.7	1	1.1	0	0	3.6	213	30	11	22	0.5	0	1.3	32
Cheerios, Honey Nut, General Mills™	250mL	35	134	561	3	28	12	2.1	1	N/A	0	128	4.7	252	99	38	115	0	0.06	1.6	41
Cheerios, regular General Mills™	250mL	24	95	396	3	18	1	2.2	2	N/A	0	44	3.2	219	78	32	105	tr	0.04	1.1	28
Cinnamon Toast Crunch, General Mills™	175mL	28	123	514	1	22	9	1.0	3	N/A	0	103	3.8	193	41	12	93	0	0.01	1.3	33
Corn Bran, Quaker™	250mL	38	124	520	3	30	8	6.1	2	0.8	0	0	5.0	349	91	N/A	42	0.8	0.02	1.7	45
Corn Flakes, Kellogg's™	250mL	26	103	430	2	23	2	0.7	tr	0	0	1	3.5	190	28	2	12	0.5	0.71	1.6	32
Corn Pops, Kellogg's™	250mL	33	130	544	1	30	12	0.4	tr	0	0	2	4.4	192	26	3	13	0.7	0.01	1.8	40
Fibre 1, General Mills™	125mL	30	79	329	3	24	0	14.1	1	0.1	0	110	4.1	130	239	68	188	0.1	0.06	1.4	36
Froot Loops, Kellogg's™	250mL	30	116	485	1	26	14	0.6	1	N/A	0	3	3.9	121	30	7	31	0.6	0.02	1.7	36
Frosted Flakes, Kellogg's™	250mL	37	142	595	2	33	15	0.6	tr	0	0	1	4.9	196	28	2	9	0.7	0.67	2.1	45
Fruit & Fibre, Dates/Raisins/Walnuts, Post™	125mL	29	93	389	3	22	7	4.3	1	N/A	0	16	3.9	134	145	55	126	0.6	0.05	1.9	35

Food Name	Measure	Weight	Energy	Energy	Protein	Carbohydrate	Total Sugar	Total Dietary Fibre	Total Fat	Saturated Fat	Cholesterol	Calcium	Iron	Sodium	Potassium	Magnesium	Phosphorus	Thiamin	Riboflavin	Niacin	Folate
		g	kcal	kJ	g	g	g	g	g	g	mg	mg	mg	mg	mg	mg	mg	mg	mg	NE	DFE
Breads, Cereals and Other Grain Products																					
Granola with Raisins, low fat, Kellogg's™	125mL	59	226	944	5	46	17	3.5	3	N/A	0	24	7.8	147	173	47	135	1.2	0.14	3.7	71
Granola with Raisins, Rogers™	125mL	59	245	1023	5	41	N/A	5.3	8	N/A	0	28	1.9	95	198	N/A	157	0.4	0.06	1.8	N/A
Grape-Nuts, Post™	125mL	58	208	872	6	46	5	6.0	1	N/A	0	24	2.0	348	253	59	241	0.2	0.09	4.5	68
Harvest Crunch, regular, Quaker™	125mL	47	218	911	5	31	12	3.3	9	6.7	1	51	1.1	45	226	N/A	N/A	0.1	0.07	1.5	14
Honeycomb, Post™	250mL	23	92	384	1	21	8	0.2	tr	N/A	0	8	3.7	93	46	7	36	0.5	tr	1.4	28
Just Right, Kellogg's™	250mL	45	172	720	4	38	10	2.2	1	N/A	0	11	6.0	250	105	28	93	0.9	0.10	2.9	55
Life, Quaker™	175mL	33	124	518	5	23	7	2.9	2	0.3	0	24	4.3	195	188	10	160	0.6	0.03	1.5	19
Lucky Charms, General Mills™	250mL	34	132	550	2	28	15	1.7	1	N/A	0	124	4.6	227	64	28	87	0	0.02	1.6	40
Mini-Wheats with White Frosting, Kellogg's™	175mL	35	121	505	3	29	3	3.6	1	N/A	0	14	4.7	4	135	31	102	0.7	0.02	2.3	42
Muesli, President's Choice™	75mL	40	144	603	5	28	10	3.5	2	N/A	0	9	1.6	24	228	13	40	0.1	0.10	1.4	N/A
Nesquik, General Mills™	250mL	30	120	502	1	27	14	0.6	1	N/A	0	33	4.1	192	49	8	44	0	0	1.4	36
Oatmeal Crisp Almond, General Mills™	125mL	32	131	546	3	23	8	2.3	3	N/A	0	81	4.3	108	93	34	93	0.6	0.05	1.5	38
Oatmeal Crisp Maple Walnut, General Mills™	125mL	32	133	557	3	25	9	2.3	2	0.3	0	81	4.3	142	101	29	81	0.6	0.05	1.5	38
Puffed Wheat, Quaker™	250mL	13	45	188	2	9	tr	1.4	tr	0.1	0	9	0.5	0	60	18	40	0.1	0.01	1.0	1
Raisin Bran, Kellogg's™	250mL	59	187	782	5	47	17	6.7	1	N/A	0	22	7.9	367	334	75	189	1.2	0.08	4.5	72
Reese's Puffs, General Mills™	175mL	30	128	533	2	24	13	0.6	3	0.6	0	98	4.0	178	43	2	11	0	0	1.4	35
Rice Krispies, Kellogg's™	250mL	29	110	458	2	24	3	0.3	tr	0	0	4	3.8	315	31	11	41	0.6	0.01	1.7	30
Shredded Wheat, Post™	1 biscuit	25	91	379	3	21	tr	3.5	1	0.1	0	9	1.5	1	92	31	83	0.1	0.06	2.3	11
Shreddies, Post™	175mL	38	138	579	4	32	6	4.4	1	N/A	0	14	5.1	241	143	38	109	0.8	0.01	2.5	N/A
Special K, Kellogg's™	250mL	24	94	392	4	18	2	0.3	tr	N/A	0	tr	3.2	226	34	13	49	0.5	0.03	1.9	29
Sugar Crisp, Post™	250mL	26	103	432	1	24	14	0.8	1	N/A	0	3	0.3	33	1	11	44	0.5	tr	1.5	32
Trix, General Mills™	250mL	30	117	491	1	27	13	1.0	1	N/A	0	98	4.0	195	16	2	22	0	0	1.4	35
Weetabix™	2 biscuits	35	130	543	4	29	2	4.4	1	0.1	0	14	1.1	126	141	58	144	0.7	N/A	2.6	13
Crackers																					
Cheese crackers, small	15	15	75	316	2	9	tr	0.4	4	1.4	2	23	0.7	149	22	5	33	0.1	0.06	1.0	36
Melba toast, plain	2	10	39	163	1	8	tr	0.6	tr	tr	0	9	0.4	83	20	6	20	tr	0.03	0.6	19

Food Name	Measure	Weight	Energy	Energy	Protein	Carbohydrate	Total Sugar	Total Dietary Fibre	Total Fat	Saturated Fat	Cholesterol	Calcium	Iron	Sodium	Potassium	Magnesium	Phosphorus	Thiamin	Riboflavin	Niacin	Folate
		g	kcal	kJ	g	g	g	g	g	g	mg	mg	mg	mg	mg	mg	mg	mg	mg	NE	DFE
Breads, Cereals and Other Grain Products																					
Milk crackers	2	24	109	457	2	17	4	0.5	4	0.6	3	41	0.9	142	27	5	73	0.1	0.10	1.5	34
Rusk toast	1	10	41	170	1	7	N/A	0.6	1	0.1	0	3	0.3	25	25	4	15	tr	0.04	0.7	10
Rye wafers, plain	2	20	67	279	2	16	tr	4.6	tr	tr	0	8	1.2	159	99	24	67	0.1	0.06	0.7	9
Saltine (oyster, soda, soup)	4	12	51	215	1	9	tr	0.4	1	0.2	0	8	0.7	129	18	3	12	tr	0.05	0.9	26
Saltine (oyster, soda, soup), unsalted top	4	12	52	218	1	9	0	0.4	1	0.4	0	14	0.6	92	15	3	13	0.1	0.06	0.9	23
Standard-type (snack-type) (Ritz™)	4	12	60	252	1	7	tr	0.2	3	0.5	0	14	0.4	102	16	3	27	tr	0.04	0.7	17
Standard-type, reduced sodium (Ritz™)	4	12	60	252	1	7	tr	0.2	3	0.5	0	14	0.4	45	43	3	27	tr	0.04	0.7	17
Wheat crackers	4	20	95	396	2	13	1	1.4	3	2.0	0	10	1.0	173	60	12	44	0.1	0.07	1.4	37
Wheat crackers, low fat	4	18	79	330	2	12	2	0.9	2	1.2	tr	34	0.7	112	72	13	52	0.1	0.10	1.3	28
Whole wheat crackers	4	16	71	296	1	11	tr	1.7	3	0.5	0	8	0.5	105	48	16	47	tr	0.02	1.1	4

Serving sizes for ready-to-eat cereals vary.
Be sure to check the amount specified for 1 serving on the Nutrition Facts table
(i.e., 1 serving of All Bran™ is 125mL but 1 serving of Cheerios™ is 250mL)

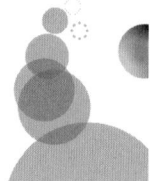

Baked Goods

Food Name	Measure	Weight	Energy	Energy	Protein	Carbohydrate	Total Sugar	Total Dietary Fibre	Total Fat	Saturated Fat	Cholesterol	Calcium	Iron	Sodium	Potassium	Magnesium	Phosphorus	Thiamin	Riboflavin	Niacin	Folate
		g	kcal	kJ	g	g	g	g	g	g	mg	mg	mg	mg	mg	mg	mg	mg	mg	NE	DFE
Baked Goods																					
Biscuits, Croissants, and Muffins																					
Biscuit, plain or buttermilk, fast food	1	51	186	776	3	25	2	0.7	8	1.3	1	25	1.7	537	114	9	219	0.2	0.15	2.4	58
Biscuit, plain or buttermilk, from mix, baked	1	30	97	404	2	14	3	0.4	4	1.0	2	54	0.6	273	55	7	136	0.1	0.11	1.4	31
Biscuit, plain or buttermilk, homemade	1	60	212	888	4	27	1	0.9	10	2.6	2	141	1.7	348	73	11	98	0.2	0.19	2.6	57
Biscuit, plain, refrigerated dough, baked	1	27	93	391	2	13	tr	0.4	4	1.0	0	5	0.7	325	42	4	104	0.1	0.06	1.2	37
Croissant, butter	1	57	231	968	5	26	6	1.5	12	6.6	38	21	1.2	424	67	9	60	0.2	0.14	2.2	74
Muffin, blueberry, from mix, prepared	1	54	149	623	3	24	N/A	N/A	5	1.2	32	14	0.6	216	41	6	93	0.1	0.17	1.9	61
Muffin, bran, from mix, prepared	1	55	159	666	4	27	N/A	N/A	5	1.4	32	18	1.5	271	84	33	189	0.1	0.13	2.9	38
Muffin, bran, homemade	1	57	199	833	4	32	13	3.7	8	0.9	23	82	2.3	242	363	80	129	0.1	0.16	3.0	37
Muffin, carrot, commercial	1	113	344	1439	7	49	17	1.9	14	1.6	34	100	2.2	396	208	18	117	0.3	0.31	4.1	90
Muffin, chocolate chip, commercial	1	113	366	1530	8	53	16	2.4	14	5.3	37	116	2.9	341	192	34	147	0.3	0.35	4.6	102
Muffin, fruit, commercial	1	113	313	1309	6	54	22	2.9	7	1.6	34	64	1.8	505	139	18	223	0.2	0.14	2.5	129
Muffin, fruit, homemade	1	57	162	679	4	23	N/A	0.9	6	1.2	21	108	1.3	251	70	9	83	0.2	0.16	2.0	42
Cookies, Granola Bars and Other Bars																					
Bars																					
Breakfast bar, Oatmeal to Go™	1	47	197	825	3	33	10	2.4	5	0.9	tr	17	4.2	202	102	N/A	N/A	0.7	N/A	1.7	N/A
Cereal bar, fruit filled (Nutri-Grain™)	1	37	135	566	2	26	14	1.2	3	0.5	tr	17	0.6	96	72	3	43	0.1	0.04	0.8	N/A
Granola bar, hard, chocolate chip	1	24	105	440	2	17	N/A	1.1	4	2.7	0	18	0.7	83	60	17	49	tr	0.02	0.7	3
Granola bar, hard, plain	1	25	118	493	3	16	N/A	1.3	5	0.6	0	15	0.7	74	84	24	69	0.1	0.03	1.1	6
Granola bar, soft, chocolate chip, graham and marshmallow	1	26	109	454	1	20	6	1.0	3	0.6	0	6	0.6	90	48	18	53	tr	0.04	0.5	3
Granola bar, soft, nuts and raisins	1	28	127	532	2	18	N/A	1.6	6	2.7	tr	24	0.6	71	110	25	67	0.1	0.05	1.2	8
Granola bar, soft, peanut butter, chocolate coated	1	37	188	788	4	20	N/A	1.0	12	6.3	4	40	0.5	71	125	25	84	tr	0.08	2.0	9
Granola bar, soft, plain	1	28	124	519	2	19	N/A	1.3	5	2.0	tr	29	0.7	78	91	21	64	0.1	0.05	0.6	7
Muffin bar (Hop&Go™, Sweet Mornings™)	1	50	178	746	2	30	18	0.6	6	1.0	20	7	0.8	175	64	7	26	0.1	0.10	1.4	33

Food Name	Measure	Weight	Energy	Energy	Protein	Carbohydrate	Total Sugar	Total Dietary Fibre	Total Fat	Saturated Fat	Cholesterol	Calcium	Iron	Sodium	Potassium	Magnesium	Phosphorus	Thiamin	Riboflavin	Niacin	Folate
		g	kcal	kJ	g	g	g	g	g	g	mg	mg	mg	mg	mg	mg	mg	mg	mg	NE	DFE
Baked Goods																					
Cookies																					
Chocolate chip, commercial	2	20	98	409	1	13	7	0.6	5	1.5	N/A	7	0.7	59	30	10	23	tr	0.05	0.7	20
Chocolate chip, homemade	2	32	156	653	2	19	N/A	0.9	9	2.6	10	12	0.8	116	72	18	32	0.1	0.06	0.8	15
Chocolate chip, refrigerated dough, baked	2	24	118	494	1	16	N/A	0.4	5	1.9	6	7	0.6	56	48	6	18	tr	0.05	0.7	17
Chocolate coated marshmallow	2	30	129	541	1	21	14	0.6	4	2.2	tr	6	0.9	46	43	11	29	tr	0.06	0.4	11
Chocolate sandwich	2	20	93	390	1	14	8	0.6	4	1.8	0	4	2.1	97	37	10	18	tr	0.03	0.8	17
Coconut macaroons, homemade	2	48	194	811	2	35	34	0.9	6	5.4	0	3	0.4	119	75	10	21	tr	0.05	0.4	2
Fig	2	32	111	466	1	23	15	1.5	2	0.4	0	20	0.9	112	66	9	20	0.1	0.07	0.8	17
Ginger snaps	2	14	58	244	1	11	3	0.3	1	0.3	0	11	0.9	92	48	7	12	tr	0.04	0.6	20
Graham crackers, plain or honey	2	14	59	248	1	11	4	0.4	1	0.2	0	3	0.5	85	19	4	15	tr	0.04	0.8	9
Molasses	2	30	129	539	2	22	5	0.3	4	1.0	0	22	1.9	138	104	16	29	0.1	0.08	1.3	44
Oatmeal, with raisins, commercial	2	26	117	489	2	18	6	0.7	5	1.2	0	10	0.7	100	37	9	36	0.1	0.06	1.0	19
Oatmeal, without raisins, homemade	2	30	134	561	2	20	N/A	0.7	5	1.1	11	32	0.8	179	55	13	50	0.1	0.05	0.8	14
Peanut butter sandwich	2	28	134	560	2	18	10	0.5	6	1.4	0	15	0.7	103	54	14	53	0.1	0.07	1.6	26
Peanut butter, homemade	2	40	190	794	4	24	N/A	1.5	10	1.8	12	16	0.9	207	92	16	46	0.1	0.08	2.1	32
Shortbread, commercial, plain	2	16	80	336	1	10	2	0.3	4	1.0	3	6	0.4	73	16	3	17	0.1	0.05	0.8	18
Shortbread, homemade	2	33	185	773	2	19	7	0.5	12	7.3	31	6	0.7	130	20	4	20	0.1	0.08	1.3	32
Animal crackers (arrowroot, social tea)	2	10	45	187	1	7	1	0.2	1	0.3	0	4	0.3	39	10	2	11	tr	0.03	0.5	17
Sugar cookies, commercial	2	30	143	600	2	20	11	0.2	6	1.6	15	6	0.6	107	19	4	24	0.1	0.06	1.2	25
Sugar cookies, homemade	2	32	142	592	2	25	16	0.4	4	1.1	8	18	0.6	72	23	3	23	0.1	0.07	1.0	24
Vanilla wafers	2	12	57	237	1	9	N/A	0.2	2	0.6	0	3	0.3	37	13	1	8	tr	0.03	0.5	8
Cakes																					
Angelfood, commercial (25cm diam)	1/12	28	73	306	2	16	N/A	0.4	tr	tr	0	40	0.1	212	26	3	9	tr	0.14	0.6	16
Angelfood, from mix (25cm diam)	1/12	50	129	538	3	29	15	0.1	tr	tr	0	42	0.1	255	68	4	116	tr	0.10	0.7	14
Banana bread, homemade (11cm X 6cm X 1cm)	1 slice	60	196	818	3	33	N/A	0.7	6	1.3	26	13	0.8	181	80	8	35	0.1	0.12	1.4	29
Boston cream pie, commercial	1/6	92	232	970	2	39	33	1.3	8	2.2	34	21	0.3	132	36	6	45	0.4	0.25	0.7	17
Brownies, commercial (5cm X 5cm)	1 square	34	138	576	2	22	12	0.7	6	1.4	6	10	0.8	106	51	11	34	0	0.07	0.9	24
Brownies, homemade (5cm X 5cm)	1 square	36	168	702	2	18	N/A	0.8	10	2.6	26	21	0.7	123	63	19	48	0.1	0.07	0.8	14
Carrot, homemade with cream cheese icing (2 layer, 23cm diam)	1/12	133	542	2266	5	70	52	1.5	28	3.8	73	49	1.6	201	131	10	70	0.2	0.22	2.7	57

Food Name	Measure	Weight	Energy	Energy	Protein	Carbohydrate	Total Sugar	Total Dietary Fibre	Total Fat	Saturated Fat	Cholesterol	Calcium	Iron	Sodium	Potassium	Magnesium	Phosphorus	Thiamin	Riboflavin	Niacin	Folate
		g	kcal	kJ	g	g	g	g	g	g	mg	mg	mg	mg	mg	mg	mg	mg	mg	NE	DFE
Baked Goods																					
Cheesecake, commercial (15 cm diam)	1/6	100	321	1342	6	26	N/A	0.4	23	9.9	55	51	0.6	207	90	11	93	tr	0.19	1.3	20
Cheesecake, from mix, no-bake type (20cm diam)	1/8	149	407	1702	8	53	N/A	2.8	19	9.9	43	255	0.7	564	313	28	347	0.2	0.39	2.4	57
Cheesecake, plain, homemade with cherry topping (20cm diam)	1/8	168	459	1920	11	55	45	0.8	23	8.8	75	65	1.6	496	146	12	124	tr	0.24	2.8	23
Chocolate, from mix, with icing (23cm diam)	1/12	109	362	1513	4	61	47	2.0	13	1.9	43	63	1.6	396	177	27	141	0.1	0.13	1.9	26
Chocolate, frozen, commercial, with chocolate icing (1 layer, 5cm X 20cm diam)	1/6	85	282	1180	3	48	37	2.0	10	1.0	33	49	1.0	309	138	21	110	N/A	N/A	1.0	20
Chocolate, homemade, with icing (2 layer, 23cm diam)	1/12	109	408	1706	4	67	52	1.9	16	5.0	28	66	2.5	253	138	34	91	0.1	0.15	2.0	36
Coffee cake, cinnamon with crumb topping, commercial	1/10	57	237	991	4	26	N/A	1.1	13	3.3	18	31	1.1	199	70	12	61	0.1	0.13	1.7	46
Coffee cake, cinnamon with crumb topping, from mix (20cm X 15cm)	1/10	45	142	596	2	24	13	0.5	4	0.8	22	61	0.6	189	50	8	96	0.1	0.08	1.2	33
Fruitcake, commercial	1 piece	43	139	583	1	26	13	1.6	4	0.5	2	14	0.9	116	66	7	22	tr	0.04	0.6	14
Gingerbread, from mix (23cm X 23cm)	1/9	69	212	889	3	35	22	0.8	7	1.8	22	47	2.3	315	166	11	113	0.1	0.13	1.9	28
Pound cake, homemade (23cm X 13cm X 7.5cm)	1/10	91	391	1633	5	42	22	0.4	23	4.1	96	22	2.1	368	66	7	59	0.2	0.23	3.0	62
Shortcake, biscuit-type, homemade (4cm X 7.5cm diam)	1	75	234	978	5	34	8	1.0	8	2.4	28	106	1.7	459	96	12	100	0.2	0.24	3.1	72
Sponge, commercial, individual shell	1	25	72	302	1	15	9	0.1	1	0.2	26	18	0.7	61	25	3	34	0	0.07	0.8	18
Sponge, homemade (25cm diam)	1/12	63	187	782	5	36	N/A	0.2	3	0.8	107	26	1.0	144	89	6	63	0.1	0.19	1.7	33
White, from mix, with icing (2 layer, 23cm diam)	1/12	109	363	1518	3	66	51	0.9	10	1.6	N/A	41	0.9	342	76	15	138	0.1	0.12	1.9	47
White, homemade, with icing (2 layer, 23cm diam)	1/12	109	371	1553	3	70	56	0.3	9	2.5	1	50	1.3	205	55	5	41	0.1	0.14	1.9	33
White, frozen, commercial, with icing (1 layer, 5cm X 20cm diam)	1/6	85	283	1184	2	52	40	1.0	8	1.0	0	32	1.0	266	59	12	108	N/A	N/A	1.0	37
Yellow, from mix, with icing (2 layer, 23cm diam)	1/12	109	363	1519	4	64	47	0.9	11	2.0	46	60	1.1	338	74	15	137	0.1	0.14	2.0	57
Pies																					
Apple, commercial, 2 crust (23cm diam)	1/8	125	296	1239	2	43	20	2.0	14	4.7	0	14	0.6	333	81	9	30	tr	0.03	0.9	54
Apple, homemade, 2 crust (23cm diam)	1/8	155	411	1717	4	58	N/A	2.3	19	4.7	0	11	1.7	327	122	11	43	0.2	0.17	2.7	59
Banana cream, from mix, no-bake type (23cm diam)	1/8	92	231	966	3	29	N/A	0.6	12	6.4	27	67	0.4	267	104	11	154	0.1	0.13	1.4	28
Butter tart	1	54	248	1038	2	29	15	0.7	14	5.6	30	22	1.1	164	109	10	35	0.1	0.10	1.5	35
Cherry, commercial, 2 crust (23cm diam)	1/8	125	325	1359	3	50	18	1.0	14	3.2	0	15	2.0	308	101	10	36	0.2	0.16	2.5	50
Chocolate cream, commercial (20cm diam)	1/6	113	344	1436	3	38	N/A	2.3	22	5.6	6	41	1.2	154	144	24	77	tr	0.12	1.4	19
Coconut cream, commercial (20cm diam)	1/6	64	191	797	1	24	23	0.8	11	4.5	0	19	0.5	163	42	13	54	tr	0.05	0.4	5
Fried pie, fruit (13cm X 10cm)	1	128	404	1692	4	55	27	3.3	21	3.1	0	28	1.6	479	83	13	55	0.2	0.14	2.7	36

Food Name	Measure	Weight	Energy	Energy	Protein	Carbohydrate	Total Sugar	Total Dietary Fibre	Total Fat	Saturated Fat	Cholesterol	Calcium	Iron	Sodium	Potassium	Magnesium	Phosphorus	Thiamin	Riboflavin	Niacin	Folate
		g	kcal	kJ	g	g	g	g	g	g	mg	mg	mg	mg	mg	mg	mg	mg	mg	NE	DFE
Baked Goods																					
Lemon meringue, commercial (20cm diam)	1/6	113	303	1267	2	53	27	1.4	10	2.0	51	63	0.7	165	101	17	119	0.1	0.24	1.1	40
Mincemeat pie, homemade, 2 crust (23cm diam)	1/8	165	477	1995	4	79	47	4.3	18	4.4	0	36	2.5	419	335	23	69	0.2	0.17	2.7	59
Pecan, commercial (20cm diam)	1/6	113	452	1890	5	65	32	4.0	21	4.0	36	19	1.2	479	84	20	87	0.1	0.14	1.5	61
Pumpkin, commercial (20cm diam)	1/6	109	229	957	4	30	15	2.9	10	1.9	22	65	1.5	307	168	16	77	0.2	0.22	1.9	35
Sugar pie, homemade, 1 crust	1/8	88	407	1703	3	31	18	0.5	31	17.3	84	61	1.1	81	139	13	59	0.1	0.15	1.6	34
Other Baked Goods																					
Apple crisp, homemade	125mL	128	206	863	2	39	25	1.8	4	0.9	0	45	1.0	449	100	10	36	0.1	0.10	N/A	31
Bread pudding with raisins, homemade	125mL	106	162	677	6	24	15	0.9	5	1.8	61	124	1.2	252	228	18	111	0.1	0.26	2.1	31
Danish pastry, cinnamon (11cm diam)	1	65	262	1095	5	29	13	0.8	15	3.7	14	46	1.3	241	81	12	70	0.2	0.17	2.8	60
Danish pastry, fruit (11cm diam)	1	71	263	1102	4	34	20	1.3	13	3.5	81	33	1.3	251	59	11	63	0.2	0.16	2.2	49
Date squares, homemade	1 square	61	226	944	3	37	N/A	2.3	8	4.7	20	21	2.0	241	154	23	61	0.2	0.08	1.7	31
Doughnut, cake-type, plain (8cm diam)	1	47	198	828	2	23	11	0.7	11	1.7	17	21	0.9	257	60	9	126	0.1	0.11	1.4	39
Doughnut, cake-type, plain, chocolate coated (9cm diam)	1	57	270	1130	3	27	13	1.1	18	4.6	35	20	1.4	245	112	23	115	0.1	0.06	1.4	39
Doughnut, yeast-leavened, honey bun, glazed (9cm x 6cm)	1	60	242	1011	4	27	14	0.7	14	3.5	4	26	1.2	205	65	13	56	0.2	0.13	2.5	41
Doughnut, yeast-leavened, jelly filled (9cm X 6cm)	1	85	289	1209	5	33	18	0.8	16	4.1	22	21	1.5	249	67	17	72	0.3	0.12	2.8	88
Eclairs, custard filled, chocolate glaze	1	100	262	1096	6	24	7	0.6	16	4.1	127	63	1.2	337	117	15	107	0.1	0.27	2.1	63
Rice Krispies Squares™, commercial	1 square	22	91	381	1	18	N/A	0.1	2	0.3	0	1	0.3	77	9	3	9	0.3	0.30	3.7	38
Toaster pastries (Pop-Tarts™), brown sugar & cinnamon	1	50	206	862	3	34	N/A	0.5	7	1.8	0	17	2.0	212	57	12	67	0.2	0.29	2.8	21
Toaster pastries (Pop-Tarts™), fruit, frosted	1	55	215	900	2	39	20	0.4	6	1.5	0	16	3.9	387	81	13	75	0.2	0.20	N/A	39

You may wonder why the nutrition label of a food reports 0 grams of trans fat when hydrogenated oil, partly hydrogenated oil or shortening are listed as ingredients. If the amount of trans fat is lower than 0.2g per serving, it can be rounded down to 0g per serving.

Vegetables and Vegetable Products

Food Name	Measure	Weight	Energy	Energy	Protein	Carbohydrate	Total Sugar	Total Dietary Fibre	Total Fat	Calcium	Iron	Sodium	Potassium	Magnesium	Phosphorus	Vitamin A	Beta-carotene	Lycopene	Folate	Vitamin C	Vitamin B12
		g	kcal	kJ	g	g	g	g	g	mg	mg	mg	mg	mg	mg	RAE	mcg	mcg	DFE	mg	mcg
Vegetables and Vegetable Products																					
Vegetables																					
Alfalfa sprouts, raw	60mL	8	2	10	tr	tr	tr	0.2	tr	3	0.1	1	7	2	6	1	7	0	3	1	0
Artichoke hearts, canned in water	1 heart	27	13	56	1	3	tr	1.0	tr	12	0.3	74	95	16	23	2	28	0	14	3	0
Artichoke hearts, marinated in oil	1 heart	28	27	111	1	3	tr	1.0	2	12	0.3	79	93	16	23	2	28	0	13	3	0
Artichoke, boiled, drained	1 medium	120	60	251	4	13	1	4.7	tr	54	1.5	114	425	72	103	11	127	0	61	12	0
Asparagus, canned, drained	6 spears	108	21	85	2	3	1	1.5	1	17	2.0	310	186	11	46	44	532	26	104	20	0
Asparagus, fresh or frozen, boiled, drained	6 spears	90	18	75	2	3	1	1.6	tr	18	0.7	8	178	11	46	41	489	24	128	14	0
Bean sprouts, stir-fried	125mL	66	33	137	3	7	N/A	1.2	tr	9	1.2	6	143	22	52	1	12	N/A	46	10	0
Beans, lima, frozen, boiled, drained	125mL	95	100	417	6	18	1	4.0	tr	27	1.9	28	391	53	107	8	95	0	15	6	0
Beans, snap (green, yellow, Italian), canned, drained	125mL	71	14	60	1	3	1	1.5	tr	19	0.6	187	78	9	14	16	186	0	23	2	0
Beans, snap (green, yellow, Italian), fresh or frozen, boiled, drained	125mL	71	22	94	1	5	1	1.9	tr	33	0.5	4	97	15	21	22	269	0	20	5	0
Beets, pickled, sliced, not drained	125mL	120	78	326	1	20	N/A	2.2	tr	13	0.5	317	177	18	20	1	7	N/A	32	3	0
Beets, sliced, boiled, drained	125mL	90	40	165	2	9	7	1.8	tr	14	0.7	69	274	21	34	2	19	0	72	3	0
Beets, sliced, canned, drained	125mL	90	28	117	1	6	5	1.9	tr	13	1.6	174	133	15	15	1	13	0	27	6	0
Belgium endive, raw	1 endive	53	9	38	tr	2	N/A	1.6	tr	10	0.1	1	112	5	14	1	9	N/A	20	1	0
Bok Choy, Pak-Choi, shredded, boiled, drained	125mL	90	11	45	1	2	1	0.9	tr	84	0.9	31	333	10	26	190	2289	0	37	23	0
Broccoli, chopped, boiled, drained	125mL	82	29	120	2	6	1	2.0	tr	33	0.6	34	241	17	55	81	973	0	89	53	0
Broccoli, chopped, raw	125mL	46	16	66	1	3	1	1.1	tr	22	0.3	15	147	10	31	15	178	0	29	41	0
Broccoli, frozen spears, boiled, drained	125mL	97	27	114	3	5	1	2.3	tr	50	0.6	23	175	19	53	54	645	0	29	39	0
Brussels sprouts, fresh or frozen, boiled, drained	4 sprouts	84	33	137	3	6	2	3.2	tr	26	0.7	15	255	16	47	36	428	0	68	45	0
Cabbage, green, shredded, boiled, drained	125mL	79	17	73	1	4	2	1.3	tr	25	0.1	6	77	6	12	6	59	0	16	16	0
Cabbage, green, shredded, raw	125mL	37	9	37	1	2	1	0.7	tr	17	0.2	7	91	6	9	3	33	0	16	12	0
Cabbage, napa, shredded, boiled, drained	125mL	58	7	29	1	1	N/A	N/A	tr	17	0.4	6	50	5	11	7	77	0	25	2	0
Cabbage, red, shredded, raw	125mL	37	11	48	1	3	1	0.8	tr	17	0.3	10	90	6	11	21	248	7	7	21	0

Food Name	Measure	Weight	Energy	Energy	Protein	Carbohydrate	Total Sugar	Total Dietary Fibre	Total Fat	Calcium	Iron	Sodium	Potassium	Magnesium	Phosphorus	Vitamin A	Beta-carotene	Lycopene	Folate	Vitamin C	Vitamin B12
		g	kcal	kJ	g	g	g	g	g	mg	mg	mg	mg	mg	mg	RAE	mcg	mcg	DFE	mg	mcg
Vegetables and Vegetable Products																					
Carrots, baby, raw	8	80	28	117	1	7	4	1.4	tr	26	0.7	62	190	8	22	552	5113	0	26	7	0
Carrots, fresh or frozen, boiled, drained	125mL	77	28	116	1	6	3	1.9	tr	25	0.3	45	165	8	24	652	6333	1	10	2	0
Carrots, raw	1 medium	61	25	104	1	6	3	1.5	tr	20	0.2	42	195	7	21	367	3522	1	12	4	0
Cauliflower, pieces, boiled, drained	125mL	66	15	63	1	3	1	1.8	tr	10	0.2	10	93	6	21	1	5	0	29	29	0
Cauliflower, pieces, raw	125mL	53	13	55	1	3	1	0.9	tr	12	0.2	16	160	8	23	1	4	0	30	25	0
Celery, raw	1 stalk	40	6	24	tr	1	1	0.6	tr	16	0.1	32	104	4	10	9	108	0	14	1	0
Corn, sweet, canned, cream style	125mL	135	97	407	2	25	4	1.8	1	4	0.5	385	181	23	69	5	41	0	61	6	0
Corn, sweet, canned, niblets	125mL	111	88	366	3	22	4	2.3	1	6	0.5	302	206	26	71	4	37	0	54	6	0
Corn, sweet, on or off cob, fresh or frozen, boiled, drained	125mL	87	82	343	3	19	3	2.0	1	2	0.5	8	209	26	79	7	50	0	35	4	0
Cucumber, peeled, raw	4 slices	28	3	14	tr	1	tr	0.2	tr	4	0.1	1	38	3	6	1	9	0	4	1	0
Edamame	125mL	82	100	417	9	8	2	4.3	4	52	1.9	5	357	52	138	N/A	N/A	N/A	255	5	0
Eggplant, pieces, boiled, drained	125mL	52	18	76	tr	5	2	1.3	tr	3	0.1	1	64	6	8	1	12	0	7	1	0
Fiddleheads, frozen, boiled	125mL	98	33	139	4	6	N/A	0.9	tr	27	1.0	tr	244	26	78	171	1911	N/A	N/A	22	0
Fireweed leaves, raw	125mL	12	13	52	1	2	N/A	1.3	tr	52	0.3	4	60	19	13	22	262	N/A	14	tr	0
Hearts of palm, canned	2	66	18	77	2	3	N/A	1.6	tr	38	2.1	281	117	25	43	0	0	N/A	26	5	0
Kale, chopped, boiled, drained	125mL	69	19	80	1	4	1	1.4	tr	49	0.6	16	157	12	19	468	5613	0	9	28	0
Leeks, chopped, boiled, drained	125mL	55	17	71	tr	4	N/A	0.5	tr	16	0.6	5	48	8	9	1	15	N/A	13	2	0
Lettuce, Boston, shredded	250mL	58	8	31	1	1	1	0.6	tr	20	0.7	3	138	8	19	96	1155	0	42	2	0
Lettuce, iceberg, shredded	250mL	58	8	34	1	2	1	0.7	tr	10	0.2	6	82	4	12	15	174	0	17	2	0
Lettuce, looseleaf, shredded	250mL	59	9	37	1	2	tr	0.8	tr	21	0.5	17	115	8	17	219	2629	0	22	11	0
Lettuce, romaine, shredded	250mL	59	10	42	1	2	1	1.2	tr	20	0.6	5	146	8	18	172	2062	0	80	14	0
Lettuce, spring mix (mesclun)	250mL	58	12	50	1	2	tr	1.1	tr	43	0.7	21	202	19	23	124	1489	0	62	9	0
Mushrooms, pieces, canned, drained	125mL	82	21	87	2	4	2	2.3	tr	9	0.7	350	106	12	54	0	0	0	10	1	0
Mushrooms, portobello, grilled	125mL	85	30	124	4	4	0	1.9	1	3	0.5	9	443	13	128	0	0	0	16	0	0
Mushrooms, raw	3 medium	54	12	50	2	2	1	0.6	tr	2	0.3	2	170	5	46	0	0	0	9	1	0.02
Mushrooms, shiitake, sliced, stir-fried	125mL	57	27	115	2	4	tr	2.1	tr	1	0.3	3	186	11	63	0	0	0	8	0	0
Mushrooms, white, sliced, stir-fried	125mL	57	15	62	2	2	0	1.0	tr	2	0.1	7	226	6	60	0	0	0	11	0	0
Onions, green (scallion), raw	1 medium	15	5	20	tr	1	tr	0.4	tr	11	0.2	2	41	3	6	8	90	0	10	3	0
Onions, yellow, chopped, raw	60mL	41	17	71	tr	4	2	0.6	tr	9	0.1	1	58	4	11	0	tr	0	8	3	0

Food Name	Measure	Weight	Energy	Energy	Protein	Carbohydrate	Total Sugar	Total Dietary Fibre	Total Fat	Calcium	Iron	Sodium	Potassium	Magnesium	Phosphorus	Vitamin A	Beta-carotene	Lycopene	Folate	Vitamin C	Vitamin B12
		g	kcal	kJ	g	g	g	g	g	mg	mg	mg	mg	mg	mg	RAE	mcg	mcg	DFE	mg	mcg
Vegetables and Vegetable Products																					
Onions, yellow, chopped, sauteed	125mL	46	61	254	tr	4	2	0.8	5	9	0.1	6	61	4	15	N/A	N/A	N/A	N/A	1	0
Parsnip, sliced, boiled, drained	125mL	82	59	245	1	14	4	2.7	tr	30	0.5	8	302	24	57	0	0	0	48	11	0
Peas, green, canned, drained	125mL	90	62	260	4	11	4	4.0	tr	18	0.9	226	155	15	60	24	287	0	40	9	0
Peas, green, frozen, boiled, drained	125mL	85	66	276	4	12	4	3.7	tr	20	1.3	61	93	19	65	89	1057	0	50	8	0
Peas, snowpeas, boiled, drained	125mL	85	36	149	3	6	3	2.4	tr	36	1.7	3	203	22	46	44	505	0	25	40	0
Peas, snowpeas, raw	10	34	14	60	1	3	1	0.6	tr	15	0.7	1	68	8	18	18	214	0	14	20	0
Pepper, jalapeno, raw	1	14	4	18	tr	1	tr	0.4	tr	1	0.1	tr	30	3	4	6	64	0	7	6	0
Pepper, sweet, green, raw	1/2	82	16	69	1	4	2	1.2	tr	8	0.3	2	144	8	16	15	171	0	9	66	0
Pepper, sweet, green, sauteed	125mL	74	95	396	1	3	2	1.3	9	6	0.2	13	100	6	11	8	101	0	1	132	0
Pepper, sweet, red, raw	1/2	60	15	65	1	4	2	0.8	tr	4	0.3	1	126	7	15	93	966	183	11	113	0
Pepper, sweet, red, sauteed	125mL	74	99	413	1	5	3	1.3	9	5	0.4	16	144	9	17	98	1169	361	1	121	0
Pepper, sweet, yellow, raw	1/2	93	25	105	1	6	N/A	0.8	tr	10	0.4	2	197	11	22	9	112	N/A	24	171	0
Pepper, sweet, yellow, sauteed	125mL	74	36	149	1	5	0	0.6	2	9	0.3	175	153	9	18	30	86	0	19	132	tr
Potato, baked, flesh	1	156	145	607	3	34	3	3.4	tr	8	0.5	8	610	39	78	0	0	0	14	20	0
Potato, baked, flesh and skin	1	173	161	673	4	37	2	3.8	tr	26	1.9	17	926	48	121	2	10	0	48	17	0
Potato, boiled without skin	1	135	116	486	2	27	1	1.9	tr	11	0.4	7	443	27	54	0	3	0	12	10	0
Potato, boiled, flesh and skin	1	150	129	540	3	30	1	2.5	tr	13	1.3	7	572	34	67	0	0	0	15	18	0
Potato, canned, drained	4	140	84	351	2	19	N/A	1.3	tr	7	1.8	307	321	20	39	0	0	0	8	7	0
Potato, microwaved, flesh and skin	1	202	212	887	5	49	N/A	5.1	tr	22	2.5	16	903	55	212	0	0	0	24	31	0
Potato, microwaved, peeled after cooking	1	156	156	652	3	36	N/A	3.4	tr	8	0.6	11	641	39	170	0	0	0	19	24	0
Potatoes, French fried, frozen, home-prepared in oven	20 strips	48	96	403	2	15	tr	1.6	4	4	0.6	14	201	11	40	0	1	0	6	5	0
Potatoes, hashed brown, plain, frozen, heated	125mL	82	180	752	3	23	1	1.8	9	12	1.2	28	359	14	59	0	0	0	6	5	0
Potatoes, mashed, dried, with 2% milk and margarine	125mL	111	107	447	3	15	2	1.1	4	46	0.2	284	235	15	59	61	2	0	8	14	0.13
Potatoes, mashed, homemade with 2% milk and margarine	125mL	111	116	487	2	19	N/A	2.2	4	29	0.3	327	321	20	51	19	N/A	0	9	7	0.06
Potatoes, scalloped, from mix with water, with 2% milk and margarine	125mL	129	120	502	3	16	2	1.0	5	66	0.4	420	243	17	81	64	1	0	8	3	0.11
Potatoes, scalloped, homemade	125mL	129	111	466	4	14	N/A	2.5	5	74	0.7	434	489	25	82	N/A	83	0	16	14	0
Pumpkin, canned	125mL	129	44	184	1	10	4	3.8	tr	34	1.8	6	267	30	45	1007	8983	0	16	5	0
Radicchio, chopped	125mL	21	5	20	tr	1	tr	0.2	tr	4	0.1	5	64	3	8	tr	3	0	13	2	0

Food Name	Measure	Weight	Energy	Energy	Protein	Carbohydrate	Total Sugar	Total Dietary Fibre	Total Fat	Calcium	Iron	Sodium	Potassium	Magnesium	Phosphorus	Vitamin A	Beta-carotene	Lycopene	Folate	Vitamin C	Vitamin B12
		g	kcal	kJ	g	g	g	g	g	mg	mg	mg	mg	mg	mg	RAE	mcg	mcg	DFE	mg	mcg
Vegetables and Vegetable Products																					
Radishes	3 medium	14	2	9	tr	tr	tr	0.2	tr	3	tr	5	31	1	3	0	1	0	3	2	0
Rutabaga (yellow turnip), diced, boiled, drained	125mL	90	35	146	1	8	5	1.6	tr	43	0.5	18	293	21	50	13	1	0	13	17	0
Sauerkraut, canned, not drained	125mL	75	14	59	1	3	1	1.9	tr	23	1.1	496	128	10	15	1	6	0	18	11	0
Seaweed, dulse, dried	60mL	4	8	35	1	1	tr	0.1	tr	17	0.4	11	84	tr	14	62	740	N/A	35	9	0
Spinach, boiled, drained	125mL	95	22	91	3	4	tr	2.3	tr	129	3.4	67	443	83	53	498	5980	0	139	9	0
Spinach, chopped, raw	250mL	32	7	30	1	1	tr	0.7	tr	31	0.9	25	177	25	16	149	1783	0	61	9	0
Squash, acorn, cubed, baked	125mL	108	61	253	1	16	N/A	2.1	tr	48	1.0	4	473	47	49	23	277	N/A	21	12	0
Squash, butternut, cubed, baked	125mL	108	43	181	1	11	2	1.8	tr	44	0.6	4	308	31	29	413	4950	0	21	16	0
Squash, spaghetti, baked	125mL	82	22	93	1	5	2	0.9	tr	17	0.3	15	96	9	11	5	48	0	7	3	0
Sweet potato, baked, peeled after cooking	1/2	57	51	214	1	12	5	1.9	tr	22	0.4	21	271	15	31	548	6560	0	3	11	0
Sweet potato, boiled without skin	1/2	76	57	240	1	13	4	1.9	tr	20	0.5	20	174	14	24	594	7130	0	5	10	0
Swiss chard, chopped, boiled, drained	125mL	92	18	78	2	4	1	1.9	tr	54	2.1	165	508	80	31	283	3376	0	8	17	0
Tomatoes, canned, stewed	125mL	135	35	147	1	8	6	1.4	tr	46	1.8	298	279	16	27	12	140	5436	7	11	0
Tomatoes, canned, whole	125mL	127	22	90	1	5	3	1.0	tr	39	1.2	162	238	14	24	8	89	3423	10	18	0
Tomatoes, raw	1	123	22	92	1	5	3	1.5	tr	12	0.3	6	292	14	30	52	552	3165	18	16	0
Tomatoes, sun-dried	1 piece	2	5	22	tr	1	1	0.2	tr	2	0.2	42	69	4	7	1	10	815	1	1	0
Tomatoes, sun-dried, packed in oil, drained	1 piece	3	6	27	tr	1	N/A	0.2	tr	1	0.1	8	47	2	4	2	23	N/A	1	3	0
Turnip (white turnip), cubed, boiled, drained	125mL	82	18	76	1	4	2	1.6	tr	27	0.1	13	146	7	21	0	0	0	7	10	0
Vegetables, Asian mix (broccoli, carrots, green beans, "mini corn", snow peas, sweet red pepper), frozen, boiled, drained	125mL	74	29	122	1	6	2	1.8	tr	24	0.5	15	128	13	32	192	1878	tr	23	22	0
Vegetables, broccoli and cauliflower, frozen, boiled, drained	125mL	95	22	93	2	4	1	2.4	tr	33	0.5	20	152	14	38	27	322	0	34	34	0
Vegetables, mixed (corn, lima beans, snap beans, peas, carrots), frozen, boiled, drained	125mL	96	63	262	3	13	3	2.8	tr	24	0.8	34	163	21	49	206	2002	0	18	3	0
Vegetables, peas and carrots, canned, not drained	125mL	135	51	214	3	11	N/A	2.7	tr	31	1.0	350	135	19	62	389	0	N/A	24	9	0
Zucchini, raw, slices	4	40	6	27	tr	1	1	0.4	tr	6	0.1	4	104	7	15	4	48	0	11	7	0
Zucchini, sliced, boiled, drained	125mL	95	15	64	1	4	2	1.3	tr	12	0.3	3	241	21	38	53	637	0	16	4	0
Vegetable Juices and Other Products																					
Carrot juice	125mL	125	50	208	1	12	5	1.0	tr	30	0.6	36	364	17	52	966	11599	2	5	11	0
Coleslaw with dressing, homemade	125mL	63	44	183	1	8	N/A	1.0	2	29	0.4	15	115	6	20	34	87	N/A	17	21	0

Food Name	Measure	Weight	Energy	Energy	Protein	Carbohydrate	Total Sugar	Total Dietary Fibre	Total Fat	Calcium	Iron	Sodium	Potassium	Magnesium	Phosphorus	Vitamin A	Beta-carotene	Lycopene	Folate	Vitamin C	Vitamin B12
		g	kcal	kJ	g	g	g	g	g	mg	mg	mg	mg	mg	mg	RAE	mcg	mcg	DFE	mg	mcg
Vegetables and Vegetable Products																					
Potato salad, homemade	125mL	132	205	858	4	14	3	1.4	15	28	0.7	579	276	17	66	57	183	0	22	17	0.20
Tomato clam cocktail	125mL	128	61	257	1	14	4	0.5	tr	10	0.2	462	114	6	14	9	163	3807	10	6	0.04
Tomato juice	125mL	128	22	91	1	5	5	0.9	tr	13	0.6	345	294	14	23	30	347	11602	26	10	0
Tomato juice, without added salt	125mL	184	31	131	1	8	7	0.7	tr	18	0.8	18	421	20	33	42	N/A	16611	37	34	0
Tomato sauce for spaghetti, canned	125mL	132	143	600	2	21	N/A	1.9	6	37	0.9	652	505	32	47	82	967	N/A	28	15	0
Tomato sauce, canned	125mL	129	41	173	2	10	6	1.9	tr	17	1.3	678	428	21	34	22	271	19612	12	8	0
Vegetable juice cocktail	125mL	128	24	101	1	6	4	0.7	tr	14	0.5	345	247	14	22	100	1061	12351	27	35	0
Vegetable juice cocktail, low sodium	125mL	128	28	118	1	6	5	1.0	tr	14	0.5	89	247	14	22	66	1061	12350	27	35	0

Lycopene is a pigment responsible for the red colour of tomatoes, guava, papaya and a few other fruits. Processed tomato products like juice, sauce, paste and ketchup contain high amounts of lycopene.

Fruit and Fruit Juices

Food Name	Measure	Weight	Energy	Energy	Protein	Carbohydrate	Total Sugar	Total Dietary Fibre	Total Fat	Calcium	Iron	Sodium	Potassium	Magnesium	Phosphorus	Vitamin A	Beta-carotene	Lycopene	Folate	Vitamin C	Vitamin B12
		g	kcal	kJ	g	g	g	g	g	mg	mg	mg	mg	mg	mg	RAE	mcg	mcg	DFE	mg	mcg
Fruit and Fruit Juices																					
Fruit																					
Apple with skin (7cm.diam)	1	138	72	300	tr	19	14	2.6	tr	8	0.2	1	148	7	15	4	37	0	4	6	0
Applesauce, unsweetened	125mL	129	55	232	tr	15	13	1.5	tr	4	0.2	3	97	4	9	1	17	0	1	13	0
Apricots, dried	3	21	67	281	1	17	N/A	1.2	tr	13	1.3	3	389	13	33	133	0	0	1	2	0
Apricots, raw	3	105	50	211	1	12	10	2.1	tr	14	0.4	1	272	11	24	101	1149	0	9	11	0
Avocado	1/2	101	161	672	2	9	1	6.7	15	12	0.6	7	487	29	52	7	62	0	81	10	0
Banana	1	118	105	439	1	27	14	2.1	tr	6	0.3	1	422	32	26	4	31	0	24	10	0
Blackberries	125mL	76	33	137	1	7	4	4.0	tr	22	0.5	1	123	15	17	8	97	0	19	16	0
Blueberries, frozen, unsweetened	125mL	82	42	174	tr	10	7	2.6	1	7	0.1	1	44	4	9	2	23	0	6	2	0
Blueberries, raw	125mL	77	44	182	1	11	8	2.0	tr	5	0.2	1	59	5	9	2	25	0	5	7	0
Cherries, sweet	10	68	43	179	1	11	9	1.4	tr	9	0.2	0	151	7	14	2	26	0	3	5	0
Clementine	1	74	35	146	1	9	7	1.3	tr	22	0.1	1	131	7	16	N/A	N/A	N/A	18	36	0
Cranberries, dried, sweetened	60mL	31	95	396	tr	25	20	1.8	tr	3	0.2	1	12	2	2	0	0	0	0	tr	0
Dates, dried	3	25	70	294	1	19	16	2.0	tr	10	0.3	tr	163	11	15	0	1	0	5	tr	0
Figs, dried	2	17	42	175	1	11	8	1.6	tr	27	0.3	2	114	11	11	tr	1	0	2	tr	0
Figs, raw	1	50	37	155	tr	10	8	1.5	tr	18	0.2	1	116	9	7	4	43	0	3	1	0
Fruit cocktail, canned, juice pack	125mL	125	58	240	1	15	14	1.3	tr	10	0.3	5	119	9	18	19	193	0	4	3	0
Fruit cocktail, canned, light syrup pack	125mL	128	73	304	1	19	18	1.3	tr	8	0.4	8	114	6	14	13	133	0	4	2	0
Fruit salad, tropical, canned, heavy syrup pack	125mL	136	117	489	1	30	N/A	1.8	tr	18	0.7	3	178	18	10	8	102	N/A	12	24	0
Fruit salad, tropical, canned, juice pack	125mL	131	70	272	1	18	16	1.1	tr	17	0.3	4	160	14	10	8	96	0	4	16	0
Grapefruit, pink or red	1/2	123	52	216	1	13	8	2.0	tr	27	0.1	0	166	11	22	71	844	1745	16	38	0
Grapefruit, white	1/2	118	39	163	1	10	9	2.1	tr	14	0.1	0	175	11	9	2	17	0	12	39	0
Grapes	20	100	69	289	1	18	15	1.2	tr	10	0.4	2	191	7	20	3	39	0	2	11	0
Groundcherries	10	49	26	108	1	5	N/A	N/A	tr	4	0.5	tr	75	N/A	19	17	210	N/A	3	5	0
Kiwifruit	1	76	46	194	1	11	7	2.3	tr	26	0.2	2	237	13	26	3	40	0	19	70	0
Lychees (litchis)	10	96	63	265	1	16	15	1.2	tr	5	0.3	1	164	10	30	0	0	0	13	69	0

Food Name	Measure	Weight	Energy	Energy	Protein	Carbohydrate	Total Sugar	Total Dietary Fibre	Total Fat	Calcium	Iron	Sodium	Potassium	Magnesium	Phosphorus	Vitamin A	Beta-carotene	Lycopene	Folate	Vitamin C	Vitamin B12
		g	kcal	kJ	g	g	g	g	g	mg	mg	mg	mg	mg	mg	RAE	mcg	mcg	DFE	mg	mcg
Fruit and Fruit Juices																					
Mango	1/2	104	67	282	1	18	15	1.9	tr	10	0.1	2	161	9	11	39	461	0	14	29	0
Melon, cantaloupe, cubes	125mL	85	29	120	1	7	7	0.6	tr	8	0.2	14	226	10	13	143	1708	0	18	31	0
Melon, honeydew, cubes	125mL	90	32	136	tr	8	7	0.7	tr	5	0.2	16	205	9	10	3	27	0	17	16	0
Melon, watermelon, cubes	125mL	80	24	100	tr	6	5	0.3	tr	6	0.2	1	90	8	9	22	243	3639	2	7	0
Nectarine	1	136	60	250	1	14	11	2.3	tr	8	0.4	0	273	12	35	18	204	0	7	7	0
Orange	1	131	62	258	1	15	12	2.3	tr	52	0.1	0	237	13	18	8	93	0	39	70	0
Papaya, cubes	125mL	74	29	121	tr	7	4	1.3	tr	18	0.1	2	190	7	4	17	204	0	28	46	0
Peach	1	98	38	160	1	9	8	1.9	tr	6	0.2	0	186	9	20	16	159	0	3	6	0
Peach, canned halves or slices, juice pack	125mL	132	58	243	1	15	14	1.7	tr	8	0.4	5	169	9	22	25	250	0	4	5	0
Peach, canned halves or slices, light syrup pack	125mL	133	72	300	1	19	18	1.7	tr	4	0.5	7	129	7	15	24	233	0	4	9	0
Peach, canned halves or slices, water pack	125mL	129	31	129	1	8	6	1.7	tr	3	0.4	4	128	6	13	35	340	0	4	4	0
Pear with skin	1	166	96	403	1	26	16	5.0	tr	15	0.3	2	198	12	18	2	22	0	12	7	0
Pear, canned halves, juice pack	125mL	131	66	274	tr	17	13	2.1	tr	12	0.4	5	126	9	16	0	4	0	1	2	0
Pear, canned halves, light syrup pack	125mL	133	76	316	tr	20	16	2.1	tr	7	0.4	7	88	5	9	0	0	0	1	2	0
Pear, canned halves, water pack	125mL	128	37	155	tr	10	8	2.0	tr	5	0.3	3	68	5	9	0	0	0	1	1	0
Pineapple, canned, juice pack	125mL	132	79	330	1	21	19	1.2	tr	18	0.4	1	160	18	8	3	30	0	7	12	0
Pineapple, cubes	125mL	82	42	174	tr	11	8	1.1	tr	11	0.2	1	88	10	7	2	28	0	16	46	0
Plantain, baked or boiled, sliced	125mL	81	94	395	1	25	11	1.9	tr	2	0.5	4	378	26	23	37	300	0	21	9	0
Plum	1	66	30	127	tr	8	7	1.1	tr	4	0.1	0	104	5	11	11	125	0	3	6	0
Pomegranate (9.5cm diam)	1/2	77	53	220	1	13	13	0.5	tr	2	0.2	2	200	2	6	2	31	0	5	5	0
Prunes, dried	3	25	60	253	1	16	10	1.8	tr	11	0.2	1	184	10	17	10	99	0	1	tr	0
Prunes, dried, cooked, without added sugar	60mL	63	67	281	1	18	16	3.6	tr	12	0.3	1	202	11	19	11	109	0	0	2	0
Raisins	60mL	37	110	460	1	29	22	1.3	tr	18	0.7	4	275	12	37	0	0	0	2	1	0
Raspberries	125mL	65	34	141	1	8	3	4.2	tr	16	0.4	1	98	14	19	1	8	0	14	17	0
Rhubarb, frozen, cooked, with added sugar	125mL	127	147	615	tr	40	36	2.5	tr	184	0.3	1	122	15	10	5	56	0	6	4	0
Strawberries	7	84	27	113	1	6	4	1.9	tr	13	0.4	1	129	11	20	1	6	0	20	49	0
Strawberries, frozen, unsweetened	125mL	117	41	170	1	11	5	1.8	tr	19	0.9	2	173	13	15	2	32	0	20	48	0
Tangerine (mandarin)	1	84	45	186	1	11	9	1.5	tr	31	0.1	2	139	10	17	11	130	0	13	22	0
Tangerine (mandarin), canned, juice pack, drained	125mL	100	38	159	1	9	8	1.2	tr	12	0.3	5	136	11	11	25	298	0	5	34	0

Food Name	Measure	Weight	Energy	Energy	Protein	Carbohydrate	Total Sugar	Total Dietary Fibre	Total Fat	Calcium	Iron	Sodium	Potassium	Magnesium	Phosphorus	Vitamin A	Beta-carotene	Lycopene	Folate	Vitamin C	Vitamin B12
		g	kcal	kJ	g	g	g	g	g	mg	mg	mg	mg	mg	mg	RAE	mcg	mcg	DFE	mg	mcg
Fruit and Fruit Juices																					
Fruit Juices																					
Apple juice, ready-to-drink, vitamin C added	125mL	126	59	249	tr	15	14	0.1	tr	9	0.5	4	150	4	9	0	0	0	tr	52	0
Cranberry juice cocktail, ready-to-drink, vitamin C added	125mL	134	76	318	0	19	16	0.1	tr	4	0.2	3	24	3	3	0	0	0	0	48	0
Cranberry juice, unsweetened, ready-to-drink	125mL	134	61	257	1	16	16	0.1	tr	11	0.3	3	103	8	17	3	36	0	1	12	0
Cranberry-apple juice-drink, ready-to-drink, low Calorie, vitamin C added	125mL	127	24	100	tr	6	6	0.1	0	13	0.1	6	57	4	1	1	8	0	0	41	0
Grape juice, frozen, sweetened, diluted, vitamin C added	125mL	132	67	281	tr	17	17	0.1	tr	5	0.1	3	28	5	5	0	7	0	1	20	0
Grape juice, ready-to-drink, vitamin C added	125mL	132	81	337	1	20	20	0.1	tr	12	0.3	4	174	13	15	0	7	0	4	32	0
Grapefruit juice, ready-to-drink unsweetened or freshly squeezed	125mL	130	50	210	1	12	12	0.4	tr	10	0.3	1	206	14	17	1	11	0	13	44	0
Grapefruit juice, ready-to-drink, sweetened	125mL	132	61	254	1	15	15	0.1	tr	11	0.5	3	214	13	15	0	4	0	13	36	0
Lemon juice, canned or bottled	15mL	15	3	14	tr	1	tr	0.1	tr	2	tr	3	16	1	1	tr	tr	0	2	4	0
Lime juice, canned or bottled	15mL	16	3	14	tr	1	tr	0.1	tr	2	tr	2	12	1	2	tr	2	0	1	1	0
Nectar, apricot	125mL	133	74	310	tr	19	18	0.8	tr	9	0.5	4	151	7	12	88	1042	0	1	44	0
Nectar, mango	125mL	133	68	281	tr	17	17	0.4	tr	23	0.5	7	32	4	3	46	533	0	9	20	0
Orange and grapefruit juice, ready-to-drink	125mL	130	56	235	1	13	13	0.1	tr	10	0.6	4	206	13	18	8	26	0	18	38	0
Orange juice, frozen, diluted	125mL	132	59	247	1	14	11	0.3	tr	12	0.1	1	250	13	21	7	22	0	58	51	0
Orange juice, ready-to-drink	125mL	132	58	242	1	13	N/A	0.3	tr	13	0.2	1	250	14	14	5	61	0	24	43	0
Orange juice, ready-to-drink, refrigerated, vitamin D and calcium added	125mL	132	58	242	1	13	N/A	0.3	tr	185	0.2	1	250	14	14	5	N/A	0	N/A	43	0
Orange, strawberry and banana juice, ready-to-drink	125mL	124	57	237	1	15	13	0.2	tr	14	0.3	5	124	12	15	1	21	0	21	31	0
Pineapple juice, ready-to-drink, vitamin C added	125mL	132	74	309	tr	18	13	0.3	tr	22	0.3	1	177	17	11	0	4	0	30	32	0
Pomegranate juice, ready-to-drink	125mL	128	72	300	0	20	17	0	0	0	0	5	215	N/A	N/A	0	N/A	N/A	N/A	0	0
Prune juice, ready-to-drink	125mL	135	96	402	1	24	22	1.4	tr	16	1.6	5	373	19	34	0	3	0	0	6	0

Did you know that fruit «juice» does not contain added sugar?
You can tell if sugar or sweeteners have been added to a product by looking for the words «drink», «beverage», «cocktail» or «punch».

Dairy Foods and Other Related Products

Food Name	Measure	Weight	Energy	Energy	Protein	Carbohydrate	Total Sugar	Total Fat	Saturated Fat	Cholesterol	Calcium	Iron	Sodium	Potassium	Magnesium	Phosphorus	Vitamin A	Vitamin D	Folate	Vitamin B12	Riboflavin
		g	kcal	kJ	g	g	g	g	g	mg	mg	mg	mg	mg	mg	mg	RAE	mcg	DFE	mcg	mg
Dairy Foods and Other Related Products																					
Milk and Substitutes																					
Buttermilk	250mL	259	104	432	9	12	12	2	1.4	10	300	0.1	272	391	28	230	18	0.2	13	0.57	0.40
Milk, chocolate, 1% M.F.	250mL	264	166	695	9	28	26	3	1.6	8	304	0.6	161	449	34	272	153	2.6	13	0.90	0.44
Milk, chocolate, 2% M.F.	250mL	264	190	795	8	27	26	5	3.3	18	301	0.6	158	446	34	269	145	2.6	13	0.90	0.43
Milk, skim	250mL	259	88	368	9	13	13	tr	0.2	5	324	0.1	109	404	28	261	158	2.7	13	1.37	0.47
Milk, partly skimmed, 1% M.F.	250mL	258	108	454	9	13	13	3	1.6	13	307	0.1	113	387	28	245	150	2.6	13	1.13	0.48
Milk, partly skimmed, 2% M.F.	250mL	258	129	539	9	12	13	5	3.3	21	302	0.1	106	387	28	242	142	2.8	13	1.19	0.48
Milk, partly skimmed, 2% M.F., with added milk solids	250mL	260	146	608	10	14	14	5	3.2	21	372	0.2	153	473	42	291	143	2.6	16	1.12	0.50
Milk, whole, 3.3% M.F.	250mL	258	155	647	8	12	14	8	5.4	26	291	0.1	103	369	26	235	72	2.7	13	1.13	0.47
Rice beverage, flavoured and unflavoured, enriched	250mL	259	127	531	tr	26	N/A	2	0.2	0	319	0.2	91	72	10	36	52	2.2	96	1.03	0.03
Soy beverage, chocolate, enriched	250mL	257	162	673	6	26	20	4	0.6	0	323	1.2	136	367	38	131	180	2.6	29	1.80	0.67
Soy beverage, original and vanilla, enriched	250mL	257	110	465	7	13	9	4	0.5	0	316	1.1	120	313	38	110	142	2.7	23	2.19	0.47
Soy beverage, unsweetened, enriched	250mL	257	85	354	7	4	1	4	0.5	0	318	1.2	95	308	41	82	160	3.1	18	2.85	0.53
Processed Milk																					
Milk, condensed, sweetened, canned (Eagle Brand™)	15mL	19	62	260	2	11	11	2	1.1	7	55	tr	25	72	5	49	14	N/A	2	0.09	0.08
Milk, evaporated, partly skimmed, canned, diluted, 2% M.F.	250mL	258	122	512	10	15	13	3	1.6	10	369	0.3	149	422	35	264	104	2.9	11	0.28	0.41
Milk, evaporated, partly skimmed, canned, undiluted, 2% M.F.	15mL	16	15	62	1	2	2	tr	0.2	1	44	tr	18	51	4	32	12	0.3	1	0.03	0.05
Milk, evaporated, skim, canned, diluted, 0.2% M.F.	250mL	259	105	438	10	15	15	tr	0.2	5	392	0.4	157	446	38	262	159	2.9	12	0.32	0.42
Milk, evaporated, skim, canned, undiluted, 0.2% M.F.	15mL	16	13	53	1	2	2	tr	tr	1	47	tr	19	54	4	32	19	0.4	1	0.04	0.05
Milk, evaporated, whole, canned, diluted, 7.8% M.F.	250mL	258	178	744	9	13	13	10	6.3	39	349	0.3	143	403	33	270	86	2.9	11	0.21	0.42
Milk, evaporated, whole, canned, undiluted, 7.8% M.F.	15mL	16	21	89	1	2	2	1	0.8	5	42	tr	17	48	4	32	10	0.3	1	0.03	0.05
Milk, reconstituted, from skim milk powder	250mL	259	86	360	8	13	13	tr	0.1	4	301	0.1	137	410	30	237	170	2.6	12	0.96	0.42
Skim milk powder	5mL	1	5	22	1	1	1	tr	tr	tr	18	tr	8	25	2	14	10	0.2	1	0.06	0.03

Food Name	Measure	Weight	Energy	Energy	Protein	Carbohydrate	Total Sugar	Total Fat	Saturated Fat	Cholesterol	Calcium	Iron	Sodium	Potassium	Magnesium	Phosphorus	Vitamin A	Vitamin D	Folate	Vitamin B12	Riboflavin
		g	kcal	kJ	g	g	g	g	g	mg	mg	mg	mg	mg	mg	mg	RAE	mcg	DFE	mcg	mg
Dairy Foods and Other Related Products																					
Milk Beverages																					
Chocolate milk, chocolate flavour powder + 2% milk	250mL	279	207	863	9	33	N/A	6	3.4	20	321	0.8	176	531	59	274	143	2.8	N/A	0.92	0.46
Chocolate milk, syrup + 2% milk	250mL	298	238	998	10	38	N/A	5	3.3	21	319	1.0	158	489	60	298	146	2.8	15	0.95	0.45
Eggnog	250mL	268	362	1516	10	36	23	20	11.9	158	349	0.5	145	443	51	293	121	1.1	3	1.21	0.51
Hot chocolate, aspartame sweetened, powder + water	250mL	270	78	326	3	15	9	1	0	0	127	1.1	240	569	46	189	38	N/A	3	0.35	0.29
Hot chocolate, homemade with cocoa + 2% milk	250mL	264	203	851	9	28	26	6	3.8	21	277	1.3	116	520	61	277	135	2.6	13	1.11	0.48
Hot chocolate, powder + 2% milk	250mL	264	255	1068	10	41	37	6	3.8	20	318	0.5	272	595	55	327	126	2.5	11	1.52	0.62
Hot chocolate, powder + water	250mL	291	160	669	2	34	30	2	0.9	3	64	0.5	206	285	35	125	0	N/A	0	0.52	0.23
Instant breakfast powder + 2% milk	250mL	280	260	1087	16	36	12	5	3.1	24	555	3.9	286	811	61	459	444	2.6	12	2.21	1.41
Milk shake, chocolate	250mL	249	296	1240	8	53	52	7	4.2	27	329	0.8	276	558	40	314	45	1.0	12	0.80	0.55
Milk shake, vanilla	250mL	249	279	1166	10	44	44	8	4.7	30	364	0.2	237	456	30	286	62	0.5	17	1.30	0.49
Yogourts and Fermented Milk Products																					
Drinkable yogourt	200mL	207	145	607	5	24	24	3	2.1	12	191	0.2	81	257	23	157	N/A	0.2	25	0.58	0.23
Fresh cheese (Danimal™, Minigo™)	1	60	68	286	3	10	10	2	1.1	6	138	0.1	32	84	7	50	N/A	N/A	N/A	N/A	N/A
Kefir, plain	175mL	165	104	433	6	7	6	6	3.8	25	187	0.1	70	250	19	148	58	0.2	23	0.33	0.30
Yogourt parfait with berries and granola	175mL	188	233	973	7	40	3	5	2.7	14	208	2.2	119	337	36	201	23	0	40	0.59	0.31
Yogourt, plain, 1-2% M.F.	175mL	181	114	477	10	13	13	3	1.8	11	332	0.1	127	424	31	261	25	N/A	20	1.01	0.39
Yogourt, plain, 2-4% M.F.	175mL	181	129	538	9	12	8	5	3.3	17	292	0.1	111	412	28	246	31	N/A	21	1.03	0.42
Yogourt, plain, fat-free	175mL	189	79	332	8	11	9	tr	0	6	253	0.1	113	368	26	215	N/A	1.8	N/A	0.89	0.32
Yogourt, vanilla or fruit, 1-2% M.F.	175mL	185	183	767	7	30	25	4	2.3	17	227	0.1	98	335	20	167	N/A	N/A	N/A	0.31	0.15
Yogourt, vanilla or fruit, fat-free	175mL	181	116	484	8	21	19	tr	tr	4	229	0.2	103	349	20	163	N/A	N/A	N/A	0.59	N/A
Yogourt, vanilla or fruit, fat-free with sugar substitute	175mL	189	94	394	7	16	14	tr	0	6	205	0.2	92	311	22	179	N/A	1.4	N/A	0.72	0.27
Cheese																					
Blue	50g	50	177	738	11	1	tr	14	9.3	38	264	0.2	698	128	12	194	99	0.2	18	0.61	0.19
Brick	50g	50	186	776	12	1	tr	15	9.4	47	337	0.2	280	68	12	226	146	0.2	10	0.63	0.18
Brie	50g	50	167	699	10	tr	tr	14	8.7	50	92	0.3	315	76	10	94	87	0.2	33	0.83	0.26
Camembert	50g	50	150	628	10	tr	tr	12	7.6	36	194	0.2	421	94	10	174	121	0.2	31	0.65	0.24
Cheddar	50g	50	202	843	12	1	tr	17	10.5	53	361	0.3	311	49	14	256	133	0.1	9	0.42	0.19
Cheddar, low fat (18% M.F.)	50g	50	141	590	14	1	N/A	9	5.8	28	453	0.1	363	47	18	292	75	N/A	10	0.83	0.15

Food Name	Measure	Weight	Energy	Energy	Protein	Carbohydrate	Total Sugar	Total Fat	Saturated Fat	Cholesterol	Calcium	Iron	Sodium	Potassium	Magnesium	Phosphorus	Vitamin A	Vitamin D	Folate	Vitamin B12	Riboflavin
		g	kcal	kJ	g	g	g	g	g	mg	mg	mg	mg	mg	mg	mg	RAE	mcg	DFE	mcg	mg
Dairy Foods and Other Related Products																					
Cottage cheese (1% M.F.)	125mL	119	86	359	15	3	3	1	0.8	5	73	0.2	500	103	6	160	13	N/A	14	0.75	0.20
Cream cheese, light	30mL	30	70	294	3	2	tr	5	3.4	17	34	0.5	90	51	2	44	56	N/A	5	0.18	0.09
Cream cheese, regular	30mL	29	103	430	2	1	tr	10	6.5	32	24	0.4	87	35	2	31	108	N/A	4	0.12	0.06
Edam	50g	50	179	747	12	1	1	14	8.8	45	366	0.2	483	94	15	268	122	0.5	8	0.77	0.19
Feta	50g	50	132	552	7	2	2	11	7.7	46	247	0.3	558	31	10	169	63	0.2	16	0.87	0.44
Goat cheese, soft	50g	50	134	561	9	tr	tr	11	7.3	23	70	1.0	184	13	8	128	144	0.2	6	0.10	0.19
Gouda	50g	50	178	745	13	1	1	14	9.0	58	350	0.1	410	61	15	273	83	0.2	11	0.78	0.17
Gruyere	50g	50	207	864	15	tr	tr	16	9.5	55	506	0.1	168	41	18	303	136	0.2	5	0.80	0.14
Imitation cheese	50g	50	120	500	8	6	4	7	4.4	18	281	0.2	673	121	15	356	57	0	4	0.20	0.22
Mozzarella (22.5% M.F.)	50g	50	141	588	10	1	1	11	6.8	39	269	0.1	187	34	10	186	90	0.1	4	0.33	0.13
Mozzarella, partially skimmed (16.5% M.F.)	50g	50	127	531	13	1	1	8	5.2	29	323	0.1	241	42	12	239	64	0.1	5	0.41	0.16
Parmesan, grated	15mL	6	27	114	2	tr	tr	2	1.1	6	70	0.1	97	8	2	46	8	tr	1	0.14	0.03
Processed cheese food, thin slices	1	21	78	327	5	tr	tr	7	4.1	20	115	tr	310	35	6	107	53	tr	2	0.15	0.07
Processed cheese food, thin slices, light	1	21	50	209	4	2	2	3	1.8	11	110	tr	331	69	7	173	53	tr	4	0.23	0.10
Processed cheese spread (Cheez Whiz™)	30mL	31	90	375	5	3	N/A	7	4.1	17	174	0.1	503	75	9	271	N/A	0.1	2	0.12	0.13
Processed cheese spread, light (Light Cheez Whiz™)	30mL	31	69	287	6	4	3	3	2.2	13	178	tr	491	107	9	317	91	N/A	N/A	N/A	0.20
Ricotta cheese, partly skimmed milk	125mL	131	181	756	15	7	tr	10	6.5	41	356	0.6	164	164	20	240	140	N/A	17	0.38	0.24
Romano, grated	15mL	6	25	103	2	tr	tr	2	1.1	7	67	tr	76	5	3	48	6	tr	tr	0.07	0.02
Swiss (Emmental)	50g	50	190	795	13	3	1	14	8.9	46	396	0.1	96	39	19	284	110	0.6	3	1.67	0.15
Swiss, processed, thin slices	1	21	70	291	5	tr	tr	5	3.3	18	161	0.1	285	45	6	159	41	0.2	1	0.26	0.06
Cream																					
Half and half, 10% M.F.	15mL	15	18	76	tr	1	tr	2	1.0	5	16	tr	6	20	2	15	15	tr	tr	0.05	0.02
Sour cream, 14% M.F.	15mL	15	22	93	tr	1	tr	2	1.3	6	16	tr	6	19	1	14	17	0.1	2	0.04	0.02
Sour cream, light, 5% M.F.	15mL	16	21	89	1	1	tr	2	1.0	6	22	tr	11	33	2	11	14	N/A	2	0.07	0.02
Table cream (coffee cream), 18% M.F.	15mL	15	28	118	tr	1	tr	3	1.7	9	15	tr	6	19	1	13	25	0.1	tr	0.04	0.02
Whipped, pressurized	60mL	15	39	164	tr	2	1	3	2.1	12	15	tr	20	22	2	14	29	0.1	tr	0.04	0.01
Whipping cream, 35% M.F., not whipped	15mL	15	49	207	tr	tr	tr	5	3.3	19	10	tr	5	12	1	9	62	0.1	1	0.03	0.02
Whipping cream, 35% M.F., sweetened, whipped	60mL	30	100	419	1	3	2	10	6.2	36	19	tr	10	23	2	17	117	0.2	1	0.05	0.03

Food Name	Measure	Weight	Energy	Energy	Protein	Carbohydrate	Total Sugar	Total Fat	Saturated Fat	Cholesterol	Calcium	Iron	Sodium	Potassium	Magnesium	Phosphorus	Vitamin A	Vitamin D	Folate	Vitamin B12	Riboflavin
		g	kcal	kJ	g	g	g	g	g	mg	mg	mg	mg	mg	mg	mg	RAE	mcg	DFE	mcg	mg
Dairy Foods and Other Related Products																					
Imitation Cream Products																					
Coffee whitener, frozen liquid	15mL	15	21	87	tr	2	2	2	0.3	0	1	tr	12	29	0	10	tr	0	0	0	0
Coffee whitener, powdered	5mL	2	11	45	tr	1	1	1	0.6	0	tr	tr	4	16	tr	8	tr	0	0	0	tr
Coffee whitener, powdered, light	5mL	2	9	36	tr	1	1	tr	0.1	0	tr	tr	5	18	0	3	tr	0	tr	0	0
Dessert topping, frozen	60mL	19	60	253	tr	4	4	5	4.1	0	1	tr	5	3	tr	2	1	0	0	0	0
Dessert topping, frozen, low fat	60mL	19	42	175	1	4	4	2	2.1	tr	14	tr	14	19	1	14	1	N/A	1	0.04	0.02
Dessert topping, powdered, prepared with 2% milk	60mL	20	37	153	1	3	3	2	2.0	1	19	tr	12	31	2	18	9	0.2	1	0.07	0.03
Dessert topping, pressurized	60mL	18	47	196	tr	3	3	4	3.4	0	1	tr	11	3	tr	3	1	0	0	0	0
Pudding																					
All flavours, instant, from mix, prepared with 2% milk	125mL	139	149	623	4	27	23	3	1.6	9	141	0.2	391	206	18	307	65	1.3	6	0.54	0.23
Chocolate, ready-to-eat	1 unit	99	138	575	3	23	18	4	0.7	3	89	0.5	128	178	21	79	10	N/A	3	0	0.15
Chocolate, ready-to-eat, fat-free	1 unit	99	96	402	3	20	15	tr	0.2	1	72	0.8	168	139	19	75	47	N/A	4	0.22	0.15
Rice, homemade	125mL	119	160	669	4	32	19	2	1.2	7	115	0.3	55	211	18	112	51	1.0	5	0.24	0.19
Rice, ready-to-eat	1 unit	99	161	675	2	22	N/A	7	1.2	1	51	0.3	84	59	8	67	25	0.1	3	0.21	0.07
Tapioca, ready-to-eat	1 unit	99	118	493	2	19	18	4	0.6	1	83	0.2	157	95	8	78	0	N/A	3	0.21	0.10
Tapioca, ready-to-eat, fat-free	1 unit	99	88	368	2	20	16	tr	0	1	50	0.3	210	52	5	40	32	N/A	2	0.15	0.10
Vanilla, ready-to-eat	1 unit	99	128	534	2	22	20	4	0.6	7	87	0.1	134	112	8	67	6	N/A	0	0.10	0.14
Vanilla, ready-to-eat, fat-free	1 unit	99	92	385	2	22	16	tr	tr	1	59	0.4	211	71	7	49	40	N/A	3	0.19	0.12

Fortified soy beverages can be an important source of calcium and vitamin D for people who do not drink milk.

Eggs and Egg Dishes

Food Name	Measure	Weight	Energy	Energy	Protein	Carbohydrate	Total Fat	Saturated Fat	Monounsaturated Fat	Polyunsaturated Fat	Cholesterol	Calcium	Iron	Sodium	Potassium	Phosphorus	Vitamin A	Vitamin D	Folate	Vitamin B12	Vitamin E
		g	kcal	kJ	g	g	g	g	g	g	mg	mg	mg	mg	mg	mg	RAE	mcg	DFE	mcg	mg
Eggs and Egg Dishes																					
Egg substitute, frozen (yolk replaced), cooked	2 eggs	111	226	947	14	4	17	2.9	4.6	8.8	2	89	2.4	291	258	88	60	1.9	14	0.35	2.2
Egg white, cooked	1 large	33	16	66	3	tr	0	0	0	0	0	3	tr	106	39	4	0	0	0	0.01	0
Egg yolk, cooked	1 large	17	59	249	3	1	6	1.7	2.3	0.8	202	22	0.7	34	17	64	106	0.8	30	0.88	1.4
Egg, fried	2 large	92	173	726	12	2	14	3.6	5.8	2.7	367	46	1.4	322	116	127	236	1.9	54	1.62	2.7
Egg, hard-boiled	1 large	50	78	324	6	1	5	1.6	2.0	0.7	216	25	0.6	62	63	86	85	0.7	22	0.56	0.5
Egg, poached	1 large	50	74	308	6	tr	5	1.5	1.9	0.7	215	27	0.9	147	67	95	70	0.4	24	0.64	0.5
Eggs benedict	2 eggs	310	572	2393	34	30	35	12.5	14.2	4.9	458	189	4.0	2015	456	453	265	2.1	113	1.96	1.7
Eggs, scrambled, made with 2 eggs	2 eggs	124	189	792	13	4	14	4.1	5.9	2.7	363	90	1.4	476	171	160	253	2.3	55	1.73	2.6
Omelet, cheese, made with 2 eggs	1 omelet	150	273	1142	18	5	20	8.0	7.8	2.8	376	238	1.6	890	241	356	304	2.3	56	1.99	2.7
Omelet, spanish, made with 2 eggs (mushrooms, onions, green peppers, tomatoes)	1 omelet	290	319	1336	15	13	24	5.7	10.4	6.3	353	111	1.8	607	514	211	403	4.3	72	1.70	3.7
Omelet, western, made with 2 eggs (green peppers, ham, onions)	1 omelet	158	237	993	17	5	17	5.1	7.3	2.9	346	86	1.5	720	258	202	231	2.2	53	1.72	2.5

There are no nutritional differences between brown eggs and white eggs.

Fish and Shellfish

Food Name	Measure	Weight	Energy	Energy	Protein	Carbohydrate	Total Fat	Saturated Fat	Polyunsaturated Fat	DHA	EPA	Cholesterol	Calcium	Iron	Sodium	Potassium	Phosphorus	Vitamin A	Vitamin D	Vitamin B12	Vitamin E
		g	kcal	kJ	g	g	g	g	g	g	g	mg	mg	mg	mg	mg	mg	RAE	mcg	mcg	mg
Fish and Shellfish																					
Fish																					
Anchovies, canned in oil, drained solids	2	8	17	70	2	0	1	0.2	0.2	0.10	0.06	7	19	0.4	293	44	20	1	0.1	0.07	0.3
Arctic char, cooked	75g	75	119	496	20	0	4	0.7	0.9	0.30	0.38	N/A	23	0.4	38	N/A	188	68	2.8	N/A	N/A
Bass, mixed species, baked or broiled	75g	75	110	458	18	0	4	0.8	1.0	0.34	0.23	65	77	1.4	68	342	192	26	N/A	1.73	N/A
Burbot (loche), raw	90g	90	71	297	16	0	1	0.1	0.3	0.09	0.06	54	22	0.3	63	288	171	5	0.5	0.72	N/A
Catfish, channel, farmed, baked or broiled	75g	75	114	477	14	0	6	1.3	1.0	0.10	0.04	48	7	0.6	60	241	184	11	N/A	2.10	1.0
Cisco (lake herring, tullibee), baked or broiled	75g	75	98	408	17	0	3	N/A	N/A	N/A	N/A	N/A	38	0.5	38	312	188	0	N/A	N/A	N/A
Cisco (lake herring, tullibee), raw	90g	90	88	369	17	0	2	1.1	1.2	0.46	0.11	45	10	0.4	50	319	137	27	N/A	0.90	N/A
Cod, Atlantic, baked or broiled	75g	75	79	329	17	0	1	0.1	0.2	0.12	tr	41	11	0.4	59	183	104	11	0.5	0.79	0.6
Cod, Atlantic, dried and salted, soaked in water	75g	75	62	259	13	0	1	0.1	0.2	0.09	tr	32	35	0.5	1353	265	183	9	0.5	1.82	0.6
Gefiltefish	75g	75	63	263	7	6	1	0.3	0.2	0.03	0.06	23	17	1.9	393	68	55	20	N/A	0.63	N/A
Grayling, baked or broiled	75g	75	80	332	17	0	1	N/A	N/A	N/A	N/A	N/A	29	0.5	N/A	N/A	N/A	N/A	N/A	N/A	N/A
Haddock, baked or broiled	75g	75	84	351	18	0	1	0.1	0.2	0.12	0.06	56	32	1.0	65	299	181	14	0.2	1.04	0.4
Halibut, Atlantic and Pacific, baked or broiled	75g	75	105	439	20	0	2	0.3	0.7	0.28	0.07	31	45	0.8	52	432	214	41	3.6	1.03	2.2
Herring, Atlantic, kippered	75g	75	163	680	18	0	9	2.1	2.2	0.88	0.73	62	63	1.1	689	335	244	30	1.6	14.03	1.2
Mackerel, Atlantic, baked or broiled	75g	75	197	822	18	0	13	3.1	3.2	0.52	0.38	56	11	1.2	62	301	209	41	2.0	14.25	1.5
Ocean Perch, Atlantic, baked or broiled	75g	75	91	380	18	0	2	0.2	0.4	0.20	0.08	41	103	0.9	72	263	208	11	N/A	0.86	1.2
Pickerel (Walleye), baked or broiled	75g	75	89	374	18	0	1	0.2	0.4	0.22	0.08	83	106	1.3	49	374	202	18	3.5	1.73	N/A
Pike, northern, baked or broiled	75g	75	71	298	16	0	1	0.2	0.2	0.08	0.08	38	33	0.3	23	323	180	1	2.4	1.73	0.2
Pollock, Atlantic, baked or broiled	75g	75	89	370	19	0	1	0.1	0.5	0.34	0.07	68	58	0.4	83	342	212	9	1.4	2.76	0.2
Salmon, Atlantic, farmed, baked or broiled	75g	75	155	646	17	0	9	1.9	3.3	1.09	0.52	47	11	0.3	46	288	189	11	5.1	2.10	N/A
Salmon, chum (keta), baked or broiled	75g	75	116	483	19	0	4	0.8	0.9	0.38	0.22	71	11	0.5	48	413	272	26	14.0	2.60	1.1
Salmon, chum (keta), canned, drained solids with bone, salted	75g	75	106	443	16	0	4	1.1	1.1	0.53	0.35	29	187	0.5	365	225	266	14	5.0	3.30	1.2
Salmon, chum (keta), canned, drained solids with bone, unsalted	75g	75	106	443	16	0	4	1.1	1.1	0.53	0.35	29	187	0.5	56	225	266	14	4.2	3.30	1.2
Salmon, coho, farmed, baked or broiled	75g	75	134	558	18	0	6	1.5	1.5	0.65	0.31	47	9	0.3	39	345	249	44	N/A	2.38	0.7

Food Name	Measure	Weight	Energy	Energy	Protein	Carbohydrate	Total Fat	Saturated Fat	Polyunsaturated Fat	DHA	EPA	Cholesterol	Calcium	Iron	Sodium	Potassium	Phosphorus	Vitamin A	Vitamin D	Vitamin B12	Vitamin E
		g	kcal	kJ	g	g	g	g	g	g	g	mg	mg	mg	mg	mg	mg	RAE	mcg	mcg	mg
Fish and Shellfish																					
Salmon, eggs, raw	90g	90	116	485	24	0	9	2.1	2.3	1.17	0.99	N/A	11	0.6	45	369	198	N/A	N/A	N/A	N/A
Salmon, king or chinook, smoked, canned	75g	75	113	470	17	1	4	N/A	N/A	N/A	N/A	N/A	45	1.4	N/A	N/A	N/A	72	N/A	N/A	N/A
Salmon, pink, canned, drained with bones	75g	75	102	427	17	0	4	0.6	1.1	0.52	0.27	62	208	0.7	299	233	274	17	N/A	3.71	1.0
Salmon, smoked	2 pieces	40	47	196	7	0	2	0.4	0.4	0.11	0.07	9	4	0.3	314	70	66	10	4.2	1.30	0.5
Salmon, smoked, lox	2 pieces	40	47	196	7	0	2	0.4	0.4	0.11	0.07	9	4	0.3	800	70	66	10	4.2	1.30	N/A
Salmon, sockeye, baked or broiled	75g	75	162	677	20	0	8	1.4	1.8	0.53	0.40	65	5	0.4	50	281	207	47	17.0	4.35	2.3
Sardines, Atlantic, canned in oil, drained with bones	1 can	106	220	922	26	0	12	1.6	5.5	0.54	0.50	151	405	3.1	535	421	519	34	2.5	9.48	2.2
Sardines, Pacific, canned in tomato sauce, drained with bones	1 can	106	197	825	22	1	11	2.8	2.2	0.92	0.56	65	254	2.4	439	361	388	36	12.7	9.54	1.5
Smelt, breaded and fried	5	80	201	840	17	10	10	2.5	2.7	N/A	N/A	79	31	1.0	N/A	332	246	20	N/A	N/A	N/A
Snapper, mixed species, baked or broiled	75g	75	96	401	20	0	1	0.3	0.4	0.20	0.04	35	30	0.2	43	392	151	26	2.2	2.63	0.5
Sole (flatfish), baked or broiled	75g	75	88	367	18	0	1	0.3	0.5	0.19	0.18	51	14	0.3	79	258	217	10	1.1	1.88	0.5
Trout, rainbow, farmed, baked or broiled	75g	75	127	530	18	0	5	1.6	1.7	0.62	0.25	51	65	0.2	32	331	200	65	4.8	3.73	0
Tuna, light, canned in water, drained, salted	75g	75	87	364	19	0	1	0.2	0.3	0.17	0.04	23	8	1.1	254	178	122	13	0.9	2.24	0.3
Tuna, light, canned with oil, drained, salted	75g	75	149	621	22	0	6	1.2	2.2	0.08	0.02	14	10	1.0	266	155	233	17	0.7	1.65	0.7
Turbot, baked or broiled	75g	75	92	383	15	0	3	N/A	N/A	N/A	N/A	47	17	0.3	144	229	124	9	N/A	1.91	N/A
Whitefish, lake, native, baked	75g	75	100	417	17	0	3	0.9	2.1	0.90	0.30	58	12	0.3	33	294	168	8	11.3	0.72	N/A
Shellfish																					
Clams, mixed species, boiled or steamed	5 large	60	89	371	15	3	1	0.1	0.3	0.09	0.08	40	55	16.8	67	377	203	103	0.1	59.33	0.4
Clams, mixed species, canned, drained solids	125mL	85	125	523	22	4	2	0.2	0.5	0.12	0.12	57	78	23.6	95	531	286	153	0.1	83.59	0.5
Crab, canned, drained	125mL	71	71	295	15	0	1	0.2	0.3	0.12	0.14	63	72	0.6	238	267	185	1	N/A	0.33	1.3
Crab, snow, boiled or steamed	125mL	62	72	300	15	0	1	0.1	0.3	0.09	0.21	44	21	1.8	431	125	80	32	N/A	6.47	N/A
Crayfish, mixed species, farmed, boiled or steamed	4 medium	60	52	218	11	0	1	0.1	0.2	0.02	0.07	82	31	0.7	58	143	145	9	N/A	1.86	N/A
Lobster, boiled or steamed	125mL	77	75	314	16	1	tr	0.1	0.1	0.02	0.04	55	47	0.3	291	270	142	20	N/A	2.38	0.8
Mussels, boiled or steamed	15 small	75	129	539	18	6	3	0.6	0.9	0.38	0.21	42	25	5.0	277	201	214	68	0.2	18.00	0.8
Oysters, boiled or steamed	6 medium	42	58	241	6	3	2	0.6	0.8	0.25	0.23	44	38	5.0	177	118	85	23	3.4	14.71	0.7
Oysters, canned, solids and liquid	125mL	131	90	379	9	5	3	0.8	1.0	0.30	0.28	72	59	8.8	147	300	182	118	N/A	25.06	1.1
Oysters, raw	6 medium	84	50	207	4	5	1	0.4	0.5	0.17	0.16	21	37	4.9	150	104	78	7	N/A	13.61	0.5
Scallops, cooked, steamed	6 medium	78	87	365	18	0	1	0.1	0.4	0.16	0.13	41	90	2.3	207	371	264	23	0	1.01	1.2
Shrimp, boiled or steamed	6 medium	30	30	124	6	0	tr	0.1	0.1	0.04	0.05	59	12	0.9	67	55	41	20	N/A	0.45	0.4

Food Name	Measure	Weight	Energy	Energy	Protein	Carbohydrate	Total Fat	Saturated Fat	Polyunsaturated Fat	DHA	EPA	Cholesterol	Calcium	Iron	Sodium	Potassium	Phosphorus	Vitamin A	Vitamin D	Vitamin B12	Vitamin E
		g	kcal	kJ	g	g	g	g	g	g	g	mg	mg	mg	mg	mg	mg	RAE	mcg	mcg	mg
Fish and Shellfish																					
Fish Products																					
Calamari, breaded and fried	125mL	79	156	651	14	9	7	1.7	1.6	0.27	0.11	197	45	1.0	303	216	194	17	0.1	1.02	1.0
Caviar, black or red	15mL	16	41	171	4	1	3	0.7	1.2	0.62	0.44	95	45	1.9	243	29	58	91	0.5	3.25	1.1
Crab cake	1	60	93	389	12	tr	5	0.9	1.4	0.13	0.14	90	63	0.6	198	194	128	34	N/A	3.56	N/A
Crab, imitation, made from surimi	125mL	67	68	284	8	7	1	0.2	0.4	0.24	0.16	13	9	0.3	560	60	188	13	1.2	1.07	0.1
Fish cake	1	120	240	1004	16	15	12	3.3	2.6	0.10	tr	63	30	0.8	290	526	201	28	1.5	0.73	0.7
Fish fillet, battered and fried	1	134	265	1108	22	9	15	3.6	3.4	0.14	0.08	71	42	1.0	133	508	266	23	0.8	1.02	1.0
Fish sticks, frozen, heated (10cm x 2.5cm x 1.3cm)	3 sticks	83	227	948	13	20	10	2.6	2.6	0.11	0.07	93	17	0.6	485	217	151	26	0.1	1.50	0.4
Shrimp, breaded and fried	6 medium	66	160	668	14	8	8	1.4	3.4	0.08	0.07	117	44	0.8	227	149	144	N/A	N/A	1.23	N/A
Tuna salad	125mL	108	203	847	17	10	10	1.7	4.5	0.06	0.02	14	18	1.1	435	193	193	26	3.6	1.30	N/A

DHA and EPA are omega-3 fatty acids which appear to have many health benefits.
Good sources of DHA and EPA are fatty fish
such as salmon, mackerel, herring, sardines and trout.

Meat and Poultry

Food Name	Measure	Weight	Energy	Energy	Protein	Carbohydrate	Total Fat	Saturated Fat	Monounsaturated Fat	Polyunsaturated Fat	Cholesterol	Iron	Sodium	Potassium	Magnesium	Phosphorus	Vitamin A	Vitamin D	Vitamin B12	Folate	Vitamin E
		g	kcal	kJ	g	g	g	g	g	g	mg	mg	mg	mg	mg	mg	RAE	mcg	mcg	DFE	mg
Meat and Poultry																					
Beef																					
Blade roast, lean + fat, braised	75g	75	200	834	26	0	10	4.0	5.0	0.4	71	2.5	46	202	18	142	0	0.5	2.38	4	0.1
Blade steak, lean + fat, braised	75g	75	227	947	23	0	14	5.7	7.1	0.5	71	2.4	49	178	17	138	0	0.5	2.00	4	0.2
Composite, roast, lean + fat, cooked	75g	75	181	756	24	0	8	3.5	4.2	0.4	61	2.3	40	230	19	155	0	0.5	1.89	4	0.1
Composite, steak, lean + fat, cooked	75g	75	196	819	25	0	9	3.9	4.9	0.4	64	2.4	40	200	18	148	0	0.5	1.78	4	0.1
Cross rib roast, lean + fat, braised	75g	75	197	825	27	0	9	3.6	4.5	0.5	70	2.6	52	242	21	164	0	0.5	1.89	5	0.6
Eye of round roast, lean + fat, roasted	75g	75	148	618	24	0	5	2.1	2.5	0.2	50	1.5	40	243	19	152	0	0.5	1.44	5	0.2
Eye of round steak, lean + fat, braised	75g	75	171	715	28	0	5	2.2	2.8	0.3	61	1.8	35	243	19	152	0	0.5	1.38	5	0.2
Flank steak, lean + fat, braised	75g	75	184	769	25	0	8	3.6	4.1	0.3	54	2.2	45	243	19	152	0	0.5	2.15	5	0.3
Ground, extra lean, crumbled, pan-fried	75g	75	167	696	23	0	8	3.2	3.3	0.3	59	2.1	65	311	22	180	0	0.3	2.06	5	N/A
Ground, lean, crumbled, pan-fried	75g	75	194	809	22	0	11	4.5	5.1	0.3	59	2.1	70	293	21	174	0	0.5	2.16	0	N/A
Ground, medium, crumbled, pan-fried	75g	75	214	894	22	0	13	5.6	6.0	0.4	61	2.0	68	303	21	173	0	0.6	1.88	6	N/A
Ground, regular, crumbled, pan-fried	75g	75	243	1016	22	0	17	7.0	7.9	0.4	63	2.2	78	301	21	178	0	0.8	2.72	0	N/A
Inside (top) round roast, lean + fat, roasted	75g	75	133	555	24	0	3	1.4	1.6	0.2	53	2.1	48	253	20	163	0	0.5	1.68	5	0.1
Inside (top) round steak, lean + fat, braised	75g	75	175	731	30	0	5	2.1	2.6	0.3	68	2.4	38	204	20	157	0	0.5	1.43	5	0.4
Outside (bottom) round roast, lean + fat, roasted	75g	75	158	659	25	0	5	2.1	2.8	0.3	58	2.9	42	243	19	152	0	0.5	1.67	5	0.2
Outside (bottom) round steak, lean + fat, braised	75g	75	195	815	29	0	8	3.0	4.2	0.4	72	3.1	43	243	19	152	0	0.5	1.41	5	0.3
Rib eye steak, lean + fat, broiled	75g	75	230	963	20	0	16	6.7	8.0	0.5	53	2.4	40	243	19	152	0	0.5	1.54	5	0.8
Rib steak, lean + fat, broiled	75g	75	232	969	23	0	15	6.4	7.3	0.5	58	1.9	56	243	19	152	0	0.5	1.80	5	0.5
Rump roast, lean + fat, broiled	75g	75	164	684	21	0	8	3.2	3.6	0.3	59	1.9	47	296	20	180	0	0.3	2.27	7	N/A
Short ribs, lean + fat, simmered	75g	75	309	1292	17	0	26	11.2	11.8	1.0	57	1.4	29	146	10	86	0	1.7	1.97	4	N/A
Sirloin tip roast, lean + fat, roasted	75g	75	156	653	25	0	5	2.2	2.8	0.3	58	2.7	44	243	19	152	0	0.5	1.85	5	0.1
Standing rib roast, lean + fat, roasted	75g	75	237	992	21	0	16	6.9	8.0	0.5	55	1.7	53	243	19	152	0	0.5	1.73	5	0.5
Stewing beef, lean, simmered	75g	75	183	765	28	0	7	2.9	N/A	N/A	68	2.6	45	214	19	150	0	0.5	1.80	4	0.2

Food Name	Measure	Weight	Energy	Energy	Protein	Carbohydrate	Total Fat	Saturated Fat	Monounsaturated Fat	Polyunsaturated Fat	Cholesterol	Iron	Sodium	Potassium	Magnesium	Phosphorus	Vitamin A	Vitamin D	Vitamin B12	Folate	Vitamin E
		g	kcal	kJ	g	g	g	g	g	g	mg	mg	mg	mg	mg	mg	RAE	mcg	mcg	DFE	mg
Meat and Poultry																					
Strip loin (New York) steak, lean + fat, broiled	75g	75	191	797	23	0	10	4.3	5.2	0.4	55	2.1	43	243	19	152	0	0.5	1.72	5	0.3
T-Bone (Porterhouse) steak, lean + fat, broiled	75g	75	216	903	22	0	13	5.6	6.6	0.4	54	2.1	51	243	19	152	0	0.5	1.89	5	0.1
Tenderloin, steak, lean + fat, broiled	75g	75	170	709	24	0	7	3.2	3.6	0.3	59	2.9	50	243	19	152	0	0.5	2.04	5	0.2
Top sirloin steak, lean + fat, broiled	75g	75	146	611	21	0	6	2.6	3.1	0.3	52	2.0	43	257	20	160	0	0.5	2.33	5	0.2
Veal																					
Composite cuts, lean + fat, cooked	75g	75	173	725	23	0	9	3.2	3.3	0.6	86	0.9	65	244	20	179	0	1.1	1.18	11	0.3
Cutlets, grain-fed, pan-fried	75g	75	136	568	27	0	2	0.7	0.8	0.6	78	1.5	33	266	21	171	0	0.5	2.46	N/A	0.3
Cutlets, milk-fed, pan-fried	75g	75	142	593	28	0	2	0.6	0.8	1.0	78	0.5	58	332	16	218	0	0.5	1.27	12	0.3
Ground, broiled	75g	75	129	539	18	0	6	2.3	2.1	0.4	77	0.7	62	253	18	163	0	0.8	0.95	8	0.1
Leg, lean + fat, breaded, pan-fried	75g	75	171	715	20	7	7	2.3	2.5	1.1	84	1.2	341	278	23	188	8	0.9	0.93	24	0.4
Leg, lean + fat, roasted	75g	75	120	502	21	0	3	1.4	1.3	0.3	77	0.7	51	292	21	176	0	0.5	0.88	12	0.4
Loin, lean + fat, roasted	75g	75	163	680	19	0	9	3.9	3.6	0.6	77	0.7	70	244	19	159	0	1.3	0.93	11	0.3
Shoulder, whole, lean + fat, roasted	75g	75	142	593	23	0	5	2.2	1.8	0.3	65	0.7	56	266	17	140	0	0.7	2.50	N/A	0.4
Stewing meat, lean, braised	75g	75	141	590	26	0	3	1.0	1.0	0.3	109	1.1	70	257	21	179	0	0.7	1.25	12	0.3
Pork																					
Back ribs, lean + fat, roasted	75g	75	274	1145	21	0	20	7.9	8.9	2.6	85	0.9	100	251	18	147	2	0.8	0.83	2	N/A
Centre cut, loin, chop, lean + fat, broiled	75g	75	180	753	22	0	10	3.6	4.4	0.7	62	0.6	44	269	19	174	2	0.4	0.55	5	0.1
Centre cut, loin, chop, lean + fat, pan-fried	75g	75	208	869	22	0	12	4.5	5.3	1.4	69	0.7	60	319	22	194	2	0.5	0.55	5	0.2
Ground, lean, pan-fried	75g	75	175	731	19	0	11	4.1	5.0	1.3	60	0.9	60	278	20	166	2	0.5	0.80	5	0.2
Ground, medium, pan-fried	75g	75	224	938	18	0	16	6.0	7.3	2.2	66	0.8	68	275	19	164	2	0.5	0.86	5	0.2
Leg, butt end, lean + fat, roasted	75g	75	189	791	22	0	11	3.9	4.8	1.0	72	0.8	47	281	20	204	2	0.4	0.54	2	0.2
Loin, rib end, lean + fat, broiled	75g	75	197	825	22	0	12	4.3	5.2	0.9	62	0.6	47	301	20	178	2	0.4	0.55	2	0.3
Loin, rib end, lean + fat, pan-fried	75g	75	199	831	20	0	13	4.8	5.6	1.4	55	0.5	38	323	19	177	2	0.5	0.53	2	0.2
Shoulder, butt, lean + fat, roasted	75g	75	198	828	19	0	13	5.0	5.9	1.9	67	1.1	50	245	18	153	2	0.6	0.92	4	0.2
Shoulder, whole, lean + fat, roasted	75g	75	219	916	17	0	16	5.9	7.1	1.5	68	1.0	51	247	14	159	2	0.5	0.60	4	0.1
Spareribs, lean + fat, braised	75g	75	251	1048	20	0	18	7.0	7.8	2.5	74	1.1	49	118	14	107	2	0.6	0.68	3	N/A
Tenderloin, lean, roasted	75g	75	108	452	21	0	2	0.8	0.9	0.4	52	1.0	44	302	23	184	2	0.1	0.41	5	0.2

Food Name	Measure	Weight	Energy	Energy	Protein	Carbohydrate	Total Fat	Saturated Fat	Monounsaturated Fat	Polyunsaturated Fat	Cholesterol	Iron	Sodium	Potassium	Magnesium	Phosphorus	Vitamin A	Vitamin D	Vitamin B12	Folate	Vitamin E
		g	kcal	kJ	g	g	g	g	g	g	mg	mg	mg	mg	mg	mg	RAE	mcg	mcg	DFE	mg
Meat and Poultry																					
Lamb																					
American, fresh, foreshank, lean + fat, cooked	75g	75	182	762	21	0	10	4.2	4.3	0.7	80	1.6	54	193	17	125	0	0.2	1.71	13	0.1
American, fresh, ground, cooked	75g	75	212	888	19	0	15	6.1	6.2	1.1	73	1.3	61	254	18	151	0	0.6	1.96	14	0.1
American, fresh, leg, whole, lean + fat, cooked	75g	75	194	809	19	0	12	5.2	5.2	0.9	70	1.5	50	235	18	143	0	0.5	1.94	15	0.1
American, fresh, loin, lean + fat, cooked	75g	75	232	969	17	0	18	7.7	7.3	1.4	71	1.6	48	185	17	135	0	0.5	1.66	14	0.1
American, fresh, rib, lean + fat, cooked	75g	75	269	1126	16	0	22	9.6	9.4	1.6	73	1.2	55	203	15	125	0	0.5	1.67	11	0.1
American, fresh, shoulder, whole, lean+ fat, cooked	75g	75	207	866	17	0	15	6.3	6.1	1.2	69	1.5	50	188	17	138	0	0.5	1.98	16	0.1
New Zealand, frozen, composite, lean + fat, cooked	75g	75	203	847	19	0	13	6.6	5.2	0.7	80	1.6	35	121	14	158	0	0.5	2.03	1	0.1
New Zealand, frozen, foreshank, lean + fat, braised	75g	75	194	809	20	0	12	5.9	4.6	0.5	77	1.6	35	89	11	131	0	0.3	1.83	1	0.1
New Zealand, frozen, leg, whole, lean + fat, roasted	75g	75	176	734	19	0	10	5.1	4.1	0.5	76	1.6	33	128	15	166	0	0.5	1.96	1	0.1
New Zealand, frozen, loin, lean + fat, broiled	75g	75	222	929	18	0	16	7.9	6.2	0.7	85	1.6	38	123	15	160	0	0.5	1.91	1	0.1
New Zealand, frozen, rib, lean + fat, roasted	75g	75	238	995	15	0	19	9.6	7.4	0.9	74	1.3	33	96	11	130	0	0.4	1.74	1	0.1
New Zealand, frozen, shoulder, whole, lean + fat, braised	75g	75	257	1073	22	0	18	8.6	7.0	0.9	92	1.6	39	113	14	150	0	0.4	2.60	1	0.2
Poultry and Game Birds																					
Chicken, broiler, breast, meat and skin, roasted	75g	75	142	593	19	0	7	1.8	2.6	1.4	63	0.4	45	241	20	N/A	20	0.2	0.24	3	0.2
Chicken, broiler, breast, meat, roasted	75g	75	119	499	25	0	2	0.4	0.5	0.3	64	0.4	56	301	22	N/A	5	0.2	0.26	3	0.2
Chicken, broiler, drumstick, meat and skin, roasted	75g	75	161	671	16	0	10	2.8	3.8	2.3	68	1.0	68	172	17	131	23	0.2	0.24	6	0.2
Chicken, broiler, drumstick, meat, roasted	75g	75	127	530	19	0	5	1.4	1.7	1.3	70	1.0	71	185	18	N/A	14	0.2	0.26	7	0.2
Chicken, broiler, flesh and skin, roasted	75g	75	179	749	20	0	10	2.8	4.0	2.2	66	0.9	62	167	17	137	35	0.2	0.23	4	0.2
Chicken, broiler, flesh, roasted	75g	75	143	596	22	0	6	1.5	2.0	1.3	67	0.9	65	182	19	146	12	0.2	0.25	5	0.2
Chicken, broiler, thigh, meat and skin, roasted	75g	75	187	781	15	0	14	3.8	5.4	3.0	70	1.0	63	167	17	131	36	0.2	0.22	5	0.2
Chicken, broiler, thigh, meat, roasted	75g	75	127	530	19	0	5	1.5	2.0	1.2	71	1.0	66	179	18	N/A	15	0.1	0.23	6	0.2
Chicken, broiler, wing, meat and skin, roasted	75g	75	218	910	20	0	15	4.1	5.7	3.1	63	1.0	62	138	14	113	35	0.5	0.22	2	0.2
Chicken, cornish game hens, flesh and skin, roasted	75g	75	195	815	17	0	14	3.8	6.0	2.7	98	0.7	48	184	14	110	24	0.3	0.21	2	0.3
Chicken, ground, lean, cooked	75g	75	153	640	16	0	9	N/A	N/A	N/A	59	1.2	51	212	N/A	N/A	9	0.2	N/A	N/A	N/A
Duck, domesticated, roasted	75g	75	253	1057	14	0	21	7.3	9.7	2.7	63	2.0	44	153	12	117	47	4.1	0.23	5	0.5
Duck, wild, cooked	75g	75	128	533	23	0	3	1.0	1.4	0.4	N/A	7.4	40	197	23	187	12	N/A	N/A	N/A	N/A
Goose, domesticated, flesh, roasted	75g	75	179	746	22	0	10	3.4	3.3	1.2	72	2.2	57	291	19	232	9	0.1	0.37	9	N/A
Goose, wild (Canada goose), flesh, roasted	75g	75	150	627	23	0	6	0.7	1.9	1.1	72	7.4	57	291	19	232	9	0.1	0.37	9	N/A

Food Name	Measure	Weight	Energy	Energy	Protein	Carbohydrate	Total Fat	Saturated Fat	Monounsaturated Fat	Polyunsaturated Fat	Cholesterol	Iron	Sodium	Potassium	Magnesium	Phosphorus	Vitamin A	Vitamin D	Vitamin B12	Folate	Vitamin E
		g	kcal	kJ	g	g	g	g	g	g	mg	mg	mg	mg	mg	mg	RAE	mcg	mcg	DFE	mg
Meat and Poultry																					
Ptarmigan, flesh, cooked	75g	75	116	483	23	0	2	N/A	N/A	N/A	N/A	6.5	37	247	27	190	N/A	N/A	N/A	N/A	N/A
Spruce grouse, flesh, cooked	75g	75	99	414	20	0	2	N/A	N/A	N/A	N/A	3.3	38	204	25	152	N/A	N/A	N/A	N/A	N/A
Turkey, dark meat and skin, roasted	75g	75	162	677	17	0	9	2.0	2.6	1.4	82	1.7	60	207	17	148	0	0.5	0.28	7	N/A
Turkey, dark meat, roasted	75g	75	139	581	19	0	6	1.6	2.0	1.0	82	1.7	62	220	17	154	0	0.2	0.29	8	N/A
Turkey, ground, cooked	75g	75	176	737	21	0	10	2.5	3.7	2.4	77	1.4	80	203	18	147	0	0.8	0.25	5	0.3
Turkey, light meat and skin, roasted	75g	75	143	599	21	0	4	0.9	1.2	0.6	58	1.1	50	215	20	157	0	0.2	0.27	5	N/A
Turkey, light meat, roasted	75g	75	116	483	21	0	2	0.7	0.9	0.5	55	1.0	51	231	21	165	0	0.2	0.29	5	N/A
Game Meats and Other Meats																					
Bear, simmered	75g	75	194	812	24	0	10	2.7	4.2	1.8	74	8.0	53	197	17	128	14	N/A	1.85	5	0.4
Beaver, roasted	75g	75	95	398	20	0	1	1.6	1.4	1.0	88	3.6	68	255	17	135	N/A	N/A	6.23	8	0.3
Bison, roasted	75g	75	107	449	21	0	2	0.7	0.7	0.2	62	2.6	43	271	20	157	0	N/A	2.15	6	0.3
Caribou (reindeer), roasted	75g	75	122	512	24	0	2	1.9	1.4	0.9	82	4.2	35	268	23	168	4	0.2	4.98	4	0.3
Deer (venison), roasted	75g	75	119	496	23	0	2	0.9	0.7	0.5	84	3.4	41	251	18	170	0	N/A	N/A	N/A	N/A
Emu, inside drum, broiled	75g	75	117	489	24	0	2	0.5	0.6	0.3	68	5.5	89	234	25	230	2	N/A	1.80	8	0.2
Goat, roasted	75g	75	107	449	20	0	2	0.7	1.0	0.2	56	2.8	65	304	0	151	0	N/A	0.89	4	0.3
Horsemeat, roasted	75g	75	131	549	21	0	5	1.4	1.6	0.6	51	3.8	41	284	19	185	0	N/A	2.37	N/A	N/A
Moose, roasted	75g	75	121	505	26	0	1	0.2	0.2	0.2	59	3.8	38	375	23	188	0	N/A	4.73	3	0.2
Narwhal skin (muktuk), raw	90g	90	119	497	20	0	4	0.6	2.7	0.3	N/A	0.3	91	332	14	146	126	N/A	N/A	N/A	N/A
Ostrich, inside strip, cooked	75g	75	123	515	22	0	3	1.3	1.3	0.6	73	3.6	55	275	20	190	0	N/A	4.83	12	0.2
Rabbit, composite cuts, roasted	75g	75	148	618	22	0	6	1.8	1.6	1.2	62	1.7	35	287	16	197	0	0.1	6.23	8	N/A
Seal meat, boiled	75g	75	129	539	26	0	2	0.8	1.6	0.3	133	17.6	33	212	20	139	11	N/A	N/A	N/A	N/A
Liver and Organ Meats																					
Heart, beef, simmered	75g	75	124	518	21	tr	4	1.1	0.8	0.7	159	4.8	44	164	16	191	0	1.3	8.10	4	0.2
Kidney, beef, simmered	75g	75	119	496	20	0	3	0.8	0.5	0.6	537	4.4	71	101	9	228	0	1.3	N/A	62	0.1
Liver, beef, pan-fried	75g	75	131	549	20	4	4	1.1	0.5	0.4	286	4.6	58	263	17	364	5808	0.5	N/A	195	0.4
Liver, chicken, pan-fried	75g	75	129	539	19	1	5	1.5	1.0	1.0	423	9.7	69	236	20	332	3972	N/A	N/A	420	0.6
Liver, veal, pan-fried	75g	75	145	605	21	3	5	1.6	0.9	0.8	364	4.5	64	265	17	362	N/A	0.2	N/A	263	0.5
Thymus, veal, braised	75g	75	94	392	17	0	2	0.7	0.7	0.2	263	0.9	44	326	18	470	0	N/A	2.14	15	0.1
Tongue, beef, canned or pickled	75g	75	200	838	14	tr	15	7.5	6.8	0	71	1.6	55	148	11	137	0	N/A	N/A	4	0.3

Food Name	Measure	Weight	Energy	Energy	Protein	Carbohydrate	Total Fat	Saturated Fat	Monounsaturated Fat	Polyunsaturated Fat	Cholesterol	Iron	Sodium	Potassium	Magnesium	Phosphorus	Vitamin A	Vitamin D	Vitamin B12	Folate	Vitamin E
		g	kcal	kJ	g	g	g	g	g	g	mg	mg	mg	mg	mg	mg	RAE	mcg	mcg	DFE	mg
Meat and Poultry																					
Processed Meat Products																					
Back bacon, pork, grilled	2 slices	47	87	364	11	1	4	1.3	1.9	0.4	27	0.4	727	183	10	139	0	0.1	0.37	2	0.2
Bacon, pork, broiled, pan-fried or roasted	3 slices	24	130	543	9	tr	10	3.3	4.4	1.1	26	0.3	554	136	8	128	3	0.4	0.30	tr	tr
Bacon, pork, broiled, pan-fried or roasted, reduced sodium	3 slices	24	130	543	9	tr	10	3.3	4.4	1.1	26	0.3	247	136	8	128	3	0.1	0.30	tr	0.1
Bologna (baloney), beef and pork	2 slices	56	153	640	7	3	13	4.7	5.9	1.1	31	0.8	549	132	6	51	14	0.6	0.74	3	0.2
Bologna (baloney), beef and pork, light	2 slices	56	129	539	6	1	11	4.1	5.1	0.9	22	0.4	620	87	7	101	0	0.4	0.73	3	0.1
Bologna (baloney), chicken	2 slices	56	127	531	7	4	9	3.0	2.8	2.5	55	0.9	492	111	8	73	0	0.3	0.15	4	N/A
Chicken, canned, flaked	60mL	52	89	372	9	tr	5	1.5	2.1	1.2	32	0.8	374	135	6	58	18	0.2	0.15	2	N/A
Corned beef, brisket, cooked	2 slices	56	101	422	11	1	6	2.0	2.9	0.2	55	1.0	653	112	7	70	0	0.2	0.91	3	0.1
Cottage roll, pork, lean and fat, roasted	2 slices	56	69	291	9	1	3	1.0	1.3	0.3	38	0.5	642	152	7	87	0	0.1	0.59	2	0.2
Creton	30mL	34	193	808	5	tr	19	8.3	7.7	1.6	36	0.3	129	96	6	56	1	0.3	0.19	1	0.1
Deli meat, beef, thin sliced	4 slices	56	83	349	11	tr	4	1.6	1.7	0.2	39	1.2	791	240	11	94	0	0	1.44	6	0.1
Deli meat, chicken breast roll	2 slices	56	75	314	8	1	4	1.4	1.6	0.8	22	0.2	494	181	10	68	0	0.3	0.13	2	tr
Deli meat, chicken breast, low fat	2 slices	56	48	199	10	1	tr	0.1	0.1	tr	25	0.7	696	177	20	143	0	0	N/A	N/A	tr
Deli meat, ham, extra lean (5% fat)	2 slices	56	62	258	10	1	2	0.5	0.7	0.2	27	0.4	619	196	10	122	0	0.1	0.42	2	0.2
Deli meat, ham, regular (11% fat)	2 slices	56	91	382	9	2	5	1.6	2.4	0.4	32	0.6	730	161	12	86	0	0.1	0.24	4	tr
Deli meat, mock chicken, loaved	2 slices	56	147	616	7	2	12	7.4	N/A	1.7	33	N/A	536	129	N/A	N/A	0	0.4	N/A	N/A	0.1
Deli meat, turkey breast	2 slices	56	63	262	8	4	2	0.1	0.3	0.2	31	1.2	672	195	11	88	0	0	0.12	2	0.1
Ham, extra lean, canned	2 slices	56	62	260	9	tr	2	0.8	1.2	0.2	21	0.5	638	151	10	125	0	0.1	0.46	3	0.1
Ham, lean, canned	2 slices	56	81	337	10	0	4	1.4	2.0	0.4	21	0.5	715	187	9	116	0	0.2	0.45	3	0.1
Ham, flaked, canned	60mL	35	48	199	6	tr	3	0.9	1.3	0.3	16	0.3	367	87	5	49	0	0.1	0.24	tr	0.1
Ham, lean and regular, roasted	75g	75	124	518	16	tr	6	2.0	2.8	0.8	43	1.1	1039	272	14	186	0	0.2	0.51	2	0.2
Ham, lean, roasted	75g	75	118	493	19	1	4	1.4	1.9	0.5	41	0.7	995	237	17	170	0	0.2	0.53	3	0.2
Kielbasa (Kolbassa), pork and beef	1 piece	56	124	517	9	2	9	3.1	4.1	1.0	38	0.8	520	155	9	83	0	0	0.90	3	0.1
Liver sausage (liverwurst), pork	30mL	27	93	388	4	1	8	3.0	3.8	0.7	43	1.7	191	41	3	62	2248	0.2	3.64	8	0.1
Pastrami, beef	2 slices	56	74	309	10	1	3	1.3	1.8	0.1	52	1.1	694	121	10	84	0	0.2	0.99	4	N/A
Pate, liver, canned	30mL	26	84	352	4	tr	7	2.5	3.3	0.8	67	1.4	184	36	3	53	261	0.2	0.84	16	N/A
Pepperoni, pork, beef	10 slices	55	252	1053	11	2	22	8.7	10.3	1.4	64	0.8	966	170	10	95	0	0	0.85	3	tr
Salami, beef and pork	2 slices	46	118	495	6	2	9	3.7	4.2	0.9	30	1.2	490	105	7	53	0	0.2	1.68	1	0.1

Food Name	Measure	Weight	Energy	Energy	Protein	Carbohydrate	Total Fat	Saturated Fat	Monounsaturated Fat	Polyunsaturated Fat	Cholesterol	Iron	Sodium	Potassium	Magnesium	Phosphorus	Vitamin A	Vitamin D	Vitamin B12	Folate	Vitamin E
		g	kcal	kJ	g	g	g	g	g	g	mg	mg	mg	mg	mg	mg	RAE	mcg	mcg	DFE	mg
Meat and Poultry																					
Salami, pork and beef, dry or hard	5 slices	50	185	774	12	1	15	5.1	7.2	1.4	40	0.8	900	194	9	71	0	0.4	0.95	1	0.1
Salami, pork and beef, reduced salt	2 slices	46	182	762	7	7	14	4.9	6.1	1.4	41	0.7	287	631	14	125	tr	0.4	0.81	4	0.1
Sausage, Bratwurst, pork, cooked	1	75	184	769	11	2	14	5.2	6.8	1.5	45	1.0	418	159	11	112	0	0.8	0.71	2	0
Sausage, Italian, pork, cooked	1	75	258	1079	14	3	20	7.2	9.0	2.5	43	1.1	905	228	14	128	8	0.8	0.98	4	0.2
Sausage, breakfast, pork and beef, cooked	1	13	51	215	2	tr	5	1.7	2.2	0.5	9	0.1	105	25	2	14	0	0.1	0.06	tr	tr
Sausage, breakfast, pork, cooked	1	13	35	145	2	tr	3	0.9	1.2	0.3	11	0.2	102	28	2	24	2	0.1	0.22	tr	0.1
Sausage, turkey, cooked	1	75	147	588	18	0	8	1.7	2.2	2.0	69	1.1	499	224	16	152	9	0.1	0.92	1	tr
Summer sausage, beef	2 slices	56	188	785	9	tr	17	6.7	7.3	0.7	42	1.4	696	152	8	62	0	0.5	3.08	1	N/A
Turkey, canned, flaked	60mL	34	50	207	6	tr	3	0.8	0.9	0.7	23	0.6	229	92	7	55	0	0.2	0.10	2	N/A
Vienna sausage (cocktail), beef and pork, canned	3	48	110	462	5	1	9	3.4	4.6	0.6	42	0.4	465	48	3	24	0	0.4	0.49	2	0.1
Wiener (frankfurter), beef	1	38	104	436	5	2	8	3.3	4.0	0.5	23	0.6	343	54	5	60	0	0.3	0.65	2	0.1
Wiener (frankfurter), beef and pork	1	38	107	449	5	2	9	3.4	4.3	0.9	19	0.4	374	69	4	32	0	0.3	0.49	2	0.1
Wiener (frankfurter), beef and pork, light	1	38	58	242	4	2	4	1.4	1.8	0.4	17	0.5	471	56	4	53	0	0.1	0.49	2	tr
Wiener (frankfurter), chicken	1	38	93	390	4	2	7	2.1	3.2	1.5	38	0.8	514	32	4	40	14	0.2	0.09	2	0.1

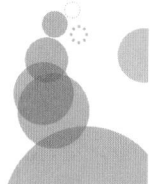

Deli meats, wieners and sausages are often high in salt and saturated fats

Legumes, Nuts and Seeds

Food Name	Measure	Weight	Energy	Energy	Protein	Carbohydrate	Total Sugar	Total Daietary Fibre	Total Fat	Saturated Fat	Monounsaturated Fat	Polyunsaturated Fat	Calcium	Iron	Sodium	Potassium	Magnesium	Phosphorus	Folate	Vitamin B12	Vitamin E
		g	kcal	kJ	g	g	g	g	g	g	g	g	mg	mg	mg	mg	mg	mg	DFE	mcg	mg
Legumes, Nuts and Seeds																					
Meatless Products																					
Meatless breaded chicken nuggets	2	72	168	705	15	6	0	3.1	9	0.8	2.3	3.3	30	2.8	288	216	9	176	40	3.68	1.4
Meatless ground beef	75g	75	148	618	16	6	1	3.5	7	1.1	1.6	3.5	22	1.6	413	135	14	258	59	1.80	1.3
Soy patty	1	70	136	568	15	5	1	3.2	6	0.8	1.2	2.5	20	1.5	385	126	13	241	55	1.68	1.2
Tofu, regular, firm and extra firm	150g	150	189	791	21	3	1	0	11	1.3	1.8	2.7	234	2.4	26	222	56	182	29	0	tr
Tofu, silken, soft	150g	150	83	345	7	4	2	0.2	4	0.5	0.8	2.3	47	1.2	8	270	44	93	N/A	0	tr
Vegetable patty	1	90	138	576	18	7	N/A	5.7	4	1.0	2.1	0.3	102	3.9	411	432	70	225	22	0	N/A
Vegetarian luncheon meat	4 slices	56	106	442	10	2	1	0	6	0.7	1.2	2.5	23	1.0	398	112	13	248	56	2.24	1.7
Wiener, meatless	1	46	107	448	9	4	0	1.8	6	0.9	1.8	3.6	15	0.6	217	45	8	158	36	1.08	0.9
Beans, Peas and Lentils																					
Beans, baked, homemade	175mL	187	283	1181	10	40	N/A	10.3	10	3.6	4.0	1.4	114	3.7	790	670	80	204	90	0	N/A
Beans, baked, plain or vegetarian, canned	175mL	188	177	738	9	40	17	7.7	1	0.2	0.2	0.2	64	2.2	633	408	49	135	23	0	0.3
Beans, baked, with pork, canned	175mL	187	198	829	10	37	N/A	10.4	3	1.1	1.3	0.4	99	3.2	775	578	64	202	67	0	N/A
Beans, black, canned, not drained	175mL	178	162	676	11	29	N/A	12.2	1	0.1	tr	0.2	62	3.4	682	547	62	192	108	0	1.3
Beans, kidney, dark red, canned, not drained	175mL	189	161	672	10	30	tr	12.1	1	0.1	0.1	0.4	45	2.4	646	487	53	178	97	0	1.1
Beans, navy, canned, not drained	175mL	194	219	917	15	40	1	9.9	1	0.2	0.1	0.4	91	3.6	868	558	91	260	120	0	1.5
Beans, pinto, canned, not drained	175mL	178	153	639	9	27	tr	8.2	1	0.3	0.3	0.5	76	2.6	522	431	48	163	107	0	1.1
Beans, refried, canned	175mL	186	175	733	10	29	tr	9.9	2	0.9	1.0	0.3	65	3.1	557	498	62	160	21	0	N/A
Beans, white, canned, not drained	175mL	194	227	948	14	43	N/A	9.3	1	0.1	tr	0.2	141	5.8	315	880	99	176	126	0	1.6
Black-eyed peas, canned, not drained	175mL	178	137	572	8	24	N/A	5.9	1	0.3	0.1	0.4	36	1.7	531	305	50	124	91	0	0.5
Chickpeas (garbanzo beans), canned, not drained	175mL	178	211	884	9	40	N/A	7.8	2	0.2	0.5	0.9	57	2.4	531	305	51	160	119	0	0.3
Falafel, homemade	1 ball	17	57	237	2	5	N/A	1.3	3	0.4	1.7	0.7	9	0.6	50	99	14	33	18	0	N/A
Hummus, commercial	60mL	57	94	394	4	8	N/A	3.4	5	0.8	2.3	2.1	22	1.4	215	129	40	100	47	0	N/A
Lentils, boiled, salted	175mL	146	170	710	13	29	3	6.2	1	0.1	0.1	0.3	28	4.9	349	540	53	264	265	0	N/A

Food Name	Measure	Weight	Energy	Energy	Protein	Carbohydrate	Total Sugar	Total Daietary Fibre	Total Fat	Saturated Fat	Monounsaturated Fat	Polyunsaturated Fat	Calcium	Iron	Sodium	Potassium	Magnesium	Phosphorus	Folate	Vitamin B12	Vitamin E
		g	kcal	kJ	g	g	g	g	g	g	g	g	mg	mg	mg	mg	mg	mg	DFE	mcg	mg
Legumes, Nuts and Seeds																					
Lentils, pink, boiled	175mL	179	190	793	14	32	N/A	5.9	1	0.2	0.3	0.6	22	4.1	4	317	39	161	112	0	N/A
Peas, split, boiled	175mL	145	171	715	12	31	4	4.2	1	0.1	0.1	0.2	20	1.9	3	525	52	144	94	0	N/A
Soybeans, boiled	175mL	127	220	920	21	13	4	8.0	11	1.7	2.5	6.4	130	6.5	1	655	109	312	69	0	N/A
Peanuts																					
Peanut butter, chunk type, fat, sugar and salt added	30mL	32	191	799	8	7	3	2.6	16	2.6	8.0	4.8	15	0.6	158	242	52	103	30	0	2.0
Peanut butter, natural	30mL	31	184	770	7	7	1	2.5	16	2.2	7.8	4.9	17	0.7	2	207	55	113	46	0	2.2
Peanut butter, smooth type, fat, sugar and salt added	30mL	32	191	798	8	6	3	1.8	16	3.3	7.7	4.5	14	0.6	149	210	50	116	24	0	2.9
Peanut butter, smooth type, light	30mL	36	190	794	9	13	3	1.9	12	2.7	5.9	3.7	13	0.7	197	244	62	135	22	0	2.4
Peanuts, all types, shelled, oil-roasted, salted	60mL	37	219	915	10	6	2	2.7	19	3.2	9.5	5.6	22	0.6	117	265	64	145	44	0	2.5
Peanuts, all types, shelled, roasted	60mL	37	217	906	9	8	2	3.0	18	2.6	9.1	5.8	20	0.8	2	244	65	133	54	0	2.6
Nuts																					
Almonds, dried	60mL	36	208	870	8	7	2	4.2	18	1.4	11.6	4.4	89	1.5	tr	262	99	171	10	0	9.3
Almonds, oil roasted	60mL	40	242	1010	8	7	2	4.2	22	1.7	13.9	5.4	116	1.5	tr	278	109	186	11	0	10.3
Almonds, roasted, salted	60mL	35	209	874	8	7	2	4.1	18	1.4	11.8	4.4	93	1.6	119	261	100	171	12	0	9.1
Brazil nuts, dried	60mL	36	233	974	5	4	1	2.7	24	5.4	8.7	7.3	57	0.9	1	234	133	257	8	0	2.0
Cashews, roasted, salted	60mL	35	199	834	5	11	2	1.0	16	3.2	9.5	2.7	16	2.1	222	196	90	170	24	0	0.3
Hazelnuts or filberts, dried	60mL	34	215	899	5	6	1	3.3	21	1.5	15.6	2.7	39	1.6	0	233	56	99	39	0	5.2
Macadamia nuts, roasted, salted	60mL	34	243	1017	3	4	1	2.7	26	4.1	20.1	0.5	24	0.9	90	123	40	67	3	0	0.2
Mixed nuts, oil roasted, salted	60mL	36	222	929	6	8	2	3.2	20	3.1	11.4	4.8	39	1.2	151	209	85	167	30	0	2.6
Mixed nuts, roasted	60mL	35	206	863	6	9	N/A	3.1	18	2.4	10.9	3.7	24	1.3	4	207	78	151	17	0	N/A
Mixed nuts, roasted, salted	60mL	35	206	863	6	9	2	3.1	18	2.4	10.9	3.7	24	1.3	232	207	78	151	17	0	3.8
Pecans, dried	60mL	25	173	726	2	3	1	2.4	18	1.6	10.2	5.4	18	0.6	0	103	30	70	6	0	0.4
Pine nuts, pignolia, dried	60mL	34	230	963	5	4	1	1.3	23	1.7	6.4	11.7	5	1.9	1	204	86	197	12	0	3.2
Pistachios, shelled, roasted, salted	60mL	31	177	741	7	8	2	3.2	14	1.7	7.6	4.3	34	1.3	126	325	37	151	16	0	0.6
Walnuts, dried	60mL	25	166	694	4	3	1	1.7	17	1.6	2.3	12.0	25	0.7	1	112	40	88	25	0	0.2
Nut Butters																					
Almond butter	30mL	32	205	858	5	7	N/A	1.2	19	1.8	12.4	4.0	88	1.2	4	246	98	170	21	0	N/A
Cashew butter	30mL	32	190	796	6	9	N/A	0.6	16	3.2	9.4	2.7	14	1.6	5	177	84	148	22	0	0.5
Sesame butter, tahini	30mL	30	181	757	5	6	tr	2.8	16	2.3	6.2	7.2	130	2.7	35	126	29	223	30	0	0.1

Food Name	Measure	Weight	Energy	Energy	Protein	Carbohydrate	Total Sugar	Total Daietary Fibre	Total Fat	Saturated Fat	Monounsaturated Fat	Polyunsaturated Fat	Calcium	Iron	Sodium	Potassium	Magnesium	Phosphorus	Folate	Vitamin B12	Vitamin E
		g	kcal	kJ	g	g	g	g	g	g	g	g	mg	mg	mg	mg	mg	mg	DFE	mcg	mg
Legumes, Nuts and Seeds																					
Seeds																					
Flaxseeds, whole and ground	15mL	11	56	235	2	3	tr	3.0	4	0.4	0.8	3.2	36	0.5	3	89	39	53	30	0	tr
Pumpkin and squash seeds, kernels, dried	60mL	35	189	792	9	6	tr	1.4	16	3.0	5.0	7.3	15	5.2	6	282	187	411	20	0	N/A
Sunflower seed kernels, roasted, salted	60mL	32	189	790	6	8	1	2.9	16	1.7	3.1	10.7	23	1.2	133	276	42	375	77	0	8.5

You would need approximately 170mL of peanuts in the shell to give you a 60mL serving.

Fast Foods

Food Name	Measure	Weight	Energy	Energy	Protein	Carbohydrate	Total Sugar	Total Dietary Fibre	Total Fat	Saturated Fat	Cholesterol	Calcium	Iron	Sodium	Potassium	Magnesium	Phosphorus	Vitamin A	Folate	Vitamin C	Vitamin B12
		g	kcal	kJ	g	g	g	g	g	g	mg	mg	mg	mg	mg	mg	mg	RAE	DFE	mg	mcg
Fast Foods																					
Beverages																					
Milk shake, chocolate	250mL	175	223	931	6	36	33	3.3	6	4.1	23	198	0.5	170	351	30	179	46	9	1	0.60
Milk shake, vanilla	250mL	175	195	814	6	31	31	0.2	5	3.3	19	214	0.2	144	305	21	179	65	9	1	0.63
Side Dishes																					
French fries	20-25 fries	76	236	989	3	29	N/A	2.5	12	5.0	11	12	1.0	124	541	25	101	2	25	4	0.09
Garlic bread	2 slices	52	192	801	5	26	tr	1.5	8	1.3	0	40	1.3	384	65	14	56	74	97	tr	0.01
Onion rings, breaded and fried	8-9	83	276	1152	4	31	N/A	1.7	16	7.0	14	73	0.8	430	129	16	86	1	85	1	0.12
Zucchini, breaded and fried, sticks	4	36	60	250	1	3	1	0.3	5	0.5	5	18	0.2	44	81	6	36	8	9	3	0.05
Sandwiches																					
Breakfast bagel, with ham, egg and cheese	1	191	483	2019	27	52	7	0.4	18	7.8	243	185	4.1	1259	262	40	397	181	172	0	1.39
Breakfast biscuit with egg, cheese and bacon	1	144	477	1993	16	33	3	1.1	31	11.4	261	164	2.5	1260	230	20	459	N/A	64	2	1.05
Breakfast English muffin with egg, cheese and bacon	1	137	289	1208	17	27	3	1.5	13	4.7	234	151	2.4	729	199	23	270	177	86	2	0.67
Cheeseburger, double patty + condiments + vegetables	1	228	650	2718	30	53	N/A	1.8	35	12.8	93	169	4.7	921	390	36	349	N/A	131	3	2.07
Cheeseburger, single patty, plain	1	102	319	1335	15	32	6	1.3	15	6.5	50	141	2.4	500	164	21	196	N/A	N/A	0	0.97
Chicken sandwich, breaded chicken + condiments + vegetables	1	228	632	2640	29	42	N/A	2.2	39	12.4	78	258	3.6	1238	333	43	406	164	154	3	0.46
Chicken sandwich, grilled chicken + condiments + vegetables	1	169	335	1402	33	23	3	1.2	12	2.2	78	70	2.1	330	449	37	36	23	83	2	0.41
Donair / Gyro	1	195	310	1295	22	37	3	2.0	7	2.8	49	98	3.1	361	404	40	223	22	115	6	1.82
Fish sandwich with breaded fish	1	183	523	2189	21	48	N/A	2.4	29	8.1	68	185	3.5	939	353	37	311	N/A	134	3	1.08
Hamburger, double patty + condiments	1	215	576	2410	32	39	N/A	1.9	32	12.0	103	92	5.5	742	527	45	284	N/A	111	1	3.33
Hamburger, single patty, plain	1	90	275	1148	12	31	5	1.3	12	4.1	35	63	2.4	387	145	19	103	0	N/A	0	0.89
Submarine sandwich (6 inches), vegetarian	1	167	216	904	7	38	3	3.4	4	0.8	0	77	2.7	529	236	27	88	25	213	20	0
Submarine sandwich (6 inches), with cold cuts	1	228	456	1906	22	51	N/A	3.0	19	6.8	36	189	2.5	1651	394	68	287	71	109	12	1.09
Submarine sandwich (6 inches), with grilled/roasted chicken	1	229	417	1742	24	44	3	3.3	16	2.8	47	81	3.0	722	437	44	104	37	255	12	0.20
Submarine sandwich (6 inches), with tuna	1	256	584	2440	30	55	N/A	2.9	28	5.3	49	74	2.6	1293	335	79	220	46	135	4	1.61

Food Name	Measure	Weight	Energy	Energy	Protein	Carbohydrate	Total Sugar	Total Dietary Fibre	Total Fat	Saturated Fat	Cholesterol	Calcium	Iron	Sodium	Potassium	Magnesium	Phosphorus	Vitamin A	Folate	Vitamin C	Vitamin B12
		g	kcal	kJ	g	g	g	g	g	g	mg	mg	mg	mg	mg	mg	mg	RAE	DFE	mg	mcg
Fast Foods																					
Veggie burger, single patty + condiments + vegetables	1	157	359	1504	19	28	4	4.5	19	2.9	5	86	3.1	671	233	25	278	22	135	3	1.80
Wrap sandwich, chicken ranch	1	249	532	2227	32	44	3	3.5	25	6.7	77	134	3.3	847	544	50	235	50	146	12	0.47
Chinese																					
Beef and broccoli stir fry	250mL	229	266	1111	24	9	1	2.2	15	3.5	58	48	2.8	433	473	35	189	90	104	59	2.00
Chicken almond guy ding	250mL	256	295	1232	22	18	3	2.6	15	1.6	42	58	1.7	510	591	61	123	14	27	7	0.29
Chicken chow mein	250mL	232	200	837	21	10	7	2.2	9	1.6	51	38	1.7	982	423	35	191	17	50	8	0.26
Chicken fried rice	250mL	209	343	1436	12	44	1	1.3	13	1.8	99	36	1.3	797	169	28	139	59	30	4	0.42
Egg roll	1	64	113	472	5	9	1	0.7	6	1.2	35	14	0.8	249	121	9	53	17	27	2	0.19
General Tao/Tso chicken	250mL	258	806	3371	50	8	3	0.6	62	11.0	163	39	2.2	1285	476	47	340	38	13	11	0.56
Hot and sour soup	250mL	258	167	697	17	5	1	0.5	8	2.8	36	45	1.8	1596	383	20	192	2	12	1	0.45
Sweet and sour chicken balls	3	75	199	831	9	17	7	0.5	10	2.7	46	24	1.0	390	90	13	23	18	19	1	0.17
Won ton soup	250mL	255	191	798	15	15	1	1.0	7	2.4	53	37	1.8	810	339	23	159	74	55	2	0.49
Pizza																					
Pizza with cheese (medium - 12 inches)	1/6	84	210	880	9	25	2	1.5	8	3.4	14	171	2.0	515	180	19	161	32	70	4	0.13
Pizza with cheese and pepperoni (medium - 12 inches)	1/6	85	219	916	11	23	1	1.4	9	4.2	21	187	1.7	340	157	18	182	37	74	2	0.20
Pizza with cheese and vegetables (medium - 12 inches)	1/6	93	193	809	8	24	3	1.8	7	3.0	12	154	1.9	482	201	19	147	31	63	11	0.11
Pizza with cheese, meat and vegetables (medium - 12 inches)	1/6	105	250	1044	11	24	3	1.9	12	4.8	24	159	2.1	629	237	21	168	31	65	11	0.24
Other																					
Chicken, breaded and fried (pieces)	2 pieces	98	283	1184	22	9	0	0.3	17	4.6	85	20	1.3	286	181	20	151	0	N/A	0	0.27
Chicken, breaded and fried, boneless (nuggets)	6	96	285	1192	15	16	1	0.9	18	3.9	53	13	0.8	551	251	24	277	5	14	1	0.32
Chili con carne	250mL	267	270	1128	26	23	N/A	4.9	9	3.6	142	72	5.5	1064	730	48	209	88	59	2	1.20
Corndog (Pogo™)	1	75	197	825	7	24	N/A	1.1	8	2.2	34	44	2.6	417	113	8	71	16	57	0	0.19
Hot-dog, plain	1	98	242	1012	10	18	N/A	0.9	15	5.1	44	24	2.3	670	143	13	97	0	61	tr	0.51

Mixed Dishes

Food Name	Measure	Weight	Energy	Energy	Protein	Carbohydrate	Total Sugar	Total Dietary Fibre	Total Fat	Saturated Fat	Cholesterol	Calcium	Iron	Sodium	Potassium	Magnesium	Phosphorus	Vitamin A	Folate	Vitamin C	Vitamin B12
		g	kcal	kJ	g	g	g	g	g	g	mg	mg	mg	mg	mg	mg	mg	RAE	DFE	mg	mcg
Mixed Dishes																					
Mexican																					
Burrito with beans and cheese	1	93	189	790	8	27	N/A	3.8	6	3.4	14	107	1.1	583	248	40	90	49	52	1	0.45
Burrito with beef, cheese and chilli	1	152	316	1322	20	32	N/A	2.2	12	5.2	85	111	3.9	1046	333	35	158	99	99	2	1.03
Nachos with cheese	15-20 nachos	113	346	1446	9	36	N/A	4.1	19	7.8	18	272	1.3	816	172	55	276	N/A	N/A	1	0.82
Quesadilla with meat	1	184	627	2622	31	40	tr	2.5	38	17.3	95	442	3.9	1265	319	44	457	167	104	6	1.03
Taco salad	250mL	129	193	807	12	13	2	2.0	11	4.1	35	92	1.3	452	275	29	138	40	18	4	0.58
Taco with beef, cheese, salsa + vegetables	1	78	168	704	9	12	N/A	N/A	9	5.2	26	101	1.1	366	216	32	93	N/A	45	1	0.48
Sandwiches																					
Club sandwich	1	246	558	2335	32	47	5	2.8	26	5.8	76	152	4.5	1152	480	47	347	43	163	6	0.48
Egg salad	1	157	479	2003	14	27	3	1.2	35	6.6	335	119	2.9	693	155	19	187	153	121	0	0.92
Hot chicken sandwich	1	284	388	1621	40	31	2	1.7	10	3.0	89	109	4.7	1344	519	43	327	0	96	0	0.54
Ham	1	121	260	1089	13	28	2	2.1	10	2.6	32	92	2.5	1132	229	25	139	49	93	3	0.24
Roast beef	1	139	346	1447	22	33	N/A	2.5	14	3.6	51	54	4.2	792	316	31	239	11	69	2	1.22
Salmon salad	1	162	340	1422	16	33	5	1.7	16	2.9	27	222	2.5	818	271	31	257	27	105	1	2.45
Tuna salad	1	162	371	1552	20	33	5	1.7	18	2.9	15	93	2.9	745	220	32	233	30	97	1	1.25
Salads																					
Caesar	250mL	114	179	751	5	7	1	1.7	15	2.0	39	92	1.3	268	233	17	81	234	118	20	0.30
Caesar salad with chicken	500mL	327	491	2055	41	12	3	3.7	31	4.3	137	147	2.9	718	890	61	146	504	249	42	0.76
Garden	250mL	77	47	198	1	4	3	0.9	4	0.6	0	13	0.3	216	135	6	16	48	15	4	0
Greek	250mL	111	139	580	4	4	2	1.1	13	3.9	19	121	0.6	315	130	12	85	43	20	11	0.36
Pasta salad with vegetables	250mL	187	245	1001	5	33	5	2.2	10	1.6	0	27	1.8	1273	173	25	69	98	129	10	0
Pasta																					
Lasagna with meat (7.5cm x 9cm)	1 piece	232	364	1523	22	37	6	2.4	14	7.4	50	251	3.2	623	428	46	280	83	99	11	0.65
Lasagna, vegetarian (7.5cm x 9cm)	1 piece	256	355	1485	19	46	7	2.9	11	6.6	38	304	3.2	737	423	49	290	102	119	13	0.21
Macaroni and cheese (Kraft Dinner™)	250mL	202	395	1653	11	49	6	2.0	17	4.1	9	158	2.2	784	162	36	194	165	191	tr	0.22

Food Name	Measure	Weight	Energy	Energy	Protein	Carbohydrate	Total Sugar	Total Dietary Fibre	Total Fat	Saturated Fat	Cholesterol	Calcium	Iron	Sodium	Potassium	Magnesium	Phosphorus	Vitamin A	Folate	Vitamin C	Vitamin B12
		g	kcal	kJ	g	g	g	g	g	g	mg	mg	mg	mg	mg	mg	mg	RAE	DFE	mg	mcg
Mixed Dishes																					
Macaroni casserole with beef and tomato soup	250mL	263	319	1334	23	32	6	1.9	10	4.0	52	31	3.5	376	399	40	186	14	112	2	1.30
Spaghetti with cream sauce	250mL	211	250	1047	9	47	4	1.9	2	0.9	5	81	2.2	111	140	34	140	33	192	tr	0.22
Spaghetti with meat sauce	250mL	262	401	1678	19	50	9	4.9	14	4.5	56	101	4.7	1008	761	60	216	68	162	13	0.89
Other																					
Beef pot pie, commercial, individual	1 serving	227	638	2667	18	57	N/A	2.0	38	11.4	41	45	2.3	1203	293	N/A	109	279	88	0	N/A
Beef stew	250mL	259	168	701	18	14	3	1.8	4	1.6	39	29	2.2	604	496	33	183	132	26	9	1.52
Butter chicken	250mL	258	368	1538	28	13	4	1.5	23	9.9	116	125	2.4	740	669	54	307	147	15	11	0.44
Chicken fajita	1 fajita	223	350	1462	19	50	3	4.1	8	2.1	33	52	3.4	540	405	41	183	28	153	26	0.09
Chicken pot pie, commercial, individual	1 serving	227	494	2065	21	37	3	3.1	29	9.5	62	59	3.0	347	349	34	195	222	102	9	0.20
Pad Thaï	250mL	171	220	920	15	26	4	1.5	6	0.9	68	26	0.9	344	258	30	56	36	24	5	0.23
Poutine	250mL	165	380	1587	13	25	1	1.9	26	9.9	40	282	1.4	755	387	26	261	97	16	7	0.38
Samosa, vegetarian	2	100	306	1280	5	32	1	2.1	18	5.6	8	33	1.8	795	178	17	70	36	68	3	0.06
Shepherd's pie	250mL	257	389	1628	17	40	5	3.1	17	5.0	41	52	1.9	584	766	54	213	94	42	14	1.23
Stir fry with beef	250mL	229	290	1213	22	20	11	2.2	14	2.3	46	45	2.7	888	534	37	211	30	43	69	1.77
Stir fry with chicken	250mL	171	255	1067	18	8	2	1.5	17	4.0	63	27	1.3	552	387	25	165	109	16	22	0.19
Stir fry with tofu	250mL	171	183	767	14	10	3	1.4	10	1.1	tr	142	1.8	493	326	36	141	72	22	20	0.02
Sushi with fish	4	104	164	684	5	35	7	0.8	tr	0.1	3	20	0.5	666	142	21	66	52	15	2	0.11
Sushi with vegetables, no fish	4	104	122	510	2	27	5	0.5	tr	0.1	0	13	0.2	100	60	13	38	16	7	2	tr
Sweet and sour meatballs	6	258	472	2322	26	33	19	0.7	26	10.6	95	76	3.3	931	409	37	243	33	34	1	2.60
Tourtiere, homemade (20cm diam)	1/6	113	307	1283	15	23	1	1.2	17	6.4	47	28	1.9	352	273	22	157	1	59	1	0.30

New frozen dinners are being introduced on the market regularly.
Please refer to the Nutrition Facts table on the package for nutritional information.
For help understanding the Nutrition Facts table, visit the Health Canada website at
www.healthcanada.gc.ca/nutritionlabelling

Soups

Food Name	Measure	Weight	Energy	Energy	Protein	Carbohydrate	Total Sugar	Total Dietary Fibre	Total Fat	Saturated Fat	Cholesterol	Calcium	Iron	Sodium	Potassium	Magnesium	Phosphorus	Vitamin A	Folate	Vitamin C	Vitamin B12
		g	kcal	kJ	g	g	g	g	g	g	mg	mg	mg	mg	mg	mg	mg	RAE	DFE	mg	mcg
Soups																					
Ready-to-serve																					
Beef or chicken, broth/bouillon	250mL	254	18	74	3	tr	0	0	1	0.3	0	15	0.4	827	137	5	33	0	5	0	0.18
Beef, chunky	250mL	254	180	753	12	21	2	1.5	5	2.7	15	33	2.5	915	355	5	127	137	15	7	0.66
Chicken noodle, chunky	250mL	254	185	773	13	18	2	4.1	6	1.5	20	25	1.5	898	114	10	76	71	65	0	0.33
Chicken noodle, low fat, reduced salt	250mL	257	105	444	9	13	1	2.1	2	1.0	13	21	0	501	N/A	N/A	N/A	N/A	N/A	0	N/A
Chicken vegetable, chunky	250mL	254	175	733	13	20	N/A	0.9	5	1.5	18	28	1.5	1128	388	10	112	317	13	6	0.25
Clam chowder, Manhattan	250mL	254	142	593	8	20	4	3.0	4	2.2	15	71	2.8	1057	406	20	89	178	10	13	8.37
Minestrone, chunky	250mL	254	134	563	5	22	6	6.1	3	1.6	5	63	1.9	913	647	15	117	226	72	5	0
Split pea with ham, chunky	250mL	254	195	817	12	28	5	4.1	4	1.7	8	36	2.3	1019	322	41	188	259	5	7	0.25
Vegetable, chunky	250mL	254	129	540	4	20	4	1.3	4	0.6	0	58	1.7	1068	418	8	76	307	18	6	0
Condensed, prepared with water																					
Beef noodle	250mL	258	88	366	5	9	2	0.8	3	1.2	5	15	1.2	1005	106	5	49	8	31	tr	0.21
Chicken broth	250mL	254	41	170	5	1	1	0	1	0.4	0	10	0.5	806	218	3	76	0	5	0	0.25
Chicken noodle	250mL	255	79	331	4	10	N/A	0.8	3	0.7	8	18	0.8	1169	59	5	38	38	37	tr	0.15
Cream of mushroom	250mL	258	137	572	2	10	2	0.5	9	2.6	3	49	0.5	931	106	5	52	15	5	1	0.05
Tomato	250mL	258	90	376	2	18	9	1.2	2	0.4	0	13	1.9	735	278	8	36	26	15	3	0
Tomato, reduced salt	250mL	258	90	376	2	19	8	0.5	2	0.4	0	13	1.9	52	278	8	36	44	18	70	0
Vegetables with beef	250mL	258	83	345	6	11	1	0.7	2	0.9	5	18	1.2	835	183	5	44	101	10	1	0.34
Vegetarian vegetable	250mL	255	76	318	2	13	4	0.5	2	0.3	0	23	1.1	868	222	8	36	122	10	2	0
Condensed, prepared with 2% milk																					
Clam chowder, New England	250mL	262	157	658	10	18	N/A	1.6	5	1.9	16	202	1.6	1051	320	26	168	71	10	4	10.85
Cream of chicken	250mL	262	189	789	8	16	7	0.3	10	3.7	21	194	0.7	1108	293	21	162	86	N/A	1	0.58
Cream of mushroom	250mL	262	202	844	6	16	N/A	0.5	13	4.2	10	191	0.6	983	288	24	168	86	10	2	0.52
Cream of mushroom, reduced salt	250mL	262	134	558	6	17	9	0.8	5	2.4	14	168	0.7	562	691	21	189	74	21	tr	0.50
Cream of tomato	250mL	262	155	647	6	24	16	1.3	5	1.9	10	173	1.9	802	480	26	160	69	22	4	0.47

Food Name	Measure	Weight	Energy	Energy	Protein	Carbohydrate	Total Sugar	Total Dietary Fibre	Total Fat	Saturated Fat	Cholesterol	Calcium	Iron	Sodium	Potassium	Magnesium	Phosphorus	Vitamin A	Folate	Vitamin C	Vitamin B12
		g	kcal	kJ	g	g	g	g	g	g	mg	mg	mg	mg	mg	mg	mg	RAE	DFE	mg	mcg
Soups																					
Dehydrated, prepared with water																					
Chicken noodle	250mL	254	58	243	2	9	1	0.3	1	0.3	10	5	0.5	581	33	8	30	3	28	0	0.05
Minestrone	250mL	268	83	349	5	13	N/A	0.8	2	0.9	3	40	1.1	1084	360	8	64	16	51	1	0
Onion	250mL	260	29	120	1	5	2	0.8	1	0.1	0	13	0.2	897	68	5	31	0	3	tr	0
Ramen noodles, chicken flavour, cooked	250mL	258	162	678	3	20	N/A	6.2	8	3.5	0	N/A	1.2	792	N/A	N/A	N/A	72	N/A	0	N/A
Tomato vegetable	250mL	255	56	234	2	10	2	0.5	1	0.4	0	8	0.6	1154	104	20	31	10	10	6	0
Homemade																					
Chicken noodle	250mL	255	135	564	19	7	2	0.9	3	0.7	64	26	1.1	336	302	30	168	136	28	3	0.22
Cream of vegetable	250mL	251	62	262	5	7	3	0.8	2	0.7	2	53	0.6	586	287	11	95	99	11	3	0.31
French onion	250mL	255	204	852	10	28	3	1.9	6	2.9	13	159	1.5	904	204	25	157	30	69	2	0.58
Lentil	250mL	262	193	805	12	27	3	5.1	5	0.4	0	41	3.3	654	365	41	171	45	69	6	0
Split pea with ham	250mL	267	190	797	13	31	5	3.8	2	0.6	7	39	1.9	312	437	50	176	56	70	2	0.04
Vegetable	250mL	252	49	204	3	8	2	1.4	1	0.2	0	34	0.7	692	336	16	58	93	20	11	0.14

Many broths and canned soups now have a reduced salt version.

Fats and Oils

Food Name	Measure	Weight	Energy	Energy	Protein	Carbohydrate	Total Fat	Saturated Fat	Monounsaturated Fat	Polyunsaturated Fat	Trans Fat	Cholesterol	Calcium	Iron	Sodium	Potassium	Magnesium	Phosphorus	Vitamin A	Vitamin D	Vitamin E
		g	kcal	kJ	g	g	g	g	g	g	g	mg	mg	mg	mg	mg	mg	mg	RAE	mcg	mg
Fats and Oils																					
Butter and Margarine																					
Becel™, tub, calorie-reduced, canola and safflower oils (non-hydrogenated)	5mL	5	17	70	tr	tr	2	0.3	0.8	0.6	tr	0	1	0	46	1	tr	1	48	0.6	0.2
Becel™, tub, canola and safflower oils (non-hydrogenated)	5mL	5	34	144	tr	tr	4	0.5	1.7	1.2	tr	0	1	0	52	2	tr	1	48	0.6	0.2
Butter	5mL	5	34	144	tr	tr	4	2.5	1.0	0.1	0.2	10	1	tr	28	1	tr	1	33	tr	0.1
Chefmaster™, tub, unspecified vegetable oils (hydrogenated)	5mL	5	34	144	tr	tr	4	0.5	1.6	0.9	0.5	0	1	0	52	2	tr	1	48	0.6	0.2
Imperial™, stick, soy and canola oils (hydrogenated)	5mL	5	34	141	tr	tr	4	0.5	2.5	0.4	1.5	0	tr	tr	31	1	tr	tr	48	0.6	0.3
Imperial™, tub, soya oil (non-hydrogenated)	5mL	5	34	144	tr	tr	4	0.9	0.7	1.8	tr	0	1	0	52	2	tr	1	48	0.6	0.2
Lactantia™, tub, soya oil (hydrogenated)	5mL	5	34	144	tr	tr	4	0.7	1.3	1.4	0.6	0	1	0	52	2	tr	1	48	0.6	0.2
Margarine, tub, composite	5mL	5	34	144	tr	tr	4	0.6	1.7	1.3		0	1	0	52	2	tr	1	48	0.6	0.2
Spread (20% butter / 80% margarine)	5mL	5	34	141	tr	tr	4	1.0	2.2	0.4	1.0	2	1	tr	43	2	tr	1	47	N/A	0.4
Spread (50% butter / 50% margarine)	5mL	5	33	137	tr	tr	4	1.5	1.8	0.2	0.7	5	1	tr	40	2	tr	1	16	0	0.2
Oils																					
Canola	15mL	14	125	525	0	0	14	1.0	8.4	4.2	0.3	0	0	0	0	0	0	0	0	0	2.4
Corn	15mL	14	122	510	0	0	14	1.8	3.8	7.5	0.1	0	0	0	0	0	0	0	0	0	2.0
Flaxseed	15mL	14	122	511	0	0	14	1.4	2.5	9.9	tr	0	0	0	0	0	0	0	0	0	2.4
Grapeseed	15mL	14	122	510	0	0	14	1.3	2.2	9.6	N/A	0	0	0	0	0	0	0	0	0	4.0
Olive	15mL	14	121	506	0	0	14	1.8	10.1	1.4	tr	0	tr	0.1	tr	0	0	0	0	0	2.0
Peanut	15mL	14	121	506	0	0	14	2.3	6.3	4.4	N/A	0	0	tr	0	0	0	0	0	0	2.2
Sesame	15mL	14	122	510	0	0	14	2.0	5.5	5.7	N/A	0	0	0	0	0	0	0	0	0	0.2
Soybean	15mL	14	122	510	0	0	14	2.0	3.2	8.0	0.2	0	0	tr	0	0	0	0	0	0	1.3
Sunflower	15mL	14	122	510	0	0	14	1.4	2.7	9.1	0.1	0	0	0	0	0	0	0	0	0	5.7
Other																					
Bacon grease	15mL	12	110	459	0	0	12	4.8	5.5	1.4	N/A	12	0	0	18	0	0	0	0	0	0.1
Lard	15mL	13	117	489	0	0	13	5.2	5.9	1.5	0.2	12	0	0	0	0	0	0	0	0	0.1

Food Name	Measure	Weight	Energy	Energy	Protein	Carbohydrate	Total Fat	Saturated Fat	Monounsaturated Fat	Polyunsaturated Fat	Trans Fat	Cholesterol	Calcium	Iron	Sodium	Potassium	Magnesium	Phosphorus	Vitamin A	Vitamin D	Vitamin E
		g	kcal	kJ	g	g	g	g	g	g	g	mg	mg	mg	mg	mg	mg	mg	RAE	mcg	mg
Fats and Oils																					
Shortening	15mL	13	115	481	0	0	13	3.2	5.4	3.7	N/A	0	tr	tr	1	0	0	0	0	0	0.1
Salad Dressings																					
Blue cheese	15mL	16	78	327	1	1	8	1.5	1.9	4.3	N/A	3	13	tr	170	6	0	11	10	N/A	0.9
Blue cheese, low Calorie	15mL	16	15	64	1	tr	1	0.4	0.3	0.4	N/A	tr	14	0.1	186	1	1	13	N/A	N/A	tr
Creamy Caesar	15mL	15	79	329	tr	tr	9	1.3	2.0	4.9	N/A	tr	4	tr	161	4	tr	3	tr	tr	0.8
Creamy Caesar, low Calorie	15mL	15	17	70	tr	3	1	0.1	0.2	0.4	N/A	tr	4	tr	164	4	tr	3	tr	0	0.1
Creamy dressing, fat-free	15mL	16	21	90	tr	5	tr	tr	tr	tr	N/A	0	1	0.1	130	14	tr	0	tr	0	tr
French	15mL	16	72	303	tr	2	7	0.9	1.3	3.3	N/A	0	4	0.1	133	11	1	3	4	0	0.8
French, low fat	15mL	16	33	138	tr	4	2	0.3	0.5	1.2	N/A	0	2	0.1	165	13	0	2	2	0	0.5
Italian	15mL	15	43	181	tr	2	4	0.7	0.9	1.9	N/A	0	1	0.1	246	7	tr	1	2	0	0.7
Italian, low Calorie	15mL	15	11	48	tr	1	1	0.1	0.3	0.3	N/A	1	1	0.1	208	13	1	2	tr	0	tr
Mayonnaise	15mL	14	100	419	tr	1	11	1.7	2.7	6.0	tr	5	3	0.1	79	5	tr	4	11	tr	0.7
Mayonnaise, light	15mL	16	51	215	tr	1	5	0.8	1.3	2.8	tr	6	1	0.1	107	6	tr	6	3	N/A	0.5
Non creamy dressing, fat-free	15mL	15	7	29	tr	1	tr	tr	tr	tr	N/A	tr	4	0.1	165	15	1	16	tr	0	0.1
Oil and vinegar	15mL	16	73	305	0	tr	8	1.5	2.4	3.9	N/A	0	0	0	tr	1	0	0	0	0	0.8
Ranch	15mL	15	71	297	tr	1	8	1.2	1.7	4.2	0	5	5	0.1	120	9	1	24	1	tr	0.7
Ranch, low fat	15mL	16	36	149	tr	3	3	0.2	0.9	0.7	0	3	20	0.1	151	21	1	31	3	tr	0.3
Salad dressing, mayonnaise type	15mL	15	58	243	tr	4	5	0.7	1.3	2.7	0.4	4	2	tr	106	1	tr	4	3	tr	0.3
Salad dressing, mayonnaise type, fat-free	15mL	16	14	57	tr	3	tr	0.1	0.3	tr	N/A	1	1	tr	128	8	tr	1	0	N/A	tr
Salad dressing, mayonnaise type, light	15mL	15	44	184	0	2	4	0.2	2.2	1.1	N/A	0	tr	0	117	0	0	N/A	3	N/A	tr
Thousand Island	15mL	16	59	245	tr	2	6	0.8	1.2	2.9	N/A	4	3	0.2	137	17	1	4	2	N/A	0.6
Thousand Island, low Calorie	15mL	16	32	132	tr	3	2	0.1	1.0	0.4	N/A	tr	2	0.1	129	31	1	2	2	N/A	0.2

When cooking with oil, remember that 5mL (1 teaspoon) of oil contains 40 calories and approximately 5 grams of fat

Nutrient Value of Some Common Foods

Sweets and Sugars

Food Name	Measure	Weight	Energy	Energy	Protein	Carbohydrate	Total Sugar	Total Dietary Fibre	Total Fat	Saturated Fat	Cholesterol	Calcium	Iron	Sodium	Potassium	Magnesium	Phosphorus	Vitamin A	Vitamin C	Vitamin B12	Caffeine
		g	kcal	kJ	g	g	g	g	g	g	mg	mg	mg	mg	mg	mg	mg	RAE	mg	mcg	mg
Sweets and Sugars																					
Sugar, Honey and Substitutes																					
Brown sugar	5mL	5	18	73	0	5	4	0	0	0	0	4	0.1	2	16	1	1	0	0	0	0
Honey	5mL	7	22	91	tr	6	6	tr	0	0	0	tr	tr	tr	4	tr	tr	0	tr	0	0
Icing sugar (powdered)	5mL	3	10	41	0	2	2	0	tr	0	0	tr	tr	tr	0	0	0	0	0	0	0
Sugar substitute, aspartame (Equal™)	1 packet	1	4	15	tr	1	1	0	0	0	0	0	0	0	0	0	0	0	0	0	0
Sugar substitute, sucralose (Splenda™)	5mL	1	2	7	0	tr	tr	0	0	0	0	0	0	0	0	0	0	0	0	0	0
White sugar (granulated)	5mL	4	16	68	0	4	4	0	0	0	0	tr	0	0	0	0	0	0	0	0	0
Syrup and Molasses																					
Chocolate syrup, thin type	15mL	20	110	461	1	26	20	1.0	tr	0.2	0	6	0.8	28	89	26	51	tr	tr	0	6
Corn syrup	15mL	21	59	249	0	16	6	0	0	0	0	4	0.1	32	9	2	2	0	0	0	0
Maple syrup	15mL	20	55	230	0	14	12	0	tr	tr	0	22	0.2	2	46	4	tr	0	0	0	0
Molasses	15mL	21	62	257	0	16	12	0	tr	tr	0	44	1.0	8	311	51	7	0	0	0	0
Pancake syrup	15mL	20	47	195	0	12	7	0.1	0	0	0	1	tr	16	3	tr	2	0	0	0	0
Preserves																					
Double fruit jam type spread	15mL	19	42	177	tr	10	9	0.5	tr	0	0	2	0.1	6	N/A	N/A	N/A	N/A	tr	N/A	N/A
Double fruit jam type spread, reduced sugar	15mL	17	23	95	tr	5	5	0.4	tr	0	0	3	0.1	3	N/A	N/A	N/A	N/A	tr	N/A	N/A
Jams and preserves	15mL	20	56	234	tr	14	10	0.2	tr	tr	0	4	0.1	6	16	1	4	tr	2	0	0
Jelly	15mL	21	56	235	tr	15	11	0.2	tr	tr	0	1	tr	6	11	1	1	0	tr	0	0
Marmalade	15mL	20	50	207	tr	13	12	0.1	0	0	0	8	tr	11	7	tr	1	1	1	0	0
Toppings and Spreads																					
Chocolate topping, fudge-type	30mL	39	135	564	2	24	13	1.1	3	1.5	1	39	0.6	133	174	25	65	2	tr	0.11	3
Pie filling, cherry, canned	30mL	25	29	121	tr	7	N/A	0.2	tr	tr	0	3	0.1	5	26	2	4	3	1	0	0
Spread, chocolate hazelnut (Nutella™)	30mL	38	203	848	2	23	21	2.0	11	2.0	0	41	1.6	15	153	24	57	tr	0	0.11	3
Topping or spread, butterscotch	30mL	42	105	438	1	27	N/A	0.4	tr	tr	tr	22	0.1	145	35	3	20	11	tr	0.04	0
Topping, strawberry	30mL	43	110	458	tr	29	12	0.3	tr	tr	0	3	0.1	9	22	2	2	tr	6	0	0

Food Name	Measure	Weight	Energy	Energy	Protein	Carbohydrate	Total Sugar	Total Dietary Fibre	Total Fat	Saturated Fat	Cholesterol	Calcium	Iron	Sodium	Potassium	Magnesium	Phosphorus	Vitamin A	Vitamin C	Vitamin B12	Caffeine
		g	kcal	kJ	g	g	g	g	g	g	mg	mg	mg	mg	mg	mg	mg	RAE	mg	mcg	mg
Sweets and Sugars																					
Candies																					
Butterscotch	1 piece	5	21	87	tr	5	4	0	tr	0.1	tr	tr	tr	21	0	tr	tr	1	0	0	0
Candy, chocolate covered, sweetened with sorbitol	1 piece	5	29	120	1	2	1	0.2	2	1.1	1	15	0.1	5	30	5	17	3	tr	0.04	tr
Caramel	4	40	154	646	2	31	26	0.5	3	2.7	3	56	0.1	99	86	7	46	tr	tr	0	0
Chewing gum	1 stick	3	7	31	0	2	2	0.1	tr	tr	0	0	0	tr	0	0	0	0	0	0	0
Chewing gum, sugarless	1 stick	2	5	22	0	2	0	tr	tr	tr	0	tr	0	tr	0	0	0	0	0	0	0
Fruit leather	1 roll	14	52	217	tr	12	7	0.5	tr	0.1	0	4	0.1	44	41	3	4	1	17	0	0
Fudge, chocolate, homemade	1 piece	17	70	292	tr	13	13	0.3	2	1.0	2	8	0.3	8	22	6	12	7	0	0.02	1
Fudge, vanilla, homemade	1 piece	22	84	353	tr	18	18	0	1	0.6	3	7	tr	11	10	1	6	10	0	0.02	0
Gumdrops	10 pieces	36	143	596	0	36	21	tr	0	0	0	1	0.1	16	2	tr	tr	0	0	0	0
Hard candy	1	6	24	99	0	6	4	0	tr	0	0	tr	tr	2	0	tr	tr	0	0	0	0
Hard candy, reduced sugar	1	3	11	47	0	3	3	0	0	0	0	0	0	0	0	0	0	0	0	0	0
Jellybeans	10 beans	28	105	439	0	26	20	0.1	tr	0	0	1	tr	14	10	1	1	0	0	0	0
Licorice, strawberry (Twizzlers™)	3 strips	38	132	553	1	30	15	0	1	0	0	0	0.2	108	N/A	N/A	N/A	0	0	0	0
Marshmallows	1	7	23	96	tr	6	4	tr	tr	tr	0	tr	tr	6	0	tr	1	0	0	0	0
Sesame crunch (sesame snap)	4 pieces	35	181	757	4	18	11	2.8	12	1.6	0	229	1.5	58	113	88	148	0	tr	0	0
Skittles™	10 candies	11	43	181	tr	10	8	0	tr	0.1	0	0	tr	2	1	tr	tr	0	7	0	0
Toffee	1 piece	12	67	281	tr	8	8	0	4	2.5	12	4	tr	16	6	tr	4	38	tr	0.01	0
Chocolate Bars																					
Almonds, chocolate covered	10	32	180	752	4	15	12	1.4	12	4.8	4	64	0.8	16	N/A	N/A	N/A	0	0	N/A	N/A
Caramel coated cookies, chocolate covered (Twix™)	1 package	58	289	1210	3	38	28	0.6	14	5.2	3	52	0.5	112	110	19	63	13	tr	0.17	2
Caramel with nuts, chocolate covered (Turtles™)	2	28	132	550	3	17	12	1.2	6	1.3	0	22	0.5	7	125	23	46	12	tr	0	5
Caramel, chocolate covered (Rolo™, Caramilk™)	1 bar	52	246	1031	3	35	33	0.5	11	7.5	6	75	0.2	98	98	0	37	18	tr	0.14	2
Chocolate covered wafer (Kit Kat™, Coffee Crisp™)	1 bar	42	218	910	3	27	20	0.4	11	7.5	5	53	0.4	23	97	16	57	10	0	0.24	6
Chocolate malt-nougat and caramel, chocolate covered (Mars™)	1 bar	58	245	1026	3	42	35	1.0	9	4.5	8	75	0.4	139	140	20	84	10	1	0.19	5
Chocolate, candy coated (M&M'S™ , Smarties™)	1 package	40	201	841	2	27	25	1.1	9	5.8	6	46	0.5	27	117	18	66	16	tr	0.12	N/A
Chocolate, semisweet, bars or chips	60mL	43	204	853	2	27	23	2.5	13	7.6	0	14	1.3	5	156	49	56	0	0	0	26
Coconut candy, chocolate covered (Bounty™, Almond Joy™)	1 bar	49	235	981	2	29	24	2.5	13	8.6	2	31	0.6	70	124	N/A	55	N/A	tr	N/A	N/A

Food Name	Measure	Weight	Energy	Energy	Protein	Carbohydrate	Total Sugar	Total Dietary Fibre	Total Fat	Saturated Fat	Cholesterol	Calcium	Iron	Sodium	Potassium	Magnesium	Phosphorus	Vitamin A	Vitamin C	Vitamin B12	Caffeine
		g	kcal	kJ	g	g	g	g	g	g	mg	mg	mg	mg	mg	mg	mg	RAE	mg	mcg	mg
Sweets and Sugars																					
Fondant, chocolate covered (After Eight™)	2 pieces	16	59	246	tr	13	11	0.3	2	1.3	0	4	0.3	2	N/A	N/A	N/A	tr	0	N/A	N/A
Fudge, caramel and nuts, chocolate covered (Oh Henry!™)	1 bar	63	289	1208	5	41	31	1.3	14	4.2	6	51	0.4	144	203	32	88	6	tr	0.13	3
Milk chocolate and crisped rice (Nestle Crunch™)	1 bar	40	209	873	2	26	22	1.0	11	6.1	5	68	0.2	53	138	23	81	8	tr	0.15	10
Milk chocolate, bars or chips	1 bar	50	268	1119	4	30	26	1.7	15	7.1	12	95	1.2	40	186	32	104	25	0	0.31	10
Peanut butter cups (Reese's™)	3 cups	51	263	1099	5	28	24	1.8	16	5.5	3	40	0.6	160	175	32	82	9	tr	0.29	9
Peanuts, chocolate covered	10	40	208	868	5	20	15	1.9	13	5.8	4	42	0.5	16	201	38	85	14	0	0.18	9
Raisins, chocolate covered (Glosette™)	10 pieces	10	39	163	tr	7	6	0.4	1	0.9	tr	9	0.2	4	51	5	14	2	tr	0.02	3
Toffee, chocolate covered (Skor™)	1 bar	39	209	872	1	24	23	0.5	13	7.3	21	51	0.2	124	60	4	24	60	tr	N/A	N/A
Frozen Desserts																					
Chocolate ice milk bar (Fudgesicle™)	1	51	65	271	3	14	10	0.9	tr	0.2	2	81	0.5	48	N/A	N/A	N/A	N/A	1	N/A	N/A
Frozen yogourt, chocolate	125mL	91	116	484	3	20	20	1.2	3	2.1	12	91	0.4	57	213	23	81	36	6	0.06	3
Frozen yogourt, vanilla	125mL	76	124	519	3	18	18	0	4	2.6	2	109	0.2	66	161	11	98	45	1	0.22	0
Fruit and juice bar	1	77	63	264	1	16	13	0.8	tr	0	0	4	0.1	3	41	3	5	1	7	0	0
Ice cream cone, vanilla, chocolate covered, with nuts	1	78	222	928	5	23	16	1.9	14	5.4	25	105	0.8	54	208	42	117	68	tr	0.23	4
Ice cream cone, vanilla, soft serve	1	150	266	1110	7	43	32	0.6	7	4.3	39	232	0.5	116	305	22	154	90	2	0.67	0
Ice cream sandwich	1	59	143	598	3	22	14	0.9	6	3.2	20	60	0.6	36	122	13	63	53	tr	0.18	1
Ice cream, chocolate	125mL	70	151	630	3	20	18	0.8	8	4.7	24	76	0.6	53	174	20	75	82	tr	0.20	2
Ice cream, dairy free	125mL	87	237	990	4	21	N/A	0.8	16	2.0	0	36	1.2	216	64	19	59	tr	tr	0	0
Ice cream, strawberry	125mL	70	134	560	2	19	N/A	0.6	6	3.6	20	84	0.1	42	131	10	70	67	5	0.21	0
Ice cream, vanilla, low fat	125mL	93	117	490	5	20	10	0	2	1.5	11	146	0.1	65	205	13	113	27	1	0.46	0
Ice cream, vanilla, low fat, aspartame sweetened	125mL	69	106	445	3	15	4	0.5	5	2.8	19	93	0.1	66	135	6	52	1	1	0.36	0
Ice cream, vanilla, premium	125mL	113	282	1177	4	25	23	0	18	11.7	104	132	0.4	69	178	12	119	206	0	0.44	0
Ice cream, vanilla, regular	125mL	76	153	640	3	18	16	0.5	8	5.2	33	97	0.1	61	151	11	80	90	tr	0.30	0
Popsicles	1	75	54	226	0	14	10	0	0	0	0	0	0	9	3	1	0	0	0	0	0
Sherbet, orange	125mL	78	113	471	1	24	19	2.6	2	0.9	0	42	0.1	36	75	6	31	8	5	0.09	0
Soft serve ice cream with Oreo™ cookies (Blizzard™, McFlurry™)	1 small	275	575	2404	13	89	68	1.9	20	10.5	63	386	4.7	368	564	52	279	148	3	1.12	5

Food Name	Measure	Weight	Energy	Energy	Protein	Carbohydrate	Total Sugar	Total Dietary Fibre	Total Fat	Saturated Fat	Cholesterol	Calcium	Iron	Sodium	Potassium	Magnesium	Phosphorus	Vitamin A	Vitamin C	Vitamin B12	Caffeine
		g	kcal	kJ	g	g	g	g	g	g	mg	mg	mg	mg	mg	mg	mg	RAE	mg	mcg	mg
Sweets and Sugars																					
Other Desserts																					
Chocolate mousse, homemade	125mL	90	203	847	4	14	13	0.5	14	8.2	126	86	0.5	34	129	18	105	126	tr	0.42	6
Gelatin dessert, calorie-reduced, prepared (Jello™)	125mL	124	25	104	1	5	0	0	0	0	0	4	tr	59	1	1	84	0	0	0	0
Gelatin dessert, prepared (Jello™)	125mL	143	88	369	2	20	19	0	0	0	0	4	tr	107	1	1	31	0	0	0	0

Brown sugar is white sugar combined with molasses

Snacks

Food Name	Measure	Weight	Energy	Energy	Protein	Carbohydrate	Total Sugar	Total Dietary Fibre	Total Fat	Saturated Fat	Cholesterol	Calcium	Iron	Sodium	Potassium	Magnesium	Phosphorus	Vitamin A	Folate	Vitamin C	Vitamin B12
		g	kcal	kJ	g	g	g	g	g	g	mg	mg	mg	mg	mg	mg	mg	RAE	DFE	mg	mcg
Snacks																					
Popcorn																					
Air-popped	250mL	8	32	135	1	7	tr	1.3	tr	tr	0	1	0.2	tr	25	11	25	1	2	0	0
Caramel-coated	250mL	37	160	670	1	29	20	1.9	5	1.3	2	16	0.6	77	41	13	31	1	2	0	tr
Microwave, low fat and reduced salt	250mL	8	34	144	1	6	tr	1.1	1	0.1	0	1	0.2	39	19	12	21	tr	1	0	0
Oil-popped, regular and microwaved	250mL	12	58	243	1	7	tr	1.2	3	0.6	0	1	0.3	103	26	13	29	1	2	tr	0
Chips																					
Corn-based puffs or twists, cheese (Cheesies™)	250mL	37	205	857	3	20	1	0.4	13	2.4	1	21	0.9	388	61	7	40	2	67	tr	0.05
Potato chips made from dried potatoes, plain (Pringles™)	17 chips	28	156	654	2	14	1	1.0	11	2.6	0	7	0.4	184	282	16	44	0	2	2	0
Potato chips, baked, plain	1 small bag	43	202	843	2	31	2	2.1	8	1.1	0	54	0.3	394	310	18	118	0	0	0	0
Potato chips, flavoured	1 small bag	43	211	883	3	23	N/A	1.9	14	3.5	0	22	0.8	323	542	32	80	5	36	15	0
Potato chips, plain	1 small bag	43	230	964	3	21	tr	1.6	15	1.8	0	9	0.7	229	571	30	65	0	20	25	0
Tortilla chips, nacho flavoured (Doritos™)	1 small bag	50	249	1042	4	31	2	2.7	13	2.5	2	74	0.7	354	108	41	122	12	7	1	0
Tortilla chips, plain	26 small	47	234	980	3	29	tr	3.0	12	2.3	0	72	0.7	247	92	41	96	2	5	0	0
Other Snacks																					
Banana chips	10 chips	14	73	304	tr	8	5	1.1	5	4.1	0	3	0.2	1	75	11	8	1	2	1	0
Beef jerky (22cm long)	1 stick	20	81	340	7	2	2	0.4	5	2.1	10	4	1.1	438	118	10	81	0	27	0	0.20
Beer nuts	10 nuts	34	186	779	8	10	5	2.2	14	2.0	0	26	0.6	2	203	54	152	0	37	tr	0
Bits and bites snack bites (Bits & Bites™)	125mL	31	132	554	4	21	3	1.9	4	1.0	1	18	2.6	263	92	24	71	2	37	tr	0.03
Fruit leather bar (Fruit to Go™)	1 bar	14	49	206	tr	11	N/A	0.5	1	0.6	0	4	0.1	11	19	3	8	1	1	1	0
Pretzels, hard, plain, salted	10 sticks	5	19	80	tr	4	tr	0.2	tr	tr	0	2	0.2	86	7	2	6	0	12	0	0
Pretzels, hard, plain, unsalted	10 sticks	5	19	80	tr	4	tr	0.2	tr	tr	0	2	0.2	15	7	2	6	0	12	0	0
Rice cakes, plain	1	9	35	146	1	7	tr	0.4	tr	0.1	0	1	0.1	29	26	12	32	0	2	0	0
Sesame sticks, salted	60mL	14	75	316	2	6	tr	0.4	5	0.9	0	24	0.1	208	25	6	19	0	3	0	0
Soybeans, roasted, salted	60mL	44	205	859	15	15	2	7.7	11	1.6	0	60	1.7	71	641	63	158	4	92	1	0
Trail mix, regular	60mL	38	176	735	5	17	N/A	2.5	11	2.1	0	30	1.2	87	261	60	131	tr	27	1	0
Trail mix, tropical	60mL	36	144	604	2	23	N/A	2.4	6	3.0	0	20	0.9	4	252	34	66	1	15	3	0

Beverages

Food Name	Measure	Weight	Energy	Energy	Protein	Carbohydrate	Total Sugar	Total Dietary Fibre	Total Fat	Saturated Fat	Cholesterol	Calcium	Iron	Sodium	Potassium	Magnesium	Phosphorus	Vitamin A	Vitamin C	Alcohol	Caffeine
		g	kcal	kJ	g	g	g	g	g	g	mg	mg	mg	mg	mg	mg	mg	RAE	mg	g	mg
Beverages																					
Coffee, Tea and Substitutes																					
Chai, latte	250mL	242	149	624	5	26	26	0	3	2.0	13	186	0.1	67	263	19	150	88	tr	0	13
Coffee, brewed	250mL	250	3	10	tr	0	0	0	tr	tr	0	5	tr	5	123	8	8	0	0	0	100
Coffee, brewed, decaffeinated	250mL	251	3	10	tr	0	0	0	0	0	0	5	0.1	5	135	13	3	0	0	0	3
Coffee, instant, regular, powder + water	250mL	253	5	20	tr	1	0	0	tr	tr	0	10	0.1	5	76	8	8	0	0	0	66
Coffee, latte	250mL	256	101	420	5	7	9	0	6	3.5	16	188	0.2	79	340	89	156	46	tr	0	193
Coffee, substitute, powder + water	250mL	254	13	53	tr	3	tr	0.8	tr	tr	0	8	0.2	8	79	10	18	0	0	0	0
Iced cappuccino - original - with cream (Tim Hortons™)	250mL	N/A	211	886	2	28	28	0	9	5.0	38	80	0.3	42	N/A	N/A	N/A	N/A	0	N/A	N/A
Iced cappuccino - with 2% milk (Tim Hortons™)	250mL	N/A	127	533	3	27	27	0	1	1.0	4	70	0.3	30	N/A	N/A	N/A	N/A	0	N/A	N/A
Iced coffee, Frappuccino (Starbucks™)	250mL	N/A	127	533	3	26	22	0	2	1.0	7	110	0	120	N/A	N/A	N/A	N/A	0	N/A	60
Iced tea, lemon flavor, ready-to-drink	250mL	254	91	383	0	23	23	0	0	0	0	N/A	N/A	53	N/A	N/A	N/A	0	N/A	0	N/A
Iced tea, lemon flavour, powder + water	250mL	274	93	389	tr	23	23	0	tr	tr	0	5	0.1	8	52	5	3	0	tr	0	30
Tea, brewed	250mL	250	3	10	0	1	0	0	tr	tr	0	0	0.1	8	93	8	3	0	0	0	50
Tea, brewed, herbal	250mL	250	3	10	0	1	0	0	tr	tr	0	5	0.2	3	23	3	0	0	0	0	0
Carbonated Drinks																					
Club soda	250mL	250	0	0	0	0	0	0	0	0	0	13	tr	53	5	3	0	0	0	0	0
Cola	250mL	262	110	461	tr	28	24	0	0	0	0	8	0.1	10	3	3	34	0	0	0	26
Cola, aspartame sweetened	250mL	250	3	10	tr	tr	0	0	0	0	0	8	0.1	13	15	3	28	0	0	0	35
Cola, decaffeinated	250mL	262	107	448	0	28	28	0	0	0	0	5	0.1	10	8	0	29	0	0	0	0
Ginger ale	250mL	258	88	366	0	23	22	0	0	0	0	8	0.5	18	3	3	0	0	0	0	0
Lemon-lime soda	250mL	260	104	433	0	27	23	0	0	0	0	5	0.2	29	3	3	0	0	0	0	0
Non cola soda, aspartame sweetened	250mL	250	0	0	0	tr	0	0	0	0	0	10	0.1	40	5	3	0	0	0	0	0
Orange soda	250mL	262	126	527	0	32	N/A	0	0	0	0	13	0.2	31	5	3	3	0	0	0	0
Tonic water	250mL	258	124	520	0	32	32	0	0	0	0	4	tr	15	0	0	0	0	0	0	0

Food Name	Measure	Weight	Energy	Energy	Protein	Carbohydrate	Total Sugar	Total Dietary Fibre	Total Fat	Saturated Fat	Cholesterol	Calcium	Iron	Sodium	Potassium	Magnesium	Phosphorus	Vitamin A	Vitamin C	Alcohol	Caffeine
		g	kcal	kJ	g	g	g	g	g	g	mg	mg	mg	mg	mg	mg	mg	RAE	mg	g	mg
Beverages																					
Fruit Flavoured Drinks																					
Citrus juice drink, frozen, diluted (Five Alive™)	250mL	262	131	548	tr	32	30	0.3	tr	0	0	13	1.8	5	128	10	10	N/A	38	0	0
Fruit flavour drink, low Calorie, powder + water (Crystal Light™)	250mL	254	3	14	0	1	0	0	tr	0	0	6	tr	6	0	3	2	tr	0	0	0
Fruit punch flavour drink, powder (Kool-Aid™) + water	250mL	276	102	427	0	26	N/A	0	tr	tr	0	44	0.1	39	3	3	55	0	0	0	0
Fruit punch flavour drink, vitamin C added, powder + water	250mL	277	102	429	0	26	N/A	0	tr	tr	0	44	0.1	39	3	3	55	0	100	0	0
Fruit punch juice drink, ready-to-drink (Sunny D™)	250mL	262	123	516	0	33	31	0	0	0	0	3	0.1	26	31	N/A	3	0	3	0	0
Lemonade, pink or white, frozen, diluted	250mL	262	105	440	tr	27	13	0.2	tr	tr	0	8	0.4	6	39	5	5	0	10	0	0
Mixed vegetable and fruit juice drink, ready-to-drink (V8 Splash™)	250mL	257	113	472	tr	29	5	0.3	tr	0	0	10	0.2	41	62	5	8	N/A	81	0	0
Orange drink, vitamin C added (Hi-C™), ready-to-drink	250mL	262	134	558	0	34	29	0	tr	tr	0	16	0.7	42	47	5	3	N/A	94	0	0
Orange drink, vitamin C added (Tang™, Quench™, Rise'n Shine™), powder + water	250mL	286	135	564	0	34	34	0	0	0	0	140	0.1	11	69	3	63	N/A	88	0	0
Other Beverages																					
Sports drink, fruit flavour, low Calorie, ready-to-drink (Gatorade™, Powerade™)	250mL	261	29	120	0	8	0	0	0	0	0	0	0.1	91	26	3	23	0	16	0	0
Sports drink, fruit flavour, ready-to-drink (Gatorade™, Powerade™)	250mL	258	67	281	0	16	14	0	tr	0	0	3	0.5	101	36	3	23	0	1	N/A	N/A
Water, mineral (Perrier™)	250mL	250	0	0	0	0	0	0	0	0	0	35	0	3	0	0	0	0	0	0	0
Water, municipal	250mL	250	0	0	0	0	0	0	0	0	0	5	0	5	0	3	0	0	0	0	0
Alcoholic																					
Beer, de-alcoholized, (Labbat .5™)	1 can	350	210	878	1	47	28	0	tr	0.1	0	24	0.2	45	28	24	56	0	2	1	0
Beer, high alcohol (7%alcohol by volume)	1 bottle	342	183	766	1	10	N/A	0.7	0	0	0	17	0.1	17	86	21	41	0	0	20	0
Beer, light (4% alcohol by volume)	1 bottle	340	99	412	1	5	tr	0	0	0	0	14	0.1	14	71	17	41	0	0	11	0
Beer, regular (5% alcohol by volume)	1 bottle	342	140	586	1	10	0	0	0	0	0	14	0.1	14	92	21	48	0	0	14	0
Cocktail, daiquiri	125mL	128	237	993	tr	9	7	0.1	tr	tr	0	4	0.1	6	27	3	6	0	2	29	0
Cocktail, margarita	125mL	131	246	1031	tr	6	4	0.1	tr	tr	0	4	0.1	527	23	2	7	tr	2	33	0
Liqueur, coffee and cream	45mL	53	172	719	1	11	10	0	8	5.1	31	8	0.1	48	17	1	26	91	tr	7	4
Sangria	125mL	123	87	365	tr	12	10	0.1	tr	tr	0	9	0.2	13	80	8	10	1	6	6	0
Spirits (gin, rum, vodka, whisky)	50mL	47	109	456	0	0	0	0	0	0	0	0	tr	1	1	0	2	0	0	16	0
Vodka cooler	1 bottle	390	220	799	tr	33	12	0.3	1	tr	0	20	0.9	12	211	23	19	tr	11	13	0

Food Name	Measure	Weight	Energy	Energy	Protein	Carbohydrate	Total Sugar	Total Dietary Fibre	Total Fat	Saturated Fat	Cholesterol	Calcium	Iron	Sodium	Potassium	Magnesium	Phosphorus	Vitamin A	Vitamin C	Alcohol	Caffeine
		g	kcal	kJ	g	g	g	g	g	g	mg	mg	mg	mg	mg	mg	mg	RAE	mg	g	mg
Beverages																					
Wine, dessert, sweet	125mL	127	203	848	tr	17	10	0	0	0	0	10	0.3	11	117	11	11	0	0	19	0
Wine, table, red	125mL	125	90	375	tr	2	1	0	0	0	0	10	0.5	6	140	16	17	0	0	12	0
Wine, table, white	125mL	125	85	354	tr	1	1	0	0	0	0	11	0.4	6	100	12	17	0	0	12	0

Miscellaneous

Food Name	Measure	Weight	Energy	Energy	Protein	Carbohydrate	Total Sugar	Total Fat	Saturated Fat	Monounsaturated Fat	Polyunsaturated Fat	Cholesterol	Calcium	Iron	Sodium	Potassium	Magnesium	Phosphorus	Vitamin A	Lycopene	Folate
		g	kcal	kJ	g	g	g	g	g	g	g	mg	mg	mg	mg	mg	mg	mg	RAE	mcg	DFE
Miscellaneous																					
Condiments																					
Bacon bits, simulated meat	15mL	7	34	141	2	2	0	2	0.3	0.4	1.0	0	7	0.1	126	10	7	15	0	0	9
Ketchup	15mL	15	15	64	tr	4	3	tr	tr	tr	tr	0	3	0.1	169	57	3	5	7	2586	2
Mustard	15mL	16	11	44	1	1	tr	1	tr	0.4	0.2	0	9	0.2	180	22	8	17	1	0	1
Olives, pickled, canned or bottled	4	16	23	97	tr	1	tr	2	0.3	1.8	0.2	0	8	0.1	249	7	2	1	3	0	tr
Olives, ripe, canned, jumbo	2	16	13	54	tr	1	0	1	0.1	0.8	0.1	0	15	0.5	144	1	1	tr	3	0	0
Pickle relish, sweet	15mL	15	20	83	tr	5	2	tr	tr	tr	tr	0	tr	0.1	123	4	1	2	1	0	tr
Pickles, cucumber, dill	1 medium pickle	65	12	49	tr	3	1	tr	tr	tr	0.1	0	6	0.3	833	75	7	14	6	0	1
Pickles, cucumber, sweet, slices	4	28	33	137	tr	9	5	tr	tr	tr	tr	0	1	0.2	263	9	1	3	3	0	tr
Salsa	15mL	17	5	19	tr	1	1	tr	tr	tr	tr	0	5	0.1	100	50	3	5	3	1758	1
Dips																					
Cream cheese dip	30mL	30	108	451	2	1	tr	11	5.8	3.0	1.6	28	23	0.3	176	39	2	28	92	0	4
Onion dip	30mL	31	50	211	1	3	tr	4	2.5	1.2	0.2	11	34	0.1	206	60	4	31	33	0	3
Spinach dip	30mL	30	74	309	1	2	tr	7	1.6	1.9	3.3	6	26	0.3	84	57	8	17	75	tr	15
Gravies and Sauces																					
Gravy, beef, canned	60mL	59	31	131	2	3	tr	1	0.7	0.6	tr	2	4	0.4	331	48	1	18	1	0	1
Gravy, beef, dehydrated, prepared with water	60mL	65	20	85	1	3	0	1	0.2	0.2	tr	tr	9	0.1	271	15	2	11	tr	0	2
Gravy, chicken, canned	60mL	60	48	199	1	3	tr	3	0.9	1.5	0.9	1	12	0.3	348	66	1	18	1	0	1
Gravy, chicken, dehydrated, prepared with water	60mL	66	22	93	1	4	0	1	0.2	0.3	0.1	1	10	0.1	244	24	3	15	2	0	8
Gravy, turkey, canned	60mL	61	31	130	2	3	tr	1	0.4	0.6	0.3	1	2	0.4	353	67	1	18	0	0	1
Gravy, unspecified, dehydrated, prepared with water	60mL	66	22	91	1	4	0	1	0.2	0.2	0.1	tr	11	0.1	362	16	3	13	0	0	3
Sauce, barbecue	15mL	16	12	50	tr	2	4	tr	tr	0.1	0.1	0	3	0.1	129	28	3	3	tr	68	1
Sauce, cheese, dehydrated, prepared with 2% milk	60mL	71	81	337	5	7	6	4	2.1	1.3	0.4	11	163	0.1	445	158	12	127	45	0	4
Sauce, cranberry, canned, sweetened	60mL	70	106	443	tr	27	27	tr	tr	tr	tr	0	3	0.2	20	18	2	4	1	0	1
Sauce, nacho cheese, ready-to-serve	60mL	64	121	505	5	3	0	10	4.3	3.1	2.1	20	120	0.2	499	20	6	107	66	N/A	3

Food Name	Measure	Weight	Energy	Energy	Protein	Carbohydrate	Total Sugar	Total Fat	Saturated Fat	Monounsaturated Fat	Polyunsaturated Fat	Cholesterol	Calcium	Iron	Sodium	Potassium	Magnesium	Phosphorus	Vitamin A	Lycopene	Folate
		g	kcal	kJ	g	g	g	g	g	g	g	mg	mg	mg	mg	mg	mg	mg	RAE	mcg	DFE
Miscellaneous																					
Sauce, soy	15mL	18	7	30	tr	1	tr	tr	tr	tr	tr	0	1	0.3	1038	28	1	17	0	0	2
Sauce, steak (HP™, A1™)	15mL	15	9	39	tr	2	N/A	tr	tr	tr	tr	0	4	0.2	218	60	2	6	7	N/A	1
Sauce, sweet and sour	15mL	17	20	85	tr	4	3	tr	0.1	0.1	0.2	0	3	0.1	59	11	1	2	1	N/A	tr
Sauce, teriyaki	15mL	18	15	64	1	3	2	0	0	0	0	0	5	0.3	700	41	11	28	0	0	4
Sauce, white, medium, homemade with 2% milk	60mL	61	89	374	2	6	3	6	1.7	2.7	1.7	4	72	0.2	215	95	9	60	55	0	6

Index

Nutrient Value of Some Common Foods

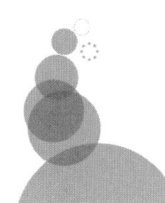

WHO: Nutrition Recommendations, United States Dietary Guidelines and Meal Planning

CONTENTS

This appendix presents nutrition recommendations from the World Health Organization (WHO) and details for Americans on the *USDA Dietary Guidelines for Americans, 2010*, USDA Food Patterns, and USDA MyPlate resources.

Nutrition Recommendations from WHO

The World Health Organization (WHO) has assessed the relationships between diet and the development of chronic diseases. Its recommendations include:

- Energy: sufficient to support growth, physical activity, and a healthy body weight (BMI between 18.5 and 24.9) and to avoid weight gain greater than 5 kilograms (11 pounds) during adult life
- Total fat: 15 to 30 percent of total energy
- Saturated fatty acids: <10 percent of total energy
- Polyunsaturated fatty acids: 6 to 10 percent of total energy
- Omega-6 polyunsaturated fatty acids: 5 to 8 percent of total energy
- Omega-3 polyunsaturated fatty acids: 1 to 2 percent of total energy
- *Trans*-fatty acids: <1 percent of total energy
- Total carbohydrate: 55 to 75 percent of total energy
- Sugars: <10 percent of total energy
- Protein: 10 to 15 percent of total energy
- Cholesterol: <300 mg per day
- Salt (sodium): <5 g salt per day (<2 g sodium per day), appropriately iodized
- Fruits and vegetables: ≥400 g per day (about 0.5 kilogram or 1 pound)
- Total dietary fibre: >25 g per day from foods
- Physical activity: one hour of moderate-intensity activity, such as walking, on most days of the week

USDA Dietary Guidelines for Americans, 2010

What should a person eat to stay healthy? The answers can be found in the *Dietary Guidelines for Americans, 2010.* The guidelines provide science-based advice to promote health and to reduce risk of chronic diseases through diet and physical activity. Figure I-1 presents 20 key recommendations for the general population in three main areas: balancing kcalories with physical activity; consuming more healthy foods; and consuming less sodium, saturated and *trans* fats, added sugars, and refined grains. Figure I-1 also includes three key recommendations for building healthy eating patterns in the general population and six recommendations for specific population groups, such as pregnant women. The recommendations for the first area of balancing kcalories focus on eating the right amount of kcalories balanced with regular physical activity to achieve and maintain a healthy body weight; for the second area, the recommendations focus on selecting more of a variety of vegetables and fruits, whole grains, fat-free and low-fat dairy products, and plant-based, seafood, and lean animal-based protein foods; and recommendations for the third area focus on selecting less of foods high in solid fats, added sugars, and salt. In building healthy eating patterns, consumers are reminded to choose healthful foods that will meet their nutrient needs and to handle foods safely during food preparation and eating. The key recommendations for specific population groups address nutrients of concern during certain life stages. Together, the Dietary Guidelines point the way toward better health through practicing healthy patterns of eating and physical activity behaviours.

USDA Food Patterns

The USDA Food Patterns quantify the types of foods an individual should eat for health. Figure I-2 (p. I-5) shows guidance for making healthful food choices from the five basic food groups for 12 different kcalorie levels. Specific information is also provided for making selections in the subgroups of fruits, vegetables, and protein-based foods. The amounts recommended are based on a person's age, sex, and activity level.

FIGURE I-1 Key Recommendations from the *Dietary Guidelines for Americans, 2010*

Key
Recommendations

BALANCING CALORIES TO MANAGE WEIGHT

- Prevent and/or reduce overweight and obesity through improved eating and physical activity behaviors.
- Control total calorie intake to manage body weight. For people who are overweight or obese, this will mean consuming fewer calories from foods and beverages.
- Increase physical activity and reduce time spent in sedentary behaviors.
- Maintain appropriate calorie balance during each stage of life—childhood, adolescence, adulthood, pregnancy and breastfeeding, and older age.

FOODS AND FOOD COMPONENTS TO REDUCE

- Reduce daily sodium intake to less than 2,300 milligrams (mg) and further reduce intake to 1,500 mg among persons who are 51 and older and those of any age who are African American or have hypertension, diabetes, or chronic kidney disease. The 1,500 mg recommendation applies to about half of the U.S. population, including children, and the majority of adults.
- Consume less than 10 percent of calories from saturated fatty acids by replacing them with monounsaturated and polyunsaturated fatty acids.
- Consume less than 300 mg per day of dietary cholesterol.
- Keep *trans* fatty acid consumption as low as possible by limiting foods that contain synthetic sources of *trans* fats, such as partially hydrogenated oils, and by limiting other solid fats.
- Reduce the intake of calories from solid fats and added sugars.
- Limit the consumption of foods that contain refined grains, especially refined grain foods that contain solid fats, added sugars, and sodium.
- If alcohol is consumed, it should be consumed in moderation—up to one drink per day for women and two drinks per day for men—and only by adults of legal drinking age.[5]

(*continued*)

FIGURE I-1 Key Recommendations from the *Dietary Guidelines for Americans, 2010* (continued)

FOODS AND NUTRIENTS TO INCREASE

Individuals should meet the following recommendations as part of a healthy eating pattern while staying within their calorie needs.

- Increase vegetable and fruit intake.
- Eat a variety of vegetables, especially dark-green and red and orange vegetables and beans and peas.
- Consume at least half of all grains as whole grains. Increase whole-grain intake by replacing refined grains with whole grains.
- Increase intake of fat-free or low-fat milk and milk products, such as milk, yogurt, cheese, or fortified soy beverages.[6]
- Choose a variety of protein foods, which include seafood, lean meat and poultry, eggs, beans and peas, soy products, and unsalted nuts and seeds.
- Increase the amount and variety of seafood consumed by choosing seafood in place of some meat and poultry.
- Replace protein foods that are higher in solid fats with choices that are lower in solid fats and calories and/or are sources of oils.
- Use oils to replace solid fats where possible.
- Choose foods that provide more potassium, dietary fiber, calcium, and vitamin D, which are nutrients of concern in American diets. These foods include vegetables, fruits, whole grains, and milk and milk products.

Recommendations for specific population groups

Women capable of becoming pregnant[7]

- Choose foods that supply heme iron, which is more readily absorbed by the body, additional iron sources, and enhancers of iron absorption such as vitamin C-rich foods.
- Consume 400 micrograms (mcg) per day of synthetic folic acid (from fortified foods and/or supplements) in addition to food forms of folate from a varied diet.[8]

Women who are pregnant or breastfeeding[7]

- Consume 8 to 12 ounces of seafood per week from a variety of seafood types.
- Due to their high methyl mercury content, limit white (albacore) tuna to 6 ounces per week and do not eat the following four types of fish: tilefish, shark, swordfish, and king mackerel.
- If pregnant, take an iron supplement, as recommended by an obstetrician or other health care provider.

Individuals ages 50 years and older

- Consume foods fortified with vitamin B_{12}, such as fortified cereals, or dietary supplements.

BUILDING HEALTHY EATING PATTERNS

- Select an eating pattern that meets nutrient needs over time at an appropriate calorie level.
- Account for all foods and beverages consumed and assess how they fit within a total healthy eating pattern.
- Follow food safety recommendations when preparing and eating foods to reduce the risk of foodborne illnesses.

U.S. Department of Agriculture

FIGURE I-2 **USDA Food Patterns**

The Food Patterns suggest amounts of food to consume from the basic food groups, subgroups, and oils to meet recommended nutrient intakes at 12 different calorie levels. Nutrient and energy contributions from each group are calculated according to the nutrient-dense forms of foods in each group (e.g., lean meats and fat-free milk). The table also shows the number of calories from solid fats and added sugars (SoFAS) that can be accommodated within each calorie level, in addition to the suggested amounts of nutrient-dense forms of foods in each group.

Daily Amount of Food From Each Group

Calorie Level[1]	1,000	1,200	1,400	1,600	1,800	2,000	2,200	2,400	2,600	2,800	3,000	3,200
Fruits[2]	1 cup	1 cup	1½ cups	1½ cups	1½ cups	2 cups	2 cups	2 cups	2 cups	2½ cups	2½ cups	2½ cups
Vegetables[3]	1 cup	1½ cups	1½ cups	2 cups	2½ cups	2½ cups	3 cups	3 cups	3½ cups	3½ cups	4 cups	4 cups
Grains[4]	3 oz-eq	4 oz-eq	5 oz-eq	5 oz-eq	6 oz-eq	6 oz-eq	7 oz-eq	8 oz-eq	9 oz-eq	10 oz-eq	10 oz-eq	10 oz-eq
Protein Foods[5]	2 oz-eq	3 oz-eq	4 oz-eq	5 oz-eq	5 oz-eq	5½ oz-eq	6 oz-eq	6½ oz-eq	6½ oz-eq	7 oz-eq	7 oz-eq	7 oz-eq
Dairy[6]	2 cups	2½ cups	2½ cups	3 cups	3 cups	3 cups	3 cups	3 cups	3 cups	3 cups	3 cups	3 cups
Oils[7]	15 g	17 g	17 g	22 g	24 g	27 g	29 g	31 g	34 g	36 g	44 g	51 g
Limit on calories from SoFAS[8]	137	121	121	121	161	258	266	330	362	395	459	596

1 **Calorie Levels** are set across a wide range to accommodate the needs of different individuals. The attached table "Estimated Daily Calorie Needs" can be used to help assign individuals to the food pattern at a particular calorie level.

2 **Fruit Group** includes all fresh, frozen, canned, and dried fruits and fruit juices. In general, 1 cup of fruit or 100% fruit juice, or ½ cup of dried fruit can be considered as 1 cup from the fruit group.

3 **Vegetable Group** includes all fresh, frozen, canned, and dried vegetables and vegetable juices. In general, 1 cup of raw or cooked vegetables or vegetable juice, or 2 cups of raw leafy greens can be considered as 1 cup from the vegetable group.

Vegetable Subgroup Amounts Per Week

Calorie Level	1,000	1,200	1,400	1,600	1,800	2,000	2,200	2,400	2,600	2,800	3,000	3,200
Dark-green vegetables	½ c/wk	1 c/wk	1 c/wk	1½ c/wk	1½ c/wk	1½ c/wk	2 c/wk	2 c/wk	2½ c/wk	2½ c/wk	2½ c/wk	2½ c/wk
Red and orange vegetables	2½ c/wk	3 c/wk	3 c/wk	4 c/wk	5½ c/wk	5½ c/wk	6 c/wk	6 c/wk	7 c/wk	7 c/wk	7½ c/wk	7½ c/wk
Beans and peas (e.g. pintos, lentils, split peas)	½ c/wk	½ c/wk	½ c/wk	1 c/wk	1½ c/wk	1½ c/wk	2 c/wk	2 c/wk	2½ c/wk	2½ c/wk	3 c/wk	3 c/wk
Starchy vegetables	2 c/wk	3½ c/wk	3½ c/wk	4 c/wk	5 c/wk	5 c/wk	6 c/wk	6 c/wk	7 c/wk	7 c/wk	8 c/wk	8 c/wk
Other vegetables	1½ c/wk	2½ c/wk	2½ c/wk	3½ c/wk	4 c/wk	4 c/wk	5 c/wk	5 c/wk	5½ c/wk	5½ c/wk	7 c/wk	7 c/wk

4 **Grains Group** includes all foods made from wheat, rice, oats, cornmeal, barley, such as bread, pasta, oatmeal, breakfast cereals, tortillas, and grits. In general, 1 slice of bread, 1 cup of ready-to-eat cereal, or ½ cup of cooked rice, pasta, or cooked cereal can be considered as 1 ounce-equivalent from the grains group. **At least half of all grains consumed should be whole grains.**

(continued)

FIGURE I-2 **USDA Food Patterns (*continued*)**

5 **Protein Foods Group** includes meat, poultry, seafood, eggs, processed soy products, and nuts and seeds. In general, 1 ounce of lean meat, poultry, or seafood, 1 egg, 1 Tbsp peanut butter, or ½ ounce of nuts or seeds can be considered as 1 ounce-equivalent from the protein foods group. Also, ¼ cup of beans or peas may be counted as 1 ounce-equivalent in this group.

Protein Foods Subgroup Amounts Per Week

Calorie Level	1,000	1,200	1,400	1,600	1,800	2,000	2,200	2,400	2,600	2,800	3,000	3,200
Seafood	3 oz/wk	5 oz/wk	6 oz/wk	8 oz/wk	8 oz/wk	8 oz/wk	9 oz/wk	10 oz/wk	10 oz/wk	11 oz/wk	11 oz/wk	11 oz/wk
Meat, poultry, eggs	10 oz/wk	14 oz/wk	19 oz/wk	24 oz/wk	24 oz/wk	26 oz/wk	29 oz/wk	31 oz/wk	31 oz/wk	34 oz/wk	34 oz/wk	34 oz/wk
Nuts, seeds, soy	1 oz/wk	2 oz/wk	3 oz/wk	4 oz/wk	4 oz/wk	4 oz/wk	4 oz/wk	5 oz/wk	5 oz/wk	5 oz/wk	5 oz/wk	5 oz/wk

6 **Dairy Group** includes all milks, including lactose-free products and fortified soymilk (soy beverage), and foods made from milk that retain their calcium content, such as yogurt and cheese. Foods made from milk that have little to no calcium, such as cream cheese, cream, and butter, are not part of the group. Most dairy group choices should be fat-free or low-fat. In general, 1 cup of milk or yogurt, 1½ ounces of natural cheese, or 2 ounces of processed cheese can be considered as 1 cup from the dairy group.

7 **Oils** include fats from many different plants and from fish that are liquid at room temperature, such as canola, corn, olive, soybean, and sunflower oil. Some foods are naturally high in oils, like nuts, olives, some fish, and avocados. Foods that are mainly oil include mayonnaise, certain salad dressings, and soft margarine.

8 **SoFAS** are solid fats and added sugars. The limits for calories from SoFAS are the remaining amount of calories in each food pattern after selecting the specified amounts in each food group in nutrient-dense forms (forms that are fat-free or low-fat and with no added sugars).

Estimated Daily Calorie Needs

To determine which food intake pattern to use for an individual, the following chart gives an estimate of individual calorie needs. The calorie range for each age/sex group is based on physical activity level, from sedentary to active.

	Calorie Range		
Children	**Sedentary**	→	**Active**
2–3 years	1,000	→	1,400
Females			
4–8 years	1,200	→	1,800
9–13	1,600	→	2,200
14–18	1,800	→	2,400
19–30	2,000	→	2,400
31–50	1,800	→	2,200
51+	1,600	→	2,200
Males			
4–8 years	1,400	→	2,000
9–13	1,800	→	2,600
14–18	2,200	→	3,200
19–30	2,400	→	3,000
31–50	2,400	→	3,000
51+	2,200	→	2,800

U.S. Department of Agriculture

Sedentary means a lifestyle that includes only the light physical activity associated with typical day-to-day life.

Active means a lifestyle that includes physical activity equivalent to walking more than 3 miles per day at 3 to 4 miles per hour, in addition to light physical activity associated with typical day-to-day life.

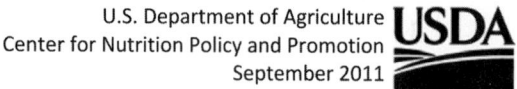

U.S. Department of Agriculture
Center for Nutrition Policy and Promotion
September 2011
USDA

USDA MyPlate

The MyPlate icon that was introduced in Chapter 2 (pp. 43–44) is repeated in Figure I-3 below. MyPlate is a visual reminder to Americans to choose healthy foods from the five basic food groups. The proportionality of food groups found in the icon is based on the USDA Food Patterns.

FIGURE I-3 MyPlate

The USDA MyPlate icon reminds Americans to choose healthy foods from five food groups.

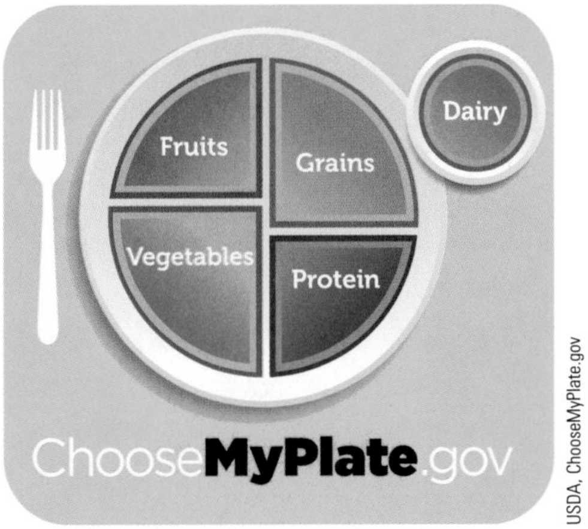
Fruits
Grains
Dairy
Vegetables
Protein
ChooseMyPlate.gov
USDA, ChooseMyPlate.gov

Using the familiar place setting, MyPlate reminds Americans how to eat healthfully from the five food groups.

Glossary

Many medical terms have their origins in Latin or Greek. By learning a few common derivations, you can glean the meaning of words you have never heard of before. For example, once you know that "hyper" means above normal, "glyc" means glucose, and "emia" means blood, you can easily determine that "hyperglycemia" means high blood glucose. The derivations under General, Body, and Chemistry will help you to learn many terms presented in this glossary.

GENERAL

a- or *an-* = not or without
ana- = up
ant- or *anti-* = against
ante- or *pre-* or *pro-* = before
bi- or *di-* = two, twice
cata- = down
co- = with or together
dys- or *mal-* = bad, difficult, painful
endo- = inner or within
epi- = upon
exo- = outside of or without
extra- = outside of, beyond, or in addition
gen- or *-gen* = gives rise to, producing
homeo- = like, similar, constant unchanging state
hyper- = over, above, excessive
hypo- = below, under, beneath
in- = not
inter- = between, in the midst
intra- = within
-itis = infection or inflammation
-lysis = break
macro- = large or long
micro- = small
mono- = one, single
neo- = new, recent
oligo- = few or small
-osis or *-asis* = condition
para- = near
peri- = around, about
poly- = many or much
semi- = half
-stat or *-stasis-* = stationary
tri- = three

BODY

angi- or *vaso-* = vessel
arterio- = artery
cardiac or *cardio-* = heart
-cyte = cell
enteron = intestine
gastro- = stomach
hema- or *-emia* = blood
hepatic = liver
myo- or *sarco-* = muscle
nephr- or *renal* = kidney
neuro- = nerve
osteo- = bone
pulmo- = lung
ure- or *-uria* = urine
vena = vein

CHEMISTRY

-al = aldehyde
-ase = enzyme
-ate = salt
glyc- or *gluc-* = sweet (glucose)
hydro- or *hydrate* = water
lipo- = lipid
-ol = alcohol
-ose = carbohydrate
saccha- = sugar

1,25-dihydroxyvitamin D: vitamin D that is made from the hydroxylation of calcidiol in the kidneys; the biologically active hormone; also called **calcitriol** or **active vitamin D.**

24-hour recall: a record of foods eaten by a person for one 24-hour period.

25-hydroxyvitamin D: vitamin D found in the blood that is made from the hydroxylation of cholecalciferol in the liver; also called **calcidiol.**

A

absorption: the uptake of nutrients by the cells of the small intestine for transport into either the blood or the lymph.

Acceptable Daily Intake (ADI): the estimated amount of a sweetener that individuals can safely consume each day over the course of a lifetime without adverse effect.

Acceptable Macronutrient Distribution Ranges (AMDR): ranges of intakes for the energy-yielding nutrients that provide adequate energy and nutrients and reduce the risk of chronic diseases.

accredited: approved; in the case of dietetic programs, certified by Dietitians of Canada.

acetaldehyde (ass-et-AL-duh-hide): an intermediate in alcohol metabolism.

acetyl CoA (ASS-eh-teel, or ah-SEET-il, coh-AY): a 2-carbon compound (*acetate,* or *acetic acid*) to which a molecule of CoA is attached.

acid controllers: medications used to prevent or relieve indigestion by suppressing production of acid in the stomach; also called *H2 blockers.*

acid–base balance: the equilibrium in the body between acid and base concentrations.

acidosis (assi-DOE-sis): above-normal acidity in the blood and body fluids.

acids: compounds that release hydrogen ions in a solution.

acne: a chronic inflammation of the skin's follicles and oil-producing glands, which leads to an accumulation of oils inside the ducts that surround hairs; usually associated with the maturation of young adults.

active vitamin D: vitamin D that is made from the hydroxylation of calcidiol in the kidneys; the biologically active hormone; also called **1,25-dihydroxyvitamin D** or **calcitriol.**

acupuncture (AK-you-PUNK-cher): a technique that involves piercing the skin with long thin needles at specific anatomical points to relieve pain or illness. Acupuncture sometimes uses heat, pressure, friction, suction, or electromagnetic energy to stimulate the points.

acute PEM: protein-energy malnutrition caused by recent severe food restriction; characterized in children by thinness for height (wasting).

adaptive thermogenesis: adjustments in energy expenditure related to changes in environment such as extreme cold and to physiological events such as overfeeding, trauma, and changes in hormone status.

added sugars: sugars and syrups used as an ingredient in the processing and preparation of foods such as breads, cakes, beverages, jellies, and ice cream as well as sugars eaten separately or added to foods at the table.

additives: substances not normally consumed as foods but added to food either intentionally or by accident.

adequacy (dietary): providing all the essential nutrients, fibre, and energy in amounts sufficient to maintain health.

Adequate Intake (AI): the average daily amount of a nutrient that appears sufficient to maintain a specified criterion; a value used as a guide for nutrient intake when an RDA cannot be determined.

adipokines: proteins synthesized and secreted by adipose cells.

adiponectin: a protein produced by the fat cells that inhibits inflammation and protects against insulin resistance, type 2 diabetes, and cardiovascular disease.

adipose (ADD-ih-poce) **tissue:** the body's fat tissue; consists of masses of triglyceride-storing cells.

adipose tissue lipase: an enzyme involved in the breakdown of body fat.

adolescence: the period from the beginning of puberty until maturity.

adrenal glands: glands adjacent to, and just above, each kidney.

adrenocorticotropin (ad-REE-noh-KORE-tee-koh-TROP-in) or **ATCH:** a hormone, so named because it stimulates *(trope)* the adrenal cortex. The adrenal gland, like the pituitary, has two parts, in this case the outer portion *(cortex)* and an inner core *(medulla)*. The release of ACTH is mediated by *corticotropin-releasing hormone (CRH)*.

adverse reactions: unusual responses to food (including intolerances and allergies).

aerobic (air-ROE-bic): requiring oxygen.

aerobic physical activity: activity in which the body's large muscles move in a rhythmic manner for a sustained period of time. Aerobic activity, also called *endurance activity*, improves cardiorespiratory fitness. Brisk walking, running, swimming, and bicycling are examples.

Agriculture and Agri-Food Canada (AAFC): A federal agency that provides information, research and technology, and policies and programs to achieve an environmentally sustainable/competitive/innovative agriculture, agri-food and agri-based products sector. **www.agr.gc.ca**

AIDS (acquired immune deficiency syndrome): the late stage of HIV infection, in which severe complications develop.

alcohol: a class of organic compounds containing hydroxyl (OH) groups.

alcohol abuse: a pattern of drinking that includes failure to fulfill work, school, or home responsibilities; drinking in situations that are physically dangerous (as in driving while intoxicated); recurring alcohol-related legal problems (as in aggravated assault charges); or continued drinking despite ongoing social problems that are caused by or worsened by alcohol.

alcohol dehydrogenase (dee-high-DROJ-eh-nayz): an enzyme active in the stomach and the liver that converts ethanol to acetaldehyde.

alcoholism: a pattern of drinking that includes a strong craving for alcohol, a loss of control and an inability to stop drinking once begun, withdrawal symptoms (nausea, sweating, shakiness, and anxiety) after heavy drinking, and the need for increasing amounts of alcohol to feel "high."

alcohol-related birth defects (ARBD): malformations in the skeletal and organ systems (heart, kidneys, eyes, ears) associated with prenatal alcohol exposure.

alcohol-related neurodevelopmental disorder (ARND): abnormalities in the central nervous system and cognitive development associated with prenatal alcohol exposure.

aldosterone (al-DOS-ter-own): a hormone secreted by the adrenal glands that regulates blood pressure by increasing the reabsorption of sodium by the kidneys. Aldosterone also regulates chloride and potassium concentrations.

alkalosis (alka-LOE-sis): above-normal alkalinity (base) in the blood and body fluids.

alpha-lactalbumin (lact-AL-byoo-min): a major protein in human breast milk, as opposed to *casein* (CAY-seen), a major protein in cow's milk.

alpha-tocopherol: the active vitamin E compound.

Alzheimer's disease: a degenerative disease of the brain involving memory loss and major structural changes in neuron networks; also known as *senile dementia of the Alzheimer's type (SDAT), primary degenerative dementia of senile onset*, or *chronic brain syndrome*.

amenorrhea (ay-MEN-oh-REE-ah): the absence of or cessation of menstruation. *Primary amenorrhea* is menarche delayed beyond 16 years of age. *Secondary amenorrhea* is the absence of three to six consecutive menstrual cycles.

amino (a-MEEN-oh) **acids:** building blocks of proteins. Each contains an amino group, an acid group, a hydrogen atom, and a distinctive side group, all attached to a central carbon atom.

amino acid pool: the supply of amino acids derived from either food proteins or body proteins that collect in the cells and circulating blood and stand ready to be incorporated in proteins and other compounds or used for energy.

amino acid scoring: a measure of protein quality assessed by comparing a protein's amino acid pattern with that of a reference protein; sometimes called *chemical scoring*.

ammonia: a compound with the chemical formula NH_3; produced during the deamination of amino acids.

amniotic (am-nee-OTT-ic) **sac:** the "bag of waters" in the uterus, in which the fetus floats.

amylase (AM-ih-lace): an enzyme that hydrolyzes amylose (a form of starch). Amylase is a **carbohydrase**, an enzyme that breaks down carbohydrates.

anabolic: building up reactions.

anabolic steroids: drugs related to the male sex hormone, testosterone, that stimulate the development of lean body mass.

anabolism (an-AB-o-lism): reactions in which small molecules are put together to build larger ones. Anabolic reactions require energy.

anaerobic (AN-air-ROE-bic): not requiring oxygen.

anaphylactic (ana-fill-LAC-tic) **shock:** a life-threatening, whole-body allergic reaction to an offending substance.

androstenedione: a hormone made in the adrenal glands that serves as a precursor to the male hormone testosterone; falsely promoted as burning fat, building muscle, and slowing aging. Side effects include acne, aggressiveness, and liver enlargement. See also **DHEA**.

anecdote: a personal account of an experience or event; not reliable scientific information.

anemia (ah-NEE-me-ah): literally, "too little blood." Anemia is any condition in which too few red blood cells are present, or the red blood cells are immature (and therefore large) or too small or contain too little hemoglobin to carry the normal amount of oxygen to the tissues. It is not a disease itself but can be a symptom of many different disease conditions, including many nutrient deficiencies, bleeding, excessive red blood cell destruction, and defective red blood cell formation.

anencephaly (AN-en-SEF-a-lee): an uncommon and always fatal type of neural tube defect; characterized by the absence of a brain.

aneurysm (AN-you-rizm): an abnormal enlargement or bulging of a blood vessel (usually an artery) caused by damage to or weakness in the blood vessel wall.

angina (an-JYE-nah or AN-ji-nah): a painful feeling of tightness or pressure in and around the heart, often radiating to the back, neck, jaw, and arms; caused by a lack of oxygen to an area of heart muscle.

angiotensin: a hormone involved in blood pressure regulation that is activated by renin, an enzyme from the kidneys.

angiotensin I (AN-gee-oh-TEN-sin): an inactive precursor that is converted by an enzyme to yield active angiotensin II.

angiotensin II: a hormone involved in blood pressure regulation.

anions (AN-eye-uns): negatively charged ions.

anorexia (an-oh-RECK-see-ah) **nervosa:** an eating disorder characterized by a refusal to maintain a minimally normal body weight and a distortion in perception of body shape and weight.

antacids: medications used to relieve indigestion by neutralizing acid in the stomach.

antagonist: a competing factor that counteracts the action of another factor. When a drug displaces a vitamin from its site of action, the drug renders the vitamin ineffective and thus acts as a vitamin antagonist.

anthropometric (AN-throw-poe-MET-rick): relating to measurement of the physical characteristics of the body, such as height and weight.

antibodies: large proteins of the blood and body fluids, produced by the immune system in response to the invasion of the body by foreign molecules (usually proteins called *antigens*). Antibodies combine with and inactivate the foreign invaders, thus protecting the body.

antidiuretic hormone (ADH): a hormone produced by the pituitary gland in response to dehydration (or a high sodium concentration in the blood). It stimulates the kidneys to reabsorb more water and therefore prevents water loss in urine (also called **vasopressin**).

antigens: substances that elicit the formation of antibodies or an inflammation reaction from the immune system. A bacterium, a virus, a toxin, and a protein in food that causes allergy are all examples of antigens.

antioxidant: a substance that significantly decreases the adverse effects of free radicals on normal physiological functions.

antioxidants (food additive): preservatives that delay or prevent rancidity of fats in foods and other damage to food caused by oxygen.

antipromoters: factors that oppose the development of cancer.

antiscorbutic (AN-tee-skor-BUE-tik) **factor:** the original name for vitamin C.

anus (AY-nus): the terminal outlet of the GI tract.

aorta (ay-OR-tuh): the large, primary artery that conducts blood from the heart to the body's smaller arteries.

apoptosis: cell death.

appendix: a narrow blind sac extending from the beginning of the colon that stores lymph cells.

appetite: the integrated response to the sight, smell, thought, or taste of food that initiates or delays eating.

appropriate for gestational age (AGA): term describing an infant whose birth weight is normal compared with the number of weeks in utero.

aquaculture: the practice of fish farming.

arachidonic (a-RACK-ih-DON-ic) **acid:** an omega-6 polyunsaturated fatty acid with 20 carbons and four double bonds; present in small amounts in meat and other animal products and synthesized in the body from linoleic acid.

ariboflavinosis (ay-RYE-boh-FLAY-vin-oh-sis): riboflavin deficiency.

aroma therapy: a technique that uses oil extracts from plants and flowers (usually applied by massage or baths) to enhance physical, psychological, and spiritual health.

arteries: vessels that carry blood from the heart to the tissues.

artesian water: water drawn from a well that taps a confined aquifer in which the water is under pressure.

arthritis: inflammation of a joint, usually accompanied by pain, swelling, and structural changes.

artificial fats: zero-energy fat replacers that are chemically synthesized to mimic the sensory and cooking qualities of naturally occurring fats but are totally or partially resistant to digestion.

artificial sweeteners: sugar substitutes that provide negligible, if any, energy; sometimes called *nonnutritive sweeteners*.

ascorbic acid: one of the two active forms of vitamin C.

-ase (AZE): a word ending denoting an enzyme. The word beginning often identifies the compounds the enzyme works on.

aspartame (ah-SPAR-tame or ASS-par-tame): an artificial sweetener composed of two amino acids (phenylalanine and aspartic acid); approved for use in both Canada and the United States.

asymptomatic allergy: an immune response that produces antibodies but no symptoms.

atheromatous (ATH-er-OH-ma-tus) **plaque:** plaque associated with atherosclerosis.

atherosclerosis (ATH-er-oh-scler-OH-sis): a type of artery disease characterized by plaques (accumulations of lipid-containing material) on the inner walls of the arteries.

atoms: the smallest components of an element that have all of the properties of the element.

ATP or **adenosine** (ah-DEN-oh-seen) **triphosphate** (try-FOS-fate): a common high-energy compound composed of a purine (adenine), a sugar (ribose), and three phosphate groups.

atrophic (a-TRO-fik) **gastritis** (gas-TRY-tis): chronic inflammation of the stomach accompanied by a diminished size and functioning of the mucous membrane and glands.

atrophy (AT-ro-fee): becoming smaller; with regard to muscles, a decrease in size (and strength) because of disuse, undernutrition, or wasting diseases.

autoimmune disorder: a condition in which the body develops antibodies to its own proteins and then proceeds to destroy cells containing these proteins. In type 1 diabetes, the body develops antibodies to its insulin and destroys the pancreatic cells that produce the insulin, creating an insulin deficiency.

autonomic nervous system: the division of the nervous system that controls the body's automatic responses. Its two branches are the sympathetic branch, which helps the body respond to stressors from the outside environment, and the parasympathetic branch, which regulates normal body activities between stressful times.

avidin (AV-eh-din): the protein in egg whites that binds biotin.

ayurveda (AH-your-VAY-dah): a traditional Hindu system of improving health by using herbs, diet, meditation, massage, and yoga to stimulate the body, mind, and spirit to prevent and treat disease.

B

bacteriophages (bak-TIR-ee-oh-fayjz): viruses that infect bacteria.

balance (dietary): providing foods in proportion to one another and in proportion to the body's needs.

bariatrics: the field of medicine that specializes in treating obesity.

basal metabolic rate (BMR): the rate of energy use for metabolism under specified conditions: after a 12-hour fast and restful sleep, without any physical activity or emotional excitement, and in a comfortable setting. It is usually expressed as kcalories per kilogram body weight per hour.

basal metabolism: the energy needed to maintain life when a body is at complete digestive, physical, and emotional rest.

bases: compounds that accept hydrogen ions in a solution.

B-cells: lymphocytes that produce antibodies. B stands for bone marrow where the B-cells develop and mature.

beer: an alcoholic beverage traditionally brewed by fermenting malted barley and adding hops for flavour.

behaviour modification: the changing of behaviour by the manipulation of antecedents (cues or environmental factors that trigger behavior), the behaviour itself, and consequences (the penalties or rewards attached to behaviour).

belching: the expulsion of gas from the stomach through the mouth.

benign: an abnormal mass of cells that is noncancerous.

beriberi: the thiamin-deficiency disease.

beta-carotene (BAY-tah KARE-oh-teen): one of the carotenoids; an orange pigment and vitamin A precursor found in plants.

BHA and BHT: preservatives commonly used to slow the development of off-flavours, odours, and colour changes caused by oxidation.

bicarbonate: an alkaline compound with the formula HCO_3 that is secreted from the pancreas as part of the pancreatic juice. (Bicarbonate is also produced in all cell fluids from the dissociation of cabonic acid to help maintain the body's acid–base balance.)

bifidus (BIFF-id-us, by-FEED-us) **factors:** factors in colostrum and breast milk that favour the growth of the "friendly" bacterium *Lactobacillus* (lack-toh-ba-SILL-us) *bifidus* in the infant's intestinal tract, so that other, less desirable intestinal inhabitants will not flourish.

bile: an emulsifier that prepares fats and oils for digestion; an exocrine secretion made by the liver, stored in the gallbladder, and released into the small intestine when needed.

binders: chemical compounds in foods that combine with nutrients (especially minerals) to form complexes the body cannot absorb. Examples include *phytates* (FYE-tates) and *oxalates* (OCK-sa-lates).

binge drinking: four or more drinks for women and five or more drinks for men of alcohol in a row (within a couple of hours).

binge-eating disorder: an eating disorder with criteria similar to those of bulimia nervosa, excluding purging or other compensatory behaviours.

bioaccumulation: the accumulation of contaminants in the flesh of animals high on the food chain.

bioavailability: the rate at and the extent to which a nutrient is absorbed and used.

bioelectromagnetic medical applications: the use of electrical energy, magnetic energy, or both to stimulate bone repair, wound healing, and tissue regeneration.

biofeedback: the use of special devices to convey information about heart rate, blood pressure, skin temperature, muscle relaxation, and the like to enable a person to learn how to consciously control these medically important functions.

biofield therapeutics: a manual healing method that directs a healing force from an outside source (commonly God or another supernatural being) through the practitioner and into the client's body; commonly known as "laying on of hands."

biological value (BV): a measure of protein quality assessed by measuring the amount of protein nitrogen that is retained from a given amount of protein nitrogen absorbed.

biotechnology: the use of biological systems or organisms to create or modify products. Examples include the use of bacteria to make yogurt, yeast to make beer, and cross-breeding to enhance crop production.

biotin (BY-oh-tin): a B vitamin that functions as a coenzyme in metabolism.

blastocyst (BLASS-toe-sist): the developmental stage of the zygote when it is about five days old and ready for implantation.

blind experiment: an experiment in which the subjects do not know whether they are members of the experimental group or the control group.

blood lipid profile: results of blood tests that reveal a person's total cholesterol, triglycerides, and various lipoproteins.

body composition: the proportions of muscle, bone, fat, and other tissue that make up a person's total body weight.

body mass index (BMI): an index of a person's weight in relation to height; determined by dividing the weight (in kilograms) by the square of the height (in metres).

bolus (BOH-lus): a portion; with respect to food, the amount swallowed at one time.

bomb calorimeter (KAL-oh-RIM-eh-ter): an instrument that measures the heat energy released when foods are burned, thus providing an estimate of the potential energy of the foods.

bone meal or **powdered bone:** crushed or ground bone preparations intended to supply calcium to the diet. Calcium from bone is not well absorbed and is often contaminated with toxic minerals such as arsenic, mercury, lead, and cadmium.

bone mineral density: a measure of bone strength. When minerals fill the bone matrix (making it dense), they give it strength.

bottled water: drinking water sold in bottles.

botulism (BOT-chew-lism): an often fatal food-borne illness caused by the ingestion of foods containing a toxin produced by bacteria that grow without oxygen.

bovine growth hormone (BGH): a hormone produced naturally in the pituitary gland of a cow that promotes growth and milk production; now produced for agricultural use by bacteria.

bowel: an alternative term for *intestine*, the *small bowel* refers to the small intestine, and the *large bowel* refers to the large intestine or colon.

bran: the protective coating around the kernel of grain, rich in nutrients and fibre.

branched-chain amino acids: the essential amino acids leucine, isoleucine, and valine, which are present in large amounts in skeletal muscle tissue; falsely promoted as fuel for exercising muscles.

breast milk bank: a service that collects, screens, processes, and distributes donated human milk.

brown adipose tissue: masses of specialized fat cells packed with pigmented mitochondria that produce heat instead of ATP.

brown sugar: refined white sugar crystals to which manufacturers have added molasses syrup with natural flavour and colour; 91 to 96 percent pure sucrose.

buffers: compounds that keep a solution's pH constant when acids or bases are added.

bulimia (byoo-LEEM-ee-ah) **nervosa:** an eating disorder characterized by repeated episodes of binge eating usually followed by self-induced vomiting, misuse of laxatives or diuretics, fasting, or excessive exercise.

C

caffeine: a natural stimulant found in many common foods and beverages, including coffee, tea, and chocolate; may enhance endurance by stimulating fatty acid release. High doses cause headaches, trembling, rapid heart rate, and other undesirable side effects.

calbindin: a calcium-binding transport protein.

calcidiol: vitamin D found in the blood that is made from the hydroxylation of cholecalciferol in the liver; also called **25-hydroxyvitamin D.**

calciol: derived from animals in the diet and made in the skin from 7-dehydrocholesterol, a precursor of cholesterol, with the help of sunlight; also called **cholecalciferol** or **vitamin D_3**.

calcitonin (KAL-seh-TOE-nin): a hormone secreted by the thyroid gland that regulates blood calcium by lowering it when levels rise too high.

calcitriol: vitamin D that is made from the hydroxylation of calcidiol in the kidneys; the biologically active hormone; also called **1,25-dihydroxyvitamin D** or **active vitamin D.**

calcium: the most abundant mineral in the body; found primarily in the body's bones and teeth.

calcium-binding protein: a protein in the intestinal cells, made with the help of vitamin D, that facilitates calcium absorption.

calcium rigour: hardness or stiffness of the muscles caused by high blood calcium concentrations.

calcium tetany (TET-ah-nee): intermittent spasm of the extremities due to nervous and muscular excitability caused by low blood calcium concentrations.

calmodulin (cal-MOD-you-lin): a protein that binds with and activates calcium.

calories: units by which energy is measured. Food energy is measured in kilocalories (1000 calories equal 1 kilocalorie), abbreviated **kcalories** or **kcal.** One kcalorie is the amount of energy necessary to raise the temperature of 1 kilogram (kg) of water 1°C. The scientific use of the term *kcalorie* is the same as the popular use of the term *calorie.* On food labels, the energy content of a food is listed as Calories (with a captial "C"), meaning kcalories.

Canadian Food Inspection Agency: This federal agency works with other agencies from the farm gate to the consumer's plate to protect public health and the safety of Canada's food supply is central to everything they do. **www.inspection.gc.ca**

cancers: malignant growths or tumours that result from abnormal and uncontrolled cell division.

capillaries (CAP-ill-aries): small vessels that branch from an artery. Capillaries connect arteries to veins. Exchange of oxygen, nutrients, and waste materials takes place across capillary walls.

carbohydrase (KAR-boe-HIGH-drase): an enzyme that hydrolyzes carbohydrates.

carbohydrate loading: a regimen of moderate exercise followed by the consumption of a high-carbohydrate diet that enables muscles to store glycogen beyond their normal capacities; also called *glycogen loading* or *glycogen super compensation.*

carbohydrates: compounds composed of carbon, oxygen, and hydrogen arranged as monosaccharides or multiples of monosaccharides. Most, but not all, carbohydrates have a ratio of one carbon molecule to one water molecule: $(CH_2O)_n$.

carbonated water: water that contains carbon dioxide gas, either naturally occurring or added, that causes bubbles to form in it; also called *bubbling* or *sparkling water.*

carbonic acid: a compound with the formula H_2CO_3 that results from the combination of carbon dioxide (CO_2) and water (H_2O); of particular importance in maintaining the body's acid–base balance.

carcinogenesis (CAR-sin-oh-JEN-eh-sis): the process of cancer development.

carcinogens (CAR-sin-oh-jenz or car-SIN-oh-jenz): substances that can cause cancer (the adjective is *carcinogenic*).

cardiac output: the volume of blood discharged by the heart each minute; determined by multiplying the stroke volume by the heart rate. The stroke volume is the amount of oxygenated blood the heart ejects toward the tissues at each beat. Cardiac output (volume/minute) = stroke volume (volume/beat) × heart rate (beats/minute).

cardiorespiratory conditioning: improvements in heart and lung function and increased blood volume, brought about by aerobic training.

cardiorespiratory endurance: the ability to perform large-muscle, dynamic exercise of moderate to high intensity for prolonged periods.

cardiovascular disease (CVD): a general term for all diseases of the heart and blood vessels. Atherosclerosis is the main cause of CVD. When the arteries that carry blood to the heart muscle become blocked, the heart suffers damage known as **coronary heart disease (CHD).**

carnitine (CAR-neh-teen): a nonessential, nonprotein amino acid made in the body from lysine that helps transport fatty acids across the mitochondrial membrane.

carotenoids (kah-ROT-eh-noyds): pigments commonly found in plants and animals, some of which have vitamin A activity. The carotenoid with the greatest vitamin A activity is beta-carotene.

carpal tunnel syndrome: a pinched nerve at the wrist, causing pain or numbness in the hand. It is often caused by repetitive motion of the wrist.

cartilage therapy: the use of cleaned and powdered connective tissue, such as collagen, to improve health.

catabolic: breaking down reactions.

catabolism (ca-TAB-o-lism): reactions in which large molecules are broken down to smaller ones. Catabolic reactions release energy.

catalyst (CAT-uh-list): a compound that facilitates chemical reactions without itself being changed in the process.

cataracts (KAT-ah-rakts): thickenings of the eye lenses that impair vision and can lead to blindness.

cathartic (ka-THAR-tik): a strong laxative.

cations (CAT-eye-uns): positively charged ions.

celiac disease: a sensitivity to gluten, a protein found in wheat, rye, triticale, and barley that damages the villi and increases risk for malnutrition.

cell: the basic structural unit of all living things.

cell differentiation (DIF-er-EN-she-AY-shun): the process by which immature cells develop specific functions different from those of the original that are characteristic of their mature cell type.

cell membrane: the thin layer of tissue that surrounds the cell and encloses its contents; made primarily of lipid and protein.

cellulite (SELL-you-light or SELL-you-leet): supposedly, a lumpy form of fat; actually, a fraud. Fatty areas of the body may appear lumpy when the strands of connective tissue that attach the skin to underlying muscles pull tight where the fat is thick. The fat itself is the same as fat anywhere else in the body. If the fat in these areas is lost, the lumpy appearance disappears.

central nervous system: the central part of the nervous system; the brain and spinal cord.

central obesity: excess fat around the trunk of the body; also called *abdominal fat* or *upper-body fat.*

cerebral thrombosis: a clot that blocks blood flow through an artery that feeds the brain.

certified lactation consultants: health-care providers who specialize in helping new mothers establish a healthy breastfeeding relationship with their newborn. These consultants are often registered nurses and dietitians with specialized training in breast and infant anatomy and physiology.

cesarean (si-ZAIR-ee-un) section: a surgically assisted birth involving removal of the fetus by an incision into the uterus, usually by way of the abdominal wall.

chaff: the outer inedible part of a grain; also called the *husk.*

CHD risk equivalents: disorders that raise the risk of heart attacks, strokes, and other complications associated with cardiovascular disease to the same degree as existing CHD. These disorders include symptomatic carotid artery disease, peripheral arterial disease, abdominal aortic aneurysm, and diabetes mellitus.

cheilosis (kye-LOH-sis or kee-LOH-sis): a condition of reddened lips with cracks at the corners of the mouth.

chelate (KEY-late): a substance that can grasp the positive ions of a mineral.

chelation (kee-LAY-shun) **therapy:** the use of ethylene diamine tetraacetic acid (EDTA) to bind with metallic ions, thus healing the body by removing toxic metals.

chiropractic (KYE-roh-PRAK-tik): a manual healing method of manipulating the spine to restore health.

chloride (KLO-ride): the major anion in the extracellular fluids of the body. Chloride is the ionic form of chlorine, Cl^-.

chlorophyll (KLO-row-fil): the green pigment of plants, which absorbs light and transfers the energy to other molecules, thereby initiating photosynthesis.

cholecalciferol (KO-lee-kal-SIF-er-ol): vitamin D derived from animals in the diet and made in the skin from 7-dehydrocholesterol, a precursor of cholesterol, with the help of sunlight; also called **vitamin D_3** or **calciol.**

cholecystokinin (COAL-ee-SIS-toe-KINE-in), or **CCK:** a hormone produced by cells of the intestinal wall. Target organ: the gallbladder. Response: release of bile and slowing of GI motility.

cholesterol (koh-LESS-ter-ol): one of the sterols containing a four-ring carbon structure with a carbon side chain.

cholesterol-free: less than 2 milligrams cholesterol per serving and *low in saturated fat* per serving.

choline (KOH-leen): a nitrogen-containing compound found in foods and made in the body from the amino acid methionine. Choline is part of the phospholipid lecithin and the neurotransmitter acetylcholine.

chromium picolinate (CROW-mee-um pick-oh-LYN-ate): a trace mineral supplement; falsely promoted as building muscle, enhancing energy, and burning fat. Picolinate is a derivative of the amino acid tryptophan, which seems to enhance chromium absorption.

chromosomes: structures within the nucleus of a cell made of DNA and associated proteins. Human beings have 46 chromosomes in 23 pairs. Each chromosome has many genes.

chronic diseases: diseases characterized by a slow progression and long duration.

chronic PEM: protein-energy malnutrition caused by long-term food deprivation; characterized in children by short height for age (stunting).

chronological age: a person's age in years from his or her date of birth.

chylomicrons (kye-lo-MY-cronz): the class of lipoproteins that transport lipids from the intestinal cells to the rest of the body.

chyme (KIME): the semiliquid mass of partly digested food released by the stomach into the duodenum.

cirrhosis (seer-OH-sis): advanced liver disease in which liver cells turn orange, die, and harden, permanently losing their function; often associated with alcoholism.

***cis*:** on the near side of; refers to a chemical configuration in which the hydrogen atoms are located on the same side of a double bond.

citric acid cycle: a series of metabolic reactions that break down molecules of acetyl CoA to carbon dioxide and hydrogen atoms; also called the *TCA cycle* or the *Kreb's cycle.*

clinically severe obesity: a BMI of 40 or greater or a BMI of 35 or greater with additional medical problems. A less preferred term used to describe the same condition is *morbid obesity.*

clone: a genetic copy of an animal, similar to identical twins but born at different times.

CoA (coh-AY): coenzyme A; the coenzyme derived from the B vitamin pantothenic acid and central to energy metabolism.

coenzymes: complex organic molecules that work with enzymes to facilitate the enzymes' activity. Many coenzymes have B vitamins as part of their structures.

cofactor: a small, inorganic or organic substance that facilitates enzyme action; includes both organic coenzymes made from vitamins and inorganic substances such as minerals.

collagen (KOL-ah-jen): the protein from which connective tissues such as scars, tendons, ligaments, and the foundations of bones and teeth are made.

colonic irrigation: the popular, but potentially harmful practice of "washing" the large intestine with a powerful enema machine.

colostrum (ko-LAHS-trum): a milklike secretion from the breast, present during the first day or so after delivery before milk appears; rich in protective factors.

complementary and alternative medicine (CAM): diverse medical and health-care systems, practices, and products that are not currently considered part of conventional medicine; also called adjunctive, unconventional, or unorthodox therapies.

complementary medicine: an approach that uses alternative therapies as an adjunct to, and not simply a replacement for, conventional medicine.

complementary proteins: two or more dietary proteins whose amino acid assortments complement each other in such a way that the essential amino acids missing from one are supplied by the other.

complex carbohydrates: polysaccharides composed of straight or branched chains of monosaccharides.

compound: a substance composed of two or more different atoms—for example, water (H_2O).

conception: the union of the male sperm and the female ovum; fertilization.

condensation: a chemical reaction in which two reactants combine to yield one larger product.

conditionally essential amino acid: an amino acid that is normally nonessential, but must be supplied by the diet in special circumstances when the need for it exceeds the body's ability to produce it.

conditionally essential nutrient: a nutrient that is normally nonessential, but must be supplied by the diet in special circumstances when the need for it exceeds the body's ability to produce it.

conditioning: the physical effect of training; improved flexibility, strength, and endurance.

confectioners' sugar: finely powdered sucrose, 99.9 percent pure.

congenital hypothyroidism: decreased thyroid hormone production in a newborn.

conjugated linoleic acid: several fatty acids that have the same chemical formula as linoleic acid (18 carbons, two double bonds) but with different configurations (the double bonds occur on adjacent carbons). (These can occur naturally in milk and meat from cows.) Sometimes taken as a supplement to improve body composition.

constipation: the condition of having infrequent or difficult bowel movements.

contaminants: substances that make a food impure and unsuitable for ingestion.

contamination iron: iron found in foods as the result of contamination by inorganic iron salts from iron cookware, iron-containing soils, and the like.

control group: a group of individuals similar in all possible respects to the experimental group except for the treatment. Ideally, the control group receives a placebo while the experimental group receives a real treatment.

conventional medicine: diagnosis and treatment of diseases as practised by medical doctors (M.D.) and doctors of osteopathy (D.O.) and allied health professionals such as physical therapists and registered dietitians; also called *allopathy; Western, mainstream, orthodox,* or *regular medicine;* and *biomedicine.*

cool-down: 5 to 10 minutes of light activity, such as walking or stretching, following a vigorous workout to gradually return the body's core to near-normal temperature.

coral: the skeleton of marine polyps, comprised mostly of calcium carbonate.

Cori cycle: the path from muscle glycogen to glucose to pyruvate to lactate (which travels to the liver) to glucose (which can travel back to the muscle) to glycogen; named after the scientist who elucidated this pathway.

corn sweeteners: corn syrup and sugars derived from corn.

corn syrup: a syrup made from cornstarch that has been treated with acid, high temperatures, and enzymes that produce glucose, maltose, and dextrins. See also *high-fructose corn syrup (HFCS).*

cornea (KOR-nee-uh): the transparent membrane covering the outside of the eye.

coronary arteries: blood vessels that supply blood to the heart.

coronary heart disease (CHD): the damage that occurs when the blood vessels carrying blood to the heart (the coronary arteries) become narrow and occluded.

coronary thrombosis: a clot that blocks blood flow through an artery that feeds the heart muscle.

correlation (CORE-ee-LAY-shun): the simultaneous increase, decrease, or change in two variables. If A increases as B increases, or if A decreases as B decreases, the correlation is positive. (This does not mean that A causes B or vice versa.) If A increases as B decreases, or if A decreases as B increases, the correlation is negative. (This does not mean that A prevents B or vice versa.) Some third factor may account for both A and B.

cortical bone: the very dense bone tissue that forms the outer shell surrounding trabecular bone and comprises the shaft of a long bone.

coupled reactions: pairs of chemical reactions in which some of the energy released from the breakdown of one compound is used to create a bond in the formation of another compound.

covert (KOH-vert): hidden, as if under covers.

CP, creatine phosphate (also called **phosphocreatine**): a high-energy compound in muscle cells that acts as a reservoir of energy that can maintain a steady supply of ATP. CP provides the energy for short bursts of activity.

C-reactive protein (CRP): a protein released during the acute phase of infection or inflammation that enhances immunity by promoting phagocytosis and activating platelets. Its presence may be used to assess a person's risk of an impending heart attack or stroke.

creatine (KREE-ah-tin): a nitrogen-containing compound that combines with phosphate to form the high-energy compound creatine phosphate (or phosphocreatine) in muscles. Claims that creatine enhances energy use and muscle strength need further confirmation.

cretinism (KREE-tin-ism): a congenital disease characterized by mental and physical retardation and commonly caused by maternal iodine deficiency during pregnancy.

critical periods: finite periods during development in which certain events occur that will have irreversible effects on later developmental stages; usually a period of rapid cell division.

Crohn's disease: a type of inflammatory bowel disease of unknown cause resulting abdominal pain, cramping, diarrhea, constipation, and bloody stools. Managed with medication and a dietary plan, but has no cure.

cross-contamination: the contamination of food by bacteria that occurs when the food comes into contact with surfaces previously touched by raw meat, poultry, or seafood.

cruciferous vegetables: vegetables of the cabbage family, including cauliflower, broccoli, and brussels sprouts.

crypt (KRIPT) **glands:** tubular glands that lie between the intestinal villi and secrete intestinal juices into the small intestine.

cytokines (SIGH-toe-kines): special proteins that direct immune and inflammatory responses.

cytoplasm (SIGH-toh-plazm): the cell contents, except for the nucleus.

cytosol: the fluid of cytoplasm; contains water, ions, nutrients, and enzymes.

D

Daily Values (DV): reference values developed specifically for use on food labels.

deamination (dee-AM-ih-NAY-shun): removal of the amino (NH_2) group from a compound such as an amino acid.

defecate (DEF-uh-cate): to move the bowels and eliminate waste.

deficient: the amount of a nutrient below which almost all healthy people can be expected, over time, to experience deficiency symptoms.

dehydration: the condition in which body water output exceeds water input. Symptoms include thirst, dry skin and mucous membranes, rapid heartbeat, low blood pressure, and weakness.

Delaney Clause: a clause in the Food Additive Amendment to the Food, Drug, and Cosmetic Act that states that no substance that is known to cause cancer in animals or human beings at any dose level shall be added to foods.

denaturation (dee-NAY-chur-AY-shun): the change in a protein's shape and consequent loss of its function brought about by heat, agitation, acid, base, alcohol, heavy metals, or other agents.

dental caries: decay of teeth.

dental plaque: a gummy mass of bacteria that grows on teeth and can lead to dental caries and gum disease.

dextrose: an older name for glucose.

DHEA (dehydroepiandrosterone) and **androstenedione:** hormones made in the adrenal glands that serve as precursors to the male hormone testosterone; falsely promoted as burning fat, building muscle, and slowing aging. Side effects include acne, aggressiveness, and liver enlargement.

DHF (dihydrofolate): a coenzyme form of folate.

diabetes (DYE-uh-BEET-eez) **mellitus:** a chronic disorder of carbohydrate metabolism, usually resulting from insufficient or ineffective insulin.

diarrhea: the frequent passage of watery bowel movements.

diet: the foods and beverages a person eats and drinks.

diet history: a record of eating behaviours and the foods a person eats.

dietary fibres: in plant foods, the *nonstarch polysaccharides* that are not digested by human digestive enzymes, although some are digested by GI tract bacteria. Dietary fibres include cellulose, hemicelluloses, pectins, gums, and mucilages and the nonpolysaccharides lignins, cutins, and tannins.

dietary folate equivalents (DFE): the amount of folate available to the body from naturally occurring sources, fortified foods, and supplements, accounting for differences in the bioavailability from each source.

Dietary Reference Intakes (DRI): a set of nutrient intake values for healthy people in Canada and the United States. These values are used for planning and assessing diets and include: Estimated Average Requirements (EAR), Recommended Dietary Allowances (RDA), Adequate Intakes (AI), Tolerable Upper Intake Levels (UL).

dietary supplement: any pill, capsule, tablet, liquid, or powder that contains vitamins, minerals, herbs, or amino acids; intended to increase dietary intake of these substances.

dietetic technician: a person who often works under the supervision of a dietitian. Qualifications for a dietetic technician vary; many require a four-year undergraduate degree in human nutrition or a community college diploma in food service management.

dietitian: a person trained in nutrition, food science, and diet planning. See also *registered dietitian*.

Dietitians of Canada (DC): the professional organization of dietitians in Canada. The American equivalent is the American Dietetic Association.

digestion: the process by which food is broken down into absorbable units.

digestive enzymes: proteins found in digestive juices that act on food substances, causing them to break down into simpler compounds.

digestive system: all the organs and glands associated with the ingestion and digestion of food.

dioxins (dye-OCK-sins): a class of chemical pollutants created as by-products of chemical manufacturing, incineration, chlorine bleaching of paper pulp, and other industrial processes. Dioxins persist in the environment and accumulate in the food chain.

dipeptide (dye-PEP-tide): two amino acids bonded together.

direct calorimetry: a means of estimating energy expenditure by measuring the amount of heat released.

disaccharides (dye-SACK-uh-rides): pairs of monosaccharides linked together. See APPENDIX C for the chemical structures of the disaccharides.

discretionary kcalories: the kcalories remaining in a person's energy allowance after consuming enough nutrient-dense foods to meet all nutrient needs for a day.

disordered eating: eating behaviours that are neither normal nor healthy, including restrained eating, fasting, binge eating, and purging.

dispensable amino acids: nonessential amino acids.

dissociates (dis-SO-see-aites): physically separates.

distilled liquor or **hard liquor:** an alcoholic beverage traditionally made by fermenting and distilling a carbohydrate source such as molasses, potatoes, rye, beets, barley, or corn; sometimes called *distilled spirits*.

distilled water: water that has been vaporized and recondensed, leaving it free of dissolved minerals.

diverticula (dye-ver-TIC-you-la): sacs or pouches that develop in the weakened areas of the intestinal wall (like bulges in an inner tube where the tire wall is weak).

diverticulitis (DYE-ver-tic-you-LYE-tis): infected or inflamed diverticula.

diverticulosis (DYE-ver-tic-you-LOH-sis): the condition of having diverticula.

DNA (deoxyribonucleic acid): the double helix molecules of which genes are made.

docosahexaenoic (DOE-cossa-HEXA-ee-NO-ick) **acid (DHA):** an omega-3 polyunsaturated fatty acid with 22 carbons and six double bonds; present in fatty fish and synthesized in limited amounts in the body from linolenic acid.

dolomite: a compound of minerals (calcium magnesium carbonate) found in limestone and marble. Dolomite is powdered and is sold as a calcium-magnesium supplement. However, it may be contaminated with toxic minerals, is not well absorbed, and interacts adversely with absorption of other esssential minerals.

double-blind experiment: an experiment in which neither the subjects nor the researchers know which subjects are members of the experimental group and which are serving as control subjects, until after the experiment is over.

Down syndrome: a genetic abnormality that causes mental retardation, short stature, and flattened facial features.

drink: a dose of any alcoholic beverage that delivers 15 mL of pure ethanol: 150 mL of wine, 300 mL of wine cooler, 340 mL of beer, or 50 mL of hard liquor.

drug: a substance that can modify one or more of the body's functions.

drug history: a record of all the drugs, over-the-counter and prescribed, that a person takes routinely.

duodenum (doo-oh-DEEN-um, doo-ODD-num): the top portion of the small intestine (about "12 fingers' breadth" long in ancient terminology).

duration: length of time (e.g., the time spent in each activity session).

dysentery (DISS-en-terry): an infection of the digestive tract that causes diarrhea.

dysphagia (dis-FAY-jah): a common term used to describe problems with swallowing.

E

eating disorders: disturbances in eating behaviour that jeopardize a person's physical or psychological health.

eclampsia (eh-KLAMP-see-ah): a severe stage of preeclampsia characterized by convulsions.

edema (eh-DEEM-uh): the swelling of body tissue caused by excessive amounts of fluid in the interstitial spaces; seen in protein deficiency (among other conditions).

edentulous (ee-DENT-you-lus): lack of teeth.

eicosanoids (eye-COSS-uh-noyds): derivatives of 20-carbon fatty acids; biologically active compounds that help to regulate blood pressure, blood clotting, and other body functions. They include *prostaglandins* (PROS-tah-GLAND-ins), *thromboxanes* (throm-BOX-ains), and *leukotrienes* (LOO-ko-TRY-eens).

eicosapentaenoic (EYE-cossa-PENTA-ee-NO-ick) **acid (EPA):** an omega-3 polyunsaturated fatty acid with 20 carbons and five double bonds; present in fatty fish and synthesized in limited amounts in the body from linolenic acid.

electrolyte solutions: solutions that can conduct electricity.

electrolytes: salts that dissolve in water and dissociate into charged particles called ions.

electron transport chain: the final pathway in energy metabolism that transports electrons from hydrogen to oxygen and captures about half the energy released by breaking C—C bonds in the high-energy bonds of ATP.

element: a substance composed of atoms that are alike—for example, iron (Fe).

embolism (EM-boh-lizm): the obstruction of a blood vessel by an embolus (EM-boh-luss), or travelling clot, causing sudden tissue death.

embryo (EM-bree-oh): the developing infant from two to eight weeks after conception.

emergency shelters: facilities that are used to provide temporary housing.

emerging risk factors: recently identified factors that enhance the ability to predict disease risk in an individual.

emetic (em-ETT-ic): an agent that causes vomiting.

empty-kcalorie foods: a popular term used to denote foods that contribute energy but lack protein, vitamins, and minerals.

emulsifier (ee-MUL-sih-fire): a substance with both water-soluble and fat-soluble portions that promotes the mixing of oils and fats in a watery solution.

endogenous (en-DODGE-eh-nus): compounds that derive from within the body.

endoplasmic reticulum (en-doh-PLAZ-mic reh-TIC-you-lum): a complex network of intracellular membranes. The rough endoplasmic reticulum is dotted with ribosomes, where protein synthesis takes place. The smooth endoplasmic reticulum bears no ribosomes.

endosperm: the inner edible part of a grain, rich in starch and proteins.

enemas: solutions inserted into the rectum and colon to stimulate a bowel movement and empty the lower large intestine.

energy: the capacity to do work. The energy in food is chemical energy. The body can convert this chemical energy to mechanical, electrical, or heat energy.

energy density: a measure of the energy a food provides relative to the amount of food (kcalories per gram).

energy-free: fewer than 5 kcalories per serving; synonyms include *Calorie-free* and *zero energy*.

energy-yielding nutrients: the nutrients that break down to yield energy the body can use: carbohydrate, fat, and protein.

enhanced water: water that is fortified with ingredients such as vitamins, minerals, protein, oxygen, or herbs. Enhanced water is marketed as *vitamin water, sports water, oxygenated water,* and *protein water.*

enriched: the addition to a food of nutrients that were lost during processing so that the food will meet a specified standard.

enterogastrone (EN-ter-oh-GAS-trone): a general term for any gastrointestinal hormone; sometimes used to refer specifically to *gastric inhibitory peptide.*

enteropancreatic (EN-ter-oh-PAN-kree-AT-ik) **circulation:** the circulatory route from the pancreas to the intestine and back to the pancreas.

Environment Bureau of Agriculture and Agri-Food Canada: a federal agency that is an integration of three existing components—Prairie Farm Rehabilitation Administration (PFRA), National Land and Water Information Service (NLWIS), and Agri-Environmental Policy Bureau (AEPB)—to address Agriculture and Agri-Food Canada (AAFC)'s agri-environmental issues. **www.agr.gc.ca/policy/environment/**

Environment Canada: is a science-based agency that provides the science and technology information needed so that Canadians can make informed decisions about the environment. In addition, their science and technology work helps us to protect and conserve our air, water, wildlife and spaces. **www.ec.gc.ca**

enzymes: proteins that facilitate chemical reactions without being changed in the process; protein catalysts.

epidemic (ep-ih-DEM-ick): the appearance of a disease (usually infectious) or condition that attacks many people at the same time in the same region.

epigenetics: the study of heritable changes in gene function that occur without a change in the DNA sequence.

epiglottis (epp-ih-GLOTT-iss): cartilage in the throat that guards the entrance to the trachea and prevents fluid or food from entering it when a person swallows.

epinephrine (EP-ih-NEFF-rin): a hormone of the adrenal gland that modulates the stress response; formerly called *adrenaline.* When administered by injection, epinephrine counteracts anaphylactic shock by opening the airways and maintaining heartbeat and blood pressure.

epithelial (ep-i-THEE-lee-ul) **cells:** cells on the surface of the skin and mucous membranes.

epithelial tissue: the layer of the body that serves as a selective barrier between the body's interior and the environment. (Examples are the cornea of the eyes, the skin, the respiratory lining of the lungs, and the lining of the digestive tract.)

ergocalciferol (ER-go-kal-SIF-er-ol): vitamin D derived from plants in the diet and made from the yeast and plant sterol ergosterol; also called **vitamin D_2.**

ergogenic (ER-go-JEN-ick) **aids:** substances or techniques used in an attempt to enhance physical performance.

erythrocyte (eh-RITH-ro-cite) **hemolysis** (he-MOLL-uh-sis): the breaking open of red blood cells (erythrocytes); a symptom of vitamin E–deficiency disease in human beings.

erythrocyte protoporphyrin (PRO-toe-PORE-fe-rin): a precursor to hemoglobin.

erythropoietin (eh-RITH-ro-POY-eh-tin): a hormone that stimulates red blood cell production.

esophageal (ee-SOF-ah-GEE-al) **sphincter:** a sphincter muscle at the upper or lower end of the esophagus. The lower esophageal sphincter is also called the *cardiac sphincter.*

esophagus (ee-SOFF-ah-gus): the food pipe; the conduit from the mouth to the stomach.

essential amino acids: amino acids that the body cannot synthesize in amounts sufficient to meet physiological needs.

essential fatty acids: fatty acids needed by the body that must be supplied by the diet because the body cannot make them. These are linoleic acid and linolenic acid.

essential nutrients: nutrients a person must obtain from food because the body cannot make them for itself in sufficient quantity to meet physiological needs; also called *indispensable nutrients.* About 40 nutrients are currently known to be essential for human beings.

Estimated Average Requirement (EAR): the average daily amount of a nutrient that will maintain a specific biochemical or physiological function in half the healthy people of a given age and gender group.

Estimated Energy Requirement (EER): the average dietary energy intake that maintains energy balance and good health in a person of a given age, gender, weight, height, and level of physical activity.

estrogens: hormones responsible for the menstrual cycle and other female characteristics.

ethanol: a particular type of alcohol found in beer, wine, and distilled liquor; also called *ethyl alcohol.*

excessive drinking: heavy drinking, binge drinking, or both.

exchange lists: diet-planning tools that organize foods by their proportions of carbohydrate, fat, and protein. Foods on any single list can be used interchangeably.

exercise: planned, structured, and repetitive body movements that promote or maintain physical fitness.

exogenous (eks-ODGE-eh-nus): compounds that derive from foods.

experimental group: a group of individuals similar in all possible respects to the control group except for the treatment. The experimental group receives the real treatment.

extra lean: meat or poultry that has not been ground or aquatic animal that contains 7.5 percent or less fat by weight; ground meat or poultry can contain a maximum of 10 percent fat.

extracellular fluid: fluid outside the cells. Extracellular fluid includes two main components—the interstitial fluid and plasma. Extracellular fluid accounts for approximately one-third of the body's water.

F

FAD (flavin adenine dinucleotide): a coenzyme form of riboflavin.

fad diets: popular eating plans that promise quick weight loss. Most fad diets severely limit certain foods or overemphasize others (e.g., never eat potatoes or pasta or eat cabbage soup daily).

faith healing: healing by invoking divine intervention without the use of medical, surgical, or other traditional therapy.

false negative: a test result indicating that a condition is not present (negative) when in fact it is present (therefore false).

false positive: a test result indicating that a condition is present (positive) when in fact it is not (therefore false).

famine: widespread and extreme scarcity of food in an area that causes starvation and death in a large portion of the population.

FAO (Food and Agriculture Organization): an international agency (part of the United Nations) that has adopted standards to regulate pesticide use among other responsibilities.

fat replacers: ingredients that replace some or all of the functions of fat and may or may not provide energy.

fat-free: less than 0.5 grams of fat per serving; synonyms include *zero-fat, no fat,* and *nonfat.*

fats: lipids that are solid at room temperature (77°F or 25°C).

fatty acid: an organic compound composed of a carbon chain with hydrogens attached and an acid group (COOH) at one end and a methyl group (CH_3) at the other end.

fatty acid oxidation: the metabolic breakdown of fatty acids to acetyl CoA; also called *beta oxidation.*

fatty liver: an early stage of liver deterioration seen in several diseases, including kwashiorkor and alcoholic liver disease. Fatty liver is characterized by an accumulation of fat in the liver cells.

fatty streaks: accumulations of cholesterol and other lipids along the walls of the arteries.

female athlete triad: a potentially fatal combination of three medical problems—disordered eating, amenorrhea, and osteoporosis.

fermentable: the extent to which bacteria in the GI tract can break down fibres to fragments that the body can use.

ferritin (FAIR-ih-tin): the iron-storage protein.

fertility: the capacity of a woman to produce a normal ovum periodically and of a man to produce normal sperm; the ability to reproduce.

fetal alcohol spectrum disorder (FASD): a range of physical, behavioural, and cognitive abnormalities caused by prenatal alcohol exposure.

fetal alcohol syndrome (FAS): a cluster of physical, behavioural, and cognitive abnormalities associated with prenatal alcohol exposure, including facial malformations, growth retardation, and central nervous disorders.

fetal programming: the influence of substances during fetal growth on the development of diseases in later life.

fetus (FEET-us): the developing infant from eight weeks after conception until term.

fibrocystic (FYE-bro-SIS-tik) **breast disease:** a harmless condition in which the breasts develop lumps, sometimes associated with caffeine consumption. In some, it responds to abstinence from caffeine; in others, it can be treated with vitamin E.

fibrosis (fye-BROH-sis): an intermediate stage of liver deterioration seen in several diseases, including viral hepatitis and alcoholic liver disease. In fibrosis, the liver cells lose their function and assume the characteristics of connective tissue cells (fibres).

field gleaning: collecting crops from fields that either have already been harvested or are not profitable to harvest.

filtered water: water treated by filtration, usually through activated carbon filters that reduce the lead in tap water, or by reverse osmosis units that force pressurized water across a membrane removing lead, arsenic, and some microorganisms from tap water.

fitness: the characteristics that enable the body to perform physical activity; more broadly, the ability to meet routine physical demands with enough reserve energy to rise to a physical challenge; or the body's ability to withstand stress of all kinds.

flavonoids (FLAY-von-oyds): yellow pigments in foods; phytochemicals that may exert physiological effects on the body.

flaxseeds: the small brown seeds of the flax plant; valued as a source of linseed oil, fibre, and omega-3 fatty acids.

flexibility: the capacity of the joints to move through a full range of motion; the ability to bend and recover without injury.

flora: bacteria within a given environment, such as the intestines.

fluid balance: maintenance of the proper types and amounts of fluid in each compartment of the body fluids.

fluorapatite (floor-APP-uh-tite): the stabilized form of bone and tooth crystal, in which fluoride has replaced the hydroxyl groups of hydroxyapatite.

fluorosis (floor-OH-sis): discolouration and pitting of tooth enamel caused by excess fluoride during tooth development.

FMN (flavin mononucleotide): a coenzyme form of riboflavin.

folate (FOLE-ate): a B vitamin; also known as folic acid, folacin, or pteroylglutamic (tare-o-EEL-glue-TAM-ick) acid (PGA). The coenzyme forms are **DHF (dihydrofolate)** and **THF (tetrahydrofolate).**

follicle-stimulating hormone (FSH): a hormone that stimulates maturation of the ovarian follicles in females and the production of sperm in males. (The ovarian follicles are part of the female reproductive system where the eggs are produced.) The release of FSH is mediated by follicle-stimulating hormone releasing hormone (FSH–RH).

food allergy: an adverse reaction to food that involves an immune response; also called *food-hypersensitivity reaction.*

food aversions: strong desires to avoid particular foods.

food bank: a facility that collects and distributes food donations to authorized organizations feeding the hungry.

food chain: the sequence in which living things depend on other living things for food.

food cravings: strong desires to eat particular foods.

food frequency questionnaire: a checklist of foods on which a person can record the frequency with which he or she eats each food.

food group plans: diet-planning tools that sort foods into groups based on nutrient content and other common attributes (e.g., commodity group, common use) and then specify that people should eat certain amounts of foods from each group.

food insecurity: limited or uncertain access to foods of sufficient quality or quantity to sustain a healthy and active life.

food insufficiency: an inadequate amount of food due to a lack of resources.

food intolerances: adverse reactions to foods that do not involve the immune system.

food pantries: programs that provide groceries to be prepared and eaten at home.

food poverty: hunger resulting from inadequate access to available food for various reasons, including inadequate resources, political obstacles, social disruptions, poor weather conditions, and lack of transportation.

food record: an extensive, accurate log of all foods eaten over a period of several days or weeks. A food record that includes associated information such as when, where, and with whom each food is eaten is sometimes called a food diary.

food recovery: collecting wholesome food for distribution to low-income people who are hungry.

food security: access to enough food to sustain a healthy and active life.

foodborne illness: illness transmitted to human beings through food and water, caused by either an infectious agent (foodborne infection) or a poisonous substance (food intoxication); commonly known as *food poisoning.*

foods: products derived from plants or animals that can be taken into the body to yield energy and nutrients for the maintenance of life and the growth and repair of tissues.

fortified: the addition to a food of nutrients that were either not originally present or present in insignificant amounts. Fortification can be used to correct or prevent a widespread nutrient deficiency or to balance the total nutrient profile of a food.

fossil fuels: coal, oil, and natural gas.

fraudulent: the promotion, for financial gain, of devices, treatments, services, plans, or products (including diets and supplements) that alter or claim to alter a human condition without proof of safety or effectiveness.

free: "nutritionally trivial" and unlikely to have a physiological consequence; synonyms include *without, no,* and *zero.* A food that does not contain a nutrient naturally may make such a claim, but only as it applies to all similar foods (e.g., "applesauce, a fat-free food").

free radical: unstable and highly reactive atom or molecule that has one or more unpaired electrons in the outer orbital.

frequency: the number of occurrences per unit of time (e.g., the number of activity sessions per week).

fructose (FRUK-tose or FROOK-tose): a monosaccharide; sometimes known as *fruit sugar* or *levulose.* Fructose is found abundantly in fruits, honey, and saps.

fuel: compounds that cells can use for energy. The major fuels include glucose, fatty acids, and amino acids; other fuels include ketone bodies, lactate, glycerol, and alcohol.

full term: between the thirty-eighth and forty-second week of pregnancy.

functional foods: foods that contain physiologically active compounds that provide health benefits beyond their nutrient contributions; sometimes called *designer foods* or *nutraceuticals*.

G

g: grams; a unit of weight equivalent to about 0.03 ounces.

galactose (ga-LAK-tose): a monosaccharide; part of the disaccharide lactose.

gallbladder: the organ that stores and concentrates bile. When it receives the signal that fat is present in the duodenum, the gallbladder contracts and squirts bile through the bile duct into the duodenum.

gangrene (GANG-green): death of tissue, usually due to insufficient blood supply.

gastric glands: exocrine glands in the stomach wall that secrete gastric juice into the stomach.

gastric inhibitory peptide: a gastrointestinal hormone that slows motility and inhibits gastric secretions.

gastric juice: the digestive secretion of the gastric glands of the stomach.

gastrin: a hormone secreted by cells in the stomach wall. Target organ: the glands of the stomach. Response: secretion of gastric acid.

gastroesophageal reflux: the backflow of stomach acid into the esophagus, causing damage to the cells of the esophagus and the sensation of heartburn.

gastroesophageal reflux disease (GERD): a condition characterized by the backflow of stomach acid into the esophagus two or more times a week.

gastrointestinal (GI) tract: the digestive tract. The principal organs are the stomach and intestines.

gatekeepers: with respect to nutrition, key people who control other people's access to foods and thereby exert profound impacts on their nutrition. Examples are the spouse who buys and cooks the food, the parent who feeds the children, and the caregiver in a day care centre.

gene expression: the process by which a cell converts the genetic code into RNA and protein.

gene pool: all the genetic information of a population at a given time.

generally recognized as safe (GRAS): food additives that have long been in use and are believed to be safe. First established by the U.S. FDA in 1958, the GRAS list is subject to revision as new facts become known.

genes: sections of chromosomes that contain the instructions needed to make one or more proteins.

genetic engineering: the use of biotechnology to modify the genetic material of living cells so that they will produce new substances or perform new functions. Foods produced via this technology are called *genetically modified (GM)* or *genetically engineered (GE) foods*.

genetics: the study of genes and inheritance.

genome (GEE-nome): the complete set of genetic material (DNA) in an organism or a cell. The study of genomes is called **genomics.**

genomics: the study of all the genes in an organism and their interactions with environmental factors.

genotoxicant: a substance that mutates or damages genetic material.

geophagia: the specific craving for nonfood items that come from the earth, such as clay or dirt.

germ: the seed that grows into a mature plant, especially rich in vitamins and minerals.

gestation (jes-TAY-shun): the period from conception to birth. For human beings, the average length of a healthy gestation is 40 weeks. Pregnancy is often divided into three-month periods, called *trimesters*.

gestational diabetes: glucose intolerance with onset or first recognition during pregnancy.

gestational hypertension: high blood pressure that develops in the second half of pregnancy and resolves after childbirth, usually without affecting the outcome of the pregnancy.

ghrelin (GRELL-in): a protein produced by the stomach cells that enhances appetite and decreases energy expenditure.

glands: cells or groups of cells that secrete materials for special uses in the body. Glands may be exocrine (EKS-oh-crin) glands, secreting their materials "out" (into the digestive tract or onto the surface of the skin), or endocrine (EN-doe-crin) glands, secreting their materials "in" (into the blood).

glossitis (gloss-EYE-tis): an inflammation of the tongue.

glucagon (GLOO-ka-gon): a hormone that is secreted by special cells in the pancreas in response to low blood glucose concentration and elicits release of glucose from liver glycogen stores.

glucocorticoids: hormones from the adrenal cortex that affect the body's management of glucose.

glucogenic amino acids: amino acids that can make glucose via either pyruvate or TCA cycle intermediates.

gluconeogenesis (gloo-ko-nee-oh-JEN-ih-sis): the making of glucose from a noncarbohydrate source.

glucose (GLOO-kose): a monosaccharide; sometimes known as *blood sugar* or *dextrose*.

glucose polymers: compounds that supply glucose, not as single molecules, but linked in chains somewhat like starch. The objective is to attract less water from the body into the digestive tract (osmotic attraction depends on the number, not the size, of particles).

glucose tolerance factors (GTF): small organic compounds that enhance insulin's action.

glycemic index: a method of classifying foods according to their potential for raising blood glucose.

glycemic load: a mathematical expression of both the glycemic index and the carbohydrate content of a food, meal, or diet (glycemic index multiplied by grams carbohydrate).

glycemic (gly-SEEM-ic) **response:** the extent to which a food raises the blood glucose concentration and elicits an insulin response.

glycerol (GLISS-er-ol): produced during carbohydrate metabolism is an alcohol composed of a three-carbon chain, which can serve as the backbone for a triglyceride.

glycogen (GLY-ko-jen): an animal polysaccharide composed of glucose; manufactured and stored in the liver and muscles as a storage form of glucose. Glycogen is not a significant food source of carbohydrate and is not counted as one of the complex carbohydrates in foods.

glycolysis (gly-COLL-ih-sis): the metabolic breakdown of glucose to pyruvate. Glycolysis can operate in both the presence (aerobic) or absence (anaerobic) of oxygen.

goblet cells: cells of the GI tract (and lungs) that secrete mucus.

goiter (GOY-ter): an enlargement of the thyroid gland due to an iodine deficiency, malfunction of the gland, or overconsumption of a goitrogen. Goiter caused by iodine deficiency is *simple goiter.*

goitrogen (GOY-troh-jen): a substance that enlarges the thyroid gland and causes *toxic goiter.* Goitrogens occur naturally in such foods as cabbage, kale, Brussels sprouts, cauliflower, broccoli, and kohlrabi.

Golgi (GOAL-gee) **apparatus:** a set of membranes within the cell where secretory materials are packaged for export.

good source of: the product provides 15 percent or more of the Daily Value for a given nutrient per serving; synonymous with *high in.*

gout (GOWT): a common form of arthritis characterized by deposits of uric acid crystals in the joints.

granulated sugar: crystalline sucrose; 99.9 percent pure.

growth hormone (GH): a hormone secreted by the pituitary that regulates the cell division and protein synthesis needed for normal growth. The release of GH is mediated by GH-releasing hormone (GHRH).

H

hard water: water with a high calcium and magnesium content.

hazard: a source of danger; used to refer to circumstances in which harm is possible under normal conditions of use.

Hazard Analysis Critical Control Points (HACCP): a systematic plan to identify and correct potential microbial hazards in the manufacturing, distribution, and commercial use of food products; commonly referred to as "HASS-ip."

HDL (high-density lipoprotein): the type of lipoprotein that transports cholesterol back to the liver from the cells; composed primarily of protein.

Health Canada: is the Federal agency responsible for helping Canadians maintain and improve their health, while respecting individual choices and circumstances. **www.hc-sc.gc.ca**

Health Canada, Natural Health Products Directorate: authority that ensures Canadians have access to safe, high quality, and effective natural health products; includes vitamins and minerals, herbal remedies, homeopathic medicines, traditional Chinese medicines, probiotics, and other products such as amino acids and essential fatty acids.

health claims: statements that characterize the relationship between a nutrient or other components in a food and a disease or health-related condition.

health history: an account of a client's current and past health status and disease risks.

heart attack: sudden tissue death caused by blockages of vessels that feed the heart muscle; also called *myocardial* (my-oh-KAR-dee-al) *infarction* (in-FARK-shun) or *cardiac arrest.*

heartburn: a burning sensation in the chest area caused by backflow of stomach acid into the esophagus.

heat stroke: a dangerous accumulation of body heat with accompanying loss of body fluid.

heavy drinking: more than one drink per day on average for women and more than two drinks per day on average for men.

heavy metals: mineral ions such as mercury and lead, so called because they are of relatively high atomic weight. Many heavy metals are poisonous.

Heimlich (HIME-lick) **manoeuvre (abdominal thrust manoeuvre):** a technique for dislodging an object from the trachea of a choking person; also known as *abdominal thrust manoeuvre.*

hematocrit (hee-MAT-oh-krit): measurement of the volume of the red blood cells packed by centrifuge in a given volume of blood.

heme (HEEM) **iron:** the iron in foods that is bound to the hemoglobin and myoglobin proteins; found only in meat, fish, poultry, and eggs.

hemochromatosis (HE-moh-KRO-ma-toe-sis): a genetically determined failure to prevent absorption of unneeded dietary iron that is characterized by iron overload and tissue damage.

hemoglobin (HE-moh-GLO-bin): the globular protein of the red blood cells that carries oxygen from the lungs to the cells throughout the body.

hemolytic (HE-moh-LIT-ick) **anemia:** the condition of having too few red blood cells as a result of erythrocyte hemolysis.

hemorrhoids (HEM-oh-royds): painful swelling of the veins surrounding the rectum.

hemosiderin (heem-oh-SID-er-in): an iron-storage protein primarily made in times of iron overload.

hemosiderosis (HE-moh-sid-er-OH-sis): a condition characterized by the deposition of hemosiderin in the liver and other tissues.

hepatic portal vein: the vein that collects blood from the GI tract and conducts it to capillaries in the liver.

hepatic vein: the vein that collects blood from the liver capillaries and returns it to the heart.

hepcidin: a hormone produced by the liver that regulates iron balance.

herbal (ERB-al) **medicine:** the use of plants to treat disease or improve health; also known as *botanical medicine* or *phytotherapy.*

hGH (human growth hormone): a hormone produced by the brain's pituitary gland that regulates normal growth and development; also called *somatotropin.* Some athletes misuse this hormone to increase their height and strength.

hiccups (HICK-ups): repeated cough-like sounds and jerks that are produced when an involuntary spasm of the diaphragm muscle sucks air down the windpipe; also spelled hiccoughs.

high in: 15 percent or more of the Daily Value for a given nutrient per serving; synonymous with *good source.*

high source of fibre: 4 grams or more fibre per serving.

high food security: no indications of food-access problems or limitations.

high potency: one hundred percent or more of the Daily Value for the nutrient in a single supplement and for at least two-thirds of the nutrients in a multinutrient supplement.

high-fructose corn syrup (HFCS): a syrup made from cornstarch that has been treated with an enzyme that converts some of the glucose to the sweeter fructose; made especially for use in processed foods and beverages, where it is the predominant sweetener.

high-quality proteins: dietary proteins containing all the indispensible/essential amino acids in relatively the same amounts that human beings require. They may also contain dispensible/nonessential amino acids.

high-risk pregnancy: a pregnancy characterized by indicators that make it likely the birth will be surrounded by problems such as premature delivery, difficult birth, retarded growth, birth defects, and early infant death.

histamine (HISS-tah-mean or HISS-tah-men): a substance produced by cells of the immune system as part of a local immune reaction to an antigen; participates in causing inflammation.

HIV (human immunodeficiency virus): the virus that causes AIDS. The infection progresses to become an immune system disorder that leaves its victims defenceless against numerous infections.

homeopathy (hoh-me-OP-ah-thee): a practice based on the theory that "like cures like," that is, that substances that cause symptoms in healthy people can cure those symptoms when given in very dilute amounts.

homeostasis (HOME-ee-oh-STAY-sis): the maintenance of constant internal conditions (such as blood chemistry, temperature, and blood pressure) by the body's control systems. A homeostatic system is constantly reacting to external forces to maintain limits set by the body's needs.

honey: sugar (mostly sucrose) formed from nectar gathered by bees. An enzyme splits the sucrose into glucose and fructose. Composition and flavour vary, but honey always contains a mixture of sucrose, fructose, and glucose.

hormones: chemical messengers. Hormones are secreted by a variety of glands in response to altered conditions in the body. Each hormone travels to one or more specific target tissues or organs, where it elicits a specific response to maintain homeostasis.

hormone-sensitive lipase: an enzyme inside adipose cells that responds to the body's need for fuel by hydrolyzing triglycerides so that their parts (glycerol and fatty acids) escape into the general circulation and thus become available to other cells for fuel. The signals to which this enzyme responds include epinephrine and glucagon, which oppose insulin.

hourly sweat rate: the amount of weight lost plus fluid consumed during exercise per hour.

human carrying capacity: the maximum number of people the Earth can support over time.

human genome (GEE-nome): the full complement of genetic material in the chromosomes of a person's cells.

hunger: the painful sensation caused by a lack of food that initiates food-seeking behaviour; consequence of food insecurity that, because of prolonged, involuntary lack of food, results in discomfort, illness, weakness, or pain that goes beyond the usual uneasy sensation.

husk: the outer inedible part of a grain; also called the *chaff.*

hydrochloric acid: an acid composed of hydrogen and chloride atoms (HCl) that is normally produced by the gastric glands.

hydrogenation (HIGH-dro-jen-AY-shun or high-DROJ-eh-NAY-shun): a chemical process by which hydrogens are added to monounsaturated or polyunsaturated fatty acids to reduce the number of double bonds, making the fats more saturated (solid) and more resistant to oxidation (protecting against rancidity). Hydrogenation produces *trans*-fatty acids.

hydrolysis (high-DROL-ih-sis): a chemical reaction in which a major reactant is split into two products, with the addition of a hydrogen atom (H) to one and a hydroxyl group (OH) to the other (from water, H_2O). (The noun is *hydrolysis;* the verb is *hydrolyze.*)

hydrophilic (high-dro-FIL-ick): a term referring to water-loving, or water-soluble, substances.

hydrophobic (high-dro-FOE-bick): a term referring to water-fearing, or non-water-soluble, substances; also known as *lipophilic* (fat loving).

hydrotherapy: the use of water (in whirlpools, as douches, or packed as ice, for example) to promote relaxation and healing.

hydroxyapatite (high-drox-ee-APP-ah-tite): crystals made of calcium and phosphorus.

hyperactivity: inattentive and impulsive behaviour that is more frequent and severe than is typical of others a similar age; professionally called *attention-deficit/hyperactivity disorder (ADHD).*

hypercalcemia: high blood calcium that may develop from a variety of disorders, including vitamin D toxicity. It does *not* develop from a high calcium intake.

hyperglycemia: elevated blood glucose concentrations.

hyperplastic obesity: obesity due to an increase in the *number* of fat cells.

hypertension: higher-than-normal blood pressure. Hypertension that develops without an identifiable cause is known as *essential* or *primary hypertension;* hypertension that is caused by a specific disorder such as kidney disease is known as *secondary hypertension.*

hyperthermia: an above-normal body temperature.

hypertrophic obesity: obesity due to an increase in the *size* of fat cells.

hypertrophy (high-PER-tro-fee): growing larger; with regard to muscles, an increase in size (and strength) in response to use.

hypnotherapy: a technique that uses hypnosis and the power of suggestion to improve health behaviours, relieve pain, and heal.

hypoglycemia (HIGH-po-gly-SEE-me-ah): an abnormally low blood glucose concentration.

hyponatremia (HIGH-poe-na-TREE-mee-ah): a decreased concentration of sodium in the blood.

hypothalamus (high-po-THAL-ah-mus): a brain centre that controls activities such as maintenance of water balance, regulation of body temperature, and control of appetite.

hypothermia: a below-normal body temperature.

hypothesis (hi-POTH-eh-sis): an unproven statement that tentatively explains the relationships between two or more variables.

hypothyroidism: underactivity of the thyroid gland that may be caused by iodine deficiency or any number of other causes.

I

ileocecal (ill-ee-oh-SEEK-ul) **sphincter**: the sphincter separating the small and large intestines.

ileum (ILL-ee-um): the last segment of the small intestine.

imagery: a technique that guides clients to achieve a desired physical, emotional, or spiritual state by visualizing themselves in that state.

imitation foods: foods that substitute for and resemble another food in flavour, texture, appearance, and nutritional values. On food labels, the word "imitation" must appear as part of the common name, such as "imitation crab."

immune system: the body's natural defence against foreign materials that have penetrated the skin or mucous membranes.

immunity: the body's ability to defend itself against diseases.

immunoglobulins (IM-you-noh-GLOB-you-linz): proteins capable of acting as antibodies.

implantation (IM-plan-TAY-shun): the embedding of the blastocyst in the inner lining of the uterus.

indigestion: incomplete or uncomfortable digestion, usually accompanied by pain, nausea, vomiting, heartburn, intestinal gas, or belching.

indirect calorimetry: a means of estimating energy expenditure by measuring the amount of oxygen consumed.

indirect or **incidental additives**: substances that can get into food as a result of contact during growing, processing, packaging, storing, cooking, or some other stage before the foods are consumed; sometimes called *accidental additives.*

indispensable amino acids: essential amino acids.

indispensable nutrients: nutrients a person must obtain from food because the body cannot make them for itself in sufficient quantity to meet physiological needs; also called **essential nutrients.**

infectious diseases: diseases caused by bacteria, viruses, parasites, or other microorganisms that can be transmitted from one person to another through air, water, or food; by contact; or through vector organisms such as mosquitoes.

inflammation: an immunological response to cellular injury characterized by an increase in white blood cells.

inflammatory bowel disease: immune-engaged intestinal diseases of unknown causes, including *Crohn's disease* and *ulcerative colitis.*

initiators: factors that cause mutations that give rise to cancer, such as radiation and carcinogens.

inorganic: not containing carbon or pertaining to living things.

inositol (in-OSS-ih-tall): a nonessential nutrient that can be made in the body from glucose. Inositol is a part of cell membrane structures.

insoluble fibres: nonstarch polysaccharides that do not dissolve in water. Examples include the tough, fibrous structures found in the strings of celery and the skins of corn kernels.

insulin (IN-suh-lin): a hormone secreted by special cells in the pancreas in response to (among other things) increased blood glucose concentration. The primary role of insulin is to control the transport of glucose from the bloodstream into the muscle and fat cells.

insulin resistance: the condition in which a normal amount of insulin produces a subnormal effect in muscle, adipose, and liver cells, resulting in an elevated fasting glucose; a metabolic consequence of obesity that precedes type 2 diabetes.

integrative medicine: care that combines conventional and complementary therapies for which there is some high-quality scientific evidence of safety and effectiveness. Integrative medicine emphasizes the importance of the relationship between the practitioner and the patient and focuses on wellness, healing, and the whole person.

intensity: the degree of exertion while exercising (e.g., the amount of weight lifted or the speed of running).

intentional food additives: additives intentionally added to foods, such as nutrients, colours, and preservatives.

intermittent claudication (klaw-dih-KAY-shun): severe calf pain caused by inadequate blood supply. It occurs when walking and subsides during rest.

Internet (the Net): a worldwide network of millions of computers linked together to share information.

interstitial (IN-ter-STISH-al) **fluid**: fluid between the cells (intercellular), usually high in sodium and chloride. Interstitial fluid is a large component of extracellular fluid.

intestinal ischemia (is-KEY-me-ah): a diminished blood flow to the intestines that is characterized by abdominal pain, forceful bowel movements, and blood in the stool.

intracellular fluid: fluid within the cells, usually high in potassium and phosphate. Intracellular fluid accounts for approximately two-thirds of the body's water.

intrinsic factor: a glycoprotein (a protein with short polysaccharide chains attached) secreted by the stomach cells that binds with vitamin B_{12} in the small intestine to aid in the absorption of vitamin B_{12}.

invert sugar: a mixture of glucose and fructose formed by the hydrolysis of sucrose in a chemical process; sold only in liquid form and sweeter than sucrose. Invert sugar is used as a food additive to help preserve freshness and prevent shrinkage.

iodide: the ion form of iodine.

ions (EYE-uns): atoms or molecules that have gained or lost electrons and therefore have electrical charges. Examples include the positively charged sodium ion ($Na+$) and the negatively charged chloride ion (Cl^-). For a closer look at ions, see APPENDIX B.

iridology: the study of changes in the iris of the eye and their relationships to disease.

iron deficiency: the state of having depleted iron stores.

iron overload: toxicity from excess iron.

iron-deficiency anemia: severe depletion of iron stores that results in low hemoglobin and small, pale red blood cells. Anemias that impair hemoglobin synthesis are *microcytic* (small cell).

irradiation: sterilizing a food by exposure to energy waves, similar to ultraviolet light and microwaves; sometimes called *ionizing radiation.*

irritable bowel syndrome: an intestinal disorder of unknown cause. Symptoms include abdominal discomfort and cramping, diarrhea, constipation, or alternating diarrhea and constipation.

J

jejunum (je-JOON-um): the first two-fifths of the small intestine beyond the duodenum.

joule: a measure of *work* energy; the international unit for measuring food energy.

K

kcal: abbreviation of **kcalories;** a unit by which energy is measured.

kcalorie: a unit by which energy is measured. One kcalorie is the amount of energy necessary to raise the temperature of 1 kilogram (kg) of water 1°C. The scientific use of the term *kcalorie* is the same as the popular use of the term *calorie.*

kcalorie (energy) control: management of food energy intake.

kefir (keh-FUR): a fermented milk created by adding *Lactobacillus acidophilus* and other bacteria that break down lactose to glucose and galactose, producing a sweet, lactose-free product.

keratin (KARE-uh-tin): a water-insoluble protein; the normal protein of hair and nails.

keratinization: accumulation of keratin in a tissue; a sign of vitamin A deficiency.

keratomalacia (KARE-ah-toe-ma-LAY-shuh): softening of the cornea that leads to irreversible blindness; seen in severe vitamin A deficiency.

Keshan (KESH-an or ka-SHAWN) **disease:** the heart disease associated with selenium deficiency named for one of the provinces of China where it was first studied. Keshan disease is characterized by heart enlargement and insufficiency; fibrous tissue replaces the muscle tissue that normally composes the middle layer of the walls of the heart.

keto (KEY-toe) **acid:** an organic acid that contains a carbonyl group (C=O).

ketogenic amino acids: amino acids that are degraded to acetyl CoA.

ketone (KEE-tone) **bodies:** the metabolic products of the incomplete breakdown of fat when glucose is not available in the cells.

ketosis (kee-TOE-sis): an undesirably high concentration of ketone bodies in the blood and urine.

Kreb's cycle: named after the scientist who elucidated this biochemistry, a series of metabolic reactions that break down molecules of acetyl CoA to carbon dioxide and hydrogen atoms; also called the *citric acid cycle* or the *TCA cycle.*

kwashiorkor (kwash-ee-OR-core or kwash-ee-or-CORE): a form of PEM that results either from inadequate protein intake or infections.

L

lactadherin (lack-tad-HAIR-in): a protein in breast milk that attacks diarrhea-causing viruses.

lactase: an enzyme that hydrolyzes lactose.

lactase deficiency: a lack of the enzyme required to digest the disaccharide lactose into its component monosaccharides (glucose and galactose).

lactate: a 3-carbon compound produced from pyruvate during both aerobic and anaerobic metabolism.

lactation: production and secretion of breast milk for the purpose of nourishing an infant.

lacteals (LACK-tee-als): the lymphatic vessels of the intestine that take up nutrients and pass them to the lymph circulation.

lactoferrin (lack-toh-FERR-in): a protein in breast milk that binds iron and keeps it from supporting the growth of the infant's intestinal bacteria.

lacto-ovo-vegetarians: people who include milk, milk products, and eggs, but exclude meat, poultry, fish, and seafood from their diets.

lactose (LAK-tose): a disaccharide composed of glucose and galactose; commonly known as *milk sugar.*

lactose intolerance: a condition that results from inability to digest the milk sugar lactose; characterized by bloating, gas, abdominal discomfort, and diarrhea. Lactose intolerance differs from milk allergy, which is caused by an immune reaction to the protein in milk.

lacto-vegetarians: people who include milk and milk products, but exclude meat, poultry, fish, seafood, and eggs from their diets.

large intestine or **colon** (COAL-un): about 1.5 metres of large diameter intestine; the lower portion of intestine that completes the digestive process. Its segments are the ascending colon, the transverse colon, the descending colon, and the sigmoid colon.

larynx: the upper part of the air passageway that contains the vocal cords; also called the *voice box.*

laxatives: substances that loosen the bowels and thereby prevent or treat constipation.

LDL (low-density lipoprotein): the type of lipoprotein derived from very-low-density lipoproteins (VLDL) as VLDL triglycerides are removed and broken down; composed primarily of cholesterol.

lean: meat or poultry that has not been ground or aquatic animal that contains 10 percent or less fat by weight; ground meat or poultry can contain a maximum of 17 percent fat.

lean body mass: the body minus its fat.

lecithin (LESS-uh-thin): one of the phospholipids. Both nature and the food industry use lecithin as an emulsifier to combine water-soluble and fat-soluble ingredients that do not ordinarily mix, such as water and oil.

legumes (lay-GYOOMS or LEG-yooms): plants of the bean and pea family, with seeds that are rich in protein compared with other plant-derived foods.

leptin: a protein produced by fat cells under direction of the *ob* gene that decreases appetite and increases energy expenditure; sometimes called the *ob protein.*

less: at least 25 percent less of a given nutrient or kcalories than the comparison food (see individual nutrients); synonymous with *reduced.*

less saturated fat: at least 25 percent less saturated fat and the content of *trans* fat is not higher than the reference amount of the comparison food.

let-down reflex: the reflex that forces milk to the front of the breast when the infant begins to nurse.

levulose: an older name for fructose.

licence to practise: permission under provincial law, granted on meeting specified criteria, to use a certain title (such as dietitian) and offer certain services.

life expectancy: the average number of years lived by people in a given society.

life span: the maximum number of years of life attainable by a member of a species.

light or lite: restricted to foods that meet the criteria for "reduced in fat" or "reduced in energy"; any use of the term other than as defined must specify what it is referring to (e.g., "light in colour" or "light in texture").

lightly salted: contains at least 50 percent less sodium than the sodium added to a similar reference food.

lignans: phytochemicals present in flaxseed, but not in flax oil, that are converted to phytosterols by intestinal bacteria and are under study as possible anticancer agents.

limiting amino acid: the indispensible/essential amino acid found in the shortest supply relative to the amounts needed for protein synthesis in the body. Four amino acids are most likely to be limiting: lysine, methionine, threonine, tryptophan.

lingual: pertaining to the tongue.

linoleic (lin-oh-LAY-ick) **acid:** an essential fatty acid with 18 carbons and two double bonds.

linolenic (lin-oh-LEN-ick) **acid:** an essential fatty acid with 18 carbons and three double bonds.

lipase (LYE-paze): an enzyme that hydrolyzes lipids.

lipids: a family of compounds that includes triglycerides, phospholipids, and sterols. Lipids are characterized by their insolubility in water. (Lipids also include the fat-soluble vitamins.)

lipoprotein lipase (LPL): an enzyme that hydrolyzes triglycerides passing by in the bloodstream, the resulting fatty acids can then enter the cells, where they can be metabolized for energy or reassembled for storage.

lipoprotein-associated phospholipase A(2) or **Lp-PLA(2):** a lipoprotein-bound enzyme that generates potent proinflammatory and proatherogenic products such as oxidized free fatty acids and lysophosphatidylcholine. Lp-PLA(2) is a specific marker of plaque inflammation.

lipoproteins (LIP-oh-PRO-teenz): clusters of lipids associated with proteins that serve as transport vehicles for lipids in the lymph and blood.

lipotoxicity: the adverse effects of fat in nonadipose tissues.

listeriosis: an infection caused by eating food contaminated with the bacterium *Listeria monocytogenes,* which can be killed by pasteurization and cooking but can survive at refrigerated temperatures; certain ready-to-eat foods, such as hot dogs and deli meats, may become contaminated after cooking or processing, but before packaging.

liver: the organ that manufactures bile.

longevity: long duration of life.

low birthweight (LBW): a birthweight of 2500 grams (5½ pounds) or less; indicates probable poor health in the newborn and poor nutrition status in the mother during pregnancy, before pregnancy, or both. Optimal birthweight for a full-term baby is about 3100 to 3600 grams (6.8 to 7.9 pounds).

low cholesterol: 20 milligrams or less cholesterol per serving and is low in saturated fat.

low in energy: 40 kcalories or less per serving; synonyms include *low calorie* and *little energy.*

low food security: reduced quality of life with little or no indication of reduced food intake; formerly known as *food insecurity without hunger.*

low in fat: 3 grams or less fat per serving; synonyms include *low fat* and *little fat.*

low saturated fat: 2 grams or less saturated and *trans* fat combined per serving.

low sodium: 140 milligrams or less per serving.

low-risk pregnancy: a pregnancy characterized by factors that make it likely the birth will be normal and the infant healthy.

lumen (LOO-men): the space within a vessel, such as the intestine.

lutein (LOO-teen): a plant pigment of yellow hue; a phytochemical believed to play roles in eye functioning and health.

luteinizing (LOO-tee-in-EYE-zing) **hormone (LH):** a hormone that stimulates ovulation and the development of the corpus luteum (the small tissue that develops from a ruptured ovarian follicle and secretes hormones); so called because the follicle turns yellow as it matures. In men, LH stimulates testosterone secretion. The release of LH is mediated by luteinizing hormone–releasing hormone (LH–RH).

lycopene (LYE-koh-peen): a pigment responsible for the red colour of tomatoes and other red-hued vegetables; a phytochemical that may act as an antioxidant in the body.

lymph (LIMF): a clear yellowish fluid that is similar to blood except that it contains no red blood cells or platelets. Lymph from the GI tract transports fat and fat-soluble vitamins to the bloodstream via lymphatic vessels.

lymphatic (lim-FAT-ic) **system:** a loosely organized system of vessels and ducts that convey fluids toward the heart. The GI part of the lymphatic system carries the products of fat digestion into the bloodstream.

lymphocytes (LIM-foh-sites): white blood cells that participate in acquired immunity; B-cells and T-cells.

lysosomes (LYE-so-zomes): cellular organelles; membrane-enclosed sacs of degradative enzymes.

M

macrobiotic diets: a philosophical approach of eating mostly plant foods such as whole grains, legumes, and vegetables, with small amounts of fish, fruit, nuts, and seeds.

macrocytic: abnormally large blood cells.

macronutrients: carbohydrate, fat, and protein; the nutrients the body requires in relatively large amounts (many grams daily).

macrophages: large immune system cells that ingest and destroy foreign antigens by phagocytosis.

macular (MACK-you-lar) **degeneration:** deterioration of the macular area of the eye that can lead to loss of central vision and eventual blindness. The *macula* is a small, oval, yellowish region in the centre of the retina that provides the sharp, straight-ahead vision so critical to reading and driving.

magnesium: a cation within the body's cells, active in many enzyme systems.

major minerals: essential mineral nutrients the human body requires in relatively large amounts (greater than 100 milligrams per day); sometimes called *macrominerals.*

malignant (ma-LIG-nant): describes a cancerous cell or tumour, which can injure healthy tissue and spread cancer to other regions of the body.

malnutrition: any condition caused by excess or deficient food energy or nutrient intake or by an imbalance of nutrients.

maltase: an enzyme that hydrolyzes maltose.

maltose (MAWL-tose): a disaccharide composed of two glucose units; sometimes known as *malt sugar.*

mammary glands: glands of the female breast that secrete milk.

maple sugar: a sugar (mostly sucrose) purified from the concentrated sap of the sugar maple tree.

marasmus (ma-RAZ-mus): a form of PEM that results from a severe deprivation, or impaired absorption, of energy, protein, vitamins, and minerals.

margin of safety: when speaking of food additives, a zone between the concentration normally used and that at which a hazard exists. For common table salt, for example, the margin of safety is 1/5 (five times the amount normally used would be hazardous).

marginal food security: one or two indications of food-access problems but with little or no change in food intake.

massage therapy: a healing method in which the therapist manually kneads muscles to reduce tension, increase blood circulation, improve joint mobility, and promote healing of injuries.

mastication: the process of chewing.

matrix (MAY-tricks): the basic substance that gives form to a developing structure; in the body, the formative cells from which teeth and bones grow.

matter: anything that takes up space and has mass.

Meals on Wheels: a nutrition program that delivers food for the elderly to their homes.

meat replacements: products formulated to look and taste like meat, fish, or poultry; usually made of textured vegetable protein.

meditation: a self-directed technique of relaxing the body and calming the mind.

megaloblastic: abnormally large blood cells.

menadione (men-uh-DYE-own): the synthetic form of vitamin K.

MEOS or **microsomal** (my-krow-SO-mal) **ethanol oxidizing system:** a system of enzymes in the liver that oxidize not only alcohol but also several classes of drugs.

metabolic syndrome: a combination of risk factors—insulin resistance, hypertension, abnormal blood lipids, and abdominal obesity—that greatly increase a person's risk of developing coronary heart disease; also called *Syndrome X, insulin resistance syndrome,* or *dysmetabolic syndrome.*

metabolic water: water generated during metabolism.

metabolism: the sum total of all the chemical reactions that go on in living cells. Energy metabolism includes all the reactions by which the body obtains and expends the energy from food.

metalloenzymes (meh-TAL-oh-EN-zimes): enzymes that contain one or more minerals as part of their structures.

metallothionein (meh-TAL-oh-THIGH-oh-neen): a sulphur-rich protein that avidly binds with and transports metals such as zinc.

metastasize (me-TAS-tah-size): the spread of cancer from one part of the body to another.

methylation: the addition of a methyl group (CH_3).

MFP factor: a peptide released during the digestion of meat, fish, and poultry that enhances nonheme iron absorption.

micelles (MY-cells): tiny spherical complexes of emulsified fat that arise during digestion; most contain bile salts and the products of lipid digestion, including fatty acids, monoglycerides, and cholesterol.

microangiopathies: disorders of the small blood vessels.

microarray technology: research tools that analyze the expression of thousands of genes simultaneously and search for particular gene changes associated with a disease. DNA microarrays are also called *DNA chips*.

microcytic (my-cro-SIT-ic) **hypochromic** (high-po-KROME-ic) **anemia:** small, pale red blood cells that develop in iron-deficiency anemia.

micronutrients: vitamins and minerals; the nutrients the body requires in relatively small amounts (milligrams or micrograms daily).

microvilli (MY-cro-VILL-ee, MY-cro-VILL-eye): tiny, hairlike projections on each intestinal cell of every villus that can trap nutrient particles and transport them into the cells; singular *microvillus*.

milk anemia: iron-deficiency anemia that develops when an excessive milk intake displaces iron-rich foods from the diet.

milliequivalents per litre (mEq/L): a measure of the concentration of electrolytes in a volume of solution.

mineral oil: a purified liquid derived from petroleum and used to treat constipation.

mineral water: water from a spring or well that naturally contains dissolved minerals. Minerals give water a distinctive flavour. Many mineral waters are high in sodium.

mineralization: the process in which calcium, phosphorus, and other minerals crystallize on the collagen matrix of a growing bone, hardening the bone.

minerals: inorganic elements. Some minerals are essential nutrients required in small amounts by the body for health.

misinformation: false or misleading information.

mitochondria (my-toh-KON-dree-uh): the cellular organelles responsible for producing ATP aerobically; made of membranes (lipid and protein) with enzymes mounted on them. (The singular is *mitochondrion*.)

moderate-intensity physical activity: physical activity that requires some increase in breathing and/or heart rate and expends 3.5 to 7 kcalories per minute. Walking at a speed of 5 to 7 kilometres per hour (about 8 to 12 minutes to walk 1 kilometre) is an example.

moderation: in relation to alcohol consumption, not more than two drinks a day for the average-size man and not more than one drink a day for the average-size woman.

moderation (dietary): providing enough but not too much of a substance.

molasses: the thick brown syrup produced during sugar refining. Molasses retains residual sugar and other by-products and a few minerals; blackstrap molasses contains significant amounts of calcium and iron.

molecule: two or more atoms of the same or different elements joined by chemical bonds. Examples are molecules of the element oxygen, composed of two oxygen atoms (O_2), and molecules of the compound water, composed of two hydrogen atoms and one oxygen atom (H_2O).

monoglycerides: molecules of glycerol with one fatty acid attached. A molecule of glycerol with two fatty acids attached is a *diglyceride*.

monosaccharides (mon-oh-SACK-uh-rides): carbohydrates of the general formula $C_nH_{2n}O_n$ that typically form a single ring. See APPENDIX C for the chemical structures of the monosaccharides.

monosodium glutamate (MSG): a sodium salt of the amino acid glutamic acid commonly used as a flavour enhancer. The FDA classifies MSG as a "generally recognized as safe" ingredient.

monounsaturated fatty acid (MUFA): a fatty acid that lacks two hydrogen atoms and has one double bond between carbons—for example, oleic acid.

motility: the ability of the GI tract muscles to move.

mouth: the oral cavity containing the tongue and teeth.

MSG symptom complex: an acute, temporary intolerance reaction that may occur after the ingestion of the additive MSG (monosodium glutamate). Symptoms include burning sensations, chest and facial flushing and pain, and throbbing headaches.

mucous (MYOO-kus) **membranes:** the membranes, composed of mucus-secreting cells, that line the surfaces of body tissues.

mucus (MYOO-kus): a slippery substance secreted by cells of the GI lining (and other body linings) that protects the cells from exposure to digestive juices (and other destructive agents).

muscle dysmorphia (dis-MORE-fee-ah): a psychiatric disorder characterized by a preoccupation with building body mass.

muscle endurance: the ability of a muscle to contract repeatedly without becoming exhausted.

muscle power: the product of force generation (strength) and movement velocity (speed); the speed at which a given amount of exertion is completed.

muscle strength: the ability of muscles to work against resistance.

mutations: permanent changes in the DNA that can be inherited.

myoglobin: the oxygen-holding protein of the muscle cells.

N

NAD (nicotinamide adenine dinucleotide): the main coenzyme form of the vitamin niacin. Its reduced form is NADH.

NADP (the phosphate form of NAD): a coenzyme form of niacin.

narcotic (nar-KOT-ic): a drug that dulls the senses, induces sleep, and becomes addictive with prolonged use.

natural water: water obtained from a spring or well that is certified to be safe and sanitary. The mineral content may not be changed, but the water may be treated in other ways such as with ozone or by filtration.

naturopathic (nay-chur-oh-PATH-ick) **medicine:** a system that taps the natural healing forces within the body by integrating several practices, including traditional medicine, herbal medicine, clinical nutrition, homeopathy, acupuncture, East Asian medicine, hydrotherapy, and manipulative therapy.

neotame (NEE-oh-tame): an artificial sweetener composed of two amino acids (phenylalanine and aspartic acid); approved for use in Canada.

net protein utilization (NPU): a measure of protein quality assessed by measuring the amount of protein nitrogen that is retained from a given amount of protein nitrogen eaten.

neural tube: the embryonic tissue that forms the brain and spinal cord.

neural tube defects: malformations of the brain, spinal cord, or both during embryonic development that often result in lifelong disability or death.

neurofibrillary tangles: snarls of the thread-like strands that extend from the nerve cells, commonly found in the brains of people with Alzheimer's dementia.

neurons: nerve cells; the structural and functional units of the nervous system. Neurons initiate and conduct nerve impulse transmissions.

neuropeptide Y: a chemical produced in the brain that stimulates appetite, diminishes energy expenditure, and increases fat storage.

neurotransmitters: chemicals that are released at the end of a nerve cell when a nerve impulse arrives there. They diffuse across the gap to the next cell and alter the membrane of that second cell to either inhibit or excite it.

neutrophils: the most common of the immune system cells, they ingest and destroy foreign antigens by phagocytosis.

niacin (NIGH-a-sin): a B vitamin. The coenzyme forms are **NAD (nicotinamide adenine dinucleotide)** and **NADP (the phosphate form of NAD)**. Niacin can be eaten preformed or made in the body from its precursor, tryptophan, an essential amino acid.

niacin equivalents (NE): the amount of niacin present in food, including the niacin that can theoretically be made from its precursor, tryptophan, present in the food.

niacin flush: a temporary burning, tingling, and itching sensation that occurs when a person takes a large dose of nicotinic acid; often accompanied by a headache and reddened face, arms, and chest.

night blindness: slow recovery of vision after flashes of bright light at night or an inability to see in dim light; an early symptom of vitamin A deficiency.

nitrites (NYE-trites): salts added to food to prevent botulism. One example is sodium nitrite, which is used to preserve meats.

nitrogen balance: the amount of nitrogen consumed (N in) as compared with the amount of nitrogen excreted (N out) in a given period of time.

nitrosamines (nye-TROHS-uh-meens): derivatives of nitrites that may be formed in the stomach when nitrites combine with amines. Nitrosamines are carcinogenic in animals.

nonessential amino acids: amino acids that the body can synthesize.

nonexercise activity thermogenesis (NEAT): energy expenditure associated with everyday spontaneous activities.

nonheme iron: the iron in foods that is not bound to proteins; found in both plant-derived and animal-derived foods.

nonnutritive sweeteners: sweeteners that yield no energy (or insignificant energy in the case of aspartame).

nonpoint water pollution: water pollution caused by runoff from all over an area rather than from discrete "point" sources. An example is the pollution caused by runoff from agricultural fields.

nucleotide bases: the nitrogen-containing building blocks of DNA and RNA—cytosine (C), thymine (T), uracil (U), guanine (G), and adenine (A). In DNA, the base pairs are A–T and C–G and in RNA, the base pairs are A–U and C–G.

nucleotides: the subunits of DNA and RNA molecules, composed of a phosphate group, a 5-carbon sugar (deoxyribose for DNA and ribose for RNA), and a nitrogen-containing base.

nucleus: a major membrane-enclosed body within every cell, which contains the cell's genetic material, DNA, embedded in chromosomes.

nursing bottle tooth decay: extensive tooth decay due to prolonged tooth contact with formula, milk, fruit juice, or other carbohydrate-rich liquid offered to an infant in a bottle.

nutrient claims: statements that characterize the quantity of a nutrient in a food.

nutrient density: a measure of the nutrients a food provides relative to the energy it provides. The more nutrients and the fewer kcalories, the higher the nutrient density.

nutrient profiling: ranking foods based on their nutrient composition.

nutrients: chemical substances obtained from food and used in the body to provide energy, structural materials, and regulating agents to support growth, maintenance, and repair of the body's tissues. Nutrients may also reduce the risks of some diseases.

nutrigenetics: the science of how genes affect the interactions between diet and disease.

nutrigenomics: the science of how nutrients affect the activities of genes.

nutrition: the science of foods and the nutrients they contain, and of their actions within the body (including ingestion, digestion, absorption, transport, metabolism, and excretion). A broader definition includes the social, economic, cultural, and psychological implications of food and eating.

nutrition assessment: a comprehensive analysis of a person's nutrition status that uses health, socioeconomic, drug, and diet histories; anthropometric measurements; physical examinations; and laboratory tests.

nutrition screening: the use of preliminary nutrition assessment techniques to identify people who are malnourished or are at risk for malnutrition.

nutritional genomics: the science of how nutrients affect the activities of genes **(nutrigenomics)** and how genes affect the interactions between diet and disease **(nutrigenetics)**.

nutritionist: a person who specializes in the study of nutrition. Note that this definition does not specify qualifications and may apply not only to registered dietitians but also to self-described experts whose training is questionable.

nutritive sweeteners: sweeteners that yield energy, including both sugars and sugar replacers.

O

obese: overweight with adverse health effects; class I: BMI 30 to 34.9; class II: BMI 35 to 39.9; class III: BMI 40 or higher.

obligatory (ah-BLIG-ah-TORE-ee) **water excretion:** the amount of water the body has to excrete each day to dispose of its wastes—about 500 millilitres (2 cups).

oils: lipids that are liquid at room temperature (77°F or 25°C).

olestra: a synthetic fat made from sucrose and fatty acids that provides 0 kcalories per gram; also known as *sucrose polyester.*

oligopeptide (OL-ee-go-PEP-tide): string of four to nine amino acids.

omega: the last letter of the Greek alphabet (ω), used by chemists to refer to the position of the first double bond from the methyl (CH_3) end of a fatty acid.

omega-3 fatty acid: a polyunsaturated fatty acid in which the first double bond is three carbons away from the methyl (CH_3) end of the carbon chain.

omega-6 fatty acid: a polyunsaturated fatty acid in which the first double bond is six carbons from the methyl (CH_3) end of the carbon chain.

omnivores: people who have no formal restriction on the eating of any foods.

opsin (OP-sin): the protein portion of the visual pigment molecule.

oral rehydration therapy (ORT): the administration of a simple solution of sugar, salt, and water, taken by mouth, to treat dehydration caused by diarrhea. A simple ORT recipe: ½ litre boiling water, 20 mL (4 tsp) sugar, 2 mL (1/2 tsp) salt.

organelles: subcellular structures such as ribosomes, mitochondria, and lysosomes.

organic: in agriculture, crops grown and processed according to Canada's Organic Product Regulations defining the use of fertilizers, herbicides, insecticides, fungicides, preservatives, and other chemical ingredients.

organic: in chemistry, a substance or molecule containing carbon-carbon bonds or carbon-hydrogen bonds. This definition excludes coal, diamonds, and a few carbon-containing compounds that contain only a single carbon and no hydrogen, such as carbon dioxide (CO_2), calcium carbonate ($CaCO_3$), magnesium carbonate ($MgCO_3$), and sodium cyanide (NaCN).

organic (on food labels): at least 95 percent of the product's ingredients have been grown and processed according to the Canadian Organic Products Regulations.

organic halogens: an organic compound containing one or more atoms of a halogen—fluorine, chlorine, iodine, or bromine.

orlistat (OR-leh-stat): a drug used in the treatment of obesity that inhibits the absorption of fat in the GI tract, thus limiting kcaloric intake.

orthomolecular medicine: the use of large doses of vitamins to treat chronic disease.

osmosis: the movement of water across a membrane *toward* the side where the solutes are more concentrated.

osmotic pressure: the amount of pressure needed to prevent the movement of water across a membrane.

osteoarthritis: a painful, degenerative disease of the joints that occurs when the cartilage in a joint deteriorates; joint structure is damaged, with loss of function; also called *degenerative arthritis.*

osteoblasts: cells that build bone during growth.

osteocalcin (os-teo-KAL-sen): a calcium-binding protein in bones, essential for normal mineralization.

osteoclasts: cells that destroy bone during growth.

osteomalacia (OS-tee-oh-ma-LAY-shuh): a bone disease characterized by softening of the bones. Symptoms include bending of the spine and bowing of the legs. The disease occurs most often in adult women.

osteoporosis (OS-tee-oh-pore-OH-sis): a disease in which the bones become porous and fragile due to a loss of minerals; also called *adult bone loss.*

outbreaks: two or more cases of a similar illness resulting from the ingestion of a common food.

overfishing: catching fish at a faster rate than they can reproduce.

overnutrition: excess energy or nutrients.

overt (oh-VERT): out in the open and easy to observe.

overweight: body weight above some standard of acceptable weight that is usually defined in relation to height (such as BMI); BMI 25 to 29.9.

ovum (OH-vum): the female reproductive cell, capable of developing into a new organism upon fertilization; commonly referred to as an egg.

oxaloacetate (OKS-ah-low-AS-eh-tate): a carbohydrate intermediate of the TCA cycle.

oxidants (OKS-ih-dants): compounds (such as oxygen itself) that oxidize other compounds. Compounds that prevent oxidation are called *antioxidants,* whereas those that promote it are called *pro-oxidants.*

oxidation (OKS-ee-day-shun): the process of a substance combining with oxygen; oxidation reactions involve the loss of electrons.

oxidative stress: a condition in which the production of oxidants and free radicals exceeds the body's ability to handle them and prevent damage.

oxytocin (OCK-see-TOH-sin): a hormone that stimulates the mammary glands to eject milk during lactation and the uterus to contract during and after childbirth.

oyster shell: a product made from the powdered shells of oysters that is sold as a calcium supplement, but it is not well absorbed by the digestive system.

ozone therapy: the use of ozone gas to enhance the body's immune system.

P

pancreas: a gland that secretes digestive enzymes and juices into the duodenum. (The pancreas also secretes hormones into the blood that help to maintain glucose homeostasis.)

pancreatic (pank-ree-AT-ic) **juice:** the exocrine secretion of the pancreas, containing enzymes for the digestion of carbohydrate, fat, and protein as well as bicarbonate, a neutralizing agent. The juice flows from the pancreas into the small intestine through the pancreatic duct. (The pancreas also has an endocrine function, the secretion of insulin and other hormones.)

pantothenic (PAN-toe-THEN-ick) **acid:** a B vitamin. The principal active form is part of coenzyme A, called "CoA" throughout Chapter 7.

parathyroid hormone: a hormone from the parathyroid glands that regulates blood calcium by raising it when levels fall too low; also known as *parathormone* (PAIR-ah-THOR-moan).

pasteurization: heat processing of food that inactivates some, but not all, microorganisms in the food; not a sterilization process. Bacteria that cause spoilage are still present.

pathogen (PATH-oh-jen): a microorganism capable of producing disease.

PBB (polybrominated biphenyl) and **PCB (polychlorinated biphenyl):** toxic organic compounds used in pesticides, paints, and flame retardants.

peak bone mass: the highest attainable bone density for an individual, developed during the first three decades of life.

peer review: a process in which a panel of scientists rigorously evaluates a research study to assure that the scientific method was followed.

pellagra (pell-AY-gra): the niacin-deficiency disease.

pepsin: a gastric enzyme that hydrolyzes protein. Pepsin is secreted in an inactive form, **pepsinogen,** which is activated by hydrochloric acid in the stomach.

pepsinogen: an inactive compound that is activated by hydrochloric acid in the stomach to form pepsin.

peptic ulcer: a lesion in the mucous membrane of either the stomach (a gastric ulcer) or the duodenum (a duodenal ulcer).

peptidase: a digestive enzyme that hydrolyzes peptide bonds. *Tripeptidases* cleave tripeptides; *dipeptidases* cleave dipeptides. *Endopeptidases* cleave peptide bonds within the chain to create smaller fragments, whereas *exopeptidases* cleave bonds at the ends to release free amino acids.

peptide bond: a bond that connects the acid end of one amino acid with the amino end of another, forming a link in a protein chain.

percent Daily Value (%DV): the percentage of a Daily Value recommendation found in a specified serving of food for key nutrients based on a 2000-kcalorie diet.

percent fat-free: may be used only if the product meets the definition of *low fat* or *fat-free* and must reflect the amount of fat in 100 grams (e.g., a food that contains 2.5 grams of fat per 50 grams can claim to be "95 percent fat-free").

peripheral (puh-RIFF-er-ul) **nervous system:** the peripheral (outermost) part of the nervous system; the vast complex of wiring that extends from the central nervous system to the body's outermost areas. It contains both somatic and autonomic components.

peripheral resistance: the resistance to pumped blood in the small arterial branches (arterioles) that carry blood to tissues.

peristalsis (per-ih-STALL-sis): wavelike muscular contractions of the GI tract that push its contents along.

pernicious (per-NISH-us) **anemia:** a blood disorder that reflects a vitamin B_{12} deficiency caused by lack of intrinsic factor and characterized by abnormally large and immature red blood cells. Other symptoms include muscle weakness and irreversible neurological damage.

persistence: stubborn or enduring continuance; with respect to food contaminants, the quality of persisting, rather than breaking down, in the bodies of animals and human beings.

pesticides: chemicals used to control insects, weeds, fungi, and other pests on plants, vegetables, fruits, and animals. Used broadly, the term includes herbicides (to kill weeds), insecticides (to kill insects), and fungicides (to kill fungi).

pH: the unit of measure expressing a substance's acidity or alkalinity.

phagocytes (FAG-oh-sites): white blood cells (neutrophils and macrophages) that have the ability to ingest and destroy foreign substances.

phagocytosis (FAG-oh-sigh-TOH-sis): the process by which phagocytes engulf and destroy foreign materials.

pharmacological effect: a large dose of a nutrient (levels commonly available only from supplements) that overwhelms some body system and acts like a drug.

pharynx (FAIR-inks): the passageway leading from the nose and mouth to the larynx and esophagus, respectively.

phenylketonuria (FEN-il-KEY-toe-NEW-ree-ah) or **PKU:** an inherited disorder characterized by failure to metabolize the amino acid phenylalanine to tyrosine.

phosphocreatine (PC): a high-energy compound in muscle cells that acts as a reservoir of energy that can maintain a steady supply of ATP; also called *creatine phosphate.*

phospholipid (FOS-foe-LIP-id): a compound similar to a triglyceride but having a phosphate group (a phosphorus-containing salt) and choline (or another nitrogen-containing compound) in place of one of the fatty acids.

phosphorus: a major mineral found mostly in the body's bones and teeth.

photosynthesis: the process by which green plants use the sun's energy to make carbohydrates from carbon dioxide and water.

physical activity: bodily movement produced by muscle contractions that substantially increase energy expenditure.

physiological age: a person's age as estimated from her or his body's health and probable life expectancy.

physiological effect: a normal dose of a nutrient (levels commonly found in foods) that provides a normal blood concentration.

physiological fuel value: the number of kcalories that the body derives from a food, in contrast to the number of kcalories determined by calorimetry.

phytic (FYE-tick) **acid:** a nonnutrient component of plant seeds; also called *phytate* (FYE-tate). Phytic acid occurs in the husks of grains, legumes, and seeds and is capable of binding minerals such as zinc, iron, calcium, magnesium, and copper in insoluble complexes in the intestine, which the body excretes unused.

phytochemicals (FIE-toe-KEM-ih-cals): nonnutrient compounds found in plant-derived foods that have biological activity in the body.

phytoestrogens: plant-derived compounds that have structural and functional similarities to human estrogen. Phytoestrogens include the isoflavones genistein, daidzein, and glycitein.

phytosterols: plant-derived compounds that have structural similarities to cholesterol and lower blood cholesterol by competing with cholesterol for absorption. Phytosterols include sterol esters and stanol esters.

pica (PIE-ka): a craving for and consumption of nonfood substances. Also known as *geophagia* (gee-oh-FAY-gee-uh) when referring to eating clay, baby powder, chalk, ash, ceramics, paper, paint chips, or charcoal; *pagophagia* (pag-oh-FAY-gee-uh) when referring to eating large quantities of ice; and *amylophagia* (AM-ee-low-FAY-gee-ah) when referring to eating uncooked starch (flour, laundry starch, or raw rice).

pigment: a molecule capable of absorbing certain wavelengths of light so that it reflects only those that we perceive as a certain colour.

placebo (pla-see-bo): an inert, harmless medication given to provide comfort and hope; a sham treatment used in controlled research studies.

placebo effect: a change that occurs in response to expectations in the effectiveness of a treatment that actually has no pharmaceutical effects.

placenta (plah-SEN-tuh): the organ that develops inside the uterus early in pregnancy, through which the fetus receives nutrients and oxygen and returns carbon dioxide and other waste products to be excreted.

plant-pesticides: pesticides made by the plants themselves.

plaque (PLACK): an accumulation of fatty deposits, smooth muscle cells, calcium, and fibrous connective tissue that develops in the artery walls in atherosclerosis. Plaque associated with atherosclerosis is known as *atheromatous* (ATH-er-OH-ma-tus) *plaque*.

platelets: tiny, disc-shaped bodies in the blood, important in blood clot formation.

PLP (pyridoxal phosphate): the primary active coenzyme form of vitamin B_6.

point of unsaturation: the double bond of a fatty acid, where hydrogen atoms can easily be added to the structure.

polar: characteristic of a neutral molecule, such as water, that has opposite charges spatially separated within the molecule.

polypeptide: many (ten or more) amino acids bonded together.

polysaccharides: compounds composed of many monosaccharides linked together. An intermediate string of three to ten monosaccharides is an *oligosaccharide*.

polyunsaturated fatty acid (PUFA): a fatty acid that lacks four or more hydrogen atoms and has two or more double bonds between carbons—for example, linoleic acid (two double bonds) and linolenic acid (three double bonds).

post term: an infant born after the forty-second week of pregnancy.

postpartum amenorrhea: the normal temporary absence of menstrual periods immediately following childbirth.

potable (POT-ah-bul): water that is suitable for drinking.

potassium: the principal cation within the body's cells; critical to the maintenance of fluid balance, nerve impulse transmissions, and muscle contractions.

prebiotics: food components (such as fibres) that are not digested in the small intestine, but are used instead as food by bacteria to encourage their growth or activity.

precursors: substances that precede others; with regard to vitamins, compounds that can be converted into active vitamins; also known as *provitamins*.

prediabetes: condition in which blood glucose levels are higher than normal but not high enough to be diagnosed as diabetes; considered a major risk factor for future diabetes and cardiovascular diseases; formerly called *impaired glucose tolerance*.

preeclampsia (PRE-ee-KLAMP-see-ah): a condition characterized by hypertension and protein in the urine.

preformed vitamin A: dietary vitamin A in its active form.

prehypertension: slightly higher-than-normal blood pressure, but not as high as hypertension.

prenatal alcohol exposure: subjecting a fetus to a pattern of excessive alcohol intake characterized by substantial regular use or heavy episodic drinking.

preservatives: antimicrobial agents, antioxidants, and other additives that retard spoilage or maintain desired qualities, such as softness in baked goods.

pressure ulcers: damage to the skin and underlying tissues as a result of compression and poor circulation; commonly seen in people who are bedridden or chairbound.

preterm (premature): an infant born prior to the thirty-eighth week of pregnancy; also called a *premature infant*. A *term* infant is born between the thirty-eighth and forty-second week of pregnancy.

primary deficiency: a nutrient deficiency caused by inadequate dietary intake of a nutrient.

probiotics: living microorganisms found in foods that, when consumed in sufficient quantities, are beneficial to health.

processed foods: foods that have been treated to change their physical, chemical, microbiological, or sensory properties.

proenzyme: the inactive form of an enzyme; also called a *zymogen*.

progesterone: the hormone of gestation (pregnancy).

progressive overload principle: the training principle that a body system, in order to improve, must be worked at frequencies, durations, or intensities that gradually increase physical demands.

prolactin (pro-LAK-tin): a hormone secreted from the anterior pituitary gland that acts on the mammary glands to promote the production of milk. The release of prolactin is mediated by *prolactin-inhibiting hormone (PIH)*.

promoters: factors that favour the development of cancers once they have begun.

proof: a way of stating the percentage of alcohol in distilled liquor. Liquor that is 100 proof is 50 percent alcohol; 90 proof is 45 percent; and so forth.

pro-oxidants: substances that significantly induce oxidative stress.

protease (PRO-tee-azes): an enzyme that hydrolyzes protein.

protein digestibility: a measure of the amount of amino acids absorbed from a given protein intake.

protein digestibility–corrected amino acid score (PDCAAS): a measuring tool used to determine protein quality. The PSCAAS reflects a protein's digestibility as well as the proportions of amino acids that it provides.

protein efficiency ratio (PER): a measure of protein quality assessed by determining how well a given protein supports weight gain in growing rats; used to establish the protein quality for infant formulas and baby foods.

protein turnover: the degradation and synthesis of protein.

protein-energy malnutrition (PEM): a deficiency of protein, energy, or both, including kwashiorkor, marasmus, and instances in which they overlap; also called *protein-kcalorie malnutrition (PCM)*.

protein-sparing action: the action of carbohydrate (and fat) in providing energy that allows protein to be used for other purposes.

proteins: compounds composed of carbon, hydrogen, oxygen, and nitrogen atoms, arranged into amino acids linked in a chain. Some amino acids also contain sulphur atoms.

proteome: all of the proteins synthesized by our cells.

proteomics: the study of the body's proteins.

puberty: the period in life in which a person becomes physically capable of reproduction.

public health dietitians: dietitians who specialize in providing nutrition services through organized community efforts.

public water: water from a municipal system that has been treated and disinfected.

purified water: water that has been treated by distillation or other physical or chemical processes that remove dissolved solids. Because purified water contains no minerals or contaminants, it is useful for medical and research purposes.

purines: compounds of nitrogen-containing bases such as adenine, guanine, and caffeine. Purines that originate from the body are *endogenous* and those that derive from foods are *exogenous*.

pyloric (pie-LORE-ic) **sphincter:** the circular muscle that separates the stomach from the small intestine and regulates the flow of partially digested food into the small intestine; also called *pylorus* or *pyloric valve*.

pyruvate (PIE-roo-vate): a 3-carbon compound that plays a key role in energy metabolism.

Q

qi gong (chée GUNG): a Chinese system that combines movement, meditation, and breathing techniques to enhance the flow of qi (vital energy) in the body.

quality of life: a person's perceived physical and mental well-being.

R

rachitic (ra-KIT-ik) **rosary:** the poorly formed rib attachments that may develop in a vitamin D deficiency; literally, "the rosary of rickets."

radura: an international symbol used to identify retail foods that have been irradiated.

randomization (ran-dom-ih-zay-shun): a process of choosing the members of the experimental and control groups without bias.

raw sugar: the first crop of crystals harvested during sugar processing. Raw sugar cannot be sold in Canada and the United States because it contains too much filth (dirt, insect fragments, and the like). Sugar sold as "raw sugar" domestically has actually gone through more than half of the refining steps.

RD: see *registered dietitian.*

Recommended Dietary Allowance (RDA): the average daily amount of a nutrient considered adequate to meet the known nutrient needs of practically all healthy people; a goal for dietary intake by individuals.

rectum: the muscular terminal part of the intestine, extending from the sigmoid colon to the anus.

reduced cholesterol: foods contains 25 percent less cholesterol than the comparison food, and is low in saturated fat; synonyms include *lower in cholesterol* and *less cholesterol.*

reduced in energy: at least 25 percent fewer kcalories per reference amount than the comparison food; synonyms include *reduced Calories, less energy,* and *lower in energy.*

reduced in fat: food contains at least 25 percent less fat than the comparison food; synonyms include *fat-reduced, less fat,* and *lower fat.*

reduced in sugar: food contains at least 25 percent less sugars totalling at least 5 grams per serving compared to a similar food.

reduced in sodium or salt: contains at least 25 percent less sodium per serving than a similar reference food.

reference protein: a standard against which to measure the quality of other proteins.

refined: the process by which the coarse parts of a food are removed. When wheat is refined into flour, the bran, germ, and husk are removed, leaving only the endosperm.

refined flour: finely ground endosperm that is usually enriched with nutrients and bleached for whiteness; sometimes called *white flour.*

reflux: a backward flow.

registered dietitian (RD): a person who has completed a minimum of a bachelor's degree from an accredited university, has completed approved course work and a supervised practice program, has passed a national examination, and maintains registration through continuing professional education.

registration: listing; with respect to health professionals, listing with a professional organization that requires specific course work, experience, and passing of an examination.

relaxin: the hormone of late pregnancy.

remodelling: the dismantling and re-formation of a structure.

renin (REN-in): an enzyme from the kidneys that hydrolyzes the protein angiotensinogen to angiotensin I.

rennin: an enzyme that coagulates milk; found in the gastric juice of cows, but not human beings.

replication (REP-lih-KAY-shun): repeating an experiment and getting the same results.

requirement: the lowest continuing intake of a nutrient that will maintain a specified criterion of adequacy.

residues: whatever remains. In the case of pesticides, those amounts that remain on or in foods when people buy and use them.

resistance training: the use of free weights or weight machines to provide resistance for developing muscle strength, power, and endurance; also called *weight training.* A person's own body weight may also be used to provide resistance as when a person does push-ups, pull-ups, or abdominal crunches.

resistant starches: starches that escape digestion and absorption in the small intestine of healthy people.

respiratory chain: the final pathway in energy metabolism that transports electrons from hydrogen to oxygen and captures the energy released in the bonds of ATP; also called the *electron transport chain.*

resting metabolic rate (RMR): similar to the basal metabolic rate (BMR), a measure of the energy use of a person at rest in a comfortable setting, but with less stringent criteria for recent food intake and physical activity. Consequently, the RMR is slightly higher than the BMR.

retina (RET-in-uh): the innermost membrane of the eye, composed of several layers including one that contains the rods and cones.

retinoids (RET-ih-noyds): chemically related compounds with biological activity similar to that of retinol; metabolites of retinol.

retinol (RET-ih-nol): the alcohol form of vitamin A.

retinol activity equivalents (RAE): a measure of vitamin A activity; the amount of retinol that the body will derive from a food containing preformed retinol or its precursor beta-carotene.

retinol-binding protein (RBP): the specific protein responsible for transporting retinol.

rheumatoid (ROO-ma-toyd) **arthritis:** a disease of the immune system involving painful inflammation of the joints and related structures.

rhodopsin (ro-DOP-sin): a light-sensitive pigment of the retina; contains the retinal form of vitamin A and the protein opsin.

riboflavin (RYE-boh-flay-vin): a B vitamin. The coenzyme forms are **FMN (flavin mononucleotide)** and **FAD (flavin adenine dinucleotide).**

ribosomes (RYE-boh-zomes): protein-making organelles in cells; composed of RNA and protein.

rickets: the vitamin D–deficiency disease in children characterized by inadequate mineralization of bone (manifested in bowed legs or knock-knees, outward-bowed chest, and knobs on ribs). A rare type of rickets, not caused by vitamin D deficiency, is known as *vitamin D–refractory rickets.*

risk: a measure of the probability and severity of harm.

risk factor: a condition or behaviour associated with an elevated frequency of a disease but not proved to be causal. Leading risk factors for chronic diseases include obesity, cigarette smoking, high blood pressure, high blood cholesterol, physical inactivity, and a diet high in saturated fats and low in vegetables, fruits, and whole grains.

RNA (ribonucleic acid): a compound similar to DNA, but RNA is a single strand with a ribose sugar instead of a deoxyribose sugar and uracil instead of thymine as one of its bases.

S

saccharin (SAK-ah-ren): an artificial sweetener that has been approved for use in the United States. In Canada, approval for use in foods and beverages is pending; currently available only in pharmacies and only as a tabletop sweetener, not as an additive.

safety: the condition of being free from harm or danger.

saliva: the secretion of the salivary glands. Its principal enzyme begins carbohydrate digestion.

salivary glands: exocrine glands that secrete saliva into the mouth.

salt: a compound composed of a positive ion other than H^+ and a negative ion other than OH^-. An example is sodium chloride (Na^+Cl^-).

salt sensitivity: a characteristic of individuals who respond to a high salt intake with an increase in blood pressure or to a low salt intake with a decrease in blood pressure.

sarcopenia (SAR-koh-PEE-nee-ah): loss of skeletal muscle mass, strength, and quality.

satiating: having the power to suppress hunger and inhibit eating.

satiation (say-she-AY-shun): the feeling of satisfaction and fullness that occurs during a meal and halts eating. Satiation determines how much food is consumed during a meal.

satiety (sah-TIE-eh-tee): the feeling of fullness and satisfaction that occurs after a meal and inhibits eating until the next meal. Satiety determines how much time passes between meals.

saturated fat-free: less than 0.2 grams of saturated fat and 0.2 grams of *trans* fat per serving.

saturated fatty acid: a fatty acid carrying the maximum possible number of hydrogen atoms—for example, stearic acid.

scurvy: the vitamin C–deficiency disease.

secondary deficiency: a nutrient deficiency caused by something other than an inadequate intake such as a disease condition or drug interaction that reduces absorption, accelerates use, hastens excretion, or destroys the nutrient.

secretin (see-CREET-in): a hormone produced by cells in the duodenum wall. Target organ: the pancreas. Response: secretion of bicarbonate-rich pancreatic juice.

sedentary: physically inactive (literally, "sitting down a lot").

segmentation (SEG-men-TAY-shun): a periodic squeezing or partitioning of the intestine at intervals along its length by its circular muscles.

selenium (se-LEEN-ee-um): a trace element.

senile dementia: the loss of brain function beyond the normal loss of physical adeptness and memory that occurs with aging.

senile plaques: clumps of the protein fragment beta-amyloid on the nerve cells, commonly found in the brains of people with Alzheimer's dementia.

serotonin (SER-oh-TONE-in): a neurotransmitter important in sleep regulation, appetite control, and sensory perception, among other roles. Serotonin is synthesized in the body from the amino acid tryptophan with the help of vitamin B_6.

set point: the point at which controls are set (e.g., on a thermostat). The set-point theory that relates to body weight proposes that the body tends to maintain a certain weight by means of its own internal controls.

sickle-cell anemia: a hereditary form of anemia characterized by abnormal sickle- or crescent-shaped red blood cells. Sickled cells interfere with oxygen transport and blood flow. Symptoms are precipitated by dehydration and insufficient oxygen (as may occur at high altitudes) and include hemolytic anemia (red blood cells burst), fever, and severe pain in the joints and abdomen.

simple carbohydrates: monosaccharides and disaccharides.

small for gestational age (SGA): term describing an infant whose birth weight is low compared with the number of weeks in utero, often reflecting malnutrition.

small intestine: a 3 metre length of small-diameter intestine that extends from the stomach to the ileocecal sphincter and is the major site of digestion of food and absorption of nutrients. Its segments are the duodenum, jejunum, and ileum.

socio-economic history: a record of a person's social and economic background, including such factors as education, income, and ethnic identity.

sodium: the principal cation in the extracellular fluids of the body; critical to the maintenance of fluid balance, nerve impulse transmissions, and muscle contractions.

sodium-free and **salt-free:** less than 5 milligrams of sodium per serving.

soft water: water with a high sodium or potassium content.

solanine (SOH-lah-neen): a poisonous narcotic-like substance present in potato peels and sprouts.

soluble fibres: nonstarch polysaccharides that dissolve in water to form a gel. An example is pectin from fruit, which is used to thicken jellies.

solutes (SOLL-yutes): the substances that are dissolved in a solution. The number of molecules in a given volume of fluid is the *solute concentration*.

somatic (so-MAT-ick) **nervous system:** the division of the nervous system that controls the voluntary muscles, as distinguished from the autonomic nervous system, which controls involuntary functions.

somatostatin (GHIH): a hormone that inhibits the release of growth hormone; the opposite of somatotropin (GH).

soup kitchens: programs that provide prepared meals to be eaten on site.

source of fibre: 2 grams or more of fibre.

sperm: the male reproductive cell, capable of fertilizing an ovum.

sphincter (SFINK-ter): a circular muscle surrounding, and able to close, a body opening. Sphincters are found at specific points along the GI tract and regulate the flow of food particles.

spina (SPY-nah) **bifida** (BIFF-ih-dah): one of the most common types of neural tube defects; characterized by the incomplete closure of the spinal cord and its bony encasement.

sports anemia: a transient condition of low hemoglobin in the blood, associated with the early stages of sports training or other strenuous activity.

spring water: water originating from an underground spring or well. It may be bubbly (carbonated), or "flat" or "still," meaning not carbonated. Brand names such as "Spring Pure" do not necessarily mean that the water comes from a spring.

starches: plant polysaccharides composed of glucose.

sterols (STARE-ols or STEER-ols): compounds containing a four-ring carbon structure with any of a variety of side chains attached.

stomach: a muscular, elastic, saclike portion of the digestive tract that grinds and churns swallowed food, mixing it with acid and enzymes to form chyme.

stools: waste matter discharged from the colon; also called *feces* (FEE-seez).

stress: any threat to a person's well-being; a demand placed on the body to adapt.

stress eating: eating in response to arousal.

stress fractures: bone damage or breaks caused by stress on bone surfaces during exercise.

stress response: the body's response to stress, mediated by both nerves and hormones.

stressors: environmental elements, physical or psychological, that cause stress.

stroke: an event in which the blood flow to a part of the brain is cut off; also called *cerebrovascular accident (CVA).*

subclavian (sub-KLAY-vee-an) **vein:** the vein that provides passage from the lymphatic system to the vascular system.

subclinical deficiency: a deficiency in the early stages, before the outward signs have appeared.

subcutaneous fat: fat stored directly under the skin.

subjects: the people or animals participating in a research project.

substitute foods: foods that have the same nutritional value as another food, but are not physically similar, such as simulated whole egg products.

successful weight-loss maintenance: achieving a weight loss of at least 10 percent of initial body weight and maintaining the loss for at least one year.

sucralose (SUE-kra-lose): an artificial sweetener approved for use in Canada and the United States.

sucrase: an enzyme that hydrolyzes sucrose.

sucrose (SUE-krose): a disaccharide composed of glucose and fructose; commonly known as *table sugar, beet sugar,* or *cane sugar.* Sucrose also occurs in many fruits and some vegetables and grains.

sudden infant death syndrome (SIDS): the unexpected and unexplained death of an apparently well infant; the most common cause of death of infants between the second week and the end of the first year of life; also called *crib death.*

sugar alcohols: sugarlike compounds that can be derived from fruits or commercially produced from dextrose; also called *polyols.* Sugar alcohols are absorbed more slowly than other sugars and metabolized differently in the human body; they are not readily utilized by ordinary mouth bacteria. Examples are maltitol, mannitol, sorbitol, xylitol, isomalt, and lactitol.

sugar-free: less than 0.5 grams of sugar per serving and is energy-free.

sugars: monosaccharides and disaccharides.

sulphate: the oxidized form of sulphur.

sulphites: salts containing sulphur that are added to foods to prevent spoilage.

sulphur: a mineral present in the body as part of some proteins.

sushi: vinegar-flavoured rice and seafood, typically wrapped in seaweed and stuffed with colourful vegetables. Some sushi is stuffed with raw fish; other varieties contain cooked seafood.

sustainable: able to continue indefinitely; using resources at such a rate that the Earth can keep on replacing them and producing pollutants at a rate with which the environment and human cleanup efforts can keep pace, so that no net accumulation of pollution occurs.

sustainable agriculture: ability to produce food indefinitely, with little or no harm to the environment.

symptomatic allergy: an immune response that produces antibodies and symptoms.

synbiotic: a mixture of probiotics and prebiotics.

synergistic (SIN-er-JIS-tick): multiple factors operating together in such a way that their combined effects are greater than the sum of their individual effects.

T

TCA cycle or **tricarboxylic** (try-car-box-ILL-ick) **acid cycle:** a series of metabolic reactions that break down molecules of acetyl CoA to carbon dioxide and hydrogen atoms; also called the *citric acid cycle* or the *Kreb's cycle* after the biochemist who elucidated its reactions.

T-cells: lymphocytes that attack antigens. T stands for the thymus gland, where the T-cells mature.

tempeh (TEM-pay): a fermented soybean food, rich in protein and fibre.

teratogen (ter-AT-oh-jen): a substance that causes abnormal fetal development and birth defects.

testosterone: a steroid hormone from the testicles, or testes. The steroids are chemically related to, and some are derived from, the lipid cholesterol.

textured vegetable protein: processed soybean protein used in vegetarian products such as soy burgers.

theory: a tentative explanation that integrates many and diverse findings to further the understanding of a defined topic.

thermic effect of food (TEF): an estimation of the energy required to process food (digest, absorb, transport, metabolize, and store ingested nutrients); also called the *specific dynamic effect (SDE) of food* or the *specific dynamic activity (SDA) of food*. The sum of the TEF and any increase in the metabolic rate due to overeating is known as *diet-induced thermogenesis (DIT)*.

thermogenesis: the generation of heat; used in physiology and nutrition studies as an index of how much energy the body is expending.

THF (tetrahydrofolate): a coenzyme form of folate.

thiamin (THIGH-ah-min): a B vitamin. The coenzyme form is **TPP (thiamin pyrophosphate).**

thirst: a conscious desire to drink.

thoracic (thor-ASS-ic) **duct:** the main lymphatic vessel that collects lymph and drains into the left subclavian vein.

thrombosis (throm-BOH-sis): the formation of a *thrombus* (THROM-bus), or a blood clot, that may obstruct a blood vessel, causing gradual tissue death.

thyroid-stimulating hormone (TSH): a hormone secreted by the pituitary that stimulates the thyroid gland to secrete its hormones—thyroxine and triiodothyronine. The release of TSH is mediated by TSH-releasing hormone (TRH).

thyrotropin: another name for thyroid-stimulating hormone (TSH).

tocopherol (tuh-KOFF-er-ol): a general term for several chemically related compounds, one of which has vitamin E activity. (See APPENDIX C for chemical structures.)

tofu (TOE-foo): a curd made from soybeans, rich in protein and often fortified with calcium; used in many Asian and vegetarian dishes in place of meat.

Tolerable Upper Intake Level (UL): the maximum daily amount of a nutrient that appears safe for most healthy people and beyond which there is an increased risk of adverse health effects.

tolerance level: the maximum amount of residue permitted in a food when a pesticide is used according to the label directions.

toxicity: the ability of a substance to harm living organisms. All substances are toxic if high enough concentrations are used.

TPP (thiamin pyrophosphate): the coenzyme form of thiamin.

trabecular (tra-BECK-you-lar) **bone:** the lacy inner structure of calcium crystals that supports the bone's structure and provides a calcium storage bank.

trace minerals: essential mineral nutrients the human body requires in relatively small amounts (less than 100 milligrams per day); sometimes called *microminerals*.

trachea (TRAKE-ee-uh): the air passageway from the larynx to the lungs; also called the *windpipe*.

training: practising an activity regularly, which leads to conditioning. (Training is what you do; conditioning is what you get.)

trans: on the other side of; refers to a chemical configuration in which the hydrogen atoms are located on opposite sides of a double bond.

***trans* fat-free:** less than 0.2 grams of *trans* fat per serving and is low in saturated fat.

transamination (TRANS-am-ih-NAY-shun): the transfer of an amino group from one amino acid to a keto acid, producing a new dipensible/nonessential amino acid and a new keto acid.

transcription: the process of messenger RNA being made from a template of DNA.

***trans*-fatty acids:** fatty acids with hydrogens on opposite sides of the double bond.

transferrin (trans-FAIR-in): the iron transport protein.

transient ischemic (is-KEY-mik) **attack (TIA):** a temporary reduction in blood flow to the brain, which causes temporary symptoms that vary depending on the part of the brain affected. Common symptoms include light-headedness, visual disturbances, paralysis, staggering, numbness, and inability to swallow.

translation: the process of messenger RNA directing the sequence of amino acids and synthesis of proteins.

travellers' diarrhea: nausea, vomiting, and diarrhea caused by consuming food or water contaminated by any of several organisms, most commonly, *E. coli, Shigella, Campylobacter jejuni,* and *Salmonella.*

triglycerides (try-GLISS-er-rides): the chief form of fat in the diet and the major storage form of fat in the body; composed of a molecule of glycerol with three fatty acids attached; also called *triacylglycerols* (try-ay-seel-GLISS-er-ols).

tripeptide: three amino acids bonded together.

tumour: an abnormal tissue mass with no physiological function; also called a *neoplasm* (NEE-oh-plazm).

turbinado (ter-bih-NOD-oh) **sugar:** sugar produced using the same refining process as white sugar, but without the bleaching and anti-caking treatment. Traces of molasses give turbinado its sandy colour.

type 1 diabetes: the less common type of diabetes in which the pancreas fails to produce insulin.

type 2 diabetes: the more common type of diabetes in which the cells fail to respond to insulin.

type I osteoporosis: osteoporosis characterized by rapid bone losses, primarily of trabecular bone.

type II osteoporosis: osteoporosis characterized by gradual losses of both trabecular and cortical bone.

U

ulcer: a lesion of the skin or mucous membranes characterized by inflammation and damaged tissues.

ulcerative colitis (ko-LYE-tis): a type of *inflammatory bowel* disease of unknown cause resulting in sores and inflammation of the rectum and colon. Abdominal pain and cramping, diarrhea, and frequent false urges to defecate often restricts people's activities.

ultrahigh temperature (UHT) treatment: sterilizing a food by brief exposure to temperatures above those normally used.

umbilical (um-BILL-ih-cul) **cord:** the ropelike structure through which the fetus's veins and arteries reach the placenta; the route of nourishment and oxygen to the fetus and the route of waste disposal from the fetus. The scar in the middle of the abdomen that marks the former attachment of the umbilical cord is the *umbilicus* (um-BILL-ih-cus), commonly known as the "belly button."

uncoupled reactions: chemical reactions in which energy is released as heat.

undernutrition: deficient energy or nutrients.

underweight: body weight below some standard of acceptable weight that is usually defined in relation to height (such as BMI); BMI below 18.5.

unsaturated fatty acid: a fatty acid that lacks two or more hydrogen atoms and has at least one double bond between carbons (includes monounsaturated and polyunsaturated fatty acids).

unspecified eating disorders: eating disorders that do not meet the defined criteria for specific eating disorders.

urea (you-REE-uh): the principal nitrogen-excretion product of protein metabolism. Two ammonia fragments are combined with carbon dioxide to form urea.

uterus (YOU-ter-us): the muscular organ within which the infant develops before birth.

V

validity (va-lid-ih-tee): having the quality of being founded on fact or evidence.

variables: factors that change. A variable may depend on another variable (e.g., a child's height depends on his age), or it may be independent (e.g., a child's height does not depend on the colour of her eyes). Sometimes both variables correlate with a third variable (a child's height and eye colour both depend on genetics).

variety (dietary): eating a wide selection of foods within and among the major food groups.

vasoconstrictor (VAS-oh-kon-STRIK-tor): a substance that constricts or narrows the blood vessels.

vasopressin (VAS-oh-PRES-in): another name for antidiuretic hormone, so called because it elevates blood pressure.

vegans (VEE-gans): people who exclude all animal-derived foods (including meat, poultry, fish, eggs, and dairy products) from their diets; also called *pure vegetarians, strict vegetarians,* or *total vegetarians.*

vegetarians: a general term used to describe people who exclude meat, poultry, fish, or other animal-derived foods from their diets.

veins (VANES): vessels that carry blood to the heart.

very high source of fibre: 6 grams or more fibre per serving.

very low food security: multiple indications of disrupted eating patterns and reduced food intake; formerly known as *food insecurity with hunger.*

very low sodium: 35 milligrams or less per serving.

vigorous-intensity physical activity: physical activity that requires a large increase in breathing and/or heart rate and expends more than 7 kcalories per minute. Walking at a very brisk pace (>7 kilometres/4.5 miles per hour) or running at a pace of at least 8 kilometres/5 miles per hour are examples.

villi (VILL-ee, VILL-eye): fingerlike projections from the folds of the small intestine; singular *villus.*

visceral fat: fat stored within the abdominal cavity in association with the internal abdominal organs; also called *intra-abdominal fat.*

viscous: a gel-like consistency.

vitamin A: all naturally occurring compounds with the biological activity of **retinol** (RET-ih-nol), the alcohol form of vitamin A.

vitamin A activity: a term referring to both the active forms of vitamin A and the precursor forms in foods without distinguishing between them.

vitamin B_6: a family of compounds—pyridoxal, pyridoxine, and pyridoxamine. The primary active coenzyme form is PLP (pyridoxal phosphate).

vitamin B_{12}: a B vitamin characterized by the presence of cobalt. The active forms of coenzyme B_{12} are methylcobalamin and deoxyadenosylcobalamin.

vitamin D_2: vitamin D derived from plants in the diet and made from the yeast and plant sterol ergosterol; also called **ergocalciferol.**

vitamin D_3: vitamin D derived from animals in the diet and made in the skin from 7-dehydrocholesterol, a precursor of cholesterol, with the help of sunlight; also called **cholecalciferol** or **calciol.**

vitamins: organic, essential nutrients required in small amounts by the body for health.

VLDL (very-low-density lipoprotein): the type of lipoprotein made primarily by liver cells to transport lipids to various tissues in the body; composed primarily of triglycerides (i.e., those derived from the diet and those synthesized by the liver from excess energy).

VO_2max: the maximum rate of oxygen consumption by an individual at sea level.

vomiting: expulsion of the contents of the stomach up through the esophagus to the mouth.

vulnerable plaque: plaque that is susceptible to rupture because it has only a thin fibrous barrier between its lipid-rich core and the artery lining.

W

waist circumference: an anthropometric measurement used to assess a person's abdominal fat.

warm-up: 5 to 10 minutes of light activity, such as easy jogging or cycling, prior to a workout to prepare the body for more vigorous activity.

water balance: the balance between water intake and output (losses).

water intoxication: the rare condition in which body water contents are too high in all body fluid compartments.

wean: to gradually replace breast milk with infant formula or other foods appropriate to an infant's diet.

websites: Internet resources composed of text and graphic files, each with a unique URL (Uniform Resource Locator) that names the site (e.g., www.dietitians.ca).

weight management: maintaining body weight in a healthy range by preventing gradual weight gain over time and losing weight if overweight.

well water: water drawn from groundwater by tapping into an aquifer.

Wernicke–Korsakoff (VER-nee-key KORE-sah-kof) **syndrome:** a neurological disorder typically associated with chronic alcoholism and caused by a deficiency of the B vitamin thiamin; also called *alcohol-related dementia.*

wheat flour: any flour made from the endosperm of the wheat kernel.

whey protein: a by-product of cheese production; falsely promoted as increasing muscle mass. Whey is the watery part of milk that separates from the curds.

white sugar: pure sucrose or "table sugar," produced by dissolving, concentrating, and recrystallizing raw sugar.

WHO (World Health Organization): an international agency concerned with promoting health and eradicating disease.

whole grain: a grain that maintains the same relative proportions of starchy endosperm, germ, and bran as the original (all but the husk); not refined.

whole-wheat flour: any flour made from the entire wheat kernel.

wine: an alcoholic beverage traditionally made by fermenting a sugar source such as grape juice.

World Wide Web (the Web, commonly abbreviated www): a graphical subset of the Internet.

X

xanthophylls (ZAN-tho-fills): pigments found in plants; responsible for the colour changes seen in autumn leaves.

xerophthalmia (zer-off-THAL-mee-uh): progressive blindness caused by inadequate tear production due to severe vitamin A deficiency.

xerosis (zee-ROW-sis): abnormal drying of the skin and mucous membranes; a sign of vitamin A deficiency.

Y

yields: production per acre.

yogurt: milk product that results from the fermentation of lactic acid in milk by *Lactobacillus bulgaricus* and *Streptococcus thermophilus.*

Z

zygote (ZY-goat): the initial product of the union of ovum and sperm; a fertilized ovum.

zymogen (ZYE-mo-jen): the inactive precursor of an enzyme; sometimes called a *proenzyme.*

Index

NOTE: Page letters in bold indicate definition of terms. Page references followed by the letter "f" indicate figures or photographs. Page references followed by the letter "t" indicate tables. Page references with combined letter and number (A-1) refer to the appendices.

C

D

G

H

I

N

Aids to Calculation

Many mathematical problems have been worked out in the "How To" sections of the text. These pages offer additional help and examples.

Conversions

A conversion factor is a fraction that converts a measurement expressed in one unit to another unit—for example, from pounds to kilograms or from feet to metres. To create a conversion factor, an equality (such as 1 kilogram = 2.2 pounds) is expressed as a fraction:

$$\frac{1\text{ kg}}{2.2\text{ lb}} \text{ and } \frac{2.2\text{ lb}}{1\text{ kg}}$$

To convert the units of a measurement, use the fraction with the desired unit in the numerator.

Example 1: Convert a weight of 130 pounds to kilograms. Multiply 130 pounds by the conversion factor that includes both pounds and kilograms, with the desired unit (kilograms) in the numerator:

$$130\text{ lb} \times \frac{1\text{ kg}}{2.2\text{ lb}} = \frac{130\text{ kg}}{2.2} = 59\text{ kg}$$

Alternatively, to convert a measurement from one unit of measure to another, multiply the given measurement by the appropriate equivalent found on the next page of Weights and Measures.

Example 2: Convert 64 fluid ounces to litres.
Locate the equivalent measure from the next page (1 ounce = 0.03 litre) and multiply the number of ounces by 0.03:

$$64\text{ oz} \times 0.03\text{ oz/L} = 1.9\text{ L}$$

Percentages

A percentage is a fraction whose denominator is 100. For example:

$$50\% = \frac{50}{100}$$

Like other fractions, percentages are used to express a portion of a quantity. Fractions whose denominators are numbers other than 100 can be converted to percentages by first dividing the numerator by the denominator and then multiplying the result by 100.

Example 3: Express $5/8$ as a percent.

$$\frac{5}{8} = 5 \div 8 = 0.625$$

$$0.625 \times 100 = 62.5\%$$

The following examples show how to calculate specific percentages.

Example 4: Suppose your energy intake for the day is 2000 kcalories (kcal) and your recommended energy intake is 2400 kcalories. What percent of the recommended energy intake did you consume?

Divide your intake by the recommended intake.
2000 kcal (intake) ÷ 2400 kcal (recommended) = 0.83
Multiply by 100 to express the decimal as a percent.
0.83 × 100 = 83%

Example 5: Suppose a man's intake of vitamin C is 120 milligrams and his RDA is 90 milligrams. What percent of the RDA for vitamin C did he consume?

Divide the intake by the recommended intake.
120 mg (intake) ÷ 90 mg (RDA) = 1.33
Multiply by 100 to express the decimal as a percent.
1.33 × 100 = 133%

Example 6: Dietary recommendations suggest that carbohydrates provide 45 to 65 percent of the day's energy intake. If your energy intake is 2000 kcalories, how much carbohydrate should you eat?

Because this question has a range of acceptable answers, work the problem twice. First, use 45 percent to find the least amount you should eat.

Divide 45 by 100 to convert to a decimal.
45 ÷ 100 = 0.45
Multiply kcalories by 0.45.
2000 kcal × 0.45 = 900 kcal
Divide kcalories by 4 to convert carbohydrate kcal to grams.
900 kcal ÷ 4 kcal/g = 225 g

Now repeat the process using 65 percent to find the maximum number of grams of carbohydrates you should eat.

Divide 65 by 100 to convert it to a decimal.
65 ÷ 100 = 0.65
Multiply kcalories by 0.65.
2000 kcal × 0.65 = 1300 kcal
Divide kcalories by 4 to convert carbohydrate kcal to grams.
1300 kcal ÷ 4 kcal/g = 325 g

If you plan for between 45 and 65 percent of your 2000-kcalorie intake to be from carbohydrates, you should eat between 225 and 325 grams of carbohydrates.

Weights and Measures

Length

1 centimetre (cm) = 0.39 inches (in)
1 foot (ft) = 30 centimetres (cm)
1 inch (in) = 2.54 centimetres (cm)
1 metre (m) = 39.37 inches (in)

Weight

1 gram (g) = 0.001 kilograms (kg)
= 1000 milligrams (mg)
= 0.035 ounces (oz)
1 kilogram (kg) = 1000 grams (g)
= 2.2 pounds (lb)
1 microgram (μg) = 0.001 milligrams (mg)
1 milligram (mg) = 0.001 grams (g)
= 1000 micrograms (μg)
1 ounce (oz) = 28 grams (g)
= 0.03 kilograms (kg)
1 pound (lb) = 454 grams (g)
= 0.45 kilograms (kg)
= 16 ounces (oz)

Volume

1 cup = 16 tablespoons (Tbsp)
= 0.25 litres (L)
= 236 millilitres (mL; commonly rounded to 250 mL)
= 8 ounces (oz)
1 litre (L) = 33.8 fluid ounces (fl oz)
= 0.26 gallons (gal)
= 2.1 pints (pt)
= 1.06 quarts (qt)
= 1000 millilitres (mL)
1 millilitre (mL) = 0.001 litres (L)
= 0.03 fluid ounces (fl oz)
1 ounce (oz) = 0.03 litres (L)
= 30 millilitres (mL)
1 pint (pt) = 2 cups (c)
= 0.47 litres (L)
= 16 ounces (oz)
1 quart (qt) = 4 cups (c)
= 0.95 litres (L)
= 32 ounces (oz)
1 tablespoon (Tbsp) = 3 teaspoons (tsp)
= 15 millilitres (mL)
1 teaspoon (tsp) = 5 millilitres (mL)
1 gallon (gal) = 16 cups (c)
= 3.8 litres (L)
= 128 ounces (oz)

Energy

1 millijoule (mJ) = 240 kcalories (kcal)
1 kilojoule (kJ) = 0.24 kcalories (kcal)
1 kcalorie (kcal) = 4.2 kilojoule (kJ)
1 g alcohol = 7 kcal = 29 kJ
1 g carbohydrate = 4 kcal = 17 kJ
1 g fat = 9 kcal = 37 kJ
1 g protein = 4 kcal = 17 kJ

Temperature

To change from Fahrenheit (°F) to Celsius (°C), subtract 32 from the Fahrenheit measure and then multiply that result by 0.56.

To change from Celsius (°C) to Fahrenheit (°F), multiply the Celsius measure by 1.8 and add 32 to that result.

A comparison of some useful temperatures is given below.

	Celsius	Fahrenheit
Boiling point	100°C	212°F
Body temperature	37°C	98.6°F
Freezing point	0°C	32°F

STUDY CARD 1

To help you succeed, we've designed a study card for each chapter.

An Overview of Nutrition

Food Choices

- People select foods based on such factors as taste and convenience, but selections bas… edge may better support good he…
- Individual foods are neither "goo… choices made over a lifetime m… person's health.

Each study card presents a review list of the chapter's core concepts by chapter section.

The Nutrients

- Foods provide nutrients—substances that provide energy, structural materials, and regulating agents to support the growth, maintenance, and repair of the body's tissues. Essential nutrients *must* be obtained from foods.
- The six classes of nutrients include carbohydrates, lipids (fats), proteins, vitamins, minerals, and water. Carbohydrates, lipids, proteins, and vitamins are organic, meaning they contain carbon; minerals and water are inorganic.
- Energy is measured in kcalories—a measure of heat energy. One kcalorie is the amount of heat necessary to raise the temperature of 1 kg water 1°C.
- The energy-yielding nutrients are carbohydrate (4 kcal/g), fat (9 kcal/g), and protein (4 kcal/g).

The Science of Nutrition

- The science of nutrition is the study of nutrients and other substances in foods and the body's handling of them.
- Researchers follow the scientific method (review Figure 1-3, p. 12). They randomly assign control and experimental groups, use large sample sizes, provide placebos, and are blind to treatments. Their findings are reviewed and replicated by other scientists before being accepted as valid.
- Correlations indicate an association between variables, not a cause.
- Qualitative research seeks to gain a deep understanding of *why* and *how* certain phenomena occur.

Dietary Reference Intakes

- Dietary Reference Intakes (DRI) are a set of nutrient intake values used to plan and evaluate diets for healthy people.
- Estimated Average Requirement (EAR) defines the amount of a nutrient that supports a specific function in the body for half of the population. Recommended Dietary Allowance (RDA) is based on the EAR and establishes a goal for dietary intake that will meet the needs of almost all healthy people. Adequate Intake (AI) serves a similar purpose when an RDA cannot be determined.
- Estimated Energy Requirement (EER) defines the average amount of energy intake needed to maintain energy bal… …ronutrient Distribution Ranges … …rtions contributed by carbohy… … healthy diet.
- … …vel (UL) establishes the highest … for regular consumption.

Nutrition Assessment

- Malnutrition develops when people get too little, too much, or an imbalance of energy or nutrients.
- Four nutrition assessment methods include historical information on diet and health, anthropometric measurements, physical examinations, and laboratory tests. Together, these methods reveal the stages of a nutrient deficiency (review Figure 1-8, p. 23).
- A primary deficiency is caused by an inadequate intake of a nutrient; a secondary deficiency is caused by a condition that reduces absorption, accelerates use, increases excretion, or destroys the nutrient.

Diet and Health

- Risk factors such as obesity and cigarette smoking increase the likelihood of disease development.
- Some risk factors, such as genetics, are important but cannot be changed. Recommendations focus on changeable, personal life choices such as diet and activity habits.
- D… …ses but is linked

Select tables and figures are included to remind you of key points.

TABLE 1-6 Ten Lead… of Death, Canada, 200…

	Percentage of Total Deaths
1. Cancer	**29.3**
2. Heart disease	**22.4**
3. Stroke	**6.1**
4. Respiratory disease	4.6
5. Accidents	4.1
6. Diabetes	**3.4**
7. Influenza and pneumonia	2.5
8. Alzheimer's disease	2.5
9. Suicide	1.6
10. Kidney disease	1.6

NOTE: The diseases highlighted in bold have relationships with diet.
SOURCE: Statistics Canada, Leading Causes of Death in Canada, 84-215-XWE2009000, March 2009; http://www.statcan.gc.ca/bsolc/olc-cel/olc-cel?catno=84-215-x&lang=eng

TABLE 1-7 Risk Factors for Chronic Disease in Canada

Factors
Daily/occasional smoking
Heavy drinking
Low fruit/vegetable consumption
Inactivity
Obesity

SOURCE: Adapted from Statistics Canada, Leading Causes of Death in Canada, 84-215-XWE2009000, March 2009; http://www.statcan.gc.ca/bsolc/olc-cel/olc-cel?catno=84-215-x&lang=eng

Food Choices (pp. 3–5)

1. Give several reasons (and examples) why people make the food choices they do.

The Nutrients (pp. 5–11)

2. What is a nutrient? Name the six classes of … found in foods. What is an essential nutrient?
3. Which nutrients are inorganic, and which are organic? Discuss the significance of that distinction.
4. Which nutrients yield energy, and how much energy do they yield per gram? How is energy measured?
5. Describe how alcohol resembles nutrients. Why is alcohol not considered a nutrient?
6. Which is the most abundant nutrient in both the human body and most foods?
   a. fat b. water c. minerals d. proteins
7. Which nutrients are inorganic?
   a. proteins and fats c. minerals and water
   b. vitamins and minerals d. vitamins and proteins
8. Which nutrients yield energy?
   a. fats, minerals, and water
   b. minerals, proteins, and vitamins
   c. carbohydrates, fats, and vitamins
   d. carbohydrates, fats, and proteins

The Science of Nutrition (pp. 11–17)

9. What is the science of nutrition? Describe the types of research studies and methods used in acquiring nutrition information.
10. Explain how variables might be correlational but not causal.
11. Which term refers to studies of populations that reveal correlations between dietary habits and disease incidence?
    a. clinical trials c. case-control studies
    b. laboratory studies d. epidemiological studies
12. Which term refers to an experiment i… the researchers nor the subjects know… the treatment?
    a. double blind c. blind …
    b. double control d. placebo control
13. The type of research that studies reasons why people make certain food choices is an example of:
    a. quantitative research b. qualitative research

Dietary Reference Intakes (pp. 17–21)

14. What are the DRI? To whom do they apply? How are they used? In your description, identify the categories of DRI and indicate how they are related.
15. What judgement factors are involved in setting the energy and nutrient recommendations?
16. … that appears safe … hat will maintain a …
    c. the average amount of a nutrient considered adequate to meet the known nutrient needs of practically all healthy people
    d. the average amount of a nutrient that will maintain a specific biochemical or physiological function in half the people

> The back side of the study card provides essay and multiple-choice questions to help you prepare for your exams.

Nutrition Assessment (pp. 21–24)

17. What happens when people get either too little or too much energy or nutrients? Define *malnutrition, undernutrition,* and *overnutrition.* Describe the four methods used to detect energy and nutrient deficiencies and excesses.
18. What methods are used in nutrition surveys? What kinds of information can these surveys provide?
19. Which of the following involves gathering historical information, performing physical examinations, doing laboratory tests, and making anthropometric measurements?
    a. techniques used in diet planning
    b. steps used in the scientific method
    c. approaches used in disease prevention
    d. methods used in a nutrition assessment
20. Which term refers to a deficiency caused by an inadequate dietary intake?
    a. overt deficiency c. primary deficiency
    b. covert deficiency d. secondary deficiency

Diet and Health (pp. 24–26)

21. Describe risk factors and their relationships to disease.
22. … ours that influence the … s smoking, dietary hab- …
    … preventive agents
    b. chronic causes d. disease descriptors

> Solutions to the multiple-choice questions are provided at the end of the study card.

Study Questions (multiple choice)
6. b 7. c 8. d 11. d 12. a 13. b 16. c 19. d 20. c 22. a

CENGAGENOW™ For additional study questions and activities, go to **www.cengage.com/sso** and complete the Personalized Study Plan for this chapter.

STUDY CARD 1

An Overview of Nutrition

Food Choices

- People select foods based on such factors as taste and convenience, but selections based on nutrition knowledge may better support good health.
- Individual foods are neither "good" nor "bad"; daily food choices made over a lifetime may improve or impair a person's health.

The Nutrients

- Foods provide nutrients—substances that provide energy, structural materials, and regulating agents to support the growth, maintenance, and repair of the body's tissues. Essential nutrients *must* be obtained from foods.
- The six classes of nutrients include carbohydrates, lipids (fats), proteins, vitamins, minerals, and water. Carbohydrates, lipids, proteins, and vitamins are organic, meaning they contain carbon; minerals and water are inorganic.
- Energy is measured in kcalories—a measure of heat energy. One kcalorie is the amount of heat necessary to raise the temperature of 1 kg water 1°C.
- The energy-yielding nutrients are carbohydrate (4 kcal/g), fat (9 kcal/g), and protein (4 kcal/g).

The Science of Nutrition

- The science of nutrition is the study of nutrients and other substances in foods and the body's handling of them.
- Researchers follow the scientific method (review Figure 1-3, p. 12). They randomly assign control and experimental groups, use large sample sizes, provide placebos, and are blind to treatments. Their findings are reviewed and replicated by other scientists before being accepted as valid.
- Correlations indicate an association between variables, not a cause.
- Qualitative research seeks to gain a deep understanding of *why* and *how* certain phenomena occur.

Dietary Reference Intakes

- Dietary Reference Intakes (DRI) are a set of nutrient intake values used to plan and evaluate diets for healthy people.
- Estimated Average Requirement (EAR) defines the amount of a nutrient that supports a specific function in the body for half of the population. Recommended Dietary Allowance (RDA) is based on the EAR and establishes a goal for dietary intake that will meet the needs of almost all healthy people. Adequate Intake (AI) serves a similar purpose when an RDA cannot be determined.
- Estimated Energy Requirement (EER) defines the average amount of energy intake needed to maintain energy balance, and Acceptable Macronutrient Distribution Ranges (AMDR) define the proportions contributed by carbohydrate, fat, and protein to a healthy diet.
- Tolerable Upper Intake Level (UL) establishes the highest amount that appears safe for regular consumption.

Nutrition Assessment

- Malnutrition develops when people get too little, too much, or an imbalance of energy or nutrients.
- Four nutrition assessment methods include historical information on diet and health, anthropometric measurements, physical examinations, and laboratory tests. Together, these methods reveal the stages of a nutrient deficiency (review Figure 1-8, p. 23).
- A primary deficiency is caused by an inadequate intake of a nutrient; a secondary deficiency is caused by a condition that reduces absorption, accelerates use, increases excretion, or destroys the nutrient.

Diet and Health

- Risk factors such as obesity and cigarette smoking increase the likelihood of disease development.
- Some risk factors, such as genetics, are important but cannot be changed. Recommendations focus on changeable, personal life choices such as diet and activity habits.
- Diet has no influence on some diseases but is linked closely to others.

TABLE 1-6 Ten Leading Causes of Death, Canada, 2005

	Percentage of Total Deaths
1. Cancer	**29.3**
2. Heart disease	**22.4**
3. Stroke	**6.1**
4. Respiratory disease	4.6
5. Accidents	4.1
6. Diabetes	**3.4**
7. Influenza and pneumonia	2.5
8. Alzheimer's disease	2.5
9. Suicide	1.6
10. Kidney disease	1.6

NOTE: The diseases highlighted in bold have relationships with diet.
SOURCE: Statistics Canada, Leading Causes of Death in Canada, 84-215-XWE2009000, March 2009; http://www.statcan.gc.ca/bsolc/olc-cel/olc-cel?catno=84-215-x&lang=eng

TABLE 1-7 Risk Factors for Chronic Disease in Canada

Factors
Daily/occasional smoking
Heavy drinking
Low fruit/vegetable consumption
Inactivity
Obesity

SOURCE: Adapted from Statistics Canada, Leading Causes of Death in Canada, 84-215-XWE2009000, March 2009; http://www.statcan.gc.ca/bsolc/olc-cel/olc-cel?catno=84-215-x&lang=eng

Food Choices (pp. 3–5)

1. Give several reasons (and examples) why people make the food choices they do.

The Nutrients (pp. 5–11)

2. What is a nutrient? Name the six classes of nutrients found in foods. What is an essential nutrient?
3. Which nutrients are inorganic, and which are organic? Discuss the significance of that distinction.
4. Which nutrients yield energy, and how much energy do they yield per gram? How is energy measured?
5. Describe how alcohol resembles nutrients. Why is alcohol not considered a nutrient?
6. Which is the most abundant nutrient in both the human body and most foods?
   a. fat b. water c. minerals d. proteins
7. Which nutrients are inorganic?
   a. proteins and fats
   b. vitamins and minerals
   c. minerals and water
   d. vitamins and proteins
8. Which nutrients yield energy?
   a. fats, minerals, and water
   b. minerals, proteins, and vitamins
   c. carbohydrates, fats, and vitamins
   d. carbohydrates, fats, and proteins

The Science of Nutrition (pp. 11–17)

9. What is the science of nutrition? Describe the types of research studies and methods used in acquiring nutrition information.
10. Explain how variables might be correlational but not causal.
11. Which term refers to studies of populations that reveal correlations between dietary habits and disease incidence?
    a. clinical trials
    b. laboratory studies
    c. case-control studies
    d. epidemiological studies
12. Which term refers to an experiment in which neither the researchers nor the subjects know who is receiving the treatment?
    a. double blind
    b. double control
    c. blind variable
    d. placebo control
13. The type of research that studies reasons why people make certain food choices is an example of:
    a. quantitative research b. qualitative research

Dietary Reference Intakes (pp. 17–21)

14. What are the DRI? To whom do they apply? How are they used? In your description, identify the categories of DRI and indicate how they are related.
15. What judgement factors are involved in setting the energy and nutrient recommendations?
16. What does an RDA represent?
    a. the highest amount of a nutrient that appears safe for most healthy people
    b. the lowest amount of a nutrient that will maintain a specified criterion of adequacy
    c. the average amount of a nutrient considered adequate to meet the known nutrient needs of practically all healthy people
    d. the average amount of a nutrient that will maintain a specific biochemical or physiological function in half the people

Nutrition Assessment (pp. 21–24)

17. What happens when people get either too little or too much energy or nutrients? Define *malnutrition, undernutrition,* and *overnutrition.* Describe the four methods used to detect energy and nutrient deficiencies and excesses.
18. What methods are used in nutrition surveys? What kinds of information can these surveys provide?
19. Which of the following involves gathering historical information, performing physical examinations, doing laboratory tests, and making anthropometric measurements?
    a. techniques used in diet planning
    b. steps used in the scientific method
    c. approaches used in disease prevention
    d. methods used in a nutrition assessment
20. Which term refers to a deficiency caused by an inadequate dietary intake?
    a. overt deficiency
    b. covert deficiency
    c. primary deficiency
    d. secondary deficiency

Diet and Health (pp. 24–26)

21. Describe risk factors and their relationships to disease.
22. Which term is given to behaviours that influence the development of disease, such as smoking, dietary habits, and physical activity?
    a. risk factors
    b. chronic causes
    c. preventive agents
    d. disease descriptors

Study Questions (multiple choice)
6. b 7. c 8. d 11. d 12. a 13. b 16. c 19. d 20. c 22. a

CENGAGENOW™ For additional study questions and activities, go to **www.cengage.com/sso** and complete the Personalized Study Plan for this chapter.

STUDY CARD 2

Planning a Healthy Diet

Diet-Planning Principles

- A well-planned diet delivers *adequate* nutrients, a *balanced* array of nutrients, and an appropriate amount of *energy (kcalories)*. It is based on *nutrient-dense* foods, *moderate* in substances that can be detrimental to health, and *varied* in its selections.

Diet-Planning Guides

- *Eating Well with Canada's Food Guide* suggests the amounts to eat from each of four food groups—Vegetables and Fruits, Grain Products, Milk and Alternatives, and Meat and Alternatives (review Figure 2-1, p. 38).
- *Eating Well with Canada's Food Guide* encourages consumption of a variety of foods to provide an assortment of nutrients (review Table 2-1, p. 38).

Food Labels

- Food labels provide Nutrition Facts tables including Daily Values based on a 2000-kcalorie diet and a specified serving size of food (review Figure 2-11, p. 50). Ingredients are listed in descending order of predominance by weight. Nutrient claims reflect the quantity of a nutrient in a food (*e.g., excellent source, low fat*). Health claims reflect relationships between a nutrient and health (*e.g., A healthy diet low in saturated and trans fats may reduce the risk of heart disease. [Naming the food] is low in saturated and trans fats.*).

FIGURE 2-11 **Example of a Food Label**

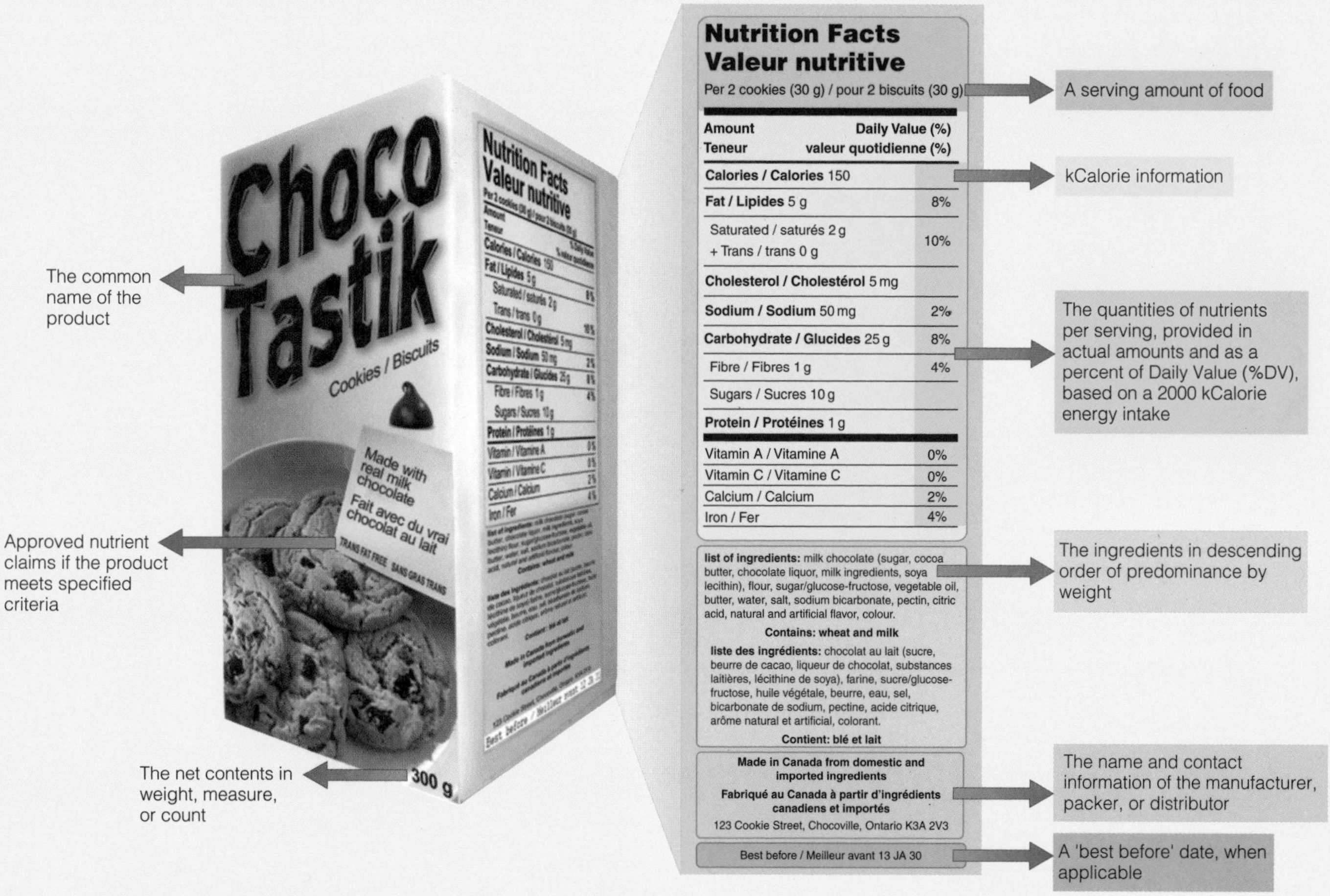

Choco Tastik
Cookies / Biscuits
Made with real milk chocolate
Fait avec du vrai chocolat au lait
TRANS FAT FREE SANS GRAS TRANS
300 g
The common name of the product
Approved nutrient claims if the product meets specified criteria
The net contents in weight, measure, or count
Nutrition Facts
Valeur nutritive
Per 2 cookies (30 g) / pour 2 biscuits (30 g)
Amount / Teneur — Daily Value (%) / valeur quotidienne (%)
Calories / Calories 150
Fat / Lipides 5 g — 8%
Saturated / saturés 2 g + Trans / trans 0 g — 10%
Cholesterol / Cholestérol 5 mg
Sodium / Sodium 50 mg — 2%
Carbohydrate / Glucides 25 g — 8%
Fibre / Fibres 1 g — 4%
Sugars / Sucres 10 g
Protein / Protéines 1 g
Vitamin A / Vitamine A — 0%
Vitamin C / Vitamine C — 0%
Calcium / Calcium — 2%
Iron / Fer — 4%
list of ingredients: milk chocolate (sugar, cocoa butter, chocolate liquor, milk ingredients, soya lecithin), flour, sugar/glucose-fructose, vegetable oil, butter, water, salt, sodium bicarbonate, pectin, citric acid, natural and artificial flavor, colour.
Contains: wheat and milk
liste des ingrédients: chocolat au lait (sucre, beurre de cacao, liqueur de chocolat, substances laitières, lécithine de soya), farine, sucre/glucose-fructose, huile végétale, beurre, eau, sel, bicarbonate de sodium, pectine, acide citrique, arôme natural et artificial, colorant.
Contient: blé et lait
Made in Canada from domestic and imported ingredients
Fabriqué au Canada à partir d'ingrédients canadiens et importés
123 Cookie Street, Chocoville, Ontario K3A 2V3
Best before / Meilleur avant 13 JA 30
A serving amount of food
kCalorie information
The quantities of nutrients per serving, provided in actual amounts and as a percent of Daily Value (%DV), based on a 2000 kCalorie energy intake
The ingredients in descending order of predominance by weight
The name and contact information of the manufacturer, packer, or distributor
A 'best before' date, when applicable

Diet-Planning Principles (pp. 35–38)

1. Name the diet-planning principles and briefly describe how each principle helps in diet planning.
2. Which diet-planning principle provides all of the essential nutrients in sufficient amounts to support health?
   a. balance
   b. variety
   c. adequacy
   d. moderation
3. Suppose a person chooses to eat a chicken leg that provides 0.5 milligram of iron and 95 kcalories instead of eating 2 tablespoons of peanut butter that also provide 0.5 milligram of iron but 188 kcalories. What principle is the person using?
   a. balance
   b. nutrient density
   c. adequacy
   d. moderation

Diet-Planning Guides (pp. 38–50)

4. Name the four food groups in *Eating Well with Canada's Food Guide* and identify several foods typical of each group. Explain how such plans group foods and what diet-planning principles the plans best accommodate. How are food group plans used, and what are some of their strengths and weaknesses?
5. Which statement is a key message in *Eating Well with Canada's Food Guide*?
   a. Have meat alternatives such as beans, lentils, and tofu often.
   b. At least one-third of the grain products you eat each day should be whole grain products.
   c. Eat at least two dark green vegetables each day.
   d. Eat at least one *Food Guide* serving of fish each week.
6. What types of grocery selections would you make to meet the key messages in *Eating Well with Canada's Food Guide*?
7. Which type of fat does *Eating Well with Canada's Food Guide* recommend you eat each day?
   a. *trans* fat
   b. unsaturated fat
   c. dietary cholesterol
   d. saturated fat
8. Which supplement does *Eating Well with Canada's Food Guide* advise women and men over the age of 50 years to take?
   a. calcium
   b. vitamin D
   c. vitamin C
   d. iron
9. On any given list in the exchange system of diet planning, what does each portion of food provide about the same amount of?
   a. energy
   b. satiety
   c. vitamins
   d. minerals
10. What are enriched grain products fortified with?
    a. fibre, folate, iron, niacin, and zinc
    b. thiamin, iron, calcium, zinc, and sodium
    c. iron, thiamin, riboflavin, niacin, and folate
    d. folate, magnesium, vitamin B_6, zinc, and fibre

Food Labels (pp. 50–55)

11. What information can you expect to find on a food label? How can this information help you choose between two similar products?
12. What are the Daily Values? How can they help you meet health recommendations?
13. What are Daily Values on food labels based on?
    a. a 1500-kcalorie diet
    b. a 2000-kcalorie diet
    c. a 2500-kcalorie diet
    d. a 3000-kcalorie diet
14. What are the core vitamins and minerals found in the Nutrition Facts table?
    a. calcium, sodium, vitamin D, vitamin C
    b. vitamin A, vitamin C, calcium, iron
    c. potassium, sodium, vitamin E, vitamin A
    d. calcium, iron, vitamin D, vitamin A
15. How are ingredients listed on food labels?
    a. in alphabetical order
    b. in ascending order of predominance by weight
    c. in descending order of predominance by weight
    d. in manufacturer's order of preference
16. Describe the difference between nutrient claims and health claims.
17. Explain why it is important to regulate the information found on food labels.

Study Questions (multiple choice)
2. c 3. b 5. a 7. b 8. b 9. a 10. c 13. b 14. d 15. c

STUDY CARD 3

FIGURE 3-1 **The Gastrointestinal Tract**

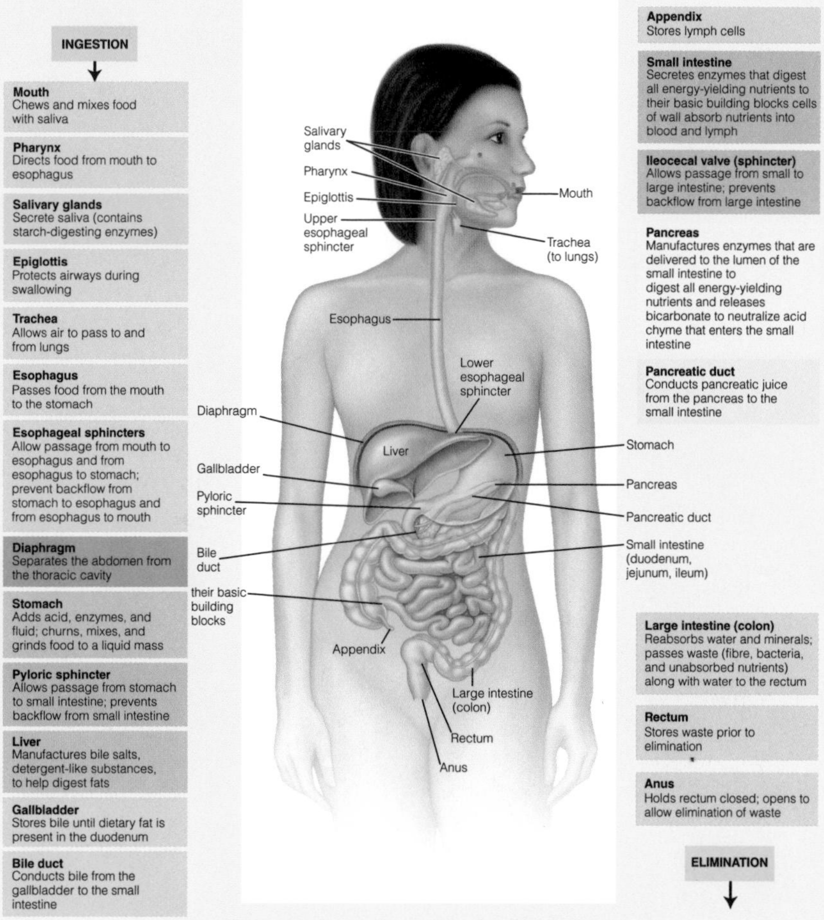

INGESTION
Mouth
Chews and mixes food with saliva
Pharynx
Directs food from mouth to esophagus
Salivary glands
Secrete saliva (contains starch-digesting enzymes)
Epiglottis
Protects airways during swallowing
Trachea
Allows air to pass to and from lungs
Esophagus
Passes food from the mouth to the stomach
Esophageal sphincters
Allow passage from mouth to esophagus and from esophagus to stomach; prevent backflow from stomach to esophagus and from esophagus to mouth
Diaphragm
Separates the abdomen from the thoracic cavity
Stomach
Adds acid, enzymes, and fluid; churns, mixes, and grinds food to a liquid mass
Pyloric sphincter
Allows passage from stomach to small intestine; prevents backflow from small intestine
Liver
Manufactures bile salts, detergent-like substances, to help digest fats
Gallbladder
Stores bile until dietary fat is present in the duodenum
Bile duct
Conducts bile from the gallbladder to the small intestine
Salivary glands
Pharynx
Epiglottis
Upper esophageal sphincter
Mouth
Trachea (to lungs)
Esophagus
Lower esophageal sphincter
Diaphragm
Liver
Gallbladder
Pyloric sphincter
Bile duct
their basic building blocks
Appendix
Large intestine (colon)
Rectum
Anus
Stomach
Pancreas
Pancreatic duct
Small intestine (duodenum, jejunum, ileum)
Appendix
Stores lymph cells
Small intestine
Secretes enzymes that digest all energy-yielding nutrients to their basic building blocks cells of wall absorb nutrients into blood and lymph
Ileocecal valve (sphincter)
Allows passage from small to large intestine; prevents backflow from large intestine
Pancreas
Manufactures enzymes that are delivered to the lumen of the small intestine to digest all energy-yielding nutrients and releases bicarbonate to neutralize acid chyme that enters the small intestine
Pancreatic duct
Conducts pancreatic juice from the pancreas to the small intestine
Large intestine (colon)
Reabsorbs water and minerals; passes waste (fibre, bacteria, and unabsorbed nutrients) along with water to the rectum
Rectum
Stores waste prior to elimination
Anus
Holds rectum closed; opens to allow elimination of waste
ELIMINATION

Digestion, Absorption, and Transport

Digestion

- Digestion breaks down foods into nutrients. Absorption brings the nutrients into the cells of the small intestine for transport to the body's cells.
- Food enters the mouth and travels down the esophagus and through the upper and lower esophageal sphincters to the stomach, then through the pyloric sphincter to the small intestine, on through the ileocecal valve to the large intestine, past the appendix to the rectum, ending at the anus (review Figure 3-1, p. 67).
- The wavelike contractions of peristalsis and the periodic squeezing of segmentation keep things moving at a reasonable pace. Along the way, secretions from the salivary glands, stomach, pancreas, liver (via the gallbladder), and small intestine deliver fluids and digestive enzymes.

Absorption

- The many folds and villi of the small intestine increase its surface area, making nutrient absorption efficient.
- Nutrients pass through the cells of the intestinal villi and enter either the blood (if they are water soluble or small fat fragments) or the lymph (if they are fat soluble).

The Circulatory Systems

- Nutrients leaving the digestive system via the blood are routed directly to the liver before being transported to the body's cells.
- Nutrients leaving via the lymphatic system bypass the liver at first, but eventually enter the vascular system via the thoracic duct, which opens into the subclavian vein.

The Health and Regulation of the GI Tract

- A diverse and abundant bacteria population supports GI health.
- The regulation of GI processes depends on the coordinated efforts of the hormonal system and the nervous system.

Summary of Digestive Secretions and Their Major Actions

Organ or Gland	Target Organ	Secretion	Action
Salivary glands	Mouth	Saliva	Fluid eases swallowing; salivary enzyme breaks down some ***carbohydrate.****
Gastric glands	Stomach	Gastric juice	Fluid mixes with bolus; hydrochloric acid uncoils ***proteins;*** enzymes break down proteins; mucus protects stomach cells.*
Pancreas	Small intestine	Pancreatic juice	Bicarbonate neutralizes acidic gastric juices; pancreatic enzymes break down ***carbohydrates, fats,*** and ***proteins.***
Liver	Gallbladder	Bile	Bile stored until needed.
Gallbladder	Small intestine	Bile	Bile emulsifies ***fat*** so that enzymes can have access to break it down.
Intestinal glands	Small intestine	Intestinal juice	Intestinal enzymes break down ***carbohydrate, fat,*** and ***protein*** fragments; mucus protects the intestinal wall.

*Saliva and gastric juice also contain lipases, but most fat breakdown occurs in the small intestine.

Digestion (pp. 65–73)

1. Describe the challenges associated with digesting food and the solutions offered by the human body.
2. Describe the path food follows as it travels through the digestive system. Summarize the muscular actions that take place along the way.
3. Name five organs that secrete digestive juices. How do the juices and enzymes facilitate digestion?
4. What is the name of the semiliquid, partially digested food that travels through the intestinal tract?
   a. bile
   b. lymph
   c. chyme
   d. secretin
5. What are the muscular contractions that propel food through the GI tract called?
   a. hydrolysis
   b. sphincters
   c. peristalsis
   d. bowel movements
6. What is the main function of bile?
   a. to emulsify fats
   b. to catalyze hydrolysis
   c. to slow protein digestion
   d. to neutralize stomach acidity
7. What does the pancreas secrete in order to neutralize stomach acid in the small intestine?
   a. bil
   b. mucus
   c. enzymes
   d. bicarbonate
8. Which nutrient passes through the GI tract mostly undigested and unabsorbed?
   a. fat
   b. fibre
   c. protein
   d. carbohydrate

Absorption (pp. 74–76)

9. Describe the problems associated with absorbing nutrients and the solutions offered by the small intestine.
10. Where dose absorption primarily occur?
    a. in the mouth
    b. in the stomach
    c. in the small intestine
    d. in the large intestine
11. Describe three common processes used for absorbing nutrients.

The Circulatory Systems (pp. 76–79)

12. How is blood routed through the digestive system? Which nutrients enter the bloodstream directly? Which are first absorbed into the lymph?
13. Where does all blood leaving the GI tract travel to first?
    a. the heart
    b. the liver
    c. the kidneys
    d. the pancreas
14. Which nutrients leave the GI tract by way of the lymphatic system?
    a. water and minerals
    b. proteins and minerals
    c. all vitamins and minerals
    d. fats and fat-soluble vitamins

The Health and Regulation of the GI Tract (pp. 79–82)

15. Describe how the body coordinates and regulates the processes of digestion and absorption.
16. How does the composition of the diet influence the functioning of the GI tract?
17. What steps can you take to help your GI tract function at its best?
18. What systems coordinate digestion and absorption?
    a. the pancreas and kidneys
    b. the liver and gallbladder
    c. the hormonal system and the nervous system
    d. the vascular system and the lymphatic system
19. What are gastrin, secretin, and cholecystokinin examples of?
    a. crypts
    b. enzymes
    c. hormones
    d. goblet cells

Study Questions (multiple choice)
4. c 5. c 6. a 7. d 8. b 10. c 13. b 14. d 18. c 19. c

CENGAGENOW™ For additional study questions and activities, go to **www.cengage.com/sso** and complete the Personalized Study Plan for this chapter.

STUDY CARD 4

The Carbohydrates: Sugars, Starches, and Fibres

The Chemist's View of Carbohydrates

- Carbohydrates are made of carbon (C), oxygen (O), and hydrogen (H); each atom forms a specified number of chemical bonds: carbon forms four, oxygen forms two, and hydrogen forms one (review Figure 4-1, p. 94).
- Monosaccharides (glucose, fructose, and galactose) all have the same chemical formula ($C_6H_{12}O_6$), but their structures differ. Disaccharides (maltose, sucrose, and lactose) each contain a glucose paired with one of the three monosaccharides.
- A condensation reaction can bond two monosaccharides together to form a disaccharide and water (review Figure 4-6, p. 96). A hydrolysis reaction can use water to split a disaccharide into its two monosaccharides (review Figure 4-7, p. 96).
- Chains of monosaccharides are called polysaccharides and include glycogen, starches, and dietary fibres. Both glycogen and starch are storage forms of glucose—glycogen in the body, and starch in plants—and both yield energy.
- Dietary fibres contain glucose (and other monosaccharides), but their bonds cannot be broken by human digestive enzymes; they yield little, if any, energy.

The Carbohydrate Family

- *Monosaccharides* (single sugars)
  - Glucose
  - Fructose
  - Galactose
- *Disaccharides* (pairs of monosaccharides)
  - Maltose (glucose + glucose)
  - Sucrose (glucose + fructose)
  - Lactose (glucose + galactose)
- *Polysaccharides* (chains of monosaccharides)
  - Glycogen (a polysaccharide, but not a dietary carbohydrate)
  - Starches (amylose and amylopectin)
  - Fibres (soluble and insoluble)

Digestion and Absorption of Carbohydrates

- The body digests starches into the disaccharide maltose. Maltose and the other disaccharides (lactose and sucrose) from foods are broken down into monosaccharides, which are absorbed.
- Monosaccharides arriving at the liver are converted mostly to glucose (review Figure 4-11, p. 101).
- Fibres help to regulate the passage of food through the GI system and slow the absorption of glucose.
- Lactose intolerance occurs when there is insufficient lactase to digest the disaccharide lactose found in milk and milk products. Symptoms include GI distress.

Glucose in the Body

- Dietary carbohydrates provide glucose that can be used by the cells for energy, stored by the liver and muscles as glycogen, or converted into fat if intakes exceed needs.
- All of the body's cells depend on glucose; those of the central nervous system as well as RBCs are especially dependent on it.
- Without glucose, the body is forced to break down its protein tissues to make glucose and to alter energy metabolism to make ketone bodies from fats.
- Blood glucose regulation depends on two pancreatic hormones: insulin to move glucose from the blood into the muscle and adipose tissue cells when levels are high and glucagon to free glucose from liver glycogen stores and release it into the blood when levels are low (review Figure 4-12, p. 105).

Health Effects and Recommended Intakes of Sugars

- Excessive intakes of sugars may increase the risk of dental caries, displace needed nutrients and fibre, increase plasma triglycerides and contribute to obesity when energy intake exceeds needs.
- Concentrated sweets are relatively low in nutrients, high in kcalories, and may need to be limited; sugars that occur naturally in fruits, vegetables, and milk are more nutrient-dense.

Alternative Sweeteners

- To control weight gain, blood glucose, and dental caries, consumers may use alternative sweeteners (artificial sweeteners, herbal products, and sugar alcohols) to limit kcalories and minimize sugar intake (review Table 4-2, pp. 113–114).

Health Effects and Recommended Intakes of Starch and Fibres

- Adequate intake of fibre fosters weight management, lowers blood cholesterol, and may help prevent colon cancer, diabetes, hemorrhoids, appendicitis, and diverticulosis.
- Excessive intake of fibre displaces energy- and nutrient-dense foods, causes intestinal discomfort and distention, and may interfere with mineral absorption.
- Because starches and fibres help control body weight and prevent heart disease, cancer, diabetes, and GI disorders,

guidelines suggest plenty of whole grains, vegetables, legumes, and fruits—enough to provide 45 to 65 percent of the daily energy intake from carbohydrate.

The Chemist's View of Carbohydrates (pp. 93–99)

1. Describe the structure of a monosaccharide and name the three monosaccharides important in nutrition. Name the three disaccharides commonly found in foods and their component monosaccharides. In what foods are these sugars found?
2. What happens in a condensation reaction? In a hydrolysis reaction?
3. Describe the structure of polysaccharides and name the ones important in nutrition. How are starch and glycogen similar, and how do they differ? How do the fibres differ from the other polysaccharides?
4. Which set of terms fits into the category of disaccharides?
   a. starch, glycogen, and fibre
   b. amylose, pectin, and dextrose
   c. sucrose, maltose, and lactose
   d. glucose, galactose, and fructose
5. During which metabolic process is a disaccharide made from two monosaccharides?
   a. digestion
   b. hydrolysis
   c. condensation
   d. gluconeogenesis
6. What is a significant difference between starch and cellulose?
   a. Starch is a polysaccharide, but cellulose is not.
   b. Animals can store glucose as starch, but not as cellulose.
   c. Hormones can make glucose from cellulose, but not from starch.
   d. Digestive enzymes can break the bonds in starch, but not in cellulose.

Digestion and Absorption of Carbohydrates (pp. 99–103)

7. Describe carbohydrate digestion and absorption. What role does fibre play in the process?
8. What is the ultimate goal of carbohydrate digestion and absorption?
   a. to yield fibres
   b. to yield glucose
   c. to yield enzymes
   d. to yield amylase
9. Which enzyme breaks a disaccharide into glucose and galactose?
   a. amylase
   b. maltase
   c. sucrase
   d. lactase

Glucose in the Body (pp. 103–108)

10. What are the possible fates of glucose in the body? What is the protein-sparing action of carbohydrate?
11. How does the body maintain its blood glucose concentration? What happens when the blood glucose concentration rises too high or falls too low?
12. What is the storage form of glucose in the body?
    a. insulin
    b. maltose
    c. glucagon
    d. glycogen
13. When glucose is insufficient in metabolism, what do fat fragments combine to form?
    a. dextrins
    b. mucilages
    c. phytic acids
    d. ketone bodies
14. What does the pancreas secrete when blood glucose rises? When blood glucose falls?
    a. insulin; glucagon
    b. glucagon; insulin
    c. insulin; glycogen
    d. glycogen; epinephrine

Health Effects and Recommended Intakes of Sugars (pp. 108–112)

15. What are the health effects of sugars? What are the dietary recommendations regarding concentrated sugar intakes?

Alternative Sweeteners (pp. 112–114)

16. Describe the risks and benefits of using alternative sweeteners.

Health Effects and Recommended Intakes of Starch and Fibres (pp. 115–119)

17. What are the health effects of starches and fibres? What are the dietary recommendations regarding these complex carbohydrates?
18. What foods provide starches and fibres?
19. Which type of food does NOT contain carbohydrates?
    a. milks
    b. meats
    c. breads
    d. fruits
20. For young adults, what percentage of the daily energy intake should come from carbohydrates?
    a. 15 to 20
    b. 25 to 30
    c. 45 to 50
    d. 45 to 65

Study Questions (multiple choice)
4. c 5. c 6. d 8. b 9. d 12. d 13. d 14. a 19. b 20. d

CENGAGENOW™ For additional study questions and activities, go to **www.cengage.com/sso** and complete the Personalized Study Plan for this chapter.

STUDY CARD 5

The Lipids: Triglycerides, Phospholipids, and Sterols

The Chemist's View of Fatty Acids and Triglycerides

- The predominant storage lipids both in foods and in the body are triglycerides: glycerol with three fatty acids attached by way of condensation reactions (review Figure 5-4, p. 133). Other lipids include cell membrane phospholipids and sterols.
- Fatty acids vary in the length of their carbon chains, their degrees of unsaturation, and the location of their double bond(s). Saturated fatty acids are fully loaded with hydrogens; unsaturated (monounsaturated or polyunsaturated) fatty acids are missing hydrogens and have double bonds.
- Hydrogenation makes polyunsaturated fats more saturated and creates *trans*-fatty acids.

The Chemist's View of Phospholipids and Sterols

- The chemical structure of phospholipids, including lecithin, allows them to be soluble in both water and fat. In the body, phospholipids are part of cell membranes; in foods, phospholipids act as emulsifiers to mix fats with water.
- Sterols have a multiple-ring structure that differs from the structure of other lipids. In the body, sterols include cholesterol, bile, vitamin D, and some hormones. Animal-derived foods contain cholesterol.

The Lipid Family

- *Triglycerides* (fats and oils), which are made of:
  - *Glycerol* (1 per triglyceride) and
  - *Fatty acids* (3 per triglyceride); depending on the number of double bonds, fatty acids may be:
    - *Saturated* (no double bonds)
    - *Monounsaturated* (one double bond)
    - *Polyunsaturated* (more than one double bond); depending on the location of the double bonds, polyunsaturated fatty acids may be:
      - *Omega-3* (first double bond 3 carbons away from methyl end)
      - *Omega-6* (first double bond 6 carbons away from methyl end)
- *Phospholipids* (such as lecithin)
- *Sterols* (such as cholesterol)

Digestion, Absorption, and Transport of Lipids

- Bile emulsifies fats, making them accessible to the lipases that dismantle triglycerides to monoglycerides and free fatty acids for absorption (review Figure 5-14, p. 139).
- Four types of lipoproteins carry triglycerides, phospholipids, and cholesterol throughout the body: *chylomicrons* are the largest and contain mostly dietary triglycerides, *VLDL* are smaller and are about half triglycerides, *LDL* are smaller still and contain mostly cholesterol, and *HDL* are the densest and are rich in protein (review Figure 5-18, p. 142).

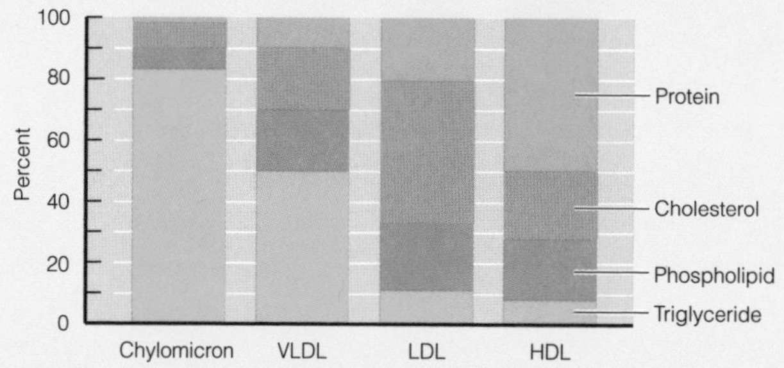

100
80
60
40
20
0
Percent
Chylomicron
VLDL
LDL
HDL
Protein
Cholesterol
Phospholipid
Triglyceride

Lipids in the Body

- In the body, triglycerides provide energy, insulate against temperature extremes, protect against shock, and help the body use carbohydrate and protein efficiently.
- Linoleic acid (18 carbons, omega-6) and linolenic acid (18 carbons, omega-3) are essential fatty acids, serving as structural parts of cell membranes and as precursors to the longer fatty acids that can make eicosanoids.
- The body stores fat if given excesses, and uses body fat for energy when needed. (The liver can also convert excess carbohydrate and protein into fat.) Fat breakdown requires carbohydrate for maximum efficiency; without carbohydrate, fatty acids break down to ketone bodies.

Health Effects and Recommended Intakes of Lipids

- High blood LDL cholesterol increases the risk of heart disease, and high intakes of saturated and *trans* fats contribute most to high LDL. Omega-3 fatty acids appear to be protective.
- In foods, triglycerides deliver fat-soluble vitamins, energy, and essential fatty acids; contribute to the sensory appeal of foods and stimulate appetite.
- Some fat in the diet is necessary; ideally, a diet is moderate in total fat and low in saturated fat, *trans* fat, and cholesterol. Recommendations include replacing saturated and *trans* fats with monounsaturated and polyunsaturated fats, particularly omega-3 fatty acids from foods such as fatty fish, not from supplements.

The Chemist's View of Fatty Acids and Triglycerides (pp. 129–135)

1. Name three classes of lipids found in the body and in foods. What are some of their functions in the body? What features do fats bring to foods?
2. What features distinguish fatty acids from each other?
3. What does the term *omega* mean with respect to fatty acids? Describe the roles of the omega fatty acids in disease prevention.
4. What are the differences between saturated, unsaturated, monounsaturated, and polyunsaturated fatty acids? Describe the structure of a triglyceride.
5. What does hydrogenation do to fats? What are *trans*-fatty acids, and how do they influence heart disease?
6. Which of the following statements about saturated fatty acids is correct?
   a. Saturated fatty acids are always 18 carbons long.
   b. Saturated fatty acids have at least one double bond.
   c. Saturated fatty acids are fully loaded with hydrogens.
   d. Saturated fatty acids are always liquid at room temperature.
7. What does a triglyceride consists of?
   a. three glycerols attached to a lipid
   b. three fatty acids attached to a glucose
   c. three fatty acids attached to a glycerol
   d. three phospholipids attached to a cholesterol
8. What is the difference between *cis*- and *trans*-fatty acids?
   a. the number of double bonds
   b. the length of their carbon chains
   c. the location of the first double bond
   d. the configuration around the double bond

The Chemist's View of Phospholipids and Sterols (pp. 135–137)

9. How do phospholipids differ from triglycerides in structure? How does cholesterol differ? How do these differences in structure affect function?
10. What roles do phospholipids perform in the body? What roles does cholesterol play in the body?
11. Which of the following statements about lecithin is NOT true?
    a. Lecithin is an emulsifier.
    b. Lecithin is a phospholipid.
    c. Lecithin is an essential nutrient.
    d. Lecithin is a constituent of cell membranes.

Digestion, Absorption, and Transport of Lipids (pp. 138–144)

12. Trace the steps in fat digestion, absorption, and transport. Describe the routes cholesterol takes in the body.
13. What do lipoproteins do? What are the differences among the chylomicrons, VLDL, LDL, and HDL?
14. Where are chylomicrons produced?
    a. in the liver
    b. in the pancreas
    c. in the gallbladder
    d. in the small intestine
15. What are the vehicles that transport lipids called?
    a. micelles
    b. lipoproteins
    c. blood vessels
    d. monoglycerides

Lipids in the Body (pp. 144–147)

16. Which of the fatty acids are essential? Name their chief dietary sources.
17. Which of the following statements about fats is NOT true?
    a. Fats contain glucose.
    b. Fats provide energy.
    c. Fats protect against organ shock.
    d. Fats carry vitamins A, D, E, and K.
18. Which of the following pairs of acids are among the essential fatty acids?
    a. stearic acid and oleic acid
    b. oleic acid and linoleic acid
    c. palmitic acid and linolenic acid
    d. linoleic acid and linolenic acid

Health Effects and Recommended Intakes of Lipids (pp. 147–157)

19. How does excessive fat intake influence health? What factors influence LDL, HDL, and total blood cholesterol?
20. What are the dietary recommendations regarding fat and cholesterol intake? List ways to reduce intake.
21. What is the Daily Value for fat (for a 2000-kcalorie diet)? What does this number represent?
22. Which lipoprotein is most associated with a high risk of heart disease?
    a. CHD
    b. HDL
    c. LDL
    d. LPL
23. Suppose that a person consuming 2200 kcalories a day wants to meet health recommendations. What should he limit his daily fat intake to?
    a. 20 to 35 grams
    b. 50 to 85 grams
    c. 75 to 100 grams
    d. 90 to 130 grams

Study Questions (multiple choice)
6. c 7. c 8. d 11. c 14. d 15. b 17. a 18. d 22. c 23. b

CENGAGENOW™ For additional study questions and activities, go to **www.cengage.com/sso** and complete the Personalized Study Plan for this chapter.

STUDY CARD 6

Protein: Amino Acids

The Chemist's View of Proteins

- Proteins are more chemically complex than carbohydrates or lipids; they are made of 20 different amino acids, 9 of which the body cannot make. These 9 are the indispensable/essential amino acids—histidine, isoleucine, leucine, lysine, methionine, phenylalanine, threonine, tryptophan, and valine.
- Each amino acid contains an amino group, an acid group, a hydrogen atom, and a distinctive side group, all attached to a central carbon atom.
- Cells link amino acids together in a series of condensation reactions to create proteins (review Figure 6-3, p. 173). The distinctive sequence of amino acids in each protein determines its unique shape and function.

Digestion and Absorption of Proteins

- The stomach's acid first denatures dietary proteins, then enzymes cleave them into smaller polypeptides and some amino acids. Pancreatic and intestinal enzymes split polypeptides further, to oligo-, tri-, and dipeptides, and then split most of these to single amino acids that can be absorbed.

Proteins in the Body

- Cells synthesize proteins according to the genetic information provided by the DNA in the nucleus of each cell (review Figure 6-7, p. 177). This information dictates the sequence in which amino acids are linked together to form a given protein. Genetic sequencing errors occasionally occur, sometimes with significant consequences.
- A sampling of protein functions are summarized in the accompanying table.
- Proteins are constantly being synthesized and broken down as needed.
- The body's assimilation of amino acids into proteins and its release of amino acids via protein degradation and excretion can be tracked by measuring nitrogen balance, which should be positive during growth and steady in adulthood. An energy deficit or an inadequate protein intake may force the body to use amino acids as fuel, creating a negative nitrogen balance.
- Protein eaten in excess of need is degraded, converted to glucose, and stored as body fat.

Protein in Foods

- High-quality proteins deliver all of the indispensable/essential amino acids in adequate amounts, which ensures protein synthesis. Mixtures of foods containing complementary proteins can each supply the amino acids missing in the other.
- In addition to its amino acid content, the quality of protein is measured by its digestibility and its ability to support growth.

Health Effects and Recommended Intakes of Protein and Amino Acids

- Protein deficiencies arise from both energy-poor and protein-poor diets and lead to marasmus and kwashiorkor. Together, these diseases are known as PEM (protein-energy malnutrition), a major form of malnutrition causing death in children worldwide.
- Excess protein offers no advantage and may incur health problems as well.
- The optimal diet for a sedentary or slightly active adult is adequate in energy from carbohydrate and fat and delivers 0.8 grams of protein per kilogram of healthy body weight each day.
- Normal, healthy people who consume the diet described above do not need protein or amino acid supplements.

Growth and maintenance	Proteins form integral parts of most body structures such as skin, tendons, membranes, muscles, organs, and bones. As such, they support the growth and repair of body tissues.
Enzymes	Proteins facilitate chemical reactions.
Hormones	Proteins regulate body processes. (Some, but not all, hormones are proteins.)
Fluid balance	Proteins help to maintain the volume and composition of body fluids.
Acid–base balance	Proteins help to maintain the acid-base balance of body fluids by acting as buffers.
Transportation	Proteins transport substances, such as lipids, vitamins, minerals, and oxygen, around the body.
Antibodies	Proteins inactivate foreign invaders, thus protecting the body against diseases.
Energy and glucose	Proteins provide some fuel, and glucose if needed, for the body's energy needs.

The Chemist's View of Proteins (pp. 171–174)

1. How does the chemical structure of proteins differ from the structures of carbohydrates and fats?
2. Describe the structure of amino acids, and explain how their sequence in proteins affects the proteins' shapes. What are indispensable/essential amino acids?
3. Which part of its chemical structure differentiates one amino acid from another?
   a. its side group
   b. its acid group
   c. its amino group
   d. its double bonds
4. What are isoleucine, leucine, and lysine?
   a. proteases
   b. polypeptides
   c. indispensable/essential amino acids
   d. complementary proteins

Digestion and Absorption of Proteins (pp. 174–176)

5. Describe protein digestion and absorption.
6. What does hydrochloric acid do in the stomach?
   a. it denatures proteins and activates pepsin
   b. it hydrolyzes proteins and denatures pepsin
   c. it emulsifies proteins and releases peptidase
   d. it condenses proteins and facilitates digestion

Proteins in the Body (pp. 176–185)

7. Describe protein synthesis.
8. Describe some of the roles proteins play in the human body.
9. What are enzymes? What roles do they play in chemical reactions? Describe the differences between enzymes and hormones.
10. How does the body use amino acids? What is deamination? Define nitrogen balance. What conditions are associated with zero, positive, and negative balance?
11. What are proteins that facilitate chemical reactions?
    a. buffers
    b. enzymes
    c. hormones
    d. antigens
12. What must the cells do if an indispensable/essential amino acid that is needed to make a protein is unavailable?
    a. deaminate another amino acid
    b. substitute a similar amino acid
    c. cease synthesis of that particular protein
    d. synthesize the amino acid from glucose and nitrogen
13. What does protein turnover describe?
    a. the amount of protein found in foods and the body
    b. the amount of protein absorbed from the diet
    c. the amount of protein synthesized and degraded
    d. the amount of protein used to make glucose

Protein in Foods (pp. 185–186)

14. What factors affect the quality of dietary protein? What is a high-quality protein?
15. How can vegetarians meet their protein needs without eating meat?
16. Which of the following foods provides the highest quality protein?
    a. an egg
    b. corn
    c. gelatin
    d. whole grains

Health Effects and Recommended Intakes of Protein and Amino Acids (pp. 187–194)

17. What are the health consequences of ingesting inadequate protein and energy? Describe marasmus and kwashiorkor. How can the two conditions be distinguished, and in what ways do they overlap?
18. How might protein excess, or the type of protein eaten, influence health?
19. What factors are considered in establishing recommended protein intakes?
20. What are the benefits and risks of taking protein and amino acid supplements?
21. What does marasmus develop from?
    a. too much fat clogging the liver
    b. megadoses of amino acid supplements
    c. inadequate protein and energy intake
    d. excessive fluid intake causing edema
22. What is the protein RDA for a healthy, sedentary to slightly active adult who weighs 82 kilograms (180 pounds)?
    a. 50 milligrams/day
    b. 65 grams/day
    c. 180 grams/day
    d. 2000 milligrams/day
23. Which of these foods contains the least protein per 125 millilitres (½ cup)?
    a. rice
    b. broccoli
    c. pinto beans
    d. orange juice

Study Questions (multiple choice)
3. a 4. c 6. a 11. b 12. c 13. c 16. a 21. c 22. b 23. d

CENGAGENOW™ For additional study questions and activities, go to **www.cengage.com/sso** and complete the Personalized Study Plan for this chapter.

STUDY CARD 7

Metabolism: Transformations and Interactions

Chemical Reactions in the Body

- During digestion, the energy-yielding nutrients—carbohydrates, lipids, and proteins—are broken down to glucose (and other monosaccharides), glycerol, fatty acids, and amino acids.
- Enzymes with their coenzymes help cells use nutrients to build compounds (anabolism) or break them down to release energy (catabolism)—review Figure 7-2, p. 207.
- ATP—a high-energy compound—captures about half the energy released during catabolism (review Figure 7-4, p. 208).

Breaking Down Nutrients for Energy

- Glucose breakdown begins with glycolysis, a pathway that produces pyruvate (review Figure 7-6, p. 212).
- Pyruvate may be converted to lactate anaerobically (without oxygen) or to acetyl CoA aerobically (with oxygen).
- Pyruvate and lactate can be used make glucose; acetyl CoA cannot make glucose (review Figure 7-9, p. 214).
- The glycerol part of a triglyceride can make either pyruvate (and then glucose) or acetyl CoA. The fatty acids of a triglyceride *cannot* make glucose; they can provide abundant acetyl CoA (review Figure 7-11, p. 216).
- Some amino acids can be used to make glucose; others can be used either to provide energy or to make fat. Before an amino acid enters these metabolic pathways, its nitrogen-containing amino group must be removed through deamination.
- The digestion of carbohydrate yields glucose (and other monosaccharides); some glucose is stored as glycogen, and some is broken down to pyruvate and acetyl CoA.
- The digestion of fat yields glycerol and fatty acids; some are reassembled and stored as body fat, and others are broken down to acetyl CoA.
- The digestion of protein yields amino acids; most amino acids are used to build body protein or other nitrogen-containing compounds, some are broken down to acetyl CoA, while the carbon skeletons of others enter the TCA cycle directly.
- Acetyl CoA may enter the TCA cycle to release energy (review Figure 7-16, p. 220) or combine with with other molecules of acetyl CoA to make body fat.

FIGURE 7-5 Simplified Overview of Energy-Yielding Pathways

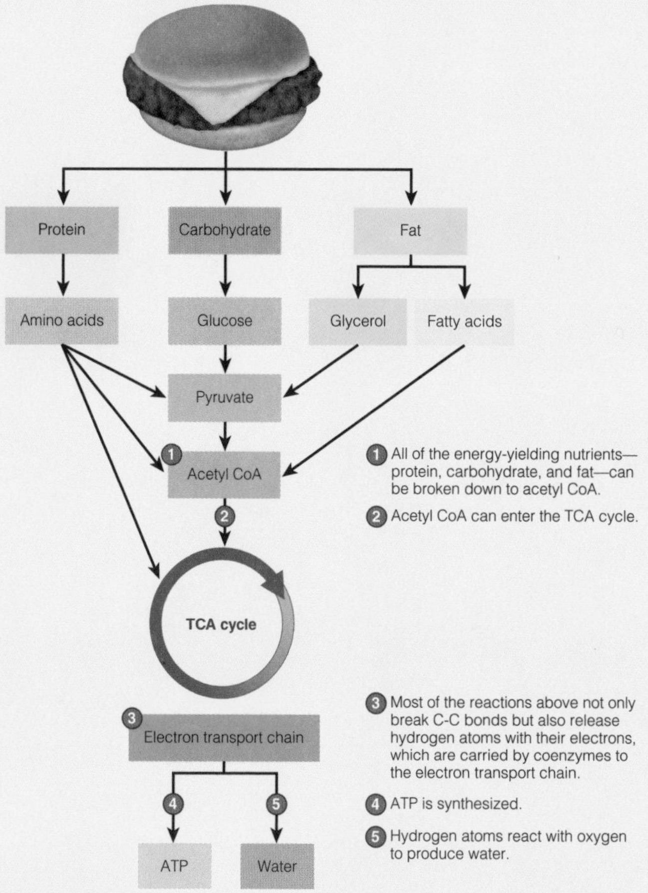

Protein
Carbohydrate
Fat
Amino acids
Glucose
Glycerol
Fatty acids
Pyruvate
Acetyl CoA
TCA cycle
Electron transport chain
ATP
Water
1 All of the energy-yielding nutrients—protein, carbohydrate, and fat—can be broken down to acetyl CoA.
2 Acetyl CoA can enter the TCA cycle.
3 Most of the reactions above not only break C-C bonds but also release hydrogen atoms with their electrons, which are carried by coenzymes to the electron transport chain.
4 ATP is synthesized.
5 Hydrogen atoms react with oxygen to produce water.

Energy Balance

- If energy intake exceeds energy needs, the result will be weight gain—regardless of whether the excess is from protein, carbohydrate, or fat. The body is most efficient at storing excess energy from dietary fat.
- When fasting, the body adapts to conserve energy and minimize losses by increasing fat breakdown to fuel most

In Summary

Nutrient	Yields Energy?	Yields Glucose?	Yields Amino Acids and Body Proteins?	Yields Fat Stores?
Carbohydrates (glucose)	Yes	Yes	Yes—when nitrogen is available, can yield *nonessential/dispensable* amino acids	Yes
Lipids (fatty acids)	Yes	No	No	Yes
Lipids (glycerol)	Yes	Yes—when carbohydrate is unavailable	Yes—when nitrogen is available, can yield *nonessential/dispensable* amino acids	Yes
Proteins (amino acids)	Yes	Yes—when carbohydrate is unavailable	Yes	Yes

cells, using glycerol and amino acids to make glucose for the brain and red blood cells, producing ketones for the brain, suppressing appetite, and slowing metabolism.

Chemical Reactions in the Body (pp. 206–209)

1. Define metabolism, anabolism, and catabolism; give an example of each.
2. Name one of the body's high-energy molecules, and describe how it is used.
3. What are coenzymes, and what service do they provide in metabolism?
4. Name the four basic units, derived from foods, that are used by the body in metabolic transformations. How many carbons are in the "backbones" of each?
5. What is hydrolysis an example of?
   a. a coupled reaction
   b. an anabolic reaction
   c. a catabolic reaction
   d. a synthesis reaction
6. During metabolism, how is released energy captured and transferred?
   a. by enzymes
   b. by pyruvate
   c. by acetyl CoA
   d. by adenosine triphosphate

Breaking Down Nutrients for Energy (pp. 209–222)

7. Define aerobic and anaerobic metabolism. How does insufficient oxygen influence metabolism?
8. How does the body dispose of excess nitrogen?
9. Summarize the main steps in the metabolism of glucose, glycerol, fatty acids, and amino acids.
10. Which of the following statements about glycolysis is correct?
    a. Glycolysis requires oxygen.
    b. Glycolysis generates abundant energy.
    c. Glycolysis converts glucose to pyruvate.
    d. Glycolysis produces ammonia as a by-product.
11. Which of the following is correct about the pathway from pyruvate to acetyl CoA?
    a. it produces lactate
    b. it is known as gluconeogenesis
    c. it is metabolically irreversible
    d. it requires more energy than it produces
12. For complete oxidation, which process does acetyl CoA enter?
    a. glycolysis
    b. the TCA cycle
    c. the Cori cycle
    d. the electron transport chain
13. What does deamination of an amino acid produce?
    a. vitamin B_6 and energy
    b. pyruvate and acetyl CoA
    c. ammonia and a keto acid
    d. carbon dioxide and water
14. What may each of the energy-yielding nutrients first be metabolized to before entering the TCA cycle?
    a. ammonia
    b. pyruvate
    c. electrons
    d. acetyl CoA

Energy Balance (pp. 222–228)

15. Describe how a surplus of the three energy nutrients contributes to body fat stores.
16. What adaptations does the body make during a fast? What are ketone bodies? Define ketosis.
17. Distinguish between a loss of *fat* and a loss of *weight*, and describe how each might happen.
18. In what form does the body store energy for future use?
    a. in proteins
    b. in acetyl CoA
    c. in triglycerides
    d. in ketone bodies
19. During a fast, when glycogen stores have been depleted, what does the body then use to synthesize glucose?
    a. acetyl CoA
    b. amino acids
    c. fatty acids
    d. ketone bodies
20. During a fast, how does the body produce ketone bodies?
    a. hydrolyzing glycogen
    b. condensing acetyl CoA units
    c. transaminating keto acids
    d. converting ammonia to urea

Study Questions (multiple choice)
5. c 6. d 10. c 11. c 12. b 13. c 14. d 18. c 19. b 20. b

For additional study questions and activities, go to **www.cengage.com/sso** and complete the Personalized Study Plan for this chapter.

STUDY CARD 8

Energy Balance and Body Composition

Energy Balance

- When energy consumed equals energy expended, a person is in energy balance and body weight is stable.
- If more energy is taken in than is expended, a person gains weight. If more energy is expended than is taken in, a person loses weight.

Energy In: The kCalories Foods Provide

- Hunger and appetite initiate eating, whereas satiation and satiety stop and delay eating, respectively (review Figure 8-2, p. 244).

Energy Out: The kCalories the Body Expends

- A person in energy balance takes in energy from food and expends much of it on basal metabolic activities, some of it on physical activities, and a little on the thermic effect of food (review Figure 8-4).
- Energy requirements vary from person to person based on such factors as gender, age, weight, and height as well as the intensity and duration of physical activity.

Body Weight, Body Composition, and Health

- Body weight standards are based on a person's weight in relation to height, called the body mass index (BMI), and reflect disease risks. BMI does not identify body fat or its distribution, and it may misclassify muscular people as overweight.
- $\text{BMI} = \dfrac{\text{weight (kg)}}{\text{height (m)}^2}$ or $\dfrac{\text{weight (lb)}}{\text{height (in)}^2} \times 703.$

  Healthy: BMI 18.5 to 24.9
  Underweight: BMI <18.5
  Overweight: BMI 25 to 29.9
  Obese Class I: BMI 30.0 to 34.9
  Obese Class II: BMI 35.0 to 39.9
  Obese Class III: BMI ≥40.
- Almost six in ten Canadian adults have a BMI greater than 25 (review Figure 8-5).
- The ideal amount of body fat varies from person to person, but body fat in excess of 22 percent for young men and 32 percent for young women (the levels rise slightly with age) poses health risks.
- Central obesity—excess abdominal fat distributed around the trunk of the body—presents greater health risks than excess fat distributed on the lower body (review Figures 8-7 and 8-8, p. 255).

FIGURE 8-5 Distribution of Body Weights in Canadian Adults

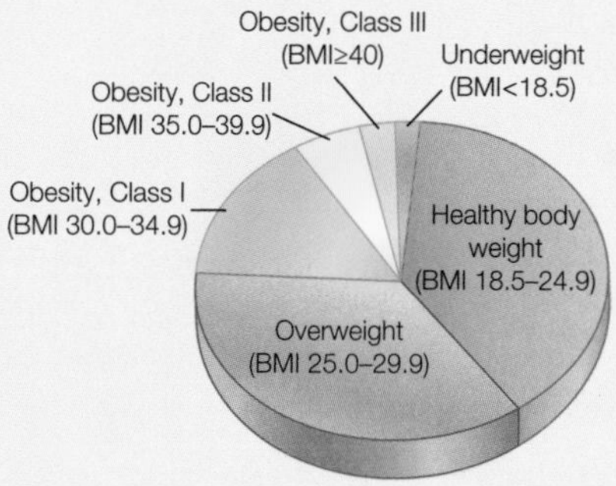
Obesity, Class III
(BMI≥40)
Underweight
(BMI<18.5)
Obesity, Class II
(BMI 35.0–39.9)
Obesity, Class I
(BMI 30.0–34.9)
Healthy body
weight
(BMI 18.5–24.9)
Overweight
(BMI 25.0–29.9)

FIGURE 8-4 Components of Energy Expenditure

The amount of energy spent in a day differs for each individual, but in general, basal metabolism is the largest component of energy expenditure and the thermic effect of food is the smallest. The amount spent in voluntary physical activities has the greatest variability, depending on a person's activity patterns. For a sedentary person, physical activities may account for less than half as much energy as basal metabolism, whereas an extremely active person may expend as much on activity as for basal metabolism.

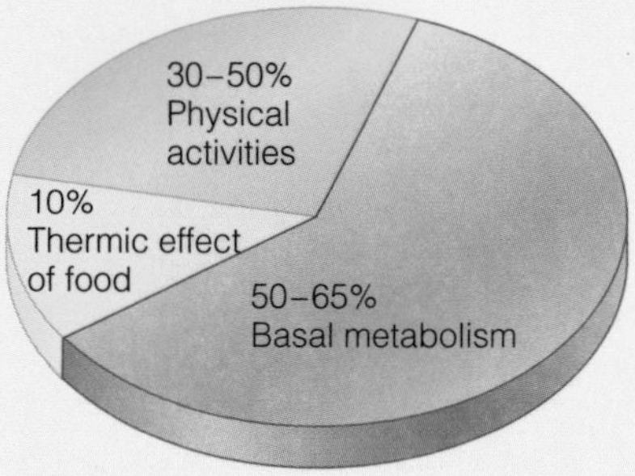
30–50%
Physical
activities
10%
Thermic effect
of food
50–65%
Basal metabolism

FIGURE 8-10 BMI and Mortality

This J-shaped curve describes the relationship between body mass index (BMI) and mortality and shows that both underweight and overweight present risks of a premature death.

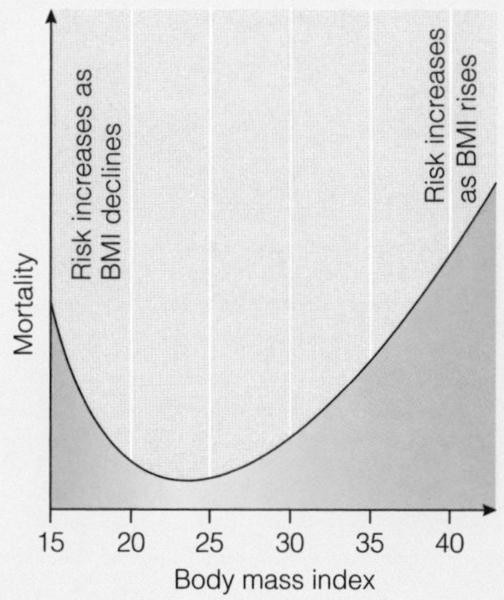
Risk increases as
BMI declines
Risk increases
as BMI rises
Mortality
15
20
25
30
35
40
Body mass index

- The healthiest weight for an individual depends on personal factors such as body fat distribution, family health history, and current health status. At the extremes, both overweight and underweight impose health risks (review Figure 8-10).

Energy Balance (pp. 241–242)

1. What are the consequences of an unbalanced energy budget?
2. Suppose that a person consistently consumes 1700 kcalories a day and spends 2200 kcalories a day. After one month, what would you expect this person's change in weight to be?
   a. lose $\frac{1}{4}$ to $\frac{1}{2}$ kilogram ($\frac{1}{2}$ to 1 pound)
   b. gain $\frac{1}{4}$ to $\frac{1}{2}$ kilogram ($\frac{1}{2}$ to 1 pound)
   c. lose 1.8 to 2.3 kilograms (4 to 5 pounds)
   d. gain 1.8 to 2.3 kilograms (4 to 5 pounds)

Energy In: The kCalories Foods Provide (pp. 242–245)

3. Define hunger, appetite, satiation, and satiety and describe how each influences food intake.
4. What does a bomb calorimeter measure?
   a. physiological fuel
   b. energy available from foods
   c. kcalories a person derives from foods
   d. heat a person releases in basal metabolism
5. Which term refers to the psychological desire to eat that accompanies the sight, smell, or thought of food?
   a. hunger
   b. satiety
   c. appetite
   d. palatability
6. Suppose that a person watching television after dinner reaches for a snack during a commercial. What is the person responding to?
   a. external cues
   b. hunger signals
   c. stress arousal
   d. satiety factors

Energy Out: The kCalories the Body Expends (pp. 245–249)

7. Describe each component of energy expenditure. What factors influence each? How can energy expenditure be estimated?
8. What is the largest component of energy expenditure?
   a. basal metabolism
   b. physical activity
   c. thermic effect of food
9. Which of the following is a major factor influencing BMR?
   a. hunger
   b. food intake
   c. body composition
   d. physical activity
10. What is the thermic effect of an 800-kcalorie meal?
    a. about 8 kcalories
    b. about 80 kcalories
    c. about 160 kcalories
    d. about 200 kcalories

Body Weight, Body Composition, and Health (pp. 249–258)

11. Distinguish between body weight and body composition. What assessment techniques are used to measure each?
12. What problems are involved in defining "ideal" body weight?
13. What is central obesity, and what is its relationship to disease?
14. What risks are associated with excess body weight and excess body fat?
15. What might a person with a BMI of 21 want to do for the sake of their health?
    a. lose weight
    b. maintain weight
    c. gain weight
16. Which of the following reflects height and weight?
    a. body mass index
    b. central obesity
    c. waist circumference
    d. body composition
17. Which of the following increases disease risks?
    a. BMI 19–21
    b. BMI 22–25
    c. lower-body fat
    d. central obesity

Study Questions (multiple choice)
2. c 4. b 5. c 6. a 8. a 9. c 10. b 15. b 16. a 17. d

For additional study questions and activities, go to **www.cengage.com/sso** and complete the Personalized Study Plan for this chapter.

STUDY CARD 9

Weight Management: Overweight, Obesity, and Underweight

Overweight and Obesity

- Fat cells develop by increasing in number (hyperplasia) and size (hypertrophy).
- Preventing weight gain depends on limiting the number of fat cells; weight loss depends on decreasing the size of fat cells.
- With weight gains or losses, the body adjusts in an attempt to return to its previous weight (set-point theory).

Causes of Overweight and Obesity

- Obesity has multiple causes and different combinations of causes in different people.
- Some environmental causes, such as overeating and physical inactivity, may be within a person's control, and some, such as genetics, may be beyond it.
- Proteins such as adiponectin, ghrelin, and leptin regulate food intake and energy homeostasis.

Problems of Overweight and Obesity

- Whether a person should lose weight depends on factors such as the extent of overweight, age, health risks, and genetic makeup.
- Not all obesity will cause disease or shorten life expectancy. Just as there are unhealthy, normal-weight people, there are healthy, overweight people.
- Some people risk more in the process of losing weight than in remaining overweight.
- Fad diets and weight-loss supplements can be as physically and psychologically damaging as excess body weight.

Aggressive Treatments for Obesity

- Obese people with high risks of medical problems may need aggressive treatment, including drugs or surgery.
- Others may benefit most from improving eating and physical activity habits.

Weight-Loss Strategies

- A person who adopts a lifelong "eating plan for good health" rather than a "diet for weight loss" will be more likely to keep the lost weight off.

FIGURE 9-8 Influence of Physical Activity on Discretionary kCalories

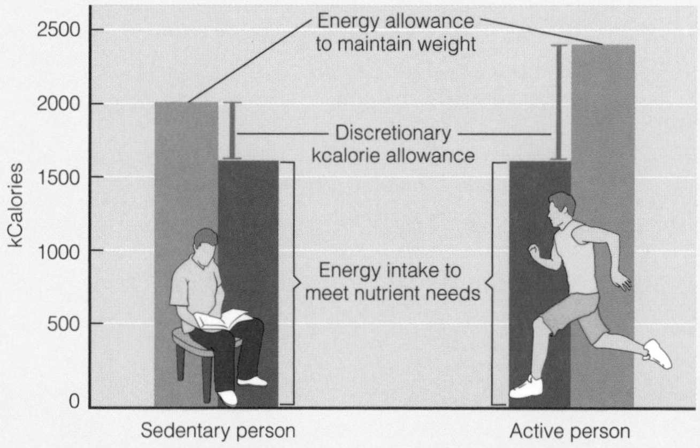

kCalories
2500
2000
1500
1000
500
0
Energy allowance to maintain weight
Discretionary kcalorie allowance
Energy intake to meet nutrient needs
Sedentary person
Active person

- Table 9-5 (p. 290) provides several tips for successful weight management.
- Physical activity can increase energy expenditure, improve body composition, help control appetite, reduce stress and stress eating, and enhance physical and psychological well-being.
- A surefire remedy for obesity has yet to be found; a combination of approaches is most effective.
- Weight loss depends on adjusting diet and physical activity so that more energy is expended than is taken in.
- For weight loss, energy intake should be reduced by 500 to 1000 kcalories per day, depending on starting body weight and usual food intake.
- Safe rate for weight loss is ¼ to 1 kilogram (½ to 2 pounds) per week or 10 percent body weight per 6 months.
- Behaviour modification and cognitive restructuring retrain habits to support a healthy eating and activity plan.
- Treatment requires time, individualization, and sometimes the assistance of a registered dietitian or support group.
- Preventing weight gains and maintaining weight losses require vigilant attention to diet and physical activity; taking care of oneself is a lifelong responsibility.

Underweight

- Both the incidence of underweight and the health problems associated with it are less prevalent than overweight and its associated problems.
- To gain weight, a person must train physically and increase energy intake by selecting energy-dense foods, eating regular meals, taking larger portions, and consuming extra snacks and beverages.
- Table 9-5 (p. 290) includes a summary of weight-gain strategies.

Overweight and Obesity (pp. 271–273)

1. Describe how body fat develops, and suggest some reasons why it is difficult for an obese person to maintain weight loss.
2. What do fat cells do as a person loses weight?
   a. they decrease in size only
   b. they decrease in number only
   c. they decrease in both number and size
   d. they decrease in number, but increase in size

Causes of Overweight and Obesity (pp. 273–278)

3. What factors contribute to obesity?
4. What causes obesity?
   a. overeating
   b. inactivity
   c. defective genes
   d. multiple factors
5. What is the name of the protein produced by the fat cells under the direction of the *ob* gene?
   a. leptin
   b. serotonin
   c. sibutramine
   d. phentermine

Problems of Overweight and Obesity (pp. 279–282)

6. Describe the physical, social, and psychological consequences of overweight and obesity.

Aggressive Treatments for Obesity (pp. 282–284)

7. List several aggressive ways to treat obesity, and explain why such methods are not recommended for every overweight person.

Weight-Loss Strategies (pp. 284–297)

8. Discuss reasonable dietary strategies for achieving and maintaining a healthy body weight.
9. What are the benefits of increased physical activity in a weight-loss program?
10. Describe the behavioural strategies for changing an individual's dietary habits. What role does personal attitude play?
11. Which of the following is a realistic weight-loss goal?
    a. drop down to the weight a person was at age 25
    b. drop down to the ideal weight in the weight-for-height tables
    c. drop down by 10 percent over six months
    d. drop down by 15 percent over three months
12. What is the rate of daily energy restriction required to lose one kilogram of body weight per week?
    a. a 100-kcalorie-per-day deficit
    b. a 500-kcalorie-per-day deficit
    c. a 1000-kcalorie-per-day deficit
    d. a 3500-kcalorie-per-day deficit
13. What does successful weight loss depend on?
    a. avoiding fats and limiting water
    b. taking supplements and drinking water
    c. increasing proteins and restricting carbohydrates
    d. reducing energy intake and increasing physical activity
14. Which of the following is NOT likely to be improved by physical activity?
    a. weight loss
    b. muscle retention
    c. maintenance of weight loss
    d. loss of fat in trouble spots
15. Which strategy would NOT help an overweight person to lose weight?
    a. exercise
    b. eat slowly
    c. limit intake of high-fat foods
    d. eat energy-dense foods regularly

Underweight (pp. 297–299)

16. Describe strategies for successful weight gain.
17. Which strategy would NOT help an underweight person gain weight?
    a. exercise
    b. drink plenty of water
    c. eat snacks between meals
    d. eat large portions of foods

Study Questions (multiple choice)
2.a 4.d 5.a 11.c 12.c 13.d 14.d 15.d 17.b

CENGAGENOW™ For additional study questions and activities, go to **www.cengage.com/sso** and complete the Personalized Study Plan for this chapter.

STUDY CARD 10

FIGURE 10-3 Coenzyme Action

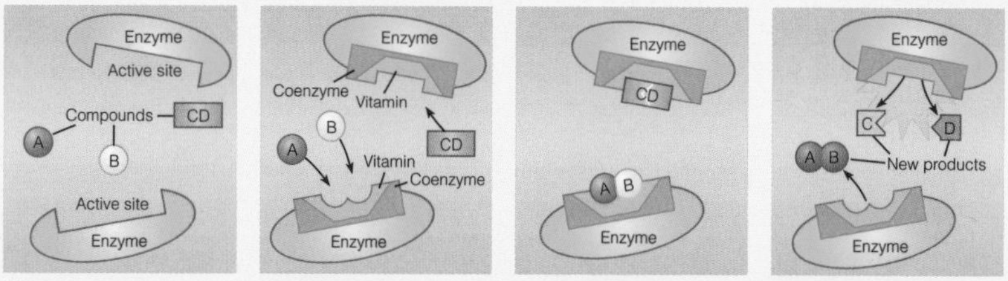
Enzyme
Active site
Compounds
CD
A
B
Active site
Enzyme
Enzyme
Coenzyme
Vitamin
B
A
CD
Vitamin
Coenzyme
Enzyme
Enzyme
CD
A
B
Enzyme
Enzyme
C
D
A
B
New products
Enzyme

Without coenzymes, compounds A, B, and CD don't respond to their enzymes.

With the coenzymes in place, compounds are attracted to their sites on the enzymes . . .

. . . and the reactions proceed instantaneously. The coenzymes often donate or accept electrons, atoms, or groups of atoms.

The reactions are completed with either the formation of a new product, AB, or the breaking apart of a compound into two new products, C and D, and the release of energy.

Nutrients for Energy Metabolism

The Vitamins and Minerals—An Overview

- The vitamins are organic, essential nutrients needed in small amounts in the diet both to prevent deficiency diseases and to support optimal health. The fat-soluble vitamins are vitamins A, D, E, and K; the water-soluble vitamins are vitamin C and the B vitamins, which are thiamin, niacin, riboflavin, vitamin B_6, folate, vitamin B_{12}, pantothenic acid, and biotin.
- The minerals are inorganic, essential nutrients needed in varying amounts. The major minerals sodium, chloride, potassium, phosphorus, calcium, magnesium, and sulphur are needed in larger quantities than the trace minerals, which include iodide, manganese, chromium, selenium, fluoride, iron, zinc, and copper.

Nutrients for Energy Metabolism

- The macronutrients contain energy in their bonds, but it's the roles of the micronutrients that allow us to extract the energy found in carbohydrates, fats, and proteins. The B vitamins exert their greatest effect as coenzymes and the trace minerals often interact with hormones involved in energy metabolism.

Introducing the B Vitamins

- Of notable interest are the interdependent roles of the B vitamins in energy metabolism. Although overt deficiencies of these nutrients are uncommon, there is concern when people overuse supplements.

The B Vitamins—As Individuals

- Thiamin is part of the coenzyme TPP, which assists in energy metabolism. Deficiency can result in beriberi. Thiamin occurs in small quantities in many nutritious foods; pork is an exceptionally good source.
- Riboflavin is part of the coenzymes FMN and FAD that accept and donate hydrogens during energy metabolism. Milk and milk products are rich sources.
- Niacin is part of the coenzymes NAD and NADP that participate in many metabolic reactions. The deficiency disease, pellagra, causes diarrhea, dermatitis, dementia, and eventually death ("the 4 Ds"). Toxicity produces "niacin flush"—a tingling, painful sensation. The amino acid tryptophan can be converted to niacin in the body: 60 mg tryptophan = 1 NE (niacin equivalent). Good sources of niacin are protein-rich foods.
- Biotin plays a critical role in energy metabolism, replenishing oxaloacetate in the TCA cycle. Biotin is widespread in foods; deficiencies and toxicities are rare.
- Pantothenic acid is part of coenzyme A that forms acetyl CoA found in many metabolic pathways. Pantothenic acid is widespread in foods; deficiencies and toxicities are rare.
- Vitamin B_6 occurs as pyridoxal, pyridoxine, and pyridoxamine; all can become part of the coenzyme PLP, which is active in amino acid metabolism. Deficiency causes convulsions; toxicity causes nerve damage.
- Folate is part of the coenzyme THF that activates vitamin B_{12}, synthesizes DNA, and regenerates the amino acid methionine from homocysteine. Folate helps prevent neural tube defects. Excessive folate can mask the anemia of a vitamin B_{12} deficiency, but it will not prevent the associated nerve damage. Folate is abundant in legumes, fruits, and vegetables.
- Vitamin B_{12} activates folate, synthesizes DNA, regenerates methionine from homocysteine, and maintains the sheath that protects nerve fibres. Deficiencies typically occur when either hydrochloric acid or intrinsic factor is lacking. Vitamin B_{12} is found primarily in foods derived from animals.

The B Vitamins—In Concert

- The B vitamins serve as coenzymes—small organic molecules closely associated with enzymes that facilitate the work of cells, participating in metabolism and in DNA synthesis.
- Grain products are enriched with thiamin, riboflavin, niacin, and folate; a variety of foods from each food group provides an adequate supply of all B vitamins.

Minerals for Energy Metabolism

- Sulphur is mostly consumed as amino acids, methionine and cysteine, in food proteins. Sulphur helps stabilize the three-dimensional structure of body proteins. No recommended intake exists for sulphur as Canadians' protein intake makes deficiencies rare.
- Iodide, the iodine ion, is an essential component of the thyroid hormone. A deficiency can lead to goiter (enlargement of the thyroid gland) and can impair fetal development, causing cretinism. Iodization of salt has largely eliminated iodine deficiency in Canada.

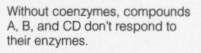

- Manganese-dependent enzymes are involved in bone formation and various metabolic processes. Manganese is widespread in plant foods and deficiencies are rare.
- Chromium enhances the action of insulin. Deficiency can result in a diabetes-like condition. Chromium is widely available in unrefined foods including whole grains and liver.

The Vitamins and Minerals—An Overview

(pp. 311–315)

1. How do the vitamins and minerals differ from the energy nutrients?
2. Which of the statements about vitamins is correct?
   a. Vitamins are inorganic compounds.
   b. Vitamins yield energy when broken down.
   c. Vitamins are soluble in either water or fat.
   d. Vitamins perform best when linked in long chains.
3. Which of the statements about minerals is correct?
   a. Minerals are used primarily for structural functions and regulatory processes.
   b. Minerals are needed in tiny amounts.
   c. Minerals are fat soluble.
   d. Minerals are nontoxic at higher intakes.

Nutrients for Energy Metabolism

(pp. 315–316)

4. Which terms refers to the rate at and the extent to which a vitamin or mineral is absorbed and used in the body?
   a. bioavailability
   b. intrinsic factor
   c. physiological effect
   d. pharmacological effect
5. In what role do many of the B vitamins serve?
   a. as antagonists
   b. as coenzymes
   c. as antioxidants
   d. as serotonin precursors

Introducing the B Vitamins (pp. 316–317)

6. Name the B vitamins involved in energy metabolism.
7. Describe the interdependence between a pair of B vitamins.

The B Vitamins—As Individuals

(pp. 318–335)

8. For each of thiamin, riboflavin, niacin, biotin, pantothenic acid, vitamin B_6, folate, and vitamin B_{12}, state:
   - its chief function in the body.
   - its characteristic deficiency symptoms.
   - its significant food sources.
9. Describe the relationship between folate and vitamin B_{12}.
10. What risks are associated with high doses of niacin? Vitamin B_6?
11. With respect to thiamin, which of the following is the most nutrient dense?
    a. 1 slice whole-wheat bread (69 kcalories and 0.1 milligram thiamin)
    b. 250 millilitres (1 cup) yogurt (144 kcalories and 0.1 milligram thiamin)
    c. 250 millilitres (1 cup) snow peas (69 kcalories and 0.22 milligram thiamin)
    d. 1 chicken breast (141 kcalories and 0.06 milligram thiamin)
12. What can the body make niacin from?
    a. tyrosine
    b. serotonin
    c. carnitine
    d. tryptophan
13. Which of the following is a B vitamin?
    a. inositol
    b. carnitine
    c. vitamin B_{15}
    d. pantothenic acid
14. Which vitamin protects against neural tube defects?
    a. niacin
    b. folate
    c. riboflavin
    d. vitamin B_{12}
15. What may a lack of intrinsic factor lead to?
    a. pernicious anemia
    b. beriberi
    c. pellagra
    d. atrophic gastritis

Minerals for Energy Metabolism

(pp. 339–343)

16. Explain why no DRI exists for sulphur.
17. What can a lack of iodide result in?
    a. anemia
    b. goiter
    c. diabetes
    d. osteoporosis
18. Which of the following supplements can limit manganese absorption?
    a. folate
    b. vitamin B_6
    c. niacin
    d. calcium
19. Which hormone depends on chromium for optimal activity?
    a. cholecystokinin
    b. glucagon
    c. insulin
    d. gastrin

Study Questions (multiple choice)
2. c 3. a 4. a 5. b 11. c 12. d 13. d 14. b 15. a 17. b
18. d 19. c

For additional study questions and activities, go to **www.cengage.com/sso** and complete the Personalized Study Plan for this chapter.

STUDY CARD 11

Water and the Electrolytes

Water and the Body Fluids

- Water makes up about 60 percent of the adult body's weight.
- Water assists with the transport of nutrients and waste products throughout the body, participates in chemical reactions, acts as a solvent, serves as a shock absorber, and regulates body temperature.
- To maintain water balance, intake from liquids, foods, and metabolism must equal losses from the kidneys, skin, lungs, and GI tract (review Table 11-2, p. 357).
- To restore homeostasis, the body responds to low blood volume, low blood pressure, or highly concentrated body fluids by producing ADH to stimulate the kidneys to reabsorb water, renin to initiate the pathway that leads to the production of angiotensin II, angiotensin II to constrict blood vessels and stimulate the release of aldosterone and ADH, and aldosterone to regulate potassium and sodium levels.

FIGURE 11-4 How the Body Regulates Blood Volume

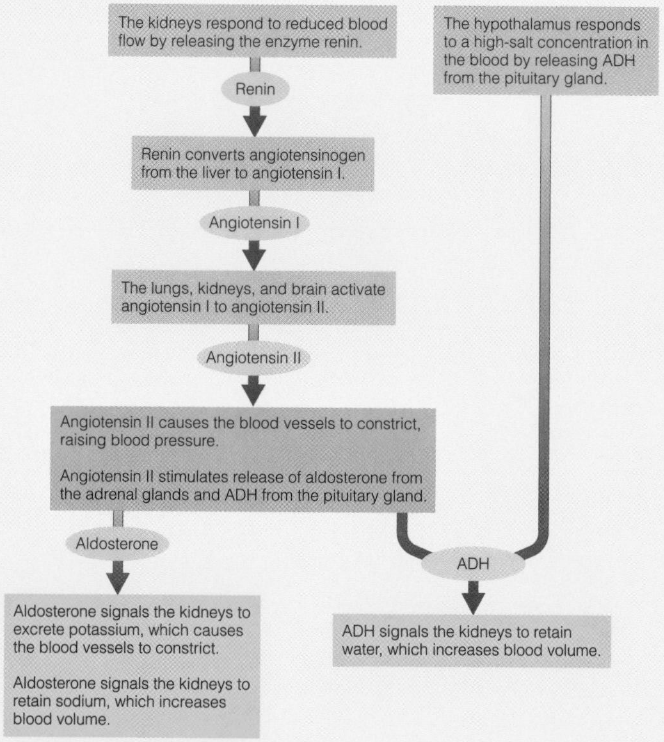

The kidneys respond to reduced blood flow by releasing the enzyme renin.
Renin
Renin converts angiotensinogen from the liver to angiotensin I.
Angiotensin I
The lungs, kidneys, and brain activate angiotensin I to angiotensin II.
Angiotensin II
Angiotensin II causes the blood vessels to constrict, raising blood pressure.
Angiotensin II stimulates release of aldosterone from the adrenal glands and ADH from the pituitary gland.
Aldosterone
Aldosterone signals the kidneys to excrete potassium, which causes the blood vessels to constrict.
Aldosterone signals the kidneys to retain sodium, which increases blood volume.
The hypothalamus responds to a high-salt concentration in the blood by releasing ADH from the pituitary gland.
ADH
ADH signals the kidneys to retain water, which increases blood volume.

- Electrolytes (charged minerals) in body fluids help distribute the fluids inside and outside the cells, thus ensuring the appropriate water balance and acid–base balance to support all life processes.
- Excessive losses of fluids and electrolytes upset these balances, and the kidneys play a key role in restoring homeostasis.
- The major minerals, especially sodium, chloride, and potassium, influence the body's fluid balance; whenever an anion moves, a cation moves—always maintaining homeostasis.

Sodium

- Sodium is the main cation outside cells and one of the primary electrolytes responsible for maintaining fluid balance. Dietary deficiency is rare; excesses may aggravate hypertension in some people, and so health-care professionals advise a diet moderate in salt and sodium.

Chloride

- Chloride is the major anion outside cells, and it associates closely with sodium. In addition to its role in fluid balance, chloride is part of the stomach's hydrochloric acid.

Potassium

- Potassium is the primary cation inside cells and plays an important role in maintaining fluid balance. Fresh foods, notably fruits and vegetables, are its best sources.

Phosphorus

- Phosphorus is important as part of ATP used in energy metabolism, as part of phospholipids found in cell membranes and lipoproteins, and as part of the genetic materials DNA and RNA.

Summary

- Consuming water throughout the day and enough of the major minerals to maintain fluid balance is easy when choosing a balanced, nutrient-dense, and varied diet.

Water and the Body Fluids (pp. 355–365)

1. List the roles of water in the body.
2. List the sources of water intake and routes of water excretion.
3. What is ADH? Where does it exert its action? What is aldosterone? How does it work?

4. How does the body use electrolytes to regulate fluid balance?

5. When does the body generate water?
   a. during the buffering of acids
   b. during the dismantling of bone
   c. during the metabolism of minerals
   d. during the oxidation of energy-yielding nutrients

6. Which part of the body does the regulation of fluid and electrolyte balance and acid–base balance primarily depend on?
   a. the kidneys
   b. the intestines
   c. the sweat glands
   d. the specialized tear ducts

7. Which is a trigger for the thirst mechanism?
   a. decreased salt concentration in blood
   b. increased blood pressure
   c. dry mouth and throat
   d. increased blood volume

Sodium (pp. 365–368)

8. What is the major function of sodium in the body? Describe how the kidneys regulate blood sodium. Is a dietary deficiency of sodium likely? Why or why not?

9. How much sodium is in five millilitres (1 tsp; ~6 g) of salt?
   a. about 1500 mg
   b. about 2000 mg
   c. about 2300 mg
   d. about 3000 mg

Chloride (p. 369)

10. What is the role of chloride in the stomach?
    a. to help support nerve impulses
    b. to help convey hormonal messages
    c. to help maintain a strong acidity
    d. to help assist in muscular contractions

Potassium (pp. 369–371)

11. Which food would provide the most potassium?
    a. bologna
    b. potatoes
    c. pickles
    d. whole-wheat bread

Phosphorus (pp. 371–372)

12. Which of the following is NOT a role for phosphorus?
    a. being a constituent of cell membranes
    b. being part of ATP
    c. acting as a buffer
    d. activating the enzyme pepsin

13. What does phosphorus team with inside cells to maintain fluid balance?
    a. sodium
    b. protein
    c. potassium
    d. chloride

Summary (pp. 373–374)

14. What is the principal cation in extracellular fluids?
    a. sodium
    b. chloride
    c. potassium
    d. phosphorus

15. What is the principal cation in intracellular fluids?
    a. sodium
    b. chloride
    c. potassium
    d. phosphorus

16. State the major functions of chloride, potassium, and phosphorus in the body. Are deficiencies of these nutrients likely to occur in your own diet? Why or why not?

Study Questions (multiple choice)
5. d 6. a 7. c 9. c 10. c 11. b 12. d 13. c 14. a 15. c

For additional study questions and activities, go to **www.cengage.com/sso** and complete the Personalized Study Plan for this chapter.

STUDY CARD 12

The Antioxidant Nutrients

The Antioxidant Nutrients—An Overview

- Normal body processes and environmental factors generate free radicals that damage cellular constituents including proteins, polyunsaturated fatty acids, DNA, and RNA.
- The vitamin antioxidants donate electrons to quench free radicals.
- The trace mineral antioxidants are cofactors for enzyme systems that protect against oxidative damage caused by free radicals.

Vitamin A and Beta-Carotene

- Vitamin A is found in the body in three forms: retinol, retinal, and retinoic acid. Together, they are essential to reproduction, vision, and growth.
- Vitamin A deficiency is a major health problem worldwide, leading to infections, blindness, and keratinization.
- Toxicity can also cause problems and is most often associated with supplement abuse.
- Animal-derived foods such as liver and whole or fortified milk provide retinoids, whereas brightly coloured plant-derived foods such as spinach, carrots, and pumpkins provide beta-carotene and other carotenoids.
- In addition to serving as a precursor for vitamin A, beta-carotene may act as an antioxidant in the body.

Vitamin E

- Vitamin E (alpha-tocopherol) acts as an antioxidant, defending lipids and other components of the cells against oxidative damage.
- Deficiencies are rare, but they do occur in premature infants, the primary symptom being erythrocyte hemolysis.
- Vitamin E is found predominantly in vegetable oils and appears to be one of the least toxic of the fat-soluble vitamins.

Vitamin C

- Vitamin C acts as an antioxidant to decrease the adverse effects of free radicals in the body.
- Vitamin C works as a cofactor in the synthesis of collagen, neurotransmitters (serotonin and norepinephrine), hormones (thyroxin), and other compounds.
- Vitamin C deficiency causes scurvy.

Selenium

- Selenium is a trace mineral cofactor for the antioxidant enzyme glutathione peroxidase, and works in tandem with vitamin E. Selenium is found with proteins in food. Deficiencies are associated with a predisposition to a type of heart abnormality known as Keshan disease.

FIGURE H12-1 Free-Radical Damage

Free radicals are highly reactive. They might attack the polyunsaturated fatty acids in a cell membrane, which generates lipid radicals that damage cells and accelerate disease progression. Free radicals might also attack and damage DNA, RNA, and proteins, which interferes with the body's ability to maintain normal cell function, causing disease and premature aging.

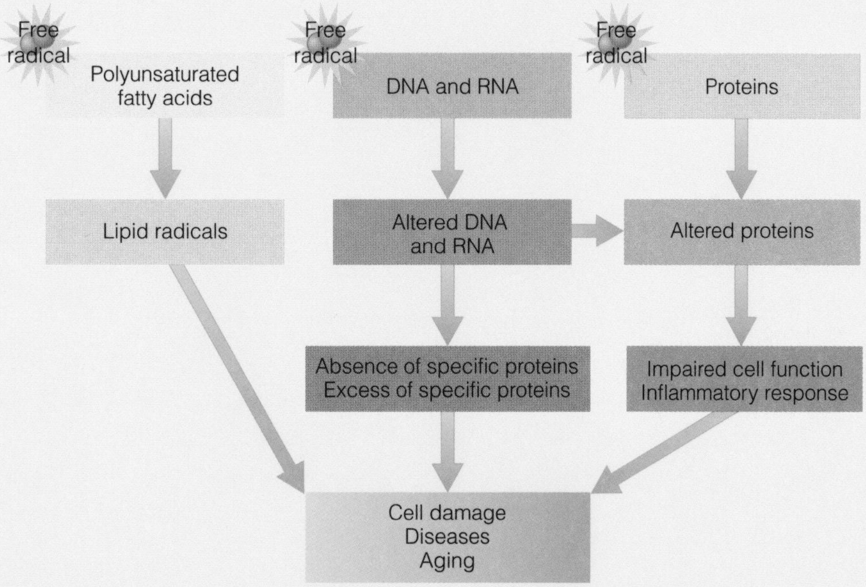

Free radical
Polyunsaturated fatty acids
Free radical
DNA and RNA
Free radical
Proteins
Lipid radicals
Altered DNA and RNA
Altered proteins
Absence of specific proteins
Excess of specific proteins
Impaired cell function
Inflammatory response
Cell damage
Diseases
Aging

The Antioxidant Nutrients—An Overview (pp. 381–382)

1. Which of the following is NOT damaged by free radicals?
   a. cell membranes
   b. DNA
   c. cell proteins
   d. glycogen
2. Which of the following antioxidant nutrients also has pro-oxidant effects?
   a. vitamin C
   b. vitamin E
   c. selenium
   d. beta-carotene

Vitamin A and Beta-Carotene (pp. 382–389)

3. Summarize the roles of vitamin A and the symptoms of its deficiency.
4. What are vitamin precursors? Name the precursors of vitamin A. Identify foods with high vitamin A activity.
5. Which form of vitamin A is active in vision?
   a. retinal
   b. retinol
   c. rhodopsin
   d. retinoic acid
6. What of the following are among the symptoms of vitamin A–deficiency?
   a. rickets and osteomalacia
   b. hemorrhaging and jaundice
   c. night blindness and keratomalacia
   d. fibrocystic breast disease and erythrocyte hemolysis
7. Which of the following itemizes foods that are good sources of vitamin A?
   a. oatmeal, pinto beans, and ham
   b. apricots, turnip greens, and liver
   c. whole-wheat bread, green peas, and tuna
   d. corn, grapefruit juice, and sunflower seeds

Vitamin E (pp. 390–391)

8. Describe vitamin E's role as an antioxidant. What are the chief symptoms of vitamin E deficiency?
9. What is vitamin E's most notable role?
   a. to protect lipids against oxidation
   b. to activate blood-clotting proteins
   c. to support protein and DNA synthesis
   d. to enhance calcium deposits in the bones
10. What is the classic sign of vitamin E deficiency?
    a. rickets
    b. xerophthalmia
    c. muscular dystrophy
    d. erythrocyte hemolysis

Vitamin C (pp. 391–396)

11. Which group has the highest requirement for vitamin C?
    a. smokers
    b. athletes
    c. alcoholics
    d. the elderly
12. Which is a rich source of vitamin C?
    a. squash
    b. kiwi
    c. spinach
    d. banana

Selenium (pp. 397–398)

13. Which of the following antioxidant enzyme systems uses selenium as a cofactor?
    a. superoxide dismutase
    b. catalase
    c. glutathione peroxidase
    d. nitric oxide synthase
14. What vitamin does selenium work in harmony with?
    a. vitamin E
    b. vitamin A
    c. vitamin C
    d. vitamin B_6

Study Questions (multiple choice)
1. d 2. a 5. a 6. c 7. b 9. a 10. d 11. a 12. b 13. c 14. a

CENGAGENOW™ For additional study questions and activities, go to **www.cengage.com/sso** and complete the Personalized Study Plan for this chapter.

STUDY CARD 13

Nutrients for Bone Health

About Bones

- Strength and flexibility are key characteristics of bones. Inorganic minerals provide strength and structural support; the organic protein portion of bone provides flexibility, especially important during times of applied stress.
- Calcium, phosphorus, magnesium, and fluoride form mineral crystals; vitamins D and K are associated with proteins that aid mineral absorption in the GI tract and bind minerals to the protein-based matrix of bone.
- Cortical bone tissue is dense and ivory-like; trabecular bone is less dense with a lace-like architecture.
- The relative activities of osteoblast cells that build bone and osteoclast cells that degrade bone changes throughout life. A lifetime commitment to diet, exercise, and lifestyle factors is important for optimizing bone health.

Calcium

- Calcium is found primarily in the bones where it provides a rigid structure and a reservoir of calcium for the blood. Blood calcium participates in muscle contraction, blood clotting, and nerve impulses, and it is closely regulated by a system of hormones and vitamin D. Milk and milk products are good sources of calcium, but certain vegetables and calcium-set tofu are also sources.
- Blood calcium remains normal even when calcium intake is inadequate; this is at the expense of bone loss, which can lead to osteoporosis.

Phosphorus

- Phosphorus accompanies calcium both in the hydroxyapatite crystals of bone and in many foods such as milk.

Vitamin D

- Vitamin D can be synthesized in the body with the help of sunlight. Few foods are naturally rich sources of vitamin D (e.g., salmon); fortified foods are more common sources (e.g., milk).
- Vitamin D sends signals to three primary target sites: the GI tract to absorb more calcium and phosphorus, the bones to release more, and the kidneys to retain more. These actions maintain blood calcium concentrations and support bone formation.
- A deficiency of vitamin D causes rickets in childhood and osteomalacia in later life.

FIGURE 13-2 Maintaining Blood Calcium from the Diet and from the Bones

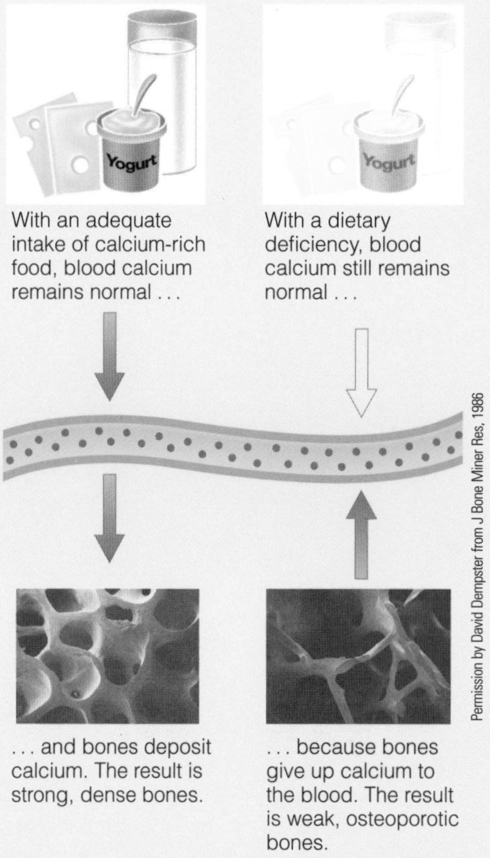
Yogurt
Yogurt
With an adequate intake of calcium-rich food, blood calcium remains normal . . .
With a dietary deficiency, blood calcium still remains normal . . .
. . . and bones deposit calcium. The result is strong, dense bones.
. . . because bones give up calcium to the blood. The result is weak, osteoporotic bones.
Permission by David Dempster from J Bone Miner Res, 1986

Magnesium

- Magnesium supports bone mineralization and participates in numerous enzyme systems and in heart function. It is found abundantly in legumes and leafy green vegetables and, in some areas, in water.
- Magnesium works in opposition to calcium in muscle contraction and blood clotting; calcium promotes these processes and magnesium inhibits them.

Fluoride

- Fluoride makes bones stronger and teeth more resistant to decay. Fluoridation of public water reduces the incidence of dental caries; excess fluoride during tooth development can discolour and pit tooth enamel (fluorosis).

Vitamin K

- Vitamin K is required for the protein osteocalcin to mineralize bones.
- Bacteria in the GI tract can make vitamin K; people typically receive about half of their requirements from bacterial synthesis and half from foods such as green vegetables and vegetable oils.

Nutrients for Bone Health—In Summary

- The minerals—calcium, magnesium, phosphorus, and fluoride—provide structural support for your bones, whereas the vitamins—vitamin D and vitamin K—perform more functional roles in maintaining bone health.

About Bones (pp. 409–410)

1. Describe how osteoblast and osteoclast activities change over the lifespan.
2. Discuss differences in the processes of bone growth, bone modelling, and bone remodelling.

Calcium (pp. 410–416)

3. List calcium's roles in the body. How does the body keep blood calcium constant regardless of intake?
4. Name significant food sources of calcium. What are the consequences of inadequate intakes?
5. What does calcium homeostasis depends on?
   a. vitamin K, aldosterone, and renin
   b. vitamin K, parathyroid hormone, and renin
   c. vitamin D, aldosterone, and calcitonin
   d. vitamin D, calcitonin, and parathyroid hormone
6. What hinders calcium absorption?
   a. lactose
   b. oxalates
   c. vitamin D
   d. stomach acid

Phosphorus (pp. 416–417)

7. List the roles of phosphorus in bone health. Discuss the relationships between calcium and phosphorus. Is a dietary deficiency of phosphorus likely? Why or why not?
8. Where is phosphorus predominately found?
   a. in the blood
   b. in the liver
   c. in bone
   d. in the kidneys

Vitamin D (pp. 417–422)

9. How is vitamin D unique among the vitamins? What is its chief function? What are the richest sources of this vitamin?
10. What does vitamin D target in order to keep minerals available in the blood?
    a. the skin, the muscles, and the bones
    b. the kidneys, the liver, and the bones
    c. the intestines, the kidneys, and the bones
    d. the intestines, the pancreas, and the liver
11. Vitamin D can be synthesized from a precursor. What does the body make the precursor from?
    a. bilirubin
    b. cholesterol
    c. tocopherol
    d. beta-carotene

Magnesium (pp. 422–424)

12. Where is most of the body's magnesium found?
    a. in the bones
    b. in the nerves
    c. in the muscles
    d. in the extracellular fluids
13. Which of the following statements does NOT apply to magnesium?
    a. It is required for protein synthesis.
    b. It is necessary for the production of ATP.
    c. It aids in the absorption of dietary calcium.
    d. It is needed for the synthesis of nucleic acids.

Fluoride (pp. 424–425)

14. When does fluorosis occur?
    a. when fluoride is excessive
    b. when fluoride is inadequate
    c. when fluoride binds with phosphorus
    d. when fluoride interacts with calcium

Vitamin K (p. 425)

15. What is vitamin K's primary role in bone health?
16. What conditions may lead to vitamin K deficiency?

Nutrients for Bone Health—In Summary (pp. 426–427)

17. What is the mineral that is present in the greatest proportion in bone?
    a. magnesium
    b. fluoride
    c. phosphorus
    d. calcium

Study Questions (multiple choice)
5. d 6. b 8. c 10. c 11. b 12. a 13. c 14. a 17. d

CENGAGENOW™ For additional study questions and activities, go to **www.cengage.com/sso** and complete the Personalized Study Plan for this chapter.

STUDY CARD 14

Nutrients for Blood Health

About Blood

- Blood is the only fluid tissue in the body.
- Blood transports nutrients and oxygen to cells and carries waste products away.
- Plasma accounts for about 55 percent of whole blood and red blood cells about 45 percent. Less than 1 percent contains white blood cells and platelets.

Vitamin K

- Vitamin K activates proteins required for blood clotting, and its deficiency causes hemorrhagic disease (uncontrolled bleeding).
- Because people depend on bacterial synthesis in the GI tract for vitamin K, deficiency is most likely in newborn infants (sterile GI tract) and in people taking antibiotics. About half of vitamin K comes from foods such as green vegetables and vegetable oils and the other half from bacterial synthesis.

Iron

- Iron is found in hemoglobin and myoglobin where it carries oxygen for energy metabolism; iron also acts as a cofactor for some enzymes. Iron deficiency is most common among infants and young children, teenagers, women of childbearing age, and pregnant women. Symptoms include fatigue and anemia. Iron overload is most common in men. Heme iron, which is found only in meat, fish, and poultry, is better absorbed than nonheme iron, which occurs in most foods. Nonheme iron absorption is improved by eating iron-containing foods with foods containing the MFP factor and vitamin C; absorption is limited by phytates and oxalates.

Zinc

- Zinc-requiring enzymes participate in reactions affecting growth, vitamin A activity, and pancreatic digestive enzyme synthesis. Both dietary zinc and zinc-rich pancreatic secretions (via enteropancreatic circulation) are available for absorption. Absorption is monitored by a special binding protein (metallothionein) in the small intestine. Protein-rich foods derived from animals are the best sources of bioavailable zinc. Fibre and phytates in cereals bind zinc, limiting absorption. Symptoms of deficiency include growth retardation and sexual immaturity.

Copper

- Copper is a component of several enzymes, all of which are involved with oxygen or oxidation. Some act as antioxidants; others are essential to iron metabolism. Legumes, whole grains, and shellfish are good sources of copper.

Other Trace Minerals

- Other trace minerals may prove to be essential nutrients, but we will not know until we can detect their minute presence in tissues, determine discrete functional roles, and see symptoms of deficiency corrected when the mineral is added in sufficient quantities back into the diet.

Contaminant Minerals

- Avoiding the ingestion or inhalation of contaminant minerals—heavy metals like lead, mercury, and cadmium—protects the body from harmful effects that impair general health.

Closing Thoughts on the Nutrients

- Learning about the nutrients individually and grouped by functional role is a good start to understanding why we ought to choose nutrient-dense foods containing an array of nutrients. As you have seen in the first 14 chapters, nutrients affect metabolism throughout the body, and their interactions more so than individual actions illustrate the importance of consuming an adequate, balanced, and varied diet to support good health.

FIGURE 14-3 **Heme and Nonheme Iron in Foods**

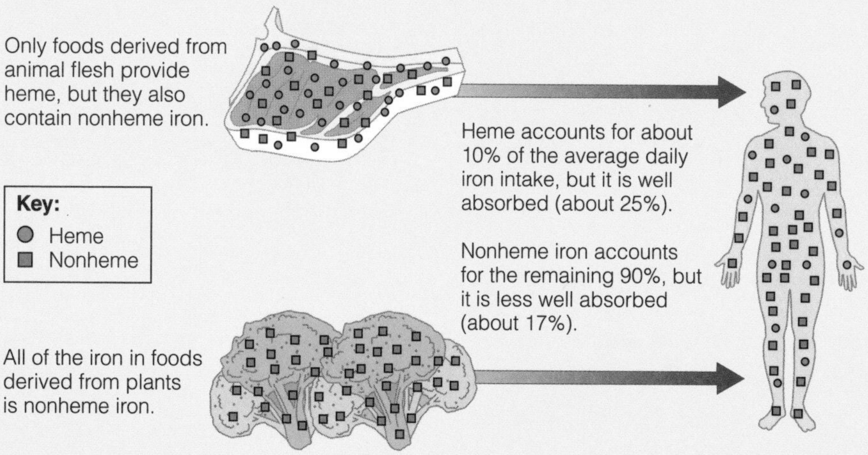

Only foods derived from animal flesh provide heme, but they also contain nonheme iron.
Key:
Heme
Nonheme
Heme accounts for about 10% of the average daily iron intake, but it is well absorbed (about 25%).
Nonheme iron accounts for the remaining 90%, but it is less well absorbed (about 17%).
All of the iron in foods derived from plants is nonheme iron.

About Blood (p. 441)

1. Describe the unique features of blood and its importance to health.

Vitamin K (pp. 441–442)

2. A significant amount of vitamin K comes from:
   a. plant oils.
   b. sunlight exposure.
   c. orange vegetables.
   d. fortified grain products.

Iron (pp. 442–451)

3. Distinguish between heme and nonheme iron. Discuss the factors that enhance iron absorption.
4. Differentiate between iron deficiency and iron-deficiency anemia. What are the symptoms of iron-deficiency anemia?
5. Describe the similarities and differences in the absorption and regulation of iron and zinc.
6. What impairs iron absorption?
   a. heme
   b. phytates
   c. vitamin C
   d. MFP factor
7. Which of these people is *least* likely to develop an iron deficiency?
   a. a 3-year-old boy
   b. a 52-year-old man
   c. a 17-year-old girl
   d. a 24-year-old woman
8. Which of the following would NOT describe the blood cells of a severe iron deficiency?
   a. anemic
   b. microcytic
   c. pernicious
   d. hypochromic
9. Which of the following foods provides the most absorbable iron?
   a. 1 medium apple
   b. 250 millilitres (1 cup) milk
   c. 90 grams (3 ounces) steak
   d. 125 millilitres (½ cup) spinach

Zinc (pp. 451–454)

10. Discuss possible reasons for a low intake of zinc. What factors affect the bioavailability of zinc?
11. Which intestinal protein helps regulate zinc absorption?
    a. albumin
    b. ferritin
    c. hemosiderin
    d. metallothionein
12. Which of the following contains high amounts of zinc?
    a. foods high in polyunsaturated fat
    b. foods high in fibre
    c. foods high in carbohydrate
    d. foods high in protein
13. What is a classic sign of zinc deficiency?
    a. anemia
    b. goitre
    c. mottled teeth
    d. growth retardation

Copper (pp. 455–456)

14. What is copper required for?
    a. for iron to bind to transferrin
    b. for zinc to bind to metallothionein
    c. for iron to bind to metallothionein
    d. for zinc to bind to transferrin

Other Trace Minerals (p. 456)

15. Describe two challenges faced in discovering the roles of other trace minerals in the human body.

Contaminant Minerals (p. 456)

16. Describe two examples of how lead can displace mineral nutrients to cause ill health effects.

Closing Thoughts on the Nutrients (p. 460)

17. Explain why it is important to think about nutrients as a whole when learning about them individually and by function.

Study Questions (multiple choice)
2. a 6. b 7. b 8. c 9. c 11. d 12. d 13. d 14. a

STUDY CARD 15

Fitness: Physical Activity, Nutrients, and Body Adaptations

Fitness

- Physical activity brings good health and long quality of life.
- The components of fitness are flexibility, muscle strength and endurance, and cardiorespiratory endurance; these are obtained by conditioning the body, through training, to adapt to the activity performed.
- Participating in cardiorespiratory endurance and resistance activities improves fitness and benefits health (review Table 15-2, p. 472).

Energy Systems and Fuels to Support Activity

- Fuel mixture during physical activity depends on diet, the intensity and duration of activity, and training (review Table 15-4).
- During intense activity, the fuel mix is mostly glucose; during less intense activity, fat makes a greater contribution.
- With endurance training, muscle cells adapt to store more glycogen and to rely less on glucose and more on fat for energy.
- Active athletes may need more protein than sedentary people do; they typically eat more food and therefore obtain enough protein without supplements.

Vitamins and Minerals to Support Activity

- With the possible exception of iron for women, well-nourished active people and athletes do not need dietary supplements.

Fluids and Electrolytes to Support Activity

- Active people need to drink plenty of water (review Table 15-6, p. 488).
- Symptoms of dehydration and heat stroke:
  - Headache
  - Nausea
  - Dizziness
  - Clumsiness
  - Stumbling
  - Sudden cessation of sweating (hot, dry skin)
  - Confusion or other mental changes
- Endurance athletes need to drink both water and carbohydrate-containing beverages, especially during training and competition.
- During events of long duration, athletes may need to replace sodium losses to prevent hyponatremia.

Diets for Physically Active People

- To enhance athletic performance and overall health, a diet should provide ample fluid and a variety of nutrient-dense foods in quantities to meet energy needs.
- Carbohydrate-rich foods that are light and easy to digest are best for pregame and postgame meals.
- Athletes in heavy training need 8 to 10 grams carbohydrate per kilogram body weight.

TABLE 15-4 Fuels Used for Activities of Different Intensities and Durations

Activity Intensity	Activity Duration	Preferred Fuel Source	Oxygen Needed?	Activity Example
Extreme[a]	8 to 10 sec	ATP-CP (immediate availability)	No (anaerobic)	100 metre dash, shot put
Very high	20 sec to 3 min	ATP from carbohydrate (lactate)	No (anaerobic)	400 metre run at maximal speed
High	3 min to 20 min	ATP from carbohydrate	Yes (aerobic)	Cycling, swimming, or running
Moderate	More than 20 min	ATP from fat	Yes (aerobic)	Hiking

[a]All levels of activity intensity use the ATP-CP system initially; extremely intense short-term activities rely solely on the ATP-CP system.

Fitness (pp. 469–476)

1. Define fitness, and list its benefits.
2. Explain the overload principle.
3. Define cardiorespiratory conditioning and list some of its benefits.
4. Which disease is NOT linked to physical inactivity?
   a. cancer
   b. diabetes
   c. emphysema
   d. hypertension
5. How is the progressive overload principle applied?
   a. by performing an activity less often
   b. by performing an activity with more intensity
   c. by performing an activity in a different setting
   d. by performing a different activity each day of the week

Energy Systems and Fuels to Support Activity (pp. 476–484)

6. What types of activity are anaerobic? Which are aerobic? Describe the relationships among energy expenditure, type of activity, and oxygen use.
7. What factors influence the body's use of glucose during physical activity? How?
8. What factors influence the body's use of fat during physical activity? How?
9. What factors influence the body's use of protein during physical activity? How?
10. What is the process that regenerates glucose from lactate?
    a. the Cori cycle
    b. the ATP-CP cycle
    c. the adaptation cycle
    d. the cardiac output cycle
11. "Hitting the wall" is a term that runners sometimes use. What does it describe?
    a. dehydration
    b. competition
    c. indigestion
    d. the glucose depletion
12. Which term refers to the technique endurance athletes use to maximize glycogen stores?
    a. aerobic training
    b. muscle conditioning
    c. carbohydrate loading
    d. progressive overloading
13. Which of the following fuels do conditioned muscles burn more efficiently over a longer period of time?
    a. protein
    b. fat
    c. glycogen

Vitamins and Minerals to Support Activity (pp. 484–487)

14. Why are some athletes likely to develop iron-deficiency anemia? Compare iron-deficiency anemia and sports anemia, explaining the differences.
15. Why are vitamin or mineral supplements taken just before an event useless for improving performance?
    a. because an athlete sweats the nutrients out during the event
    b. because the stomach can't digest supplements during physical activity
    c. because the nutrients are diluted by all the fluids the athlete drinks
    d. because the body needs hours or days for the nutrients to do their work
16. Which of the following are physically active young women, especially those who are endurance athletes, prone to?
    a. energy excess
    b. iron deficiency
    c. protein overload
    d. vitamin A toxicity

Fluids and Electrolytes to Support Activity (pp. 487–491)

17. Discuss the importance of hydration during training, and list recommendations to maintain fluid balance.
18. Which nutrient does the body have the greatest need for?
    a. water
    b. protein
    c. vitamins
    d. carbohydrate

Diets for Physically Active People (pp. 491–494)

19. Describe the components of a healthy diet for athletic performance.
20. Which of the following is a recommended pregame meal that includes plenty of fluids?
    a. between 50 and 100 kcalories, mostly from fibre-rich foods
    b. between 300 and 800 kcalories, mostly from fat-rich foods
    c. between 300 and 800 kcalories, mostly from carbohydrate-rich foods
    d. between 1000 and 2000 kcalories, mostly from protein-rich foods

Study Questions (multiple choice)
4. c 5. b 10. a 11. d 12. c 13. b 15. d 16. b 18. a 20. c

CENGAGENOW™ For additional study questions and activities, go to **www.cengage.com/sso** and complete the Personalized Study Plan for this chapter.

STUDY CARD 16

Life Cycle Nutrition: Pregnancy and Lactation

Nutrition prior to Pregnancy

- Maternal nutrition before and during pregnancy supports the mother's health and the infant's growth.

Growth and Development during Pregnancy

- The infant develops through three stages—the zygote, embryo, and fetus (review Figure 16-2, p. 507). Each organ and tissue grows on its own schedule (review Figure 16-4, p. 508).
- Times of intense development are critical periods that depend on nutrients (review Figure 16-3, p. 508).
- Without folate, the neural tube fails to develop completely during the first month of pregnancy; all women of childbearing age should take supplemental folate daily.

Maternal Weight

- A healthy pregnancy depends on a sufficient weight gain.
- Women who begin their pregnancies at a healthy weight need to gain about 13.5 kilograms (30 pounds) to cover the growth and development of the placenta, uterus, blood, breasts, and infant (review Figure 16-8, p. 514).
- Physical activity throughout pregnancy can help a woman develop the strength she needs to carry the extra weight and maintain habits that will help her lose it after the birth.

Nutrition during Pregnancy

- Energy and nutrient needs are high during pregnancy; the diet should include an extra serving from each of the four food groups.
- Supplements of iron and folate are recommended.
- Nausea, constipation, and heartburn commonly accompany pregnancy and can usually be alleviated with a few simple strategies (review Table 16-2, p. 520). Food cravings do not typically reflect physiological needs.

High-Risk Pregnancies

- High-risk pregnancies threaten the life and health of both mother and infant.
- Proper nutrition and abstinence from smoking, alcohol, and other drugs improve the outcome as can prenatal care to monitor for gestational diabetes and preeclampsia.

Nutrition during Lactation

- Lactating women need extra fluid and enough energy and nutrients to produce about 750 millilitres (25 ounces) of milk a day.
- Breastfeeding is contraindicated for those with HIV/AIDS.
- Alcohol, other drugs, smoking, and contaminants may reduce milk production or enter breast milk and impair infant development.

TABLE 16-3 High-Risk Pregnancy Factors

Factor	Condition that Raises Risk
Maternal weight	
• Prior to pregnancy	Prepregnancy BMI either <18.5 or ≥ 25
• During pregnancy	Insufficient or excessive pregnancy weight gain
Maternal nutrition	Nutrient deficiencies or toxicities; eating disorders
Socioeconomic status	Poverty, lack of family support, low level of education, limited food available
Lifestyle habits	Smoking, alcohol, or other drug use
Age	Teens, especially 15 years or younger; women 35 years or older
Previous pregnancies	
• Number	Many previous pregnancies (3 or more to mothers under age 20; 4 or more to mothers age 20 or older)
• Interval	Short or long intervals between pregnancies (<18 months or >59 months)
• Outcomes	Previous history of problems
• Multiple births	Twins or triplets
• Birthweight	Low- or high-birthweight infants
Maternal health	
• High blood pressure	Development of gestational hypertension
• Diabetes	Development of gestational diabetes
• Chronic diseases	Diabetes; heart, respiratory, and kidney disease; certain genetic disorders; special diets and medications

Nutrition prior to Pregnancy (pp. 505–506)

1. Describe how men and women can prepare for a healthy pregnancy.

Growth and Development during Pregnancy (pp. 506–511)

2. Describe the placenta and its function.
3. Describe the normal events of fetal development. How does malnutrition impair fetal development?
4. Define the term *critical period.* How do adverse influences during critical periods affect later health?
5. Explain why women of childbearing age need folate in their diets. How much is recommended, and how can women ensure that these needs are met?
6. What is the name of the spongy structure that delivers nutrients to the fetus and returns waste products to the mother?
   a. the embryo
   b. the uterus
   c. the placenta
   d. the amniotic sac

Maternal Weight (pp. 511–515)

7. What is the recommended pattern of weight gain during pregnancy for a woman at a healthy weight? For an underweight woman? For an overweight woman?
8. What does a pregnant woman need to know about exercise?
9. Which of these strategies is NOT a healthy option for an overweight woman?
   a. Limit weight gain during pregnancy.
   b. Postpone weight loss until after pregnancy.
   c. Follow a weight-loss diet during pregnancy.
   d. Try to achieve a healthy weight before becoming pregnant.
10. What is a reasonable weight gain during pregnancy for a normal-weight woman?
    a. about 4.5 kilograms
    b. about 9 kilograms
    c. about 13.5 kilograms
    d. about 18 kilograms

Nutrition during Pregnancy (pp. 515–520)

11. Which nutrients are needed in the greatest amounts during pregnancy? Why are they so important? Describe wise food choices for the pregnant woman.
12. How much do energy needs increase during pregnancy?
    a. about 100 kcalories/day
    b. about 300 kcalories/day
    c. about 500 kcalories/day
    d. about 700 kcalories/day

High-Risk Pregnancies (pp. 521–527)

13. Define low-risk and high-risk pregnancies. What is the significance of infant birthweight in terms of the child's future health?
14. Describe some of the special problems of the pregnant adolescent. Which nutrients are needed in increased amounts?
15. What practices should be avoided during pregnancy? Why?
16. To help prevent neural tube defects, what are wheat-based grain products now fortified with?
    a. iron
    b. folate
    c. protein
    d. vitamin C
17. Which supplements should NOT be taken by pregnant women?
    a. iron
    b. folate
    c. vitamin A
    d. vitamin C
18. What is signalled by the combination of high blood pressure, protein in the urine, and edema?
    a. jaundice
    b. preeclampsia
    c. gestational diabetes
    d. gestational hypertension

Nutrition during Lactation (pp. 527–533)

19. How do nutrient needs during lactation differ from nutrient needs during pregnancy?
20. What does a mother need to facilitate lactation?
    a. about 5000 kcalories a day
    b. adequate nutrition and rest
    c. vitamin and mineral supplements
    d. a glass of wine or beer before each feeding
21. Why should a breastfeeding woman drink plenty of water?
    a. to produce more milk
    b. to suppress lactation
    c. to prevent dehydration
    d. to dilute nutrient concentration
22. Why might a woman need iron supplements during lactation?
    a. to enhance the iron in her breast milk
    b. to provide iron for the infant's growth
    c. to replace the iron in her body's stores
    d. to support the increase in her blood volume

Study Questions (multiple choice)
6. c 9. c 10. c 12. b 16. b 17. c 18. b 20. b 21. c 22. c

CENGAGENOW™ For additional study questions and activities, go to **www.cengage.com/sso** and complete the Personalized Study Plan for this chapter.

STUDY CARD 17

Life Cycle Nutrition: Infancy, Childhood, and Adolescence

Nutrition during Infancy

- The primary food for infants during the first 12 months is either breast milk or iron-fortified formula.
- Breast milk offers both nutrients and immunological protection.
- At 4 to 6 months of age, infants should gradually begin eating solid foods, including iron-fortified cereals, vitamin-C rich vegetables and fruits, and pureed meats.
- By 1 year, infants are drinking from a cup and eating a variety of foods.
- Infants may benefit from supplements containing vitamin D, iron, and fluoride (review Table 17-2, p. 548).

Nutrition during Childhood

- Children's appetites and nutrient needs reflect their stage of growth.
- Children who are chronically hungry and malnourished suffer growth retardation; temporary hunger and mild nutrient deficiencies produce more subtle problems—such as poor academic performance.
- Iron deficiency has many physical and behavioural consequences.
- "Hyper" behaviour is mistakenly blamed on sweets and candy; misbehaviour may be due to lack of sleep, too little physical activity, or too much television, among other factors.
- Childhood overweight and obesity is a major health problem (review Figure 17-8, p. 563, and Table 17-7 for strategies to help prevent obesity).
- Children need to eat nutrient-dense foods and learn how to make healthful diet and activity choices.
- Some children have food allergies—adverse reactions that involve an immune response—most often caused by peanuts, tree nuts, milk, eggs, wheat, soybeans, fish, or shellfish.

Nutrition during Adolescence

- The need for iron increases during adolescence for both males and females; blood losses incurred through menstruation further increase iron needs for females.
- Sufficient calcium intake during adolescence supports optimal bone growth and density.
- The adolescent growth spurt increases the need for energy and nutrients.
- Adolescents who drink soft drinks regularly have a higher energy intake and a lower calcium intake; they are also more likely to be overweight.

Nutrition during Infancy (pp. 543–554)

1. Describe some of the nutrient and immunological attributes of breast milk.
2. What are the appropriate uses of formula feeding? What criteria would you use in selecting an infant formula?
3. Why are solid foods not recommended for an infant during the first few months of life? When is an infant ready to start eating solid food?
4. Identify foods that are inappropriate for infants and explain why they are inappropriate.
5. What is a reasonable weight for a healthy 5-month-old infant who weighed 3.5 kilograms at birth?
   a. about 5.5 kilograms
   b. about 7.5 kilograms
   c. about 9 kilograms
   d. about 11 kilograms

TABLE 17-7 Recommended Eating and Physical Activity Behaviours to Prevent Obesity

The Expert Committee of the American Medical Association recommends the following healthy habits for children 2 to 18 years of age to help prevent childhood obesity:

- Limit consumption of sugar-sweetened beverages, such as soft drinks and fruit flavoured punches.
- Eat the recommended amounts of fruits and vegetables every day (500 to 1125 mL/2 to 4.5 cups per day based on age).
- Learn to eat age-appropriate portions of foods.
- Eat foods low in energy density such as those high in fibre and/or water and modest in fat.
- Eat a nutritious breakfast every day.
- Eat a diet rich in calcium.
- Eat a diet balanced in recommended proportions for carbohydrate, fat, and protein.
- Eat a diet high in fibre.
- Eat together as a family as often as possible.
- Limit the frequency of restaurant meals.
- Limit television watching or other screen time to no more than 2 hours per day and do not have televisions or computers in bedrooms.
- Engage in at least 60 minutes of moderate to vigorous physical activity every day.

SOURCES: D. C. W. Lau and co-authors, 2006 Canadian clinical practice guidelines on the management and prevention of obesity in adults and children. http://www.cmaj.ca/content/176/8/S1.full; Canadian Paediatric Society, Healthy active living for children and youth. http://www.cps.ca/english/statements/HAL/HAL02-01.htm; Canadian Society for Exercise Physiology (CSEP), 2011 Canadian Physical Activity and Sedentary Behaviour Guidelines. http://www.csep.ca/english/view.asp?x=804; S. E. Barlow, Expert Committee recommendations regarding the prevention, assessment, and treatment of child and adolescent overweight and obesity: Summary report, *Pediatrics* 120 (2007): S164–S192.

6. Why can dehydration develop quickly in infants?
   a. because much of their body water is extracellular.
   b. because they lose a lot of water through urination and tears
   c. because only a small percentage of their body weight is water
   d. because they drink lots of breast milk or formula, but little water
7. When should an infant begin eating solid food?
   a. between 2 and 4 weeks old
   b. between 1 and 3 months old
   c. between 4 and 6 months old
   d. between 8 and 10 months old

Nutrition during Childhood (pp. 554–571)

8. What nutrition problems are most common in children? What strategies can help prevent these problems?
9. Describe the relationships between nutrition and behaviour. How can television influence nutrition?
10. Describe a true food allergy. Which foods most often cause allergic reactions? How do food allergies influence nutrition status?
11. Describe the problems associated with childhood obesity and the strategies for prevention and treatment.
12. List strategies for introducing nutritious foods to children.
13. What impact can school meal programs have on the nutrition status of children?
14. What is the most prevalent nutrient deficiency among Canadian and U.S. children?
   a. iron
   b. folate
   c. protein
   d. vitamin C
15. Which of the following statements about a true food allergy is correct?
   a. A true food allergy always elicits an immune response.
   b. A true food allergy always causes an immediate reaction.
   c. A true food allergy always creates an aversion to the offending food.
   d. A true food allergy always involves symptoms such as headaches or hives.
16. Which of the following strategies is NOT effective for promoting healthy eating habits in children ?
   a. Play first, eat later.
   b. Provide small portions.
   c. Encourage children to help prepare meals.
   d. Use dessert as a reward for eating vegetables.

Nutrition during Adolescence (pp. 571–575)

17. Describe the changes in nutrient needs from childhood to adolescence. Why is an adolescent girl more likely to develop an iron deficiency than is a boy?
18. How do adolescents' eating habits influence their nutrient intakes?
19. How does the use of illicit drugs influence nutrition status?
20. How do the nutrient intakes of smokers differ from those of nonsmokers? What impacts can those differences exert on health?
21. What can parents do to help teenagers consume a balanced diet?
   a. Monitor the teens' food intake.
   b. Give up—parents cannot influence teenagers.
   c. Keep the cupboard and refrigerator well stocked healthy food choices.
   d. Forbid snacking and insist on regular, well-balanced meals.
22. What happens to energy and nutrient needs during adolescence?
   a. They reach a peak.
   b. They fall dramatically.
   c. They rise, but do not peak until adulthood.
   d. They fluctuate so much that generalizations can't be made.
23. Which nutrients are most likely to be inadequate in an adolescent's diet?
   a. sodium and fat
   b. folate and zinc
   c. iron and calcium
   d. protein and vitamin A
24. Suppose an adolescent eats a hamburger, some fries, and a cola at lunch. To balance the day's intake, which dinner would benefit him most?
   a. fried chicken, rice, and banana
   b. ribeye steak, baked potato, and salad
   c. pork chop, mashed potatoes, and apple juice
   d. spaghetti with meat sauce, broccoli, and milk

Study Questions (multiple choice)
5. b 6. a 7. c 14. a 15. a 16. d 21. c 22. a 23. c 24. d

CENGAGENOW™ For additional study questions and activities, go to **www.cengage.com/sso** and complete the Personalized Study Plan for this chapter.

STUDY CARD 18

Life Cycle Nutrition: Adulthood and the Later Years

Seniors in the Community: Risk Evaluation For Eating and Nutrition (SCREEN)

A tool called Seniors in the Community: Risk Evaluation For Eating and Nutrition (SCREEN) was developed recently to assess "weight change, food intake and risk factors for impaired food intake." For the latest developments in terms of research, SCREEN tool applications (i.e., SCREEN™ I & SCREEN™ II) and copyright licence for your site or community, see Dr Keller's SCREEN website at www.drheatherkeller.com/SCREEN.htm.

NOTE: An abbreviated version (SCREEN II-AB) was used with permission by Statistics Canada in their 2008–2009 Canadian Community Health Survey (CCHS) - Healthy Aging (www.statcan.gc.ca/daily-quotidien/100512/dq100512f-eng.htm).

SOURCE: H. H. Keller, M. R. Hedley, and S. Wong-Brownlee, The development of Seniors in the Community: Risk Evaluation for Eating and Nutrition (SCREEN), *Canadian Journal of Dietetic Practice and Research* 61 (2000): 62–72.

Nutrition and Longevity

- Life expectancy in Canada increased dramatically in the 20th century.
- Factors that enhance longevity include limited or no alcohol use, regular balanced meals, weight control, abstinence from smoking, regular physical activity, and adequate sleep.
- Energy restriction in animals seems to lengthen their lives; whether such dietary intervention in human beings is beneficial remains unknown.
- Nutrition—especially when combined with regular physical activity—can influence aging and longevity by supporting good health and preventing disease.

The Aging Process

- Changes that accompany aging can impair nutrition status. Among physiological changes, hormone activity alters body composition, immune system changes raise the risk of infections, atrophic gastritis interferes with digestion and absorption, and tooth loss limits food choices.
- Psychological changes such as depression, economic changes such as loss of income, and social changes such as loneliness contribute to poor food intake.

Energy and Nutrient Needs of Older Adults

- Some nutrients need special attention in the diet, but aside from supplemental vitamin D for those 50 years and older, for otherwise nonpregnant and nonlactating healthy adults supplements are not routinely recommended.

Nutrition-Related Concerns of Older Adults

- Senile dementia and cognitive losses afflict many older adults; some face loss of vision due to cataracts or macular degeneration or cope with the pain of arthritis.
- The table below provides a summary of the nutrient concerns of aging.
- Some problems may be inevitable, but others are preventable and good nutrition may play a key role.

Food Choices and Eating Habits of Older Adults

- Congregate meals provide older adults with both nutrients and social interactions; those who are homebound receive delivered meals.
- Adults living alone can prepare nutritious, inexpensive meals with a little creativity and careful shopping.

Nutrient	Effect of Aging	Comments
Water	Lack of thirst and decreased total body water make dehydration likely.	Mild dehydration is a common cause of confusion. Difficulty obtaining water or getting to the bathroom may compound the problem.
Energy	Need decreases as muscle mass decreases (sarcopenia).	Physical activity moderates the decline.
Fibre	Likelihood of constipation increases with low intakes and changes in the GI tract.	Inadequate water intakes and lack of physical activity, along with some medications, compound the problem.
Protein	Needs may stay the same or increase slightly.	Low-fat, high-fibre legumes and grains meet both protein and other nutrient needs.
Vitamin B_{12}	Atrophic gastritis is common.	Deficiency causes neurological damage; supplements may be needed.
Vitamin D	Increased likelihood of inadequate intake; skin synthesis declines.	Daily sunlight exposure in moderation from mid-spring to mid-fall and a daily vitamin D supplement is recommended for all those 50 years and older.
Calcium	Intakes may be low; osteoporosis is common.	Stomach discomfort commonly limits milk intake; calcium substitutes or supplements may be needed.
Iron	In women, status improves after menopause; deficiencies are linked to chronic blood losses and low stomach acid output.	Adequate stomach acid is required for absorption; antacid or other medicine use may aggravate iron deficiency; vitamin C and meat increase absorption.

Nutrition and Longevity (pp. 588–592)

1. What roles does nutrition play in aging, and what roles can it play in retarding aging?
2. What is life expectancy in Canada?
   a. about 48 to 60 years
   b. about 58 to 70 years
   c. about 79 to 83 years
   d. about 85 to 90 years
3. How long is the human life span?
   a. about 85 years
   b. about 100 years
   c. about 115 years
   d. about 130 years
4. Suppose a 72-year-old person has physical health that is similar to that of a person 10 years younger. What is another way to describe the age of this person?
   a. chronological age is 62
   b. physiological age is 72
   c. physiological age is 62
   d. absolute age is minus 10
5. Which diet will allow a rat to live the longest?
   a. a no-fat diet
   b. a high-protein diet
   c. an unrestricted diet
   d. an energy-restricted diet

The Aging Process (pp. 592–595)

6. What are some of the physiological changes that occur in the body's systems with aging? To what extent can aging be prevented?
7. Which characteristic is NOT commonly associated with atrophic gastritis?
   a. inflamed stomach
   b. vitamin B_{12} toxicity
   c. bacterial overgrowth
   d. lack of intrinsic factor

Energy and Nutrient Needs of Older Adults (pp. 595–599)

8. Why does the risk of dehydration increase as people age?
9. Why do energy needs usually decline with advancing age?
10. Which vitamins and minerals need special consideration for the elderly? Explain why. Identify some factors that complicate the task of setting nutrient standards for older adults.
11. On average, what happens to adult energy needs over time?
    a. energy needs decline 5 percent per year
    b. energy needs decline 5 percent per decade
    c. energy needs remain stable throughout life
    d. energy needs rise gradually throughout life

Nutrition-Related Concerns of Older Adults (pp. 600–603)

12. Discuss the relationships between nutrition and cataracts and between nutrition and arthritis.
13. Which nutrients seem to protect against cataract development?
    a. minerals
    b. lecithins
    c. antioxidants
    d. amino acids
14. Which is the best lifestyle advice for a person with osteoarthritis?
    a. avoid milk products
    b. take fish oil supplements
    c. take vitamin E supplements
    d. lose weight, if overweight

Food Choices and Eating Habits of Older Adults (pp. 603–606)

15. What characteristics contribute to malnutrition in older people?
16. Why are congregate meal programs preferable to Meals on Wheels?
    a. because they provide nutritious meals
    b. because they provide referral services
    c. because they provide social interactions
    d. because they provide financial assistance
17. Who is eligible for the Old Age Security?
    a. only women 65 years and older
    b. all Canadians 65 years and older
    c. homebound people only, 60 years and older
    d. low-income people only, at any age

Study Questions (multiple choice)
2. c 3. d 4. c 5. d 7. b 11. b 13. c 14. d 16. c 17. b

CENGAGENOW™ For additional study questions and activities, go to **www.cengage.com/sso** and complete the Personalized Study Plan for this chapter.

STUDY CARD 19

Diet and Health

Nutrition and Infectious Diseases

- Public health measures such as purification of water and safe handling of food help prevent the spread of infection in populations; immunizations and antibiotics protect individuals.
- Nutrition cannot prevent or cure infectious diseases, but adequate intakes of all the nutrients can help support the immune system as the body defends against disease-causing agents.
- If the immune system is impaired because of malnutrition or diseases such as AIDS, a person becomes vulnerable to infectious disease.
- Inflammation underlies many chronic diseases.

Nutrition and Chronic Diseases

- Cancers, heart disease, and strokes are the three leading causes of death in Canada; diabetes also ranks among the top 10.
- These four chronic diseases have significant links with nutrition and with one another (see Figure 19-3, p. 621, and Table 19-12); other lifestyle risk factors and genetics also play a role.

TABLE 19-12 Recommendations for the Prevention and Treatment of Chronic Diseases Compared

Dietary Guidelines	Heart Disease	Hypertension	Diabetes	Cancer
Maintain a healthy body weight.	✓	✓	✓	✓
Engage in regular physical activity.	✓	✓	✓	✓
Keep total fat 20–35%.	✓			
Limit saturated and *trans* fats.	✓			
Select fibre-rich fruits, vegetables, and whole grains.	✓	✓	✓	✓
Use little added sugars.	✓		✓	
Use little salt.	✓	✓		✓
Drink alcohol in moderation.	✓	✓	✓	✓

Cardiovascular Disease

- Atherosclerosis is characterized by a build-up of plaque in an artery wall.
- Rupture of plaque or abnormal blood clotting can cause heart attacks and strokes.
- Dietary recommendations to lower the risks of cardiovascular disease are summarized in Table 19-6 (p. 627); quitting smoking and engaging in regular physical activity also improve heart health.

Hypertension

- The most effective dietary strategy for preventing hypertension is weight control.
- The DASH eating plan is rich in fruits, vegetables, nuts, and low-fat milk products and low in fat, saturated fat, and sodium.

FIGURE 19-3 Interrelationships among Chronic Diseases

Notice that many chronic diseases are themselves risk factors for other chronic diseases and that all of them are linked to obesity. The risk factors highlighted in blue define the metabolic syndrome.

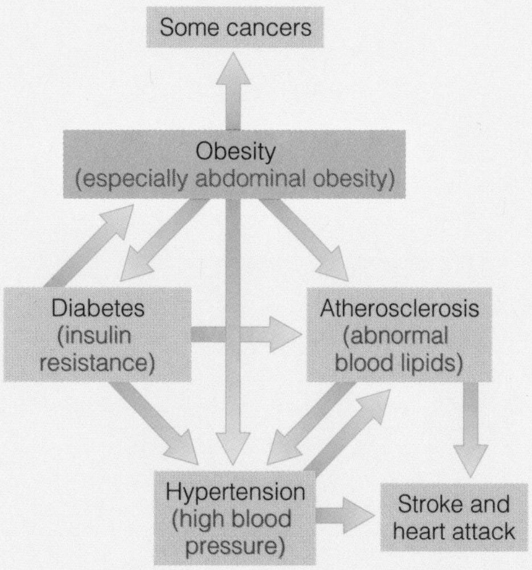

Some cancers
Obesity (especially abdominal obesity)
Diabetes (insulin resistance)
Atherosclerosis (abnormal blood lipids)
Hypertension (high blood pressure)
Stroke and heart attack

Diabetes Mellitus

- Diabetes is characterized by high blood glucose and either insufficient insulin, reduced insulin sensitivity, or a combination of the two.
- People with type 1 diabetes coordinate diet, insulin, and physical activity to help control their blood glucose.
- People with type 2 diabetes benefit most from a diet and physical activity program that controls glucose fluctuations and promotes weight loss.

Cancer

- Some dietary factors, such as alcohol and heavily smoked foods, may initiate cancer development; others, such as animal fats, may promote cancer once it develops; and still others, such as fibre, antioxidant nutrients, and phytochemicals, may serve as antipromoters that protect against its development.
- To obtain the best possible nutrition at the lowest possible cancer risk, eat many fruits, vegetables, legumes, and whole grains and little saturated fat; minimize weight gain through regular physical activity and a healthy diet.

Recommendations for Chronic Diseases

- Optimal nutrition keeps people healthy and reduces the risk of chronic diseases.
- Dietary recommendations are aimed at populations and focus on controlling weight; limiting saturated and *trans* fat; increasing fibre-rich fruits, vegetables, and whole grains; and balancing food intake with physical activity.

Nutrition and Infectious Diseases
(pp. 617–620)

1. How do the major diseases of today as a group differ from those of several decades ago as a group? Why is nutrition considered so important in connection with today's major diseases?
2. Which of the following are NOT included in the immune cells of the body?
   a. B-cells
   b. T-cells
   c. antigens
   d. phagocytes
3. Which of the following produce antibodies?
   a. phagocytes
   b. T-cells
   c. antigens
   d. B-cells

Nutrition and Chronic Diseases (pp. 620–622)

4. Identify the major diet-related risk factors for atherosclerosis, hypertension, diabetes, and cancer.
5. What is the leading cause of death in Canada?
   a. AIDS
   b. heart disease
   c. diabetes
   d. cancer

Cardiovascular Disease (pp. 622–629)

6. Describe some ways in which people can alter their diets to lower their blood cholesterol levels.
7. What do plaques in the arteries contribute to the development of?
   a. cancer
   b. diabetes
   c. atherosclerosis
   d. infectious diseases
8. Which blood lipid correlates in a positive manner with heart disease?
   a. HDL
   b. LDL
   c. VLDL
   d. triglycerides
9. How mights weight loss and physical activity protect against heart disease?
   a. by raising LDL and insulin levels
   b. by raising HDL and lowering blood pressure
   c. by lowering LDL and increasing clot formation
   d. by improving insulin sensitivity and raising blood pressure

Hypertension (pp. 630–632)

10. Describe some steps that people with hypertension can take to lower their blood pressure.
11. What is the most effective strategy for most people to lower their blood pressure?
    a. lose weight
    b. restrict salt
    c. monitor glucose
    d. supplement protein

Diabetes Mellitus (pp. 632–637)

12. Name the two major types of diabetes and describe some differences between them. How do dietary recommendations for diabetes compare with the healthy diet recommended for all people?
13. Which factor does NOT increase the risk of type 2 diabetes?
    a. aging
    b. inactivity
    c. obesity
    d. smoking
14. What is the most important dietary strategy in diabetes?
    a. provide for a consistent carbohydrate intake
    b. restrict fat to 30 percent of daily kcalories
    c. limit carbohydrate intake to 300 milligrams a day
    d. take multiple vitamin and mineral supplements daily

Cancer (pp. 637–640)

15. Differentiate between cancer initiators, promoters, and antipromoters. Which nutrients or foods fit into each of these categories?
16. Describe the characteristics of a diet that might offer the best protection against the onset of cancer.
17. Which of the following helps to protect against cancer?
    a. alcohol
    b. pickled foods
    c. phytochemicals
    d. omega-6 fatty acids

Recommendations for Chronic Diseases
(pp. 640–643)

18. Describe the dietary choices that best protect against the development of most chronic diseases.

Study Questions (multiple choice)
2. c 3. d 5. d 7. c 8. b 9. b 11. a 13. d 14. a 17. c

CENGAGENOW™ For additional study questions and activities, go to **www.cengage.com/sso** and complete the Personalized Study Plan for this chapter.

STUDY CARD 20

Consumer Concerns about Foods and Water

Foodborne Illnesses

- Millions of people suffer mild to life-threatening symptoms caused by foodborne illnesses (review Table 20-1, pp. 662–663, and Figure 20-2).
- The "How To" (pp. 666–667) describes how these illnesses can be prevented by storing and cooking foods at their proper temperatures and by preparing them in sanitary conditions.

Nutritional Adequacy of Foods and Diets

- In the marketplace, food labels and *Eating Well with Canada's Food Guide* help consumers learn about nutrition and how to plan healthy diets.
- At home, consumers can minimize nutrient losses from fruits and vegetables by refrigerating them, washing them before cutting them, storing them in airtight containers, and cooking them for short times in minimal water.

Environmental Contaminants

- Environmental contamination of foods is a concern, but so far, the hazards appear relatively small.
- Remain alert to the possibility of contamination, and keep an eye and ear open for public health announcements and advice.
- Eat a variety of foods to protect against the accumulation of toxins in the body. Each food eaten dilutes contaminants that may be present in other components of the diet.

Natural Toxicants in Foods

- Natural toxicants include the goitrogens in cabbage, cyanogens in lima beans, and solanine in potatoes.
- Any substance can be toxic when consumed in excess.
- Poisons are poisons, whether made by people or by nature. The source of a chemical does not make it hazardous; its chemical structure and the quantity consumed do.

Pesticides

- The Canadian Food Inspection Agency (CFIA) tests both domestic and imported foods for pesticide residues in the fields and in market basket surveys of foods prepared table ready.
- Consumers can minimize their ingestion of pesticide residues on foods by following the suggestions in Table 20-4 (p. 676).
- Alternative farming methods may allow farmers to grow crops using fewer or natural pesticides.

Food Additives

- The benefits of food additives seem to justify the risks associated with their use.
- Health Canada regulates the use of these intentional additives: antimicrobial agents (such as nitrites) to prevent microbial spoilage; antioxidants (such as vitamins C and E, sulphites, and BHA and BHT) to prevent oxidative changes; colours (such as tartrazine) and flavour enhancers (such as MSG) to appeal to senses; and nutrients (such as iodine in salt) to enrich or fortify foods.
- Incidental additives sometimes get into foods during processing, but rarely present a hazard; some processes such as treating livestock with hormones and antibiotics raise consumer concerns—for example, Bovine Somatotropin (rBST, a growth hormone) is not approved for use or sale in Canada.

Consumer Concerns about Water

- Like foods, water may contain infectious microorganisms, environmental contaminants, pesticide residues, and additives.
- Safe drinking water is the shared responsibility of the federal, provincial/territorial, and municipal governments.

FIGURE 20-2 Food Safety from Farms to Consumers

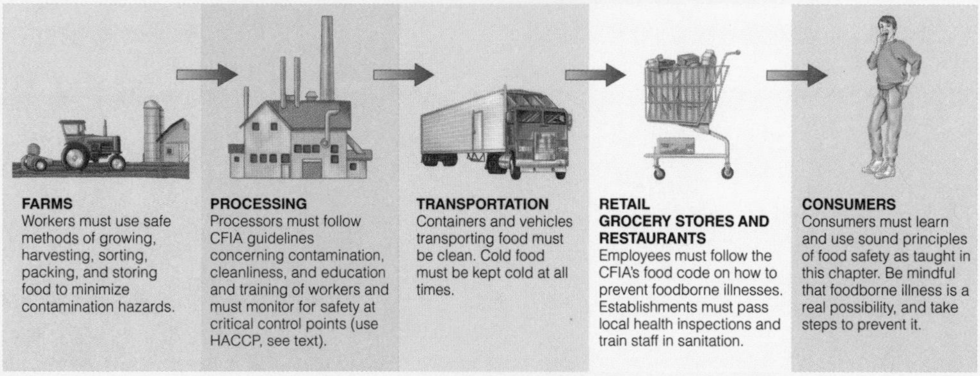
FARMS
Workers must use safe methods of growing, harvesting, sorting, packing, and storing food to minimize contamination hazards.
PROCESSING
Processors must follow CFIA guidelines concerning contamination, cleanliness, and education and training of workers and must monitor for safety at critical control points (use HACCP, see text).
TRANSPORTATION
Containers and vehicles transporting food must be clean. Cold food must be kept cold at all times.
RETAIL
GROCERY STORES AND RESTAURANTS
Employees must follow the CFIA's food code on how to prevent foodborne illnesses. Establishments must pass local health inspections and train staff in sanitation.
CONSUMERS
Consumers must learn and use sound principles of food safety as taught in this chapter. Be mindful that foodborne illness is a real possibility, and take steps to prevent it.

Foodborne Illnesses (pp. 661–670)

1. To what extent does food poisoning present a real hazard to consumers eating Canadian foods? How often does it occur?
2. Distinguish between the two types of foodborne illnesses and provide an example of each. Describe measures that help prevent foodborne illnesses.
3. What special precautions apply to meats? To seafood?
4. What might be the result of eating a contaminated food such as undercooked poultry or unpasteurized milk?
   a. a food allergy
   b. a food infection
   c. a food intoxication
   d. a botulinum reaction
5. What is the range of the temperature danger zone for foods?
   a. from –30°C to 50°C
   b. from 0°C to 100°C
   c. from –10°C to 50°C
   d. from 4°C to 60°C
6. Which foods frequently cause foodborne illness?
   a. canned foods
   b. steaming-hot foods
   c. fresh fruits and vegetables
   d. raw milk, seafood, meat, and eggs
7. How can irradiation help improve our food supply?
   a. by cooking foods quickly
   b. by killing microorganisms
   c. by minimizing the use of preservatives
   d. by improving the nutrient content of foods

Nutritional Adequacy of Foods and Diets (p. 670)

8. Describe which nutrients are most vulnerable and what consumers can do to minimize nutrient losses when storing and preparing foods.

Environmental Contaminants (pp. 671–673)

9. What is meant by a "persistent" contaminant of foods? Describe how contaminants get into foods and build up in the food chain.

Natural Toxicants in Foods (pp. 673–674)

10. What dangers do natural toxicants present?
11. What is solanine an example of?
    a. a heavy metal
    b. an artificial colour
    c. a natural toxicant
    d. an animal hormone

Pesticides (pp. 674–678)

12. How do pesticides become a hazard to the food supply, and how are they monitored? In what ways can people reduce the concentrations of pesticides in and on foods that they prepare?

Food Additives (pp. 678–685)

13. What is the difference between a substance added according to Good Manufacturing Practice (GMP) and one regulated as a food additive? Give examples of each, along with an example of intentional and incidental food additives. Name and describe the different classes of additives.
14. Which of the following is NOT used as an intentional food additive?
    a. antimicrobial agents
    b. antioxidants
    c. emulsifiers
    d. Bisphenol A
15. Which of the following are among the common antimicrobial additives?
    a. salt and nitrites
    b. carrageenan and MSG
    c. dioxins and sulphites
    d. vitamin C and vitamin E
16. Which of the following are among the common antioxidants?
    a. BHA and BHT
    b. tartrazine and MSG
    c. sugar and vitamin E
    d. nitrosamines and salt
17. Which of the following are among the incidental additives that may enter foods during processing?
    a. dioxins and acrylamide
    b. dioxins and folate
    c. beta-carotene and agar
    d. nitrites and irradiation

Consumer Concerns about Water (pp. 685–687)

18. Why is chlorine added to water?
    a. to protect against dental caries
    b. to destroy harmful minerals such as lead and mercury.
    c. to kill pathogenic microorganisms
    d. to remove the sulphur that produces a "rotten egg" odour

Study Questions (multiple choice)
4.b 5.d 6.d 7.b 11.c 14.d 15.a 16.a 17.a 18.c

CENGAGENOW™ For additional study questions and activities, go to **www.cengage.com/sso** and complete the Personalized Study Plan for this chapter.

STUDY CARD 21

Hunger and the Global Environment

Hunger in Canada

- Food insecurity and hunger are widespread in Canada among those living in poverty (review Figure 21-1).
- Ironically, hunger and malnutrition can occur among obese people (review Figure 21-2).
- Government assistance programs help to relieve poverty and hunger; food recovery programs and other community efforts are equally important.

World Hunger

- Natural causes such as drought, flood, and pests and political causes such as armed conflicts and government policies all contribute to the extreme hunger and poverty seen in the developing countries.
- To meet future demands for food, technology must improve food production, and nations must control overpopulation.

Poverty and Overpopulation

- More people means more mouths to feed, which worsens the problems of poverty and hunger.
- In some developing countries poverty and hunger encourage parents to have more children; breaking this cycle requires improving the economic status of the people and providing them with health care, education, and family planning.

The Global Environment

- The global environment is deteriorating, largely because of our irresponsible use of arable land and water resources and energy.
- Environmental degradation reduces our ability to produce enough food to feed the world's people.
- The rapid increase in the world's population exacerbates the situation.
- Governments, businesses, and all individuals can make environmentally conscious choices to help solve the hunger problem, improve the quality of life, and generate jobs.
- Personal choices, made by many people, can have a great impact.

FIGURE 21-1 Household Food Insecurity in Canada, 2007–2008

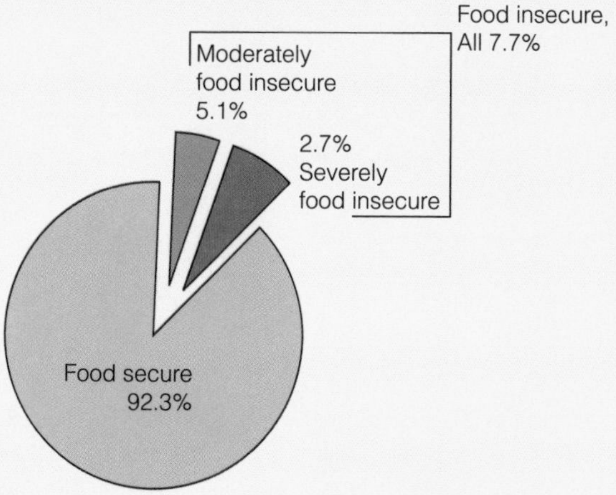
Food insecure, All 7.7%
Moderately food insecure 5.1%
2.7% Severely food insecure
Food secure 92.3%

SOURCE: Health Canada, Food & Nutrition - Household Food Insecurity in Canada 2007–2008. http://www.hc-sc.gc.ca/fn-an/surveill/nutrition/commun/insecurit/key-stats-cles-2007-2008-eng.php

FIGURE 21-2 The Poverty-Obesity Paradox

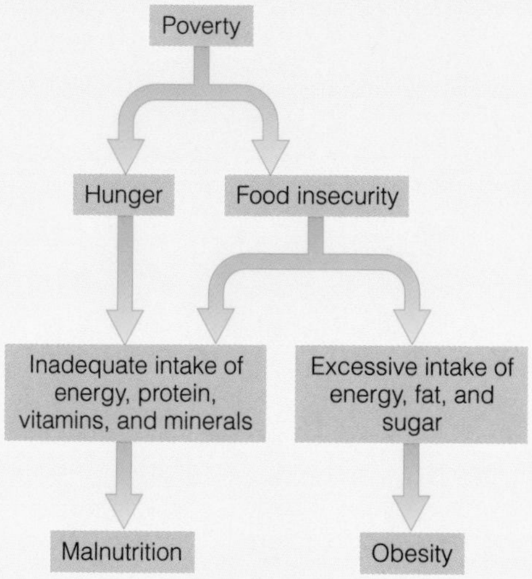
Poverty
Hunger
Food insecurity
Inadequate intake of energy, protein, vitamins, and minerals
Excessive intake of energy, fat, and sugar
Malnutrition
Obesity

Hunger in Canada (pp. 698–700)

1. Identify some reasons why hunger is present in a country as wealthy as Canada.
2. What does food insecurity refer to?
   a. the uncertainty of foods' safety
   b. the fear of eating too much food
   c. the limited availability of foods
   d. the reliability of food production
3. What is the most common cause of hunger in Canada?
   a. poverty
   b. alcohol abuse
   c. mental illness
   d. lack of education
4. Which region of the world has the largest ecological footprint?
   a. Europe
   b. Latin America and the Caribbean
   c. the United Kingdom
   d. Canada and the United States
5. Which action is NOT typical of a food recovery program?
   a. gathering potatoes from a harvested field
   b. collecting overripe tomatoes from a wholesaler
   c. offering a Guaranteed Income Supplement (GIS) to low-income people
   d. delivering restaurant leftovers to a community shelter

World Hunger (pp. 700–703)

6. Identify some reasons why hunger is present in the developing countries of the world.
7. What was the primary cause of the worst famine in the 20th century?
   a. armed conflicts
   b. natural disasters
   c. food contaminations
   d. government policies
8. What is the most likely cause of death in malnourished children?
   a. growth failure
   b. diarrheal disease
   c. simple starvation
   d. vitamin A deficiency

Poverty and Overpopulation (pp. 703–705)

9. Which of the following is most critical in providing food to all the world's people?
   a. decreasing air pollution
   b. increasing water supplies
   c. decreasing population growth
   d. increasing agricultural land

The Global Environment (pp. 705–710)

10. Explain why relieving environmental problems will also help to alleviate hunger and poverty.
11. Discuss the different paths by which rich and poor countries can attack the problems of world hunger and the environment.

Study Questions (multiple choice)
2. c 3. a 4. d 5. c 7. d 8. b 9. c

CENGAGENOW™ For additional study questions and activities, go to **www.cengage.com/sso** and complete the Personalized Study Plan for this chapter.